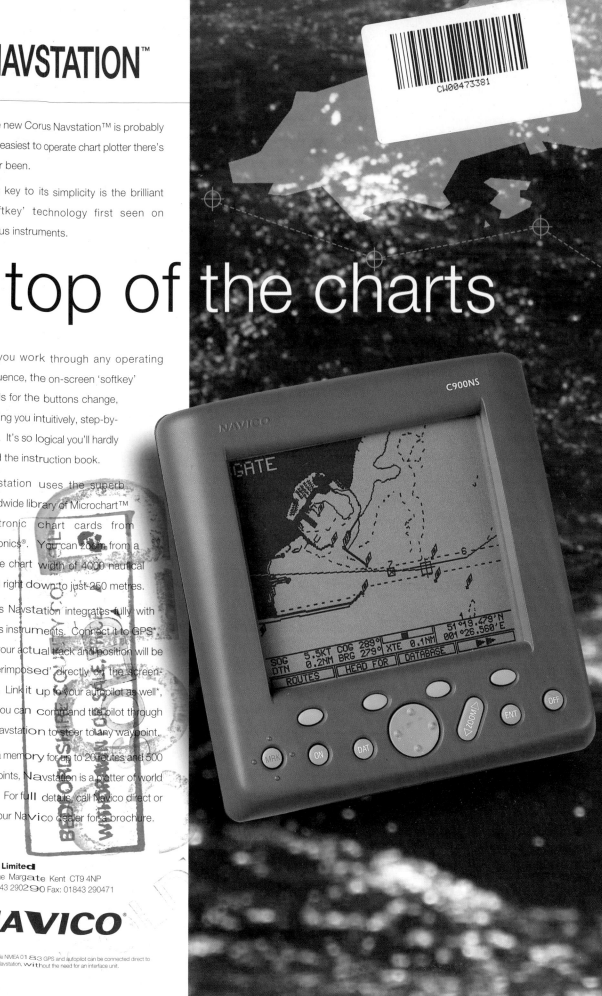

NAVSTATION™

The new Corus Navstation™ is probably the easiest to operate chart plotter there's ever been.

The key to its simplicity is the brilliant 'softkey' technology first seen on Corus instruments.

top of the charts

As you work through any operating sequence, the on-screen 'softkey' labels for the buttons change, guiding you intuitively, step-by-step. It's so logical you'll hardly need the instruction book.

Navstation uses the superb worldwide library of Microchart™ electronic chart cards from Navionics®. You can zoom from a visible chart width of 4000 nautical miles right down to just 250 metres.

Corus Navstation integrates fully with Corus instruments. Connect it to GPS* and your actual track and position will be 'superimposed' directly on the screen chart. Link it up to your autopilot as well*, and you can command the pilot through the Navstation to steer to any waypoint.

With a memory for up to 20 routes and 500 waypoints, Navstation is a plotter of world class. For full details, call Navico direct or ask your Navico dealer for a brochure.

Navico Limited
Star Lane Margate Kent CT9 4NP
Tel: 01843 290290 Fax: 01843 290471

NAVICO®

*A compatible NMEA 0183 GPS and autopilot can be connected direct to the Navico Navstation, without the need for an interface unit.

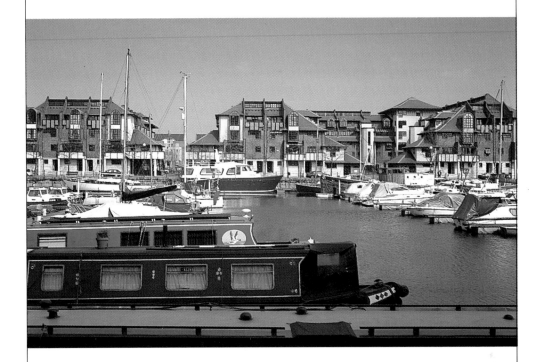

The Macmillan and Silk Cut Nautical Almanac
(Incorporating *Reed's Nautical Almanac*)

IMPROVEMENTS FOR THE 1996 EDITION

GENERAL IMPROVEMENTS

❏ **Waypoints:** The Almanac now contains over 3,600 waypoint coordinates for use with electronic navigation equipment. The tabulated listings of Waypoints for East Anglia and the southern North Sea are now combined in Area 4. The Clyde area listing has also been expanded.

❏ **Updating:** Once published the Almanac is kept up to date by the issue of a free Supplement which includes, when necessary, replacement pages or chartlet blocks. A later printing date this year has allowed more recent data to be included within the Almanac in the Late Corrections pages.

❏ **Directory of Marine Services and Supplies:**
Responding to requests for a simple and easy-to-use guide to services, supplies and equipment, this year the commercial section has been formalised in the pink pages at the front of the book. The directory is split into two parts, the first listing types of service or supply and the second showing geographical locations in line with the 21 areas in Chapter 10.

Both will be an invaluable addition to those carrying out maintenance and repairs at leisure – but especially useful in emergencies. Section One in the current edition has over 60 different services to offer and will grow year by year. Section Two contains many harbours and marinas with details of their facilities.

IMPROVEMENTS IN CHAPTERS ONE TO NINE

CHAPTER FIVE
ASTRO-NAVIGATION

The information given in the Almanac now consists of a new two page tabulated listing of Sunrise and Sunset times for selected Ports and calendar information. All other data for Astro has been transferred to a self-contained Astro-Supplement.

The information required for astro-navigation has been produced separately in a forty-eight page supplement which is available at a cost of £4.00. The Astro-Supplement contains the ephemerides of the Sun, Moon, GHA Aries, 57 navigational stars and the Pole star together with tables for interpolating the ephemerides, sextant altitude, sunrise, sunset, twilight, moonrise and moonset set and conversions. Supporting text explains the general principles of astro-navigation. Details of how to apply for the Astro-Supplement are contained in Chapter 1.

CHAPTER SIX
COMMUNICATIONS

The layout of radio communications has been extensively revised and improved. The listing of UK and European Coast Radio Stations is all in tabular form. A larger type size makes the data more readable and easier to use in difficult light conditions.

CHAPTER SEVEN
WEATHER

Revised to include new maps of the Marinecall and Metfax forecast areas, and a selected broadcast schedule for the radio fax transmissions from Bracknell and Northwood. Details of latest weather reports from Marinecall have also been included.

CHAPTER EIGHT
SAFETY

Information on the Global Maritime Distress and Safety System (GMDSS) and Emergency Position Indicator Beacons (EPIRBs) has been extensively updated. Details of the French CROSS Search and Rescue Centres, together with a map showing the CROSS boundaries, are also included.

❏ **The Thames Estuary** is now covered wholly in one Area (4) which runs from North Foreland to Great Yarmouth. A full page chart of the Estuary much assists passage planning.

❏ **French Areas between the Spanish border and Cherbourg** have been reversed so as to flow westward from Cherbourg to Brest; thence southward to the Spanish border. This more closely fits the movements of yachts cruising the popular North Brittany coast; whilst progress southward from Brest is a more natural orientation. (Areas 19 to 21 are unchanged: Cherbourg to Danish border).

❏ **Special notes for France** have been re-located more conveniently alongside the much-used arrival port of Cherbourg.

❏ **The cost of an overnight berth** for a visiting 30ft/9m yacht is shown for most ports and marinas.

❏ **Portland Tidal predictions** and curves have been included.

❏ **West coast of Ireland tidal streams** are shown, courtesy of the Irish Cruising Club.

❏ **Tidal stream chartlets** in 5 Areas are more legible, with larger type size.

❏ **Historic Wrecks:** 40 sites are listed.

❏ **A bibliography of relevant** Pilot and guide books is included at the start of all the fully revised Passage Information sections.

❏ **Ferry services** around the west coast of Scotland and Western Isles are tabulated in more detail.

❏ **New ports and anchorages,** or much enhanced chartlets of existing entries, are shown below by geographic areas:

England, South coast
Isles of Scilly, Fowey, Plymouth, Dartmouth, Needles Channel, Langstone hbr entrance, Weymouth, Southampton.

England and Scotland, East coast
Thames Estuary chartlet, Queenborough, Herne Bay, Gallions Pt marina, Limehouse Yacht Basin, Beadnell Bay, Avoch.

Scotland, West coast
Port Ellen, Clyde Area chartlet and twenty-eight new minor harbours and anchorages on the mainland and among the islands.

England, West coast and Wales
Holyhead, Lynmouth, Clovelly, Boscastle.

Ireland
Skerries, Balbriggan, Annalong, Dundrum Bay, Courtmacsherry, Glandore, Barloge Creek, Horseshoe Harbour, Clear Island, Goleen, Dunmanus Bay, Bantry Bay and six local anchorages, Valentia, Smerwick, Brandon Bay.

France, Channel coast
Dielette, Portbail, Carteret, St Malo.

France, Atlantic coast
Chenal du Four, Hendaye.

Belgium and Netherlands
Blankenberge, Lauwersoog, Zeegat van Terschelling.

Germany
Emden, Rüstersiel, Büsum, Pellworm.

THE MACMILLAN & SILK CUT NAUTICAL ALMANAC

1996

EDITORS

Wing Commander B. D'Oliveira OBE, FRIN
Commander N. L. Featherstone RN

CONSULTANT EDITORS

Commander R. L. Hewitt LVO, RN MIMechE, MRINA, FRIN
Dr. B. D. Yallop PhD, BSc, ARCS

MACMILLAN

First published 1980
This edition published 1995 by Macmillan Reference Books
London and Basingstoke

Associated Companies in Auckland, Delhi, Dublin, Gaborone, Hamburg, Harare, Hong Kong, Johannesburg, Kuala Lumpur, Lagos, Manzini, Melbourne, Mexico City, Nairobi, New York, Singapore and Tokyo.

British Cataloguing In Publication Data
A CIP catalogue record for this book is available from the British Library.

ISBN 0-333-63824-7

IMPORTANT NOTE

Whilst every care has been taken in compiling the information contained in this Almanac, the Publishers and Editors accept no responsibility for any errors or omissions, or for any accidents or mishaps which may arise from its use.

CORRESPONDENCE

Letters on nautical matters should be addressed to:

The Editor, The Macmillan & Silk Cut Nautical Almanac
41 Arbor Lane, Winnersh, Wokingham, Berks RG41 5JE
or The Editor, The Macmillan & Silk Cut Nautical Almanac
Edington House, Trent, Sherborne, Dorset DT9 4SR.
See also Chapter 1 paragraph 1.2.1.

Enquiries about despatch, invoicing or commercial matters should be addressed to:

Customer Services Department,
Macmillan Press Ltd, Houndmills, Basingstoke,
Hampshire RG21 2XS

Enquiries about advertising space should be addressed to:

Communications Management International,
Chiltern House, 120 Eskdale Avenue, Chesham,
Buckinghamshire HP5 3BD

Chapters 1-9   Page preparation by
              Wyvern Typesetting Limited, Bristol
Chapter 10   Cartography and page preparation by
              Lovell Johns Ltd, Oxford

Colour artwork by Dick Vine

Printed and bound in Great Britain by
              BPC Hazell Books Limited, a member of
              The British Printing Company Limited

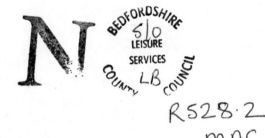

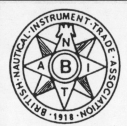

The symbol of the **BRITISH NAUTICAL INSTRUMENT TRADE ASSOCIATION**, founded in 1918. With the full support of the Hydrographer of the Navy and leading manufacturers of nautical instruments, members of the Association are able to place their experience and service at the disposal of the shipping industry and all navigators.

CHART SUPPLY AND CORRECTION SERVICES

The BNITA counts among its members many of the leading Admiralty Chart Agents who can supply your requirements from a single chart or publication to a worldwide outfit and special folio requirements from comprehensive stocks in all the major ports. Carefully trained chart correctors are available to examine and correct all Admiralty charts.

THE BNITA TRACING SERVICE

Although tracings have been in use by the Royal Navy and Admiralty Chart Agents for many years, it was the Chart Committee of the British Nautical Instrument Trade Association that successfully negotiated with the Hydrographer of the Navy for them to become available to the merchant navigator and private user.

The BNITA tracing overlay correction service is available from all Admiralty Chart Agents who are members of the Association, and is now supplied to more than 5,000 vessels each week. Each tracing wallet contains the weekly "Notices to Mariners" and the tracings printed with much of the relevant details of the area surrounding the correction, making the correction of each chart a simpler operation. All that the user has to do is match the tracing to the chart, pierce through the small circle showing the exact position of the correction, in conjunction with the "Notices to Mariners", and then transfer the information onto the chart. Navigating Officers welcome the tracings systems for its accuracy and speed. Onboard chart correction time can be cut by up to 80% and Masters can now rest assured that their charts can be kept continually up to date. Reasonably priced, these tracings are an economical and invaluable contribution to safety at sea.

COMPASS ADJUSTING AND NAUTICAL INSTRUMENTS

The BNITA insists that its Compass Adjusters are thoroughly trained to its own high standards, and independently examined by the Department of Trade. For yacht or super tanker our compass adjusters can advise you on the type of compass you need, its siting, and any adjustments needed. BNITA Compass Adjusters are based in all the major ports and are available day and night to "swing" ships.

Members of the BNITA, many with a life long experience in this field, can advise you when purchasing all your nautical instruments. Most suppliers provide an instrument repair service combining traditional craftsmanship with modern methods to ensure that instruments are serviced and tested to a high standard.

ARE YOU COMPLYING WITH THE LATEST INTERNATIONAL REGULATIONS?

British Nautical Instrument Trade Association members established in most UK ports and overseas are able to advise you. For full details of the Association, its activities and its services to the Navigator, write to:

The Secretaries,
BRITISH NAUTICAL INSTRUMENT TRADE ASSOCIATION,
105 West George Street, GLASGOW G2 1QP.

PORTS WHERE SHIPS' COMPASSES ARE ADJUSTED

Names of member firms. Those marked * have DoT Certified Compass Adjusters available for Adjustment of Compasses, day or night.

Port or District	Name and Address	Telephone
ABERDEEN	*Thomas Gunn Navigation Services, 62 Marischal Street, Aberdeen AB1 2AL.	01224 595045
AVONMOUTH	*Severnside Consultants, Imperial Chambers, 2nd Floor, Gloucester Road, Avonmouth BS11 9AQ.	0117-982 7184
BANGOR (N Ireland)	Todd Chart Agency Ltd., 4 Seacliff Road, The Harbour, Bangor, N Ireland BT20 5EY.	01247 466640
BRISTOL	*W F Price & Co Ltd., Northpoint House, Wapping Wharf, Bristol BS1 6UD.	0117-929 2229
CARDIFF	*T J Williams & Son (Cardiff) Ltd., 15-17 Harrowby Street, Cardiff CF1 6HA.	01222 487676
FALMOUTH	*Marine Instruments, The Bosun's Locker, Upton Slip, Falmouth TR11 3DQ.	01326 312414
GLASGOW	Brown, Son & Ferguson, Ltd., 4-10 Darnley Street, Glasgow G41 2SD.	0141-429 1234
HULL	*B Cooke & Son, Ltd., Kingston Observatory, 58-59 Market Place, Hull HU1 1RH.	01482 223454
KENT	*SIRS Navigation Ltd., 186a Milton Road, Swanscombe, Kent DA10 0LX.	01322.383672
LIVERPOOL	Dubois-Phillips & McCallum Ltd. Oriel Chambers, Covent Garden, Liverpool L2 8UD.	0151-236 2776
LONDON	*Kelvin Hughes Charts and Maritime Supplies New North Road, Hainault, Ilford, Essex IG6 2UR.	0181-500 6166
	A M Smith (Marine) Ltd., 33 Epping Way, Chingford, London E4 7PB.	0181-529 6988
LOWESTOFT	*Seath Instruments (1992) Ltd., Unit 30, Colville Road Works, Colville Road, Lowestoft NR33 9QS.	01502 573811

Port or District	Name and Address	Telephone
NORTH SHIELDS (Newcastle)	*John Lilley & Gillie Ltd., Clive Street, North Shields, Tyne & Wear NE29 6LF.	0191-257 2217
SOUTHAMPTON	*R J Muir, 22 Seymour Close, Chandlers Ford, Eastleigh, Southampton SO5 2JE.	01703 261042
	Wessex Marine Equipment Ltd., Logistics House, 2nd Avenue Business Park, Millbrook Road East, Southampton SO1 0LP.	01703 510570

OVERSEAS MEMBERS

Port or District	Name and Address	Telephone
ANTWERP	Bogerd Navtec NV, Oude Leenwnrui 37 Antwerp 2000.	
	*Martin & Co. Oude Leewenrui 37, Antwerp 2000.	
COPENHAGEN	Iver C Weilbach & Co. A/S, 35 Toldbodgade, Postbox 1560, DK-1253 Copenhagen K.	
GOTHENBURG	A B Ramantenn, Knipplagatan 12 S-414 74, Gothenburg.	
HONG KONG	George Falconer (Nautical) Ltd., The Hong Kong Jewellery Building, 178-180 Queen's Road, Central Hong Kong.	
	Hong Kong Ship's Supplies Co. Room 1614, Melbourne Plaza,33 Queen's Road, Central Hong Kong.	
LISBON	J Garraio & Co. Ltd., Avenida 24 de Julho, 2-1°, D-1200, Lisbon.	
ROTTERDAM	*Kelvin Hughes Observator, Nieuwe Langeweg 41, 3194 DC, Hoogliet.	
SINGAPORE	Motion Smith, 78 Shenton Way #01-03, Singapore 0207.	
SKYTTA	A/S Navicharts, Masteveien 3, N-1483 Skytta, Norway.	
URUGUAY	Captain Stephan Nedelchev Soc. Col. Port of Montevideo, Florida 1562, 11100 Montevideo.	
VARNA	Captain Lyudmil N. Jordanov, 13A Han Omurtag Str. 9000 Bulgaria.	

  1918 - 1996
78 YEARS OF SERVING THE MARINER

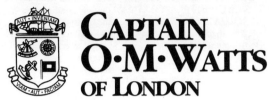

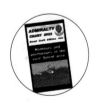

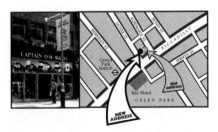

Contents

PERSONAL INDEX OF IMPORTANT PAGES

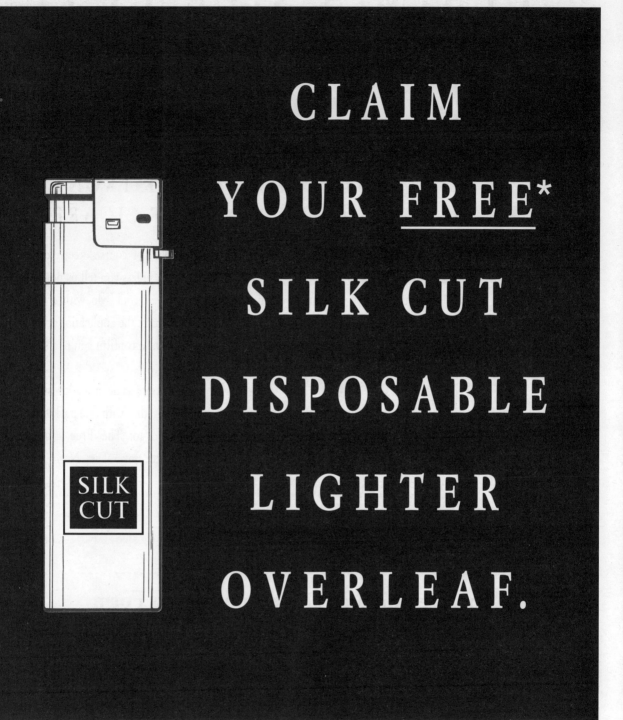

CLAIM YOUR FREE* SILK CUT DISPOSABLE LIGHTER OVERLEAF.

SILK CUT

SMOKING WHEN PREGNANT HARMS YOUR BABY

Chief Medical Officers' Warning
5mg Tar 0.5 mg Nicotine

CLAIM A SILK CUT DISPOSABLE LIGHTER ABSOLUTELY FREE*

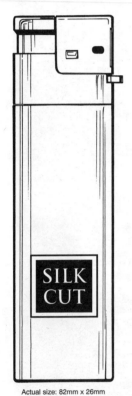

Actual size: 82mm x 26mm

*JUST SEND ONE PACK FRONT OF YOUR USUAL BRAND OF CIGARETTES.

Yes, claiming your free lighter really is as easy as that.

Just send us one pack front of your usual brand of cigarettes and in return we'll send you your free Silk Cut lighter. And it won't even cost you a penny in postage if you use our Freepost address.

The free lighter is just one of many special prizes, discounts and free gifts that we offer from time to time to smokers aged 18 or over.

And we will, of course, keep you informed about them, unless you tell us not to.

So if you could do with a free lighter, please complete the application form ensuring that you sign to confirm you're a smoker aged 18 or over.

Fill in your name and address and post it off today together with one pack front of your usual brand to: The Free Lighter Offer, FREEPOST, P.O. Box 3, Diss, Norfolk 1P22 3BR.

TERMS AND CONDITIONS 1. **Open only to UK resident smokers aged 18 or over.** 2. All applications must be signed. Unsigned applications will be deemed invalid. 3. Only one application is permitted per person. 4. **The closing date for receipt of applications is 31/12/96.** 5. All applications must be on an official application form and accompanied by a cigarette pack front. Photocopies will not be accepted. 6 No responsibility will be accepted for applications lost, delayed or damaged in the post. Proof of posting will not be accepted as proof of delivery. 7. Please allow 28 days for delivery from receipt of your application. 8. The colour and style of the lighter may differ from that illustrated. 9. Applications should be sent to: The Free Lighter Offer, FREEPOST, P.O. Box 3, Diss, Norfolk 1P22 3BR.

Promoter (Please DO NOT send your application to this address) Benson & Hedges Limited, Registered Office: 13, Old Bond Street, London W1X 4 QP.

The Free Lighter Offer Application Form

CLOSING DATE FOR RECEIPT OF APPLICATIONS IS 31 DECEMBER 1996

Please fill in the details below and send to: The Free Lighter Offer, FREEPOST, P.O. Box 3, Diss, Norfolk 1P22 3BR.

Applications can only be accepted from UK resident smokers aged 18 or over. Only one application per person. Applications cannot be accepted after 31/12/96.

I enclose a pack front of my usual brand. Please send me my free disposable lighter.

I am a smoker aged 18 or over.

Signature X _____ X

(Unsigned applications will be deemed invalid and returned)

On average, how many cigarettes do you currently smoke a day?

1-5 ☐   6-10 ☐   11-15 ☐   16-20 ☐
21-25 ☐   26-30 ☐   31-35 ☐   36+ ☐

Title: Mr/Mrs/Miss/Ms/Other* _____ Initials _____
*(*Please delete as applicable)*

Surname _____

Address _____

_____

_____

Postcode _____

If you DO NOT wish to receive news of future special offers, prize draws and discounts from Gallaher Ltd., please mark a cross here ☐

SCNA/95

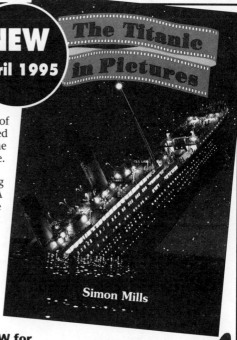
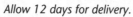

Quick Reference Marine Supplies and Services Guide
Coastal & Waterways Services
Directory - area by area

This section provides readers with a quick reference to harbours, marinas, companies and organisations currently delivering services - including emergency services, equipment and supplies to boat owners and the boating industry. Each entry carries concise information for guidance.

Pages i-xxvii lists by types of service and products and xxviii-li by coastal location.

LANGSTONE HARBOUR BOARD
Ferry Road, Hayling Island,
Hampshire PO11 0DG.
Tel (01705) 463419 Fax (01705) 467144
All boatyard facilities. Deep water and
tidal moorings available. Water, electricity
and diesel. Summer and winter storage.
Public slipways. 6-ton crane. Landrover
vessel and trailer recovery services.

MALDON BOAT YARD
(formerly Dan Webb & Feesey)
North Street, Maldon,
Essex CM9 7HN.
Tel (01621) 854280
Full chandlery, slipway, stage berths,
winter storage, diesel. Based in the historic
town of Maldon.

MANOR OF BOSHAM LTD
Bosham Quay, Old Bosham,
West Sussex PO18 8HR.
Tel (01243) 573336 Fax (01243) 576285
Deep water moorings up to 14 metres in
length in picturesque Bosham Channel -
Chichester Harbour, also includes some
tidal moorings. Services available at quay.
Also scrubbing off grids including pressure
washers. **Contact Name: M McGrail.**

MELFORT PIER & HARBOUR
Kilmelford, By Oban,
Argyll PA34 4XD.
Tel (01852) 200333 Fax (01852) 200329
A small pretty harbour set up, surrounded
by top quality holiday houses each with
private sauna/spa, tel/fax. All shoreside
facilities for the cruising yachtsman;
moorings and pontoon berthing, showers,
laundry, tel/fax, B & B, diesel, water,
electricity, gas, provisions. Restaurant, bar,
hotel, bikes, watersports, horseriding and
much more. Call sign: Melfort Pier 16/12.

OBAN YACHTS & MARINE
SERVICES LTD
Ardentrive, Kerrera,
By Oban, Argyll PA34 4SX.
Tel (01631)565333 Fax (01631) 565888
Moorings, visitor pontoon, toilets, showers,
drying room, diesel, gas. water, chandlery,
slipway, 18-ton hoist, full workshop
facilities, undercover storage, hardstanding. Regular ferry to Oban town centre
less than 10 minutes across the bay.

PORT OF TRURO
Harbour Office, Town Quay,
Truro, Cornwall.
Tel (01872) 72130 Fax (01872) 225346
Facilities for the yachtsman include
visitors' pontoons located at Turnaware
Bar near Ruan Creek, Boscawen Park.
Visitors' moorings at Woodbury. Quay
facilities at Truro with free showers and
toilets. Chemical toilet disposal, fresh water
and garbage disposal.

R.I.B.S. MARINE
Little Avon Marina,
Stony Lane South,
Christchurch,
Dorset BH23 1HW.
Tel (01202) 477327 Fax (01202) 471456
Full boatyard facilities. Mooring, slipping
and dry boat storage. Marine engineers for
all makes of outboard and inboard. Petrol
and diesel. Specialist repairs in wood and
GRP. Main agents for Mariner and Force
outboards and Mercruiser stern drives.
Brokerage facilities.

RAMSGATE ROYAL HARBOUR
Harbour Office, Military Road,
Ramsgate, Kent CT11 9LG.
Tel (01843) 592277 Fax (01843) 590941
One of south east England's premier leisure
areas. Ideal for crossing to the Continent.
24-hour access to finger pontoons.
Comprehensive security systems.
Amenities: launderette, repairs, slipways,
boatpark. Competitive rates for permanent
berths and visiting vessels.

SHELL BAY MARINE
Ferry Road, Studland,
Dorset BH19 3BA.
Tel (01929) 450340 Fax (01929) 450570
Sensibly priced moorings immediately
inside Poole harbour entrance. Slipway,
boat hoist, winter storage, repairs. Good
security, open all year, terms available by
day, week or season. Parking, licensed bar,
cafe and RYA recognised watersports
centre.

SHOTLEY MARINA LTD
Shotley Gate, Ipswich,
Suffolk IP9 1QJ.
Tel (01473) 788982 Fax (01473) 788868
A modern state of the art marina with 350
berths offering all the services expected.
Open 24-hours with full security. Access
all states of tide, ideal cruising base. Well
stocked chandlery and general store, repair
facilities, laundry and ironing centre,
showers/baths and toilets. Restaurants, bar,
children's room, TV/video and function
rooms with dance floor and bar. Disabled
facilities.

SPARKES YACHT HARBOUR
& BOATYARD
38 Wittering Road,
Sandy Point, Hayling Island,
Hampshire PO11 9SR.
Tel (01705) 463572 Fax (01705) 465741
Sparkes Marina - a small friendly, family
run business offering all the facilities you
require including access at all states of the
tide to a depth of 2 metres at lowest low
water springs. In addition to marina berths,
accessible through a security gate, we also
offer dry boat sailing, moorings, storage
ashore plus full maintenance facilities, new
boat sales and brokerage, chandlery and
restaurant.

WEIR QUAY BOATYARD
Heron's Reach, Bere Alston,
Devon PL20 7BT.
Tel (01822) 840474 Fax (01822) 840948
Deepwater swinging moorings, shore
storage, full boatyard facilities and services,
cranage to 12 tons, repairs, maintenance,
slipway. A traditional boatyard 'in a superb
setting' on the Tamar, with excellent
security at affordable rates.

WORCESTER YACHT
CHANDLERS LTD
Unit 7, 75 Waterworks Road,
Barbourne, Worcester WR1 3EZ.
Tel (01905) 22522 & 27949
Chandlery, paints, ropes, cables, chain,
clothing, footwear, shackles, books, bottled
gas, anti-foul, fastenings, oakam, fenders.
Hard storage, crane, haulage, engine
service, oils, navigation aids, buoyancy
aids, life jackets, distress flares, small boat
hire.

YARMOUTH MARINE SERVICE
River Yar Boatyard,
Yarmouth, Isle of Wight PO41 0SE.
Tel (01983) 760521 Fax (01983) 760096
All boatyard facilities and commercial
charter. Slipway to 20 tons. Boat repairs,
wood and GRP, osmosis and painting.
Annual and visitors' moorings. Two
workboats available with loadline
exemption for all types of commercial
work.

BOAT BUILDERS & REPAIRS

ARDFERN YACHT CENTRE
Ardfern By Lochgilphead,
Argyll PA31 8QN.
Tel (01852) 500247/636
Fax (01852) 500624
Boatyard with full repair and maintenance
facilities. Timber and GRP repairs, painting and engineering. Sheltered moorings
and pontoon berthing. Winter storage,
chandlery, showers, fuel, Calor, brokerage, 20-ton boat hoist. Hotel, bars and
restaurant.

ARUNCRAFT LTD
Littlehampton Marina,
Ferry Road, Littlehampton,
West Sussex BN17 5DS.
Tel (01903) 723667 Fax (01903) 730983
Mobile 0836 703006. Family business
based at Littlehampton Marina for 11 years.
Large workshop for boat maintenance,
GRP repairs, engine work, rigging,
electronic systems and propeller repairs.
In-house paint spraying and osmosis
treatments by Arunspray. Chandlery and
comprehensive range of craft in the
brokerage department.

BLACKWATER MARINA
Marine Parade, Maylandsea,
Essex CM3 6AN.
Tel (01621) 740264 Fax (01621) 742122
Refurbished tidal marina on the Blackwater estuary. New pontoons, new clubhouse, bar and restaurant, toilets and showers. 18-ton slipway hoist, 70-ton winch, 130' workshop with full services. Full chandlery, brokerage/boat sales. Car parking and on-site security. Full tide swinging moorings, half tide moorings and half tide pontoon berths. A few long-term berths available.

BOATWORKS + LTD
Castle Emplacement,
St Peter Port, Guernsey,
Channel Islands GY1 1AU.
Tel (01481) 726071 Fax (01481) 714224
Boatworks+ provides a comprehensive range of services including electronics, chandlery, boatbuilding and repairs, engine sales and services, yacht brokerage, clothing and fuel supplies.

BRUNDALL BAY MARINA - SALES
Riverside Estate, Brundall,
Norwich, Norfolk NR13 5PN.
Tel (01603) 716606 Fax (01603) 715666
New and used boat sales, brokerage, full workshop services. Agents for Faircraft river cruisers. Hardy, Seawings sports cruisers, Evinrude outboard motors. 200-berth marina with full facilities.

CLEDDAU BOATYARD
Cleddau House, Milford Marina,
Milford Haven, Dyfed SA73 3AF.
Tel (01646) 697834 Fax (01646) 697834
Travel hoist, storage, inboard and outboard. Repairs, spares and service. General leisurecraft repairs, wood and fibreglass work. Chandlery and breakdown service.

DARTHAVEN MARINA LTD
Brixham Road, Kingswear,
Dartmouth, Devon TQ6 0SG.
Tel (01803) 752242 Fax (01803) 752722
Marina Office: (01803) 752545 Chandlery: (01803) 752733 Fax (01803) 752790. All types of repair facilities available. Fully trained staff. 30-ton mobile hoist available all states of tide. Extensive chandlery open 7 days a week. Agents for Autohelm/ Raytheon, Cetrek, Simpson Lawrence, Vetus and Webasto. Visitors welcome. 24-hour engineering call-out service. Mobile Nos: 0860 873553 Engineering; 0589 340609 Electronics.

ELKINS BOATYARD
Tidesreach, 18 Convent Meadow,
The Quay, Christchurch,
Dorset BH23 1BD.
Tel (01202) 483141
All boatyard facilities. Moorings alongside, water and electricity, storage ashore, repairs. Boats up to 45', 10 tons maximum, haul out.

GAVIN POOLE YACHT BROKERS
14 Hooke Close, Canford Heath,
Dorset BH17 8BB.
Tel (01202) 604068 Fax (01202) 659680
The motor cruiser and Fairey boat specialist for modern diesel and classic boats. Sales, service, finance. Open every day. Mobile number 0860 236389

GWEEK QUAY BOATYARD
Gweek Quay (Helford River),
Helston, Cornwall TR12 6UF.
Tel (01326) 221657 Fax (01326) 221685
Head of the Helford river. Yacht repair yard, 30-ton crane, chandlery, brokerage, coffee shop, toilets and showers. Boat storage and all boat repair and service facilities. Access approximately 2 hours either side of highwater.

HAMOAZE MARINE SERVICES
Calstock Boatyard, Lower Kelly,
Calstock, Cornwall PL18 9RY.
Tel (01822) 834024 & (01752) 823118
High class yacht and boat repairs, especially wood. Sheltered moorings up to 4' draught in upper Tamar river. Showers, fuel, winter storage. Also agents for Avon inflatable boats and Heyland Marine fibreglass dinghies.

HOO MARINA (MEDWAY) LTD
Vicarage Lane, Hoo,
Rochester, Kent ME3 9LE.
Tel (01634) 250311 Fax (01634) 251761
An established marina with fully serviced pontoon berths, winter lay-up on concrete hardstanding. 20-ton lifting capacity. Chandlery and brokerage as well as full workshop facilities for yacht repair and maintenance.

HULL MARINA LTD
Warehouse 13, Kingston Street,
Hull HU1 2DQ.
Tel (01482) 593451 Fax (01482) 224148
Five Anchor Marina. Situated 5 minues from the centre of Hull and all national and international transport systems. First class leisure, boatyard and brokerage facilities. 4-Star hotel and quayside restaurants. Professional and caring staff. Competitive rates.

LANGNEY MARINE SERVICES LTD
Sovereign Harbour Marina,
Pevensey Bay Road, Eastbourne,
East Sussex BN23 6JH.
Tel (01323) 470244 Fax (01323) 470255
We offer a complete service to the boat owner offering repairs on all types of engines, GRP, steel, wood, electronics, rigging, cleaning, etc. We are also contractors to the R.N.L.I.

MARINE & GENERAL ENGINEERS LTD
The Shipyard,
St Sampson's Harbour, Guernsey,
Channel Islands GY1 6AT.
Tel (01481) 45808 Fax (01481) 48765
High standard boat building and yacht repair yard supported by slipway with two cradles. Comprehensive on-site support facilities - fabrication, carpentry, welding. 24-hour Emergency Support on 0860 741217.

OBAN YACHTS & MARINE SERVICES LTD
Ardentrive, Kerrera, By Oban,
Argyll PA34 4SX.
Tel (01631) 565333 Fax (01631) 565888
Moorings, visitor pontoon, toilets, showers, drying room, diesel, gas, water, chandlery, slipway, 18-ton hoist, full workshop facilities, undercover storage, hardstanding. Regular ferry to Oban town centre less than 10 minutes across the bay.

R J P FABRICATIONS
83B Sterte Avenue West, Poole,
Dorset BH15 2AL.
Tel (01202) 660205 Mobile 0860 678326
Aluminium and stainless steel custom made ladders and handrails. General light fabrication and repairs.

R.I.B.S. MARINE
Little Avon Marina,
Stony Lane South, Christchurch,
Dorset BH23 1HW.
Tel (01202) 477327 Fax (01202) 471456
Full boatyard facilities. Mooring, slipping and dry boat storage. Marine engineers for all makes of outboard and inboard. Petrol and diesel. Specialist repairs in wood and GRP. Main agents for Mariner and Force outboards and Mercruiser stern drives. Brokerage facilities.

SHOTLEY MARINA LTD
Shotley Gate, Ipswich,
Suffolk IP9 1QJ.
Tel (01473) 788982 Fax (01473) 788868
A modern state of the art marina with 350 berths offering all the services expected. Open 24-hours with full security. Access all states of tide, ideal cruising base. Well stocked chandlery and general store, repair facilities, laundry and ironing centre, showers/baths and toilets. Restaurants, bar, children's room, TV/video and function rooms with dance floor and bar. Disabled facilities.

SLEAT MARINE SERVICES
Ardvasar, Isle of Skye IV45 8RU.
Tel (01471) 844 216/387
Yacht charter (bareboat and skippered) from Armadale Bay, Isle of Skye. Six yachts 34' to 40' LOA. All medium to heavy displacement blue water cruisers. Fuel, water and emergency services for passing yachts with problems.

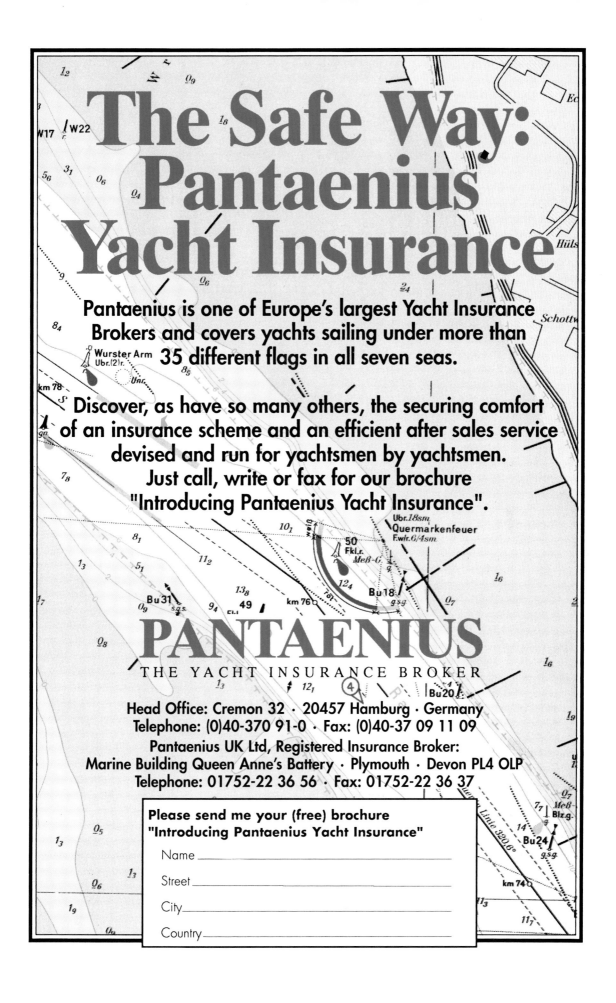

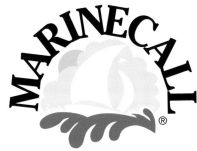

THE SPECIALIST WEATHER SERVICE
KEEPING SAILORS IN THE PICTURE

FOR A DETAILED 2 DAY LOCAL FORECAST
PHONE 0891·500·PLUS AREA NUMBER

FOR A 2 DAY LOCAL FORECAST AND CHARTS
FAX 0336·400·PLUS AREA NUMBER

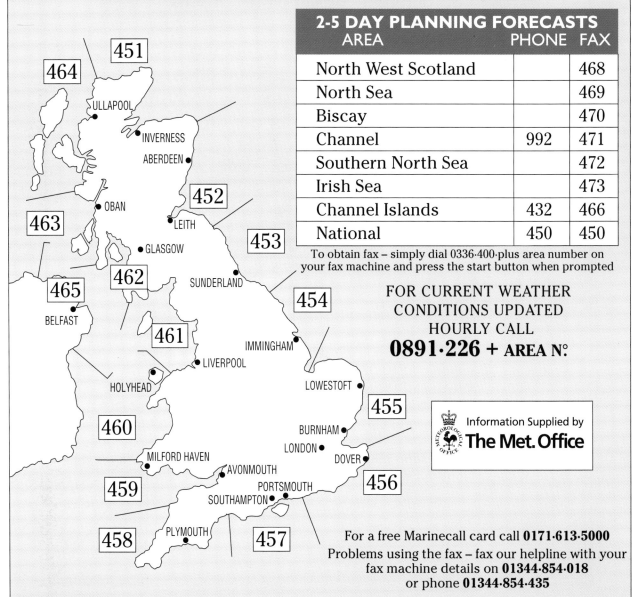

2-5 DAY PLANNING FORECASTS		
AREA	PHONE	FAX
North West Scotland		468
North Sea		469
Biscay		470
Channel	992	471
Southern North Sea		472
Irish Sea		473
Channel Islands	432	466
National	450	450

To obtain fax – simply dial 0336·400·plus area number on your fax machine and press the start button when prompted

FOR CURRENT WEATHER
CONDITIONS UPDATED
HOURLY CALL
0891·226 + AREA Nº

Information Supplied by
The Met. Office

For a free Marinecall card call **0171·613·5000**
Problems using the fax – fax our helpline with your fax machine details on **01344·854·018**
or phone **01344·854·435**

Telephone Information Services plc, Avalon House, London EC2A 4PJ. Tel: 0171 613 5000. Calls cost 39p per minute cheap rate and 49p per minute at all other times (as at April '95).

SOUTHDOWN MARINA
**Southdown Quay, Millbrook,
Cornwall PL10 1EZ.**
Tel/Fax (01752) 823084
32-berth marina on edge of river Tamar in quiet location behind Rame Peninsula. Plymouth is just across the river. Quayside berths available for large vessels. Winter storage. Good security. DIY facilities available.

THAMES (DITTON) MARINA LTD
**Portsmouth Road,
Thames Ditton, Surrey KT6 5QD.**
Tel 0181-398 6159 Fax 0181-398 6438
Over 120 berths and moorings. All main services, diesel, Calor Gas, repairs and service. Large chandlery with comprehensive stock of safety equipment, paint, charts and books. Very large car park for convenience of customers. Open 7 days a week.

THORNHAM MARINA
**Thornham Lane, Prinsted,
Nr Emsworth,
Hampshire PO10 8DD.**
Tel (01243) 375335
First class serviced hardstanding, 12-ton slipway hoist. Tidal pontoons, deep water gated pool, modern workshop, bar, restaurant, showers and toilets. Visitors welcome - club rallies etc. A very few long-term berths available. Brokerage service.

TOLLESBURY MARINA
**The Yacht Harbour, Tollesbury,
Maldon, Essex CM9 8SE.**
Tel (01621) 869202
Fax (01621) 868489
VHF Channel 37/80 Tollesbury Marina can offer 260 marina berths with water and electricty on all pontoons. Clubhouse with bar, restaurant, swimming pool and tennis courts. Repair workshops with West Osmosis Treatment Centre. Full brokerage service listing over 200 boats, with friendly professional service.

WEST COUNTRY GAFFERS BOAT TRANSPORT
**3 Tregrehan Mills, Tregrehan,
St Austell PL25 3TH.**
Tel (01726) 816516/63188
Fax (01726) 817636
Established 1984 by ex-shipmaster/ yachtsman. Transportation by road up to 18 tons. Approved MoD boat transporter. Boat repairs - wood and GRP. Main agent for B P Dory.

WINTERS MARINE LTD
**(Lincombe Boatyard)
Lincombe,
Salcombe, Devon TQ8 8NQ.**
Tel (01548) 843580
Deep water pontoon moorings. Winter storage for 150 boats. All maintenance and repair facilities. Slipway capacity 30 tonnes. Inflatable craft sales and service. Lifecraft surveys and repairs. Short and long-term lifecraft hire.

BOATYARD SERVICES

CHICHESTER MARINA
**Birdham, Chichester,
West Sussex PO20 7EJ.**
Tel (01243) 512731 Fax (01243) 513472
A very attractive marina offering superb services and shore installations, welcoming long and short-term visitors. Chandlery, bar, restaurant and boatyard facilities. Ring for further details.

CLARKE & CARTER BOATYARD
**128 Coast Road, West Mersea,
Nr Colchester, Essex.**
Tel (01206) 382244 Fax (01206) 384455
The Clarke & Carter Boatyard is a division of West Mersea Marine Ltd. The yard is situated on the main waterfront at West Mersea. The anchorage, which has retained its traditional character, offers both swinging and post moorings for vessels up to about 50' LOA. Access is at all states of the tide to the river Blackwater. There are also some edge moorings available.

CRAOBH MARINA
By Lochgilphead, Argyll PA31 8UD.
Tel (01852) 500222 Fax (01852) 500252
250-berth marina on Loch Shuna. Water, electricity, diesel and gas. Full boatyard services. Chandlery. Brokerage. Insurance. Shops, bar, sailing centre and dive centre. Hotel and self-catering accommodation close by. 24-hour access. VHF channels 37(M) & 80.

DOVER YACHT COMPANY
**Cambridge Road, Dover,
Kent CT17 9BY.**
Tel (01304) 201073 Fax (01304) 207458
The boat centre of the South East where all your small craft and yacht maintenance and refit needs can be carried out. Established 50 years, the company offers traditional craftsmanship and skills working in GRP, metal and wood. Full rigging service. Kemp agents. West System Osmosis Centre. Volvo parts centre. Bukh agents. Avon inflatable repair centre.

ESSEX MARINA LTD
**Wallasea Island,
Nr Rochford, Essex SS4 2HG.**
Tel (01702) 258531 Fax (01702) 258227
Deep water marina berths for yachts up to 150'. Full marina shipyard services. NO locks or sills. One hour from London. Also swinging moorings available. Visiting yachtsmen welcome. Luxury toilets, laundry and shower block. Bar and restaurant.

FIDDLERS FERRY YACHT HAVEN
**Off Station Road, Penketh,
Warrington, Cheshire WA5 2UJ.**
Tel (01925) 727519
Sheltered moorings upto 6'6" draught, 50' long. Access through lock from river Mersey 1¹/₂ hours either side of high tide. Signed from A652. Boatyard and lift-out facilities. Annual rate per foot £8.

ISLAND HARBOUR MARINA
**Mill Lane, Binfield,
Newport, Isle of Wight PO30 2LA.**
Tel (01983) 526020 & 822999
Locked marina on Medina river. Tidal access HW ± 3¹/₂ hrs. 150 visitors' berths. Services include - water, electricity, showers, launderette, gas, diesel, chandlery, restaurant and bar. Full boatyard facilities with 12-ton hoist and 30-ton cradle.

KIP MARINA
**The Yacht Harbour, Inverkip,
Renfrewshire PA16 0AS.**
Tel (01475) 521485 (01475) 521298
Marina berths for vessels up to 65' LOA. Full boatyard facilities including travel hoist, crane, on-site engineers, GRP repairs etc. Bar, restaurant, saunas, launderette and chandlery.

LANGSTONE HARBOUR BOARD
**Ferry Road, Hayling Island,
Hampshire PO11 0DG.**
Tel (01705) 463419 Fax (01705) 467144
All boatyard facilities. Deep water and tidal moorings available. Water, electricity and diesel. Summer and winter storage. Public slipways. 6-ton crane. Landrover vessel and trailer recovery services.

SALTERNS MARINA
**40 Salterns Way, Lilliput,
Poole, Dorset BH14 8JR.**
Tel (01202) 707321/709971
Fax (01202) 700398
Pontoon Berths - Swinging Moorings - 24-hour Security - Visitors Welcome - Full Boatyard Facilities - Osmosis Treatment - 5 & 45 Tonne Hoists - Engine & Boat Sales - Award Winning Hotel, Restaurant and Bar - Chandlery - 24-hour Fuelling.

SPARKES YACHT HARBOUR & BOATYARD
**38 Wittering Road,
Sandy Point, Hayling Island,
Hampshire PO11 9SR.**
Tel (01705) 463572 Fax (01705) 465741
Sparkes Marina - a small friendly, family run business offering all the facilities you require including access at all states of the tide to a depth of 2 metres at lowest low water springs. In addition to marina berths, accessible through a security gate, we also offer dry boat sailing, moorings, storage ashore plus full maintenance facilities, new boat sales and brokerage, chandlery and restaurant.

TOLLESBURY MARINA
The Yacht Harbour, Tollesbury,
Maldon, Essex CM9 8SE.
Tel (01621) 869202
Fax (01621) 868489
VHF Channel 37/80 Tollesbury Marina
can offer 260 marina berths with water
and electricty on all pontoons.
Clubhouse with bar, restaurant,
swimming pool and tennis courts.
Repair workshops with West Osmosis
Treatment Centre. Full brokerage
service listing over 200 boats, with
friendly professional service.

WEIR QUAY BOATYARD
Heron's Reach,
Bere Alston, Devon PL20 7BT.
Tel (01822) 840474 Fax (01822) 840948
Deepwater swinging moorings, shore
storage, full boatyard facilities and services,
cranage to 12 tons, repairs, maintenance,
slipway. A traditional boatyard 'in a superb
setting' on the Tamar, with excellent
security at affordable rates.

YARMOUTH MARINE SERVICE
River Yar Boatyard, Yarmouth,
Isle of Wight PO41 0SE.
Tel (01983) 760521 Fax (01983) 760096
All boatyard facilities and commercial
charter. Slipway to 20 tons. Boat repairs,
wood and GRP, osmosis and painting.
Annual and visitors' moorings. Two
workboats available with loadline
exemption for all types of commercial
work.

BOOKS & CHARTS

A M SMITH (MARINE) LTD
33 Epping Way, Chingford E4 7PB.
Tel 0181-529 6988

B COOKE & SON LTD
Kingston Observatory,
58-59 Market Place, Hull HU1 1RH.
Tel (01482) 223454
DTp Certificated.

BOGERD NAVTEC NV
Oude Leeuwenrui 37,
Antwerp 20000, Germany.

BROWN SON & FERGUSON LTD
4-10 Darnley Street,
Glasgow G41 2SD.
Tel 0141-429 1234

CAPTAIN O M WATTS
7 Dover Street, London W1X 3PJ.
Tel 0171-493 4633 Fax 0171-495 0755
Admiralty charts, navigational instruments,
technical and leisure clothing, flags, books,
antiques and gifts, clocks and barometers,
lifejackets, paint and rope.

**DUBOIS-PHILLIPS
& McCALLUM LTD**
Oriel Chambers, Covent Garden,
Liverpool L2 8UD.
Tel 0151-236 2776

HYDROGRAPHIC OFFICE
Taunton, Somerset TA1 2DN.
Tel (01823) 337900 Fax (01823) 323753
Admiralty charts and hydrographic
publications - worldwide coverage
corrected to date of issue, available from
appointed Admiralty agents together with
notices to mariners. Products designed
specifically for the small craft user also
available from good chandlers.

IVER C WEILBACH & CO., A/S
35 Toldbodgade, Postbox 1560,
DK-1253 Copenhagen K, Denmark.

JOHN LILLIE & GILLIE LTD
Clive Street, North Shields,
Tyne & Wear NE29 6LF.
Tel 0191-257 2217
DTp Certificated.

**KELVIN HUGHES CHARTS
& MARITIME SUPPLIES**
Royal Crescent Road,
Southampton, Hampshire.
Tel (01703) 634911 Fax (01703) 330014
Charts, books, chandlery, safety equipment
and clothing. Liferaft hire, sales and
servicing. Also in London with worldwide
mail order service.

**KELVIN HUGHES CHARTS
& MARITIME SUPPLIES**
New North Road, Hainault,
Ilford, Essex IG6 2UR.
Tel 0181-500 6166
DTp Certificated.

**KELVIN HUGHES
OBSERVATOR**
Nieuwe Longowed 41, 3199 DC,
Hoogliet, The Netherlands.
DTp Certificated.

MARINE INSTRUMENTS
The Bosun's Locker,
Upton Slip, Falmouth TR11 3DQ.
Tel (01326) 312414
DTp Certificated.

MARTIN & CO
Oude Leewenrui 37,
Antwerp 2000, Germany.
DTp Certificated.

OCEAN LEISURE LTD
11-14 Northumberland Avenue,
London WC2N 5AQ.
Tel 0171-930 5050 Fax 0171-930 3032
Complete range of sailing clothing and
leisure wear stocked all year round.
Chandlery includes marine electronic

equipment, marine antiques, books and
charts and yachting holiday travel agent.
Also canoeing, underwater photography,
diving and waterskiing specialists.

R J MUIR
22 Seymour Close, Chandlers Ford,
Eastleigh, Southampton SO5 2JE.
Tel (01703) 261042
DTp Certificated.

S I R S NAVIGATION LTD
186a Milton Road, Swanscombe,
Kent DA10 0LX.
Tel (01322) 383672
DTp Certificated.

SEATH INSTRUMENTS (1992) LTD
Unit 30, Colville Road Works,
Colville Road, Lowestoft NR33 9QS.
Tel (01502) 573811
DTp Certificated.

SEVERNSIDE CONSULTANTS
Imperial Chambers,
2nd Floor, Gloucester Road,
Avonmouth BS11 9AQ.
Tel 0117-982 7184
DTp Certificated.

SIMPSON LAWRENCE LTD
218-228 Edmiston Drive,
Glasgow G51 2YT.
Tel 0141-427 5331 Fax 0141-427 5419
Simpson Lawrence are manufacturers and
the UK's largest wholesale distributors of
quality marine equipment.

**T J WILLIAMS & SON
(CARDIFF) LTD**
15-17 Harrowby Street,
Cardiff CF1 6HA.
Tel (01222) 487676
DTp Certificated.

**THOMAS GUNN
NAVIGATION SERVICES**
62 Marischal Street,
Aberdeen AB1 2AL.
Tel (01224) 595045
DTp Certificated.

TODD CHART AGENCY LTD
4 Seacliff Road, The Harbour,
Bangor, N Ireland BT20 5EY.
Tel (01247) 466640 Fax (01247) 471070
Admiralty Class 'A' chart agent for
Northern Ireland. Chart correction service
and nautical booksellers. Stockist of
navigation and chartroom instruments,
binoculars, clocks etc. Mail order service
available. Visa, Access and American
Express accepted.

W & H CHINA
Howley Properties Ltd.,
PO Box 149, Warrington,
Lancashire WA1 2DW.
Tel (01925) 634621 Fax (01925) 418009
Manufacturers of China chart dividers.

W F PRICE & CO LTD
Northpoint House, Wapping Wharf,
Bristol BS1 6UD.
Tel 0117-929 2229
DTp Certificated.

WARSASH NAUTICAL
BOOKSHOP
6 Dibles Road, Warsash,
Southampton SO31 9HZ.
Tel (01489) 572384 Fax (01489) 885756
Email: wnbooks@aladdin.co.uk Nautical
bookseller and chart agent. Callers and
mail order. New and secondhand.
Catalogues free also on Internet: http://
www.aladdin.co.uk/wnbooks.

WESSEX MARINE
EQUIPMENT LTD
Logistics House,
2nd Avenue Business Park,
Millbrook Road East,
Southampton SO1 0LP.
Tel (01703) 510570

CAPELLES MARINE LTD
Camp du Roi,
St Sampsons, Guernsey,
Channel Islands GY2 4XG.
Tel (01481) 57010 Fax (01481) 53590
Cellnet 0860 741245. Out of town - we are
only a phone call away and happy to find
YOU. Mercury and Mercruiser dealers on
the island. We also service all makes of
outboards. Petrol and diesel sterndrives
and diesel inboards. Perry's Guide Ref:
9F 4G3.

CLEDDAU BOATYARD
Cleddau House, Milford Marina,
Milford Haven, Dyfed SA73 3AF.
Tel (01646) 697834 Fax (01646) 697834
Travel hoist, storage, inboard and outboard.
Repairs, spares and service. General
leisurecraft repairs, wood and fibreglass
work. Chandlery and breakdown service.

DARTHAVEN MARINA LTD
Brixham Road, Kingswear,
Dartmouth, Devon TQ6 0SG.
Tel (01803) 752242 Fax (01803) 752722
Marina Office: (01803) 752545 Chandlery:
(01803) 752733 Fax (01803) 752790 All
types of repair facilities available. Fully
trained staff. 30-ton mobile hoist available
all states of tide. Extensive chandlery open
7 days a week. Agents for Autohelm/
Raytheon, Cetrek, Simpson Lawrence,
Vetus and Webasto. Visitors welcome.
24-hour engineering call-out service.
Mobile Nos: 0860 873553 Engineering;
0589 340609 Electronics.

SEA START
Unit 13 Hamble Point Marina,
School Lane, Hamble,
Southampton SO3 4JD.
Tel (01703) 457245 Fax (01703) 458000
Sea Start is the 24-hour marine breakdown

service with a 24-hour Area Update and
Helpline. A fast and effective solution for
boat owners in need of assistance, whether
on a mooring or underway. Freephone
0800 885500.

SMYE-RUMSBY LTD
123 Snargate Street, Dover,
Kent CT17 9AP.
Tel (01304) 201187 Fax (01304) 240135
Established since 1948, our company
welcomes visitors to Dover Port requiring
excellent marine electronic maintenance
services. We have comprehensive knowledge of current navigational equipment,
and can provide a 24-hour call-out repair
facility.

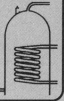
A R K MARINE LTD
1 Clifton Road, Isleworth,
Middlesex TW7 4HN.
Tel 0181-568 2778 Fax 0181-569 7503
We specialise in marine hot water systems
using the inboard engine as the heat source.
A full range are ex-stock, single or twin
coil, vertical or horizontal. Also 1, 2 and
3kw immersion heaters. Technical and
price lists free.

ARDFERN YACHT CENTRE
Ardfern By Lochgilphead,
Argyll PA31 8QN.
Tel (01852) 500247/636
Fax (01852) 500624 Boatyard with full
repair and maintenance facilities. Timber
and GRP repairs, painting and engineering.
Sheltered moorings and pontoon berthing.
Winter storage, chandlery, showers, fuel,
Calor, brokerage, 20-ton boat hoist. Hotel,
bars and restaurant.

ARUNCRAFT LTD
Littlehampton Marina,
Ferry Road, Littlehampton,
West Sussex BN17 5DS.
Tel (01903) 723667 Fax (01903) 730983
Mobile 0836 703006 Family business
based at Littlehampton Marina for 11 years.
Large workshop for boat maintenance,
GRP repairs, engine work, rigging,
electronic systems and propeller repairs.
In-house paint spraying and osmosis

treatments by Arunspray. Chandlery and
comprehensive range of craft in the
brokerage department.

THE BOAT SHOP
9 The Colonnade,
Woolston, Southampton,
Hampshire SO19 7QT.
Tel (01703) 449338 Fax (01703) 447791
Yacht and dinghy chandlery, fibreglass
products, Strand West & SP, Indespension
agent, Seagull, Force, Mariner and Mercury
outboards, spares, servicing (mobile 0860
232930), ropes, electronics, International
and Blakes paints, Perception canoes, laser
spares, Topper agents, resident surveyor.

BOATWORKS + LTD
Castle Emplacement,
St Peter Port, Guernsey,
Channel Islands GY1 1AU.
Tel (01481) 726071 Fax (01481) 714224
Boatworks+ provides a comprehensive
range of services including electronics,
chandlery, boatbuilding and repairs, engine
sales and services, yacht brokerage,
clothing and fuel supplies.

BOSUN'S LOCKER
10 Military Road, Royal Harbour,
Ramsgate, Kent CT11 9LG.
Tel/Fax (01843) 597158
The Bosun's Locker, a friendly, family
owned business, caters for a wide range of
boat owners and is staffed by experienced
yachtsmen. The stock is extensive,
including paint, ropes, quality clothing for
foul weather and fashion, electronics,
inflatables and charts.

BRIXHAM YACHT
SUPPLIES LTD
72 Middle Street,
Brixham, Devon TQ5 8EJ.
Tel (01803) 882290
We stock a complete range of sailing and
leisure clothing. English and continental
pure wool traditional knitwear. Camping
accessories.

CALEY MARINA
Canal Road, Inverness IV3 6NF.
Tel (01463) 236539 Fax (01463) 238323
Open 08.30 - 17.30. Berths: 50 Pontoons
(visitors available). Facilities: Fuel, water,
pump-out facilities, provisions (nearby
shops), repair, cranage, secure storage
afloat and ashore. Comprehensive chandlery, showers, workshop. Situated at
eastern end of Caledonian canal above
Muirtown locks. Access via sea locks 4
hours either side of highwater.

CAPTAIN O M WATTS
7 Dover Street, London W1X 3PJ.
Tel 0171-493 4633 Fax 0171-495 0755
Admiralty charts, navigational instruments,
technical and leisure clothing, flags, books,
antiques and gifts, clocks and barometers,
lifejackets, paint and rope.

CAVENHAM MARINE
15 Abbey Road, Billericay,
Essex CM12 9NF.
Tel (01277) 654788 Fax (01277) 631343
Boat chandlers and small new boats.

CLEDDAU BOATYARD
Cleddau House, Milford Marina,
Milford Haven, Dyfed SA73 3AF.
Tel (01646) 697834 Fax (01646) 697834
Travel hoist, storage, inboard and outboard.
Repairs, spares and service. General
leisurecraft repairs, wood and fibreglass
work. Chandlery and breakdown service.

COMPASS POINT CHANDLERY
The Quay, High Street,
Hamble, Hampshire SO31 4HA.
Tel (01703) 452388 Fax (01703) 456942
Compass Point is adjacent to the new quay
at Hamble. It stocks an attractive selection
of leisure clothing and foulweather gear as
well as a wide range of chandlery.

CRAOBH MARINA
By Lochgilphead, Argyll PA31 8UD.
Tel (01852) 500222 Fax (01852) 500252
250-berth marina on Loch Shuna. Water,
electricity, diesel and gas. Full boatyard
services. Chandlery. Brokerage. Insurance.
Shops, bar, sailing centre and dive centre.
Hotel and self-catering accommodation
close by. 24-hour access. VHF channels
37(M) & 80.

DARTHAVEN MARINA LTD
Brixham Road, Kingswear,
Dartmouth, Devon TQ6 0SG.
Tel (01803) 752242 Fax (01803) 752722
Marina Office: (01803) 752545 Chandlery:
(01803) 752733 Fax (01803) 752790 All
types of repair facilities available. Fully
trained staff. 30-ton mobile hoist available
all states of tide. Extensive chandlery open
7 days a week. Agents for Autohelm/
Raytheon, Cetrek, Simpson Lawrence,
Vetus and Webasto. Visitors welcome.
24-hour engineering call-out service.
Mobile Nos: 0860 873553 Engineering;
0589 340609 Electronics.

FALMOUTH YACHT MARINA
North Parade, Falmouth,
Cornwall TR11 2TD.
(01326) 316620 Fax (01326) 313939
The most westerly marina in England.
Strategically placed for transatlantic
departures and arrivals. Fully serviced
permanent and visitor berths. Diesel fuel,
chandlery, 30-ton hoist. Famous friendly
service.

GUY RYDER LEISURE
Dorset Lake Shipyard,
Lake Drive, Hamworthy,
Poole, Dorset BH15 4DT.
Tel/Fax (01202) 661052
The A-Z chandlery for sports boats. Boston
Whaler accessories, safety and security
equipment, Blakes paints, Pro-Rainer
clothing, life jackets and buoyancy aids,
navigational equipment, Ritchie

compasses, Tempo products. Mail order
available.

GWEEK QUAY BOATYARD
Gweek Quay (Helford River),
Helston, Cornwall TR12 6UF.
Tel (01326) 221657 Fax (01326) 221685
Head of the Helford river. Yacht repair
yard, 30-ton crane, chandlery, brokerage,
coffee shop, toilets and showers. Boat
storage and all boat repair and service
facilities. Access approximately 2 hours
either side of highwater.

HULL MARINA LTD
Warehouse 13,
Kingston Street, Hull HU1 2DQ.
Tel (01482) 593451 Fax (01482) 224148
Four Anchor Marina. Situated 5 minues
from the centre of Hull and all national and
international transport systems. First class
leisure, boatyard and brokerage facilities.
4-Star hotel and quayside restaurants.
Professional and caring staff. Competitive
rates.

ISLAND MARINE POWER
(ELECTRICAL) LTD
East Cowes Marina,
Clarence Road, Cowes Marina,
Isle of Wight PO32 6HA.
Tel/Fax (01983) 280011
Island Marine Power (Electrical) Ltd now
in our new premises facing the river at East
Cowes. The workshop - as always - open
for major, minor and emergency electrical
works. The shop - stocking practical
chandlery and hardware is still growing.
Tel/Fax 01983 280011 East Cowes Marina.

JOSEPH P LAMB & SONS
Maritime Building
(opposite Albert Dock),
Wapping, Liverpool L1 8DQ.
Tel 0151-709 4861 Fax 0151-709 2786
Situated in the centre of Liverpool, J P
Lamb have provided a service to world
shipping for over 200 years. All chandlery
supplies, clothing, rope, paint and flags are
available, together with a full sailmaking,
repair and rigging service. Open Mon to
Fri 8am to 6pm - Sat to Sun 9am to 1pm.

LANGSTONE YACHTING PLC
Fort Cumberland Road,
Southsea, Hampshire PO4 9RJ.
Tel (01705) 822719 Fax (01705) 822220
Langstone Marina with over 300 berths is
on the western side of the entrance to
Langstone Harbour. Facilities include:
hoist, brokerage, restaurant, bar, chandlery,
hard standing. Access over the sill is
available approximately 3 hours either side
of highwater.

LIVERPOOL MARINA
Coburg Dock, Sefton Street,
Liverpool L3 4BP.
Tel 0151-709 0578/(2683 after 5pm)
Fax 0151-709 8731.
300-berth yacht harbour. All serviced
pontoons. Tidal access HW ±2½ hrs

approximately, depending on draft. 60-ton
hoist, workshops, bar and restaurant, toilets
and showers. City centre one mile. Open
all year. Active yacht club and yacht
brokerage.

MALDON BOAT YARD
(formerly Dan Webb & Feesey)
North Street,
Maldon, Essex CM9 7HN.
Tel (01621) 854280
Full chandlery, slipway, stage berths,
winter storage, diesel. Based in the historic
town of Maldon.

MANX MARINE
35 North Quay,
Douglas, Isle of Man IM1 4LB.
Tel/Fax (01624) 674842
The Island's leading and most established
yacht chandlery. Stockists of quality foul
weather clothing and Thermalware. Large
stock holdings of stainless steel fixtures
and fittings and a comprehensive range of
general chandlery. Agents for Mariner.
Rigging facilities.

MARINE & GENERAL
ENGINEERS LTD
The Shipyard,
St Sampson's Harbour, Guernsey,
Channel Islands GY1 6AT.
Tel (01481) 45808 Fax (01481) 48765
Comprehensive marine hardware stores
stocking products from Caterpiller,
International, Sikaflex, Racor, MGDuff.
Excellent rigging facilities - rope/wire
splicing, lifting tackle and wire stops. 24-
hour Emergency Support on 0860 741217.

MARQUAND BROS LTD
North Quay, St Peter Port,
Guernsey, Channel Islands.
Tel (01481) 720962 Fax (01481) 713974
Yacht chandlers, stockists of a
comprehensive range of marine products.
Guernsey distributor for International
Yacht Paint. Extensive leisure and marine
clothing department including Barbour,
Driza-Bone, Dubarry and Quayside.

THE MAYFLOWER
INTERNATIONAL MARINA
Ocean Quay, Richmond Walk,
Plymouth PL1 4LS.
Tel (01752) 556633 Fax (01752) 606896
Marina operators with boat-hoist (25 ton)
facility. Restaurant, clubroom, launderette,
fuel, chandlery, shop and off-licence.
Winter storage. Owned by berth holders
and operated to a very high standard.

NORTH QUAY MARINE
North Side, St Sampson's Harbour,
Guernsey, Channel Islands.
Tel (01481) 46561 Fax (01481) 43488
The complete boating centre. Orkney and
Fletcher boats - Mariner outboards - Full
range of chandlery, rope, chain, lubricants,
paint, boatwear and shoes. Fishing tackle
for onshore and onboard. Inflatables and
safety equipment. Electronics.

OCEAN LEISURE LTD
**11-14 Northumberland Avenue,
London WC2N 5AQ.**
Tel 0171-930 5050 Fax 0171-930 3032
Complete range of sailing clothing and leisure wear stocked all year round. Chandlery includes marine electronic equipment, marine antiques, books and charts and yachting holiday travel agent. Also canoeing, underwater photography, diving and waterskiing specialists.

SEAQUEST MARINE LTD
**13 Fountain Street,
St Peter Port, Guernsey,
Channel Islands GY1 1BX.**
Tel (01481) 721773 Fax (01481) 716738
Seaquest Marine have a fully stocked chandlery. Agents for Sowester and Simpson Lawrence. Sole agents for Avon, Typhoon and Compass inflatables. Splashdown clothing. Electronics specialising in GPS. Inflatable specialists. Official Avon service station. VAT free friendly advice.

SHAMROCK CHANDLERY
**Shamrock Quay, William Street,
Northam, Southampton SO14 5QL.**
Tel (01703) 632725 Fax (01703) 225611
Situated on Shamrock Quay, a busy working yard with a pub, restaurant and boutiques. Shamrock Chandlery is renowned for extensive quality stocks and service and is widely used by both the trade and boat owners.

SHELL BAY MARINE
**Ferry Road, Studland,
Dorset BH19 3BA.**
Tel (01929) 450340 Fax (01929) 450570
Sensibly priced moorings immediately inside Poole harbour entrance. Slipway, boat hoist, winter storage, repairs. Good security, open all year, terms available by day, week or season. Parking, licensed bar, cafe and RYA recognised watersports centre.

THAMES (DITTON) MARINA LTD
**Portsmouth Road, Thames Ditton,
Surrey KT6 5QD.**
Tel 0181-398 6159 Fax 0181-398 6438
Over 120 berths and moorings. All main services, diesel, Calor Gas, repairs and service. Large chandlery with comprehensive stock of safety equipment, paint, charts and books. Very large car park for convenience of customers. Open 7 days a week.

UPPER DECK MARINE
**Albert Quay, Fowey,
Cornwall PL23 1AQ.**
Tel (01726) 832287 Fax (01726) 833265
Chandlery, fastenings, paints, cords, fenders, anchors, compasses, lifejackets, Gaz. Leading names in waterproofs and warm wear.

WEYMOUTH OLD HARBOUR
Weymouth & Portland Borough Council,
Borough Engineers Department,
**Municipal Offices, North Quay,
Weymouth, Dorset DT4 8TA.**
Tel (01305) 206278/206423
Fax (01305) 206276
Access at all stages of tide. Visitors' berths in the centre of prime tourist resort with shops, restaurants and night life all at hand. Diesel fuelling from pontoon or tanker. Chandlery and repair facilities available.

WORCESTER YACHT CHANDLERS LTD
**Unit 7, 75 Waterworks Road,
Barbourne, Worcester WR1 3EZ.**
Tel (01905) 22522 & 27949
Chandlery, paints, ropes, cables, chain, clothing, footwear, shackles, books, bottled gas, anti-foul, fastenings, oakam, fenders. Hard storage, crane, haulage, engine service, oils, navigation aids, buoyancy aids, life jackets, distress flares, small boat hire.

WYATTS CHANDLERY
**128 Coast Road, West Mersea,
Nr Colchester, Essex.**
Tel (01206) 384745 Fax (01206) 384455
Wyatts Chandlery, well stocked and competitively priced.

CLOTHING

OCEAN LEISURE LTD
**11-14 Northumberland Avenue,
London WC2N 5AQ.**
Tel 0171-930 5050 Fax 0171-930 3032
Complete range of sailing clothing and leisure wear stocked all year round. Chandlery includes marine electronic equipment, marine antiques, books and charts and yachting holiday travel agent. Also canoeing, underwater photography, diving and waterskiing specialists.

UPPER DECK MARINE (OUTRIGGERS)
**Albert Quay, Fowey,
Cornwall PL23 1AQ.**
Tel (01726) 833233 Fax (01726) 833265
'Outriggers' casual and marine clothing, footwear, nautical gifts, Admiralty chart agent and marine books.

COMMUNICATIONS EQUIPMENT

COMMUNICATION AERIALS LTD
**Unit 1A,
Woodland Industrial Estate,
Eden Vale Road, Westbury,
Wiltshire BA13 3QS.**
Tel (01373) 822835 Fax (01373) 858081
We have antennae and accessories to meet most applications. We use high quality cable and connectors to ensure your antenna operates efficiently. Ask for details on the comprehensive range of products that we now have to offer for VHF, cellular and Active Antenna installations.

ICS ELECTRONICS LTD
**Unit V, Rudford Industrial Estate,
Ford, Arundel,
West Sussex BN18 0BD.**
Tel (01903) 731101 Fax (01903) 731105
The manufacturer of data communication products - DSC, MSI, Navtex, radio telex modems, weatherfax and weather satellite receivers and software programmes - electronic charting. Weatherfax and Synop. UK distributor for Davis weather stations.

NAVICO LTD
Star Lane, Margate, Kent CT9 4NP.
Tel (01843) 290290 Fax (01843) 290471
Manufacturers of high quality VHF radios, yacht instrumentation systems, and advanced cockpit and below deck autopilots for sail, power and commercial applications. Leaders in onboard VHF radio telephones and the exclusive waterproof, handheld AXIS radio, also approved for commercial and military use. Autopilot models cover tiller and wheel, direct and hydraulic steering configurations. The CORUS instrumentation system is the most technically advanced to be found, offering significant advantages in ease of installation and use, and subsequent system expansion.

NORTH QUAY MARINE
**North Side, St Sampson's Harbour,
Guernsey, Channel Islands.**
Tel (01481) 46561 Fax (01481) 43488
The complete boating centre. Orkney and Fletcher boats - Mariner outboards - Full range of chandlery, rope, chain, lubricants, paint, boatwear and shoes. Fishing tackle for onshore and onboard. Inflatables and safety equipment. Electronics.

R T TRAINING
**286 Sea Front, Hayling Island,
Hampshire PO11 0AZ.**
Tel/Fax (01705) 462122
Weekend radio courses at Southampton and Port Solent for leisure and professional yachtsmen. SSB - 3-day Restricted Course/ Exam. Long Range Certificate - contact us for details of this new certificate. VHF - 1- day Course/Exam.

ROWLANDS MARINE ELECTRONICS LTD
**Unit 4, Glandon Industrial Estate,
Pwllheli, Gwynedd LL53 5YT**
Tel/Fax (01758) 613193
BEMA and BMIF members, dealer for Autohelm, B & G, Cetrek, ICOM, Kelvin Hughes, Marconi, Nasa, Navico, Navstar, Neco, Seafarer, Shipmate, Stowe, Racal-Decca, V-Tronix, Ampro, Walker. Equipment supplied installed and serviced.

COMPASS ADJUSTERS/ MANUFACTURERS

B COOKE & SON LTD
Kingston Observatory,
58-59 Market Place, Hull HU1 1RH.
Tel (01482) 223454
DTp Certificated.

JOHN LILLIE & GILLIE LTD
Clive Street, North Shields,
Tyne & Wear NE29 6LF.
Tel 0191-257 2217
DTp Certificated.

**KELVIN HUGHES CHARTS
& MARITIME SUPPLIES**
New North Road, Hainault,
Ilford, Essex IG6 2UR.
Tel 0181-500 6166
DTp Certificated.

**KELVIN HUGHES
OBSERVATOR**
Nieuwe Longowed 41, 3199 DC,
Hoogliet, The Netherlands.
DTp Certificated.

MARINE INSTRUMENTS
The Bosun's Locker,
Upton Slip, Falmouth TR11 3DQ.
Tel (01326) 312414
DTp Certificated.

MARTIN & CO
Oude Leewenrui 37,
Antwerp 2000, Germany.
DTp Certificated.

R J MUIR
22 Seymour Close, Chandlers Ford,
Eastleigh, Southampton SO5 2JE.
Tel (01703) 261042
DTp Certificated.

S I R S NAVIGATION LTD
186a Milton Road, Swanscombe,
Kent DA10 0LX.
Tel (01322) 383672
DTp Certificated.

SEATH INSTRUMENTS (1992) LTD
Unit 30, Colville Road Works,
Colville Road, Lowestoft NR33 9QS.
Tel (01502) 573811
DTp Certificated.

SEVERNSIDE CONSULTANTS
Imperial Chambers,
2nd Floor, Gloucester Road,
Avonmouth BS11 9AQ.
Tel 0117-982 7184
DTp Certificated.

**T J WILLIAMS & SON
(CARDIFF) LTD**
15-17 Harrowby Street,
Cardiff CF1 6HA.
Tel (01222) 487676
DTp Certificated.

**THOMAS GUNN
NAVIGATION SERVICES**
62 Marischal Street,
Aberdeen AB1 2AL.
Tel (01224) 595045
DTp Certificated.

W F PRICE & CO LTD
Northpoint House,
Wapping Wharf, Bristol BS1 6UD.
Tel 0117-929 2229
DTp Certificated.

COMPUTERS & SOFTWARE

**DOLPHIN MARITIME
SOFTWARE LTD**
25 Roosevelt Avenue,
Lancaster LA1 5EJ.
Tel/Fax (01524) 841946
Marine computer programs for IBM PC,
Psion and Sharp pocket computers.
Specialists in navigation, tidal prediction
and other programs for both yachting and
commercial uses.

MARITEK LTD
1-D7 Templeton Centre,
Glasgow G40 1DA.
Tel 0141-554 2492 Fax 0141-639 1910
Computer programs for coastal/celestial
navigation/tidal height prediction, using
Psion pocket computer. Large computer
systems and projects using 4th generation
languages.

**PROSSER SCIENTIFIC
INSTRUMENTS LTD**
Lady Lane Industrial Estate,
Hadleigh, Ipswich, Suffolk IP7 6BQ.
Tel (01473) 823005 Fax (01473) 824095
Manufacturer of a range of marine
instruments, including the WEATHER-
TREND digital barometer, with full 24-
hour history, the unique TIDECLOCK tidal
data predictor and tidal software.

CORRESPONDENCE COURSES/SCHOOLS

**NORTHUMBRIA SCHOOL
OF NAVIGATION**
53 High Street, Amble,
Northumberland NE65 0LE.
Tel (01665) 713437
Whatever your experience we have an RYA
accredited course for you. The Day Skipper
Course will suit the inexperienced while
those ready for an offshore passage should
enrol for the Yachtmaster Offshore. Our
Ocean Yachtmaster Course provides a
fascinating guide through astro-navigation,
world meteorolgy and ocean currents.
GCSE Navigation includes sections from
both yachtmaster courses.

CREW FINDER SERVICE

WORLD CREWS
52 York Place,
Bournemouth BH7 6JN.
Tel/Fax (01202) 431520
An International crewfinder service
providing amateur and professional crew
for yachts cruising in home and overseas
waters. Files contain delivery skippers,
engineers, cook/hostess, chefs and various
marine tradesmen.

DECK EQUIPMENT

BASELINE LTD
Unit 10 Apple Industrial Estate,
Segensworth West,
Fareham, Hampshire PO15 5SX.
Tel (014895) 76349 Fax (014895) 78835
Extensive range of marine hardware for all
boats including many difficult to find
articles. Fastenings, canopy fittings, vents,
hinges - stainless steel available - fittings
for sails and rigging, rails and boarding
ladders. Efficient mail order service
available.

**HARKEN - DISTRIBUTED BY
SIMPSON LAWRENCE**
218-228 Edmiston Drive,
Glasgow G51 2YT.
Tel 0141-427 5331/8 Fax 0141-427 5419
Distributors of Harken deck hardware, ball
bearing blocks in all sizes from micros to
maxis, jib reefing and furling systems,
from dinghies to 150 footers, winches,
backstay tensioners, power sheet jammers
and deck shoes. We also distribute Head
Foil plastic luff groove systems, and Edson
steering and pump-out systems.

**SOUTHERN SPAR SERVICES
& EQUIPMENT**
Shamrock Quay, William Street,
Northam, Southampton,
Hampshire SO14 5QL.
Tel (01703) 331714 Fax (01703) 230559
Mobile 0850 736540 Mast manufacturer,
all spars, Toerails, stanchions, bases. Deck
equipment. Rigging and Furlex headsail
reefing systems.

DIESEL MARINE FUEL ADDITIVES

CHICKS MARINE LTD
Collings Road, St Peter Port,
Guernsey, Channel Islands.
Tel (01481) 723716 Fax (01481) 713632
Distributors of diesel fuel biocide used to
treat and protect contamination in fuel
tanks where an algae (bug) is present.
Most owners do not realise what the
problem is, loss of power, blocked fuel
filter, exhaust smoking, resulting in
expensive repairs to injectors - fuel pump
- or complete engine overhaul. Marine
engineers, engines, spares, service - VAT
free. Honda outboards, pumps and
generators. Volvo Penta specialists.

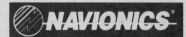
NAVIONICS UK
Oak Wood House,
Gospel Oak Lane,
Stratford-upon-Avon,
Warwickshire CV37 0JA.
Tel (01789) 269891 Fax (01789) 262717
Navionics UK, the exclusive UK and Irish
distributor for Navionics electronic charts.
Charts suitable in chart plotters from
Furuno, Koden, Geonav, Trimble,
Panasonic, B & G, Philips etc. 24-hour
despatch service for any Navionics chart
worldwide.

REGIS ELECTRONICS LTD
Regis House, Quay Hill, Lymington,
Hampshire SO41 3AR.
Tel (01590) 679251/679176
Fax (01590) 679910
(also at COWES, SOUTHAMPTON &
CHICHESTER). Sales, service and ins-
tallation of marine electronic equipment.
Leading south coast agents for AUTO-
HELM, FURUNO, RAYTHEON,
CETREK, STOWE, ROBERTSON, A.P.
NAVIGATOR, GARMIN, KELVIN
HUGHES and other manufacturers of
quality marine electronic equipment.
Competitively priced quotations (including
owner familiarisation and sea trials)
forwarded by return of post.

SEAQUEST MARINE LTD
13 Fountain Street,
St Peter Port, Guernsey,
Channel Islands GY1 1BX.
Tel (01481) 721773 Fax (01481) 716738
Seaquest Marine have a fully stocked
chandlery. Agents for Sowester and
Simpson Lawrence. Sole agents for Avon,
Typhoon and Compass inflatables.
Splashdown clothing. Electronics
specialising in GPS. Inflatable specialists.
Official Avon service station. VAT free
friendly advice.

SIMPSON LAWRENCE LTD
218-228 Edmiston Drive,
Glasgow G51 2YT.
Tel 0141-427 5331 Fax 0141-427 5419
Simpson Lawrence are manufacturers and
the UK's largest wholesale distributors of
quality marine equipment.

TOLLEY MARINE LTD
Unit 7, Blackhill Road West,
Holton Heath Trading Park,
Poole, Dorset BH16 6LS.
Tel (01202) 632644 Fax (01202) 632622
(also at: Plymouth - Tel (01752) 222530;
Brighton - Tel (01273) 424224 and London
- 0171-930 3237. Agents of sales and
service for Autohelm, B & G, Cetrek,
Furuno, Garmin, Icom, Koden, Lo-Kata,
MLR, Magnavox, Navico, Panasonic,
Raytheon, Robertson, Sailor, Shipmate,
Trimble.

ENGINES

BOSUN'S LOCKER
10 Military Road, Royal Harbour,
Ramsgate, Kent CT11 9LG.
Tel/Fax (01843) 597158
The Bosun's Locker, a friendly, family
owned business, caters for a wide range of
boat owners and is staffed by experienced
yachtsmen. The stock is extensive,
including paint, ropes, quality clothing for
foul weather and fashion, electronics,
inflatables and charts.

CAPELLES MARINE LTD
Camp du Roi, St Sampsons,
Guernsey, GY2 4XG.
Tel (01481) 57010 Fax (01481) 53590
Cellnet 0860 741245 Out of town - we are
only a phone call away and happy to find
YOU. Mercury and Mercruiser dealers on
the island. We also service all makes of
outboards. Petrol and diesel sterndrives
and diesel inboards. Perry's Guide Ref: 9F
4G3.

CHICKS MARINE LTD
Collings Road, St Peter Port,
Guernsey, Channel Islands.
Tel (01481) 723716 Fax (01481) 713632
Distributors of diesel fuel biocide used to
treat and protect contamination in fuel
tanks where an algae (bug) is present.
Most owners do not realise what the
problem is, loss of power, blocked fuel
filter, exhaust smoking, resulting in
expensive repairs to injectors - fuel pump
- or complete engine overhaul. Marine
engineers, engines, spares, service - VAT
free. Honda outboards, pumps and
generators. Volvo Penta specialists.

CLEDDAU BOATYARD
Cleddau House, Milford Marina,
Milford Haven, Dyfed SA73 3AF.
Tel (01646) 697834 Fax (01646) 697834
Travel hoist, storage, inboard and outboard.
Repairs, spares and service. General
leisurecraft repairs, wood and fibreglass
work. Chandlery and breakdown service.

DARTMOUTH YACHT
CRUISE SCHOOL
103 High Street,
Totnes, Devon TQ9 5SN.
Ans/Fax (01803) 864027
Tel (01803) 722226
Home: 55 The Old Common, Bussage,
Stroud, Gloucestershire GL6 8HH. Tel
(01453) 731142. RYA recognised teaching
establishment since 1990. Skipper charter;
Bareboat charter; Youth training, Duke of
Edinburgh's Scheme; Sail training all RYA
recognised courses including First Aid;
Diesel engine courses; Sea survival;
Helmsman's certificates to Yachtmaster
offshore preparation.

LANGNEY MARINE
SERVICES LTD
Sovereign Harbour Marina,
Pevensey Bay Road, Eastbourne,
East Sussex BN23 6JH.
Tel (01323) 470244 Fax (01323 470255
We offer a complete service to the boat
owner offering repairs on all types of
engines, GRP, steel, wood, electronics,
rigging, cleaning, etc. We are also
contractors to the R.N.L.I.

MARINE & AUTO SERVICES
Bridge Boathouse, River Road,
Maidenhead, Berkshire SL6 0BE.
Tel/Fax (01628) 36435
Marine consultant and engineers.
Condition, survey and valuation reports
undertaken on fibreglass craft - Thames
and nationwide. Engines sold and
delivered. Repairs, overhauls and servicing
on all types of engines. Mail order for parts
available. 35 years experience in the marine
industry.

R.I.B.S. MARINE
Little Avon Marina,
Stony Lane South,
Christchurch, Dorset BH23 1HW.
Tel (01202) 477327 Fax (01202) 471456
Full boatyard facilities. Mooring, slipping
and dry boat storage. Marine engineers for
all makes of outboard and inboard. Petrol
and diesel. Specialist repairs in wood and
GRP. Main agents for Mariner and Force
outboards and Mercruiser stern drives.
Brokerage facilities.

ROBIN CURNOW MARINE
ENGINEERS
Commercial Road,
Penryn, Cornwall TR10 8AG.
Tel (01326) 373438 Fax (01326) 376534
Outboard motor sales and service. Morse
controls service centre. British Seagull/
Selva - Evinrude - Honda - Mercury -
Yamaha.

VOLVO PENTA LTD
Otterspool Way, Watford,
Hertfordshire WD2 8HW.
Tel (01923) 28544
Volvo Penta's leading marine power-petrol and diesel for leisurecraft and workboats - is supported by an extensive network of parts and service dealers.

FABRICATIONS & REPAIRS

R J P FABRICATIONS
83B Sterte Avenue West,
Poole, Dorset BH15 2AL.
Tel (01202) 660205 Mobile 0860 678326
Aluminium and stainless steel custom made ladders and handrails. General light fabrication and repairs.

FIRST AID

D G I MEDICAL SERVICES
Hyfrydle, Capel Curig,
Gwynedd LL24 0EU.
Tel/Fax (01690) 720344
Providers of H&SE and Rescue and Emergency Care (REC). Our instructors can provide the full REC training programme for first aid at sea. If you would like to learn how to handle emergency situations, we have a programme to suit your needs. (Department of DGI Mountaineering Ltd.)

FLAGS & PENNANTS

JOSEPH P LAMB & SONS
Maritime Building
(opposite Albert Dock),
Wapping, Liverpool L1 8DQ.
Tel 0151-709 4861 Fax 0151-709 2786
Situated in the centre of Liverpool, J P Lamb have provided a service to world shipping for over 200 years. All chandlery supplies, clothing, rope, paint and flags are available, together with a full sailmaking, repair and rigging service. Open Mon to Fri 8am to 6pm - Sat to Sun 9am to 1pm.

SARNIA FLAGS
8 Belmont Road,
St Peter Port, Guernsey,
Channel Islands GY1 1PY.
Tel (01481) 725995 Fax (01481) 729335
Flags and pennants made to order. National flags, house, club and battle flags, and burgees made to order. Any size, shape or design. Prices on request.

GENERAL MARINE EQUIPMENT

A B MARINE LTD
Castle Walk, St Peter Port,
Guernsey, Channel Islands.
Tel (01481) 722378
We specialise in safety and survival equipment and are a D.O.T. approved service station for liferafts including R.F.D.

Beaufort/Dunlop, Zodiac, Plastimo and Lifeguard. We also carry a full range of new liferafts, dinghies, and lifejackets and are agents for Bukh marine engines.

AQUA-MARINE
MANUFACTURING (UK) LTD
216 Fair Oak Road, Bishopstoke,
Eastleigh, Hampshire SO50 8NJ.
Tel (01703) 694949 Fax (01703) 601381
Manufacturers and distributors of chandlery, including: Engel refrigeration, Dutton-Lainson winches, Anchor fenders, Rule pumps, Aquaflow water systems, SeaStar steering and controls, Skyblazer flares, Admiralty small craft charts, Aquameter compasses, RWO and Holt fittings, Danforth anchors, Aqua-Signal lights.

CHICKS MARINE LTD
Collings Road, St Peter Port,
Guernsey, Channel Islands.
Tel (01481) 723716 Fax (01481) 713632
Distributors of diesel fuel biocide used to treat and protect contamination in fuel tanks where an algae (bug) is present. Most owners do not realise what the problem is, loss of power, blocked fuel filter, exhaust smoking, resulting in expensive repairs to injectors - fuel pump - or complete engine overhaul. Marine engineers, engines, spares, service - VAT free. Honda outboards, pumps and generators. Volvo Penta specialists.

HAMOAZE MARINE SERVICES
Calstock Boatyard, Lower Kelly,
Calstock, Cornwall PL18 9RY.
Tel (01822) 834024 & (01752) 823118
High class yacht and boat repairs, especially wood. Sheltered moorings up to 4' draught in upper Tamar river. Showers, fuel, winter storage. Also agents for Avon inflatable boats and Heyland Marine fibreglass dinghies.

LEWMAR MARINE LTD
Southmoor Lane, Havant,
Hampshire PO9 1JJ.
Tel (01705) 471841 Fax (01705) 476043
Manufacturers of winches, windlasses, hatches, hardware, hydraulics and marine thrusters for boats ranging in size from 25' to 300' LOA.

SIMPSON LAWRENCE LTD
218-228 Edmiston Drive,
Glasgow G51 2YT.
Tel 0141-427 5331 Fax 0141-427 5419
Simpson Lawrence are manufacturers and the UK's largest wholesale distributors of quality marine equipment.

VETUS DEN OUDEN LTD
38 South Hants Industrial Park,
Totton, Southampton,
Hampshire SO40 3SA.
Tel (01703) 861033 Fax (01703) 663142
Suppliers of marine diesel equipment, exhaust systems, steering systems, bow propellers, propellers and shafts, hatches, portlights, windows, electronic instru-

ments, batteries, ventilators, windlasses, water and fuel tanks, chandlery items and much much more.

WORCESTER YACHT
CHANDLERS LTD
Unit 7, 75 Waterworks Road,
Barbourne, Worcester WR1 3EZ.
Tel (01905) 22522 & 27949
Chandlery, paints, ropes, cables, chain, clothing, footwear, shackles, books, bottled gas, anti-foul, fastenings, oakam, fenders. Hard storage, crane, haulage, engine service, oils, navigation aids, buoyancy aids, life jackets, distress flares, small boat hire.

HARBOURS

ABERYSTWYTH
MARINA - Y LANFA
Trefechan, Aberystwyth,
Dyfed SY23 1AS.
Tel (01970) 611422 Fax (01970) 624122
NEW fully serviced marina. Diesel, gas, water, toilets, hot showers. Launching facilities, winter storage and dry boat sailing. Car parking and security. Town centre 5 minutes' walk with excellent restaurants, shops, pubs and full recreational leisure facilities. Waterside apartments available.

BALTIC WHARF WATER
LEISURE CENTRE
Bristol Harbour,
Underfall Yard, Bristol.
Tel 0117-929 7608 Fax 0117-929 4454
Sailing school and centre, with qualified instruction in most watersports. Also moorings available throughout the Bristol Harbour for all types of leisurecraft at extremely competitive rates.

CHICHESTER HARBOUR
CONSERVANCY
The Harbour Office,
Itchenor, Chichester,
West Sussex PO20 7AW.
Tel (01243) 512301 Fax (01243) 513026
We offer a full range of swinging moorings, at affordable prices in this area of outstanding natural beauty, combining 11 square miles of water, with easy access to the Solent. Visitors welcome.

DOVER HARBOUR BOARD -
DOVER MARINA
Harbour House, Dover,
Kent CT17 9BU.
Tel (01304) 241663/240400
Fax (01304) 240465
Providing 24-hour sailing from expanded facilities. Over 100 new pontoon berths in Tidal Harbour with minimum depth of 2.5 metres. 147 berths in adjacent Wellington Dock. Closest marina to Continental Europe. Excellent new road access. Many tourist attractions. Free marina guide with berth maps, navigational information and distance charts for cruising available. Boatyard and repair services available.

HAFAN PWLLHELI
Glan Don, Pwllheli,
Gwynedd LL53 5YT.
Tel (01758) 701219 Fax (01758) 701443
Hafan Pwllheli has over 400 pontoon berths and offers access at virtually all states of the tide. Ashore, its modern purpose-built facilities include luxury toilets, showers, landerette, a secure boat park for winter storage, 40-ton travel hoist, mobile crane and plenty of space for car parking. Open 24-hours a day, 7 days a week.

LANGSTONE HARBOUR BOARD
Ferry Road, Hayling Island,
Hampshire PO11 0DG.
Tel (01705) 463419 Fax (01705) 467144
All boatyard facilities. Deep water and tidal moorings available. Water, electricity and diesel. Summer and winter storage. Public slipways. 6-ton crane. Landrover vessel and trailer recovery services.

MERSEYSIDE DEVELOPMENT CORPORATION
4th Floor, Royal Liver Building,
Pierhead, Liverpool L3 1JH.
Tel 0151-236 6090 Fax 0151-227 3174
Albert Dock welcomes vessels for short or long-term visits to what is now one of the north west's most popular maritime locations. Maximum length 55m. Concessionary rates (details on application). Access by prior agreement.

PETERHEAD BAY AUTHORITY
Bath House, Bath Street,
Peterhead AB42 6DX.
Tel (01779) 474020 Fax (01779) 475712
Contact: Stephen Paterson. Opened in April 1994, Peterhead Bay Marina offers a comprehensive range of services and facilities for local and visiting boat owners. Ideal stopover marina for vessels heading to/from Scandinavia or the Caledonian canal.

PORT OF TRURO
Harbour Office,
Town Quay, Truro, Cornwall.
Tel (01872) 72130 Fax (01872) 225346
Facilities for the yachtsman include visitors' pontoons located at Turnaware Bar near Ruan Creek, Boscawen Park. Visitors' moorings at Woodbury. Quay facilities at Truro with free showers and toilets. Chemical toilet disposal, fresh water and garbage disposal.

RAMSGATE ROYAL HARBOUR
Harbour Office,
Military Road,
Ramsgate, Kent CT11 9LG.
Tel (01843) 592277 Fax (01843) 590941
One of south east England's premier leisure areas. Ideal for crossing to the Continent. 24-hour access to finger pontoons. Comprehensive security systems. Amenities: launderette, repairs, slipways, boatpark. Competitive rates for permanent berths and visiting vessels.

SOVEREIGN HARBOUR MARINA LTD
Pevensey Bay Road,
Eastbourne, Sussex BN23 6JH.
Tel (01323) 470099 Fax (01323) 470077
Situated at Langney Point, Eastbourne, Sovereign Harbour is centred around twin harbours, one tidal and one accessed by two high capacity locks. A full service marina with diesel, petrol and unleaded petrol available 24-hours daily.

WEYMOUTH OLD HARBOUR
Weymouth & Portland Borough Council, Borough Engineers Department,
Municipal Offices, North Quay,
Weymouth, Dorset DT4 8TA.
Tel (01305) 206278/206423
Fax (01305) 206276
Access at all stages of tide. Visitors' berths in the centre of prime tourist resort with shops, restaurants and night life all at hand. Diesel fuelling from pontoon or tanker. Chandlery and repair facilities available.

NELSON STOVES
Chequers, Wainfleet Road,
Irby in the Marsh, Skegness,
Lincolnshire PE24 5AY.
Tel (01754) 810799
The unique Nelson stove is 9" square by 21" high, finished in matt black with brass trim. Heat output range 750 to 3000 watts. Designed to burn only smokeless fuels. Only available from Nelson Stoves.

COWES YACHTING
Britannia House, 2 & 3 High Street,
Cowes, Isle of Wight PO31 7SA.
Tel (01983) 280770 Fax (01983) 280766
The complete information and liaison service for yachting in and around Cowes. Cowes Yachting can provide all the information that regatta or rally organisers or individual yachtsmen need to plan a visit to Cowes.

AMPRO NAVIGATION LTD
PO Box 373A,
Surbiton, Surrey KT6 5YL.
Tel 0181-398 1169 Fax 0181-398 6184
Tel (01734) 820337 Fax (01734) 820338
UK agents for Philips Navigation AP range of marine electronic equipment including GPS and Decca Navigators, Chart Plotters, Instruments, hand portable and Differential GPS units. Full sales and technical support available.

AUTOHELM - RAYTHEON MARINE EUROPE
Anchorage Park, Portsmouth,
Hampshire PO3 5TD.
Tel (01705) 693611 Fax (01705) 694642
Telex: 86384 Nautec G. Manufacturers of the Autohelm range of instruments, compasses, GPS, chart plotters and autopilots for power and sail craft from 22' to 125'. Manufacturer of the Autohelm personal compass.

DIVERSE YACHT SERVICES
Unit 12,
Hamble Yacht Services,
Port Hamble, Hamble,
Hampshire SO31 4NN.
Tel (01703) 453399 Fax (01703) 455288
Marine electronics and electrics. Supplied and installed. Specialists in racing yachts. Suppliers of 'Loadsense' Loadcells for marine applications.

GREENHAM MARINE LTD
King's Saltern Road, Lymington,
Hampshire SO41 9QD.
Tel (01590) 671144 Fax (01590) 679517
Greenham Marine can offer yachtsmen one of the most comprehensive selections of marine electronic equipment currently available.

NAVICO LTD
Star Lane, Margate, Kent CT9 4NP.
Tel (01843) 290290 Fax (01843) 290471
Manufacturers of high quality VHF radios, yacht instrumentation systems, and advanced cockpit and below deck autopilots for sail, power and commercial applications. Leaders in onboard VHF radio telephones and the exclusive waterproof, handheld AXIS radio, also approved for commercial and military use. Autopilot models cover tiller and wheel, direct and hydraulic steering configurations. The CORUS instrumentation system is the most technically advanced to be found, offering significant advantages in ease of installation and use, and subsequent system expansion.

PROSSER SCIENTIFIC INSTRUMENTS LTD
Lady Lane Industrial Estate,
Hadleigh, Ipswich, Suffolk IP7 6BQ.
Tel (01473) 823005 Fax (01473) 824095
Manufacturer of a range of marine instruments, including the WEATHER-TREND digital barometer, with full 24-hour history, the unique TIDECLOCK tidal data predictor and tidal software.

**ROWLANDS MARINE
ELECTRONICS LTD**
Unit 4, Glandon Industrial Estate,
Pwllheli, Gwynedd LL53 5YT
Tel/Fax (01758) 613193
BEMA and BMIF members, dealer for
Autohelm, B & G, Cetrek, ICOM, Kelvin
Hughes, Marconi, Nasa, Navico, Navstar,
Neco, Seafarer, Shipmate, Stowe, Racal-
Decca, V-Tronix, Ampro, Walker.
Equipment supplied installed and serviced.

W & H CHINA
Howley Properties Ltd.,
PO Box 149, Warrington,
Lancashire WA1 2DW.
Tel (01925) 634621 Fax (01925) 418009
Manufacturers of China chart dividers.

**BOWRING MARSH
& McLENNAN LTD**
Yacht Division,
Havelock Chambers,
Queens Terrace, Southampton,
Hampshire SO14 3PP.
Tel (01703) 318300 Fax (01703) 318391
A member of the largest insurance broking
firm in the world with associated offices in
Antibes and Fort Lauderdale. Specialists
in yacht insurance for craft cruising
Mediterranean, Caribbean and US waters.

**CRAVEN HODGSON
ASSOCIATES**
Suite 15, 30-38 Dock Street,
Leeds LS10 1JF.
Tel 0113-243 8443
As an independent intermediary, we
recommend and advise in relation to all
major experienced marine insurers and act
as your agent.

**DESMOND CHEERS
& PARTNERS**
44 High Street, Hampton Hill,
Middlesex TW12 1PD.
Tel 0181-943 5333 Fax 0181-943 5444
Marine insurance specialists with over 30
years' experience in arranging tailor-made
policies through leading marine
underwriters. For all your insurance and
finance enquiries for yachts, motorcruisers
and speedboats call Tim Cheers or Daphne
Bamberger.

**GAVIN POOLE YACHT
BROKERS**
14 Hooke Close,
Canford Heath, Dorset BH17 8BB.
Tel (01202) 604068 Fax (01202) 659680
The motor cruiser and Fairey boat specialist
for modern diesel and classic boats. Sales,
service, finance. Open every day. Mobile
number 0860 236389

**GENERAL ACCIDENT FIRE
& LIFE ASSURANCE
CORPORATION plc**
Head Office: Pitheavlis,
Perth PH2 0NH.
Tel (01738) 621202 Fax (01738) 621843
Pleasurecraft insurance for small craft,
yachts and motor boats. Contact your local
GA office for details of our Sailplan
policies.

**GILES INSURANCE
BROKERS LTD**
22 Portland Road,
Kilmarnock KA1 2BS.
Tel (01563) 520554 Fax (01563) 528345
Scotland's marine insurance experts.
Established 1967. Registered insurance
brokers. Rates from the top 25 insurers are
compared before quotations are sent out in
an easy to read format with a copy of the

policy wording. Staff are very efficient
and friendly.

**INDEPENDENT INSURANCE
BROKERS LTD**
PO Box 285, Esplanade House,
29 Glategny Esplanade,
St Peter Port, Guernsey,
Channel Islands GY1 1WR.
Tel (01481) 722868 Fax (01481) 714234
Marine insurance brokers with a
comprehensive portfolio of insurance
products and services, extending to home,
personal, etc. Our reputation is built on
thoroughness, active client support and
communication.

PANTAENIUS UK LTD
Registered Insurance Broker:
Marine Building,
Queen Anne's Battery,
Plymouth, Devon PL4 0LP.
Tel (01752) 223656 Fax (01752) 223637
Head Office: Cremon 32.20457 Hamburg,
Germany. Tel: +49 40 370 910 Fax +49 40
3709 1109. Pantaenius is one of Europe's
largest yacht insurance brokers and covers
yachts sailing under more than 35 different
flags in all seven seas.

K C POWELL & PARTNERS LTD
50 The Broadway,
Leigh-on-Sea, Essex SS9 1AG.
Tel (01702) 470035 Fax (01702) 715344
Yacht and motor yacht brokers and
underwriters since 1970. Underwriters are
RYA Yachtmasters Offshore. You can feel
safe in your choice knowing you are talking
to kindred spirits. Non-marine accounts
also placed in the British market.

SHAMROCK CHANDLERY
Shamrock Quay, William Street,
Northam, Southampton S014 5QL.
Tel (01703) 632725 Fax (01703) 225611
Situated on Shamrock Quay, a busy
working yard with a pub, restaurant and
boutiques. Shamrock Chandlery is
renowned for extensive quality stocks and
service and is widely used by both the
trade and boat owners.

**ST MARGARETS
INSURANCES LTD**
153-155 High Street,
Penge, London SE20 7DL.
Tel 0181-778 6161 Fax 0181-659 1968
Marine insurance. Over 25 years dedicated
to insuring yachts and pleasurecraft. Many
unique policies available only through St
Margarets. Immediate quotations and cover
available.

ARDFERN YACHT CENTRE
Ardfern By Lochgilphead,
Argyll PA31 8QN.
Tel (01852) 500247/636
Fax (01852) 500624
Boatyard with full repair and maintenance facilities. Timber and GRP repairs, painting and engineering. Sheltered moorings and pontoon berthing. Winter storage, chandlery, showers, fuel, Calor, brokerage, 20-ton boat hoist, rigging. Hotel, bars and restaurant.

BLACKWATER MARINA
Marine Parade,
Maylandsea, Essex CM3 6AN.
Tel (01621) 740264 Fax (01621) 742122
Refurbished tidal marina on the Blackwater estuary. New pontoons, new clubhouse, bar and restaurant, toilets and showers. 18-ton slipway hoist, 70-ton winch, 130' workshop with full services. Full chandlery, brokerage/boat sales. Car parking and on-site security. Full tide swinging moorings, half tide moorings and half tide pontoon berths. A few long-term berths available.

BRAY MARINA
Monkey Island Lane, Bray,
Berkshire SL6 2EB.
Tel (01628) 23654 Fax (01628) 773484
400 berths many with 240v electricity. Shower and toilet facilities, car park, petrol, diesel and Calor gas. Chandlery, shops and cafe. Hardstanding, brokerage, refuse and chemical toilet disposal. Ample restaurants close by. Part of the MDL Group.

THE BRIGHTON MARINA COMPANY LTD
Brighton Marina Village,
Brighton, East Sussex BN2 5UF.
Tel (01273) 693636 Fax (01273) 675082
Britain's largest marina (1800 pontoon berths) with marina village under development. TYHA Five Gold Anchors. Full boatyard and shore facilities. Brokerage and boat sales. Club racing throughout the year. Group visits, rallies welcome.

BRIXHAM MARINA
Berry Head Road,
Brixham, Devon TQ5 9BW.
Tel (01803) 882929 Fax (01803) 882737
Contact: Mrs Amanda Pledger. Sheltered 480-berth marina in Torbay. Pontoon fully serviced berths up to 18 metres. Larger vessel by arrangement. 24-hour dockmaster. Diesel 24 hours, car park, toilet and launderette facilities, chandlery. Part of the MDL Group.

BRUNDALL BAY MARINA - SALES
Riverside Estate, Brundall,
Norwich, Norfolk NR13 5PN.
Tel (01603) 716606 Fax (01603) 715666
New and used boat sales, brokerage, full workshop services. Agents for Faircraft river cruisers. Hardy, Seawings sports cruisers, Evinrude outboard motors. 200-berth marina with full facilities.

BURNHAM YACHT HARBOUR MARINA LTD
Burnham Yacht Harbour,
Burnham-on-Crouch,
Essex CM0 8BL.
Tel (01621) 782150
The only Five Gold Anchor marina in Essex. 350 fully serviced pontoon berths and 120 deep water swing moorings. Marina access at all states of tide with minimum 2.5 metres depth at low water.

CALEY MARINA
Canal Road, Inverness IV3 6NF.
Tel (01463) 236539 Fax (01463) 238323
Open 08.30 - 17.30. Berths: 50 Pontoons (visitors available). Facilities: Fuel, water, pump-out facilities, provisions (nearby shops), repair, cranage, secure storage afloat and ashore. Comprehensive chandlery, showers, workshop. Situated at eastern end of Caledonian canal above Muirtown locks. Access via sea locks 4 hours either side of highwater.

CARRICKFERGUS MARINA
Rodger's Quay, Carrickfergus,
Co Antrim, N Ireland BT38 8BE.
Tel (01960) 366666 Fax (01960) 350505
300 fully serviced pontoon berths with full on-shore facilities (half a mile from town centre). Steeped in a wealth of historical legend, Carrickfergus has excellent restaurants, hotels, pubs, shops and a host of recreational leisure facilities.

CASTLEPARK MARINA
Kinsale, Co Cork, Eire.
Tel +353 21 774959 Fax +353 21 774958
100-berth fully serviced marina. Access at all stages of the tide. Located within picturesque Kinsale harbour with ferry service to town. New marina centre with accommodation, restaurant, laundry, showers and toilets.

CHICHESTER MARINA
Birdham, Chichester,
West Sussex PO20 7EJ.
Tel (01243) 512731 Fax (01243) 513472
A very attractive marina offering superb services and shore installations, welcoming long and short-term visitors. Chandlery, bar, restaurant and boatyard facilities. Ring for further details.

CHISWICK QUAY MARINA LTD
Marina Office,
Chiswick Quay, London W4 3UR.
Tel 0181-994 8743
Small, secluded, peaceful marina on tidal Thames at Chiswick. Slipway, marine engineers and electricians, power, water, toilets and sluice.

CLARKE & CARTER BOATYARD
128 Coast Road,
West Mersea, Nr Colchester, Essex.
Tel (01206) 382244 Fax (01206) 384455
The Clarke & Carter Boatyard is a division of West Mersea Marine Ltd. The yard is situated on the main waterfront at West Mersea. The anchorage, which has retained its traditional character, offers both swinging and post moorings for vessels up to about 50' LOA. Access is at all states of the tide to the river Blackwater. There are also some edge moorings available.

CLOVELLY BAY MARINA
The Quay, Turnchapel,
Plymouth PL9 9TF.
Tel (01752) 404231 Fax (01752) 484177
Position: Southern side of cattewater, sheltered from prevailing winds by Mountbatten Peninsula. Open: All year, 24 hours. Radio: VHF channel 37 and 80. Callsign: Clovelly Bay. Berths: 180 berths, vessels up to 150', some fore and afts, visitors welcome. Facilities: electricity, water, 24-hour security, workshop, chandlery, brokerage, showers, laundry, diesel. Calor gas, payphone, refuse, water taxi, two local pubs

COBB'S QUAY
Hamworthy, Poole,
Dorset BH15 4EL.
Tel (01202) 674299 Fax (01202) 665217
Contact: Eileen Browne. 850-berth marina. Access to superb sailing. Fully serviced pontoon berths. Ample hardstanding for maintenance and storage ashore. 24-hour security. Shower and toilet facilities, petrol and diesel fuel, car park, lift out and slipping, chandlers, repairs and restaurant. Yacht club. Part of the MDL Group.

COWES MARINA
Clarence Road, East Cowes,
Isle of Wight PO32 6HA.
Tel (01983) 293983 Fax (01983) 299276
Cowes Marina lies just 300 metres upstream of the floating bridge in East Cowes. Fully sheltered pontoons with water and power can accommodate up to 200 visiting craft as well as 100 resident yachts.

COWES YACHT HAVEN
Vectis Yard, High Street,
Cowes, Isle of Wight PO31 7BD.
Tel (01983) 299975 Fax (01983) 200332
Cowes Yacht Haven is the Solent's premier sailing event centre offering 200 fully serviced berths right in the heart of Cowes. Our improved facilities, capability and location ensures the perfect venue and profile for every kind of boating event.

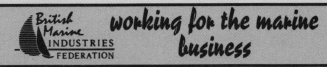

CRAOBH MARINA
By Lochgilphead, Argyll PA31 8UD.
Tel (01852) 500222 Fax (01852) 500252
250-berth marina on Loch Shuna. Water, electricity, diesel and gas. Full boatyard services. Chandlery. Brokerage. Insurance. Shops, bar, sailing centre and dive centre. Hotel and self-catering accommodation close by. 24-hour access. VHF channels 37(M) & 80.

DARTHAVEN MARINA LTD
Brixham Road, Kingswear,
Dartmouth, Devon TQ6 0SG.
Tel (01803) 752242 Fax (01803) 752722
Marina Office: (01803) 752545 Chandlery: (01803) 752733 Fax (01803) 752790 All types of repair facilities available. Fully trained staff. 30-ton mobile hoist available all states of tide. Extensive chandlery open 7 days a week. Agents for Autohelm/Raytheon, Cetrek, Simpson Lawrence, Vetus and Webasto. Visitors welcome. 24-hour engineering call-out service. Mobile Nos: 0860 873553 Engineering; 0589 340609 Electronics.

DARTSIDE QUAY
Galmpton Creek, Galmpton,
Brixham, South Devon TQ5 0EH.
Tel (01803) 845445 Fax (01803) 843558
Contact: Brian Speechly. 53-ton hoist and 9-acre storage facility. Fully serviced with power and water plus 16-ton trailer hoist. Pressure washing service. half tide moorings. Diesel fuel. Part of the MDL Group.

DOVER HARBOUR BOARD - DOVER MARINA
Harbour House,
Dover, Kent CT17 9BU.
Tel (01304) 241663/240400
Fax (01304) 240465
Providing 24-hour sailing from expanded facilities. Over 100 new pontoon berths in Tidal Harbour with minimum depth of 2.5 metres. 147 berths in adjacent Wellington Dock. Closest marina to Continental Europe. Excellent new road access. Many tourist attractions. Free marina guide with berth maps, navigational information and distance charts for cruising available. Boatyard and repair services available.

DUNSTAFFNAGE YACHT HAVEN LTD
Oban, Argyll PA37 1PX.
Tel (01631) 566555 Fax (01631) 565620
Dunstaffnage Yacht Haven is an idyllic natural harbour and centrally situated base for sailing the Western Isles offering pontoon berths, swinging moorings, bar, restaurant, holiday flats, chandlery, slip, travel hoist, storage ashore, repair and maintenance facilities.

ELMHAVEN MARINA
Rochester Road, Halling, Kent.
Tel (01634) 240489
Elmhaven provides a peaceful setting combined with good facilities including toilets, showers, power on pontoons, mud

berths, hard standing, boat lifting up to 5 tons maximum with repairs by Nigel Taylor on-site. Competitive rates and good security.

ESSEX MARINA LTD
Wallasea Island,
Nr Rochford, Essex SS4 2HG.
Tel (01702) 258531 Fax (01702) 258227
Deep water marina berths for yachts up to 150'. Full marina shipyard services. NO locks or sills. One hour from London. Also swinging moorings available. Visiting yachtsmen welcome. Luxury toilets, laundry and shower block. Bar and restaurant.

FALMOUTH YACHT MARINA
North Parade, Falmouth,
Cornwall TR11 2TD.
(01326) 316620 Fax (01326) 313939
The most westerly marina in England. Strategically placed for transatlantic departures and arrivals. Fully serviced permanent and visitor berths. Diesel fuel, chandlery, 30-ton hoist. Famous friendly service.

FIDDLERS FERRY YACHT HAVEN
Off Station Road, Penketh,
Warrington, Cheshire WA5 2UJ.
Tel (01925) 727519
Sheltered moorings upto 6'6" draught, 50' long. Access through lock from river Mersey $1\frac{1}{2}$ hours either side of high tide. Signed from A652. Boatyard and lift-out facilities. Annual rate per foot £8.

HAFAN PWLLHELI
Glan Don, Pwllheli,
Gwynedd LL53 5YT.
Tel (01758) 701219 Fax (01758) 701443
Hafan Pwllheli has over 400 pontoon berths and offers access at virtually all states of the tide. Ashore, its modern purpose-built facilities include luxury toilets, showers, landerette, a secure boat park for winter storage, 40-ton travel hoist, mobile crane and plenty of space for car parking. Open 24-hours a day, 7 days a week.

HAMBLE POINT MARINA
School Lane,
Hamble, Southampton,
Hampshire SO31 4NB.
Tel (01703) 452464 Fax (01703) 456440
Contact: Chris Hibbs. Mouth of river Hamble. 220 fully serviced berths. Toilet and shower facilities. Yacht repair yard, lifting for boats up to 65 tons, boat storage. Licensed members' club. 7-ton crane, diesel fuel, Calor gas and ice. 24-hour security. Chandlery and all boat repair/service facilities. Part of the MDL Group.

HOO MARINA (MEDWAY) LTD
Vicarage Lane, Hoo,
Rochester, Kent ME3 9LE.
Tel (01634) 250311 Fax (01634) 251761
An established marina with fully serviced pontoon berths, winter lay-up on concrete

hardstanding. 20-ton lifting capacity. Chandlery and brokerage as well as full workshop facilities for yacht repair and maintenance.

HULL MARINA LTD
Warehouse 13,
Kingston Street, Hull HU1 2DQ.
Tel (01482) 593451 Fax (01482) 224148
Four Anchor Marina. Situated 5 minues from the centre of Hull and all national and international transport systems. First class leisure, boatyard and brokerage facilities. 4-Star hotel and quayside restaurants. Professional and caring staff. Competitive rates.

HYTHE MARINA
Shamrock Way,
Hythe, Southampton,
Hampshire SO45 6DY.
Tel (01703) 207073/849263
Fax (01703) 842424
Contact: Peter Bedwell. Three marina basins surrounded by character homes and miniature village square 210 fully serviced berths. Chandlery, shops. Fully serviced pontoons. Access by lock manned 24 hours. Shower and toilet facilities. Petrol and diesel fuel. 30-ton hoist, car park. Part of the MDL Group.

ISLAND HARBOUR MARINA
Mill Lane, Binfield, Newport,
Isle of Wight PO30 2LA.
Tel (01983) 526020 & 822999
Locked marina on Medina river. Tidal access HW ± 3$\frac{1}{2}$ hrs. 150 visitors' berths. Services include - water, electricity, showers, launderette, gas, diesel, chandlery, restaurant and bar. Full boatyard facilities with 12-ton hoist and 30-ton cradle.

KINNEGO MARINA
- Lough Neagh
Oxford Island, Lurgan,
Co Armagh, N Ireland.
Tel (01762) 327573 Fax (01762) 347438
90 berths 10 moorings, Kinnego Marina is based in the south east corner of Lough Neagh, close to the M1 motorway. Mullen Marine offers chandlery, engine repairs on-site, and we offer RYA powerboat, keelboat and dinghy courses all year round. Access to the Lough via the Lower Bann at Coleraine. Lough Neagh - 154 sq mile 77 mile of shoreline.

KINSALE YACHT CLUB MARINA
Kinsale, Co Cork, Eire.
Tel +353 21 772196 Fax +353 21 774426
Magnificent deep water yacht club marina offering Kinsale hospitality to visiting yachtsmen. Full facilities include berths up to 20 metres, fresh water, electricity, diesel on pier. Club bar and wealth of pubs and restaurants in Kinsale. Enter Kinsale Harbour - lit at night - no restrictions.

KIP MARINA
The Yacht Harbour,
Inverkip, Renfrewshire PA16 0AS.
Tel (01475) 521485 Fax (01475) 521298
Marina berths for vessels up to 65' LOA.
Full boatyard facilities including travel
hoist, crane, on-site engineers, GRP repairs
etc. Bar, restaurant, sauna launderette and
chandlery.

LANGSTONE YACHTING PLC
Fort Cumberland Road,
Southsea, Hampshire PO4 9RJ.
Tel (01705) 822719 Fax (01705) 822220
Langstone Marina with over 300 berths is
on the western side of the entrance to
Langstone Harbour. Facilities include:
hoist, brokerage, restaurant, bar, chandlery,
hard standing. Access over the sill is
available approximately 3 hours either side
of highwater.

LARGS YACHT HAVEN
Irvine Road,
Largs, Ayrshire KA30 8EZ.
Tel (01475) 675333 Fax (01475) 672245
Perfectly located 600-berth marina with
full services afloat and ashore. 45-ton travel
hoist operational 7 days; fuel (diesel and
petrol); gas and ice on sale 24-hours. Bar,
coffee shop, dive shop plus usual marine
services.

LITTLEHAMPTON
MARINA LTD
Ferry Road, Littlehampton,
West Sussex BN17 5DS.
Tel (01903) 713553 Fax (01903) 732264
Only 2 miles upstream of harbour entrance,
we have deep water pontoon berths with
electricity and lighting. Showers, toilets,
changing rooms, cafe, and floating pub.
Petrol, marine diesel, slipway with tractor
launch, recovery service, and storage
compounds. 30 miles from Isle of Wight,
18 miles from Brighton and 14 miles of
navigable river which flows through the
historic town of Arundel. Good diving and
fishing available.

LIVERPOOL MARINA
Coburg Dock,
Sefton Street, Liverpool L3 4BP.
Tel 0151-709 0578/(2683 after 5pm)
Fax 0151-709 8731
300-berth yacht harbour. All serviced
pontoons. Tidal access HW ± 2½ hrs
approximately, depending on draft. 60-ton
hoist, workshops, bar and restaurant, toilets
and showers. City centre one mile. Open
all year. Active yacht club and yacht
brokerage.

THE MAYFLOWER
INTERNATIONAL MARINA
Ocean Quay, Richmond Walk,
Plymouth PL1 4LS.
Tel (01752) 556633 Fax (01752) 606896
Marina operators with boat-hoist (25 ton)
facility. Restaurant, clubroom, launderette,
fuel, chandlery, shop and off-licence.
Winter storage. Owned by berth holders
and operated to a very high standard.

MELFORT PIER & HARBOUR
Kilmelford,
By Oban, Argyll PA34 4XD.
Tel (01852) 200333 Fax (01852) 200329
A small pretty harbour set up, surrounded
by top quality holiday houses each with
private sauna/spa, tel/fax. All shoreside
facilities for the cruising yachtsman;
moorings and pontoon berthing, showers,
laundry, tel/fax, B & B, diesel, water,
electricity, gas, provisions. Restaurant, bar,
hotel, bikes, watersports, horseriding and
much more. Call sign: Melfort Pier 16/12.

MERCURY YACHT HARBOUR
Satchell Lane, Hamble,
Southampton,
Hampshire SO31 4HQ.
Tel (01703) 455994 Fax (01703) 457369
Contact: Paul Keast. Peaceful, 350 fully
serviced berths. Car park. 24-hour staff.
Toilet and shower facilities. Yacht repairs,
10-ton lifting, chandlery, yacht brokerage,
sailmakers, electronics. Licensed
members' club. Sailing school. Part of the
MDL Group.

MERSEYSIDE DEVELOPMENT
CORPORATION
4th Floor, Royal Liver Building,
Pierhead, Liverpool L3 1JH.
Tel 0151-236 6090 Fax 0151-227 3174
Albert Dock welcomes vessels for short or
long-term visits to what is now one of the
north west's most popular maritime
locations. Maximum length 55m.
Concessionary rates (details on
application). Access by prior agreement.

MILLBAY MARINA
Millbay Docks,
Great Western Road,
Plymouth PL1 3EQ.
Tel/Fax (01752) 226785
Contact: Alan Smith. Sheltered 86-berth
marina adjacent to Plymouth Hoe. Fully
serviced berths. Car park. Advance booking
essential. Part of the MDL Group.

NEYLAND YACHT HAVEN LTD
Brunel Quay, Neyland,
Pembrokeshire SA73 1PY.
Tel (01646) 601601 Fax (01646) 600713
Marina operators with all facilities. 420
fully serviced pontoon berths in a sheltered,
tree lined marina. On-site services include
boatyard, sailmaker, sailing school,
chandlery, cafe, launderette, showers and
toilets. 30 visitors' berths. 24-hour access
and security.

NORTHNEY MARINA
Northney Road, Hayling Island,
Hampshire PO11 0NH.
Tel (01705) 466321/2 Fax (01705) 461467
Contact: Tony Barker. Chichester
harbour. 228-berth marina. Fully serviced
pontoon berths. Diesel fuel, car park.
Shower and toilet facilities. Brokerage,
yacht repair, lifting to 35 tons, chandlery.
Licensed club. Sailing and wind surfing
school. Part of the MDL Group.

OBAN YACHTS & MARINE
SERVICES LTD
Ardentrive, Kerrera,
By Oban, Argyll PA34 4SX.
Tel (01631) 565333 Fax (01631) 565888
Moorings, visitor pontoon, toilets, showers,
drying room, diesel, gas, water, chandlery,
slipway, 18-ton hoist, full workshop
facilities, undercover storage, hardstanding. Regular ferry to Oban town centre
less than 10 minutes across the bay.

OCEAN VILLAGE MARINA
Channel Way,
Canute Road, Southampton,
Hampshire SO14 3TG.
Tel (01703) 229385 Fax (01703) 233515
Contact: Adrian Smith. Modern city
centre marina with 450 fully serviced
pontoon berths up to 75 metres. 24-hour
security. Royal Southampton Yacht Club.
Toilet and shower facilities. Car park.
Adjacent shopping and entertainment
complex. Part of the MDL Group.

PENTON HOOK MARINA
Staines Road,
Chertsey, Surrey KT16 8PY.
Tel (01932) 568681 Fax (01932) 567423
Largest inland harbour, access to river
Thames. 610 fully serviced berths, craning,
engineering and repairs, hardstanding,
petrol, diesel and Calor gas. Shower and
toilet facilities, refuse and chemical toilet
disposal, car park, pumpout, chandlery.
Yacht club. Part of the MDL Group.

PETERHEAD BAY AUTHORITY
Bath House,
Bath Street, Peterhead AB42 6DX.
Tel (01779) 474020 Fax (01779) 475712
Contact Stephen Paterson. Opened in
April 1994, Peterhead Bay Marina offers a
comprehensive range of services and
facilities for local and visiting boatowners.
Ideal stopover marina for vessels heading
to/from Scandinavia or the Caledonian
canal.

PORT FLAIR LTD
Bradwell Marina, Waterside,
Bradwell-on-Sea, Essex CM0 7RB.
Tel (01621) 776235/776391
300 pontoon berths with water and
electricity, petrol and diesel, chandlery,
marine slip/hoistage to 20 tons. Repairs,
winter lay-ups, licensed club, yacht
brokerage.

PORT HAMBLE
Satchell Lane,
Hamble, Southampton,
Hampshire SO31 4QD.
Tel (01703) 452741 Fax (01703) 455206
Close to Hamble village. 310 fully serviced
marina berths. Shower and toilet facilities.
Car park, petrol and diesel fuel, yacht
repair yard. Lifting to 100 tons, chandlery,
brokerage, sailmakers. Members' licensed
club. 24-hour staff. Part of the MDL Group.

PORT OF TRURO
Harbour Office,
Town Quay, Truro, Cornwall.
Tel (01872) 72130 Fax (01872) 225346
Facilities for the yachtsman include visitors' pontoons located at Turnaware Bar near Ruan Creek, Boscawen Park. Visitors' moorings at Woodbury. Quay facilities at Truro with free showers and toilets. Chemical toilet disposal, fresh water and garbage disposal.

PORT SOLENT
South Lockside, Port Solent,
Portsmouth, Hampshire PO6 4TJ.
Tel (01705) 210765 Fax (01705) 324241
Port Solent is a community of houses, apartments, restaurants, shops and a cinema encompassing 900 berths. This includes 400 public berths with excellent facilities for visitors, including luxury showers and club.

RAMSGATE ROYAL HARBOUR
Harbour Office, Military Road,
Ramsgate, Kent CT11 9LG.
Tel (01843) 592277 Fax (01843) 590941
One of south east England's premier leisure areas. Ideal for crossing to the Continent. 24-hour access to finger pontoons. Comprehensive security systems. Amenities: launderette, repairs, slipways, boatpark. Competitive rates for permanent berths and visiting vessels.

SALTERNS MARINA
40 Salterns Way,
Lilliput, Poole, Dorset BH14 8JR.
Tel (01202) 707321/709971
Fax (01202) 700398
Pontoon Berths - Swinging Moorings - 24-hour Security - Visitors Welcome - Full Boatyard Facilities - Osmosis Treatment - 5 & 45 Tonne Hoists - Engine & Boat Sales - Award Winning Hotel, Restaurant and Bar - Chandlery - 24-hour Fuelling.

SHAMROCK QUAY
William Street, Southampton,
Hampshire SO14 5QL.
Tel (01703) 229461 Fax (01703) 333384
250-berth marina on river Itchen, access to Solent. Pontoons fully serviced. Shower, toilet and laundry facilities. 62-ton hoist and 12-ton mobile crane. 24-hour harbour staff. Chandlery, shops and restaurants. Part of the MDL Group.

SHOTLEY MARINA LTD
Shotley Gate,
Ipswich, Suffolk IP9 1QJ.
Tel (01473) 788982 Fax (01473) 788868
A modern state of the art marina with 350 berths offering all the services expected. Open 24-hours with full security. Access all states of tide, ideal cruising base. Well stocked chandlery and general store, repair facilities, laundry and ironing centre, showers/baths and toilets. Restaurants, bar, children's room, TV/video and function rooms with dance floor and bar. Disabled facilities.

SOUTH DOCK MARINA
South Lock Office, Rope Street,
Plough Way, London SE16 1TX.
Tel 0171-252 2244 Fax 0171-237 3806
London's largest marina. 200+ berths. Spacious tranquil setting. Manned 24 hours. Lift-out to 20 tonnes. Competitive mooring rates.

SOUTHDOWN MARINA
Southdown Quay,
Millbrook, Cornwall PL10 1EZ.
Tel/Fax (01752) 823084
32-berth marina on edge of river Tamar in quiet location behind Rame Peninsula. Plymouth is just across the river. Quayside berths available for large vessels. Winter storage. Good security. DIY facilities available.

SOVEREIGN HARBOUR MARINA LTD
Pevensey Bay Road,
Eastbourne, Sussex BN23 6JH.
Tel (01323) 470099 Fax (01323) 470077
Situated at Langney Point, Eastbourne, Sovereign Harbour is centred around twin harbours, one tidal and one accessed by two high capacity locks. A full service marina with diesel, petrol and unleaded petrol available 24-hours daily.

SPARKES YACHT HARBOUR & BOATYARD
38 Wittering Road,
Sandy Point, Hayling Island,
Hampshire PO11 9SR.
Tel (01705) 463572 Fax (01705) 465741
Sparkes Marina - a small friendly, family run business offering all the facilities you require including access at all states of the tide to a depth of 2 metres at lowest low water springs. In addition to marina berths, accessible through a security gate, we also offer dry boat sailing, moorings, storage ashore plus full maintenance facilities, new boat sales and brokerage, chandlery and restaurant.

ST KATHARINE HAVEN
50 St Katharine's Way,
London E1 9LB.
Tel 0171-488 2400 Fax 0171-702 2252
In the heart of London, St Katharine's 200-berth Haven offers facilities for 100+ vessels, access to the West End and City, its own shops, restaurants, health club and yacht club, plus water, electric, showers and sewerage disposal. Entry via a lock. Operational HW - 2hrs to HW + 1^1/$_2$ hrs London Bridge. October-March 0800-1800. April-August 0600-2030.

THAMES (DITTON) MARINA LTD
Portsmouth Road,
Thames Ditton, Surrey KT6 5QD.
Tel 0181-398 6159 Fax 0181-398 6438
Over 120 berths and moorings. All main

services, diesel, Calor Gas, repairs and service. Large chandlery with comprehensive stock of safety equipment, paint, charts and books. Very large car park for convenience of customers. Open 7 days a week.

THORNHAM MARINA
Thornham Lane,
Prinsted,
Nr Emsworth,
Hampshire PO10 8DD.
Tel (01243) 375335
First class serviced hardstanding, 12-ton slipway hoist. Tidal pontoons, deep water gated pool, modern workshop, bar, restaurant, showers and toilets. Visitors welcome - club rallies etc. A very few long-term berths available. Brokerage service.

TOLLESBURY MARINA
The Yacht Harbour,
Tollesbury,
Maldon, Essex CM9 8SE.
Tel (01621) 869202
Fax (01621) 868489
VHF Channel 37/80 Tollesbury Marina can offer 260 marina berths with water and electricty on all pontoons. Clubhouse with bar, restaurant, swimming pool and tennis courts. Repair workshops with West Osmosis Treatment Centre. Full brokerage service listing over 200 boats, with a friendly professional service.

TORQUAY MARINA
Torquay, Devon TQ2 5EQ.
Tel (01803) 214624 Fax (01803) 291634
Contact: Wendy-Jane Latham. Lively 500-berth marina adjacent town centre. Pontoon fully serviced berths. 24-hour dockmaster. Superb shower and toilet facilities, launderette, private car park, fuel, boat repair facilities, chandlery. Cafe/bar, restaurant. Part of the MDL Group.

TOWN QUAY MARINA
Town Quay, The Waterfront,
Southampton, Hampshire.
Tel (01703) 234397
Town Quay is a growing development of bars and restaurants on an attractive waterfront environment just Minutes away from the city centre. A number of attractions occur on the quay throughout the year.

TROON YACHT HAVEN
The Harbour, Troon,
Ayrshire KA10 6DJ.
Tel (01292) 315553 Fax (01292) 312836
Sheltered harbour for 350 berths. Well placed for those on passage to and from the Clyde. Bar, restaurant, marine services. Attractive seafront town with good beaches and championship golf.

WEYMOUTH OLD HARBOUR
Weymouth & Portland Borough Council,
Borough Engineers Department,
Municipal Offices, North Quay,
Weymouth, Dorset DT4 8TA.
Tel (01305) 206278/206423
Fax (01305) 206276
Access at all stages of tide. Visitors' berths in the centre of prime tourist resort with shops, restaurants and night life all at hand. Diesel fuelling from pontoon or tanker. Chandlery and repair facilities available.

WINDSOR MARINA
Maidenhead Road, Oakley Green,
Windsor, Berkshire SL4 5TZ.
Tel (01753) 853911 Fax (01753) 868195
Small pastoral 200-berth marina. Showers and toilet facilities, petrol, diesel and Calor gas, car parking, dry berthing and hardstanding. Private yacht club. Repair services and mobile crane, refuse and chemical toilet disposal, pumpout, chandlery and boat sales. 240v electricity. Part of the MDL Group.

WOOLVERSTONE MARINA
Woolverstone,
Ipswich, Suffolk IP9 1AS.
Tel (01473) 780206/780354
Fax (01473) 780273
Contact: Judy Cracknell. Easy access through Harwich harbour. 200 fully serviced berths, 120 swinging moorings, diesel fuel, car park, toilet and shower facilities, repair yard with 20-ton mobile crane. Foodstore, clubhouse, restaurant and bar. Part of the MDL Group.

MARINE ENGINEERS

CAPELLES MARINE LTD
Camp du Roi,
St Sampsons, Guernsey,
Channel Islands GY2 4XG.
Tel (01481) 57010 Fax (01481) 53590
Cellnet 0860 741245 Out of town - we are only a phone call away and happy to find YOU. Mercury and Mercruiser dealers on the island. We also service all makes of outboards. Petrol and diesel sterndrives and diesel inboards. Perry's Guide Ref: 9F 4G3.

GWEEK QUAY BOATYARD
Gweek Quay (Helford River),
Helston, Cornwall TR12 6UF.
Tel (01326) 221657 Fax (01326) 221685
Head of the Helford river. Yacht repair yard, 30-ton crane, chandlery, brokerage, coffee shop, toilets and showers. Boat storage and all boat repair and service facilities. Access approximately 2 hours either side of highwater.

HOO MARINA (MEDWAY) LTD
Vicarage Lane, Hoo,
Rochester, Kent ME3 9LE.
Tel (01634) 250311 Fax (01634) 251761
An established marina with fully serviced pontoon berths, winter lay-up on concrete hardstanding. 20-ton lifting capacity.

Chandlery and brokerage as well as full workshop facilities for yacht repair and maintenance.

ISLAND MARINE POWER (ELECTRICAL) LTD
East Cowes Marina,
Clarence Road, Cowes Marina,
Isle of Wight PO32 6HA.
Tel/Fax (01983) 280011
Island Marine Power (Electrical) Ltd now in our new premises facing the river at East Cowes. The workshop - as always - open for major, minor and emergency electrical works. The shop - stocking practical chandlery and hardware is still growing. Tel/Fax 01983 280011 East Cowes Marina.

MARINE & AUTO SERVICES
Bridge Boathouse, River Road,
Maidenhead, Berkshire SL6 0BE.
Tel/Fax (01628) 36435
Marine consultant and engineers. Condition, survey and valuation reports undertaken on fibreglass craft - Thames and nationwide. Engines sold and delivered. Repairs, overhauls and servicing on all types of engines. Mail order for parts available. 35 years' experience in the marine industry.

MARINE & GENERAL ENGINEERS LTD
The Shipyard,
St Sampson's Harbour, Guernsey,
Channel Islands GY1 6AT.
Tel (01481) 45808 Fax (01481) 48765
High standard boat building and yacht repair yard supported by slipway with two cradles. Appointed service and repair agents for Caterpiller, MTU, Mermaid, DAF, Lombardini, Mariner, Tohatsu and Evinrude engines. Also, Bosch fuel injection service centre. 24-hour Emergency Support on 0860 741217.

R.I.B.S. MARINE
Little Avon Marina,
Stony Lane South,
Christchurch, Dorset BH23 1HW.
Tel (01202) 477327 Fax (01202) 471456
Full boatyard facilities. Mooring, slipping and dry boat storage. Marine engineers for all makes of outboard and inboard. Petrol and diesel. Specialist repairs in wood and GRP. Main agents for Mariner and Force outboards and Mercruiser stern drives. Brokerage facilities.

SHELL BAY MARINE
Ferry Road,
Studland, Dorset BH19 3BA.
Tel (01929) 450340 Fax (01929) 450570
Sensibly priced moorings immediately inside Poole harbour entrance. Slipway, boat hoist, winter storage, repairs. Good security, open all year, terms available by day, week or season. Parking, licensed bar, cafe and RYA recognised watersports centre.

NAVIGATION EQUIPMENT

AMPRO NAVIGATION LTD
PO Box 373A,
Surbiton, Surrey KT6 5YL.
Tel 0181-398 1169 Fax 0181-398 6184
Tel (01734) 820337 Fax (01734) 820338
UK agents for Philips Navigation AP range of marine electronic equipment including GPS and Decca Navigators, Chart Plotters, Instruments, hand portable and Differential GPS units. Full sales and technical support available.

DOLPHIN MARITIME SOFTWARE LTD
25 Roosevelt Avenue,
Lancaster LA1 5EJ.
Tel/Fax (01524) 841946
Marine computer programs for IBM PC, Psion and Sharp pocket computers. Specialists in navigation, tidal prediction and other programs for both yachting and commercial uses.

MARITEK LTD
1-D7 Templeton Centre,
Glasgow G40 1DA.
Tel 0141-554 2492 Fax 0141-639 1910
Computer programs for coastal/celestial navigation/tidal height prediction, using Psion pocket computer. Large computer systems and projects using 4th generation languages.

NAVIONICS UK
Oak Wood House,
Gospel Oak Lane,
Stratford-upon-Avon,
Warwickshire CV37 0JA.
Tel (01789) 269891 Fax (01789) 262717
Navioncs UK, the exclusive UK and Irish distributor for Navionics electronic charts. Charts suitable in chart plotters from Furuno, Koden, Geonav, Trimble, Panasonic, B & G, Philips etc. 24-hour despatch service for any Navionics chart worlwide.

SMYE-RUMSBY LTD
123 Snargate Street,
Dover, Kent CT17 9AP.
Tel (01304) 201187 Fax (01304) 240135
Established since 1948, our company welcomes visitors to Dover Port requiring excellent marine electronic maintenance services. We have comprehensive knowledge of current navigational equipment, and can provide a 24-hour call-out repair facility.

NAVIGATION LIGHT SWITCHES & MONITORS

MECTRONICS MARINE
PO Box 8, Newton Abbot,
Devon TQ12 1FF.
Tel (01626) 334453
LIGHT ACTIVATED SWITCHES, rugged solid state devices to automatically switch anchor lights at sunset and sunrise. NAVLIGHT SELECTORS, protected enclosed rotary switches internally connected to ensure approved navigation light combination on auxiliary sailing vessels. NAVLIGHT STATUS MONITORS, diagnostic displays on which the appropriate indicator flashes quickly or slowly in the event of a short or open circuit fault. Also drives an optional audible warning device.

OUTBOARD MOTORS

ROBIN CURNOW MARINE ENGINEERS
Commercial Road,
Penryn, Cornwall TR10 8AG.
Tel (01326) 373438 Fax (01326) 376534
Outboard motor sales and service. Morse controls service centre. British Seagull/ Selva - Evinrude - Honda - Mercury - Yamaha.

PAINT & OSMOSIS

ARUNCRAFT LTD
Littlehampton Marina,
Ferry Road, Littlehampton,
West Sussex BN17 5DS.
Tel (01903) 723667 Fax (01903) 730983
Mobile 0836 703006 Family business based at Littlehampton Marina for 11 years. Large workshop for boat maintenance, GRP repairs, engine work, rigging, electronic systems and propeller repairs. In-house paint spraying and osmosis treatments by Arunspray. Chandlery and comprehensive range of craft in the brokerage department.

INTERNATIONAL PAINT
24-30 Canute Road, Southampton,
Hampshire SO14 3PB.
Tel (01703) 226722 Fax (01703) 335975
International Paint is the leading supplier of quality paints, epoxies, varnishes and anti-foulings to the marine industry. Over half the world's pleasure craft are protected by International products.

NORTH QUAY MARINE
North Side, St Sampson's Harbour,
Guernsey, Channel Islands.
Tel (01481) 46561 Fax (01481) 43488
The complete boating centre. Orkney and Fletcher boats - Mariner outboards - Full range of chandlery, rope, chain, lubricants, paint, boatwear and shoes. Fishing tackle for on-shore and onboard. Inflatables and safety equipment. Electronics.

S P SYSTEMS
Love Lane, Cowes,
Isle of Wight PO31 7EU.
Tel (01983) 298451 Fax (01983) 298453
Epoxy resins for laminating, bonding, coating and filling. Usable with wood, GRP, concrete. GRP/FRP materials including glass, carbon and Kevlar fibres. Structural engineering of GRP and composite materials. Technical advice service.

V C SYSTEMS
24-30 Canute Road, Southampton,
Hampshire SO14 3PB.
Tel (01703) 226722 Fax (01703) 335975
VC Systems provides a comprehensive range of yacht paint products designed for first class boat maintenance. This range includes the Teflon anti-foulings, VC17m and VC Offshore Extra and a range of epoxies, fillers, varnishes and accessory paint products.

PUBLISHERS

HYDROGRAPHIC OFFICE
Taunton, Somerset TA1 2DN.
Tel (01823) 337900 Fax (01823) 323753
Admiralty charts and hydrographic publications - worldwide coverage corrected to date of issue, available from appointed Admiralty agents together with notices to mariners. Products designed specifically for the small craft user also available from good chandlers.

WORDSMITH PUBLICATIONS
Chiltern House,
120 Eskdale Avenue, Chesham,
Buckinghamshire HP5 3BD.
Tel (01494) 782376 Fax (01494) 791322
Specialising in nautical books Wordsmith Publications can offer professional advice to authors wishing to publish their own book at an affordable cost.

QUAY SERVICES

GWEEK QUAY BOATYARD
Gweek Quay (Helford River),
Helston, Cornwall TR12 6UF.
Tel (01326) 221657 Fax (01326) 221685
Head of the Helford river. Yacht repair yard, 30-ton crane, chandlery, brokerage, coffee shop, toilets and showers. Boat storage and all boat repair and service facilities. Access approximately 2 hours either side of highwater.

MANOR OF BOSHAM LTD
Bosham Quay, Old Bosham,
West Sussex PO18 8HR.
Tel (01243) 573336 Fax (01243) 576285
Deep water moorings up to 14 metres in length in picturesque Bosham Channel - Chichester Harbour, also includes some tidal moorings. Services available at quay. Also scrubbing off grids including pressure washers. **Contact Name: M McGrail.**

RADIO COURSES/SCHOOLS

DARTMOUTH YACHT CRUISE SCHOOL
103 High Street,
Totnes, Devon TQ9 5SN.
Ans/Fax (01803) 864027
Tel (01803) 722226
Home: 55 The Old Common, Bussage, Stroud, Gloucestershire GL6 8HH. Tel (01453) 731142. RYA recognised teaching establishment since 1990. Skipper charter; Bareboat charter; Youth training, Duke of Edinburgh's Scheme; Sail training all RYA recognised courses including First Aid; Diesel engine courses; Sea survival; Helmsman's certificates to Yachtmaster offshore preparation.

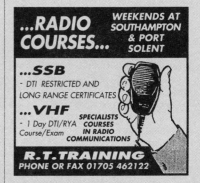
R T TRAINING
286 Sea Front, Hayling Island,
Hampshire PO11 0AZ.
Tel/Fax (01705) 462122
Weekend radio courses at Southampton and Port Solent for leisure and professional yachtsmen. SSB - 3-day Restricted Course/ Exam. Long Range Certificate - contact us for details of this new certificate. VHF - 1- day Course/Exam.

RADIO SCHOOL LTD
33 Island Close, Hayling Island,
Hampshire PO11 0NJ.
Tel (01705) 466450 Fax (01705) 461449
Weekend integrated courses/exams for Marine VHF and SSB Radiotelephone Operator's Certificates in Britain's only permanent, fully equipped classroom soley dedicated to training leisure sailors in radio operation on a full-time, professional basis.

REEFING SYSTEMS

SOUTHERN SPAR SERVICES & EQUIPMENT
Shamrock Quay, William Street,
Northam, Southampton, SO14 5QL.
Tel (01703) 331714 Fax (01703) 230559
Mobile 0850 736540 Mast manufacturer, all spars, Toerails, stanchions, bases. Deck equipment. Rigging and Furlex headsail reefing systems.

JOSEPH P LAMB & SONS
Maritime Building
(opposite Albert Dock), Wapping,
Liverpool L1 8DQ.
Tel 0151-709 4861 Fax 0151-709 2786
Situated in the centre of Liverpool, J P
Lamb have provided a service to world
shipping for over 200 years. All chandlery
supplies, clothing, rope, paint and flags are
available, together with a full sailmaking,
repair and rigging service. Open Mon to
Fri 8am to 6pm - Sat to Sun 9am to 1pm.

MANX MARINE
35 North Quay,
Douglas, Isle of Man IM1 4LB.
Tel/Fax (01624) 674842
The Island's leading and most established
yacht chandlery. Stockists of quality foul
weather clothing and Thermalware. Large
stock holdings of stainless steel fixtures
and fittings and a comprehensive range of
general chandlery. Agents for Mariner.
Rigging facilities.

MINERVA RIGGING LTD
Kip Marina, Inverkip,
Renfrewshire PA16 0AS.
Tel (01475) 522700 Fax (01475) 522800
THE name for rigging services, based at
Kip Marina. Stockists of high tech Spectra/
Dyneeman and Vectran ropes. Roll
swaging up to 14mm rod and 16mm wire.
We are the Kemp service centre for
Scotland.

SIMPSON LAWRENCE LTD
218-228 Edmiston Drive,
Glasgow G51 2YT.
Tel 0141-427 5331 Fax 0141-427 5419
Simpson Lawrence are manufacturers and
the UK's largest wholesale distributors of
quality marine equipment.

SMALLCRAFT RIGGING
East Cowes Marina,
Clarence Road, East Cowes,
Isle of Wight PO32 6HA.
Tel (01983) 298269 Fax (01983) 299276
Service and repair of masts - rigging and
reefing systems. Manufacture and repair
of sprayhoods, covers and dodgers. Repair
of inflatable dinghies and other yacht
services.

**SOUTHERN SPAR SERVICES
& EQUIPMENT**
Shamrock Quay, William Street,
Northam, Southampton,
Hampshire SO14 5QL.
Tel (01703) 331714 Fax (01703) 230559
Mobile 0850 736540 Mast manufacturer,
all spars, Toerails, stanchions, bases. Deck
equipment. Rigging and Furlex headsail
reefing systems.

**TUBBY LEE
YACHTING SERVICES**
Kings Road, Burnham-on-Crouch,
Essex CM0 8HJ.
Tel (01621) 783562 Fax (01621) 785119
A complete yacht rigging service for

standing and running rigging. Large stocks
of wire and rope. Taluriting, swaging, wire
to rope splicing, deck layout advice. Rig
tuning a speciality. Yacht deliveries.

SPEED LOGS

THOMAS WALKER GROUP LTD
37-41 Bissell Street,
Birmingham B5 7HR.
Tel 0121-622 4475 Fax 0121-622 4478
Manufacturers of marine instruments
including, Neco Autopilots, Walker Logs
and Towing Logs, Walker Anemometers,
Chernikeeff Logs.

SPRAYHOODS & DODGERS

MARTELLO YACHT SERVICES
Mulberry House, Mulberry Road,
Canvey Island, Essex SS8 0PR.
Tel/Fax (01268) 681970
Manufacturers and suppliers of made-to-
measure upholstery, covers, hoods,
dodgers, sailcovers, curtains and cushions
etc. Repairs undertaken. DIY materials,
chandlery and fitting-supplies.

SMALLCRAFT RIGGING
East Cowes Marina,
Clarence Road, East Cowes,
Isle of Wight PO32 6HA.
Tel (01983) 298269 Fax (01983) 299276
Service and repair of masts - rigging and
reefing systems. Manufacture and repair
of sprayhoods, covers and dodgers. Repair
of inflatable dinghies and other yacht
services.

STAINLESS STEEL HARDWARE

BASELINE LTD
Unit 10 Apple Industrial Estate,
Segensworth West,
Fareham, Hampshire PO15 5SX.
Tel (014895) 76349 Fax (014895) 78835
Extensive range of marine hardware for all
boats including many difficult to find
articles. Fastenings, canopy fittings, vents,
hinges - stainless steel available - fittings
for sails and rigging, rails and boarding
ladders. Efficient mail order service
available.

MANX MARINE
35 North Quay, Douglas,
Isle of Man IM1 4LB.
Tel/Fax (01624) 674842
The Island's leading and most established
yacht chandlery. Stockists of quality foul
weather clothing and Thermalware. Large
stock holdings of stainless steel fixtures
and fittings and a comprehensive range of
general chandlery. Agents for Mariner.
Rigging facilities.

SURVEYORS

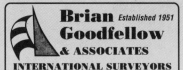
**BRIAN GOODFELLOW
& ASSOCIATES** INTERNATIONAL SURVEYORS
15 Chaseside Gardens,
Chertsey, Surrey KT16 8JP.
Tel/Fax 01932 567634
Mobile 0860 446982 (24 hours) Approved
by British Waterways and the Marine
Safety Agency, Brian Goodfellow &
Associates can offer very competitive
quotations for surveys, insurance and
valuations. We act for most leading
companies and major builders. Companion
RINA, Ass Member YDSA, Member of
BMIF.

MARINE & AUTO SERVICES
Bridge Boathouse, River Road,
Maidenhead, Berkshire SL6 0BE.
Tel/Fax (01628) 36435
Marine consultant and engineers.
Condition, survey and valuation reports
undertaken on fibreglass craft - Thames
and nationwide. Engines sold and
delivered. Repairs, overhauls and servicing
on all types of engines. Mail order for parts
available. 35 years' experience in the
marine industry.

TANKS

TEK-TANKS
The Ridings, The Shrave,
Four Marks,
Alton, Hampshire GU34 5BH.
Tel (01420) 564359 Fax (01962) 772563
Email: 100010.3172@compuserve.com
Manufacturers of high quality made-to-
measure polypropylene water, waste and
diesel tanks. Also suppliers of tank sensors,
pumps, deck fittings and hoses.

TRANSPORT/YACHT DELIVERIES

BOB SALMON & ASSOCIATES
112 Mewstone Avenue,
Wembury, Plymouth PL9 0HT.
Tel (01752) 862558 Fax (01752) 862557
Worldwide delivery of power and sailing
craft by sea. Established 1972. We offer
personal attention and very experienced
professional service. Non smoking skippers
and crews. No obligation advice.
Quotations and draft contracts with
pleasure.

BRIAN FENTON MARINE TRANSPORT SERVICES
17 Weatherdon Drive,
Ivybridge, South Devon PL21 0DD.
Tel/Fax (01752) 690373
Specialist yacht, motor cruiser and catamaran transporters to all areas in UK and Europe. 25 years' experience. Purpose-built vehicles, single and multiple loads. Trade references available if required. Plymouth based.

MAX WALKER YACHT DELIVERIES
Zinderneuf Sailing, PO Box 105,
Macclesfield, Cheshire SK10 2EY.
Tel (01625) 431712 Fax (01625) 619704
Fixed price deliveries. Sailing yachts delivered with care in north west European, UK and Eire waters by RYA/DoT yachtmaster and crew; 30 years' experience. Owners welcome. Tuition if required. References available. Your enquiries welcome 24 hours.

SEALAND BOAT DELIVERIES
133 Corn Exchange Buildings,
Manchester M4 3BW.
Tel (01254) 705225 Fax (01254) 776582
Nationwide and European road transporters of all craft. No weight limit. Irish service. Worldwide shipping agents. Extrication of yachts from workshops and building yards. Salvage contractors. Established over 21 years. We never close.

TUBBY LEE YACHTING SERVICES
Kings Road, Burnham-on-Crouch,
Essex CM0 8HJ.
Tel (01621) 783562 Fax (01621) 785119
A complete yacht rigging service for standing and running rigging. Large stocks of wire and rope. Taluriting, swaging, wire to rope splicing, deck layout advice. Rig tuning a speciality. Yacht deliveries.

WEST COUNTRY GAFFERS BOAT TRANSPORT
3 Tregrehan Mills,
Tregrehan, St Austell PL25 3TH.
Tel (01726) 816516/63188
Fax (01726) 817636
Established 1984 by ex-shipmaster/yachtsman. Transportation by road up to 18 tons. Approved MoD boat transporter. Boat repairs - wood and GRP. Main agent for B P Dory.

TUITION/SAILING SCHOOLS

BALTIC WHARF WATER LEISURE CENTRE
Bristol Harbour,
Underfall Yard, Bristol.
Tel 0ll7-929 7608 Fax 0117-929 4454
Sailing school and centre, with qualified instruction in most watersports. Also moorings available throughout the Bristol Harbour for all types of leisurecraft at extremely competitive rates.

DARTMOUTH YACHT CRUISE SCHOOL
103 High Street,
Totnes, Devon TQ9 5SN.
Ans/Fax (01803) 864027
Tel (01803) 722226
Home: 55 The Old Common, Bussage, Stroud, Gloucestershire GL6 8HH. Tel (01453) 731142. RYA recognised teaching establishment since 1990. Skipper charter; Bareboat charter; Youth training, Duke of Edinburgh's Scheme; Sail training all RYA recognised courses including First Aid; Diesel engine courses; Sea survival; Helmsman's certificates to Yachtmaster offshore preparation.

FOWEY CRUISING SCHOOL
32 Fore Street,
Fowey, Cornwall PL23 1AQ.
Tel (01726) 832129
All RYA cruising courses and shore-based exam courses plus skippered charters and cruises available in the West Country.

KINNEGO MARINA
- Lough Neagh
Oxford Island, Lurgan,
Co Armagh, N Ireland.
Tel (01762) 327573 Fax (01762) 347438
90 berths 10 moorings, Kinnego Marina is based in the south east corner of Lough Neagh, close to the M1 motorway. Mullen Marine offers chandlery, engine repairs on-site, and we offer RYA powerboat, keelboat and dinghy courses all year round. Access to the Lough via the Lower Bann at Coleraine. Lough Neagh - 154 sq mile 77 mile of shoreline.

MAX WALKER YACHT DELIVERIES
Zinderneuf Sailing, PO Box 105,
Macclesfield, Cheshire SK10 2EY.
Tel (01625) 431712 Fax (01625) 619704
Fixed price deliveries. Sailing yachts delivered with care in north west European, UK and Eire waters by RYA/DoT yachtmaster and crew; 30 years' experience. Owners welcome. Tuition if required. References available. Your enquiries welcome 24 hours.

THE SCOTTISH NATIONAL SPORTS CENTRE: CUMBRAE
Burnside Road, Largs, Ayrshire.
Tel (01475) 674666 Fax (01475) 674720
Scotland's national watersports centre offers RYA Dinghy Courses at all levels in Lasers, 470s, Toppers, Wayfarers. Instructor courses. Coastal Skipper/Yachtmaster in Sigma and Westerly Fulmar Cruiser/Racers. Catamaran sailing. Fully qualified expert instructors.

TRYSAIL
Falmouth Marina, North Parade,
Falmouth, Cornwall TR11 2TD.
Tel (01326) 212320
RYA motor cruising and sailing courses conducted in relaxed holiday atmosphere,

while encouraging a responsible attitude towards seamanship and safety at sea. Shore-based and practical courses for all, from novice to experienced sailor.

UPHOLSTERY & COVERS

MARTELLO YACHT SERVICES
Mulberry House, Mulberry Road,
Canvey Island, Essex SS8 0PR.
Tel/Fax (01268) 681970
Manufacturers and suppliers of made-to-measure upholstery, covers, hoods, dodgers, sailcovers, curtains and cushions etc. Repairs undertaken. DIY materials, chandlery and fitting-supplies.

WATERSIDE ACCOMMODATION

ABERYSTWYTH MARINA - Y LANFA
Trefechan,
Aberystwyth, Dyfed SY23 1AS.
Tel (01970) 611422 Fax (01970) 624122
Quality waterside apartments (1, 2 and 3 bedrooms) overlooking the new fully serviced marina and Cardigan Bay. All are served by balconies, gardens and car park spaces. A pub, restaurant, cafe and shops are presently under construction. Town centre 5 minutes' walk with excellent restaurants, shops, pubs and full recreational leisure facilities.

ARDFERN YACHT CENTRE
Ardfern By Lochgilphead,
Argyll PA31 8QN.
Tel (01852) 500247/636
Fax (01852) 500624
Boatyard with full repair and maintenance facilities. Timber and GRP repairs, painting and engineering. Sheltered moorings and pontoon berthing. Winter storage, chandlery, showers, fuel, Calor, brokerage, 20-ton boat hoist. Hotel, bars and restaurant.

CASTLEPARK MARINA
Kinsale, Co Cork, Eire.
Tel +353 21 774959 Fax +353 21 774958
100-berth fully serviced marina. Access at all stages of the tide. Located within picturesque Kinsale harbour with ferry service to town. New marina centre with accommodation, restaurant, laundry, showers and toilets.

GIGHA HOTEL
Isle of Gigha, Argyll PA41 7AA.
Tel (01583) 505254 Fax (01583) 505244
Beautiful island, good food, lots of booze and friendly folk. Ideal to pick up or leave your family when sailing around the Mull of Kintyre. Moorings, water, fuel, showers and laundry facilities. Self-catering cottages also available. Achamor Gardens and 9-hole golf course.

MELFORT PIER & HARBOUR
Kilmelford,
By Oban, Argyll PA34 4XD.
Tel (01852) 200333 Fax (01852) 200329
A small pretty harbour set up, surrounded by top quality holiday houses each with private sauna/spa, tel/fax. All shoreside facilities for the cruising yachtsman; moorings and pontoon berthing, showers, laundry, tel/fax, B & B, diesel, water, electricity, gas, provisions. Restaurant, bar, hotel, bikes, watersports, horseriding and much more. Call sign: Melfort Pier 16/12.

SALTERNS MARINA
40 Salterns Way,
Lilliput, Poole, Dorset BH14 8JR.
Tel (01202) 707321/709971
Fax (01202) 700398
Pontoon Berths - Swinging Moorings - 24-hour Security - Visitors Welcome - Full Boatyard Facilities - Osmosis Treatment - 5 & 45 Tonne Hoists - Engine & Boat Sales - Award Winning Hotel, Restaurant and Bar - Chandlery - 24-hour Fuelling.

SHOTLEY MARINA LTD
Shotley Gate,
Ipswich, Suffolk IP9 1QJ.
Tel (01473) 788982 Fax (01473) 788868
A modern state of the art marina with 350 berths offering all the services expected. Open 24-hours with full security. Access all states of tide, ideal cruising base. Well stocked chandlery and general store, repair facilities, laundry and ironing centre, showers/baths and toilets. Restaurants, bar, children's room, TV/video and function rooms with dance floor and bar. Disabled facilities.

TRIDENT HOTEL - KINSALE
World's End,
Kinsale, Co Cork, Eire.
Tel +353 21 772301 Fax +353 21 774173
Recently refurbished the Trident has 56 comfortable bedrooms and two luxurious suites with delightful views of Kinsale harbour. The Savannah Restaurant, a member of the Good Food Circle, offers appetising meals complemented by efficient service from our friendly staff. Bar food available in our Fishermans Wharf bar. Leisure facilities include sauna, steamroom, gym, jacuzzi and games room.

WEATHER INFORMATION

ICS ELECTRONICS LTD
Unit V, Rudford Industrial Estate,
Ford, Arundel,
West Sussex BN18 0BD.
Tel (01903) 731101 Fax (01903) 731105
The manufacturer of data communication products - DSC, MSI, Navtex, radio telex modems, weatherfax and weather satellite receivers and software programmes - electronic charting. Weatherfax and Synop. UK distributor for Davis weather stations.

MARINECALL -
Telephone Information Services plc
Avalon House, London EC2A 4PJ.
Tel 0171-631 5000
Marinecall offers detailed coastal weather forecasts for 17 different regions, for up to 5 days ahead, from the Met Office. Current weather conditions, updated hourly 0891 226 + Area Number; Fax 0336 400 + Area Number for 2-day local forecasts and charts.

NORTHUMBRIA SCHOOL OF NAVIGATION
53 High Street, Amble,
Northumberland NE65 0LE.
Tel (01665) 713437
Two courses that bring weather and the oceans to life. Learn all there is to know about wind and pressure. Discover how to use the sky, shipping forecasts, fax and satellite images to predict the weather. Find out about the weather in major cruising areas. Follow the Oceanography Course to discover how waves develop and how to survive heavy seas. Learn about ocean currents and the need to conserve the marine environment.

WOOD FITTINGS

SHERATON MARINE CABINET
White Oak Green, Hailey,
Witney, Oxfordshire OX8 5XP.
Tel/Fax (01993) 868275
Manufacturers of quality teak and mahogany marine fittings, louvre doors, gratings and tables. Special fitting out items to customer specification. Colour catalogue available on request.

YACHT BROKERS

BOATWORKS + LTD
Castle Emplacement,
St Peter Port, Guernsey,
Channel Islands GY1 1AU.
Tel (01481) 726071 Fax (01481) 714224
Boatworks+ provides a comprehensive range of services including electronics, chandlery, boatbuilding and repairs, engine sales and services, yacht brokerage, clothing and fuel supplies.

BRIAN FENTON MARINE TRANSPORT SERVICES
17 Weatherdon Drive,
Ivybridge, South Devon PL21 0DD.
Tel/Fax (01752) 690373
Specialist yacht, motor cruiser and catamaran transporters to all areas in UK and Europe. 25 years' experience. Purpose-built vehicles, single and multiple loads. Trade references available if required. Plymouth based.

BRUNDALL BAY MARINA - SALES
Riverside Estate, Brundall,
Norwich, Norfolk NR13 5PN.
Tel (01603) 716606 Fax (01603) 715666
New and used boat sales, brokerage, full workshop services. Agents for Faircraft river cruisers. Hardy, Seawings sports cruisers, Evinrude outboard motors. 200-berth marina with full facilities.

CRAOBH MARINA
By Lochgilphead, Argyll PA31 8UD.
Tel (01852) 500222 Fax (01852) 500252
250-berth marina on Loch Shuna. Water, electricity, diesel and gas. Full boatyard services. Chandlery. Brokerage. Insurance. Shops, bar, sailing centre and dive centre. Hotel and self-catering accommodation close by. 24-hour access. VHF channels 37(M) & 80.

GAVIN POOLE YACHT BROKERS
14 Hooke Close,
Canford Heath, Dorset BH17 8BB.
Tel (01202) 604068 Fax (01202) 659680
The motor cruiser and Fairey boat specialist for modern diesel and classic boats. Sales, service, finance. Open every day. Mobile number 0860 236389

INDEPENDENT INSURANCE BROKERS LTD
PO Box 285, Esplanade House,
29 Glategny Esplanade,
St Peter Port, Guernsey,
Channel Islands GY1 1WR.
Tel (01481) 722868 Fax (01481) 714234
Marine insurance brokers supporting yacht sales procedures. Boast a comprehensive portfolio of insurance products and services, extending to home, personal, etc. Our reputation is built on thoroughness, active client support and communication.

LANGSTONE YACHTING plc
Fort Cumberland Road,
Southsea, Hampshire PO4 9RJ.
Tel (01705) 822719 Fax (01705) 822220
Langstone Marina with over 300 berths is on the western side of the entrance to Langstone Harbour. Facilities include: hoist, brokerage, restaurant, bar, chandlery, hard standing. Access over the sill is available approximately 3 hours either side of highwater.

TOLLESBURY MARINA
The Yacht Harbour, Tollesbury,
Maldon, Essex CM9 8SE.
Tel (01621) 869202
Fax (01621) 868489
VHF Channel 37/80 Tollesbury Marina can offer 260 marina berths with water and electricty on all pontoons. Clubhouse with bar, restaurant, swimming pool and tennis courts. Repair workshops with West Osmosis Treatment Centre. Full brokerage service listing over 200 boats, with a friendly professional service.

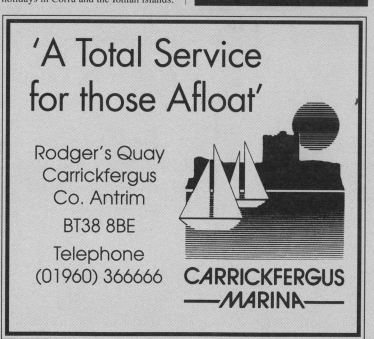

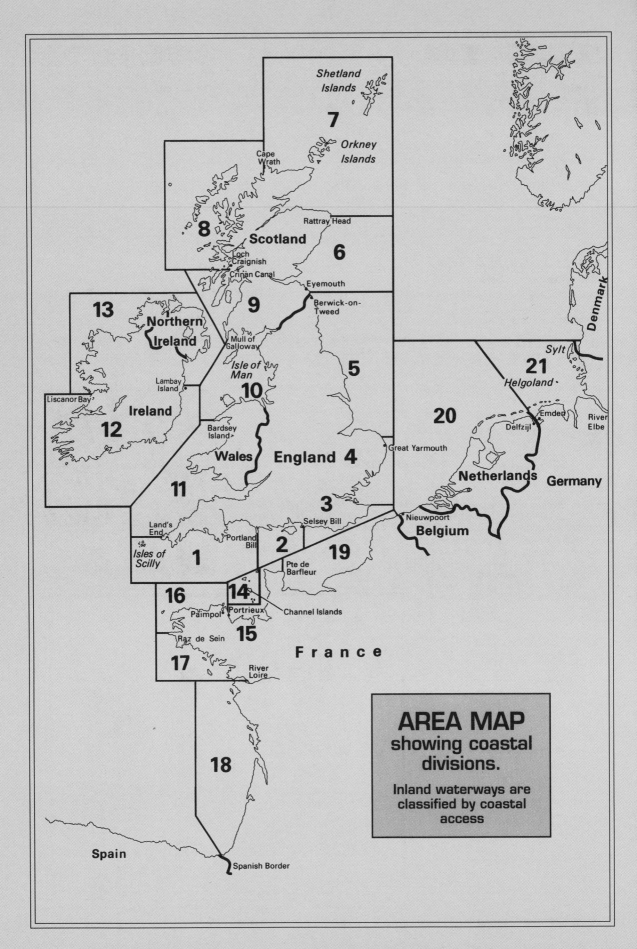

AREA MAP
showing coastal divisions.

Inland waterways are classified by coastal access

Coastal and Waterways Services Directory - Area by Area

SOUTH WEST ENGLAND (AREA 1)
Scilly Isles to Portland Bill

BOB SALMON & ASSOCIATES
112 Mewstone Avenue, Wembury, Plymouth PL9 0HT. Tel (01752) 862558 Fax (01752) 862557. Worldwide delivery of power and sailing craft by sea. Established 1972. We offer personal attention and very experienced professional service. Non smoking skippers and crews. No obligation advice. Quotations and draft contracts with pleasure.

BRIAN FENTON MARINE TRANSPORT

17 Weatherdon Drive, Ivybridge, South Devon PL21 0DD.
Tel/Fax: (01752) 690373
*Specialist yacht, motor cruiser and catamaran transporters to all areas in UK and Europe.
25 years experience. Purpose built vehicles, single and multiple loads.
Trade references available if required. Plymouth based.*

BRIAN FENTON MARINE TRANSPORT SERVICES
17 Weatherdon Drive, Ivybridge, South Devon PL21 0DD. Tel/Fax (01752) 690373. Specialist yacht, motor cruiser and catamaran transporters to all areas in UK and Europe. 25 years' experience. Purpose-built vehicles, single and multiple loads. Trade references available if required. Plymouth based.

BRIXHAM MARINA
Berry Head Road, Brixham, Devon TQ5 9BW. Tel (01803) 882929 Fax (01803) 882737. Contact: Mrs Amanda Pledger. Sheltered 480-berth marina in Torbay. Pontoon fully serviced berths up to 18 metres. Larger vessel by arrangement. 24-hour dockmaster. Diesel 24 hours, car park, toilet and launderette facilities, chandlery. Part of the MDL Group.

BRIXHAM YACHT SUPPLIES
72 MIDDLE STREET TQ5 8EJ
☎ 01803 882290

CLOTHING SPECIALISTS
BRADSPORT • GUY COTTON
REGATTA • HELLY HENSON

YACHTING AND CAMPING EQUIPMENT

BRIXHAM YACHT SUPPLIES LTD
72 Middle Street, Brixham, Devon TQ5 8EJ. Tel (01803) 882290. We stock a complete range of sailing and leisure clothing. English and continental pure wool traditional knitwear. Camping accessories.

CLOVELLY BAY MARINA
The Quay, Turnchapel, Plymouth PL9 9TF. Tel (01752) 404231 Fax (01752) 484177. Position: Southern side of cattewater, sheltered from prevailing winds by Mountbatten Peninsula. Open: All year, 24 hours. Radio: VHF channel 37 and 80. Callsign: Clovelly Bay. Berths: 180 berths, vessels up to 150', some fore and afts, visitors welcome. Facilities: electricity, water, 24-hour security, workshop, chandlery, brokerage, showers, laundry, diesel. Calor gas, payphone, refuse, water taxi, two local pubs

---

DARTHAVEN MARINA LTD
Brixham Road, Kingswear, Dartmouth, Devon TQ6 0SG
*All types of repair facilities available. Fully trained staff
30-ton mobile hoist available all states of tide.
Extensive Chandlery open 7 days a week.
Agents for Autohelm • Raytheon• Cetrek
Simpson Lawrence • Vetus• Webasto
- Visitors welcome. 24 hour Engineering call out service
- Mobile No (0860) 873553 (engineering)/ (0589) 340609 (electronics)*

Telephone - Office (01803) 752242
Fax: (01803) 752722
Marina Office: (01803) 752545
Chandlery: (01803) 752733
Fax: (01803) 752790

DARTHAVEN MARINA LTD
Brixham Road, Kingswear, Dartmouth, Devon TQ6 0SG. Tel (01803) 752242 Fax (01803) 752722 Marina Office: (01803) 752545 Chandlery: (01803) 752733 Fax 752790. All types of repair facilities available. Fully trained staff. 30-ton mobile hoist available all states of tide. Extensive chandlery open 7 days a week. Agents for Autohelm/Raytheon, Cetrek, Simpson Lawrence, Vetus and Webasto. Visitors welcome. 24-hour engineering call-out service. Mobile Nos: 0860 873553 Engineering; 0589 340609 Electronics.

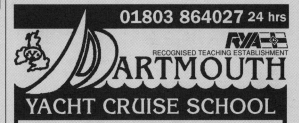

01803 864027 24 hrs

RECOGNISED TEACHING ESTABLISHMENT

DARTMOUTH
YACHT CRUISE SCHOOL

Selection of charter boats available from £180 per week 2 day or weekend - pre-flotilla; Boat handling; RYA, HOCC/ICC, VHF, First Aid, Diesel courses Sea-survival. All RYA recognised courses on request. All vessels to RYA/DPt YBDSA YCA MSA standards.

103 High Street, Totnes, Devon TQ9 5SN. Tel & Fax: 01803 864027
55 The Old Common, Bussage, Stroud, Glos GL6 8HH. Tel: 01453 731142

DARTMOUTH YACHT CRUISE SCHOOL
103 High Street, Totnes, Devon TQ9 5SN. Ans/Fax (01803) 864027 Tel (01803) 722226 Home: 55 The Old Common, Bussage, Stroud, Gloucestershire GL6 8HH. Tel (01453) 731142. RYA recognised teaching establishment since 1990. Skipper charter; Bareboat charter; Youth training, Duke of Edinburgh's Scheme; Sail training all RYA recognised courses including First Aid; Diesel engine courses; Sea survivial; Helmsman's certificates to Yachtmaster offshore preparation.

DARTSIDE QUAY
Galmpton Creek, Galmpton, Brixham, South Devon TQ5 0EH. Tel (01803) 845445 Fax (01803) 843558. Contact: Brian Speechly. 53-ton hoist and 9-acre storage facility. Fully serviced with power and water plus 16-ton trailer hoist. Pressure washing service. Half tide moorings. Diesel fuel. Part of the MDL Group.

FALMOUTH YACHT MARINA
North Parade, Falmouth, Cornwall TR11 2TD. (01326) 316620 Fax (01326) 313939. The most westerly marina in England. Strategically placed for transatlantic departures and arrivals. Fully serviced permanent and visitor berths. Diesel fuel, chandlery, 30-ton hoist. Famous friendly service.

J H FOILS
Unit 2, Woodland Yard, High Street, Market Lavington, Nr Devizes, Wiltshire SN10 4AG. Tel/Fax (01380) 818003. J H Foils for quality and precision made rudders and centreboards. Our range of blades have hardened tips. Contact us for friendly service, competitive prices and a first class range of products.

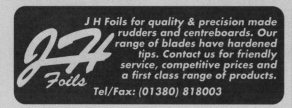
FOWEY CRUISING SCHOOL
32 Fore Street, Fowey, Cornwall PL23 1AQ. Tel (01726) 832129. All RYA cruising courses and shore based exam courses plus skippered charters and cruises available in the West Country.

GWEEK QUAY BOATYARD
Gweek Quay (Helford River), Helston, Cornwall TR12 6UF. Tel (01326) 221657 Fax (01326) 221685. Head of the Helford river. Yacht repair yard, 30-ton crane, chandlery, brokerage, coffee shop, toilets and showers. Boat storage and all boat repair and service facilities. Access approximately 2 hours either side of highwater.

HAMOAZE MARINE SERVICES
Calstock Boatyard, Lower Kelly, Calstock, Cornwall PL18 9RY. Tel (01822) 834024 & (01752) 823118. High class yacht and boat repairs, especially wood. Sheltered moorings up to 4' draught in upper Tamar river. Showers, fuel, winter storage. Also agents for Avon inflatable boats and Heyland Marine fibreglass dinghies.

HYDROGRAPHIC OFFICE
Taunton, Somerset TA1 2DN. Tel (01823) 337900 Fax (01823) 323753. Admiralty charts and hydrographic publications - worldwide coverage corrected to date of issue, available from appointed Admiralty agents together with notices to mariners. Products designed specifically for the small craft user also available from good chandlers.

MARINE INSTRUMENTS
The Bosun's Locker, Upton Slip, Falmouth TR11 3DQ. Tel (01326) 312414. DTp Certificated.

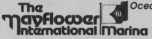
THE MAYFLOWER INTERNATIONAL MARINA
Ocean Quay, Richmond Walk, Plymouth PL1 4LS. Tel (01752) 556633 Fax (01752) 606896. Marina operators with boat-hoist (25 ton) facility. Restaurant, clubroom, launderette, fuel, chandlery, shop and off-licence. Winter storage. Owned by berth holders and operated to a very high standard.

MECTRONICS MARINE
PO Box 8, Newton Abbot, Devon TQ12 1FF. Tel (01626) 334453. LIGHT ACTIVATED SWITCHES, rugged solid state devices to automatically switch anchor lights at sunset and sunrise. NAVLIGHT SELECTORS, protected enclosed rotary switches internally connected to ensure approved navigation light combination on auxiliary sailing vessels. NAVLIGHT STATUS MONITORS, diagnostic displays on which the appropriate indicator flashes quickly or slowly in the event of a short or open circuit fault. Also drives an optional audible warning device.

MILLBAY MARINA
Millbay Docks, Great Western Road, Plymouth PL1 3EQ. Tel/Fax (01752) 226785. Contact: Alan Smith. Sheltered 86-berth marina adjacent to Plymouth Hoe. Fully serviced berths. Car park. Advance booking essential. Part of the MDL Group.

PANTAENIUS UK LTD
Registered Insurance Broker: Marine Building, Queen Anne's Battery, Plymouth, Devon PL4 0LP. Tel (01752) 223656 Fax (01752) 223637 *Head Office: Cremon 32.20457 Hamburg, Germany. Tel: +49 40 370 910 Fax +49 40 3709 1109.* Pantaenius is one of Europe's largest yacht insurance brokers and covers yachts sailing under more than 35 different flags in all seven seas.

PORT OF TRURO
Harbour Office, Town Quay, Truro, Cornwall. Tel (01872) 72130 Fax (01872) 225346. Facilities for the yachtsman include visitors' pontoons located at Turnaware Bar near Ruan Creek, Boscawen Park. Visitors' moorings at Woodbury. Quay facilities at Truro with free showers and toilets. Chemical toilet disposal, fresh water and garbage disposal.

PORTWAY YACHT CHARTERS
Falmouth Marina, North Parade, Falmouth, Cornwall TR11 2TD. Tel (01326) 212320. Wide range of sail and motor cruising yachts available for charter from the beautiful south coast of Cornwall. Tuition also available (see TRYSAIL). Owners of quality yachts are invited to contact us regarding yacht management.

ROBIN CURNOW MARINE ENGINEERS
Commercial Road, Penryn, Cornwall TR10 8AG. Tel (01326) 373438 Fax (01326) 376534. Outboard motor sales and service. Morse controls service centre. British Seagull/Selva - Evinrude - Honda - Mercury - Yamaha.

SOUTHDOWN MARINA
Southdown Quay, Millbrook, Cornwall PL10 1EZ. Tel/Fax (01752) 823084. 32-berth marina on edge of river Tamar in quiet location behind Rame Peninsula. Plymouth is just across the river. Quayside berths available for large vessels. Winter storage. Good security. DIY facilities available.

TORQUAY MARINA
Torquay, Devon TQ2 5EQ. Tel (01803) 214624 Fax (01803) 291634. Contact: Wendy-Jane Latham. Lively 500-berth marina adjacent town centre. Pontoon fully serviced berths. 24-hour dockmaster. Superb shower and toilet facilities, launderette, private car park, fuel, boat repair facilities, chandlery. Cafe/bar, restaurant. Part of the MDL Group.

TRYSAIL
Falmouth Marina, North Parade, Falmouth, Cornwall TR11 2TD. Tel (01326) 212320. RYA motor cruising and sailing courses conducted in relaxed holiday atmosphere, while encouraging a responsible attitude towards seamanship and safety at sea. Shore based and practical courses for all, from novice to experienced sailor.

UPPER DECK MARINE
Albert Quay, Fowey, Cornwall PL23 1AQ. Tel (01726) 832287 Fax (01726) 833265. Chandlery, fastenings, paints, cords, fenders, anchors, compasses, lifejackets, Gaz. Leading names in waterproofs and warm wear.

UPPER DECK MARINE (Outriggers)
Albert Quay, Fowey, Cornwall PL23 1AQ. Tel (01726) 833233 Fax (01726) 833265. 'Outriggers' casual and marine clothing, footwear, nautical gifts, Admiralty chart agent and marine books.

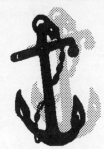
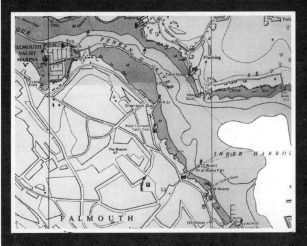

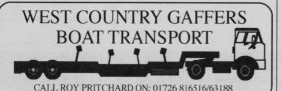
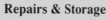
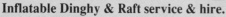

CHICHESTER MARINA

Birdham, Chichester, West Sussex PO20 7EJ. Tel **(01243) 512731 Fax (01243) 513472.** A very attractive marina offering superb services and shore installations, welcoming long and short-term visitors. Chandlery, bar, restaurant and boatyard facilities. Ring for further details.

COBB'S QUAY

Hamworthy, Poole, Dorset BH15 4EL. Tel (01202) 674299 Fax (01202) 665217. Contact: Eileen Browne. 850-berth marina. Access to superb sailing. Fully serviced pontoon berths. Ample hardstanding for maintenance and storage ashore. 24-hour security. Shower and toilet facilities, petrol and diesel fuel, car park, lift out and slipping, chandlers, repairs and restaurant. Yacht club. Part of the MDL Group.

COMMUNICATION AERIALS LTD

Unit 1A, Woodland Industrial Estate, Eden Vale Road, Westbury, Wiltshire BA13 3QS. Tel (01373) 822835 Fax (01373) 858081. We have antennae and accessories to meet most applications. We use high quality cable and connectors to ensure your antenna operates efficiently. Ask for details on the comprehensive range of products that we now have to offer for VHF, cellular and Active Antenna installations.

COMPASS POINT CHANDLERY

The Quay, High Street, Hamble, Hampshire SO31 4HA. Tel (01703) 452388 Fax (01703) 456942. Compass Point is adjacent to the new quay at Hamble. It stocks an attractive selection of leisure clothing and foulweather gear as well as a wide range of chandlery.

COWES MARINA

Clarence Road, East Cowes, Isle of Wight PO32 6HA. Tel (01983) 293983 Fax (01983) 299276. Cowes Marina lies just 300 metres upstream of the floating bridge in East Cowes. Fully sheltered pontoons with water and power can accommodate up to 200 visiting craft as well as 100 resident yachts.

COWES YACHT HAVEN

Vectis Yard, High Street, Cowes, Isle of Wight PO31 7BD. Tel (01983) 299975 Fax (01983) 200332. Cowes Yacht Haven is the Solent's premier sailing event centre offering 200 fully serviced berths right in the heart of Cowes. Our improved facilities, capability and location ensures the perfect venue and profile for every kind of boating event.

COWES YACHTING

Britannia House, 2 & 3 High Street, Cowes, Isle of Wight PO31 7SA. Tel (01983) 280770 Fax (01983) 280766. The complete information and liaison service for yachting in and around Cowes. Cowes Yachting can provide all the information that regatta or rally organisers or individual yachtsmen need to plan a visit to Cowes.

CREWSAVER LTD

Mumby Road, Gosport, Hampshire PO12 1AQ. Tel (01705) 528621. Crewsaver - leading UK manufacturers of lifejackets, buoyancy aids and personal safety equipment. Crewsaver is able to offer a complete range designed to meet your individual water sport needs.

DIVERSE YACHT SERVICES

Unit 12, Hamble Yacht Services, Port Hamble, Hamble, Hampshire SO31 4NN. Tel (01703) 453399 Fax (01703) 455288. Marine electronics and electrics. Supplied and installed. Specialists in racing yachts. Suppliers of 'Loadsense' Loadcells for marine applications.

ELKINS BOATYARD

Tidesreach, 18 Convent Meadow, The Quay, Christchurch, Dorset BH23 1BD. Tel (01202) 483141. All boatyard facilities. Moorings alongside, water and electricity, storage ashore, repairs. Boats up to 45', 10 tons maximum, haul out.

GAVIN POOLE YACHT BROKERS

14 Hooke Close, Canford Heath, Dorset BH17 8BB. Tel (01202) 604068 Fax (01202) 659680. The motor cruiser and Fairey boat specialist for modern diesel and classic boats. Sales, service, finance. Open every day. Mobile number 0860 236389

GREENHAM MARINE LTD

King's Saltern Road, Lymington, Hampshire SO41 9QD. Tel (01590) 671144 Fax (01590) 679517. Greenham Marine can offer yachtsmen one of the most comprehensive selections of marine electronic equipment currently available.

GUY RYDER LEISURE

Dorset Lake Shipyard, Lake Drive, Hamworthy, Poole, Dorset BH15 4DT. Tel/Fax (01202) 661052. The A-Z chandlery for sports boats. Boston Whaler accessories, safety and security equipment, Blakes paints, Pro-Rainer clothing, life jackets and buoyancy aids, navigational equipment, Ritchie compasses, Tempo products. Mail order available.

HAMBLE POINT MARINA

School Lane, Hamble, Southampton, Hampshire SO31 4NB. Tel (01703) 452464 Fax (01703) 456440. Contact: Chris Hibbs. Mouth of river Hamble. 220 fully serviced berths. Toilet and shower facilities. Yacht repair yard, lifting for boats up to 65 tons, boat storage. Licensed members' club. 7-ton crane, diesel fuel, Calor gas and ice. 24-hour security. Chandlery and all boat repair/service facilities. Part of the MDL Group.

HYTHE MARINA

Shamrock Way, Hythe, Southampton, Hampshire SO45 6DY. Tel (01703) 207073/849263 Fax (01703) 842424. Contact: Peter Bedwell. Three marina basins surrounded by character homes and miniature village square 210 fully serviced berths. Chandlery, shops. Fully serviced pontoons. Access by lock manned 24 hours. Shower and toilet facilities. Petrol and diesel fuel. 30-ton hoist, car park. Part of the MDL Group.

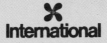
INTERNATIONAL PAINT

24-30 Canute Road, Southampton, Hampshire SO14 3PB. Tel (01703) 226722 Fax (01703) 335975. International Paint is the leading supplier of quality paints, epoxies, varnishes and anti-foulings to the marine industry. Over half the world's pleasure craft are protected by International products.

ISLAND HARBOUR MARINA

Mill Lane, Binfield, Newport, Isle of Wight PO30 2LA. Tel (01983) 526020 & 822999. Locked marina on Medina river. Tidal access HW ±3½ hrs. 150 visitors' berths. Services include - water, electricity, showers, launderette, gas, diesel, chandlery, restaurant and bar. Full boatyard facilities with 12-ton hoist and 30-ton cradle.

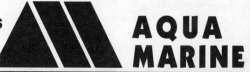
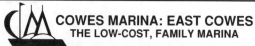
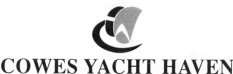

ISLAND MARINE POWER (ELECTRICAL) LTD

East Cowes Marina, Clarence Road, Cowes Marina, Isle of Wight PO32 6HA. Tel/Fax (01983) 280011. Island Marine Power (Electrical) Ltd now in our new premises facing the river at East Cowes. The workshop - as always - open for major, minor and emergency electrical works. The shop - stocking practical chandlery and hardware is still growing. Tel/Fax 01983 280011 East Cowes Marina.

KELVIN HUGHES CHARTS & MARITIME SUPPLIES

Royal Crescent Road, Southampton, Hampshire. Tel (01703) 634911 Fax (01703) 330014. Charts, books, chandlery, safety equipment and clothing. Liferaft hire, sales and servicing. Also in London with worldwide mail order service.

LANGSTONE HARBOUR BOARD

Ferry Road, Hayling Island, Hampshire PO11 0DG. Tel (01705) 463419 Fax (01705) 467144. All boatyard facilities. Deep water and tidal moorings available. Water, electricity and diesel. Summer and winter storage. Public slipways. 6-ton crane. Landrover vessel and trailer recovery services.

LANGSTONE YACHTING PLC

Fort Cumberland Road, Southsea, Hampshire PO4 9RJ. Tel (01705) 822719 Fax (01705) 822220. Langstone Marina with over 300 berths is on the western side of the entrance to Langstone Harbour. Facilities include: hoist, brokerage, restaurant, bar, chandlery, hard standing. Access over the sill is available approximately 3 hours either side of highwater.

LEWMAR MARINE LTD

Southmoor Lane, Havant, Hampshire PO9 1JJ. Tel (01705) 471841 Fax (01705) 476043. Manufacturers of winches, windlasses, hatches, hardware, hydraulics and marine thrusters for boats ranging in size from 25' to 300' LOA.

MANOR OF BOSHAM LTD

Bosham Quay, Old Bosham, West Sussex PO18 8HR. Tel (01243) 573336 Fax (01243) 576285. Deep water moorings up to 14 metres in length in picturesque Bosham Channel - Chichester Harbour, also includes some tidal moorings. Services available at quay. Also scrubbing off grids including pressure washers.
Contact Name: M McGrail.

MERCURY YACHT HARBOUR

Satchell Lane, Hamble, Southampton, Hampshire SO31 4HQ. Tel (01703) 455994 Fax (01703) 457369. Contact: Paul Keast. Peaceful, 350 fully serviced berths. Car park. 24-hour staff. Toilet and shower facilities. Yacht repairs, 10-ton lifting, chandlery, yacht brokerage, sailmakers, electronics. Licensed members' club. Sailing school. Part of the MDL Group.

R J MUIR

22 Seymour Close, Chandlers Ford, Eastleigh, Southampton SO5 2JE. Tel (01703) 261042. DTp Certifcated.

NORTHNEY MARINA

Northney Road, Hayling Island, Hampshire PO11 0NH. Tel (01705) 466321/2 Fax (01705) 461467. Contact: Tony Barker. Chichester harbour. 228-berth marina. Fully serviced pontoon berths. Diesel fuel, car park. Shower and toilet facilities. Brokerage, yacht repair, lifting to 35 tons, chandlery. Licensed club. Sailing and wind surfing school. Part of the MDL Group.

OCEAN VILLAGE MARINA

Channel Way, Canute Road, Southampton, Hampshire SO14 3TG. Tel (01703) 229385 Fax (01703) 233515. Contact: Adrian Smith. Modern city centre marina with 450 fully serviced pontoon berths up to 75 metres. 24-hour security. Royal Southampton Yacht Club. Toilet and shower facilities. Car park. Adjacent shopping and entertainment complex. Part of the MDL Group.

PORT HAMBLE

Satchell Lane, Hamble, Southampton, Hampshire SO31 4QD. Tel (01703) 452741 Fax (01703) 455206. Close to Hamble village. 310 fully serviced marina berths. Shower and toilet facilities. Car park, petrol and diesel fuel, yacht repair yard. Lifting to 100 tons, chandlery, brokerage, sailmakers. Members' licensed club. 24-hour staff. Part of the MDL Group.

PORT SOLENT

South Lockside, Port Solent, Portsmouth, Hampshire PO6 4TJ. Tel (01705) 210765 Fax (01705) 324241. Port Solent is a community of houses, apartments, restaurants, shops and a cinema encompassing 900 berths. This includes 400 public berths with excellent facilities for visitors, including luxury showers and club.

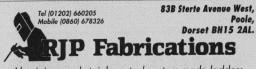
R J P FABRICATIONS

83B Sterte Avenue West, Poole, Dorset BH15 2AL. Tel (01202) 660205 Mobile 0860 678326. Aluminium and stainless steel custom made ladders and handrails. General light fabrication and repairs.

R T TRAINING

286 Sea Front, Hayling Island, Hampshire PO11 0AZ. Tel/Fax (01705) 462122. Weekend radio courses at Southampton and Port Solent for leisure and professional yachtsmen. SSB - 3-day Restricted Course/Exam. Long Range Certificate - contact us for details of this new certificate. VHF - 1-day Course/Exam.

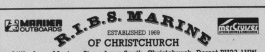
R.I.B.S. MARINE

Little Avon Marina, Stony Lane South, Christchurch, Dorset BH23 1HW. Tel (01202) 477327 Fax (01202) 471456.

RADIO SCHOOL LTD

33 Island Close, Hayling Island, Hampshire PO11 0NJ. Tel (01705) 466450 Fax (01705) 461449. Weekend integrated courses/exams for Marine VHF and SSB Radiotelephone Operator's Certificates in Britain's only permanent, fully equipped classroom soley dedicated to training leisure sailors in radio operation on a full-time, professional basis.

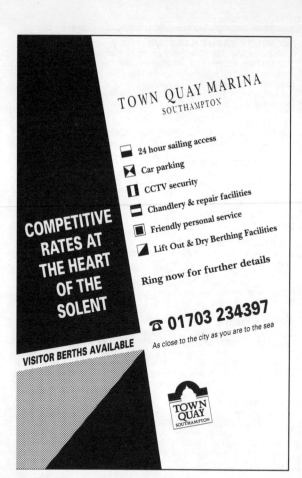

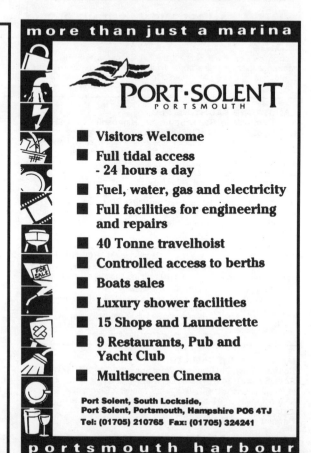

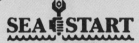
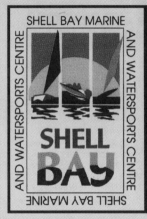

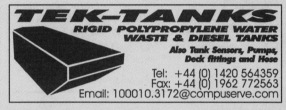

THORNHAM MARINA
Thornham Lane, Prinsted, Nr Emsworth, Hampshire PO10 8DD. Tel (01243) 375335. First class serviced hardstanding, 12-ton slipway hoist. Tidal pontoons, deep water gated pool, modern workshop, bar, restaurant, showers and toilets. Visitors welcome - club rallies etc. A very few long-term berths available. Brokerage service.

TOLLEY MARINE LTD
Unit 7, Blackhill Road West, Holton Heath Trading Park, Poole, Dorset BH16 6LS. Tel (01202) 632644 Fax (01202) 632622. (also at: Plymouth - Tel (01752) 222530; Brighton - Tel (01273) 424224 and London - 0171-930 3237. Agents of sales and service for Autohelm, B & G, Cetrek, Furuno, Garmin, Icom, Koden, Lo-Kata, MLR, Magnavox, Navico, Panasonic, Raytheon, Robertson, Sailor, Shipmate, Trimble.

TOWN QUAY MARINA
Town Quay, The Waterfront, Southampton, Hampshire. Tel (01703) 234397. Town Quay is a growing development of bars and restaurants on an attractive waterfront environment just minutes away from the city centre. A number of attractions occur on the quay throughout the year.

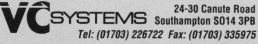
V C SYSTEMS
24-30 Canute Road, Southampton, Hampshire SO14 3PB. Tel (01703) 226722 Fax (01703) 335975. VC Systems provides a comprehensive range of yacht paint products designed for first class boat maintenance. This range includes the Teflon anti-foulings, VC17m and VC Offshore Extra and a range of epoxies, fillers, varnishes and accessory paint products.

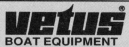
VETUS DEN OUDEN LTD
38 South Hants Industrial Park, Totton, Southampton, Hampshire SO40 3SA. Tel (01703) 861033 Fax (01703) 663142. Suppliers of marine diesel equipment, exhaust systems, steering systems, bow propellers, propellers and shafts, hatches, portlights, windows, electronic instruments, batteries, ventilators, windlasses, water and fuel tanks, chandlery items and much much more.

WARSASH NAUTICAL BOOKS
6 Dibles Road, Warsash, Southampton SO31 9HZ. Tel (01489) 572384 Fax (01489) 885756. Nautical bookseller and chart agent. Callers and mail order. Free new and secondhand book lists. Credit cards taken. Publishers of the Bibliography of Nautical books.

WESSEX MARINE EQUIPMENT LTD
Logistics House, 2nd Avenue Business Park, Millbrook Road East, Southampton SO1 0LP. Tel (01703) 510570.

WEYMOUTH OLD HARBOUR
Weymouth & Portland Borough Council, Borough Engineers Department, Municipal Offices, North Quay, Weymouth, Dorset DT4 8TA. Tel (01305) 206278/206423 Fax (01305) 206276. Access at all stages of tide. Visitors' berths in the centre of prime tourist resort with shops, restaurants and night life all at hand. Diesel fuelling from pontoon or tanker. Chandlery and repair facilities available.

WORLD CREWS
52 York Place, Bournemouth BH7 6JN. Tel/Fax (01202) 431520. WORLD CREWS is an International crewfinder service providing amateur and professional crew for yachts cruising in home and overseas waters. Files contain delivery skippers, engineers, cook/hostess, chefs and various marine tradesmen.

YARMOUTH MARINE SERVICE
River Yar Boatyard, Yarmouth, Isle of Wight PO41 0SE. Tel (01983) 760521 Fax (01983) 760096. All boatyard facilities and commercial charter. Slipway to 20 tons. Boat repairs, wood and GRP, osmosis and painting. Annual and visitors' moorings. Two workboats available with loadline exemption for all types of commercial work.

SOUTH EAST ENGLAND   (AREA 3)
Selsey Bill to North Foreland

ADEC MARINE LTD
4 Masons Avenue, Croydon, Surrey CR0 1EH. Tel 0181-686 9717 Fax 0181-680 9912. Approved liferaft service station for south east UK. Additionally we hire and sell new rafts and sell a complete range of safety equipment for yachts including pyrotechnics, fire extinguishers, lifejackets, buoys and a buoyancy bag system.

AMPRO NAVIGATION LTD
PO Box 373A, Surbiton, Surrey KT6 5YL. Tel 0181-398 1169 Fax 0181-398 6184 Tel (01734) 820337 Fax (01734) 820338. UK agents for Philips Navigation AP range of marine electronic equipment including GPS and Decca Navigators, Chart Plotters, Instruments, hand portable and Differential GPS units. Full sales and technical support available.

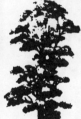
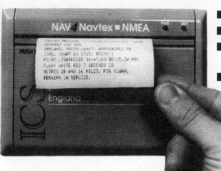

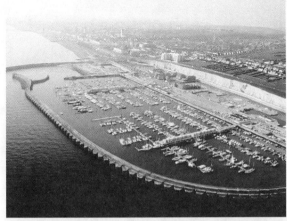
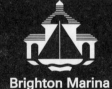

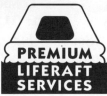
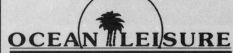
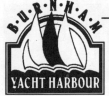
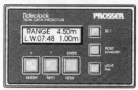
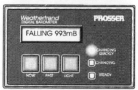

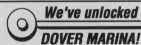
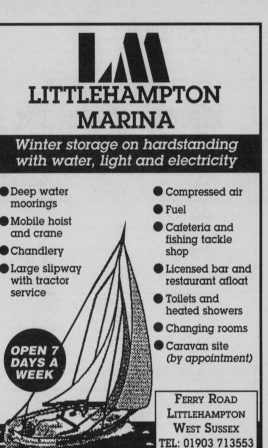

ODYSSEUS YACHTING HOLIDAYS
33 Grand Parade, Brighton, Sussex BN2 2QA. Tel (01273) 695094 Fax (01273) 688855. Templecraft Yacht Charters are bonded tour operators specialising in independent yacht charter holidays in the Mediterranean and in the Caribbean, and as Odysseus Yachting Holidays in flotilla sailing holidays in Corfu and the Ionian islands.

RAMSGATE ROYAL HARBOUR
Harbour Office, Military Road, Ramsgate, Kent CT11 9LG. Tel (01843) 592277 Fax (01843) 590941. One of south east England's premier leisure areas. Ideal for crossing to the Continent. 24-hour access to finger pontoons. Comprehensive security systems. Amenities: launderette, repairs, slipways, boatpark. Competitive rates for permanent berths and visiting vessels.

SMYE-RUMSBY LTD
123 Snargate Street, Dover, Kent CT17 9AP. Tel (01304) 201187 Fax (01304) 240135. Established since 1948, our company welcomes visitors to Dover Port requiring excellent marine electronic maintenance services. We have comprehensive knowledge of current navigational equipment, and can provide a 24-hour call-out repair facility.

SOVEREIGN HARBOUR MARINA LTD
Pevensey Bay Road, Eastbourne, Sussex BN23 6JH. Tel (01323) 470099 Fax (01323) 470077. Situated at Langney Point, Eastbourne, Sovereign Harbour is centred around twin harbours, one tidal and one accessed by two high capacity locks. A full service marina with diesel, petrol and unleaded petrol available 24-hours daily.

TEMPLECRAFT YACHT CHARTERS
33 Grand Parade, Brighton BN2 2QA. Tel (01273) 695094 Fax (01273) 688855. Templecraft Yacht Charters are bonded tour operators specialising in independent yacht charter holidays in the Mediterranean and in the Caribbean, and as Odysseus Yachting Holidays in flotilla sailing holidays in Corfu and the Ionian islands.

THAMES ESTUARY (AREA 4)
North Foreland to Great Yarmouth

A M SMITH (MARINE) LTD
33 Epping Way, Chingford E4 7PB. Tel 0181-529 6988.

BLACKWATER MARINA
Marine Parade, Maylandsea, Essex CM3 6AN. Tel (01621) 740264 Fax (01621) 742122. Refurbished tidal marina on the Blackwater estuary. New pontoons, new clubhouse, bar and restaurant, toilets and showers. 18-ton slipway hoist, 70-ton winch, 130' workshop with full services. Full chandlery, brokerage/boat sales. Car parking and on-site security. Full tide swinging moorings, half tide moorings and half tide pontoon berths. A few long-term berths available.

BRUNDALL BAY MARINA - SALES
Riverside Estate, Brundall, Norwich, Norfolk NR13 5PN. Tel (01603) 716606 Fax (01603) 715666. New and used boat sales, brokerage, full workshop services. Agents for Faircraft river cruisers. Hardy, Seawings sports cruisers, Evinrude outboard motors. 200-berth marina with full facilities.

BURNHAM YACHT HARBOUR MARINA LTD
Burnham Yacht Harbour, Burnham-on-Crouch, Essex CM0 8BL. Tel (01621) 782150. The only Five Gold Anchor marina in Essex. 350 fully serviced pontoon berths and 120 deep water swing moorings. Marina access at all states of tide with minimum 2.5 metres depth at low water.

CAPTAIN O M WATTS
7 Dover Street, London W1X 3PJ. Tel 0171-493 4633 Fax 0171-495 0755. Admiralty charts, navigational instruments, technical and leisure clothing, flags, books, antiques and gifts, clocks and barometers, lifejackets, paint and rope.

CAVENHAM MARINE
15 Abbey Road, Billericay, Essex CM12 9NF. Tel (01277) 654788 Fax (01277) 631343. Boat chandlers and small new boats.

CLARKE & CARTER BOATYARD
128 Coast Road, West Mersea, Nr Colchester, Essex. Tel (01206) 382244 Fax (01206) 384455. The Clarke & Carter Boatyard is a division of West Mersea Marine Ltd. The yard is situated on the main waterfront at West Mersea. The anchorage, which has retained its traditional character, offers both swinging and post moorings for vessels up to about 50' LOA. Access is at all states of the tide to the river Blackwater. There are also some edge moorings available.

ELMHAVEN MARINA
Rochester Road, Halling, Kent. Tel (01634) 240489. Elmhaven provides a peaceful setting combined with good facilities including toilets, showers, power on pontoons, mud berths, hard standing, boat lifting up to 5 tons maximum with repairs by Nigel Taylor on-site. Competitive rates and good security.

ESSEX MARINA LTD
Wallasea Island, Nr Rochford, Essex SS4 2HG. Tel (01702) 258531 Fax (01702) 258227. Deep water marina berths for yachts up to 150'. Full marina shipyard services. NO locks or sills. One hour from London. Also swinging moorings available. Visiting yachtsmen welcome. Luxury toilets, laundry and shower block. Bar and restaurant.

HOO MARINA (MEDWAY) LTD
Vicarage Lane, Hoo, Rochester, Kent ME3 9LE. Tel (01634) 250311 Fax (01634) 251761. An established marina with fully serviced pontoon berths, winter lay-up on concrete hardstanding. 20-ton lifting capacity. Chandlery and brokerage as well as full workshop facilities for yacht repair and maintenance.

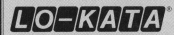
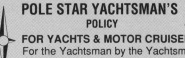
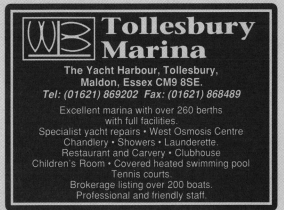

TOLLESBURY MARINA
The Yacht Harbour, Tollesbury, Maldon, Essex CM9 8SE. Tel (01621) 869202 Fax (01621) 868489. VHF Channel 37/80 Tollesbury Marina can offer 260 marina berths with water and electricty on all pontoons. Clubouse with bar, restaurant, swimming pool and tennis courts. Repair workshops with West Osmosis Treatment Centre. Full brokerage service listing over 200 boats, with friendly professional service.

TUBBY LEE YACHTING SERVICES
Kings Road, Burnham-on-Crouch, Essex CM0 8HJ. Tel (01621) 783562 Fax (01621) 785119. A complete yacht rigging service for standing and running rigging. Large stocks of wire and rope. Taluriting, swaging, wire to rope splicing, deck layout advice. Rig tuning a speciality. Yacht deliveries.

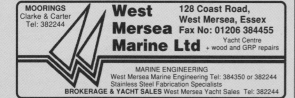

MOORINGS Clarke & Carter Tel: 382244

West Mersea Marine Ltd

128 Coast Road, West Mersea, Essex Fax No: 01206 384455 Yacht Centre + wood and GRP repairs

MARINE ENGINEERING West Mersea Marine Engineering Tel: 384350 or 382244 Stainless Steel Fabrication Specialists BROKERAGE & YACHT SALES West Mersea Yacht Sales Tel: 382244

WEST MERSEA MARINE ENGINEERING
128 Coast Road, West Mersea, Nr Colchester, Essex. Tel (01206) 384350 Fax (01206) 384455. Providing full marine engineering facilities. There are also undercover facilities for those vessels being worked on by our staff. Shipwrights, GRP specialists, painters and riggers are also available. There is a sailmaker and an outboard repair and service workshop nearby, and liferaft hire, sales and service, together with inflatable dinghy repairs and service also available locally.

WOOLVERSTONE MARINA
Woolverstone, Ipswich, Suffolk IP9 1AS. Tel (01473) 780206/780354 Fax (01473) 780273. Contact: Judy Cracknell. Easy access through Harwich harbour. 200 fully serviced berths, 120 swinging moorings, diesel fuel, car park, toilet and shower facilities, repair yard with 20-ton mobile crane. Foodstore, clubhouse, restaurant and bar. Part of the MDL Group.

WYATTS CHANDLERY
128 Coast Road, West Mersea, Nr Colchester, Essex. Tel (01206) 384745 Fax (01206) 384455. Wyatts Chandlery, well stocked and competitively priced.

UPPER THAMES (AREA 4)
Navigable west of Westminster Bridge

A R K MARINE LTD
1 Clifton Road, Isleworth, Middlesex TW7 4HN. Tel 0181-568 2778 Fax 0181-569 7503. We specialise in marine hot water systems using the inboard engine as the heat source. A full range are ex-stock, single or twin coil, vertical or horizontal. Also 1, 2 and 3kw immersion heaters. Technical and price lists free.

BRAY MARINA
Monkey Island Lane, Bray, Berkshire SL6 2EB. Tel (01628) 23654 Fax (01628) 773484. 400 berths many with 240v electricity. Shower and toilet facilities, car park, petrol, diesel and Calor gas. Chandlery, shops and cafe. Hardstanding, brokerage, refuse and chemical toilet disposal. Ample restaurants close by. Part of the MDL Group.

BRIAN GOODFELLOW & ASSOCIATES
International Surveyors
15 Chaseside Gardens, Chertsey, Surrey KT16 8JP. Tel/Fax 01932 567634 Mobile 0860 446982 (24 hours). Approved by British Waterways and the Marine Safety Agency, Brian Goodfellow & Associates can offer very competitive quotations for surveys, insurance and valuations. We act for most leading companies and major builders. Companion RINA, Ass Member YDSA, Member of BMIF.

CHISWICK QUAY MARINA LTD
Marina Office, Chiswick Quay, London W4 3UR. Tel 0181-994 8743. Small, secluded, peaceful marina on tidal Thames at Chiswick. Slipway, marine engineers and electricians, power, water, toilets and sluice.

DESMOND CHEERS & PARTNERS
44 High Street, Hampton Hill, Middlesex TW12 1PD. Tel 0181-943 5333 Fax 0181-943 5444. Marine insurance specialists with over 30 years' experience in arranging tailor-made policies through leading marine underwriters. For all your insurance and finance enquiries for yachts, motorcruisers and speedboats call Tim Cheers or Daphne Bamberger.

MARINE & AUTO SERVICES
Bridge Boathouse, River Road, Maidenhead, Berkshire SL6 0BE. Tel/Fax (01628) 36435. Marine consultant and engineers. Condition, survey and valuation reports undertaken on fibreglass craft - Thames and nationwide. Engines sold and delivered. Repairs, overhauls and servicing on all types of engines. Mail order for parts available. 35 years' experience in the marine industry.

PENTON HOOK MARINA
Staines Road, Chertsey, Surrey KT16 8PY. Tel (01932) 568681 Fax (01932) 567423. Largest inland harbour, access to river Thames. 610 fully serviced berths, craning, engineering and repairs, hardstanding, petrol, diesel and Calor gas. Shower and toilet facilities, refuse and chemical toilet disposal, car park, pumpout, chandlery. Yacht club. Part of the MDL Group.

SHERATON MARINE CABINET
White Oak Green, Hailey, Witney, Oxfordshire OX8 5XP. Tel/Fax (01993) 868275. Manufacturers of quality teak and mahogany marine fittings, louvre doors, gratings and tables. Special fitting out items to customer specification. Colour catalogue available on request.

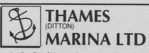
THAMES (DITTON) MARINA LTD
Portsmouth Road, Thames Ditton, Surrey KT6 5QD. Tel 0181-398 6159 Fax 0181-398 6438. Over 120 berths and moorings. All main services, diesel, Calor Gas, repairs and service. Large chandlery with comprehensive stock of safety equipment, paint, charts and books. Very large car park for convenience of customers. Open 7 days a week.

WINDSOR MARINA
Maidenhead Road, Oakley Green, Windsor, Berkshire SL4 5TZ. Tel (01753) 853911 Fax (01753) 868195. Small pastoral 200-berth marina. Showers and toilet facilities, petrol, diesel and Calor gas, car parking, dry berthing and hardstanding. Private yacht club. Repair services and mobile crane, refuse and chemical toilet disposal, pumpout, chandlery and boat sales. 240v electricity. Part of the MDL Group.

EAST ENGLAND   (AREA 5)
Blakeney to Berwick-on-Tweed

B COOKE & SON LTD
Kingston Observatory, 58-59 Market Place, Hull HU1 1RH. Tel (01482) 223454. DTp Certificated.

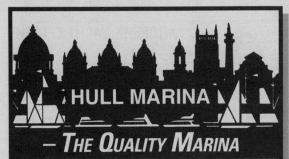
HULL MARINA LTD
Warehouse 13, Kingston Street, Hull HU1 2DQ. Tel (01482) 593451 Fax (01482) 224148. Four Anchor Marina. Situated 5 minutes from the centre of Hull and all national and international transport systems. First class leisure, boatyard and brokerage facilities. 4-Star hotel and quayside restaurants. Professional and caring staff. Competitive rates.

JOHN LILLIE & GILLIE LTD
Clive Street, North Shields, Tyne & Wear NE29 6LF. Tel 0191-257 2217. DTp Certifcated.

NELSON STOVES
Chequers, Wainfleet Road, Irby in the Marsh, Skegness, Lincolnshire PE24 5AY. Tel (01754) 810799. The unique Nelson stove is 9" square by 21" high, finished in matt black with brass trim. Heat output range 750 to 3000 watts. Designed to burn only smokeless fuels. Only available from Nelson Stoves.

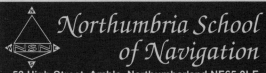
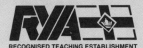
NORTHUMBRIA SCHOOL OF NAVIGATION
53 High Street, Amble, Northumberland NE65 0LE. Tel (01665) 713437. Whatever your experience we have an RYA accredited course for you. The Day Skipper Course will suit the inexperienced while those ready for an offshore passage should enrol for the Yachtmaster Offshore. Our Ocean Yachtmaster Course provides a fascinating guide through astro-navigation, world meteorolgy and ocean currents. GCSE Navigation includes sections from both yachtmaster courses.

SOUTH EAST SCOTLAND   (AREA 6)
Eyemouth to Rattray Head

PETERHEAD BAY AUTHORITY
Bath House, Bath Street, Peterhead AB42 6DX. Tel (01779) 474020 Fax (01779) 475712. Contact: Stephen Paterson. Opened in April 1994, Peterhead Bay Marina offers a comprehensive range of services and facilities for local and visiting boat owners. Ideal stopover marina for vessels heading to/from Scandinavia or the Caledonian canal.

THOMAS GUNN NAVIGATION SERVICES
62 Marischal Street, Aberdeen AB1 2AL. Tel (01224) 595045. DTp Certificated.

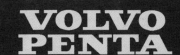

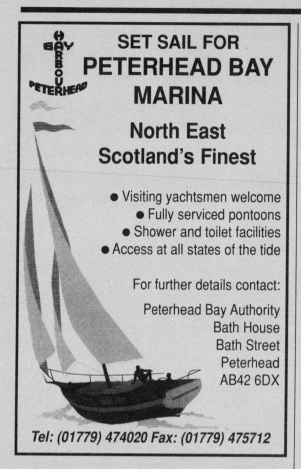

OBAN YACHTS & MARINE SERVICES LTD

Ardentrive, Kerrera, By Oban, Argyll PA34 4SX. Tel (01631) 565333 Fax (01631) 565888. Moorings, visitor pontoon, toilets, showers, drying room, diesel, gas, water, chandlery, slipway, 18-ton hoist, full workshop facilities, undercover storage, hardstanding. Regular ferry to Oban town centre less than 10 minutes across the bay.

SLEAT MARINE SERVICES

Ardvasar, Isle of Skye IV45 8RU. Tel (01471) 844 216/387. Yacht charter (bareboat and skippered) from Armadale Bay, Isle of Skye. Six yachts 34' to 40' LOA. All medium to heavy displacement blue water cruisers. Fuel, water and emergency services for passing yachts with problems.

SOUTH WEST SCOTLAND   (AREA 9)
Crinan Canal to Mull of Galloway

BROWN SON & FERGUSON LTD
4-10 Darnley Street, Glasgow G41 2SD. Tel 0141-429 1234.

GILES INSURANCE BROKERS LTD
22 Portland Road, Kilmarnock KA1 2BS. Tel (01563) 520554 Fax (01563) 528345. Scotland's marine insurance experts. Established 1967. Registered insurance brokers. Rates from the top 25 insurers are compared before quotations are sent out in an easy to read format with a copy of the policy wording. Staff are very efficient and friendly.

HARKEN - DISTRIBUTED BY SIMPSON LAWRENCE
218-228 Edmiston Drive, Glasgow G51 2YT. Tel 0141-427 5331/8 Fax 0141-427 5419. Distributors of Harken deck hardware, ball bearing blocks in all sizes from micros to maxis, jib reefing and furling systems, from dinghies to 150 footers, winches, backstay tensioners, power sheet jammers and deck shoes. We also distribute Head Foil plastic luff groove systems, and Edson steering and pump-out systems.

KIP MARINA
The Yacht Harbour, Inverkip, Renfrewshire PA16 0AS. Tel (01475) 521485 (01475) 521298. Marina berths for vessels up to 65' LOA. Full boatyard facilities including travel hoist, crane, on-site engineers, GRP repairs etc. Bar, restaurant, saunas, launderette and chandlery.

LARGS YACHT HAVEN
Irvine Road, Largs, Ayrshire KA30 8EZ. Tel (01475) 675333 Fax (01475) 672245. Perfectly located 600-berth marina with full services afloat and ashore. 45-ton travel hoist operational 7 days; fuel (diesel and petrol); gas and ice on sale 24-hours. Bar, coffee shop, dive shop plus usual marine services.

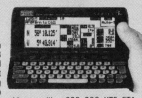

MARITEK LTD
1-D7 Templeton Centre, Glasgow G40 1DA. Tel 0141-554 2492 Fax 0141-639 1910. Computer programs for coastal/celestial navigation/tidal height prediction, using Psion pocket computer. Large computer systems and projects using 4th generation languages.

MINERVA RIGGING LTD
Kip Marina, Inverkip, Renfrewshire PA16 0AS. Tel (01475) 522700 Fax (01475) 522800. THE name for rigging services, based at Kip Marina. Stockists of high tech Spectra/Dyneeman and Vectran ropes. Roll swaging up to 14mm rod and 16mm wire. We are the Kemp service centre for Scotland.

THE SCOTTISH NATIONAL SPORTS CENTRE: CUMBRAE
Burnside Road, Largs, Ayrshire. Tel (01475) 674666 Fax (01475) 674720. Scotland's national watersports centre offers RYA Dinghy Courses at all levels in Lasers, 470s, Toppers, Wayfarers. Instructor courses. Coastal Skipper/Yachtmaster in Sigma and Westerly Fulmar Cruiser/Racers. Catamaran sailing. Fully qualified expert instructors.

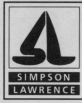

218-228 Edmiston Drive, Glasgow, Scotland G51 2YT

Tel 0141-427 5331 Fax 0141-427 5419

Simpson Lawrence are manufacturers and the UK's largest wholesale distributors of quality marine equipment.

SIMPSON LAWRENCE LTD
218-228 Edmiston Drive, Glasgow G51 2YT. Tel 0141-427 5331 Fax 0141-427 5419. Simpson Lawrence are manufacturers and the UK's largest wholesale distributors of quality marine equipment.

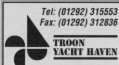

Tel: (01292) 315553
Fax: (01292) 312836

TROON YACHT HAVEN
THE HARBOUR, TROON, AYRSHIRE KA10 6DJ

Sheltered harbour for 350 berths. Well placed for those on passage to/from the Clyde. Bar and restaurant. Marine services. Attractive seafront town with good beaches and championship golf.

TROON YACHT HAVEN
The Harbour, Troon, Ayrshire KA10 6DJ. Tel (01292) 315553 Fax (01292) 312836. Sheltered harbour for 350 berths. Well placed for those on passage to and from the Clyde. Bar, restaurant, marine services. Attractive seafront town with good beaches and championship golf.

NORTH WEST ENGLAND (AREA 10)
Isle of Man and North Wales, Mull of Galloway to Bardsey Island

D G I MEDICAL SERVICES
Hyfrydle, Capel Curig, Gwynedd LL24 0EU. Tel/Fax (01690) 720344. Providers of H&SE and Rescue and Emergency Care (REC). Our instructors can provide the full REC training programme for first aid at sea. If you would like to learn how to handle emergency situations, we have a programme to suit your needs. (Department of DGI Mountaineering Ltd.)

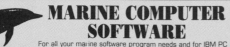

DGI MEDICAL SERVICES
PROVIDERS OF RESCUE EMERGENCY CARE (REC)

FIRST AID COURSES

Telephone or Fax on 01690 720344

DOLPHIN MARITIME SOFTWARE LTD
25 Roosevelt Avenue, Lancaster LA1 5EJ. Tel/Fax (01524) 841946. Marine computer programs for IBM PC, Psion and Sharp pocket computers. Specialists in navigation, tidal prediction and other programs for both yachting and commercial uses.

MARINE COMPUTER SOFTWARE

For all your marine software program needs and for IBM PC compatible, Psion Series 3 or 3a pocket computers, ruggedised Workabout handheld computers at affordable prices. We are specialists in both Navigation and Tidal prediction programs for yachtsmen and also offer a large number of commercial shipping programs. Free lifetime support is included with all programs. Please contact us for our latest catalogue. We deliver worldwide.

DUBOIS-PHILLIPS & McCALLUM LTD
Oriel Chambers, Covent Garden, Liverpool L2 8UD. Tel 0151-236 2776.

FIDDLERS FERRY YACHT HAVEN
Off Station Road, Penketh, Warrington, Cheshire WA5 2UJ. Tel (01925) 727519. Sheltered moorings upto 6'6" draught, 50' long. Access through lock from river Mersey 1½ hours either side of high tide. Signed from A652. Boatyard and lift-out facilities. Annual rate per foot £8.

JOSEPH P LAMB & SONS
Maritime Building (opposite Albert Dock), Wapping, Liverpool L1 8DQ. Tel 0151-709 4861 Fax 0151-709 2786. Situated in the centre of Liverpool, J P Lamb have provided a service to world shipping for over 200 years. All chandlery supplies, clothing, rope, paint and flags are available, together with a full sailmaking, repair and rigging service. Open Mon to Fri 8am to 6pm - Sat to Sun 9am to 1pm.

J P LAMB, Maritime Building
(opposite Albert Dock), Wapping, Liverpool L1 8DQ.
Tel: 0151-709 4861 Fax: 0151-709 2786
Open Mon-Fri: 8am to 6pm Sat-Sun: 9am to 1pm
Situated in the centre of Liverpool J P Lamb have provided a service to world shipping for over 200 years. All chandlery supplies, clothing, rope, paint, flags etc are available together with a full sail making, repair and rigging service

LIVERPOOL MARINA
Coburg Dock, Sefton Street, Liverpool L3 4BP. Tel 0151-709 0578/(2683 after 5pm) Fax 0151-709 8731. 300-berth yacht harbour. All serviced pontoons. Tidal access HW + or - 2½hrs approximately, depending on draft. 60-ton hoist, workshops, bar and restaurant, toilets and showers. City centre one mile. Open all year. Active yacht club and yacht brokerage.

LIVERPOOL MARINA
Coburg Dock, Sefton Street, Liverpool L3 4BP
Tel: 0151-709 0578 & 0151-709 2683 (after 5 pm)
Fax: 0151-709 8731
300 berth yacht harbour. All serviced pontoons.
Tidal access HW ± 2½ hrs. approx. depending on draft.
60 ton hoist•Workshops•Bar and Restaurant•Toilets and showers
CITY CENTRE ONE MILE OPEN ALL YEAR ACTIVE YACHT CLUB

MANX MARINE
35 North Quay, Douglas, Isle of Man IM1 4LB. Tel/Fax (01624) 674842. The Island's leading and most established yacht chandlery. Stockists of quality foul weather clothing and Thermalware. Large stock holdings of stainless steel fixtures and fittings and a comprehensive range of general chandlery. Agents for Mariner. Rigging facilities.

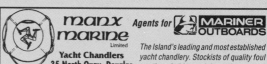

manx marine Limited
Yacht Chandlers
35 North Quay, Douglas, Isle of Man IM1 4LB
Tel: 01624 674842
Fax: 01624 674842
Agents for MARINER OUTBOARDS

The Island's leading and most established yacht chandlery. Stockists of quality foul weather clothing and thermal wear. Large stock holdings of s/steel fixtures and fittings and a comprehensive range of general chandlery including rigging facilities.

MAX WALKER YACHT DELIVERIES
Zinderneuf Sailing, PO Box 105, Macclesfield, Cheshire SK10 2EY. Tel (01625) 431712 Fax (01625) 619704. Fixed price deliveries. Sailing yachts delivered with care in north west European, UK and Eire waters by RYA/DoT yachtmaster and crew; 30 years' experience. Owners welcome. Tuition if required. References available. Your enquiries welcome 24 hours.

MERSEYSIDE DEVELOPMENT CORPORATION
4th Floor, Royal Liver Building, Pierhead, Liverpool L3 1JH. Tel 0151-236 6090 Fax 0151-227 3174. Albert Dock welcomes vessels for short or long-term visits to what is now one of the north west's most popular maritime locations. Maximum length 55m. Concessionary rates (details on application). Access by prior agreement.

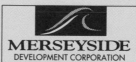

MERSEYSIDE DEVELOPMENT CORPORATION
4th Floor, Royal Liver Building, Pier Head, Liverpool L3 1JH
Tel: 0151-236 6090 Fax: 0151-227 3174
Albert Dock welcomes vessels for short or long term visits to what is now one of the north west's most popular locations. Maximum length 55m. Concessionary rates (details on application). Access by prior agreement.

SEALAND BOAT DELIVERIES
133 Corn Exchange Buildings, Manchester M4 3BW. Tel (01254) 705225 Fax (01254) 776582. Nationwide and European road transporters of all craft. No weight limit. Irish service. Worldwide shipping agents. Extrication of yachts from workshops and building yards. Salvage contractors. Established over 21 years. We never close.

WEST WALES, SOUTH WALES AND BRISTOL CHANNEL (AREA 11)
Bardsey Island to Lands End

ABERYSTWYTH MARINA - Y LANFA
Trefechan, Aberystwyth, Dyfed SY23 1AS.
Tel: 01970 611422 Fax: 01970 624122

NEW FULLY-SERVICED MARINA. Diesel, gas, water, toilets, hot showers. Launching facilities, winter storage and dry boat sailing. Car parking and security. Town centre five minutes' walk with excellent restaurants, shops, pubs and full recreational leisure facilities. Quality waterside apartments available overlooking the marina and Cardigan Bay.

ABERYSTWYTH MARINA - Y LANFA
Trefechan, Aberystwyth, Dyfed SY23 1AS. Tel (01970) 611422 Fax (01970) 624122. NEW fully serviced marina. Diesel, gas, water, toilets, hot showers. Launching facilities, winter storage and dry boat sailing. Car parking and security. Town centre 5 minutes' walk with excellent restaurants, shops, pubs and full recreational leisure facilities. Waterside apartments available.

BALTIC WHARF WATER LEISURE CENTRE
Bristol Harbour, Underfall Yard, Bristol. Tel 0ll7-929 7608 Fax 0117-929 4454. Sailing school and centre, with qualified instruction in most watersports. Also moorings available throughout the Bristol Harbour for all types of leisurecraft at extremely competitive rates.

Cleddau House, Milford Marina, Milford Haven, Dyfed SA73 3AF
Tel: 01646 697834 Fax: 01646 697834
Travel Hoist Storage • Inboard and outboard • Repairs, spares and service • General leisure craft repairs • Wood and fibreglass work • Chandlery and Breakdown Service

CLEDDAU BOATYARD
& Bosuns Locker Chandlery

CLEDDAU BOATYARD
Cleddau House, Milford Marina, Milford Haven, Dyfed SA73 3AF. Tel (01646) 697834 Fax (01646) 697834. Travel hoist, storage, inboard and outboard. Repairs, spares and service. General leisurecraft repairs, wood and fibreglass work. Chandlery and breakdown service.

HAFAN PWLLHELI
Glan Don, Pwllheli, Gwynedd LL53 5YT. Tel (01758) 701219 Fax (01758) 701443. Hafan Pwllheli has over 400 pontoon berths and offers access at virtually all states of the tide. Ashore, its modern purpose-built facilities include luxury toilets, showers, landerette, a secure boat park for winter storage, 40-ton travel hoist, mobile crane and plenty of space for car parking. Open 24-hours a day, 7 days a week.

420 fully serviced pontoon berths in a sheltered, tree-lined marina. On-site services include boatyard, sailmaker, sailing school, chandlery, cafe, launderette, showers and toilets. 30 visitors' berths - 24 hour access - security.
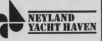
NEYLAND YACHT HAVEN
Neyland Yacht Haven Ltd, Brunel Quay, Neyland, Pembrokeshire SA73 1PY.
Tel: 01646 601601 Fax: 01646 600713

NEYLAND YACHT HAVEN LTD
Brunel Quay, Neyland, Pembrokeshire SA73 1PY. Tel (01646) 601601 Fax (01646) 600713. Marina operators with all facilities. 420 fully serviced pontoon berths in a sheltered, tree lined marina. On-site services include boatyard, sailmaker, sailing school, chandlery, cafe, launderette, showers and toilets. 30 visitors' berths. 24-hour access and security.

W F PRICE & CO LTD
Northpoint House, Wapping Wharf, Bristol BS1 6UD. Tel 0117-929 2229. DTp Certificated.

ROWLANDS MARINE ELECTRONICS LTD
Unit 4, Glandon Industrial Estate, Pwllheli, Gwynedd LL53 5YT Tel/Fax (01758) 613193. BEMA and BMIF members, dealer for Autohelm, B & G, Cetrek, ICOM, Kelvin Hughes, Marconi, Nasa, Navico, Navstar, Neco, Seafarer, Shipmate, Stowe, Racal-Decca, V-Tronix, Ampro, Walker. Equipment supplied installed and serviced.

SEVERNSIDE CONSULTANTS
Imperial Chambers, 2nd Floor, Gloucester Road, Avonmouth BS11 9AQ. Tel 0117-982 7184. DTp Certificated.

T J WILLIAMS & SON (CARDIFF) LTD
15-17 Harrowby Street, Cardiff CF1 6HA. Tel (01222) 487676. DTp Certificated.

WORCESTER YACHT CHANDLERS LTD
Unit 7, 75 Waterworks Road, Barbourne, Worcester WR1 3EZ
We stock paints, ropes, clothing, footwear, bottled gas, navigation and buoyancy aids. Engine service, oils, crane, haulage. Motor boats and rowing boats available. Travel upstream on the river Severn and discover idyllic picnic spots.

Tel: 01905 22522/27949

WORCESTER YACHT CHANDLERS LTD
Unit 7, 75 Waterworks Road, Barbourne, Worcester WR1 3EZ. Tel (01905) 22522 & 27949. Chandlery, paints, ropes, cables, chain, clothing, footwear, shackles, books, bottled gas, anti-foul, fastenings, oakam, fenders. Hard storage, crane, haulage, engine service, oils, navigation aids, buoyancy aids, life jackets, distress flares, small boat hire.

SOUTHERN IRELAND (AREA 12)
Malahide , south to Liscanor Bay

CASTLEPARK MARINA
Kinsale, Co Cork, Eire.
Tel: +353 21 774959
Fax: +353 21 774958
100 berth fully serviced marina. Access at all stages of tide. Located within picturesque Kinsale Harbour with ferry service to town. New marina centre located next to Dock pub. Facilities include hot showers, toilets, laundry, waterside hostel accommodation and restaurant open all day.
MARITIME TOURISM LIMITED

CASTLEPARK MARINA
Kinsale, Co Cork, Eire. Tel +353 21 774959 Fax +353 21 774958. 100-berth fully serviced marina with restaurant, laundry, showers and toilets. Waterside hostel-type accommodation available. New restaurant catering for both breakfast and evening meals. Access at all stages of the tide.

KILRUSH CREEK MARINA
Kilrush, Co Clare, Eire. Tel +353 65 52072 Fax +353 65 51692. Kilrush Creek Marina on Ireland's beautiful west coast, is a new marina with 120 fully serviced berths with 24-hour access. The marina has all shore facilities including a modern boatyard with 45-ton hoist. It adjoins the busy market town of Kilrush which has every facility required by the visiting yachtsman.

KILRUSH CREEK MARINA
Kilrush, Co Clare, Ireland. Tel: +353 65-52072 Fax: +353 65 51692

A new marina with 120 fully serviced berths with 24 hour access, having all shore facilities including modern boatyard and 45 ton hoist.
Situated on Ireland's beautiful west coast in the busy market town of Kilrush which has all the visiting yachtsman's needs.

KINSALE YACHT CLUB MARINA

Kinsale, Co Cork, Eire. Tel +353 21 772196 Fax +353 21 774426. Magnificent deep water yacht club marina offering Kinsale hospitality to visiting yachtsmen. Full facilities include berths up to 20 metres, fresh water, electricity, diesel on pier. Club bar and wealth of pubs and restaurants in Kinsale. Enter Kinsale Harbour - lit at night - no restrictions.

SAIL IRELAND CHARTERS

Trident Hotel, Kinsale, Co Cork, Eire. Tel +353 21 772927 Fax +353 21 774170. Sail Ireland Charters is Ireland's premier yacht charter company. Yachts varying in size from 35' to 45' Beneteau's, Sigma's, Roberts 45. Based in the picturesque village of Kinsale, an ideal place to commence your cruise of Europe's secret paradise of uncrowded sailing.

TRIDENT HOTEL - KINSALE

World's End, Kinsale, Co Cork, Eire. Tel +353 21 772301 Fax +353 21 774173. Recently refurbished the Trident has 56 comfortable bedrooms and two luxurious suites with delightful views of Kinsale harbour. The Savannah Restaurant, a member of the Good Food Circle, offers appetising meals complemented by efficient service from our friendly staff. Bar food available in our Fishermans Wharf bar. Leisure facilities include sauna, steamroom, gym, jacuzzi and games room.

NORTHERN IRELAND   (AREA 13)
Lambay Island, north to Liscanor Bay

CARRICKFERGUS MARINA

Rodger's Quay, Carrickfergus, Co Antrim, N Ireland BT38 8BE. Tel (01960) 366666 Fax (01960) 350505. 300 fully serviced pontoon berths with full onshore facilities (half a mile from town centre). Steeped in a wealth of historical legend, Carrickfergus has excellent restaurants, hotels, pubs, shops and a host of recreational leisure facilities.

KINNEGO MARINA - LOUGH NEAGH

Oxford Island, Lurgan, Co Armagh, N Ireland. Tel (01762) 327573 Fax (01762) 347438. 90 berths 10 moorings, Kinnego Marina is based in the south east corner of Lough Neagh, close to the M1 motorway. Mullen Marine offers chandlery, engine repairs on-site, and we offer RYA powerboat, keelboat and dinghy courses all year round. Access to the Lough via the Lower Bann at Coleraine. Lough Neagh - 154 sq mile 77 mile of shoreline.

TODD CHART AGENCY LTD

4 Seacliff Road, The Harbour, Bangor, N Ireland BT20 5EY. Tel (01247) 466640 Fax (01247) 471070. Admiralty Class 'A' chart agent for Northern Ireland. Chart correction service and nautical booksellers. Stockist of navigation and chartroom instruments, binoculars, clocks etc. Mail order service available. Visa, Access and American Express accepted.

CHANNEL ISLANDS   (AREA 14)
Guernsey, Jersey, Alderney.

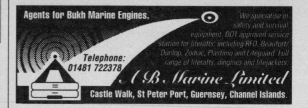
A B MARINE LTD

Castle Walk, St Peter Port, Guernsey, Channel Islands. Tel (01481) 722378. We specialise in safety and survival equipment and are a D.O.T. approved service station for liferafts including R.F.D. Beaufort/Dunlop, Zodiac, Plastimo and Lifeguard. We also carry a full range of new liferafts, dinghies, and lifejackets and are agents for Bukh marine engines.

BOATWORKS + LTD

Castle Emplacement, St Peter Port, Guernsey, Channel Islands GY1 1AU. Tel (01481) 726071 Fax (01481) 714224. Boatworks+ provides a comprehensive range of services including electronics, chandlery, boatbuilding and repairs, engine sales and services, yacht brokerage, clothing and fuel supplies.

CAPELLES MARINE LTD

Camp du Roi, St Sampsons, Guernsey, Channel Islands GY2 4XG. Tel (01481) 57010 Fax (01481) 53590 Cellnet 0860 741245. Out of town - we are only a phone call away and happy to find YOU. Mercury and Mercruiser dealers on the island. We also service all makes of outboards. Petrol and diesel sterndrives and diesel inboards. Perry's Guide Ref: 9F 4G3.

CHICKS MARINE LTD

Collings Road, St Peter Port, Guernsey, Channel Islands. Tel (01481) 723716 Fax (01481) 713632. Distributors of diesel fuel biocide used to treat and protect contamination in fuel tanks where an algae (bug) is present. Most owners do not realise what the problem is, loss of power, blocked fuel filter, exhaust smoking, resulting in expensive repairs to injectors - fuel pump - or complete engine overhaul. Marine engineers, engines, spares, service - VAT free. Honda outboards, pumps and generators. Volvo Penta specialists.

DARTMOUTH YACHT CRUISE SCHOOL
103 High Street, Totnes, Devon TQ9 5SN. Ans/Fax (01803) 864027 Tel/Fax (01803) 722226. Regular trips to and from Channel Islands.

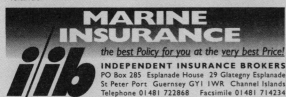
INDEPENDENT INSURANCE BROKERS LTD
PO Box 285, Esplanade House, 29 Glategny Esplanade, St Peter Port, Guernsey, Channel Islands GY1 1WR. Tel (01481) 722868 Fax (01481) 714234. Marine insurance brokers with a comprehensive portfolio of insurance products and services, extending to home, personal, etc. Our reputation is built on thoroughness, active client support and communication.

MARINE & GENERAL ENGINEERS LTD
The Shipyard, St Sampson's Harbour, Guernsey GY1 6AT. Tel (01481) 45808 Fax (01481) 48765. Comprehensive service to the yachting fraternity. Building, repairs, engine sales and repairs, marine hardware stores, rigging, chandlery, boat lifting, transport and winter lay-up. Popular call-in point for craft sailing to mainland Europe. 24-hour Emergency Support on 0860 741217.

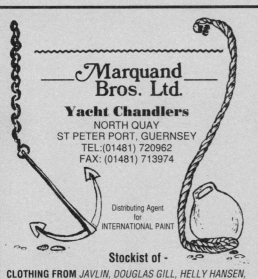
MARQUAND BROS LTD
North Quay, St Peter Port, Guernsey, Channel Islands. Tel (01481) 720962 Fax (01481) 713974. Yacht chandlers, stockists of a comprehensive range of marine products. Guernsey distributor for International Yacht Paint. Extensive leisure and marine clothing department including Barbour, Driza-Bone, Dubarry and Quayside.

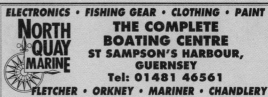
NORTH QUAY MARINE
North Side, St Sampson's Harbour, Guernsey, Channel Islands. Tel (01481) 46561 Fax (01481) 43488. The complete boating centre. Orkney and Fletcher boats - Mariner outboards - Full range of chandlery, rope, chain, lubricants, paint, boatwear and shoes. Fishing tackle for onshore and onboard. Inflatables and safety equipment. Electronics.

SARNIA FLAGS
8 Belmont Road, St Peter Port, Guernsey, Channel Islands GY1 1PY. Tel (01481) 725995 Fax (01481) 729335. Flags and pennants made to order. National flags, house, club and battle flags, and burgees made to order. Any size, shape or design. Prices on request.

SEAQUEST MARINE LTD
13 Fountain Street, St Peter Port, Guernsey, Channel Islands GY1 1BX. Tel (01481) 721773 Fax (01481) 716738. Seaquest Marine have a fully stocked chandlery. Agents for Sowester and Simpson Lawrence. Sole agents for Avon, Typhoon and Compass inflatables. Splashdown clothing. Electronics specialising in GPS. Inflatable specialists. Official Avon service station. VAT free friendly advice.

BELGIUM AND THE NETHERLANDS   (AREA 20)
Nieuwpoort to Delfzijl

KELVIN HUGHES OBSERVATOR
Nieuwe Longowed 41, 3199 DC, Hoogliet, The Netherlands. DTp Certificated.

GERMANY   (AREA 21)
Emden (new port) to the Danish Border

BOGERD NAVTEC NV
Oude Leeuwenrui 37, Antwerp 20000, Germany.

MARTIN & CO
Oude Leewenrui 37, Antwerp 2000, Germany. DTp Certificated.

PANTAENIUS UK LTD
Head Office: Cremon 32.20457 Hamburg, Germany. Tel +49 40 370 910 Fax +49 40 3709 1109. Registered Insurance Broker: Marine Building, Queen Anne's Battery, Plymouth, Devon PL4 0LP. Tel (01752) 223656 Fax (01752) 223637 Pantaenius is one of Europe's largest yacht insurance brokers and covers yachts sailing under more than 35 different flags in all seven seas.

IVER C WEILBACH & CO., A/S
35 Toldbodgade, Postbox 1560, DK-1253 Copenhagen K, Denmark.

Chapter 1

About this Almanac

Contents

1

Explanation

The Almanac contains important data which is subject to frequent and detailed correction (see 1.3). The 1996 Almanac is a stand-alone compendium of the essential navigational data needed by yachtsmen for the waters around the United Kingdom, Ireland and the coast of Europe from the Franco-Spanish Atlantic border to the North Sea border of Germany and Denmark. Important information is kept updated by the issue of a correcting Supplement. Much data of a permanent or semi-permanent nature has been tranferred from the Almanac to the Handbook. It is therefore essential that both books are used together and should be carried on-board at all times.

Chapter 5 in the Almanac now contains only Sunrise and Sunset data and calendar information. The information required for astro-navigation has been produced separately in a forty-eight page Astro-Supplement. This can be obtained by ticking the relevant box on the Supplement request card and enclosing a cheque for £4·00 made out to *Macmillan Publishers Ltd.*

The 1996 edition of *The Macmillan & Silk Cut Nautical Almanac* continues the pattern set up in 1985, when much of the standing information which does not alter from year to year was transferred to a new companion volume – *The Macmillan & Silk Cut Yachtsman's Handbook.* The Handbook is an enduring and valuable reference work which covers matters of a semi-permanent nature in as much detail as a single volume permits. The Handbook is not published on an annual basis, but is revised as necessary: a new third edition was published in 1993.

For convenience, Chapters 2–9 in the Almanac deal with the same subjects as Chapters 2–9 in the Handbook, whilst Chapter 10 contains harbour, coastal and tidal information, arranged area by area. A map of the twenty-one geographical areas covered in the Almanac is on page 146. Chapters 2–9 of the Almanac and the Handbook are cross-referenced where this is helpful to the user. Chapters 10–19 in the Handbook cover additional subjects.

1.1   INTRODUCTION

1.1.1   Numbering system

There are ten chapters. For ease of reference each chapter is divided into numbered sections, prefaced by the number of the chapter. Thus the sections in Chapter 7, for example, are numbered 7.1, 7.2 etc.

Within each section the key paragraphs are numbered. Thus in section 7.2 (say) the main paragraphs are numbered 7.2.1, 7.2.2, 7.2.3 etc.

Diagrams carry the chapter number and a figure in brackets, thus: Fig. 7(1), Fig. 7(2), Fig. 7(3) etc.

Tables carry the chapter number and a figure in brackets, thus Table 3(1), Table 3(2) etc.

1.1.2   Index

The main paragraph headings and the page number of each section are listed on the contents page at the start of each chapter. At the back of the book is a full index, while at the front is a quick reference and personal index for important items.

1.1.3   General acknowledgments

The Editors wish to record their thanks to the many individuals and official bodies who have assisted by providing essential information and much advice in the preparation of this Almanac. They include the Hydrographic Office at Taunton, HM Nautical Almanac Office, HM Stationery Office, HM Customs, the Meteorological Office, the Coastguard, British Telecom, Trinity House, the Northern Lighthouse Board, the Commissioners of Irish Lights, the National Maritime Museum, the BBC and IBA, the Marine Safety Agency, the Royal National Lifeboat Institution, Koninklijke Nederlandse Redding Maatschappij (KNRM), Deutsche Gesellschaft zur Rettung Schiffbrüchiger (DGzRS), the Port of London Authority, Associated British Ports, countless Harbour Masters, and our many individual agents.

Chartlets, tidal stream diagrams and tidal curves are produced from British Admiralty Charts and Hydrographic Publications with the permission of the Controller of HM Stationery Office and of the Hydrographer of the Navy, and from French publications by permission of the Service Hydrographique et Océanographique de la Marine.

The tidal stream arrows on the S and W coasts of Ireland are printed in 10.12.3 and 10.13.3 by kind permission of the Irish Cruising Club.

Information from the *Admiralty Lists of Lights, Admiralty Sailing Directions* and from the *Admiralty List of Radio Signals* is reproduced with the sanction of the Controller of HM Stationery Office, and of the Hydrographer of the Navy.

Extracts from the following are published by permission of the Controller of HM Stationery Office: *International Code of Signals, 1969*; *Meteorological Office Weather Services for Shipping*.

Astronomical data in the Astro Supplement is derived from the current edition of the *The Nautical Almanac*, and is included by permission of HM Nautical Almanac Office and of the Particle Physics and Astronomy Research Council.

1.1.4   Acknowledgments – tidal information

Tidal predictions for all UK ports including Dover Range and HW data (on the bookmark) are Crown Copyright and are supplied by permission of the Controller of HM Stationery Office and the Hydrographer of the Navy.

Phases of the Moon are supplied by the Particle Physics and Astronomy Research Council.

Acknowledgment is made to the following authorities for permission to use tidal predictions stated: Rijkswaterstaat, Netherlands: Vlissingen (Flushing), Hoek van Holland. Bundesamt für Seeschiffahrt und Hydrographie: Helgoland, Wilhelmshaven and Cuxhaven. Predictions for French ports are reproduced from *L'annuaire des Marées*, Vol. 1 by kind permission of Service Hydrographique et Océanographique de la Marine, France (No. 788/94).

1.1.5   Standard terms

All bearings given in this Almanac are 'True'. For example, the sector of a light shown as G (Green) 090°–180° is visible over an arc of 90° to any observer between due West and due North of that light.

Dimensions, in general, are stated in metric terms, the Imperial equivalent being included where appropriate. Distances, unless otherwise stated, are in International nautical (sea) miles, abbreviated as M. All depths and heights are shown in metres (m) unless otherwise indicated.

The 24-hour clock convention is used throughout, i.e. 0001 to 2359. Unless otherwise stated, times are in Universal Time (UT). Local times, if quoted, are indicated by LT.

The UK and Republic of Ireland, alone of the European countries, use UT as their standard time. During the specified summer months, the UK uses British Summer Time (BST) which is UT+1 hour. In France, Belgium, Netherlands and Germany the Standard Time is UT+1 hour; during the summer months these countries use UT+2, as Daylight Saving Time (DST).

For 1996, in the UK and Republic of Ireland BST will apply from 31 Mar to 27 Oct. In other EU countries DST will also apply from 31 Mar to 27 Oct.

VHF frequencies are identified throughout by their International Maritime VHF series channel (Ch) designator. Frequencies used for calling and working may be separated by a semi-colon, i.e. Ch 16; 12.

1.2   IMPROVING THE ALMANAC

1.2.1   Suggestions for improvements

The Editors always welcome suggestions for improving the content or layout of the Almanac. Ideas based on experience and practical use afloat are especially welcome. It is not always feasible to implement suggestions received, but all will be very carefully considered. Even minor ideas are welcome.

If you have any comments, please write them on the Supplement application card, or alternatively send your ideas or comments by letter or fax direct to the appropriate Editor. Correspondence on nautical matters should always be sent direct to the Editors at one of the addresses below and not to the Publisher's address.

For Chapters 1 to 9 inclusive, and for those pages in Chapter 10 covering Area Maps; Coastal Lights, Fog Signals, and Waypoints; Area Waypoints; and Supplements:

The Editor, The Macmillan & Silk Cut Nautical Almanac, 41 Arbor Lane, Winnersh, Wokingham, Berks RG41 5JE. (Fax 01734 772717.)

For Chapter 10, Areas 1 to 21 inclusive and for the Passage Information pages: The Editor, The Macmillan & Silk Cut Nautical Almanac, Edington House, Trent, Sherborne, Dorset DT9 4SR. (Fax 01935 850737.)

1.2.2   Notification of errors

Although very great care has been taken in compiling all the information from innumerable sources, it is recognised that in a publication of this nature some errors may occur. The Editors would be extremely grateful if their attention could be called to any such lapses, by writing to them at the appropriate address in 1.2.1 above.

1.3   KEEPING IT UP TO DATE

1.3.1   Late corrections

Late corrections are given at the back of the Almanac, before the index.

1.3.2   Sources of amendments

It is most important that charts and other navigational publications – such as this Almanac – are kept up to date. Corrections to Admiralty charts and publications are issued weekly in *Admiralty Notices to Mariners*. These are obtainable from Admiralty Chart Agents (by post if required), or they can be sighted at Customs Houses or Mercantile Marine Offices.

An alternative, but less frequent, service is given by the *Admiralty Notices to Mariners, Small Craft Edition*. This contains reprinted Notices for the British Isles and the European coast from the Gironde to the Elbe. Notices concerning depths greater in general than 7 metres (23ft), or which do not affect small craft for some other reason, are not included. They are available from Admiralty Chart Agents, or through the Royal Yachting Association.

1.3.3   Our free Supplement

This Almanac contains corrections up to and including Admiralty Notices to Mariners, Weekly Edition No. 13/95. Subsequent corrections up to mid April 1996 are contained in a free Supplement, published in May 1996.

As information contained in this Almanac is subject to constant change throughout the year, it is essential that users should **immediately** apply for the correcting Supplement in order to bring the Almanac fully up to date before using operationally.

To obtain the free Supplement please complete and return the enclosed postcard, duly stamped, to: Dominic Taylor, *The Macmillan & Silk Cut Nautical Almanac*, Macmillan Reference Books, 25 Eccleston Place, London SW1W 9NF. (☎ 0171-373 6070).

The Supplement will be sent to you free, postage paid, as soon as possible after publication. The Supplement also includes important corrections to *The Macmillan & Silk Cut Yachtsman's Handbook*.

1.3.4   Record of amendments

The amendment sheet below is intended to assist you in keeping the Almanac up to date, although it can also be used to record corrections to charts or other publications. Tick where indicated when the appropriate amendments have been made.

Weekly Notices to Mariners		Small Craft Editions	
1	27	1 Feb 1995	....
2	28		
3	29	1 May 1995	....
4	30		
5	31	1 July 1995	....
6	32		
7	33	1 Sept 1995	....
8	34		
9	35	1 Feb 1996	....
10	36		
11	37	1 May 1996	....
12	38		
13	39	1 July 1996	....
14	40		
15	41	1 Sept 1996	....
16	42		
17	43	**Late corrections**	
18	44	(see back of Almanac,	
19	45	before index)	
20	46		
21	47	**Macmillan**	
22	48	**Supplement**	
23	49	May 1996	....
24	50		
25	51		
26	52		

1.4   ABBREVIATIONS/GLOSSARY

1.4.1   Abbreviations and symbols

The following selected abbreviations and symbols may be encountered in this Almanac, in Supplements, in Admiralty Publications, or on Charts. Abbreviations for harbour facilities in Chapter 10 are also printed for convenience on the loose leaf card bookmark for HW Dover and Range.

NOTE: *	Not shown for Marinas
AB*	Alongside berth
ABP	Associated British Ports
abt	About
AC	220v AC electrical supplies
AC	Admiralty Chart
ACA	Admiralty Chart Agent
✈	Airport
Aff Mar	Affaires Maritimes
ALL	Admiralty List of Lights
ALRS	Admiralty List of Radio Signals
Alt	Altitude
Al	Alternating Lt
AM	Amplitude Modulation
anch, ⚓	Anchorage
annly	Annually
ANWB	Dutch Association of Road & Waterway Users
App	Apparent
Appr.	Approaches
approx	Approximate
ATT	Admiralty Tide Tables
Auto	Météo Répondeur Automatique
Az	Azimuth
B.	Bay
B	Black
Ⓑ	Bank (£)
Bar	Licensed bar
Bcst	Broadcast
BFO	Beat Frequency Oscillator
BH	Boat Hoist (tons)
Bk.	Bank (shoal)
bk	Broken
Bkwtr	Breakwater
Bldg	Building
Bn(s)	Beacon, beacon(s)
Bol	Bollard
brg	Bearing
BS	British Standard
BSH	German Hydrographic chart(s)
BST	British Summer Time
Bu	Blue
BWB	British Waterways Board
By(s)	Buoy, buoys
BY	Boatyard

C.	Cape
C	Crane (tons)
c	Coarse
ca	Cable
Calib	Calibration
Cas	Castle
CD	Chart datum
CEVNI	Code Européen de Voies de la Navigation Intérieure
CG	Coastguard station
CG, ⌂	Coastguard MRCC, MRSC
CH	Chandlery
Ch	Channel (VHF)
Ch, ✠	Church, chapel
chan.	Channel (navigational)
Chy	Chimney
cm	Centimetre(s)
Col, I	Column, pillar, obelisk
conspic	Conspicuous
const	Construction
cont	Continuous
Corr	Correction
cov	Covers
Cr.	Creek
CROSS	Centre Régional Opérationnel de Surveillance et Sauvetage
CRS, ☏	Coast Radio Station
CS	Calibration Station
Cup	Cupola
⌗	Customs (see HMC)
Cy	Clay
D	Diesel fuel
Dec	Declination
decrg	Decreasing
dest	Destroyed
DF	Direction finding
DG Range	Degaussing Range
DGPS	Differential GPS
Dia	Diaphone
◆ ◇	Diamond
Dir Lt	Directional light
discont	Discontinued
dist	Distance, Distant
Dk	Dock
dm	Decimetre(s)
Dn(s)	Dolphin(s)
DOP	Dilution of Precision (GPS)
Dr	Doctor
dr	Dries
DSC	Digital Selective Calling system
DST	Daylight Saving Time
DW	Deep Water, Deep-draught Route
DYC	Dutch Yacht Chart(s)
DZ	Danger Zone (buoy)

E	East
EC	Early closing
ECM	East Cardinal Mark
ECM	Éditions Cartographiques Maritimes
ED	Existence doubtful, European datum
El	Electrical repairs
Ⓔ	Electronics repairs
Ent.	Entrance
Est.	Estuary
ETA	Estimated Time of Arrival
ETD	Estimated Time of Departure
exper	Experimental
explos	Explosive
ext	Extension
(fog signal symbol)	Fog signal
F	Fixed Light
f	Fine
Fcst	Forecast
FFL	Fixed and Flashing light
Fl	Flashing light
FM	Frequency Modulation
Fog Det Lt	Fog Detector Light
Freq, Fx	Frequency
FS	Flagstaff, Flagpole
ft	Foot, feet
Ft	Fort
FV(s)	Fishing vessel(s)
FW, (tap symbol)	Fresh water supply
G	Gravel
G, Ⓖ	Green, Green Fixed light
Gas	Calor Gas
Gaz	Camping Gaz
GC	Great-circle
GDOP (GPS)	Geometrical Dilution of Precision
GHA	Greenwich Hour Angle
GMDSS	Global Maritime Distress and Safety System
GPS	Global Positioning System
grt	Gross Registered Tonnage
Gt	Great
Gy	Grey
h	Hard, Hour
H+, H-	Minutes past/before each hour
H24	Continuous
HAT	Highest Astronomical Tide
Hd.	Head, Headland
HF	High Frequency
HFP	High Focal Plane Buoy
HIE	Highlands & Islands Enterprise
HJ	Day Service only, Sunrise to Sunset
HMC, #	HM Customs
HMSO	Her Majesty's Stationery Office
HN	Night Service only, Sunset to Sunrise
Hn.	Haven

Ho	House
HO	Office hours, Hydrographic Office
(hor)	Horizontally disposed
[H]	Hospital
Hr(s)	Harbour(s)
Hrs	Hours
Hr Mr, ⚓	Harbour Master
ht	Height
HW	High Water
HX	No fixed hrs
Hz	Hertz
[i]	Harbour information/tidal data
I	Island, islet
IALA	International Association of Lighthouse Authorities
Ident	Identification signal
IDM	Isolated Danger Mark
IHO	International Hydrographic Organisation
(illum)	Illuminated
IMO	International Maritime Organisation
incrg	Increasing
info	Information
INMARSAT	International Maritime Satellite Organisation
inop	Inoperative
INT	International
intens	Intensified
IPTS	International Port Traffic Signals
IQ	Interrupted quick flashing light
IRPCS	International Regulations for Prevention of Collision at Sea
Iso	Isophase light
ITU	International Telecommunications Union
ITZ	Inshore Traffic Zone
IUQ	Interrupted ultra quick flashing light
IVQ	Interrupted very quick flashing light
kHz	Kilohertz
km	Kilometre(s)
kn	knot(s)
Kos	Kosangas
kW	Kilowatts
L	Lake, Loch, Lough
L*, Lndg, (landing symbol)	Landing place
(launderette symbol)	Launderette
Lat	Latitude
LAT	Lowest Astronomical Tide
Lanby	Large Automatic Navigational Buoy
LB, [LB], (ILB symbol)	Lifeboat, inshore lifeboat
Ldg	Leading
L Fl	Long-flashing light
Le.	Ledge
LF	Low frequency

LHA	Local Hour Angle		(occas)	Occasional
LH	Left hand		Off	Office
LL	List of Lights		Or	Orange
Lndg	Landing place		OSGB	Ordnance Survey GB Datum (1936)
LOA	Length overall		OT	Other times
Long	Longitude			
LT	Local time			
Lt(s)	Light(s)		P	Petrol
Lt By	Light buoy		P.	Port (harbour)
Lt F	Light float		P	Pebbles
Lt Ho	Lighthouse		(P)	Preliminary (NM)
Lt V	Light vessel		PA	Position approximate
LW	Low Water		Pass.	Passage
			PD	Position doubtful
M*	Moorings available		PHM	Port-hand Mark
M	Marinecall ☎ No		Pk.	Peak
M	Sea mile(s)		⌇ ⌇	Perch, Stake (PHM & SHM)
M	Mud		📞	Port Radio
m	Metre(s)		PO, ✉	Post Office
mm	Millimetre(s)		pos	Position
Mag	Magnetic, magnitude (of Star)		PPS	Precise Positioning Service (GPS)
ME	Marine engineering repairs		⚠	Precautionary Area
Météo	Météorologie/Weather		(priv)	Private
MF	Medium Frequency		Prog	Prognosis (weather charts)
MHWN	Mean High Water Neaps		prohib	Prohibited
MHWS	Mean High Water Springs		proj	Projected
MHz	Megahertz		prom	Prominent
min(s)	Minute(s) of time		Pt.	Point
Mk	Mark		PV	Pilot Vessel
ML	Mean Level		Pyl	Pylon
MLWN	Mean Low Water Neaps			
MLWS	Mean Low Water Springs		Q	Quick-flashing light
Mo	Morse			
Mon	Monument, Monday			
MRCC	Maritime Rescue Co-ordination Centre		R, Ⓡ	Red, Red Fixed light, Rock
			R.	River
MRSC	Maritime Rescue Sub-Centre		R, Rk(s),Rky	Rock(s), Rocky
ms	Millisecond(s); minutes seconds		Ra	Coast Radar Station
µs	Microseconds		Ⓡⓒ	Marine RDF Beacon
MSL	Mean Sea Level		Ⓡⓒ Aero	Aeronautical RDF Beacon
Mt.	Mountain, Mount		Racon	Radar Transponder Beacon
			Radome	Radar dome
N	North		Ramark	Radar Beacon
n.mile	International Nautical mile		RC	Non-directional radiobeacon
NAVTEX	Navigational telex service		RDF	Radio direction-finding
NB	Notice Board		Rds.	Roads, Roadstead
NCM	North Cardinal Mark		Rep	Reported
NM	Notice(s) to Mariners		R, ✕	Restaurant
No	Number		Rf.	Reef
NON	Unmodulated continuous wave emission		RG	Radio Direction-Finding Station
np	Neap tides		RH	Right hand
NP	Naval Publication		⇌	Railway station
NRT	Net registered tonnage		RNLI	Royal National Lifeboat Institution
NT	National Trust		Ro Ro	Roll-on Roll-off (ferry terminal)
			● ○	Round, circular; Ball
Obscd	Obscured		RT	Radiotelephony
Obstn	Obstruction		Ru	Ruins
Oc	Occulting Light		Rx	Receiver

S	South
S	Sand
S, St, Ste	Saint(s)
SAR	Search and Rescue
☛	SAR helicopter base
SC	Sailing Club
Sch	School
SCM	South Cardinal Mark
Sd.	Sound
SD	Sailing Directions, Semi-Diameter
SD	Sounding of doubtful depth
sec(s)	Second(s) (of time)
Sem	Semaphore
Seq	Sequence
sf	Stiff
Sh	Shells, Shoal
Sh	Shipwright, hull repairs etc
SHA	Sidereal Hour Angle (Stars)
SHM	Starboard-hand Mark
SHOM	French Hydrographic Charts
Si	Silt
Sig	Signal
SIGNI	Signalisation de Navigation Intérieure (Dutch inland buoyage)
SM	Sailmaker
➤	Slip for launching, scrubbing
SNSM	Société Nationale de Sauvetage en Mer (Lifeboats)
so	Soft
Sp	Spire
sp	Spring tides
SPM	Special Mark, Single Point Mooring
SPS	Standard Positioning Service (GPS)
■ □	Square
SR	Sunrise
SS	Sunset, Signal Station
SSB	Single Sideband
St	Stones
Stbd	Starboard
Sta	Station
Str.	Strait
subm	Submerged
sum	Summer
SWM	Safe Water Mark
sy	Sticky
sync	Synchronised
(T), (temp)	Temporary (NM)
t	Ton, tonne
TD	Fog signal temp discontinued
TE	Light temp extinguished

☎, Tel	Telephone
Tfc	Traffic
Tr	Tower
▼ ▲ ▽ △	Triangle, cone
TSS	Traffic Separation Scheme
Twi	Twilight
≠	In transit with
Tx	Transmitter, Transmission
ufn	Until further notice
uncov	Uncovers
Unintens	Unintesified
unexam	Unexamined
UQ	Ultra quick-flashing light
UT	Universal Time
V	Victuals, food stores etc
Ⓥ, ⓥ	Visitors berth/mooring
Var	Variation
Vel	Velocity
(vert)	Vertically disposed
VHF	Very High Frequency
Vi	Violet
vis	Visibility, visible
Volmet	Weather broadcasts for aviation
VTM	Vessel Traffic Management
VTS	Vessel Traffic Service
VQ	Very quick flashing light
☼, Wx	Weather (☎ or times)
W	West
W, Ⓦ	White, White Fixed light
WCM	West Cardinal Mark
Wd	Weed
wef	With effect from
WGS	World Geodetic System (datum)
Whf	Wharf
Whis	Whistle
win	Winter
WIP	Work in progress
⚓ ⚓	Withy (SHM & PHM)
Wk	Wreck
WMO	World Meteorological Organisation
WPT, ⊕	Waypoint
Y, Ⓨ	Yellow, Amber, Orange, Yellow Fixed Light
YC, ⚑	Yacht Club
⚓	Yacht harbour, Marina
⚓	Where to report, or yacht berths without facilities

1.4.2

GLOSSARY	GLOSSAIRE	WOORDENLIJST	GLOSSAR
English	**Français**	**Nederlands**	**Deutsch**

A. NAVIGATION	NAVIGATION	NAVIGATIE	NAVIGATION
Marks, Buoys, Beacons	**Bouées et Balises**	**Merken, Tonnen, Bakens**	**Tonnen, Baken**
Buoy	Bouée	Boei	Tonne
Topmark	Voyant	Topteken	Toppzeichen
Starboard (Stbd)	Tribord	Stuurboord	Steuerbord
Cone, conical (SHM buoy)	Cone, conique	Spitse ton	Kegel, kegelförmig
Port (side)	Bâbord	Bakboord	Backbord
Can (PHM buoy)	Plate, cylindrique	Stompe ton	Kanne, (Stumpftonne)
Landfall (SWM buoy)	Atterrisage	Verkenningston	Ansteuerungstonne
Isolated danger (IDM buoy)	Danger isolé	Losliggend gevaar	Einzellgenfar-Zeichen
Special mark (SPM buoy)	Marque spéciale	Bijzondere betonning	Sonder-Zeichen
Diamond (◊ shape)	Losange	Ruit (◊ vorm)	Rautenförmig
Chequered	A damier	Geblokt	Gewürfelt
Beacon (Bn)	Balise	Baken	Bake
Perch	Perche, pieu	Prikk	Prick
Leading line, transit	Alignement	Geleidelijn	Leitlinie
Landmark	Amer	Markatiepunt	Landmarke
Square (□)	Carré	Vierkant	Viereck
Framework Tower	Charpente	Traliemast	Gittermast
Tower (Tr)	Tour, tourelle	Toren	Turm
Column	Colonne	Zuil, kolom	Laternenträger
Radio beacon	Radiobalise	Radiobaken	Funkfeuer
Signal station	Sémaphore	Seinstation	Signalstelle
Pilot Station	Station de pilotage	Loodsstation	Lotsenstation
Watch Tr, lookout	Vigie	Uitkijk	Beobachtungsstelle
Log Book	Livre de Bord	Journaal	Logbuch, Schiffstagebuch
Dividers	Compas une main	Steekpasser	Kartenzirkel, Stechzirkel

Colours	**Couleurs**	**Kleuren**	**Farben**
Red, (R)	Rouge	Rood (r)	Rot (R)
White (W)	Blanc, (B)	Wit (W)	Weiß (W)
Blue (Bu)	Bleu, (Bl)	Blauw (B)	Blau (Bl)
Black (B)	Noir	Zwart (Z)	Schwarz (S)
Grey	Gris	Grijs	Grau (Gr)
Yellow (Y)	Jaune, (J)	Geel (gl)	Gelb (G)
Green (G)	Vert, (V)	Groen (Gn)	Grün (Gn)
Stripe	Raie	Streep	Streifen

Lights	**Feux**	**Lichten**	**Leuchtfeuer**
Lighthouse	Phare	Vuurtoren	Leuchtturm
Lightship	Bateau-phare	Lichtschip	Feuerschiff
Fixed (F)	Feu fixe	Vast licht (V)	Festfeuer (F)
Alternating (Al)	Feu alternatif	Alternerend (Alt)	Wechselfeuer (Wchs)
Flashing	Éclat (É)	Schitterlicht (S)	Blitz (Blz)
Quick flashing (Q)	Feu scintillant, (Scint)	Flikkerlicht (Fl)	Funkel (Fkl)
Very quick flashing (VQ)	Feu scintillant rapide	Snelflikkerlicht	Schnelles Funkel (S Ful)
Interrupted quick flashing (IQ)	Scintillant, interrompu	Onderbroken flikkerlicht (Int Fl)	Funkel unterbrochen
Fixed and Flashing (F Fl)	Fixe É	Vast en schitterend (V & S)	Mischfeuer (F & Blz)
Occulting (Oc)	Feu à occultations (Oc)	Onderbroken (GO)	Unterbrochen (Ubr)
Isophase (Iso)	Feu isophase (Iso)	Isofase (Iso)	Gleichtakt (Glt)
Leading Light	Feu d'alignement	Geleidelicht	Richtfeuer
Obscured	Masqué	Verduisterd	Verdunkelt
Extinguished (Lt)	Éteint	Gedoofd	Verlöscht
Temporary	Temporaire	Tijdelijk	Zeitweilig

Fog Signals	**Signaux de brume**	**Mistseinen**	**Nebelsignale**
Whistle	Sifflet	Fluit	Heuler/Nebelhorn
Siren	Sirène	Sirene	Sirene
Reed (horn)	Trompette	Hoorn	Zungenhorn
Bell	Cloche	Bel/klok	Glocke
Explosive (fog)	Explosif	Knalmistsein	Knallkörper
Foghorn	Corne de brume	Misthoorn	Horn

Compass	**Compas**	**Kompas**	**Kompaß**
Compass, hand-bearing	Compas de relèvement	Handpeilkompas	Handpeilkompaß
North (N)	Nord	Noord	Nord

South (S)	Sud	Zuid	Süd
East (E)	Est	Oost	Ost
West (W)	Ouest	West	West

Tides/Depths	**Marées/Profondeur**	**Getij/Diepten**	**Gezeiten/Tiefen**
Mean Sea level	Niveau de la mer moyen	Zeespiegel	Wasserstand
Chart Datum (CD)	Zéro des cartes	Reductievlak	Kartennull
High Water (HW)	Pleine Mer	Hoogwater	Hochwasser
Low Water (LW)	Basse Mer	Laagwater	Niedrigwasser
Mean (tide)	Mi-marée	Gemiddeld	Mittlere/Mittelwasser
Neaps (np)	Morte eau	Doodtij	Nipptide
Springs (sp)	Vive eau	Springtij	Springtide
Slack water, stand	Etale	Kentering (hoog of laag)	Stauwasser
Range	Amplitude	Verval	Tidenhub
Tide Tables	Annuaire des Marées	Getijtafel	Gezeitentafeln
Tidal stream atlas	Atlas des Marées	Stroomatlas	Stromatlas
Flood/ebb stream	Courant de flot de jusant	Vloed/eb stroom	Flutstrom/Ebbstrom
Rate (tide)	Vitesse	Snelheid	Geschwindigkeit
Knots (kn)	Nœuds	Knopen	Knoten
Height, headroom, clearance	Tirant d'air	Doorvaarthoogte	Durchfahrtshöhe
Draught	Tirant d'eau	Diepgang	Tiefgang
Echosounder	Échosondeur	Dieptemeter	Echolot
Coastline	Contour de la côte	Geul, vaarwater	Küstenlinien
Bay	Anse	Baai, inham	Bucht
Sandhill, dunes	Dunes	Duinen	Sandhügel, Dünen
Channel	Chenal, Passe	Kanaal	Fahrwasser
Cliff	Falaise	Klip	Kliff
Estuary	Estuaire	Riviermond	Flußmündung
River	Fleuve, rivière	Rivier	Fluß
Gulf	Golfe	Golf	Golf, Haff
Narrows	Goulet	Zeeëngte	Enge
Strait(s)	Pertuis	Straat	Straße
Point, headland	Pointe, pte	Punt	Huk, Landspitze
Peninsula	Presqu'île	Schiereiland	Halbinsel
Beach, sandy	Grève, plage	Zandstrand	Strand
Island	Ile	Eiland	Insel

Features	**Marques distinctives**	**Kenmerken**	**Merkmale**
Bridge	Pont	Brug	Brücke
Castle	Château	Kasteel	Schloß
Railway	Chemin de fer	Spoorweg	Eisenbahn
Steeple, spire	Clocher, flèche	Toren, spits	Kirchturm
Water tower	Château d'eau	Watertoren	Wasserturm
Windmill	Moulin à vent	Windmolen	Windmühle
Conspicuous (conspic)	Visible (vis)	Opvallend	Auffällig (auff)

Dangers/Seabed	**Dangers/Fonds**	**Gevaren/Zeebodem**	**Gefahren/Meeresboden**
Prohibited area	Zone interdite	Verboden gebied	Verbotenes Gebiet
Wreck	Épave	Wrak	Wrack
Shoal	Haut fond, Basse	Droogte	Untiefe
Bank	Chaussée, rive	Bank	Bank
Reef	Récif	Rif	Riff
Breakers	Brisants	Branding	Brandung
Aground	Dérive, Échoué	Aan de grond	Auf Grund sitzen
Clay	Argile	Klei	Lehm/Ton
Mud (M)	Vase (V)	Modder (M)	Schlick (Sk)
Sand (S)	Sable (S)	Zand (Z)	Sand (Sd)
Stony, shingly	Cailloux, galets	Grind of kiezel	Stein-oder Kiesküste
Rock, stone	Roche, pierre	Rots, steen	Fels
Sea-weed, kelp	Algues	Zeewier	Seetang

Ports/Harbours	**Ports**	**Havens**	**Häfen**
Roadstead	Rade	Rede	Reede
Breakwater, mole	Digue	Havendam	Mole
Breakwater, wave-break	Brise-lames	Golfbreker	Wellenbrecher
Outer harbour	Avant Port	Buitenhaven	Aussenhafen
Inner harbour	Arrière Port	Binnenhaven	Innerer Hafen
Basin	Darse, bassin	Bassin, dok	Becken
Yacht harbour, marina	Port de plaisance	Jachthaven	Yachthafen
Fishing harbour	Port de pêche	Vissershaven	Fischereihafen
Alongside berth (AB)	Accostage	Aanlegplaats	Liegeplatz, Anleger
Drying berth	Assèchage	Droogvalling	Trockenplatz
Finger berth/pontoon	Catway	Box/Ponton	Liegeplatz/Ponton

1

Mooring buoy	Corps-mort	Meerboei	Festmachetonne
Mooring	Coffre d'amarrage	Ligplaats	Ligenplatz
Dolphin	Bouée de corps mort	Dukdalf	Dalben
Post, pile (mooring)	Poteau	Paal, meerpaal	Festmachepfahl
Anchorage (⚓)	Mouillage	Ankerplaats	Ankerplatz
Dredged	Dragué	Gebaggerd	Gebaggert
Landing (L)	Escalier du quai	Haventrap	Landungstreppe
Jetty	Jetée	Pier	Anlegestelle
Harbour Master	Maitre de Port	Havenmeester	Hafenmeister
Harbour dues	Taxes portuaires	Havengeld	Hafengebühr
Ferry	Bac	Veer	Fähre
Upstream	Amont	Stroomopwaarts	Stromauf
Downstream	Aval	Stroomafwaarts	Stromab
Slipway (slip)	Cale	Scheepshelling	Slip/Aufschleppe
Concrete	Béton	Beton	Beton
Stone	Maçonnerie	Steen	Stein
Lock	Écluse, Sas	Sluis	Schleuse
Lifting bridge	Pont basculant	Hefbrug	Hubbrücke
Swing bridge	Pont tournant	Draaibrug	Drehbrücke
Fixed bridge	Pont fixe	Vaste brug	Feste Brücke
Lifeboat (LB)	Canot de sauvetage	Reddingsboot	Rettungsboot

B. METEOROLOGY — MÉTÉO — METEOROLOGIE — METEOROLOGIE

Pressure	**Pression**	**Drukgebied**	**Druck**
Ridge (high)	Crête	Rug	Rücken
Trough (low)	Creux	Trog	Trog
High Pressure	Haute pression, anticyclone	Hogedrukgebied	Hochdruck
To fill	Se combler	Opvullen	Auffüllen
Low pressure	Dépression, bas	Depressie	Tiefdruck
To deepen	Se creuser	Dieper worden	Sich vertiefen
Front, warm/cold	Front, chaud/froid	Front, warm/koud	Front, warm/kalt
Rise/fall	Monter/baisser	Rijⅉen/vallen	Steigen/fallen
Settled	Temps établi	Vast	Beständig
Forecast	Prévision	Weervoorspelling	Wettervorhersage

Wind	**Vent**	**Wind**	**Wind**
Light airs (F1)	Très légère brise	Flauw en stil	Leiser Zug
Calm (F0)	Calme	Windstil	Ruhig
Light breeze (F2)	Légère brise	Flauwe koelte	Leichte Brise
Gentle breeze (F3)	Petite brise	Lichte koelte	Schwache Brise
Moderate breeze (F4)	Jolie brise	Matige koelte	Mäßige Brise
Fresh breeze (F5)	Bonne brise	Frisse bries	Frische Brise
Strong breeze (F6)	Vent frais	Stijve bries	Starker Wind
Near gale (F7)	Grand frais	Harde wind	Steifer Wind
Gale (F8)	Coup de vent	Stormachtig	Stürmischer Wind
Severe gale (F9)	Fort coup de vent	Storm	Sturm
Storm (F10)	Tempête	Zware storm	Schwerer Sturm
Squall	Grain	Bui	Bö
Gust	Rafale	Windvlaag	Windstoß
Lull	Accalmie	Luwte	Vorübergehendes Abflauen
Freshening	Fraîchissant	Toenemend	Zunehmend
Moderating	Décroissant	Afnemend	Abnehmend
Veer	Vire au...	Ruimen	Rechtsdrehen
Back	Adonner...	Krimpen	Zurückdrehen

Precipitation	**Précipitation**	**Neerslag**	**Niederschlag**
Drizzle	Bruine. crachin	Motregen	Sprühregen
Shower	Averse	Stortbui	Schauer
Rain	Pluie	Regen	Regen
Hail	Grêle	Hagel	Hagel
Sleet	Neige et pluie	Natte sneeuw	Schneeregen
Thunderstorm	Orage	Onweer	Gewitter

Cloud & Visibility	**Ciel et Visibilité**	**Hemel en Zicht**	**Himmel und Sichtweite**
Overcast	Couvert	Betrokken	Bedeckt
Cloudy	Nuageux	Bewolkt	Bewölkt
Clearing up	Éclaircie	Opklarend	Aufklarend
Mist	Brume	Nevel	Feuchter Dunst
Fog	Brouillard	Mist	Nebel
Sea state	**Mer**	**Zee**	**See (-gaug)**
Swell	Houle	Deining	Dünung

Rough	Forte	Ruw	Grob
Moderate	Agitée,	Aanschietende zee	Bewegt
Smooth	Belle	Vlak	Glatt
Choppy	Croisée	Kort	Kabbelig
Overfalls (tide race)	Remous (violents)	Stroomrafeling	Stromkabbelung

C THE BOAT   LE BATEAU   HET JACHT   DAS BOOT

Sails/Spars/Rigging   Voiles/Mâts/Gréement   Zeilen/Masten/Tuigage   Segel/Masten und Spieren/Rigg

Mainsail	Grand voile	Grootzeil	Grossegel
Genoa	Génois	Genua	Genua
Staysail	Trinquette	Stagfok	Fock
Batten (sail)	Latte	Zeillat	Latte
Mast	Mât	Mast	Mast
Mast, to step/unstep	Mâter/démâter	Mast plaatsen/verwijderen	Mast setzen/legen
Halyard	Drisse	Val	Fall
Sheet	Ecoute	Schoot	Schot
Topping lift	Balancine	Kraanlijn	Dirk
Boom	Bôme	Giek	Baum
Forestay	Etai	Voorstag	Vorstag
Backstay	Pataras	Achterstag	Achterstag
Turnbuckle, bottle-screw	Ridoir	Wantspanner	Wantenspanner
Spinnaker boom	Tangon de spi	Spinnakerboom	Spinnakerbaum
Splice	Epissure	Splits	Spleiß
Whipping twine	Fil à surlier	Garen	Takelgarn
Bosun's chair	Chaise de gabier	Bootsmanstoel	Bootsmannsstuhl
Stainless steel	Acier inoxydable	Roestvast staal (RVS)	Rostfreier Stahl
Shackle	Manille	Sluiting	Schäkel
Ensign	Pavillon	Scheepsvlag	Nationalflagge

On deck   Sur le pont   Aan dek   An deck

Pulpit/pushpit	Balcon avant/arrière	Preekstoel/Hekstoel	Bugkorb/Heckkorb
Anchor	Ancre	Anker	Anker
Oar	Aviron	Riemen	Riemen
Fender	Défense	Stootkussen	Fender
Boat hook	Gaffe	Pikhaak	Peekhaken
Life jacket	Gilet de sauvetage	Reddingvest	Rettungsweste
Tiller	Barre	Helmstok	Ruderpinne
Rudder	Gouvernail, safran	Roer	Ruder
Beam, breadth	Largeur	Breedte	Breite
Winch handle	Manivelle	Zwengel	Winschenkurbel
Bilge pump	Pompe de cale	Lenspomp	Lenzpumpe
Bucket	Seau	Emmer, puts	Pütz
Glass fibre (GRP)	Fibre de verre	Fiberglas	Fiberglas (GFK)
Varnish	Vernis	Lak, vernis	Lack
Tender	Annexe		

Below deck   Sous le pont   Onderdeks   Unter Deck

Galley	Cuisine	Kombuis	Kombüse
Gas cooker	Réchaud à gaz	Gastoestel	Gasherd
Plug	Bouchon	Stop	Stöpsel
Tap	Robinet	Kraan	Hahn
Saucepan	Casserole	Steelpan	Kochtopf
Corkscrew	Tire-bouchon	Kurketrekker	Korkenzieher
Matches	Allumettes	Lucifers	Streichhölzer

Electrics   Électrique   Elektrisch   Elektrik

Battery (ships)	Batterie	Accu	Batterie
Navigation lights	Feux de bord	Navigatielichten	Positions laternen
Bulb, lamp	Ampoule	Lamp	Glühlampe
Switch	Interrupteur	Schakelaar	Schalter
Fuse	Fusible	Zekering	Sicherung
Solder	Soudure	Soldeer	Lötmetall
Insulating tape	Chatterton	Isolatieband	Isolierband
Distilled water	Eau distillée	Gedestilleerd water	Destilliertes Wasser

Engine   Moteur   Motor   Motor

Drive-belt	Courroie	V-snaar	Keilriemen
Starter motor	Démarreur	Startmotor	Anlasser
Alternator	Alternateur	Wisselstroom-dynamo	Lichtmaschine
Split pin	Goupille fendue	Splitpen	Splint
Nut and bolt	Ecrou et boulon	Moer en bout	Mutter und Schraube

Washer	Rondelle	Vulring	Unterlegscheibe
Injector	Injecteur	Verstuiver	Einspritzdüse
Fuel filter	Filtre à combustible	Brandstoffilter	Brenstoffilter
To bleed (air)	Purger l'air	Ontluchten	Entlüften
Gasket	Garniture, joint	Pakking	Dichtung, Packungsring
Grease	Graisse	Vet	Fett
Propeller	Hélice	Schroef	Schraube/Propeller
Oil, lubricating	Huile	Smeerolie	Schmieröl
Sea-cock	Vanne	Buitenboordkraan	Seeventil
Spark plug	Bougie	Bougie	Zündkerze

Tools	**Outils**	**Gereedschappen**	**Werkzeug**
Spanner, adjustable	Clé anglaise	Sleutel	Schlüssel, (Engländer)
File (wood/metal)	Lime	Vijl	Feile
Hammer	Marteau	Hamer	Hammer
Feeler gauge	Calibre d'épaisseur	Voelermaat	Fühlerlshre (Spion)
Pliers	Pince	Buigtang	Kneifzange
Hacksaw	Scie à métaux	Metaalzaag	Metallsäge, Bügelsäge
Screwdriver	Tournevis	Schroevedraaier	Schraubenzieher
Vice	Étau	Bankschroef	Schraubstock, Feilkloben

D. ASHORE	**A TERRE**	**AAN LAND**	**AN LAND**
Nautical	**Nautique**	**Nautisch**	**Nautisch**
Chandlery (CH)	Accastillage	Scheepsleverancier	Jachtausrüster
Crane (C)	Grue	Hijskraan	Kran
Boatyard (BY)	Chantier naval	Jachtwerf	Yachtwerft
Shipwright (Sh)	Constructeur	Scheepsbouwmeester	Bootsbauer
Sailmaker (SM)	Voilier	Zeilmaker	Segelmacher
Engineer (ME)	Mécanicien	mecanicien/elektricien	Mechaniker
Boat hoist (BH)	Élévateur	Botenlift	Bootswinde/ Bootskran
Fresh water (FW)	Eau douce, potable	Drinkwater	Trinkwasser
Fuel	Carburant	Brandstof	Kraftstoff
Diesel (D)	Gas-oil, diesel	Dieselolie	Dieselöl
Petrol (P)	Essence	Benzine	Benzin
Paraffin	Petrole	Petroleum	Petroleum
Methylated spirits	Alcool à brûler	Spiritus	Brennspiritus
Dustbin	Poubelle	Vuilniscontainer	Mülltonne
Power point (AC)	Prise d'électricité	Stopcontact	Steckdose
Coastguard (CG)	Garde-Côte	Kustwacht	Küstenwacht
Customs (#)	Douane	Douane	Zoll

Non-nautical, Shopping	**Avitaillement**	**Niet nautisch, winkelen**	**Einkaufen/Shopping**
Butcher	Boucherie	Slager	Schlachter/Fleischer
Bakery	Boulangerie	Bakker	Bäcker
Ironmonger	Quincaillerie	Yerwarenwinkel	Eisenwarenhändler
Chemist	Pharmacie	Apotheek	Apotheke
Dentist	Dentiste	Tandarts	Zahnarzt
Doctor	Médecin	Dokter, huisarts	Arzt
Post Office (✉)	Bureau de Poste	Postkantoor	Postamt
Stamps	Timbres	Postzegels	Briefmarken
Railway station (⇌)	Gare	Spoorwegstation	Bahnhof
Airport (✈)	Aéroport	Vliegveld	Flughafen
Hospital (Ⓗ)	Hôpital	Ziekenhuis	Krankenhaus
Launderette (◎)	Laverie	Wasserette	Wäscherei
Market, food (V)	Marché	Supermarkt	Markt

E. FIRST AID	**PREMIERS SOINS**	**EERSTE HULP**	**ERSTE-HILFE**
Heart attack	Crise cardiaque	Hartaanval	Herzanfall
Haemorrhage	Hémorragie	Bloeding	Blutung
Coma	dans le coma	Coma	Koma
Fracture	Fracture	Breuk	Fraktur
Head injury	Traumisme cranien	Hoofdwond	Kopfverletzung
Laceration	Déchirure	Scheuring	Schürfwunde, Verletzung
Appendicitis	Appendicite	Blindedarmontsteking	Blinddarmentzündung
Vomiting blood	Vomir du sang	Bloed braken	Bluterbrechen
Coughing blood	Cracher le sang	Bloed ophoesten	Bluthusten
Perforated ulcer	Ulcère perforé	Opengebarsten zweer	Magendurchbruch
Delirium	Delirium	Delirium, geest-verwarring	Delirium
Burn	Brûlure	Brandwond	Brandwunde
Acute infection	Infection aiguë	Acute infectie	akute Infektion
Sting (insect, jellyfish)	Piqûre	Steek (insect, kwal)	Stich, Stachel (Insekt)
Poisoning	Empoisonnement	Vergiftig	Vergiftung
Drowning	Noyade	Verdrinken	Ertrinkend

Chapter 2

General Information

Contents

General information – introduction

Here in the Almanac are given brief notes on the *International Regulations for Preventing Collisions at Sea*, useful conversion factors, a summary of documentation, Customs procedures and useful addresses. For further details of these items, and of the subjects listed above, reference should be made to *The Macmillan & Silk Cut Yachtsman's Handbook*.

The following subjects are described in detail in Chapter 2 of *The Macmillan & Silk Cut Yachtsman's Handbook*:

Limits and dangers – e.g. territorial waters; fishing limits; measured distances; hovercraft; warships on exercises; practice and exercise areas; submarines; minefields; wrecks; offshore oil and gas fields; power cables; traffic schemes. HM Customs – notice of departure; immigration; full and quick reports. Customs regulations in European countries. Yacht tonnage measurement – Net and Gross Tonnages; Lloyd's Register Tonnage; Deadweight Tonnage; One Ton Cup etc. Units and conversions. Glossaries of nautical terms. Yachting organisations – Royal Yachting Association; Seamanship Foundation; British Marine Industries Federation; Trinity House; useful addresses.

2.1 INTERNATIONAL REGULATIONS FOR PREVENTING COLLISIONS AT SEA

2.1.1 General

a.   The 1972 International Regulations for Preventing Collisions at Sea (IRPCS), occasionally referred to as Colregs or Rule of the Road, are given in full in *The Macmillan & Silk Cut Yachtsman's Handbook* (2.1), together with supporting diagrams and explanatory notes. The following are notes on some of the provisions of special concern to yachtsmen. It is important that these shortened notes should only be used in conjunction with the complete IRPCS and not in isolation. The numbers of the rules quoted are given for reference.

b.   The rules must be interpreted in a seamanlike way if collisions are to be avoided (Rule 2). A vessel does not have right of way over another regardless of special factors – such as other vessels under way or at anchor, shallow water or other hazards, poor visibility, traffic separation schemes, fishing boats etc. – or the handling characteristics of the vessels concerned in the prevailing conditions. Sometimes vessels must depart from the rules to avoid a collision.

c.   A sailing vessel is so defined (Rule 3) when she is under sail only. When under power she must show the lights for a power-driven vessel, and when under sail and power a cone point down forward (Rule 25).

d.   Keep a good lookout at all times, using eyes and ears as well as by Radar and VHF, particularly at night or in poor visibility (Rule 5).

e.   Safe speed is dictated by visibility, traffic density, including concentrations of fishing or other vessels, depth of water, the state of wind, sea and current, proximity of navigational dangers, and the manoeuvrability of the boat with special reference to stopping distance and turning ability in the prevailing conditions (Rule 6). Excessive speed gives less time to appreciate the situation, less time to take avoiding action, and produces a worse collision if such action fails.

f.   When faced with converging vessel(s), a skipper/crew must always answer the following 3 questions and take action if required.

    1.   Is there a risk of collision?
    2.   If there is, am I the give way vessel?
    3.   If I am, what action must I take?

g.   If there is any doubt assume there is a risk (Rule 7). A yacht should take a series of compass bearings on a converging ship – see Fig 2(1). Unless the bearings change appreciably, there is risk of collision. If fitted, use radar to obtain early warning of risk of collision. Take special care with large ships.

Take early and positive action to avoid collision (Rule 8). Large alterations of course and/or speed are more evident to the other skipper, particularly at night

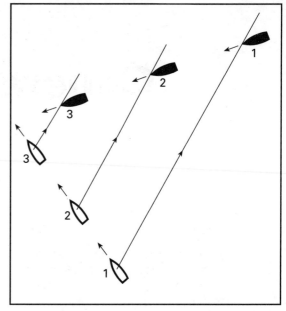

Fig. 2(1) Rule 7. *The bearing of black from white is steady. White should have taken action long before position 2 by altering course to starboard by at least 45° to pass under black's stern.*

or on radar. Do not hesitate to slow down, stop (or even go astern, under power). While keeping clear of one vessel, watch out for others.

h.   In narrow channels, keep to starboard and as near to the outer limit of the channel or fairway as is safe and practical whether under power or sail (Rule 9). A yacht under 20m in length must not impede larger vessels confined to a channel. A yacht should not cross a narrow channel if such crossing would impede a vessel which can only safely navigate within the channel, and should avoid anchoring in such channels.

2.1.2 Vessels in sight of each other

a.   When two sailing vessels are in risk of collision and on opposite tacks, the one on the port tack keeps clear. If on the same tack, the windward yacht keeps clear. If a yacht with the wind on the port side sees a yacht to windward and cannot determine with certainty whether the other yacht has the wind on the port or starboard side, then keep out of the way of the other. For the purpose of this rule the windward side is deemed to be the side opposite to that on which the mainsail is carried (Rule 12). Rule 12 does not apply when either yacht is motor sailing. Fig. 2(2) illustrates the practical application of the rules in the three cases mentioned above. There are other practical situations which might give cause for doubt about the application of Rule 12. The first is when running downwind under spinnaker alone. In this case windward would be the side on which the spinnaker boom is set (normally opposite to the mainsail). The second case is when hove-to. This would have to be determined by the most likely position of the mainsail if it were set.

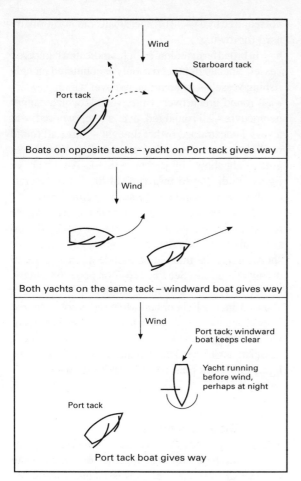

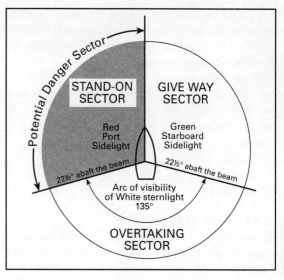

Fig. 2(3) Rules 11 to 17. *These rules apply only to vessels in sight of one another and do not apply when vessels can only see each other on radar.*

Fig. 2(2) Rule 12. *Conduct between sailing vessels. In all cases the yacht on the port tack keeps clear; if both yachts are on the same tack the windward boat keeps clear. If in doubt, always keep clear.*

2

b.   Any overtaking vessel, whether power or sail, shall keep out of the way of the vessel being overtaken (Rule 13). Overtaking means approaching the other vessel from a direction more than 22½° abaft her beam (in the sector of her sternlight by night). An overtaken vessel must not hamper one overtaking: always look astern before altering course to ensure another vessel is not coming up on either quarter.

c.   When two power-driven vessels approach head-on, each must alter course to starboard, to pass port to port (Rule 14). A substantial alteration may be needed, with the appropriate sound signal (see page 16 and Rule 34), to make intentions clear.

d.   When two power-driven vessels are crossing and in risk of collision, the one with the other on her starboard side must keep clear and, if possible, avoid passing ahead of the other (Rule 15). The give-way vessel should normally alter to starboard; exceptionally, an alteration to port may be justified, in which case a large alteration may be needed to avoid crossing ahead of the other.

e.   When one vessel has to keep clear, the other shall maintain her course and speed (Rule 17a). But if she realises that the give-way vessel is failing to keep clear, she must take independent action to avoid collision (Rule 17b).

f.   Using the arcs of visibility of the sidelights and stern light to illustrate the rules, Fig. 2(3) allocates names to each arc. The arc of the sternlight is called the "overtaking sector"; the arc of the starboard (Green) sidelight is called the "giving way sector"; and the arc covered by the port (Red) sidelight is called the "stand-on sector". The stand-on sector is sometimes referred to as the "potential danger sector" because, under Rule 17b, if it becomes apparent that the giving way vessel is not going to alter course, the stand-on vessel shall take action to avoid it by making a substantial alteration to starboard to keep clear under Rule 17b and Rule 2. In taking such action, you should avoid any risk of the two vessels turning towards each other.

g.   Under Rule 18, except where Rules 9 (Narrow Channels), 10 (Traffic Schemes) and 13 (Overtaking) otherwise require:

(a)   A power-driven vessel underway keeps clear of:
   (i)   a vessel not under command;
  (ii)   a vessel restricted in manoeuvrability;
 (iii)   a vessel engaged in fishing;
 (iv)   a sailing vessel.

(b)   A sailing vessel underway keeps clear of:
   (i)-(iii) in (a) above.

(c)   A vessel engaged in fishing, underway, keeps clear of: (i) and (ii) in (a) above.

(d)   (i) Any vessel, except one not under command or one restricted in her ability to manoeuvre, shall if possible avoid impeding a vessel constrained by her draught, showing the signals prescribed in Rule 28 (see page 66).

(ii) A vessel constrained by her draught shall navigate with particular caution.

2.1.3   Traffic Separation Schemes

Under Rule 10 all vessels, including yachts, must conform to Traffic Separation Schemes (TSS). Full details of the procedures involved are given in Chapter 10 (10.0.9).

2.1.4   Restricted visibility

In poor visibility vessels must proceed at a safe speed (Rule 19). On hearing a fog signal ahead of the beam, be prepared to reduce speed or stop. If a vessel is detected by radar, take early action to avoid collision: if the other vessel is ahead of the beam, avoid altering course to port, unless the other vessel is being overtaken: if the other vessel is abaft the beam, do not alter course towards it. Sound the appropriate fog signal; keep a good lookout; have an efficient radar reflector; keep clear of shipping lanes; and be ready to take avoiding action. In thick fog it is best to anchor in shallow water, out of the shipping channels.

2.1.5 Lights and shapes

a.   The required lights must be shown from sunset to sunrise, and by day in restricted visibility. The required shapes must be shown by day (Rule 20).
b.   The types of navigation light are defined in Rule 21, and are shown in Plate 1 on page 63, together with illustrations of the lights to be shown by power-driven vessels and sailing vessels underway. A summary of further lights and shapes to be shown by various classes of vessel is given in Plate 4 on page 66.
c.   A yacht, even with sails set, which is under engine must show the lights of a power-driven vessel, and by day, a cone, point down, forward.
d.   In a sailing yacht up to 20m in length, the sidelights and sternlight may be combined in one tricolour lantern at the masthead. This gives excellent visibility for the lights, and maximum brightness for minimum battery drain. A tricolour light should not be switched on at the same time as the normal sidelights and sternlight, and must not be used when under power.
e.   A sailing vessel underway may, in addition to her normal sidelights and sternlight, show near the masthead two all-round lights in a vertical line, red over green. But these lights must not be shown in conjunction with the tricolour lantern described in the previous paragraph (Rule 25).
f.   A power-driven vessel under 12m in length may combine her masthead light and sternlight in one all-round white light (Rule 23).
g.   Lights required for vessels towing and being towed (Rule 24) include a special yellow towing light above the sternlight of the towing vessel. But this is not required by a yacht or other small craft not normally used for towing.
h.   In broad terms coloured lights indicate a hampered vessel. Special lights commonly encountered include fishing vessels – an all round red over white; trawlers – all round green over white; vessels which cannot manoeuvre – all round red, over white, over red; and a vessel constrained by her draught – three all round red lights; and not least the optional all round red over green light shown by yachts so fitted. All the above lights are displayed in a vertical line. A hovercraft exhibits an all round rapid flashing yellow light.
j.   The rules for vessels not under command, or restricted in their ability to manoeuvre (Rule 27), do not apply to vessels under 12m in length, except for showing flag 'A' International Code when engaged in diving operations. See Plates 6–7 on pages 68 and 69.
k.   A yacht less than 7m in length is not required to show an anchor light or ball when she is not anchored in or near a narrow channel, fairway or anchorage, or where other vessels normally navigate (Rule 30). A vessel under 12m in length is not required to show the lights or shapes prescribed by that rule when she is aground.

2.1.6   Distress signals

The IRPCS, Annex IV, gives details of all the signals which may be used either together or separately to indicate distress and need of assistance. These are described in more detail in Chapter 8 (8.2). For those flag and sound signals having a special meaning under IRPCS, see also Plates 6 and 7 on pages 68 and 69. For lesser emergencies use 'V' International Code – 'I require assistance'.

Distress signals must only be used when a vessel or person is in serious and immediate danger and urgent help is needed.

2.1.7   Sound signals

Sound signals required (by Rules 34 and 35) are summarised in the table below. Vessels over 12m in length must be provided with a whistle (foghorn) and a bell. A boat under 12m is not obliged to carry these sound signalling appliances, but must have some means of making an efficient sound signal. The effectiveness of a yacht's sound signal should be judged against its audibility from the bridge of a large ship, with conflicting noises from other sources. Note that a short blast is about one second, and a prolonged blast four to six seconds in duration. A sailing vessel underway in fog sounds one prolonged blast, followed by two short blasts ('D'). The maximum interval between sound signals for vessels underway in restricted visibility is two minutes, but they should be sounded more frequently if other craft are near.

SUMMARY OF IMPORTANT SOUND SIGNALS, RULES 34 AND 35

Note: •   indicates a short blast of foghorn, of about one second's duration.
     —   indicates a prolonged blast of foghorn, of four to six seconds' duration.

Vessels in sight of each other (Rule 34)

•	I am altering course to starboard (power-driven vessel).
••	I am altering course to port (power-driven vessel).
•••	I am operating astern propulsion (power-driven vessel).
— — •	(In a narrow channel) I intend to overtake you on your starboard side.
— — ••	(In a narrow channel) I intend to overtake you on your port side.
— • — •	Agreement with the overtaking signal above.
•••••	I fail to understand your intentions or actions/I doubt if you are taking sufficient action to avoid collision.
—	Warning signal by vessel(s) approaching a bend in channel.

Sound signals in restricted visibility (Rule 35)

—	Power-driven vessel making way through the water.
— —	Power-driven vessel under way, but stopped and not making way through the water.
— ••	Vessel not under command, or restricted in her ability to manoeuvre, or constrained by her draught, or engaged in fishing, or towing or pushing, or a sailing vessel.
— •••	Vessel being towed, or if more than one vessel is towed, the last vessel in the tow.
••••	Pilot vessel engaged on pilotage duties.

Bell rung rapidly for about 5 seconds, every minute.	Vessel at anchor.
Gong rung rapidly for about 5 seconds following above signal, every minute.	Vessel of 100m or more in length at anchor: the bell being sounded in the fore part of the vessel and the gong aft.
• — •	Vessel at anchor (optional additional signal).
Bell rung rapidly for about 5 seconds, with three separate and distinct strokes before and after.	Vessel aground.

2.2   DOCUMENTATION

2. 2.1   Registration

Two forms of registration are available for British owned yachts. Both are described more fully in section 1.5 of *The Macmillan & Silk Cut Yachtsman's Handbook*.

Full registration, under the Merchant Shipping (Registration, etc.) Act 1993 and the Merchant Shipping (Registration of Ships) Regulations 1993 is a relatively complex and expensive business, since a yacht has to follow the same procedure as for a large merchant vessel. It does however have the advantage of establishing title (ownership), and is also useful for recording a marine mortgage. The register is in four parts:

Part I	for Merchant Ships and pleasure vessels
Part II	for fishing vessels
Part III	for small ships
Part IV	for bareboat charter ships

The procedure for Part 1 registrations is fully described in a pamphlet issued by the Department of Transport titled *"Registering British Ships in the United Kingdom"* obtainable from Registry of Shipping and Seamen (RSS), PO Box 165, Cardiff CF4 5FU.

☎: 01222 747333. Fax: 01222 747877. There is a ☎ help line available on 0891 615353 .

The Small Ships Register, established in 1983, is sufficient for most purposes. A small ship is deemed to be less than 24 metres in overall length and is, or applying to be, registered on Part III of the Register of British Ships. It satisfies the law that a British yacht proceeding abroad must be registered, and it also meets the registration requirement for a privileged ensign. Part III registration does not register "Title" and you cannot register mortgages. The cost is only £10 for a five-year period, and measurement is a simple matter of taking the overall length of the boat – well described in the instructions which accompany the application form, obtainable from the Small Ships Register, Driver and Vehicle Licensing Centre, Swansea SA 99 1BX (☎ (01792) 783355, Fax: (01792) 783401).

2.2.2   International Certificate for Pleasure Navigation

With the introduction of the Small Ships Register, this certificate has no relevance for yachts owned by UK or Commonwealth citizens resident in the UK. It is however available for European citizens established in the UK.

2.2.3 International Certificate of Competence

The former Helmsman's Overseas Certificate of Competence (HOCC) is replaced by the International Certificate of Competence (ICC) (Pleasure Craft). If a suitable RYA Certificate (e.g. Yachtmaster offshore) is not held, the ICC will be issued by the RYA to UK residents who pass a test at an RYA recognised teaching establishment or participating Club, who already hold a HOCC, or a professional or services seagoing qualification. The ICC period of validity is 5 years. Holders of existing HOCC can be renewed on expiry without the requirement of a practical test.

2.2.4 Licences

A licence is required to operate a boat on most inland waterways (e.g. the River Thames above Teddington Lock, the Norfolk Broads, Yorkshire Ouse above Naburn Lock, and canals or rivers controlled by the British Waterways Board).

2.2.5 Insurance

Any cruising boat represents a large capital investment, which should be protected against possible loss or damage by adequate insurance. It is also essential to insure against third-party risks, and cover for at least £500,000 is recommended.

The value for which a boat is insured should be the replacement cost of the boat and all equipment. Read the proposal form carefully, and fill in the details required as accurately as possible. Take care to abide by the nominated period in commission and cruising area. Note the various warranties which are implied or expressed in the policy. For example, the owner is required to keep the boat in good, seaworthy condition; insurance does not cover charter, unless specially arranged; prompt notice must be given of any claim; a reduction may be made for fair wear and tear for items such as outboards, sails and rigging; theft is only covered if forcible entry or removal can be shown; engines and other mechanical items are only covered in exceptional circumstances; personal effects are not covered, unless specially arranged; and motor boats with speeds of 17 knots or more are subject to special clauses and often to extra premiums.

2.2.6 Classification

Lloyd's Register of Shipping provides an advisory and consultancy service to owners, builders, moulders and designers, and publishes rules for the construction of yachts in various materials. Experienced surveyors approve drawings, supervise moulding, inspect fitting out, check the machinery, and certify the completed yacht. To remain 'in class' a yacht must be subjected to periodical surveys.

As an alternative to full classification, Lloyd's Register Building Certificate is provided to newly-built yachts which have been constructed of any approved material in accordance with the Society's rules, and under the supervision of its surveyors, without the requirement for periodical survey.

2.2.7 Cruising formalities

Before, or while cruising abroad, certain formalities are necessary, as summarised below:

(1) Conform to HM Customs regulations, see 2.3.
(2) The yacht must be registered, see 2.2.1.
(3) Take valid passports for all the crew, and conform to health regulations (e.g. by reporting any infectious disease): exceptionally, vaccination certificates may be needed.
(4) Conform to Customs regulations in countries visited. Brief notes are given in section 2.4, but if in doubt about specific items or procedures, ask. All countries are sensitive to the importation (including carriage on board) of illegal quantities of alcohol and tobacco, and drugs of any kind.
(5) Make sure the yacht is covered by insurance for the intended cruising area, including third-party cover.
(6) It is wise for the skipper to carry a Certificate of Competence or similar document (e.g. Yachtmaster Certificate).
(7) The yacht should wear the Red Ensign (or a Special Ensign, if so authorised), and fly a courtesy ensign of the country concerned at starboard crosstree. Flag 'Q' must be carried to comply with Customs procedures.
(8) In most countries it is illegal to use a visiting cruising yacht for any commercial purpose (e.g. charter).

2.3 HM CUSTOMS

2.3.1 General information

All yachts sailing outside UK Territorial Waters must conform to Customs Notice No. 8B summarised below. This Notice, Form C1331, and further information may be obtained from any Customs and Excise Office, or from HM Customs and Excise, OAS, 5th Floor East, New King's Beam House, 22 Upper Ground, London SE1 9PJ (☎ 0171-865 4742). Most yacht clubs and marinas hold stocks of Form C1331.

On 1st January 1993 the European Union (EU) became a single market and EU yachtsmen can now enjoy unhindered movement within the EU, provided that all taxes due, such as customs duty, VAT, or any other customs charges, have been paid in one of the EU countries.

Countries of the EU are: Austria, Belgium, Denmark, France, Finland, Germany, Greece, the Republic of Ireland, Italy, Luxembourg, the Netherlands, Portugal (including the Azores and Madeira), Spain (including the Balearic Islands, but not the Canary Islands), Sweden, and the United Kingdom (including the Isle of Man, but not the Channel Islands).

It is important to note that the Channel Islands and the Canary Islands do not operate a VAT system under Community rules, and for practical purposes are therefore treated as being outside the EU single market.

Yachtsmen are warned that a boat may be searched at any time. There are severe penalties for non-declaration of prohibited or restricted goods, and the carriage and non-declaration of prohibited drugs and firearms will incur the forfeiture of your boat and all its equipment. A separate Form C1331 will be required for each voyage to or from a non-EU country. In addition yachtsmen arriving from outside the EU, including the Channel Islands need to remember to fly flag 'Q'. Failure to clear outwards and inwards in this way may result in a fine. It is clearly in the yachtsman's best interests to have a copy of Customs Notice No. 8B aboard.

2.3.2 Notice of departure

It is not necessary to report any voyage planned to another EU country, unless asked to do so by a Customs officer. Each intended departure to a place outside the EU must be notified to HM Customs on Part I of Form C1331, copies of which are available at Customs offices and from most yacht clubs, etc. The form is in two parts. When completed Part I should be handed to a Customs officer, taken to the Customs office nearest the place of departure, or put in a Customs post box, so the form arrives before departure. Retain Part II on board as evidence of your notification of departure. Form C1331 is valid for up to 48 hours after the stated time of departure. Should the voyage be abandoned, Part II should be delivered to the same office marked 'voyage abandoned'. Failure to give notice of departure may result in delay and inconvenience on return, and possible prosecution.

2.3.3 Stores

In general there is no restriction on taking reasonable quantities of food, fuel and other stores on which all duties and VAT have been paid elsewhere in the EU. Duty-free stores may be allowed on vessels proceeding south of Brest (France) or north of the north bank of the Eider (Germany), but you will need to apply to a Customs office in advance, and will have to meet certain conditions. Details on how to ship stores, or to re-ship previously landed surplus duty-free stores, can be obtained from any Customs office. You cannot take duty-free stores to the Republic of Ireland or the Channel Islands. If you are shipping stores under bond, or on which you are claiming repayment of customs charges, the goods must be placed under a customs seal on board. Such goods cannot be used in UK waters without paying duty, and you may be liable to duty if you abandon or interrupt the voyage. Further details may be obtained from any Customs office.

2.3.4 Immigration

Anyone who is not an EU national must get the Immigration officer's permission to enter the UK. In most yachting centres the Customs officer acts as the Immigration officer as well. It is a skipper's responsibility to inform a Customs or Immigration officer if there is any person on board who is not a national of the EU and who is arriving in the UK from any country other than the Isle of Man, the Channel Islands, or the Republic of Ireland.

2.3.5 Arrivals from an EC country

If arriving directly from another EU country there is no need to fly flag 'Q', complete any paperwork, or contact Customs. You must, however, contact Customs if you have goods to declare, or have non-EC nationals on board. You must declare any animals or birds; any prohibited or restricted goods such as controlled drugs,

firearms, or radio transmitters not approved for use in UK; counterfeit goods; any duty-free stores; or the boat itself if duty and VAT are owed on it. Further details on which goods are classified as prohibited or restricted are given in Notice 8B.

2.3.6 Arrival from countries outside the EC

If arriving directly from a country outside the EC (including the Channel Islands), yachts are subject to Customs control and on arrival you must contact a Customs officer in person or by telephone. As soon as UK Territorial Waters are entered, i.e. the 12-mile limit, complete Form C1331 and fly the flag 'Q' where it can easily be seen until formalities are complete. If an officer boards your vessel, you must hand Form C1331 to him. You must declare any tobacco goods, alcoholic drinks, perfumes and toilet waters in excess of your duty-free allowance; animals or birds; prohibited or restricted goods; duty-free stores; or the boat itself if duty and VAT are owed on it. You must also declare any goods that are to be left in the UK. You must not land any persons or goods, or transfer them to another vessel until a Customs officer says so.

2.3.7 Customs offices – telephone numbers

The telephone number of the appropriate Customs office (#) is given under the heading 'Telephone' for each British harbour in Chapter 10.

2.4 FOREIGN CUSTOMS – PROCEDURES

2.4.1 General

Other EU countries should follow the same regulations as described in 2.3.1 to 2.3.6 above, and any customs formalities are likely to be minimal. However, before departure, skippers are recommended to check the procedures in force in their destination country. Currently, both the Netherlands and Belgium require a vessel to report on arrival even if coming from another EU country. If you are going directly to a country outside the EU you must inform UK Customs before departure by filling in Form C1331.

2.5. VAT AND THE SINGLE MARKET

2.5.1 General

An EU resident can move a yacht between Member States without restriction, providing VAT has been paid.

All queries on this complex subject should be directed to HM Customs and Excise at the address given in 2.3.1, or any Customs office. The RYA may also be able to provide useful advice.

2.5.2 Temporary importation (TI)

A boat can only be permitted into an EU country under temporary import arrangements if:

(1) The owner is not an EU resident (i.e. lives outside the EU for at least 185 days in any 12 month period), and

(2) The owner does not keep the boat in the EU for more than six months in a continuous twelve month period, within the EU as a whole. The period of TI cannot be extended by moving the boat to another EU member state.

2.6 USEFUL ADDRESSES

British Marine Industries Federation (BMIF).
Boating Industry House, Mead Lake Place, Thorpe Lea Road, Egham, Surrey TW20 8HE.
☎: 01784 473377. Fax: 01784 439678.

British Sub-Aqua Club.
Telford's Quay, Ellesmere Port, South Wirral, Cheshire L65 4FY.
☎: 0151-357 1951. Fax: 0151-357 1250.

British Telecom Maritime Radio Services.
43 Bartholomew Close, London EC1A 7HP.
☎: 0171-583 9416. Fax: 0171-726 8123.

British Waterways Board.
Willow Grange, Church Road, Watford, Herts WD1 3QA.
☎: 01923 226422. Fax: 01923 226081.

Clyde Cruising Club.
Suite 408, The Pentagon Centre, 36 Washington Street, Glasgow G3 8AZ.
☎: 0141-221 2774. Fax: 0141-221 2775.

Cowes Combined Clubs.
Secretary, 18 Bath Road, Cowes, Isle of Wight PO31 7QN.
☎: 01983 295744. Fax: 01983 295329.

Cruising Association (CA).
CA House, 1 Northey Street, Limehouse Basin, London E14 8BT.
☎: 0171-537 2828. Fax: 0171-537 2266.

Coastguard Headquarters.
Spring Place, 105 Commercial Road, Southampton SO1 0ZD.
☎: 01703 329486. Fax: 01703 329351.

HM Customs and Excise.
OAS, 5th Floor East, New King's Beam House, 22 Upper Ground, London SE1 9PJ.
☎: 0171-865 4742. Fax: 0171-865 4744.

Hydrographic Office.
Ministry of Defence, Taunton, Somerset TA1 2DN.
☎: 01823 337900. Fax: 01823 284077.

International Maritime Organisation (IMO).
4 Albert Embankment, London SE1 7SR.
☎: 0171-735 7611. Fax: 0171-587 3210.

International Maritime Satellite Organisation (INMARSAT).
99 City Road, London EC1Y 1AX.
☎: 0171-728 1000. Fax: 0171-728 1044.

Junior Offshore Group.
43 Parklands Ave, Cowes, Isle of Wight PO31 7NH.
☎: 01983 280279. Fax: 01983 292962.

Little Ship Club.
Bell Wharf Lane, Upper Thames Street, London EC4R 3TB..
☎: 0171-236 7729. Fax: 0171-236 9100.

Lloyd's Register of Shipping.
Yacht and Small Craft Services, 71 Fenchurch Street, LONDON EC3M 4BS.
☎: 0171 709 9166. Fax: 0171 423 2016.

Maritime Trust.
2 Greenwich Church Street, London SE10 9BG.
☎: 0181-858 2698. Fax: 0181-858 6976.

Meteorological Office.
London Road, Bracknell, Berks RG12 2SZ.
☎: 01344 420242. Fax: 01344 855921.

Radiocommunication Agency
Waterloo Bridge House, Waterloo Road, London SE1 8UA.
☎: 0171 215 2150. Fax: 0171 928 4309

Radio Licensing Centre.
Subscription Service Ltd, PO Box 885, Bristol BS99 5LG.
☎: 0117 9258333. Fax: 0117 9219026.

Registry of Shipping and Seamen (RSS).
PO Box 165, Cardiff CF4 5FU.
☎: 01222 747333. Fax: 01222 747877.
☎: RSS Helpline 0891 615353.

Royal Cruising Club (RCC).
At the Royal Thames Yacht Club (see below).

Royal Institute of Navigation.
At the Royal Geographical Society, 1 Kensington Gore, London SW7 2AT.
☎ 0171-589 5021. Fax: 0171-823 8671.

Royal National Lifeboat Institution (RNLI).
West Quay Road, Poole, Dorset BH15 1HZ.
☎: 01202 671133. Fax: 01202 670128.

Royal Naval Sailing Association (RNSA).
17 Pembroke Road, Portsmouth, Hants PO1 2NT.
☎: 01705 823524. Fax: 01705 870654.

Royal Ocean Racing Club (RORC).
20 St James Place, London SW1A 1NN.
☎: 0171-493 2248. Fax: 0171-493 5252.

Royal Thames Yacht Club (RTYC).
60 Knightsbridge, London SW1A 7LF.
☎: 0171-235 2121. Fax: 0171-235 5672.

Royal Yachting Association (RYA).
RYA House, Romsey Road, Eastleigh, Hants SO5 9YA.
☎: 01703 629962. Fax: 01703 629924.

Royal Yachting Association (Scotland).
Caledonia House, South Gyle, Edinburgh EH12 9DQ.
☎: 0131-317 7388. Fax: 0131-317 8566.

Ship Radio Licensing Unit.
Radiocommunications Agency, Room 613, Waterloo Bridge House, Waterloo Road, London SE1 8UA.
☎ 0171-215 2047. Fax: 0171-928 4309.

Small Ships Register.
DVLA, Swansea SA99 1BX.
☎: 01792 783355 Fax: 01792 783401
☎: RSS Helpline 01891 615353.

Solent Cruising and Racing Association.
18 Bath Road, Cowes, Isle of Wight PO31 7QN.
☎: 01983 295744. Fax: 01983 295329.

Sports Council.
16 Upper Woburn Place, London WC1H 0QP.
☎: 0171-388 1277. Fax: 0171-383 5740.

Trinity House, Corporation of.
Trinity House, Tower Hill, London EC3N 4DH.
☎: 0171-480 6601. Fax: 0171-480 7662.

UK Civil Satnav Group (UK CSG).
c/o The Royal Institute of Navigation, at the Royal Geographical Society, 1 Kensington Gore, London SW7 2AT.
☎: 0171-589 5021. Fax: 0171-823 8671.

UK Offshore Boating Association.
1 Carbis Close, Port Solent, Portsmouth PO6 4TW.
☎: 01705 219949. Fax: 01705 219969.

2.7 CONVERSION FACTORS

2.7.1 Conversion factors

To convert	Multiply by	To convert	Multiply by
sq in to sq mm	645·16	sq mm to sq in	0·00155
sq ft to sq m	0·0929	sq m to sq ft	10·76
in to mm	25·40	mm to in	0·0394
ft to m	0·3048	m to ft	3·2808
fathoms to m	1·8288	m to fathoms	0·5468
nautical miles to statute miles	1·1515	statute miles to nautical miles	0·8684
lb to kg	0·4536	kg to lb	2·205
tons to tonnes (1000 kg)	1·016	tonnes to tons (2240 lb)	0·9842
kilometres to nautical miles	0·539957	nautical miles to kilometres	1·852
millibars to inches	0·0295	inches to millibars	33·86
lb/sq in to kg/sq cm	0·0703	kg/sq cm to lb/sq in	14·22
lb/sq in to atmospheres	0·0680	atmospheres to lb/sq in	14·7
ft/sec to m/sec	0·3048	m/sec to ft/sec	3·281
ft/sec to miles/hr	0·682	miles/hr to ft/sec	1·467
ft/min to m/sec	0·0051	m/sec to ft/min	196·8
knots to miles/hr	1·1515	miles/hr to knots	0·868
knots to km/hr	1·8520	km/hr to knots	0·5400
cu ft to galls	6·25	galls to cu ft	0·16
cu ft to litres	28·33	litres to cu ft	0·035
pints to litres	0·568	litres to pints	1·76
galls to litres	4·546	litres to galls	0·22
Imp galls to US galls	1·2	US galls to Imp galls	0·833

2.7.2 Speed conversions

Knots	Kilometres per Hour	Metres per Second	Knots	Kilometres per Hour	Metres per Second
0 – 1	0 – 1·8	0 – 0·5	28 – 33	51·9 – 61·1	14·4 – 17·0
1 – 3	1·8 – 5·6	0·5 – 1·5	34 – 40	63·0 – 74·1	17·5 – 20·6
4 – 6	7·4 – 11·1	2·1 – 3·1	41 – 47	76·0 – 87·0	21·1 – 24·2
7 – 10	13·0 – 18·5	3·6 – 5·1	48 – 55	88·9 – 101·9	24·7 – 28·3
11 – 16	20·4 – 29·6	5·7 – 8·2	56 – 63	103·7 – 116·7	28·8 – 32·4
17 – 21	31·5 – 39·0	8·7 – 10·8	64+	119+	32·9+
22 – 27	40·8 – 50·0	11·3 – 13·9			

2.7.3 Feet to metres, metres to feet

Explanation: The central columns of figures in **bold** type can be referred in either direction. To the left to convert metres into feet, or to the right to convert feet into metres.

For example, five lines down: 5 feet = 1·52 metres, and 5 metres = 16·40 feet.

Feet		Metres	Feet		Metres	Feet		Metres	Feet		Metres
3·28	**1**	0·30	45·93	**14**	4·27	88·58	**27**	8·23	131·23	**40**	12·19
6·56	**2**	0·61	49·21	**15**	4·57	91·86	**28**	8·53	134·51	**41**	12·50
9·84	**3**	0·91	52·49	**16**	4·88	95·14	**29**	8·84	137·80	**42**	12·80
13·12	**4**	1·22	55·77	**17**	5·18	98·43	**30**	9·14	141·08	**43**	13·11
16·40	**5**	1·52	59·06	**18**	5·49	101·71	**31**	9·45	144·36	**44**	13·41
19·69	**6**	1·83	62·34	**19**	5·79	104·99	**32**	9·75	147·64	**45**	13·72
22·97	**7**	2·13	65·62	**20**	6·10	108·27	**33**	10·06	150·92	**46**	14·02
26·25	**8**	2·44	68·90	**21**	6·40	111·55	**34**	10·36	154·20	**47**	14·33
29·53	**9**	2·74	72·18	**22**	6·71	114·83	**35**	10·67	157·48	**48**	14·63
32·81	**10**	3·05	75·46	**23**	7·01	118·11	**36**	10·97	160·76	**49**	14·94
36·09	**11**	3·35	78·74	**24**	7·32	121·39	**37**	11·28	164·04	**50**	15·24
39·37	**12**	3·66	82·02	**25**	7·62	124·67	**38**	11·58			
42·65	**13**	3·96	85·30	**26**	7·92	127·95	**39**	11·89			

IN AN EMERGENCY
Look in The Pink
and don't be in the doldrums

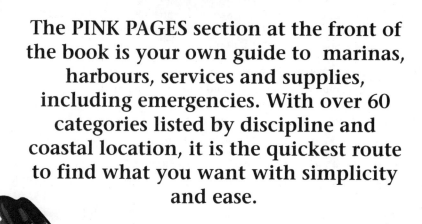

The PINK PAGES section at the front of the book is your own guide to marinas, harbours, services and supplies, including emergencies. With over 60 categories listed by discipline and coastal location, it is the quickest route to find what you want with simplicity and ease.

The MACMILLAN & SILK CUT *incorporating* REED'S
NAUTICAL ALMANAC

Chapter 3

Coastal Navigation

Contents

3

Coastal navigation – introduction

The following subjects are described in more detail in Chapters 3 and 15 of *The Macmillan & Silk Cut Yachtsman's Handbook:*

The terms and definitions used in coastal navigation; magnetic variation and deviation: compass checks; compass adjusting and compass swinging; charts and their symbols; lights and fog signals; methods of laying off courses and position fixing; time, speed and distance; measured mile table; pilotage; IALA buoyage system; passage planning; the use of calculators; practical passage making; sailing directions.

3.1 DEFINITIONS AND TERMS

3.1.1 General

The information given in this chapter covers a few of the more important aspects of basic coastal navigation in simplified form, together with useful tables.

The Macmillan and Silk Cut Yachtsman's Handbook provides a more extensive reference on Coastal Navigation covering terms and definitions, charts, chartwork and pilotage.

3.1.2 Position

Position on the Earth's surface can be expressed in two ways. By Latitude and Longitude, or by a bearing and distance from a known position.

The latitude of a place is its distance North or South of the Equator. It is measured in degrees (°), minutes (') and decimals of a minute from 0° to 90° north or south of the equator.

The longitude of a place is measured in degrees (°), minutes ('), and decimals of a minute from 0° to 180° east or west from the Greenwich meridian.

3.1.3 Direction

Direction is measured clockwise from North in a three figure group, i.e. 000° to 359°. Thus East is written as 090°, and West 270°.

There are three different Norths from which direction is measured. It is imperative for a navigator to distinguish clearly between each. These are:

(1) **True** North measured from the North Geographic Pole.

(2) **Magnetic** North measured from the Magnetic North Pole, which does not coincide with the geographic pole.

(3) **Compass** North measured from the north seeking end of the compass needle.

Wind direction is normally given in points of the compass clockwise from a cardinal or quadrantal point rather than in degrees i.e. N, NNE, NE by N etc. There are 32 points of the compass, with each point equal to 11¼°.

Tidal streams are always expressed in the direction towards which they are running.

3.1.4 Compass variation and deviation

The magnetic compass is the most vital navigational instrument in a cruising boat. It is affected by **variation** (the angular difference between True North and Magnetic North), which alters from place to place, and by **deviation** which is the angular difference between the direction of magnetic North and the direction indicated by a compass needle (caused by the boat's local magnetic field).

Variation, which alters slightly from year to year, is shown on the chart – normally at the compass rose.

Deviation varies according to the boat's heading: it should be shown, for different headings, on a deviation card – produced as a result of swinging and adjusting the compass. With a properly adjusted compass, deviation should not be more than about 2° on any heading – in which case it can often be ignored except on long passages.

When converting a True course or a True bearing to Magnetic: add Westerly variation or deviation and subtract Easterly.

When converting a Magnetic course or bearing to True: subtract Westerly variation or deviation, and add Easterly.

Bearings given on charts, or quoted in Sailing Directions, are normally True bearings, from seaward.

3.1.5 Distance

Distance at sea is measured in nautical miles (M). A nautical mile is defined as the length of one minute of latitude.

The length of a nautical mile varies with latitude and measures 6108 feet at the Pole and 6046 at the Equator. For practical purposes the International nautical mile is taken as being 6076 feet or 1852 metres.

Short distances are measured in cables. A cable is one tenth of a nautical mile, and for practical purposes approximates to 200 yards, 600 feet or 100 fathoms in length and is always used for navigational purposes irrespective of the latitude.

Distances must always be measured from the latitude scale of a chart, never from the longitude scale because the length of one minute of longitude on the earth varies from being roughly equal to a minute of latitude at the Equator, to zero length at the Pole. The longitude scale is therefore of no value as a measure of distance.

3.1.6 Speed

Speed at sea is measured in knots. A knot is one nautical mile per hour. There is an important relationship between speed, time and distance. A convenient Time, Speed and Distance table is given in Table 3(5), (see also 3.4.1 for basic formulae used to find speed when time and distance are known, or to find distance when speed and time are known).

A log measures distance run through the water and most logs today also incorporate a speed indicator. Course and speed made good over the ground can be obtained directly from electronic position-fixing receivers such as GPS, Decca or Loran.

3.1.7 Depth

One of the most important functions of a navigator is to ensure he keeps the boat safely afloat in sufficient water. The depth of water is therefore highly important and is measured by echo sounder (or lead line). Chart Datum (CD) is the level below which the tide never, or very rarely, falls. Soundings and drying heights shown on charts are always referred to CD. The height of tide is the height of the sea surface above chart datum at any given instant. It is important that you should know whether the reading of the echo sounder gives the below keel or the true depth of the water. Tidal height calculations are fully covered in Chapter 9.

3.1.8 Light sectors, arcs of visibility

The abbreviations and characteristics for lights are shown in Fig 3.5.2 or on *Admiralty Chart 5011*.
The limits of light sectors and arcs of visibility, and the alignment of directional and leading lights, are given as seen from seaward by an observer aboard ship looking towards the light. All bearings are given in °True, starting from 000°, and going clockwise to 359°.

A typical example of a simple sectored light occurs with the Ouistreham main light, which is an Oc WR 4s 37m **W17M**, R13M having visibility sectors R115°-151°,W151°-115°. This is depicted in Fig 3(1) below. **Bold** type indicates a light with a nominal range of >15M which is 37 metres above the level of MHWS, occulting every 4s and has red and white sectors. The red sector of the light has a nominal range of 13 M; it is visible over an arc of 36°, i.e. between 115° (WNW of the light) and 151° (NW of the light). The white sector of the light is visible from 151° clockwise right round to 115°, an angular coverage of the remaining 324°; the white sector has a nominal range of 17M.

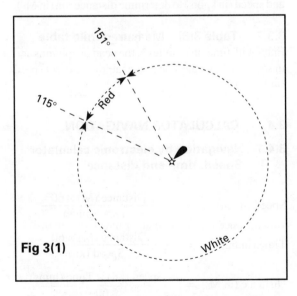

Fig 3(1)

Coloured sector lights often mean there are special navigation problems. Sometimes they show you where the channel is so if you stray to port you see red and if you stray to starboard you see green. Or alternatively, the lights are used to cover a dangerous area. Details are always shown on charts. A slightly more complex example of a sectored light listed as Q WRG 9m 10M, vis G015°-058°(43°), W058°-065°(7°), R065°-103°(38°), G103°-143·5°(40·5°), W143·5°-145·5°(3°), R146·5°-015° (129·5°) is shown in Fig. 3(2).

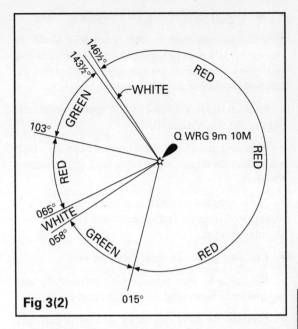

Fig 3(2)

It is a quick flashing light, with an elevation of 9 metres above MHWS, with a nominal range of 10M. It has White, Red and Green sectors – in fact two sectors of each colour. After plotting these sectors, it will be seen that there are two sets of WRG directional sectors, such that in each case a narrow White sector is flanked by a Red sector to port and a Green sector to starboard. The White sector defines the navigable channel; deviation out of the White sector is immediately obvious as the light changes colour to red or green as appropriate.

3.2 PASSAGE PLANNING

3.2.1 General

Detailed guidance on practical passage making and planning is contained in Chapter 15 of the *Macmillan and Silk Cut Nautical Handbook*.

Before commencing any passage it is necessary to undertake some form of basic planning. Having decided where you want to go, the next step is to study the charts and read any relevant yachtsman's sailing directions or cruising guides.

You also need to prepare a check-list of those items that need further detailed planning. Much of the required work such as laying off courses on the chart, measuring distances, selecting waypoints and making the necessary tidal calculations can all be done at home well before you start the passage.   If you possess or have access to a computer then all the tidal predictions for your entire trip can be done.

3.2.2 Passage planning checklist

The following is a suggested list of navigational items which need to be considered before departure. Other more general items such as the boat, crew and feeding arrangements may also need to be taken into account.

• Note the times of HW at the reference port(s).

• Tidal streams tend to form gates to a yacht on passage so you need to know the critical points of any tidal gates which affect your passage together with the times of favourable and adverse tides.

• Insert the dates and times of HW applicable on each page of the tidal stream atlas.

• Note the critical heights and times of any tides which may affect the departure, crossing bars, or destination harbours.

• Note potential dangers en-route: clearing lines, distances off dangers, Traffic Separation Schemes, busy shipping lanes etc.

• Consider visual and radio aids to be used.

• Prepare a detailed pilotage plan for entry to any unfamiliar harbour, final destination or refuge port.

• Consider the entry criteria for alternative harbours which might be required during the planned passage.

• Ensure that charts covering the intended route and alternative harbours that might be used are up to date and on board together with a copy of the current Almanac, Yachtsmans Handbook, and correcting Supplement, or the relevant lists of lights, radio and communication aids, and pilotage information.

Having completed all the necessary planning the weather is a major factor which is likely to have considerable impact and may well cause you to alter your original plans.

3.3   NAVIGATION TABLES

3.3.1   Tables - explanations
The tables listed below are given on pages 30-37. Here are brief explanations of their use. For greater detail see Chapter 3 in *The Macmillan & Silk Cut Yachtsman's Handbook.*

3.3.2   Table 3(1) – True bearing of Sun at sunrise and sunset
A compass can always be checked against the Sun's azimuth when rising or setting. In order to do so you only require to know the approximate latitude and the Sun's declination.

Enter with the approximate latitude and declination (extracted from the ephemeris in the Astro Supplement). The tabulated figure is the True bearing, measured from North if declination is North or from South if declination is South, towards the East if rising or towards the West if setting. Having extracted the True bearing, apply variation before comparing with the compass to determine deviation on course steered. The bearing of the Sun should be taken when its lower limb is a little over half a diameter above the horizon.

3.3.3   Table 3(2) – Distance off by Vertical Sextant Angle
Enter with the height of the body (in metres) and read across the page until the required sextant angle (corrected for index error) is met. Take out the distance of the object (in miles) at the head of the column. Caution is needed when the base of the object (e.g. a lighthouse) is below the horizon. For precise ranges the distance that sea level is below MHWS must be added to the height of the object (above MHWS) before entering the table.

3.3.4   Table 3(3) – Distance of horizon for various heights of eye
Enter with height of eye (in metres), and extract distance of horizon (in Miles). The actual distance may be affected by abnormal refraction.

3.3.5   Table 3(4) – Lights – distance off when rising or dipping
This table combines selected heights of eye with selected heights of lights, to give the range at which a light dips below or rises above the horizon.

3.3.6   Table 3(5) – Distance for a given speed and time
Enter with time (in decimals of an hour, or in minutes) and speed (in knots) to determine distance run (in Ms).

3.3.7   Table 3(6) – Measured mile table
Enter with time (in minutes at the head of columns and in seconds down the side of the table) to extract speed (in knots).

3.4   CALCULATOR NAVIGATION

3.4.1   Navigation by electronic calculator Speed, time and distance

$$\text{Speed (in kn)} = \frac{\text{Distance (M)} \times 60}{\text{Time (mins)}}$$

$$\text{Time (in mins)} = \frac{\text{Distance (M)} \times 60}{\text{Speed (kn)}}$$

$$\text{Distance (in M)} = \frac{\text{Speed (kn)} \times \text{Time (mins)}}{60}$$

Distances and speed

Distance of horizon (in M) = $2 \cdot 072 \times \sqrt{\text{Ht of eye (m)}}$

Distance a light is visible (M) = $2 \cdot 072 \times (\sqrt{h_o} + \sqrt{h_e})$ where heights are in metres.

Distance of mountains etc. beyond horizon, in

$M = \sqrt{3 \cdot 71}(h_o - h_e) + (a - 1 \cdot 76 \times \sqrt{h_e})^2 - (a - 1 \cdot 76 \times \sqrt{h_e})$ where both heights are in metres, and a is the sextant angle in minutes.

Distance to radar horizon (M)
$$= 2{\cdot}21 \times \sqrt{\text{Ht of scanner (m)}}$$

Boat speed over measured distance of lM =
$$\frac{3600}{\text{time in seconds}} \text{ (knots)}$$

Horizontal sextant angle

Radius of position circle (in M) =
$$\frac{D}{2 \times \sin A}$$
where D is distance between objects in M, and A is the angle between them in degrees.

Vertical sextant angle

Distance off = $\dfrac{\text{Ht of object (above MHWS in m)}}{1852 \times \tan \text{ (sextant angle)}}$

Note: sextant angle above is in degrees and minutes, and must be corrected for index error.

An approximate distance off, in Ms, adequate for most purposes is given by:

Distance = $\dfrac{\text{Ht of object (in metres)} \times 1{\cdot}854}{\text{Sextant angle (in minutes)}}$

Coastal navigation

To find the DR/EP, as bearing and distance from start position; example using algebraic calculator. Key in:

1st distance run	5.2	x < > t
1st course (°T)	230	→R STO 0 x< >t STO 6
2nd distance run	1.9	x< >t
2nd course (°T)	255	→R SUM 0 x< >t SUM 6

Repeat for each subsequent Co(°T) and distance. For EP, treat Set/Drift as for Co(°T) and distance.

To display bearing and distance from start:

RCL 6 x < >t RCL 0 → P	236.6	(°T)	
x< >t	6.97	(M)	

Note: To find EP, treat Set/Drift as for Co(°T) and distance run.
Example: Using RPN calculator. Key in:

1st course (°T)	230 ENTER	
1st distance run	5.2	→R Σ+
2nd course (°T)	255 ENTER	
2nd distance run	1.9	→R Σ+

Repeat for each subsequent Co(°T) and distance.

To display distance and bearing from start:

RCL 13[1] RCL 11[1]	→P	6.97	M
x ↔ y		236.6[2]	(°T)

Notes: (1) Check the actual stores used for vector summation in your calculator.
(2) If display negative (–), add 360.

To find EP, treat Set/Drift as for Co(°T) and distance run.
Distance (D, in M) of object at second bearing
$$= \frac{R \times \sin A}{\sin (B - A)}$$

Predicted distance (in Ms) object will be off when abeam = D x sin B, where R is distance run (M) between two relative bearings of an object, first A degrees and then B degrees.

Course to steer and speed made good

Co (°T) = Tr (°T) – sin⁻¹ – ((Drift ÷ Speed) × sin (Set – Track))
SMG = Speed × cos (Co.T – Track) + Drift × cos (Set – Track)

Note: The Drift must be less than the yacht's speed.

Conversion angle (half convergency)

Radio bearings follow great circles, and become curved lines when plotted on a Mercator chart. A correction may be needed for bearings of beacons more than about 60Ms away, and can be calculated from the formula:
Conversion angle = ½ d.Long × sin mid Latitude
A great circle always lies on the polar side of the rhumb line, and conversion angle is applied towards the equator. Further information is given in Chapter 4 in *The Macmillan & Silk Cut Yachtsman's Handbook*.

Short distance sailing

(Note: These formulae should not be used for distances over 600M).

Departure	=	Distance × sin Course
	=	d.Long × cos Mean Latitude
	=	tan Course × d.Lat
d.Lat	=	Distance × cos Course
d.Long	=	Departure ÷ cos Mean Latitude
Distance	=	Departure ÷ sin Course
	=	d.Lat × sec Course
sin Course	=	Departure ÷ Distance
cos Course	=	d.Lat ÷ Distance
tan Course	=	Departure ÷ d.Lat

Further explanation of the use of calculators, and formulae for the calculation of tracks and distances for distances over 600Ms are contained in Chapter 3 of *The Macmillan & Silk Cut Yachtsman's Handbook*.

3

3.5   IALA BUOYAGE

3.5.1   IALA Buoyage System (Region A)
(See also Plate 5 on page 67.)

International buoyage is harmonised into a single system which, applied to Regions A and B, differs only in the use of red and green lateral marks. In Region A (which includes all Europe) lateral marks are red on the port hand, and in Region B red on the starboard hand, related to direction of buoyage. Five types of marks are used, as illustrated in Plate 5, on page 67.

(1) *Lateral marks* are used in conjunction with a direction of buoyage, shown by a special arrow on the chart. In and around the British Isles its general direction is from SW to NE in open waters, but from seaward when approaching a harbour, river or estuary. Where port or starboard lateral marks do not rely on can or conical buoy shapes for identification, they carry, where practicable, the appropriate topmarks. Any numbering or lettering follows the direction of buoyage, evens to port and odds to starboard.

In Region A, port-hand marks are coloured red, and port-hand buoys are can or spar shaped. Any topmark fitted is a single red can. Any light fitted is red, any rhythm. Starboard-hand marks are coloured green, and starboard-hand buoys are conical or spar shaped. Any topmark fitted is a single green cone, point up. Any light fitted is green, any rhythm. In exceptional cases starboard-hand marks may be coloured black.

At a division, the preferred channel may be shown by lateral marks with red or green bands:

Preferred channel	Indicated by	Light (if any)
To starboard	Port lateral mark with green band	Flashing red (2 + 1)
To port	Starboard lateral mark with red band	Flashing green (2 + 1)

(2) *Cardinal marks* are used in conjunction with a compass to show where dangers exist or where the mariner may find navigable water. They are named after the quadrant in which the mark is placed, in relation to the danger or point indicated. The four quadrants (North, East, South and West) are bounded by the true bearings NW-NE, NE-SE, SE-SW and SW-NW, taken from the point of interest. The name of a cardinal mark indicates that it should be passed on the named side.

A cardinal mark may indicate the safe side on which to pass a danger, or that the deepest water is on the named side of the mark, or it may draw attention to a feature in a channel such as a bend, junction or fork, or the end of a shoal.

Cardinal marks are pillar or spar shaped, painted black and yellow, and always carry black double cone topmarks, one cone above the other. Their lights are white, either very quick flashing (Q or VQ) 100 to 120 flashes per minute, or quick flashing (Q or VQ) 50 to 60 flashes per minute. A long flash is one of not less than two seconds duration.

North cardinal mark

Two black cones	— Points up
Colour	— Black above yellow
Light (if fitted)	— White; Q or VQ

East cardinal mark

Two black cones	— Base to base
Colour	— Black, with horizontal yellow band
Light (if fitted)	— White; Q (3) 10 sec or VQ (3) 5 sec

South cardinal mark

Two black cones	— Points down
Colour	— Yellow above black
Light (if fitted)	— White; VQ (6) plus long flash 10 sec or Q (6) plus long flash 15 sec

West cardinal mark

Two black cones	— Point to point
Colour	— Yellow, with horizontal black band
Light (if fitted)	— White; VQ (9) 10 sec or Q (9) 15 sec

(3) *Isolated danger marks* are placed on or above an isolated danger such as a rock or a wreck which has navigable water all around it. The marks are black, with one or more broad horizontal red bands. Buoys are pillar or spar shaped. Any light is white, flashing twice. Topmark – two black spheres.

(4) *Safe water marks* indicate that there is navigable water all round the mark, and are used for mid-channel or landfall marks. Buoys are spherical, pillar, with spherical topmark or spar, and are coloured with red and white vertical stripes. Any topmark fitted is a single red sphere. Any light fitted is white - either isophase, occulting or long flash every 10 seconds.

(5) *Special marks* do not primarily assist navigation, but indicate a special area or feature (e.g. spoil grounds, exercise areas, water ski areas, cable or pipeline marks, outfalls, Ocean Data Acquisition Systems (ODAS), or traffic separation marks where conventional channel marks may cause confusion). Special marks are yellow, and any shape not conflicting with lateral or safe water marks. If can, spherical or conical are used they indicate the side on which to pass. Any topmark fitted is a yellow X. Any light fitted is yellow, and may have any rhythm not used for white lights.

New dangers (which may be natural obstructions such as a sandbank, or a wreck for example) are marked in accordance with the rules above, and lit accordingly. For a very grave danger one of the marks may be duplicated.

3.5.2 Light Characteristics (Metric and Fathoms Charts)

Reproduced by kind permission of H.M. Stationery Office and the Hydrographer of the Navy

CLASS OF LIGHT	International abbreviations	National abbreviations	Illustration Period shown ⊢————⊣
Fixed	F		
Occulting *(total duration of light more than dark)*			
Single-occulting	Oc	Occ	
Group-occulting e.g.	Oc(2)	Gp Occ(2)	
Composite group-occulting e.g.	Oc(2+3)	Gp Occ(2+3)	
Isophase *(light and dark equal)*	Iso		
Flashing *(total duration of light less than dark)*			
Single-flashing	Fl		
Long-flashing *(flash 2s or longer)*	L Fl		
Group-flashing e.g.	Fl(3)	Gp Fl(3)	
Composite group-flashing e.g.	Fl(2+1)	Gp Fl(2+1)	
Quick *(50 to 79 – usually either 50 or 60 – flashes per minute)*			
Continuous quick	Q	Qk Fl	
Group quick e.g.	Q(3)	Qk Fl(3)	
Interrupted quick	IQ	Int Qk Fl	
Very Quick *(80 to 159 – usually either 100 or 120 - flashes per minute)*			
Continuous very quick	VQ	V Qk Fl	
Group very quick e.g.	VQ(3)	V Qk Fl(3)	
Interrupted very quick	IVQ	Int V Qk Fl	
Ultra Quick *(160 or more – usually 240 to 300 – flashes per minute)*			
Continuous ultra quick	UQ		
Interrupted ultra quick	IUQ		
Morse Code e.g.	Mo(K)		
Fixed and Flashing	F Fl		
Alternating e.g.	Al.WR	Alt.WR	

COLOUR	International abbreviations	NOMINAL RANGE in miles		International abbreviations
White	W *(may be omitted)*	Light with single range	e.g.	15M
Red	R			
Green	G	Light with two different ranges	e.g.	15/10M
Blue	Bu			
Violet	Vi	Light with three or more ranges	e.g.	15-7M
Yellow	Y			
Orange	Y	**PERIOD** is given in seconds	e.g.	90s
Amber	Y			
ELEVATION is given in metres (m) or feet (ft) above MHWS		**DISPOSITION** horizontally disposed vertically disposed		(hor) (vert)

Coastal Navigation

TABLE 3(1) True bearing of sun at sunrise and sunset

DECLINATION

LAT	0°	1°	2°	3°	4°	5°	6°	7°	8°	9°	10°	11°	LAT
30°	90	88·8	87·7	86·5	85·4	84·2	83·1	81·9	80·7	79·6	78·4	77·3	30°
31°	90	88·8	87·7	86·5	85·3	84·2	83·0	81·9	80·6	79·5	78·3	77·1	31°
32°	90	88·8	87·6	86·5	85·3	84·1	82·9	81·7	80·5	79·4	78·2	77·0	32°
33°	90	88·8	87·6	86·4	85·2	84·0	82·8	81·6	80·4	79·2	78·0	76·8	33°
34°	90	88·8	87·6	86·4	85·2	84·0	82·7	81·5	80·3	79·1	77·9	76·7	34°
35°	90	88·8	87·5	86·3	85·1	83·9	82·7	81·4	80·2	79·0	77·8	76·5	35°
36°	90	88·8	87·5	86·3	85·0	83·8	82·6	81·3	80·1	78·8	77·6	76·3	36°
37°	90	88·7	87·5	86·2	85·0	83·7	82·5	81·2	80·0	78·7	77·4	76·2	37°
38°	90	88·7	87·5	86·2	84·9	83·6	82·4	81·1	79·8	78·5	77·3	76·0	38°
39°	90	88·7	87·4	86·1	84·8	83·6	82·3	81·0	79·7	78·4	77·1	75·8	39°
40°	90	88·7	87·4	86·1	84·8	83·5	82·1	80·8	79·5	78·2	76·9	75·6	40°
41°	90	88·7	87·3	86·0	84·7	83·4	82·0	80·7	79·4	78·0	76·7	75·3	41°
42°	90	88·6	87·3	86·0	84·6	83·3	81·9	80·6	79·2	77·8	76·5	75·1	42°
43°	90	88·6	87·3	85·9	84·5	83·1	81·8	80·4	79·0	77·6	76·3	74·9	43°
44°	90	88·6	87·2	85·8	84·4	83·0	81·6	80·2	78·8	77·4	76·0	74·6	44°
45°	90	88·6	87·2	85·7	84·3	82·9	81·5	80·1	78·6	77·2	75·8	74·3	45°
46°	90	88·6	87·1	85·7	84·2	82·8	81·3	79·9	78·4	77·0	75·5	74·0	46°
47°	90	88·5	87·1	85·6	84·1	82·6	81·2	79·7	78·2	76·7	75·2	73·7	47°
48°	90	88·5	87·0	85·5	84·0	82·5	81·0	79·5	78·0	76·5	75·0	73·4	48°
49°	90	88·5	86·9	85·4	83·9	82·4	80·8	79·3	77·7	76·2	74·6	73·1	49°
50°	90	88·4	86·9	85·3	83·8	82·2	80·6	79·1	77·5	75·9	74·3	72·7	50°
51°	90	88·4	86·8	85·2	83·6	82·0	80·4	78·8	77·2	75·6	74·0	72·4	51°
52°	90	88·4	86·7	85·1	83·5	81·9	80·2	78·6	76·9	75·3	73·6	71·9	52°
53°	90	88·3	86·7	85·0	83·3	81·7	80·0	78·3	76·6	74·9	73·2	71·5	53°
54°	90	88·3	86·6	84·9	83·2	81·5	79·8	78·0	76·3	74·6	72·8	71·1	54°
55°	90	88·2	86·5	84·8	83·0	81·3	79·5	77·7	76·0	74·2	72·4	70·6	55°
56°	90	88·2	86·4	84·6	82·8	81·0	79·2	77·4	75·6	73·8	71·9	70·0	56°
57°	90	88·2	86·3	84·5	82·6	80·8	78·9	77·0	75·2	73·3	71·4	69·5	57°
58°	90	88·1	86·2	84·3	82·4	80·5	78·6	76·7	74·8	72·8	70·9	68·9	58°
59°	90	88·1	86·1	84·2	82·2	80·3	78·3	76·3	74·3	72·3	70·3	68·3	59°
60°	90	88·0	86·0	84·0	82·0	80·0	77·9	75·9	73·8	71·8	69·7	67·6	60°

DECLINATION

LAT	12°	13°	14°	15°	16°	17°	18°	19°	20°	21°	22°	23°	LAT
30°	76·1	74·9	73·8	72·6	71·4	70·3	69·1	67·9	66·7	65·5	64·4	63·2	30°
31°	76·0	74·8	73·6	72·4	71·2	70·0	68·9	67·7	66·5	65·3	64·1	62·9	31°
32°	75·8	74·6	73·4	72·2	71·0	69·8	68·6	67·4	66·2	65·0	63·8	62·6	32°
33°	75·6	74·4	73·2	72·1	70·8	69·6	68·4	67·1	65·9	64·7	63·5	62·2	33°
34°	75·5	74·2	73·0	71·8	70·6	69·3	68·1	66·9	65·6	64·4	63·1	61·9	34°
35°	75·3	74·1	72·8	71·6	70·3	69·1	67·8	66·6	65·3	64·1	62·8	61·5	35°
36°	75·1	73·8	72·6	71·3	70·1	68·8	67·5	66·3	65·0	63·7	62·4	61·1	36°
37°	74·9	73·6	72·4	71·1	69·8	68·5	67·2	65·9	64·6	63·3	62·0	60·7	37°
38°	74·7	73·4	72·0	70·8	69·5	68·2	66·9	65·6	64·3	62·9	61·6	60·3	38°
39°	74·5	73·2	71·9	70·5	69·2	67·9	66·6	65·2	63·9	62·5	61·2	59·8	39°
40°	74·2	72·9	71·6	70·2	68·9	67·6	66·2	64·8	63·5	62·1	60·7	59·3	40°
41°	74·0	72·7	71·3	69·9	68·6	67·2	65·8	64·4	63·0	61·6	60·2	58·8	41°
42°	73·7	72·4	71·0	69·6	68·2	66·8	65·4	64·0	62·6	61·2	59·7	58·3	42°
43°	73·5	72·1	70·7	69·3	67·9	66·4	65·0	63·6	62·1	60·7	59·2	57·7	43°
44°	73·2	71·8	70·3	68·9	67·5	66·0	64·6	63·1	61·6	60·1	58·6	57·1	44°
45°	72·9	71·4	70·0	68·5	67·0	65·6	64·1	62·6	61·1	59·5	58·0	56·4	45°
46°	72·6	71·1	69·6	68·1	66·6	65·1	63·6	62·0	60·5	58·9	57·4	55·8	46°
47°	72·2	70·7	69·2	67·7	66·2	64·6	63·1	61·5	59·9	58·3	56·7	55·0	47°
48°	71·9	70·3	68·8	67·2	65·7	64·1	62·5	60·9	59·3	57·6	55·9	54·3	48°
49°	71·5	69·9	68·4	66·8	65·1	63·5	61·9	60·2	58·6	56·9	55·2	53·4	49°
50°	71·1	69·5	67·9	66·2	64·6	62·9	61·3	59·6	57·8	56·1	54·3	52·6	50°
51°	70·7	69·1	67·4	65·7	64·0	62·3	60·6	58·8	57·1	55·3	53·5	51·6	51°
52°	70·3	68·6	66·9	65·1	63·4	61·6	59·9	58·1	56·3	54·4	52·5	50·6	52°
53°	69·8	68·1	66·3	64·5	62·7	60·9	59·1	57·3	55·4	53·5	51·5	49·5	53°
54°	69·3	67·5	65·7	63·9	62·0	60·2	58·3	56·4	54·4	52·4	50·4	48·3	54°
55°	68·7	66·9	65·1	63·2	61·3	59·4	57·4	55·4	53·4	51·3	49·2	47·1	55°
56°	68·2	66·3	64·4	62·4	60·5	58·5	56·5	54·4	52·3	50·1	47·9	45·7	56°
57°	67·6	65·6	63·6	61·6	59·6	57·5	55·4	53·3	51·1	48·9	46·5	44·2	57°
58°	66·9	64·9	62·8	60·8	58·7	56·5	54·3	52·1	49·8	47·4	45·0	42·5	58°
59°	66·2	64·1	62·0	59·8	57·6	55·4	53·1	50·8	48·4	45·9	43·3	40·7	59°
60°	65·4	63·3	61·1	58·8	56·5	54·2	51·8	49·4	46·8	44·2	41·5	38·6	60°

TABLE 3(2)   Distance off by Vertical Sextant Angle

Height of object ft	m	0·1	0·2	0·3	0·4	0·5	0·6	0·7	0·8	0·9	1·0	1·1	1·2	1·3	1·4	1·5	m	ft
		° ′	° ′	° ′	° ′	° ′	° ′	° ′	° ′	° ′	° ′	° ′	° ′	° ′	° ′	° ′		
33	10	3 05	1 33	1 02	0 46	0 37	0 31	0 27	0 23	0 21	0 19	0 17	0 15	0 14	0 13	0 12	10	33
39	12	3 42	1 51	1 14	0 56	0 45	0 37	0 32	0 28	0 25	0 22	0 20	0 19	0 17	0 16	0 15	12	39
46	14	4 19	2 10	1 27	1 05	0 52	0 43	0 37	0 32	0 29	0 26	0 24	0 22	0 20	0 19	0 17	14	46
53	16	4 56	2 28	1 39	1 14	0 59	0 49	0 42	0 37	0 33	0 30	0 27	0 25	0 23	0 21	0 20	16	53
59	18	5 33	2 47	1 51	1 24	1 07	0 56	0 48	0 42	0 37	0 33	0 30	0 28	0 26	0 24	0 22	18	59
66	20	6 10	3 05	2 04	1 33	1 14	1 02	0 53	0 46	0 41	0 37	0 34	0 31	0 29	0 27	0 25	20	66
72	22	6 46	3 24	2 16	1 42	1 22	1 08	0 58	0 51	0 45	0 41	0 37	0 34	0 31	0 29	0 27	22	72
79	24	7 23	3 42	2 28	1 51	1 29	1 14	1 04	0 56	0 49	0 45	0 40	0 37	0 34	0 32	0 30	24	79
85	26	7 59	4 01	2 41	2 01	1 36	1 20	1 09	1 00	0 54	0 48	0 44	0 40	0 37	0 34	0 32	26	85
92	28	8 36	4 19	2 53	2 10	1 44	1 27	1 14	1 05	0 58	0 52	0 47	0 43	0 40	0 37	0 35	28	92
98	30	9 12	4 38	3 05	2 19	1 51	1 33	1 20	1 10	1 02	0 56	0 51	0 46	0 43	0 40	0 37	30	98
105	32	9 48	4 56	3 18	2 28	1 58	1 39	1 25	1 14	1 06	0 59	0 54	0 49	0 46	0 42	0 40	32	105
112	34	10 24	5 15	3 30	2 38	2 06	1 45	1 30	1 19	1 10	1 03	0 57	0 53	0 49	0 45	0 42	34	112
118	36	11 00	5 33	3 42	2 47	2 14	1 51	1 35	1 24	1 14	1 07	1 01	0 56	0 51	0 48	0 45	36	118
125	38	11 36	5 41	3 55	2 56	2 21	1 58	1 41	1 28	1 18	1 11	1 04	0 59	0 54	0 50	0 47	38	125
131	40	12 11	6 10	4 07	3 05	2 28	2 04	1 46	1 33	1 22	1 14	1 07	1 02	0 57	0 53	0 49	40	131
138	42	12 47	6 28	4 19	3 15	2 36	2 10	1 51	1 37	1 27	1 18	1 11	1 05	1 00	0 56	0 52	42	138
144	44	13 22	6 46	4 32	3 24	2 43	2 16	1 57	1 42	1 31	1 22	1 14	1 08	1 03	0 58	0 54	44	144
151	46	13 57	7 05	4 44	3 33	2 51	2 22	2 02	1 47	1 35	1 25	1 18	1 11	1 06	1 01	0 57	46	151
157	48	14 32	7 23	4 56	3 42	2 58	2 28	2 07	1 51	1 39	1 29	1 21	1 14	1 09	1 04	0 59	48	157
164	50	15 07	7 41	5 09	3 52	3 05	2 35	2 13	1 56	1 43	1 33	1 24	1 17	1 11	1 06	1 02	50	164
171	52	15 41	7 59	5 21	4 01	3 13	2 41	2 18	2 01	1 47	1 36	1 28	1 20	1 14	1 09	1 04	52	171
177	54	16 15	8 18	5 33	4 10	3 20	2 47	2 23	2 05	1 51	1 40	1 31	1 23	1 17	1 12	1 07	54	177
184	56	16 49	8 36	5 45	4 19	3 28	2 53	2 28	2 10	1 55	1 44	1 34	1 27	1 20	1 14	1 09	56	184
190	58	17 23	8 54	5 58	4 29	3 35	2 59	2 34	2 15	2 00	1 48	1 38	1 30	1 23	1 17	1 12	58	190
197	60	17 57	9 12	6 10	4 38	3 42	3 05	2 39	2 19	2 04	1 51	1 41	1 33	1 26	1 20	1 14	60	197
203	62	18 31	9 30	6 22	4 47	3 50	3 12	2 44	2 24	2 08	1 55	1 45	1 36	1 29	1 22	1 17	62	203
210	64	19 04	9 48	6 34	4 56	3 57	3 18	2 50	2 28	2 12	1 59	1 48	1 39	1 31	1 25	1 19	64	210
217	66	19 37	10 06	6 46	5 05	4 05	3 24	2 53	2 33	2 16	2 02	1 51	1 42	1 34	1 27	1 22	66	217
223	68	20 10	10 24	6 59	5 15	4 12	3 30	3 00	2 38	2 20	2 06	1 55	1 45	1 37	1 30	1 24	68	223
230	70	20 42	10 42	7 11	5 24	4 19	3 36	3 05	2 42	2 24	2 09	1 58	1 48	1 40	1 33	1 27	70	230
236	72	21 15	11 00	7 23	5 33	4 27	3 42	3 11	2 47	2 28	2 14	2 01	1 51	1 43	1 35	1 29	72	236
246	75	22 03	11 27	7 41	5 47	4 38	3 52	3 19	2 54	2 35	2 19	2 07	1 56	1 47	1 39	1 33	75	246
256	78	22 50	11 54	7 59	6 01	4 49	4 01	3 27	3 01	2 41	2 24	2 12	2 01	1 51	1 43	1 36	78	256
266	81	23 37	12 20	8 18	6 14	5 00	4 10	3 35	3 08	2 47	2 30	2 17	2 05	1 56	1 47	1 40	81	266
276	84	24 24	12 47	8 36	6 28	5 11	4 19	3 42	3 15	2 53	2 36	2 22	2 10	2 00	1 51	1 44	84	276
289	88	25 25	13 22	9 00	6 46	5 26	4 32	3 53	3 24	3 01	2 43	2 28	2 16	2 06	1 57	1 49	88	289
302	92	26 25	13 57	9 24	7 05	5 40	4 44	4 04	3 33	3 10	2 51	2 35	2 22	2 11	2 02	1 54	92	302
315	96	27 24	14 32	9 48	7 23	5 55	4 56	4 14	3 42	3 18	2 58	2 42	2 28	2 17	2 07	1 59	96	315
328	100	28 22	15 07	10 12	7 41	6 10	5 09	4 25	3 52	3 26	3 05	2 49	2 35	2 23	2 13	2 04	100	328
341	104	29 19	15 41	10 36	7 59	6 24	5 21	4 35	4 01	3 34	3 13	2 55	2 41	2 28	2 18	2 09	104	341
358	109	30 29	16 24	11 06	8 22	6 43	5 36	4 48	4 12	3 44	3 22	3 04	2 48	2 36	2 24	2 15	109	358
374	114	31 37	17 06	11 36	8 45	7 01	5 51	5 02	4 24	3 55	3 31	3 12	2 56	2 43	2 31	2 21	114	374
394	120	32 56	17 57	12 11	9 12	7 23	6 10	5 17	4 38	4 07	3 42	3 22	3 05	2 51	2 39	2 28	120	394
427	130	35 04	19 20	13 10	9 57	8 00	6 40	5 44	5 01	4 28	4 01	3 39	3 21	3 05	2 52	2 41	130	427
459	140	37 05	20 42	14 09	10 42	8 36	7 11	6 10	5 24	4 48	4 19	3 56	3 36	3 20	3 05	2 53	140	459
492	150	39 00	22 03	15 07	11 27	9 12	7 41	6 36	5 47	5 09	4 38	4 13	3 52	3 34	3 19	3 05	150	492
574	175		25 17	17 29	13 17	10 42	8 57	7 41	6 44	6 00	5 24	4 55	4 30	4 09	3 52	3 36	175	574
656	200		28 22	19 48	15 07	12 11	10 12	8 46	7 41	6 51	6 10	5 36	5 09	4 45	4 25	4 07	200	656
738	225			22 03	16 54	13 39	11 27	9 51	8 38	7 41	6 56	6 18	5 47	5 20	4 58	4 38	225	738
820	250			24 14	18 39	15 07	12 41	10 55	9 35	8 32	7 41	7 00	6 25	5 56	5 30	5 09	250	820
902	275			26 20	20 22	16 32	13 54	11 59	10 31	9 22	8 27	7 41	7 03	6 31	6 03	5 39	275	902
984	300				22 03	17 57	15 07	13 02	11 27	10 12	9 12	8 23	7 41	7 06	6 36	6 10	300	984
1148	350					20 42	17 29	15 07	13 17	11 51	10 42	9 45	8 57	8 16	7 41	7 11	350	1148
1312	400						19 48	17 09	15 07	13 30	12 11	11 07	10 12	9 26	8 46	8 12	400	1312
ft m Height of object		0·1	0·2	0·3	0·4	0·5	0·6	0·7	0·8	0·9	1·0	1·1	1·2	1·3	1·4	1·5	m ft Height of object	

Distance of object (miles)

TABLE 3(2) Distance off by Vertical Sextant Angle (continued)

ft	m	1·6	1·7	1·8	1·9	2·0	2·1	2·2	2·3	2·4	2·5	2·6	2·7	2·8	2·9	3·0	m	ft
		o ′	o ′	o ′	o ′	o ′	o ′	o ′	o ′	o ′	o ′	o ′	o ′	o ′	o ′	o ′		
33	10	0 12	0 11	0 10	0 10												10	33
39	12	0 14	0 13	0 12	0 12	0 11	0 11	0 10	0 10	0 10							12	39
46	14	0 16	0 15	0 14	0 14	0 13	0 12	0 12	0 11	0 11	0 10	0 10	0 10				14	46
53	16	0 19	0 17	0 16	0 16	0 15	0 14	0 13	0 13	0 12	0 12	0 11	0 11	0 11	0 10	0 10	16	53
59	18	0 21	0 20	0 19	0 18	0 17	0 16	0 15	0 15	0 14	0 13	0 13	0 12	0 12	0 12	0 11	18	59
66	20	0 23	0 22	0 21	0 20	0 19	0 18	0 17	0 16	0 15	0 15	0 14	0 14	0 13	0 13	0 12	20	66
72	22	0 26	0 24	0 23	0 21	0 20	0 19	0 19	0 18	0 17	0 16	0 16	0 15	0 15	0 14	0 14	22	72
79	24	0 28	0 26	0 25	0 23	0 22	0 21	0 20	0 19	0 19	0 18	0 17	0 16	0 16	0 15	0 15	24	79
85	26	0 30	0 28	0 27	0 25	0 24	0 23	0 22	0 21	0 20	0 19	0 19	0 18	0 17	0 17	0 16	26	85
92	28	0 32	0 31	0 29	0 27	0 26	0 25	0 24	0 23	0 22	0 21	0 20	0 19	0 19	0 18	0 17	28	92
98	30	0 35	0 33	0 31	0 29	0 28	0 27	0 25	0 24	0 23	0 22	0 21	0 21	0 20	0 19	0 19	30	98
105	32	0 37	0 35	0 33	0 31	0 30	0 28	0 27	0 26	0 25	0 24	0 23	0 22	0 21	0 20	0 20	32	105
112	34	0 39	0 37	0 35	0 33	0 31	0 30	0 29	0 27	0 26	0 25	0 24	0 23	0 23	0 22	0 21	34	112
118	36	0 42	0 39	0 37	0 35	0 33	0 32	0 30	0 29	0 28	0 27	0 26	0 25	0 24	0 23	0 22	36	118
125	38	0 44	0 41	0 39	0 37	0 35	0 34	0 32	0 31	0 29	0 28	0 27	0 26	0 25	0 24	0 24	38	125
131	40	0 46	0 44	0 41	0 39	0 37	0 35	0 34	0 32	0 31	0 30	0 29	0 27	0 27	0 26	0 25	40	131
138	42	0 49	0 46	0 43	0 41	0 40	0 37	0 35	0 34	0 32	0 31	0 30	0 29	0 28	0 27	0 26	42	138
144	44	0 51	0 48	0 45	0 43	0 41	0 39	0 37	0 36	0 34	0 33	0 31	0 30	0 29	0 28	0 27	44	144
151	46	0 53	0 50	0 47	0 45	0 43	0 41	0 39	0 37	0 36	0 34	0 33	0 32	0 30	0 29	0 28	46	151
157	48	0 56	0 52	0 49	0 47	0 45	0 42	0 40	0 39	0 37	0 36	0 34	0 33	0 32	0 31	0 30	48	1 57
164	50	0 58	0 55	0 52	0 49	0 46	0 44	0 42	0 40	0 39	0 37	0 36	0 34	0 33	0 32	0 31	50	164
171	52	1 00	0 57	0 54	0 51	0 48	0 46	0 44	0 42	0 40	0 39	0 37	0 36	0 34	0 33	0 32	52	171
177	54	1 03	0 59	0 56	0 53	0 50	0 48	0 46	0 44	0 42	0 40	0 39	0 37	0 36	0 35	0 33	54	177
184	56	1 05	1 01	0 58	0 55	0 52	0 49	0 47	0 45	0 43	0 42	0 40	0 38	0 37	0 36	0 35	56	184
190	58	1 07	1 03	1 00	0 57	0 54	0 51	0 49	0 47	0 45	0 43	0 41	0 40	0 38	0 37	0 36	58	190
197	60	1 10	1 06	1 02	0 59	0 56	0 53	0 51	0 48	0 46	0 45	0 43	0 41	0 40	0 38	0 37	60	197
203	62	1 12	1 08	1 04	1 01	0 58	0 55	0 52	0 50	0 48	0 46	0 44	0 43	0 41	0 40	0 38	62	203
210	64	1 14	1 10	1 06	1 03	0 59	0 57	0 54	0 52	0 49	0 48	0 46	0 44	0 42	0 41	0 40	64	210
217	66	1 17	1 12	1 08	1 05	1 01	0 58	0 56	0 53	0 51	0 49	0 47	0 45	0 44	0 42	0 41	66	217
223	68	1 19	1 14	1 10	1 06	1 03	1 00	0 57	0 55	0 53	0 50	0 49	0 47	0 45	0 44	0 42	68	223
230	70	1 21	1 16	1 12	1 08	1 05	1 02	0 59	0 56	0 54	0 52	0 50	0 48	0 46	0 45	0 43	70	230
236	72	1 24	1 19	1 14	1 10	1 07	1 04	1 01	0 58	0 56	0 53	0 51	0 49	0 48	0 46	0 45	72	236
246	75	1 27	1 22	1 17	1 13	1 10	1 06	1 03	1 01	0 58	0 56	0 54	0 51	0 50	0 48	0 46	75	246
256	78	1 30	1 25	1 20	1 16	1 12	1 09	1 06	1 03	1 00	0 58	0 56	0 54	0 52	0 50	0 48	78	256
266	81	1 34	1 28	1 23	1 19	1 15	1 12	1 08	1 05	1 03	1 00	0 58	0 56	0 54	0 52	0 50	81	266
276	84	1 37	1 32	1 27	1 22	1 18	1 14	1 11	1 08	1 05	1 02	1 00	0 58	0 56	0 54	0 52	84	276
289	88	1 42	1 36	1 31	1 26	1 22	1 18	1 14	1 11	1 08	1 05	1 03	1 00	0 58	0 56	0 54	88	289
302	92	1 47	1 40	1 35	1 30	1 25	1 21	1 18	1 14	1 11	1 08	1 06	1 03	1 01	0 59	0 57	92	302
315	96	1 51	1 45	1 39	1 34	1 29	1 25	1 21	1 17	1 14	1 11	1 09	1 06	1 04	1 01	0 59	96	315
328	100	1 56	1 49	1 43	1 38	1 33	1 28	1 24	1 21	1 17	1 14	1 11	1 09	1 06	1 04	1 02	100	328
341	104	2 01	1 54	1 47	1 42	1 36	1 32	1 28	1 24	1 20	1 17	1 14	1 11	1 09	1 07	1 04	104	341
358	109	2 06	1 59	1 52	1 46	1 41	1 36	1 32	1 28	1 24	1 21	1 18	1 15	1 12	1 10	1 07	109	358
374	114	2 12	2 04	1 58	1 51	1 46	1 41	1 36	1 32	1 28	1 25	1 21	1 18	1 16	1 13	1 11	114	374
394	120	2 19	2 11	2 04	1 57	1 51	1 46	1 41	1 37	1 33	1 29	1 26	1 22	1 20	1 17	1 14	120	394
427	130	2 31	2 22	2 14	2 07	2 01	1 55	1 50	1 45	1 41	1 36	1 33	1 29	1 26	1 23	1 20	130	427
459	140	2 42	2 33	2 24	2 17	2 10	2 04	1 58	1 53	1 48	1 44	1 40	1 36	1 33	1 30	1 27	140	459
492	150	2 54	2 44	2 35	2 26	2 19	2 13	2 07	2 01	1 56	1 51	1 47	1 43	1 39	1 36	1 33	150	492
574	175	3 23	3 11	3 00	2 51	2 42	2 35	2 28	2 21	2 15	2 10	2 05	2 00	1 56	1 52	1 48	175	574
656	200	3 52	3 38	3 26	3 15	3 05	2 57	2 49	2 41	2 35	2 28	2 23	2 17	2 13	2 08	2 04	200	656
738	225	4 21	4 05	3 52	3 40	3 29	3 19	3 10	3 01	2 54	2 47	2 41	2 36	2 29	2 24	2 19	225	738
820	250	4 49	4 32	4 17	4 04	3 52	3 41	3 31	3 22	3 13	3 05	2 58	2 52	2 46	2 40	2 35	250	820
902	275	5 18	5 00	4 43	4 28	4 15	4 03	3 52	3 42	3 32	3 24	3 16	3 09	3 02	2 56	2 50	275	902
984	300	5 47	5 27	5 09	4 52	4 38	4 25	4 13	4 02	3 52	3 42	3 34	3 26	3 19	3 12	3 05	300	984
1148	350	6 44	6 21	6 00	5 41	5 24	5 09	4 55	4 42	4 30	4 19	4 09	4 00	3 52	3 44	3 36	350	1148
1312	400	7 41	7 14	6 51	6 29	6 10	5 52	5 36	5 22	5 09	4 56	4 45	4 34	4 25	4 16	4 07	400	1312
ft m		1·6	1·7	1·8	1·9	2·0	2·1	2·2	2·3	2·4	2·5	2·6	2·7	2·8	2·9	3·0	m ft	

Height of object

Distance of object (miles)

TABLE 3(2) Distance off by Vertical Sextant Angle (continued)

Height of object ft	m	3·1	3·2	3·3	3·4	3·5	3·6	3·7	3·8	3·9	4·0	4·2	4·4	4·6	4·8	5·0	Height of object m	ft
		o '	o '	o '	o '	o '	o '	o '	o '	o '	o '	o '	o '	o '	o '	o '		
33	10																10	33
39	12																12	39
46	14																14	46
53	16	0 01															16	53
59	18	0 11	0 10	0 10	0 10	0 10											18	59
66	20	0 12	0 12	0 11	0 11	0 11	0 10	0 10	0 10	0 10							20	66
72	22	0 13	0 13	0 12	0 12	0 12	0 11	0 11	0 11	0 10	0 10						22	72
79	24	0 14	0 14	0 13	0 13	0 13	0 12	0 12	0 12	0 11	0 11	0 11	0 10				24	79
85	26	0 16	0 15	0 15	0 14	0 14	0 13	0 13	0 13	0 12	0 12	0 11	0 11	0 10	0 10		26	85
92	28	0 17	0 16	0 16	0 15	0 15	0 14	0 14	0 14	0 13	0 13	0 12	0 12	0 11	0 11	0 10	28	92
98	30	0 18	0 17	0 17	0 16	0 16	0 15	0 15	0 15	0 14	0 14	0 13	0 13	0 12	0 12	0 11	30	98
105	32	0 19	0 19	0 18	0 17	0 17	0 16	0 16	0 16	0 15	0 15	0 14	0 13	0 13	0 12	0 12	32	105
112	34	0 20	0 20	0 19	0 19	0 18	0 17	0 17	0 17	0 16	0 16	0 15	0 14	0 14	0 13	0 13	34	112
118	36	0 22	0 21	0 20	0 20	0 19	0 19	0 18	0 18	0 17	0 17	0 16	0 15	0 14	0 14	0 13	36	118
125	38	0 23	0 22	0 21	0 21	0 20	0 20	0 19	0 19	0 18	0 18	0 17	0 16	0 15	0 15	0 14	38	125
131	40	0 24	0 23	0 22	0 22	0 21	0 21	0 20	0 20	0 19	0 19	0 18	0 17	0 16	0 15	0 15	40	131
138	42	0 25	0 24	0 24	0 23	0 22	0 22	0 21	0 21	0 20	0 19	0 19	0 18	0 17	0 16	0 16	42	138
144	44	0 26	0 25	0 25	0 24	0 23	0 23	0 22	0 22	0 21	0 20	0 19	0 19	0 18	0 17	0 16	44	144
151	46	0 28	0 27	0 26	0 25	0 24	0 24	0 23	0 22	0 22	0 21	0 20	0 19	0 19	0 18	0 17	46	151
157	48	0 29	0 28	0 27	0 26	0 25	0 25	0 24	0 23	0 23	0 22	0 21	0 20	0 19	0 19	0 18	48	157
164	50	0 30	0 29	0 28	0 27	0 27	0 26	0 25	0 24	0 24	0 23	0 22	0 21	0 20	0 19	0 19	50	164
171	52	0 31	0 30	0 29	0 28	0 28	0 27	0 26	0 25	0 25	0 24	0 23	0 22	0 21	0 20	0 19	52	171
177	54	0 32	0 31	0 30	0 29	0 29	0 28	0 27	0 26	0 26	0 25	0 24	0 23	0 22	0 21	0 20	54	177
184	56	0 34	0 32	0 31	0 31	0 30	0 29	0 28	0 27	0 27	0 26	0 25	0 24	0 23	0 22	0 21	56	184
190	58	0 35	0 34	0 33	0 32	0 31	0 30	0 29	0 28	0 28	0 27	0 26	0 24	0 23	0 22	0 21	58	190
197	60	0 36	0 35	0 34	0 33	0 32	0 31	0 30	0 29	0 29	0 28	0 26	0 25	0 24	0 23	0 22	60	197
203	62	0 37	0 36	0 35	0 34	0 33	0 32	0 31	0 30	0 30	0 29	0 27	0 26	0 25	0 24	0 23	62	203
210	64	0 38	0 37	0 36	0 35	0 34	0 33	0 32	0 31	0 30	0 30	0 28	0 27	0 26	0 25	0 24	64	210
217	66	0 40	0 38	0 37	0 36	0 35	0 34	0 33	0 32	0 31	0 31	0 29	0 28	0 27	0 26	0 25	66	217
223	68	0 41	0 39	0 38	0 37	0 36	0 35	0 34	0 33	0 32	0 32	0 30	0 29	0 27	0 26	0 25	68	223
230	70	0 42	0 41	0 39	0 38	0 37	0 36	0 35	0 34	0 33	0 32	0 31	0 29	0 28	0 27	0 26	70	230
236	72	0 43	0 42	0 40	0 39	0 38	0 37	0 36	0 35	0 34	0 33	0 32	0 30	0 29	0 28	0 27	72	236
246	75	0 45	0 44	0 42	0 41	0 40	0 39	0 38	0 37	0 36	0 35	0 33	0 32	0 30	0 29	0 28	75	246
256	78	0 47	0 45	0 44	0 43	0 41	0 40	0 39	0 38	0 37	0 36	0 34	0 33	0 31	0 30	0 29	78	256
266	81	0 48	0 47	0 46	0 44	0 43	0 42	0 41	0 40	0 39	0 38	0 36	0 34	0 33	0 31	0 30	81	266
276	84	0 50	0 49	0 47	0 46	0 45	0 43	0 42	0 41	0 40	0 39	0 37	0 35	0 34	0 32	0 31	84	276
289	88	0 53	0 51	0 49	0 48	0 47	0 45	0 44	0 43	0 42	0 41	0 39	0 37	0 36	0 34	0 33	88	289
302	92	0 55	0 53	0 52	0 50	0 49	0 47	0 46	0 45	0 44	0 43	0 41	0 39	0 37	0 36	0 34	92	302
315	96	0 57	0 56	0 54	0 52	0 51	0 49	0 48	0 47	0 46	0 45	0 42	0 41	0 39	0 37	0 36	96	315
328	100	1 00	0 58	0 56	0 55	0 53	0 52	0 50	0 49	0 48	0 46	0 44	0 42	0 40	0 39	0 37	100	328
341	104	1 02	1 00	0·58	0 57	0 55	0 54	0 52	0 51	0 49	0 48	0 46	0 44	0 42	0 40	0 39	104	341
358	109	1 05	1 03	1 01	1 00	0 58	0 56	0 55	0 53	0 52	0 51	0 48	0 46	0 44	0 42	0 40	109	358
374	114	1 08	1 06	1 04	1 02	1 00	0 59	0 57	0 56	0 54	0 53	0 50	0 48	0 46	0 44	0 42	114	374
394	120	1 12	1 10	1 07	1 06	1 04	1 02	1 00	0 59	0 57	0 56	0 53	0 51	0 48	0 46	0 45	120	394
427	130	1 18	1 15	1 13	1 11	1 09	1 07	1 05	1 03	1 02	1 00	0 57	0 55	0 52	0 50	0 48	130	427
459	140	1 24	1 21	1 19	1 16	1 14	1 12	1 10	1 08	1 07	1 05	1 02	0 59	0 56	0 54	0 52	140	459
492	150	1 30	1 27	1 24	1 22	1 20	1 17	1 15	1 13	1 11	1 10	1 06	1 03	1 01	0 58	0 56	150	492
574	175	1 45	1 41	1 38	1 36	1 33	1 30	1 28	1 25	1 23	1 21	1 17	1 14	1 11	1 08	1 05	175	574
656	200	2 00	1 56	1 52	1 49	1 46	1 43	1 40	1 38	1 35	1 33	1 28	1 24	1 21	1 17	1 14	200	656
738	225	2 15	2 10	2 06	2 03	1 59	1 56	1 53	1 50	1 47	1 44	1 39	1 35	1 31	1 27	1 24	225	738
820	250	2 30	2 25	2 20	2 16	2 13	2 09	2 05	2 02	1 59	1 56	1 50	1 45	1 41	1 37	1 33	250	820
902	275	2 45	2 39	2 34	2 30	2 26	2 22	2 18	2 14	2 11	2 08	2 01	1 56	1 51	1 46	1 42	275	902
984	300	2 59	2 54	2 48	2 44	2 39	2 35	2 30	2 26	2 23	2 19	2 13	2 07	2 01	1 56	1 51	300	984
1148	350	3 29	3 23	3 16	3 11	3 05	3 00	2 55	2 51	2 46	2 42	2 35	2 28	2 21	2 15	2 10	350	1148
1312	400	3 59	3 52	3 44	3 38	3 32	3 26	3 20	3 15	3 10	3 05	2 57	2 49	2 41	2 35	2 28	400	1312
ft m Height of object		3·1	3·2	3·3	3·4	3·5	3·6	3·7	3·8	3·9	4·0	4·2	4·4	4·6	4·8	5·0	m ft Height of object	

Distance of object (miles)

3

TABLE 3(3)   Distance of horizon for various heights of eye

Height of eye		Horizon distance	Height of eye		Horizon distance	Height of eye		Horizon distance
metres	feet	M	metres	feet	M	metres	feet	M
1	3·3	2·1	21	68·9	9·5	41	134·5	13·3
2	6·6	2·9	22	72·2	9·8	42	137·8	13·5
3	9·8	3·6	23	75·5	10·0	43	141·1	13·7
4	13·1	4·1	24	78·7	10·2	44	144·4	13·8
5	16·4	4·7	25	82·0	10·4	45	147·6	14·0
6	19·7	5·1	26	85·3	10·6	46	150·9	14·1
7	23·0	5·5	27	88·6	10·8	47	154·2	14·3
8	26·2	5·9	28	91·9	11·0	48	157·5	14·4
9	29·6	6·2	29	95·1	11·2	49	160·8	14·6
10	32·8	6·6	30	98·4	11·4	50	164·0	14·7
11	36·1	6·9	31	101·7	11·6	51	167·3	14·9
12	39·4	7·2	32	105·0	11·8	52	170·6	15·0
13	42·7	7·5	33	108·3	12·0	53	173·9	15·2
14	45·9	7·8	34	111·6	12·1	54	177·2	15·3
15	49·2	8·1	35	114·8	12·3	55	180·4	15·4
16	52·5	8·3	36	118·1	12·5	56	183·7	15·6
17	55·8	8·6	37	121·4	12·7	57	187·0	15·7
18	59·1	8·8	38	124·7	12·8	58	190·3	15·9
19	62·3	9·1	39	128·0	13·0	59	193·6	16·0
20	65·6	9·3	40	131·2	13·2	60	196·9	16·1

TABLE 3 (4) Lights – distance off when rising or dipping (M)

Height of light		Height of eye									
		metres	1	2	3	4	5	6	7	8	9	10
metres	feet	feet	3	7	10	13	16	20	23	26	30	33
10	33		8·7	9·5	10·2	10·8	11·3	11·7	12·1	12·5	12·8	13·2
12	39		9·3	10·1	10·8	11·4	11·9	12·3	12·7	13·1	13·4	13·8
14	46		9·9	10·7	11·4	12·0	12·5	12·9	13·3	13·7	14·0	14·4
16	53		10·4	11·2	11·9	12·5	13·0	13·4	13·8	14·2	14·5	14·9
18	59		10·9	11·7	12·4	13·0	13·5	13·9	14·3	14·7	15·0	15·4
20	66		11·4	12·2	12·9	13·5	14·0	14·4	14·8	15·2	15·5	15·9
22	72		11·9	12·7	13·4	14·0	14·5	14·9	15·3	15·7	16·0	16·4
24	79		12·3	13·1	13·8	14·4	14·9	15·3	15·7	16·1	16·4	17·0
26	85		12·7	13·5	14·2	14·8	15·3	15·7	16·1	16·5	16·8	17·2
28	92		13·1	13·9	14·6	15·2	15·7	16·1	16·5	16·9	17·2	17·6
30	98		13·5	14·3	15·0	15·6	16·1	16·5	16·9	17·3	17·6	18·0
32	105		13·9	14·7	15·4	16·0	16·5	16·9	17·3	17·7	18·0	18·4
34	112		14·2	15·0	15·7	16·3	16·8	17·2	17·6	18·0	18·3	18·7
36	118		14·6	15·4	16·1	16·7	17·2	17·6	18·0	18·4	18·7	19·1
38	125		14·9	15·7	16·4	17·0	17·5	17·9	18·3	18·7	19·0	19·4
40	131		15·3	16·1	16·8	17·4	17·9	18·3	18·7	19·1	19·4	19·8
42	138		15·6	16·4	17·1	17·7	18·2	18·6	19·0	19·4	19·7	20·1
44	144		15·9	16·7	17·4	18·0	18·5	18·9	19·3	19·7	20·0	20·4
46	151		16·2	17·0	17·7	18·3	18·8	19·2	19·6	20·0	20·3	20·7
48	157		16·5	17·3	18·0	18·6	19·1	19·5	19·9	20·3	20·6	21·0
50	164		16·8	17·6	18·3	18·9	19·4	19·8	20·2	20·6	20·9	21·3
55	180		17·5	18·3	19·0	19·6	20·1	20·5	20·9	21·3	21·6	22·0
60	197		18·2	19·0	19·7	20·3	20·8	21·2	21·6	22·0	22·3	22·7
65	213		18·9	19·7	20·4	21·0	21·5	21·9	22·3	22·7	23·0	23·4
70	230		19·5	20·3	21·0	21·6	22·1	22·5	22·9	23·2	23·6	24·0
75	246		20·1	20·9	21·6	22·2	22·7	23·1	23·5	23·9	24·2	24·6
80	262		20·7	21·5	22·2	22·8	23·3	23·7	24·1	24·5	24·8	25·2
85	279		21·3	22·1	22·8	23·4	23·9	24·3	24·7	25·1	25·4	25·8
90	295		21·8	22·6	23·3	23·9	24·4	24·8	25·2	25·6	25·9	26·3
95	312		22·4	23·2	23·9	24·5	25·0	25·4	25·8	26·2	26·5	26·9
metres	feet	metres	1	2	3	4	5	6	7	8	9	10
Height of light		feet	3	7	10	13	16	20	23	26	30	33
							Height of eye					

Table 3(5) Distance for a given speed and time

Time Decimal of hr	Mins	2·5	3·0	3·5	4·0	4·5	5·0	5·5	6·0	6·5	7·0	7·5	8·0	8·5	9·0	9·5	10·0	Mins	Time Decimal of hr
													Speed in knots						
·0167	1				0·1	0·1	0·1	0·1	0·1	0·1	0·1	0·1	0·1	0·1	0·2	0·2	0·2	1	·0167
·0333	2	0·1	0·1	0·1	0·1	0·1	0·2	0·2	0·2	0·2	0·2	0·2	0·3	0·3	0·3	0·3	0·3	2	·0333
·0500	3	0·1	0·1	0·2	0·2	0·2	0·2	0·3	0·3	0·3	0·3	0·4	0·4	0·4	0·4	0·5	0·5	3	·0500
·0667	4	0·1	0·2	0·2	0·3	0·3	0·3	0·4	0·4	0·4	0·5	0·5	0·5	0·6	0·6	0·6	0·7	4	·0667
·0833	5	0·2	0·2	0·3	0·3	0·4	0·4	0·5	0·5	0·5	0·6	0·6	0·7	0·7	0·7	0·8	0·8	5	·0833
·1000	6	0·2	0·3	0·3	0·4	0·4	0·5	0·5	0·6	0·6	0·7	0·7	0·8	0·8	0·9	0·9	1·0	6	·1000
·1167	7	0·3	0·4	0·4	0·5	0·5	0·6	0·6	0·7	0·8	0·8	0·9	0·9	1·0	1·1	1·1	1·2	7	·1167
·1333	8	0·3	0·4	0·5	0·5	0·6	0·7	0·7	0·8	0·9	0·9	1·0	1·1	1·1	1·2	1·3	1·3	8	·1333
·1500	9	0·4	0·4	0·5	0·6	0·7	0·7	0·8	0·9	1·0	1·0	1·1	1·2	1·3	1·3	1·4	1·5	9	·1500
·1667	10	0·4	0·5	0·6	0·7	0·8	0·8	0·9	1·0	1·1	1·2	1·3	1·3	1·4	1·5	1·6	1·7	10	·1667
·1833	11	0·5	0·5	0·6	0·7	0·8	0·9	1·0	1·1	1·2	1·3	1·4	1·5	1·6	1·6	1·7	1·8	11	·1833
·2000	12	0·5	0·6	0·7	0·8	0·9	1·0	1·1	1·2	1·3	1·4	1·5	1·6	1·7	1·8	1·9	2·0	12	·2000
·2167	13	0·5	0·6	0·8	0·9	1·0	1·1	1·2	1·3	1·4	1·5	1·6	1·7	1·8	2·0	2·0	2·2	13	·2167
·2333	14	0·6	0·7	0·8	0·9	1·0	1·2	1·3	1·4	1·5	1·6	1·7	1·9	2·0	2·1	2·2	2·3	14	·2333
·2500	15	0·6	0·7	0·9	1·0	1·1	1·2	1·4	1·5	1·6	1·8	1·9	2·0	2·1	2·2	2·4	2·5	15	·2500
·2667	16	0·7	0·8	0·9	1·1	1·2	1·3	1·5	1·6	1·7	1·9	2·0	2·1	2·3	2·4	2·5	2·7	16	·2667
·2833	17	0·7	0·8	1·0	1·1	1·3	1·4	1·6	1·7	1·8	2·0	2·1	2·3	2·4	2·5	2·7	2·8	17	·2833
·3000	18	0·7	0·9	1·0	1·2	1·3	1·5	1·6	1·8	1·9	2·1	2·2	2·4	2·5	2·7	2·8	3·0	18	·3000
·3167	19	0·8	1·0	1·1	1·3	1·4	1·6	1·7	1·9	2·1	2·1	2·4	2·5	2·7	2·9	3·0	3·2	19	·3167
·3333	20	0·8	1·0	1·2	1·3	1·5	1·7	1·8	2·0	2·2	2·3	2·5	2·7	2·8	3·0	3·2	3·3	20	3333
·3500	21	0·9	1·0	1·2	1·4	1·6	1·7	1·9	2·1	2·3	2·4	2·6	2·8	3·0	3·1	3·3	3·5	21	·3500
·3667	22	0·9	1·1	1·3	1·5	1·7	1·8	2·1	2·2	2·4	2·6	2·8	2·9	3·1	3·3	3·5	3·7	22	·3667
·3833	23	1·0	1·1	1·3	1·5	1·7	1·9	2·1	2·3	2·5	2·7	2·9	3·1	3·3	3·4	3·6	3·8	23	·3833
·4000	24	1·0	1·2	1·4	1·6	1·8	2·0	2·2	2·4	2·6	2·8	3·0	3·2	3·4	3·6	3·8	4·0	24	·4000
·4167	25	1·0	1·3	1·5	1·7	1·9	2·1	2·3	2·5	2·7	2·9	3·1	3·3	3·5	3·8	4·0	4·2	25	·4167
·4333	26	1·1	1·3	1·5	1·7	1·9	2·2	2·4	2·6	2·8	3·0	3·2	3·5	3·7	3·9	4·1	4·3	26	·4333
·4500	27	1·1	1·3	1·6	1·8	2·0	2·2	2·5	2·7	2·9	3·1	3·4	3·6	3·8	4·0	4·3	4·5	27	·4500
·4667	28	1·2	1·4	1·6	1·9	2·1	2·3	2·6	2·8	3·0	3·3	3·5	3·7	4·0	4·2	4·4	4·7	28	·4667
·4833	29	1·2	1·5	1·7	1·9	2·2	2·4	2·7	2·9	3·1	3·4	3·6	3·9	4·1	4·3	4·6	4·8	29	·4833
·5000	30	1·2	1·5	1·7	2·0	2·2	2·5	2·7	3·0	3·2	3·5	3·7	4·0	4·2	4·5	4·7	5·0	30	·5000
·5167	31	1·3	1·6	1·8	2·1	2·3	2·6	2·8	3·1	3·4	3·6	3·9	4·1	4·4	4·7	4·9	5·2	31	·5167
·5333	32	1·3	1·6	1·9	2·1	2·4	2·7	2·9	3·2	3·5	3·7	4·0	4·3	4·5	4·8	5·1	5·3	32	·5333
·5500	33	1·4	1·6	1·9	2·2	2·5	2·7	3·0	3·3	3·6	3·8	4·1	4·4	4·7	4·9	5·2	5·5	33	·5500
·5667	34	1·4	1·7	2·0	2·3	2·6	2·8	3·1	3·4	3·7	4·0	4·3	4·5	4·8	5·1	5·4	5·7	34	·5667
·5833	35	1·5	1·7	2·0	2·3	2·6	2·9	3·2	3·5	3·8	4·1	4·4	4·7	5·0	5·2	5·5	5·8	35	·5833
·6000	36	1·5	1·8	2·1	2·4	2·7	3·0	3·3	3·6	3·9	4·2	4·5	4·8	5·1	5·4	5·7	6·0	36	·6000
·6117	37	1·6	1·8	2·1	2·4	2·8	3·1	3·4	3·7	4·0	4·3	4·6	4·9	5·2	5·5	5·8	6·1	37	·6117
·6333	38	1·6	1·9	2·2	2·5	2·8	3·2	3·5	3·8	4·1	4·4	4·7	5·1	5·4	5·7	6·0	6·3	38	·6333
·6500	39	1·6	1·9	2·3	2·6	2·9	3·2	3·6	3·9	4·2	4·5	4·9	5·2	5·5	5·8	6·2	6·5	39	·6500
·6667	40	1·7	2·0	2·3	2·7	3·0	3·3	3·7	4·0	4·3	4·7	5·0	5·3	5·7	6·0	6·3	6·7	40	·6667
·6833	41	1·7	2·0	2·4	2·7	3·1	3·4	3·8	4·1	4·4	4·8	5·1	5·5	5·8	6·1	6·5	6·8	41	·6833
·7000	42	1·7	2·1	2·4	2·8	3·1	3·5	3·8	4·2	4·5	4·9	5·2	5·6	5·9	6·3	6·6	7·0	42	·7000
·7167	43	1·8	2·2	2·5	2·9	3·2	3·6	3·9	4·3	4·7	5·0	5·4	5·7	6·1	6·5	6·8	7·2	43	·7167
·7333	44	1·8	2·2	2·6	2·9	3·3	3·7	4·0	4·4	4·8	5·1	5·5	5·9	6·2	6·6	7·0	7·3	44	·7333
·7500	45	1·9	2·2	2·6	3·0	3·4	3·7	4·1	4·5	4·9	5·2	5·6	6·0	6·4	6·7	7·1	7·5	45	·7500
·7667	46	1·9	2·3	2·7	3·1	3·5	3·8	4·2	4·6	5·0	5·4	5·8	6·1	6·5	6·9	7·3	7·7	46	·7667
·7833	47	2·0	2·3	2·7	3·1	3·5	3·9	4·3	4·7	5·1	5·5	5·9	6·3	6·7	7·0	7·4	7·8	47	·7833
·8000	48	2·0	2·4	2·8	3·2	3·6	4·0	4·4	4·8	5·2	5·6	6·0	6·4	6·8	7·2	7·6	8·0	48	·8000
·8167	49	2·0	2·5	2·9	3·3	3·7	4·1	4·5	4·9	5·3	5·7	6·1	6·5	6·9	7·4	7·8	8·2	49	·8167
·8333	50	2·1	2·5	2·9	3·3	3·7	4·2	4·6	5·0	5·4	5·8	6·2	6·7	7·1	7·5	7·9	8·3	50	·8333
·8500	51	2·1	2·5	3·0	3·4	3·8	4·2	4·7	5·1	5·5	5·9	6·4	6·8	7·2	7·6	8·1	8·5	51	·8500
·8667	52	2·2	2·6	3·0	3·5	3·9	4·3	4·8	5·2	5·6	6·1	6·5	6·9	7·4	7·8	8·2	8·7	52	·8667
·8833	53	2·2	2·6	3·1	3·5	4·0	4·4	4·9	5·3	5·7	6·2	6·6	7·1	7·5	7·9	8·4	8·8	53	·8833
·9000	54	2·2	2·7	3·1	3·6	4·0	4·5	4·9	5·4	5·8	6·3	6·7	7·2	7·6	8·1	8·5	9·0	54	·9000
·9167	55	2·3	2·8	3·2	3·7	4·1	4·6	5·0	5·5	6·0	6·4	6·9	7·3	7·8	8·3	8·7	9·2	55	·9167
·9333	56	2·3	2·8	3·3	3·7	4·2	4·7	5·1	5·6	6·1	6·5	7·0	7·5	7·9	8·4	8·9	9·3	56	·9333
·9500	57	2·4	2·8	3·3	3·8	4·3	4·7	5·2	5·7	6·2	6·6	7·1	7·6	8·1	8·5	9·0	9·5	57	·9500
·9667	58	2·4	2·9	3·4	3·9	4·4	4·8	5·3	5·8	6·3	6·8	7·3	7·7	8·2	8·7	9·2	9·7	58	·9667
·9833	59	2·5	2·9	3·4	3·9	4·4	4·9	5·4	5·9	6·4	6·9	7·4	7·9	8·4	8·8	9·3	9·8	59	·9833
1·0000	60	2·5	3·0	3·5	4·0	4·5	5·0	5·5	6·0	6·5	7·0	7·5	8·0	8·5	9·0	9·5	10·0	60	1·0000
Decimal of hr	Mins	2·5	3·0	3·5	4·0	4·5	5·0	5·5	6·0	6·5	7·0	7·5	8·0	8·5	9·0	9·5	10·0	Mins	Decimal of hr
Time								Speed in knots											Time

3

Table 3(5)   Distance for a given speed and time (continued)

Decimal of hr	Mins	10·5	11·0	11·5	12·0	12·5	13·0	13·5	14·0	14·5	15·0	15·5	16·0	17·0	18·0	19·0	20·0	Mins	Decimal of hr
·0167	1	0·2	0·2	0·2	0·2	0·2	0·2	0·2	0·2	0·2	0·3	0·3	0·3	0·3	0·3	0·3	0·3	1	·0167
·0333	2	0·3	0·4	0·4	0·4	0·4	0·4	0·4	0·5	0·5	0·5	0·5	0·5	0·6	0·6	0·6	0·7	2	·0333
·0500	3	0·5	0·5	0·6	0·6	0·6	0·6	0·7	0·7	0·7	0·7	0·8	0·8	0·8	0·8	0·9	1·0	3	·0500
·0667	4	0·7	0·7	0·8	0·8	0·8	0·9	0·9	0·9	1·0	1·0	1·0	1·1	1·1	1·2	1·3	1·3	4	·0667
·0833	5	0·9	0·9	1·0	1·0	1·0	1·1	1·1	1·2	1·2	1·2	1·3	1·3	1·4	1·5	1·6	1·7	5	·0833
·1000	6	1·0	1·1	1·1	1·2	1·2	1·3	1·3	1·4	1·4	1·5	1·5	1·6	1·7	1·8	1·9	2·0	6	·1000
·1167	7	1·2	1·3	1·3	1·4	1·5	1·5	1·6	1·6	1·7	1·8	1·8	1·9	2·0	2·1	2·2	2·3	7	·1167
·1333	8	1·4	1·5	1·5	1·6	1·7	1·7	1·8	1·9	1·9	2·0	2·1	2·1	2·3	2·4	2·5	2·7	8	·1333
·1500	9	1·6	1·6	1·7	1·8	1·9	1·9	2·0	2·1	2·1	2·2	2·3	2·4	2·5	2·7	2·8	3·0	9	·1500
·1667	10	1·8	1·8	1·9	2·0	2·1	2·2	2·3	2·3	2·4	2·5	2·6	2·7	2·8	3·0	3·2	3·3	10	·1667
·1833	11	1·9	2·0	2·1	2·2	2·3	2·4	2·5	2·6	2·7	2·7	2·8	2·9	3·1	3·3	3·5	3·7	11	·1833
·2000	12	2·1	2·2	2·3	2·4	2·5	2·6	2·7	2·8	2·9	3·0	3·1	3·2	3·4	3·6	3·8	4·0	12	·2000
·2167	13	2·3	2·4	2·5	2·6	2·7	2·8	2·9	3·0	3·1	3·2	3·3	3·5	3·7	3·9	4·1	4·3	13	·2167
·2333	14	2·4	2·6	2·7	2·8	2·9	3·0	3·1	3·3	3·4	3·5	3·6	3·7	4·0	4·2	4·4	4·7	14	·2333
·2500	15	2·6	2·7	2·9	3·0	3·1	3·2	3·4	3·5	3·6	3·7	3·9	4·0	4·2	4·5	4·7	5·0	15	·2500
·2667	16	2·8	2·9	3·1	3·2	3·3	3·5	3·6	3·7	3·9	4·0	4·1	4·3	4·5	4·8	5·1	5·3	16	·2667
·2833	17	3·0	3·1	3·3	3·4	3·5	3·7	3·8	4·0	4·1	4·2	4·4	4·5	4·8	5·1	5·4	5·7	17	·2833
·3000	18	3·1	3·3	3·4	3·6	3·7	3·9	4·0	4·2	4·3	4·5	4·6	4·8	5·1	5·4	5·7	6·0	18	·3000
·3167	19	3·3	3·5	3·6	3·8	4·0	4·1	4·3	4·4	4·6	4·8	4·9	5·1	5·4	5·7	6·0	6·3	19	·3167
·3333	20	3·5	3·7	3·8	4·0	4·2	4·3	4·5	4·7	4·8	5·0	5·2	5·3	5·7	6·0	6·3	6·7	20	·3333
·3500	21	3·7	3·8	4·0	4·2	4·4	4·5	4·7	4·9	5·1	5·2	5·4	5·6	5·9	6·3	6·6	7·0	21	·3500
·3667	22	3·9	4·0	4·2	4·4	4·6	4·8	5·0	5·1	5·3	5·5	5·7	5·9	6·2	6·6	7·0	7·3	22	·3667
·3833	23	4·0	4·2	4·4	4·6	4·8	5·0	5·2	5·4	5·6	5·7	5·9	6·1	6·5	6·9	7·3	7·7	23	·3833
·4000	24	4·2	4·4	4·6	4·8	5·0	5·2	5·4	5·6	5·8	6·0	6·2	6·4	6·8	7·2	7·6	8·0	24	·4000
·4167	25	4·4	4·6	4·8	5·0	5·2	5·4	5·6	5·8	6·0	6·3	6·5	6·7	7·1	7·5	7·9	8·3	25	·4167
·4333	26	4·5	4·8	5·0	5·2	5·4	5·6	5·8	6·1	6·3	6·5	6·7	6·9	7·4	7·8	8·2	8·7	26	·4333
·4500	27	4·7	4·9	5·2	5·4	5·6	5·8	6·1	6·3	6·5	6·7	7·0	7·2	7·6	8·1	8·5	9·0	27	·4500
·4667	28	4·9	5·1	5·4	5·6	5·8	6·1	6·3	6·5	6·8	7·0	7·2	7·5	7·9	8·4	8·9	9·3	28	·4667
·4833	29	5·1	5·3	5·6	5·8	6·0	6·3	6·5	6·8	7·0	7·2	7·5	7·7	8·2	8·7	9·2	9·7	29	·4833
·5000	30	5·2	5·5	5·7	6·0	6·2	6·5	6·7	7·0	7·2	7·5	7·7	8·0	8·5	9·0	9·5	10·0	30	·5000
·5167	31	5·4	5·7	5·9	6·2	6·5	6·7	7·0	7·2	7·5	7·8	8·0	8·3	8·8	9·3	9·8	10·3	31	·5167
·5333	32	5·6	5·9	6·1	6·4	6·7	6·9	7·2	7·5	7·7	8·0	8·3	8·5	9·1	9·6	10·1	10·7	32	·5333
·5500	33	5·8	6·0	6·3	6·6	6·9	7·1	7·4	7·7	8·0	8·2	8·5	8·8	9·3	9·9	10·4	11·0	33	·5500
·5667	34	6·0	6·2	6·5	6·8	7·1	7·4	7·7	7·9	8·2	8·5	8·8	9·1	9·6	10·2	10·8	11·3	34	·5667
·5833	35	6·1	6·4	6·7	7·0	7·3	7·6	7·9	8·2	8·5	8·7	9·0	9·3	9·9	10·5	11·1	11·7	35	·5833
·6000	36	6·3	6·6	6·9	7·2	7·5	7·8	8·1	8·4	8·7	9·0	9·3	9·6	10·2	10·8	11·4	12·0	36	·6000
·6117	37	6·4	6·7	7·0	7·3	7·6	8·0	8·3	8·6	8·9	9·2	9·5	9·8	10·4	11·0	11·6	12·2	37	·6117
·6333	38	6·6	7·0	7·3	7·6	7·9	8·2	8·5	8·9	9·2	9·5	9·8	10·1	10·8	11·4	12·0	12·7	38	·6333
·6500	39	6·8	7·1	7·5	7·8	8·1	8·4	8·8	9·1	9·4	9·7	10·1	10·4	11·0	11·7	12·3	13·0	39	·6500
·6667	40	7·0	7·3	7·7	8·0	8·3	8·7	9·0	9·3	9·7	10·0	10·3	10·7	11·3	12·0	12·7	13·3	40	·6667
·6833	41	7·2	7·5	7·9	8·2	8·5	8·9	9·2	9·6	9·9	10·2	10·6	10·9	11·6	12·3	13·0	13·7	41	·6833
·7000	42	7·3	7·7	8·0	8·4	8·7	9·1	9·4	9·8	10·1	10·5	10·8	11·2	11·9	12·6	13·3	14·0	42	·7000
·7167	43	7·5	7·9	8·2	8·6	9·0	9·3	9·7	10·0	10·4	10·8	11·1	11·5	12·2	12·9	13·6	14·3	43	·7167
·7333	44	7·7	8·1	8·4	8·8	9·2	9·5	10·0	10·3	10·6	11·0	11·4	11·7	12·5	13·2	13·9	14·7	44	·7333
·7500	45	7·9	8·2	8·6	9·0	9·4	9·7	10·1	10·5	10·9	11·2	11·6	12·0	12·7	13·5	14·2	15·0	45	·7500
·7667	46	8·1	8·4	8·8	9·2	9·6	10·0	10·4	10·7	11·1	11·5	11·9	12·3	13·0	13·8	14·6	15·3	46	·7667
·7833	47	8·2	8·6	9·0	9·4	9·8	10·2	10·6	11·0	11·4	11·7	12·1	12·5	13·3	14·1	14·9	15·7	47	·7833
·8000	48	8·4	8·8	9·2	9·6	10·0	10·4	10·8	11·2	11·6	12·0	12·4	12·8	13·6	14·4	15·2	16·0	48	·8000
·8167	49	8·6	9·0	9·4	9·8	10·2	10·6	11·0	11·4	11·8	12·2	12·7	13·1	13·9	14·7	15·5	16·3	49	·8167
·8333	50	8·7	9·2	9·6	10·0	10·4	10·8	11·2	11·7	12·1	12·5	12·9	13·3	14·2	15·0	15·8	16·7	50	·8333
·8500	51	8·9	9·3	9·8	10·2	10·6	11·0	11·5	11·9	12·3	12·7	13·2	13·6	14·4	15·3	16·1	17·0	51	·8500
·8667	52	9·1	9·5	10·0	10·4	10·8	11·3	11·7	12·1	12·6	13·0	13·4	13·9	14·7	15·6	16·5	17·3	52	·8667
·8833	53	9·3	9·7	10·2	10·6	11·0	11·5	11·9	12·4	12·8	13·2	13·7	14·1	15·0	15·9	16·8	17·7	53	·8833
·9000	54	9·4	9·9	10·3	10·8	11·2	11·7	12·1	12·6	13·0	13·5	13·9	14·4	15·3	16·2	17·1	18·0	54	·9000
·9167	55	9·6	10·1	10·5	11·0	11·5	11·9	12·4	12·8	13·3	13·8	14·2	14·7	15·6	16·5	17·4	18·3	55	·9167
·9333	56	9·8	10·3	10·7	11·2	11·7	12·1	12·6	13·1	13·5	14·0	14·5	14·9	15·9	16·8	17·7	18·7	56	·9333
·9500	57	10·0	10·4	10·9	11·4	11·9	12·3	12·8	13·3	13·8	14·2	14·7	15·2	16·1	17·1	18·0	19·0	57	·9500
·9667	58	10·2	10·6	11·1	11·6	12·1	12·6	13·1	13·5	14·0	14·5	15·0	15·5	16·4	17·4	18·4	19·3	58	·9667
·9833	59	10·3	10·8	11·3	11·8	12·3	12·8	13·3	13·8	14·3	14·7	15·2	15·7	16·7	17·7	18·7	19·7	59	·9833
1·0000	60	10·5	11·0	11·5	12·0	12·5	13·0	13·5	14·0	14·5	15·0	15·5	16·0	17·0	18·0	19·0	20·0	60	1·0000
Decimal of hr	Mins	10·5	11·0	11·5	12·0	12·5	13·0	13·5	14·0	14·5	15·0	15·5	16·0	17·0	18·0	19·0	20·0	Mins	Decimal of hr

Table 3(6)   Measured Mile Table – Knots related to time over one mile

Secs	1 min	2 min	3 min	4 min	5 min	6 min	7 min	8 min	9 min	10 min	11 min
	60·00	30·00	20·00	15·00	12·00	10·00	8·57	7·50	6·67	6·00	5·45
1	59·02	29·75	19·89	14·94	11·96	9·97	8·55	7·48	6·66	5·99	5·45
2	58·06	29·51	19·78	14·88	11·92	9·94	8·53	7·47	6·64	5·98	5·44
3	57·14	29·27	19·67	14·81	11·88	9·92	8·51	7·45	6·63	5·97	5·43
4	56·25	29·03	19·57	14·75	11·84	9·89	8·49	7·44	6·62	5·96	5·42
5	55·38	28·80	19·46	14·69	11·80	9·86	8·47	7·42	6·61	5·95	5·41
6	54·55	28·57	19·35	14·63	11·76	9·84	8·45	7·41	6·59	5·94	5·41
7	53·73	28·35	19·25	14·57	11·73	9·81	8·43	7·39	6·58	5·93	5·40
8	52·94	28·12	19·15	14·52	11·69	9·78	8·41	7·38	6·57	5·92	5·39
9	52·17	27·91	19·05	14·46	11·65	9·76	8·39	7·36	6·56	5·91	5·38
10	51·43	27·69	18·95	14·40	11·61	9·73	8·37	7·35	6·55	5·90	5·37
11	50·70	27·48	18·85	14·34	11·58	9·70	8·35	7·33	6·53	5·89	5·37
12	50·00	27·27	18·75	14·29	11·54	9·68	8·33	7·32	6·52	5·88	5·36
13	49·32	27·07	18·65	14·23	11·50	9·65	8·31	7·30	6·51	5·87	5·35
14	48·65	26·87	18·56	14·17	11·46	9·63	8·29	7·29	6·50	5·86	5·34
15	48·00	26·67	18·46	14·12	11·43	9·60	8·28	7·27	6·49	5·85	5·33
16	47·37	26·47	18·37	14·06	11·39	9·58	8·26	7·26	6·47	5·84	5·33
17	46·75	26·28	18·27	14·01	11·36	9·55	8·24	7·24	6·46	5·83	5·32
18	46·15	26·09	18·18	13·95	11·32	9·52	8·22	7·23	6·45	5·83	5·31
19	45·57	25·90	18·09	13·90	11·29	9·50	8·20	7·21	6·44	5·82	5·30
20	45·00	25·71	18·00	13·85	11·25	9·47	8·18	7·20	6·43	5·81	5·29
21	44·44	25·53	17·91	13·79	11·21	9·45	8·16	7·19	6·42	5·80	5·29
22	43·90	25·35	17·82	13·74	11·18	9·42	8·14	7·17	6·41	5·79	5·28
23	43·37	25·17	17·73	13·69	11·15	9·40	8·13	7·16	6·39	5·78	5·27
24	42·86	25·00	17·65	13·64	11·11	9·37	8·11	7·14	6·38	5·77	5·26
25	42·35	24·83	17·56	13·58	11·08	9·35	8·09	7·13	6·37	5·76	5·26
26	41·86	24·66	17·48	13·53	11·04	9·33	8·07	7·11	6·36	5·75	5·25
27	41·38	24·49	17·39	13·48	11·01	9·30	8·05	7·10	6·35	5·74	5·24
28	40·91	24·32	17·31	13·43	10·98	9·28	8·04	7·09	6·34	5·73	5·23
29	40·45	24·16	17·22	13·38	10·94	9·25	8·02	7·07	6·33	5·72	5·22
30	40·00	24·00	17·14	13·33	10·91	9·23	8·00	7·06	6·32	5·71	5·22
31	39·56	23·84	17·06	13·28	10·88	9·21	7·98	7·04	6·30	5·71	5·21
32	39·13	23·68	16·98	13·24	10·84	9·18	7·96	7·03	6·29	5·70	5·20
33	38·71	23·53	16·90	13·19	10·81	9·16	7·95	7·02	6·28	5·69	5·19
34	38·30	23·38	16·82	13·14	10·78	9·14	7·93	7·00	6·27	5·68	5·19
35	37·89	23·23	16·74	13·09	10·75	9·11	7·91	6·99	6·26	5·67	5·18
36	37·50	23·08	16·67	13·04	10·71	9·09	7·89	6·98	6·25	5·66	5·17
37	37·11	22·93	16·59	13·00	10·68	9·07	7·88	6·96	6·24	5·65	5·16
38	36·73	22·78	16·51	12·95	10·65	9·05	7·86	6·95	6·23	5·64	5·16
39	36·36	22·64	16·44	12·90	10·62	9·02	7·84	6·94	6·22	5·63	5·15
40	36·00	22·50	16·36	12·86	10·59	9·00	7·83	6·92	6·21	5·62	5·14
41	35·64	22·36	16·29	12·81	10·56	8·98	7·81	6·91	6·20	5·62	5·13
42	35·29	22·22	16·22	12·77	10·53	8·96	7·79	6·90	6·19	5·61	5·13
43	34·95	22·09	16·14	12·72	10·50	8·93	7·78	6·89	6·17	5·60	5·12
44	34·62	21·95	16·07	12·68	10·47	8·91	7·76	6·87	6·16	5·59	5·11
45	34·29	21·82	16·00	12·63	10·43	8·89	7·74	6·86	6·15	5·58	5·10
46	33·96	21·69	15·93	12·59	10·40	8·87	7·72	6·84	6·14	5·57	5·10
47	33·64	21·56	15·86	12·54	10·37	8·85	7·71	6·83	6·13	5·56	5·09
48	33·33	21·43	15·79	12·50	10·34	8·82	7·69	6·82	6·12	5·56	5·08
49	33·03	21·30	15·72	12·46	10·32	8·80	7·68	6·80	6·11	5·55	5·08
50	32·73	21·18	15·65	12·41	10·29	8·78	7·66	6·79	6·10	5·54	5·07
51	32·43	21·05	15·58	12·37	10·26	8·76	7·64	6·78	6·09	5·53	5·06
52	32·14	20·93	15·52	12·33	10·23	8·74	7·63	6·77	6·08	5·52	5·06
53	31·86	20·81	15·45	12·29	10·20	8·72	7·61	6·75	6·07	5·51	5·05
54	31·58	20·69	15·38	12·24	10·17	8·70	7·59	6·74	6·06	5·50	5·04
55	31·30	20·57	15·32	12·20	10·14	8·67	7·58	6·73	6·05	5·50	5·04
56	31·03	20·45	15·25	12·16	10·11	8·65	7·56	6·72	6·04	5·49	5·03
57	30·77	20·34	15·19	12·12	10·08	8·63	7·55	6·70	6·03	5·48	5·02
58	30·51	20·22	15·13	12·08	10·06	8·61	7·53	6·69	6·02	5·47	5·01
59	30·25	20·11	15·06	12·04	10·03	8·59	7·52	6·68	6·01	5·46	5·00
Secs	1 min	2 min	3 min	4 min	5 min	6 min	7 min	8 min	9 min	10 min	11 min

3

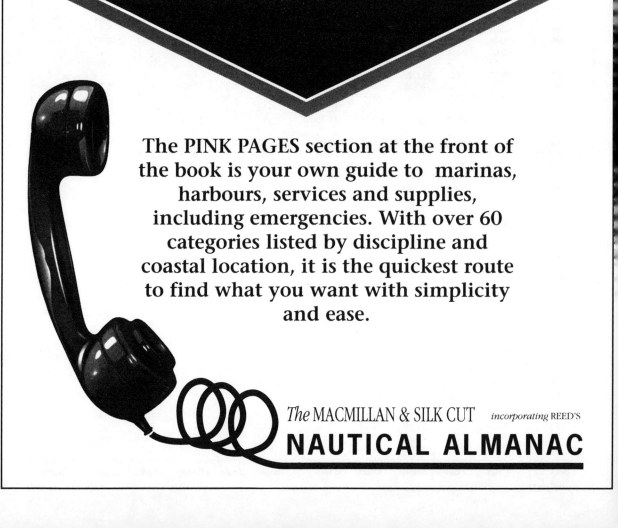

Radio Navigational Aids

Contents

4

Radio navigational aids – introduction

Basic information on position fixing systems such as GPS, Decca, Loran C and the use of Waypoints, together with details of individual RDF beacons and Racons, for navigational use is given in this Almanac. Further information on procedures and possible errors, together with the other subjects listed below, is given in Chapter 4 of *The Macmillan & Silk Cut Yachtsman's Handbook:*

Aids to navigation; Developments; Navigational aids and position fixing systems; satellite position fixing systems; Transit system; Global positioning system (GPS); differential GPS; hyperbolic position fixing systems; Decca; Loran-C; Omega; differential Omega; radar in yachts; how radar works; radar for collision avoidance; radar as a navigational aid; radar beacons (Racons); marine and aeronautical RDF beacons; DF receiving sets; directional radiobeacons; beacons incorporating distance finding; aero RDF beacons operating procedures; Errors in radio bearings; Calibration; Radio direction finding; Half convergency; VHF emergency direction finding; QTG service from Coast Radio Stations.

4.1 INTRODUCTION

4.1.1   Types of systems

Five position fixing systems are currently available to yachtsmen. Satellite navigation is provided by the Global Positioning System (GPS) and Transit, and the hyperbolic area navigation systems by Decca, Loran-C and Omega. The Transit satnav system will cease operation on 31 December 1996. Radio Direction Finding (RDF) is now obsolescent having been superseded by easier to use and more accurate systems such as GPS, Loran-C, and Decca. Each aid has its merits for particular applications and geographical areas. These aids are more fully described in *The Macmillan & Silk Cut Yachtsman's Handbook.*

The choice of navigation aids for a yacht largely depends on the usage of the boat, the owner's requirements and interests, and the particular waters sailed. Broadly speaking Satnav provides high accuracy global fixes in any weather. GPS provides continuous high accuracy fixes of approximately 100m, whilst Transit provides intermittent fixes to a basic system accuracy of 0·25M. Loran-C and Decca provide continuous fixes within coverage areas, albeit with less accuracy and reliability. Omega provides global coverage, but the accuracy is not as good as Loran-C or Decca.

4.2 SATELLITE SYSTEMS

4.2.1   Global Positioning System (GPS)

GPS provides highly accurate worldwide continuous three dimensional position fixing (latitude, longitude and altitude), together with velocity and time information in all weather conditions.

The GPS constellation, shown in Fig. 4(1), consists of 21 operational satellites plus three operational hot spares configured in six orbital planes. The satellites circle the earth in 12 hour orbits at a height of about 10,900M.

GPS provides two levels of service. These are:-

(1)   **Standard Positioning Service (SPS)**.
(2)   **Precise Positioning Service (PPS)**.

It is the SPS service which is of interest to yachtsmen. SPS is available to all civil users at no cost. PPS provides higher accuracy but, at present, is reserved solely for military purposes and is only made available to selected civil users when specially authorised.

The principle on which GPS works is the accurate measurement of the range, or distance, from the receiver to a number of satellites transmitting accurately timed signals together with information on their accurate position in space. In very simplistic terms each satellite transmits a PPS and SPS code saying 'this is my position and this is the time'.

By accurately knowing the times of transmission and reception of the signal it is possible to establish the transit time. Multiply the transit time by the speed of light (161,829 miles per second) to get the range to the satellite. If similar measurements are made on three satellites, three intersecting range circles, each centred on the satellite's position at the time of transmission, are obtained. If no other errors are present, the intersection of the three range circles represents the yacht's position.

GPS basic system errors are relatively small and are of the order of 19-20m using SPS. Current US plans for the use of SPS are based on a denial of full system accuracy by the use of cryptology. This is called Selective Availability (SA). The imposition of SA means there is no guarantee that a standard GPS yacht receiver will give a horizontal fix of better than ±100m, 140m vertically, and time to 340 nanoseconds for 95% of the time. Accuracy will be ±300m for 99·99% of the time. As fix accuracy continually varies when SA is switched on, no assumptions should be made about fix accuracy at any given time. SPS accuracy can be significantly improved by access to a differential (DGPS) service, but a user charge may be applicable.

GPS receivers vary from single channel to multi-channel receivers. Better quality positioning is obtained by tracking more than the minimum three satellites required to produce a two dimensional fix (latitude and longitude). A receiver with at least six channels is the most suitable for use on a yacht.

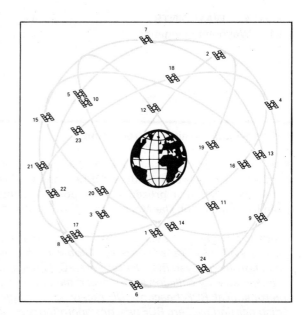

Fig. 4(1) The GPS constellation consists of 21 operational and three operational hot spares at heights of 11,000M arranged in six orbital planes inclined to the equator at 55°. The configuration is planned to have at least four satellites in view from a receiver anywhere on earth.

In conventional coastal navigation it is generally recommended to avoid using any visual position lines where the angle of cut is less than 30°. The accuracy of GPS fixes equally depends on the angle of cut of its position lines, but this is more difficult to appreciate because the geometry of the satellites is constantly changing. The receiver, rather than the navigator, selects those satellites which offer the best fix geometry.

4.2.2   Dilution of precision

The efficiency of the satellite geometry is indicated by the Dilution of Precision (DOP) factor which is computed from the angular separation between various satellites. The greater the separation the better the fix geometry is, and the lower the DOP value.

Performance is most likely to be degraded when there are less than 5 satellites visible, or when DOP is greater than 5. Since high DOP is caused by poor satellite geometry, these events usually coincide.

The potential inaccuracy of a 2D GPS fix resulting from poor geometry is expressed by a factor called the Horizontal Dilution of Precision (HDOP). The accuracy of a GPS fix varies with the capability of the user's receiver and receiver-to-satellite geometry. Receivers are programmed to select satellites which give the lowest HDOP value. Should the HDOP value exceed a certain figure, usually 4 or 5, then receivers give a warning, or cease computing fixes until satellite geometry improves.

4.2.3   Datum

GPS satellites are referenced to the World Geodetic System 84 (WGS 84) datum. This means that satellite fixes cannot be directly plotted on Admiralty charts, which are usually referenced to a local datum. If the full potential benefit of GPS accuracy is to be achieved, then suitable corrections need to be applied.

UK Admiralty charts are based on the Ordnance Survey Great Britain 1936 (OSGB 36) datum. Admiralty charts covering the NW European Coastline are based on the European 1950 Datum (ED 50). Admiralty charts always show which datum is used under the chart title. Admiralty charts also show the amount of correction required between satellite and chart positions.

In the Dover Strait the approximate difference between WGS 84 and OSGB 36 amounts to 140m, and between WGS 84 and ED 50, 135m. The difference between OSGB 36 and ED 50 is 165m. The amount of the error varies at each location and can be substantial in some parts of the world such as the Pacific.

Good GPS receivers generally allow users a choice of many different chart datums. Navigators should always ensure that their receiver chart datum is set to the same datum as the chart in use.

4.2.4   Differential GPS

Differential GPS (DGPS) is a method of considerably improving the basic accuracy of GPS SPS locally. Initially, DGPS is only likely to appeal to a limited number of yacht users such as those engaged in racing, or having special requirements for high accuracy.

When fully operational, a DGPS ground monitoring station compares its known position to the computed position using a GPS monitor receiver and determines the cumulative error. The DGPS reference station then transmits corrections back to the on-board GPS receiver via a data link. A radio receiver capable of receiving selected marine radiobeacons, and equipped with a suitable demodulator for the DGPS messages is required and is interfaced to the GPS receiver. It will then automatically apply the transmitted corrections to the navigational data. Once the errors at a particular time and place have been established, differential corrections can be applied to achieve an accuracy of better than ± 10m for a limited period of time.

The UK and Ireland are alone in being the only countries so far to make a charge for the DGPS service. The charge for the service is £950 per annum. The commercial firm responsible for providing the UK DGPS service on behalf of Trinity House is Scorpio Marine Electronics Limited, Bennett House, 1 High Street, Edgware, Middlesex HA8 7DF. (☎ 0181-951 4446, Fax: 0181-951 5650.)

4.2.5   GPS integrity monitoring

Information on the current status and performance of GPS can be obtained in the UK by fax. The status information is updated every Friday afternoon. The number to call is 0336-400 599. Urgent information on GPS is also given in BT Coast Radio Station navigation warning broadcasts on VHF or MF, and by any NAVTEX station under message category J.

Information is also obtainable from the US Coast Guard GPS Information Centre (GPSIC) on ☎ 0001 703 313 5907 which gives a pre-recorded daily status message. GPSIC duty personnel can be contacted on ☎ 0001 703 313 5900.

4.2.6   The Transit satellite system

The 'Transit' satellite navigation system comprises 7 to 9 operational satellites circling the Earth in low polar orbits at heights of about 600M and provides an accurate fix every 70 to 90 minutes according to latitude. There are a further 10 satellites in orbital storage which can be switched on at short notice in the event of satellite failure occurring. It is a worldwide system which is unaffected by weather conditions. Transit is easy to use, and produces a basic fix accuracy of 0·25M. An additional error of up to 0·2M per knot due to a vessel's speed occurs. Transit's limitation is that it does not provide continuous fixing.

4

The receiver's calculation of a fix takes about 10-15 minutes to complete and is based on the measurement of the doppler effect on the frequency as the slant distance between the satellite and the receiver decreases and increases due to their relative movement. It is important to ensure during a satellite pass that no changes to the yacht's heading and speed are made. The 'Transit' system will cease operation on 31 December 1996.

4.3 HYPERBOLIC SYSTEMS

4.3.1 Decca
The Decca Navigator System is a very accurate short to medium range hyperbolic fixing system ideally suited to coastal and landfall navigation. Good coverage is available over the UK and the European coastline to a range of approximately 400M by day, and 250M by night. The six UK Decca chains will remain operational until at least 31 March 1998. Decca chains available in the UK and NW Europe are shown on Fig. 4(2).

The general principle on which Decca works is the accurate measurement of the difference in time taken by radio waves travelling between at least two sets of transmitters. This is achieved by measuring the phase differences.

The propagation of radio waves is affected by weather, season, radio noise, time of day and night, terrain over which the radio waves pass, and range from transmitters. Decca errors are mostly quite small but are present and can have navigational significance. A good tip is to treat all Decca positions with extreme caution whenever your TV picture at home is distorted by abnormal radio propagation conditions. Such conditions are quite frequent whenever atmospheric pressure is approximately 10 Millibars (Mbs) higher than the average. Average Mean Sea Level pressure during the month of July would be approximately 1017 Mbs in the English Channel and 1012 Mbs in Scotland. Therefore, if the barometer reads 1030 Mbs abnormal radio propagation is likely to occur.

There are two main types of error:

(1) *Fixed errors* resulting from variations in the velocity of radio waves over different types of terrain, or the presence of land between transmitter and receiver. The effect of fixed errors can be very pronounced when close to the coast. Fixed errors are constant at any given location. Racal-Decca publishes data sheets giving fixed error corrections for each Decca chain but unfortunately these are in a form which can only be applied to large ship receivers using Decca coordinates, rather than latitude/longitude. It is not possible to apply fixed error corrections to yacht receivers which only give a latitude/longitude read-out.

(2) *Variable errors* are due to the effect of skywave/groundwave interference and to the other factors mentioned above. Generally speaking, conditions are worse on winter nights than in summer and errors are bigger at the extremities of the coverage area than in the centre.

For practical navigation purposes it is unwise to assume an accuracy of better than 0·25M at ranges of 50-100M from transmitters, and up to 1·5M or more at the limits of coverage, especially when abnormal propagation conditions are present.

4.3.2 Loran-C
Loran-C is a long range hyperbolic system suitable for coastal and offshore navigation within coverage. It provides continuous fixing and the ground wave can be received at ranges of 800-1200M. Loran-C pulses also propagate as skywaves which may be received at much greater range, but with much less accuracy.
Four new Loran-C chains provide extensive coverage over North-West Europe, and the British Isles. See Fig. 4(3).

The general principle on which Loran-C works is the accurate measurement of the time difference in the arrival of pulse signals transmitted from a Master and Secondary station. Loran chains consist of three to five transmitters and operate in sequenced pairs. The time difference obtained from each pair of transmitters determines an exclusive hyperbolic curve of constant time difference and the intersection of two or more curves produces the fix. Loran-C radio wave propagation is affected by conditions similar to those already described for Decca. Several factors can affect overall system accuracy such as the type of terrain over which the radio waves pass, range from transmitters, system geometry, weather, electronic noise, angle of cut of position lines and gradient, and synchronisation errors between transmitters. Using the groundwave system, accuracy varies from about 100m at a range of 200M from transmitters, to 250m to 1M or more at 500M range.

4.4 WAYPOINTS

4.4.1 Waypoint navigation
A waypoint can be any point chosen by a navigator such as a departure point or destination, any selected position along the intended route where it is proposed to alter course, a point at a selected distance off a headland or lighthouse, a buoy, or any other position in the open sea. Always study the chart first and plot the position of any planned Waypoint before loading the coordinates into electronic equipment. This ensures that any projected route will not take you across shallows, into danger, or even across land. It is usual to tag either a number or name to waypoint coordinates.

Fig. 4(2)   DECCA CHAINS – NORTH-WEST EUROPE

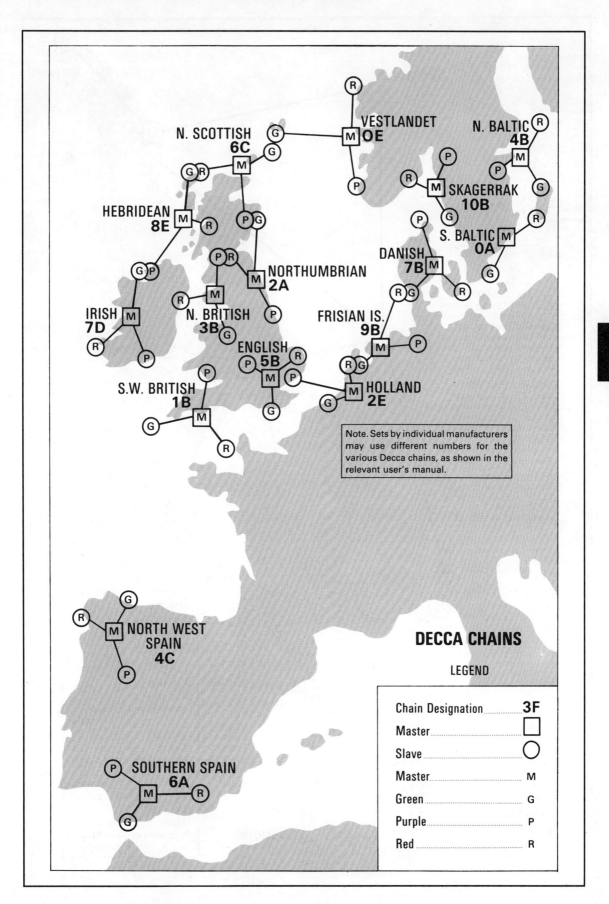

Note. Sets by individual manufacturers may use different numbers for the various Decca chains, as shown in the relevant user's manual.

DECCA CHAINS

LEGEND

Chain Designation	**3F**
Master	□
Slave	○
Master	M
Green	G
Purple	P
Red	R

Fig. 4(3)   LORAN-C CHAINS – NORTH-WEST EUROPE

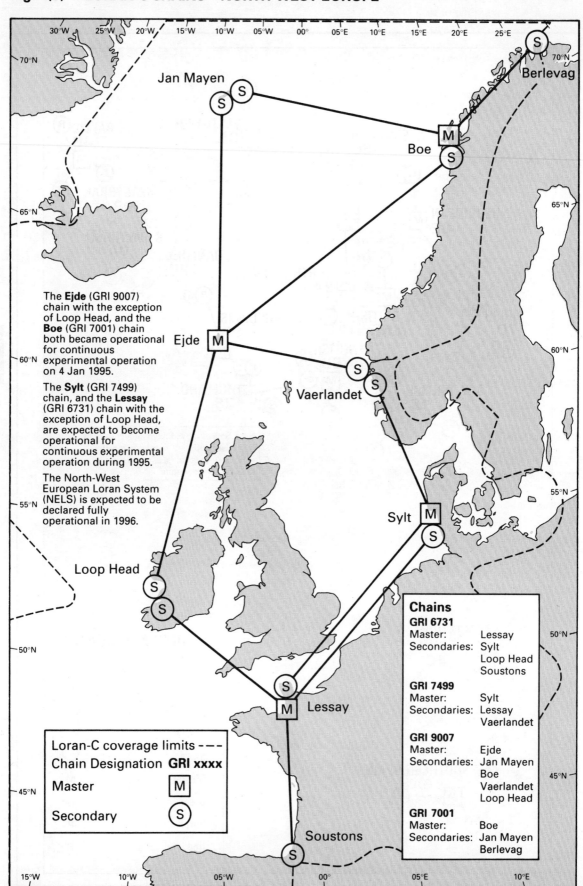

The **Ejde** (GRI 9007) chain with the exception of Loop Head, and the **Boe** (GRI 7001) chain both became operational for continuous experimental operation on 4 Jan 1995.

The **Sylt** (GRI 7499) chain, and the **Lessay** (GRI 6731) chain with the exception of Loop Head, are expected to become operational for continuous experimental operation during 1995.

The North-West European Loran System (NELS) is expected to be declared fully operational in 1996.

Loran-C coverage limits – – –
Chain Designation **GRI xxxx**

Master   M

Secondary   S

Chains

GRI 6731
Master: Lessay
Secondaries: Sylt
                     Loop Head
                     Soustons

GRI 7499
Master: Sylt
Secondaries: Lessay
                     Vaerlandet

GRI 9007
Master: Ejde
Secondaries: Jan Mayen
                     Boe
                     Vaerlandet
                     Loop Head

GRI 7001
Master: Boe
Secondaries: Jan Mayen
                     Berlevag

A waypoint listing may be assembled in any order required to form a route or sailing plan.

Approximately 3500 waypoints are given in Chapter 10 for navigational use. They are shown for individual harbour entrances after the harbour name and county (or equivalent abroad) which provides a good final waypoint, and also for harbour approaches under the heading of 'Navigation'. A list of selected Waypoints is given in section 4 of each Area (where they are underlined in the lists of 'Coastal Lights, Fog Signals and Waypoints'). A convenient tabulated listing of waypoints is also given for cross-Channel passages (10.1.7), the Solent area (10.2.21), SE England (10.3.8), East Anglian (10.4.7), and the Clyde (10.9.15).

Latitudes and longitudes are normally stated to one-hundredth of a minute, as taken from a large scale chart. But it should be realised that a chart using a different datum or based on another survey may give a slightly different position. Charts may also contain small errors, just like the read-out from an electronic instrument.

The greatest care needs to be taken when loading waypoint coordinates into electronic equipment. Always check that you have taken the position off the chart correctly. Any error in the entry of latitude/ longitude coordinates into the receiver will result in navigational error if undetected. It is particularly important to understand the format required to enter data into the receiver. For example, the incorrect placing of the decimal point can result in considerable errors in the calculation of bearing and distance. Another point to watch is whether East or West longitude is assumed by the receiver. Use the ± or other designated key to change the sign from East to West if necessary.

Following the precautions listed below can assist in preventing errors being made when loading waypoints:

(1)   Check that you have taken the latitude/longitude coordinates off the chart correctly.

(2)   Check the intended route between Waypoints for navigational safety.

(2)   Measure the tracks and distances on the chart and record the results in a simplified passage plan.

(3)   Check that the waypoints have been keyed into the receiver memory correctly.

(4)   Get an independent check if possible.

After loading waypoints check the track and distances between waypoints computed by the receiver against those measured off the chart and shown in the passage plan.

One of the major advantages of modern waypoint navigation technology is its ability to present navigators with a continuous read-out of valuable navigational information in addition to position, such as course and speed made good, along and across-track error, distance and time to go to next waypoint etc. Probably the most useful of the additional displays, especially with GPS, is the course and speed made good facility where the continuous read-out can be directly compared to the required track. By comparison with course and speed through the water, the same data can also be used to calculate set and drift quickly. Some receivers allow the presentation of both position and course and speed made good on the same display.

Electronic systems are only aids to navigation and are subject to fixed and variable errors, or on rare occasions even total failure. It is therefore essential to maintain a record in the log of the yacht's position, course and speed from the receiver display and to plot a position on the chart at regular intervals so that you can quickly work up a DR/EP not only to cover the case of equipment failure, but also to ensure that the boat's track is keeping well clear of all dangers. Take great care when using waypoints on shore.

4.5   RDF BEACONS

4.5.1   RDF beacons – general

Radio direction finding (RDF) is a relatively simple, but generally inaccurate, method whereby yachtsmen can establish an approximate position using marine or aeronautical RDF beacons and a radio receiver with a directional antenna. With the increasing use of aids such as GPS, Decca and Loran, RDF is now little used and rapidly becoming obsolescent. A number of strategically placed marine RDF beacons have been retained solely to provide a Differential GPS service (DGPS).

Marine and Aeronautical RDF beacons are non-directional and transmit on medium frequencies on a continuous basis. The navigator tunes to the listed frequency, identifies the beacon by its Morse ident (13 secs) followed by a long dash (47 secs) during which time the DF antenna is rotated until it registers the minimum or null signal. The antenna position, usually associated with a compass, then indicates the direction of the beacon.

4.5.2   Types of emission (Modes)

All marine RDF beacons transmit using A1A emission. This means transmissions are unmodulated and need a DF receiver with a built in oscillator, called a Beat Frequency Oscillator (BFO), to be switched ON in order to receive the A1A transmissions and identify the beacon.

Aeronautical RDF beacons mostly use Non A2A type emissions and require the BFO to be switched ON for DF use, and OFF to identify the station. As individual RDF receivers vary it is necessary to consult the manufacturer's handbook for precise instructions on the use of the BFO switch.

4

4.5.3 RDF beacons incorporating distance finding

The RDF beacons at St Peter Port and St Helier allow radio and sound signals to be synchronised for distance finding. The two signals are synchronised at an easily identifiable point in the cycle, e.g. at the start or end of a long dash.

Using a stopwatch, the difference between the two times in seconds, multiplied by 0·18, gives the distance from the horn in miles.

The system at St Helier involves the transmission of a number of measuring signals or pips, started when the fog signal is sounded. The number of pips received before the horn is heard indicates the distance. Each pip received corresponds to a distance of 335m from the Light.

4.5.4   Errors in radio bearings

The various errors to which radio bearings are subject are described in Chapter 4 of *The Macmillan & Silk Cut Yachtsman's Handbook*. They fall into two categories – signal errors (caused by distance from the beacon, night or sky-wave effect particularly near sunset and sunrise, land effect or coastal refraction where the beam passes over high ground or along the coast, and synchronised transmissions of two beacons), and errors on board the boat (caused by quadrantal error due to magnetic objects re-radiating the incoming signal, compass error, the possibility of inadvertently taking a reciprocal bearing, and operating error due to inexperience or bad weather). Do not rely on radio bearings exclusively, unless three or more give an acceptable cocked hat.

4.5.5   RDF beacons – calibration

A DF set can be calibrated for quadrantal error by taking simultaneous radio and visual bearings of a beacon on different headings. Alternatively radio bearings may be taken from a known position, and the bearing of the beacon taken from the chart. To save time it is helpful if the beacon transmits continuously. A selection of RDF beacons which provide a calibration service are shown in Table 4(1).

4.6   VHF DIRECTION FINDING

4.6.1   VHF emergency DF service

The stations below operate a VHF DF service for emergency use only (see Fig. 4 (3)). UK stations are controlled by a Coastguard MRCC or MRSC as shown in brackets. On request from a yacht in distress, the station transmits her bearing *from the DF site*. Watch is kept on Ch 16. A yacht should transmit on Ch 16 (Distress only) or on Ch 67 (Ch 67 or 82 for Jersey, and Ch 11 for French stations) to allow the station to obtain a bearing, which is then passed to the vessel on the same frequency.

In France, CROSS stations keep watch on Ch 16, 11; 67. Other Signal or Lookout stations equipped with VHF DF keep watch on Ch 16 and other continuously scanned frequencies which include Ch 36, 39, 48, 50, 52, 55, and 56.

St Mary's	(Falmouth)	49°55'·9N 06°18'·2W
Pendeen	(Falmouth)	50°07'·9N 05°39'·0W
Pendennis	(Falmouth)	50°08'·7N 05°01'·7W
Rame Head	(Brixham)	50°19'·2N 04°13'·0W
East Prawle	(Brixham)	50°13'·1N 03°42'·5W
Berry Head	(Brixham)	50°23'·9N 03°29'·3W
Grove Point	(Portland)	50°32'·9N 02°25'·2W
Hengistbury Head	(Portland)	50°42'·9N 01°45'·6W
Boniface Down	(Solent)	50°36'·1N 01°12'·0W
Selsey Bill	(Solent)	50°43'·8N 00°48'·1W
Newhaven	(Solent)	50°46'·8N 00°03'·0E
Fairlight	(Dover)	50°52'·2N 00°40'·0E
Dover	(Dover)	51°07'·9N 01°20'·7E
North Foreland	(Dover)	51°22'·5N 01°24'·8E
Shoeburyness	(Thames)	51°31'·4N 00°46'·7E
Bawdsey	(Thames)	51°59'·5N 01°24'·6E
Trimingham	(Yarmouth)	52°54'·7N 01°20'·5E
Hunstanton	(Yarmouth)	52°56'·8N 00°29'·8E
Caister	(Yarmouth)	52°39'·6N 01°43'·0E
Easington	(Humber)	53°39'·1N 00°05'·9E
Flamborough	(Humber)	54°07'·6N 00°06'·0W
Whitby	(Humber)	54°29'·0N 00°36'·0W
Hartlepool	(Tyne Tees)	54°41'·8N 01°10'·5W
Tyne/Tees	(Tyne Tees)	55°01'·1N 01°25'·0W
Newton-by-the-Sea	(Tyne Tees)	55°31'·1N 01°37'·2W
St Abb's (Crosslaw)	(Forth)	55°54'·0N 02°12'·1W
Fife Ness	(Forth)	56°16'·7N 02°35'·0W
Inverbervie	(Aberdeen)	56°51'·5N 02°15'·7W
Windy Head Hill	(Aberdeen)	57°38'·9N 02°14'·5W
Compass Head	(Shetland)	59°52'·0N 01°16'·3W
Thrumster	(Pentland)	58°23'·6N 03°07'·5W
Dunnett Head	(Pentland)	58°40'·3N 03°22'·5W
Wideford Hill	(Pentland)	58°59'·3N 03°01'·4W
Sandwick	(Stornoway)	58°12'·6N 06°21'·2W
Barra	(Stornoway)	57°00'·8N 07°30'·4W
Rodel	(Stornoway)	57°44'·9N 06°57'·5W
Tiree	(Oban)	56°30'·5N 06°56'·7W
Kilchiaran	(Clyde)	55°45'·9N 06°27'·2W
Lawhill	(Clyde)	55°41'·8N 04°50'·0W
Snaefell	(Liverpool)	54°16'·1N 04°28'·2W
Walney Island	(Liverpool)	54°06'·5N 03°15'·9W
Great Ormes Head	(Holyhead)	53°20'·0N 03°51'·2W
Mynydd Rhiw	(Holyhead)	52°49'·1N 04°37'·8W
St Ann's Head	(Milford Haven)	51°41'·0N 05°10'·5W
Hartland	(Swansea)	51°01'·3N 04°31'·3W
Trevose Head	(Falmouth)	50°32'·7N 05°02'·6W
Orlock Point	(Belfast)	54°40'·4N 05°35'·0W
West Torr	(Belfast)	55°11'·7N 06°05'·2W
Guernsey	–	49°26'·3N 02°35'·8W
Jersey	–	49°10'·8N 02°14'·3W
Étel	(CROSS)	47°39'·8N 03°12'·0W
Créac'h	(CROSS)	48°27'·6N 05°07'·7W
Roches Douvres	(CROSS)	49°06'·5N 02°48'·8W
Jobourg	(CROSS)	49°41'·1N 01°54'·6W
Gris Nez	(CROSS)	50°52'·1N 01°35'·0E

Fig. 4(4) VHF EMERGENCY DF SERVICE

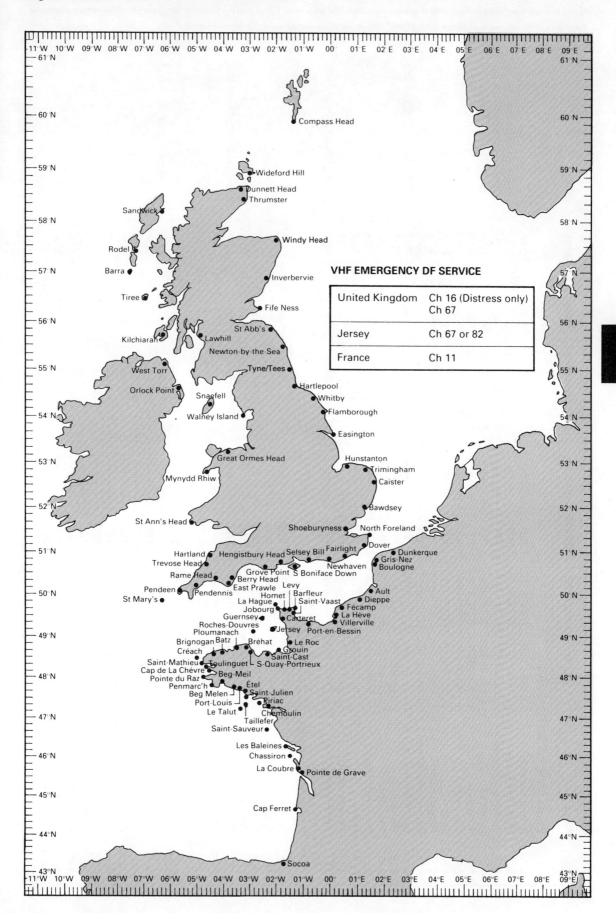

VHF EMERGENCY DF SERVICE

United Kingdom	Ch 16 (Distress only) Ch 67
Jersey	Ch 67 or 82
France	Ch 11

Compass Head

Wideford Hill
Dunnett Head
Thrumster

Sandwick

Windy Head

Rodel
Barra

Inverbervie

Tiree

Fife Ness

Kilchiaran
Lawhill
St Abb's
Newton-by-the-Sea
West Torr
Tyne/Tees
Orlock Point
Snaefell
Hartlepool
Walney Island
Whitby
Flamborough

Easington

Great Ormes Head
Hunstanton
Trimingham
Mynydd Rhiw
Caister

Bawdsey

St Ann's Head
Shoeburyness
North Foreland
Fairlight
Dover
Hartland
Hengistbury Head Selsey Bill
Dunkerque
Trevose Head
Newhaven
Gris-Nez
Rame Head
Grove Point S Boniface Down
Boulogne
Berry Head
Pendeen
East Prawle
Levy
Ault
Pendennis
Homet Barfleur
Dieppe
St Mary's
La Hague Saint-Vaast
Fécamp
Jobourg
La Hève
Guernsey
Carteret
Villerville
Roches-Douvres
Port-en-Bessin
Ploumanach
Jersey
Brignogan Batz
Bréhat
Le Roc
Créach
Grouin
Saint-Mathieu
Saint-Cast
Toulinguet S-Quay-Portrieux
Cap de La Chèvre
Beg-Meil
Pointe du Raz
Penmarc'h
Étel
Beg Melen
Saint-Julien
Port-Louis
Piriac
Le Talut
Chemoulin
Taillefer
Saint-Sauveur

Les Baleines
Chassiron
La Coubre
Pointe de Grave

Cap Ferret

Socoa

TABLE 4(1)   MARINE AND AERONAUTICAL RDF BEACONS

Note: Beacon numbers prefixed with A are Aeronautical RDF beacons. Some marine beacons also provide differential corrections for the satellite navigation system GPS (DGPS) which are transmitted on an additional signal.

No	Name	Latitude	Longitude	Morse Ident	Frequency	Mode	Range	Notes
	ENGLAND – SOUTH COAST							
1	Round Island Lt	49°58'·70N	06°19'·33W	RR	298·50	A1A	150M	
A2	St Mary's, Scilly	49°54'·81N	06°17'·41W	STM	321·00	Non A2A	15M	Day service: Mon-Sat
A4	Penzance Heliport	50°07'·67N	05°31'·00W	PH	333·00	Non A2A	15M	Day service: Mon-Sat
3	Lizard Lt	49°57'·58N	05°12'·07W	LZ	284·50	A1A	70M	
A6	Plymouth	50°25'·37N	04°06'·67W	PY	396·50	Non A2A	20M	
A8	Berry Head	50°23'·89N	03°29'·56W	BHD	318·00	Non A2A	25M	
A10	Exeter	50°45'·12N	03°17'·62W	EX	337·00	Non A2A	25M	Day service
5	Portland Bill	50°30'·82N	02°27'·30W	PB	309·50	A1A	50M	
A12	Bournemouth/Hurn	50°46'·03N	01°50'·47W	BIA	339·00	Non A2A	20M	
7	St Catherine's Pt	50°34'·52N	01°17'·80W	CP	293·00	A1A	50M	DGPS service 293·50 kHz 40M
A16	Bembridge	50°40'·78N	01°06'·18W	IW	426·00	Non A2A	15M	
A18	Shoreham	50°49'·89N	00°17'·75W	SHM	332·00	Non A2A	10M	Day service
9	Brighton Marina	50°48'·67N	00°05'·95W	BM	294·50	A1A	10M	
A20	Lydd	50°58'·23N	00°57'·30E	LYX	397·00	Non A2A	15M	
11.	Dungeness Lt	50°54'·77N	00°58'·67E	DU	300·50	A1A	50M	
13	North Foreland Lt	51°22'·49N	01°26'·85E	NF	311·00	A1A	50M	DGPS service 310·50 kHz 40M
	ENGLAND – EAST COAST							
A22	Southend	51°34'·55N	00°42'·12E	SND	362·50	Non A2A	20M	
15	Sunk Lt F	51°51'·00N	01°35'·00E	UK	294·50	A1A	10M	
A24	Great Yarmouth	52°38'·21N	01°43'·52E	ND	397·00	Non A2A	15M	Calibration station
17	Cromer Lt	52°55'·45N	01°19'·10E	CM	313·50	A1A	50M	
19	Flamborough Head Lt	54°06'·95N	00°04'·87W	FB	302·00	A1A	70M	DGPS service 303·00 kHz 40M
A26	Teeside	54°33'·57N	01°20'·03W	TD	347·50	Non A2A	25M	
	SCOTLAND – EAST COAST							
21	Souter Point Lt	54°58'·23N	01°21'·80W	SJ	292·00	A1A	50M	
				PT	294·50	A1A	5M	Calibration station
A28	Edinburgh	55°58'·72N	03°17'·03W	EDN	341·00	Non A2A	35M	
23	Inchkeith	56°02'·02N	03°08'·08W	NK	286·50	A1A	10M	
25	Fidra Lt	56°04'·40N	02°46'·98W	FD	290·00	A1A	15M	
27	Fife Ness Lt	56°16'·73N	02°35'·10W	FP	305·00	A1A	50M	
A30	Dundee	56°27'·30N	03°06'·83W	DND	394·00	Non A2A	25M	
29	Girdle Ness	57°08'·32N	02°02'·83W	GD	311·00	A1A	50M	
A32	Aberdeen	57°16'·13N	02°24'·18W	AOS	377·00	Non A2A	50M	
A34	Scotstown Head	57°33'·56N	01°48'·94W	SHD	383·00	Non A2A	80M	
A36	Kinloss	57°39'·00N	03°35'·00W	KS	370·00	Non A2A	20M	

No.	Name	Lat	Long	Call	Freq (kHz)	Emission	Range	Notes
A38	**Wick**	58°26'.83N	03°03'.70W	WIK	344.00	Non A2A	40M	
33	**Duncansby Head**	58°38'.67N	03°01'.42W	DY	290.50	A1A	50M	
A40	**Kirkwall**	58°58'.67N	02°54'.62W	KW	395.00	Non A2A	30M	
35	**Sumburgh Head**	59°51'.30N	01°16'.37W	SB	304.00	A1A	70M	DGPS service 304·50 kHz 56M
A42	**Lerwick/Tingwall**	60°11'.33N	01°14'.67W	TL	376.00	Non A2A	25M	
A44	**Scatsa**	60°27'.68N	01°12'.78W	SS	315.50	Non A2A	25M	
A46	**Unst**	60°44'.33N	00°49'.17W	UT	325.00	Non A2A	20M	

SCOTLAND – WEST COAST

No.	Name	Lat	Long	Call	Freq (kHz)	Emission	Range	Notes
37	**Butt of Lewis**	58°30'.93N	06°15'.72W	BL	289.00	A1A	70M	DGPS service 289·50 kHz 40M
A52	**Stornoway**	58°12'.86N	06°19'.49W	SAY	669.50	Non A2A	20M	
A54	**St Kilda**	57°49'.00N	08°35'.00W	KL	338.00	Non A2A	30M	
A56	**Barra**	57°01'.40N	07°26'.40W	BRR	316.00	Non A2A	20M	Occasl
A58	**North Connel/Oban**	56°27'.83N	05°23'.62W	CNL	404.00	Non A2A	15M	
39	**Rhinns of Islay**	55°40'.38N	06°30'.70W	RN	293.00	A1A	70M	DGPS service 293·50 kHz 56M
A60	**Islay/Port Ellen**	55°40'.98N	06°14'.90W	LAY	395.00	Non A2A	20M	
41	**Cloch Point Lt**	55°56'.53N	04°52'.67W	CL	300.00	A1A	8M	Calibration station. On request
A62	**Turnberry**	55°18'.80N	04°46'.96W	TRN	355.00	Non A2A	25M	
A64	**New Galloway**	55°10'.63N	04°10'.03W	NGY	399.00	Non A2A	35M	

ENGLAND (WEST COAST), ISLE OF MAN, WALES

No.	Name	Lat	Long	Call	Freq (kHz)	Emission	Range	Notes
A66	**Carnane**	54°08'.46N	04°29'.42W	CAR	366.50	Non A2A	25M	
A68	**Ronaldsway/IOM**	54°05'.15N	04°36'.45W	RWY	359.00	Non A2A	20M	
43	**Walney Island**	54°02'.92N	03°10'.55W	FN	306.00	A1A	50M	
A70	**Barrow/Walney Island**	54°07'.64N	03°15'.80W	WL	385.00	Non A2A	15M	
A72	**Blackpool**	53°46'.36N	03°01'.59W	BPL	420.00	Non A2A	15M	
A74	**Warton**	53°45'.09N	02°51'.05W	WTN	337.00	Non A2A	15M	Day service
45	**Point Lynas Lt**	53°24'.97N	04°17'.30W	PS	304.00	A1A	50M	DGPS service 304·50 kHz 40M
A76	**Aberporth**	52°06'.98N	04°33'.57W	AP	370.50	Non A2	20M	
47	**South Bishop Lt**	51°51'.15N	05°24'.65W	SB	290.50	A1A	70M	
A78	**Swansea**	51°36'.10N	04°03'.88W	SWN	320.50	Non A2A	15M	Day service
A80	**Cardiff/Rhoose**	51°23'.57N	03°20'.23W	CDF	388.50	Non A2A	20M	
49	**Nash Point Lt**	51°24'.03N	03°33'.06W	NP	299.50	A1A	50M	
51	**Lynemouth Foreland Lt**	51°14'.70N	03°47'.13W	FP	294.50	A1A	5M	Calibration station. SR+1 to SS−1 hr
A82	**St Mawgan**	50°26'.51N	04°59'.36W	SM	365.5	Non A2A	20M	

4

CHANNEL ISLANDS

No.	Station	Call	Position	Freq (kHz)	Emission	Range	Remarks
A92	Alderney	ALD	49°42'.58N 02°11'.90W	383·00	Non A2A	50M	
55	Castle Breakwater St Peter Port❶	GY	49°27'.37N 02°31'.37W	304·50	A1A	10M	

❶ Synchronised with horn for distance finding. Horn begins simultaneously with 27 sec long dash after the four GY ident signals. Time in secs from start of long dash until horn is heard, multiplied by 0·18 gives dist in M.

No.	Station	Call	Position	Freq (kHz)	Emission	Range	Remarks
A94	Guernsey	GRB	49°26'.12N 02°38'.30W	361·00	Non A2A	30M	
57	La Corbière Lt❶❷	CB	49°10'.85N 02°14'.90W	295·50	A1A	20M	

❶ For details of coded wind information see 7.2.15.
❷ Synchronised for distance finding. The beacon transmits on a 6 min cycle. The 6th minute signal consists of: CB 3 times, 26 sec long dash, followed by a series of pips. Horn blast (Morse 'C') begins with end of 26 sec long dash. Each pip heard before the blast corresponds to a distance of 335m from the light.

No.	Station	Call	Position	Freq (kHz)	Emission	Range	Remarks
59	Elizabeth Castle, St Helier	EC	49°10'.62N 02°07'.50W	306·00	A1A	10MM	
A96	Jersey West	JW	49°12'.37N 02°13'.30W	329·00	Non A2A	25M	

IRELAND

No.	Station	Call	Position	Freq (kHz)	Emission	Range	Remarks
63	Mizen Head Lt	MZ	51°27'.05N 09°48'.80W	300·00	A1A	100M	DGPS service 300·50 kHz 56M
65	Old Head of Kinsale Lt	OH	51°36'.26N 08°31'.98W	288·00	A1A	50M	
		KC		294·50	A1A	5M	Calibration station. On request
A100	Waterford	WTD	52°11'.19N 07°04'.57W	368·00	Non A2A	25M	
67	Tuskar Rock Lt	TR	52°12'.17N 06°12'.40W	286·00	A1A	50M	
A102	Killiney/Dublin	KLY	53°16'.17N 06°06'.33W	378·00	Non A2A	50M	
69	Baily	BY	53°21'.68N 06°03'.08W	289·00	A1A	50M	
		BY		286·50	A1A	5M	Calibration station. On request
A104	Rush/Dublin	RSH	53°30'.73N 06°06'.60W	326·00	Non A2A	30M	
71	South Rock Lt F	SU	54°21'.47N 05°21'.92W	291·50	A1A	50M	
A106	Belfast City	HB	54°36'.94N 05°52'.86W	420·00	Non A2A	15M	
73	Black Head (Antrim)	BA	54°46'.05N 05°41'.30W	294·50	A1A	5M	Calibration station. On request
A108	Eglinton/Londonderry	EGT	55°02'.70N 07°09'.25W	328·50	Non A2A	25M	
75	Tory Island Lt	TY	55°16'.36N 08°14'.91W	313·00	A1A	100M	
77	Eagle Island Lt	GL	54°16'.98N 10°05'.52W	307·00	A1A	100M	
A110	Sligo	SLG	54°16'.83N 08°36'.00W	384·00	Non A2A	25M	
A112	Galway/Carnmore	CRN	53°18'.05N 08°56'.50W	321·00	Non A2A	25M	
A114	Ennis	ENS	52°54'.27N 08°55'.62W	352·00	Non A2A	80M	
A116	Foynes	FOY	52°33'.97N 09°11'.67W	395·00	Non A2A	50M	DGPS service 313·50 kHz 56M
79	Loop Head Lt	LP	52°33'.65N 09°55'.90W	311·50	A1A	50M	

Fig. 4(5)   RDF BEACONS
– BRITISH ISLES

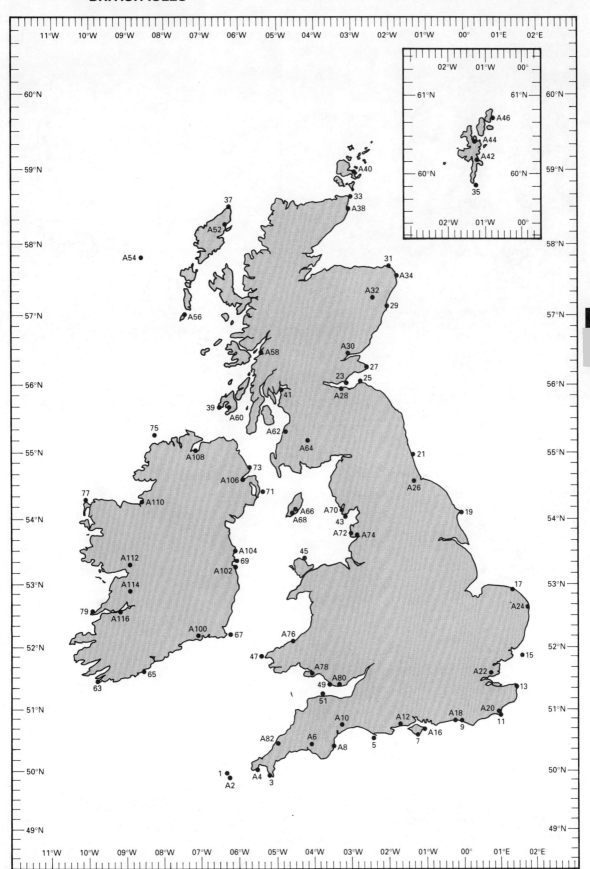

Fig. 4(6) RDF BEACONS
– CHANNEL ISLES AND EUROPE

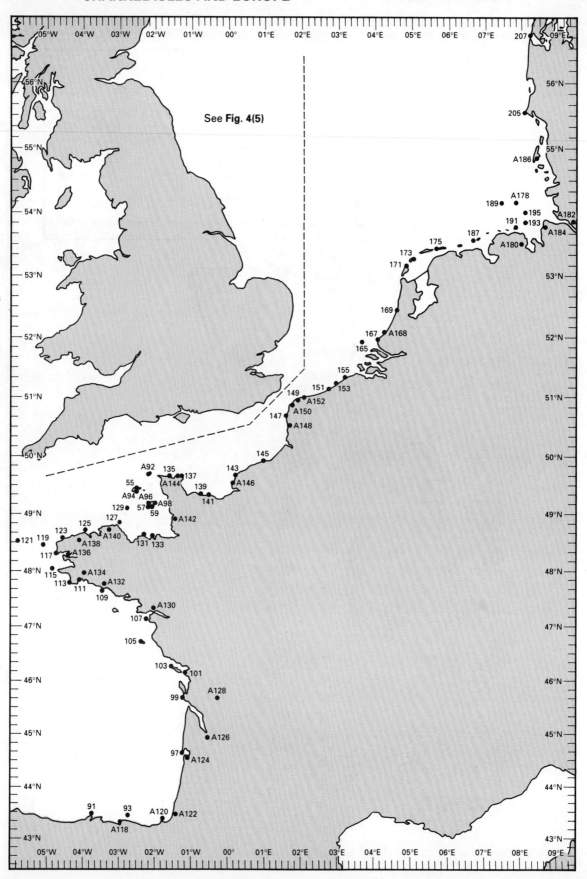

SPAIN – NORTH COAST

No.	Name	Lat	Long	Ident	Freq (kHz)	Type	Range	Notes
91	Cabo Mayor Lt	43°29'·48N	03°47'·37W	MY	304·50	A1A	100M	
A118	Bilbao	43°19'·52N	02°58'·32W	BLO	370·00	Non A2A	70M	
93	Cabo Machichaco Lt	43°27'·45N	02°45'·08W	MA	284·50	A1A	100M	
A120	San Sebastian	43°23'·25N	01°47'·65W	HIG	328·00	Non A2A	50M	

FRANCE – WEST COAST

No.	Name	Lat	Long	Ident	Freq (kHz)	Type	Range	Notes
A122	Biarritz	43°28'·25N	01°24'·18W	BZ	341·00	A1A	35M	Day service
A124	Cazaux	44°33'·08N	01°07'·13W	CAA	382·00	A1A	80M	DGPS service 287·00 kHz 40M
97	Cap Ferret Lt	44°38'·77N	01°14'·81W	FT	286·50	A1A	100M	
A126	Bordeaux/Mérignac	44°55'·92N	00°33'·88W	BD	393·00	A1A	30M	
A128	Cognac/Châteaubernard	45°40'·13N	00°18'·53W	CGC	354·00	A1A	75M	
99	Pointe de la Coubre	45°41'·87N	01°13'·93W	LK	292·00	A1A	100M	
101	La Rochelle	46°08'·97N	01°10'·27W	RE	295·50	A1A	25M	
103	Les Balines Lt (île de Ré)	46:14'·70N	01°33'·60W	BN	299·50	A1A	40M	DGPS service 299·50 kHz 40M
105	île d'Yeu Main Lt	46°43'·10N	02°22'·90W	YE	303·00	A1A	100M	
107	Pointe de St Gildas	47°08'·10N	02°14'·67W	NZ	308·50	A1A	40M	
A130	St Nazaire/Montoir	47°20'·02N	02°02'·57W	MT	398·00	A1A	50M	
A132	Lorient/Lann–Bihoué	47°45'·75N	03°26'·43W	LOR	359·00	A1A	80M	
109	Pen Men Lt, île de Groix	47°38'·97N	03°30'·36W	GX	298·00	A1A	50M	
A134	Quimper/Pluguffan	47°58'·10N	03°59'·80W	QR	380·00	A1A	20M	
111	Pointe de Combrit Lt	47°51'·92N	04°06'·70W	CT	288·50	A1A	50M	
113	Eckmühl Lt	47°47'·95N	04°22'·35W	ÜH	312·00	A1A	70M	
115	île de Sein NW Lt	48°02'·70N	04°51'·95W	SN	289·50	A1A	80M	
A136	Lanvéoc, Poulmic	48°17'·07N	04°26'·00W	BST	316·00	A1A	50M	
117	Pointe St Mathieu Lt	48°19'·85N	04°46'·17W	SM	292·50	A1A	100M	DGPS service 312·50 kHz 40M
119	île d'Ouessant	48°27'·63N	05°07'·57W	CA	301·00	A1A	100M	

FRANCE – NORTH COAST

No.	Name	Lat	Long	Ident	Freq (kHz)	Type	Range	Notes
121	Ouessant SW Lanby	48°31'·68N	05°49'·10W	SW	305·50	A1A	10M	
123	île Vierge Lt	48°38'·38N	04°33'·97W	VG	314·00	A1A	70M	
A138	Landivisiau	48°32'·80N	04°08'·25W	LDV	324·00	A1A	60M	
125	Roscoff–Bloscon Jetty Lt	48°43'·29N	03°57'·62W	BC	304·50	A1A	10M	
A140	Lannion	48°43'·25N	03°18'·45W	LN	345·00	A1A	50M	
127	Rosédo Lt, île Bréhat	48°51'·50N	03°00'·32W	DO	287·50	A1A	10M	
129	Roches–Douvres Lt	49°06'·47N	02°48'·65W	RD	308·00	A1A	70M	
131	Cap Fréhel Lt	48°41'·10N	02°19'·07W	FÉ	286·50	A1A	20M	
133	Le Grand Jardin Lt	48°40'·27N	02°04'·90W	GJ	306·50	A1A	10M	
A142	Granville	48°55'·10N	01°28'·87W	GV	321·00	A1A	25M	
135	Cherbourg W Fort Lt	49°40'·50N	01°38'·87W	RB	302·00	A1A	20M	

4

No.	Name	Latitude	Longitude	Ident	Frequency	Emission	Range	Remarks
137	**Pointe de Barfleur Lt**	49°41'·87N	01°15'·87W	FG	297·00	A1A	70M	
139	**Port en Bessin Rear Lt**	49°21'·00N	00°45'·60W	BS	290·00	A1A	5M	
A144	**Cherbourg/Maupertus**	49°38'·30N	01°22'·28W	MP	373·00	A1A	20M	
141	**Pointe de Ver Lt**	49°20'·47N	00°31'·15W	ÉR	310·00	A1A	15M	
A146	**Le Havre/Octeville**	49°35'·70N	00°11'·00E	LHO	346·00	A1A	50M	
143	**Cap d'Antifer Lt**	49°41'·07N	00°10'·00E	TI	300·00	A1A	50M	
145	**Pointe d'Ailly Lt**	49°55'·00N	00°57'·55E	AL	305·50	A1A	20M	
A148	**Le Touquet/Paris Plage**	50°32'·23N	01°35'·38E	LT	358·00	A2A	20M	
147	**Cap d'Alprech Lt**	50°41'·95N	01°33'·83E	PH	294·00	A1A	20M	
149	**Calais Main Lt**	50°57'·73N	01°51'·30E	CS	312·50	A1A	50M	
A150	**St Inglevert**	50°52'·98N	01°44'·55E	ING	387·50	A1A	50M	Day service
A152	**Calais/Dunkirk**	50°59'·85N	02°03'·33E	MK	418·00	A1A	15M	

BELGIUM

No.	Name	Latitude	Longitude	Ident	Frequency	Emission	Range	Remarks
151	**Nieuwpoort W Pier Lt**	51°09'·40N	02°43'·08E	NP	285·00	A1A	5M	
153	**Oostende Rear Lt**	51°14'·36N	02°55'·97E	OE	312·00	A1A	40M	
155	**Zeebrugge**	51°21'·66N	03°11'·33E	ZB	289·00	A1A	5M	

NETHERLANDS

No.	Name	Latitude	Longitude	Ident	Frequency	Emission	Range	Remarks
165	**Goeree Lt**	51°55'·53N	03°40'·18E	GR	296·00	A1A	48M	
167	**Hoek van Holland**	51°58'·90N	04°06'·83E	HH	288·00	A1A	50M	DGPS service 287·50 kHz 40M
A69	**IJmuiden Front Lt**	52°27'·78N	04°34'·57E	YM	288·50	A1A	20M	
171	**Eierland Lt**	53°10'·97N	04°51'·40E	ER	301·00	A1A	20M	
173	**Vlieland Lt**	53°17'·80N	05°03'·57E	VL	303·50	A1A	20M	
175	**Ameland Lt**	53°27'·02N	05°37'·60E	AD	299·00	A1A	50M	DGPS service 299·50 kHz 40M

GERMANY

No.	Name	Latitude	Longitude	Ident	Frequency	Emission	Range	Remarks
187	**Borkum, Kleiner Lt**	53°34'·78N	06°40'·09E	BE	302·00	A1A	20M	
189	**German Bight Lt V**	54°10'·80N	07°26'·10E	GB	312·00	A1A	10M	
191	**Wangerooge Lt**	53°47'·45N	07°51'·52E	WE	309·50	A1A	20M	
A178	**Helgoland Lt**	54°11'·00N	07°53'·00E	DHE	397·20	A1A/A2A	100M	
193	**Alte Weser Lt**	53°51'·85N	08°07'·72E	AR	309·00	A1A	20M	
195	**Elbe Lt F**	54°00'·00N	08°06'·58E	EL	298·00	A1A	20M	
A180	**Jever**	53°31'·18N	08°00'·92E	JEV	390·00	A1A	50M	
A182	**Glukstadt**	53°51'·07N	09°27'·32E	GLX	365·00	Non A2A	30M	
A184	**Nordholz**	53°47'·18N	08°48'·47E	NDO	372·00	Non A2A	30M	
A186	**Westerland/Sylt**	54°51'·40N	08°24'·67E	SLT	387·00	Non A2A	25M	

4.7   RADAR

4.7.1   Radar in yachts
Radar is useful both for navigation and for collision avoidance, but to take full advantage of it and to use it in safety demands a proper understanding of its operation and of its limitations. Read the instruction book carefully, and practise using and adjusting the set so as to get optimum performance in different conditions. It is important to learn how to interpret what is seen on the display.

Radar beams do not discriminate so well in bearing as they do in range — so an accurate fix is sometimes best obtained by a radar range and a visual bearing of the same object.

The effective range of radar is approximately line of sight, but this can be decreased or increased by abnormal conditions. It is necessary to be aware that radar will not detect a low-lying coastline which is over the radar horizon.

The details of radar, and its use are described in *The Macmillan & Silk Cut Yachtsman's Handbook* (4.6).

4.7.2   Radar for collision avoidance
Yacht radars invariably have a ship's head up display, with the boat at the centre, apparently stationary. If a target is moving in the same direction and at the same speed, it is stationary relative to own ship, and its echo should be sharp and well defined. If it is on a reciprocal course, it paints an echo with a long tail.

If an echo is on a steady bearing, and the range is decreasing, there is risk of collision. But to determine the proper action to take it is necessary to plot an approaching echo three or four times, in order to determine her actual course and speed, and how close she will actually approach.

4.7.3   Radar as a navigation aid
Radar cannot see behind other objects, or round corners; it may not pick up small objects, or differentiate between two targets that are close together. As already stated, radar ranges are more accurate than radar bearings. Objects with sharp features such as buildings give a better reflection than those with curved or sloping surfaces. High cliffs make a good target, but low coastlines should be approached with extreme caution as the first thing to show on radar may be hills some distance inland.

4.7.4   Radar beacons (Racons)
A Racon is a transponder beacon which, when triggered by a transmission from a vessel's radar, sends back a distinctive signal which appears on the vessel's radar display. Racons are fitted to some light-vessels, buoys and lighthouses, and are marked on charts by a magenta circle and the word Racon.™

In most cases the Racon flash on the display is a line extending radially outwards from a point slightly beyond the actual position of the Racon, due to the slight delay in the response of the beacon apparatus. Thus the distance to the mark of the Racon flash is a little more than the vessel's real distance from the Racon. Some Racons give a flash composed of a Morse identification signal, often with a tail to it, the length of the tail depending on the number of Morse characters.

The maximum range of a radar beacon is usually about 10 nautical miles, but may be more. In practice, picking up a Racon at greater distances depends also on the effective range of the boat's radar. With abnormal radio propagation, a spurious Racon flash may be seen at much greater distances than the beacon's normal range, appearing at any random position along the correct bearing on the display. Only rely on a Racon flash if its appearance is consistent, and the boat is believed to be within its range. At short range a Racon sometimes causes unwelcome interference on the radar display, and this may be reduced by adjusting the rain clutter control on the set.

The characteristics of radar beacons around the coasts of Great Britain are given in Table 4(2). Details are arranged in the following columns:

(1)   Reference number.
(2)   The type of radar beacon. Unless otherwise stated, all radar beacons sweep the frequency range of marine 3cm (X-band) radar emissions. The older type of radar beacon (swept frequency Racons) take 30 to 90 seconds to sweep the band and the period of sweep is adjusted during installation to suit the individual location.

The newer type of radar beacon (agile frequency Racon) responds immediately to radar interrogations. However, in order that wanted echoes should not be obscured by the Racon signal, the agile response is switched 'on' and 'off' at a pre-determined rate to suit the installation. Where indicated, radar beacons respond to both 10cm (S-band) and 3cm (X-band) emissions and are usually agile frequency Racons.
(3)   Name of the station.
(4)   Latitude and longitude.
(5)   The sector within which signals may be received, bearings being towards the beacon, clockwise from 000° to 359°. 360° indicates all round operation.
(6)   Approximate range, in nautical miles. This also depends on the range of the yacht's radar set.
(7)   The form of the beacon's flash on the radar display. Morse signals are shown alphabetically, and are often followed by a 'tail'. Racons coded 'D' are used to mark new dangers.

Table 4(2) LIST OF RADAR BEACONS

(For heading details see 4.6.4)

(1) No	(2) Type	(3) Name	(4) Lat	Long	(5) Sector	(6) Approx range	(7) Ident
GREAT BRITAIN							
1	3 & 10 cm	**Bishop Rock Lt**	49°52'·33N	06°26'·68W	245°-215°	**18M**	T
3	3 & 10 cm	**Seven Stones Lt V**	50°03'·58N	06°04'·28W	360°	**15M**	O
5	3 & 10 cm	**Wolf Rock Lt**	49°56'·67N	05°48'·48W	360°	**10M**	T
7	3 & 10 cm	**Eddystone Lt**	50°10'·81N	04°15'·87W	360°	**10M**	T
9	3 cm	**West Bramble Lt By**	50°47'·17N	01°18'·57W	360°	**3M**	T
11	3 & 10 cm	**Nab Tower Lt**	50°40'·05N	00°57'·07W	360°	**10M**	T
13	3 & 10 cm	**Greenwich Lt V**	50°24'·50N	00°00'·00	360°	**10M**	T
15	3 & 10 cm	**Varne Lanby**	51°01'·26N	01°24'·01E	360°	**10M**	T
17	3 & 10 cm	**Sandettié Lt V**	51°09'·40N	01°47'·20E	360°	**10M**	T
19	3 & 10 cm	**East Goodwin Lt F**	51°13'·05N	01°36'·32E	360°	**10M**	T
21	3 & 10 cm	**Inter Bank Lt By**	51°16'·45N	01°52'·33E	360°	**10M**	M
23	3 & 10 cm	**NE Goodwin Lt By**	51°20'·28N	01°34'·27E	360°	**10M**	M
25	3 & 10 cm	**Dover Strait TSS, F3 Lanby**	51°23'·82N	02°00'·62E	360°	**10M**	T
27	3 cm	**Thames Sea Reach Lt By No 1**	51°29'·42N	00°52'·67E	360°	**10M**	T
29	3 cm	**Thames Sea Reach Lt By No 7**	51°30'·08N	00°37'·15E	360°	**10M**	T
31	3 & 10 cm	**Outer Tongue Lt By**	51°30'·78N	01°26'·47E	360°	**10M**	T
33	3 & 10 cm	**Barrow Lt By No 3**	51°41'·99N	01°20'·35E	360°	**10M**	M
35	3 & 10 cm	**South Galloper Lt By**	51°43'·95N	01°56'·50E	360°	**10M**	T
37	3 & 10 cm	**Sunk Lt F**	51°51'·00N	01°35'·00E	360°	**10M**	T
39	3 & 10 cm	**Harwich Channel Lt By No 1**	51°56'·11N	01°27'·30E	360°	**10M**	T
41	3 & 10 cm	**Outer Gabbard Lt By**	51°57'·80N	02°04'·30E	360°	**10M**	O
43	3 & 10 cm	**N Shipwash Lt By**	52°01'·38N	01°38'·38W	360°	**10M**	M
45	3 & 10 cm	**Orfordness Lt**	52°05'·01N	01°34'·60E		**18M**	T
47	3 cm	**Cross Sand Lt By**	52°37'·00N	01°59'·25E	360°	**10M**	T
49	3 & 10 cm	**Winterton Old Lt Ho**	52°42'·75N	01°41'·82E	360°	**10M**	T
51	3 & 10 cm	**Smiths Knoll Lt By**	53°43'·50N	02°18'·00E	360°	**10M**	T
53	3 & 10 cm	**Newarp Lt By**	52°48'·35N	01°55'·80E	360°	**10M**	O
55	3 & 10 cm	**Cromer Lt**	52°55'·45N	01°19'·10E	360°	**25M**	T
55	3 & 10 cm	**North Haisbro Lt By**	53°00'·20N	01°32'·40E	360°	**10M**	T
59	3 & 10 cm	**North Well Lt By**	53°03'·00N	00°28'·00E	360°	**10M**	T
61	3 & 10 cm	**Dudgeon Lt By**	53°16'·60N	01°17'·00E	360°	**10M**	O
63	3 & 10 cm	**Anglia Field Platform A48/19**	53°22'·03N	01°39'·21W	360°	**15M**	Q
65	3 & 10 cm	**Inner Dowsing Lt**	53°19'·70N	00°33'·98E	360°	**25M**	T
67	3 & 10 cm	**Spurn Lt F**	53°33'·53N	00°14'·33E	360°	**5M**	M
69	3 & 10 cm	**Amethyst B1D Platform**	53°33'·65N	00°52'·75E	360°	**10M**	T
71	3 & 10 cm	**Humber Lt By**	53°36'·72N	01°21'·60E	360°	**7M**	T
73	3 cm	**Tees Fairway By**	54°40'·93N	01°06'·37W	360°		B
75	3 & 10 cm	**St Abb's Head Lt**	55°54'·97N	02°08'·20W	360°	**18M**	T
77	3 cm	**Inchkeith Fairway By**	56°03'·50N	03°00'·00W	360°	**5M**	T
79	3 cm	**Forth North Channel Lt By No 7**	56°02'·80N	03°10'·87W	360°	**5M**	T
81	3 & 10 cm	**Bell Rock Lt**	56°26'·05N	02°23'·07W	360°	**18M**	M
83	3 & 10 cm	**Abertay Lt By**	56°27'·41N	02°40'·65W	360°	**8M**	T
85	3 cm	**Scurdie Ness Lt**	56°42'·12N	02°26'·15W	360°	**15M**	T
87	3 & 10 cm	**Girdle Ness Lt**	57°08'·35N	02°02'·82W	165°-055°[1]	**25M**	G
	[1] Reduced coverage within sector 055°-165°.						
89	3 cm	**Aberdeen Fairway By**	57°09'·33N	02°01'·85W	360°	**7M**	T
91		**Carragh Rocks Lt By**					
93	3 cm	**Buchan Ness Lt**	57°28'·23N	01°46'·37W	155°-045°[1]	**25M**	O
	[1] Reduced coverage within sector 045°-155°.						
95	3 & 10 cm	**Rattray Head Lt**	57°36'·62N	01°48'·83W	110°-340°	**15M**	M
97	3 cm	**Cromarty Firth Fairway By**	57°39'·98N	03°54'·10W	360°	**5M**	M
99	3 cm	**Tarbert Ness Lt**	57°51'·92N	03°46'·52W	360°	**12M**	T

(1) No	(2) Type	(3) Name	(4) Lat	Long	(5) Sector	(6) Approx range	(7) Ident
101	3 & 10cm	Alba Oilfield, Platform Alba	58°03'·52N	01°04'·88E	360°		C
103	3 & 10 cm	Saltire Oil Field, Platform Alpha	58°25'·05N	00°19'·85E	360°		N
105	3 & 10 cm	Piper Oil Field, Platform Bravo	58°27'·68N	00°15'·07E	360°		N
107	3 & 10 cm	Duncansby Head Lt	58°38'·67N	03°01'·44W	360°	20M	T
109	3 & 10 cm	Lother Rock Lt	58°43'·82N	02°58'·59W	360°	10M	M
111	3 &10cm	North Ronaldsay Lt	59°23'·40N	02°22'·80W	360°	10M	T
113	3 cm	Rumble Rock Bn	60°28'·22N	01°07'·13W	360°	10M	O
115	3 & 10 cm	Gruney Island Lt	60°39'·20N	01°18'·03W	360°	14M	T
117	3 & 10 cm	Ve Skerries Lt	60°22'·40N	01°48'·67W	360°	15M	T
119	3 & 10 cm	Sule Skerry Lt	59°05'·10N	04°24'·30W	360°	20M	T
121	3 cm	Eilean Glas Lt	57°51'·43N	06°38'·45W	360°	12M	T
123	3 cm	Castlebay South By	56°56'·10N	07°27'·17W	360°	7M	T
125	3 cm	Monach Lt Ho	57°31'·55N	07°41'·63W	360°	16M	T
127	3 & 10 cm	Bo Vic Chuan By	56°56'·17N	07°23'·25W	360°	5M	M
129	3 & 10 cm	Skerryvore Lt	56°19'·40N	07°06'·90W	360°	18M	M
131	3 cm	Sanda Lt	55°16'·50N	05°34'·90W	360°	20M	T
133	3 cm	Point of Ayre Lt	54°24'·95N	04°22'·03W	360°	13M	M
135	3 & 10 cm	Lune Deep Lt By	53°55'·80N	03°11'·00W	360°	10M	T
137	3 & 10 cm	Halfway Shoal Lt Bn	54°01'·46N	03°11'·80W	360°	10M	B
139	3 cm	Bar Lanby	53°32'·00N	03°20'·90W	360°	10M	T
141	3 & 10 cm	The Skerries Lt	53°25'·27N	04°36'·44W	360°	25M	T
143	3 & 10 cm	The Smalls Lt	51°43'·23N	05°40'·10W	360°	25M	T
145	3 & 10 cm	St Gowan Lt By	51°31'·90N	04°59'·70W	360°	10M	T
147	3 & 10 cm	West Helwick Lt By W. HWK	51°31'·37N	04°23'·58W	360°	10M	T
149	3 & 10 cm	West Scar Lt By (Swansea Bay)	51°28'·28N	03°55'·50W	360°	10M	T
151	3 & 10 cm	English & Welsh Grounds Lt By	51°26'·90N	03°00'·10W	360°	7M	O
153	3 & 10 cm	Breaksea Lt F	51°19'·85N	03°19'·00W	360°	10M	T

CHANNEL/CHANNEL ISLANDS (see also No. 13)

(1) No	(2) Type	(3) Name	(4) Lat	Long	(5) Sector	(6) Approx range	(7) Ident
171	3 & 10 cm	English Channel Lt By EC 1	50°05'·90N	01°48'·35W	360°	10M	T
173	3 & 10 cm	English Channel Lt By EC 2	50°12'·10N	01°12'·40W	360°	10M	T
175	3 & 10 cm	English Channel Lt By EC 3	50°18'·30N	00°36'·10W	360°	10M	T
177	3 & 10 cm	East Channel Lt By	49°58'·67N	02°28'·87W	360°	10M	T
179	3 & 10 cm	Channel Lt V	49°54'·42N	02°53'·67W	360°	15M	O
181	3 & 10 cm	Casquets Lt	49°43'·38N	02°22'·55W	360°	25M	T
183	3 cm	Platte Fougère Lt	49°30'·88N	02°29'·05W	360°	–	P
185	3 cm	St Helier, Demie de Pas Lt	49°09'·07N	02°06'·05W	360°	10M	T
187	3 cm	St Helier, Mont Ubé Ldg Lt	49°10'·35N	02°03'·53W	360°	14M	T

IRELAND

(1) No	(2) Type	(3) Name	(4) Lat	Long	(5) Sector	(6) Approx range	(7) Ident
199	3 & 10 cm	Inishtearaght Lt	52°04'·51N	10°39'·66W	313°-221°	18M	O
201	3 & 10 cm	Rathlin O'Birne Lt	54°39'·80N	08°49'·90W	284°-203°	13M	O
203	3 & 10 cm	Inisheer Lt	53°02'·78N	09°31'·57 W	216°-144°	13M	K
205	3 & 10 cm	Ballybunnion Lt By	52°32'·50N	09°46'·92W	360°	6M	M
207	3 & 10 cm	Mizen Head Lt	51°26'·97N	09°49'·18W	360°	24M	T
209	3 & 10 cm	Fastnet Lt	51°23'·33N	09°36'·14W	360°	18M	G
211	3 cm	Cork Lt By	51°42'·90N	08°15'·50W	360°	7M	T
213	3 & 10 cm	Hook Head Lt	52°07'·40N	06°55'·72W	237°–177°	10M	K
215	3 & 10 cm	Coningbeg Lt V	52°02'·38N	06°39'·45W	360°	13M	M
217	3 cm	Tuskar Rock Lt	52°12'·15N	06°12'·38W	360°	18M	T
219	3 & 10 cm	Arklow Lt By	52°39'·50N	05°58'·10W	360°	10M	O
221	3 cm	Codling Lanby	53°03'·02N	05°40'·70W	360°	10M	G
223	3 & 10 cm	Kish Bank Lt	53°18'·68N	05°55'·38W	360°	15M	T
225	3 cm	South Rock Lt V	54°24'·47N	05°21'·92W	360°	13M	T
227	3 & 10 cm	Mew Island Lt	54°41'·91N	05°30'·73W	360°	14M	O
229	3 & 10 cm	Inishtrahull Lt	55°25'·85N	07°14'·60W	060°–310°[1]	24M	T

[1] Reduced or no signal 310°–060°.

4

(1) No	(2) Type	(3) Name	(4) Lat	Long	(5) Sector	(6) Approx range	(7) Ident

FRANCE

No	Type	Name	Lat	Long	Sector	Approx range	Ident
301	3 cm	**BXA Lanby**	45°37'·60N	01°28'·60W	360°		**B**
303	3 cm	**St Nazaire, La Couronnée Lt By**	47°07'·67N	02°20'·00W	360°	**3–5M**	See [1]

[1] Signals appear as a series of dots, the distance between each dot corresponding to 0·2M.

No	Type	Name	Lat	Long	Sector	Approx range	Ident
305	3 cm	**St Nazaire Lt By SN 1**	47°00'·12N	02°39'·75W	360°	**3–8M**	**Z**
307	3 cm	**Chausée de Sein Lt By**	48°03'·80N	05°07'·70W	360°	**10M**	**0**
309	3 cm	**Pointe de Créac'h Lt**	48°27'·62N	05°07'·65W	030°–248°	**20M**	**C**
311	3 & 10 cm	**Ouessant SW Lanby**	48°31'·68N	05°49'·10W	360°	**20M**	**M**
313	3 cm	**Ouessant NE Lt By**	48°45'·90N	05°11'·60W	360°	**20M**	**B**
315	3 & 10 cm	**Le Havre LHA Lanby**	49°31'·67N	00°09'·80W	360°	**8–10M**	See [1]

[1] Signals appear as a series of 8 dots or 8 groups of dots. The distance between each dot or group of dots corresponds to 0·3M.

No	Type	Name	Lat	Long	Sector	Approx range	Ident
317	3 cm	**Antifer Approach Lt By A5**	49°45'·89N	00°17'·40W	360°	**–**	**K**
319	3 cm	**Bassurelle Lt By**	50°32'·70N	00°57'·80E	360°	**5–8M**	**B**
321	3 cm	**Vergoyer Lt By N**	50°39'·70N	01°22'·30E	360°	**5– 8M**	**C**
323	3 cm	**Dunkerque Lanby**	51°02'·96N	01°51'·86E	360°	**–**	See [1]

[1] Signal appears as a succession of 8 dots. The distance between each dot corresponds to 0·3M.

BELGIUM AND NETHERLANDS

No	Type	Name	Lat	Long	Sector	Approx range	Ident
351	3 & 10 cm	**Wandelaar Lt MOW 0**	51°23'·70N	03°02'·80E	360°	**10M**	**S**
353	3 & 10 cm	**Bol Van Heist Lt MOW 3**	51°23'·43N	03°11'·98E	360°	**10M**	**H**
355	3 & 10 cm	**Keeten B Lt By**	51°36'·40N	03°58'·12E	360°	**–**	**K**
357	3 & 10 cm	**Zuid Vilije Lt By ZV11/SRK 4**	51°38'·23N	04°14'·56E	360°	**–**	**K**
359	3 & 10 cm	**Noord Hinder Lt By NHR–SE**	51°45'·50N	02°40'·00E	360°	**10M**	**N**
361	3 & 10 cm	**Noord Hinder Lt By**	52°00'·15N	02°51'·20E	360°	**12–15M**	**T**
363	3 cm	**Noord Hinder N Lt By**	52°08'·25N	03°01'·38E	360°	**10M**	**K**
365		**West Hinder Lt**	51°23'·36N	02°26'·35E			**W**
367	3 cm	**Schouwenbank Lt By**	51°45'·00N	03°14'·40E	360°	**10M**	**0**
369	3 & 10 cm	**Goeree Lt**	51°55'·53N	03°40'·18E	360°	**12–15M**	**T**
371	3 & 10 cm	**Maas Centre Lt By MC**	52°01'·18N	03°53'·57E	360°	**10M**	**M**
373	3 & 10 cm	**Rijn Field Platform P15–B**	52°18'·48N	03°46'·72E	030°–270°	**12–15M**	**B**
375	3 & 10 cm	**IJmuiden Lt By**	52°28'·70N	04°23'·93E	360°	**10M**	**Y**
377		**Horizon P9-6 Platform**	52°33'·20N	03°44'·54E			**Q**
379	3 & 10 cm	**Helm Veld A Platform**	52°52'·39N	04°08'·58E	360°	**–**	**T**
381	3 & 10 cm	**Logger Platform**	53°00'·90N	04°13'·05E	060°–270°	**12–15M**	**X**
383	3 cm	**Schulpengat Fairway Lt By SG**	52°52'·95N	04°38'·00E			**Z**
385	3 & 10 cm	**NAM Field Platform K14–FA–1**	53°16'·17N	03°37'·66E	360°	**7M**	
387	3 & 10 cm	**Vlieland Lanby VL–Center**	53°27'·00N	04°40'·00E	360°	**12–15M**	**C**
389	3 & 10 cm	**Wintershall Platform L8–G**	53°34'·92N	04°36'·32E	000°–340°	**12–15M**	**G**
391	3 & 10 cm	**Placid Field Platform PL–K9C–PA**	53°39'·20N	03°52'·45E	360°	**8M**	**B**
393	3 & 10 cm	**West Friesland Platform L2–FA–1**	53°57'·65N	04°29'·85E		**9M**	
395	3 cm	**DW Route Lt By FR/A**	54°00'·35N	04°21'·41E	360°	**6–10M**	**M**
397	3cm	**Elf Petroland Platform F15-A**	54°12'·98N	04°49'·71E	360°		**U**
399	3cm	**DW Route Lt By EF**	54°03'·30N	04°59'·80E			**T**
401	3cm	**DW Route Lt By EF/B**	54°06'·65N	05°40'·00E			**M**

GERMANY (North Sea Coast)

No	Type	Name	Lat	Long	Sector	Approx range	Ident
411	3 cm	**Westerems Lt By**	53°36'·97N	06°19'·48E	360°	**8M**	**T**
413	3 cm	**Borkumriff Lt By**	53°47'·50N	06°22'·13E	360°	**8M**	**T**
415	3 cm	**GW/Ems Lt F**	54°10'·00N	06°20'·80E	360°	**8M**	**T**
417	3 cm	**German Bight Lt V**	54°10'·80N	07°27'·60E	360°	**8M**	**T**
419	3 cm	**Jade/Weser Lt By**	53°58'·33N	07°38'·83E	360°	**8M**	**T**
421	3 & 10 cm	**Weser 1/Jade 2 Lt By**	53°52'·12N	07°47'·33E	360°	**8M**	**T**
423	3 cm	**Elbe Lt F**	54°00'·00N	08°06'·58E	360°	**8M**	**T**

Chapter 5

Astro-Navigation

Contents

The Astro-Supplement

The information required for astro-navigation has been produced separately in a forty-eight page Astro-Supplement. This can be obtained on request by ticking the relevant box on the Supplement request card and enclosing a cheque for £4·00 made out to Macmillan Publishers Ltd.

The middle section of the Astro-Supplement, comprising thirty pages of tables, contains the ephemerides of the Sun and Moon, GHA Aries and the 57 navigational stars, the Pole star, tables for interpolating the ephemerides, sextant altitude correction tables, rise set tables and conversion tables. Many of the tables are unique; they have all been designed to be compact and simple to use, and are intended to provide the GHA and Dec of all the bodies to within ±0'·3, which will be sufficient for most purposes.

The tables of sunrise, sunset and twilight, moonrise and moonset, and phases of the Moon enable the degree of darkness around twilight and throughout the night to be estimated.

The text that precedes the tables explains the general principles of astro-navigation, the role of the position line and how it is used to obtain position from astronomical sights. In this section it is assumed that the calculations are done manually, and that the intercept and azimuth are obtained using the *Sight Reduction Tables for Air Navigation*, AP3270, volume 1, for selected stars, and AP3270 volume 3, for the Sun, Moon and stars within 30° of the equator. A Sun-run-Sun example for obtaining position using volume 3 is included.

The final section of the Astro-Supplement contains algorithms for making some or all of the manual calculations required for a sight reduction with a micro-processor, such as a lap-top computer or a programmable calculator. Thus for example, algorithms for altitude correction may be used instead of the altitude correction tables themselves, which avoids interpolation, and increases the precision of the reduction. If the intercept and azimuth are determined manually from AP3270, a method is given for calculating the position, that is based on the standard plotting procedure. A method is also given for calculating the transit times of the Sun, Moon or a navigation star.

For a general introduction to the main principles and practices of astro-navigation Chapter 5 of the *Macmillan & Silk Cut Yachtsman's Handbook* is recommended. In particular it contains practical information on the use of a marine sextant, explaining how sextant errors are determined and how to take sights of the Sun, Moon and stars at sea.

5.1.1 TIMES OF SUNRISE (UT)

	JAN 1	15	FEB 1	15	MAR 1	15	APR 1	15	MAY 1	15	JUN 1	15	JUL 1	15	AUG 1	15	SEP 1	15	OCT 1	15	NOV 1	15	DEC 1	15
ABERDOVEY	0827	0820	0759	0733	0703	0631	0551	0519	0445	0420	0359	0352	0357	0411	0435	0458	0527	0550	0617	0641	0712	0738	0804	0821
ARCACHON	0742	0738	0724	0706	0643	0617	0546	0521	0455	0437	0422	0419	0423	0433	0451	0507	0527	0543	0602	0620	0642	0701	0721	0735
BELFAST	0846	0838	0813	0746	0713	0639	0556	0522	0445	0418	0355	0347	0352	0407	0434	0459	0530	0556	0626	0652	0726	0754	0822	0840
BERGEN	0845	0830	0756	0719	0638	0556	0504	0421	0335	0259	0224	0211	0216	0238	0316	0351	0432	0506	0544	0618	0702	0739	0817	0839
BREST	0809	0805	0747	0726	0700	0632	0556	0528	0459	0438	0421	0416	0421	0432	0453	0512	0535	0555	0617	0637	0704	0725	0748	0803
BURNHAM (Crouch)	0810	0803	0743	0718	0649	0618	0539	0508	0435	0411	0351	0345	0349	0403	0426	0448	0515	0538	0604	0627	0657	0722	0747	0803
CORK	0825	0819	0758	0733	0704	0633	0554	0522	0449	0425	0405	0359	0403	0417	0440	0502	0530	0552	0619	0642	0712	0737	0803	0819
CHERBOURG	0804	0758	0740	0717	0650	0621	0544	0515	0444	0422	0404	0358	0403	0415	0437	0457	0522	0542	0606	0628	0655	0718	0742	0757
CRAOBH HAVEN	0855	0845	0819	0749	0714	0638	0553	0517	0438	0409	0343	0334	0339	0355	0425	0452	0526	0553	0625	0654	0730	0800	0830	0849
CUXHAVEN	0853	0845	0822	0755	0723	0650	0608	0535	0459	0433	0411	0403	0408	0423	0449	0513	0543	0608	0636	0702	0735	0802	0830	0847
DARTMOUTH	0814	0809	0749	0726	0658	0628	0551	0521	0450	0427	0409	0403	0407	0420	0442	0503	0528	0550	0614	0636	0705	0728	0752	0808
EASTBOURNE	0801	0755	0735	0712	0643	0613	0535	0505	0433	0410	0351	0345	0349	0402	0425	0446	0512	0534	0559	0621	0650	0714	0739	0754
FALMOUTH	0819	0814	0755	0732	0704	0634	0557	0527	0456	0434	0415	0410	0414	0427	0449	0509	0535	0556	0620	0642	0710	0733	0757	0813
FLEETWOOD	0831	0823	0759	0733	0701	0627	0545	0512	0436	0410	0347	0340	0345	0359	0425	0450	0520	0545	0613	0639	0712	0739	0807	0824
GALWAY	0851	0843	0821	0755	0724	0651	0610	0537	0503	0437	0415	0408	0413	0427	0452	0516	0545	0610	0637	0703	0734	0801	0828	0845
GT YARMOUTH	0804	0757	0736	0710	0640	0608	0528	0456	0422	0357	0336	0329	0334	0348	0412	0435	0503	0527	0554	0618	0649	0715	0741	0758
HAMBURG	0737	0729	0706	0640	0609	0535	0454	0421	0346	0320	0258	0251	0256	0310	0336	0359	0429	0453	0522	0547	0619	0646	0713	0730
HARTLEPOOL	0828	0819	0755	0727	0655	0620	0537	0503	0426	0359	0336	0327	0332	0348	0415	0440	0511	0537	0607	0633	0707	0735	0804	0822
HARWICH	0803	0756	0735	0710	0641	0609	0530	0459	0426	0401	0341	0335	0339	0353	0416	0439	0506	0529	0555	0619	0649	0714	0740	0756
HELGOLAND	0748	0740	0717	0650	0618	0544	0502	0428	0352	0325	0302	0254	0259	0314	0341	0405	0436	0501	0530	0556	0629	0656	0725	0742
HOLYHEAD	0834	0826	0804	0737	0706	0633	0552	0519	0445	0419	0357	0350	0355	0409	0434	0458	0528	0552	0620	0645	0717	0743	0810	0827
IJMUIDEN	0752	0745	0724	0659	0629	0557	0517	0445	0411	0346	0325	0319	0323	0337	0401	0424	0452	0516	0543	0607	0638	0703	0729	0746
KIEL	0742	0734	0711	0644	0612	0539	0457	0423	0348	0321	0259	0251	0256	0311	0337	0401	0431	0456	0525	0551	0623	0650	0718	0735
KIRKWALL	0903	0850	0819	0745	0707	0627	0537	0457	0413	0340	0309	0257	0302	0322	0357	0428	0507	0538	0614	0647	0727	0801	0837	0858
LA CORUÑA	0806	0803	0750	0732	0710	0646	0616	0551	0527	0509	0456	0452	0457	0506	0523	0538	0557	0613	0631	0647	0708	0727	0746	0759
LEITH	0844	0834	0808	0739	0704	0628	0544	0508	0429	0400	0335	0326	0331	0347	0416	0443	0517	0544	0615	0644	0719	0749	0819	0838
LÉZARDRIEUX	0806	0801	0743	0721	0655	0626	0551	0522	0452	0431	0414	0409	0413	0425	0446	0505	0529	0549	0612	0632	0659	0721	0744	0759
LISBON	0755	0753	0743	0728	0709	0648	0622	0601	0539	0525	0514	0511	0515	0524	0538	0550	0605	0618	0632	0646	0703	0719	0735	0747
LONDON	0806	0800	0739	0715	0646	0615	0536	0505	0432	0409	0349	0342	0347	0400	0424	0445	0512	0535	0601	0624	0654	0718	0743	0759
MILFORD HAVEN	0827	0820	0800	0736	0706	0635	0556	0525	0452	0428	0408	0402	0407	0420	0443	0505	0533	0555	0621	0644	0714	0739	0804	0820
NIEUWPOORT	0753	0747	0727	0703	0634	0604	0525	0455	0422	0359	0339	0333	0338	0351	0414	0435	0502	0524	0549	0612	0641	0706	0731	0747
OBAN	0911	0859	0828	0755	0718	0639	0550	0510	0428	0355	0326	0315	0320	0339	0412	0443	0520	0551	0626	0657	0737	0810	0844	0905
OUISTREHAM	0756	0751	0733	0711	0644	0615	0539	0510	0440	0418	0400	0355	0359	0411	0433	0452	0517	0537	0600	0622	0649	0711	0735	0750
PETERHEAD	0849	0838	0809	0738	0701	0623	0536	0458	0417	0346	0318	0308	0313	0331	0403	0432	0508	0537	0611	0641	0719	0751	0823	0843
POOLE	0810	0804	0744	0721	0652	0622	0544	0514	0443	0420	0401	0354	0359	0412	0434	0455	0521	0543	0608	0630	0659	0723	0747	0803
PORT LA FORÊT	0805	0801	0744	0723	0657	0629	0555	0527	0458	0438	0421	0416	0421	0432	0452	0511	0534	0553	0615	0635	0700	0722	0744	0758
PORTSMOUTH	0807	0801	0741	0717	0649	0619	0541	0511	0439	0416	0357	0351	0355	0408	0431	0452	0518	0539	0604	0627	0656	0720	0744	0800
RAMSGATE	0759	0753	0733	0709	0640	0609	0530	0459	0427	0403	0344	0337	0342	0355	0418	0440	0507	0529	0554	0618	0647	0711	0737	0752
ST MALO	0801	0756	0738	0717	0650	0622	0546	0518	0449	0427	0410	0405	0410	0421	0442	0501	0525	0544	0607	0628	0654	0716	0739	0754
ST MARY'S (Scilly)	0823	0818	0759	0736	0709	0639	0602	0533	0502	0440	0422	0416	0421	0433	0455	0515	0540	0601	0625	0647	0714	0738	0801	0817
ST NAZAIRE	0756	0752	0735	0715	0650	0622	0548	0521	0453	0433	0417	0412	0417	0428	0447	0505	0528	0546	0608	0627	0652	0713	0735	0749
ST PETER PORT	0806	0801	0743	0720	0653	0624	0548	0519	0448	0426	0409	0403	0408	0420	0441	0501	0526	0546	0610	0631	0658	0721	0744	0800
STORNOWAY	0913	0901	0831	0758	0721	0642	0554	0515	0433	0400	0331	0320	0325	0344	0417	0447	0524	0555	0629	0701	0740	0813	0846	0907
SYLT	0750	0742	0717	0650	0617	0542	0459	0425	0348	0321	0257	0249	0254	0309	0336	0402	0433	0459	0529	0555	0629	0657	0726	0744
TERSCHELLING	0754	0747	0724	0658	0627	0554	0513	0440	0405	0340	0318	0310	0315	0330	0355	0419	0448	0512	0540	0606	0637	0704	0731	0748
TROON	0847	0838	0812	0744	0710	0634	0550	0515	0437	0409	0344	0335	0340	0356	0425	0451	0524	0550	0621	0649	0724	0753	0823	0841

5.1.2 TIMES OF SUNSET (UT)

	JAN 1	JAN 15	FEB 1	FEB 15	MAR 1	MAR 15	APR 1	APR 15	MAY 1	MAY 15	JUN 1	JUN 15	JUL 1	JUL 15	AUG 1	AUG 15	SEP 1	SEP 15	OCT 1	OCT 15	NOV 1	NOV 15	DEC 1	DEC 15
ABERDOVEY	1612	1631	1702	1728	1755	1820	1850	1915	1943	2006	2029	2041	2042	2032	2008	1942	1905	1832	1754	1722	1647	1623	1606	1602
ARCACHON	1635	1650	1713	1733	1752	1810	1832	1849	1909	1926	1943	1952	1954	1947	1930	1911	1842	1816	1746	1720	1654	1637	1626	1625
BELFAST	1608	1629	1702	1731	1800	1827	1900	1927	1957	2023	2049	2102	2103	2051	2025	1956	1916	1841	1800	1726	1648	1622	1603	1558
BERGEN	1440	1507	1550	1628	1705	1741	1823	1858	1938	2013	2050	2108	2108	2050	2012	1934	1844	1801	1712	1629	1542	1507	1438	1428
BREST	1634	1650	1716	1739	1802	1823	1848	1909	1932	1951	2011	2021	2023	2015	1955	1932	1900	1831	1757	1729	1659	1639	1626	1624
BURNHAM (Crouch)	1604	1623	1652	1717	1743	1808	1836	1900	1927	1949	2012	2023	2024	2015	1952	1926	1850	1818	1741	1710	1636	1614	1557	1554
CORK	1618	1637	1706	1732	1758	1822	1851	1915	1942	2005	2027	2039	2040	2030	2007	1942	1905	1833	1756	1725	1650	1628	1611	1608
CHERBOURG	1617	1634	1701	1725	1749	1811	1838	1859	1924	1944	2005	2016	2017	2009	1948	1924	1850	1820	1745	1716	1645	1624	1609	1606
CRAOBH HAVEN	1557	1619	1654	1725	1756	1825	1901	1929	2002	2030	2058	2112	2113	2100	2031	2000	1917	1840	1758	1722	1641	1614	1552	1546
CUXHAVEN	1624	1644	1716	1744	1812	1839	1910	1936	2006	2031	2056	2108	2109	2058	2033	2005	1926	1851	1812	1738	1701	1637	1618	1613
DARTMOUTH	1621	1639	1707	1731	1756	1819	1846	1909	1934	1955	2016	2027	2029	2020	1958	1934	1859	1828	1753	1723	1650	1629	1614	1611
EASTBOURNE	1604	1622	1650	1715	1740	1803	1831	1854	1919	1941	2003	2014	2015	2006	1944	1919	1844	1813	1737	1707	1634	1612	1556	1553
FALMOUTH	1628	1646	1713	1738	1802	1825	1852	1914	1939	2000	2021	2032	2033	2025	2003	1939	1905	1834	1759	1729	1657	1636	1621	1618
FLEETWOOD	1601	1621	1652	1721	1749	1816	1848	1914	1943	2008	2033	2045	2047	2036	2010	1942	1903	1828	1749	1715	1638	1613	1555	1550
GALWAY	1628	1648	1719	1747	1814	1840	1911	1936	2005	2029	2053	2105	2107	2056	2031	2004	1926	1852	1813	1741	1704	1640	1622	1618
GT YARMOUTH	1549	1608	1638	1705	1732	1757	1827	1852	1920	1943	2006	2018	2020	2009	1946	1919	1842	1809	1731	1659	1623	1600	1543	1539
HAMBURG	1511	1531	1602	1630	1658	1724	1755	1821	1850	1914	1939	1951	1952	1942	1917	1849	1810	1737	1657	1624	1548	1524	1505	1501
HARTLEPOOL	1549	1610	1642	1711	1741	1808	1841	1908	1939	2004	2030	2043	2044	2033	2006	1937	1857	1822	1741	1707	1629	1603	1543	1538
HARWICH	1554	1613	1642	1708	1734	1759	1828	1852	1919	1942	2005	2016	2018	2008	1945	1919	1842	1810	1733	1701	1627	1604	1547	1544
HELGOLAND	1516	1536	1608	1636	1705	1732	1804	1831	1900	1925	1951	2003	2005	1953	1928	1859	1820	1745	1705	1631	1554	1529	1510	1505
HOLYHEAD	1610	1630	1701	1729	1756	1822	1853	1919	1948	2012	2036	2048	2049	2039	2014	1947	1908	1834	1756	1723	1647	1622	1604	1600
IJMUIDEN	1538	1557	1628	1654	1721	1746	1816	1840	1908	1931	1955	2006	2008	1958	1934	1907	1830	1757	1719	1648	1612	1549	1532	1528
KIEL	1512	1532	1604	1632	1700	1727	1759	1825	1854	1919	1944	1957	1958	1947	1921	1853	1814	1740	1700	1627	1550	1525	1506	1501
KIRKWALL	1524	1548	1629	1704	1739	1812	1852	1925	2002	2034	2108	2124	2124	2108	2034	1959	1911	1830	1744	1704	1619	1547	1521	1512
LA CORUÑA	1708	1723	1745	1804	1822	1840	1900	1916	1935	1951	2007	2016	2018	2012	1956	1937	1909	1844	1815	1751	1725	1709	1659	1658
LEITH	1549	1610	1645	1716	1747	1816	1851	1919	1952	2019	2047	2101	2101	2049	2020	1950	1907	1831	1748	1712	1632	1605	1544	1538
LÉZARDRIEUX	1626	1643	1710	1733	1756	1817	1843	1904	1927	1947	2007	2017	2019	2011	1951	1928	1855	1826	1752	1723	1652	1632	1618	1616
LISBON	1726	1739	1758	1814	1829	1843	1900	1913	1929	1942	1955	2003	2005	2001	1947	1931	1907	1845	1820	1759	1737	1723	1715	1716
LONDON	1602	1620	1649	1715	1740	1805	1833	1857	1923	1946	2008	2019	2021	2011	1949	1923	1847	1815	1738	1707	1633	1611	1555	1551
MILFORD HAVEN	1621	1640	1709	1735	1800	1825	1854	1917	1944	2006	2029	2040	2042	2032	2009	1944	1907	1835	1758	1727	1653	1631	1614	1611
NIEUWPOORT	1552	1610	1639	1704	1730	1754	1822	1845	1911	1933	1955	2006	2008	1958	1936	1911	1835	1804	1727	1657	1623	1601	1545	1542
OBAN	1540	1604	1643	1718	1752	1824	1903	1935	2012	2043	2115	2131	2131	2116	2043	2008	1922	1842	1756	1717	1633	1602	1537	1529
OUISTREHAM	1613	1630	1657	1720	1744	1806	1832	1853	1917	1938	1958	2008	2010	2002	1941	1918	1844	1815	1740	1711	1640	1620	1605	1603
PETERHEAD	1532	1556	1633	1706	1739	1810	1847	1918	1953	2022	2052	2107	2108	2054	2023	1950	1905	1826	1742	1704	1621	1552	1529	1521
POOLE	1613	1631	1659	1724	1749	1812	1840	1903	1928	1950	2011	2022	2024	2015	1953	1928	1853	1822	1746	1716	1643	1622	1606	1603
PORT LA FORÊT	1633	1650	1716	1738	1800	1821	1846	1906	1928	1947	2007	2017	2018	2011	1951	1929	1857	1829	1756	1728	1658	1639	1625	1623
PORTSMOUTH	1609	1627	1656	1721	1745	1809	1837	1900	1925	1947	2009	2019	2021	2012	1950	1925	1850	1819	1743	1713	1640	1618	1602	1559
RAMSGATE	1557	1615	1644	1709	1735	1759	1827	1850	1917	1939	2001	2012	2014	2004	1942	1916	1841	1809	1732	1702	1628	1606	1550	1546
ST MALO	1623	1640	1706	1729	1752	1813	1839	1859	1923	1942	2002	2012	2014	2006	1946	1923	1850	1821	1748	1719	1649	1629	1615	1613
ST MARY'S (Scilly)	1634	1652	1719	1743	1807	1830	1857	1919	1944	2004	2025	2036	2037	2029	2008	1944	1909	1839	1804	1735	1703	1642	1627	1624
ST NAZAIRE	1629	1646	1711	1732	1754	1814	1838	1858	1920	1938	1957	2007	2009	2001	1943	1921	1849	1821	1749	1722	1653	1634	1621	1619
ST PETER PORT	1621	1638	1705	1729	1753	1815	1841	1903	1927	1947	2008	2018	2020	2012	1951	1927	1854	1824	1749	1720	1649	1628	1614	1611
STORNOWAY	1546	1609	1648	1722	1756	1828	1906	1938	2014	2045	2116	2132	2132	2117	2045	2011	1925	1845	1800	1721	1637	1607	1542	1534
SYLT	1510	1531	1604	1633	1703	1730	1803	1830	1901	1927	1953	2006	2007	1955	1929	1900	1819	1744	1703	1629	1551	1525	1505	1500
TERSCHELLING	1531	1551	1622	1649	1717	1743	1814	1839	1908	1932	1957	2009	2010	2000	1935	1907	1829	1755	1716	1643	1607	1543	1525	1520
TROON	1557	1619	1653	1723	1753	1822	1856	1924	1956	2023	2050	2103	2104	2052	2024	1954	1913	1836	1755	1719	1640	1613	1552	1547

5

5.2.1   UK PUBLIC HOLIDAYS 1996

ENGLAND & WALES: Jan 1†, Apr 5, Apr 8, May 6†, May 27, Aug 26, Dec 25, Dec 26

NORTHERN IRELAND: Jan 1†, Mar 18, Apr 5, Apr 8, May 6†, May 27, July 12† Aug 26, Dec 25, Dec 26

SCOTLAND: Jan 1, Jan 2, Apr 5, May 6, May 27†, Aug 5, Dec 25, Dec 26†

† Subject to confirmation.

5.2.2   PHASES OF THE MOON 1996

New Moon				First Quarter				Full Moon				Last Quarter			
	d	h	m		d	h	m		d	h	m		d	h	m
								Jan	05	20	51	Jan	13	20	45
Jan	20	12	50	Jan	27	11	14	Feb	04	15	58	Feb	12	08	37
Feb	18	23	30	Feb	26	05	52	Mar	05	09	23	Mar	12	17	15
Mar	19	10	45	Mar	27	01	31	Apr	04	00	07	Apr	10	23	36
Apr	17	22	49	Apr	25	20	40	May	03	11	48	May	10	05	04
May	17	11	46	May	25	14	13	June	01	20	47	June	08	11	05
June	16	01	36	June	24	05	23	July	01	03	58	July	07	18	55
July	15	16	15	July	23	17	49	July	30	10	35	Aug	06	05	25
Aug	14	07	34	Aug	22	03	36	Aug	28	17	52	Sept	04	19	06
Sept	12	23	07	Sept	20	11	23	Sept	27	02	51	Oct	04	12	04
Oct	12	14	14	Oct	19	18	09	Oct	26	14	11	Nov	03	07	50
Nov	11	04	16	Nov	18	01	09	Nov	25	04	10	Dec	03	05	06
Dec	10	16	56	Dec	17	09	31	Dec	24	20	41				

Note: All times UT.

5.2.3   ECLIPSE NOTES 1996

1. Total Eclipse of the Moon, 3-4 April.   Visible from Europe, including the British Isles.
2. Partial Eclipse of the Sun, 17-18 April.   Not visible from Europe.
3. Total Eclipse of the Moon, 27 September.   Visible from Europe, including the British Isles.
4. Partial Eclipse of the Sun, 12 October.   Visible from Europe, including the British Isles.

5.2.4   STANDARD TIMES
(Corrected to September 1994)

PLACES NORMALLY KEEPING UT

Canary Islands*	Great Britain*	Irish Republic*
Channel Islands**	Iceland	Morocco
Faeroes, The*	Ireland, Northern**	

PLACES FAST ON UT

Algeria	01	Germany*	01	Norway*	01
Balearic Islands*	01	Gibraltar*	01	Poland*	01
Belgium*	01	Italy*	01	Portugal*	01
Corsica*	01	Latvia*	02	Russia, W of 40°*	03
Denmark*	01	Lithuania*	02	Sardinia*	01
Estonia*	02	Malta*	01	Spain*	01
Finland*	02	Monaco*	01	Sweden*	01
France*	01	Netherlands, The*	01	Tunisia	01

The times should be *added* to UT to give Standard Time
        subtracted from Standard Time to give UT

*   Summer time may be kept in these places
**   Summer time, one hour in advance of UT, is kept from March 31 01h UT to October 27 01h UT in 1996.

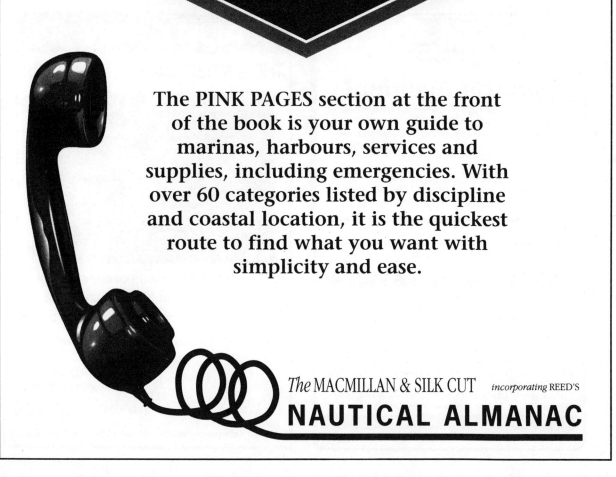

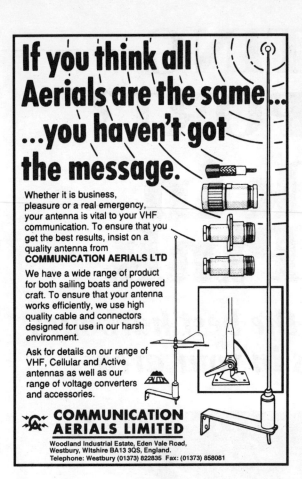
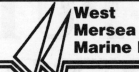

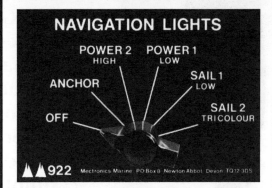

PLATE 1 – NAVIGATION LIGHTS (SEE ALSO PLATE 4)

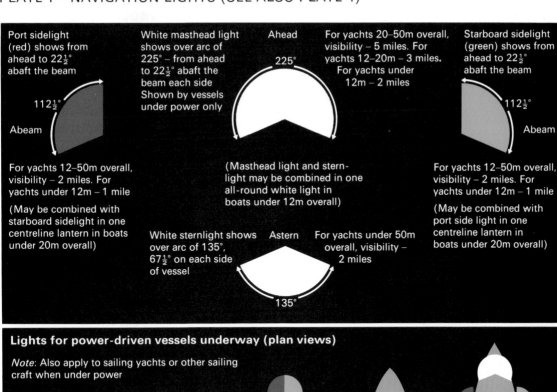

Port sidelight (red) shows from ahead to 22½° abaft the beam

White masthead light shows over arc of 225° – from ahead to 22½° abaft the beam each side Shown by vessels under power only

Ahead

225°

For yachts 20–50m overall, visibility – 5 miles. For yachts 12–20m – 3 miles. For yachts under 12m – 2 miles

Starboard sidelight (green) shows from ahead to 22½° abaft the beam

Abeam

112½°

112½°

Abeam

For yachts 12–50m overall, visibility – 2 miles. For yachts under 12m – 1 mile

(May be combined with starboard sidelight in one centreline lantern in boats under 20m overall)

(Masthead light and stern-light may be combined in one all-round white light in boats under 12m overall)

For yachts 12–50m overall, visibility – 2 miles. For yachts under 12m – 1 mile

(May be combined with port side light in one centreline lantern in boats under 20m overall)

White sternlight shows over arc of 135°, 67½° on each side of vessel

Astern

For yachts under 50m overall, visibility – 2 miles

135°

Lights for power-driven vessels underway (plan views)

Note: Also apply to sailing yachts or other sailing craft when under power

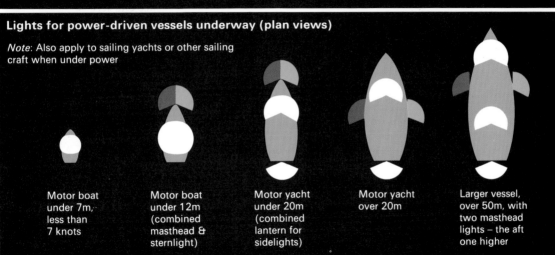

Motor boat under 7m, less than 7 knots

Motor boat under 12m (combined masthead & sternlight)

Motor yacht under 20m (combined lantern for sidelights)

Motor yacht over 20m

Larger vessel, over 50m, with two masthead lights – the aft one higher

Lights for sailing vessels underway (plan views)

Note: These lights apply to sailing craft when under sail ONLY. If motor-sailing the appropriate lights for a power-driven vessel must be shown, as above

Bow view

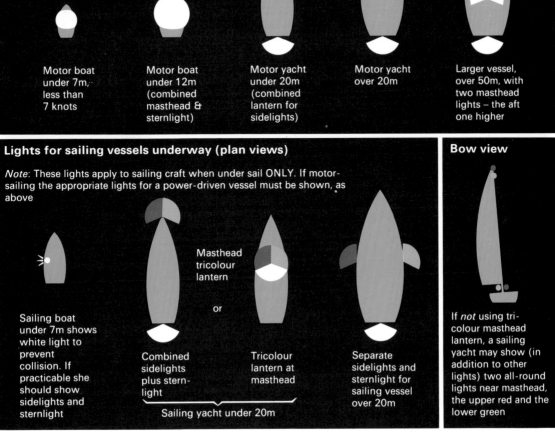

Sailing boat under 7m shows white light to prevent collision. If practicable she should show sidelights and sternlight

Masthead tricolour lantern

or

Combined sidelights plus stern-light

Tricolour lantern at masthead

Sailing yacht under 20m

Separate sidelights and sternlight for sailing vessel over 20m

If *not* using tri-colour masthead lantern, a sailing yacht may show (in addition to other lights) two all-round lights near masthead, the upper red and the lower green

PLATE 2 – ADMIRALTY METRIC CHART SYMBOLS

A selection of the more common symbols from Admiralty Publication 5011

Reproduced by kind permission of H.M. Stationery Office and the Hydrographer of the Navy.

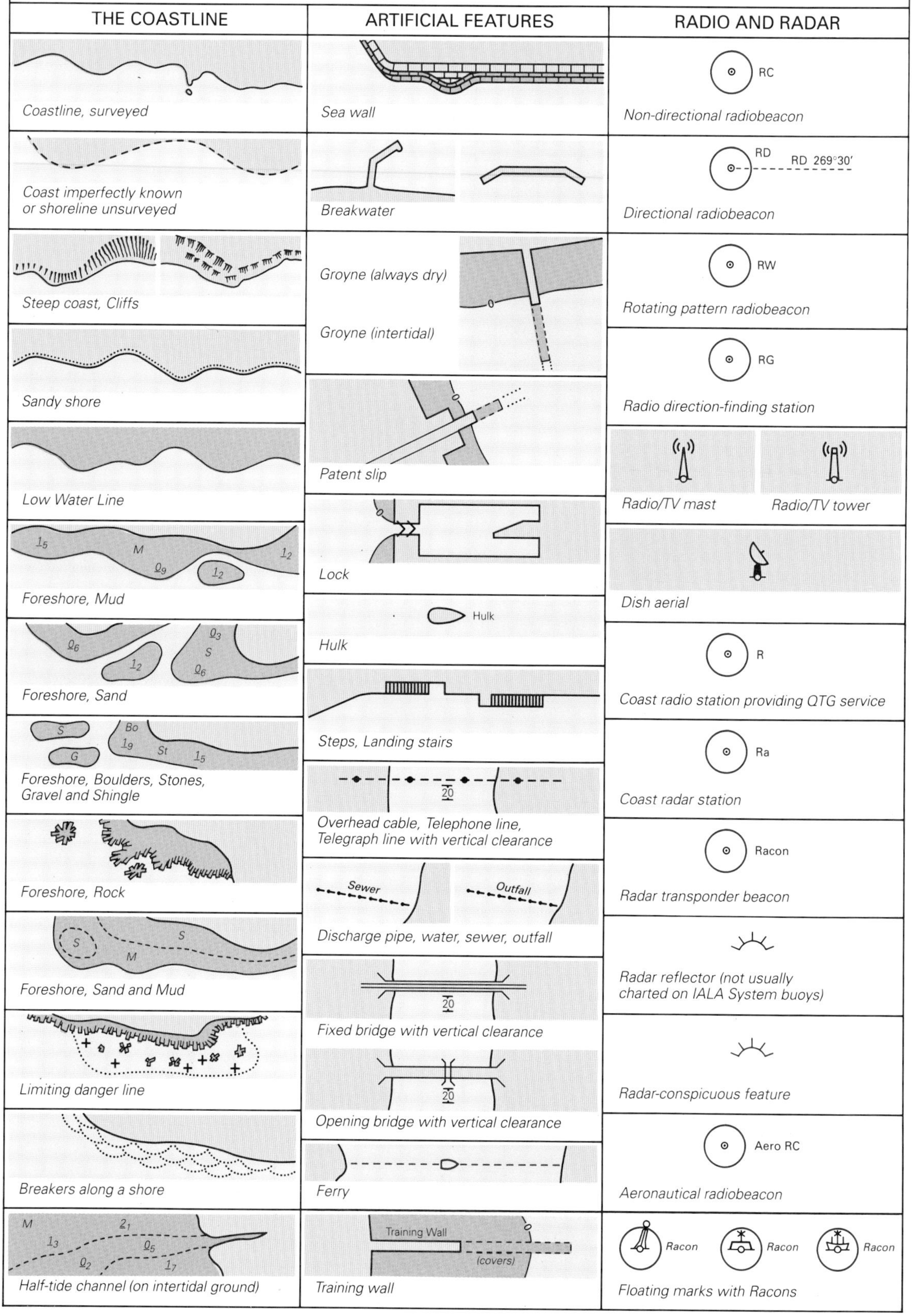
THE COASTLINE
Coastline, surveyed
Coast imperfectly known or shoreline unsurveyed
Steep coast, Cliffs
Sandy shore
Low Water Line
Foreshore, Mud
Foreshore, Sand
Foreshore, Boulders, Stones, Gravel and Shingle
Foreshore, Rock
Foreshore, Sand and Mud
Limiting danger line
Breakers along a shore
Half-tide channel (on intertidal ground)
ARTIFICIAL FEATURES
Sea wall
Breakwater
Groyne (always dry)
Groyne (intertidal)
Patent slip
Lock
Hulk
Hulk
Steps, Landing stairs
Overhead cable, Telephone line, Telegraph line with vertical clearance
Sewer
Outfall
Discharge pipe, water, sewer, outfall
Fixed bridge with vertical clearance
Opening bridge with vertical clearance
Ferry
Training Wall
(covers)
Training wall
RADIO AND RADAR
RC
Non-directional radiobeacon
RD
RD 269°30′
Directional radiobeacon
RW
Rotating pattern radiobeacon
RG
Radio direction-finding station
Radio/TV mast
Radio/TV tower
Dish aerial
R
Coast radio station providing QTG service
Ra
Coast radar station
Racon
Radar transponder beacon
Radar reflector (not usually charted on IALA System buoys)
Radar-conspicuous feature
Aero RC
Aeronautical radiobeacon
Racon
Racon
Racon
Floating marks with Racons

PLATE 3 – ADMIRALTY METRIC CHART SYMBOLS

A selection of the more common symbols from Admiralty Publication 5011

Reproduced by kind permission of H.M. Stationery Office and the Hydrographer of the Navy.

DANGERS	DANGERS	LIMITS
Rock which does not cover, height above High Water	Wreck over which the depth has been obtained by sounding, but not by wire sweep	Leading line (the firm line is the track to be followed)
Rock which covers and uncovers, height above Chart Datum	Wreck over which the exact depth is unknown, but which is considered to have a safe clearance at the depth shown	Limit of sector
Rock awash at the level of Chart Datum	The remains of a wreck, or other foul area no longer dangerous to surface navigation, but to be avoided by vessels anchoring, trawling, etc.	Traffic separation scheme: one-way traffic lanes (separated by zone)
A rock or rock ledge over which the exact depth is unknown but which is considered to be dangerous to surface navigation	Obstruction, depth known	Submarine cable (telegraph & telephone)
Shoal sounding on isolated rock	Obstruction which has been swept by wire to the depth shown	Submarine cable (power)
Submerged rock not dangerous to surface navigation	Overfalls, tide rips, races	Limits of national fishing zones
Wreck which has been swept by wire to the depth shown	Eddies	Anchorage area in general. Type of anchorage may be specified, e.g. by number or name, DW (deep water), tanker, 24h (for periods up to 24 hours), small craft etc.
Wreck showing any part of hull or superstructure at the level of Chart Datum — *Large scale charts*	Kelp	
(Masts) *(Mast 3m)* *(Funnel)* *(Mast dries 2.1m)* — *Large scale charts* Wreck of which the mast(s) only are visible	Breakers	Anchoring prohibited
Wrecks, depths unknown. On left considered dangerous to surface navigation, and on right not considered dangerous	Fish haven, depth known	Fishing prohibited

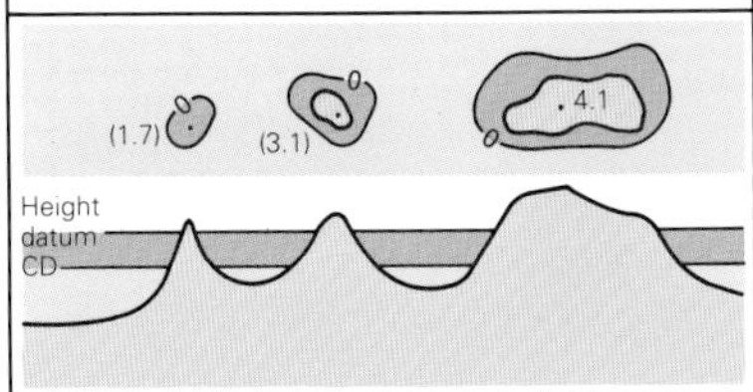

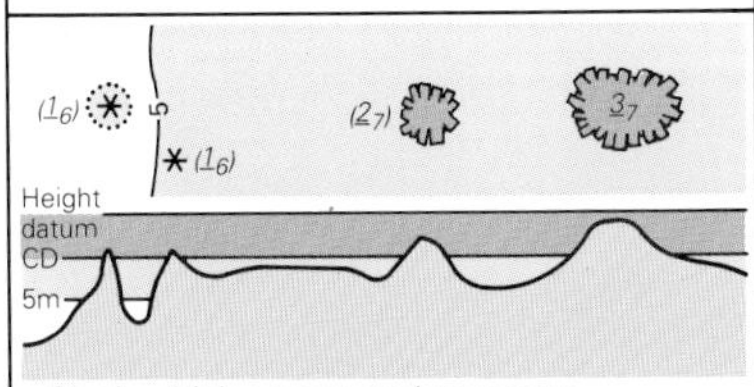

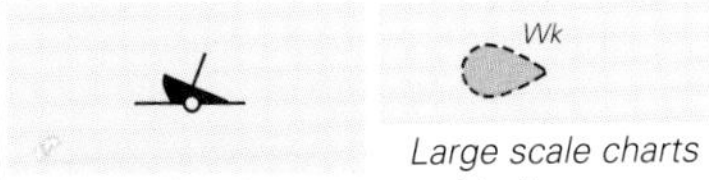

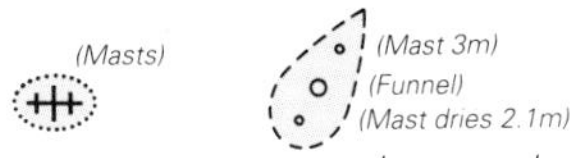

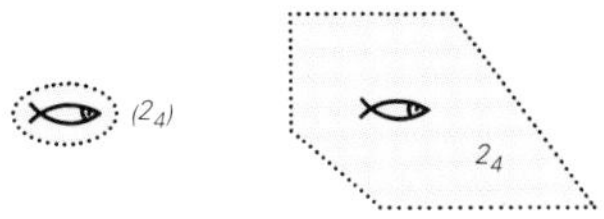

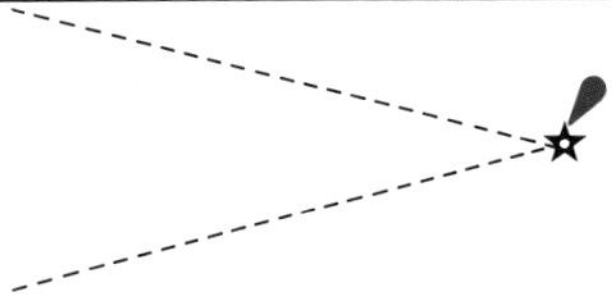

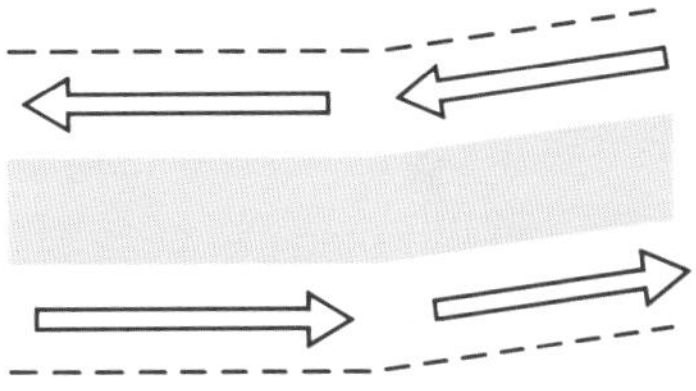

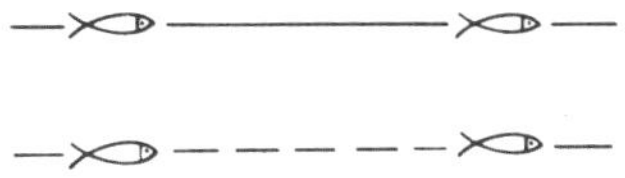

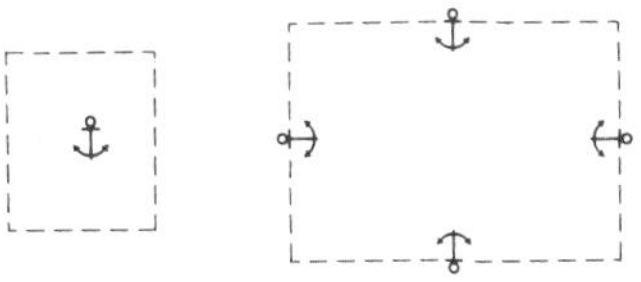

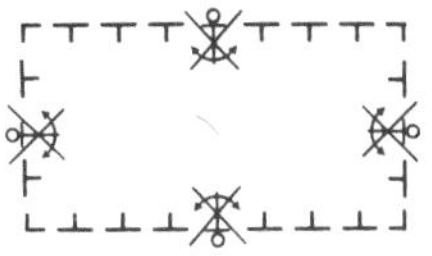

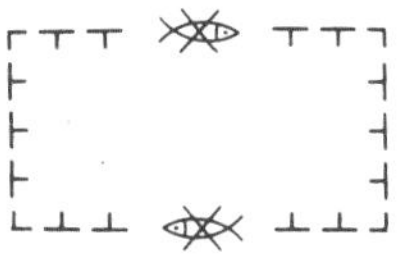

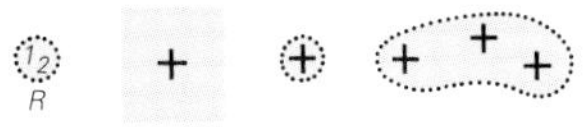

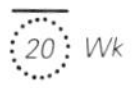

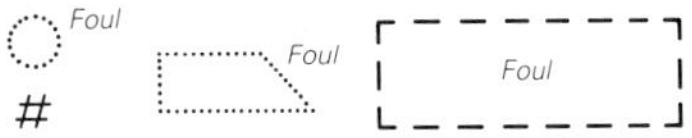

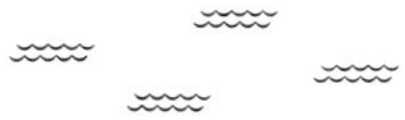

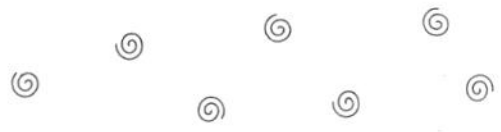

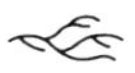

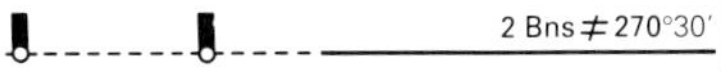

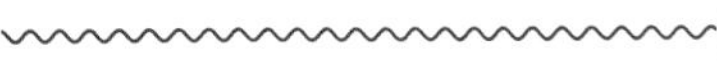

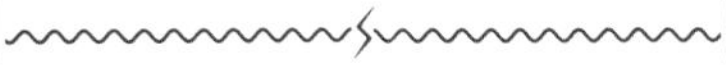

PLATE 4 – PRINCIPAL NAVIGATION LIGHTS AND SHAPES

(*Note*: All vessels seen from starboard beam)

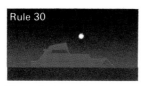

Vessel at anchor

All-round white light: if over 50m, a second light aft and lower

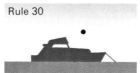

Black ball forward

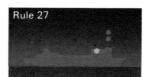

Not under command

Two all-round red lights, plus sidelights and sternlight when making way

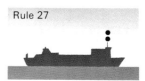

Two black balls vertically

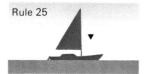

Motor sailing

Cone point down, forward

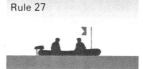

Divers down

Letter 'A' International Code

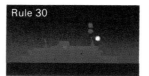

Vessel aground

Anchor light(s), plus two all-round red lights in a vertical line

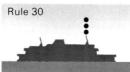

Three black balls in a vertical line

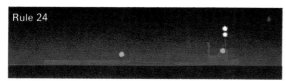

Vessels being towed and towing

Vessel towed shows side-lights (forward) and sternlight

Tug shows two masthead lights, sidelights, stern-light, yellow towing light

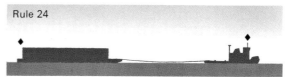

Towing by day – Length of tow more than 200m

Towing vessel and tow display diamond shapes. By night, the towing vessel shows three masthead lights instead of two as for shorter tows

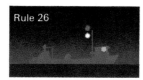

Vessel fishing

All-round red light over all-round white, plus side-lights and sternlight when underway

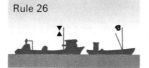

Fishing/trawling

Two cones point to point, or a basket if fishing vessel is less than 20m

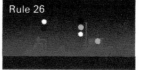

Vessel trawling

All-round green light over all-round white, plus side-lights and sternlight when underway

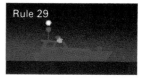

Pilot boat

All-round white light over all-round red; plus side-lights and sternlight when underway, or anchor light

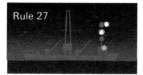

Vessel restricted in her ability to manoeuvre

All-round red, white, red lights vertically; plus normal steaming lights when under way

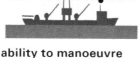

Three shapes in a vertical line – ball, diamond, ball

Dredger

As left, plus two all-round red lights (or two balls) on foul side, and two all-round green (or two diamonds) on clear side

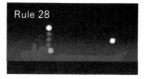

Constrained by draught

Three all-round red lights in a vertical line, plus normal steaming lights. By day – a cylinder

PLATE 5 – IALA BUOYAGE

Lateral marks

Used generally to mark the sides of well defined navigable channels.

Port Hand marks

Light:
Colour – red
Rhythm – any

Navigable channel

Direction of buoyage

Starboard Hand marks

Light:
Colour – green
Rhythm – any

Cardinal marks

Used to indicate the direction from the mark in which the best navigable water lies, or to draw attention to a bend, junction or fork in a channel, or to mark the end of a shoal.

Lights: Always white

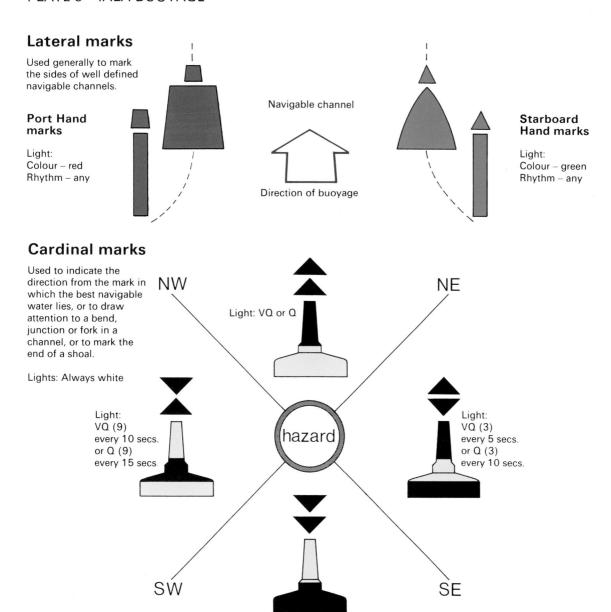

NW

NE

Light: VQ or Q

Light:
VQ (9)
every 10 secs.
or Q (9)
every 15 secs.

hazard

Light:
VQ (3)
every 5 secs.
or Q (3)
every 10 secs.

SW

SE

Light: VQ (6) + LFl every 10 secs. or Q (6) + LFl every 15 secs.

Other marks

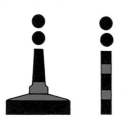

Isolated danger marks

Use: To mark a small isolated danger with navigable water all round.
Light: Colour – white
Rhythm – group flashing (2)

Safe water marks

Use: Mid-channel or landfall.
Light: Colour – white
Rhythm – Isophase, occulting or 1 long flash every 10 seconds.

Special marks

Any shape not conflicting with lateral or safe water marks.
Light: Colour – yellow
Rhythm – different from other white lights used on buoys.

PLATES 6-7 – INTERNATIONAL CODE OF SIGNALS
CODE FLAGS, PHONETIC ALPHABET, MORSE SYMBOLS AND SINGLE-LETTER SIGNALS

Notes:
1. Single letter signals may be made by any method of signalling. Those marked * when made by sound must comply with the *International Regulations for Preventing Collisions at Sea*, Rules 34 and 35.
2. Signals 'K' and 'S' have special meanings as landing signals for small boats with persons in distress.
3. In the phonetic alphabet, the syllables to be emphasised are in italics.

A   Alfa   (*AL* FAH)

I have a diver down; keep well clear at slow speed

*B   Bravo   (*BRAH* VOH)

I am taking in, or discharging, or carrying dangerous goods

*C   Charlie   (*CHAR* LEE)

Yes (affirmative or 'The significance of the previous group should be read in the affirmative)

*D   Delta   (*DELL* TAH)

Keep clear of me; I am manoeuvring with difficulty

*E   Echo   (*ECK* OH)

I am altering my course to starboard

F   Foxtrot   (*FOKS* TROT)

I am disabled; communicate with me

*G   Golf   (*GOLF*)
I require a pilot. When made by fishing vessels operating in close proximity on the fishing grounds it means: I am hauling nets

*H   Hotel   (HOH *TELL*)

I have a pilot on board

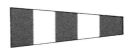
Code and Answering Pendant

*I   India   (*IN* DEE AH)

I am altering my course to port

J   Juliett   (*JEW* LEE *ETT*)
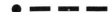
I am on fire and have dangerous cargo on board: keep well clear of me

K   Kilo   (*KEY* LOH)
I wish to communicate with you

L   Lima   (*LEE* MAH)

You should stop your vessel instantly

*M   Mike   (MIKE)
My vessel is stopped and making no way through the water

N   November   (NO *VEM* BER)
No (negative or 'The significance of the previous group should be read in the negative'). This signal may be given only visually or by sound

O   Oscar   (*OSS* CAH)
Man overboard

P   Papa   (PAH *PAH*)
In harbour, all persons should report on board as the vessel is about to proceed to sea. **At sea**: it may be used by fishing vessels to mean 'My nets have come fast upon an obstruction'

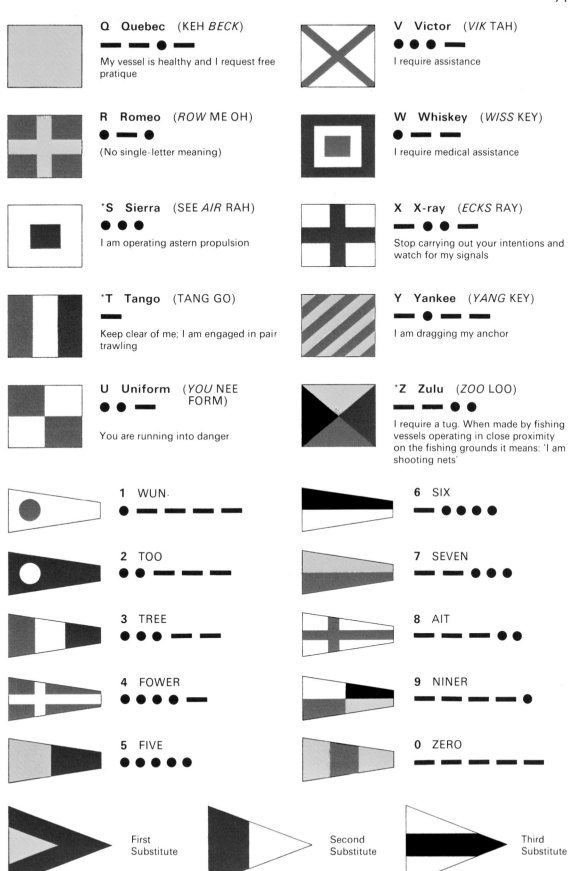

Q Quebec (KEH *BECK*)
— — ●
My vessel is healthy and I request free pratique

V Victor (*VIK* TAH)
● ● ● —
I require assistance

R Romeo (*ROW* ME OH)
● — ●
(No single-letter meaning)

W Whiskey (*WISS* KEY)
● — — —
I require medical assistance

*S Sierra (SEE *AIR* RAH)
● ● ●
I am operating astern propulsion

X X-ray (*ECKS* RAY)
— ● ● —
Stop carrying out your intentions and watch for my signals

*T Tango (TANG GO)
—
Keep clear of me; I am engaged in pair trawling

Y Yankee (*YANG* KEY)
— ● — —
I am dragging my anchor

U Uniform (*YOU* NEE FORM)
● ● —
You are running into danger

*Z Zulu (*ZOO* LOO)
— — ● ●
I require a tug. When made by fishing vessels operating in close proximity on the fishing grounds it means: 'I am shooting nets'

1 WUN.
● — — — —

6 SIX
— ● ● ● ●

2 TOO
● ● — — —

7 SEVEN
— — ● ● ●

3 TREE
● ● ● — —

8 AIT
— — — ● ●

4 FOWER
● ● ● ● —

9 NINER
— — — — ●

5 FIVE
● ● ● ● ●

0 ZERO
— — — — —

First Substitute

Second Substitute

Third Substitute

72

PLATE 8 – NATIONAL ENSIGNS

UK WHITE ENSIGN

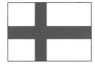

FINLAND

UK BLUE ENSIGN

SWEDEN

UK RED ENSIGN

NORWAY

IRELAND

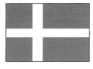

DENMARK

GUERNSEY

GERMANY

FRANCE

NETHERLANDS

SPAIN

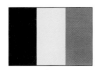

BELGIUM

PORTUGAL

GREECE

PANAMA

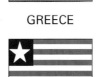

LIBERIA

PLATE 9 – INTERNATIONAL PORT TRAFFIC SIGNALS

No	Lights		Main message
1	● ● ●	Flashing	Serious emergency – all vessels to stop or divert according to instructions
2	● ● ●	Fixed or Slow Occulting	Vessels shall not proceed (*Note*: Some ports may use an exemption signal, as in 2a below)
3	● ● ●	Fixed or Slow Occulting	Vessels may proceed. One way traffic
4	● ● ○	Fixed or Slow Occulting	Vessels may proceed. Two way traffic
5	● ○ ●	Fixed or Slow Occulting	A vessel may proceed only when she has received specific orders to do so (*Note*: Some ports may use an exemption signal, as in 5a below)
			Exemption signals and messages
2a	○ ● ● ●	Fixed or Slow Occulting	Vessels shall not proceed, except that vessels which navigate outside the main channel need not comply with the main message
5a	○ ● ○ ●	Fixed or Slow Occulting	A vessel may proceed only when she has received specific orders to do so, except that vessels which navigate outside the main channel need not comply with the main message
			Auxiliary signals and messages
	White and/or yellow lights, displayed to the right of the main lights		Local meanings, as promulgated in local port orders

Chapter 6

Communications

Contents

6

Communications – introduction

Yachts may often need to communicate with other vessels and with shore stations. This is now commonly done by Very High Frequency (VHF) radiotelephone, so emphasis is placed on this method in this chapter. Radio broadcasts of gale warnings and weather messages are described in Chapter 7, while detailed information on Distress, Urgency and Safety signals is given in Chapter 8.

A full description of the various methods of signalling and the procedures that are involved, including an explanation of the *International Code of Signals,* is given in Chapter 6 of *The Macmillan & Silk Cut Yachtsman's Handook.* This also contains more detailed notes on flag etiquette, with colour plates showing the burgees of 217 selected yacht clubs and the maritime flags of 165 nations.

6.1   INTERNATIONAL CODE

6.1.1   International Code of Signals

Most communication afloat by pleasure craft is now by radiotelephone, in plain language and mostly using Very High Frequency (VHF) equipment, providing short range services up to 30-40 miles depending on the heights of the aerials concerned. Other forms of radiotelephony are described in section 6.3.

In more general terms marine communication is based on the *International Code of Signals* (HMSO), which provides for safety of navigation and of persons particularly where there are language problems. The code can be used by alphabetical flags and numeral pendants, by flashing light and sound signalling using the Morse code, by voice using radiotelephony or loud hailer, by radiotelegraphy, or by hand flags.

Signals consist of: single-letter signals which are very urgent or very common; two-letter signals in the General Section; and three-letter signals starting with 'M' in the Medical Section.

6.1.2   Using the International Code

The present International Code came into force in 1969 and is presented in nine editorial languages – English, French, Italian, German, Japanese, Spanish, Norwegian, Russian and Greek. Ships, aircraft and shore stations can communicate with each other in these languages without knowing a foreign tongue if a copy of the appropriate *International Code of Signals* is held. The English language edition is published by HMSO.

An explanation of the use of the International Code is given in Chapter 6 of *The Macmillan & Silk Cut Yachtsman's Handbook*, which also contains a few selected code groups which can be useful in emergency situations.

Plates 6 and 7 on pages 68–69 of this Almanac show the International Code flags for the alphabet and for numerals, the phonetic alphabet, the phonetic figure-spelling table, the Morse symbols for letters and numerals, and the meanings of important or common single-letter signals.

6.2   MISCELLANEOUS SIGNALS

6.2.1   Radio time signals

The BBC broadcast time signals at the local times and on the frequencies indicated in the table below. The start of the final, longer pulse marks the minute.

BBC Radio 1   97·6–99·8 MHz
(97·1MHz for Channel Islands)
BBC Radio 2   88–90·2 MHz
(89·6 MHz for Channel Islands)
BBC Radio 3   90·2–92·4 MHz
(91·1 MHz for Channel Islands)

BBC Radio 4   198 kHz
92·4–94·6 MHz
(94·8 MHz for Channel Islands)
Also 603 kHz (Tyneside)
720 kHz   (N Ireland & London)
756 kHz   (Redruth)
774 kHz   (Plymouth & Enniskillen)
1449 kHz (Aberdeen)
1485 kHz (Carlisle)

Local time	Mon-Fri Radio	Sat Radio	Sun Radio
0000	2,4*	2,4*	2,4*
0600	4	3	4
0700	1,2,3,4	2,3,4	4
0800	1,2,3,4	2,4	2,4
0900	4	4	2,4
1000	4	4	
1100	4	4	
1200	4		
1300	2,4	1,4	4
1400	4	4	
1500	4		
1600	4	4	
1700	2,4		1,4
1800	4*	4*	4*
1900	4		2
2100			4
2200	4	4*	4*

* indicates Big Ben (first hour strike)

6.2.2   Pratique messages

All vessels arriving directly from outside the European Union must fly the yellow 'Q' flag where it can easily be seen, and illuminated at night, on entering the 12 mile limit. It must be kept hoisted until Customs formalities are completed.

Other pratique messages from the International Code are given in *The Macmillan & Silk Cut Yachtsman's Handbook*.

6.2.3   Distress signals and emergencies

Details of distress signals, visual signals between shore and ships in distress, signals used by SAR aircraft, and directing signals used by aircraft are given in Chapter 8 (8.2 and 8.3).

6.2.4   Port Traffic signals

Traffic signals etc for individual harbours are shown in Chapter 10. On the Continent traffic signals are to some extent standardised – see 10. 15 . 8 for France, 10.20.7 for Belgium and the Netherlands, and 10. 21.7 for Germany.

International Port Traffic Signals are shown in Plate 9 and described on page 70. These are being increasingly used. Local variations are shown under individual harbours in Chapter 10.

For Port Operations and Vessel Traffic Services (VTS) on VHF RT see 6.3.19.

6.2.5 Visual storm signals

An International System of visual storm signals is used in France, the Netherlands and Germany. This is illustrated in 10.15.8. Official storm signals are no longer displayed in the British Isles.

6.2.6 Tidal signals

Tidal signals are shown for individual harbours in Chapter 10. There is no standard system for British ports, nor for the Netherlands and Germany. France uses a system as described in 10.15.8.

6.3 RADIO COMMUNICATIONS

6.3.1 Radiotelephones – general

Many yachts are fitted with radiotelephones, mostly Very High Frequency (VHF) sets with ranges of about 20 miles. Medium Frequency (MF) sets give much greater ranges, but must be Single Sideband (SSB). Double Sideband (DSB) transmissions are prohibited except for emergency transmissions on 2182 kHz, the international MF distress frequency. Full details of the various licences and operating procedures are given in Chapter 6 of *The Macmillan & Silk Cut Yachtsman's Handbook*. The brief notes which follow cover only the most important points.

For a yacht which requires to maintain radio contact with shore on ocean passages it is necessary to use High Frequency (HF) radio, which is more powerful and gives a much longer range than MF, as described below.

6.3.2 Licensing requirements

A Ship Radio License is required for any VHF, UHF, MF, HF equipment, satellite communication or EPIRB on board. It is obtained from Wray Castle, Ship Radio Licensing, PO Box 5, Ambleside, LA22 0BF. Tel: 015394 34662. Fax: 015394 34663. This allows the use, afloat in the UK, of Ch M and Ch M2 for communications between yachts, yacht harbours and clubs, and for race control.

A Certificate of Competence and an Authority to Operate are required by the person in charge of a set. For yachtsmen this is likely to be the Certificate of Competence, Restricted VHF Only. The Royal Yachting Association (RYA) is responsible for the conduct of this examination. Details of the syllabus and examination are in RYA booklet G26, available (with application form for the examination) from the RYA.

6.3.3 Radiotelephones–regulations

For details see the *Handbook for Marine Radio Communication* (Lloyds of London Press). Briefly: operators must not divulge the contents of messages heard; stations must identify themselves when transmitting; except in cases of distress, coast radio stations control communications in their areas; at sea a yacht may call other vessels or shore stations, but messages must not be sent to an address ashore except through a coast radio station; in harbour a yacht may not use inter-ship channels except for safety, and may only communicate with the local Port Operations Service, British Telecom (BT) coast stations, or with stations on Ch M or M2; do not interfere with the working of other stations – before transmitting, listen to see that the channel is free; it is forbidden to transmit unnecessary or superfluous signals; priority must be given to distress calls; the transmission of bad language is forbidden; a log must be kept, recording all transmissions, etc.

6.3.4 VHF radio

Very High Frequency (VHF) radio has a range slightly better than the line of sight between the aerials. It pays to fit a good aerial, as high as possible. Maximum power output is 25 watts, and a lower power (usually one watt) is used for short ranges. Most UK coast stations and many harbours now have VHF, as do the principal Coastguard stations and other rescue services.

Marine VHF frequencies are in the band 156·00–174·00 MHz. Ch 16 (156·80 MHz) is for distress and safety purposes, and for calling and answering. Once contact has been made, the stations concerned must switch to a working channel, except for safety matters. Yachts at sea are encouraged to listen on Ch 16.

Basic VHF sets are 'simplex', transmitting and receiving on the same frequency, so that it is not possible to speak and listen simultaneously. 'Semi-duplex' sets transmit and receive on different frequencies, while fully 'duplex' sets can do this simultaneously so that conversation is normal.

There are three main groups of frequencies, but certain channels can be used for more than one purpose. *They are shown in order of preference.*
(1) *Public correspondence* (through coast radio stations). All can be used for duplex. Ch 26, 27, 25, 24, 23, 28, 04, 01, 03, 02, 07, 05, 84, 87, 86, 83, 85, 88, 61, 64, 65, 62, 66, 63, 60, 82.
(2) *Inter-ship*. These are all simplex. Ch 06, 08, 10, 13, 09, 72, 73, 69, 67, 77, 15, 17.
(3) *Port operations*. Simplex: Ch 12, 14, 11, 13, 09, 68, 71, 74, 10, 67, 69, 73, 17, 15. Duplex: Ch 20, 22, 18, 19, 21, 05, 07, 02, 03, 01, 04, 78, 82, 79, 81, 80, 60, 63, 66, 62, 65, 64, 61, 84.

Ch 80 (Tx 161·625 MHz Rx 157·025 MHz) is the primary working channel for yachts with yacht harbours, plus Ch M (157·85 MHz) as a stand-by. Yacht clubs may use Ch M2 (161·425 MHz) for race control with Ch M as stand-by (see 6.3.2). Ch 67 (156·375 MHz) is operated in the UK by principal Coastguard stations as the Small Craft Safety Channel, accessed via Ch 16 (see 8.2.4).

Ch 70 is reserved exclusively for digital selective calling for distress and safety purposes.

6.3.5 MF radio

MF radiotelephones operate in the 1605–4200 kHz wavebands. Unlike VHF and HF, MF transmissions tend to follow the curve of the earth, which makes them suitable for direction finding equipment. For this reason, and because of their good range, the marine distress radiotelephone frequency is in the MF band

(2182 kHz). Silence periods are observed on this frequency for three minutes commencing every hour and half hour.

During these silence periods only Distress and Urgency messages may be transmitted (see 8.2.5). MF radio equipment must be single sideband (SSB). Double sideband (DSB) transmissions are prohibited except for emergency-only sets operating on 2182 kHz. As for VHF, both the operator and the set must be licensed. MF sets are more complex and more expensive than VHF, and are subject to more regulations.

6.3.6   HF radio

HF radiotelephones use wave bands that are chosen, according to prevailing propagation conditions, from 4, 8, 12, 16 and 22 MHz bands (short wave). HF is more expensive than MF and absorbs more power, but it can provide worldwide coverage – although good installation and correct operation are essential for satisfactory results.

Whereas MF transmissions follow the curve of the earth, HF waves travel upwards and bounce off the ionosphere back to earth. Reception is better at night when the ionosphere is more dense. The directional properties of HF transmissions are poor, and there is no radiotelephone HF distress frequency.

6.3.7   RT procedures

Except for distress, urgency or safety messages, communications between a ship and a coast station are controlled by the latter. Between two ship stations, the station called controls the working. A calling station must use a frequency on which the station called is keeping watch. After making contact, communication can continue on an agreed working channel. For VHF the name of the station called need normally only be given once, and that of the calling station twice. Once contact is made, each name need only be transmitted once. If a station does not reply, check the settings on the transmitter and repeat the call at three-minute intervals (if the channel is clear).

Prowords

It is important to understand the following:

ACKNOWLEDGE	'Have you received and understood?'
CONFIRM	'My version is … is that correct?'
CORRECTION	'An error has been made; the correct version is …'
I SAY AGAIN	'I repeat … (e.g. important words)'
I SPELL	'What follows is spelt phonetically'
OUT	End of work
OVER	'I have completed this part of my message, and am inviting you to reply'
RECEIVED	'Receipt acknowledged'
SAY AGAIN	'Repeat your message (or part indicated)'
STATION CALLING	Used when a station is uncertain of the identity of a station which is calling

Before making a call, decide exactly what needs to be said. It may help to write the message down. Speak clearly and distinctly. Names or important words can be repeated or spelt phonetically.

For a position, give latitude and longitude, or the yacht's bearing and distance from a charted object. For bearings use 360° True notation. For times use 24 hour notation, and specify UT, BST etc.

6.3.8   Coast Radio Stations – general

Maritime countries operate Coast Radio Stations which control communications and link ship stations with the telephone network ashore. These coast stations operate on nominated frequencies – for European waters see 6.3.26–6.3.31.

At scheduled times they transmit traffic lists, navigation warnings, weather bulletins, and (as required) gale warnings. They play an important part in Distress, Urgency and Safety Messages (see 8.2).

6.3.9   Coast Radio Stations – United Kingdom

In the United Kingdom Coast Radio Stations are operated by BT Maritime Services, and details are shown in 6.3.26.

There are nine MF stations and a larger number of VHF stations, the latter providing VHF coverage for most inshore waters.

For commercial telephone (link) calls the MF and VHF stations form one big network, and any call that comes in through any station within the UK will be answered by the first available Radio Officer, wherever he may be. A call to Land's End Radio might well be answered by an operator at Portpatrick.

For Distress and Safety, including medical advice and assistance, and for broadcasting Navigational Warnings, Weather Forecasts, Gale Warnings etc, the stations are divided into Northern and Southern Regions. The MF stations in the Southern Region comprise Land's End, Niton, North Foreland and Humber Radios. The Northern Region comprises Cullercoats, Stonehaven, Wick/Shetland, Hebrides, and Portpatrick Radios. The Southern Region controlling station is Land's End, and the Northern Region station is Stonehaven. The Commercial and Broadcasting systems are separate to reduce problems in the event of equipment or line failure.

Broadcasts are on dedicated MF frequencies and on selected VHF channels (also used for link calls). The Officer in each region making the broadcast can engage and speak over the broadcast frequencies and channels of all regional stations.

VHF stations may keep watch on Ch 16, but distress cover for this primarily rests with HM Coastguard.

Long range service is provided by Portishead Radio on High Frequency (HF). See 6.3.13 and 6.3.26.

6.3.10   VHF link calls to UK Coast Stations

When within range (about 40 miles) you are likely to be able to call a Coast Station. This allows you to make ordinary telephone calls, reverse charge calls, YTD calls (see below), or send telegrams. There is also free access to navigational warnings, weather bulletins and gale warnings.

Except in emergency, vessels should call a UK Coast Station on one of the working frequencies shown in 6.3.26. For a Distress or Urgency Call (only) use Ch 16. Avoid using the station's designated broadcast channel at about the time of a scheduled broadcast. Proceed as follows:

(1) Listen for a 'clear' channel, with no transmission at all. A busy channel will have either carrier noise, speech or the engaged signal (a series of pips).

(2) Having located a free channel, the initial call must last at least six seconds in order to activate the Coast Station's ship-call latch equipment. For example: 'Land's End Radio, Land's End Radio, this is Yacht Seabird, Seabird Golf Oscar Romeo India – Channel 85, Over'.

(3) When the call is accepted by the Coast Station you will hear engaged pips, indicating that you have activated and engaged the channel. Wait for the operator to speak. If you are not answered, do not change channel since you may lose your turn. If you do not hear the pips you have not activated the station's transmitter and may be out of range. Try another station or call again when you get closer.

(4) When you are answered by the Radio Officer be ready to give the following: Vessel's callsign, name, type of call and billing details (see below), and for a link call the telephone number required (and the name of the person in the case of a personal call).

It is possible to make personal calls to certain countries and collect (transferred charge) calls to the UK. Worldwide accounting for calls is arranged by quoting the 'Accounting Authority Indicator Code' (AAIC) if this has been arranged with one of the several ITU-recognised authorities such as BT. VHF link calls through BT coast stations to the UK, or Isle of Man can be charged to the owner's home telephone by yacht telephone debit (YTD). Be prepared to advise the operator accordingly. Payment can also be made by transfer charge or by BT Chargecard, which also applies to foreign calls. The operator makes the connection. Timing is automatic.

Note: St Peter Port and Jersey CRS are regarded as foreign stations by BT who add a handling charge of £4 – £7 on the bill. For Jersey, calls may be billed to a UK address. See page 83.

For receiving calls, you are called on Ch 16 when a message or phone call is ready for you, but it is recommended to listen to the regular traffic lists broadcast from the nearest Coast Station. If your vessel is equipped with a selective call device, you can be alerted by a Coast Station transmitting your Selcall number on Ch 16. Some Selcall equipment displays the number of the station calling you (see 6.3.26). In practice, when responding to a call, contact the nearest station to you.

6.3.11   VHF calls to foreign Coast Stations

French, German and Irish stations are called on a working channel, similarly Belgian and Dutch stations but depending on the position of the yacht. VHF calls to Scheveningen Radio should last several seconds and state the calling channel. A four-tone signal indicates temporary delay but you will be answered when an operator is free.

6.3.12   MF calls to/from UK Coast Stations

Calls should be made on 2182 kHz. The Coast Station will answer on 2182 kHz, allocate a working channel, and queue you into the system.

Distress and Urgency calls should always be made on 2182 kHz, and will be answered on the same frequency. This includes urgent medical calls which should be preceded by the Urgency Signal 'PAN PAN MEDICO' (see 6.3.17). For full details of radio distress procedures see Chapter 8.

Should a coast station be operating distress traffic on 2182 kHz, call on 2191 kHz and listen for a reply on the station's broadcast frequency. You will then be allocated a channel. The Radio Officer will then request the following information: Vessel's callsign, name, Accounting Code (AAIC – see 6.3.10), and category of traffic (e.g. telegram, telephone call).

For receiving MF calls, you will be called by a coast station on 2182 kHz when a message or telephone call booking is received from a shore number, but it is important (especially if expecting a call) to listen to the regular broadcast traffic lists, the times of which are shown in 6.3.26. Selective calling from BT coast stations operates on MF in a similar way to VHF described in 6.3.10 above, the Selcall number being transmitted on 2170·5 kHz.

6.3.13   HF calls – Portishead Radio

The long-range service in the United Kingdom is provided by Portishead Radio, operated by BT Maritime Radio. Watch is kept on the higher bands during daylight, and on the lower bands at night. A 24-hour watch is kept on the 8 MHz band.

The bands in use are announced after the traffic lists, broadcast every H+00, and major changes are notified during the previous week. Channels assigned to Portishead Radio are listed in 6.3.26. R3E (SSB reduced carrier) or J3E (SSB suppressed carrier) are the modes of transmission that are mandatory in both directions, but on channel 1201 J3E should be used whenever possible and this is the preferred mode for all transmissions.

An *Optimum Transmitting Frequency Guide*, is available on radiotelex from Portishead Radio Databank facility. It predicts the best band for contacting Portishead worldwide. It is only a guide, and bands should be monitored to get the best signal.

Equipment must be correctly tuned before calling, and interference not caused to calls in progress. Do not call until a channel is clear, which is announced by Portishead Radio after each period of working.

6

6.3.14 Link calls to a yacht

Telephone call bookings to vessels via BT Coast Stations are handled by Portishead Radio. By dialling 0800 378389 you will be connected free of charge to the ship's radiotelephone service. This number should be used to book calls on VHF, Short Range; the MF, Medium Range; or the HF, Long Range services. You will be asked for the name of the vessel, station through which vessel normally communicates, voyage details, caller's telephone number (or number to be charged if different), person to whom you wish to speak, and caller's name. Portishead Radio will route the call to the appropriate Coast Station. If the vessel is subsequently contacted by other means (e.g. landline) a call via a coast station should be cancelled.

6.3.15 Autolink RT

Autolink RT gives direct dialling from ship to shore into national and international telephone networks without going through a coast station operator. It functions through an onboard unit which is easily connected to the radio, and which does not interfere with normal manual operation. This service on VHF, MF and HF gives quicker access, cheaper calls, call scrambling on some units where privacy is required, and simplified accounting. Last number redial and a ten number memory store are available.

To make an Autolink call, switch on the radio and the Autolink unit. Select a working channel and enter your PIN number (see below) as prompted. Key in or recall from memory the required telephone number in response to the prompt. If the channel is free, press the Send key on the Autolink unit, and connection is automatic. If the radio channel is already in use, either wait until it is free or select another channel if available. Then press the Send key again.

With full duplex radios press the PTT key throughout the conversation. With semi-duplex sets press the PTT key only when speaking. The connection is ended and charging stops when the receiver is replaced on the telephone ashore, but it is best to press the Send button at the end of each call.

To obtain manual assistance from a BT coast station, key in one of these two-digit codes instead of a telephone number: 00 for high priority assistance, 11 for low priority assistance.

For the local weather forecast, key in the code 12 instead of the full Marinecall telephone number. To obtain Marinecall numbers for other areas you must dial the full 0898 numbers.

For Distress, Urgency and Safety (including medical) calls use the normal manual procedure on VHF Ch 16 or 2182 kHz.

If you own an Autolink unit, on registering with BT you may elect to pay for calls by one of three methods: (1) A nominated UK telephone number (UK stations only), (2) a BT Chargecard, or (3) a ship's Accounting Authority. There is no registration or subscription charge, and you may change your method of payment on request. For charging you are identified by the PIN number allocated. Up to 99 different PIN numbers can be issued with the serial number of each Autolink unit, so 99 people can be charged individually.

6.3.16 Weather information by RT

See Chapter 7 – for example 7.2.5 (ships at sea), 7.2.16 (broadcasts by coast stations), 7.2.17 (present weather), 7.2.18 (broadcasts by HM Coastguard).

6.3.17 Medical help by RT

Medical advice can be obtained through any UK (BT) coast station by calling on a working channel and asking for a Medico call. In emergency call on Ch 16 using the Urgency Signal PAN PAN, followed by the word MEDICO. Urgent requests for advice should be made on Ch 16 direct to HM Coastguard who will arrange with the coast station for a priority working channel so that your call is connected to a doctor.

Calls for medical assistance (i.e. the presence of a doctor or a casualty to be off-lifted) should be made direct to HM Coastguard on Ch 16. If such a call is received by a coast station it will be referred to HM Coastguard. A Medico message should contain:

(1)   Yacht's name, callsign and nationality
(2)   Yacht's position, next port of call (with ETA) and nearest harbour if required to divert
(3)   Patient's details - name, age, sex, medical history
(4)   Present symptoms and advice required
(5)   What medication is carried on board

When out of VHF range call on 2182 kHz. There is no charge for medical calls.

Similar arrangements apply in other countries. For France call: PAN PAN Radiomédical (name of station) in French. For Belgium call: Radiomédical Oostende, in French, Dutch, English or German. For Netherlands call: Radiomédical Scheveningen, in Dutch, English, French or German. For Germany call: Funkarzt (name of station) in German or English.

6.3.18 Flotilla reporting schemes

Where numbers of yachts are required to report on a regular basis to a control centre, BT offer two schemes. (1) Where vessels are given a window during which to report, and (2) Where vessels report at fixed times. Details from BT Maritime Radio, 43 Bartholomew Close, London EC1A 7HP.

6.3.19 Port Operations and Vessel Traffic Services

Most harbours and marinas now have VHF RT facilities, while a few harbours also operate on MF (mostly for pilotage). The nominated channels are only for messages concerning port operations or, in emergency, the safety of persons, and not for public correspondence. For details of harbour RT information in Chapter 10, see 10.0.3.

An increasing number of ports are implementing Vessel Traffic Services (VTS) schemes, to improve the safety and efficiency of traffic and to protect the environment. VTS may range from the provision of information messages to the extensive management of traffic within a port or waterway, and is aimed primarily at commercial vessels which must comply with the laid down procedures.

Yachts are not normally expected to comply with VTS radio and reporting procedures, except in certain ports and waterways where larger yachts may fall within the stipulated minimum length or tonnage.

When navigating in areas covered by VTS or Port Operations Service, especially in poor visibility or at night, yachts can gain valuable information about the movement of ships by listening on the nominated working channel.

Most VTS (and some Port Operations) schemes have information broadcasts at scheduled times, typically covering traffic, weather, tidal details, and local navigational warnings. VTS radio channels are shown in Chapter 10 on Area Maps, Traffic Separation Scheme diagrams, or under RADIO TELEPHONE in port entries.

6.3.20   Distress, Urgency and Safety traffic by radiotelephone

There are agreed international procedures for passing radiotelephone messages concerning vessels in distress – or for lesser emergencies or situations where Urgency or Safety Messages are appropriate. These are fully described in 8.2. For the Global Maritime Distress and Safety System (GMDSS) see 8.3.1.

If you hear a distress call, you must cease all transmissions that might interfere with it or other distress traffic, and continue listening on the frequency concerned. Write down what you hear. You may have responsibilities for assisting the casualty or for relaying the distress messages. This, and the general control of distress traffic, are discussed in 8.2.5 and 8.2.7.

6.3.21   INMARSAT

Worldwide satellite communication (Satcom) is provided by the International Maritime Satellite Organisation (INMARSAT), through satellites in geostationary orbits above the equator over the Atlantic, Pacific and Indian Oceans. These satellites are the links between the Coast Earth Stations (CESs), operated by organisations such as BT, and the onboard terminals called Ship Earth Stations (SESs). Satcom is more reliable and gives better reception than HF SSB radio.

A CES connects the satellite system with the landbased communication network. A message to a ship originating on land is transmitted by the CES to one of the satellites, and thence to the ship. A call from a ship is received via the satellite by the CES, which then transmits it onwards over landbased networks.

Standard 'A' terminals, with a big antenna only suitable for larger vessels, have direct dialling telephone, Telex, data and fax facilities.

Standard 'C' are smaller, and are for sending and receiving data or text (but not voice). Both 'A' and 'C' offer speedy connection to HM Coastguard's MRCC at Falmouth for Distress, Safety etc.

More recently, Inmarsat 'B' was launched as an improved successor to Inmarsat 'A', while Standard 'M' now makes satellite telephone, fax and data services available to a wide range of yachts, using smaller and cheaper equipment.

6.3.22   Navigational Warnings – General

The worldwide Navigational Warning Service covers 16 sea areas (NAVAREAS) numbered I–XVI, each with a country nominated as Area Co-ordinator responsible for issuing long range warnings. These are numbered consecutively through the year and are transmitted in English and in one or more other languages at scheduled times by WT. Other forms of transmission (RT, radiotelex and fax) may also be used. Warnings cover items such as failures or changes to navigational aids, wrecks and navigational dangers of all kinds, SAR operations, cable or pipe laying, naval exercises etc.

Within each NAVAREA, Coastal Warnings and Local Warnings may also be issued. Coastal Warnings, up to 100 or 200 miles offshore, are broadcast in English and in the national language by coast radio stations. Local Warnings are issued by harbour authorities in the national language.

6.3.23   Navigational Warnings – Europe

United Kingdom

The United Kingdom (together with Northern Europe and Scandinavia) comes within NAVAREA I, with Britain as the Area Co-ordinator for long range navigational warnings which are broadcast by Portishead Radio (GKA). Messages are numbered and are published in the weekly *Notices to Mariners* together with a list of warnings still in force.

NAVTEX warnings (see 6.3.25) are broadcast by Niton, Cullercoats and Portpatrick Radio for the areas shown in Fig. 6(1).

Coastal Warnings are broadcast by RT at scheduled times from coast radio stations for the Sea Regions lettered A–N in Fig.6(2). Important warnings are broadcast at any time on the distress frequencies of 500 kHz, 2182 kHz and VHF Ch 16.

Local warnings from harbour authorities are broadcast by nearby coast radio stations. HM Coastguard broadcasts local warnings for inshore waters outside of harbour limits, on VHF Ch 67 after an announcement on Ch 16.

Vessels which encounter dangers to navigation should notify other craft and the nearest coast radio station, prefacing the message by the safety signal (see 8.2.6).

BT coast radio stations and HM Coastguard in areas concerned make scheduled SUBFACTS broadcasts of submarine activity in specified exercise areas. For details see 8.5.1.

France

Long range warnings are broadcast in English and French for NAVAREA II, which includes the west coast of France, by St Lys Radio. The north coast comes within NAVAREA I.

AVURNAVS (AVis URgents aux NAVigateurs) are coastal and local warnings issued by regional authorities:

(1) Avurnavs Brest for the west coast of France and the western Channel (to Mont St Michel).

(2) Avurnavs Cherbourg for the eastern Channel and the North Sea (Mont St Michel to the Belgian frontier).

Avurnavs are broadcast by the appropriate coast radio station, urgent ones on receipt and at the end of the next silence period as well as at scheduled times (see 6.3.28). RT warnings are prefixed by 'Sécurité Avurnav', followed by the name of the station.

Belgium
Navigational warnings are broadcast by Oostende Radio on receipt on 2761 kHz and VHF Ch 27 and at scheduled times (see 6.3.29) on 2761 kHz MF, 518 kHz (NAVTEX) and on Ch 27.

Netherlands
Navigational warnings are broadcast by Scheveningen Radio on receipt and at scheduled times (see 6.3.30) on 1713 kHz (Nes) and 1890 kHz and VHF (after announcement on Ch 16). Netherlands Coast Guard broadcasts warnings on 518 kHz (NAVTEX) on receipt and at scheduled times (see 6.3.25).

Germany
Navigational warnings are broadcast by Norddeich Radio on 2614 kHz on receipt, after the next silence period, and at scheduled times. Broadcasts commence with the safety signal, the words *Nautische Warnnachricht*, and the serial number; they are in English and German. Decca Warnings for the German and Frisian Islands chains (*Decca Warnnachricht*) are included. Dangers to navigation should be reported to Seewarn Cuxhaven.

6.3.24   Other Maritime Radio Services
Apart from Coast Radio Stations, Port Operations, and Vessel Traffic Services, some countries operate other radio services connected with Search and Rescue (SAR) and Maritime Safety Information (MSI).

United Kingdom
HM Coastguard MRCCs and MRSCs (see 8.4.2) keep a constant watch on VHF Ch 16 through 96 remote radio sites around the coast. Ch 67 is the Small Craft Safety Frequency, and safety information can be exchanged with HM Coastguard after an initial call on Ch 16. Other channels held by MRCCs and MRSCs include Ch 0 10 73. Local Navigational Warnings are broadcast on Ch 67 after an announcement on Ch 16.

Local Strong Wind Warnings are broadcast on receipt, and local Weather Messages every four hours (every two hours in bad weather) - both on Ch 67 after announcement on Ch 16. For details see 7.2.19.

The Channel Navigation Information Service (CNIS) provides a 24-hour radio safety service and radar coverage in the Dover Strait. Liaison is established with the Belgian Sea Rescue Service at Oostende, the (French) MRSC at Cap Gris-Nez, and the Air Traffic Control Centre (ATCC) at West Drayton.

France
Five Centres Régionaux Opérationnels de Surveillance et de Sauvetage (CROSS) cover the Atlantic Coast, situated at Gris-Nez, Jobourg, Corsen, Étel and Soulac. They keep constant watch and cooperate with foreign MRCCs and MRSCs. Their main tasks are:
(1) Surveillance of marine traffic, especially within the 12 mile limit.
(2) Maritime Search and Rescue.
(3) Fishery surveillance out to 200M.
(4) Monitoring of pollution.
(5) Collecting and organising data for future use.

CROSS Étel specialises in medical advice and also responds to alerts from COSPAS/SARSAT satellites.

All CROSS stations keep watch on Ch 16 and broadcast Navigational Warnings, Storm Warnings and Weather Messages through a number of remote VHF relay stations.

Netherlands
Netherlands Coastguard (at IJmuiden) keeps watch (H24) on 2182 kHz and on VHF Ch 16 (H24) through Scheveningen Radio VHF sites listed on page 97 (Coastal and Inland). Digital Selective Calling (DSC) is provided on 2187·5 kHz and VHF Ch 70. MMSI N0. 002442000. Telephone (alarm) number: 02550 34344.

Germany
Digital Selective Calling is operated on 2187·5 kHz from Norddeich Radio, and on Ch 70 from Norddeich, Bremen, Helgoland, Elbe-Weser, Hamburg, Eiderstedt and Nordfriesland Radios.

6.3.25   NAVTEX
NAVTEX provides navigational and meteorological warnings and other safety information by automatic print-outs from a dedicated receiver, and is a component of the International Maritime Organization (IMO) Global Maritime Distress and Safety System (GMDSS) (see 8.3.1).

At present, broadcasts are all in English on a single frequency of 518 kHz, with excellent coverage of coastal waters in areas such as NW Europe where the scheme originated. Interference between stations is avoided by time sharing and by limiting the range of transmitters to about 300 miles, so that three stations cover the United Kingdom. IMO is expected to make a second NAVTEX channel available for broadcasts in the local national language.

The use of a single frequency allows a simple receiver with a printer using cash-roll paper, although some yacht receivers have a video screen. The user programmes the receiver for the vessel's area and for the types of messages required. For example, if Decca is not carried, Decca Warnings can be rejected. The receiver automatically rejects messages which are corrupt or ones that have already been printed.

Each message is prefixed by a four character group. The first character is the code letter of the transmitting station (in the United Kingdom: S for Niton, G for Cullercoats and O for Portpatrick). The second character indicates the category of the message as in the code below. The third and fourth are message serial numbers, from 01 to 99. The serial number 00 denotes urgent traffic such as gale warnings and SAR alerts, and messages with this prefix are always printed.

NAVTEX stations
The table below shows the NAVTEX stations in NAVAREAS I and II with their identity codes and transmission times (UT). The times of weather bulletins are shown in bold. (P) indicates that the station is provisional or projected.

Message categories
A   Navigational warnings
B   Gale warnings
C   Ice reports (unlikely to apply in UK)
D   SAR information and pirate attack warnings
E   Weather forecasts
F   Pilot Service messages
G   Decca messages
H   Loran-C messages
I   Omega messages
J   Satnav messages
K   Other electronic navaid messages
L   Navigational warnings additional to letter A
Z   No messages on hand at scheduled time

Information in a NAVTEX broadcast applies only to the area for which the broadcast station is responsible, as shown in Fig.6(1). A user may accept messages from one or more stations.

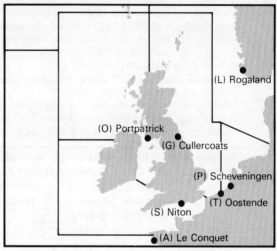

Fig. 6(1)   NAVTEX areas – NW Europe

NAVAREA I

	Station							
R –	**Reykjavik,** Iceland	0318	**0718**	1118	1518	**1918**	**2318**	
B –	**Bodø,** Norway	**0018**	0418	0900	**1218**	1618	2100	
J –	**Gislövshammar,** (Stockholm Radio), Sweden	0330	**0730**	1130	1530	**1930**	2330	
H –	**Bjuröklubb,** (Stockholm Radio), Sweden	0000	0400	**0800**	1200	1600	**2000**	
U –	**Stavsnäs,** (Stockholm Radio), Sweden	0030	0430	**0830**	1230	1630	**2030**	
P –	**Netherlands Coast Guard** (IJmuiden), Netherlands	0348	0748	1148	1548	1948	2348	
T –	**Oostende,** Belgium	0248	**0648**	1048	1448	**1848**	2248	
G –	**Cullercoats,** UK	0048	0448	**0848**	1248	1648	**2048**	
S –	**Niton,** UK	0018	0418	**0818**	1218	1618	**2018**	
O –	**Portpatrick,** UK	0130	0530	**0930**	1330	1730	**2130**	
V –	**Vardø,** Norway	0300	0700	**1100**	1500	1900	**2300**	
L –	**Rogaland,** Norway	**0148**	0548	**0948**	**1348**	1748	**2148**	
W –	(No information),Ireland	0340	0740	1140	1540	1940	2340	(Planned – no date)

NAVAREA II

	Station							
A –	**Le Stiff,** Corsen (CROSS), France	**0000**	0400	0800	**1200**	1600	2000	
G –	**Tarifa,** Spain	0100	0500	0900	1300	1700	2100	
R –	**Lisboa,** Portugal	**0250**	**0650**	**1050**	**1450**	**1850**	**2250**	
F –	**Horta,** Azores	**0050**	**0450**	**0850**	**1250**	**1650**	**2050**	
D –	**La Coruña,** Spain	0030	0430	**0830**	1230	1630	**2030**	(On trial 1995)
I –	**Las Palmas,** Islas Canarias, Spain	0100	0500	0900	1300	1700	2100	(Planned Summer 1995)

6

6.3.26 UK Coast Radio Stations (HF, MF and VHF)

Notes:

a)   Except for St. Peter Port Radio and Jersey Radio, services are provided by BT.

b)   MF calls to BT coast stations are made and answered on 2182 kHz. During distress working, call on 2191 kHz and listen for reply on the station's broadcast frequency.

c)   Channel letters and frequencies in *italics* are for Autolink RT only. Most working VHF channels at BT stations are available for manual or Autolink calls.

d)   Gale warnings are broadcast by BT stations after the first silence period after receipt, and at the next of the following times: 0303 0903 1503 2103 (UT), or if first broadcast at a scheduled time the warning is repeated after the next silence period. In the Southern Region, Weather Bulletins are broadcast at 0733 1933 (UT) or on request. In the Northern Region at 0703 1903 (UT) or on request. For further details of Gale Warnings and Weather Bulletins see Table 7(4) on page 116.

e)   Traffic Lists are sent by BT stations at all scheduled broadcast times (Navigation Warnings, Gale Warnings and Weather Bulletins).

f)   SUBFACTS and GUNFACTS are sent on the broadcast frequencies of certain stations as detailed in 8.5.1 and 8.5.2 on page 133.

g)   Telephone numbers marked by an asterisk (*) are not continually manned.

h)   Where so indicated stations operate 2187·5 kHz and/or VHF Ch 70 for distress alerts and safety calls using digital selective calling (DSC).

Coast Station Name Position	VHF Ch other than Ch 16	Station details with MF frequencies where relevant as shown below				Navigation and Decca Warning Times (UT) For Weather Bulletins and Gale Warnings see page 112-113 Note: Traffic Lists are sent with all scheduled broadcasts
		Distress, Urgency, Safety (kHz)	Working paired MF frequencies (kHz)			
			MF Ch	Coast Station		
				Transmit	Receive	

SOUTHERN REGION

Coast Station Name Position	VHF Ch	Station details with MF frequencies				Navigation and Decca Warning Times
CELTIC RADIO 51°41'N 05°11'W	24	VHF station remotely controlled Selcall (3218): Ch 16				Broadcasts on Ch 24 at same times as Land's End below
BURNHAM RADIO 51°13'N 02°59'W	25	VHF station remotely controlled				For commercial traffic in Severn Estuary. No broadcasts
ILFRACOMBE RADIO 51°11'N 04°07'W	05 07	VHF station remotely controlled Selcall (3205): Ch 16				Broadcasts on Ch 05 at same times as Land's End below
LAND'S END RADIO 50°07'N 05°40'W Tel: 01736 871363	27 64[1] 85 88	2182 Note (1) VHF Ch 64 directed to Scillies Selcall (3204): 2170·5 kHz Ch 16	W X	2782 3610	2111 2120	Broadcasts on 2670 kHz and Ch 27 and Ch 64 at: 0233 0633 1033 1433 1833 2233 (Decca chains 1B 7D)
PENDENNIS RADIO 50°09'N 05°03'W	62 66	VHF station remotely controlled Selcall (3238): Ch 16				Broadcasts on Ch 62 at same times as Land's End above
START POINT RADIO 50°21'N 03°43'W	26 60 65	VHF station remotely controlled Selcall (3224): Ch 16				Broadcasts on Ch 26 at same times as Land's End above
WEYMOUTH BAY RADIO 50°36'N 02°27'W	05	VHF station remotely controlled Selcall (3242): Ch 16				Broadcasts on Ch 05 at same times as Lands End above

CHANNEL ISLANDS

Coast Station Name Position	VHF Ch	Station details				Navigation Warning Times
ST PETER PORT RADIO 49°27'N 02°32'W Note: Commercial calls only. Link calls available on VHF Ch 62 only.	20[1] 62[2] 67[3] 78	Ship calls on 2182 kHz Station replies on 1764kHz	1662.5[4] 2182 1764	1662.5[4] 2182[5] 2381[6] 2108 2056		Broadcasts on 1764 kHz and Ch 20 62: *Navigation Warnings* followed by *Traffic Lists* at: 0133 0533 0933 1333 1733 2133. Ships are also called for Traffic on 2182 kHz and Ch 16.

Notes: (1) Direct calling on Ch 20
(2) Link calls on Ch 62 only
(3) Ch 67 for small craft safety

(4) Trinity House and SAR only
(5) H24
(6) When 2182 is distress working

Tel: 01481 720672

6.3.26   UK Coast Radio Stations (HF, MF and VHF) *continued*

CHANNEL ISLANDS continued

JERSEY RADIO 49°11'N 02°14'W Note: Link calls available on VHF Ch 25 82 only. Pay by credit card, or direct bill to UK address, or to a Jersey Harbour Office account, or on arrival through contact address. *Tel: 01534 41121*	25 67[1] 82[2]	Ship calls on 2182 kHz Station replies on 1659 kHz (British ships) or 2182 kHz (foreign ships)	2182 1659	2182[3] 2084[4] 2045[5] 2048[5] 2534[4]	Broadcasts on 1659 kHz and Ch 25 82: *Navigation Warnings:* 0433 UT, 0645 0745 LT,1245 2245 UT. *Decca Warnings:* On receipt and H+03 for next two hours (Chain 1B).
	Notes: (1) Ch 67 for yacht safety messages. Call on Ch 16 (2) Direct calling for UK ships (3) H24. When distress working call on 2191 and listen on 1659 kHz (4) UK registered vessels (5) Foreign vessels (6) DSC (H24) on Ch 70 (GMDSS A1)				*Traffic Lists:* After *Weather Messages* at 0645 0745 LT 1245 1845 2245 UT. Ships are also called for traffic on 2182 kHz and Ch 16. *Gale Warnings:* On receipt, after next silence period, and at 0307 0907 1507 2107 UT.

SOUTHERN REGION continued

NITON RADIO 50°35'N 01°18'W VHF service at: 50°36'N 01°12'W For NAVTEX see 6.3.25 – page 80 *Tel: 01983 730495**	04 28 64 85 87	2182	U	2628	2009	Broadcasts on 1641 kHz and Ch 28 at: 0233 0633 1033 1433 1833 2233 (Decca chains 1B 5B)
		Note (1) VHF Ch 64 directed to Brighton area Selcall (3203): 2170·5 kHz Ch 16				
HASTINGS RADIO 50°52'N 00°37'E	07 66	VHF station remotely controlled Selcall (3225): Ch 16				Broadcasts on Ch 07 at same times as North Foreland below
NORTH FORELAND RADIO 51°22'N 01°25'E	05 26 65	2182		1707	2132	Broadcasts on 1707 kHz and Ch 26 at: 0133 0533 0933 1333 1733 2133 (Decca chains 1B 5B 2E)
		Selcall (3201): 2170·5 kHz Ch16				
THAMES RADIO 51°20'N 00°20'E	02 83	VHF station remotely controlled Selcall (3202): Ch 16				Broadcasts on Ch 02 at same times as North Foreland above
ORFORDNESS RADIO 52°00'N 01°25'E	62 82	VHF station remotely controlled Selcall (3235): Ch 16				Broadcasts on Ch 62 at same times as North Foreland above
BACTON RADIO 52°51'N 01°28'E	03 07	VHF station remotely controlled Selcall (3214): Ch 16				Broadcasts on Ch 07 at same times as Humber below
HUMBER RADIO 53°20'N 00°17'E *Tel: 01507 473447**	24 26 85	2182	Q R S 5	1925 2684 2810 *3624*	2105 2002 2562 *3324*	Broadcasts on 1869 kHz and Ch 26 at: 0133 0533 0933 1333 1733 2133 (Decca chains 5B 2A 2E 9B)
		Note (1) VHF Ch 64 directed to The Wash Selcall (3212): 2170.5 kHz Ch 16				
GRIMSBY RADIO 53°34'N 00°05'W	04 27	VHF station remotely controlled Selcall (3239): Ch 16				Broadcasts on Ch 27 at same times as Humber above

6

6.3.26   UK Coast Radio Stations (HF, MF and VHF) *continued*

Notes:

a)   Except for St. Peter Port Radio and Jersey Radio, services are provided by BT.

b)   MF calls to BT coast stations are made and answered on 2182 kHz. During distress working, call on 2191 kHz and listen for reply on the station's broadcast frequency.

c)   Channel letters and frequencies in *italics* are for Autolink RT only. Most working VHF channels at BT stations are available for manual or Autolink calls.

d)   Gale warnings are broadcast by BT stations after the first silence period after receipt, and at the next of the following times: 0303 0903 1503 2103 (UT), or if first broadcast at a scheduled time the warning is repeated after the next silence period. In the Southern Region, Weather Bulletins are broadcast at 0733 1933 (UT) or on request. In the Northern Region at 0703 1903 (UT) or on request. For further details of Gale Warnings and Weather Bulletins see Table 7(4) on page 116.

e)   Traffic Lists are sent by BT stations at all scheduled broadcast times (Navigation Warnings, Gale Warnings and Weather Bulletins).

f)   SUBFACTS and GUNFACTS are sent on the broadcast frequencies of certain stations as detailed in 8.5.1 and 8.5.2 on page 133.

g)   Telephone numbers marked by an asterisk (*) are not continually manned.

h)   Where so indicated stations operate 2187·5 kHz and/or VHF Ch 70 for distress alerts and safety calls using digital selective calling (DSC).

Coast Station Name Position	VHF Ch other than Ch 16	Station details with MF frequencies where relevant as shown below				Navigation and Decca Warning Times (UT) For Weather Bulletins and Gale Warnings see page 112-113 Note: Traffic Lists are sent with all scheduled broadcasts
		Distress, Urgency, Safety (kHz)	Working paired MF frequencies (kHz)			
			MF Ch	Coast Station		
				Transmit	Receive	

NORTHERN REGION

WHITBY RADIO 54°29'N 00°36'W	25 28	VHF station remotely controlled Selcall (3231): Ch 16				Broadcasts on Ch 25 at same times as Cullercoats below
CULLERCOATS RADIO 55°04'N 01°28'W For NAVTEX see 6.3.25 – page 80 *Tel: 0191 297 0301**	26	2182	N *O* P	1731 *2828* 3750	2527 *1953* 2123	Broadcasts on 2719 kHz and Ch 26 at: 0233 0633 1033 1433 1833 2233 (Decca chain 2A)
		Selcall (3211): 2170·5 kHz Ch 16				
STONEHAVEN RADIO 56°57'N 02°13'W	26	2182	I J K L M T *1* *3*	1856 1650 1946 2607 3617 2698 *1722* *3666*	2555 2075 2566 1999 3249 2016 *2066* *3252*	Broadcasts on 2691 kHz and Ch 26 at: 0233 0633 1033 1433 1833 2233 (Decca chains 2A 6C 0E)
Tel: 01569 762917		Selcall (3222): 2170·5 kHz Ch 16				
FORTH RADIO 55°57'N 02°27'W	24 62	VHF station remotely controlled Selcall (3228): Ch 16				Broadcasts on Ch 24 at same times as Stonehaven above
BUCHAN RADIO 57°36'N 02°03'W	25	VHF station remotely controlled Selcall (3237): Ch 16				Broadcasts on Ch 25 at same times as Stonehaven above
WICK RADIO 58°26'N 03°06'W Located at Norwick, Shetland 60°49'N 00°49'W (Controlled by Wick Radio)		2182	E F G H *4* A B C D *2*	2705 1797 1755 2625 *3775* 2751 2840.6 2604 1659 *3528*	2524 2060 2099 2108 *3355* 2006 2277 2013 2084 *3338*	Broadcasts on 1764 kHz (Wick) and 1770 kHz (Norwick, Shetland) at: 0233 0633 1033 1433 1833 2233
Tel: 01955 602271*		Selcall (3221): 2170·5 kHz				

Fig. 6(2) *Coast Radio Stations*

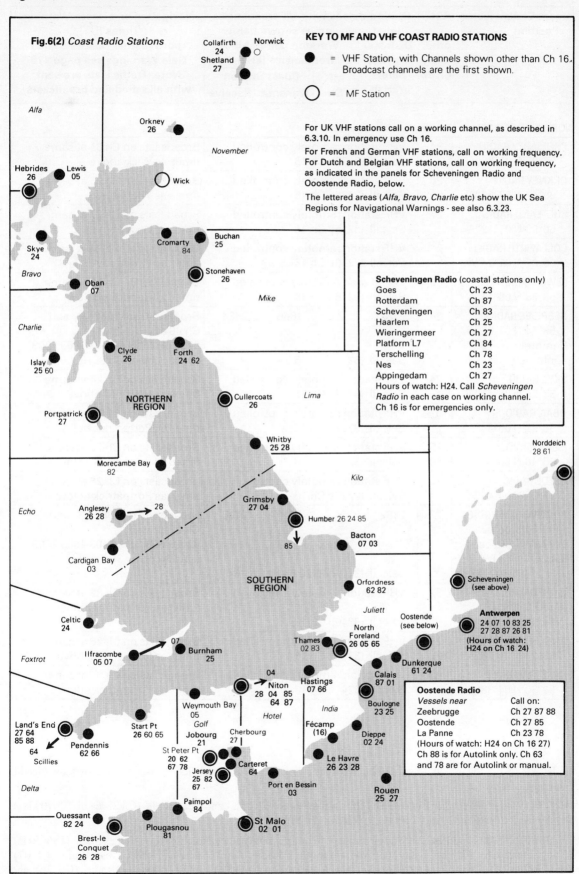

Fig.6(2) *Coast Radio Stations*

KEY TO MF AND VHF COAST RADIO STATIONS

● = VHF Station, with Channels shown other than Ch 16. Broadcast channels are the first shown.

○ = MF Station

For UK VHF stations call on a working channel, as described in 6.3.10. In emergency use Ch 16.

For French and German VHF stations, call on working frequency. For Dutch and Belgian VHF stations, call on working frequency, as indicated in the panels for Scheveningen Radio and Ooostende Radio, below.

The lettered areas (*Alfa, Bravo, Charlie* etc) show the UK Sea Regions for Navigational Warnings - see also 6.3.23.

Scheveningen Radio (coastal stations only)

Goes	Ch 23
Rotterdam	Ch 87
Scheveningen	Ch 83
Haarlem	Ch 25
Wieringermeer	Ch 27
Platform L7	Ch 84
Terschelling	Ch 78
Nes	Ch 23
Appingedam	Ch 27

Hours of watch: H24. Call *Scheveningen Radio* in each case on working channel. Ch 16 is for emergencies only.

Oostende Radio

Vessels near	Call on:
Zeebrugge	Ch 27 87 88
Oostende	Ch 27 85
La Panne	Ch 23 78

(Hours of watch: H24 on Ch 16 27) Ch 88 is for Autolink only. Ch 63 and 78 are for Autolink or manual.

Collafirth 24 Shetland 27
Norwick

Alfa

Orkney 26

November

Hebrides 26
Lewis 05

Wick

Skye 24

Bravo

Oban 07

Cromarty 84
Buchan 25

Stonehaven 26

Mike

Charlie

Islay 25 60

Clyde 26
Forth 24 62

Portpatrick 27

NORTHERN REGION

Cullercoats 26

Lima

Whitby 25 28

Morecambe Bay 82

Kilo

Echo

Anglesey 26 28
28

Grimsby 27 04

Humber 26 24 85

Bacton 07 03

Cardigan Bay 03

SOUTHERN REGION

Orfordness 62 82

Juliett

Scheveningen (see above)

Norddeich 28 61

Antwerpen 24 07 10 83 25 27 28 87 26 81 (Hours of watch: H24 on Ch 16 24)

Celtic 24

Oostende (see below)

Ilfracombe 05 07
07

Burnham 25

Thames 02 83
North Foreland 26 05 65

Dunkerque 61 24

Foxtrot

04

Niton 28 04 85 64 87

Hastings 07 66

Calais 87 01

Weymouth Bay 05

Golf

Cherbourg 27

Jobourg 21

Hotel

Fécamp (16)

Boulogne 23 25

India

Dieppe 02 24

Land's End 27 64 85 88

64

Scillies

Start Pt 26 60 65

Pendennis 62 66

St Peter Pt 20 62 67 78

Jersey 25 82 67

Carteret 64

Le Havre 26 23 28

Rouen 25 27

Port en Bessin 03

Delta

Paimpol 84

Ouessant 82 24

Plougasnou 81

St Malo 02 01

Brest-le Conquet 26 28

continued

6.3.26   UK Coast Radio Stations *continued*

Coast Station Name Position	VHF Ch other than Ch 16	Station details with MF frequencies where relevant as shown below				Navigation and Decca Warning Times (UT) For Weather Bulletins and Gale Warnings see page 116 Note: Traffic Lists are sent with all scheduled broadcasts
		Distress, Urgency, Safety (kHz)	Working paired MF frequencies (kHz)			
			MF Ch	Coast Station		
				Transmit	Receive	

NORTHERN REGION (continued)

Coast Station Name Position	VHF Ch	Distress (kHz)	MF Ch	Transmit	Receive	Navigation and Decca Warning Times
CROMARTY RADIO 57°37'N 02°58'W	84	VHF station remotely controlled Selcall (3227): Ch 16				Broadcasts on Ch 84 at same times as Wick above
ORKNEY RADIO 58°47'N 02°57'W	26	VHF station remotely controlled Selcall (3226): Ch 16				Broadcasts on Ch 26 at same times as Wick above
SHETLAND RADIO 60°09'N 01°12'W	27	VHF station remotely controlled Selcall (3215): Ch 16				Broadcasts on Ch 27 at same times as Wick above
COLLAFIRTH RADIO 60°32'N 01°24'W	24	VHF station remotely controlled Selcall (3230): Ch 16				Broadcasts on Ch 24 at same times as Wick above
LEWIS RADIO 58°28'N 06°14'W	05	VHF station remotely controlled Selcall (3216): Ch 16				Broadcasts on Ch 05 at same times as Hebrides below
HEBRIDES RADIO 58°14'N 07°02'W Remotely controlled	26	2182 Selcall (3234): Ch 16	Z	1866	2534	Broadcasts on 1866 kHz and Ch 26 at: 0203 0603 1003 1403 1803 2203 (Decca chains 6C 8E)
SKYE RADIO 57°28'N 06°41'W	24	VHF station remotely controlled Selcall (3232): Ch 16				Broadcasts on Ch 24 at same times as Hebrides above
OBAN RADIO 56°27'N 05°44'W	07	VHF station remotely controlled Selcall (3207): Ch 16				Broadcasts on Ch 07 at same times as Portpatrick below
ISLAY RADIO 55°46'N 06°27'W	25 60	VHF station remotely controlled Selcall (3233): Ch 16				Broadcasts on Ch 25 at same times as Portpatrick below
CLYDE RADIO 55°38'N 04°47'W	26	VHF station remotely controlled Selcall (3213): Ch 16				Broadcasts on Ch 26 at same times as Portpatrick below
PORTPATRICK RADIO 54°51'N 05°07'W For NAVTEX see 6.3.25 – page 80 *Tel: 01766 810312**	27	2182 Selcall (3207): 2170·5 kHz Ch 16	Y	1710	2135	Broadcasts on 1883 kHz and Ch 27 at: 0203 0603 1003 1403 1803 2203 (Decca chains 3B 7D 8E)
MORECAMBE BAY RADIO 54°10'N 03°12'W	82	VHF station remotely controlled Selcall (3240): Ch 16				Broadcasts on Ch 82 at same times as Portpatrick above
ANGLESEY RADIO 53°24'N 04°18'W	26 28	VHF station remotely controlled Selcall (3206): Ch 16				Broadcasts on Ch 26 at same times as Portpatrick above
CARDIGAN BAY RADIO 52°50'N 04°38'W	03	VHF station remotely controlled Selcall (3241): Ch 16				Broadcasts on Ch 03 at same times as Portpatrick above

SUBFACTS broadcasts announcing planned submarine activity in specified areas are made by Coast Radio Stations as follows:

At **0733 1933** (after Weather Bulletins) by Ilfracombe Radio (Ch 05), Land's End Radio (Ch 27 64 and 2670 kHz), Pendennis Radio (Ch 62) and Start Point Radio (Ch 26).

At **0303 0703 1103 1503 1903 2303** (after any Gale Warnings or Weather Bulletins) by Hebrides Radio (1866 kHz), Lewis Radio (Ch 05), Skye Radio (Ch 24), Portpatrick Radio (Ch 27 and 1883 kHz), Oban Radio (Ch 07), Islay Radio (Ch 25), Clyde Radio (Ch 26), Morecambe Radio (Ch 82), Anglesey Radio (Ch 26) and Cardigan Bay Radio (Ch 03).

6.3.26 UK Coast Radio Stations *continued*

Portishead Radio – High Frequency (HF) Long Range RT service

51°29'N 02°48'W	☎:	(44) 1278 772200 or 0800 378389
52°22'N 01°11'W	Fax:	(44) 1278 792145
50°43'N 02°29'W	Telex:	46441 BTGKA G

For description of service and operation see under HF radio in 6.3.13 (page 77).

Radiotelephone HF duplex channels (carrier frequencies)

Callsign	International channel	Portishead carrier (kHz)	Ship Station carrier (kHz)	
GKT20	410	**4384**	4092	Main channel
GKT22	402	4360	4068	HF Autolink
GKT26	406	4372	4080	
GKV26	426	4432	4140	
GKU46	816	**8764**	8240	Main channel
GKT42	802	8722	8198	
GKU49	819	8773	8249	HF Autolink
GKV42	822	8782	8258	
GKV46	826	8794	8270	
GKW41	831	8809	8285	HF Autolink
GKV54	1224	**13146**	12299	Main channel
GKT51	1201	13077	12230	
GKT52	1202	13080	12233	
GKT56	1206	13092	12245	HF Autolink
GKV58	1228	13158	12311	
GKV50	1230	13164	12317	
GKW52	1232	13170	12323	
GKT62	1602	**17245**	16363	Main channel
GKT66	1606	17257	16375	
GKU61	1611	17272	16390	
GKU65	1615	17284	16402	HF Autolink
GKU68	1618	17293	16411	
GKV63	1623	17308	16426	
GKW62	1632	17335	16453	
GKW67	1637	17350	16468	
GKW60	1640	17359	16477	
GKT18	1801	**19755**	18780	Main channel
GKU18	1803	19761	18786	
GKT76	2206	**22711**	22015	Main channel
GKU72	2212	22729	22033	
GKU74	2214	22735	22039	
GKU70	2220	22753	22057	
GKV77	2227	22774	22078	
GKV79	2229	22780	22084	
GKX70	2240	22813	22117	
GKU25	2502	**26148**	25073	Main channel

NOTES:

(1) Assigned frequencies are 1·4 kHz above carrier frequencies shown.

(2) Portishead Radio monitors the main channel frequencies above, where vessels should make their initial call. These channels are also used for the broadcast of traffic lists, distress, urgency and safety signals. Traffic Lists every H+00 on frequencies in use at the time. All frequencies are J3E and R3E, power 10kW. H24 frequencies are announced after the traffic lists. Channels marked HF Autolink are for Autolink only.

6.3.27   Irish Coast Radio Stations

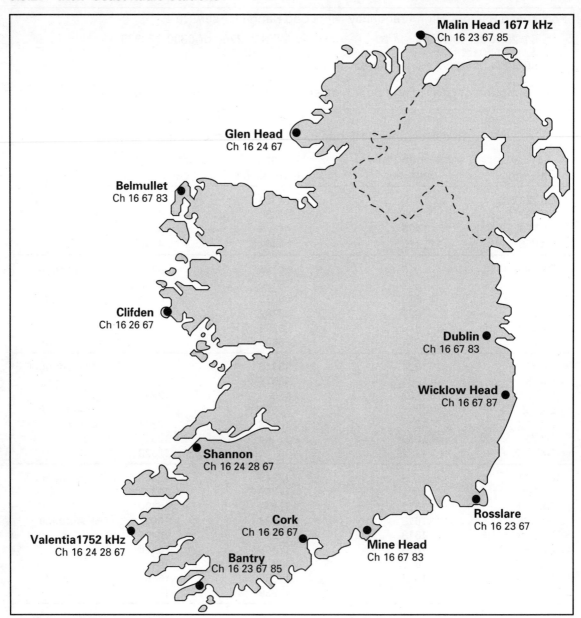

Fig. 6(3) Irish Coast Radio Stations

Irish Coast Radio Service

This service is provided by the Department of the Marine, Leeson Lane, Dublin 2. ☎ 01-785444. Traffic lists, navigational warnings, Decca warnings, weather forecasts and gale warnings are broadcast at the scheduled times shown in the table. Broadcasts are made on a working channel/frequency following a preliminary announcement on channel 16 and 2182 kHz. Ch 67 is used for safety messages only.

VHF calls to a coast station should be made on a working channel. Only use Ch 16 in case of difficulty, or for emergency situations. Malin Head and Valentia Radios are equipped with digital selective calling (DSC) on 2187·5 kHz for automatic reception of distress calls from suitably fitted ships (H24).

Link calls are available through any of the stations on VHF or MF. Telephone calls from shore subscribers can be set up with ships at sea. Contact Malin Head or Valentia Radio by telephone or telex, giving information about the vessel's voyage or whereabouts. Ships at sea should call the nearest coast radio station giving particulars of their voyage at regular intervals (track report, or TR), and listen to traffic list broadcasts.

Malin Head. ☎ 077-70103. Fax: 077-70221. Telex: 42072 MALR EI.

Valentia. ☎ 0667-6109. Fax: 0667-6289. Telex: 73968 VALR EI.

The Irish Aviation and Marine Communication Service on ☎ 01-785444 Ext 670 will be pleased to help with enquiries about the service.

6.3.27 Irish Coast Radio Stations

Notes:

a)   For VHF calls, direct call on working channel preferred, except in emergency.

b)   VHF Ch 67 is for safety communications with ships, yachts, fishing vessels, etc.

c)   Decca warnings are broadcast at scheduled times shown, and may also be broadcast on receipt and at other times after announcement on Ch 16 and/or 2182 kHz.

d)   H+... means commencing at ... minutes past the hour.

e)   For medical advice/assistance use the Urgency Signal when necessary, and ask for 'Medico Service'.

f)   Normal primary working frequencies are printed in **bold** type.

g)   Irish coast stations broadcast gale warnings on the respective VHF channels shown in the table on receipt and at the next of 0033 0633 1233 1833 (local time). Similarly weather bulletins every three hours from 0103 (local time). See Table 7(4) on page 116.

h)   For further information on the Irish Coast Radio Service see page 88 opposite.

Coast Station Name Position	VHF Ch other than Ch 16	Station Details with MF frequencies where relevant as shown below		Broadcast Services (Traffic Lists, Navigation Warnings, etc). For Details of Gale Warnings and Weather Bulletins see Table 7(4) – page 116
		Transmits (kHz)	Receives (kHz)	
MALIN HEAD RADIO 55°22'N 07°21'W (VHF Service at Crockalough 55° 21'N 07°16'W) Tel: 35377 70103	23 67 85	2182 **1677**[1] 1644 Notes: (1) Watches on 2045 and replies on 1677 kHz when 2182 kHz is distress working DSC: 2187·5 kHz No. 002500100	2182 (H24) 2045[1] (H24) 2102 (Ch 255) 2069 (Ch 244)	Broadcasts on 1677 kHz and Ch 23. *Traffic Lists:* Every odd H+03 (not 0303 0703) *Navigation/Decca Warnings:* Every four hours from 0033. May also be broadcast on receipt and at other times after announcement on 2182 kHz/Ch 16. (Decca chains 3B 7D 8E)
GLEN HEAD RADIO 54°44'N 08°43'W	24 67	VHF station remotely controlled		Broadcasts on Ch 24 at same times as Malin Head above
BELMULLET RADIO 54°16'N 10°03'W	67 83	VHF station remotely controlled		Broadcasts on Ch 83 at same times as Malin Head above
CLIFDEN RADIO 53°30'N 09°56'W	26 67	VHF station remotely controlled		Broadcasts on Ch 26 at same times as Malin Head above
DUBLIN RADIO 53°23'N 06°04'W	67 83	VHF station		Broadcasts on Ch 83 at same times as Malin Head above
MINE HEAD RADIO 52°00'N 07°35'W	67 83	VHF station remotely controlled		Broadcasts on Ch 83 at same times as Malin Head above
ROSSLARE RADIO 52°15'N 06°20'W	23 67	VHF station remotely controlled		Broadcasts on Ch 23 at same times as Malin Head above
WICKLOW HEAD RADIO 52°58'N 06°00'W	67 87	VHF station remotely controlled		Broadcasts on Ch 87 at same time as Malin Head above
VALENTIA RADIO 51°56'N 10°21'W (VHF service at Kilkeaveragh 51°52'N 10°20'W) Tel: 0667 6109	24 28 67	2182 1746 **1752**[1] Notes: (1) Watches on 2045 and replies on 1752 kHz when 2182 kHz is distress working DSC: 2187·5 kHz No. 002500200	2182 (H24) 2045[1] (H24) 2090 (Ch 278) 2096 (Ch 280)	Broadcasts on 1752 kHz and Ch 24. *Traffic Lists:* Every odd H+33 (not 0133 0533) *Navigation/Decca Warnings:* Every four hours from 0233. May also be broadcast on receipt and at other times after announcement on 2182 kHz/Ch 16. (Decca chains 1B 7D)
SHANNON RADIO 52°31'N 09°36'W	24 28 67	VHF station remotely controlled		Broadcasts on Ch 28 at same times as Valentia above
BANTRY BAY RADIO 51°38'N 10°00'W	23 67 85	VHF station remotely controlled		Broadcasts on Ch 23 at same times as Valentia above
CORK RADIO 51°51'N 08°29'W	26 67	VHF station remotely controlled		Broadcasts on Ch 26 at same times as Valentia above

6

6.3.28   French Coast Radio Stations and CROSS Stations

Notes:
a)   At French coast stations VHF Ch 16 operates H24 and is reserved for distress and safety traffic only. Normally calls must be made on working channels, which operate 0700-2200 LT.
b)   VHF channels shown in brackets are for Automatic VHF for suitably equipped ships (H24).
c)   VHF channels of coast radio stations do not broadcast Traffic Lists or Navigation Warnings. They do broadcast local coastal weather bulletins at 0733 1533 LT, in French, on the channels indicated. For details see Table 7(5).
d)   Included below are stations operated by Centres Régionaux Opérationnels de Surveillance et de Sauvetage (CROSS). These keep watch on Ch 16, and broadcast local navigation warnings, weather messages and storm warnings. They have no public correspondence role.
e)   MF coast stations broadcast coastal and local Navigation Warnings as AVURNAVS (see 6.3.23) after announcements on 2182 kHz.

Coast Station Name Position	VHF Ch other than Ch 16	Station Details with MF frequencies where relevant as shown below		Broadcast Services (Traffic Lists, Navigation Warnings, etc). For Details of Gale Warnings and Weather Bulletins see Table 7(5) – page 117
		Transmits (kHz)	Receives (kHz)	
DUNKERQUE RADIO 51°02'N 02°24'E	24 61 (86)	VHF station remotely controlled See notes (a) and (b) above		*Local coastal weather messages:* Ch 61 at 0733 1533 LT, in French. See Table 7(5).
CALAIS RADIO 50°55'N 01°43'E	01 87 (60) (62)	VHF station remotely controlled See notes (a) and (b) above		*Local coastal weather messages:* Ch 87 at 0733 1533 LT, in French. See Table 7(5).
BOULOGNE-SUR-MER RADIO 50°43'N 01°37'E *Tel: 21·33·25·26*	23 25 (see note (a)) (64) (81) (see note (b))	**1692**[1] **1770** 2744 2747 3722 3792 3795[1] 2182 (H24) Notes: (1) For fishing vessels (2) For French vessels (3) For foreign vessels Selcall (1641): 2170.5 kHz	2045[3] 2048[1] 2051 2054 2057 2093[2] 2117[1] 3168 3314 2182 (H24)	*Traffic Lists:* 1770 kHz every odd H+03. *Navigation Warnings:* 1692 1770 kHz on receipt. 1692 kHz every 4h from 0133 (Cherbourg AVURNAVS in French and English). 1692 1770 kHz at 0730 1733 (Cherbourg Local AVURNAVS in French). For weather see Table 7(5).
CROSS GRIS-NEZ 50°52'N 01°35'E (For notes on CROSS organisation see 6.3.24) *Tel: 21·87·21·87*	Ch 16 (H24) Ch 11 (HX) Ch 15 (HX) Ch 67 (HX) Ch 73 (HX) 2182 kHz (H24)	Call is 'CROSS Gris-Nez'. Covers area from Belgian border to Cap d'Antifer. Accepts distress/safety/ emergency calls only. No link calls. Transmits and receives on VHF from: Dunkerque 51°03'N 02°21'E Gris-Nez 50°52'N 01°35'E St Freiux 50°37'N 01°36'E Ailly 49°55'N 00°58'E		*Navigation Warnings:* Dover Strait bulletins from Gris-Nez Ch 11 every H+10, in French and English (includes ship move-ments, dangers to navigation, special weather bulletins). *Fog Warnings:* Ch 11 every H+25 when visibility is less than 2 n miles. *Gale Warnings:* Ch 11 on receipt every H+10, and on request. Local weather on request after call on Ch16.
DIEPPE RADIO 49°55'N 01°03'E	02 24 (61)	VHF station remotely controlled See notes (a) and (b) above		*Local coastal weather messages:* Ch 02 at 0733 1533 LT, in French. See Table 7(5).
FÉCAMP RADIO 49°46'N 00°22'E	(65) (78)	VHF station remotely controlled See notes (a) and (b) above		No broadcast services.

6.3.28   French Coast Radio Stations and CROSS Stations *continued*

Coast Station Name Position	VHF Ch other than Ch 16	Station Details with MF frequencies where relevant as shown below		Broadcast Services (Traffic Lists, Navigation Warnings, etc). For Details of Gale Warnings and Weather Bulletins see Table 7(5) – page 117
		Transmits (kHz)	Receives (kHz)	
LE HAVRE RADIO 49°31'N 00°04'E	23 26 28 (62) (84)	VHF station remotely controlled See notes (a) and (b) above		*Local coastal weather messages:* Ch 26 at 0733 1533 LT, in French. See Table 7(5)
ROUEN RADIO 49°27'N 01°02'E	25 27 (01) (86)	VHF station remotely controlled See notes (a) and (b) above		No broadcast services.
PORT-EN-BESSIN RADIO 49°20'N 00°42'W	03 (60) (66)	VHF station remotely controlled See notes (a) and (b) above		*Local coastal weather messages:* Ch 03 at 0733 1533 LT, in French. See Table 7(5).
CHERBOURG RADIO 49°38'N 01°36'W	27 (86)	VHF station remotely controlled See notes (a) and (b) above		*Local coastal weather messages:* Ch 27 at 0733 1533 LT, in French. See Table 7(5).
CROSS JOBOURG 49°41'N 01°54'W (For notes on CROSS organisation see 6.3.24) *Tel: 33·52·72·13*	Ch 16 (H24) Ch 15 (HX) Ch 67 (HX) Ch 73 (HX) 2182 kHz (H24)	Call is 'CROSS Jobourg'. Covers area from Cap d'Antifer to Mont St Michel. Accepts distress/safety/ emergency calls only. No link calls. Transmits and receives on VHF from: Antifer 49°41'N 00°09'E Ver-sur-Mer 49°20'N 00°34'W Gatteville 49°24'N 01°16'W Jobourg 49°44'N 01°54'W Granville 49°52'N 01°35'W Roches-Douvres 49°06'N 02°49'W		*Navigation Warnings:* Casquets TSS and area east to buoy EC 2, Ch 80 every H+20 H+50 and on request, in French and English (includes traffic information, gale warnings and visibility) Local weather on request after call on Ch 16, in French and English.
JOBOURG RADIO 49°43'N 01°56'W	21 (83)	VHF station remotely controlled See notes (a) and (b) above		No broadcast services.
CARTERET RADIO 49°23'N 01°47'W	64 (23) (88)	VHF station remotely controlled See notes (a) and (b) above		No broadcast services.
ST MALO RADIO 48°38'N 02°02'W	01 02 (78) (85)	VHF station remotely controlled See notes (a) and (b) above For MF service see Brest-le Conquet on page 92.		*Local coastal weather messages:* Ch 02 at 0733 1533 LT, in French. See Table 7(5).
PAIMPOL RADIO 48°45'N 02°59'W	84 (87)	VHF station remotely controlled See notes (a) and (b) above		*Local coastal weather messages:* Ch 84 at 0733 1533 LT, in French. See Table7(5).
PLOUGASNOU RADIO 48°42'N 03°48'W	81 (03)	VHF station remotely controlled See notes (a) and (b) above		*Local coastal weather messages:* Ch 81 at 0733 1533 LT, in French. See Table7(5).
OUESSANT RADIO 48°27'N 05°05'W	24 82 (61)	VHF station remotely controlled See notes (a) and (b) above		*Local coastal weather messages:* Ch 82 at 0733 1533 LT, in French. See Table7(5).

6

6.3.28   French Coast Radio Stations and CROSS Stations *continued*

Notes:
a)   At French coast stations VHF Ch 16 operates H24 and is reserved for distress and safety traffic only. Normally calls must be made on working channels, which operate 0700-2200 LT.
b)   VHF channels shown in brackets are for Automatic VHF for suitably equipped ships (H24).
c)   VHF channels of coast radio stations do not broadcast Traffic Lists or Navigation Warnings. They do broadcast local coastal weather bulletins at 0733 1533 LT, in French, on the channels indicated. For details see Table 7(5).
d)   Included below are stations operated by Centres Régionaux Opérationnels de Surveillance et de Sauvetage (CROSS). These keep watch on Ch 16, and broadcast local navigation warnings, weather messages and storm warnings. They have no public correspondence rôle.
e)   MF coast stations broadcast coastal and local Navigation Warnings as AVURNAVS (see 6.3.23) after announcements on 2182 kHz.

Coast Station Name Position	VHF Ch other than Ch 16	Station Details with MF frequencies where relevant as shown below		Broadcast Services (Traffic Lists, Navigation Warnings, etc). For Details of Gale Warnings and Weather Bulletins see Table 7(5) – page 118
		Transmits (kHz)	Receives (kHz)	
CROSS CORSEN 48°24'N 04°47'W (For notes on CROSS organisation see 6.3.24) For Navtex see 6.3.25 - page 80. *Tel: 98·89·31·31*	Ch 16 (H24) Ch 15 (HX) Ch 67 (HX) Ch 73 (HX)	Call is 'CROSS Corsen'. Covers area from Mont St Michel to Pointe du Raz. Accepts distress/safety/ emergency calls only. No link calls. Transmits and receives on VHF from: Cap Fréhel 48°41'N 02°19'W Île de Batz 48°45'N 04°02'W Le Stiff 48°28'N 05°03'W Corsen 48°24'N 04°47'W Île de Sein 48°03'N 04°52'W		*Navigation Warnings:* Ouessant TSS general bulletin on Ch 79 after announcement on Ch 16, every H+10 H+40, and on request, in French and English. Weather messages from Le Stiff on Ch 79 every 3h from 0150 UT, in French and English for Areas 14-16. For other details see Table 7(5).
BREST-LE CONQUET RADIO 48°20'N 04°44'W (For MF stations at St Malo and Quimperlé see column (3)) *Tel: 98·43·63·63*	26 28 (see note (a)) (23) (64) (see note (b))	**1635** 1671[1] 2723 2726 3719 3722 2182 (H24) At St Malo, 48°38N 02°02'W: 2691[1] 2182 (H24) At Quimperlé, 47°52'N 03°30'W: 1876[1] 2182 (H24) Notes: (1) For fishing vessels (2) For French vessels (3) For foreign vessels Selcall (1643): 2170.5 kHz	2045[3] 2048[3] 2051 2054 2057 **2060**[2] **2096**[1] 3168 2182 (H24) 3317[1] 2182 (H24) 1992[1] 2182 (H24)	*Traffic Lists:* 1635 2691 kHz every odd H+03 (UT). *Navigation Warnings:* 1671 1876 2691 kHz on receipt, after next silence period, and every 4h from 0333 UT. Brest AVURNAVS in French and English for English Channel approaches and Bay of Biscay. 1671 1876 2691 kHz at 0733 1803 Brest local AVURNAVS in French. *Gunfire Warnings:* for Landes firing range on 1635 kHz at 0703 1803. For weather broadcasts see Table 7(5).
PONT L'ABBÉ RADIO 47°53'N 04°13'W	86 (63) (66)	VHF station remotely controlled See notes (a) and (b) above		*Local coastal weather messages:* Ch 86 at 0733 1533 LT, in French. See Table 7(5).
LE CROUESTY RADIO (VANNES) 47°32'N 02°54'W	(02) (60)	See note (b) above		No broadcast services.
BELLE ÎLE RADIO 47°21'N 03°09'W	05 25 (65) (87)	VHF station remotely controlled See notes (a) and (b) above		*Local coastal weather messages:* Ch 25 at 0733 1533 LT, in French. See Table 7(5).

6.3.28   French Coast Radio Stations and CROSS Stations *continued*

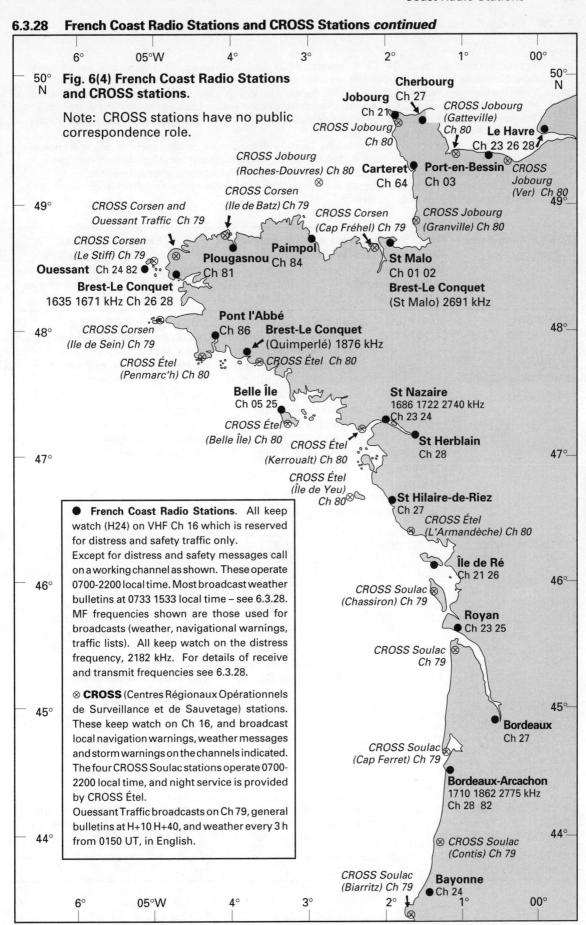

Fig. 6(4) French Coast Radio Stations and CROSS stations.

Note: CROSS stations have no public correspondence role.

Cherbourg Ch 27
Jobourg Ch 21
CROSS Jobourg (Gatteville) Ch 80
Le Havre Ch 23 26 28
CROSS Jobourg Ch 80
CROSS Jobourg (Roches-Douvres) Ch 80
Carteret Ch 64
Port-en-Bessin Ch 03
CROSS Jobourg (Ver) Ch 80
CROSS Corsen and Ouessant Traffic Ch 79
CROSS Corsen (Ile de Batz) Ch 79
CROSS Corsen (Cap Fréhel) Ch 79
CROSS Jobourg (Granville) Ch 80
CROSS Corsen (Le Stiff) Ch 79
Paimpol Ch 84
Plougasnou Ch 81
St Malo Ch 01 02
Ouessant Ch 24 82
Brest-Le Conquet 1635 1671 kHz Ch 26 28
Brest-Le Conquet (St Malo) 2691 kHz
Pont l'Abbé Ch 86
CROSS Corsen (Ile de Sein) Ch 79
Brest-Le Conquet (Quimperlé) 1876 kHz
CROSS Étel (Penmarc'h) Ch 80
CROSS Étel Ch 80
Belle Île Ch 05 25
St Nazaire 1686 1722 2740 kHz Ch 23 24
CROSS Étel (Belle Île) Ch 80
St Herblain Ch 28
CROSS Étel (Kerroualt) Ch 80
CROSS Étel (Île de Yeu) Ch 80
St Hilaire-de-Riez Ch 27
CROSS Étel (L'Armandèche) Ch 80
Île de Ré Ch 21 26
CROSS Soulac (Chassiron) Ch 79
Royan Ch 23 25
CROSS Soulac Ch 79
Bordeaux Ch 27
CROSS Soulac (Cap Ferret) Ch 79
Bordeaux-Arcachon 1710 1862 2775 kHz Ch 28 82
CROSS Soulac (Contis) Ch 79
CROSS Soulac (Biarritz) Ch 79
Bayonne Ch 24

● **French Coast Radio Stations**. All keep watch (H24) on VHF Ch 16 which is reserved for distress and safety traffic only. Except for distress and safety messages call on a working channel as shown. These operate 0700-2200 local time. Most broadcast weather bulletins at 0733 1533 local time – see 6.3.28. MF frequencies shown are those used for broadcasts (weather, navigational warnings, traffic lists). All keep watch on the distress frequency, 2182 kHz. For details of receive and transmit frequencies see 6.3.28.

⊗ **CROSS** (Centres Régionaux Opérationnels de Surveillance et de Sauvetage) stations. These keep watch on Ch 16, and broadcast local navigation warnings, weather messages and storm warnings on the channels indicated. The four CROSS Soulac stations operate 0700-2200 local time, and night service is provided by CROSS Étel. Ouessant Traffic broadcasts on Ch 79, general bulletins at H+10 H+40, and weather every 3 h from 0150 UT, in English.

6.3.28   French Coast Radio Stations and CROSS Stations *continued*

Notes:

a)   At French coast stations VHF Ch 16 operates H24 and is reserved for distress and safety traffic only. Normally calls must be made on working channels, which operate 0700-2200 LT.

b)   VHF channels shown in brackets are for Automatic VHF for suitably equipped ships (H24).

c)   VHF channels of coast radio stations do not broadcast Traffic Lists or Navigation Warnings. They do broadcast local coastal weather bulletins at 0733 1533 LT, in French, on the channels indicated. For details see Table 7(5).

d)   Included below are stations operated by Centres Régionaux Opérationnels de Surveillance et de Sauvetage (CROSS). These keep watch on Ch 16, and broadcast local navigation warnings, weather messages and storm warnings. They have no public correspondence role.

e)   MF coast stations broadcast coastal and local Navigation Warnings as AVURNAVS (see 6.3.23) after announcements on 2182 kHz.

Coast Station Name Position	VHF Ch other than Ch 16	Station Details with MF frequencies where relevant as shown below		Broadcast Services (Traffic Lists, Navigation Warnings, etc). For Details of Gale Warnings and Weather Bulletins see Table 7(5) – page 118
		Transmits (kHz)	Receives (kHz)	
CROSS ÉTEL 47°40'N 03°12'W (For notes on CROSS organisation see 6.3.24) Tel: 97·55·35·35	Ch 16 (H24) Ch 11 (HX)	Call is 'CROSSA Étel'. Covers area from Pointe du Raz to 46°20'N, and provides night cover for Sous-CROSS Soulac to Spanish border. Transmits and receives on VHF from: Penmarc'h 47°48'N 04°22'W Étel 47°40'N 03°12'W Kerroualt 47°30'N 02°21'W Belle Île 47°19'N 03°14'W Île d'Yeu 46°43'N 02°23'W L'Armandèche 46°29'N 01°48'W plus Soulac antennae 2100-0600		Station accepts distress/safety/emergency calls only. No link calls. *Navigation Warnings:* Ch 80 on receipt and repeated every 2h for urgent warnings. Warnings also broadcast on Ch 80 twice daily after weather bulletins – for details see Table 7(5).
ST NAZAIRE RADIO 47°21'N 02°06'W Tel: 98·43·63·63	23 24 (see note (a)) (04) (88) (see note (b))	**1686** **1722**[1] 2586 2740[1] 3792 3795 2182 (H24) Notes: (1) For fishing vessels (2) For French vessels (3) For foreign vessels Selcall (1645): 2170·5 kHz	1995[1] 2045[3] 2048[3] 2051 2054 2057 2066 2111[2] 3168 3314[1] 2182 (H24)	*Traffic Lists:* 1686 kHz every odd H+07 (UT). *Navigation Warnings:* 1686 1722 2740 kHz on receipt, after next silence period, and at 0803 1803 UT. Brest AVURNAVS, in French for Bay of Biscay north of 46°30'N and east of 04°00'W. For weather broadcasts see Table 7(5).
ST HERBLAIN RADIO 47°13'N 01°37'W	28 (03)	VHF station remotely controlled See notes (a) and (b) above		*Local coastal weather messages:* Ch 28 at 0733 1533 LT, in French. See Table7(5).
ÎLE D'YEU RADIO 46°43'N 02°23'W	(84)	See note (b) above		No broadcast services.
ST HILAIRE-DE-RIEZ RADIO 46°43'N 01°57'W	27 (62) (85)	VHF station remotely controlled See notes (a) and (b) above		*Local coastal weather messages:* Ch 27 at 0733 1533 LT, in French. See Table7(5).
LA ROCHELLE RADIO 46°14'N 01°33'W	(61)	See note (b) above		No broadcast services.

6.3.28   French Coast Radio Stations and CROSS Stations *continued*

Coast Station Name Position	VHF Ch other than Ch 16	Station Details with MF frequencies where relevant as shown below		Broadcast Services (Traffic Lists, Navigation Warnings, etc). For Details of Gale Warnings and Weather Bulletins see Table 7(5) – page 119
		Transmits (kHz)	Receives (kHz)	
ÎLE DE RÉ RADIO 46°12'N 01°22'W	21 26 (01) (81)	VHF station remotely controlled See notes (a) and (b) above		*Local coastal weather messages:* Ch 21 at 0733 1533 LT, in French. See Table7(5).
ROYAN RADIO 45°34'N 00°58'W	23 25 (02) (83)	VHF station remotely controlled See notes (a) and (b) above		*Local coastal weather messages:* Ch 23 at 0733 1533 LT, in French. See Table7(5).
BORDEAUX RADIO 44°53'N 00°30'W	27 (63)	VHF station. See notes (a)and (b) above		No broadcast services.
SOUS CROSS SOULAC 45°31'N 01°07'W (For notes on CROSS organisation see 6.3.24) *Tel: 56·09·82·00*	Ch 16 (H24) Ch 11 (HX)	Call is 'Sous CROSS Soulac'. Covers area from 46°20'N to Spanish border 0600-2100. NightservicebyCROSSÉtel. Transmits and receives on VHF from: Chassiron Soulac Cap Ferret Contis Biarritz	46°03'N 01°25'W 45°31'N 01°07'W 44°39'N 01°15'W 44°06'N 01°19'W 43°30'N 01°33'W	Station accepts distress/ safety/emergency calls only. No link calls. *Navigation Warnings:* Ch 79 on receipt, and repeated every 2h for urgent warnings. Warnings also broadcast on Ch 79 twice daily after weather bulletins – for details see Table 7(5).
BORDEAUX-ARCACHON RADIO 44°39'N 01°10'W (Remotely controlled from Brest Le Conquet) *Tel: 98·43·63·63*	28 82 (see note (a)) (78) (86) (see note (b))	**1710** **1862**[1] 2772 2775[1] 3719 3722 2182 (H24) Selcall (1646): 2170·5 kHz	**1995**[1] **2135**[2] 2045[3] 3168 2048[3] 3317[1] 2051 2054 2057 2182 (H24) Notes: (1) For fishing vessels (2) For French vessels (3) For foreign vessels	*Navigation Warnings:* 1862 kHz on receipt, after next silence period, and every 4h from 0333 UT. Brest AVURNAVS in French and English. 1862 kHz on receipt, after next silence period, and at 0733 1803. Brest local AVURNAVS in French. For weather see Table 7(5).
CENTRE D'ESSAIS DES LANDES (FIRING RANGE) 44°26'N 01°15'W	06	*Gunfire Warnings:* Ch 06, 0815-1615 LT (Mon-Thurs), 0815-1030. Advice and information on firings can be obtained during times given. *Tel: 58.82.22.42.*		
BAYONNE RADIO 43°16'N 01°24'W	24 (03) (64)	VHF station remotely controlled See notes (a) and (b) above		*Local coastal weather messages:* Ch 24 at 0733 1533 LT, in French. See Table7(5).

6

6.3.29 Belgian Coast Radio Stations

Coast Station Name Position	VHF Ch other than Ch 16	Station Details with MF frequencies where relevant as shown below		Broadcast Services (Traffic Lists, Navigation Warnings, etc). For Details of Gale Warnings and Weather Bulletins see Table 7(5) – page 119
		Transmits (kHz)	Receives (kHz)	
OOSTENDE RADIO 51°11'N 02°48'E 51°06'N 03°21'E See notes below for VHF Ch to be used in different areas For Navtex see 6.3.25 – page 80 Tel: 32 59 706565	23[1] 27[2 3] 63[4] 78[1 4] 85[3] 87[2] 88[2 5] (Ch16 and Ch 27 H24)	1649.5 1652.5 1665 1683 1689 1705 1708 1725 1728 1817 1820 1901 1904 1905 1908 2087 2170.5 2182 (H24) 2253 2256 2373 2376 **2484** (H24) **2761**[6] **2817**[7] 3629 **3632**[7] 3652 3655 3684[6]	2090 (Ch 251) 2108 (Ch 257) 2114 (Ch 259) 2069[5](Ch 271) 2072 (Ch 272) 2182 (H24) $\begin{Bmatrix}2484\\3178\end{Bmatrix}$ (H24) 2191[8]	*Traffic Lists:* Ch 27 every H+20. 2761 kHz every even H+20 (UT). Following Warnings are broadcast on the channel/frequency indicated after announcement on Ch 16/2182 kHz. *Navigation Warnings:* Ch 27 and 2761 kHz on receipt, after next two silence periods and at: 0233 0633 1033 1433 1833 2233 UT, in English and Dutch. *Decca Warnings:* Ch 27 and 2761 kHz after next two silence periods after receipt, in English for chains 5B 2A 6C 8E 2E 9B. *Ice Reports:* Ch 27 and 2761 kHz every 4h from 0103 UT in English. *Fog Warnings:* 2761 kHz on receipt and after next silence period, in English and Dutch, for the Schelde.
		Notes: (1) For vessels near French border (2) For vessels near Zeebrugge (3) For vessels near Oostende (4) Autolink or manual calls (5) Autolink only (6) Working frequency Belgian ships (7) Working frequency foreign ships (8) Call on 2191 kHz when 2182 is distress working		
ANTWERPEN RADIO 51°17'N 04°20'E		No Medium Frequency RT Service VHF facilities are available (H24) at the following positions. The call in each case is Antwerpen Radio.		*Traffic Lists:* Ch 24 every H+05. Following Warnings are broadcast on channel indicated after announcement on Ch 16.
Antwerpen 51°17'N 04°20'E Kortrijk 50°50'N 03°17'E Gent 51°02'N 03°44'E Vilvoorde 50°56'N 04°25'E Ronquières 50°37'N 05°13'E Mol 51°11'N 05°07'E Liège 50°34'N 05°33'E		07 16 **24** 27 **28** 83 87[1] 16 **24** 83 16 **24** 26 81 16 **24** 28 16 **24** 27 16 **24** 25 16 **24** 27		*Navigation Warnings:* Ch 24 on receipt and every H+03 H+48, in English and Dutch for the Schelde. *Fog Warnings:* Ch 24 on receipt and every H+03 H+48, in English and Dutch for the Schelde when visibility is less than 3000m.
Notes:		(1) Ch 87 is for Autolink or manual calls (2) DSC (GMDSS) on Ch 70 (3) Selcall (0486): Ch 16 24		

6.3.30 Dutch Coast Radio Stations

Notes:

a) VHF facilities, remotely controlled, are located as below. Antennae are directed to cover either the Coastal Area (seaward) or the Inland Waters. The call in each case is Scheveningen Radio. Ch 16 is remotely controlled by Netherlands Coastguard. Except in emergency, calls must be made on working channels. Watch is kept on Ch 16 and on all working channels H24. Calls must last at least three seconds.

b) Netherlands Coastguard monitors 2182 kHz for distress, urgency, safety traffic and operates DSC on 2187·5 kHz and Ch 70. Do not call Scheveningen Radio on 2182 kHz for routine traffic – call on 2520 kHz and station will reply on 2824 kHz indicating working channel to be used.

Coast Station Name Position	VHF Ch other than Ch 16	Station Details with MF frequencies where relevant as shown below: Transmits (kHz)	Receives (kHz)	Broadcast Services (Traffic Lists, Navigation Warnings, etc). For Details of Gale Warnings and Weather Bulletins see Table 7(5) – page 121
SCHEVENINGEN RADIO 52°06N 04°16'E VHF stations remotely controlled are located as below. Call Scheveningen Radio on working channel for routine traffic. Ch 16 is remotely controlled by Netherlands Coast Guard and used only for distress, urgency and safety. **Watch is kept on Ch 16 and working channels H24** *Tel: (0255) 562333*		Ch A 2824[1] B 1716 C 2600 D 1674 E – F 1713[2] I 1890 Notes: (1) Ch A is calling and answering channel (H24) (2) Located at Nes 53°24'N 06°04'E (3) Ch B C D F and I are working channels, and are indicated by Ch A operator depending on ship's position and conditions Selcall: 2170·5 kHz Ch 16.	2520 (H24) 2060 1995 2099 – 2138[2] 2045 2048 2051 2054 2057	*Traffic Lists:* VHF working channels every H+05. 1713 1890 kHz at every odd H+05 (UT). *Navigation Warnings:* Coastal area VHF working channels – see col (1) opposite – and Lelystad Ch 83 on receipt, and after next silence period, and (after anouncement on Ch 16) every 4h from 0305 UT. 1674 1713 1890 kHz on receipt and after next silence period. 1674 1890 kHz every 4h from 0333 UT. In English and Dutch. (Decca chains 2E 9B). *Ice Reports:* 1674 1890 kHz every 4h from 0333 UT. 2824 kHz at 0333 2333 UT. In English and Dutch for local waters. *Strong Breeze Warnings:* VHF working channels of coastal stations on receipt and every H+05, in Dutch. *Near Gale Warnings:* 1713 1890 kHz on recipt and after next silence period (following announcement on 2182 kHz) in English and Dutch. *Weather Messages:* VHF working channels of coastal stations and Lelystad at 0005 0705 1305 1905 LT, in Dutch.
Coastal Area – see Fig.6 (5):				
Goes	23	51°31′N 03°54′E		
Rotterdam	87	51°53′N 04°27′E		
Scheveningen	83	52°04′N 04°15′E		
Haarlem	25	52°23′N 04°40′E		
Tjerkgaast	–	52°55′N 05°42′E		
Wieringermeer	27	53°55′N 05°04′E		
Platform L7	84	53°34′N 04°12′E		
Terschelling	78	53°21′N 05°13′E		
Nes	23	53°23′N 06°03′E		
Appingedam	27	53°20′N 06°51′E		
Inland VHF stations (antennae directed inland):				
Maastricht	25	50°50′N 05°40′E		
Roermond	26	51°11′N 05°59′E		
Arcen	28	51°30′N 06°11′E		
Goes	25	51°31′N 03°54′E		
Rotterdam	24 28	51°53′N 04°27′E		
Lopic	86	52°01′N 05°03′E		
Scheveningen	26	52°04′N 04°15′E		
Markelo	23	52°14′N 06°27′E		
Haarlem	23	52°23′N 04°40′E		
Lelystad	83	53°32′N 05°26′E		
Smilde	24	52°54′N 06°24′E		
Tjerkgaast	28	52°55′N 05°42′E		

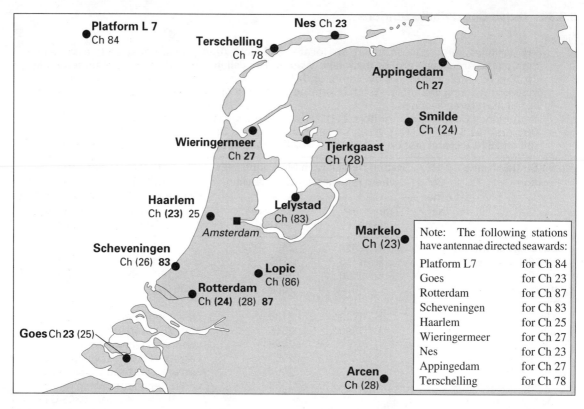

Fig. 6(5) Netherlands VHF Service (Do not call on Ch 16 except in emergency). Channels in brackets are directed to inland waters.

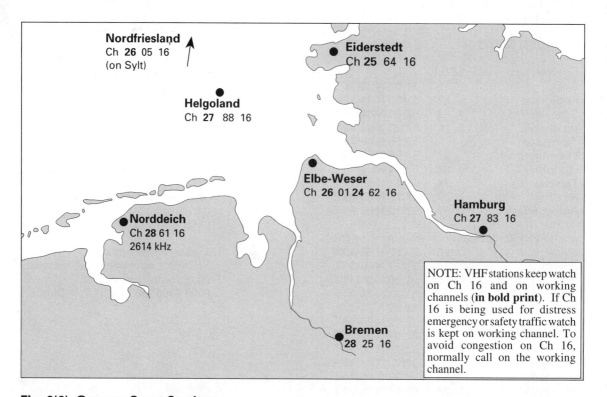

Fig. 6(6) German Coast Stations

6.3.31 German Coast Radio Stations

Notes:
a)   VHF stations keep watch (H24) on Ch 16 and on working channel(s) shown in **bold** print.
      Normally calls should be made on the indicated working channel.
b)   Ch 16 is also used for selective calling.
c)   All VHF stations operate Digital Selective Calling (DSC) on Ch 70 (GMDSS).

Coast Station Name Position	VHF Ch other than Ch 16	Station Details with MF frequencies where relevant as shown below		Broadcast Services (Traffic Lists, Navigation Warnings, etc). For Details of Gale Warnings and Weather Bulletins see Table 7(5) – page 122
		Transmits (kHz)	Receives (kHz)	
NORDDEICH RADIO 53°34'N 07°06'E 53°38'N 07°12'E 53°32'N 08°38'E 53°47'N 09°40'E *Tel: 49 4931 1831*	28 61	2182 Ch 1 **2614** 2 2799 3 1752 4 1911 5 2848 Notes: During broadcasts station replies on 2848 kHz. 3158 kHz is used if 3161 is engaged DSC (GMDSS) 2187·5 kHz Ch 70 Selcall: 217055 kHz Ch 16	2182 (H24) **2023** (0700-2300 LT) 2491 2096 2541 3161 (or 3158)	*Traffic Lists:* Ch 28 and 2614 kHz every H+45. *Navigation Warnings:* 2614 kHz on receipt, after next silence period and every 4h from 0133 UT, and on request, in English and German. (Decca chain 9B). *Ice Reports:* 2614 kHz on request and at 0910 2110 LT and 1310 UT, in English and German for German Bight, Nord-Ostsee Kanal.
BREMEN RADIO 53°05'N 08°48'E	25 **28**	VHF station remotely controlled		*Traffic Lists:* Ch 28 every H+40
HELGOLAND RADIO 54°11'N 07°53'E	27 88	VHF station remotely controlled		*Traffic Lists:* Ch 27 evey H+20
ELBE-WESER RADIO 53°50'N 08°39'E *Tel: 49 4721 22066*	01 24 26 62	Ch 24 62 for vessels in Nord-Ostsee Kanal		*Traffic Lists:* Ch 24 every H+20, Ch 26 every H+50
HAMBURG RADIO 53°33'N 09°58'E	27 83	VHF station remotely controlled		*Traffic Lists:* Ch 27 every H+40
EIDERSTEDT RADIO 54°20'N 08°47'E	25 64	VHF station remotely controlled		*Traffic Lists:* Ch 25 every H+40
NORDFRIESLAND RADIO 53°34'N 07°07'E	05 26	VHF station remotely controlled		*Traffic Lists:* Ch 26 every H+50

6

6.4 SHORT NOTES ON FLAG ETIQUETTE

6.4.1 Ensign

A yacht's ensign is the national maritime flag corresponding to the nationality of her owner. Thus a British yacht should wear the Red Ensign, unless she qualifies for a special ensign (see 6.4.2). It goes without saying that the national ensign should be kept clean and in good repair. At sea the ensign must be worn when meeting other vessels, when entering or leaving foreign ports, or when approaching forts, signal and coastguard stations etc. Increasingly it has become the practice to leave the ensign (and burgee) flying at all times in foreign waters – even at night in harbour, assuming that the boat is not unattended. In British harbours it is the custom for the ensign to be hoisted at 0800 (0900 between 1 November and 14 February) or as soon after that time as people come on board; and lowered at sunset (or 2100 local time if earlier) or before that time if the crew is leaving the boat.

The ensign should normally be worn at the stern, but if this is not possible the nearest position should be used, e.g. at the peak in a gaff-rigged boat, at the mizzen masthead in a ketch or yawl, or about two-thirds up the leech of the mainsail. In harbour or at anchor the proper position is at the stern.

The ensign should not be worn when racing (after the five minute gun). It should be hoisted on finishing or when retiring.

6.4.2 Special ensigns

Members of certain clubs may apply for permission to wear a special ensign (e.g. Blue Ensign, defaced Blue Ensign, or defaced Red Ensign). For this purpose the yacht must either be a registered ship under Part I of the Merchant Shipping Act 1894 and of at least 2 tons gross tonnage, or be registered under the Merchant Shipping Act 1983 (Small Ships Register) and of at least 7 metres overall length. The owner or owners must be British subjects, and the yacht must not be used for any professional, business or commercial purpose. Full details can be obtained from Secretaries of Clubs concerned.

A special ensign must only be worn when the owner is on board or ashore in the vicinity, and only when the yacht is flying the burgee (or a Flag Officer's flag) of the club concerned. The permit must be carried on board. When the yacht is sold, or the owner ceases to be a member of the Club, the permit must be returned to the Secretary of the Club.

6.4.3 Burgee

A burgee shows that a yacht is in the charge of a member of the club indicated, and does not necessarily indicate ownership. It should be flown at the masthead.

Should this be impossible due to wind sensors, radio antenna etc the burgee may be flown at the starboard crosstrees but this should be avoided unless absolutely necessary. A yacht should not fly more than one burgee. A burgee is not flown when a yacht is racing. If the yacht is on loan, or is chartered, it is correct to use the burgee of the skipper or charterer – not that of the absent owner. Normal practice has been to lower the burgee at night, at the same time as the ensign, but nowadays many owners leave the burgee flying if they are on board or ashore in the vicinity.

6.4.4 Flag officer's flag

Clubs authorise their flag officers to fly special swallow-tailed flags, with the same design as the club burgee and in place of it. The flags of a vice-commodore and a rear-commodore carry one and two balls respectively. A flag officer's flag is flown day and night while he is on board, or ashore nearby. A flag officer should fly his flag with the Red Ensign (or special ensign, where authorised) in preference to the burgee of some other club.

6.4.5 Choice of burgee

An owner who is not a flag officer, and who belongs to more than one club, should normally fly the burgee (and if authorised the special ensign) of the senior club in the harbour where the yacht is lying. An exception may be if another club is staging a regatta or similar function.

6.4.6 Courtesy ensign

It is customary when abroad to fly a small maritime ensign of the country concerned at the starboard crosstrees. A courtesy ensign must not be worn in a position inferior to any flag other than the yacht's own ensign and club burgee (or flag officer's flag). The correct courtesy flag for a foreign yacht in British waters is the Red Ensign (not the Union Flag). British yachts do not fly a courtesy flag in the Channel Islands since these are part of the British Isles.

6.4.7 House flag

An owner may fly his personal flag when he is on board in harbour, provided it does not conflict with the design of some existing flag. A house flag is normally rectangular, and is flown at the crosstrees in a sloop or cutter, at the mizzen masthead in a ketch or yawl, or at the foremast head in a schooner.

6.4.8 Salutes

Yachts should salute all Royal Yachts, and all warships of whatever nationality. A salute is made by dipping the ensign (only). The vessel saluted responds by dipping her ensign, and then re-hoisting it, whereupon the vessel saluting re-hoists hers. It is customary for a flag officer to be saluted (not more than once a day) by a yacht flying the burgee of that club.

Chapter 7

Weather

Contents

Weather – introduction

Here in the Almanac, emphasis is given to obtaining weather forecasts and reports.

Additional information on the weather and its interpretation can be found in Chapter 7 of *The Macmillan & Silk Cut Yachtsman's Handbook* where the following subjects are described in more detail:

Transfer of heat; world weather; air masses; atmospheric pressure; wind; humidity; clouds; depressions and fronts; the passage of a depression; anticyclones; fog; sea and land breezes; thunderstorms; tropical storms; glossary of meteorological terms; forecasting your own weather; Bibliography.

7.1 GENERAL WEATHER INFORMATION

7.1.1 Beaufort scale

Force	Wind speed			Description	State of sea	Probable wave ht (m)
	(knots)	(km/h)	(m/sec)			
0	0–1	0–2	0–0·5	Calm	Like a mirror	0
1	1–3	2–6	0·5–1·5	Light air	Ripples like scales are formed	0
2	4–6	7–11	2–3	Light breeze	Small wavelets, still short but more pronounced, not breaking	0·1
3	7–10	13–19	4–5	Gentle breeze	Large wavelets, crests begin to break; a few white horses	0·4
4	11–16	20–30	6–8	Moderate breeze	Small waves growing longer; fairly frequent white horses	1
5	17–21	31–39	8–11	Fresh breeze	Moderate waves, taking more pronounced form; many white horses, perhaps some spray	2
6	22–27	41–50	11–14	Strong breeze	Large waves forming; white foam crests more extensive; probably some spray	3
7	28–33	52–61	14–17	Near gale	Sea heaps up; white foam from breaking waves begins to blow in streaks	4
8	34–40	63–74	17–21	Gale	Moderately high waves of greater length; edge of crests break into spindrift; foam blown in well marked streaks	5·5
9	41–47	76–87	21–24	Severe gale	High waves with tumbling crests; dense streaks of foam; spray may affect visibility	7
10	48–55	89–102	25–28	Storm	Very high waves with long overhanging crests; dense streams of foam make surface of sea white. Heavy tumbling sea; visibility affected	9
11	56–63	104–117	29–32	Violent storm	Exceptionally high waves; sea completely covered with long white patches of foam; edges of wave crests blown into froth. Visibility affected	11
12	64 plus	118 plus	33 plus	Hurricane	Air filled with foam and spray; sea completely white with driving spray; visibility very seriously affected	14

Notes: (1) The state of sea and probable wave heights are a guide to what may be expected in the open sea, away from land. In enclosed waters, or near land with an offshore wind, wave heights will be less but possibly steeper – particularly with wind against tide.

(2) It should be remembered that the height of sea for a given wind strength depends upon the fetch and the duration for which the wind has been blowing. For further information on sea state, see Chapter 9 of *The Macmillan & Silk Cut Yachtsman's Handbook*.

7.1.2   Barometer and temperature conversion scales

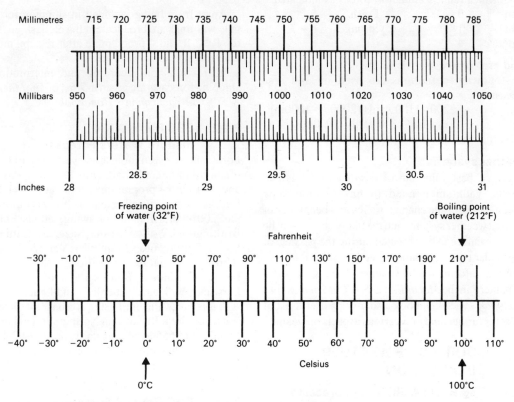

7.1.3   Meaning of terms used in weather bulletins

Speed of movement of pressure systems

Slowly	Moving at less than 15 knots
Steadily	Moving at 15 – 25 knots
Rather quickly	Moving at 25 – 35 knots
Rapidly	Moving at 35 – 45 knots
Very rapidly	Moving at more than 45 knots

Visibility

Good	More than 5 miles
Moderate	2 – 5 miles
Poor	1000 metres – 2 miles
Fog	Less than 1000 metres

Barometric pressure changes (tendency)

Rising or falling slowly: Pressure change of 0·1 to 1·5 millibars in the preceding 3 hours.

Rising or falling: Pressure change of 1·6 to 3·5 millibars in the preceding 3 hours.

Rising or falling quickly: Pressure change of 3·6 to 6 millibars in the preceding 3 hours.

Rising or falling very rapidly: Pressure change of more than 6 millibars in the preceding 3 hours.

Now rising (or falling): Pressure has been falling (rising) or steady in the preceding 3 hours, but at the time of observation was definitely rising (falling).

Gale warnings

A **'Gale'** warning indicates that winds of at least force 8 (34-40 knots) or gusts reaching 43-51 knots are expected somewhere within the area, but not necessarily over the whole area. **'Severe gale'** implies winds of at least force 9 (41- 47 knots) or gusts reaching 52-60 knots. **'Storm'** implies winds of force 10 (48-55 knots) or gusts of 61- 68 knots. **'Violent Storm'** implies winds of force 11 (56/63 kn) or gusts of 69 kn or more, and **'Hurricane Force'** implies winds of force 12 (64 knots or more).

Gale warnings remain in force until amended or cancelled ('gales now ceased'). If a gale persists for more than 24 hours the warning is re-issued.

Timing of gale warnings

Imminent	Within 6 hrs of time of issue
Soon	Within 6 – 12 hrs of time of issue
Later	Within 12 – 24 hrs of time of issue

Wind

Wind direction: Indicates the direction from which the wind is blowing.

Winds becoming cyclonic: Indicates that there will be considerable change in wind direction across the path of a depression within the forecast area.

Veering: The changing of the wind in a clockwise direction. i.e. SW to W.

Backing: The changing of the wind in an anti-clockwise direction. i.e. W to SW.

Land area forecasts – wind strength

In land area forecasts winds are given in the following terms, which relate to Beaufort forces as indicated:

Calm	0	Fresh	5
Light	1–3	Strong	6 – 7
Moderate	4	Gale	8

Land area forecasts – visibility

The following definitions are used in land area forecasts:

Mist	2200 –1100 yards (2000m –1000m)
Fog	Less than 1100 yards (1000m)
Dense fog	Less than 50 yards (46m)

Weather systems

To get the best value out of weather forecasts and reports, yachtsmen need to have some basic understanding of the characteristics and behaviour of different weather systems and the likely changes in the weather which can be expected during the passage of a particular type of weather system.

Further information on weather systems are given in Chapter 7 in the *Macmillan & Silk Cut Yachtsman's Handbook.* The Handbook also gives a useful list of books for further study on various aspects of weather.

7.2   SOURCES OF WEATHER INFORMATION

7.2.1   BBC Radio 4 Shipping Forecasts

Shipping forecasts cover large sea areas, and in a five minute bulletin it is impossible to include much detail – particularly variations that can and do occur near land – or to convey the right degree of confidence in the weather situation. Hence forecasts for 'Inshore Waters' (see 7.2.2), which extend up to 12M offshore, are often more helpful to yachtsmen cruising near the coast.

Shipping forecasts are broadcast on BBC Radio 4 on 198 kHz (1515m) 92·4-94·6 MHz, and on local MF frequencies daily at   0033–0038, 0555–0600, 1355–1400 and 1750–1755 (LT). The 0033–0038 broadcast includes sea area Trafalgar.

The 0033–0038 and 1355–1400 broadcasts Monday–Friday include a 24-hour forecast for the Minches (between Butt of Lewis and Cape Wrath in the north, and between Barra Head and Ardnamurchan Point in the south), after area Hebrides. For further details see Table 7(1).

The 0033–0038 shipping forecast is followed by a forecast, valid until 1800, for coastal waters of Great Britain up to 12M offshore, and reports from selected stations (see 7.2.2).

The bulletins include a summary of gale warnings in force; a general synopsis of the weather for the next 24 hours and expected changes within that period; forecasts for each sea area for the next 24 hours, giving wind direction and speed, weather and visibility; and the latest reports from selected stations from those shown at the foot of page 111. For each station wind direction and Beaufort force, present weather, visibility, and (if available) sea-level pressure and tendency are given. These stations are marked by their initial letters on the chart for forecast areas on page 110.

Apart from being included in shipping forecasts, gale warnings are broadcast at the earliest juncture in the BBC Radio 4 programme after receipt, and also after the next news bulletin.

Instructions on recording and interpreting the shipping forecasts are given in 7.6.4 of *The Macmillan & Silk Cut Yachtsman's Handbook.*

7.2.2   BBC Radio 3 & 4 Inshore Waters Forecast

Forecasts are given for inshore waters (up to 12 miles offshore) of Great Britain until 1800 next day at the end of Radio 4 programmes at about 0038 LT. The forecast of wind, weather and visibility is followed by the 2200 reports from the following stations: Boulmer, Bridlington, Walton-on-the-Naze, St Catherine's Point, Scilly auto, Mumbles, Valley, Liverpool (Crosby), Ronaldsway, Killough, Machrihanish, Larne, Greenock, Benbecula auto, Stornoway, Lerwick, Wick auto, Aberdeen and Leuchars.

A forecast, valid until 1800, is broadcast for inshore waters of Great Britain and Northern Ireland on BBC Radio 3, at 0655 local time daily, on 90·2-92·4 MHz.

The schedule of inshore waters forecasts for Great Britain and Ireland is included in Table 7(1) on page 112.

7.2.3   BBC General Forecasts

Land area forecasts may include the outlook period (up to 48 hours beyond the shipping forecast) and some reference to weather along the coasts. The more detailed land area forecasts are broadcast on Radio 4 on 198 kHz (1515m) and 92·4-94·6 MHz.

7.2.4   UK Local Radio stations

BBC and Commercial Local Radio stations also broadcast weather forecasts and Small Craft Warnings. Details are shown in 7.2.19 on page 114 and 115.

7.2.5   Special forecasts for ships at sea

UK weather forecasts for yachtsmen may be obtained by listening to BBC Shipping Forecasts, BT Coast Radio Stations, Marinecall or MetFax, or by contacting the local area forecasting centre shown in 7.2.8.

When telephoning a forecast office it must be realised that during busy periods, such as occasions of bad weather, the staff may be fully occupied and there is likely to be a delay.

If a forecast is required for some future occasion or period, or if the forecast is to be kept under review and updated, the request should be addressed to The Meteorological Office, Central Forecasting Office, London Road, Bracknell, Berks RG12 2SZ, ☎ (01344) 854893, or sent by telex 849801 WEABKA G, or Fax: (01344) 854412 giving full details of the service required. The charge for the service, including any transmissions costs, will be advised.

Seafarers may contact any BT CRS for the Weather Repetition Service (repeat of latest forecasts on hand). The service via Portishead Radio is the plain language section of the North Atlantic Weather Bulletin. The charge for this service is £11·50 plus VAT. Requests for repeats of forecasts should not be made direct to the Met Office.

7.2.6 Marinecall – Automatic Telephone Weather Service

(1) Telephone forecasts

Recorded inshore forecasts are provided for 16 Areas around the UK coastline. In each case dial 0891 500, followed by the three figure number of the area required (see Fig. 7(1)).

The forecasts cover the coastal waters out to 12 miles offshore and are updated twice daily except for Areas 432, 455, 456,457 and 458 which are updated three times a day.

The two day forecasts are immediately followed by forecasts for days three to five. The two day forecasts include: The general situation, warnings of gales and strong winds, wind, weather, visibility, sea state and temeperature, and the maximum air temperature.

A 2 to 5 day planning forecast for the English Channel is available on 0891 500 992, and a 3 to 5 day National forecast, covering the UK coastline is available on 0891 500 450.

The local inshore forecast for Shetland is not covered by Marinecall and is available by phoning the Coastguard at Lerwick on 01595 692976.

(2) Marinecall current weather reports

For actual weather reports from over 50 coastal locations ☎ 0891 226 plus the Marinecall inshore three figure number shown in Fig. 7(1).

Each of the 16 Marinecall areas contains three weather reports (occasionally two), and are normally updated every hour.

The reports include details of wind, weather, visibility, temperature, pressure and pressure tendency. These reports are followed by the forecast for that area.

Coastal weather reports

451	452	453
Cape Wrath	Peterhead	Boulmer
Wick	Aberdeen	Tynemouth
Lossiemouth	Fife Ness	Teesmouth

454	455	456
Bridlington	Weybourne	Dover
Easington	Sheerness	Greenwich Lt V
Holbeach	Walton-on-the Naze	Newhaven

457	458	459
Thorney Is	Brixham	Cardiff
Lee-on-Solent	Plymouth	Swansea
StCatherine's Pt	Falmouth	Milford Haven
		S. Mary's
		(Isles of Scilly)

460	461	462
Aberdaron	Rhyl	Machrihanish
Aberporth	Crosby	Prestwick
Valley	Walney Island	Greenock

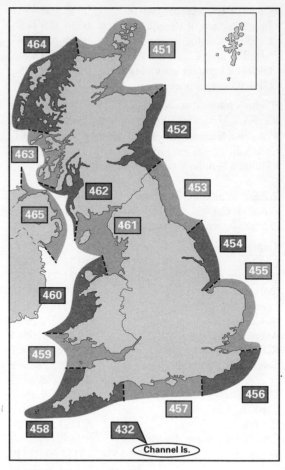

Fig. 7(1) Marinecall Areas

463	464	465
Oban	Benbecula	Ballycastle
Tiree	Altbea	Bangor Harbour
	Butt of Lewis	Malin Head

432
Channel Lt V
Guernsey
Jersey
Bréhat

7.2.7 MetFAX Marine

Weather maps, 2 day inshore forecasts, 2-5 day planning forecasts, satellite images and GPS status reports are available by facsimile. An Index for all fax products can be obtained by Fax on 0336 400 401.

2 day inshore forecasts for the Areas shown on Fig 7(1) can be obtained by dialling 0336 400 plus the three figure number of the area required. It should be noted that the Channels Islands are served by two numbers i.e. by fax on 0336 400 466 and by ☎ on 0891 500 432.

2 to 5 day planning forecasts and 48/72h forecast chart for the Areas shown on Fig. 7(2) can be obtained by dialling 0336 400 plus the three figure number of the area required.

Additional fax services available include:

24h shipping forecast	0336 400 441
Guide to surface charts	0336 400 446

7

Chart of UK weather reports   0336 400 447
Index to chart of weather reports   0336 400 448
Guide to satellite images   0336 400 498
Satellite image   0336 400 499
GPS Background information   0336 400 598
GPS Weekly Status report   0336 400 599

The charge for Marinecall, Weathercall and MetFAX Marine is 39p per minute (cheap rate) and 49p per minute at all other times, including VAT. Calls can be made through British Telecom coast stations when the VHF per minute tariff is 95p.

7.2.8   Weather Centres

Weather Centres provide a range of services at a charge. To arrange a forecast service ring:

Southampton	(01703) 228844
London	0171-696 0573 or 0171-405 4356
Birmingham	0121-717 0570
Norwich	(01603) 660779
Leeds	(0113) 2451990
Newcastle	(0191) 232 6453
Aberdeen Airport	(01224) 210574
Kirkwall Airport	(01856) 873802
Sella Ness, Scotland	(01806) 242069
Glasgow	0141-248 3451
Manchester	0161-477 1060
Cardiff	(01222) 397020
Bristol	(0117) 9279298
Belfast International Airport	(018494) 22339
Jersey	(01534) 46111 Ext 2229

Republic of Ireland

Central Forecast Office, Dublin (H24)	(01) 424655
Cork Airport Met (0900–2000)	(021) 965974
Shannon Airport Met (H24)	(061) 61333
Dublin Airport Met	(01) 379900 ext 4531

European Continent

The numbers of forecast offices and recorded weather messages are shown under 'Telephone' for individual harbours in Areas 14–21 of Chapter 10.

7.2.9   Facsimile broadcasts

Facsimile recorders that receive pictorial images such as weather maps are now available of a type that makes them suitable for use in yachts and at port locations such as marinas.

The information available is of a general meteorological nature and not all of it is relevant to the average yachtsman, but there are many items that are of direct use such as:

> Isobaric charts (actual and forecast)
> Sea and swell charts
> Representation of cloud satellite images
> Sea temperature charts
> Wind field charts.

Internationally exchanged data is processed at various centres. In NW Europe those doing such work and transmitting facsimile broadcasts are:

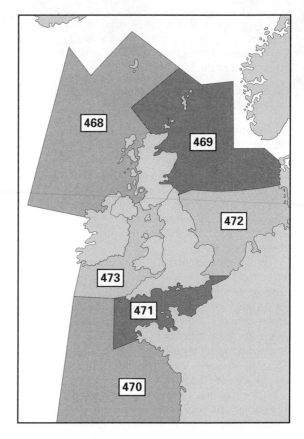

Fig. 7(2) MetFAX forecast areas

Bracknell (GFA) (England)
  2618·5*   4610   8040   14436   18261** kHz

  *   1800-0600 UT only
  **   0600-1800 UT only

Northwood (GYA) (GYZ) (GZZ) (England)
  2374*   3652   4307   6446
  8331.55   12844·5   16912** kHz

  *   1630-0730 UT 30 Sep-31 Mar
  ** 0730-1630 30 Sep-31 Mar
       H24 1 Apr- 29 Sep

Offenbach (DCF 54) (Germany)   134·2 kHz
  0100-2100 2200 2300

Selected UK Fax broadcast schedule (UT)

0230	Northwood	Schedule
0300	Northwood	Surface Wind and Wx prog
0730	Northwood	Surface Wind and Wx prog
1150	Northwood	Surface Wind and Wx prog
2025	Northwood	Surface Wind and Wx prog
0320	Northwood	Surface analysis
0341	Bracknell	Surface analysis
0431	Bracknell	24h surface analysis
0440	Northwood	Satellite pictures
0600	Northwood	Gale summary
0650	Northwood	Surface analysis
0806	Bracknell	48h & 72h surface analysis
0935	Bracknell	24h sea state prog

0941	Bracknell	Surface analysis
0950	Northwood	Surface analysis
1031	Bracknell	24h surface analysis
1040	Northwood	Satellite pictures
1045	Bracknell	48h & 72h surface analysis
1130	Northwood	Gale summary
1210	Northwood	Surface analysis
1230	Northwood	Sea and Swell state prog
1330	Northwood	Satellite pictures
1500	Northwood	Surface analysis
1541	Bracknell	Surface analysis
1631	Bracknell	24h surface analysis
1640	Northwood	Gale summary
1730	Northwood	Satellite pictures
1800	Northwood	Surface analysis
1950	Northwood	Gale summary
2018	Bracknell	24h sea state prog
2050	Northwood	Sea and Swell state prog
2120	Northwood	Surface analysis
2141	Bracknell	Surface analysis
2222	Bracknell	48h & 72h surface analysis
2320	Northwood	Surface analysis
2327	Bracknell	24h surface analysis

The quality of reception depends on the frequency used and the terrain between transmitter and receiver.

Additional frequencies to those above are also available for limited periods during any 24 hour period. Transmission frequencies and schedules are published in the *Admiralty List of Radio Signals, Vol 3* (NP 283). See also 7.6.13 of *The Macmillan & Silk Cut Yachtsman's Handbook*.

7.2.10   NAVTEX
Gale warnings are broadcast on receipt and are repeated at scheduled times. Weather messages are broadcast at scheduled times. Details of NAVTEX stations, identity codes, message categories and transmission times for NAVAREAS I and II are given in Chapter 6 (6.3.25).

7.2.11   Volmet
Volmet is a meteorological service for aviators which transmits actual weather reports and forecasts for airfields to aircraft in flight on HF SSB and/or VHF.

Yachtsmen very interested in the weather will find the information both interesting and useful. The continuously updated reports of actual weather conditions for airfields close to the UK and European coasts can also be very useful when making your own weather map.

The most useful is the Royal Air Force SSB VOLMET which continuously broadcasts actual weather reports for a number of military and civil airfields, mostly in the UK, on HF SSB on:

    4722 kHz   H24

    11200 kHz   H24

The information transmitted consists of: Airfield name, Wind direction and speed, cloud amount and height, temperature and dew point temperature, Sea level pressure (QNH), and any significant weather.

Another useful station is the HF SSB (H3E) broadcast by Shannon which operates H24 as follows:

3413 kHz	Sunset to sunrise
5505 kHz	H24
8957 kHz	H24
13264 kHz	H24

The schedule starts at H+00 at five minute intervals until all airfields are covered. Broadcasts for UK and Irish airfields are at H+05 and H+35.

7.2.12   Press forecasts
The delay between the time of issue and the time at which they are available next day make press forecasts of limited value to yachtsmen. However, the better papers publish forecasts which include a synoptic chart which, in the absence of any other chart, can be helpful when interpreting the shipping forecast on first putting to sea.

7.2.13   Television forecasts and Prestel
Some TV forecasts show a synoptic chart which, with the satellite pictures, can be a useful guide to the weather situation at the start of a passage.

Weather information is given on Ceefax (BBC) and Teletext (ITV). BBC Ceefax gives weather information on pages 400-406, and ITV (Teletext) gives details on pages 102-105 and 201-205. Antiope is the equivalent French system.

7.2.14   Visual storm signals
Visual storm signals used on the Continent are summarised in 10.15.8, 10.20.7 and 10.21.7.

7.2.15   Radiobeacon wind information
Wind information at La Corbière Lt (49°10'·85N 02°14'·92W) is transmitted by the Radiobeacon on frequency 295·50 kHz modulated as follows: Callsign CB 3 times (16 secs), a long dash of 8 secs, a series of 1 to 8 short dashes indicating average Wind Direction in eight cardinal points (one dash = NE, two dashes = E, clockwise to 8 dashes = N). Up to 8 pips indicates average wind strength on the Beaufort scale (one pip = Force 1, two pips = Force 2, up to 8 pips = Force 8 or more). One or more short dashes indicates maximum gust above average Beaufort scale. A transmission consisting of 3 dashes, followed by 5 pips, followed by 2 dashes would indicate: Wind direction SE, Force 5, Gusting 7.

7.2.16   British and Irish Coast Radio Stations – Weather Bulletins by R/T
Forecasts originating from the Meteorological Office are broadcast by BT Coast Radio Stations, as indicated in Table 7(4), by radiotelephone on VHF (where available) and simultaneously on MF, after an initial announcement on VHF Ch 16. BT CRS will also give a repeat of weather information at a charge of £11·50 on request (see 7.2.5). Weather messages comprise gale warnings, synopsis and 24-hour forecast for the sea area stated.

7

Weather broadcasts by BT Coast Radio Stations are made twice daily. There is one central Officer in each region who engages broadcast frequencies at each station from his central position, and reads the forecast for the whole of that region.

7.2.17   HM Coastguard – VHF Ch 67

Each MRCC and MRSC keeps watch on VHF Ch 16 and operates Ch 67 (see 8.4.2). They broadcast strong wind warnings for their local area (only) on receipt on Ch 67 after an announcement on Ch 16; also forecasts for their local area on Ch 67 after an announcement on Ch 16 normally every four hours (every two hours if strong wind or gale warning in force) commencing from the local times shown below. They will also respond to telephone enquiries (for the number see each harbour in Chapter 10).

7.2.18   Reports of present weather

Reports of actual local weather conditions prevailing at places around the coast of the British Isles can be obtained by telephone from the following Meteorological Office observation stations and from the Coastguard. The locations are shown in Fig. 7(3):

From Meteorological Offices

Station Name	Telephone No
Shoeburyness	01702 292271, ext 3476
Kinloss	01309 72161, ext 674
Kirkwall (Orkneys)	01856 873802
Sella Ness (Shetlands)	01806 242069
Stornoway	01851 702256 (night 702282)
Tiree	01879 2456
Ronaldsway IOM)	01624 823311 (night 823313)

(0700–1700 *Mon–Fri*, except Public Holidays)

From Coastguard stations

The following Coastguard Maritime Rescue Coordination Centres (MRCCs) and Sub-Centres (MRSCs), may provide information on actual weather conditions in their immediate locality.

Small craft which require information urgently and unable to contact a Coast Radio Station, may call Coastguard stations listed below on VHF Ch 16 to request the current local forecast.

Dover Coastguard broadcasts Gale warnings and strong wind warnings on receipt on Ch 67 following an announcement on Ch 16, and thereafter included in the next 3 routine CNIS broadcasts on VHF Ch 11.

The general synopsis and shipping forecast for local sea areas will be included in routine CNIS broadcasts on VHF Ch 11, every 4 hrs commening from 0040 UT.

Station Name	Telephone No	Fax No	Station Name (Forecasts every four (or two) hours from:)	Time
MRCC Falmouth	01326 317575	01326 318342	Falmouth	0140
MRSC Brixham	01803 882704	01803 882780	Brixham	0050
MRSC Portland	01305 760439	01305 760452	Portland	0220
MRSC Solent	01705 552100	01705 551763	Solent	0040
MRCC Dover	01304 210008	01304 210302	See CNIS broadcasts above	
MRSC Thames	01255 675518	01255 675249	Thames	0010
MRCC Yarmouth	01493 851338	01493 852307	Yarmouth	0040
MRSC Humber	01262 672317	01262 606915	Humber	0340
MRSC Tyne/Tees	0191-672317	0191 2580373	Tyne/Tees	0150
MRSC Forth	01333 450666	01333 450725	Forth	0205
MRCC Aberdeen	01224 592334	01224 575920	Aberdeen	0320
MRSC Pentland	01856 873268	01856 874202	Pentland	0135
MRSC Shetland	01595 692976	01595 694810	Shetland	0105
MRSC Stornoway	01851 702013	01851 704387	Stornoway	0110
MRSC Oban	01631 563720	01631 564917	Oban	0240
MRCC Clyde	01475 729988	01475 786955	Clyde	0020
MRSC Belfast	01247 463933	01247 465009	Belfast	0305
MRSC Liverpool	0151-931 3341	0151 931 3347	Liverpool	0210
MRSC Holyhead	01407 762051	01407 764373	Holyhead	0235
MRSC Milford Haven	01646 690909	01646 692176	Milford Haven	0335
MRCC Swansea	01792 366534	01792 369005	Swansea	0005

Fig. 7(3) Reports of present weather

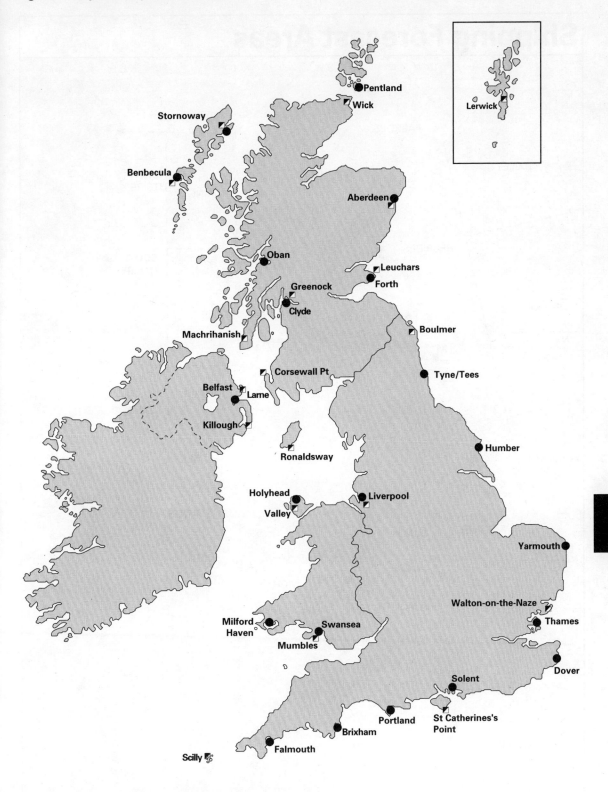

Lerwick

Pentland
Wick

Stornoway

Benbecula

Aberdeen

Oban

Leuchars
Forth

Greenock
Clyde

Machrihanish

Boulmer

Corsewall Pt

Tyne/Tees

Belfast
Larne

Killough

Humber

Ronaldsway

Holyhead
Valley

Liverpool

Yarmouth

Walton-on-the-Naze

Milford
Haven

Swansea

Mumbles

Thames

Dover

Solent

Portland

St Catherines's
Point

Brixham

Scilly

Falmouth

●   **Reports from Coastguard stations**

▰   **BBC Inshore Waters Weather Reports**

Fig 7(4) Map of Shipping Forecast Areas

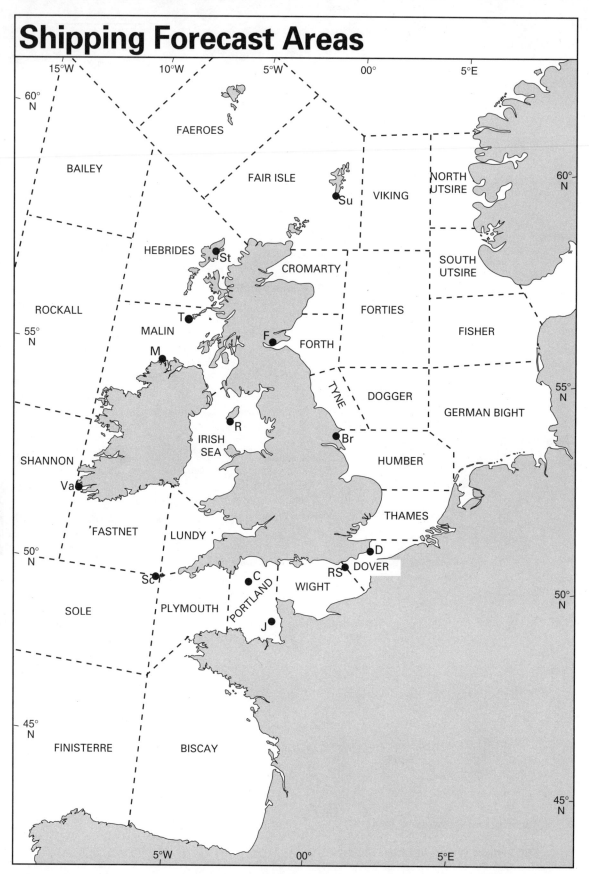

Shipping Forecast Areas

Fig 7(5) Shipping Forecast Record

Shipping Forecast Record

GENERAL SYNOPSIS   at .... UT/BST

System	Present position	Movement	Forecast position	at

Gales	SEA AREA FORECAST	Wind (At first)	(Later)	Weather	Visibility
	VIKING				
	NORTH UTSIRE				
	SOUTH UTSIRE				
	FORTIES				
	CROMARTY				
	FORTH				
	TYNE				
	DOGGER				
	FISHER				
	GERMAN BIGHT				
	HUMBER				
	THAMES				
	DOVER				
	WIGHT				
	PORTLAND				
	PLYMOUTH				
	BISCAY				
	FINISTERRE				
	SOLE				
	LUNDY				
	FASTNET				
	IRISH SEA				
	SHANNON				
	ROCKALL				
	MALIN				
	HEBRIDES				
	BAILEY				
	FAIR ISLE				
	FAEROES				
	S E ICELAND				

COASTAL REPORTS at .... BST UT	Wind Direction	Force	Weather	Visibility	Pressure	Change
Tiree (T)						
Stornoway (St)						
Sumburgh (Su)						
Fife Ness (F)						
Bridlington (Br)						
Dover (D)						

COASTAL REPORTS	Wind Direction	Force	Weather	Visibility	Pressure	Change
Royal Sovereign(RS)						
Jersey (J)						
Channel auto (C)						
Scilly auto (Sc)						
Valentia (Va)						
Ronaldsway (R)						
Malin Head (M)						

7

TABLE 7(1)   British Isles – Daily Shipping Forecasts and Forecasts for Coastal Waters
as broadcast by British Broadcasting Corporation (BBC) and Radio Telefis Eireann (RTE)

Note: All times are local times, unless otherwise stated

Time	Forecast	Contents	Stations and Frequencies
0033	Shipping Forecast – Home Waters Fcst Areas	Gale Warnings in force; synopsis; 24 hr Fcst for Home Waters (including Trafalgar, and Mon-Fri a 24 hr Fcst for Area Minch; reports from selected stations.	*BBC Radio 4:* 198 kHz, 92·4 – 94·6 MHz (England), Tyneside 603 kHz, London 720 kHz, N Ireland 720 kHz, Aberdeen 1449 kHz, Carlisle 1485 kHz, Plymouth 774 kHz, Enniskillen 774 kHz. Redruth 756 kHz, 92·4–94·6, 92·4–96·1 or 103·5–104·9 MHz (Scotland, N Ireland, Wales).
0038	Coastal Waters (Great Britain) Fcst Areas	Fcst, valid until 1800, for coastal waters of Great Britain up to 12M offshore; reports from selected stations.	*BBC Radio 4 :* as for 0033 Shipping Forecast.
0555	Shipping Forecast – Home Waters Fcst Areas	Gale warnings in force; synopsis; 24 hr Fcsts for Home Waters Fcst Areas; reports from selected stations.	*BBC Radio 4;* 198 kHz, and as for 0033 Shipping Forecast.
0633	Coastal Waters (Ireland)	Gale warnings in force; 24 hr Fcst for Irish coastal waters up to 30M offshore and the Irish Sea; and 48 hr forecast outlook.	*RTE– Radio 1:* Tullamore 567 kHz, Cork 729 kHz. FM 88·2–95·2 MHz.
0655	Coastal Waters (Great Britain)	Fcst, valid until 2400, for coastal waters of Great Britain up to 12M offshore.	*BBC Radio 3:* 90·2 – 92·4 MHz.
0755 (Mon- Sat)	Coastal Waters (Ireland)	Gale warnings in force; 24 hr Fcst for Irish coastal waters up to 30M offshore and the Irish Sea; and 48 hr forecast outlook.	*RTE– Radio 1:* Tullamore 567 kHz, Cork 729 kHz. FM 88·2–95·2 MHz.
0855 (Sun)	Coastal Waters (Ireland)	Gale warnings in force; 24 hr Fcst for Irish coastal waters up to 30M offshore and the Irish Sea; and 48 hr forecast outlook.	*RTE– Radio 1:* Tullamore 567 kHz, Cork 729 kHz. FM 88·2–95·2 MHz.
1253	Coastal Waters (Ireland)	Gale warnings in force; 24 hr Fcst for Irish coastal waters up to 30M offshore and the Irish Sea; and 48 hr forecast outlook.	*RTE – Radio 1:* Tullamore 567 kHz, FM 88·2–95·2 MHz.
1355	Shipping Forecast – Home Waters Fcst Areas	Gale warnings in force; synopsis; 24 hr Fcsts for Home Waters Fcst Areas; 24 hr Fcst for Area Minch (Mon-Fri); reports from selected stations.	*BBC Radio 4:* 198 kHz and as for 0033 Shipping Forecast.
1750	Shipping Forecast – Home Waters Fcst Areas	Gale warnings in force; synopsis; 24 hr Fcst for Home Waters Fcst Areas; reports from selected stations.	*BBC Radio 4:* 198 kHz and as for 0033 Shipping Forecast.
1823 (Sat-Sun)	Coastal Waters (Ireland)	Gale warnings in force; 24 hr Fcst for Irish coastal waters up to 30M offshore and the Irish Sea; and 48 hr forecast outlook.	*RTE – Radio 1:* Tullamore 567 kHz, Cork 729 kHz, FM 88·2–95·2 MHz.
1824 (Mon-Fri)	Coastal Waters (Ireland)	Gale warnings in force; 24 hr Fcst for Irish coastal waters up to 30M offshore and the Irish Sea; and 48 hr forecast outlook.	*RTE – Radio 1:* Tullamore 567 kHz, Cork 729 kHz, FM 88·2–95·2 MHz.
2355	Coastal Waters (Ireland)	Gale warnings in force; 24 hr Fcst for Irish coastal waters up to 30M offshore and the Irish Sea; and 48 hr forecast outlook.	*RTE – Radio 1:* Tullamore 567 kHz, Cork 729 kHz, FM 88·2–95·2 MHz.

TABLE 7(2)   Gale Warnings

Stations	Areas covered	Times
BBC Radio 4: 198 kHz, Tyneside 603 kHz, London 720 kHz, N Ireland 720 kHz, Aberdeen 1449 kHz, Carlisle 1485 kHz, Plymouth and Enniskillen 774 kHz, Redruth 756 kHz, and FM frequencies as in Table 7(1).	Home Waters Forecast Areas, including Trafalgar	At the first available programme junction after receipt and after the first news bulletin
RTE – Radio 1: Tullamore 567 kHz, Cork 729 kHz, FM 88·2–95·2 MHz.	Irish coastal waters up to 30M offshore and the Irish Sea	At first programme junction after receipt and with news bulletins (0630–2352)
RTE – Radio (2 FM): Athlone 612 kHz, Dublin and Cork 1278 kHz.		At first programme junction after receipt and with news bulletins (0630–0150)
British Coast Radio Stations broadcast gale warnings for adjacent areas at the end of the first silence period after receipt (i.e. at H+03 or H+33) and subsequently at the next of the following times: 0303, 0903, 1503, 2103 UT. For further details see 7.2.16 and Table 7(4). For Irish coast stations see 6.3.27 on pages 88-89.		

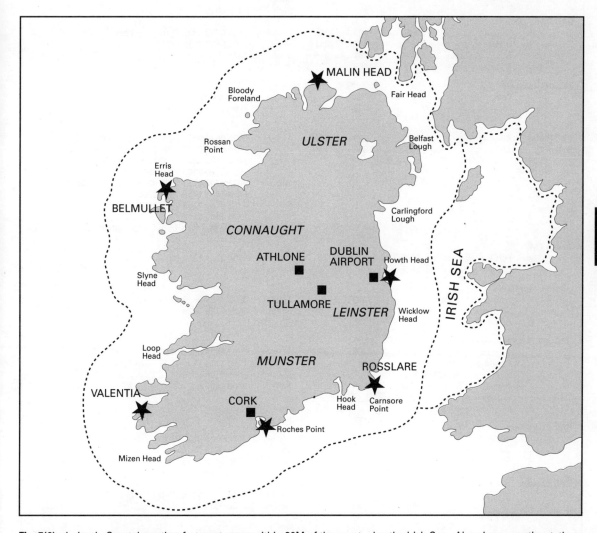

Fig. 7(6)   Ireland. Coastal weather forecast areas within 30M of the coast, plus the Irish Sea. Also shown are the stations (starred) from which reports are included and the headlands used to divide up the coastline into smaller areas, depending on the expected weather situation. RTE broadcast stations are also indicated.

7.2.19 Local Radio Stations – coastal forecasts

The details and usefulness of forecasts broadcast by local radio stations vary considerably. Some give no more than an indication of the present weather conditions, while others provide more responsible forecasts in conjunction with the local Weather Centre. The timings of weather information from local radio stations most likely to be of interest to yachtsmen in local coastal waters are shown in Table 7(3).

Many local radio stations in coastal areas participate in a scheme for broadcasting Small Craft Warning when winds of Force 6 or more are expected within the next 12 hours on the coast or up to five miles offshore. These warnings are handled in much the same way as gale warnings on Radio 4, being broadcast at the first programme junction or at the end of the first news bulletin after receipt. The stations which participate in this scheme are indicated in Table 7(3). In most cases the services operate from Good Friday until 31 October.

Table 7(3)   Local Radio Stations – Coastal Weather Forecasts

Station	VHF Transmitter(s)	Frequencies VHF (MHz)	MF (kHz)	(m)	Coastal Waters Forecasts (local times) (*summer months only)		Small Craft Warnings
BBC Radio Cornwall							
Redruth	Redruth	103·9	630	476	*Mon-Fri:*	0725 0825 1225	Yes
Bodmin	Caradon Hill	95·2	657	457			
Scilly	Scilly	96·0			*Sat:*	0725 0825 1325	
					Sun:	0825 0925	
BBC Radio Devon							
Exeter	Exeter	95·8	990	303	*Mon-Fri:*	0635 0733 0833 1310 1735 2305	Yes*
Plymouth	N Hessary Tor	103·4	855	351	*Sat:*	0605 0833 1310 2305	
N Devon	Huntshaw Cross	94·8	801	375	*Sun:*	0633 1305	
Torbay	N Hessary Tor	103·4	1458	206			
2 Counties Radio							
	Poole	102·3			*Daily:*	Every H+00	Yes
	Bournemouth		828	362	*Daily:*	Every H+30	
BBC Radio Solent	Rowridge IOW	96·1	999	300	*Mon-Fri:*	0500 0530 0600 0630 0700 0730 **0733** 0800	Yes
			1359	221		0830 **0833** 0900 1000 1100 1200 1300 **1328**	
						1400 1500 1600 1700 1730 **1733** 1800 1900	
						2000 2100 2200 2300 **2302** 2358	
					Sat:	**0632** 0709 **0732** 0809 **0832** 1104 1204 **1305**	
						1404 1504 **1758** 1804 **2300**	
					Sun:	0633 0709 **0733** 0809 **0904** 1000 1104 1204	
						1304 **1504 2302**	
					Bold times = Live forecasts from Southampton Weather Centre		
Ocean FM							
	Fort Widley	97·5			*Mon-Fri:*	0704 0804 1704 1804	
	Crabwood Farm	96·7					
South Coast Radio							
	Farlington Marshes		1170	257	*Mon-Fri:*	0629 0729 0829 1729 1829	Yes
	Southampton		1557	193	*Sat-Sun:*	0629 0729 0829	
	Brighton		1323	227			
BBC Southern Counties Radio							
	Brighton/Hove	95·3	1485	202	*Mon-Fri:*	0506 0523 0606 0706 0823 1306	Yes
	Heathfield	104·5	1161	258		1706 1723 1806 1906 1923 2206	
	Worthing	95·3			*Sat:*	0606 0706 0806	
	Reigate	104·0	1368	219	*Sun:*	0706 0806	
	Horsham	95·1					
	Newhaven/Lewes	95·0					
BBC Radio Kent							
	Wrotham	96·7			*Mon-Fri:*	0633 0733 0833 1230 1708 1808	Yes
	Swingate	104·2	774	388	*Sat:*	0745 0845 1305	
	Folkestone	97·6	1602	187	*Sun:*	0745 0845 1305	
BBC Essex							
	Mid & N Essex	103·5	729	412	*Mon-Fri:*	0740 0840 1205 1740 1840	
	SE Essex	95·3	1530	196	*SatSun:*	0720 0820 1205	1305
	All Essex		756	392			
BBC Radio Suffolk							
	East Suffolk	103·9			*Mon-Fri:*	0617 0717 0817 1328 1717 1810	Yes
	Lowestoft	95·5			*Sat-Sun:*	0707 0807 1305	
	Gt. Barton	104·6					

Table 7(3) Local Radio Stations – Coastal Weather Forecasts *Continued*

Station	VHF Transmitter(s)	Frequencies VHF (MHz)	MF (kHz)	(m)		Coastal Waters Forecasts (local times) (*summer months only)	Small Craft Warnings
BBC Radio Norfolk							
	Tacolneston	95·1	855	351	Mon-Fri:	0630 - 1600 at H+00 (0850 CG report)	Yes
	Great Massingham	104·4	873	344		1700* 1800* (* summer period only)	
					Sat:	0630-1300 at H+00	
					Sun:	0630-1400 at H+00	
BBC Radio Lincolnshire							
	Belmont	94·9	1368	219	Mon-Fri:	0615 0745 1145 1650 1810	Yes
					Sat:	0720 0845 1145 1445	
					Sun:	0845 1145	
BBC Radio Humberside							
	High Hunsley	95·9	1485	202	Mon-Fri:	0635 0735 0835 1310 1633 1733 1833	Yes
					Sat-Sun:	0733 0833 1310	
BBC Radio Cleveland							
	Bilsdale	95·0			Mon-Fri:	0645 0745 0845 1312 1645	Yes
	Whitby	95·8			Sat:	0745 0845	
					Sun:	0745 0845 0940	
BBC Radio Newcastle							
	Pentop Pike	95·4	1458	206	Mon-Fri:	0655 0755 0855 1155 1655 1755	Yes
	Chatton	96·0	in North		Sat-Sun:	0755 0855 0955	
Radio Forth	Craigkelly	97·3			Mon-Sat:	0600-1800 (every hour)	Yes
Max AM	Barns Farm		1548	194	Sun:	0600 0800 0900 1200 1500 1900	
Radio Tay	Dundee	102·8	1161	258	Sat-Sun:	0600 0700 0900 1200 1500 1800 2100	Yes
	Perth	96·4	1584	189		(April-October)	
Radio Clyde 2	Dechmont		1152	261	Daily:	H24 at H+00	Yes
BBC Radio Cumbria							
N Cumbria	Sandale	95·6	756	397	Mon-Fri:	0633 0733 0833 1710	Yes
W Cumbria	Whitehaven	95·6	1458	206	Sat-Sun:	0740 0840 1115	
S Cumbria	Morecambe Bay	96·1	837	358			
Manx Radio	Snaefell	89·0			Mon-Fri:	0710 0810 0905 1310 1740 2303	
	Carnane	97·2			Sat:	0900 1310 2303	
	Jurby	103·7			Sun:	0803 1310 2303	
	Foxdale		1368	219			
BBC Radio Merseyside	Allerton	95·8	1485	202	Mon-Fri:	0743 1143 1300	
					Sat:	0800	
					Sun:	0800	
Swansea Sound	Kilvey Hill	96·4	1170	257	Mon-Fri:	0725 0825 0925	Yes
					Sat-Sun:	0825 1003	
BBC Radio Bristol							
	Bristol	94·9	1548	194	Mon-Fri:	0605 0632 0659 0733 0759 0833 0859	Yes
	Bath	104·6				1259 1633 1755	
	Avon/Somerset	95·5			Sat:	0758 0858	
					Sun:	0758 0858	
Brunel Radio	Tor Marton		1260	238	Daily:	At H+30	Yes
Downtown Radio							
	Limavady	96·4			Mon-Fri:	0705 0805 0905 1005 1320 1403 1503	Yes
	Knockbreckon		1026			1710 2315	
	Sheriff's Mountain	102·4			Sat:	0705 0805 0905 1005 1105	
	Brougher Mountain	96·6			Sun:	1105 2303 (0003 Mon)	
BBC Radio Guernsey		93·2	1116	269	Mon-Fri:	0810 1210 1310	Yes
					Sat:	0810	
					Sun:	1010	
BBC Radio Jersey		88·8	1026	292	Mon-Fri:	0635 0810 1835	
					Sat:	0810	
					Sun:	0810	

TABLE 7(4)   Weather Broadcasts by Coast Radio Stations in the British Isles

A.   BRITISH TELECOM (BT) COAST RADIO STATIONS (for details of other services see 6.3.26)

Weather bulletins are broadcast on request and twice daily – at 0703 1903 (UT) from Northern Region stations (see below) and at 0733 1933 (UT) from Southern Region stations (see below). Bulletins include gale warnings, synopsis and 24 hour forecast for all the sea areas listed for Northern and Southern Regions respectively.

Gale warnings are broadcast on frequencies/channels listed below after an announcement on VHF Ch 16 and 2182 kHz, at the end of the first silence period after receipt (i.e. at H+03 or H+33), and at 0303 0903 1503 2103 UT. They remain in force unless amended or cancelled, but are re-issued if the gale persists for more than 24 hours.

BT NORTHERN REGION (Routine broadcasts at **0703 1903** UT)			BT SOUTHERN REGION (Routine broadcasts at **0733 1933** UT)		
Station	Channel/Frequency	For all areas below	Station	Channel/Frequency	For all areas below
Whitby	Ch 25		Celtic	Ch 24	
Cullercoats	Ch 26 2719 kHz		Ilfracombe	Ch 05	Tyne
Forth	Ch 24	Viking	Land's End	Ch 27 2670 kHz	Dogger
Stonehaven	Ch 26 2691 kHz	North Utsire		Ch 64 (to Scilly)	German Bight
Buchan	Ch 25	South Utsire	Pendennis	Ch 62	Humber
Cromarty	Ch 84	Forties	Start Point	Ch 26	Thames
Collafirth	Ch 24	Cromarty	Weymouth	Ch 05	Dover
Shetland	Ch 27 1770 kHz	Forth	Niton	Ch 28 1641 kHz	Wight
Orkney	Ch 26	Tyne	Hastings[1]	Ch 07	Portland
Wick	1764 kHz	Dogger	North Foreland[1]	Ch 26 1707 kHz	Plymouth
Lewis	Ch 05	Fisher	Thames[1]	Ch 02	Biscay
Hebrides	Ch 26 1866 kHz	German Bight	Orfordness[1]	Ch 62	Finisterre
Skye	Ch 24	Humber	Bacton	Ch 07	Sole
Oban	Ch 07	Thames	Humber	Ch 26 1869 kHz	Lundy
Islay	Ch 25	Lundy	Grimsby	Ch 27	Fastnet
Clyde	Ch 26	Irish Sea			Irish Sea
Portpatrick	Ch 27 1883 kHz	Rockall			Shannon
Morecambe Bay	Ch 82	Malin			
Anglesey	Ch 26	Hebrides			
Cardigan Bay	Ch 03	Bailey			
		Fair Isle			
		Faeroes	Note: (1) Fog warnings for River Thames broadcast when visibility falls below half a mile, at end of next silence period after receipt and repeated every two hours until amended or cancelled		
		SE Iceland			

B.   JERSEY RADIO (for details of other services see 6.3.26)

Weather bulletins are broadcast as below and comprise near gale force 7 warnings, synopsis, 12 hour forecast and outlook for a further 12 hours and reports from meteorological stations.

Near gale force 7 warnings are broadcast on receipt, at the end of the next silence period, and at 0307 0907 1507 2107 (UT).

Station	Frequency/Channel	Area	Times of weather bulletins
Jersey	Ch 25 82 1659 kHz	Channel Islands south of 50°N and east of 3°W	On request and at 0645 0745 (LT) and at 1245 1845 2245 (UT)

C.   IRISH COAST RADIO SERVICE (for details of other services see 6.3.27). See Fig. 6(3) for stations.

Weather bulletins are broadcast as below and comprise gale warnings, synopsis and 24 hour forecast.

Gale warnings are broadcast on VHF channels below on receipt and repeated at the next of the following times: 0033 0633 1233 1833 (LT) after announcement on Ch 16.

Valentia Radio broadcasts gale warnings on 1752 kHz at the end of the next silence period after receipt and at the next of following times 0303 0903 1503 2103 (UT) after announcement on 2182 kHz.

Station	Channel/Frequency	Area	Times of weather bulletins
Malin Head	Ch 23		
Glen Head	Ch 24		
Belmullet	Ch 83		
Clifden	Ch 26		
Shannon	Ch 28	Irish coastal waters up to 30 miles offshore and Irish Sea	0103 0403 0703 1003 1303 1603 1903 2203 (LT) after announcement on Ch 16
Bantry	Ch 23		
Cork	Ch 26		
Mine Head	Ch 83		
Rosslare	Ch 23		
Wicklow Head	Ch 87		
Dublin	Ch 83		
Valentia	Ch 24	Shannon, Fastnet	As above, and on request
Valentia	1752 kHz	Shannon, Fastnet	On request and at 0833 2033 (UT)

TABLE 7(5)   Western Europe – Shipping Forecasts, Coastal Waters Forecasts, and Gale Warnings

Notes:
(1) All times below are local or 'clock' times (LT) unless otherwise stated.
(2) Details of other broadcasts by Coast Radio Stations are given in Chapter 6 (6.3.28–6.3.31).
(3) Broadcasts in English are indicated in bold type, thus: in **English**.
(4) CROSS – Centres Régionaux Opérationnels de Surveillance et de Sauvetage. Broadcasts follow announcement on Ch 16. In the English Channel CROSS stations broadcast weather information on request in French or in English, after a call on Ch 16.
(5) French Coast Radio Stations make a preliminary announcement on Ch 16/2182 kHz.

Station	Frequency/ Channel	Times (LT unless stated)	Weather Bulletins	Areas for Weather Bulletins and Gale Warnings	Gale Warnings
FRANCE – NATIONAL AND REGIONAL BROADCASTS					
France Inter	162 kHz	1005 (Mon-Fri) 0650 (Sat-Sun) 2005 (daily)	Storm warnings, synopsis, 24h Fcst and outlook, in French	French Fcst areas 1-25	–
Bayonne Bordeaux	1494 kHz 1206 kHz	0655	Ditto	East Atlantic and Bay of Biscay	–
Rennes Brest	711 kHz 1404 kHz	0655	Ditto	East Atlantic and English Channel	–
Paris Lille	864 kHz 1377 kHz	0655	Ditto	English Channel and North Sea	–
FRANCE – CHANNEL COAST					
Dunkerque Calais Boulogne-sur-Mer	Ch 61 Ch 87 Ch 23	0733 1533 0733 1533 0733 1533	Strong breeze/Gale warnings synopsis & development, 12h Fcst, outlook for further 12h, observations from Signal Stations, in French	Coastal waters from Belgian border to Dieppe	Nil
Boulogne-sur-Mer	1692 kHz	0703 UT 1833 UT	Gale warnings, synopsis and development, 24h Fcst and outlook, in French	French Areas 1 to 14	Nil
	1770 kHz	–	–	Ditto	On receipt and every H+03 H+33 when imminent. Every odd H+03 (UT) while warning in force
CROSS[4] Gris-Nez	Ch 11	On receipt, every H+10 and on request	–	Coastal waters from Belgian border to Cap d'Antifer	Gale warnings and information on visibility, in French and **English**
Dunkerque Gris-Nez St Frieux Ailly	Ch 68 79 Ch 68 79 Ch 68 79 Ch 68 79	On request	Gale warnings, synopsis, 24h Fcst, outlook for 48h, in French and **English**	Coastal waters from Belgian border to Baie de Somme and areas entering Baie de Seine and Baie de Somme	Nil
Dieppe Le Havre Port-en-Bessin Cherbourg	Ch 02 Ch 26 Ch 03 Ch 27	0733 1533 0733 1533 0733 1533 0733 1533	Strong breeze/Gale warnings synopsis & development, 12h Fcst, outlook for further 12h, observations from Signal Stations, in French	Coastal waters from Baie de Somme to Baie de Seine	Nil

7

Station	Frequency/ Channel	Times (LT unless stated)	Weather Bulletins	Areas for Weather Bulletins and Gale Warnings	Gale Warnings
CROSS[4] Jobourg Broadcasts from: **Antifer** **Ver-sur-Mer** **Gatteville** **Jobourg** **Granville** **Roches Douvres**	Ch 80 Ch 80 Ch 80 Ch 80 Ch 80 Ch 80 Ch 80	Every H+20 and H+50		French Areas 13 and 14	Gale warnings and information on visibility in French and **English**
St Malo	Ch 02	0733 1533	Strong breeze/Gale warnings synopsis & development, 24h Fcst, outlook for further 24h, observations from Ouessant, in French	Coastal waters from Le Havre to Penmarc'h	Nil
Brest-Le Conquet (at St Malo)	2691 kHz	0733 UT 1803 UT	Gale warnings, synopsis and development, 24h Fcst and outlook, in French	French Areas 14 to 24	Nil
(CROSS)[4] Corsen **Ouessant Traffic**	 Ch 79	 Every 3h from 0150 UT	 Gale warnings, synopsis, 12h Fcst and outlook, in French and **English**	 French Areas 14 to 16	 On receipt and every H+10, H+40 in French and **English**
Cap Fréhel **Île de Batz** **Île de Sein**	Ch 79 Ch 79 Ch 79	0433 2133 0448 2148 0503 2203	Gale warnings, synopsis, 24h Fcst and outlook for further 48h, in French	Coastal waters from Le Havre to Penmarc'h	On receipt and every H+03 in French
Paimpol **Plougasnou** **Brest-Le Conquet** **Ouessant** **Pont l'Abbé**	Ch 84 Ch 81 Ch 26 Ch 82 Ch 86	0733 1533 0733 1533 0733 1533 0733 1533 0733 1533	Strong breeze/Gale warnings, synopsis & development, 24h Fcst, outlook for further 24h observations from Ouessant, in French	Coastal waters from Le Havre to Penmarc'h and from Pte du Raz to south of Vendée	Nil

FRANCE – ATLANTIC COAST

Station	Frequency/ Channel	Times (LT unless stated)	Weather Bulletins	Areas for Weather Bulletins and Gale Warnings	Gale Warnings
Ouessant Traffic CROSS Corsen (from Traffic Control Centre)	Ch 79	Every 3h from 0150 UT Every H+10 H+40	Gale warnings, synopsis, 12h fcst and outlook, in French and **English** General information and poor visibility	French Areas 14 to 16 Ditto	 Strong wind warnings in French and **English**
Brest-Le Conquet	1671 kHz and 3722 kHz 1635 kHz	0733 UT 1803 UT	Gale warnings, synopsis and development, 24h Fcst and outlook, in French –	French Areas 14 to 24 Ditto	Nil On receipt and every H+03 H+33 when imminent. Every even H+03 (UT) while warning in force
Paimpol **Plougasnou** **Brest-Le Conquet** **Ouessant** **Pont l'Abbé**	Ch 84 Ch 81 Ch 26 Ch 82 Ch 86	0733 1533 0733 1533 0733 1533 0733 1533 0733 1533	Strong breeze/Gale warnings, synopsis & development, 24h Fcst, outlook for further 24h, observations from Ouessant, in French	Coastal waters from Le Havre to Penmarc'h and from Pte du Raz to south of Vendée	Nil
Brest-Le Conquet (at Quimperlé)	1876 kHz	0733 UT 1803 UT	Gale warnings, synopsis and development, 24h Fcst and outlook, in French	French Areas 14 to 24	Nil
CROSS[4] Étel **Penmarc'h** **Étel** **Kerrouault** (St Nazaire) **L'Armandèche** (Sables d'Olonne)	 Ch 80 Ch 80 Ch 80 Ch 80	 0433 2133 0438 2138 0443 2143 0448 2148	 Gale warnings, synopsis, 24h Fcst and outlook for further 24h, in French. (Timings are approx)	 Coastal waters from Penmarc'h to 46°20'N	On receipt and: every H+03 every H+05 every H+07 every H+09 (In French and **English** in summer; French in winter).

Station	Frequency/Channel	Times (LT unless stated)	Weather Bulletins	Areas for Weather Bulletins and Gale Warnings	Gale Warnings
St Nazaire	1722 kHz and 2740 kHz	0803 UT 1833 UT	Gale warnings, synopsis and development, 24h Fcst and outlook, in French	French Areas 14 to 24	On 1686 kHz on receipt. Every H+03 H+33 when imminent. Every odd H+07 (UT) while warning in force
Belle Île St Nazaire St Herblain/Nantes St Hilaire-de-Riez	Ch 25 Ch 23 Ch 28 Ch 27	0733 1533 0733 1533 0733 1533 0733 1533	Strong breeze/Gale warnings, synopsis & development, 24h Fcst, outlook for further 24h, observations from Ouessant, in French	Coastal waters from Pte du Raz (48°00'N) to south of Vendée (46°20'N)	Nil
Bordeaux-Arcachon	1862 kHz	0733 UT 1803 UT	Gale warnings, synopsis and development, 24h Fcst and outlook, in French	French Areas 14 to 24	Nil
	1710 kHz	–	–	Ditto	On receipt and every H+03 H+33 (UT) when imminent, every even H+03 while while warning in force
Île de Ré Royan Bordeaux-Arcachon Bayonne	Ch 21 Ch 23 Ch 82 Ch 24	0733 1533 0733 1533 0733 1533 0733 1533	Strong breeze/Gale warnings synopsis & development, 12h Fcst, probabilities for next 12h, outlook, coastal reports, in French	Coastal waters from 46°20'N to Spanish border	Nil
CROSS[4] Soulac	(Note: Soulac operates 0700-2200 and night service is from Étel – see below)				
Chassiron Soulac Cap Ferret Contis Biarritz	Ch 79 Ch 79 Ch 79 Ch 79 Ch 79	0433 2133 0438 2138 0443 2143 0448 2148 0453 2153	Gale warnings, synopsis, 24h Fcst and outlook for further 24h, in French. (Timings are approx)	Coastal waters from 46°20'N to the Spanish border	Every H+03 in French Every H+05 in French Every H+07 in French Every H+09 in French Every H+11 in French
BELGIUM					
Belgische Radio en Televisie	927 kHz	0600 0900 0700 1200 0800	Weather report in Dutch after the news (also in special circumstances at 1700 2200)	Areas Dover, Thames, Humber, Wight, Portland	Nil
Oostende	2761 kHz and Ch 27 2256 kHz (gale warnings only)	0820 UT 1720 UT	Strong breeze warnings and Fcst, in **English** and Dutch	Areas Dover, Thames	On receipt and after next two silence periods. In **English** and Dutch. Fog warnings on 2761 kHz only, on receipt and after next silence period, in **English** and Dutch
Antwerpen	Ch 24			Schelde estuary	On receipt and every H+03, H+48. In **English**. Fog warnings for the Schelde on receipt and every H+03 H+48, in **English** and Dutch

7

Fig. 7(7) French Shipping Forecast Areas

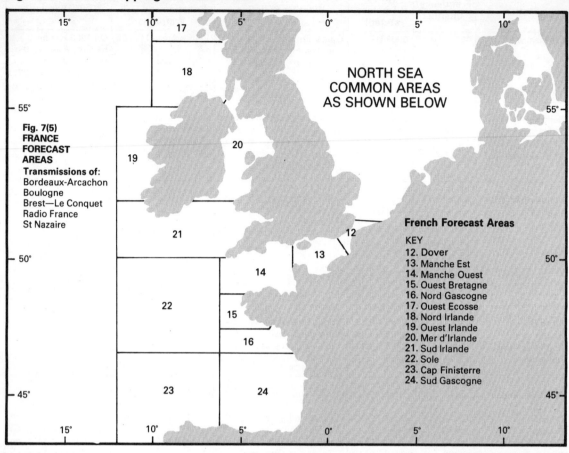

NORTH SEA
COMMON AREAS
AS SHOWN BELOW

**Fig. 7(5)
FRANCE
FORECAST
AREAS
Transmissions of:**
Bordeaux-Arcachon
Boulogne
Brest—Le Conquet
Radio France
St Nazaire

French Forecast Areas

KEY
12. Dover
13. Manche Est
14. Manche Ouest
15. Ouest Bretagne
16. Nord Gascogne
17. Ouest Ecosse
18. Nord Irlande
19. Ouest Irlande
20. Mer d'Irlande
21. Sud Irlande
22. Sole
23. Cap Finisterre
24. Sud Gascogne

Fig. 7(8)
North Sea Common
Shipping Forecast Areas

As used for forecasts from:
France
Belgium
Netherlands
Germany
Denmark
Norway
United Kingdom

Notes:
(1) Numbers are as for
French Forecast Areas.
(2) Numbers in brackets
with prefix N are as for
German Forecast Areas.

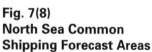

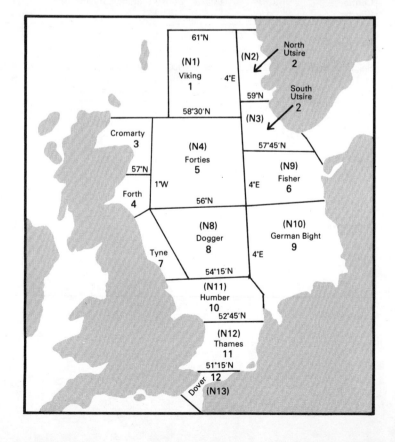

Station	Frequency/ Channel	Times (LT unless stated)	Weather Bulletins	Areas for Weather Bulletins and Gale Warnings	Gale Warnings
NETHERLANDS					
Radio 1	747 kHz	Every H+00	Near gale warnings, in Dutch	Netherlands coastal waters up to 30M offshore, and IJsselmeer	Near gale warnings, in Dutch.
Radio 5	1008 kHz	0645	Near gale warnings, Fcst situation, and reports from stations, in Dutch	Ditto	–
Scheveningen	1713 kHz (at Nes) and 1890 kHz	0340 UT 0940 UT 1540 UT 2140 UT	Near gale warnings, synopsis, 12h Fcst, outlook for further 24h, and reports from stations, in **English** and Dutch	Dutch coastal waters up to 30M offshore (including IJsselmeer) and Sea Areas for southern North Sea	On receipt and after next silence period, in **English** and Dutch. Ice reports every 4h from 0333 on 1674 and 1890 kHz in **English** and Dutch
	2824 kHz	0340 UT	Ditto	Ditto	Nil
Scheveningen VHF stations					
Goes	Ch 23	0005	Strong breeze warnings, synopsis, 12h wind Fcst, in Dutch	Dutch coastal waters up to 30M offshore (including IJsselmeer)	Strong breeze warnings on receipt and every H+05, in Dutch
Rotterdam	Ch 87	0705			
Scheveningen	Ch 83	1305			
Haarlem	Ch 25	1905			
Lelystad	Ch 83				
Wieringermeer	Ch 27				
Platform L7	Ch 84				
Terschelling	Ch 78				
Nes	Ch 23				
Appingedam	Ch 27				
GERMANY					
Norddeutscher Rundfunk Hamburg (NDR 4)	972 kHz	On receipt	Wind Fcst, in German	German Bight	Water level reports at 1000 1900, in German
		0105	Synopsis, 12h Fcst and outlook for further 12h, reports from stations, in German	German Areas N9–N12	
Radio Bremen Hansawelle Bremerhaven Bremen	936 kHz 89·3 MHz 93·8 MHz	On receipt	Wind Fcst in German for next 12 h	German Bight	Water level reports 1030 2400 (Mon-Sat), 1130 2400 (Sun and Public Holidays)
(RB1)		About 1030	Weather report, in German	German Bight	Nil
		2400	Synopsis, 12h Fcst and outlook for further 12h, reports from stations, in German	German Areas N9-N12	Nil
Deutschlandfunk	1269 kHz (Gale warnings also on 88·7 MHz)	0205 0740 1205	Synopsis, 12h Fcst and outlook for further 12h, reports from stations, and ice reports, in German. Water level reports at 0205 only.	German Areas N9-N12	On receipt in German for German Bight
Deutschlandradio	177 kHz	0205 0740 1205	Synopsis, 12h Fcst and and outlook for further 12h, in German	German Areas N9-N12	Nil

7

Station	Frequency/ Channel	Times (LT unless stated)	Weather Bulletins	Areas for Weather Bulletins and Gale Warnings	Gale Warnings
Norddeich	2614 kHz	0910 2110	Gale warnings, Synopsis, 12h Fcst and outlook for further 12h, reports from stations, in German, and in **English** for Area N10	German Areas N1-N4, N8-N12	On receipt, after next silence period, on request and every 4h from 0133 (UT). In German for Areas N3-N4, N8-N12
	Ch 28	0800 1900	Synopsis, 12h Fcst and outlook for further 12h, reports from stations, in German	German Areas N9-N12	Nil
Helgoland Eiderstedt Nordfrieseland Elbe-Weser	Ch 27 Ch 25 Ch 26 Ch 24	0800 1900	Synopsis, 12h Fcst and outlook for further 12h, in German	German Areas N9-N12	Nil

German Traffic Centres	Traffic Centres broadcast local Storm Warnings, Weather Messages, Visbility and (when appropriate) Ice Reports on VHF channels as follows:

German Bight Traffic	Ch 79 80	every H+00
Ems Traffic	Ch 15 18 20 21	every H+50
Jade Traffic	Ch 20 63	every H+10
Bremerhaven Weser Traffic	Ch 02 04 05 07 21 22 82	every H+20
Bremen Weser Traffic	Ch 19 78 81	every H+30
Hunte Traffic	Ch 63	every H+30
Cuxhaven Elbe Traffic	Ch 03 05 18 19 21	every H+55
Brunsbüttel Elbe Traffic	Ch 04 05 18 21 22 60 66 67	every H+05
Kiel Kanal II (for East going vessels)	Ch 02	every H+15 and H+45

Chapter 8

Safety

Contents

8

Safety – introduction

Here in the Almanac basic information is given about safety equipment, emergency signals, The Global Maritime Distress and Safety System (GMDSS), and SAR operations.

The following subjects are described in more detail in Chapter 8 of *The Macmillan & Silk Cut Yachtsman's Handbook*:

Safety equipment – legal requirements and recommended outfits; radar reflectors; bilge pumps; guardrails; fire prevention and fire fighting; lifejackets; safety harnesses; man overboard gear and drill; liferafts; distress signals; SAR organisation; response to distress calls; abandoning ship; helicopter rescues; first aid afloat.

8.1   SAFETY EQUIPMENT

8.1.1   Safety equipment – general

The skipper is responsible for the safety of the boat and all on board. He must ensure that:

(1) The boat is suitable in design and in construction for her intended purpose.
(2) The boat is maintained in good condition.
(3) The crew is competent and sufficiently strong.
(4) The necessary safety and emergency equipment is carried, is in good condition, and the crew know how to use it.

Individual crew members are responsible for their personal gear. Non-slip shoes or boots are essential. So is foul-weather clothing with close fastenings at neck, wrists and ankles. At least two changes of sailing clothing should be carried, including warm sweaters and towelling strips as neck scarves. Other personal items include a sailor's knife and spike on a lanyard, a waterproof torch, and a supply of anti-seasick pills. Lifejackets and safety harnesses are usually supplied on board, but if individuals bring their own, the skipper should make certain they are up to standard.

Safety guidelines for recreational boat users can be found in a useful booklet *Safety on the Sea* published jointly by the RNLI, the Coastguard Agency and the RYA.

8.1.2   Safety equipment – legal requirements

Yachts more than 45ft (13·7m) in length are required to carry safety equipment as in the *Merchant Shipping (Life Saving Appliances)* and *Merchant Shipping (Fire Appliances) Rules* (HMSO).

All yachts must carry navigation lights and sound signals which comply with the *International Regulations for Preventing Collisions at Sea*.

Racing yachts are required to carry the safety equipment specified for the class/event concerned.

8.1.3   Safety equipment recommendations for sea-going yachts 18 – 45ft (5·5 – 13·7m) overall length

Full details of recommended safety equipment are given in *The Macmillan & Silk Cut Yachtsman's Handbook*. Below are brief reminders of the minimum equipment which should be carried for (a) coastal and (b) offshore cruising.

But prevention is better than cure, and simple precautions can eliminate accidents. Be particularly careful with bottled gas and petrol. Fit a gas detector. Turn off the gas at the bottle after use. If gas or petrol is smelt – no naked lights, and do not run electrical equipment. Test systems regularly. Insist that crew wear lifejackets and harnesses when necessary, and that they do clip on. Make sure a good look-out is maintained at all times. Listen to every forecast. Double-check all navigational calculations. Take nothing for granted.

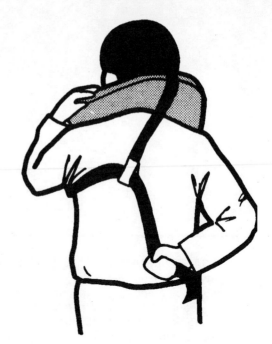

Fig. 8(1)   Putting on a lifejacket – first read the instructions. Hold the jacket up in front of you, put your head through the hole, and secure the waistband at the side or front as appropriate.

Safety equipment list

	(a) Coastal	(b) Offshore
Safety		
Lifejackets, BS3595, or CE equivalent per person	1	1
Harnesses, BS4224, or CE equivalent per person	1	1
Navigation		
Charts, almanac, pilot	Yes	Yes
Compass with deviation card	1	1
Hand bearing compass	1	1
Chart table instruments	Yes	Yes
Watch/clock	1	2
Echo sounder	1	1
Leadline	1	1
Radio direction finding set	1	1
Radio receiver (forecasts)	1	1
Barometer	1	1
Navigation lights	Yes	Yes
Radar reflector	1	1
Foghorn	1	1
Powerful waterproof torch	1	1
Anchor with warp or chain	2	2
Towline	1	1
Man overboard		
Lifebuoy, with drogue and light	2	2
Buoyant heaving line	1	1
Dan buoy	–	1
Rope (or boarding) ladder	1	1

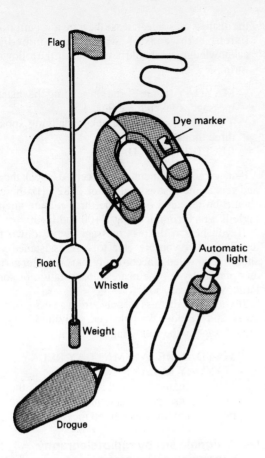

Fig. 8(2) Lifebuoy with dan buoy and flag, automatic light, whistle, dye marker and drogue.

	(a) Coastal	(b) Offshore
Fire		
Fire extinguishers	2	3
Fire blanket	1	1
Sinking		
Bilge pumps	2	2
Buckets with lanyards	2	2
Leak stopping gear	Yes	Yes
Distress signals		
Hand flares, red	2	4
Hand flares, white (warning)	4	4
Red parachute rockets	2	4
Hand smoke signals	2	–
Buoyant orange smoke signals	–	–
Emergency radio transmitter	–	1
Abandon ship		
Liferaft for whole crew	1	1
	or	
Dinghy with buoyancy, or inflated inflatable	1	–
Panic bag, extra water etc.	–	1

	(a) Coastal	(b) Offshore
Miscellaneous		
First Aid kit	1	1
Engine tool kit	1	1
Name/number prominently displayed	Yes	Yes
Storm canvas	Yes	Yes
Emergency steering arrangements	Yes	Yes

8.2   EMERGENCY SIGNALS

8.2.1   Distress
Distress is the most serious degree of Emergency. It applies to any situation where a boat or person is threatened by grave and imminent danger and requests immediate assistance. The RT prefix associated with an Distress message is MAYDAY – see 8.2.5. A Distress call has priority over all other transmissions.

8.2.2.   Urgency
Urgency is a lesser degree of emergency concerning the safety of a boat or person. Examples include man overboard (which might need to be upgraded later to Distress), vessel disabled but not sinking; medical problems (see also 6.3.17). The RT prefix associated with an Urgency message is PAN – see 8.2.8

8.2.3   Safety
Safety is the least serious degree of emergency, usually associated with a warning of hazardous navigational or meteorological circumstances. The RT prefix associated with an Safety message is SÉCURITÉ – see 8.2.9.

8.2.4   Emergency signals general
Any of the distress signals listed in 8.2.5 to 8.2.9 must only be made with the authority of the skipper, and only if the boat or a person is in grave and imminent danger, and help is urgently required; or on behalf of another vessel in distress, which for some reason is unable to make a Distress signal. If subsequently the danger is overcome, the Distress call must be cancelled by whatever means are available.

For a lesser emergency, an Urgency signal (PAN PAN) as described below may be appropriate. If help is needed, but the boat is not in immediate danger, the proper signal is 'V' (Victor) International Code, meaning 'I require assistance'. This can be sent as a flag signal (a white flag with a red St Andrew's cross), or by light or sound in Morse code (••• —). Other signals of an emergency nature in the International Code are given in Chapter 6 in the Handbook.

If medical help is required, the proper signal is 'W' (Whiskey) International Code, meaning 'I require medical assistance'.

A full list of the recognised distress signals is given in Annex IV of the *International Regulations for Preventing Collisions at Sea*. The following are those most appropriate for yachts and small craft, together with notes on their use.

8

Note that an inland 999 (or 112) call to the Coastguard by cellular radiotelephone (cellphone) is **NOT** an adequate substitute for radio communication on VHF Ch 16 or 2182 kHz from a vessel in a distress/safety situation. Cellphone coverage is limited, even in coastal waters, and is not monitored in any way – unlike Ch 16, which is monitored continuously by HM Coastguard. Nor is a cellphone call heard by other vessels nearby which may be able to help. For these and other reasons (the addition of a further link in the chain of communication, the difficulty of on-scene communication, and the impossibility of calling another vessel by cellphone unless she is so fitted and her number is known), the use of cellphone for marine distress/safety communication is very strongly discouraged.

8.2.5   Radio distress signals

(1) A signal sent by radiotelephone consisting of the spoken word MAYDAY.

This should normally be transmitted on VHF Ch 16 or 2182 kHz , but any frequency may be used if help may thereby be obtained more quickly.

Distress messages, together with Urgency and Safety messages (see below) from vessels at sea are free of charge. A distress call has priority over all other transmissions. If heard, cease all transmissions that may interfere with the distress call or messages, and listen on the frequency concerned.

Anybody in the crew should be able to pass a distress message, but this must only be done on the orders of the skipper and if the yacht or a person (or some other vessel or aircraft that cannot make a distress signal) is in serious and imminent danger and requires immediate assistance.

The full procedure is as follows:

- Check main battery switch ON
- Switch set ON, and turn power selector to HIGH
- Tune to VHF Ch 16 (or 2182 kHz for MF)
- If alarm signal generator fitted, operate for at least 30 seconds
- Press transmit button, and say slowly and distinctly:

- MAYDAY MAYDAY MAYDAY
- THIS IS (name of boat, spoken three times)
- MAYDAY (name of boat spoken once)
- MY POSITION IS (latitude and longitude, or true bearing and distance from a known point)
- Nature of distress (whether sinking, on fire etc.)
- Aid required
- Number of persons on board
- Any other important, helpful information (e.g. if the yacht is drifting, whether distress rockets are being fired)
- OVER

The yacht's position is of vital importance, and should be repeated if time allows. On completion of the distress message, release the transmit button and listen.   In coastal waters an immediate acknowledgment should be expected in the following form:

> MAYDAY (name of station sending the distress message, spoken three times)
> THIS IS (name of station acknowledging, spoken three times)
> RECEIVED MAYDAY

If an acknowledgment is not received, check the set and repeat the distress call. For 2182 kHz the call should be repeated during the three minute silence periods which commence at H+00 and H+30.

If you hear a distress message, write down the details, and if you are able to give assistance you should acknowledge accordingly, but only after giving an opportunity for the nearest coast station or some larger vessel to do so.

If you hear a distress message from a vessel further away, and it is not acknowledged, you should pass on the message in the following form:

> MAYDAY RELAY, MAYDAY RELAY, MAYDAY RELAY
> THIS IS (name of vessel re-transmitting the distress message, spoken three times)
> Followed by the intercepted message.

(2) A signal sent by radiotelegraphy consisting of the group ··· ——— ··· in the Morse Code.

The International radiotelegraph distress frequency is 500 kHz. Five British Telecom coast stations keep watch on this frequency. Larger ships are fitted with a radiotelegraph alarm signal to give notice, aurally or by triggering the auto-alarm of ships within range, of the impending transmission of a distress call and message.

8.2.6   Visual and audible distress signals

(1) Continuous sounding with any fog signalling apparatus.

In order to avoid confusion, this is best done by a succession of letters SOS in Morse (··· ——— ···).

(2) A signal made by any signalling method consisting of the group ··· ——— ··· (SOS) in the Morse Code.

For a yacht the most likely methods are by sound signal as in (1) above, or by flashing light.

(3) The International Code signal of distress 'NC'.

This can be made by flag hoist, N being a blue and white chequered flag and C one which is horizontally striped blue, white, red, white, blue.

(4) A signal consisting of a square flag having above or below it a ball or anything resembling a ball.

This is not too difficult to contrive from any square flag, and a round fender or anchor ball.

(5) A rocket parachute flare or a hand held flare showing a red light.

A red flare is the most effective distress signal at night. Flares serve two purposes – first to raise the alarm, and then to pinpoint the boat's position. Within about three miles from land a hand flare will do both. At greater distances a red parachute rocket (which projects a suspended flare to a height of more than 1,000ft, or 300m, and which burns for more than 40 seconds) is needed to raise the alarm, but hand flares are useful to indicate the boat's position. See further comments under (6) below.

(6) A smoke signal giving off orange coloured smoke.

By day orange smoke signals (hand held for short distances, or a larger buoyant type for greater ranges) are more effective than flares, although the smoke disperses quickly in a strong wind.

White flares are not distress signals, but are used to indicate the presence of a boat – to another vessel on a collision course for example. An outfit of four is suggested for boats which make night passages. Shield your eyes when using them, to protect night vision.

Pyrotechnics must be stowed where they are accessible, but protected from damp. In good storage conditions they should have a life of three years. Examine them regularly, and replace them by the expiry date. All the crew should know where the flares are stowed and how to use them. Hold hand flares firmly downwind. Rockets turn into the wind; fire them vertically in normal conditions, or aimed about 15° downwind in strong winds. Do not aim them into the wind, or they will not gain altitude. If there is low cloud, fire rockets at 45° downwind, so that the flare burns under the cloud.

(7) Slowly and repeatedly raising and lowering arms outstretched to each side.

The arms should be raised and lowered together, above and below the horizontal.

8.2.7   Control of distress traffic

A distress (MAYDAY) call imposes general radio silence, until the vessel concerned or some other authority (e.g. the nearest MRCC, MRSC or coast station) cancels the distress. If necessary the station controlling distress traffic may impose radio silence in this form:

> SEELONCE MAYDAY, followed by its name or other identification, on the distress frequency.

If some other station nearby believes it necessary to do likewise, it may transmit:

> SEELONCE DISTRESS, followed by its name or other identification.

When appropriate the station controlling distress traffic may relax radio silence so that normal working is resumed with caution on the distress frequency, with subsequent communications from the casualty prefixed by the Urgency signal (below).

When complete radio silence is no longer necessary on a frequency being used for distress traffic, the controlling station may relax radio silence as follows:

> MAYDAY
> HELLO ALL STATIONS (spoken three times)
> THIS IS (name or identification)
> The time
> The name of the station in distress
> PRUDONCE

If distress working continues on other frequencies these will be identified. For example, PRUDONCE on 500 kHz (WT distress frequency) and 2182 kHz, but SEELONCE on VHF Ch 16. When all distress traffic has ceased, normal working is authorised as follows:

> MAYDAY
> HELLO ALL STATIONS (spoken three times)
> THIS IS (name or identification)
> The time
> The name of the station which was in distress
> SEELONCE FEENEE

8.2.8   Urgency signal

The radiotelephone Urgency signal consists of the words PAN PAN, spoken three times, and indicates that the station has a very urgent message concerning the safety of a ship or person. Messages prefixed by PAN PAN take priority over all traffic except distress, and are sent on VHF Ch 16 or on 2182 kHz. The Urgency Signal is appropriate when someone is lost overboard or urgent medical advice or attention is needed. It should be cancelled when the urgency is over.

After the initial call on VHF Ch 16 or 2182 kHz, the message itself should be passed on a working frequency if it is long or if it is a medical call, or in areas of heavy traffic if the message is repeated. Where necessary this should be indicated at the end of the initial call.

Here is an example of an Urgency call and message from the yacht *Seabird*, disabled off the Needles.

> PAN PAN - PAN PAN - PAN PAN
> HELLO ALL STATIONS
> HELLO ALL STATIONS
> HELLO ALL STATIONS
> THIS IS YACHT SEABIRD SEABIRD
> SEABIRD TWO NINE ZERO DEGREES TWO
> MILES FROM NEEDLES LIGHTHOUSE
> DISMASTED AND PROPELLER FOULED
> ANCHOR DRAGGING AND DRIFTING
> EAST NORTH EAST TOWARDS SHINGLES
> BANK REQUIRE URGENT TOW OVER

The Urgency signal has priority over all messages except Distress, and should normally get an immediate response. If you hear an Urgency call you should respond in the same way as for a Distress call.

8.2.9   Safety signal

This consists of the word SÉCURITÉ (pronounced SAY-CURE-E-TAY) spoken three times, and indicates that the station is about to transmit an important navigational or meteorological warning. Such

8

messages usually originate from a coast station, and are transmitted on a working frequency after an announcement on the distress frequency.

Safety messages are usually addressed to 'all stations', and often at the end of the first available silence period (see 6.3.5 – MF radio). Always listen carefully until you are sure that the message does not affect you, and do not make any transmission that will interfere.

8.3   GMDSS

8.3.1   The Global Maritime Distress and Safety System (GMDSS)

The Global Maritime Distress and Safety System (GMDSS) is an improved maritime distress and safety communications system adopted by the International Maritime Organisation (IMO).

The GMDSS regulations apply to all passenger and cargo ships over 300 tons engaged in international voyages, but they affect all seagoing craft. GMDSS came into force in February 1992 and the system will be fully implemented world wide by February 1999. During this period existing systems will operate together with the new.

Smaller vessels may fit GMDSS equipment on a voluntary basis, but this will become an increasing necessity towards the end of the decade as the present system for sending and receiving distress calls is run down. Although not specifically designed for yachtsmen there are features of the system which are already of interest, and as the implementation period progresses yachtsmen may see an attraction in using the GMDSS.

Before the introduction of GMDSS, maritime distress and safety relied heavily on certain ships keeping a continuous radio watch on the three main international distress frequencies: i.e. Morse on 500kHz for passenger and cargo ships over 1,600 tons, RT on 2182 kHz and VHF Ch 16 on all these ships, plus cargo ships over 300 tons. A number of Coast Radio Stations (CRS) were also obliged to maintain a watch on these frequencies. Once out of range of the Coast Radio Stations any assistance could only be provided by ships in the vicinity of the distress incident.

The objective of GMDSS is to improve distress and safety radio communications, and SAR procedures,by making use of technology such as satcom and satnav. The result is that shore stations, and shipping in the vicinity of a distress incident can be alerted faster and more reliably.

In addition, GMDSS provides for urgency and safety communications, and the promulgation of Marine Safety Information (MSI) such as navigational warnings, weather warnings and forecasts. Regardless of the sea area in which they operate, vessels conforming to GMDSS must be able to perform certain functions:

- transmit ship-to-shore distress alerts by two separate means
- transmit ship-to-ship distress alerts
- transmit and receive safety information such as navigation and weather warnings
- transmit signals for locating incidents
- receive shore-to-ship distress alerts
- receive ship-to-ship distress alerts
- transmit and receive communications for SAR coordination.

Distress alerting

GMDSS caters for three independent methods of distress-alerting. These are:

1 Float-free or manually operated 406 MHz EPlRBs using the COSPAS/SARSAT satellite system or, in the 1·6 GHz band, the INMARSAT system. Both transmit distress messages which include the position of the vessel in distress and its identification. Some 406 MHz EPlRBs also transmit on 121·5 MHz to aid close-quarters homing.

2 Digital selective calling (DSC) using HF distress and alerting frequencies in the 4, 6, 8,12 and 16 MHz bands, MF 2187·5 kHz or VHF Ch70.

3 INMARSAT, via ship terminals, using voice, data or Telex.

In addition to this, GMDSS includes Navtex for receiving Marine Safety Information and Search and Rescue Transponders (SARTs). The latter are intended for operation from a lifeboat or liferaft to assist homing. When interrogated by a ship's radar, the SART responds by transmitting a series of radar pulses. Some float-free 406 MHz EPIRBs include a built-in SART.

GMDSS Communication systems

A number of terrestrial and satellite-based communications systems have been adopted for GMDSS. These are:

Digital Selective Calling. DSC is a fundamental part of GMDSS and is used to transmit distress alerts from ships, and also to receive distress acknowledgments from ships or shore stations. DSC can also be used for relay purposes and for other urgency or safety calls. Operationally, a distress call sent over VHF radio using DSC would roughly work as follows: yachtsman presses the distress button. The set automatically re-tunes itself to Ch 70 and transmits a coded distress message before re-tuning to Ch l6.

Any ship will reply directly by voice on Ch 16. However, a CRS would send a Distress Acknowledgement on Ch 70 (automatically turning off the distress transmission) before replying on Ch 16. Distress messages will be automatically repeated every four to five minutes unless already acknowledged by a CRS. Under GMDSS, every yacht will have a nine-digit identification number (referred to as an MMSCI - Maritime Mobile Selective Call Identity code) that is used in any automatically generated distress message.

INMARSAT. GMDSS communications are also provided via four geostationary satellites covering the east and west Atlantic, Pacific and Indian Ocean regions from about 70°N to 70°S. The INMARSAT system is combined with conventional Coast Radio Stations using HF, MF and VHF to provide near global coverage.

Additionally, 1·6 GHz satellite EPIRBs, operating through INMARSAT, can also be used for alerting as an alternative to 406 MHz EPIRBs which use COSPAS/SARSAT.

COSPAS/SARSAT. The US/Russian COSPAS/SARSAT satellites complement the various satcom systems available by not only providing an effective initial detection of an emergency signal transmitted by an EPIRB, but also its location to a high degree of accuracy. There are four COSPAS/SARSAT satellites operating in Polar orbits.

Marine Safety Information (MSI). MSI includes the vital meteorological, navigational and SAR messages broadcast to all vessels at sea. For this purpose the world is divided into 16 Navareas. The UK lies in Navarea I, which covers all North West Europe between 48°N and 71°N and to 35°W. Traditionally, these MSI broadcasts have been made from CRSs by Morse and RT on MF and VHF. Under GMDSS, broadcasts are made 'automatically' through INMARSAT's enhanced group calling (EGC) system; INMARSAT C, and, particularly for those broadcasts appertaining to the UK coast, Navtex on 518kHz.

Currently MSI is being broadcast on all these systems. From 1999 it is highly probable that MSI will only be broadcast using Navtex and INMARSAT. A Navtex receiver meets the requirements for coastal waters up to about 300 miles from transmitters, but an INMARSAT C Enhanced Group Calling (EGC) receiver is required when operating beyond MF coverage.

Implementation. The speed with which the shore-based side of GMDSS is introduced varies from sea area to sea area according to the policy of its controlling government. For purposes of the GMDSS, each sea area lies within one of the following classes:

• **A1** - an area within RT coverage of at least one VHF Coast Radio Station in which continuous alerting via digital selective calling (see later in text) is available. Range: approximately 40 miles of the CRS.
• **A2** - an area, excluding sea area A1, within RT coverage of at least one MF CRS in which continuous DSC alerting is available. Range: roughly 100-150 miles of the CRS.
• **A3** - an area, exccluding sea areas A1 and A2 within coverage of an INMARSAT satellite in which continuous alerting is available.
•**A4** - an area outside sea areas A1, A2 and A3. In practice this means the polar regions.

The UK intends to keep Channel 16 in operation for some time ahead and is expected to declare the UK as an A1 area. This will be implemented around the UK coastline over a three year period commencing in 1996. The Channel will be completed first, then working round the coast in an anti-clockwise direction to complete the network by 1 Feb 1999.

The French have already declared the English Channel to be an A1 Area and this came into effect in 1995. To take full advantage of GMDSS procedures it will be necessary for yachts to re-equip for operation in A1 Areas.

As most UK yachtsmen will mainly operate in an A1 area, a VHF set and a Navtex will initially suffice to meet GMDSS requirements. When suitable VHF DSC yacht sets become available it will make sense to equip your yacht with DSC equipment.

8.4   SEARCH AND RESCUE (SAR)

8.4.1   SAR – general

Various authorities are involved in SAR operations. Around the United Kingdom, the lead authority is HM Coastguard who is responsible for initiating and coordinating all civil maritime SAR. To assist them, Coast Radio Stations monitor distress frequencies and control ship/shore communications (see 6.3.9); the RNLI supplies and mans lifeboats; the Royal Navy assists with ships; and the Royal Air Force, through two Military Rescue Coordination Centres (RCC) at Edinburgh and Plymouth, controls all military helicopters and fixed wing aircraft involved in SAR. Air Traffic Control Centres (ATCC) listen out on air distress frequencies and report to the military RCCs.

The military RCC at Plymouth also mans the United Kingdom COSPAS-SARSAT Mission Control Centre (MCC) which receives satellite data on emergency distress beacons on 121·5 MHz, 243 MHz and 406 MHz. Similar organisations to the above exist in other countries in Western Europe – see 10.12.7 (Republic of Ireland), 10.15.8 (France), 10.20.7 (Belgium, Netherlands), 10.21.7 (Germany).

8.4.2   HM Coastguard

The Coastguard initiates and coordinates SAR around the United Kingdom and over a large part of the eastern Atlantic. The area is divided into six Maritime Search and Rescue Regions (SRRs), supervised by Maritime Rescue Coordination Centres (MRCCs) at Falmouth, Dover, Great Yarmouth, Aberdeen, the Clyde and Swansea. It also includes 'Shannon' area which is the responsibility of the Republic of Ireland. Each SRR is divided into Districts, each with a Maritime Rescue Sub-Centre (MRSC). Their boundaries are shown in the maps at the start of Areas 1–11 in Chapter 10. The telephone number of the nearest MRCC or MRSC (or the equivalent in other countries) is shown for each harbour.

Within each of the 21 districts thus formed there is an organisation of Auxiliary Coastguard watch and rescue stations, grouped within Sectors under the management of regular Coastguard Officers.

All MRCCs and MRSCs keep watch on VHF Ch 16, and are connected to telex and telephone. A visual look-out is maintained when necessary. The Channel Navigation Information Service (CNIS) keeps a constant radar watch on the Separation Zones and provides a 24- hour radio safety service for all shipping in the Dover Strait. CNIS broadcasts navigational and traffic information on VHF Ch 11 at 40 (and 55 minutes past each hour in periods of restricted visibility). There are about 490 Regular Coastguard Officers, backed up by more than 4400 Auxiliaries on

8

call for emergencies. The Coastguard also has a cliff and beach rescue role.

A VHF emergency direction finding service, controlled by the Coastguard, is operated from various stations round Britain (see 4.5.1).

The radiotelephony call sign of an MRCC or MRSC is the geographical name, followed by 'Coastguard' – for example 'SOLENT COASTGUARD'.

The Coastguard operates a Local Warning Service related to hazards which may affect craft in inshore waters, but outside Port and Harbour Authority limits. These local warnings are broadcast on Ch 67, after an announcement on Ch 16. There is no numerical sequence, and no specific broadcast schedule; any repetition of the broadcast is at the discretion of the originating Coastguard station. Strong wind warnings are broadcast on receipt, and forecasts for local sea areas about every four hours or on request. See also 7.2.19.

Yacht and Boat Safety Scheme
This free scheme provides useful information for the Coastguard to mount a successful SAR operation. Owners can obtain a Form CG66 from their local Coastguard station, harbour master or marina. This should be completed with details of the boat and her equipment, and then posted to the local Coastguard Rescue Centre. It is desirable to enclose a recent photograph of your craft if you have one. You should inform the Coastguard if the ownership, name of the craft, or any address given on form CG66 changes. There is a tear-off section which can be given to a friend or relative so that they know the Coastguard station to contact if they are concerned for the boat's safety.

A CG66 will remain valid for three years. If it is not renewed within that time, the old CG66 will be invalid and removed from the CG records.

It is not the function of HM Coastguard to maintain watch for boats on passage, but they will record information by phone before departure or from intermediate ports, or while on passage by visual signals or VHF Ch 67 (the Small Craft Safety Channel). When using Ch 67 for safety messages it is requested that yachts give the name of the Coastguard Rescue Centre holding the boat's Safety Scheme card. In these circumstances the Coastguard must be told of any change to the planned movements of the boat, and it is important that they are informed of the boat's safe arrival at her ultimate destination.

Raising the alarm
If an accident afloat is seen from shore, dial 999 and ask for the Coastguard. You will be asked to report on the incident, and possibly to stay near the telephone for further communications. If at sea you receive a distress signal and you are in a position to give assistance, you are obliged to do so with all speed, unless or until you are specifically released.

When alerted the Coastguard summons the most appropriate help, they may direct vessels in the vicinity

of the distress position; request the launch of an RNLI lifeboat; scramble a military or Coastguard SAR helicopter; other vessels may be alerted through Coast Radio Stations or by Satellite communications.

8.4.3   France - CROSS
France has five Regional Surveillance and Rescue Operations Centres (Centres Régionaux Opérationnels de Surveillance et de Sauvetage – CROSS).

A CROSS centre is an MRCC, and a Sous-CROSS centre is an MRSC. The areas of responsibility for each centre are shown on Fig. 8(3). All CROSS stations keep watch on Ch 16, and broadcast local navigational warnings, weather messages and strom warnings

CROSS Étel specialises in providing medical advice and also responds to alerts from COSPAS-SARSAT satellites, via the Mission Control Centre in Toulon.

CROSS stations have other functions including:

a. maritime Search and Rescue.
b. navigational surveillance, especially within the 12M limit.
c. the broadcast of meteorological information.
d. the broadcast of navigational warnings.

CROSS stations do not have any public correspondence role and should not be used as a Coast Radio Station. However, for convenience, details of CROSS station communications facilities are shown in 6.3.28 and on Fig. 6(4). Details of CROSS weather broadcasts are shown in Table 7(5).

8.4.4   Royal National Lifeboat Institution (RNLI)
The RNLI is a registered charity which exists to save life at sea. It provides, on call, a 24-hour lifeboat service up to 50M out from the coasts of the UK and Irish Republic. There are 211 stations, at which are stationed 269 lifeboats ranging from 4·9 to 16·5m in length, with a ratio of around 50% being all-weather and the other 50% inshore. There are over 100 lifeboats in reserve.

All lifeboats are capable of at least 15 knots, and new lifeboats with a speed of 25 knots are beginning to be introduced.

When launched on service lifeboats over 10m keep watch on 2182 kHz and Ch 16. They can also use alternative frequencies to contact other vessels, SAR aircraft, HM Coastguard or Coast Radio Stations or other SAR agencies. All lifeboats are fitted with VHF and show a quick-flashing blue light.

Similar organisations to the RNLI exist in other countries in Western Europe. The positions of lifeboat stations are indicated on the Area maps at the front of each Area in Chapter 10.

Yachtsmen can help support the RNLI by becoming members of the RNLI and there is also a junior club for under sixteens called 'Storm Force'. Details are available from RNLI HQ, West Quay Road, Poole, Dorset BH15 1HZ (☎ 01202 671133. Fax: 01202 670128).

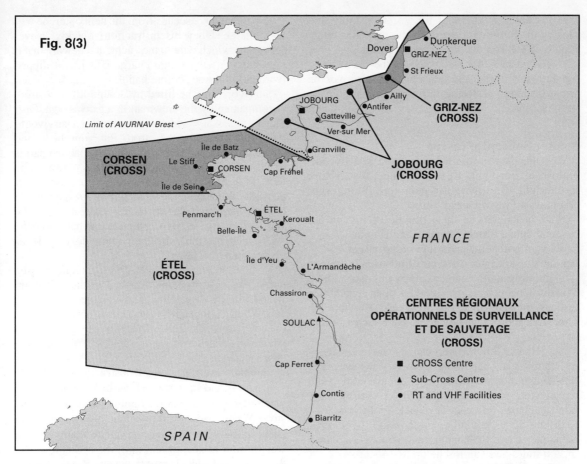

Fig. 8(3)

Limit of AVURNAV Brest

Dover
GRIZ-NEZ
Dunkerque
St Frieux
GRIZ-NEZ
(CROSS)
Ailly
Antifer
JOBOURG
Gatteville
Ver-sur-Mer
JOBOURG
(CROSS)
Granville

CORSEN
(CROSS)
Île de Batz
Le Stiff
CORSEN
Cap Fréhel
Île de Sein

ÉTEL
Penmarc'h
Keroualt
Belle-Île

ÉTEL
(CROSS)
Île d'Yeu
L'Armandèche

Chassiron

SOULAC

FRANCE

CENTRES RÉGIONAUX
OPÉRATIONNELS DE SURVEILLANCE
ET DE SAUVETAGE
(CROSS)

■ CROSS Centre
▲ Sub-Cross Centre
● RT and VHF Facilities

Cap Ferret

Contis

Biarritz

SPAIN

8.4.5   Visual signals from shore to ships in distress

The following are used to a vessel in distress or stranded off the coast of the United Kingdom.

(1) Acknowledgment of distress signal

By day: Orange smoke signal, or combined light and sound signal consisting of three signals fired at about one minute intervals.

By night: White star rocket consisting of three single signals at about one minute intervals.

(2) Landing signals for small boats

'This is the best place to land' – Vertical motion of a white flag or arms (or white light or flare by night), or signalling K (–•–) by light or sound. An indication of direction may be given by placing a steady white light or flare at a lower level.

'Landing here is highly dangerous' – Horizontal motion a white flag or arms extended horizontally (or a white light or flare by night), or signalling S (•••). In addition, a better landing place may be signalled by carrying a white flag (or flare or light), or by firing a white star signal in the direction indicated; or by signalling R (•–•) if a better landing is to the right in the direction of approach, or L (•–••) if it is to the left.

(3) Signals for shore life-saving apparatus

Affirmative or specifically 'Rocket line is held', 'Tail block is made fast', 'Hawser is made fast', 'Man is in breeches buoy' or 'Haul away' – vertical motion of a white flag or the arms (or of a white light or flare).

'Negative' or specifically 'Slack away' or 'Avast hauling' – horizontal motion of a white flag or the arms (or of a white light or flare).

(4) Warning signal

'You are running into danger' – International Code signal U (••–) or NF.

Note: Attention may be called to the above signals by a white flare, a white star rocket, or an explosive signal.

8.4.6   Signals used by SAR aircraft

A searching aircraft normally flies at about 3000–5000ft (900–1500m), or below cloud, firing a green Very light every five or ten minutes and at each turning point. On seeing a green flare, a yacht in distress should take the following action:

(1) Wait for the green flare to die out.
(2) Fire one red flare.
(3) Fire another red flare after about 20 seconds. (This enables the aircraft to line up on the bearing.)
(4) Fire a third red flare when the aircraft is overhead, or appears to be going badly off course.

8.4.7   Directing signals by aircraft

(1) To direct a yacht towards a ship or aircraft in distress –the aircraft circles the yacht at least once; it

8

then crosses low ahead of the yacht, opening and closing the throttle or changing the propeller pitch. Finally it heads in the direction of the casualty.

(2) To indicate that assistance of the yacht is no longer required – the aircraft passes low, astern of the yacht, opening and closing the throttle or changing the propeller pitch.

8.4.8   Helicopter rescue

SAR helicopters in the UK are based at Chivenor, Culdrose, Portland, Lee-on-Solent, Wattisham, Leconfield, Boulmer, Lossiemouth, Sumburgh, Stornoway, Prestwick and Valley.

SAR helicopters in the Republic of Ireland are based at Finner Camp, Shannon and Dublin.

Wessex SAR helicopters, now based only at Valley, can carry up to 10 survivors, but do not usually operate at night, or when the wind exceeds 45 knots. Whilst Wessex helicopters can be used for night searches or rescues, they are limited to night rescues where the pilot has a good visual hover reference such as a well lit vessel.

Sea King SAR helicopters can operate to a distance of 300 miles and can rescue up to 18 survivors. The Sea King has an automatic hover control system and so can effect rescues at night and in fog when there are no visual hover references available to the pilot.

In the Irish Republic a Sikorskt S61N SAR helicopter, based at Shannon, can operate to a distance of 200 miles and can rescue up to 14 survivors. A Dauphin SA 365F helicopter, based at Finner Camp, can operate to 150 miles by day and 70 miles at night.

SAR helicopters are generally fitted with VHF, FM and AM, UHF and HF SSB RT and can communicate with lifeboats etc. on VHF FM. Communications between ship and helicopter should normally be achieved on Marine band VHF FM (Ch 16 or 67). 2182 kHz SSB may also be available. If contact is difficult, communication can often be achieved through a Nimrod aircraft if one is on the scene, or through a lifeboat, a Coast Radio Station, or through HM Coastguard.

When the helicopter is sighted by a boat in distress, a flare, an orange smoke signal, dye marker or a well trained Aldis lamp will assist recognition (very important if there are other vessels in the vicinity). Dodgers with the boat's name or sail number are useful aids to identification.

While hovering, the pilot has limited vision beneath him, and relies on instructions from the winch operator. Survivors from a yacht with a mast may need to be picked up from a dinghy or liferaft streamed at least 100ft (30m) away. In a small yacht with no dinghy, survivors (wearing lifejackets) may need to be picked up from the water, at the end of a long warp. It is very important that no survivor boards a liferaft or jumps into the sea until instructed to do so by the helicopter (either by VHF Ch 16 or 67) or by the winchman (by word of mouth). Sails should be lowered and lashed and it is helpful if the drift of the boat is reduced by a sea anchor.

If a crewman descends from the helicopter, he will take charge. Obey his instructions quickly. Never secure the winch wire to the yacht, and beware that it may carry a lethal static charge if it is not dipped (earthed) in the sea before handling.

Survivors may be lifted by double lift in a strop, accompanied by the crewman in a canvas seat. Or it may be necessary, with no crewman, for a survivor to position himself in the strop. Put your head and shoulders through the strop so that the padded part is in the small of the back and the toggle is in front of the face. Pull the toggle down, as close to the chest as possible. When ready, give a thumbs up sign with an extended arm, and place both arms close down by the side of the body (resist the temptation to hang onto the strop). On reaching the helicopter, do exactly as instructed by the crew.

In some circumstances a 'Hi-line technique' may be used. This is a rope tail, attached to the helicopter winch wire by a weak link, and weighted at its lower end. When it is lowered to the yacht do not make it fast, but coil it down carefully. The helicopter pays out the winch wire and then moves to one side of the yacht and descends, while the yacht takes in the slack (keeping it outboard and clear of all obstructions) until the winch hook and strop are on board. A member of the helicopter crew may or may not be lowered with the strop. When ready to lift, the helicopter ascends and takes in the wire. Pay out the tail, keeping enough weight on it to keep it taut until the end is reached, then cast it off well clear of the yacht. But if a further lift is to be made the tail should be retained on board (not made fast) to facilitate recovery of the strop for the next lift.

Injured persons can be lifted strapped into a special stretcher carried in the helicopter.

When alighting from a helicopter, beware of the tail rotor which can be difficult to see. Obey all instructions given by the helicopter crew.

8.4.9   Abandon ship

Although preparations must be made, do not abandon a yacht until she is doomed. She is a better target for rescue craft than a liferaft, and while she is still afloat it is possible to use her resources (such as RT, for distress calls) and to select what extra equipment is put in the liferaft or lashed into the dinghy (which should be taken too, if possible).

Before entering the raft, and cutting it adrift:

(1) Send a distress message (Mayday call), saying that yacht is being abandoned, and position.

(2) Dress warmly with sweaters etc. under oilskins, and lifejackets on top. Take extra clothes.

(3) Fill any available containers with tops about 3/4 full with fresh water, so that they will float.

(4) Collect additional food – tins and tin opener.

(5) Collect navigational gear, torch, extra flares, bucket, length of line, First Aid kit, knife etc.

Once in the liferaft, plan for the worst. If there has not been time to collect items listed above, collect whatever flotsam is available.

(1) Keep the inside of the raft as dry as possible. Huddle together for warmth. Close the openings as necessary, but keep a good look-out for shipping and aircraft.

(2) Stream the drogue if necessary for stability, or if it is required to stay near the position.

(3) Ration fresh water to 3/4 pint (1/2 litre) per person per day. Do not drink sea water or urine. Collect rain water.

(4) Use flares sparingly, on the skipper's orders.

(5) Issue and commence taking anti-seasick pills.

8.4.10   Emergency Position Indicating Radio Beacons (EPIRBs)

Many yachts now carry EPIRB's which transmit on the emergency frequencies of 406 MHz and/or 121·5 MHz and 243 MHz. Transmissions on all three frequencies can be picked up by the COSPAS-SARSAT (C-S) system which uses 4 near-polar orbital satellites to detect and localise the signals. The processed positions are passed automatically to a Mission Control Centre (MCC) for assessment of any SAR action required; the UK MCC is co-located with RCC Plymouth.

C-S location accuracy is normally better than 5 km on 406 MHz and better than 20 km on 121·5 and 243 MHz. Within the North American area, the maximum waiting time (i.e. the time between EPIRB activation and satellite detection) should not exceed 90 minutes and will normally be much quicker. 121·5 MHz and 243·0 MHz are not generally monitored by ships, Coast Radio Stations or the Coastguard but are monitored by Air Traffic Control and many aircraft; survivors should switch on an EPIRB without delay.

Dedicated SAR aircraft can home on 121·5 MHz and 243·0 MHz but not on 406 MHz. Typically a helicopter at 1,000 feet can receive homing signals from about 30M range whilst a fixed wing aircraft at higher altitudes is capable of homing from about 60M. Overflying aircraft operating on normal commercial air routes often receive and relay information on alerts on 121·5 MHz EPIRBs at up to 200M range. Best results are likely to be obtained from 406 MHz EPIRBs which also transmit a 121·5 MHz signal for homing.

406 MHz EPIRBs transmit data with a unique code which identifies the individual beacon and therefore the individual yacht. However, it is absolutely essential for the integrity of the system that details of all yachts on which 406 MHz EPIRBs are carried are sent for registration to: DSG 1A, Marine Safety Agency, Spring Place, 105 Commercial Road, Southampton SO1 0ZD. Registration details should be submitted on the form provided by the EPIRB manufacturer at the point of sale. It is equally important that any changes of ownership of a 406 MHz EPIRB, or its disposal in any other way, are also notified.

The rising number of false alerts caused by inadvertent or incorrect operation of EPIRBs is putting a significant burden on SAR assets. The chances of false alerts coinciding with a real distress situation are very real and as a consequence SAR forces could be delayed in responding to a real distress – with tragic consequences.

EPIRBs must be installed and used in accordance with manufacturers' recommendations. Dependent on type, they must be installed in a proper location so they can float free and automatically activate if the yacht sinks. Many EPIRBs have lanyards intended to secure the EPIRB to a life raft or person in the water and lanyards must not be used for securing the EPIRB to the yacht. Such action will clearly prevent a float free type from activating and would be lost with the yacht should it sink.

Once an EPIRB is activated, whether accidentally or intentionally, make every reasonable attempt to communicate with SAR authorities by other means to advise them of the situation.

8.5   HAZARDS

8.5.1   Submarine hazard and broadcast warnings of submarine activity

There have been a number of incidents in which fishing vessels and occasionally yachts have been snagged or hit by submarines operating just below the surface.

The best advice available to yachts is:

(1) Listen to broadcasts of Submarine activity (SUBFACTS).

(2) Where possible avoid charted Submarine Exercise Areas.

(3) Keep clear of any surface vessel flying the International Code Flag Group 'NE2' which denotes that submarines are in the vicinity.

(4) Run your engine or generator even when under sail.

(5) Operate your echo sounder.

(6) At night show deck level navigation lights i.e. on pulpit and stern.

The risk is greatest in the W English Channel, Scottish and Irish waters, including the Clyde and North Channel and at night. Within these waters 104 geographic areas have been designated as Submarine Exercise Areas (see 10.1.18, 10.8.20 and 10.9.22 for charts).

The following BT Coast Radio Stations broadcast details of planned submarine activity in the W English Channel at 0733 and 1933 UT after gale warnings or weather forecasts:

Ilfracombe (Ch 05),
Land's End (Ch 27, 64, and 2670 kHz),
Pendennis (Ch 62),
Start Point (Ch 26).

8

The following BT Coast Radio Stations broadcast details of planned submarine activity in Scottish and Irish Waters at 0303, 0703, 1103, 1503, 1903 and 2303 UT:

Lewis (Ch 05),
Hebrides (Ch 26 and 1866 kHz),
Skye (Ch 24),
Oban (Ch 07),
Islay (Ch 25),
Clyde (Ch 26),
Portpatrick (Ch 27 and 1883 kHz),
Morecambe Bay (Ch 82),
Anglesey (Ch 26),
Cardigan Bay (Ch 03),

Information relating to submarine activity in the area between Cape Wrath and Latitude 54°N is also broadcast by Coastguard stations as follows:

Stornoway	Ch 16 on request
Oban	Ch 16 on request
Clyde	Ch 67 every 4h from 0020 LT
Belfast	Ch 16 on reques

8.5.2 Gunfacts

Gunfacts is a warning service to provide mariners with information on Naval practice firing intentions. Such warnings pose no restriction on the passage of any vessel. The onus for safety lies with the naval unit concerned.

Gunfacts includes planned or known underwater explosions; gunnery and missile firings. Broadcasts for underwater explosions only will be made on Ch 16 at H–1, –30m, and immediately prior to detonation.

No Gunfacts broadcasts are made on days when no firings are intended. Gunfacts broadcasts will include:

(1)   LT and approximate location of intended firings with a declared safe distance in M.

(2)   Whether illuminants are to be fired.

Gunfacts are promulgated by the Naval Operations room Plymouth for the English Channel areas, and for all other areas by a nominated Duty Broadcast Ship (Gunfacts - Ship).

Gunfacts – Plymouth will cover activity in the English Channel area, including the firing times only for the Portland and Portsmouth firing and practice exercise areas.

Gunfacts – Ship will cover activity in all other areas including Plymouth (outside the English Channel areas), Portsmouth, Scotland and Northern Ireland. Broadcasts will be made twice daily at 0800 and 1400 LT on Ch 16 before changing to Ch 06 or 67.

BT CRS Southern Region broadcast Gunfacts when in force at 0733 and 1933 UT following the scheduled weather forecast.

Chapter 9

Tides

Contents

9

Tides – introduction

Here in the Almanac sufficient information is given for the use of the tidal data provided in Chapter 10, but for fuller details of tides and the sea, reference should be made to Chapter 9 of *The Macmillan & Silk Cut Yachtsman's Handbook*.

The following subjects are described in detail in Chapter 9 of *The Macmillan & Silk Cut Yachtsman's Handbook*:
The theory of tides; definitions of terms; calculations of times and heights of HW and LW; calculations of depths of water at specific times; calculations of times at which tide reaches certain heights; Twelfths Rule; tidal calculations by pocket calculator; French tidal coefficients; co-tidal and co-range charts; harmonic constituents; establishment of a port; tidal stream diamonds; tidal stream information on charts and in Sailing Directions, plus: general information on the sea – how waves are formed; freak waves; wind against tide; bars; overfalls and tide races; refraction of waves; reflected waves; ocean currents etc.

9.1   GENERAL

9.1.1   Explanation

This chapter explains how to use the tidal information contained in Chapter 10, where the daily times and heights of High Water (HW) and Low Water (LW) for Standard Ports are given, together with time and height differences for many Secondary Ports. Tidal predictions are for average meteorological conditions. In abnormal weather the times and heights of HW and LW may vary considerably. (See 9.8.)

9.1.2   Times

The times of Standard Port predictions in Chapter 10 are given in the Zone Time indicated at the top left-hand corner of each page. Nearly all countries, and most ships, prefer to keep their clocks set to a whole number of hours ahead or behind UT.

The world is divided into 24 time zones. Each zone is 1 hour, or 15° of longitude wide. The zone number indicates the number of hours by which the zone time must be decreased or increased to obtain UT. Zones to the East of Greenwich are named minus (–), those to the West plus (+). Zone 0 is centred on the Greenwich meridian and extends from 7½°W to 7½°E and the time kept corresponds to UT.

Tidal predictions for Standard Ports in the UK, Channel Islands and the Republic of Ireland are given in UT (Zone 0), and those for Standard Ports in France, Belgium, Netherlands and Germany are given in UT+1 (Zone –1). To convert these Zone – 0100 times to UT, subtract one hour.

Those periods in which DST (BST in UK) applies are indicated by the absence of green tinting, and one hour must be added to obtain DST (= LT).

Under each Secondary Port listed in Chapter 10 are its Time Zone, its Standard Port and the data required to calculate time differences, which when applied to the printed times of HW and LW at the Standard Port, give the times of HW and LW at the Secondary Port in the Zone Time of that Port. If DST is required, then one hour is added after the Secondary Port time difference has been applied but not before.

9.1.3   Predicted heights

Predicted heights are given in metres and tenths of metres above chart datum (CD) (see 9.2.1). Care must be taken when using charts which show depths in fathoms/feet. A table for converting Feet to Metres and Metres to Feet is given in 2.7.3.

9.2   DEFINITIONS

Certain definitions are given below and in Fig. 9 (1). For further details see Chapter 9 of *The Macmillan & Silk Cut Yachtsman's Handbook*.

9.2.1   Chart datum

Chart datum (CD) is the reference level above which heights of tide are predicted, and below which charted depths are measured. Hence the actual depth of water is the charted depth (at that place) plus the height of tide (at that time).

Tidal predictions for most British ports use as their datum Lowest Astronomical Tide (LAT), which is the lowest sea level predicted under average meteorological conditions. All Admiralty Charts of the British Isles use LAT as chart datum, but others, particularly fathom charts, do not. Where tidal predictions and charted depths are not referenced to the same datum (e.g. LAT), errors resulting in an over estimation of depth by as much as 0·5m can occur.

9.2.2   Charted depth

Charted depth is the distance of the sea bed below chart datum, and is shown in metres and tenths of metres on metric charts, or in fathoms and/or feet on older charts. Make sure you know which units are used.

9.2.3   Drying height

Drying height is the height above chart datum of the top of any feature at times covered by water. The figures are underlined on the chart, in metres and tenths of metres on metric charts, and in fathoms and feet on older charts. The depth is the height of tide (at the time) minus the drying height. If the result is negative, then that feature is above sea level.

9.2.4   Duration

Duration is the time between LW and the next HW, normally slightly more than six hours, and can be used to calculate the approximate time of LW when only the time of HW is known.

9.2.5   Height of tide

The height of the tide is the vertical distance of sea level above (or very occasionally below) chart datum, as defined in 9.2.1.

9.2.6   Interval

The interval is the period of time between a given time and the time of HW, expressed in hours and minutes before (–) or after (+) HW. Intervals are printed in increments of one hour (–1hr and +1hr) along the bottom of each tidal curve in Chapter 10. For examples, see Figs. 9 (4) and 9 (5).

9.2.7   Mean High Water and Low Water Springs/Neaps

Mean High Water Springs (MHWS) and Mean High Water Neaps (MHWN) are the averages of the predicted heights of the Spring or Neap tides at HW over a period of 18·6 years. Similarly, Mean Low Water Springs (MLWS) and Neaps (MLWN) are the average heights of low water for the spring and neap tides respectively. Charted heights of land objects such as lights, bridges etc are referred to the level of MHWS. On French charts these charted elevations are referred to as ML rather than MHWS.

9.2.8   Mean Level

Mean Level (ML) is the average of the heights of Mean High Water Springs (MHWS), Mean High Water Neaps (MHWN), Mean Low Water Springs (MLWS) and Mean Low Water Neaps (MLWN).

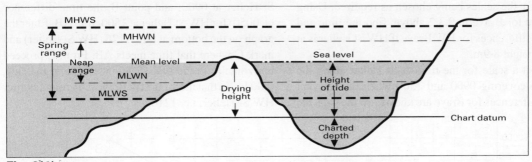

Fig. 9(1)

9.2.9   Range
The range of a tide is the difference between the heights of successive High and Low Waters.

Spring range is the difference between MHWS and MLWS, and Neap range is the difference between MHWN and MLWN.

9.2.10   Tidal coefficients
In France the size (range) of a tide and its proximity to Springs/Neaps is quantified by Tidal Coefficients which are listed and explained in 10.16.25.

9.2.11   Rise/Fall of tide
The rise of the tide is the amount the tide has risen since the earlier Low Water. The fall of the tide is the amount the tide has fallen since the last High Water.

9.3   CALCULATIONS OF TIMES AND HEIGHTS OF HIGH AND LOW WATER

9.3.1   Standard Ports
The times and heights of HW and LW are tabulated for each Standard Port in Chapter 10. The conversion of Zone – 0100 time to UT and of either Zone UT or Zone – 0100 time to Local Summer or Daylight Saving Time (DST) is dealt with in 9.1.2. See also 9.8 for the effect of wind and barometric pressure.

9.3.2   Secondary Ports – times of HW and LW
Each Secondary Port listed in Chapter 10 has a data block for the calculation of times of HW and LW as explained in 9.1.2. The following example is for Braye (Alderney):

TIDES
– 0400 Dover; ML 3·6; Duration 0545; Zone 0 (UT).

Standard Port ST HELIER (⟶)

Times				Height (metres)			
High Water		Low Water		MHWS	MHWN	MLWN	MLWS
0300	0900	0200	0900	11·0	8·1	4·0	1·4
1500	2100	1400	2100				
Differences BRAYE							
+0050	+0040	+0025	+0105	−4·8	−3·4	−1·5	−0·5

Thus – 0400 Dover indicates that, on average, HW Braye occurs 4 hours 00 minutes before HW Dover (the times of HW Dover, in UT, can be found on the bookmark). Duration 0545 indicates that LW Braye occurs 5 hours and 45 minutes before its HW. This is a very rough and ready method.

A more accurate and reliable method uses the Standard Port and Time Differences in the table. Thus when HW at St Helier occurs at 0900 and 2100, the Difference is + 0040, and HW at Braye occurs at 0940 and 2140. When HW at St Helier occurs at 0300 and 1500, the Difference is + 0050, and HW Braye then occurs at 0350 and 1550. If, as is likely, HW St Helier occurs at some other time, then the Difference for Braye must be found by interpolation – by eye, by the graphical method, or by calculator. Thus, by eye, when HW St Helier occurs at 1200, the Difference is + 0045, and HW Braye occurs at 1245. The same method is used for calculating the times of LW.

The times thus obtained are in the Zone Time indicated in the Secondary Port data block. Care must be taken when the Zone Time at the Secondary Port differs from that at the Standard Port. See 9.1.2 for converting time from one zone to another and for changing to Daylight Saving Time (DST).

9.3.3   Secondary Ports – heights of HW and LW
The Secondary Port data block also contains height Differences which are applied to the heights of HW and LW at the Standard Port. Thus when the height of HW at St Helier is 11·0m (MHWS), the Difference is – 4·8m, and the height of HW at Braye is 6·2m (MHWS). When the height of HW at St Helier is 8·1m (MHWN), the Difference is – 3·4m, and the height of HW at Braye is 4·7m (MHWN). If, as is likely, the height of tide at the Standard Port does not exactly equal the Mean Spring or Neap level, then the height Difference is found. Thus if the height of HW at St Helier is 9·55m, the Difference is – 4·1m, and the height of HW at Braye is 5·45m.

9.3.4   Graphical method for interpolating time and height differences

Any suitable squared paper can be used, see Figs. 9(2) and 9(3), the scales being chosen as required. Using the data for Braye in 9.3.2 above, find the time and height differences for HW Braye if HW St Helier is at 1126, height 8·9m.

Select a scale for the time at St Helier along the bottom covering 0900 and 1500 when the relevant time differences for Braye are known. At the side, the scale for time differences must cover + 0040 and + 0050, the two which are shown for times 0900 and 1500.

Plot point A, the time difference (+ 0040) for HW St Helier at 0900; and point B, the time difference (+ 0050) for HW St Helier at 1500. Join AB. Enter the graph on the bottom at time 1126 (HW St Helier) and mark C where that time meets AB. From C proceed horizontally to the time difference scale at the side, + 0044. So that morning HW Braye is 44 minutes after HW St Helier, i.e. 1210.

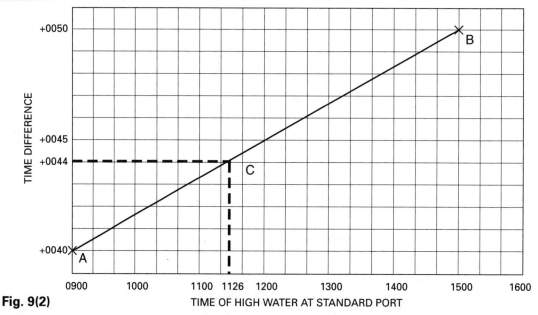

Fig. 9(2)   TIME OF HIGH WATER AT STANDARD PORT

In Fig. 9 (3), the selected scales cover the height of HW at St Helier horizontally (i.e. 8·1 to 11·0m) and the relevant height differences (− 3·4 to − 4·8m) vertically. Plot point D, the height difference (− 3·4m) at neaps when the height of HW St Helier is 8·1m; and E, the height difference (− 4·8m) at springs when the height of HW St Helier is 11·0m. Join DE. Enter the graph at 8·9m (the height of HW St Helier that morning) and mark F where that height meets DE. From F follow the horizontal line to the scale of height differences, − 3·8m. So that morning the height of HW Braye is 5·1m.

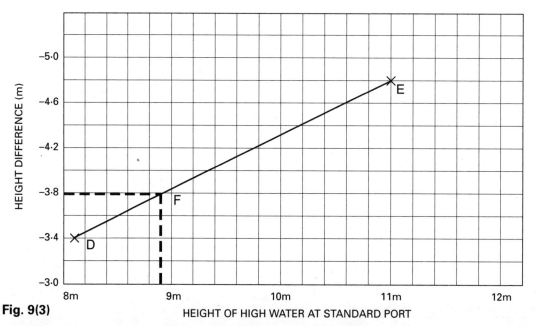

Fig. 9(3)   HEIGHT OF HIGH WATER AT STANDARD PORT

9.4   CALCULATING INTERMEDIATE TIMES AND HEIGHTS OF TIDE

9.4.1   Standard Ports

Intermediate times and heights are best calculated from the Mean Spring and Neap Curves for Standard Ports in Chapter 10. Examples below are for Leith, on a day when the predictions are:

	UT	Ht (m)
22	0202	5·3
	0752	1·0
	1417	5·4
Tu	2025	0·5

Example: Find the height of tide at Leith at 1200.

(1) On the Leith tidal diagram plot the heights of HW and LW each side of the required time, and join them by a sloping line, Fig. 9(4).

(2) Enter the HW time and other times as necessary in the boxes below the curves.

(3) From the required time, proceed vertically to the curves. The Spring curve is a solid line, and the Neap curve (where it differs) is pecked. Interpolate between the curves by comparing the actual range – 4·4m in this example – with the Mean Ranges printed beside the curves. Never extrapolate. Here the Spring curve applies.

(4) Proceed horizontally to the sloping line plotted in (1), and thence vertically to the height scale, to give 4·2m.

Example: To find the time at which the afternoon height of tide falls to 3·7m:

(1) On the Leith tidal diagram, plot the heights of HW and LW each side of the required event, and join them by a sloping line, Fig. 9(5).

(2) Enter the HW time and others to cover the required event, in the boxes below.

(3) From the required height, proceed vertically to the sloping line and thence horizontally to the curves. Interpolate between them as in the previous example and do not extrapolate. Here the actual range is 4·9m, and the Spring curve applies.

(4) Proceed vertically to the time scale, and read off the time required, 1637.

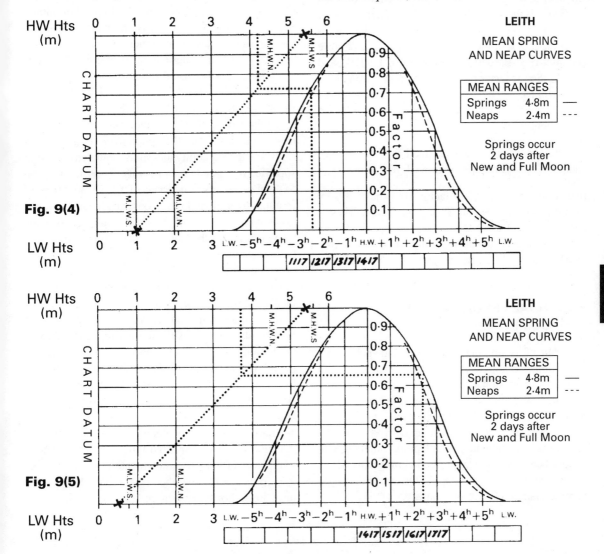

9.4.2   Secondary Ports

On coasts where there is little change of shape between tidal curves for adjacent Standard Ports, and where the duration of rise or fall at the Secondary Port is like that of the appropriate Standard Port (where the time differences for HW and LW are nearly the same), intermediate times and heights may be calculated from the tidal curves for the Standard Port in a similar manner to 9.4.1 above. The curves are entered with the times and heights of HW and LW at the Secondary Port, calculated as in 9.3.2 and 9.3.3.

Interpolation between the curves can be made by eye, using the range at the Standard Port as argument. Do not extrapolate, use the Spring curve for spring ranges or greater, and the Neap curve for neap ranges or less. With a large change in duration between springs and neaps the results may have a slight error, greater near LW.

Special curves for places between Swanage and Selsey (where the tide is very complex) are given in 10.2.12.

9.4.3   The use of factors

An alternative to the tidal curve method of tidal prediction is the use of factors which remains popular with those brought up on this method. Tidal curves show the factor of the range attained at times before and after HW. By definition a factor of 1 = HW, and 0 = LW. So the factor represents the proportion of the range (for the day in question) by which the height of tide is above the height of LW (that day) at the interval (time) concerned.

$$\text{Range} \times \text{factor} = \text{Rise above LW}$$
and $$\text{Factor} = \text{Rise above LW} \div \text{range}$$

In determining or using the factor it may be necessary to interpolate between the Spring and Neap curves as described in 9.4.2.

Factors are particularly useful when calculating hourly predicted heights for ports with special tidal problems (10.2.12).

9.5   TIDAL PREDICTION BY COMPUTER

By virtue of its simplicity, accuracy and speed, tidal prediction by computer or calculator is something no seaman – professional or amateur – with access to a computer can afford to ignore because it can do the job better and quicker than by conventional means.

Any navigator with access to an IBM PC, XT, AT or compatible computer, or a laptop computer, can choose between two tidal prediction programs which are issued by the Hydrographic Office, and several commercially produced programs.

9.5.1   Tidecalc

TIDECALC (NP 158) (version 1·0) is a version of the tidal prediction program which is used by the Hydrographic Office for computing the daily tidal predictions published in the three volumes of Admiralty Tide Tables (ATT) (NP 201 European Waters, NP 202 Atlantic and Indian Oceans, and NP 203 Pacific Ocean). This program is for use on an IBM PC and has a worldwide application.

The programme runs on IBM 286/386/486 processors and 100% compatible computers. A minimum memory size of 640k and a graphics adaptor to VGA standard is required. The program runs in colour or monochrome, and with or without a printer.

The software consists of one 720k 3·5 inch floppy disk, and a choice of 13 area disks (NP 158A1 to A13 which cover the world). Each area disk holds the relevant data for around 350-400 ports. Area 1 (v 2·0) covers the UK, Republic of Ireland and the Channel Islands, and Area 2 (v 2·0) covers Europe from Russia to Gibraltar excluding Iceland and Greenland, but including the Channel Islands and Mediterranean. Customised disks holding up to 400 sets of harmonic data can be supplied by the Hydrographic Office to meet individual user requirements.

TIDECALC includes a number of useful facilities to complement the usual presentation of times and heights of high and low water. The additional facilities include a choice of metres or feet; allowances for Daylight Saving Time; an indication of periods of daylight and twilight; the option to put in the yacht's draft, and the capability to display tabulated heights at specified times and time intervals. There is an option to display heights at intervals of 10, 20, 30, 40 or 50 minutes or one hour. Predictions can also be displayed graphically as a continuous plot of height against time.

Whichever method of tidal prediction is used, the basic accuracy will depend on the accuracy of the tidal observations made, the length of time over which the observations were undertaken, and whether the prediction method chosen is suitable for a particular port or area.

In some geographical areas better tide predictions may be obtained by using non-harmonic methods of prediction. Such areas include the upper reaches of many rivers like the Medway above Chatham; the Forth above Grangemouth; the Severn above Avonmouth, and the Crouch above Burnham. Other areas where non-harmonic methods result in more accurate predictions include many German ports.

Computations using TIDECALC are not intended to replace ATT but to supplement them, and it needs to be remembered that the official tide tables are the ultimate authority for tidal predictions.

9.5.2   NP 159 Harmonic Method

An alternative computer program issued by the Hydrographic Office is the Simplified Method of Harmonic Tidal Prediction (NP159A) (version 2·0).

The program runs on IBM PC, XT, AT and 100% compatible computers. A minimum memory size of 180k and a graphics adapter to CGA, EGA or VGA standards is required. The program runs in colour on EGA or VGA standard adaptors.

The software program consists of one 720k 3·5 inch, or one 360k 5·25 inch disk. The program automatically calculates the daily Tidal Angles and Factors which are found in Table VII in all three volumes of ATTs. The Port Harmonic Constant, and where appropriate Shallow Water Corrections and Seasonal Changes in Mean Level, are keyed in manually from data listed in Part III in all three volumes of ATTs, or from NP 160 Tidal Harmonic Constants (European Waters).

Users are required to key the relevant data into the template boxes displayed on the screen using the ENTER key to tab through the various boxes shown. A zero is entered where no value is given in ATT. For regularly used ports, up to twenty sets of port harmonic constant data can be pre-stored for later use, but remember that the date is also stored and will need to be changed before using the data for any new prediction.

As changes in Port Harmonic Constants are made from time to time, for the best results it is recommended that only the constants listed in the latest edition of the ATTs are used. NP 160 (Constants for ATT Vol 1) will be updated approximately every five years.

Predictions are displayed graphically as a continuous plot of height against time. There are options to plot and print predictions for the whole day, or part of the day, as well as the ability to continue to the next day or another date. Heights for any specified time can be added to the plot if required.

9.5.3   Commercial programs

A number of commercial firms also offer tidal prediction programs for use on computers or calculators. Most of the commercial programs are based on the NP 159 method of tidal prediction. For PCs and laptops, these include PC Maritime Ltd's PC Wayplanner; Positron Navigation's Showtide, Makeport, Moveship, and Tide Tabler; Dolphin Maritime Software Ltd also produce a tidal prediction program.

For hand-held calculators/computers such as the Psion, Pilotage Software produce a very good tidal prediction module which uses the NP 159 method.

9.6   CALCULATIONS OF CLEARANCES UNDER BRIDGES

It is sometimes necessary to calculate whether a boat can pass underneath such objects as bridges or power cables. The vertical clearance of such objects is shown on the chart above MHWS, so the actual clearance will nearly always be greater than the figure shown. The vertical clearance is shown in metres on metric charts, but in feet on older charts. It is sometimes useful to draw a diagram, as shown in Fig. 9(6), which shows how the measurements are related to chart datum.

> Clearance = (Vertical clearance of object + height of MHWS) minus (height of tide at the time + height of mast above water).

Fig. 9(6) Calculating vertical clearance

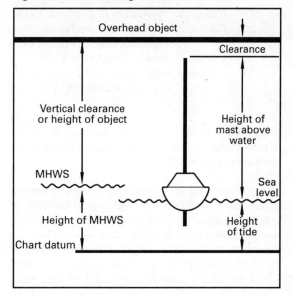

9.7   TIDAL STREAMS

9.7.1   General

Tidal streams are the horizontal movement of water caused by the vertical rise and fall of the tide. They normally change direction about every six hours. They are quite different from ocean currents, such as the Gulf Stream, which run for long periods in the same direction. Tidal streams are always expressed as the direction towards which they are running.

Tidal streams are important to yachtsmen around the British Isles because they often run at about two knots, and much more strongly in a few areas, and at spring tides. There are a few places where they can attain rates of six to eight knots.

The strength and direction of the tidal stream in the more important areas is shown in *Admiralty Tidal Stream Atlases*, as follows:

9

NP 209   Edition 4   Orkney and
                     Shetland Islands, 1986
   218   Edition 4   North Coast of Ireland, West
                     Coast of Scotland, 1983
   219   Edition 2   Portsmouth Harbour and
                     Approaches, 1991
   220   Edition 2   Rosyth Harbour and
                     Approaches, 1991
   221   Edition 2   Plymouth Harbour and
                     Approaches, 1991
   222   Edition 1   Firth of Clyde and
                     Approaches, 1992
   233   Edition 2   Dover Strait, 1975
   249   Edition 2   Thames Estuary, 1985
                     (with Co-Tidal charts)
   250   Edition 4   English Channel, 1992
   251   Edition 3   North Sea, Southern Part, 1976
   252   Edition 3   North Sea, North-Western
                     Part, 1975
   253   Edition 1   North Sea, Eastern Part, 1978
   256   Edition 4   Irish Sea and
                     Bristol Channel, 1992
   257   Edition 3   Approaches to Portland, 1973
   264   Edition 5   The Channel Islands and
                     Adjacent Coasts of France, 1993
   265   Edition 1   France, West Coast, 1978
   337   Edition 4   Solent and
                     Adjacent Waters, 1993

Extracts from the above (by permission of the Hydrographer and HMSO) are given in Chapter 10 for each area in the Almanac.

The directions of the streams are shown by arrows which are graded in weight and, where possible, in length to indicate the strength of the tidal stream. Thus ⟶ indicates a weak stream and ⟹ indicates a strong stream. The figures against the arrows give the mean neap and spring rates in tenths of a knot, thus 19,34 indicates a mean neap rate of 1·9 knots and a mean spring rate of 3·4 knots. The position of the comma on the Atlas indicates the approximate position at which the observations were taken.

It should be remembered that tidal atlases rarely show the details of inshore eddies, and the tide often sets towards the coast in bays. Along open coasts the turn of the tidal stream does not necessarily occur at HW and LW. It often occurs at about half tide. The tidal stream usually turns earlier inshore than offshore. On modern charts lettered diamonds give information on the tidal streams by reference to a table showing Set, Spring Rate and Neap Rate at hourly intervals before and after HW at a Standard Port. Where appropriate, normal river currents are included. Information on tidal streams and current streams is also included in *Admiralty Sailing Directions*.

9.7.2   Computation of tidal stream rates

Using Fig. 9(7) it is possible to predict the rate of a tidal stream at intermediate times, assuming that it varies with the range of tide at Dover.

Example

It is required to predict the rate of the tidal stream off the northerly point of the Isle of Skye at 0420 UT on a day when the heights of tide at Dover are:

UT	Ht(m)
LW 0328	1·4
HW 0819	6·3
LW 1602	1·1
HW 2054	6·4

The range of the tide is therefore 6·3 − 1·4 = 4·9m. When using either the Tidal Stream Atlas NP 218, or the Tidal Stream charts for Area 8 in Chapter 10, the appropriate chart to use is that for '4 hours before HW Dover' and this gives a mean neap and spring rate of 09 and 17 respectively (0·9 and 1·7 kn). On Fig. 9 (7), Computation of Rates, on the horizontal line marked Neaps, mark the dot above 09 on the horizontal scale; likewise on the line marked Springs, mark the dot below the figure 17 on the horizontal scale. Join these two dots with a straight line. On the vertical scale, 'Mean Range Dover', find the range 4·9. From this point follow across horizontally until the pencil line just drawn is cut; from this intersection follow the vertical line to the scale of Tidal Stream Rates, either top or bottom, and read off the predicted rate. In this example it is 14 or 1·4 knots.

A perspex sheet, or a sheet of tracing paper can be used on top of Fig. 9(7), so as to preserve it for future use.

9.7.3   Tidal streams in rivers

Tidal streams in rivers are influenced by the local topography of the river bed as well as by the phases of the Moon. At or near springs, in a river which is obstructed, for example, by sandbanks at the entrance, the time of HW gets later going up the river; the time of LW also gets later, but more rapidly so the duration of the flood becomes shorter, and duration of ebb becomes longer. At the entrance the flood stream starts at an interval after LW which increases with the degree of obstruction of the channel; this interval between local LW and the start of the flood increases with the distance up river. The ebb begins soon after local HW along the length of the river. Hence the duration of flood is less than that of the ebb and the difference increases with distance up river.

The flood stream is normally stronger than the ebb, and runs harder during the first half of the rise of tide.

At neaps the flood and ebb both start soon after local LW and HW respectively, and their durations and rates are roughly equal.

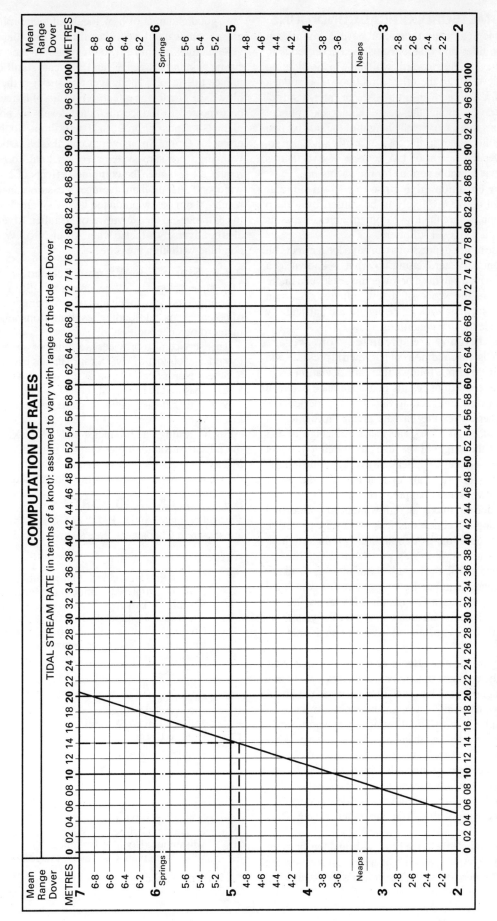

Fig. 9(7) Calculating Rates of Tidal Streams

9.8   METEOROLOGICAL CONDITIONS

Meteorological conditions can have a significant effect on tides and tidal streams. Sea level tends to rise in the direction towards which a wind is blowing and be lowered in the other direction. The sudden onset of a gale can set up a wave or 'storm surge' which travels along the coast. Under exceptional conditions this can raise the height of the tide by two or three metres, or in the case of a 'negative' surge, can lower the height of LW by one or two metres which may be more serious for the yachtsman.

Severe conditions giving rise to a storm surge as described above are likely to be caused by a deep depression, where the low barometric pressure tends to raise the sea level still more.

Intense minor depressions can have local effects on the height of water, setting up what is known as a 'seiche' which can raise or lower the sea level a metre or more in the space of a few minutes. Certain harbours such as Wick or Fishguard are particularly susceptible to such conditions.

Tidal heights are predicted for average meteorological conditions of barometric pressure and wind. It therefore follows that any deviation from 'average' conditions results in a difference between the predicted and actual tide level experienced. Atmospheric pressure has the greater influence. A change of 34 millibars can cause a change of 0·3 metres in the height of sea level, although it may not be felt immediately. Higher than average atmospheric pressure is of practical concern because the water level is always less than predictions.

In order to make an allowance for abnormal meteorological conditions it is necessary to define 'average conditions'. A good starting point is to look at the statistical tables in Admiralty Sailing Directions, or ask the local harbour master. Find out the average Mean Sea Level pressure for your local port and use this as a datum. For example, the pressure in the Solent area varies over the year from about 1014 to 1017mb, which gives an average of 1016mb.

Strong winds also affect tide levels and may alter the predicted times of high or low water by up to one hour, but are much less easy to quantify as the effect is very variable and is strongly influenced by the local topography.   In practical terms there is no need to consider winds of less than Force 5. Broadly speaking strong winds set up a current which raises the water level in the direction towards which the wind blows, and lowers the water level in the opposite direction. Although exceptionally high or low tides may occur in one place, it is not always the case that the same effect will happen in another.

Local knowledge is the best guide and the harbour master will be able to advise on how the tide levels are affected under different pressure and wind conditions.

A good example of how localised meteorological effects on water levels can differ from the more general rules occurs in Southampton Water where strong winds between N and NE can significantly reduce tide levels. The longer and stronger the wind blows, the greater the effect. NE winds of Force 5 can be expected to reduce predicted levels by about – 0·2m but winds of Force 8 to 10 will almost double the effect to –0·5m. Strong winds can also be associated with high pressure systems so the total correction required to counter the combined effects of a strong wind and higher than average pressure can easily reach – 0·6m below predicted levels. Water levels at the entrances to the Newtown or Beaulieu Rivers can also be adversely affected when strong N to NW winds combine with high pressure.

9.8.1   Storm Tide Warning Service

The Meteorological Office operates a Storm Tide Warning Service with the aim of providing warnings of potential coastal flooding resulting from abnormal meteorological conditions.

This service also provides warnings of abnormally low tidal levels in the Dover Strait, Thames Estuary and Southern North Sea. Warnings are issued when tidal levels measured at Dover, Sheerness or Lowestoft are expected to fall one metre or more below predicted levels.

Such warnings are broadcast on NAVTEX, and by the BT Coast Radio Stations on the normal VHF and MF frequencies used for navigation warnings and by the Channel Navigation Information Service.

9.9   STANDARD PORTS

The following STANDARD PORTS, listed by Areas, are shown in Chapter 10. See also 9.1.1 and 9.3.1.

AREA

1	Falmouth*, Devonport, Dartmouth*.
2	Portland, Poole*, Southampton, Portsmouth.
3	Shoreham, Dover.
4	Sheerness, London Bridge, Burnham-on-Crouch*, Walton-on-the-Naze, Lowestoft.
5	Immingham, River Tees entrance.
6	Leith, Aberdeen.
7	Lerwick.
8	Ullapool, Oban.
9	Greenock.
10	Liverpool, Holyhead.
11	Milford Haven, Avonmouth.
12	Dublin, Cobh.
13	Belfast, Galway.
14	St Peter Port*, St Helier.
15	Cherbourg, St Malo.
16	Brest.
17	Nil.
18	Pointe de Grave.
19	Le Havre, Dieppe.
20	Vlissingen, Hook of Holland.
21	Wilhelmshaven, Cuxhaven, Helgoland.

*   Daily predictions given, although not Standard Ports.

Chapter 10

Harbour, Coastal and Tidal Information

Contents

10

10.0.1 Map of areas

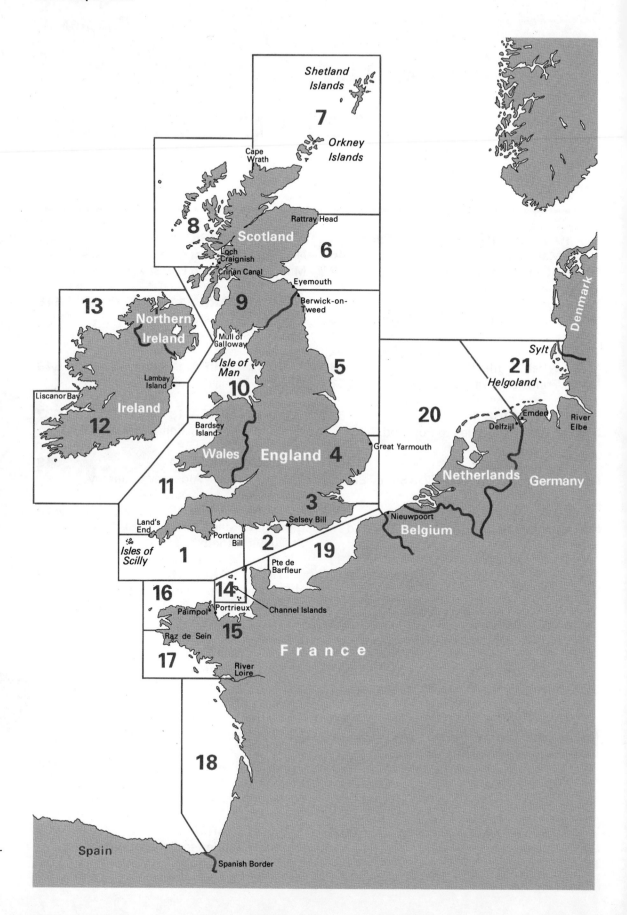

10.0.2   General information

Harbour, coastal and tidal information is given for each of the 21 Areas shown on the map at 10.0.1, with detailed text and chartlets of 375 harbours and notes on 403 lesser harbours and anchorages. The information provided enables a skipper to assess whether he can get into a harbour (tidal height, depth, wind direction etc), and whether he wants to enter the harbour (shelter, facilities available, early closing days etc). Abbreviations and symbols are in 1.4.1, and a four-language glossary is at 1.4.2.

Each Area is arranged as follows:

Index of the harbours covered in that area.

A diagram of the area showing the positions and characteristics of the harbours covered, principal lights, radiobeacons, coastal/port radio stations, weather information offices, LB stations and CG Centres with their boundaries.

Tidal stream chartlets for the area, based on Admiralty tidal stream atlases (by kind permission of the Hydrographer of the Navy and the Controller, HM Stationery Office), showing the rates and directions of tidal streams for each hour referenced to HW Dover and to HW at the relevant Standard Port. For how to use tidal stream charts see 9.6.2.

A list of principal coastal lights, fog signals and useful waypoints in the area. More powerful lights (range 15M or more) are in **bold** type; light-vessels and Lanbys are in *CAPITAL ITALICS*; fog signals are in *italics*. Latitude and longitude are shown for a selection of lights and marks, some of which are underlined as useful waypoints. Unless otherwise stated, lights are white. Elevations are in metres (m) above MHWS, and nominal ranges in nautical miles (M). Where appropriate, a brief description is given of the lighthouse or tower. Arcs of visibility, sector limits, and alignment of leading lights etc are true bearings as seen from seaward measured in a clockwise direction. Where a longitude is given (e.g. 04°12'·05W) W stands for West; W can also mean white. To avoid ambiguity, the words white or West may be written in full, except for longitude.

Passage information briefly calls attention in note form to some of the principal features of the coast, recommended routes, offlying dangers, tide races, better anchorages etc.

Table of distances in nautical miles by the most direct route, avoiding dangers, between selected places in that area and in adjacent areas. See also Tables of distances across the English Channel, Irish and North Seas at the end of this Introduction.

Special notes in certain Areas (Ireland, Channel Is, France, Belgium, Netherlands and Germany) give information specific to that country or Area.

10.0.3   Harbour information

a.   After the **harbour name**, the county (or equivalent abroad) is given, followed by the lat/long of the harbour entrance, or equivalent. This lat/long may be used as a final waypoint following the WPT given under Navigation. A published waypoint should never be used without first plotting its position on the chart.

b.   **Chart numbers** for Admiralty (AC), Imray Laurie Norie & Wilson (Imray), Stanfords or foreign charts are listed, largest scale first. The *numbers* of Admiralty Small Craft editions are shown in *italics*. The 1:50,000 Ordnance Survey (OS) Map numbers are given for UK and Eire.

c.   **Chartlets** are based on British Admiralty, French, Dutch and German charts (as acknowledged in 1.1.3).

It is emphasised that these chartlets are not designed or intended for pilotage or navigation, although every effort has been made to ensure that they accurately portray the harbour concerned. The publishers and editors disclaim any responsibility for resultant accidents or damage if they are so used.

The largest scale official chart, suitably corrected, should always be used. Due to limitations of scale, chartlets do not always cover the whole area referred to in the text nor can they show every depth, mark and feature. Depths, drying heights and elevations are in metres.The light tint shows drying areas, the dark tint indicates land.

d.   **Tidal predictions** are provided by the British, French, Dutch and German Hydrographic Offices, as acknowledged in 1.1.3.

For each Standard Port daily predictions of times and heights of HW/LW are given. Zone times are given, but no account is taken of BST or other daylight saving times (DST). In UK and Eire times are in UT.

Time and height differences for Secondary Ports are referenced to the most suitable (not always the nearest) Standard Port. An (⟵) or (⟶) points toward the Standard Port pages. The average time difference between local HW and HW Dover is given, so that the UT (±15 minutes) of local HW can be quickly found.

Times of HW Dover are in 10.3.17 and, for quick reference, on a bookmark which also shows Range. Duration (quoted for most ports), if deducted from time of HW, gives the approx time of the previous LW. Mean Level (ML) is also quoted; it should be noted, en passant, that on French charts ML is used, rather than MHWS, as the reference datum for elevations of lights, bridges etc.

Tidal Coefficients are listed and explained under Brest and are applicable to all French ports on the Channel and Atlantic coasts.

10

e.   **Tidal curves** are given for Standard Ports and those other ports for which full predictions are shown. Use the appropriate (np/sp) curve for tidal calculations (ie finding the height of tide at a given time, or the time for a given height). See Chapter 9 for tidal calculations.

HW −3 means 3 hrs before local HW; HW +2 means 2 hrs after. Secondary curves are given in 10.2.12 for ports between Swanage and Selsey Bill where special tidal conditions exist.

f.   **Shelter** assesses the degree of shelter and advises on access, berths (for charges see under Facilities), moorings and anchorages. Access· times, if quoted, are approx figures relative to mean HW. They are purely a guide for a nominal 1·5m draft, plus safety clearance, and take no account of hull form, springs/neaps, flood/ebb, swell or nature of the bottom. Their purpose is to alert a skipper to possible tidal problems. Times of lock and bridge openings etc are local (LT), unless otherwise stated.

g.   **Navigation** gives the lat/long of a waypoint (⊕) suitable for starting the approach, with its bearing/ distance from/to the hbr ent or next significant feature; some ⊕s may be off the harbour chartlet. A published waypoint should never be used without first plotting its position on the chart. Approach chans, buoyage, speed limits and hazards are outlined.

Wrecks around the UK which are of historic or archaeological interest are protected under the Protection of Wrecks Act 1973. About 40 sites, as detailed in Annual Notice to Mariners No 16 and depicted on the larger scale Admiralty charts, are listed in this almanac under the nearest harbour or in Passage Information. Unauthorised interference, including anchoring and diving on such sites, may lead to a substantial fine.

h.   **Lights and Marks** includes as much detail as space permits; some data may also be shown on the chartlet and in 10.nn.4 for that area.

j.·   **Radio Telephone** quotes VHF Channels related to each port, marina or VTS. If not obvious, the callsign of a station is shown in *italics*. Frequencies are indicated by their International Maritime Services Channel (Ch) designator. UK Marina Channels are 80 and M (formerly known as Ch 37). MF frequencies, if shown, are in kHz.

Ch 16, the Distress, Safety and Calling Ch, is monitored by most shore stations, and is shown after the working channels. Its Distress and Safety functions can be seriously jeopardised by excessive calling, test transmissions and illegal chatter. Initial contact can usually, and very desirably, be made on the listed working Ch, rather than on Ch 16.

Where known, preferred channels are shown in bold type, thus **14**. If there is a choice of calling channel, always indicate which channel you are using; eg, *'Dover Port Control, this is NONSUCH,*

NONSUCH on Channel 74, over'. This avoids confusion if the station being called is working more than one channel.

Where local times are stated, the letters LT are added. H24 means continuous watch. Times of scheduled broadcasts are shown (for example) as H +20, ie 20 minutes past the hour.

k.   **Telephone** is followed by the dialling code, which may be repeated or augmented under **Facilities** if different codes apply. For example, Portsmouth and Gosport numbers are both on (01705) as listed; but Fareham's different code (01329) is quoted separately.

In the UK the ☎s of the relevant Coastguard MRCC/MRSC (see 8.4.2) are given under each port, but dial 999 in an emergency and ask for the Coastguard.

The procedures for international calls from/to the UK are given in 10.12.7 (Ireland), 10.15.8 (France), 10.20.7 (Belgium & The Netherlands), and 10.21.7 (Germany). These sections also give ☎s for marine emergencies abroad. All EU countries use ☎ 112 for emergency calls to Fire, Police, Ambulance, in addition to their national emergency ☎s.

l.   **Facilities** available at the harbour, marinas and yacht clubs are listed first, followed by an abbreviated summary of those marine services provided commercially (see 1.4.1 and the Dover Range card for abbreviations).
Note: Facilities at Yacht Clubs are usually available to crews who arrive by sea (as opposed to trailing a dinghy by car) and belong to a recognised YC.

The overnight cost of a visitors alongside berth for a 30ft (9·1m) LOA boat is shown in local currency at the previous year's rates. Harbour dues, if applicable, and VAT are included; in the UK the cost of mains electricity is usually extra.

Town facilities are also listed, and whether there is a Post Office (✉), Bank (Ⓑ), Railway Station (⇌), or commercial Airport (✈) in or near the port. Where there is not, the nearest one may be shown in ( ). Abroad, the nearest port with a UK ferry link is given (see also 10.0.4 opposite).

10.0.4   Ferry Services

A summary is provided opposite of most of the more popular ferry routes both within UK waters and to/from the UK, together with booking or contact telephone numbers. Ferry services on the W coast of Scotland are listed in more detail in Area 8.

10.0.5/6/7   Distance Tables

In addition.to the Distance Tables in each of the 21 geographic Areas, there are three Distance Tables in this Introduction. These contain port-to-port distances for passages from/to the UK across the English Channel (10.0.5), Irish Sea (10.0.6) and North Sea (10.0.7). They may be used in conjunction with the Distance Tables in each of the 21 Areas.

FERRIES AROUND UK AND TO/FROM THE CONTINENT   10.0.4

This Table is a highly condensed version of many detailed schedules. It is intended to show broadly what is available and to help when cruise plans and/or crew movements are subject to change at short notice.

From	To	Hours	Frequency	Company	☎ Bookings
A.	**CROSS CHANNEL** (France, Belgium; and to Spain)				
Plymouth (Mar-Nov)	Santander	23½	M, W	Brittany	01752-221321
Plymouth	Roscoff	6	1 - 3	Brittany	Ditto
Poole	Cherbourg	4¼	1 - 2	Brittany (Truckline)	Ditto
Poole	St Malo	8	F, S, Su, M	Brittany	Ditto
Southampton	Cherbourg	5	2	Stena Sealink	01233-647047
Portsmouth	St Malo	8¾	1	Brittany	01705-827701
Portsmouth	Ouistreham (Caen)	6	3	Brittany	Ditto
Portsmouth (Jan-Mar)	Santander	31	Su	Brittany	Ditto
Portsmouth	Cherbourg	4¾	3	P & O	01304-203388
Portsmouth	Le Havre	5¾	3	P & O	Ditto
Portsmouth	Bilbao	33½	Su, Tu	P & O	01304-240077
Newhaven	Dieppe	4/2 (Cat)	4/NK	Stena Sealink	01233-647047
Folkestone	Boulogne	55 mins	6	Hoverspeed (Cat)	01304-240241
Dover	Calais	35 mins	14	Hoverspeed (Hovercraft)	Ditto
Dover	Calais	1½	25	Stena Sealink	01304-647047
Dover	Calais	1¼	25	P & O	01304-203388
Ramsgate	Dunkerque	2½	5	Sally	(01843-595522 and
Ramsgate	Ostend	4/1¾ (Jetfoil)	4/4 - 6	Sally/RTM	(0181-8581127
B.	**NORTH SEA**				
Felixstowe	Zeebrugge	5¾	2	P & O	01304-203388
Harwich	Hook of Holland	6½	2	Stena Sealink	01233-647047
Harwich	Hamburg	18½	4 wkly	Scandinavian Seaways	01255-240240
Harwich	Esbjerg	19½	4 wkly	Scandinavian Seaways	Ditto
Harwich	Gothenburg	23½	Su, Tu	Scandinavian Seaways	Ditto
Hull	Rotterdam	12½	1	N Sea Ferries	01482-77177
Hull	Zeebrugge	13¼	1	N Sea Ferries	Ditto
Newcastle	IJmuiden	To be announced		Scandinavian Seaways	0191-2936262
Newcastle	Hamburg	23½	2 wkly	Scandinavian Seaways	Ditto
Newcastle	Esbjerg	19½	2 wkly	Scandinavian Seaways	Ditto
Newcastle	Gothenburg	23½	F	Scandinavian Seaways	Ditto
Newcastle	Stavanger/Bergen	18½/6	M, W, S	Color	0191-296 1313
C.	**SCOTLAND**				
Aberdeen	Lerwick+Bergen	13+12½	F	P & O Scottish	01224-572615
Scrabster	Stromness	1¾	2 - 3	P & O Scottish	01856-850655
Stromness	Lerwick	8	Su, Tu	P & O Scottish	01595-5252
Ullapool	Stornoway	3½	2	Caledonian MacBrayne	01475-650000

CalMac run ferries to 23 West Scottish islands and many mainland ports; see 10.8.21 for details, inc other companies.

From	To	Hours	Frequency	Company	☎ Bookings
D.	**IRISH SEA** (and Eire-France)				
Cork	Roscoff	14	Su, Tu	Brittany	21-277801
Cork	St Malo	18	Wed	Brittany	Ditto
Cork	Cherbourg	17½	F (Jun-Aug)	Irish Ferries	01-661 0511
Cork	Le Havre	21½	Su (Jun-Aug)	Irish Ferries	Ditto
Cork	Swansea	10	1 (not Tu)	Swansea/Cork Ferries	01792-456116
Rosslare	Cherbourg	17	S, M	Irish Ferries	01-661 0511
Rosslare	Le Havre	21	Tu, W, Th	Irish Ferries	Ditto
Rosslare	Pembroke Dock	4¼	2	B & I Line	0171-734 4681
Rosslare	Fishguard	3½/1¾ (Cat)	2/4	Stena Sealink	01233-647047
Dun Laoghaire	Holyhead	3½/1¾ (Cat)	4/4	Stena Sealink	Ditto
Dublin	Holyhead	4	2	B & I Line	01-6610511 (Dublin)
Belfast	Stranraer	1½ (Cat)	4 - 5	SeaCat	01232-312002
Belfast	Liverpool	10	1	Norse Irish Ferries	01232-779090
Larne	Cairnryan	2¼	6	P & O	01304-203388
Larne	Stranraer	2h20m	10	Stena Sealink	01233-647047
Douglas, IOM*	Heysham	3¾	1 - 2	IOM Steam Packet Co	01624-661661

*Also less frequent sailings from Douglas to Belfast (4¾), Dublin (4¾), Fleetwood (3¼), Liverpool (4¼) and Ardrossan (8).

From	To	Hours	Frequency	Company	☎ Bookings
E.	**CHANNEL ISLANDS**				
Jersey/Guernsey	Weymouth	3¾/2¼	2	Condor (Cat)	01305-761551
Jersey/Guernsey	Weymouth	8/5	1	Condor (Ferry)	Ditto
Jersey	St Malo	¾	4	Condor (Cat)	Ditto
Jersey	Sark	¾	1	Condor (Cat)	Ditto
Guernsey	Alderney	¾	1	Condor (Cat)	Ditto
Jersey†	St Malo	2½/1¼ (Cat)	2/5	Emeraude	99.40.48.40 St Malo

†Also Jersey (St Helier) to Guernsey, Sark, St Quay-Portrieux, Granville; and Jersey (Gorey) to Portbail and Carteret.

10

NOTES:

1. **Hours** means approx crossing time by day.
2. **Frequency** is the number of one-way daily sailings in summer. Specific day(s) of the week may be shown, if non-daily.
3. ☎ **Bookings** may, for the larger companies, be via a centralised number applicable to all routes.

10.0.5   DISTANCES ACROSS THE ENGLISH CHANNEL

France/CI \ England	Longships	Falmouth	Fowey	Plymouth bkwtr	Salcombe	Dartmouth	Torbay	Exmouth	Weymouth	Poole Hbr Ent	Needles Lt Ho	Nab Tower	Littlehampton	Shoreham	Brighton	Newhaven	Eastbourne	Rye	Folkestone	Dover
Le Conquet	112	112	123	125	125	137	144	155	172	188	194	212	230	240	245	249	261	278	295	301
L'Aberwrac'h	102	97	106	107	105	117	124	135	153	168	174	192	211	219	224	228	239	257	275	280
Roscoff	110	97	101	97	91	100	107	117	130	144	149	165	184	193	197	200	211	229	246	252
Trébeurden	120	105	106	102	94	102	109	120	129	142	147	164	181	190	194	197	208	226	244	249
Tréguier	132	112	110	101	91	91	102	112	116	128	132	147	162	170	174	177	188	206	224	229
Lézardrieux	142	121	118	107	94	100	105	114	115	126	130	140	157	165	169	172	184	201	219	224
St Quay-Portrieux	159	137	135	124	111	115	121	129	127	135	135	146	162	171	174	178	189	207	225	230
St Malo	172	149	146	133	118	120	124	132	125	130	130	143	157	166	170	173	184	202	220	225
St Helier	155	130	123	108	93	95	100	108	99	104	104	115	132	140	144	147	158	176	194	199
St Peter Port	139	113	104	89	73	70	75	81	71	79	83	97	112	120	124	127	135	156	174	179
Braye (Alderney)	146	116	106	89	72	69	71	75	58	60	62	73	91	100	103	106	114	136	153	159
Cherbourg	168	138	125	107	92	87	88	93	66	64	63	68	81	90	92	96	102	122	140	145
St Vaast-la-Hougue	194	164	150	132	116	111	112	116	83	76	72	71	80	87	88	90	96	115	132	138
Ouistreham	229	198	185	167	151	146	147	147	117	107	100	86	91	92	91	90	92	106	125	130
Deauville	236	205	192	174	158	153	154	154	122	111	104	88	89	88	87	85	87	101	120	125
Le Havre	231	200	187	169	153	148	148	148	118	105	97	82	82	83	82	79	80	94	115	120
Fécamp	242	212	197	179	163	157	157	157	120	105	96	75	71	68	65	62	62	72	90	95
Dieppe	268	237	222	204	188	180	180	180	142	125	117	91	80	75	70	64	63	60	70	75
Boulogne	290	258	242	224	208	198	195	191	153	135	127	97	81	71	66	59	47	33	28	25
Calais	305	272	257	239	223	213	210	209	168	150	141	111	96	86	81	74	62	43	26	22

NOTES

1.   This Table applies to Areas 1 – 3, 14 – 16 and 19, each of which also contains its own internal Distance Table. Approximate distances in nautical miles are by the most direct route, while avoiding dangers and allowing for Traffic Separation Schemes.

2.   For ports within the Solent, add the appropriate distances given in 10.2.6 to those shown above under either Needles light house or Nab Tower.

3.   Distances across the Irish Sea, as applicable to Areas 9 – 13, are given in 10.0.6.

4.   Distances across the North Sea, as applicable to Areas 3 – 7 and 19 – 21, are given in 10.0.7.

5.   Some aspects of planning Cross-Channel passages are covered in Passage Information, 10.3.5 final section.

10.0.6 DISTANCES ACROSS THE IRISH SEA

Ireland \ Scotland England Wales	Port Ellen (Islay)	Campbeltown	Troon	Portpatrick	Mull of Galloway	Kirkcudbright	Maryport	Fleetwood	Pt of Ayre (IOM)	Port St Mary (IOM)	Liverpool	Holyhead	Pwllheli	Fishguard	Milford Haven	Swansea	Avonmouth	Ilfracombe	Padstow	Longships
Tory Island	75	107	132	119	134	170	185	215	156	171	238	207	260	279	307	360	406	355	372	399
Malin Head	45	76	101	88	103	139	154	184	125	140	207	176	229	248	276	329	375	324	341	368
Lough Foyle	38	61	86	73	88	124	139	169	110	125	192	161	214	233	261	314	360	309	326	353
Portrush	31	50	76	64	80	116	131	161	102	117	184	153	206	225	253	306	352	301	318	345
Carnlough	42	35	57	32	45	81	96	126	67	78	149	115	168	187	215	268	314	363	280	307
Larne	51	39	58	24	37	72	88	118	58	70	141	106	159	178	206	259	305	254	271	298
Carrickfergus	64	48	65	26	34	69	85	115	55	66	138	101	154	173	201	254	300	249	266	293
Bangor	63	48	64	22	30	65	81	111	51	62	134	97	150	169	197	250	296	245	262	289
Strangford Lough	89	72	84	36	30	63	76	97	41	37	107	69	121	141	167	219	265	214	231	258
Carlingford Lough	117	100	112	64	60	90	103	112	70	51	118	67	111	124	149	202	248	197	214	241
Dun Laoghaire	153	136	148	100	93	119	126	120	93	69	119	56	82	94	109	162	208	157	174	201
Wicklow	170	153	165	117	108	133	140	127	108	83	123	56	67	71	90	143	189	138	155	182
Arklow	182	165	177	129	120	144	149	133	117	93	131	64	71	65	79	132	179	128	144	167
Rosslare	215	202	208	161	154	179	180	164	152	125	156	90	83	55	58	109	157	110	119	137
Tuskar Rock	216	203	209	162	155	179	182	165	152	126	152	91	82	48	51	105	150	103	112	130
Dunmore East	250	237	243	196	189	213	216	199	186	160	189	127	116	79	76	130	177	124	127	136
Youghal	281	268	274	227	220	244	247	230	217	191	220	158	147	110	103	156	200	148	139	138
Crosshaven	300	287	293	246	239	263	266	249	236	210	239	177	166	131	118	170	216	163	151	144
Baltimore	346	333	339	292	285	309	312	295	282	256	285	223	212	172	160	209	254	198	178	161
Fastnet Rock	354	341	347	300	293	317	320	303	290	264	293	231	220	181	169	216	260	207	185	170

NOTES

1. This Table applies to Areas 9 – 13, each of which also contains its own internal Distance Table. Approximate distances in nautical miles are by the most direct route, whilst avoiding dangers and Traffic Separation Schemes.

2. Some aspects of planning passages across the Irish Sea are covered in Passage Information, 10.13.5 first section.

3. Distances across the English Channel, as applicable to Areas 1 – 3, 14 – 16 and 19, are given in 10.0.5.

10

10.0.7   DISTANCES ACROSS THE NORTH SEA

UK \ Norway to France	Bergen	Stavanger	Lindesnes	Skagen	Esjberg	Sylt (List)	Brunsbüttel	Helgoland	Bremerhaven	Willhelmshaven	Delfzijl	Den Helder	IJmuiden	Scheveningen	Roompotsluis	Vlissingen	Zeebrugge	Oostende	Nieuwpoort	Dunkerque
Lerwick	210	226	288	403	428	442	517	470	510	500	493	486	497	505	551	550	552	555	562	588
Kirkwall	278	275	323	438	439	452	516	467	507	497	481	460	473	481	515	514	516	519	526	545
Wick	292	283	323	437	428	440	498	449	489	479	458	433	444	451	485	484	486	489	496	514
Inverness	356	339	381	485	461	462	529	479	519	509	487	460	471	478	513	512	514	517	524	542
Fraserburgh	288	266	296	410	383	384	451	404	444	434	412	385	396	403	430	429	431	434	441	456
Aberdeen	308	279	298	411	371	378	433	382	432	412	386	353	363	369	401	400	402	405	412	426
Dundee	362	329	339	451	394	401	448	396	436	426	395	352	359	364	390	389	385	388	395	412
Port Edgar	391	355	362	472	409	413	457	405	445	435	401	355	361	366	391	390	386	389	396	413
Berwick-on-Tweed	374	325	320	431	356	361	408	355	395	385	355	310	315	320	342	341	337	340	347	364
Hartlepool	409	353	340	440	340	331	367	312	352	342	302	241	243	247	266	265	261	264	271	288
Grimsby	463	395	362	452	324	318	342	291	332	325	288	187	182	185	199	198	190	191	201	198
Kings Lynn	485	416	379	466	330	333	343	292	344	336	283	184	183	183	197	195	187	188	198	195
Lowestoft	508	431	380	453	308	300	295	262	284	271	218	118	104	98	95	99	87	87	89	106
Harwich	540	461	410	483	330	331	320	287	309	296	243	147	126	114	94	100	84	77	80	80
Brightlingsea	558	479	428	501	348	349	338	305	327	314	261	165	144	105	108	106	92	88	86	87
Burnham-on-Crouch	567	488	437	510	357	358	347	314	336	323	270	174	151	112	109	115	99	92	93	95
London Bridge	620	543	490	560	400	408	395	361	382	374	320	222	199	149	153	149	134	125	126	114
Sheerness	580	503	450	520	360	367	353	319	340	334	280	180	157	109	113	109	94	85	86	74
Ramsgate	575	498	446	516	368	346	339	305	323	315	262	161	144	121	89	85	77	65	58	42
Dover	588	511	459	529	378	359	352	328	336	328	275	174	155	132	101	92	79	65	58	44

NOTES

1.   This Table applies to Areas 3 – 7 and 19 – 21, each of which also contains its own internal Distance Table. Approximate distances in nautical miles are by the most direct route, while avoiding dangers and allowing for Traffic Separation Schemes.

2.   Some aspects of planning passages across the North Sea are covered in Passage Information, 10.4.5.

3.   Distances across the English Channel, as applicable to Areas 1 – 3, 14 – 16 and 19, are given in 10.0.5.

10.0.8 Vessel Traffic Schemes (VTS)

An increasing number of ports are implementing Vessel Traffic Services (VTS) Schemes, to improve the safety and efficiency of traffic management, and for environmental protection. Every harbour is different and has its own specific problems.

VTS may range from extensive traffic management to simple information broadcasts about shipping movements. Most VTS schemes are aimed at commercial vessels which must adhere to laid down procedures.

Yachts are not normally required to comply with port VTS radio and reporting procedures, but at some ports larger yachts may come within the stipulated minimum length or tonnage. When available, always use the recommended yacht tracks in preference to the main channels. When sailing in VTS areas valuable information about shipping movements can be obtained by listening continuously to the VTS frequency, especially in conditions of reduced visibility. Yachts should seldom need to transmit on a VTS or port operations channel. A possible exception to this rule might occur in fog, when it may be advisable to keep port operations informed before starting to cross a busy shipping channel.

Many of the larger ports operate VTS Traffic Information broadcasts which provide information about shipping movements, expected times of arrival or departure, and routes they will follow, in addition to weather and tidal information.

In some ports, such as Southampton, a launch is sent ahead of large ships to clear the channel. Obey any instructions given.

10.0.9 Traffic Separation Schemes (TSS)

Yachts, like other vessels, must conform to Traffic Separation Schemes (Rule 10). Rule 10 does not however modify the IRPCS when two vessels meet or converge in a TSS with a risk of collision. TSS are essential to the safety of larger vessels and, whilst inconvenient for yachtsmen, must be accepted as another element of passage planning, or be avoided where possible. They are shown on Admiralty charts and those around the British Isles and the continental seaboard are depicted in Figs. 10(3) to 10(7).

Craft <20m LOA, and any sailing yacht, should consider using inshore traffic zones - often the most sensible action for a yacht, rather than using the main lanes. Otherwise, join or leave a lane at its extremity, but if joining or leaving at the side, do so at as shallow an angle as possible. Proceed in the correct lane, and in the general direction of traffic.

If obliged to cross a traffic lane, do so on a heading as nearly as practicable at right angles to the lane, and do not impede vessels using a traffic lane. If under sail, start motoring if speed over the ground falls below about 3 kn or if a reasonable course cannot be maintained.

Some TSS are under surveillance by radar, aircraft or patrol vessels. There are heavy penalties for breaking the rules. 'YG' in the International Code means 'You appear not to be complying with the traffic separation scheme'. See Plates 6 and 7 on pages 68 and 69.

In summary, the best advice for yachtsmen is:

● Listen out on TSS frequencies, and to TSS information broadcasts.

● Cross TSS schemes as quickly as possible on a heading at right angles to the lane, and use the engine if that makes the crossing quicker, or the speed falls below 3kn.

● Have a good radar reflector.

● Keep a sharp lookout.

● Bear in mind that you might not easily be seen from the bridge of a big vessel, especially in a steep sea.

● Use your common sense. In poor visibility a small craft has every disadvantage imaginable.

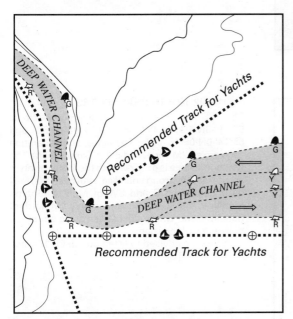

Fig 10(1) *Yachts should keep well clear of the main shipping channels and whenever possible use any recommended yachts tracks. When the main channels have to be crossed, do so at right angles. Avoid crossing the bows of oncoming commercial traffic.*

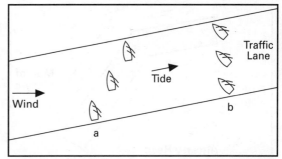

Fig. 10(2). *When crossing a traffic lane, the **heading** of the yacht must be at right angles to the traffic flow as shown in (a) above, regardless of the course made good which is affected by tidal streams. The yacht at (b) above is not heading at right angles and is therefore on an incorrect course.*

> **Fig. 10(3)**   Traffic Separation Schemes (TSS)
> and Routeing Measures

KEY TO SYMBOLS

▭ Separation zones	Cargo transhipment area	Port Hand Marks
⇐ Direction of traffic flow	VTS Vessel Traffic Service	Starboard Hand Marks
⇠⇢ Recommended direction of traffic flow	⚠ Precautionary area	Cardinal marks
▭ Boundary, Inshore Traffic Zone (ITZ)	Radio Communication Station (CRS and TSS)	Safe water marks
	● Selected Harbours and VTS/VTM Stations	Special marks
DW Deep water route	Lᴛ V Lanby Light ★	Isolated danger marks

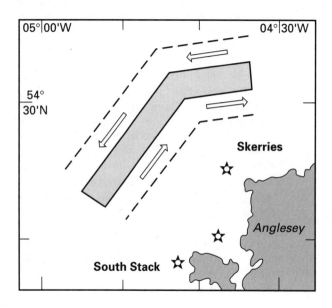

Fig. 10(3)1 OFF SKERRIES TSS

The TSS is centred upon the following positions: 53°22·8'N 04°52·0'W, 53°31'·3N 04°41'·7W and 53°32'·1N 04°31'·6W. The separation zone and the N and S bound traffic lanes are all 2M wide.

The passage outside the Skerries is preferable to the inside passage, except in strong offshore winds. The inside passage should not be used at night. When passing outside the Skerries allow a distance off of at least 1M to avoid the worst of the strong tidal stream.

Yachts are advised to listen out on Ch 16 when crossing the TSS.

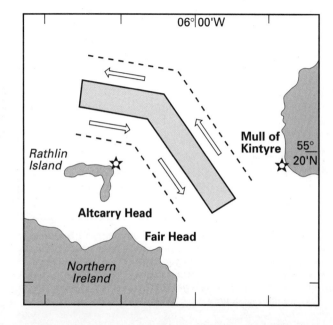

Fig. 10(3)2 NORTH CHANNEL TSS

The TSS is centred on the following positions: 55°15'·3N 05°55'·4W, 55°22'·8'N 06°04·6W and 55°24'·0N 06°15'·0W.   The lanes, and separation zone are all 2M wide. and the ITZ about 2·5M. The NW-bound lane is only 2M from the Mull of Kintyre and its race. A strong tidal race, with overfalls, may be encountered S and SW of Mull of Kintyre. Similarly, the SE bound lane is only 2M north of Rathlin Island where tidal streams are strong on both sides of the island.

Yachts are advised to listen out on Ch 16 when crossing the TSS.

Fig. 10(4)   Traffic Separation Schemes (TSS) and Routeing Measures

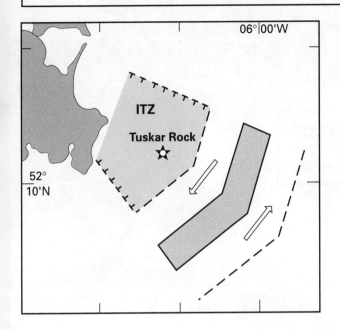

Fig. 10(4)1 TUSKAR ROCK TSS

The TSS is centred upon the following positions: 52°14'·0N, 52°08'·5N 06°03'·8W and 52°04'·7N 06°11'·5W. The separation zone is 2M wide, and the the N- and S-bound traffic lanes each side of the separation zone are 3M wide. The designated ITZ extends between Tuskar Rock and the landward boundary of the TSS.

Yachts are advised to listen out on Ch 16 when crossing the TSS or when navigating in the ITZ.

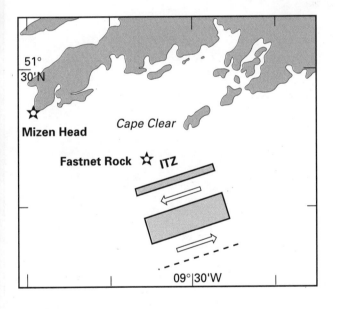

Fig. 10(4)2 FASTNET ROCK TSS

The TSS is located at approximately 51°19'N 09°31'W. The separation zone and the E- and W-bound traffic lanes are all 2M wide. The ITZ extends between Fastnet Rock and the landward boundary of the TSS which is about 2M SE of the Fastnet Rk and approx 3·5M from Cape Clear.

Yachts are advised to listen out on Ch 16 when crossing the TSS or when navigating in the ITZ.

Fig. 10(4)3 OFF SMALLS TSS

The TSS is located at approximately 51°46'N 05°52'W. The separation zone is 2M wide and the N- and S-bound traffic lanes are 3M wide.

Yachts are advised to listen out on Ch 16 when crossing the TSS.

10

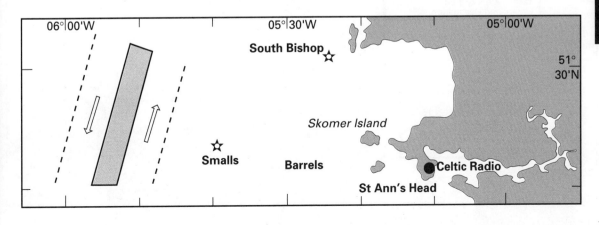

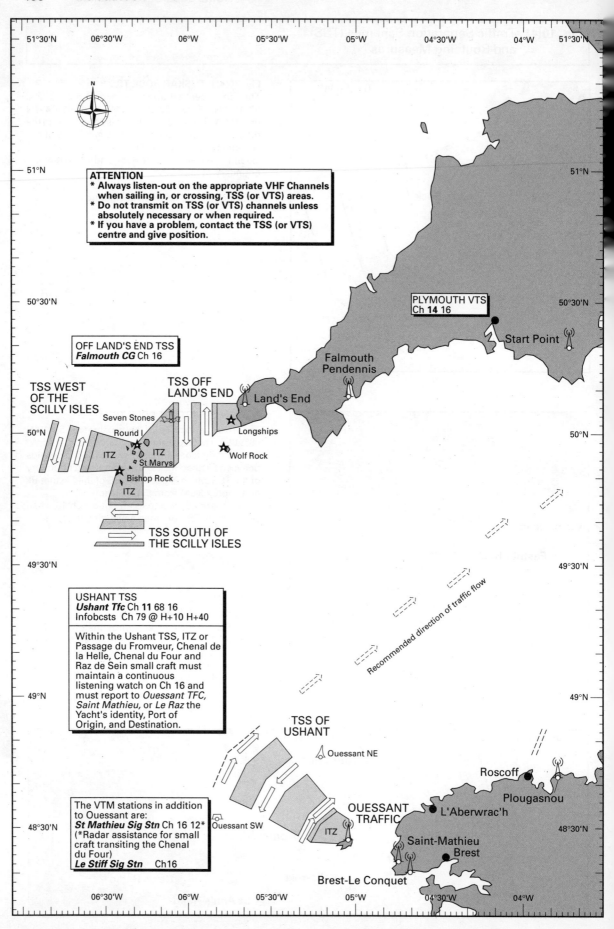

ATTENTION
* Always listen-out on the appropriate VHF Channels when sailing in, or crossing, TSS (or VTS) areas.
* Do not transmit on TSS (or VTS) channels unless absolutely necessary or when required.
* If you have a problem, contact the TSS (or VTS) centre and give position.

PLYMOUTH VTS
Ch **14** 16

Start Point

OFF LAND'S END TSS
Falmouth CG Ch 16

Falmouth
Pendennis

TSS WEST
OF THE
SCILLY ISLES

TSS OFF
LAND'S END

Land's End

Seven Stones

Round I

Longships

ITZ   ITZ

St Marys

Wolf Rock

Bishop Rock

ITZ

TSS SOUTH OF
THE SCILLY ISLES

USHANT TSS
Ushant Tfc Ch **11** 68 16
Infobcsts Ch 79 @ H+10 H+40

Within the Ushant TSS, ITZ or Passage du Fromveur, Chenal de la Helle, Chenal du Four and Raz de Sein small craft must maintain a continuous listening watch on Ch 16 and must report to *Ouessant TFC*, *Saint Mathieu*, or *Le Raz* the Yacht's identity, Port of Origin, and Destination.

TSS OF
USHANT

Ouessant NE

Recommended direction of traffic flow

The VTM stations in addition to Ouessant are:
St Mathieu Sig Stn Ch 16 12*
(*Radar assistance for small craft transiting the Chenal du Four)
Le Stiff Sig Stn   Ch16

Ouessant SW

OUESSANT
TRAFFIC

ITZ

Roscoff

Plougasnou

L'Aberwrac'h

Saint-Mathieu

Brest

Brest-Le Conquet

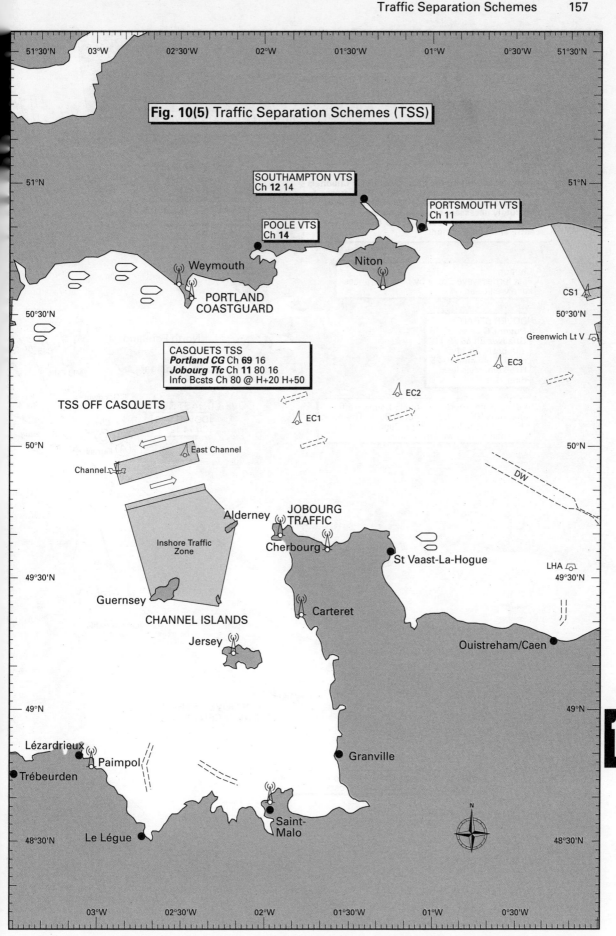

Fig. 10(5) Traffic Separation Schemes (TSS)

SOUTHAMPTON VTS
Ch **12** 14

PORTSMOUTH VTS
Ch **11**

POOLE VTS
Ch **14**

Weymouth

Niton

PORTLAND
COASTGUARD

CS1

Greenwich Lt V

CASQUETS TSS
Portland CG Ch **69** 16
Jobourg Tfc Ch **11** 80 16
Info Bcsts Ch 80 @ H+20 H+50

EC3

EC2

TSS OFF CASQUETS

EC1

East Channel

DW

Channel

JOBOURG
TRAFFIC

Alderney

Cherbourg

Inshore Traffic
Zone

St Vaast-La-Hogue

LHA

Guernsey

Carteret

CHANNEL ISLANDS

Jersey

Ouistreham/Caen

Lézardrieux

Paimpol

Granville

Trébeurden

Saint-
Malo

Le Légue

10

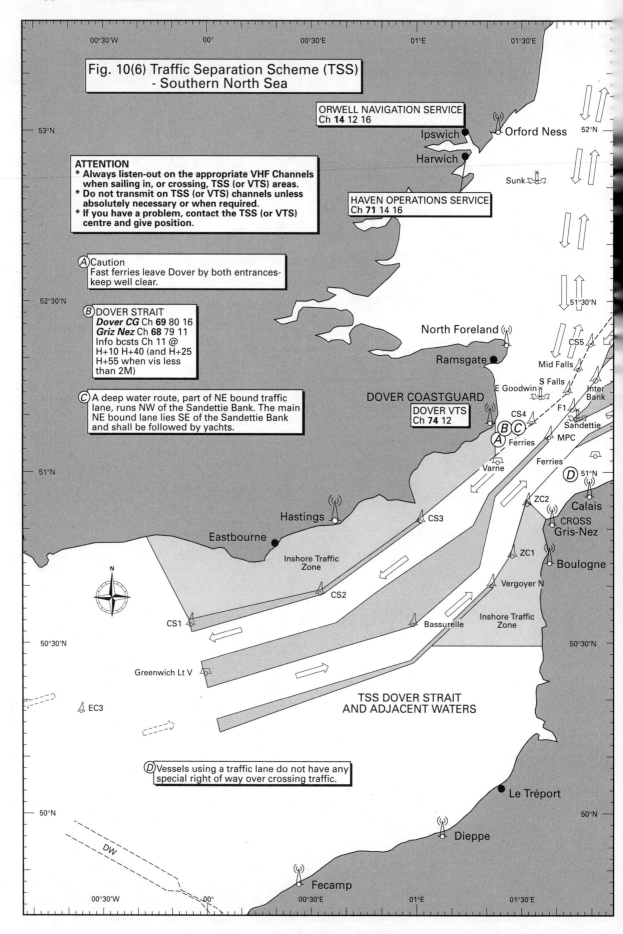

Fig. 10(6) Traffic Separation Scheme (TSS) - Southern North Sea

ORWELL NAVIGATION SERVICE
Ch **14** 12 16

ATTENTION
* Always listen-out on the appropriate VHF Channels when sailing in, or crossing, TSS (or VTS) areas.
* Do not transmit on TSS (or VTS) channels unless absolutely necessary or when required.
* If you have a problem, contact the TSS (or VTS) centre and give position.

HAVEN OPERATIONS SERVICE
Ch **71** 14 16

(A) Caution
Fast ferries leave Dover by both entrances-keep well clear.

(B) DOVER STRAIT
Dover CG Ch **69** 80 16
Griz Nez Ch **68** 79 11
Info bcsts Ch 11 @
H+10 H+40 (and H+25
H+55 when vis less
than 2M)

(C) A deep water route, part of NE bound traffic lane, runs NW of the Sandettie Bank. The main NE bound lane lies SE of the Sandettie Bank and shall be followed by yachts.

Ipswich
Orford Ness
Harwich
Sunk

North Foreland
CS5
Ramsgate
Mid Falls
E Goodwin   S Falls
Inter Bank
DOVER COASTGUARD
CS4
F1
DOVER VTS
Ch **74** 12
(B)(C)
Sandettie
(A)
Ferries
MPC
Varne
Ferries
(D) 51°N

Hastings
CS3
ZC2
Calais
Eastbourne
CROSS
Gris-Nez
Inshore Traffic Zone
ZC1
Boulogne
CS2
Vergoyer N
CS1
Bassurelle
Inshore Traffic Zone
Greenwich Lt V

TSS DOVER STRAIT AND ADJACENT WATERS

EC3

N

(D) Vessels using a traffic lane do not have any special right of way over crossing traffic.

Le Tréport

Dieppe

DW

Fecamp

53°N
52°30'N
52°N
51°30'N
51°N
50°30'N
50°N

00°30'W   00°   00°30'E   01°E   01°30'E

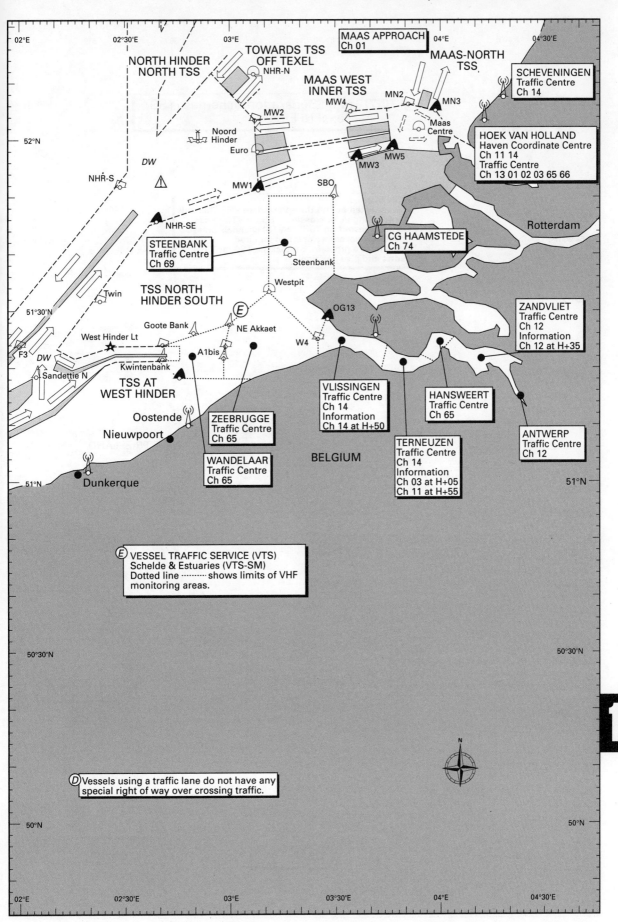

MAAS APPROACH
Ch 01

NORTH HINDER
NORTH TSS

TOWARDS TSS
OFF TEXEL
NHR-N

MAAS-NORTH
TSS.

SCHEVENINGEN
Traffic Centre
Ch 14

MAAS WEST
INNER TSS

MN2

MN3

MW4

MW2

Noord
Hinder

Euro

HOEK VAN HOLLAND
Haven Coordinate Centre
Ch 11 14
Traffic Centre
Ch 13 01 02 03 65 66

Maas
Centre

52°N

DW

MW5

MW3

NHR-S

MW1

SBO

Rotterdam

NHR-SE

CG HAAMSTEDE
Ch 74

STEENBANK
Traffic Centre
Ch 69

Steenbank

Westpit

TSS NORTH
HINDER SOUTH

Twin

OG13

ZANDVLIET
Traffic Centre
Ch 12
Information
Ch 12 at H+35

51°30'N

E

Goote Bank

NE Akkaet

West Hinder Lt

A1bis

W4

F3

DW

Sandettie N

VLISSINGEN
Traffic Centre
Ch 14
Information
Ch 14 at H+50

Kwintenbank

TSS AT
WEST HINDER

HANSWEERT
Traffic Centre
Ch 65

ANTWERP
Traffic Centre
Ch 12

Oostende

ZEEBRUGGE
Traffic Centre
Ch 65

Nieuwpoort

BELGIUM

TERNEUZEN
Traffic Centre
Ch 14
Information
Ch 03 at H+05
Ch 11 at H+55

WANDELAAR
Traffic Centre
Ch 65

51°N

51°N

Dunkerque

E VESSEL TRAFFIC SERVICE (VTS)
Schelde & Estuaries (VTS-SM)
Dotted line ········· shows limits of VHF
monitoring areas.

50°30'N

50°30'N

10

D Vessels using a traffic lane do not have any
special right of way over crossing traffic.

N

50°N

50°N

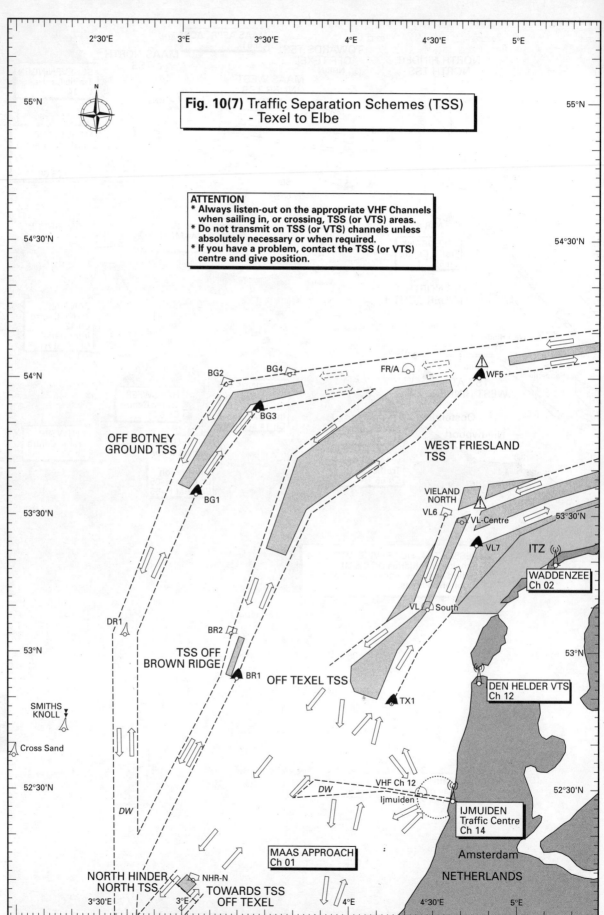

Fig. 10(7) Traffic Separation Schemes (TSS) - Texel to Elbe

ATTENTION
* Always listen-out on the appropriate VHF Channels when sailing in, or crossing, TSS (or VTS) areas.
* Do not transmit on TSS (or VTS) channels unless absolutely necessary or when required.
* If you have a problem, contact the TSS (or VTS) centre and give position.

OFF BOTNEY GROUND TSS

WEST FRIESLAND TSS

VIELAND NORTH

VL-Centre

ITZ

WADDENZEE Ch 02

DEN HELDER VTS Ch 12

TSS OFF BROWN RIDGE

OFF TEXEL TSS

SMITHS KNOLL

Cross Sand

VHF Ch 12

Ijmuiden

IJMUIDEN Traffic Centre Ch 14

Amsterdam

NETHERLANDS

MAAS APPROACH Ch 01

NORTH HINDER NORTH TSS

TOWARDS TSS OFF TEXEL

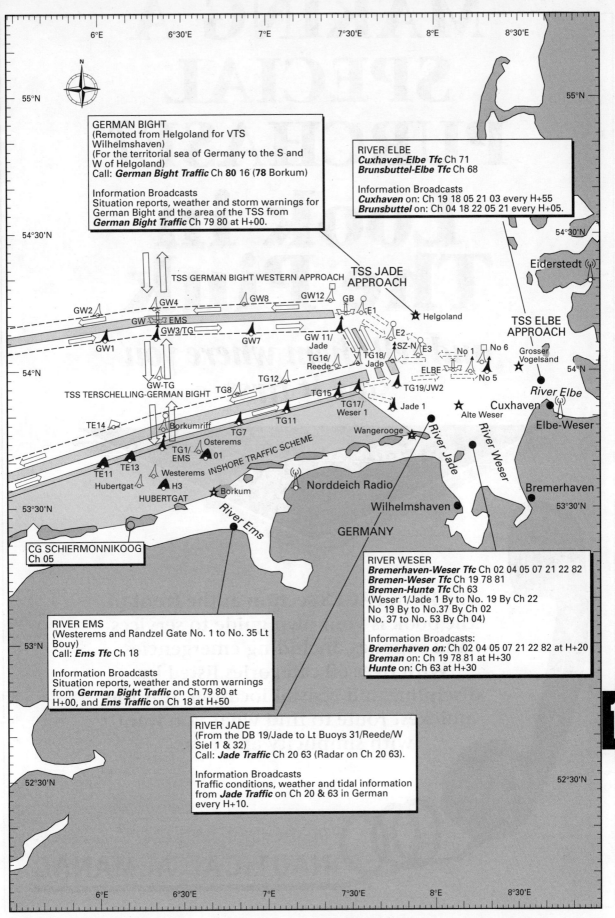

GERMAN BIGHT
(Remoted from Helgoland for VTS Wilhelmshaven)
(For the territorial sea of Germany to the S and W of Helgoland)
Call: *German Bight Traffic* Ch **80** 16 (**78** Borkum)

Information Broadcasts
Situation reports, weather and storm warnings for German Bight and the area of the TSS from *German Bight Traffic* Ch 79 80 at H+00.

RIVER ELBE
Cuxhaven-Elbe Tfc Ch 71
Brunsbuttel-Elbe Tfc Ch 68

Information Broadcasts
Cuxhaven on: Ch 19 18 05 21 03 every H+55
Brunsbuttel on: Ch 04 18 22 05 21 every H+05.

TSS GERMAN BIGHT WESTERN APPROACH

TSS JADE APPROACH

TSS ELBE APPROACH

GW2   GW4   GW8   GW12   GB   E1
GW   EMS
GW3/TG

GW1   GW7   GW 11/Jade   E2
TG16/Reede   SZ-N   E3
TG18/Jade

Helgoland

No 1   No 6
Grosser Vogelsand

ELBE
No 5
TG19/JW2

River Elbe

GW-TG

TSS TERSCHELLING-GERMAN BIGHT

TE14   TG8   TG12   TG15   TG17/Weser 1   Jade 1   Alte Weser   Cuxhaven
Borkumriff   TG7   TG11   Wangerooge   Elbe-Weser

TG1/EMS   Osterems
01

TE11   TE13   Westerems   INSHORE TRAFFIC SCHEME

Hubertgat   H3   Norddeich Radio   Bremerhaven

HUBERTGAT   Borkum

River Jade   River Weser

GERMANY

Wilhelmshaven

River Ems

CG SCHIERMONNIKOOG
Ch 05

RIVER WESER
Bremerhaven-Weser Tfc Ch 02 04 05 07 21 22 82
Bremen-Weser Tfc Ch 19 78 81
Bremen-Hunte Tfc Ch 63
(Weser 1/Jade 1 By to No. 19 By Ch 22
No 19 By to No.37 By Ch 02
No. 37 to No. 53 By Ch 04)

Information Broadcasts:
Bremerhaven on: Ch 02 04 05 07 21 22 82 at H+20
Breman on: Ch 19 78 81 at H+30
Hunte on: Ch 63 at H+30

RIVER EMS
(Westerems and Randzel Gate No. 1 to No. 35 Lt Bouy)
Call: *Ems Tfc* Ch 18

Information Broadcasts
Situation reports, weather and storm warnings from *German Bight Traffic* on Ch 79 80 at H+00, and *Ems Traffic* on Ch 18 at H+50

RIVER JADE
(From the DB 19/Jade to Lt Buoys 31/Reede/W Siel 1 & 32)
Call: *Jade Traffic* Ch 20 63 (Radar on Ch 20 63).

Information Broadcasts
Traffic conditions, weather and tidal information from *Jade Traffic* on Ch 20 & 63 in German every H+10.

Eiderstedt

10

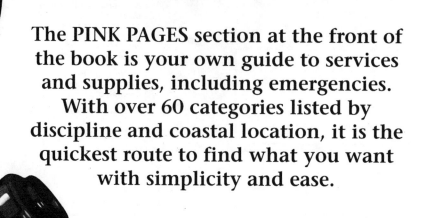

Volvo Penta service

Sales and service centres in area 1
CORNWALL Challenger Marine, Freemans Wharf, Falmouth Road, Penryn
TR10 8AS Tel (01326) 377222 Marine Engineering Looe, The Quay, East Looe
PL13 1AQ Tel (01503) 262887 & 263009 DEVON Phillip & Son Ltd, Noss
Works, Dartmouth TQ6 0EA Tel (01803) 833351 Starey Marine Services,
Lincombe Boatyard, Lincombe, Salcombe, TQ8 8NQ Tel (0154884) 3655 or
2930 Pilkington Marine Engineering, 9 Pottery Units, Forde Road, Brunel
Trading Estate, Newton Abbot TQ12 4AD Tel (01626) 52663 Retreat Boatyard
(Topsham) Ltd, Retreat Boatyard, Topsham, Exeter EX3 0LS
Tel (01392) 874720

VOLVO PENTA

Area 1

South-West England
Isles of Scilly to Portland Bill

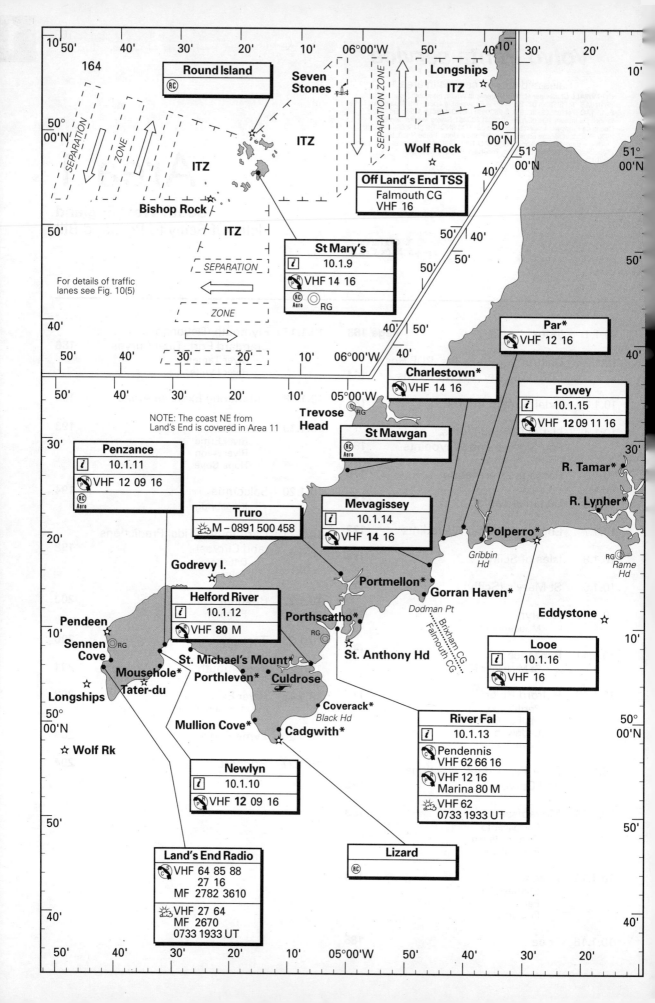

164

Round Island
(RC)

Seven Stones

Longships ITZ

SEPARATION ZONE

ITZ

ITZ

Bishop Rock

Wolf Rock

ITZ

Off Land's End TSS
Falmouth CG
VHF 16

For details of traffic lanes see Fig. 10(5)

SEPARATION

ZONE

St Mary's
(i) 10.1.9
(P)(R) VHF 14 16
(RC Aero) (RG)

Par*
(P)(R) VHF 12 16

Charlestown*
(P)(R) VHF 14 16

Fowey
(i) 10.1.15
(P)(R) VHF **12** 09 11 16

NOTE: The coast NE from
Land's End is covered in Area 11

Trevose Head (RG)

St Mawgan
(RC Aero)

R. Tamar*

R. Lynher*

Penzance
(i) 10.1.11
(P)(R) VHF 12 09 16
(RC Aero)

Truro
☂ M – 0891 500 458

Mevagissey
(i) 10.1.14
(P)(R) VHF **14** 16

Polperro*

(RG) **Rame Hd**

Godrevy I.

Gribbin Hd

Eddystone ☆

Helford River
(i) 10.1.12
(P)(R) VHF 80 M

Portmellon*

Gorran Haven*

Dodman Pt

Pendeen

Sennen Cove (RG)

Porthscatho*

(RG)

St. Anthony Hd

Brixham CG
Falmouth CG

Looe
(i) 10.1.16
(P)(R) VHF 16

Longships ☆

Mousehole*

St. Michael's Mount*

Tater-du ☆

Porthleven*

Culdrose

Coverack*
Black Hd

River Fal
(i) 10.1.13
(C)(S) Pendennis
VHF 62 66 16
(P)(R) VHF 12 16
Marina 80 M
☂ VHF 62
0733 1933 UT

☆ **Wolf Rk**

Mullion Cove*

Cadgwith*

Newlyn
(i) 10.1.10
(P)(R) VHF **12** 09 16

Land's End Radio
(C)(S) VHF 64 85 88
27 16
MF 2782 3610
☂ VHF 27 64
MF 2670
0733 1933 UT

Lizard
(RC)

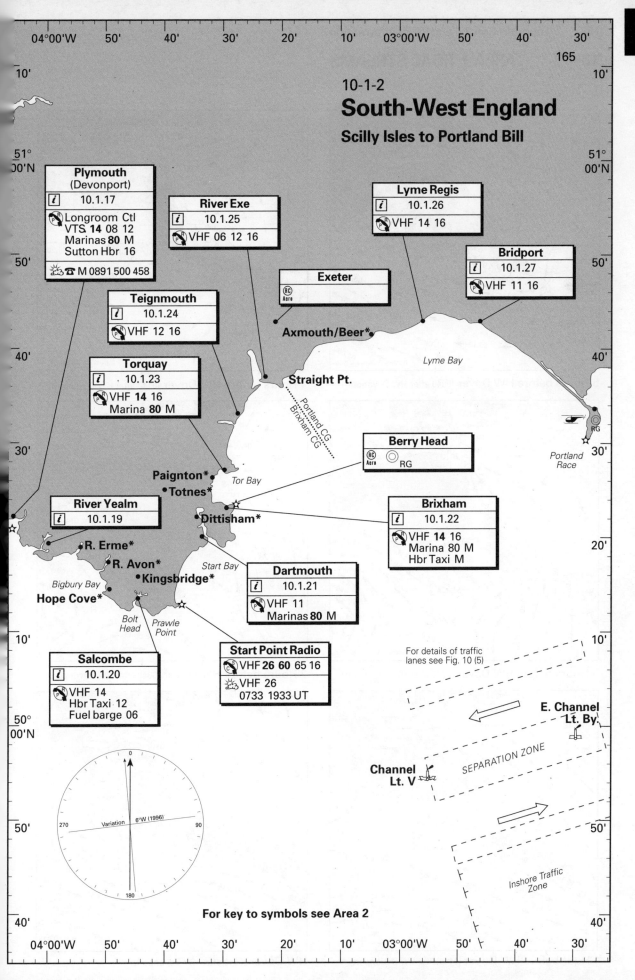

10-1-2
South-West England
Scilly Isles to Portland Bill

Plymouth
(Devonport)
i 10.1.17
Longroom Ctl
VTS **14** 08 12
Marinas **80** M
Sutton Hbr 16
☎ M 0891 500 458

River Exe
i 10.1.25
VHF 06 12 16

Exeter
RC Aero

Lyme Regis
i 10.1.26
VHF 14 16

Bridport
i 10.1.27
VHF 11 16

Teignmouth
i 10.1.24
VHF 12 16

Torquay
i 10.1.23
VHF **14** 16
Marina **80** M

Axmouth/Beer*

Lyme Bay

Straight Pt.

Portland CG
Brixham CG

Berry Head
RC Aero   RG

Portland Race

RG

Brixham
i 10.1.22
VHF **14** 16
Marina 80 M
Hbr Taxi M

Paignton*
Totnes*

Tor Bay

River Yealm
i 10.1.19

Dittisham*

R. Erme*

R. Avon*

Kingsbridge*

Start Bay

Bigbury Bay

Hope Cove*

Bolt Head   *Prawle Point*

Dartmouth
i 10.1.21
VHF 11
Marinas **80** M

Start Point Radio
VHF **26 60** 65 16
VHF 26
0733 1933 UT

For details of traffic
lanes see Fig. 10 (5)

Salcombe
i 10.1.20
VHF 14
Hbr Taxi 12
Fuel barge 06

E. Channel
Lt. By.

SEPARATION ZONE

Channel
Lt. V

Variation 6°W (1996)

Inshore Traffic Zone

For key to symbols see Area 2

10-1-3   AREA 1 TIDAL STREAMS

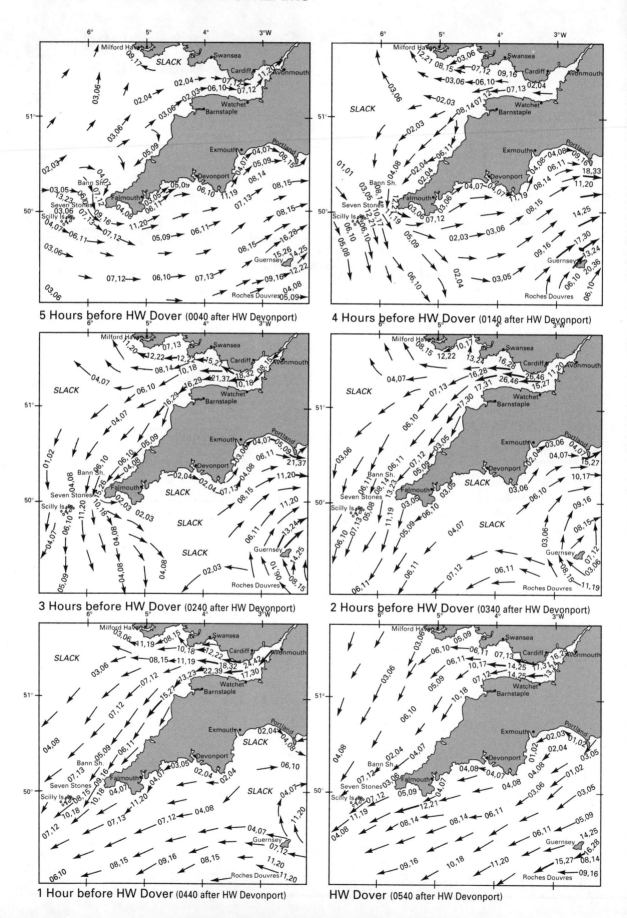

5 Hours before HW Dover (0040 after HW Devonport)

4 Hours before HW Dover (0140 after HW Devonport)

3 Hours before HW Dover (0240 after HW Devonport)

2 Hours before HW Dover (0340 after HW Devonport)

1 Hour before HW Dover (0440 after HW Devonport)

HW Dover (0540 after HW Devonport)

Eastward 10.2.3   Portland 10.2.9   Isle of Wight 10.2.26   Northward 10.11.3   Southward 10.16.3   Channel Islands 10.14.3

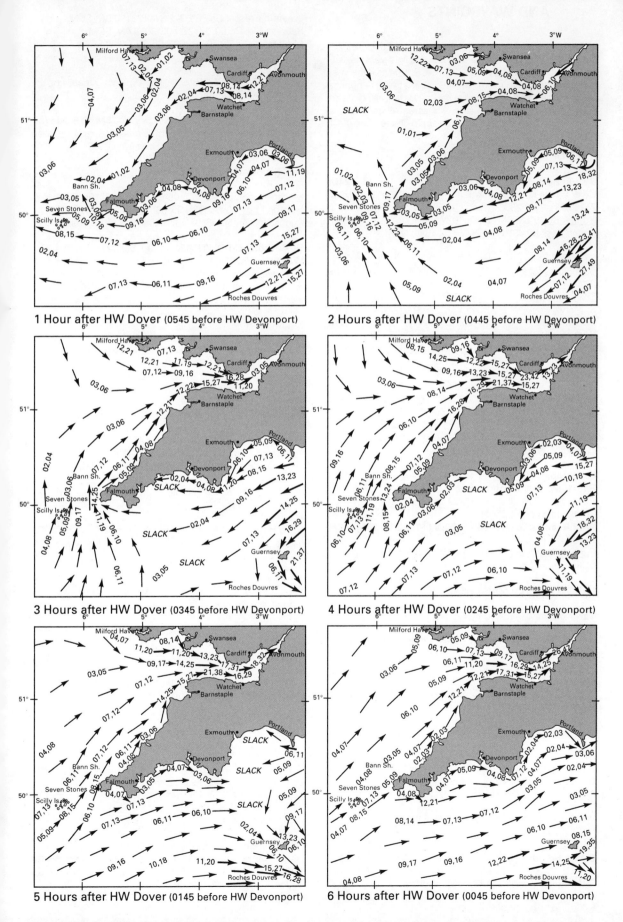

1 Hour after HW Dover (0545 before HW Devonport)

2 Hours after HW Dover (0445 before HW Devonport)

3 Hours after HW Dover (0345 before HW Devonport)

4 Hours after HW Dover (0245 before HW Devonport)

5 Hours after HW Dover (0145 before HW Devonport)

6 Hours after HW Dover (0045 before HW Devonport)

10.1.4　COASTAL LIGHTS, FOG SIGNALS AND WAYPOINTS

Abbreviations used below are given in 1.4.1. Principal lights are in **bold** print, places in CAPITALS, and light-vessels, light floats and Lanbys in *CAPITAL ITALICS*. Unless otherwise stated lights are white. m – elevation in metres; M – nominal range in miles. Fog signals are in *italics*. Useful waypoints are underlined – use those on land with care. All geographical positions should be assumed to be approximate. See 4.4.1.

ISLES OF SCILLY TO LAND'S END

Bishop Rock 49°52'·33N 06°26'·68W Fl (2) 15s 44m **24M**; Gy ● Tr with helicopter platform; part obsc 204°-211°, obsc 211°-233°, 236°-259°; Racon (T); *Horn Mo (N) 90s.*
Gunner By 49°53'·60N 06°25'·02W; SCM.
Round Rock By 49°53'·06N 06°25'·13W; NCM.

ST MARY'S
Bartholomew Ledge Lt By 49°54'·38N 06°19'·80W; Fl R 5s; PHM.
Spanish Ledge By 49°53'·90N 06°18'·80W; ECM; *Bell.*
St Mary's Pool Pier Hd FG 4m 3M; vis 072°-192°.
Peninnis Hd 49°54'·24N 06°18'·15W Fl 20s 36m **17M**; W ● metal Tr on B frame, B cupola; vis 231°-117° but part obsc 048°-083° within 5M.
FR Lts on masts to N and NE.
Hats By 49°56'·17N 06°17'·08W; SCM.

Round Is 49°58'·70N 06°19'·33W Fl 10s 55m **24M**; W ● Tr; vis 021°-288°; H24; RC; *Horn (4) 60s.*

SEVEN STONES Lt F 50°03'·58N 06°04'·28W Fl (3) 30s 12m **25M**; R hull, Lt Tr amidships; Racon (O); *Horn (3) 60s.*

Longships 50°03'·97N 05°44'·85W Iso WR 10s 35m **W19M, R18/15M**; Gy ● Tr with helicopter platform; vis R189°-208°, R (unintens) 208°-307°, R307°-327°, W327°- 189°; *Horn 10s.*
FR on radio mast 4·9M NE.
Wolf Rock 49°56'·70N 05°48'·50W Fl 15s 34m **23M** (H24); Racon (T); *Horn 30s.*
Runnel Stone Lt By 50°01'·15N 05°40'·30W Q (6) + L Fl 15s; SCM; *Bell, Whis.*

LAND'S END TO LIZARD HEAD

Tater-du 50°03'·10N 05°34'·60W Fl (3) 15s 34m **23M**; W ● Tr; vis 241°-074°. FR 31m 13M (same Tr) vis 060°-074° over Runnel stone and in places 074°-077° within 4M. *Horn (2) 30s.*

MOUSEHOLE
N Pier Hd 50°04'·94N 05°32'·21W 2 FG (vert) 8m 4M; Gy mast; replaced by FR when hbr closed.

Low Lee Lt By 50°05'·52N 05°31'·32W Q (3) 10s; ECM.

NEWLYN
S Pier Hd 50°06'·15N 05°32'·50W Fl 5s 10m 9M; W ● Tr, R base & cupola; vis 253°-336°; *Siren 60s.*
N Pier Hd F WG 4m 2M; vis G238°-248°, W over hbr.

The Gear Bn 50°06'·59N 05°31'·56W; IDM.

PENZANCE
S Pier Hd 50°07'·03N 05°31'·63W Fl WR 5s 11m **W17M**, R12M; W ● Tr, B base; vis R (unintens) 159°-224°, R224°-268°, W268°-344·5°, R344·5°-shore.

Albert Pier Hd 50°07'·06N 05°31'·72W 2 FG (vert) 11m 2M.

Western Cressar Bn 50°07'·21N 05°31'·07W; SCM.
Ryeman Rks Bn 50°07'·22N 05°30'·27W; SCM.
Mountamopus By 50°04'·60N 05°26'·20W; SCM.

PORTHLEVEN
S Pier 50°04'·87N 05°19'·03W FG 10m 4M; G metal col, Lts shown when inner hbr is open.

Lizard 49°57'·58N 05°12'·07W Fl 3s 70m **25M**; W 8-sided Tr; vis 250°-120°, part vis 235°-250°; reflection may be seen inshore of these bearings; RC; *Siren Mo (N) 60s.*

LIZARD HEAD TO START POINT

Manacles Lt By 50°02'·77N 05°01'·85W Q (3) 10s; ECM; *Bell.*
Helston Lt By 50°04'·92N 05°00'·77W Fl Y 2.5s; SPM.
August Rock By 50°06'·07N 05°04'·88W (PA); SHM (seasonal).

St Anthony Hd 50°08'·43N 05°00'·90W Oc WR 15s 22m **W22/20M, R20M**; W 8-sided Tr; vis W295°-004°, R004°-022° over Manacles, W (unintens) 022°-100°, W100°-172°; (H24); Fog Det Lt L Fl 5s 18m **16M** min vis 148·2°-151·3°; *Horn 30s.*

FALMOUTH
Black Rock Bn 50°08'·68N 05°01'·95W (unlit); IDM.
Black Rock Lt By 50°08'·65N 05°01'·68W Q (3) 10s; ECM.
Castle Lt By 50°08'·63N 05°01'·58W Fl G 10s; SHM.
The Governor 50°09'·12N 05°02'·32W; ECM.
E Bkwtr Hd 50°09'·32N 05°02'·89W Fl R 2s 20m 3M.
N Arm East Hd Q 19m 3M.
West Narrows Lt By 50°09'·35N 05°02'·03W Fl (2) R 10s; PHM.
The Vilt Lt By 50°09'·97N 05°02'·17W Fl (4) G 15s; SHM.
Northbank Lt By 50°10'·32N 05°02'·12W Fl R 4s; PHM.
No. 1 Port By 50°09'·72N 05°04'·37W QR; PHM.

Gwineas Lt By 50°14'·47N 04°45'·30W Q (3) 10s; ECM; *Bell.*

MEVAGISSEY
S Pier Hd 50°16'·11N 04°46'·85W Fl (2) 10s 9m 12M; *Horn 30s.*
Cannis Rock Lt By 50°18'·35N 04°39'·88W Q (6) + L Fl 15s; SCM; *Bell.*

FOWEY
Fowey Lt Bn Tr 50°19'·62N 04°38'·75W L Fl WR 5s 28m W11M, R9M; W 8-sided Tr, R lantern; vis R284°-295°, W295°-028°, R028°-054°.
St Catherine's Pt 50°19'·66N 04°38'·59W FR 15m 2M; vis 150°-295°.
Lamp Rk 50°19'·67N 04°38'·31W Fl G 5s 7m 2M; vis 088°-205°.
Whitehouse Pt 50°19'·95N 04°38'·22W Iso WRG 3s 11m W11M, R8M, G8M; vis G017°-022°, W022°-032°, R032°-037°.

Udder Rock By 50°18'·90N 04°33'·78W; *Bell;* SCM.

POLPERRO
Tidal basin, W Pier Hd 50°19'·83N 04°30·89W F or FR 4m 4M; R when hbr closed in bad weather.
Spy House Pt 50°19'·77N 04°30'·63W Iso WR 6s 30m 7M; vis W288°-060°, R060°-288°.

LOOE
Mid Main Bn 50°20'·53N 04°26'·87W Q (3) 10s 2M; ECM.
Banjo Pier Hd 50°21'·02N 04°27'·00W Oc WR 3s 8m **W15M** R12M; vis W013°-207°, R207°-267°, W267°-313°, R313°-332°.

Nailzee Pt 50°20'·96N 04°27'·00W *Siren (2) 30s (occas).*
Eddystone 50°10'·81N 04°15'·87W Fl (2) 10s 41m **24M**;
Gy Tr, R lantern. FR 28m 13M (same Tr) vis 112°-129° over
Hand deeps; helicopter platform, Racon (T); *Horn (3) 60s.*

PLYMOUTH SOUND
Rame Hd, S end 50°18'·63N 04°13'·31W (unlit).
Draystone Lt By 50°18'·82N 04°11'·01W Fl (2) R 5s; PHM.
Knap Lt By 50°19'·52N 04°09'·94W Fl G 5s; SHM.·
West Tinker Lt By 50°19'·22N 04°08'·57W Q (9) 15s; WCM.
Plymouth Bkwtr W Hd 50°20'·04N 04°09'·45W Fl WR 10s
19m **W15M**, R12M; W ● Tr; vis W262°-208°, R208°-262°.
Iso W 4s (same Tr) 12m 12M; vis 031°-039°; *Bell (1) 15s.*
Queens Gnd Lt By 50°20'·26N 04°10'·02W Fl (2) R 10s; PHM.
New Gnd Lt By 50°20'·44N 04°09'·37W Fl R 2s; PHM.
Melampus Lt By 50°21'·12N 04°08'·66W Fl R 4s; PHM.
S Winter Lt By 50°21'·37N 04°08'·49W Q (6) + L Fl 15s; SCM.
S Mallard Lt By 50°21'·48N 04°08'·23W VQ (6) + L Fl 10s;
SCM.
Mallard Shoal Lt Bn 50°21'·58N 04°08'·26W Q WRG 5m
W10M, R3M, G3M; W △, Or bands; vis G233°-043°, R043°-
067°, G067°-087°, W087°-099°.
Asia Lt By 50°21'·53N 04°08'·81W Fl (2) R 5s; PHM.
N Drakes Is Lt By 50°21'·49N 04°09'·31W Fl R 4s; PHM.
E Vanguard Lt By 50°21'·43N 04°10'·63W QG; SHM.
Bridge Chan SE Lt Bn 50°21'·00N 04°09'·47W QG; SHM.
W Vanguard Lt By 50°21'46N 04°09'·92W Fl G 3s; SHM.
Devils Pt Lt Bn 50°21'·55N 04°09'·97W QG 5m 3M; Fl 5s in
fog.

Duke Rk Lt By 50°20'·28N 04°08'·16W VQ (9) 10s; WCM.
Bkwtr E Hd 50°19'·98N 04°08'·18W Iso WR 5s 9m 8M;
vis R190°-353°, W353°-001°, R001°-018°, W018°-190°.
Staddon Pt Lt Bn 50°20'·13N 04°07'·47W Oc WRG 10s 15m
8M; R&W hor bands. vis R348°-012°, G012°-027°, R027°-
038°, W038°-050°, R050°-090°; obscd 090°-348°.
Whidbey 50°19'·50N 04°07'·20W Oc (2) WRG 10s 29m 5M;
Or and W col; vis G000°-137·5°, W137·5°-139·5°, R139·5°-
159°.
East Tinker Lt By 50°19'·17N 04°08'·23W Q (3) 10s; ECM.
Bovisand Pier 50°20'·21N 04°07·65W 2 FG (vert) 4m 3M.
Wembury Pt 50°18'·97N 04°06'·55W Oc Y 10s 45m; ocasl.

NGS W Lt By 50°11'·10N 04°00'·78W Fl Y 5s; SPM.
NGS E Lt By 50°11'·20N 03°58'·95W Fl Y 10s; SPM.

SALCOMBE
Sandhill Pt Dir Lt 000° 50°13'·73N 03°46'·58W Dir Fl WRG
2s 27m W10M, R7M, G7M; R&W ◆ on W mast; vis R002·5°-
182·5°, G182·5°-357·5°, W357·5°-002·5°.
Wolf Rk Lt By 50°13'·49N 03°46'·51W QG; SHM.
Blackstone Rk 50°13'·57N 03°46'·43W Q (2) G 8s 4m 2M;
G & W Bn.
Starhole By 50°12'·50N 03°46'·80W; SPM (Racing); (Apr-Sep).
Gara By 50°12'·80N 03°45'·20W; SPM (Racing); (Apr-Sep).
Gammon By 50°12'·00N 03°45'·50W; SPM (Racing); (Apr-
Sep).
Prawle By 50°12'·10N 03°43'·80W; SPM (Racing); (Apr-Sep).

Start Pt 50°13'·32N 03°38'·47W Fl (3) 10s 62m **25M**; W ● Tr;
vis 184°-068°. FR 55m 12M (same Tr) vis 210°-255° over
Skerries bank; *Horn 60s.* FR Lts on radio mast 0·9M WNW.

START POINT TO STRAIGHT POINT

Skerries Bank By 50°16'·28N 03°33'·70W; PHM; *Bell.*

DARTMOUTH
Homestone By 50°19'·57N 03°33'·48W; PHM.
Castle Ledge Lt By 50°19'·95N 03°33'·05W Fl G 5s; SHM.
Checkstone Lt By 50°20'·42N 03°33'·73W Fl (2) R 5s; PHM.

Kingswear 50°20'·78N 03°34'·02W Iso WRG 3s 9m 8M;
W ● Tr; vis G318°-325°, W325°-331°, R331°-340°, (TE 1989).
Bayards Cove Fl WRG 2s 5m 6M; vis G280°-289°, W289°-
297°, R297°-shore.
RDYC 1 By 50°18'·80N 03°35'·25W; SPM (Racing); (Apr-
Oct).
RDYC 2 By 50°18'·68N 03°33'·29W; SPM (Racing); (Apr-
Oct).
RDYC 3 By 50°20'·07N 03°31'·42W; SPM (Racing); (Apr-
Oct).

Berry Hd 50°23'·94N 03°28'·93W Fl (2) 15s 58m 14M; W Tr;
vis 100°-023°. R Lts on radio mast 5·7M NW.

BRIXHAM
Brixham Fairway Lt By 50°24'·37N 03°30'·85W Mo A 10s;
SWM.
Victoria Bkwtr Hd 50°24'·29N 03°30'·70W Oc R 15s 9m 6M.
Fairway Dir Lt 159° Dir Iso WRG 5s 4m 6M; vis G145°-157°
W157°-161°, R161°-173°
Prince William Marina SW end 2 Fl R 5s (vert) 4m 2M.

PAIGNTON
Outfall Lt Bn 50°25'·92N 03°33'·09W Q (3) 10s 5m 3M.
E Quay 50°25'·92N 03°33'·29W QR 7m 3M.

TORQUAY
Princess Pier Hd 50°27'·43N 03°31'·66W QR 9m 6M.
Haldon Pier Hd 50°27'·40N 03°31'·67W QG 9m 6M.
Marina S Pontoon E end 2 FR (vert) 2m.

TEIGNMOUTH
The Den, Lts in line 334°. Front 50°32'·51N 03°29'·74W
FR 10m 6M; Gy ● Tr; vis 225°-135°. Rear, 62m from front,
Powderham Terrace FR 11m 3M.
Den Point 50°32'·38N 03°29'·98W Oc G 5·5s FG (vert); △ on
G Bn.
Outfall Lt By 50°31'·96N 03°27'·92W Fl Y 5s; SPM.

EXMOUTH
E Exe Lt By 50°35'·97N 03°22'·30W Q (3) 10s; ECM.
Straight Pt 50°36'·45N 03°21'·67W Fl R 10s 34m 7M;
vis 246°-071°.
Ldg Lts 305°. Front FY 6m 7M. Rear, 57m from front, FY
12m 7M.
DZS Lt By 50°36'·10N 03°19'·30W Fl Y 3s; SPM.
DZN Lt By 50°36'·80N 03°19'·20W Fl Y 3s; SPM.

AXMOUTH
Pier Hd 50°42'·10N 03°03'·21W Fl 5s 7m 2M.

LYME REGIS
Ldg Lts 296°. Front, Victoria Pier Hd 50°43'·30N 02°56'·10W
Oc WR 8s 6m W9M. R7M; Bu col; vis R296°-116°, W116°.-
296°. Rear, 240m from front, FG 8m 9M.

BRIDPORT
E Pier Hd 50°42'·52N 02°45'·74W FG 3m 2M; (occas).
W Pier Hd 50°42'·52N 02°45'·77W FR 3m 2M; (occas).
W Pier Root 50°42'·61N 02°45'·76W Iso R 2s 9m 5M.

DZ Lt By 50°36'·50N 02°42'·00W Fl Y 3s; SPM.

OFFSHORE
Channel Lt F 49°54'·42N 02°53'·67W Fl 15s 12m 25M;
Horn 20s; Racon (O).
E Channel Lt By 49°58'·67N 02°28'·87W Fl Y 5s; Racon (T);
SPM.

NOTE: For English Channel Waypoints see 10.1.7.

10.1.5   PASSAGE INFORMATION

For reference, see Admiralty *Channel Pilot; West Country Cruising* (YM/Fishwick); *Shell Channel Pilot* (Imray/Cunliffe), and *Isles of Scilly Pilot* (Imray/Brandon).

NORTH CORNWALL (charts 1149, 1156)

For the coast of North Cornwall see 10.11.5. For St Ives, Hayle, Newquay, Padstow and Bude, see 10.11.25. Certain information is repeated below for continuity and convenience.

The approaches to the Bristol Chan along N coast of Cornwall are very exposed, with little shelter in bad weather. From Land's End to St Ives the coast is rugged with high cliffs. The Brisons are 27m high rky islets 5ca SW of C Cornwall; rky ledges extend inshore and to the S and SW. Vyneck Rks lie awash about 3ca NW of C Cornwall. There are overfalls SW of Pendeen Pt (lt, fog sig). St Ives (dries) is sheltered from E and S, but exposed to N. Padstow is a refuge, but in strong NW winds the sea breaks on bar and prevents entry. In these waters yachts need to be sturdy and well equipped, since if bad weather develops no shelter may be at hand. Streams are moderate W of Lundy, but strong around the island, and much stronger towards Bristol Chan proper.

ISLES OF SCILLY (10.1.8 and charts 34, 883)

There are 50 islands, extending 21-31M WSW of Land's End, with many rky outcrops and offlying dangers. Although they are all well charted, care is needed particularly in poor vis. *St Marys Harbour and Pier* is a leaflet obtainable locally. See also 10.1.8/9 for details of this rewarding cruising ground.

Several approach transits are shown on chart *34*, and these should be followed, because the tidal streams around the islands are difficult to predict with accuracy. They run harder off points and over rks, where overfalls may occur.

Conspic landmarks are Bishop Rk lt ho, Round Is lt ho, the disused lt ho on St Agnes, the daymark at the E end of St Martin's, Penninis lt ho at the S end of St Mary's, and the TV mast and CG sig stn (at the old telegraph tower) both in the NW corner of St Mary's. Yachts must expect to lie to their anchors. There is no one anch giving shelter from all winds and swell, so be prepared to move at short notice.

ISLES OF SCILLY TO LAND'S END (chart 1148)

Between Scilly and Land's End (chart 1148) streams are rotatory, clockwise. Relative to HW Devonport, they run ENE from HW – 1 (1kn at sp); SSE from HW + 2 (2kn at sp); WNW from HW + 6 (1kn at sp); and N from HW – 4 (1·75kn at sp).

The Seven Stones (rks) lie 7M NE of the Scillies and 15M W of Land's End; many of them dry, with ledges in between. They are marked by lt F (lt, fog sig) on E side. Wolf Rk (lt, fog sig) is 8M SW of Land's End, and is steep-to. The N/S lanes of Land's End TSS lie between Seven Stones and Wolf Rk; see Fig. 10 (5). The Longships (lt, fog sig) are a group of rks about 1M W of Land's End, with ledges 2ca further seaward. The inshore passage is about 4ca wide; drying rks on the W side are not marked.

LAND'S END TO LIZARD POINT (chart 777)

From Land's End to Gwennap Hd, 2M SE, rks extend up to 1½ca offshore, and depths are irregular to seaward causing a bad sea in strong W winds over a W-going tide. The Runnel Stone (dries 0·5m) lies 7ca S of Gwennap Hd, with rks closer inshore. These dangers are in R sectors of Longships and Tater-du Lts. No anch off Porth Curno, due to cables.

Entering Mount's B, the Bucks (dry) are 2ca ESE of Tater-du lt ho. Gull Rk (24m) is 9ca NE of Tater-du, close off the E point of Lamorna Cove. Little Heaver (dries) is 100m SW of Gull Rk, and Kemyel Rk (dries) is 1¾ca ENE. Mousehole (10.1.10) is a small drying hbr, sheltered from W and N, but exposed to E or S winds, when ent may be shut. Approach from SW side of St Clement's Is. In W winds there is good anch off the hbr.

Low Lee, a dangerous rk (1·1m), is 4ca NE of Penlee Pt, marked by ECM lt buoy. Carn Base Rk (1·8M) lies 3ca NNW of Low Lee. Newlyn (10.1.10) is only hbr in Mount's B safe to appr in strong onshore winds, but only near HW. From here to Penzance (10.1.11) beware Dog Rk and Gear Rk (1·9M).

From Penzance to St Michael's Mount the head of the B is shoal, drying 4ca off in places. Dangers include Cressar Rks, Long Rk, Hogus Rks, and Outer Penzeath Rk. Venton chy on with pierheads of St Michael's Mount hbr at 084° leads S of these dangers. This tiny hbr dries 2·1M, but is well sheltered, with anch about 1ca W of ent, see 10.1.11.

Two dangerous rks, Guthen Rk and Maltman Rk (0·9M), lie 2ca W and S of St Michael's Mount. 1M SE is The Greeb (7m), with rks between it and shore. The Bears (dry) lie 1¾ca E of The Greeb. The Stone (dries) is 5ca S of Cudden Pt, while offshore is Mountamopus shoal marked by SCM buoy which should be passed to seaward. Welloe Rk (dries) lies 5ca SW of Trewavas Hd.

Porthleven is a small tidal hbr, entered between Great and Little Trigg Rks and pier on S side. Dry out alongside in inner hbr, closed in bad weather when appr is dangerous. In fair weather there is good anch off Porth Mellin, about 1½ca NE of Mullion Is; Porth Mellin hbr (dries) is for temp use only.

2·5M W of Lizard Pt is The Boa, a rky shoal on which sea breaks in SW gales. The Lizard (lt, fog sig, RC) is a bold, steep headland (chart 2345). From W to E, the outer rks, all drying, are Mulvin, (2½ca SW of Lizard Pt), Taylor's Rk (2ca SSW); Clidgas Rks (5ca SW of lt ho), Men Hyr Rk (4·1m) and the Dales or Stags (5ca SSW), and Enoch Rk (3ca S). S of the rks the stream turns E at HW Devonport – 0500, and W at HW + 0155, rates up to 3kn at sp; offshore it turns an hour earlier. A dangerous race extends 2-3M S when stream is strong in either direction, worst in W'ly winds against W-going tide. Then keep at least 3M to seaward. There may be a race SE of the Point.

LIZARD POINT TO GRIBBIN HEAD (chart 1267)

E of Lizard Pt and 4ca ESE of Bass Pt, is Vrogue, a dangerous sunken rk (1·8m). Craggan Rks (1·5m) are 5ca offshore, and 1M N of Vrogue Rk. N of Black Hd rks extend at least 1ca offshore; a rk drying 1·6m lies off Chynhalls Pt. Coverack gives good anch in W winds, see 10.1.12. From Dolor Pt to E of Lowland Pt are drying rks 2½ca offshore.

The Manacles (dry), 7½ca E and SE of Manacle Pt, are marked by ECM lt buoy and are in R sector of St Anthony Hd lt. Off the Manacles the stream runs NE from HW Devonport – 0345, and SW from HW + 0200, sp rates 1·25kn. From E of the Manacles there are no offshore dangers on courses NNW to Helford River ent (10.1.12) or N to River Fal (10.1.13).

3M NNE from St Anthony Hd, Porthscatho offers safe anch in W'lies (10.1.14). Gull Rk (38m high) lies 6ca E of Nare Hd, at W side of Veryan B. The Whelps (dry) are 5ca SW of Gull Rk. There is a passage between Gull Rk and the shore. In Veryan B beware Lath Rk (2·1m) 1M SE of Portloe.

On E side of Veryan B, Dodman Pt is a 110m flat-topped cliff, with a conspic stone cross. Depths are irregular for 1M S, with heavy overfalls in strong winds over sp tide, when it is best to pass 2M off. Gorran Haven, a sandy cove with L-shaped pier which dries at sp, is a good anch in offshore winds, see 10.1.14. 2·1M NE of Dodman Pt, and 1M ENE of Gorran Haven, is Gwineas Rk (8m high) and Yaw Rk (dries 0·9m), marked by ECM lt buoy. Passage inside Gwineas Rk is possible, but not advised in strong onshore winds or poor vis. Portmellon and Mevagissey B, (10.1.14) are good anchs in offshore winds. For Charlestown and Par, see 10.1.15.

GRIBBIN HEAD TO START POINT (charts 1267, 1613)

Gribbin Hd has a conspic daymark, a ☐ tr 25m high with R & W bands. In bad weather the sea breaks on rocks round Head. Cannis Rk (dries) is 2½ca SE, marked by SCM lt buoy. 3M E of Fowey (10.1.15) is Udder Rk (dries 0·6m), 5ca offshore in E part of Lantivet B. Larrick Rk (dries 4·3m) is 1½ca off Nealand Pt.

Polperro hbr dries, but the inlet gives good anch in offshore winds, see 10.1.15. Beware E Polca Rk roughly in mid-chan. E of Polperro shoals lie 2½ca off Downend Pt, (memorial). The chan between Hannafore Pt and Looe (or St George's) Island nearly dries. The Ranneys (dry) are rks extending 2½ca E and SE of Looe Is, see 10.1.16. There are overfalls S of Looe Is in bad weather.

Eddystone rks (chart *1613*) lie 8M S of Rame Hd. Shoals extend 3ca E. Close NW of the lt ho (lt, fog sig) is the stump of old lt ho. The sea can break on Hand Deeps, sunken rks 3·5M NW of Eddystone.

Rame Hd, on W side of ent to Plymouth Sound (10.1.17), is conspic cone shaped, with small chapel on top; rks extend about 1ca off and wind-over-tide overfalls may be met 1·5M to seaward. Approaching Plymouth from the W, clear Rame Hd and Penlee Pt by about 8ca, then steer NNE for W end of the Breakwater. At the SE ent to Plymouth Sound, Great Mewstone (59m) is a conspic rky Is 4ca off Wembury Pt. Approaching from the E keep at least 1M offshore until clear of the drying Mewstone Ledge, 2½ca SW of Great Mewstone. The Slimers, which dry, lie 2ca E of Mewstone. E and W Ebb Rks (awash) lie 2½ca off Gara Pt (chart *30*). Wembury Bay gives access to R. Yealm (10.1.19).

Between Gara Pt and Stoke Pt, 2·5M to E, dangers extend about 4ca offshore in places. In Bigbury B beware Wells Rk and other dangers 5ca S of Erme Hd. From Bolt Tail to Bolt Hd keep 5ca offshore to clear Greystone Ledge, sunken rks near Ham Stone (11m), and Gregory Rks 5ca SE of Ham Stone. The Little Mew Stone and Mew Stone lie below dramatic Bolt Hd. Keep approx 7½ca SE of the Mewstones before turning N for Salcombe (10.1.20).

See 10.1.18 for submarine exercise areas offshore from Start Pt to the Scilly Isles.

START POINT TO STRAIGHT POINT (charts *1613, 3315*)

Start Pt (lt, fog sig) is 3M NE of Prawle Pt; it is a long headland with conspic radio masts and W lt ho near end. Rks lie 2½ca offshore, and the stream runs 4kn at sp, causing a race extending 1M to seaward. In fair weather the overfalls can be avoided by passing close to rks, but in bad weather keep at least 2M off. 3M S of Start the stream turns ENE at HW Devonport – 0150, and WSW at HW + 0420. Inshore it turns 30 minutes earlier.

Between Start Pt and Portland the tidal curve becomes progressively more distorted, especially on the rising tide. The rise is relatively fast for the 1st hr after LW; then slackens

noticeably for the next 1½ hrs, before resuming the rapid rate of rise. There is often a stand at HW, not very noticeable at Start Pt but lasting about 1½ hrs at Lyme Regis.

NE of Start Pt is Skerries Bank, on which sea breaks in bad weather (chart 1634). Good anch off Hallsands in offshore winds. Between Dartmouth (10.1.21) and Brixham (10.1.22) rks extend 5ca offshore.

Berry Hd (lt) is a steep, flat-topped headland (55m). Here the stream turns N at HW Devonport – 0105, and S at HW + 0440, sp rates 1·5kn. In Torbay (chart *26*) the more obvious dangers are steep-to, but beware the Sunker 100m SW of Ore Stone, and Morris Rogue 5ca W of Thatcher Rk.

There are good anchs in Babbacombe B and in Anstey's cove in W winds; beware the Three Brothers (drying rks), S side of Anstey's cove. From Long Quarry Pt for 4M N to Teignmouth (10.1.24) there are no offlying dangers. Off Teignmouth the NNE-going stream begins at HW Devonport – 0135, and the SSW-going at HW+ 0510. In the ent the flood begins at HW Devonport – 0535, and the ebb at HW +0040. The stream runs hard off Ferry Pt; the ent is dangerous in onshore winds.

Between Teignmouth and Dawlish rks extend 1ca offshore. Beware Dawlish Rk (depth 2·1m) about 5ca off N end of town. Warren Sands and Pole Sands lie W of ent to the River Exe (10.1.25), and are liable to shift. Along the NE (Exmouth) side of the chan, towards Orcomb Pt and Straight Pt (lt), drying rks and shoals extend up to 2½ca from shore. There is a firing range off Straight Pt.

LYME BAY (chart *3315*)

Start Pt is W end of Lyme B (chart *3315*), which stretches 50M ENE to Portland Bill. Tides are weak, rarely more than 0·75kn. Between Torbay and Portland there is no hbr accessible in onshore winds, and yachtsmen must take care not to be caught on a lee shore. There are no dangers offshore. In offshore winds there is a good anch NE of Beer Hd, the most W chalk cliff in England, see 10.1.25. 3·5M E of Lyme Regis (10.1.26) is Golden Cap (186m and conspic). High Ground and Pollock are rks 7ca offshore, 2M and 3M ESE of Golden Cap.

From 6M E of Bridport (10.1.27), Chesil Beach runs SE for about 8M to the N end of the Portland peninsula. From a distance Portland looks like an island, with its distinctive wedge-shaped profile sloping down from 144m at the N to the Bill at the S tip. It is mostly steep-to, but rks extend 2½ca from the Bill which is marked by a stone bn (18m) and conspic lt ho.

10.1.6   DISTANCE TABLE

Approximate distances in nautical miles are by the most direct route while avoiding dangers and allowing for Traffic Separation Schemes. Places in *italics* are in adjoining areas; places in **bold** are in 10.0.5, Cross-Channel Distances.

		1	2	3	4	5	6	7	8	9	10	11	12	13	14	15	16	17	18	19	20
1.	*Milford Haven*	**1**																			
2.	*Lundy Island*	28	**2**																		
3.	*Padstow*	67	40	**3**																	
4.	**Longships**	100	80	47	**4**																
5.	St Mary's (Scilly)	120	102	69	22	**5**															
6.	Penzance	115	95	62	15	37	**6**														
7.	Lizard Point	123	103	72	23	40	16	**7**													
8.	**Falmouth**	139	119	88	39	60	32	16	**8**												
9.	Mevagissey	152	132	99	52	69	46	28	17	**9**											
10.	**Fowey**	157	137	106	57	76	49	34	22	7	**10**										
11.	Looe	163	143	110	63	80	57	39	29	16	11	**11**									
12.	**Plymouth** (bkwtr)	170	150	117	70	92	64	49	39	25	22	11	**12**								
13.	R. Yealm (ent)	172	152	119	72	89	66	49	39	28	23	16	4	**13**							
14.	**Salcombe**	181	161	128	81	102	74	59	50	40	36	29	22	17	**14**						
15.	Start Point	186	166	135	86	103	80	63	55	45	40	33	24	22	7	**15**					
16.	**Dartmouth**	195	175	142	95	116	88	72	63	54	48	42	35	31	14	9	**16**				
17.	Torbay	201	181	150	101	118	96	78	70	62	55	50	39	38	24	15	11	**17**			
18.	Exmouth	213	193	162	113	131	107	90	82	73	67	61	51	49	33	27	24	12	**18**		
19.	Lyme Regis	226	206	173	126	144	120	104	96	86	81	74	63	62	48	41	35	30	21	**19**	
20.	*Portland Bill*	235	215	184	135	151	128	112	104	93	89	81	73	70	55	49	45	42	36	22	**20**

ENGLISH CHANNEL WAYPOINTS   10-1-7

Selected waypoints for use in English Channel crossings, are listed in order from **West** to **East** below. Those marked with an asterisk (*) are special (yellow) racing marks, and may be removed in winter. Further waypoints in coastal waters are given in section 4 of each area   (i.e. 10.1.4 to 10.3.4 on the English coast, and 10.14.4 to 10.19.4 for the French coast and the Channel Islands).

ENGLISH COAST

AREA 1

Bishop Rock Lt	49°52'·33N 06°26'·68W
Bartholomew Ledge Lt By	49°54'·38N 06°19'·80W
Seven Stones Lt F	50°03'·58N 06°04'·28W
Wolf Rock Lt	49°56'·70N 05°48'·50W
Runnel Stone Lt By	50°01'·15N 05°40'·30W
Tater Du Lt	50°03'·10N 05°34'·60W
Manacle Lt By	50°02'·77N 05°01'·85W
Low Lee Lt By	50°05'·52N 05°31'·32W
Mountamopus By	50°04'·60N 05°26'·20W
Lizard Pt Lt	49°57'·58N 05°12'·07W
August Rk By (seasonal)	50°06'·07N 05°04'·88W
Black Rk Lt By	50°08'·65N 05°01'·68W
Castle Lt By	50°08'·63N 05°01'·58W
St Anthony Hd Lt	50°08'·43N 05°00'·90W
Helston Lt By	50°04'·92N 05°00'·77W
Gwineas Lt By	50°14'·47N 04°45'·30W
Cannis Rk Lt By	50°18'·35N 04°39'·88W
Udder Rk By	50°18'·90N 04°33'·78W
Eddystone Lt	50°10'·81N 04°15'·87W
West Tinker Lt By	50°19'·22N 04°08'·57W
East Tinker Lt By	50°19'·17N 04°08'·23W
Start Point Lt	50°13'·32N 03°38'·47W
Royal Dart YC No. 1 By*	50°18'·80N 03°35'·25W
Checkstone Lt By	50°20'·42N 03°33'·73W
Royal Dart YC No. 2 By*	50°18'·68N 03°33'·29W
Castle Ledge Lt By	50°19'·95N 03°33'·05W
Royal Dart YC No. 3 By*	50°20'·07N 03°31'·42W
Brixham Fairway Lt By	50°24'·37N 03°30'·85W
Berry Head Lt	50°23'·94N 03°28'·93W
East Exe Lt By	50°35'·97N 03°22'·30W
Straight Point Lt	50°36'·45N 03°21'·67W
DZ Lt By	50°36'·50N 02°42'·00W
Portland Bill Lt	50°30'·82N 02°27'·32W

AREA 2

West Shambles Lt By	50°29'·75N 02°24'·33W
East Shambles Lt By	50°30'·75N 02°20'·00W
Anvil Point Lt	50°35'·48N 01°57'·52W
Peverill Ledge By	50°36'·38N 01°56'·02W
Poole Fairway Lt By	50°38'·95N 01°54'·78W
Needles Fairway Lt By	50°38'·20N 01°38'·90W
SW Shingles Lt By	50°39'·37N 01°37'·25W
Needles Lt	50°39'·70N 01°35'·43W
North Head Lt By	50°42'·65N 01°35'·43W
NE Shingles Lt By	50°41'·93N 01°33'·32W
St Catherine's Pt Lt	50°34'·52N 01°17'·80W
West Princessa Lt By	50°40'·12N 01°03'·57W
Bembridge Ledge Lt By	50°41'·12N 01°02'·72W
New Grounds Lt By	50°41'·97N 00°58'·53W
Nab Tower Lt	50°40'·05N 00°57'·07W

AREA 3

Boulder Lt By	50°41'·53N 00°49'·00W
Owers Lanby	50°37'·27N 00°40'·60W
East Borough Hd Lt By	50°41'·50N 00°39'·00W
Brighton Marina Lt	50°48'·47N 00°06'·30W
Newhaven Bkwtr Lt	50°46'·52N 00°03'·60E
Beachy Hd Lt	50°44'·00N 00°14'·60E
Sovereign Hbr Lt By	50°47'·38N 00°20'·45E
Royal Sovereign Lt	50°43'·42N 00°26'·18E
North Goodwin Lt By	51°17'·88N 01°30'·55E
Rye Fairway Lt By	50°54'·00N 00°48'·13E
Dungeness Lt	50°54'·77N 00°58'·67E
South Goodwin Lt F	51°07'·95N 01°28'·60E

OFFSHORE

Channel Lt F	49°54'·42N 02°53'·67W
E Channel Lt By	49°58'·67N 02°28'·87W
EC1 Lt By	50°05'·90N 01°48'·35W
EC2 Lt By	50°12'·10N 01°12'·40W
EC3 Lt By	50°18'·30N 00°36'·10W
CS1 Lt By	50°33'·67N 00°03'·83W
Greenwich Lt V	50°24'·50N 00°00'·00
CS2 Lt By	50°39'·10N 00°32'·70E
CS3 Lt By	50°52'·00N 01°02'·30E
Bullock Bank Lt By	50°46'·90N 01°07'·70E
South Varne Lt By	50°55'·60N 01°17'·40E
Varne Lanby	51°01'·25N 01°24'·00E
CS4 Lt By	51°08'·58N 01°34'·03E
MPC Lt By	51°06'·09N 01°38'·36E
Sandettié Lt F	51°09'·40N 01°47'·20E
CS5 Lt By	51°23'·00N 01°50'·00E

CHANNEL ISLANDS

AREA 14

Roches Douvres Lt	49°06'·35N 02°48'·82W
Les Hanois Lt	49°26'·16N 02°42'·02W
St Martin's Point Lt	49°25'·37N 02°31'·61W
Reffée Lt By	49°27'·80N 02°31'·18W
Platte Fougère Lt	49°30'·88N 02°29'·05W
Casquets Lt	49°43'·38N 02°22'·55W
NW Minquiers Lt By	48°59'·70N 02°20'·50W
SW Minquiers Lt By	48°54'·40N 02°19'·30W
Desormes Lt By	49°19'·00N 02°17'·90W
La Corbière Lt	49°10'·85N 02°14'·90W
Passage Rk Lt By	49°09'·59N 02°12'·18W

S Minquiers Lt By	48°53'·15N 02°10'·00W
Alderney Main Lt	49°43'·81N 02°09'·77W
Diamond Rk Lt By	49°10'·18N 02°08'·56W
N Minquiers Lt By	49°01'·70N 02°00'·50W
Canger Rk Lt By	49°07'·41N 02°00'·30W
SE Minquiers Lt By	48°53'·50N 02°00'·00W
Frouquier Aubert Lt By	49°06'·14N 01°58'·78W
NE Minquiers Lt By	49°00'·90N 01°55'·20W

FRENCH COAST

Selected waypoints in Areas 15 and 16 on the French coast are mainly listed in order from **East** to **West** below.

AREA 15

Les Équets Lt By	49°43'·68N 01°18'·28W
Basse du Rénier Lt By	49°44'·90N 01°22'·10W
La Pierre Noire Lt By	49°43'·57N 01°28'·98W
Cherbourg Fort Ouest Lt	49°40'·50N 01°38'·87W
CH1 Lt By	49°43'·30N 01°42'·10W
Basse Bréfort Lt By	49°43'·70N 01°51'·05W
Cap de la Hague Lt	49°43'·37N 01°57'·19W
Cap de Carteret Lt	49°22'·46N 01°48'·35W
Les Trois-Grunes Lt By	49°21'·88N 01°55'·12W
Écrévière Lt By	49°15'·33N 01°52'·08W
Basse Jourdan Lt By	49°06'·90N 01°44'·07W
La Catheue Lt By	48°57'·95N 01°42'·00W
Anvers Lt By	48°53'·90N 01°40'·84W
Le Videcoq Lt By	48°49'·70N 01°42'·02W
Chausey, Grand Île Lt	48°52'·25N 01°49'·27W
SW Minquiers Lt By	48°54'·40N 02°19'·30W
St Malo Fairway Lt By	48°41'·42N 02°07'·21W
Le Sou Lt By	48°40'·17N 02°05'·16W
Bassée NE Lt By	48°42'·51N 02°09'·34W
Banchenou Lt By	48°40'·52N 02°11'·42W
Cap Fréhel Lt	48°41'·10N 02°19'·07W
Caffa Lt By	48°37'·89N 02°43'·00W
Le Rohein Lt Bn	48°38'·88N 02°37'·68W
Grande Lejon Lt	48°44'·95N 02°39'·90W
Le Légué Lt By	48°34'·38N 02°41'·07W
Le Guildo Lt By	48°41'·42N 02°07'·22W
Cap Lévi Lt	49°41'·80N 01°28'·40W

AREA 16

Barnouic Lt	49°01'·70N 02°48'·33W
Roche Gautier Lt By	49°00'·49N 02°52'·92W
Les Echaudés By	48°53'·44N 02°57'·27W
Rosédo (Bréhat) Lt	48°51'·50N 03°00'·21W
Les Héaux Lt	48°54'·57N 03°05'·10W
La Jument des Héaux By	48°55'·41N 03°07'·95W

Les Sept Îles Lt	48°52'·78N 03°29'·33W
Les Triagoz Lt	48°52'·35N 03°38'·73W
Méloine By	48°45'·65N 03°50'·55W
Astan Lt By	48°44'·95N 03°57'·55W
Île de Batz Lt	48°44'·78N 04°01'·55W
Île de Batz Lt	48°44'·78N 04°01'·55W
Île Vierge Lt	48°38'·38N 04°33'·97W
Trépied By	48°37'·35N 04°37'·47W
Libenter Lt By	48°37'·57N 04°38'·35W
Ruzven Lt By	48°36'·15N 04°39'·30W
Le Relec Lt By	48°36'·05N 04°40'·76W
Basse de Portsall Lt By	48°36'·78N 04°46'·05W
Basse Paotr Bihan By	48°35'·38N 04°46'·16W
Créac'h Lt	48°27'·62N 05°07'·72W
Ouessant NE Lt By	48°45'·90N 05°11'·60W
Ouessant SW Lanby	48°31'·68N 05°49'·10W

AREA 19

Pointe de Barfleur Lt	49°41'·83N 01°15'·87W
Îles St Marcouf Lt	49°29'·90N 01°08'·70W
Norfalk Lt By	49°28'·83N 01°03'·40W
Est du Cardonnet Lt By	49°26'·97N 01°01'·00W
Broadswood Lt By	49°25'·39N 00°52'·90W
Cussy Lt By	49°29'·50N 00°43'·25W
Ver-sur-Mer Lt	49°20'·47N 00°31'·15W
Northgate Lt By	49°30'·40N 00°14'·15W
LHA Lanby	49°31'·44N 00°09'·78W
A17 Lt By	49°41'·60N 00°01'·75E
A18 Lt By	49°42'·07N 00°02'·21E
Ratier NW Lt By	49°26'·85N 00°02'·55E
Cap de la Hève Lt	49°30'·79N 00°04'·24E
Cap d'Antifer Lt	49°41'·07N 00°10'·00E
Pointe d'Ailly Lt	49°55'·13N 00°57'·56E
Bassurelle Lt By	50°32'·70N 00°57'·80E
Ecovouga Lt By	50°33'·62N 00°59'·00E
Daffodils Lt By	50°02'·52N 01°04'·10E
Vergoyer SW Lt By	50°26'·90N 01°00'·10E
ZC1 Lt By	50°44'·94N 01°27'·10E
Ault Lt	50°06'·32N 01°27'·31E
AT-SO Lt By	50°14'·00N 01°28'·50E
Ophélie Lt By	50°43'·91N 01°30'·92E
ZC2 Lt By	50°53'·50N 01°31'·00E
Pointe de Haut Blanc Lt	50°23'·90N 01°33'·75E
Cap d'Alprech Lt	50°41'·95N 01°33'·83E
Cap Gris Nez Lt	50°52'·05N 01°35'·07E
Abbeville Lt By	50°56'·05N 01°37'·70E
CA3 Lt By	50°56'·80N 01°41'·25E
CA4 Lt By	50°58'·94N 01°45'·18E
Sangatte Lt	50°57'·23N 01°46'·57E
Ruytingen SW Lt By	51°04'·94N 01°46'·90E
Dunkerque Lanby	51°03'·00N 01°51'·83E
Walde Lt	50°59'·57N 01°55'·00E
DKA Lt By	51°02'·59N 01°57'·06E

ISLES OF SCILLY   10·1·8

The Isles of Scilly are made up of 48 islands and numerous rocky outcrops, covering an area approx 10M by 7M and lying 21 – 31M WSW of Land's End. Only six islands are inhabited: St Mary's, St Martin's, Tresco, Bryher, St Agnes and Gugh. The islands belong to the Duchy of Cornwall. Arrangements for visiting uninhabited islands are given in a booklet *Duchy of Cornwall - Information for visiting craft* obtainable from Hr Mr, Hugh Town Hbr, St Mary's.There is a LB and a HM CG Sector Base at St Mary's.
Historic Wrecks (see 10.0.3g) are at: 49°52'·6N 06°26'·5N Tearing Ledge, 2ca SE of Bishop Rk Lt; and at: 49°54'·26N 06°19'·83W, Bartholomew Ledges, 5ca N of Gugh

CHARTS
AC *883, 34* (both essential); Scilly to Lands End 1148; Imray C7; Stanfords 2, 13; OS 203.
TIDES
Standard Port is Devonport. Differences for St Mary's are given in 10·1·9. Tidal heights, times, directions and rates around the islands are irregular; see AC 34 for streams.
SHELTER
The Isles of Scilly are exposed to Atlantic swell and wind. Weather can be unpredictable and fast-changing. It is not a place for inexperienced navigators or poorly equipped yachts. Normal yacht ⚓s may drag on fine sand, even with plenty of scope, but holding is mostly good. That said, the islands are attractive, interesting and rewarding.

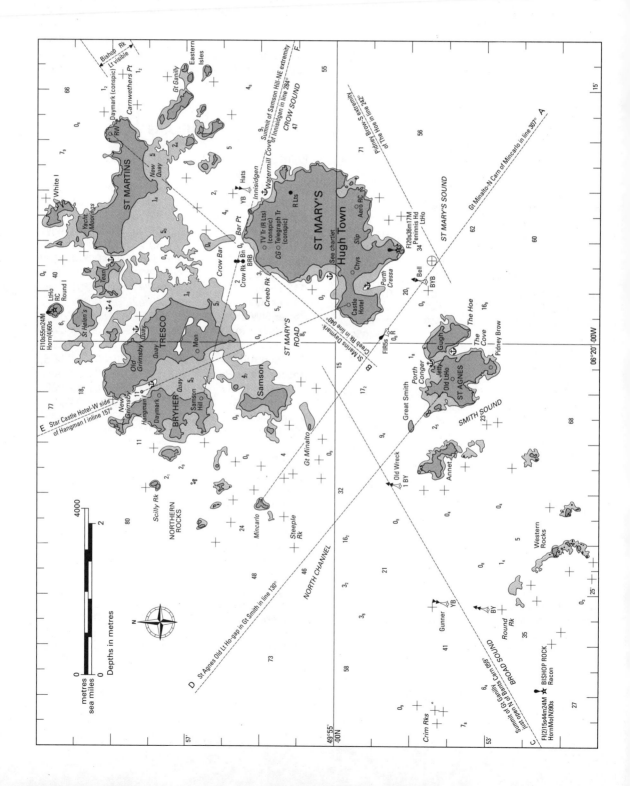

The following are some of the many ⚓s, anti-clockwise:

HUGH TOWN HBR (St Mary's). See 10·1·9 facing.

PORTH CRESSA (St. Mary's, S of Hugh Town). Beware of dangers on each side of ent and the submarine cables. Exposed to swell from SE to SW. ⚓ in approx 2m.

WATERMILL COVE (NE corner of St Mary's). Excellent shelter in winds S to NW. ⚓ in approx 5m.

TEAN SOUND (St Martin's, W end). Needs careful pilotage, but attractive ⚓ in better weather. More suitable for shoal draught boats which can ⚓ or take the ground out of main tidal stream in chan. St Martins Hotel ☎ 422092, D, FW, M (6), V, R, Bar. There are several other ⚓s which can be used in settled weather.

ST HELEN'S POOL (S of St Helen's Is). Ent via St Helen's Gap to ⚓ in 1·5m - 7m. Secure, but may be swell near HW.

OLD GRIMSBY (NE side of Tresco). Green Porth & Raven's Porth, divided by a quay, form the Old Grimsby Hbr; both dry 2·3m. Beware cable in Green Porth. ⚓ 1½ca NE of quay in 2·5m; access more difficult than New Grimsby. Well sheltered in SW winds but open to swell if wind veers N of W. Facilities: L (quay), hotel, slip (hotel).

NEW GRIMSBY (between Tresco and Bryher). Appr (line E) through New Grimsby Sound, or with sufficient rise of tide across Tresco Flats. Good shelter except in NW'lies. Popular ⚓ between Hangman Is and the quay in 1·5 to 4·5m. Beware cables. Moorings from Tresco Estate. Facilities: Bar, R, FW, V, ✉. Ferry to St Mary's.

THE COVE (St Agnes/Gugh). Well sheltered from W and N winds, except when the sand bar between the islands covers near HWS with a strong NW wind. Beware cables.

PORTH CONGER (St Agnes/Gugh). On the N side of the sandbar, sheltered in winds from E through S to W. May be uncomfortable when the bar is covered. Facilities: L (two quays), ferry to St Mary's; in Middle Town (¾M), St Agnes, V, ✉, R, Bar.

NAVIGATION
For TSS to the E, S and W, see Fig. 10 (5) and 10.1.2. If ldg lines/marks cannot be identified, then it is best to lie off. Pilotage is compulsory for all vessels, except HM Ships, trawlers <47·5m LOA and yachts <20m LOA, navigating within a radius of 6M from S tip of Samson Is excluding St Mary's Hbr. Many chans between islands have dangerous shallows, often with rky ledges. Beware lobster pots.

Line A, via St Mary's Sound, is the normal ent to St Mary's Road. Appr from the E or SE to avoid Gilstone Rk (dries 4m) 3ca E of Peninnis Hd. Spanish Ledges, off Gugh, are marked by an unlit ECM By; thence past Woolpack SCM bn and PHM By Fl R 5s (Bartholomew Ledge) to ent St Mary's Rd on 040°,

Line B, which clears Woodcock Ledge (breaks in bad wx).

Line C, from SW: Broad Sound is entered between Bishops Rk lt ho and Flemming's Ledge about 7ca to the N, then twixt Round Rk NCM and Gunner SCM buoys to Old Wreck NCM buoy; beware Jeffrey Rk, close to port. Ldg marks are more than 7M off and at first not easy to see. Smith Sound, 350° between St Agnes and Annet may also be used.

Line D, from NW: North Chan is about 7ca wide, and of easy access with good ldg marks, but beware cross tide and Steeple Rk (0·1m, 2ca to port). Intercept Line C for St Mary's Road.

Line E, from the N, leads between Bryher and Tresco, into New Grimsby Hbr (see SHELTER); thence it winds across Tresco Flats (with adequate rise of tide and good vis).

Line F, from the E & NE: Crow Sound is not difficult, with sufficient rise of tide but can be rough in strong E or S winds. From NE a yacht can pass close to Menawethan and Biggal Rk, avoiding Trinity Rk and the Ridge, which break in bad weather. Hats SCM buoy marks a shoal with an old boiler, drying 0·6m, on it. Track 254° between Bar Pt and Crow Bar (dries 0·7m), passing Crow Rk IDM bn on its N side (for best water) before altering SSW for St Mary's.

LIGHTS AND MARKS
See 10·1·4 for lts, including Seven Stones lt float, Wolf Rock lt ho and Longships lt ho. A working knowledge of the following daymarks and conspic features will greatly aid pilotage (from NE to SW):

St Martin's E end: Conical bn tr (56m) with RW bands.
Round Is: conical shaped Is with W lt ho 19/55m high.
Tresco: Abbey & FS, best seen from S. Cromwell's Castle and Hangman Is from the NW.
Bryher: Watch Hill, stone bn (43m); rounded Samson Hill.
St Mary's: TV & radio masts at N end; wind-motor to E, all with R lts. Crow Rk IDM bn, 11m on rk drying 4·6m, at N.
St. Agnes: Old lt ho, ○ W tr, visible from all directions.
Bishop Rk lt ho: Grey ○ tr, 44m; helo pad above lamp.

ST MARY'S   10-1-9
Isles of Scilly 49°55'·10N 06°18'·65W

CHARTS
AC 883, 34; Imray C7; Stanfords 2; OS 203

TIDES
+0607 Dover; ML 3·2; Duration 0600; Zone 0 (UT)

Standard Port DEVONPORT (→)

Times				Height (metres)			
High Water		Low Water		MHWS	MHWN	MLWN	MLWS
0000	0600	0000	0600	5·5	4·4	2·2	0·8
1200	1800	1200	1800				
Differences ST MARY'S							
−0050	−0100	−0045	−0045	+0·2	−0·1	−0·2	−0·1

SHELTER
Good shelter in St Mary's Pool in up to 3·5m, but it is notorious for yachts dragging in W to NW gales, when Porth Cressa (see 10·1·8) is better. ⚓ is prohib S of a line from the pier hd to the LB slip; to seaward of the LB mooring; off the pier hd where the ferry turns, and in the apprs. Speed limit 3kn. Note: Do not impede the ferry Scillonian III which arrives about 1200 and sails at 1630.

NAVIGATION
WPT via St Mary's Sound: Spanish Ledge unlit ECM buoy, 49°53'·90N 06°18'·80W, 128°/308° from/to transit line B (040°), 1·2M. See also 10·1·4 and 10·1·8. The 097° transit leads S of Bacon Ledge (0·3m); the 151° transit leads into the Pool between Bacon Ledge and the Cow & Calf (drying 0·6 and 1·8m) to the E.

LIGHTS AND MARKS
2 ldg marks, (both show FR lts for commercial ships) lead 097° into the Pool; front bn = W △ on pole on W pyramid, rear = black X on pole (hard to see). Pier hd lt is FG 4m 3M on bldg with W roof, vis 072°-192°. Buzza Hill tr and power stn chy (48m) are conspic.

RADIO TELEPHONE
St Mary's Hbr VHF Ch 14 16 (0800-1700LT). Pilot Ch 69 16. Lands End Radio Ch 64 covers Scillies. St Mary's CG Ch 16 67 (manned in bad wx only). Falmouth CG provides radio cover Ch 16 of the TSS/ITZ off Land's End. Do not hesitate to call the CG Ch 16 in emergency/gales/dragging ⚓.

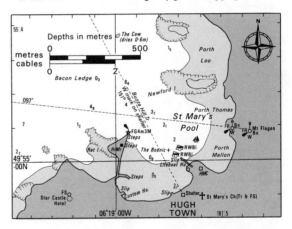

TELEPHONE (01720)
Hr Mr 422768; MRCC (01326) 317575; ⊞ (01752) 220661, or locally 422571; Marinecall 0891 500458; Police 422444; Ⓗ 422392; Dr 422628; Pilot 422066; Tourist Info 422536.

FACILITIES
Hbr ⚓ (Overnight dues: >9m LOA = £7.50; <9m = £6.50), L, M, Gas, Gaz, P (cans), D (bowser on quay), FW (⚓ on pier, 0930-1130, except Sat; see Hr Mr), Slip. Hbr Office will hold mail for visiting yachts if addressed c/o the Hr Mr.
Services: ACA, Sh, CH, ME, El; **Isles of Scilly YC** ☎ 422352, Bar, Ⓞ, R.
Hugh Town EC Wed (or Thurs according to ferry sailings); limited shopping facilities, ✉, Ⓑ, Ⓞ. Ferry bookings ☎ 01736-62009, daily (2h40m) to Penzance (⇌); ✈ Helicopter to Penzance and fixed wing to St Just, near Lands End, and Exeter (⇌). There are ✉, R, V, Bar etc. at Tresco, Bryher, St Martins and St Agnes.

NEWLYN   10-1-10

Cornwall 50°06'·15N 05°32'.52W

CHARTS
AC 2345, 777; Imray C7; Stanfords 13; OS 203
TIDES
+0600 Dover; ML 3·2; Duration 0555; Zone 0 (UT)

Standard Port DEVONPORT (→)

Times				Height (metres)			
High Water		Low Water		MHWS	MHWN	MLWN	MLWS
0000	0600	0000	0600	5·5	4·4	2·2	0·8
1200	1800	1200	1800				
Differences NEWLYN							
−0055	−0115	−0035	−0035	+0·1	0·0	−0·2	0·0

SHELTER
Good, except in SE winds when heavy swell enters hbr; access at all tides. FVs take priority. Yachts berth on SW side of Mary Williams Pier. No ⚓s, no ⚓ in hbr. Good ⚓ in Gwavas Lake in offshore winds.
NAVIGATION
WPT 50°06'·15N 05°31'·74W, 090°/270° from/to S pier, 0·5M. From NE, beware The Gear and Dog Rk 3½ca NE of hbr ent; from S beware Low Lee and Carn Base.
LIGHTS AND MARKS
S pier hd, Fl 5s 10m 9M; vis 253°-336°, W tr, R base and cupola; Siren 60s. N pier hd, F WG 4m 2M; vis G238°-248°, W over hbr. Old Quay hd, FR 3m 1M.
RADIO TELEPHONE
Call: Newlyn Hbr VHF Ch 09 12 16 (Mon-Fri 0800-1700, Sat 0800-1200LT).
TELEPHONE (01736)
Hr Mr 62523; MRCC (01326) 317575; ⌖ (10752) 220661; Marinecall 0891 500458; Police 62395; Ⓗ 62382; Dr 63866.
FACILITIES
N Pier Slip, D (cans), L, FW, C (6 ton); Mary Williams Pier £6.
Services: ME, Sh, Gas, El, Ⓔ, CH. Town EC Wed; ◌, V, R, Bar, ✉, Ⓑ (AM only), bus to Penzance for ⇌, ✈.

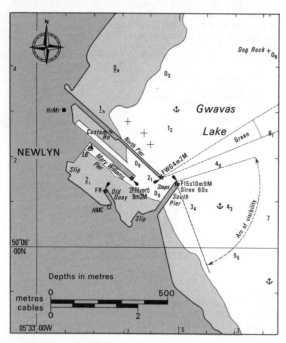

ADJACENT HARBOUR
MOUSEHOLE, Cornwall, 50°04'·93N 05°32'·20W. AC 2345. HW +0550 on Dover; Tides as Newlyn; ML 3·2m; Duration 0600. Shelter good except in NE and SE winds; protected by St Clements Is from E'lies. Best appr from S, midway between St Clements Is and bkwtr. Ent 11m wide; hbr dries 1·8m, access HW±3. Ent is closed with timber baulks from Nov-Apl. Lts N pier 2 FG (vert) 8/6m 4M; 2 FR (vert) = hbr closed. Hr Mr ☎ (01736) 731511. Facilities limited: FW, V, Slip. Buses to Penzance.

PENZANCE   10-1-11

Cornwall 50°07'·05N 05°31'·62W

CHARTS
AC 2345, 777; Imray C7; Stanfords 13; OS 203
TIDES
−0635 Dover; ML 3·2; Duration 0550; Zone 0 (UT)

Standard Port DEVONPORT (→)

Times				Height (metres)			
High Water		Low Water		MHWS	MHWN	MLWN	MLWS
0000	0600	0000	0600	5·5	4·4	2·2	0·8
1200	1800	1200	1800				
Differences PENZANCE							
−0055	−0115	−0035	−0035	+0·1	0·0	−0·2	0·0
PORTHLEVEN							
−0050	−0105	−0030	−0025	0·0	−0·1	−0·2	0·0
LIZARD POINT							
−0045	−0100	−0030	−0030	−0·2	−0·2	−0·3	−0·2

SHELTER
Excellent in the wet dock; gates open HW −1½ to HW +1. Mounts Bay is unsafe ⚓ in S or SE winds, which, if strong, also render the hbr ent dangerous.
NAVIGATION
WPT 50°06'·70N 05°31'·10W, 135°/315° from/to S pier hd, 0·48M. Beware Gear Rk 0·4M S. Cressar (5ca NE of ent) and Long Rks are marked by SCM bns. Hbr speed limit 5kn.
LIGHTS AND MARKS
There are no ldg lts/marks. S pier hd Fl WR 5s 11m 17/12M; W268°-344·5°.
Dock ent sigs, shown from FS at N side of Dock gate (may not be given for yachts).
2B ● (hor) (2FR (vert) by night) = Dock gates open.
2B ● (vert) (Ⓡ over Ⓖ by night) = Dock gates shut.
RADIO TELEPHONE
VHF Ch 09 12 16 (HW −2 to HW +1, and office hrs).
TELEPHONE (01736)
Hr Mr 66113; MRCC (01326) 317575; ⌖ (01752) 220661; Marinecall 0891 500458; Police 62395; Dr 63866, Ⓗ 62382.
FACILITIES
Wet Dock (50 visitors) ☎ 66113, Fax 66114, £9, M, D (cans), L, FW, AC, C (3 ton). S Pier ☎ 66113, AB, D, FW; Penzance YC ☎ 64989, Bar, L, FW, R; Services: Slip (dry dock), ME, El, CH, SM, Sh, Gas, Gaz.
Town EC Wed (winter only); ◌, V, R, Bar, ✉, Ⓑ, ⇌, ✈.

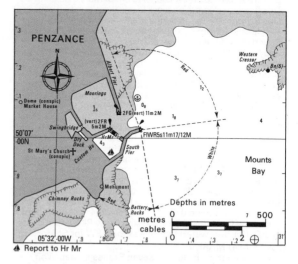

▲ Report to Hr Mr

ADJACENT HARBOUR
ST MICHAEL'S MOUNT, Cornwall, 50°07'·10N 05°28'·58W. AC 2345, 777. HW +0550 on Dover; Tides as Penzance; ML 3·2m; Duration 0550. Shelter good from N to SE, but only in fair wx. Hbr dries; it has approx 3·3m at MHWS and 1·4m at MHWN. Beware Hogus Rks to NW of hbr and Outer Penzeath Rk about 3ca WSW of Hogus Rks. Also beware Maltman Rk 1ca SSW of the Mount. There are no lts. Ent between piers is 30m wide. No facilities on the island except FW; some at Marazion, 5M to N. EC Wed.

ADJACENT HARBOURS ON THE LIZARD PENINSULA

PORTHLEVEN, Cornwall, 50°04'·88N 05°19'·07W. AC 2345, *777.* HW +0551 on Dover; ML 3·1m; Duration 0545. See 10.1.11. Hbr dries 2m above the old LB ho but has approx 2·3m in centre of ent; access HW±3. It is open to W and SW. Beware rks round pier hd and Deazle Rks to W. Lt on S pier FG 10m 4M = inner hbr open. Inside hbr FG vis 033°-067° when required for vessels entering. Visitors go alongside the Quay on E side. Hr Mr ☎ (01326) 561141; Facilities: **Inner Hbr** AB £5, FW, L, ME, P & D (cans). **Village** EC Wed; ⊠, ⎘, R, Ⓑ, V, Bar.

MULLION COVE, Cornwall, 50°00'·86N, 05°15'·48W. AC 2345, 777. Lizard HW +0552 on Dover; −0050 on Devonport; HW −0·2m on Devonport; ML 3·0m; Duration 0545. Porth Mellin hbr dries 2·4m and open to W winds. ⚓ in Mullion Cove is safer especially in lee of Mullion Island where there is approx 3·5m, but local knowledge is advised. NT owns the island and the hbr. Due to lack of space, visiting boats may only stay in hbr briefly to load/unload. There are no lts. There is a slip on E side of hbr. Hr Mr ☎ (01326) 240222. Only facilities at Mullion village (1M) EC Wed; Bar, V.

Historic Wrecks (see 10.0.3g) are located at:
50°03'·40N 05°17'·10W (*St Anthony*), 2M SE of Porthleven.
50°02'·33N 05°16'·40W (*Schiedam*), 1·5M N of Mullion Is.
49°58'·50N 05°14'·45W, Rill Cove, 1·4M NW of Lizard Pt.
49°57'·45N 05°12'·92W, (*Royal Anne*) The Stags, Lizard Pt.

CADGWITH, Cornwall, 49°59'·18N 05°10'·62W. AC 2345, *154, 777;* HW +0555 on Dover; −0030 on Devonport; −0·2m on Devonport; ML 3·0m. See Differences Lizard Pt under 10.1.11. Hbr dries; it is divided by a rky outcrop, The Todden. Beware the extension of this, rks called The Mare; also beware The Boa rks to ESE which cover at quarter tide. ⚓ off The Mare in about 2–3m, but not recommended in on-shore winds. There are no lts. Many local FVs operate from here and are hauled up on the shingle beach. Facilities: ⊠, Bar, R.

COVERACK, Cornwall, 50°01'·40N 05°05'·60W. AC *154, 777.* HW +0605 on Dover; ML 3·0m; Duration 0550. See 10.1.12. Hbr dries but has 3·3m at MHWS and 2·2m at MHWN. In good weather and off-shore winds it is better to ⚓ outside. Hbr is very small and full of FVs. From the S beware the Guthens, off Chynhalls Pt; from the N, the Dava and other rks off Lowland Pt, and Manacle Rks to the NE (ECM, Q(3) 10s bell). There are no lts. Hr Mr ☎ (01326) 280583. Facilities: EC Tues; FW (hotel) D, P (cans) from garage (2M uphill), V, ⊠.

HELFORD RIVER   10-1-12

Cornwall 50°05'·75N 05·06'·00W (Ent)

CHARTS
AC 147, *154*; Imray C6, Y57; Stanfords 13; OS 204

TIDES
−0613 Dover; ML 3·0; Duration 0550; Zone 0 (UT)

Reference Port FALMOUTH (→)

Times				Height (metres)			
High Water		Low Water		MHWS	MHWN	MLWN	MLWS
0000	0600	0000	0600	5·3	4·2	1·9	0·6
1200	1800	1200	1800				
Differences HELFORD RIVER (Ent)							
0000	−0005	−0005	0000	0·0	0·0	0·0	0·0
COVERACK							
0000	−0010	−0010	0000	0·0	0·0	0·0	0·0

SHELTER
Excellent, except in E'lies. Moorings administered by Hr Mr. ⚓s marked 'Visitors' on G can buoys or G pick-up buoys. Ferry will collect people from yachts, if requested during normal ferry operating hrs. Speed limit 6kn.
⚓ s at: Durgan Bay, good; off Helford, but tides strong; Navas Creek, good shelter, little room, YC wall dries 1·9m. Gillan Creek is good except in E'lies, but beware Car Croc rk in ent marked by ECM buoy in season.
Note: A local bye-law states that yachts must not ⚓ in the river and creeks W of Navas Creek due to oyster beds.

NAVIGATION
WPT 50°05'·70N 05°04'·50W, 093°/273° from/to The Voose NCM bn, 1·5M. From N beware August Rock (alias the Gedges), marked by SHM (seasonal). From SE keep well clear of Nare Pt and Dennis Hd. Keep Helford Pt open of Bosahan Pt to clear rky reef off E end of Bosahan Pt marked by The Voose NCM (seasonal). Avoid mud bank marked by Bar By SHM (seasonal) on N side of river opposite Helford Creek. PHM and SHM posts mark chan from Mawgan Creek to Gweek.

LIGHTS AND MARKS
Bosahan Pt on with Mawnan Shear (259°) clears August Rk (The Gedges), dangerous rks marked by unlit SHM By.

RADIO TELEPHONE
Helford River SC VHF Ch **80** M.

TELEPHONE (01326)
Moorings Officer 221265; MRCC 317575; ⚓ (01752) 220661; Marinecall 0891 500458; Police 72231; Ⓗ 572151.

FACILITIES
Moorings £4.50. Please ditch rubbish only at the Helford River SC. **Helford River SC** ☎ 231460, Slip, FW, R, Bar, ⎘; **Porth Navas YC** ☎ 40419, Gas, C (3 ton), M, AC, V, L, Bar, R, FW, P, D;
Helford Passage Slip, L, FW; **Gweek Quay** ☎ 22657, C (30 ton), M, CH, R, El, Sh, ME, FW, Ⓔ.
Services: M, FW, Gas, Gaz, Slip, L, Sh, CH, ⎘, D (cans). EC Wed; ⊠ (Helford, Gweek, Mawnan-Smith, Mawgan); Ⓑ Mawnan-Smith (Jan-Sept Mon, Wed, Fri AM only. Oct-May Tues, Fri AM only); ⇌ (bus to Falmouth); ✈ (Penzance or Newquay).

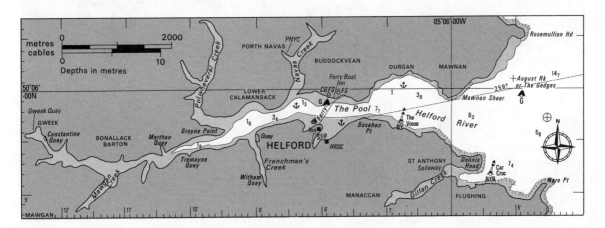

RIVER FAL   10-1-13

Cornwall 50°08'·58N 05°01'·42W (Ent)

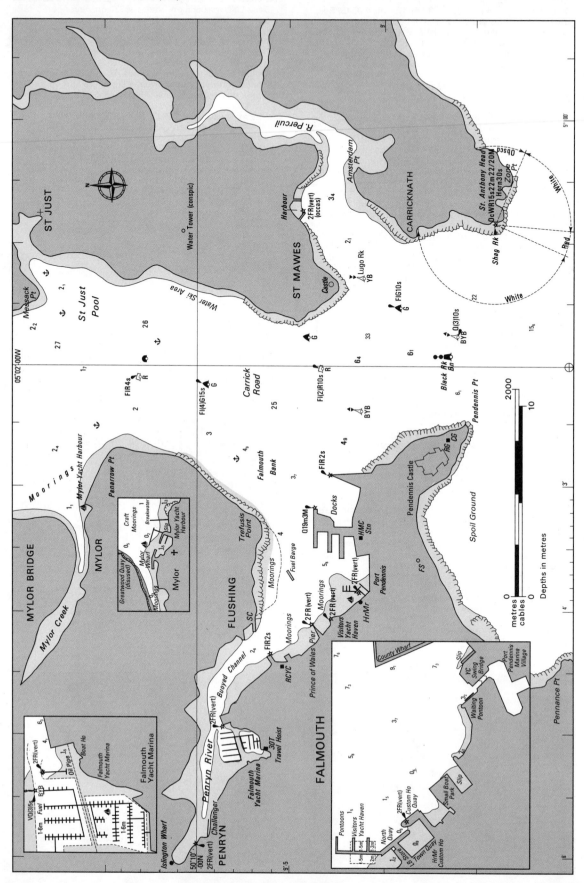

CHARTS
AC *32*, 18, *154*; Imray C6, Y58; Stanfords 13; OS 204
TIDES
–0558 Dover; ML 3·0; Duration 0550; Zone 0 (UT)
Daily Predictions and Tidal Curve are given below.
HW Truro is approx HW Falmouth +0008 and –1·8m.

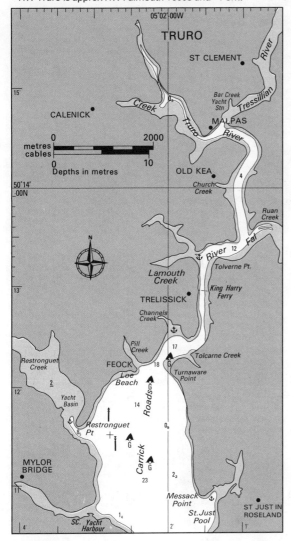

NAVIGATION
WPT 50°08'·00N 05°02'·00W, 183°/003° from/to Black Rock
IDM bn, 0·68M. Ent is 1M wide and deep. Hbr can be
entered in any weather or tide although on-shore winds
against an ebb tide make it a bit rough. The only hazard is
Black Rk in the middle of the ent; pass either side, but at
night the E chan is advised leaving the ECM buoy, Q (3)
10s, to port.
Falmouth is a deep water port, taking ships up to 90,000
tons; appropriate facilities are available. Take care not to
impede shipping or ⚓ in prohib areas. Beware oyster
beds, especially in Penryn R.
Mylor Creek is shallow, approx 1m everywhere except in
Mylor Pool itself. Restronguet Creek has as little as 0·6m
at MLWS and beware Carrick Carlys Rk just N of ent,
marked with BY posts with NCM and SCM topmarks. At
the N end of Carrick Roads, Turnaware Pt marks the start
of the river; beware strong tides and rips. Truro dries, but
can be reached on the tide; a tidal barrage 8ca NW of
Malpas, marked by 2 FR/FG (vert), is normally open. 3 Fl
R lts show when it is closed. In St Mawes Hbr ent beware
Lugo Rk, which is always covered; pass S of St Mawes
SCM buoy.

LIGHTS AND MARKS
St Anthony Hd lt (H24), R sector covers the Manacles Rks.
RADIO TELEPHONE
Call: *Falmouth Hbr Radio*, VHF Ch **12** 16 (Mon-Fri 0800-
1700LT); Hbr launch *Killigrew* Ch 12. Port Health Ch 12 16.
CG: Ch 16 67. Customs launch Ch 12 09 06 10 14 16.
Mylor Yacht Hbr, Falmouth Yacht Marina, Port Pendennis
Marina and Royal Cornwall YC Ch **80**, M (H24). Visitors
Yacht Haven Ch 12 16. Malpas Marine and St Mawes SC:
Ch M (HO). Fuel Barge Ch 16. Falmouth CG Ch 16 provides
radio coverage of the TSS/ITZ off Land's End; see Fig 10
(5) and 10.1.2.
TELEPHONE (Falmouth 01326; Truro 01872)
Hr Mr Falmouth 314379, Fax 211352; Hbr Commissioners
312285; Hr Mr Penryn 373352; Hr Mr St Mawes 270553;
MRCC 317575; ⌗ (01752) 220661; Marinecall 0891 500458;
Weather 42534; Police 72231; Dr 317317; Ⓗ Truro 74242.

FACILITIES
FALMOUTH
Port Pendennis Marina ☎ 211211, AC, FW, YC (R, Bar, ◻,
CH), visitors berths inside lock.
Falmouth Hbr Visitors Yacht Haven (40) ☎ 314379 (Apr-
Sept inc), Fax 211352, P, D, FW, Access H24.
Falmouth Yacht Marina (280+80 visitors), ☎ 316620, Fax
313939, £14.50, AC, FW, CH, V, P (cans), D, ME, El, Sh, ◻,
BH (30 ton), C (2 ton), Gas, Gaz, SM, Bar, R; access H24,
but least depths of 1·6m require caution at LWS.
Services: Slip, BH (60 ton), C (48 ton), ME, Sh, El, M, SM,
Gaz, CH, ACA, FW, C. Note: Fuel Barge all year, as chartlet,
VHF 16.
Town EC Wed (winter only); V, R, Bar, ✉, Ⓑ, ⇌, ✈
(Plymouth or Newquay).
PENRYN/FLUSHING (01326)
Challenger Marine ☎ 377222, Fax 377800, £9, VHF Ch M,
80; 46 pontoon berths, access HW±3, visitors welcome.
Services: M, FW, P & D (cans, 500m), Slip, El, ME, C (12
ton), Sh, SM, ACA, BY, CH.
MYLOR/RESTRONGUET (01326)
Mylor Yacht Hbr (250+20 visitors) ☎ 372121, Fax 372120,
BH (25 ton), CH, Gas, Gaz, AC, FW, Slip, C (4 ton), Sh, ME,
El, Ⓔ, V, D, Bar, ◻, Access HW±1. **Restronguet Yacht
Basin** ☎ 373613, Slip, M, Sh; **Pandora Inn** ☎ 372678, V, R,
Bar, pontoon dries 1·9m.
Services: Ⓔ, CH, Gas, Gaz.
ST MAWES (01326)
Inner Hbr FW, Slip. **Services:** M, ◻s (contact SC), BY, ME,
Sh, El, SM, Gas.
MALPAS/TRURO (01872)
Bar Creek Yacht Stn ☎ 73919, M; **Malpas Marine** ☎ 71260,
M, CH, ME, El, Sh, access H24 except LWS±1.
Services: CH, Gas.
YACHT CLUBS
Port of Falmouth Sailing Association ☎ 211555;
Royal Cornwall YC ☎ 311105, M, Slip, FW, R, Bar; Port
Pendennis YC ☎ 211711; Falmouth Town SC ☎ 377061;
Flushing SC ☎ 374043; Mylor YC ☎ 374391, Bar;
Restronguet SC ☎ 374536; St Mawes SC ☎ 270686.

SHELTER
Excellent. There are many Ⓥ berths, see below; also ◻s on
the S side of the main chan, clearly marked, managed by
Falmouth Hbr Commissioners or the Royal Cornwall YC.
The **Visitors Yacht Haven** operates Apr-Sept, pontoons
being connected to N Quay.
Port Pendennis marina is SW of the commercial port;
access HW±3 via lock.
Falmouth Marina, 6ca beyond RCYC up the Penryn R, is
accessible at most tides, but at LWS beware depths of
1·6m or less due silting. On near appr pass within 20m of
outside pontoon, 2FR (vert), and leave ECM lt bn, VQ (3)
5s (hard to see), close to stbd to keep within narrow chan.
Challenger Marine pontoon, 2ca up-river, has visitors'
berths; dries at LWS. Speed limit in Penryn R is 8kn.
Up-stream on the W bank is **Mylor Yacht Hbr**, sheltered
from prevailing winds but uncomfortable in strong E
winds. Further up the W bank is **Restronguet Creek**, a
good ⚓ but most of the creek dries.
On E side **is St Mawes Hbr** with 9 G ◻s (contact SC) in
excellent shelter except from SW winds, when ⚓ above
Amsterdam Pt. There is a good ⚓ at St Just but
uncomfortable in strong W/SW'lies. Further up-river
many good ⚓s include Tolcarne Creek, Tolverne, Ruan
Creek, Church Creek, Mopus Reach and Malpas (Bar
Creek Yacht Stn ¼M up Tressilian R has ◻s). Speed limit
in upper reaches and in creeks is 5kn.

ENGLAND – FALMOUTH

LAT 50°09′N   LONG 5°03′W

TIMES AND HEIGHTS OF HIGH AND LOW WATERS

YEAR **1996**

TIME ZONE (UT)
For Summer Time add ONE hour in non-shaded areas

Chart Datum: 2·91 metres below Ordnance Datum (Newlyn)

JANUARY

Day	Time	m	Day	Time	m
1 M	0130 / 0811 / 1356 / 2044	4.3 / 1.8 / 4.3 / 1.6	**16** TU	0016 / 0705 / 1247 / 1947	4.3 / 1.7 / 4.4 / 1.5
2 TU	0227 / 0915 / 1450 / 2139	4.5 / 1.6 / 4.5 / 1.4	**17** W	0134 / 0825 / 1406 / 2100	4.5 / 1.4 / 4.6 / 1.3
3 W	0314 / 1006 / 1536 / 2226	4.7 / 1.3 / 4.6 / 1.3	**18** TH	0245 / 0934 / 1513 / 2204	4.8 / 1.1 / 4.8 / 1.0
4 TH	0355 / 1051 / 1614 / 2307	4.9 / 1.2 / 4.8 / 1.1	**19** F	0343 / 1035 / 1610 / 2300	5.1 / 0.7 / 5.1 / 0.6
5 F O	0430 / 1131 / 1649 / 2344	5.0 / 1.0 / 4.8 / 1.0	**20** SA	0432 / 1129 / 1700 / ● 2353	5.4 / 0.4 / 5.2 / 0.3
6 SA	0505 / 1207 / 1726	5.1 / 1.0 / 4.9	**21** SU	0521 / 1221 / 1752	5.6 / 0.1 / 5.3
7 SU	0018 / 0542 / 1241 / 1805	1.0 / 5.1 / 0.9 / 4.9	**22** M	0042 / 0615 / 1309 / 1846	0.2 / 5.6 / 0.0 / 5.4
8 M	0049 / 0621 / 1311 / 1846	1.0 / 5.1 / 1.0 / 4.8	**23** TU	0128 / 0706 / 1353 / 1935	0.1 / 5.6 / 0.0 / 5.3
9 TU	0119 / 0701 / 1341 / 1924	1.0 / 5.0 / 1.0 / 4.8	**24** W	0210 / 0754 / 1434 / 2019	0.2 / 5.5 / 0.2 / 5.2
10 W	0149 / 0737 / 1409 / 1958	1.1 / 5.0 / 1.1 / 4.7	**25** TH	0249 / 0837 / 1512 / 2059	0.5 / 5.3 / 0.5 / 5.0
11 TH	0218 / 0809 / 1439 / 2029	1.2 / 4.9 / 1.2 / 4.6	**26** F	0326 / 0915 / 1549 / 2135	0.8 / 5.0 / 1.0 / 4.7
12 F	0251 / 0844 / 1513 / 2107	1.3 / 4.7 / 1.3 / 4.5	**27** SA	0404 / 0953 / 1628 / 2214	1.2 / 4.7 / 1.3 / 4.4
13 SA	0330 / 0927 / 1556 / 2157	1.4 / 4.6 / 1.4 / 4.4	**28** SU	0448 / 1036 / 1716 / 2311	1.5 / 4.3 / 1.7 / 4.2
14 SU	0420 / 1023 / 1655 / 2302	1.6 / 4.5 / 1.6 / 4.3	**29** M	0545 / 1152 / 1819	1.9 / 4.1 / 1.9
15 M	0533 / 1133 / 1821	1.7 / 4.4 / 1.7	**30** TU	0039 / 0702 / 1317 / 1946	4.1 / 2.0 / 4.0 / 2.0
			31 W	0150 / 0838 / 1420 / 2107	4.2 / 1.9 / 4.2 / 1.7

FEBRUARY

Day	Time	m	Day	Time	m
1 TH	0246 / 0941 / 1512 / 2201	4.4 / 1.5 / 4.4 / 1.4	**16** F	0226 / 0920 / 1501 / 2151	4.7 / 1.2 / 4.7 / 1.0
2 F	0330 / 1029 / 1553 / 2245	4.7 / 1.3 / 4.6 / 1.2	**17** SA	0328 / 1023 / 1557 / 2249	5.0 / 0.7 / 5.0 / 0.6
3 SA	0409 / 1110 / 1630 / 2324	4.9 / 1.1 / 4.8 / 1.0	**18** SU	0419 / 1117 / ● 1647 / 2339	5.3 / 0.3 / 5.2 / 0.3
4 SU O	0446 / 1147 / 1707 / 2359	5.0 / 0.9 / 4.9 / 0.9	**19** M	0506 / 1206 / 1736	5.5 / 0.0 / 5.3
5 M	0523 / 1222 / 1748	5.1 / 0.8 / 4.9	**20** TU O	0026 / 0556 / 1251 / 1825	0.0 / 5.6 / 0.0 / 5.4
6 TU	0032 / 0604 / 1254 / 1829	0.8 / 5.1 / 0.7 / 4.9	**21** W	0109 / 0646 / 1333 / 1911	0.0 / 5.6 / 0.0 / 5.4
7 W	0103 / 0645 / 1323 / 1906	0.8 / 5.1 / 0.7 / 4.9	**22** TH	0149 / 0730 / 1411 / 1950	0.1 / 5.5 / 0.1 / 5.2
8 TH	0132 / 0720 / 1352 / 1939	0.8 / 5.0 / 0.8 / 4.8	**23** F	0225 / 0808 / 1445 / 2022	0.3 / 5.3 / 0.5 / 5.0
9 F	0202 / 0751 / 1421 / 2008	0.9 / 5.0 / 0.9 / 4.8	**24** SA	0258 / 0838 / 1517 / 2047	0.7 / 5.0 / 0.9 / 4.8
10 SA	0233 / 0823 / 1453 / 2042	0.9 / 4.9 / 1.0 / 4.7	**25** SU	0331 / 0903 / 1550 / 2116	1.1 / 4.6 / 1.3 / 4.5
11 SU	0309 / 0902 / 1531 / 2126	1.1 / 4.7 / 1.2 / 4.5	**26** M	0408 / 0937 / 1630 / 2201	1.4 / 4.3 / 1.7 / 4.2
12 M	0353 / 0954 / 1620 / 2227	1.3 / 4.5 / 1.4 / 4.4	**27** TU	0457 / 1031 / 1727 / 2310	1.8 / 4.0 / 2.0 / 4.0
13 TU	0455 / 1102 / 1734 / 2344	1.6 / 4.3 / 1.6 / 4.3	**28** W	0607 / 1214 / 1843	2.1 / 3.8 / 2.1
14 W	0627 / 1223 / 1916	1.7 / 4.2 / 1.7	**29** TH	0103 / 0735 / 1348 / 2017	4.0 / 2.0 / 4.0 / 1.9
15 TH	0108 / 0748 / 1348 / 2043	4.4 / 1.5 / 4.4 / 1.4			

MARCH

Day	Time	m	Day	Time	m
1 F	0214 / 0908 / 1445 / 2130	4.2 / 1.7 / 4.2 / 1.6	**16** SA	0211 / 0907 / 1450 / 2138	4.6 / 1.2 / 4.6 / 1.1
2 SA	0304 / 1001 / 1529 / 2217	4.5 / 1.3 / 4.5 / 1.3	**17** SU	0313 / 1008 / 1544 / 2233	5.0 / 0.7 / 4.9 / 0.6
3 SU	0345 / 1042 / 1609 / 2257	4.8 / 1.1 / 4.7 / 1.0	**18** M	0402 / 1059 / 1631 / 2321	5.3 / 0.3 / 5.2 / 0.3
4 M	0424 / 1120 / 1647 / 2334	5.0 / 0.8 / 4.9 / 0.8	**19** TU	0448 / 1146 / 1715	5.4 / 0.1 / 5.3
5 TU O	0502 / 1156 / 1726	5.1 / 0.7 / 5.0	**20** W	0006 / 0534 / 1229 / 1759	0.1 / 5.5 / 0.0 / 5.4
6 W	0009 / 0541 / 1230 / 1805	0.6 / 5.1 / 0.6 / 5.0	**21** TH	0047 / 0620 / 1309 / 1841	0.0 / 5.5 / 0.0 / 5.3
7 TH	0042 / 0621 / 1302 / 1844	0.6 / 5.1 / 0.5 / 5.0	**22** F	0125 / 0702 / 1345 / 1917	0.1 / 5.4 / 0.2 / 5.2
8 F	0113 / 0659 / 1332 / 1917	0.6 / 5.1 / 0.6 / 5.0	**23** SA	0159 / 0736 / 1417 / 1943	0.3 / 5.2 / 0.5 / 5.0
9 SA	0144 / 0733 / 1403 / 1947	0.6 / 5.0 / 0.7 / 4.9	**24** SU	0231 / 0801 / 1447 / 2007	0.7 / 4.9 / 0.9 / 4.8
10 SU	0217 / 0806 / 1435 / 2022	0.7 / 4.9 / 0.8 / 4.8	**25** M	0301 / 0826 / 1517 / 2039	1.1 / 4.6 / 1.3 / 4.6
11 M	0253 / 0846 / 1513 / 2106	0.9 / 4.7 / 1.1 / 4.6	**26** TU	0334 / 0902 / 1552 / 2121	1.4 / 4.3 / 1.6 / 4.3
12 TU	0337 / 0937 / 1602 / 2204	1.2 / 4.5 / 1.3 / 4.4	**27** W	0419 / 0951 / 1645 / 2220	1.8 / 4.0 / 2.0 / 4.1
13 W	0437 / 1046 / 1712 / 2323	1.5 / 4.3 / 1.6 / 4.3	**28** TH	0526 / 1108 / 1800 / 2350	2.0 / 3.8 / 2.1 / 4.0
14 TH	0606 / 1211 / 1856	1.6 / 4.2 / 1.7	**29** F	0644 / 1307 / 1918	2.0 / 3.9 / 2.0
15 F	0052 / 0803 / 1338 / 2029	4.3 / 1.5 / 4.3 / 1.4	**30** SA	0132 / 0806 / 1412 / 2037	4.1 / 1.8 / 4.1 / 1.7
			31 SU	0230 / 0914 / 1500 / 2136	4.4 / 1.4 / 4.4 / 1.3

APRIL

Day	Time	m	Day	Time	m
1 M	0316 / 1003 / 1542 / 2221	4.7 / 1.1 / 4.7 / 1.1	**16** TU	0343 / 1037 / 1610 / 2259	5.1 / 0.4 / 5.1 / 0.4
2 TU	0357 / 1044 / 1621 / 2302	4.9 / 0.9 / 4.9 / 0.8	**17** W	0427 / 1122 / 1651 / ● 2343	5.3 / 0.2 / 5.2 / 0.2
3 W	0436 / 1124 / 1659 / 2341	5.1 / 0.6 / 5.0 / 0.6	**18** TH	0509 / 1204 / 1732	5.3 / 0.2 / 5.3
4 TH O	0514 / 1201 / 1738	5.1 / 0.5 / 5.1	**19** F	0023 / 0552 / 1243 / 1810	0.2 / 5.3 / 0.3 / 5.2
5 F	0018 / 0555 / 1238 / 1816	0.5 / 5.2 / 0.4 / 5.1	**20** SA	0100 / 0631 / 1318 / 1843	0.3 / 5.2 / 0.4 / 5.2
6 SA	0054 / 0635 / 1313 / 1853	0.4 / 5.2 / 0.5 / 5.1	**21** SU	0134 / 0703 / 1350 / 1909	0.5 / 5.0 / 0.7 / 5.0
7 SU	0129 / 0715 / 1347 / 1930	0.5 / 5.1 / 0.6 / 5.1	**22** M	0205 / 0729 / 1420 / 1938	0.8 / 4.8 / 1.0 / 4.9
8 M	0205 / 0755 / 1424 / 2009	0.6 / 5.0 / 0.8 / 5.0	**23** TU	0236 / 0800 / 1449 / 2012	1.1 / 4.6 / 1.3 / 4.7
9 TU	0244 / 0838 / 1504 / 2054	0.8 / 4.8 / 1.1 / 4.8	**24** W	0307 / 0838 / 1521 / 2053	1.3 / 4.4 / 1.6 / 4.5
10 W	0331 / 0930 / 1555 / 2153	1.1 / 4.5 / 1.3 / 4.6	**25** TH	0347 / 0925 / 1607 / 2145	1.6 / 4.1 / 1.8 / 4.1
11 TH	0431 / 1039 / 1705 / 2311	1.3 / 4.3 / 1.6 / 4.4	**26** F	0448 / 1030 / 1718 / 2256	1.9 / 3.9 / 2.0 / 4.1
12 F	0556 / 1204 / 1841	1.5 / 4.2 / 1.7	**27** SA	0602 / 1202 / 1833	1.9 / 3.9 / 2.0
13 SA	0039 / 0731 / 1325 / 2010	4.4 / 1.4 / 4.3 / 1.4	**28** SU	0026 / 0712 / 1324 / 1941	4.1 / 1.8 / 4.1 / 1.8
14 SU	0152 / 0847 / 1432 / 2117	4.6 / 1.2 / 4.6 / 1.1	**29** M	0142 / 0816 / 1421 / 2044	4.5 / 1.5 / 4.4 / 1.4
15 M	0253 / 0946 / 1525 / 2212	4.9 / 0.8 / 4.9 / 0.7	**30** TU	0237 / 0914 / 1508 / 2138	4.6 / 1.2 / 4.6 / 1.2

ENGLAND – FALMOUTH

LAT 50°09′N   LONG 5°03′W

TIMES AND HEIGHTS OF HIGH AND LOW WATERS

YEAR **1996**

TIME ZONE (UT)
For Summer Time add ONE hour in non-shaded areas

MAY

	Time	m		Time	m
1 W	0324 1004 1550 2226	4.8 0.9 4.9 0.9	**16** TH	0404 1057 1627 2318	5.0 0.6 5.1 0.6
2 TH	0406 1049 1630 2311	5.0 0.7 5.0 0.6	**17** F ●	0445 1139 1704 2359	5.1 0.5 5.1 0.5
3 F O	0447 1133 1709 2353	5.0 0.5 5.2 0.5	**18** SA	0523 1218 1739	5.0 0.6 5.1
4 SA	0529 1215 1751	5.2 0.4 5.2	**19** SU	0037 0601 1254 1812	0.6 5.0 0.7 5.1
5 SU	0036 0613 1256 1833	0.4 5.2 0.4 5.3	**20** M	0112 0635 1326 1843	0.7 4.9 0.9 5.0
6 M	0117 0659 1337 1917	0.4 5.1 0.5 5.2	**21** TU	0143 0707 1356 1917	0.9 4.7 1.1 4.9
7 TU	0159 0745 1419 2002	0.5 5.0 0.7 5.1	**22** W	0214 0742 1426 1952	1.1 4.6 1.3 4.8
8 W	0242 0834 1503 2050	0.7 4.8 1.0 5.0	**23** TH	0245 0821 1457 2032	1.3 4.4 1.4 4.6
9 TH	0332 0928 1555 2147	1.0 4.6 1.2 4.7	**24** F	0320 0904 1534 2118	1.4 4.3 1.6 4.4
10 F	0430 1035 1659 2300	1.2 4.4 1.4 4.5	**25** SA	0407 0958 1630 2213	1.6 4.1 1.8 4.3
11 SA	0544 1153 1819	1.3 4.3 1.5	**26** SU	0514 1105 1744 2322	1.7 4.0 1.9 4.2
12 SU	0020 0705 1304 1940	4.5 1.3 4.4 1.4	**27** M	0624 1220 1853	1.7 4.1 1.8
13 M	0128 0818 1406 2048	4.6 1.2 4.6 1.2	**28** TU	0037 0728 1328 1957	4.3 1.5 4.3 1.5
14 TU	0227 0919 1459 2145	4.7 1.0 4.8 1.0	**29** W	0146 0828 1426 2057	4.4 1.3 4.5 1.3
15 W	0319 1011 1545 2234	4.9 0.7 4.9 0.7	**30** TH	0244 0925 1515 2152	4.7 1.0 4.8 1.0
			31 F	0334 1017 1600 2243	4.9 0.8 5.0 0.7

JUNE

	Time	m		Time	m
1 SA O	0420 1107 1644 2332	5.0 0.6 5.2 0.5	**16** SU ●	0459 1155 1712	4.8 0.8 5.0
2 SU	0506 1155 1728	5.1 0.4 5.3	**17** M	0016 0535 1232 1748	0.8 4.8 0.8 5.0
3 M	0020 0555 1243 1816	0.3 5.2 0.4 5.4	**18** TU	0052 0612 1305 1823	0.8 4.8 0.9 5.0
4 TU	0108 0646 1330 1906	0.3 5.2 0.4 5.4	**19** W	0124 0649 1336 1900	0.9 4.7 1.0 4.9
5 W	0155 0738 1416 1956	0.3 5.1 0.5 5.3	**20** TH	0155 0727 1406 1938	1.0 4.6 1.2 4.8
6 TH	0242 0829 1503 2045	0.5 5.0 0.7 5.1	**21** F	0225 0806 1435 2015	1.2 4.5 1.3 4.7
7 F	0330 0924 1551 2140	0.7 4.8 1.0 4.9	**22** SA	0255 0844 1506 2052	1.3 4.4 1.4 4.6
8 SA	0422 1023 1645 2244	1.0 4.6 1.2 4.7	**23** SU	0329 0926 1545 2137	1.3 4.3 1.5 4.5
9 SU	0521 1132 1748 2354	1.2 4.4 1.4 4.5	**24** M	0416 1019 1641 2232	1.5 4.2 1.7 4.3
10 M	0629 1236 1901	1.3 4.4 1.4	**25** TU	0524 1119 1758 2339	1.6 4.2 1.7 4.3
11 TU	0059 0741 1335 2013	4.5 1.3 4.4 1.4	**26** W	0640 1227 1912	1.5 4.2 1.6
12 W	0158 0846 1430 2115	4.5 1.3 4.6 1.3	**27** TH	0049 0751 1337 2020	4.4 1.4 4.4 1.3
13 TH	0253 0942 1519 2208	4.6 1.1 4.7 1.1	**28** F	0201 0851 1439 2122	4.5 1.2 4.7 1.1
14 F	0340 1031 1601 2255	4.7 0.9 4.9 0.9	**29** SA	0305 0950 1533 2220	4.7 0.9 4.9 0.8
15 SA	0421 1115 1638 2337	4.8 0.8 5.0 0.8	**30** SU	0357 1046 1622 2315	4.9 0.7 5.2 0.5

JULY

	Time	m		Time	m
1 M O	0447 1139 1709	5.1 0.4 5.3	**16** TU	0511 1212 1726	4.8 0.9 5.0
2 TU	0007 0539 1231 1801	0.3 5.2 0.3 5.5	**17** W	0033 0551 1246 1804	0.8 4.8 0.9 5.0
3 W	0058 0634 1321 1854	0.2 5.2 0.3 5.5	**18** TH	0106 0631 1316 1844	0.9 4.8 0.9 5.0
4 TH	0147 0728 1408 1945	0.1 5.2 0.3 5.4	**19** F	0135 0711 1345 1922	0.9 4.7 1.0 4.9
5 F	0233 0819 1452 2034	0.2 5.1 0.4 5.3	**20** SA	0203 0748 1412 1956	1.0 4.6 1.1 4.8
6 SA	0317 0908 1535 2124	0.4 5.0 0.7 5.1	**21** SU	0230 0822 1441 2028	1.1 4.6 1.2 4.7
7 SU	0401 1000 1620 2216	0.7 4.7 1.0 4.8	**22** M	0259 0854 1513 2104	1.2 4.4 1.3 4.6
8 M	0449 1056 1711 2318	1.1 4.5 1.3 4.5	**23** TU	0335 0937 1556 2151	1.3 4.3 1.4 4.5
9 TU	0545 1159 1813	1.3 4.3 1.5	**24** W	0425 1032 1658 2255	1.4 4.3 1.6 4.3
10 W	0024 0654 1300 1930	4.3 1.5 4.3 1.6	**25** TH	0542 1142 1827	1.6 4.2 1.7
11 TH	0128 0809 1358 2044	4.2 1.5 4.3 1.5	**26** F	0008 0711 1256 1949	4.3 1.5 4.3 1.5
12 F	0226 0914 1452 2144	4.3 1.4 4.5 1.3	**27** SA	0128 0825 1411 2059	4.4 1.3 4.6 1.2
13 SA	0316 1007 1537 2233	4.5 1.2 4.7 1.2	**28** SU	0243 0931 1513 2203	4.6 1.1 4.9 0.9
14 SU	0358 1053 1615 2317	4.6 1.1 4.8 1.0	**29** M	0342 1031 1605 2301	4.9 0.7 5.2 0.5
15 M ●	0436 1134 1650 2357	4.7 0.9 5.0 0.9	**30** TU O	0433 1126 1654 2354	5.1 0.4 5.4 0.2
			31 W	0523 1218 1745	5.2 0.2 5.5

AUGUST

	Time	m		Time	m
1 TH	0045 0618 1306 1838	0.0 5.3 0.1 5.6	**16** F	0043 0610 1254 1824	0.8 4.9 0.8 5.1
2 F	0131 0711 1351 1929	0.0 5.3 0.1 5.6	**17** SA	0111 0650 1322 1902	0.8 4.9 0.8 5.0
3 SA	0215 0800 1433 2016	0.0 5.2 0.2 5.4	**18** SU	0138 0726 1349 1935	0.8 4.8 0.9 4.9
4 SU	0255 0843 1512 2058	0.3 5.1 0.5 5.1	**19** M	0205 0757 1417 2004	0.9 4.7 1.0 4.8
5 M	0334 0925 1551 2139	0.7 4.8 0.9 4.8	**20** TU	0233 0826 1448 2038	1.0 4.6 1.2 4.7
6 TU	0414 1009 1633 2222	1.1 4.5 1.3 4.4	**21** W	0307 0904 1527 2123	1.2 4.5 1.3 4.5
7 W	0500 1104 1726 2335	1.4 4.3 1.7 4.1	**22** TH	0351 0958 1621 2225	1.4 4.4 1.5 4.3
8 TH	0559 1221 1838	1.8 4.1 1.9	**23** F	0455 1109 1748 2344	1.6 4.3 1.7 4.2
9 F	0057 0723 1328 2011	4.0 1.9 4.2 1.8	**24** SA	0639 1230 1926	1.7 4.3 1.6
10 SA	0201 0846 1427 2121	4.1 1.7 4.4 1.5	**25** SU	0109 0806 1352 2045	4.3 1.5 4.6 1.3
11 SU	0254 0945 1514 2212	4.5 1.4 4.6 1.3	**26** M	0231 0918 1458 2150	4.6 1.2 4.9 0.9
12 SU	0339 1031 1554 2256	4.5 1.2 4.8 1.1	**27** TU	0330 1019 1551 2247	4.9 0.7 5.3 0.5
13 TU	0416 1112 1629 2335	4.7 1.0 5.0 0.9	**28** W O	0421 1112 1640 2339	5.2 0.4 5.5 0.1
14 W ●	0452 1150 1706 2301	4.9 0.9 5.1 0.5	**29** TH	0508 1201 1728	5.3 0.1 5.6
15 TH	0010 0529 1224 1744	0.8 5.1 0.8 5.1	**30** F	0026 0558 1247 1817	0.0 5.4 0.0 5.7
			31 SA	0111 0647 1330 1906	0.0 5.4 0.0 5.6

Chart Datum: 2·91 metres below Ordnance Datum (Newlyn)

ENGLAND – FALMOUTH

LAT 50°09′N   LONG 5°03′W

TIMES AND HEIGHTS OF HIGH AND LOW WATERS   YEAR **1996**

TIME ZONE (UT)
For Summer Time add ONE hour in non-shaded areas

SEPTEMBER

Day	Time	m	Time	m	Time	m	Time	m	Day	Time	m	Time	m	Time	m	Time	m
1 SU	0151	0.0	0731	5.3	1409	0.2	1949	5.4	16 M	0113	0.7	0700	5.0	1326	0.8	1910	5.0
2 M	0229	0.3	0811	5.1	1445	0.6	2025	5.1	17 TU	0141	0.8	0730	4.9	1356	0.9	1942	4.9
3 TU	0304	0.8	0843	4.9	1520	1.0	2054	4.8	18 W	0212	1.0	0802	4.8	1429	1.1	2019	4.8
4 W	0338	1.2	0912	4.6	1557	1.4	2123	4.4	19 TH	0246	1.2	0842	4.7	1509	1.3	2105	4.6
5 TH	0418	1.6	0950	4.3	1645	1.8	2209	4.1	20 F	0330	1.4	0935	4.5	1602	1.5	2206	4.3
6 F	0513	2.0	1056	4.1	1752	2.1			21 SA	0432	1.7	1046	4.3	1726	1.8	2328	4.2
7 SA	0016	3.9	0630	2.1	1254	4.0	1927	2.1	22 SU	0617	1.9	1212	4.4	1912	1.7		
8 SU	0137	4.0	0812	2.0	1400	4.3	2056	1.8	23 M	0101	4.3	0753	1.6	1337	4.6	2032	1.3
9 M	0233	4.2	0919	1.6	1450	4.6	2148	1.4	24 TU	0220	4.6	0905	1.3	1443	5.0	2137	0.9
10 TU	0316	4.5	1005	1.3	1531	4.8	2230	1.1	25 W	0319	5.0	1004	0.8	1536	5.3	2231	0.5
11 W	0355	4.8	1046	1.1	1608	5.0	2307	0.9	26 TH	0406	5.2	1055	0.4	1623	5.5	2319	0.2
12 TH ●	0430	4.9	1122	1.0	1644	5.1	2342	0.8	27 F O	0450	5.4	1141	0.2	1707	5.6		
13 F	0506	5.0	1156	0.8	1720	5.2			28 SA	0004	0.0	0534	5.5	1225	0.1	1754	5.6
14 SA	0014	0.7	0545	5.1	1227	0.7	1800	5.2	29 SU	0047	0.0	0619	5.5	1306	0.1	1838	5.5
15 SU	0044	0.7	0624	5.0	1257	0.7	1837	5.1	30 M	0125	0.2	0701	5.4	1343	0.4	1919	5.3

OCTOBER

Day	Time	m	Time	m	Time	m	Time	m	Day	Time	m	Time	m	Time	m	Time	m
1 TU	0201	0.5	0736	5.2	1418	0.7	1949	5.0	16 W	0122	0.8	0709	5.1	1341	0.8	1926	5.0
2 W	0234	0.9	0802	5.0	1451	1.1	2015	4.7	17 TH	0157	0.9	0746	5.0	1418	1.0	2007	4.8
3 TH	0306	1.3	0829	4.7	1526	1.5	2045	4.4	18 F	0235	1.2	0829	4.9	1501	1.3	2055	4.6
4 F	0341	1.7	0908	4.4	1609	1.9	2129	4.1	19 SA	0321	1.4	0923	4.7	1556	1.5	2157	4.4
5 SA	0431	2.1	1003	4.2	1712	2.2	2241	3.9	20 SU	0424	1.7	1032	4.5	1716	1.7	2319	4.3
6 SU	0545	2.3	1136	4.0	1834	2.2			21 M	0601	1.9	1159	4.5	1855	1.7		
7 M	0101	3.9	0712	2.2	1322	4.2	2008	2.0	22 TU	0050	4.3	0735	1.7	1320	4.6	2014	1.3
8 TU	0202	4.2	0836	1.9	1418	4.5	2109	1.6	23 W	0204	4.6	0846	1.3	1425	4.9	2117	1.0
9 W	0249	4.5	0928	1.5	1502	4.8	2153	1.3	24 TH	0301	5.0	0944	0.9	1518	5.2	2210	0.6
10 TH	0329	4.8	1010	1.2	1542	5.0	2231	1.0	25 F	0348	5.2	1034	0.6	1604	5.4	2257	0.4
11 F	0405	5.0	1048	1.0	1618	5.1	2307	0.8	26 SA O	0430	5.4	1120	0.4	1647	5.5	2341	0.3
12 SA ●	0442	5.1	1124	0.8	1655	5.2	2342	0.7	27 SU	0511	5.5	1202	0.3	1730	5.5		
13 SU	0519	5.2	1159	0.7	1734	5.2			28 M	0022	0.3	0552	5.4	1242	0.4	1812	5.4
14 M	0016	0.7	0557	5.2	1234	0.7	1812	5.2	29 TU	0100	0.5	0630	5.3	1319	0.6	1849	5.2
15 TU	0049	0.7	0634	5.2	1307	0.7	1849	5.1	30 W	0135	0.7	0702	5.2	1353	0.9	1918	5.0
									31 TH	0207	1.1	0728	5.0	1426	1.2	1945	4.7

NOVEMBER

Day	Time	m	Time	m	Time	m	Time	m	Day	Time	m	Time	m	Time	m	Time	m
1 F	0238	1.3	0801	4.8	1459	1.5	2020	4.5	16 SA	0232	1.1	0824	5.1	1501	1.1	2053	4.8
2 SA	0310	1.7	0840	4.6	1537	1.8	2104	4.2	17 SU	0321	1.3	0916	4.9	1555	1.3	2153	4.6
3 SU	0352	2.0	0930	4.4	1632	2.1	2204	4.0	18 M	0420	1.5	1022	4.7	1704	1.5	2309	4.4
4 M	0458	2.2	1037	4.2	1744	2.2	2338	4.0	19 TU	0538	1.7	1142	4.6	1828	1.5		
5 TU	0615	2.3	1210	4.2	1858	2.1			20 W	0029	4.4	0706	1.6	1255	4.7	1946	1.4
6 W	0113	4.1	0730	2.0	1329	4.4	2007	1.8	21 TH	0138	4.6	0819	1.4	1359	4.8	2051	1.2
7 TH	0210	4.4	0834	1.7	1423	4.6	2102	1.4	22 F	0236	4.8	0920	1.2	1455	5.0	2146	0.9
8 F	0255	4.7	0926	1.4	1509	4.9	2149	1.2	23 SA	0327	5.1	1012	0.9	1544	5.2	2235	0.7
9 SA	0337	4.9	1011	1.1	1550	5.1	2231	0.9	24 SU	0409	5.2	1058	0.7	1628	5.2	2319	0.6
10 SU	0415	5.1	1053	0.9	1629	5.2	2312	0.8	25 M O	0448	5.3	1141	0.6	1707	5.2	2359	0.6
11 M ●	0453	5.2	1133	0.7	1708	5.2	2351	0.7	26 TU	0527	5.3	1221	0.6	1747	5.2		
12 TU	0531	5.3	1213	0.7	1750	5.5			27 W	0038	0.7	0603	5.3	1259	0.8	1823	5.0
13 W	0031	0.7	0612	5.3	1253	0.7	1832	5.4	28 TH	0112	0.9	0635	5.2	1333	0.9	1854	4.9
14 TH	0110	0.7	0653	5.3	1333	0.7	1917	5.1	29 F	0144	1.1	0706	5.1	1405	1.2	1926	4.8
15 F	0149	0.9	0702	5.2	1415	0.9	2003	5.0	30 SA	0215	1.3	0741	4.9	1437	1.3	2003	4.6

DECEMBER

Day	Time	m	Time	m	Time	m	Time	m	Day	Time	m	Time	m	Time	m	Time	m
1 SU	0245	1.5	0820	4.7	1510	1.6	2044	4.4	16 M	0318	1.0	0910	5.1	1549	1.0	2144	4.8
2 M	0318	1.8	0904	4.6	1549	1.8	2134	4.2	17 TU	0409	1.3	1007	4.9	1644	1.3	2248	4.6
3 TU	0404	2.0	0957	4.4	1648	2.0	2238	4.1	18 W	0508	1.5	1116	4.7	1750	1.4	2359	4.5
4 W	0515	2.1	1102	4.3	1759	2.0	2356	4.1	19 TH	0623	1.6	1225	4.6	1907	1.5		
5 TH	0630	2.1	1217	4.3	1907	1.9			20 F	0105	4.5	0743	1.6	1330	4.6	2020	1.4
6 F	0111	4.3	0738	1.9	1328	4.4	2010	1.6	21 SA	0206	4.6	0852	1.4	1430	4.7	2121	1.3
7 SA	0212	4.5	0839	1.6	1428	4.6	2106	1.3	22 SU	0301	4.8	0949	1.2	1523	4.8	2213	1.1
8 SU	0302	4.8	0933	1.3	1519	4.9	2157	1.1	23 M	0347	5.0	1038	1.0	1608	4.9	2258	0.9
9 M	0346	5.0	1023	1.0	1604	5.0	2245	0.8	24 TU O	0428	5.1	1122	0.8	1647	5.0	2340	0.8
10 TU ●	0428	5.2	1111	0.8	1647	5.2	2331	0.7	25 W	0505	5.2	1204	0.8	1724	5.0		
11 W	0509	5.2	1157	0.6	1731	5.2			26 TH	0019	0.8	0539	5.2	1242	0.8	1801	4.9
12 TH	0017	0.6	0554	5.2	1244	0.5	1819	5.2	27 F	0055	0.9	0614	5.2	1316	0.9	1836	4.9
13 F	0102	0.6	0641	5.4	1330	0.5	1908	5.2	28 SA	0126	1.0	0649	5.1	1347	1.0	1911	4.8
14 SA	0147	0.6	0730	5.4	1415	0.6	1959	5.1	29 SU	0155	1.2	0726	5.0	1416	1.2	1948	4.7
15 SU	0232	0.8	0819	5.3	1501	0.8	2049	5.0	30 M	0223	1.3	0803	4.9	1444	1.3	2026	4.6
									31 TU	0251	1.4	0841	4.7	1513	1.4	2105	4.4

Chart Datum: 2·91 metres below Ordnance Datum (Newlyn)

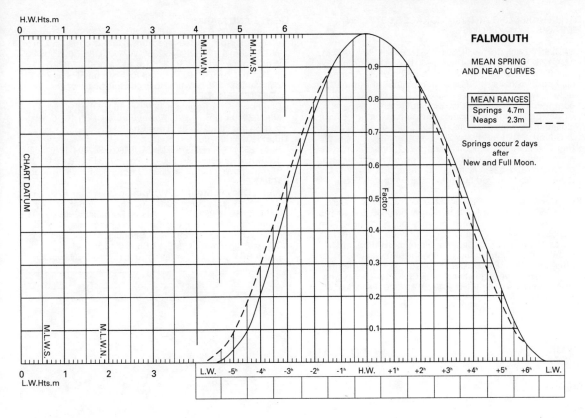

H.W.Hts.m

FALMOUTH

MEAN SPRING
AND NEAP CURVES

MEAN RANGES
Springs 4.7m
Neaps   2.3m

Springs occur 2 days
after
New and Full Moon.

L.W.Hts.m

**OTHER HARBOURS AND ANCHORAGES BETWEEN
ST.ANTHONY HEAD AND MEVAGISSEY**

PORTSCATHO, Cornwall, 50°10'·80N 04°58'·25W. AC *154*.
HW –0600 on Dover, –0025 on Devonport; HW –0·2m on
Devonport; ML 3·0m; Duration 0550. Small drying hbr,
but in settled weather and off-shore winds there is a
good ⚓ outside. There are no lts and very few facilities.
Hr Mr ☎ (01872) 58616. Facilities: BY, CH, M.

GORRAN HAVEN, Cornwall, 50°14'·45N 04°47'·09W. AC
148, *1267*. HW –0600 on Dover, –0010 on Devonport;
HW –0·1m on Devonport. Shelter good with flat sand
beach for drying out in off-shore wind; good ⚓ 100 to
500m E of Hr. Beware Gwineas Rk and Yaw Rk marked by
ECM. Beware pot markers on appr. Not suitable ⚓ when
wind is in E. Fin keels without legs should not ⚓ closer
than 300m from hbr wall where depth is 1·8m at MLWS.
Facilities: ✉, V, Bar, P & D (cans, 1M), R.

PORTMELLON, Cornwall, 50°15'·70N 04°46'·91W. AC 148,
1267. HW –0600 on Dover, –0010 on Devonport;
HW –0·1m on Devonport; ML 3·1m; Duration 0600. Shelter
good but only suitable as a temp ⚓ in settled weather and offshore winds. There are no lts and few facilities.

MEVAGISSEY   10-1-14

Cornwall 50°16'·12N 04°46'·86W

CHARTS
AC 147, 148, *1267*; Imray C6; Stanfords 13; OS 204
TIDES
–0600 Dover; ML 3·1; Duration 0600; Zone 0 (UT)

Standard Port DEVONPORT (→)

Times				Height (metres)			
High Water		Low Water		MHWS	MHWN	MLWN	MLWS
0000	0600	0000	0600	5·5	4·4	2·2	0·8
1200	1800	1200	1800				
Differences MEVAGISSEY							
–0015	–0020	–0010	–0005	–0·1	–0·1	–0·2	–0·1

SHELTER (MEVAGISSEY *continued)*
Hbr is available at all states of the tide but is exposed to
E'lies. Dangerous to appr in strong SE winds. Visitors
may find berth on S Pier (D available). Inner hbr (dries
1·5m) is reserved for FVs, except if taking on fuel or FW.
Because hbr is crowded and used by many FVs, ⚓ inside
the hbr is prohibited. ⚓ outside the S Pier is only advised
in settled weather with no E in the wind.
NAVIGATION
WPT 50°16'·11N 04°46'·54W, 090°/270° from/to pier hd lt,
0·20M. Beware rk ledges off the N Quay. Hbr ent is 46m
wide. Speed limit in the hbr is 3kn. Beware FVs.
LIGHTS AND MARKS
S Quay Fl (2) 10s 9m 12M.
RADIO TELEPHONE
Hr Mr VHF Ch 16 14 (Summer 0900-2100LT. Winter
0900-1700LT); call on 16 for berth.
TELEPHONE (01726)
Hr Mr 843305, (home 842496); MRSC (01803) 882704;
☲ (01752) 220661; Marinecall 0891 500458; Police 842262;
Dr 843701.
FACILITIES
Outer Hbr L, FW, AB (S Quay) £5, D; **Inner Hbr** Slip, M, P,
D, L, FW. **Services:** BY, Sh (wood), CH. **Village** EC Thurs;
V, R, ⌧, Gas, Bar, ✉, Ⓑ (June-Sept 1000-1430, Oct-June
1000-1300), ⇌ (bus to St. Austell), ✈ (Newquay).

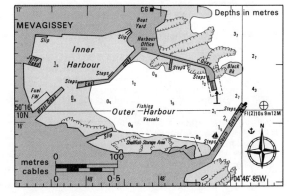

OTHER HARBOURS AND ANCHORAGES BETWEEN MEVAGISSEY AND FOWEY

CHARLESTOWN, Cornwall, 50°19′·81N 04°45′·28W. AC 31, 148, *1267*. HW −0555 on Dover, −0010 on Devonport; HW −0·1m on Devonport; ML 3·1m; Duration 0605. A china clay port; yachts should berth in the outer hbr (dries), but only in W'lies. The inner locked hbr is rarely used by commercial ships. Ent dries and should only be attempted by day and in off-shore winds with calm weather. Hbr is closed in SE winds. Waiting buoys 2ca S of hbr. N bkwtr 2FG (vert) 5m 1M; S bkwtr 2FR (vert) 5m 1M. Ent sig: Ⓡ (night) = hbr shut. VHF Ch14 16 (HW −2, only when vessel expected). Yachts should pre-arrange via Hr Mr on Ch 14 or ☎ (01726) 67526. Facilities: EC Thurs; AB, FW, P & D (cans or pre-arranged tanker), R, Bar, V at ✉, ME, Sh.

PAR, Cornwall, 50°20′·58N 04°42′·00W. AC 31, 148, *1267*. HW −0555 on Dover; ML 3·1m; Duration 0605. See 10·1·15. A china clay port, only in emergency for yachts; dries 1·2m. 4 chys are conspic 2½ca W of ent. Beware Killyvarder Rk (dries 2·4m) 3ca SE of ent, marked by a SHM bn. Ent should only be attempted by day, in calm weather with off-shore winds. Ent sigs: R shape (day) or Ⓡ lt (night) = port closed or vessel leaving. VHF Ch 12 16 (by day and HW −2 to HW +1). Hr Mr ☎ (01726) 817300. Facilities: EC Thurs; Bar, FW.

FOWEY   10-1-15

Cornwall 50°19′·62N 04°38′·47W

CHARTS
AC 31, 148, *1267*; Imray C6, Y52; Stanfords 13; OS 204

TIDES
−0540 Dover; ML 2·9; Duration 0605; Zone 0 (UT)

Standard Port DEVONPORT (→)

Times				Height (metres)			
High Water		Low Water		MHWS	MHWN	MLWN	MLWS
0000	0600	0000	0600	5·5	4·4	2·2	0·8
1200	1800	1200	1800				
Differences FOWEY							
−0010	−0015	−0010	−0005	−0·1	−0·1	−0·2	−0·2
LOSTWITHIEL							
+0005	−0010	Dries		−4·1	−4·1	Dries	
PAR							
−0005	−0015	0000	−0010	−0·4	−0·4	−0·4	−0·2

SHELTER
Good, but exposed to winds from S to SW. Gales from these directions can cause heavy swell in the lower hbr and confused seas, especially on the ebb. Entry at any tide in any conditions. Speed limit 6kn.
Pont Pill, on the E side, offers double-berth fore and aft Ⓐs and AB in 2m on a 120′ floating pontoon; there is also a refuse barge and fuel barge. Opposite Albert Quay, on the E side of the chan there is a line of single swinging Ⓐs and another 120′ pontoon.
At **Albert Quay** the 'T' shaped landing pontoon is for short stay (2 hrs), plus FW. A second short stay pontoon is 250m up-river, same side off Berrills BY.
At **Mixtow Pill** (5ca upriver) there is a quieter 120′ pontoon in 2·2m. Pontoons are in situ May to Oct. Two Ⓐs are 100m N of Wiseman's Pt. All Ⓐs are White and marked 'FHC VISITORS'. Dues £6.50 for a 30′/9m boat overnight. Vessels >12·5m LOA should berth/moor as directed by Hr Mr.

NAVIGATION
WPT 50°19′·30N 04°38′·73W, 207°/027° from/to Whitehouse Pt lt, Iso WRG 3s, 0·72M. Appr in W sector of Fowey lt ho. W sector of Whitehouse Pt lt leads 027° through hbr ent. From E beware Udder Rk (3M E of ent) marked by unlit SCM buoy. From SW beware Cannis Rk (4ca SE of Gribbin Hd) marked by SCM buoy, Q (6) + L Fl 15s. Entering hbr, keep well clear of Punch Cross Rks to stbd. Fowey is a busy commercial clay port, so take necessary precautions. Unmarked chan is navigable up to Golant, but there is little space to ⚓ due to moorings. Shoal draft boats can reach Lerryn (1·6M) and Lostwithiel (3M) on the tide. The level of CD rises upstream of Hays Pt to be 3·9m higher at Lostwithiel than at Fowey (see AC 31).

LIGHTS AND MARKS
An unlit RW tr 33m on Gribbin Hd (1·3M WSW of hbr ent) is conspic from all sea directions. Lt ho is conspic, L Fl WR 5s 28m 11/9M, R284°-295°, W295°-028°, R028°-054°. Whitehouse Pt Iso WRG 3s 11m 11/8M, G017°-022°, W022°-032°, R032°-037°. Lamp Rk SHM bn Fl G 5s 7m 2M, vis 088°-205°. White Ho is conspic 3ca E of ent.

RADIO TELEPHONE
Call *Fowey Hbr Radio* Ch 12 09 11 16 (HO). Hbr Patrol (0900-2000 LT) Ch 12 16. *Fowey Refueller* Ch 10 16. Water taxi Ch 06. Pilots Ch 09. Tugs Ch 09 12.

TELEPHONE (01726)
Hr Mr 832471, Fax 833738; MRSC (01803) 882704; ⌗ (01752) 220661; Marinecall 0891 500458; Police 72313; Ⓗ 832241; Dr 832451; Fowey Refueller 832880 or (0836) 519341 (mobile).

FACILITIES
Albert Quay Pontoon L, FW; **Polruan Quay** Slip, P, D, L, FW, C (3 ton); **Royal Fowey YC** ☎ 832245, FW, R, Bar; **Fowey Gallants SC** ☎ 832335, Bar; **Fowey Refueller** (0900-1800 LT daily; winter Mon-Fri) VHF Ch 10, 16 or ☎ as above or in emerg ☎ (01726) 870697, P, D. **Services**: M, FW, Gas, Gaz, CH, ACA, Ⓔ, BY , Slip, ME, El, Sh, C (7 ton).
Town EC Wed & Sat; ✉, Ⓑ, ⇌ (bus to Par), ✈ (Newquay).

▲ visitors moorings

POLPERRO, Cornwall, 50°19′·74N 04°30′·72W. AC 148, *1267*. HW −0554 on Dover; HW −0007 and −0·2m on Devonport; ML 3·1m; Duration 0610. Shelter good, but hbr dries about 2m. There is 3·3m at MHWS and 2·5m at MHWN. The ent is 9·8m wide (closed by gate in bad weather). AB on N quay or pick up a buoy; also temp buoys outside hbr. Beware The Ranneys to W of ent, and the rks to E. Lights: Iso WR 6s 30m 7M at Spy House Pt CG Stn, vis W288°-060°, R060°-288°. Tidal Basin, W pier hd FW 4m 4M on post; shows FR when hbr closed. Dir FW (occas) shown from measured distance bns 1M and 2·2M to ENE. Hr Mr on Fish Quay, AB £11. Facilities: EC Sat; FW on quays.

LOOE
10-1-16

Cornwall 50°21'·00N 04°26'·96W

CHARTS
AC 147, 148, *1267*; Imray C6; Stanfords 13; OS 201

TIDES
–0538 Dover; ML 3·0; Duration 0610; Zone 0 (UT)

Standard Port DEVONPORT (→)

Times				Height (metres)			
High Water		Low Water		MHWS	MHWN	MLWN	MLWS
0000	0600	0000	0600	5·5	4·4	2·2	0·8
1200	1800	1200	1800				
Differences LOOE							
–0010	–0010	–0005	–0005	–0·1	–0·2	–0·2	–0·2
WHITSAND BAY							
0000	0000	0000	0000	0·0	+0·1	–0·1	+0·2

SHELTER
Good, but uncomfortable in strong SE winds. ‡ in 2m E of the pier hd; access approx HW ±1½. Ⓥ berth, above ferry, is marked in Y on W side of hbr which dries 2·4m to the ent. The W bank has rky outcrops to S of ferry.

NAVIGATION
WPT 50°19'·73N 04°24'·60W, 130°/310° from/to pier hd lt, 2·0M. Ent dangerous in strong SE'lies, when seas break heavily on the bar. From W, beware The Ranneys, rks 2ca SE of Looe Is. Do not attempt the rky passage between Looe Is and mainland except with local knowledge and at HW. From E, beware Longstone Rks extending 1½ca from shore NE of hbr ent. At sp, ebb tide runs up to 5kn.

LIGHTS AND MARKS
Looe Island (or St George's Is) is conspic (44m), 8ca S of the ent. Mid Main bn (off Hannafore Pt, halfway between pier hd and Looe Is) Q (3) 10s 2M; ECM. At night appr in W sector (267°-313°) of pier hd lt Oc WR 3s 8m 15/12M; vis W013°-207°, R207°-267°, W267°-313°, R313°-332°. Nailzee Pt siren (2) 30s. No lts inside hbr.

RADIO TELEPHONE
VHF Ch 16 (occas).

TELEPHONE (01503)
Hr Mr 262839; CG 262138; MRSC (01803) 882704; ⌗ (01752) 220661; Marinecall 0891 500458; Police 262233; Dr 263195.

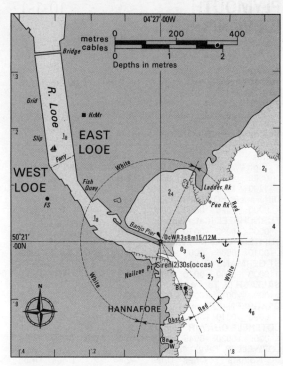

FACILITIES
W Looe Quay AB £12, Slip, M, P & D (cans), L, FW, ME, El, CH; **E Looe Quay** Access HW ±3, Slip, P & D (cans), L, FW, ME, El, C (2½ ton); **Looe SC** ☎ 262559, L, R, Bar.
Services: Sh (Wood), Ⓔ, Sh, Gas.
Town EC Thurs (winter only); P, FW, V, R, Bar, ▣, ✉, Ⓑ, ⇌, ✈ (Plymouth).

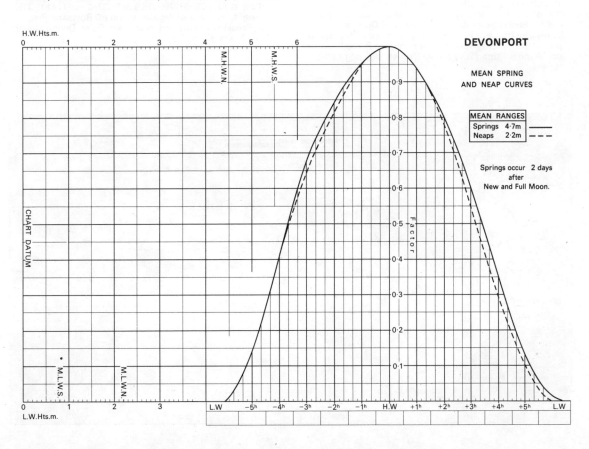

DEVONPORT

MEAN SPRING AND NEAP CURVES

MEAN RANGES	
Springs 4·7m	———
Neaps 2·2m	- - - -

Springs occur 2 days after New and Full Moon.

PLYMOUTH (DEVONPORT)

10-1-17

Devon 50°20'·00N 04°10'·00W (W Chan)
       50°20'·00N 04°08'·00W (E Chan)

CHARTS

AC 871, 1902, 1901, *30*, 1967, *1613*; Imray C14; Stanfords 13; OS 201

TIDES

–0540 Dover; ML 3·3; Duration 0610; Zone 0 (UT)

Standard Port DEVONPORT (→)

Times				Height (metres)			
High Water		Low Water		MHWS	MHWN	MLWN	MLWS
0000	0600	0000	0600	5·5	4·4	2·2	0·8
1200	1800	1200	1800				
Differences BOVISAND PIER							
0000	–0020	0000	–0010	–0·2	–0·1	0·0	+0·1
TURNCHAPEL (Cattewater)							
0000	0000	+0010	–0015	0·0	+0·1	+0·2	+0·1
JUPITER POINT (R. Lynher)							
+0010	+0005	0000	–0005	0·0	0·0	+0·1	0·0
ST GERMANS (R. Lynher)							
0000	0000	+0020	+0020	–0·3	–0·1	0·0	+0·2
SALTASH (R. Tamar)							
0000	+0010	0000	–0005	+0·1	+0·1	+0·1	+0·1
CARGREEN (R. Tamar)							
0000	+0010	+0020	+0020	0·0	0·0	–0·1	0·0
COTEHELE QUAY (R. Tamar)							
0000	+0020	+0045	+0045	–0·9	–0·9	–0·8	–0·4
LOPWELL (R. Tavy)							
No data	Dries	Dries	Dries	–2·6	–2·7	Dries	Dries

NOTE: Devonport is a Standard Port; predictions are given below. Winds from SE to W increase the flood and retard the ebb; vice versa in winds from the NW to E.

SHELTER

Excellent. Plymouth is a Naval Base, a busy commercial/ferry port principally using Mill Bay Docks, and an active fishing port based mainly on Sutton Harbour which is entered via a lock (see Facilities). There are marinas to E and W of the city centre, as well as in the Cattewater and off Torpoint (see chartlet below). Around the Sound there are ⚓s, sheltered according to the wind, in Cawsand Bay, in Barn Pool (below Mt Edgcumbe), N of Drake's Is, below The Hoe and in Jennycliff Bay to the E. Also good shelter W of Cremyll and off the Hamoaze in the R Lynher and in the R Tamar/Tavy above Saltash (see page 188).

NAVIGATION

WPT 50°19'·70N 04°09'·80W, 213°/033° from/to W bkwtr lt, 0·40M. The Sound can be entered via the W or E Chans which are well lit/buoyed with no real hazards. There are no shoal patches with less than 3·7m at MLWS. Yachts need not keep to the deep water chans.
The short cut to the Hamoaze via The Bridge (channel between Drake's Is and Mt Edgcumbe) is lit by 2 PHM and 2 SHM bns; the seaward pair show QR and QG, the inner pair Fl (4) R 10s and Fl (3) G 10s. The QR bn and the Fl (4) R 10s bn both have tide gauges calibrated to show height of tide above CD; charted depth is 2·1m. A conspic ho (3 chys) on with conspic chy (rear mark) leads 332° through The Bridge chan.
Speed limits: 10kn N of The Breakwater, 8kn in Cattewater (where oubound vessels have right of way), 4kn in Sutton Chan and 5kn in Sutton Hbr.
Historic Wrecks (see 10.0.3g) are at:
Cattewater, 50°21'·69N 04°07'·63W, 1ca N of Mount Batten. Penlee Pt, 2ca W and 7ca SW of: two sites at 50°18'·96N 04°11'·57W and 50°18'·57N 04°11'·98W.

BYE LAWS/NAVAL ACTIVITY

The whole Port is under the jurisdiction of the QHM, but certain areas are locally controlled, i.e. by Cattewater Commissioners and by ABP who operate Mill Bay Docks. Beware frequent movements of naval vessels, which have right of way in the chans. Obey MOD Police instructions. Info on Naval activities may be obtained from Naval Ops ☎ 501182 (H24) or Devonport Ops Room ☎ 563777 Ext 2182/3. Submarines may secure to a buoy close N of the Breakwater; they will show a Fl Y anti-collision lt. For Subfacts in the W English Chan see 10.1.18.
Firing Range: Wembury range extends out to 14M over an arc of 130°–245°. Firing usually occurs Mon - Fri, 0900 – 1800LT; rarely at night, weekends or public hols. No firing at Easter, Christmas and for 3 weeks in Aug. Two large R flags are flown at Wembury Pt when range active. Keep W of Eddystone lt ho if entering the Sound from S during firings. During some firings it may be safe to transit close inshore. Call *Wembury Range* VHF Ch 16 (working 11) or ☎ Freephone 0800 833608 or Range Officer ☎ (01752) 862799 (HO) or 553740 ext 77410 (OT).
Diving: Keep clear of regular diving off Bovisand Pier, The Breakwater Fort and Ravenness Point. Diving signals (Flag A) are displayed.

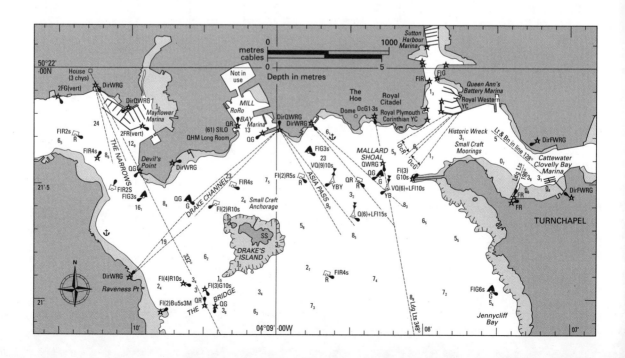

LIGHTS AND MARKS

See 10.1.4 for complete detail. Bkwtr W hd, Fl WR 10s 19m 15/12M (vis W262°-208°, R208°-262°) and Iso 4s 12m 12M (vis 031°-039°). Bkwtr E hd, Iso WR 5s 9m 8M (vis R190°-353°, W353°-001°, R001°-018°, W018°-190°). Mallard Shoal ldg lts 349°: Front Q WRG 10/3M (vis G233°-043°, R043°-067°, G067°-087°, W087°-099°, R099°-108°); rear 396m from front (on Hoe) Oc G 1·3s (vis 310°-040°).

There are Dir lts, with WRG sectors, at Whidbey (138·5°), Withyhedge (070°), W Hoe bn (315°), Mill Bay (048°30′), Western King (271°), Ravenness (225°), Mount Wise (343°), and Ocean Court (085°).

In fog the following Dir W lts operate: Mallard (front) Fl 5s (vis 232°-110°); West Hoe bn F (vis 313°-317°); Eastern King Fl 5s (vis 259°-062°); Ravenness Fl (2) 15s (vis 160 °-305°;) Mount Wise F (vis 341°-345°); Ocean Court Fl 5s (vis 270°-100°).

Notes: Principal lts in Plymouth Sound show QY if mains power fails. N of The Bkwtr, four large mooring buoys (C, D, E & F) have Fl Y lts.

Continued

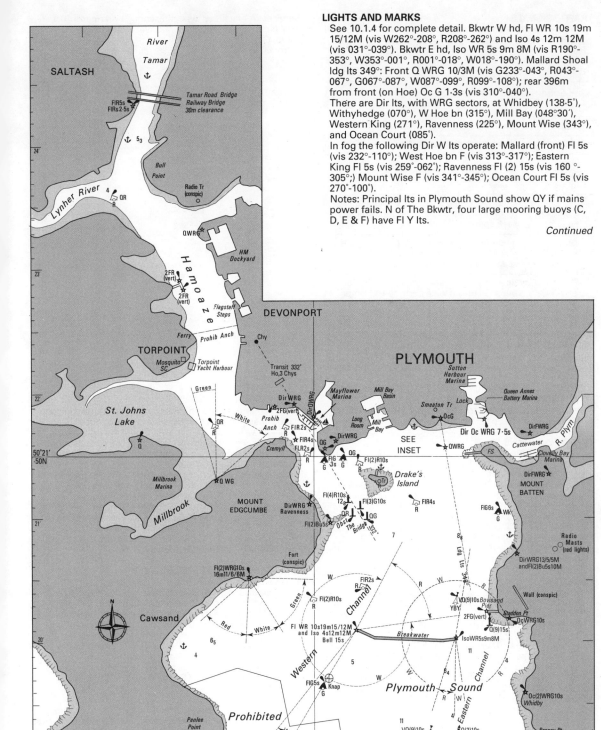

PLYMOUTH *continued*

TRAFFIC SIGNALS
Traffic is controlled H24 by the following combinations of 3 lts WRG (vert), Fl or Oc, shown from Drake's Is and at Flag Port Control Station in the Dockyard. These signals, and any hoisted by HM Ships, apply to the waters off the dockyard port and 125m either side of the deep water chan out to the W Ent. The Cattewater, Mill Bay Docks and Sutton Hbr are excluded.

Signal	Meaning
Unlit	No restrictions, unless passed on VHF
® ® ® All Fl	Serious Emergency All traffic suspended
® ⑥ ⑥ All Oc	Outgoing traffic only may proceed on the recommended track. Crossing traffic to seek approval
⑥ ⑥ ® All Oc	Incoming traffic only may proceed on the recommended track. Crossing traffic to seek approval
⑥ ⑥ ⑩ All Oc	Vessels may proceed in either direction, but shall give a wide berth to HM Ships using the recommended track

Wind Strength Warning Flags and Lights
Wind flags (R and W vert stripes) are hoisted at Queen Anne's Battery, Mayflower Marina, Sutton Hbr Marina and The Camber (HO only) to warn of strong winds as follows:

One wind flag   (1 Oc ⑩ lt)   =   Rough weather, Force 5 - 7.
Two wind flags (2 Oc ⑩ lts) =   Very rough weather, > F 7.
Note: The vert Oc ⑩ lt(s) are shown only from Drake's Island, HJ when there is no tfc sig in force.

RADIO TELEPHONE
Call: *Long Room Port Control* VHF Ch 08 12 **14** 16 (H24).
Call: *Mill Bay Docks* Ch 12 13 14 16 (only during ferry ops).
Call: *Sutton Lock* for lock opening Ch **12** 16 (H24).
Call: *Cattewater Hbr* Ch 14 16 (Mon-Fri, 0900-1700 LT).
Mayflower, Queen Anne's Battery and Clovelly Bay marinas and Torpoint Yacht Hbr: all Ch **80** M.
TELEPHONE (01752)
QHM 552047; DQHM 552701; Flagstaff Port Control 552413; Longroom Control 552411/2; Cattewater Hr Mr 665934; ABP at Mill Bay 662191; MRSC (01803) 882704; ⌗ 220661; Marinecall 0891 500458; Police 701188; Dr 663138; Ⓗ 668080.
FACILITIES
Marinas (W to E)
Torpoint Yacht Hbr (60+20 Ⓥ) ☎/Fax 813658, £10, access H24, dredged 2m. FW, AC, BY, C, ME, EI, Sh, Diver, SM.
Mayflower Marina (300+50 Ⓥ) ☎ 556633, Fax 606896, £14.50, P, D, FW, ME, EI, Sh, AC, C (2 ton), BH (25 ton), CH, Slip, Gas, Gaz, Divers, SM, BY, YC, V, R, Bar, Ⓒ.
Mill Bay Village Marina ☎ 226785, Fax 222513, No Ⓥ. Ent has Oc R 4s and Oc G 4s, not shown on chartlet.
Queen Anne's Battery Marina (240+60 Ⓥ) ☎ 671142, Fax 266527, £15.80, AC, P, D, ME, EI, Sh, FW, BH (20 ton), C (50 ton), CH, Gas, Gaz, Ⓒ, SM, Slip, V, Bar, YC.
Sutton Hbr Marina (310) ☎ 664186, Fax 223521, £16, P, D, FW, AC, EI, ME, Sh, CH, C (masts only), Slip. Note: Sutton Hbr is entered via lock gates (Barbican flood protection scheme), which maintain 3m CD in the marina. The lock, 44 x 16m, has pontoons inside and operates H24, free; call *Sutton Lock* for opening VHF Ch 12 16. When tide reaches 3m CD, gates remain open for free-flow. Tfc sigs (vert): 3 ® = Stop; 3 ⑥ = Go; 3 Fl ® = Serious hazard, wait.
Clovelly Bay Marina (180+ Ⓥ) ☎ 404231, Fax 484177, £12, D, FW, AC, CH, ME, EI, Gas, Gaz, V, Ⓒ.
Clubs
Royal Western YC of England ☎ 660077, M, Bar, R; **Royal Plymouth Corinthian YC** ☎ 664327, VHF Ch M, M, R, Bar, Slip; **Plym YC** ☎ 404991; **RNSA** c/o QHM ☎ 555581; **Mayflower SC** ☎ 662526; **Torpoint Mosquito SC** ☎ 812508, visitors welcome, R, Bar; **Saltash SC** ☎ 845988.

Services (All facilities available; consult marina/Hr Mr)
BY (several), ME, EI, Sh, SM, Divers, C (20 ton), ACA, Slip, Gas, Ⓔ.
City EC Wed; P, D, V, R, CH, ✉, Ⓑ, ⇌, ✈.

RIVER TAMAR (and TAVY)
The Tamar runs into The Hamoaze at the Tamar bridges and is navigable on the flood for 12M to Calstock. (The R Tavy flows into the Tamar 1¼ M above the bridges, but due to power lines (8m) and a bridge (7·6m) at its mouth, is only accessible to un-masted craft up to Bere Ferrers). Cargreen village is 0·7M beyond the Tavy, on the W bank, with many local moorings and ⚓ in 2m. Weir Quay on E bank has a SC, BY, M and fuel. The river S-bends, narrowing and drying, passes Cothele Quay and then turns 90° stbd to Calstock; possible AB, M, or ⚓ above the viaduct in 2m. **Tamar River SC** ☎ 362741; **Weir Quay SC** ☎ (01822) 840474, M, CH, ME; **Calstock BY** ☎ (01822) 832502, access HW ±3, M, ME, SH, C (8 ton), BH (10 ton). Facilities: P, D, V, Bar, Ⓑ (Mon a.m.), ⇌.

RIVER LYNHER (or ST GERMANS)
This river which flows into The Hamoaze about 0·8M S of the Tamar Bridge, dries extensively but is navigable on the tide for 4M up to St Germans Quay (private); but temp AB possible by prior arrangement with Quay SC. The chan, ent at Wearde Quay, is buoyed and partly lit for the first 2M. There are ⚓s, amid local moorings, at the ent to Forder Lake (N bank); SE of Ince Pt and Castle in about 3m; and at Dandy Hole, a pool with 3m, where the river bends NW and dries almost completely. Facilities: V, Bar, ✉, (½M). **Quay SC** Moorings ☎ (01503) 30531.

Our course down Channel had no doubt been tortuous. On June 2nd the visibility being poor, I reckoned we must be somewhere near the Manacles. But life is full of surprises. When the wind fell light we handed the mainsail in order to stitch a slender seam and while I was busy with this Noddy sighted through the haze a slender tower to the north-east – no doubt, the Eddystone. But when the sun went down and the lights came on it proved to be the Wolf Rock light. We were at least twenty miles and two points out in our reckoning. I concluded that Mischief knew the way down Channel better than her skipper.

Mostly Mischief: H.W.Tilman

With acknowledgements to the Executors of the estate of H.W.Tilman and to Hollis & Carter (Publishers 1966).

ENGLAND – PLYMOUTH (DEVONPORT)

LAT 50°22′N   LONG 4°11′W

TIMES AND HEIGHTS OF HIGH AND LOW WATERS   YEAR 1996

TIME ZONE (UT)
For Summer Time add ONE hour in non-shaded areas

JANUARY

Day	Time m	Time m	Time m	Time m
1 M	0202 4.5	0821 2.1	1429 4.5	2054 1.9
16 TU	0043 4.5	0715 2.0	1316 4.6	1957 1.8
2 TU	0302 4.7	0925 1.9	1526 4.7	2149 1.7
17 W	0206 4.7	0835 1.7	1440 4.8	2110 1.5
3 W	0352 4.9	1016 1.6	1615 4.8	2236 1.5
18 TH	0321 5.0	0944 1.3	1551 5.0	2214 1.2
4 TH	0435 5.1	1101 1.4	1656 5.0	2317 1.3
19 F	0422 5.3	1651 5.3	2310 0.8	
5 F O	0513 5.2	1141 1.2	1733 5.0	2354 1.2
20 SA ●	0515 5.6	1139 0.6	1744 5.4	
6 SA	0549 5.3	1217 1.2	1810 5.1	
21 SU	0003 0.5	0606 5.8	1231 0.3	1835 5.5
7 SU	0028 1.2	0626 5.3	1251 1.1	1848 5.1
22 M	0052 0.4	0657 5.8	1319 0.2	1926 5.6
8 M	0059 1.2	0703 5.3	1321 1.2	1926 5.0
23 TU	0138 0.3	0745 5.8	1403 0.2	2012 5.5
9 TU	0129 1.2	0740 5.2	1351 1.2	2002 5.0
24 W	0220 0.4	0830 5.7	1444 0.4	2054 5.4
10 W	0159 1.3	0814 5.2	1419 1.3	2034 4.9
25 TH	0259 0.7	0911 5.5	1531 0.7	2132 5.2
11 TH	0228 1.4	0845 5.1	1449 1.4	2104 4.8
26 F	0336 1.0	0948 5.2	1559 1.2	2207 4.9
12 F	0301 1.5	0918 4.9	1523 1.5	2140 4.7
27 SA	0414 1.4	1023 4.9	1638 1.6	2243 4.6
13 SA	0340 1.7	0959 4.8	1606 1.7	2227 4.6
28 SU	0458 1.8	1104 4.5	1726 2.0	2337 4.4
14 SU	0430 1.9	1052 4.7	1705 1.9	2329 4.5
29 M	0555 2.2	1218 4.3	1829 2.2	
15 M	0543 2.0	1158 4.6	1831 2.0	
30 TU	0107 4.3	0712 2.3	1348 4.2	1956 2.3
31 W	0223 4.4	0848 2.2	1455 4.4	2117 2.0

FEBRUARY

Day	Time m	Time m	Time m	Time m
1 TH	0322 4.6	0951 1.8	1549 4.6	2211 1.7
16 F	0301 4.9	0930 1.4	1538 4.9	2201 1.2
2 F	0409 4.9	1039 1.5	1633 4.8	2255 1.4
17 SA	0406 5.2	1033 0.9	1638 5.2	2259 0.8
3 SA	0450 5.1	1120 1.3	1713 5.0	2334 1.2
18 SU ●	0501 5.5	1127 0.5	1731 5.4	2349 0.5
4 SU O	0529 5.2	1157 1.1	1752 5.1	
19 M	0551 5.7	1216 0.2	1820 5.5	
5 M	0009 1.1	0608 5.3	1232 1.0	1831 5.1
20 TU	0036 0.2	0639 5.8	1301 0.1	1907 5.6
6 TU	0042 1.0	0647 5.3	1304 0.9	1910 5.1
21 W	0119 0.2	0726 5.8	1343 0.1	1950 5.6
7 W	0113 1.0	0725 5.3	1333 0.9	1945 5.1
22 TH	0159 0.3	0808 5.7	1421 0.3	2027 5.4
8 TH	0142 1.0	0758 5.2	1402 1.0	2016 5.0
23 F	0235 0.5	0844 5.5	1455 0.7	2057 5.2
9 F	0212 1.0	0828 5.2	1431 1.1	2044 5.0
24 SA	0308 0.9	0912 5.2	1527 1.1	2121 5.0
10 SA	0243 1.1	0858 5.1	1503 1.2	2116 4.9
25 SU	0341 1.3	0936 4.8	1600 1.5	2149 4.7
11 SU	0319 1.3	0935 4.9	1541 1.4	2158 4.7
26 M	0418 1.7	1008 4.5	1640 2.0	2231 4.4
12 M	0403 1.6	1024 4.7	1630 1.7	2255 4.6
27 TU	0507 2.1	1059 4.2	1737 2.3	2336 4.2
13 TU	0505 1.9	1129 4.5	1744 1.9	
28 W	0617 2.4	1241 4.0	1853 2.4	
14 W	0010 4.6	0637 2.0	1251 4.4	1926 2.0
29 TH	0133 4.2	0745 2.3	1421 4.2	2027 2.2
15 TH	0139 4.6	0813 1.8	1421 4.6	2053 1.7

MARCH

Day	Time m	Time m	Time m	Time m
1 F	0248 4.4	0918 2.0	1521 4.4	2140 1.9
16 SA	0245 4.8	0917 1.4	1526 4.8	2148 1.3
2 SA	0341 4.7	1011 1.6	1608 4.7	2227 1.5
17 SU	0350 5.2	1018 0.9	1624 5.1	2243 0.8
3 SU	0425 5.0	1052 1.3	1650 4.9	2307 1.2
18 M	0443 5.5	1109 0.5	1714 5.4	2331 0.5
4 M	0506 5.2	1130 1.0	1730 5.1	2344 1.0
19 TU ●	0532 5.6	1156 0.3	1800 5.5	
5 TU O	0546 5.3	1206 0.9	1810 5.2	
20 W	0016 0.3	0618 5.7	1239 0.1	1842 5.6
6 W	0019 0.8	0625 5.3	1240 0.8	1848 5.2
21 TH	0057 0.2	0702 5.7	1319 0.2	1922 5.5
7 TH	0052 0.8	0703 5.3	1312 0.7	1924 5.2
22 F	0135 0.3	0741 5.6	1355 0.4	1955 5.4
8 F	0123 0.8	0738 5.3	1342 0.8	1955 5.2
23 SA	0209 0.5	0813 5.4	1427 0.7	2020 5.2
9 SA	0154 0.8	0810 5.2	1413 0.9	2024 5.1
24 SU	0241 0.9	0837 5.1	1457 1.1	2043 5.0
10 SU	0227 0.9	0842 5.1	1445 1.0	2057 5.0
25 M	0311 1.3	0901 4.8	1527 1.5	2113 4.8
11 M	0303 1.1	0920 4.9	1523 1.3	2139 4.8
26 TU	0344 1.7	0935 4.5	1602 1.9	2153 4.5
12 TU	0347 1.4	1008 4.7	1612 1.6	2234 4.6
27 W	0429 2.1	1022 4.2	1655 2.3	2249 4.3
13 W	0447 1.8	1113 4.5	1722 1.9	2349 4.5
28 TH	0536 2.3	1134 4.0	1810 2.4	
14 TH	0616 2.0	1238 4.4	1906 2.0	
29 F	0016 4.2	0654 2.3	1337 4.1	1928 2.3
15 F	0121 4.5	0758 1.8	1410 4.5	2039 1.7
30 SA	0204 4.3	0816 2.1	1446 4.3	2047 2.0
31 SU	0305 4.6	0924 1.7	1537 4.6	2146 1.6

APRIL

Day	Time m	Time m	Time m	Time m
1 M	0354 4.9	1013 1.3	1621 4.9	2231 1.3
16 TU	0422 5.3	1047 0.6	1651 5.3	2309 0.6
2 TU	0437 5.1	1054 1.1	1703 5.1	2312 1.0
17 W ●	0509 5.5	1132 0.4	1735 5.4	2353 0.4
3 W	0519 5.2	1134 0.8	1743 5.2	2351 0.8
18 TH	0554 5.5	1214 0.5	1816 5.5	
4 TH O	0559 5.3	1211 0.7	1822 5.3	
19 F	0033 0.4	0635 5.5	1253 0.5	1852 5.4
5 F	0028 0.7	0638 5.4	1248 0.6	1858 5.3
20 SA	0110 0.5	0712 5.4	1328 0.6	1923 5.4
6 SA	0104 0.6	0716 5.4	1323 0.7	1933 5.3
21 SU	0144 0.7	0742 5.2	1400 0.9	1948 5.2
7 SU	0139 0.7	0753 5.3	1357 0.8	2008 5.3
22 M	0215 1.0	0807 5.0	1430 1.2	2015 5.1
8 M	0215 0.8	0831 5.2	1434 1.0	2045 5.2
23 TU	0246 1.3	0836 4.8	1459 1.5	2048 4.9
9 TU	0254 1.0	0912 5.0	1514 1.3	2128 5.0
24 W	0317 1.6	0912 4.6	1531 1.9	2127 4.7
10 W	0341 1.3	1002 4.7	1605 1.6	2223 4.8
25 TH	0357 1.9	0957 4.3	1617 2.1	2216 4.4
11 TH	0441 1.6	1107 4.5	1715 1.9	2337 4.6
26 F	0458 2.2	1058 4.1	1728 2.3	2323 4.3
12 F	0606 1.8	1231 4.4	1851 2.0	
27 SA	0612 2.2	1228 4.1	1843 2.3	
13 SA	0107 4.6	0741 1.7	1357 4.5	2020 1.7
28 SU	0054 4.3	0722 2.1	1356 4.3	1951 2.1
14 SU	0225 4.8	0857 1.4	1507 4.8	2127 1.3
29 M	0215 4.5	0826 1.8	1456 4.6	2054 1.7
15 M	0329 5.1	0956 1.0	1603 5.1	2222 0.9
30 TU	0313 4.8	0924 1.4	1545 4.8	2148 1.4

Chart Datum: 3·22 metres below Ordnance Datum (Newlyn)

ENGLAND – PLYMOUTH (DEVONPORT)

LAT 50°22′N   LONG 4°11′W

TIMES AND HEIGHTS OF HIGH AND LOW WATERS

YEAR **1996**

TIME ZONE (UT)
For Summer Time add ONE hour in non-shaded areas

MAY

Day	Time	m	Time	m	Time	m	Time	m
1 W	0402	5.0	1014	1.1	1630	5.1	2236	1.1
2 TH	0447	5.2	1059	0.9	1713	5.2	2321	0.8
3 F ○	0530	5.3	1143	0.7	1754	5.4		
4 SA	0003	0.7	0613	5.4	1225	0.6	1834	5.4
5 SU	0046	0.6	0655	5.4	1306	0.6	1914	5.5
6 M	0127	0.6	0738	5.3	1347	0.7	1955	5.4
7 TU	0209	0.7	0822	5.2	1429	0.9	2038	5.3
8 W	0252	0.9	0909	5.0	1513	1.2	2124	5.2
9 TH	0342	1.2	1000	4.8	1605	1.4	2218	4.9
10 F	0440	1.4	1103	4.6	1709	1.7	2327	4.7
11 SA	0554	1.6	1219	4.5	1829	1.8		
12 SU	0047	4.7	0715	1.6	1334	4.6	1950	1.7
13 M	0200	4.8	0828	1.4	1440	4.8	2058	1.4
14 TU	0302	4.9	0929	1.2	1536	5.0	2155	1.2
15 W	0357	5.1	1021	0.9	1625	5.1	2244	0.9
16 TH	0445	5.2	1107	0.8	1709	5.3	2328	0.8
17 F ●	0528	5.3	1149	0.7	1748	5.3		
18 SA	0009	0.7	0608	5.2	1228	0.8	1823	5.3
19 SU	0047	0.7	0644	5.2	1304	0.9	1854	5.3
20 M	0122	0.9	0716	5.1	1336	1.1	1923	5.2
21 TU	0153	1.1	0746	4.9	1406	1.3	1955	5.1
22 W	0224	1.3	0819	4.8	1436	1.5	2029	5.0
23 TH	0255	1.5	0856	4.6	1507	1.7	2107	4.8
24 F	0330	1.7	0937	4.5	1544	1.9	2150	4.6
25 SA	0417	1.9	1028	4.3	1640	2.1	2242	4.5
26 SU	0524	2.0	1131	4.2	1754	2.2	2348	4.4
27 M	0634	2.0	1247	4.3	1903	2.1		
28 TU	0105	4.5	0738	1.8	1400	4.5	2007	1.8
29 W	0219	4.6	0838	1.5	1501	4.7	2107	1.5
30 TH	0320	4.9	0935	1.2	1553	5.0	2202	1.2
31 F	0413	5.1	1027	1.0	1641	5.2	2253	0.9

JUNE

Day	Time	m	Time	m	Time	m	Time	m
1 SA ○	0502	5.2	1117	0.8	1727	5.4	2342	0.7
2 SU	0550	5.3	1205	0.6	1812	5.5		
3 M	0030	0.5	0638	5.4	1253	0.6	1858	5.6
4 TU	0118	0.5	0726	5.4	1340	0.6	1945	5.6
5 W	0205	0.5	0815	5.3	1426	0.7	2032	5.5
6 TH	0252	0.7	0904	5.2	1513	0.9	2119	5.3
7 F	0340	0.9	0956	5.0	1601	1.2	2211	5.1
8 SA	0432	1.2	1052	4.8	1655	1.4	2311	4.9
9 SU	0531	1.4	1157	4.6	1758	1.7		
10 M	0020	4.7	0639	1.6	1304	4.6	1911	1.7
11 TU	0129	4.7	0751	1.6	1407	4.6	2023	1.7
12 W	0232	4.7	0856	1.5	1505	4.8	2125	1.5
13 TH	0329	4.8	0952	1.3	1557	4.9	2218	1.3
14 F	0419	4.9	1041	1.1	1642	5.1	2305	1.1
15 SA	0503	5.0	1125	1.0	1721	5.2	2347	1.0
16 SU ●	0543	5.0	1205	1.0	1757	5.2		
17 M	0026	1.0	0619	5.0	1242	1.0	1831	5.2
18 TU	0102	1.0	0654	5.0	1315	1.1	1905	5.2
19 W	0134	1.1	0729	4.9	1346	1.2	1939	5.1
20 TH	0205	1.2	0805	4.8	1416	1.4	2015	5.0
21 F	0235	1.4	0842	4.7	1445	1.5	2050	4.9
22 SA	0305	1.5	0918	4.6	1516	1.7	2126	4.8
23 SU	0339	1.6	0958	4.5	1555	1.8	2208	4.7
24 M	0426	1.8	1046	4.4	1651	2.0	2300	4.5
25 TU	0534	1.9	1145	4.4	1808	2.0		
26 W	0004	4.5	0650	1.8	1255	4.4	1922	1.9
27 TH	0118	4.5	0758	1.7	1409	4.6	2030	1.6
28 F	0235	4.7	0901	1.4	1515	4.9	2132	1.3
29 SA	0342	4.9	1000	1.1	1612	5.1	2230	1.0
30 SU	0438	5.1	1056	0.9	1704	5.4	2325	0.7

JULY

Day	Time	m	Time	m	Time	m	Time	m
1 M ○	0531	5.3	1149	0.6	1754	5.5		
2 TU	0017	0.5	0623	5.4	1241	0.5	1844	5.7
3 W	0108	0.4	0715	5.4	1331	0.5	1934	5.7
4 TH	0157	0.3	0806	5.4	1418	0.5	2022	5.6
5 F	0243	0.4	0854	5.3	1502	0.6	2109	5.5
6 SA	0327	0.6	0941	5.2	1545	0.9	2156	5.3
7 SU	0411	0.9	1030	4.9	1630	1.2	2245	5.0
8 M	0459	1.3	1123	4.7	1721	1.6	2344	4.7
9 TU	0555	1.6	1225	4.5	1823	1.8		
10 W	0052	4.5	0704	1.8	1330	4.5	1940	1.9
11 TH	0200	4.4	0819	1.8	1432	4.5	2054	1.8
12 F	0301	4.5	0924	1.7	1528	4.7	2154	1.6
13 SA	0354	4.7	1017	1.4	1616	4.9	2243	1.4
14 SU	0439	4.8	1103	1.3	1657	5.0	2327	1.2
15 M ●	0519	4.9	1144	1.1	1734	5.2		
16 TU	0007	1.1	0556	5.0	1222	1.1	1810	5.2
17 W	0043	1.0	0634	5.0	1256	1.1	1847	5.2
18 TH	0116	1.1	0712	5.0	1326	1.1	1924	5.2
19 F	0145	1.1	0750	4.9	1355	1.2	2000	5.1
20 SA	0213	1.2	0825	4.8	1422	1.3	2032	5.0
21 SU	0240	1.3	0857	4.8	1451	1.4	2103	4.9
22 M	0309	1.4	0928	4.6	1523	1.5	2137	4.8
23 TU	0345	1.6	1008	4.5	1606	1.7	2222	4.7
24 W	0435	1.7	1100	4.5	1708	1.9	2322	4.5
25 TH	0552	1.9	1207	4.4	1837	2.0		
26 F	0035	4.5	0721	1.8	1326	4.5	1959	1.8
27 SA	0200	4.6	0835	1.6	1445	4.8	2109	1.4
28 SU	0319	4.8	0941	1.3	1550	5.1	2213	1.1
29 M	0421	5.1	1041	0.9	1646	5.4	2311	0.7
30 TU ○	0516	5.3	1136	0.6	1738	5.6		
31 W	0004	0.4	0608	5.4	1228	0.4	1829	5.7

AUGUST

Day	Time	m	Time	m	Time	m	Time	m
1 TH	0055	0.2	0700	5.5	1316	0.3	1919	5.8
2 F	0141	0.1	0750	5.5	1401	0.3	2007	5.8
3 SA	0225	0.2	0836	5.4	1443	0.4	2051	5.6
4 SU	0305	0.5	0917	5.3	1522	0.7	2131	5.3
5 M	0344	0.9	0957	5.0	1601	1.1	2210	5.0
6 TU	0424	1.3	1038	4.7	1643	1.6	2251	4.6
7 W	0510	1.7	1130	4.5	1736	2.0		
8 TH	0000	4.3	0609	2.1	1248	4.3	1848	2.2
9 F	0127	4.2	0733	2.2	1400	4.4	2021	2.1
10 SA	0235	4.3	0847	2.0	1502	4.6	2131	1.8
11 SU	0331	4.5	0955	1.7	1552	4.8	2222	1.5
12 M	0418	4.7	1041	1.4	1634	5.0	2306	1.3
13 TU	0458	4.9	1122	1.2	1712	5.2	2345	1.1
14 W ●	0536	5.0	1200	1.1	1750	5.3		
15 TH	0020	1.0	0613	5.1	1234	1.0	1828	5.3
16 F	0053	1.0	0652	5.1	1304	1.0	1906	5.3
17 SA	0121	1.0	0730	5.1	1332	1.0	1941	5.2
18 SU	0148	1.0	0804	5.0	1359	1.1	2012	5.1
19 M	0215	1.1	0833	4.9	1427	1.2	2040	5.0
20 TU	0243	1.2	0901	4.8	1458	1.4	2112	4.9
21 W	0317	1.4	0937	4.7	1537	1.6	2155	4.7
22 TH	0401	1.7	1028	4.6	1631	1.8	2253	4.5
23 F	0505	1.9	1135	4.5	1758	2.0		
24 SA	0009	4.4	0649	2.0	1258	4.5	1936	1.9
25 SU	0140	4.5	0816	1.8	1425	4.8	2055	1.5
26 M	0306	4.8	0928	1.4	1535	5.1	2200	1.1
27 TU	0409	5.1	1029	0.9	1631	5.5	2257	0.7
28 W ○	0503	5.4	1122	0.6	1723	5.7	2349	0.3
29 TH	0553	5.5	1211	0.3	1812	5.8		
30 F	0036	0.1	0641	5.6	1257	0.2	1859	5.9
31 SA	0121	0.1	0727	5.6	1340	0.2	1945	5.8

Chart Datum: 3·22 metres below Ordnance Datum (Newlyn)

ENGLAND – PLYMOUTH (DEVONPORT)

LAT 50°22′N   LONG   4°11′W

TIMES AND HEIGHTS OF HIGH AND LOW WATERS

YEAR **1996**

TIME ZONE (UT)
For Summer Time add ONE hour in non-shaded areas

SEPTEMBER

Day	Time	m	Day	Time	m
1 SU	0201 / 0809 / 1419 / 2026	0.2 / 5.5 / 0.4 / 5.6	**16** M	0123 / 0739 / 1336 / 1949	0.9 / 5.2 / 1.0 / 5.2
2 M	0239 / 0847 / 1455 / 2100	0.5 / 5.3 / 0.8 / 5.3	**17** TU	0151 / 0808 / 1406 / 2019	1.0 / 5.1 / 1.1 / 5.1
3 TU	0314 / 0917 / 1530 / 2128	1.0 / 5.1 / 1.2 / 5.0	**18** W	0222 / 0838 / 1439 / 2054	1.2 / 5.0 / 1.3 / 5.0
4 W	0348 / 0945 / 1607 / 2155	1.4 / 4.8 / 1.7 / 4.6	**19** TH	0256 / 0916 / 1519 / 2138	1.4 / 4.9 / 1.5 / 4.8
5 TH	0428 / 1021 / 1655 / 2238	1.9 / 4.5 / 2.1 / 4.3	**20** F	0340 / 1007 / 1612 / 2236	1.7 / 4.7 / 1.8 / 4.5
6 F	0523 / 1123 / 1802	2.3 / 4.3 / 2.4	**21** SA	0442 / 1113 / 1736 / 2353	2.0 / 4.5 / 2.1 / 4.4
7 SA	0043 / 0640 / 1324 / 1937	4.1 / 2.4 / 4.2 / 2.4	**22** SU	0627 / 1239 / 1922	2.2 / 4.6 / 2.0
8 SU	0209 / 0822 / 1434 / 2106	4.2 / 2.3 / 4.4 / 2.1	**23** M	0131 / 0803 / 1409 / 2042	4.5 / 1.9 / 4.8 / 1.6
9 M	0308 / 0929 / 1526 / 2158	4.4 / 1.9 / 4.8 / 1.7	**24** TU	0255 / 0915 / 1519 / 2147	4.8 / 1.5 / 5.2 / 1.1
10 TU	0354 / 1015 / 1610 / 2240	4.7 / 1.6 / 5.0 / 1.3	**25** W	0357 / 1014 / 1615 / 2241	5.2 / 1.0 / 5.5 / 0.7
11 W	0435 / 1056 / 1649 / 2317	5.0 / 1.3 / 5.2 / 1.1	**26** TH	0447 / 1105 / 1705 / 2329	5.4 / 0.6 / 5.7 / 0.4
12 TH ●	0513 / 1132 / 1727 / 2352	5.1 / 1.1 / 5.3 / 1.0	**27** F O	0534 / 1151 / 1752	5.6 / 0.4 / 5.8
13 F	0551 / 1206 / 1805	5.2 / 1.0 / 5.4	**28** SA	0014 / 0618 / 1235 / 1837	0.2 / 5.7 / 0.3 / 5.8
14 SA	0024 / 0629 / 1237 / 1843	0.9 / 5.3 / 0.9 / 5.4	**29** SU	0057 / 0701 / 1316 / 1919	0.2 / 5.7 / 0.3 / 5.7
15 SU	0054 / 0706 / 1307 / 1918	0.9 / 5.2 / 0.9 / 5.3	**30** M	0135 / 0740 / 1353 / 1957	0.4 / 5.6 / 0.6 / 5.5

OCTOBER

Day	Time	m	Day	Time	m
1 TU	0211 / 0813 / 1428 / 2026	0.7 / 5.4 / 0.9 / 5.2	**16** W	0132 / 0748 / 1351 / 2004	1.0 / 5.3 / 1.0 / 5.2
2 W	0244 / 0838 / 1501 / 2050	1.1 / 5.2 / 1.3 / 4.9	**17** TH	0207 / 0823 / 1428 / 2043	1.1 / 5.2 / 1.2 / 5.0
3 TH	0316 / 0904 / 1536 / 2119	1.6 / 4.9 / 1.8 / 4.6	**18** F	0245 / 0904 / 1511 / 2129	1.4 / 5.1 / 1.5 / 4.8
4 F	0351 / 0941 / 1619 / 2201	2.0 / 4.6 / 2.2 / 4.3	**19** SA	0331 / 0955 / 1606 / 2227	1.7 / 4.9 / 1.8 / 4.6
5 SA	0441 / 1033 / 1722 / 2309	2.4 / 4.3 / 2.5 / 4.1	**20** SU	0434 / 1100 / 1726 / 2345	2.0 / 4.7 / 2.0 / 4.5
6 SU	0555 / 1201 / 1844	2.6 / 4.2 / 2.5	**21** M	0611 / 1225 / 1905	2.2 / 4.7 / 2.0
7 M	0131 / 0722 / 1354 / 2018	4.1 / 2.5 / 4.4 / 2.3	**22** TU	0119 / 0745 / 1351 / 2024	4.5 / 2.0 / 4.8 / 1.6
8 TU	0236 / 0846 / 1453 / 2119	4.4 / 2.2 / 4.7 / 1.9	**23** W	0238 / 0856 / 1500 / 2127	4.8 / 1.6 / 5.1 / 1.2
9 W	0325 / 0938 / 1539 / 2203	4.7 / 1.8 / 5.0 / 1.5	**24** TH	0338 / 0954 / 1556 / 2220	5.2 / 1.1 / 5.4 / 0.8
10 TH	0407 / 1020 / 1621 / 2241	5.0 / 1.4 / 5.2 / 1.2	**25** F	0428 / 1044 / 1645 / 2307	5.4 / 0.8 / 5.6 / 0.6
11 F	0446 / 1058 / 1700 / 2317	5.2 / 1.0 / 5.3 / 1.0	**26** SA O	0513 / 1130 / 1731 / 2351	5.6 / 0.6 / 5.7 / 0.5
12 SA ●	0525 / 1134 / 1739 / 2352	5.3 / 1.0 / 5.4 / 0.9	**27** SU	0556 / 1212 / 1814	5.7 / 0.5 / 5.7
13 SU	0604 / 1209 / 1818	5.4 / 0.9 / 5.4	**28** M	0032 / 0635 / 1252 / 1854	0.5 / 5.7 / 0.6 / 5.6
14 M	0026 / 0640 / 1244 / 1854	0.9 / 5.4 / 0.9 / 5.4	**29** TU	0110 / 0711 / 1329 / 1929	0.7 / 5.5 / 0.8 / 5.4
15 TU	0059 / 0715 / 1317 / 1929	0.9 / 5.4 / 0.9 / 5.3	**30** W	0145 / 0741 / 1403 / 1956	0.9 / 5.4 / 1.1 / 5.2
			31 TH	0217 / 0806 / 1436 / 2022	1.3 / 5.2 / 1.4 / 4.9

NOVEMBER

Day	Time	m	Day	Time	m
1 F	0248 / 0837 / 1509 / 2055	1.6 / 5.0 / 1.8 / 4.7	**16** SA	0242 / 0859 / 1511 / 2127	1.3 / 5.3 / 1.3 / 5.0
2 SA	0320 / 0914 / 1547 / 2137	2.0 / 4.8 / 2.1 / 4.4	**17** SU	0331 / 0949 / 1605 / 2223	1.6 / 5.1 / 1.6 / 4.8
3 SU	0402 / 1002 / 1642 / 2234	2.3 / 4.6 / 2.4 / 4.2	**18** M	0430 / 1051 / 1714 / 2335	2.0 / 4.9 / 1.8 / 4.6
4 M	0508 / 1105 / 1754	2.5 / 4.4 / 2.5	**19** TU	0548 / 1207 / 1838	2.0 / 4.8 / 1.8
5 TU	0003 / 0625 / 1237 / 1908	4.2 / 2.6 / 4.4 / 2.4	**20** W	0057 / 0716 / 1325 / 1956	4.6 / 1.9 / 4.9 / 1.7
6 W	0144 / 0740 / 1401 / 2017	4.3 / 2.3 / 4.6 / 2.1	**21** TH	0210 / 0829 / 1433 / 2101	4.8 / 1.7 / 5.0 / 1.4
7 TH	0244 / 0844 / 1458 / 2112	4.6 / 2.0 / 4.8 / 1.7	**22** F	0312 / 0930 / 1532 / 2156	5.0 / 1.4 / 5.2 / 1.1
8 F	0332 / 0936 / 1546 / 2159	4.9 / 1.7 / 5.1 / 1.4	**23** SA	0405 / 1022 / 1624 / 2245	5.3 / 1.1 / 5.4 / 0.9
9 SA	0416 / 1021 / 1630 / 2241	5.1 / 1.3 / 5.3 / 1.1	**24** SU	0450 / 1108 / 1710 / 2329	5.4 / 0.9 / 5.4 / 0.8
10 SU	0457 / 1103 / 1712 / 2322	5.3 / 1.1 / 5.4 / 1.0	**25** M O	0532 / 1151 / 1752	5.5 / 0.8 / 5.4
11 M ●	0537 / 1143 / 1753	5.4 / 0.9 / 5.4	**26** TU	0009 / 0611 / 1231 / 1830	0.8 / 5.5 / 0.8 / 5.4
12 TU	0001 / 0615 / 1223 / 1833	0.9 / 5.5 / 0.9 / 5.4	**27** W	0048 / 0646 / 1309 / 1905	0.9 / 5.5 / 1.0 / 5.2
13 W	0041 / 0654 / 1303 / 1913	0.9 / 5.5 / 0.9 / 5.4	**28** TH	0122 / 0716 / 1343 / 1934	1.1 / 5.4 / 1.1 / 5.1
14 TH	0120 / 0733 / 1343 / 1955	1.1 / 5.5 / 0.9 / 5.3	**29** F	0154 / 0745 / 1415 / 2004	1.3 / 5.3 / 1.4 / 5.0
15 F	0159 / 0814 / 1425 / 2039	1.1 / 5.4 / 1.1 / 5.2	**30** SA	0225 / 0818 / 1447 / 2039	1.5 / 5.1 / 1.6 / 4.8

DECEMBER

Day	Time	m	Day	Time	m
1 SU	0255 / 0855 / 1520 / 2118	1.8 / 4.9 / 1.9 / 4.6	**16** M	0328 / 0943 / 1559 / 2215	1.2 / 5.3 / 1.2 / 5.0
2 M	0328 / 0937 / 1559 / 2206	2.1 / 4.8 / 2.1 / 4.4	**17** TU	0419 / 1037 / 1654 / 2315	1.5 / 5.1 / 1.5 / 4.8
3 TU	0414 / 1027 / 1658 / 2306	2.3 / 4.6 / 2.3 / 4.3	**18** W	0518 / 1142 / 1800	1.8 / 4.9 / 1.7
4 W	0525 / 1129 / 1809	2.4 / 4.5 / 2.3	**19** TH	0025 / 0633 / 1253 / 1917	4.7 / 1.9 / 4.8 / 1.8
5 TH	0022 / 0640 / 1244 / 1917	4.3 / 2.4 / 4.5 / 2.2	**20** F	0135 / 0753 / 1402 / 2030	4.7 / 1.9 / 4.8 / 1.7
6 F	0142 / 0748 / 1400 / 2020	4.5 / 2.2 / 4.6 / 1.9	**21** SA	0240 / 0902 / 1505 / 2131	4.8 / 1.7 / 4.9 / 1.5
7 SA	0246 / 0849 / 1503 / 2116	4.7 / 1.9 / 4.8 / 1.6	**22** SU	0338 / 0959 / 1601 / 2223	5.0 / 1.4 / 5.0 / 1.3
8 SU	0339 / 0943 / 1557 / 2207	5.0 / 1.5 / 5.1 / 1.3	**23** M	0427 / 1048 / 1649 / 2308	5.2 / 1.2 / 5.1 / 1.1
9 M	0426 / 1033 / 1645 / 2255	5.2 / 1.2 / 5.2 / 1.1	**24** TU O	0510 / 1132 / 1731 / 2350	5.3 / 1.1 / 5.2 / 1.0
10 TU ●	0510 / 1121 / 1730 / 2341	5.4 / 1.0 / 5.4 / 0.9	**25** W	0549 / 1214 / 1809	5.4 / 1.0 / 5.4
11 W	0554 / 1207 / 1815	5.5 / 0.8 / 5.4	**26** TH	0029 / 0623 / 1252 / 1844	1.0 / 5.4 / 1.0 / 5.1
12 TH	0027 / 0637 / 1254 / 1901	0.8 / 5.6 / 0.7 / 5.4	**27** F	0105 / 0656 / 1326 / 1917	1.1 / 5.4 / 1.1 / 5.1
13 F	0112 / 0722 / 1340 / 1947	0.8 / 5.6 / 0.7 / 5.4	**28** SA	0136 / 0722 / 1357 / 1950	1.2 / 5.3 / 1.2 / 5.0
14 SA	0157 / 0808 / 1425 / 2035	0.9 / 5.6 / 0.8 / 5.3	**29** SU	0205 / 0804 / 1426 / 2025	1.4 / 5.2 / 1.4 / 4.9
15 SU	0242 / 0854 / 1511 / 2123	1.1 / 5.5 / 1.0 / 5.2	**30** M	0233 / 0839 / 1454 / 2101	1.5 / 5.1 / 1.6 / 4.8
			31 TU	0301 / 0915 / 1523 / 2138	1.7 / 4.9 / 1.7 / 4.6

Chart Datum: 3·22 metres below Ordnance Datum (Newlyn)

SUBMARINE EXERCISE AREAS (SUBFACTS)

Within the SW English Channel, those areas (see below) where dived and surfaced submaries are planned to operate during all or part of the ensuing 24 hrs will be broadcast daily on VHF at 0733 and 1933UT by the four Coast Radio Stations shown below.   Further info from Naval Ops, Plymouth ☎ (01752) 557550. See also 6.3.15.

Submarines on the surface and at periscope depth will maintain constant listening watch on VHF Ch 16. The former will comply strictly with IRPCS; the latter will not close to within 1500 yds of a FV without permission from the FV. See 8.4.10 for general advice on submarine activity which also occurs in other sea areas.

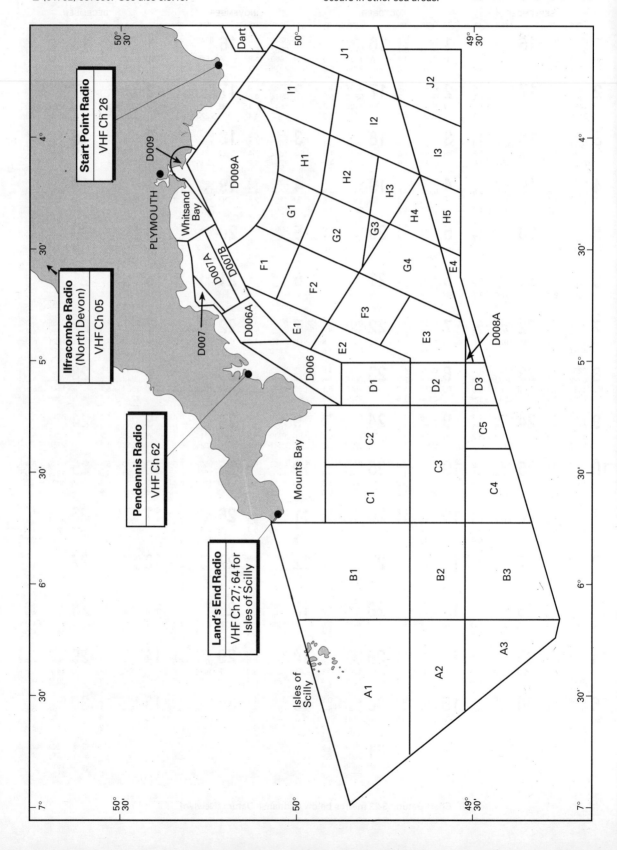

| Start Point Radio | VHF Ch 26 |

| Ilfracombe Radio (North Devon) | VHF Ch 05 |

| Pendennis Radio | VHF Ch 62 |

| Land's End Radio | VHF Ch 27; 64 for Isles of Scilly |

RIVER YEALM   10-1-19

Devon 50°18′·55N 04°04′·06W (Ent)

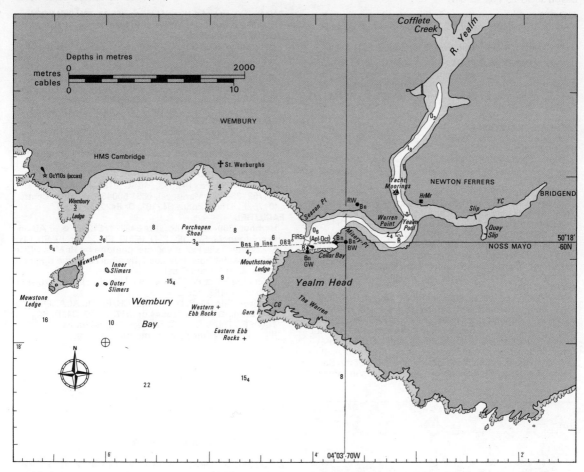

CHARTS
AC *30, 1613*; Imray C6, C14; Stanfords 13; OS 201
TIDES
−0522 Dover; ML 3·2; Duration 0615; Zone 0 (UT)

Standard Port DEVONPORT (←—)

Times				Height (metres)			
High Water		Low Water		MHWS	MHWN	MLWN	MLWS
0000	0600	0000	0600	5·5	4·4	2·2	0·8
1200	1800	1200	1800				

Differences RIVER YEALM ENTRANCE
| +0006 | +0006 | +0002 | +0002 | −0·1 | −0·1 | −0·1 | −0·1 |

Note: Strong SW winds hold up the ebb and raise levels, as does the river if in spate.

SHELTER
Very good. Ent easy except in strong onshore winds. ⚓ in Cellar Bay is open to NW winds. ♥ pontoon in The Pool.
NAVIGATION
WPT 50°18′·00N 04°06′·00W, 240°/060° from/to Season Pt, 1·4M. The W and E Ebb rks and the Inner and Outer Slimers are dangerous, lying awash on either side of Wembury B; for firing range, see 10.1.17. Ldg bns (W △, B stripe) in line at 089° clear Mouthstone Ledge, but **not** the sand bar. The PHM buoy, Fl R 5s (Apr-Oct), marks end of sand bar and **must** be left to port on entry. When abeam bn (G ▲ on W □) on S shore, turn NE toward bn (W □, R stripe) on N shore. From sand bar to Misery Pt, river carries only 1·2m at MLWS. Leave Spit PHM buoy off Warren Pt to port. It is not possible to beat in against an ebb tide. Speed limit 6kn.
LIGHTS AND MARKS
River unlit apart from PHM By Fl R 5s at ent. Bns as above.
TELEPHONE (01752)
Hr Mr 872533; MRSC (01803) 882704; ⌗ 220661; Marinecall 0891 500458; Police 701188; Dr 880392.
RADIO TELEPHONE None.

FACILITIES
Yealm Pool M, pontoon £7, L, FW; **Yealm YC** ☎ 872291, FW, R, Bar; **Services:** ME, El, Sh, SM.
Newton Ferrers Village L, Slip, FW, V, Gas, Gaz, R, Bar, ✉;
Bridgend L, Slip (HW±2½), FW; **Noss Mayo** L, Slip, FW, V, R, Bar, ✉; Nearest fuel 3M at Yealmpton. ≉ ✈ (Plymouth).

ADJACENT ANCHORAGES IN BIGBURY BAY

RIVER ERME, Devon, 50°18′·12N 03°57′·60W. AC *1613*. HW −0525 on Dover; +0015 and −0·6m on HW Devonport. Temp day ⚓ in 3m at mouth of drying river, open to SW. Access near HW, but only in offshore winds and settled wx. Beware Wells Rk (1·2m) 1M SE of ent. Appr from SW, clear of Edwards Rk. Ent between Battisborough Is and W. Mary's Rk (dries <u>1</u>·1m) keeping to the W. No facilities. Two Historic Wrecks are at 50°18′·15N 03°57′·41W and 50°18′·41N 03°57′·19W on W side of the ent; see 10.0.3g.

RIVER AVON, Devon, 50°16′·61N 03°53′·60W. AC *1613*. Tides as R. Erme, above. Enter drying river HW −1, only in N/E winds and settled wx. Appr close E of conspic Burgh Is & Murray's Rks, marked by bn. Narrow chan hugs cliffy NW shore, then turns SE and N off Bantham. A recce at LW or local knowledge would assist. Streams run hard, but able to dry out in good shelter clear of moorings. V, ✉, Bar at Bantham. Aveton Gifford accessible by dinghy, 2·5M.

HOPE COVE, Devon, 50°14′·62N 03°51′·75W. AC *1613*. Tides as R. Erme, above; ML 2·6m; Duration 0615. Popular day ⚓ in centre of cove, but poor holding ground and only safe in offshore winds. Appr with old LB ho brg 110° and ⚓ SW of pier hd. Beware rk, drying <u>2</u>·5m, ½ca offshore and 3ca E of Bolt Tail. No lts. Facilities: very limited in village, EC Thurs; but good at Kingsbridge (6M bus), or Salcombe, (4M bus).

SALCOMBE   10-1-20
Devon 50°13'·55N 03°46'·60W

CHARTS
AC *28*, 1634, *1613*; Imray C6, Y48; Stanfords 13; OS 202
TIDES
−0523 Dover; ML 3·1; Duration 0615; Zone 0 (UT)

Standard Port DEVONPORT (←)

Times				Height (metres)			
High Water		Low Water		MHWS	MHWN	MLWN	MLWS
0100	0600	0100	0600	5·5	4·4	2·2	0·8
1300	1800	1300	1800				
Differences SALCOMBE							
0000	+0010	+0005	−0005	−0·2	−0·3	−0·1	−0·1
START POINT							
+0005	+0030	−0005	+0005	−0·2	−0·4	−0·1	−0·1

SHELTER
Perfectly protected hbr but ent exposed to S winds. The estuary is 4M long and has 8 drying creeks off it. Limited ⚓ on SE side between ferry and ⚓ prohib area. Plenty of deep water ⚓s. (Hr Mr's launch will contact VHF Ch14, on duty 0600-2100 in season; 0600-2200 in peak season). S'ly winds can cause an uncomfortable swell in the ⚓ off the town. Visitors' pontoon and ⚓s in the Bag are well sheltered. Short stay pontoon (1 hour max, 0700-1900) by Hr Mr's office has 1m. Water taxi via Hr Mr, VHF Ch 12.
NAVIGATION
WPT 50°12'·40N 03°46'·60W, 180°/000° from/to Sandhill Pt lt, 1·3M. The bar (0·7m) can be dangerous at sp ebb tides with strong on-shore winds. Access HW±4½, but at springs this window applies only if swell height does not exceed 1m. The Bar is not as dangerous as rumour may have it, except in the above conditions; if in doubt, call Hr Mr Ch 14 before approaching. Rickham Rk, E of the Bar, has 3·1m depth. Speed limit 8kn; radar checks in force.

Note: The site of a Historic Wreck (50°12'·70N 03°44'·33W) is at Moor Sand, 1M WNW of Prawle Pt; see 10.0.3g.
LIGHTS AND MARKS
Outer ldg marks: Sandhill Pt bn on with Poundstone bn 000°. Sandhill Pt Dir lt 000°, Fl WRG 2s 27m 10/7M; R and W ♦ on W mast: vis R002°-182°, G182°-357°, W357°-002°. Beware unmarked Bass Rk (dries 0·8m) close W of ldg line and Wolf Rk, marked by SHM By QG, close E of ldg line. After passing Wolf Rk, pick up Inner ldg lts, Q Fl 042°, leaving Blackstone Rk Q (2) G 8s 4m 2M to stbd.
RADIO TELEPHONE
VHF Ch 14 call *Salcombe Hbr* or *Launch* (Mon-Thurs 0900-1645, Fri 0900-1615); 14 May-14 Sept Sat/Sun 0900-1615). Call *Water taxi* Ch 12. Call: *ICC Base* (clubhouse) and *Egremont* (ICC floating HQ) Ch M. *Fuel Barge* Ch 06.
TELEPHONE (01548)
Hr Mr 843791, Fax 842033; MRSC (01803) 882704; ⌗ (01752) 234600; Marinecall 0891 500458; Weather Centre (01752) 251860; Police 842107; Dr 842284.
FACILITIES
Harbour (300+150 visitors) ☎ 843791, £10 for ⚓ or AB on Ⓥ pontoon. M, Slip, Ⓔ, P, D, L, ME, EI, C (15 ton), Sh, CH, SM, Water Taxi; FW at visitors' pontoon by Hr Mr's Office or from water boat; if needed, fly a bucket in the rigging. Public ⌐ at Batson Creek.
Salcombe YC ☎ 842872/842593, L, R, Bar; **Island Cruising Club** ☎ 843483, Bar, Ⓛ.
Services: Slip, M, P, D, FW, ME, CH, EI, Sh, ACA, Ⓔ, SM; **Fuel Barge** ☎ (0836) 775644 or (01752) 223434, D, P.
Town EC Thurs; Ⓛ, ✉, Ⓑ, all facilities, ⇌ (bus to Plymouth or Totnes), ✈ (Plymouth).

ADJACENT HARBOUR UP-RIVER

KINGSBRIDGE, Devon, 50°16'·85N 03°46'·45W. AC *28*. HW = HW Salcombe +0005. Access HW±2½ for <2m draft/ bilge keelers, max LOA 11m. Berth on visitors' pontoon on E side of basin, drying 3·4m to soft mud. Best to check berth availability with Hr Mr Salcombe. The 3M chan to Kingsbridge is marked beyond Salt Stone SHM perch by R/W PHM poles with R can topmarks. 6ca N of Salt Stone a secondary chan marked by PHM buoys diverges slowly E into Balcombe Creek. There is a private ferry pontoon at New Quay, 3ca before the visitors' pontoon. Facilities: Slip, SM.
Town EC Thurs; V, R, Bar, ✉, Ⓑ, Ⓛ.

Sunset and evening star,
And one clear call for me!
And may there be no moaning of the bar,
When I put out to sea ...

Crossing the Bar: Alfred Lord Tennyson

The opening lines of Tennyson's famous poem written whilst on board a yacht at Salcombe. The description of putting out to sea on a calm evening is actually used as a metaphor for death.

ENGLAND – DARTMOUTH

LAT 50°21′N   LONG 3°34′W

TIMES AND HEIGHTS OF HIGH AND LOW WATERS   YEAR 1996

TIME ZONE (UT)
For Summer Time add ONE hour in non-shaded areas

JANUARY

Day	Time	m	Day	Time	m
1 M	0219 0817 1447 2051	3.9 1.9 3.9 1.7	**16** TU	0058 0711 1332 1953	3.9 1.8 4.0 1.6
2 TU	0321 0922 1546 2147	4.1 1.7 4.1 1.5	**17** W	0223 0832 1458 2107	4.1 1.5 4.2 1.3
3 W	0413 1014 1637 2235	4.3 1.4 4.2 1.3	**18** TH	0341 0942 1612 2212	4.4 1.1 4.4 1.0
4 TH	0457 1100 1719 2316	4.5 1.2 4.4 1.1	**19** F	0444 1044 1714 2309	4.7 0.7 4.7 0.6
5 F O	0536 1140 1757 2353	4.6 1.0 4.4 1.0	**20** SA ●	0539 1138 1808	5.0 0.4 4.8
6 SA	0614 1216 1835	4.7 1.0 4.5	**21** SU	0002 0631 1231 1859	0.3 5.2 0.1 4.9
7 SU	0027 0651 1251 1912	1.0 4.7 0.9 4.5	**22** M	0052 0721 1319 1949	0.2 5.2 0.2 5.0
8 M	0059 0727 1321 1949	1.0 4.7 1.0 4.4	**23** TU	0137 0808 1402 2034	0.1 5.2 0.0 4.9
9 TU	0129 0803 1350 2024	1.0 4.6 1.0 4.4	**24** W	0219 0852 1442 2115	0.2 5.1 0.2 4.8
10 W	0158 0836 1418 2055	1.1 4.6 1.1 4.3	**25** TH	0257 0932 1520 2152	0.5 4.9 0.5 4.6
11 TH	0227 0906 1447 2125	1.2 4.5 1.2 4.2	**26** F	0333 1007 1556 2226	0.8 4.6 1.0 4.3
12 F	0259 0938 1521 2200	1.3 4.3 1.3 4.1	**27** SA	0411 1042 1634 2301	1.2 4.3 1.4 4.0
13 SA	0337 1018 1603 2246	1.5 4.2 1.5 4.0	**28** SU	0454 1122 1722 2354	1.6 3.9 1.8 3.8
14 SU	0427 1110 1701 2346	1.7 4.1 1.7 3.9	**29** M	0550 1234 1824	2.0 3.7 2.0
15 M	0538 1214 1827	1.8 4.0 1.8	**30** TU	0122 0708 1405 1952	3.7 2.1 3.6 2.1
			31 W	0241 0845 1514 2114	3.8 2.0 3.8 1.8

FEBRUARY

Day	Time	m	Day	Time	m
1 TH	0342 0949 1610 2209	4.0 1.6 4.0 1.5	**16** F	0320 0928 1558 2159	4.3 1.2 4.3 1.0
2 F	0430 1038 1655 2254	4.3 1.3 4.2 1.2	**17** SA	0427 1032 1700 2258	4.6 0.7 4.6 0.6
3 SA	0513 1119 1736 2333	4.5 1.1 4.4 1.0	**18** SU ●	0524 1126 1755 2348	4.9 0.3 4.8 0.3
4 SU O	0553 1156 1817	4.6 0.9 4.5	**19** M	0616 1215 1845	5.1 0.0 4.9
5 M	0008 0633 1232 1855	0.9 4.7 0.8 4.5	**20** TU	0036 0703 1301 1931	0.0 5.2 -0.1 5.0
6 TU	0042 0711 1304 1934	0.8 4.7 0.7 4.5	**21** W	0119 0749 1342 2012	0.1 5.2 -0.1 5.0
7 W	0113 0748 1332 2008	0.8 4.7 0.7 4.5	**22** TH	0158 0830 1420 2049	0.1 5.1 0.1 4.8
8 TH	0141 0820 1401 2038	0.8 4.6 0.8 4.4	**23** F	0233 0905 1453 2118	0.3 4.9 0.5 4.6
9 F	0211 0850 1429 2105	0.8 4.6 0.9 4.4	**24** SA	0306 0933 1525 2141	0.7 4.6 0.9 4.4
10 SA	0241 0919 1501 2136	0.9 4.5 1.0 4.3	**25** SU	0338 0956 1557 2208	1.1 4.2 1.3 4.1
11 SU	0317 0955 1538 2217	1.1 4.3 1.2 4.1	**26** M	0415 1027 1636 2249	1.5 3.9 1.8 3.8
12 M	0400 1043 1627 2313	1.4 4.1 1.5 4.0	**27** TU	0503 1117 1732 2353	1.9 3.6 2.1 3.6
13 TU	0501 1146 1739	1.7 3.9 1.7	**28** W	0612 1256 1849	2.2 3.4 2.2
14 W	0026 0633 1306 1922	3.9 1.8 3.8 1.8	**29** TH	0149 0741 1439 2023	3.6 2.1 3.6 2.0
15 TH	0155 0809 1439 2050	4.0 1.6 4.0 1.5			

MARCH

Day	Time	m	Day	Time	m
1 F	0307 0915 1541 2138	3.8 1.8 3.8 1.7	**16** SA	0304 0914 1546 2146	4.2 1.2 4.2 1.1
2 SA	0401 1009 1629 2225	4.1 1.4 4.1 1.3	**17** SU	0411 1016 1646 2242	4.6 0.7 4.5 0.6
3 SU	0447 1051 1713 2306	4.3 1.1 4.3 1.0	**18** M	0505 1108 1737 2330	4.9 0.3 4.8 0.3
4 M	0529 1129 1754 2343	4.6 0.8 4.5 0.8	**19** TU ●	0556 1155 1825	5.0 0.1 4.9
5 TU O	0611 1205 1835	4.7 0.7 4.6	**20** W	0015 0643 1239 1906	0.1 5.1 -0.1 5.0
6 W	0018 0650 1240 1912	0.6 4.7 0.6 4.6	**21** TH	0057 0726 1319 1945	0.0 5.1 0.0 4.9
7 TH	0052 0727 1312 1947	0.6 4.7 0.6 4.6	**22** F	0134 0804 1354 2017	0.1 5.0 0.2 4.8
8 F	0123 0801 1341 2017	0.6 4.7 0.6 4.6	**23** SA	0208 0835 1426 2042	0.3 4.8 0.5 4.6
9 SA	0153 0832 1412 2046	0.6 4.6 0.7 4.5	**24** SU	0239 0858 1455 2104	0.7 4.5 0.9 4.4
10 SU	0226 0903 1443 2118	0.7 4.5 0.8 4.4	**25** M	0309 0922 1525 2134	1.1 4.2 1.3 4.2
11 M	0301 0940 1521 2159	0.9 4.3 1.1 4.2	**26** TU	0341 0955 1559 2212	1.5 3.9 1.7 3.9
12 TU	0344 1027 1609 2252	1.2 4.1 1.4 4.0	**27** W	0426 1041 1651 2307	1.9 3.6 2.1 3.7
13 W	0443 1131 1718	1.6 3.9 1.7	**28** TH	0531 1151 1805	2.1 3.4 2.2
14 TH	0005 0611 1253 1902	3.9 1.7 3.8 1.8	**29** F	0032 0650 1353 1924	3.6 2.1 3.5 2.1
15 F	0137 0754 1427 2036	3.9 1.6 3.9 1.5	**30** SA	0221 0812 1505 2044	3.7 1.9 3.7 1.8
			31 SU	0324 0921 1557 2144	4.0 1.5 4.0 1.4

APRIL

Day	Time	m	Day	Time	m
1 M	0415 1011 1643 2230	4.3 1.1 4.3 1.1	**16** TU	0444 1046 1714 2308	4.7 0.4 4.7 0.4
2 TU	0459 1053 1726 2311	4.5 0.9 4.5 0.8	**17** W ●	0532 1131 1759 2352	4.9 0.2 4.8 0.2
3 W	0543 1133 1807 2350	4.7 0.6 4.6 0.6	**18** TH	0619 1213 1841	5.0 0.2 4.9
4 TH O	0624 1210 1847	4.7 0.5 4.7	**19** F	0033 0659 1253 1916	0.2 4.9 0.3 4.8
5 F	0027 0702 1248 1922	0.5 4.8 0.4 4.7	**20** SA	0110 0736 1328 1946	0.3 4.8 0.4 4.8
6 SA	0104 0739 1323 1956	0.4 4.8 0.5 4.7	**21** SU	0143 0805 1359 2010	0.5 4.6 0.7 4.6
7 SU	0138 0815 1356 2030	0.5 4.7 0.6 4.7	**22** M	0214 0829 1429 2037	0.8 4.4 1.0 4.5
8 M	0214 0852 1432 2106	0.6 4.6 0.8 4.6	**23** TU	0244 0857 1457 2109	1.1 4.2 1.3 4.3
9 TU	0252 0933 1512 2148	0.8 4.4 1.1 4.4	**24** W	0315 0933 1528 2147	1.4 4.0 1.7 4.1
10 W	0338 1021 1602 2242	1.1 4.1 1.4 4.2	**25** TH	0354 1016 1614 2235	1.7 3.7 1.9 3.8
11 TH	0437 1125 1711 2354	1.4 3.9 1.7 4.0	**26** F	0454 1116 1724 2340	2.0 3.5 2.1 3.7
12 F	0601 1246 1847	1.6 3.8 1.8	**27** SA	0607 1244 1839	2.0 3.5 2.1
13 SA	0122 0737 1414 2016	4.0 1.5 3.9 1.5	**28** SU	0109 0718 1413 1947	3.7 1.9 3.7 1.9
14 SU	0243 0854 1526 2124	4.2 1.2 4.2 1.1	**29** M	0233 0822 1515 2051	3.9 1.6 4.0 1.5
15 M	0349 0954 1624 2220	4.5 0.8 4.5 0.7	**30** TU	0332 0921 1606 2146	4.2 1.2 4.2 1.2

Chart Datum: 2·62 metres below Ordnance Datum (Newlyn)

ENGLAND – DARTMOUTH

LAT 50°21′N   LONG 3°34′W

TIMES AND HEIGHTS OF HIGH AND LOW WATERS

YEAR **1996**

TIME ZONE (UT)
For Summer Time add ONE hour in non-shaded areas

MAY

	Time	m		Time	m
1 W	0423 1012 1652 2235	4.4 0.9 4.5 0.9	**16** TH	0508 1106 1732 2327	4.6 0.6 4.7 0.6
2 TH	0510 1058 1736 2320	4.6 0.7 4.6 0.6	**17** F ●	0552 1148 1813	4.7 0.5 4.7
3 F O	0554 1142 1819	4.7 0.5 4.8	**18** SA	0008 0633 1227 1848	0.5 4.6 0.6 4.7
4 SA	0002 0638 1224 1858	0.5 4.8 0.4 4.8	**19** SU	0047 0708 1304 1918	0.6 4.6 0.7 4.7
5 SU	0046 0719 1306 1938	0.4 4.8 0.4 4.9	**20** M	0122 0739 1335 1946	0.7 4.5 0.9 4.6
6 M	0127 0801 1346 2017	0.4 4.7 0.5 4.8	**21** TU	0152 0808 1405 2017	0.9 4.3 1.1 4.5
7 TU	0208 0844 1428 2059	0.5 4.6 0.7 4.7	**22** W	0223 0841 1434 2051	1.1 4.2 1.3 4.4
8 W	0250 0930 1511 2144	0.7 4.4 1.0 4.6	**23** TH	0253 0917 1505 2128	1.3 4.0 1.5 4.2
9 TH	0339 1019 1602 2237	1.0 4.2 1.2 4.3	**24** F	0328 0957 1541 2209	1.5 3.9 1.7 4.0
10 F	0436 1121 1705 2344	1.2 4.0 1.5 4.1	**25** SA	0414 1047 1636 2300	1.7 3.7 1.9 3.9
11 SA	0549 1235 1824	1.4 3.9 1.6	**26** SU	0520 1148 1749	1.8 3.6 2.0
12 SU	0102 0711 1350 1946	4.1 1.4 4.0 1.5	**27** M	0004 0630 1302 1859	3.8 1.8 3.7 1.9
13 M	0217 0824 1458 2055	4.2 1.2 4.2 1.2	**28** TU	0120 0734 1417 2003	3.9 1.6 3.9 1.6
14 TU	0321 0926 1556 2153	4.3 1.0 4.4 1.0	**29** W	0237 0835 1520 2104	4.0 1.3 4.1 1.3
15 W	0418 1019 1647 2243	4.5 0.7 4.5 0.7	**30** TH	0340 0933 1614 2200	4.3 1.0 4.4 1.0
			31 F	0434 1025 1703 2252	4.5 0.8 4.6 0.7

JUNE

	Time	m		Time	m
1 SA O	0525 1116 1751 2341	4.6 0.6 4.8 0.5	**16** SU ●	0607 1204 1822	4.4 0.8 4.6
2 SU	0615 1204 1837	4.7 0.4 4.9	**17** M	0025 0644 1242 1855	0.8 4.4 0.8 4.6
3 M	0030 0702 1253 1922	0.3 4.8 0.4 5.0	**18** TU	0102 0718 1315 1929	0.8 4.4 0.9 4.6
4 TU	0118 0749 1339 2008	0.3 4.8 0.4 5.0	**19** W	0133 0752 1345 2002	0.9 4.3 1.0 4.5
5 W	0204 0837 1425 2053	0.3 4.7 0.5 4.9	**20** TH	0204 0827 1415 2037	1.0 4.2 1.2 4.4
6 TH	0250 0925 1511 2139	0.5 4.6 0.7 4.7	**21** F	0233 0903 1443 2111	1.2 4.1 1.3 4.3
7 F	0337 1015 1558 2230	0.7 4.4 1.0 4.5	**22** SA	0303 0938 1514 2146	1.3 4.0 1.5 4.2
8 SA	0428 1110 1651 2329	1.0 4.2 1.2 4.3	**23** SU	0336 1017 1552 2227	1.4 3.9 1.6 4.1
9 SU	0526 1213 1753	1.2 4.0 1.5	**24** M	0423 1100 1647 2318	1.6 3.8 1.8 3.9
10 M	0036 0635 1319 1907	4.1 1.4 4.0 1.5	**25** TU	0529 1202 1803	1.7 3.8 1.8
11 TU	0145 0747 1424 2019	4.1 1.4 4.0 1.5	**26** W	0020 0646 1310 1918	3.9 1.6 3.8 1.7
12 W	0250 0853 1524 2122	4.1 1.3 4.2 1.3	**27** TH	0134 0754 1426 2027	4.0 1.5 4.0 1.4
13 TH	0349 0950 1618 2216	4.2 1.1 4.3 1.1	**28** F	0253 0858 1535 2130	4.1 1.2 4.3 1.1
14 F	0441 1040 1704 2304	4.3 0.9 4.5 0.9	**29** SA	0402 0958 1633 2229	4.3 0.9 4.5 0.8
15 SA	0526 1124 1745 2346	4.4 0.8 4.6 0.8	**30** SU	0500 1055 1727 2324	4.5 0.7 4.8 0.5

JULY

	Time	m		Time	m
1 M O	0555 1148 1819	4.7 0.4 4.9	**16** TU	0006 0621 1221 1835	0.9 4.4 0.9 4.6
2 TU	0016 0648 1241 1908	0.3 4.8 0.3 5.1	**17** W	0043 0658 1256 1911	0.8 4.4 0.9 4.6
3 W	0108 0739 1330 1957	0.3 4.8 0.3 5.1	**18** TH	0116 0736 1326 1947	0.9 4.4 0.9 4.6
4 TH	0156 0828 1417 2044	0.1 4.8 0.3 5.0	**19** F	0144 0812 1354 2022	0.9 4.3 1.0 4.5
5 F	0241 0915 1500 2130	0.2 4.7 0.4 4.9	**20** SA	0212 0847 1421 2053	1.0 4.2 1.1 4.4
6 SA	0325 1001 1542 2215	0.4 4.6 0.7 4.7	**21** SU	0238 0918 1449 2124	1.1 4.1 1.2 4.3
7 SU	0408 1049 1627 2303	0.7 4.3 1.0 4.4	**22** M	0307 0948 1521 2157	1.2 4.0 1.3 4.1
8 M	0455 1140 1717	1.1 4.1 1.4	**23** TU	0342 1027 1603 2241	1.4 3.9 1.5 4.1
9 TU	0001 0550 1241 1818	4.1 1.4 3.9 1.6	**24** W	0431 1118 1704 2339	1.5 3.9 1.7 3.9
10 W	0107 0700 1346 1936	3.9 1.6 3.9 1.7	**25** TH	0547 1223 1833	1.7 3.8 1.8
11 TH	0217 0815 1450 2051	3.8 1.6 3.9 1.6	**26** F	0050 0717 1342 1955	3.9 1.6 3.9 1.6
12 F	0320 0921 1548 2152	3.9 1.5 4.1 1.4	**27** SA	0217 0832 1504 2106	4.0 1.4 4.2 1.2
13 SA	0415 1015 1638 2242	4.1 1.2 4.3 1.2	**28** SU	0339 0939 1611 2211	4.2 1.1 4.5 0.9
14 SU	0501 1102 1720 2326	4.2 1.1 4.4 1.0	**29** M	0443 1040 1709 2310	4.5 0.7 4.8 0.5
15 M ●	0543 1143 1758	4.3 0.9 4.6	**30** TU O	0540 1135 1802 1853	4.7 0.4 5.0 4.7
			31 W	0003 0633 1227 1854	0.2 4.8 0.2 5.1

AUGUST

	Time	m		Time	m
1 TH	0055 0724 1316 1942	0.0 4.9 0.1 5.2	**16** F	0053 0716 1304 1930	0.8 4.5 0.8 4.7
2 F	0140 0812 1400 2029	-0.1 4.9 0.1 5.2	**17** SA	0121 0753 1331 2004	0.8 4.5 0.8 4.6
3 SA	0224 0857 1441 2112	0.0 4.8 0.2 5.0	**18** SU	0147 0826 1358 2034	0.8 4.4 0.9 4.5
4 SU	0303 0937 1520 2151	0.3 4.7 0.5 4.7	**19** M	0214 0854 1426 2101	0.9 4.3 1.0 4.4
5 M	0341 1016 1558 2229	0.7 4.4 0.9 4.4	**20** TU	0241 0922 1456 2133	1.0 4.2 1.2 4.3
6 TU	0421 1056 1639 2309	1.1 4.1 1.4 4.0	**21** W	0315 0957 1534 2214	1.2 4.1 1.4 4.1
7 W	0506 1147 1731	1.5 3.9 1.8	**22** TH	0358 1047 1627 2311	1.5 4.0 1.6 3.9
8 TH	0016 0604 1303 1844	3.7 1.9 3.7 2.0	**23** F	0501 1152 1753	1.7 3.9 1.8
9 F	0143 0729 1417 2017	3.6 2.0 3.8 1.9	**24** SA	0025 0645 1313 1932	3.8 1.8 3.9 1.7
10 SA	0253 0853 1521 2129	3.7 1.8 4.0 1.6	**25** SU	0156 0812 1443 2052	3.9 1.6 4.2 1.3
11 SU	0351 0953 1613 2220	3.9 1.5 4.2 1.3	**26** M	0325 0925 1555 2158	4.2 1.2 4.5 0.9
12 M	0440 1040 1656 2305	4.1 1.2 4.4 1.1	**27** TU	0430 1027 1653 2256	4.5 0.7 4.9 0.5
13 TU	0521 1121 1735 2344	4.3 1.0 4.6 0.9	**28** W O	0526 1121 1747 2348	4.8 0.3 5.1 0.1
14 W ●	0600 1159 1815	4.4 0.9 4.7	**29** TH	0618 1210 1837	4.9 0.1 5.2
15 TH	0019 0638 1234 1853	0.8 4.5 0.8 4.7	**30** F	0036 0705 1257 1923	-0.1 5.0 0.0 5.3
			31 SA	0121 0750 1339 2008	-0.1 5.0 0.0 5.2

Chart Datum: 2·62 metres below Ordnance Datum (Newlyn)

ENGLAND – DARTMOUTH

LAT 50°21′N   LONG 3°34′W

TIMES AND HEIGHTS OF HIGH AND LOW WATERS

YEAR **1996**

TIME ZONE (UT)
For Summer Time add ONE hour in non-shaded areas

SEPTEMBER

Day	Time	m		Day	Time	m
1 SU	0200 / 0831 / 1418 / 2048	0.0 / 4.9 / 0.2 / 5.0		**16** M	0123 / 0802 / 1335 / 2011	0.7 / 4.6 / 0.8 / 4.6
2 M	0237 / 0908 / 1453 / 2121	0.3 / 4.7 / 0.6 / 4.7		**17** TU	0150 / 0830 / 1405 / 2041	0.8 / 4.5 / 0.9 / 4.5
3 TU	0312 / 0937 / 1528 / 2148	0.8 / 4.5 / 1.0 / 4.4		**18** W	0221 / 0859 / 1437 / 2115	1.0 / 4.4 / 1.1 / 4.4
4 W	0345 / 1005 / 1604 / 2214	1.2 / 4.2 / 1.5 / 4.0		**19** TH	0254 / 0936 / 1517 / 2158	1.2 / 4.3 / 1.3 / 4.2
5 TH	0425 / 1040 / 1651 / 2256	1.7 / 3.9 / 1.9 / 3.7		**20** F	0337 / 1026 / 1609 / 2254	1.5 / 4.1 / 1.6 / 3.9
6 F	0519 / 1140 / 1757	2.1 / 3.7 / 2.2		**21** SA	0438 / 1131 / 1731	1.8 / 3.9 / 1.9
7 SA	0058 / 0636 / 1340 / 1933	3.5 / 2.2 / 3.6 / 2.2		**22** SU	0009 / 0622 / 1254 / 1918	3.8 / 2.0 / 4.0 / 1.8
8 SU	0226 / 0818 / 1452 / 2103	3.6 / 2.1 / 3.9 / 1.9		**23** M	0147 / 0759 / 1426 / 2039	3.9 / 1.7 / 4.2 / 1.4
9 M	0327 / 0926 / 1546 / 2156	3.8 / 1.7 / 4.2 / 1.5		**24** TU	0314 / 0912 / 1539 / 2145	4.2 / 1.3 / 4.6 / 0.9
10 TU	0415 / 1013 / 1631 / 2239	4.1 / 1.4 / 4.4 / 1.1		**25** W	0418 / 1012 / 1637 / 2240	4.6 / 0.8 / 4.9 / 0.5
11 W	0457 / 1055 / 1712 / 2316	4.4 / 1.1 / 4.6 / 0.9		**26** TH	0510 / 1104 / 1728 / 2328	4.8 / 0.4 / 5.1 / 0.2
12 TH ●	0536 / 1131 / 1751 / 2351	4.5 / 0.9 / 4.7 / 0.8		**27** F O	0558 / 1150 / 1817	5.0 / 0.2 / 5.2
13 F	0616 / 1205 / 1830	4.6 / 0.8 / 4.8		**28** SA	0013 / 0643 / 1235 / 1901	0.0 / 5.1 / 0.1 / 5.2
14 SA	0023 / 0654 / 1237 / 1907	0.7 / 4.7 / 0.7 / 4.8		**29** SU	0057 / 0725 / 1316 / 1942	0.0 / 5.1 / 0.1 / 5.1
15 SU	0054 / 0730 / 1307 / 1941	0.7 / 4.6 / 0.7 / 4.7		**30** M	0134 / 0803 / 1352 / 2019	0.2 / 5.0 / 0.4 / 4.9

OCTOBER

Day	Time	m		Day	Time	m
1 TU	0210 / 0835 / 1427 / 2048	0.5 / 4.8 / 0.7 / 4.6		**16** W	0131 / 0810 / 1350 / 2026	0.8 / 4.7 / 0.8 / 4.6
2 W	0242 / 0859 / 1459 / 2111	0.9 / 4.6 / 1.1 / 4.3		**17** TH	0206 / 0845 / 1427 / 2104	0.9 / 4.6 / 1.0 / 4.4
3 TH	0314 / 0925 / 1533 / 2139	1.4 / 4.3 / 1.6 / 4.0		**18** F	0243 / 0925 / 1509 / 2149	1.2 / 4.5 / 1.3 / 4.2
4 F	0348 / 1001 / 1616 / 2220	1.8 / 4.0 / 2.0 / 3.7		**19** SA	0328 / 1014 / 1603 / 2246	1.5 / 4.3 / 1.6 / 4.0
5 SA	0437 / 1051 / 1718 / 2327	2.2 / 3.8 / 2.3 / 3.5		**20** SU	0430 / 1118 / 1722	1.8 / 4.1 / 1.8
6 SU	0550 / 1217 / 1840	2.4 / 3.6 / 2.3		**21** M	0002 / 0606 / 1241 / 1901	3.9 / 2.0 / 4.1 / 1.8
7 M	0147 / 0718 / 1411 / 2014	3.5 / 2.3 / 3.8 / 2.1		**22** TU	0135 / 0741 / 1408 / 2020	3.9 / 1.8 / 4.2 / 1.4
8 TU	0254 / 0843 / 1512 / 2116	3.8 / 2.0 / 4.1 / 1.7		**23** W	0256 / 0853 / 1519 / 2124	4.1 / 1.4 / 4.5 / 1.0
9 W	0345 / 0936 / 1559 / 2201	4.1 / 1.6 / 4.4 / 1.3		**24** TH	0358 / 0952 / 1617 / 2218	4.6 / 0.9 / 4.8 / 0.6
10 TH	0428 / 1018 / 1643 / 2240	4.4 / 1.2 / 4.6 / 1.0		**25** F	0450 / 1043 / 1708 / 2306	4.8 / 0.6 / 5.0 / 0.4
11 F	0509 / 1057 / 1723 / 2316	4.6 / 1.0 / 4.7 / 0.8		**26** SA O	0536 / 1129 / 1755 / 2350	5.0 / 0.4 / 5.1 / 0.3
12 SA ●	0549 / 1211 / 1803 / 2351	4.7 / 0.8 / 4.8 / 0.7		**27** SU	0621 / 1211 / 1839	5.1 / 0.3 / 5.1
13 SU	0629 / 1208 / 1843	4.8 / 0.7 / 4.8		**28** M	0032 / 0659 / 1252 / 1918	0.3 / 5.0 / 0.4 / 5.0
14 M	0025 / 0704 / 1244 / 1918	0.7 / 4.8 / 0.7 / 4.8		**29** TU	0110 / 0735 / 1329 / 1952	0.5 / 4.9 / 0.6 / 4.8
15 TU	0059 / 0739 / 1317 / 1952	0.7 / 4.8 / 0.7 / 4.7		**30** W	0144 / 0804 / 1402 / 2018	0.7 / 4.8 / 0.9 / 4.6
				31 TH	0216 / 0828 / 1434 / 2044	1.1 / 4.6 / 1.2 / 4.3

NOVEMBER

Day	Time	m		Day	Time	m
1 F	0246 / 0858 / 1507 / 2116	1.4 / 4.4 / 1.6 / 4.1		**16** SA	0240 / 0920 / 1509 / 2147	1.1 / 4.7 / 1.1 / 4.4
2 SA	0318 / 0935 / 1544 / 2157	1.8 / 4.2 / 1.9 / 3.8		**17** SU	0328 / 1008 / 1602 / 2242	1.4 / 4.5 / 1.4 / 4.2
3 SU	0359 / 1021 / 1638 / 2252	2.1 / 4.0 / 2.2 / 3.6		**18** M	0427 / 1109 / 1710 / 2352	1.6 / 4.3 / 1.6 / 4.0
4 M	0504 / 1123 / 1749	2.3 / 3.8 / 2.3		**19** TU	0543 / 1223 / 1834	1.8 / 4.2 / 1.6
5 TU	0019 / 0620 / 1252 / 1904	3.6 / 2.4 / 3.8 / 2.2		**20** W	0112 / 0712 / 1341 / 1952	4.0 / 1.7 / 4.3 / 1.5
6 W	0200 / 0736 / 1418 / 2013	3.7 / 2.1 / 4.0 / 1.9		**21** TH	0227 / 0825 / 1451 / 2058	4.2 / 1.5 / 4.4 / 1.2
7 TH	0302 / 0841 / 1517 / 2109	4.0 / 1.8 / 4.2 / 1.5		**22** F	0331 / 0928 / 1552 / 2154	4.4 / 1.2 / 4.6 / 0.9
8 F	0352 / 0934 / 1607 / 2157	4.3 / 1.5 / 4.5 / 1.2		**23** SA	0426 / 1020 / 1646 / 2244	4.6 / 0.9 / 4.8 / 0.7
9 SA	0438 / 1019 / 1652 / 2240	4.5 / 1.1 / 4.7 / 0.9		**24** SU	0513 / 1107 / 1733 / 2328	4.8 / 0.7 / 4.8 / 0.6
10 SU	0520 / 1102 / 1735 / 2321	4.7 / 0.9 / 4.8 / 0.8		**25** M O	0556 / 1150 / 1817	4.9 / 0.6 / 4.8
11 M ●	0601 / 1142 / 1818	4.8 / 0.7 / 4.8		**26** TU	0008 / 0636 / 1231 / 1855	0.6 / 4.9 / 0.6 / 4.8
12 TU	0000 / 0640 / 1222 / 1857	0.7 / 4.9 / 0.7 / 4.8		**27** W	0048 / 0710 / 1309 / 1929	0.7 / 4.9 / 0.8 / 4.6
13 W	0041 / 0718 / 1303 / 1937	0.7 / 4.9 / 0.7 / 4.8		**28** TH	0122 / 0739 / 1342 / 1957	0.9 / 4.8 / 0.9 / 4.5
14 TH	0120 / 0756 / 1342 / 2017	0.7 / 4.9 / 0.7 / 4.7		**29** F	0153 / 0808 / 1414 / 2026	1.1 / 4.7 / 1.2 / 4.4
15 F	0158 / 0836 / 1424 / 2100	0.9 / 4.8 / 0.9 / 4.6		**30** SA	0224 / 0840 / 1445 / 2100	1.3 / 4.5 / 1.4 / 4.2

DECEMBER

Day	Time	m		Day	Time	m
1 SU	0253 / 0916 / 1518 / 2138	1.6 / 4.3 / 1.7 / 4.0		**16** M	0326 / 1003 / 1556 / 2234	1.0 / 4.7 / 1.0 / 4.4
2 M	0326 / 0957 / 1556 / 2225	1.9 / 4.2 / 1.9 / 3.8		**17** TU	0416 / 1055 / 1650 / 2333	1.3 / 4.5 / 1.3 / 4.2
3 TU	0411 / 1046 / 1654 / 2324	2.1 / 4.0 / 2.1 / 3.7		**18** W	0514 / 1159 / 1755	1.6 / 4.3 / 1.5
4 W	0521 / 1146 / 1804	2.2 / 3.9 / 2.1		**19** TH	0041 / 0629 / 1308 / 1913	4.1 / 1.7 / 4.2 / 1.6
5 TH	0038 / 0636 / 1259 / 1913	3.7 / 2.2 / 3.9 / 2.0		**20** F	0151 / 0749 / 1419 / 2027	4.1 / 1.7 / 4.2 / 1.5
6 F	0158 / 0744 / 1417 / 2016	3.9 / 2.0 / 4.0 / 1.7		**21** SA	0258 / 0859 / 1524 / 2129	4.2 / 1.5 / 4.3 / 1.3
7 SA	0305 / 0846 / 1522 / 2113	4.1 / 1.7 / 4.2 / 1.4		**22** SU	0358 / 0957 / 1622 / 2221	4.4 / 1.2 / 4.4 / 1.1
8 SU	0359 / 0941 / 1618 / 2205	4.4 / 1.3 / 4.5 / 1.1		**23** M	0449 / 1047 / 1712 / 2307	4.6 / 1.0 / 4.5 / 0.9
9 M	0448 / 1032 / 1708 / 2254	4.6 / 1.0 / 4.6 / 0.8		**24** TU O	0533 / 1131 / 1755 / 2349	4.7 / 0.9 / 4.6 / 0.8
10 TU ●	0533 / 1120 / 1754 / 2340	4.8 / 0.8 / 4.8 / 0.7		**25** W	0614 / 1213 / 1834	4.8 / 0.8 / 4.6
11 W	0619 / 1206 / 1840	4.9 / 0.6 / 4.8		**26** TH	0028 / 0648 / 1252 / 1908	0.8 / 4.8 / 0.8 / 4.5
12 TH	0026 / 0701 / 1254 / 1925	0.6 / 5.0 / 0.5 / 4.8		**27** F	0105 / 0720 / 1326 / 1940	0.9 / 4.8 / 0.9 / 4.5
13 F	0112 / 0745 / 1339 / 2009	0.7 / 5.0 / 0.5 / 4.8		**28** SA	0135 / 0752 / 1356 / 2012	1.0 / 4.7 / 1.0 / 4.4
14 SA	0156 / 0830 / 1424 / 2056	0.7 / 5.0 / 0.6 / 4.7		**29** SU	0204 / 0826 / 1425 / 2047	1.2 / 4.6 / 1.2 / 4.3
15 SU	0240 / 0915 / 1509 / 2143	0.8 / 4.9 / 0.8 / 4.6		**30** M	0231 / 0900 / 1452 / 2122	1.3 / 4.5 / 1.4 / 4.2
				31 TU	0259 / 0936 / 1521 / 2158	1.5 / 4.3 / 1.5 / 4.0

Chart Datum: 2·62 metres below Ordnance Datum (Newlyn)

DARTMOUTH   10-1-21

Devon 50°20'·63N 03°33'·88W

CHARTS

AC *2253*, 1634, *1613*; Imray C5, Y47, Y43; Stanfords 12, 13; OS 202

TIDES

−0510 Dover; ML 2·8; Duration 0630; Zone 0 (UT)

DARTMOUTH

High Water		Low Water		Height (metres)			
				MHWS	MHWN	MLWN	MLWS
0100	0600	0100	0600	4·9	3·8	2·0	0·6
1300	1800	1300	1800				

Differences GREENWAY QUAY (DITTISHAM)

+0015	+0020	+0025	+0010	0·0	0·0	0·0	0·0

TOTNES

+0015	+0015	+0115	+0035	−1·4	−1·5	Dries	Dries

NOTE: Dartmouth tidal predictions for each day of the year are given above.

SHELTER

Excellent protection inside the hbr, but ent can be difficult in strong winds from SE to SW. In mid-fairway there are 8 large unlit mooring buoys for commercial vessels/FVs; do not ⚓ over their ground chains, as shown on AC 2253. Only space to ⚓ is E of fairway, from Nos 3a to 5 buoys. The 3 marinas (Darthaven, Dart and Kingswear), as on the chartlet/inset, all have ♥ berths. Apart from the pontoons off the Dartmouth YC and Royal Dart YC, the extensive pontoons and mooring trots elsewhere in the hbr are run by the Hr Mr, who should be contacted by VHF/☎. The most likely ♥ berths/moorings from S to N are:

W bank: pontoon off Dartmouth YC (May-Sep); inboard side only of pontoon near Boat Camber; N end of pontoon just S of Dart marina (26'/8m max LOA).

E of fairway: (NB six pontoons N of Darthaven marina are for locals only). Some ⚓s are in the mooring trots from abeam No 5A buoy to the cable ferry. The 2 pontoons E of Nos 9/10 buoys are for visitors.

NAVIGATION

WPT 50°19'·50N 03°32'·80W, 148°/328° from/to Kingswear It, Iso WRG, 1·5M. To the E of ent, on Inner Froward Pt (153m) is a conspic obelisk (24·5m). There is no bar and the hbr is always accessible. Speed limit 6kn.

LIGHTS AND MARKS

Kingswear Main lt 328°, Iso WRG 3s 9m 8M, W 325°-331°. Bayard's Cove lt 293°, Fl WRG 2s 5m 6M, W 289°-297°. Entry buoys as on chartlet. Within hbr, all jetty/ pontoon lts to the W are 2FR (vert); and 2FG (vert) to the E.

RADIO TELEPHONE

Hr Mr call *Dartnav* VHF Ch 11 16 (Mon-Fri 0830-1800; Sat 0900-1200). Darthaven marina, Ch **80** M; Dart marina, Kingswear marina and Dart Sailing Centre, Ch 80. Fuel barge Ch 06. Water taxi: call Ch 16, work Ch 08 06 M.

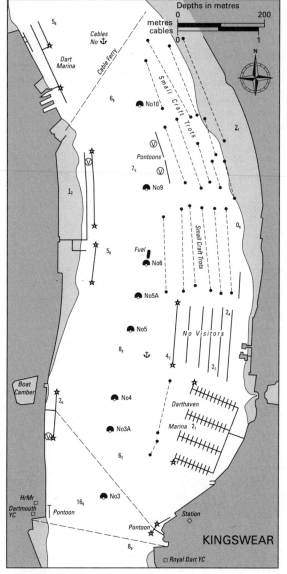

TELEPHONE (01803)

Hr Mr 832337; MRSC 882704; ⌗ (01752) 220661; Marinecall 0891 500458; Police 832288; Dr 832212; Ⓗ 832255.

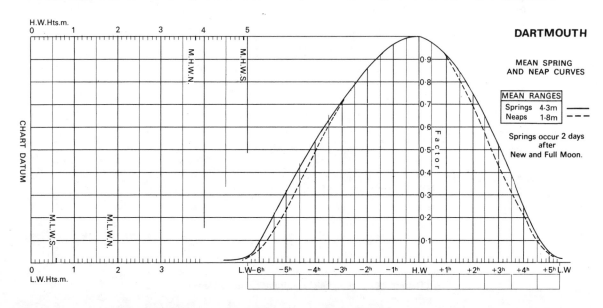

DARTMOUTH

MEAN SPRING AND NEAP CURVES

MEAN RANGES	
Springs	4·3m
Neaps	1·8m

Springs occur 2 days after New and Full Moon.

FACILITIES
Harbour/Marinas
Dart Hbr & Nav'n Authority (450+90 visitors), ☎ 832337, Fax 833631, £11.10, M, D, FW, ME, EI, Sh, CH, Slip, V, R;

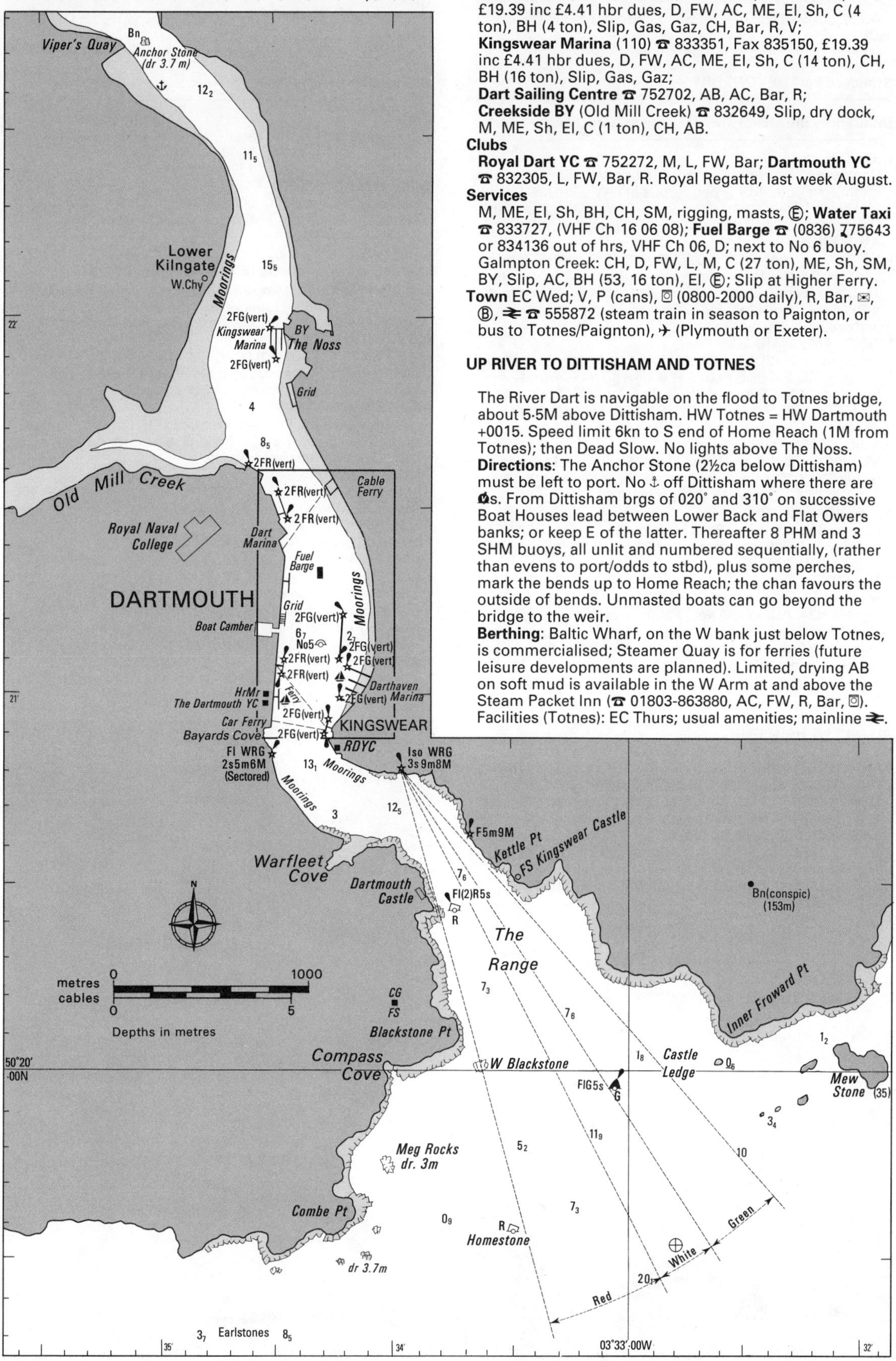

Darthaven Marina (230+12 visitors) ☎ 752242, Fax 752722, £16.04 inc £4.41 hbr dues, FW, ME, EI, Gas, Gaz, 🅞, Sh, CH, Bar, R, BH (30 ton), AC, Ⓔ;

Dart Marina (80+40 visitors) ☎ 833351, Fax 835150, £19.39 inc £4.41 hbr dues, D, FW, AC, ME, EI, Sh, C (4 ton), BH (4 ton), Slip, Gas, Gaz, CH, Bar, R, V;

Kingswear Marina (110) ☎ 833351, Fax 835150, £19.39 inc £4.41 hbr dues, D, FW, AC, ME, EI, Sh, C (14 ton), CH, BH (16 ton), Slip, Gas, Gaz;

Dart Sailing Centre ☎ 752702, AB, AC, Bar, R;

Creekside BY (Old Mill Creek) ☎ 832649, Slip, dry dock, M, ME, Sh, EI, C (1 ton), CH, AB.

Clubs
Royal Dart YC ☎ 752272, M, L, FW, Bar; **Dartmouth YC** ☎ 832305, L, FW, Bar, R. Royal Regatta, last week August.

Services
M, ME, EI, Sh, BH, CH, SM, rigging, masts, Ⓔ; **Water Taxi** ☎ 833727, (VHF Ch 16 06 08); **Fuel Barge** ☎ (0836) 775643 or 834136 out of hrs, VHF Ch 06, D; next to No 6 buoy. Galmpton Creek: CH, D, FW, L, M, C (27 ton), ME, Sh, SM, BY, Slip, AC, BH (53, 16 ton), EI, Ⓔ; Slip at Higher Ferry.

Town EC Wed; V, P (cans), 🅞 (0800-2000 daily), R, Bar, ✉, Ⓑ, ⇌ ☎ 555872 (steam train in season to Paignton, or bus to Totnes/Paignton), ✈ (Plymouth or Exeter).

UP RIVER TO DITTISHAM AND TOTNES

The River Dart is navigable on the flood to Totnes bridge, about 5·5M above Dittisham. HW Totnes = HW Dartmouth +0015. Speed limit 6kn to S end of Home Reach (1M from Totnes); then Dead Slow. No lights above The Noss.
Directions: The Anchor Stone (2½ca below Dittisham) must be left to port. No ⚓ off Dittisham where there are ⚓s. From Dittisham brgs of 020° and 310° on successive Boat Houses lead between Lower Back and Flat Owers banks; or keep E of the latter. Thereafter 8 PHM and 3 SHM buoys, all unlit and numbered sequentially, (rather than evens to port/odds to stbd), plus some perches, mark the bends up to Home Reach; the chan favours the outside of bends. Unmasted boats can go beyond the bridge to the weir.
Berthing: Baltic Wharf, on the W bank just below Totnes, is commercialised; Steamer Quay is for ferries (future leisure developments are planned). Limited, drying AB on soft mud is available in the W Arm at and above the Steam Packet Inn (☎ 01803-863880, AC, FW, R, Bar, 🅞). Facilities (Totnes): EC Thurs; usual amenities; mainline ⇌.

[Chart of Dartmouth Harbour and the River Dart, including labels: Viper's Quay, Anchor Stone (dr 3.7 m), Lower Kilngate W.Chy, Moorings, Kingswear Marina, BY The Noss, Grid, Old Mill Creek, Royal Naval College, DARTMOUTH, Dart Marina, Fuel Barge, Boat Camber, Grid, No5, HrMr, The Dartmouth YC, Car Ferry, Bayards Cove, Cable Ferry, Darthaven Marina, KINGSWEAR, RDYC, Fl WRG 2s5m6M (Sectored), Iso WRG 3s 9m8M, Moorings, Warfleet Cove, Dartmouth Castle, Kettle Pt, FS Kingswear Castle, F5m9M, Fl(2)R5s R, Bn(conspic) (153m), The Range, CG FS, Blackstone Pt, Compass Cove, W Blackstone, Castle Ledge, Fl G5s G, Mew Stone (35), Inner Froward Pt, Meg Rocks dr. 3m, Combe Pt, Homestone R, dr 3.7m, Earlstones, Red, White, Green; depth soundings; compass rose N; scale metres 0–1000, cables 0–5, Depths in metres; coordinates 50°20'·00N, 22', 21', 35', 34', 03°33'·00W, 32']

BRIXHAM   10-1-22
Devon 50°24'·28N 03°30'·79W

CHARTS
AC *26, 1613, 3315*; Imray C5, Y43; Stanfords 12; OS 202
TIDES
−0505 Dover; ML 2·9; Duration 0635; Zone 0 (UT)

Standard Port DEVONPORT (←—)

Differences **BRIXHAM** are the same as **TORQUAY** (—→)

SHELTER
Very good in marina; also pontoon below YCin SW corner
of hbr, but outer hbr is dangerous in NW winds. ⌀s (W) to
E of main fairway. Inner hbr dries. To W of hbr are ⌕s in
Fishcombe Cove and Elberry Cove (beware water skiers).
NAVIGATION
WPT 50°24'·70N 03°30'·00W, 050°/230° from/to Victoria
bkwtr lt, 0·60M. No dangers; easy access. Note: Around
Torbay are controlled areas, close inshore and marked by
Y SPM buoys, mainly for swimmers; boats may enter
with caution, speed limit 5kn.
LIGHTS AND MARKS
Berry Hd lt, Fl (2) 15s 58m 15M, is 1·2M ESE of ent. Bkwtr
hd Oc R 15s 9m 6M, W tr. 3 R ● or 3 ⓡ lts (vert) at ent =
hbr closed. At SE end of hbr a Dir lt Iso WRG 5s 4m 6M,
vis G145°-157°, W157°-161°, R161°-173° leads 159° into
the fairway, marked by two pairs of lateral lt buoys.
RADIO TELEPHONE
Marina: Ch 80. YC and Water Taxi: *Shuttle* Ch M.
Hr Mr Ch 14 16 (May-Sept 0800-1800LT; Oct-Apr 0900-
1700, Mon-Fri). Brixham CG: Ch 16 10 67 73.
TELEPHONE (01803)
Marina 882929; Hr Mr 853321; Pilot 882214; MRSC 882704;
⌗ (01752) 220661; Marinecall 0891 500458; Police 882231;
Dr 882731; Ⓗ 882153.
FACILITIES
Marina (480 inc visitors) ☎ 882929, Fax 882737, £12.70,
Access H24, AC, FW, D (0900-2000, Apr - Sep inc), Ⓞ;
Hbr Office (New Fish Quay) Slip, M, L, FW, C (2 ton), AB, D;
Brixham YC ☎ 853332, Ⓥ pontoon, M, L, Slip, FW, R, Bar;
Services: M, L, Slip, CH, ACA, ME, (H24), P (cans), El, Ⓔ.
Town EC Wed; R, Bar, Ⓞ, ✉, Ⓑ, ⇌ (bus to Paignton), ✈
(Exeter).

ADJACENT HARBOUR

PAIGNTON, Devon, 50°25'·93N 03°33'·29W. AC *26, 1613*.
HW −0500 on Dover, +0035 on Devonport; HW −0·6m on
Devonport; ML 2·9m; Duration 0640. Hbr dries 1·3m and
is only suitable for small boats. E winds cause heavy
swell in hbr. Rks extend 180m E from E wall. Black Rk has
ECM tr, Q (3) 10s 5m 3M. QR 7m 3M lt on E arm of ent. Hr
Mr (summer only) ☎ (01803) 557812. **Paignton SC**
☎ 525817; Facilities: EC Wed, M, ME, Sh, Gas, CH, ACA.

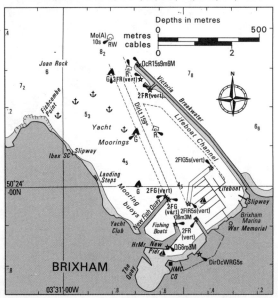

TORQUAY   10-1-23
Devon 50°27'·42N 03°31'·66W

CHARTS
AC *26, 1613, 3315*; Imray C5, Y43; Stanfords 12; OS 202
TIDES
−0500 Dover; ML 2·9; Duration 0640; Zone 0 (UT)

Standard Port DEVONPORT (←—)

Times				Height (metres)			
High Water		Low Water		MHWS	MHWN	MLWN	MLWS
0100	0600	0100	0600	5·5	4·4	2·2	0·8
1300	1800	1300	1800				
Differences TORQUAY							
+0025	+0045	+0010	0000	−0·6	−0·7	−0·2	−0·1

Note: There is often a stand of about 1 hour at HW

SHELTER
Good, but some swell in hbr with strong SE winds, which
may make the narrow ent difficult due to backwash. No ⌕
within hbr. NW of Hope's Nose there are ⌕s at Hope Cove,
Anstey's Cove and Babbacombe Bay, sheltered in W'lies.
NAVIGATION
WPT 50°27'·00N 03°31'·50W, 165°/345° from/to Haldon
pier lt, 0·40M. Access at all tides. Inner (Old) hbr dries
completely. 3 R ● or 3 R lts = hbr closed.
LIGHTS AND MARKS
No ldg marks/lts. Princess Pier head QR 9m 6M. Haldon
pier hd QG 9m 6M. S pier hd 2FG (vert) 5M. All lts may be
difficult to see against town lts.
RADIO TELEPHONE
VHF Ch 14 16 (May-Sept 0800-1800LT; Oct-Apr 0900-1700,
Mon-Fri). Marina Ch 80 (H24), M.
TELEPHONE (01803)
Hr Mr 292429; MRSC 882704; ⌗ (01752) 220661; Marinecall
0891 500458; Police 214491; Dr 298441; Ⓗ 614567.
FACILITIES
Marina (440+60 visitors) ☎ 214624, Fax 291634, £15.65,
FW, ME, Gas, Gaz, Ⓞ, AC, SM, El, Ⓔ, Sh, CH, V, R, Bar,
ACA. **S Pier** P & D by hose (Apr - Sept), L, FW, C (6 ton);
Haldon Pier FW, AB; **Princess Pier** L; **Royal Torbay YC**
☎ 292006, R, Bar.
Town V, R, Ⓞ, Bar, ✉, Ⓑ, ⇌, ✈ (Exeter or Plymouth).

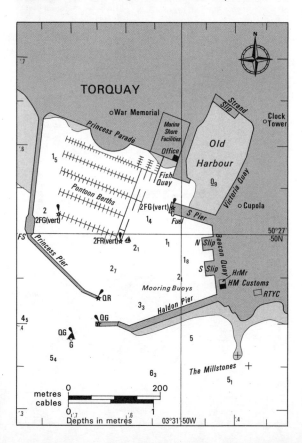

TEIGNMOUTH   10-1-24

Devon 50°32'·36N 03°30'·00W (Abeam The Point)

CHARTS
AC *26, 3315*; Imray C5, Y43; Stanfords 12; OS 192
TIDES
–0450 Dover; ML 2·7; Duration 0625; Zone 0 (UT)

Standard Port DEVONPORT (←)

Times				Height (metres)			
High Water		Low Water		MHWS	MHWN	MLWN	MLWS
0100	0600	0100	0600	5·5	4·4	2·2	0·8
1300	1800	1300	1800				
Differences TEIGNMOUTH (Approaches)							
+0025	+0040	0000	0000	–0·7	–0·8	–0·3	–0·2
SHALDON BRIDGE							
+0035	+0050	+0020	+0020	–0·9	–0·9	–0·2	0·0

SHELTER
Hbr completely sheltered, but difficult to enter especially with strong winds from NE to S when surf forms on the bar. Access HW±3. Appr chan is not buoyed so local advice is recommended. No AB, but two ⚓s just N of SHM lt buoy, Fl G 5s. Speed limit is 8kn.
NAVIGATION
WPT 50°32'·40N 03°29'·20W, 076°/256° from/to training wall lt, 0·43M. Bar shifts very frequently. Beware rks off the Ness; and variable extent of Salty flats. Clearance under Shaldon bridge is 4·2m at MHWS. Avoid a Historic wreck site (50°32'·92N 03°29'·17W; just off chartlet), close inshore by Church Rks to ENE of Ch Tr (see 10.0.3g).
LIGHTS AND MARKS
The Ness, high red sandstone headland, and Church Tr are both conspic from afar; close NE of the latter, just off N edge of chartlet, Teign Corinthian YC bldg (cream) is also conspic. From SE, 2 FR 10/11m 6/3M lead 334° clear of The Ness Rks, but not normally through the shifting chan across the bar. At seaward end of outfall, 105° The Ness 1·25M, is a Y buoy, Fl Y 5s, at 50°31'·93N 03°27'·81W. Y buoy, Fl Y 2s, marks S edge of Spratt Sand. Once round The Point, Oc G 5·5s and FG (vert), two F Bu lts on quay align 022°, but are not official ldg lts.

RADIO TELEPHONE
VHF Ch 12 16 (Mon-Fri: 0800-1700; Sat 0900-1200 LT).
TELEPHONE (01626)
Hr Mr 773165; MRSC (01803) 882704; ‡ (01752) 220661; Marinecall 0891 500458; Police 772433; Dr 774355; Ⓗ 772161.
FACILITIES
E Quay Polly Steps Slip (up to 10m); **Teign Corinthian YC** ☎ 772734, ⚓ £7.02, M, FW, Bar; **Services:** ME, CH, El, Slip, BY, Sh, D, C (8 ton), Gas, Gaz, FW, CH, Ⓔ.
Town EC Thurs; P, D, L, FW, V, R, Ⓞ, Bar, ✉, Ⓑ, ⇌, → (Exeter).

The Skipper must not only know his vessel and how to handle her, but he must be able to navigate her and must know the sea. He must be watchful and careful. He needs 'nerve', coolness and endurance, this endurance being a mental rather than a physical quality. Above all he must not be liable to panic in a sudden emergency.

I have known men who, faced with an awkward situation and knowing exactly what should be done, lose their heads and do something quite different – perhaps run for a difficult harbour on a lee shore, thereby taking a risk twenty times greater than that which they are trying to avoid. They, fortunately, are exceptions.

Of the average man R.L.Stevenson has truly said:
'It is a commonplace that we cannot answer for ourselves until we have been tried. But it is not so common a reflection, and surely more consoling, that we usually find ourselves a great deal braver and better than we thought. I believe this is every one's experience.'

Yacht Cruising: Claud Worth 1910.

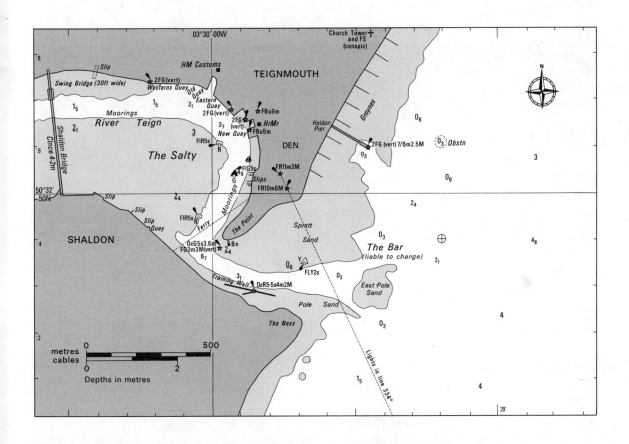

RIVER EXE   10-1-25

Devon 50°36'·91N 03°25'·33W (Abeam Exmouth)

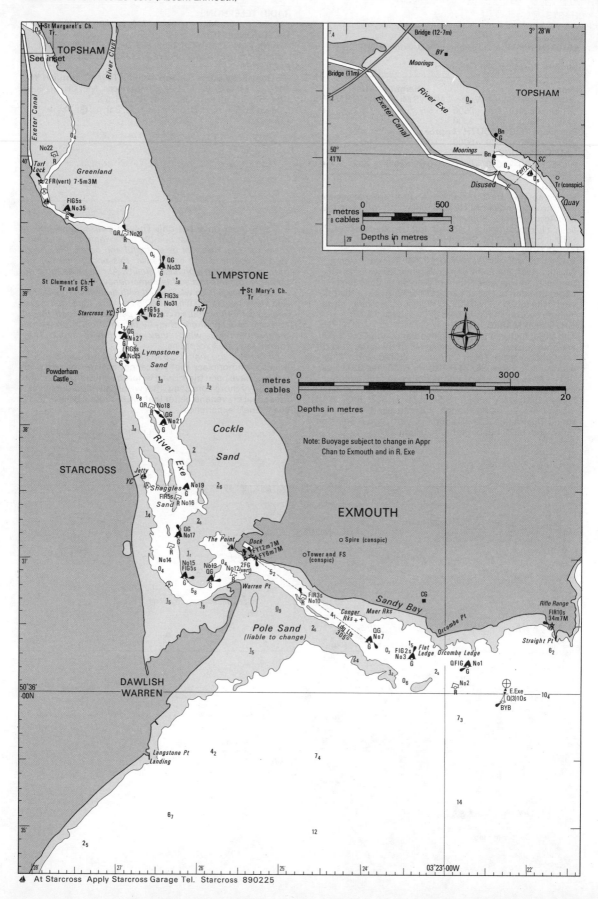

RIVER EXE *continued*

CHARTS
AC 2290, *3315*; Imray C5, Y43; Stanfords 12; OS 192

TIDES
−0445 Dover; ML 2·1; Duration 0625; Zone 0 (UT)

Standard Port DEVONPORT (◄─)

Times				Height (metres)			
High Water		Low Water		MHWS	MHWN	MLWN	MLWS
0100	0600	0100	0600	5·5	4·4	2·2	0·8
1300	1800	1300	1800				
Differences EXMOUTH (Approaches)							
+0030	+0050	+0015	+0005	−0·9	−1·0	−0·5	−0·3
EXMOUTH DOCK							
+0035	+0055	+0050	+0020	−1·5	−1·6	−0·9	−0·6
STARCROSS							
+0040	+0110	+0055	+0025	−1·4	−1·5	−0·8	−0·1
TOPSHAM							
+0045	+0105	No data		−1·5	−1·6	No data	

SHELTER
Good inside R Exe, but ent difficult in fresh winds from E and S. Exmouth Dock is not available to yachts (possible future marina). There are ⚓s in the Bight, off Starcross and off Turf Lock, but extensive moorings leave little space to ⚓. At Topsham it may be possible to dry out against The Quay or find a mooring; the river here has about 0·4m.

NAVIGATION
WPT E. Exe ECM buoy Q (3) 10s, 50°35'·97N 03°22'·30W, 111°/291° from/to No 7 SHM buoy, QG, 1·03M.

Caution: Royal Marine firing range at Straight Pt, just E of Exe buoy, has a danger area to seaward. R flags are flown when range in use and safety launch on station (callsign *Straight Pt Range* VHF Ch 08 16).

Best time to start appr is soon after LW when hazards can be seen and some shelter obtained. There are drying rky ledges to the N of chan and to the south Pole Sands which are liable to change. The long shallow bar lies NW/SE with least depth of 0·3m between Nos 3 and 6 buoys. The chan narrows to about 100m between Nos 11 and 10 buoys. It is well marked and lit, but night entry is not advised. After No 10 buoy it is important not to cut the corner round Warren Pt; stand on for 5ca to Exmouth and No 12 buoy, before altering to the WSW.

Access to Exeter via the Exeter Canal (3·7m depth) is restricted by the 10·89m clearance of the M5 bridge and passage through 4 locks and 4 swing bridges; but may be arranged with Exeter Council ☎ (01392) 74306 or Ch 12, given 2-3 days notice and about £30 total fee. The ent is at Turf Lock, 1M S of Topsham, by No 39 buoy.

LIGHTS AND MARKS
Exmouth Ch Tr and FS is conspic from seaward, almost 2M WNW of the Exe buoy. Ldg lts 305° FY 6/12m 7M by The Point; not to be used to seaward of No 6 PHM buoy.

RADIO TELEPHONE
Exeter VHF Ch 06 12 16 (Mon-Fri: 0730-1630 LT, and when vessel due). Water Taxi at Exmouth, call *Conveyance* Ch M.

TELEPHONE (01395)
Dockmaster 272009; MRSC (01803) 882704; ⌗ (01752) 220661; Pilot 264036; Marinecall 0891 500458; Police 264651; Dr 273001; Ⓗ 279684.

FACILITIES
EXMOUTH (01395)
Dockmaster ☎ 272009, L, FW, ME, D, C; **Pier** V, R, Bar, CH; **Exe SC** ☎ 264607, M, L, AB;
Services: ME, Sh, CH, El, , Gaz, ACA, SM, Ⓔ.
Town EC Wed; P, V, R, Ⓞ, Bar, ✉, Ⓑ, ⇌, ✈ (Exeter).
STARCROSS (01626)
Starcross Fishing and Cruising Club ☎ 890582; **Starcross YC** ☎ 890470; **Services:** P & D (cans), ME, M, Gas.
Village P, V, Bar, ✉, Ⓑ, ⇌, ✈ (Exeter).
TOPSHAM (01392)
Topsham SC ☎ 877524, Slip, L, FW, Bar; **Services:** BY (access HW±2), M, D, ME, El, C, Gas, CH, SM, ACA.
Village P, R, V, Ⓞ, Bar, ✉, Ⓑ, ⇌, ✈ (Exeter).
EXETER (01392)
For moorings and ⚓s apply Hr Mr Exeter City, ☎ 74306. Some moorings in estuary.
Services: CH, ME, ACA. **City** all amenities.

HARBOUR WEST OF LYME REGIS

AXMOUTH/BEER, Devon, 50°42'·10N 03°03'·20W. AC 3315. HW −0455 on Dover, +0045 and −1·1m on Devonport; ML 2·3m; Duration 0640. MHWS 4·1m, MHWN 3·1m. A small drying hbr on R Axe for boats max draught1·2m, LOA 8·5m, able to take the ground. Appr chan to bar (dries 0·5m) is unmarked and often shifts; prior knowledge from YC is essential. Enter, in settled weather only, at HW via 7m wide ent with SHM bn; turn hard port inside. A bridge (2m clearance) crosses the river 2ca from ent. Beer Roads, 1M WSW is ⚓ sheltered from prevailing W'ly, but open to S/SE winds. Landing on open beach. Facilities: **Axe YC** ☎ (01297) 20043, Slip, pontoon, M, BH, Bar; **Services:** ME CH, D (cans), CH;
Beer & Seaton: EC Thurs; R, V, P & D (cans), Bar, Gas, ✉.

AGENTS WANTED

If you are interested in becoming our agent for any of the following ports, please write to: The Editor, Edington House, Trent, Sherborne, Dorset DT9 4SR, England – and get your free copy of the almanac annually. You do not have to live in a port to be the agent, but at least a fairly regular visitor.

River Exe
Port Ellen (Islay)
Glandore/Union Hall
River Rance/Dinan
Lampaul
Port Tudy
River Etel
Le Palais (Belle Ile)
Le Pouliguen/Pornichet
L'Herbaudière
St Gilles-Croix-de-Vie
River Seudre
Royan
Anglet/Bayonne
Hendaye

Grandcamp-Maisy
Port-en-Bessin
Courseulles
Boulogne
Dunkerque
Terneuzen/Westerschelde
Oudeschild
Lauwersoog
Dornumer-Accumersiel
Hooksiel
Langeoog
Bremerhaven
Helgoland
Büsum

LYME REGIS   10-1-26

Dorset 50°43'·17N 02°56'·10W

CHARTS
AC *3315*; Imray C5; Stanfords 12; OS 193

TIDES
−0455 Dover; ML 2·4; Duration 0700; Zone 0 (UT)

Standard Port DEVONPORT (←)

Times				Height (metres)			
High Water		Low Water		MHWS	MHWN	MLWN	MLWS
0100	0600	0100	0600	5·5	4·4	2·2	0·8
1300	1800	1300	1800				

Differences LYME REGIS

| +0040 | +0100 | +0005 | −0005 | −1·2 | −1·3 | −0·5 | −0·2 |

NOTE: Rise is relatively fast for the first hour after LW, then slackens for the next 1½ hours, after which the rapid rate is resumed. There is often a stand of about 1½ hours at HW.

SHELTER
Excellent in the hbr (dries), known as The Cobb, except in strong E or SE winds. Max LOA in hbr 9m. Keel boats can dry out alongside Victoria Pier or ⚓ as shown. Five R cylindrical ⚓s are available. Access about HW±2½.

NAVIGATION
WPT 50°43'·00N 02°55'·60W, 116°/296° from/to front ldg lt 0·35M. Rock bkwtr S of ent marked by PHM bn. Beware numerous fishing floats.

LIGHTS AND MARKS
Ldg lts 296°, see chartlet. R flag on Victoria Pier = Gale warning in force.

RADIO TELEPHONE
Call: *Lyme Regis Hbr Radio* Ch14 16. (May-Sept: 0900-1200, 1600-1800 LT).

TELEPHONE (01297)
Hr Mr 442137, Fax 442137; MRSC (01305) 760439; ⌗ (01752) 220661; Marinecall 0891 500457; Police 442603; Dr 445777; Ⓗ 442254.

FACILITIES
Harbour (The Cobb) AB £8.90, Slip, M, P & D (cans), L, FW, ME, El, Ⓔ, Sh; **Lyme Regis SC** ☎ 442800, FW, R, Bar; **Lyme Regis Power Boat Club** ☎ 443788, R, Bar; **Services:** ME, El, Ⓔ, CH, ACA (5M).
Town EC Thurs; V, R, Bar, Gas, Gaz, ✉, Ⓑ, ⇌ (bus to Axminster), ✈ (Exeter).

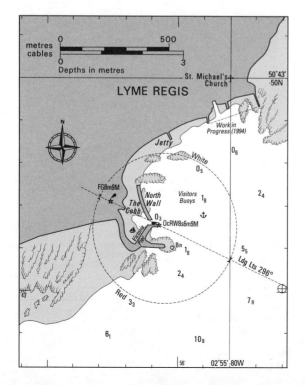

BRIDPORT   10-1-27

Dorset 50°42'·52N 02°45'·77W

CHARTS
AC *3315*; Imray C5; Stanfords 12; OS 193

TIDES
−0500 Dover; ML 2·3; Duration 0650; Zone 0 (UT)

Standard Port DEVONPORT (←)

Times				Height (metres)			
High Water		Low Water		MHWS	MHWN	MLWN	MLWS
0100	0600	0100	0600	5·5	4·4	2·2	0·8
1300	1800	1300	1800				

Differences BRIDPORT (West Bay)

| +0025 | +0040 | 0000 | 0000 | −1·4 | −1·4 | −0·6 | −0·2 |

CHESIL BEACH

| +0040 | +0055 | −0005 | +0010 | −1·6 | −1·5 | −0·5 | 0·0 |

CHESIL COVE

| +0035 | +0050 | −0010 | +0005 | −1·5 | −1·6 | −0·5 | −0·2 |

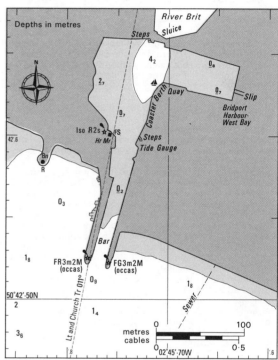

NOTE: Rise is relatively fast for first hr after LW, thence a slackening for the next 1½ hrs, after which the rapid rise is resumed. There is often a stand of about 1½ hrs at HW.

SHELTER
Good in hbr, but the narrow (12m), 180m long drying ent, is dangerous in even moderate on-shore winds; access HW±2, in favourable weather. Do not attempt entry in fresh S'lies. Hbr dries apart from pool and coaster berths (2·1m) scoured by sluice water. See Hr Mr for coaster berths if free or dry out at E end of Quay. Bridport town is 1½M inland from the hbr, known locally as West Bay.

NAVIGATION
WPT 50°41'·55N 02°46'·00W, 191°/011° from/to ent, 0·75M. No offshore dangers. SPM buoy, Fl, Y 5s, marks sewer outfall 5ca SSW of ent.

LIGHTS AND MARKS
Ldg marks 011°, church tr on with W pier hd. At night Iso R 2s 9m 5M on Hr Mr's office in line 011° with FR 3m 2M on W pier. Entry sig: B ● = hbr closed.

RADIO TELEPHONE
Call: *Bridport Radio* VHF Ch 11 16.

TELEPHONE (01308)
Hr Mr 423222, Fax 251481; MRSC (01305) 760439; ⌗ (01752) 220661; Marinecall 0891 500457; Police 422266; Dr 421109.

FACILITIES
Quay AB £8.90, M, FW, Slip, P & D (cans), Ⓞ, Sh, ME, ✉, V.
Town CH, V, R, Bar, ✉, Ⓑ, ⇌ (bus to Axminster), ✈ (Exeter).

Volvo Penta service

Area 2

Central Southern England
Portland Bill to Selsey Bill

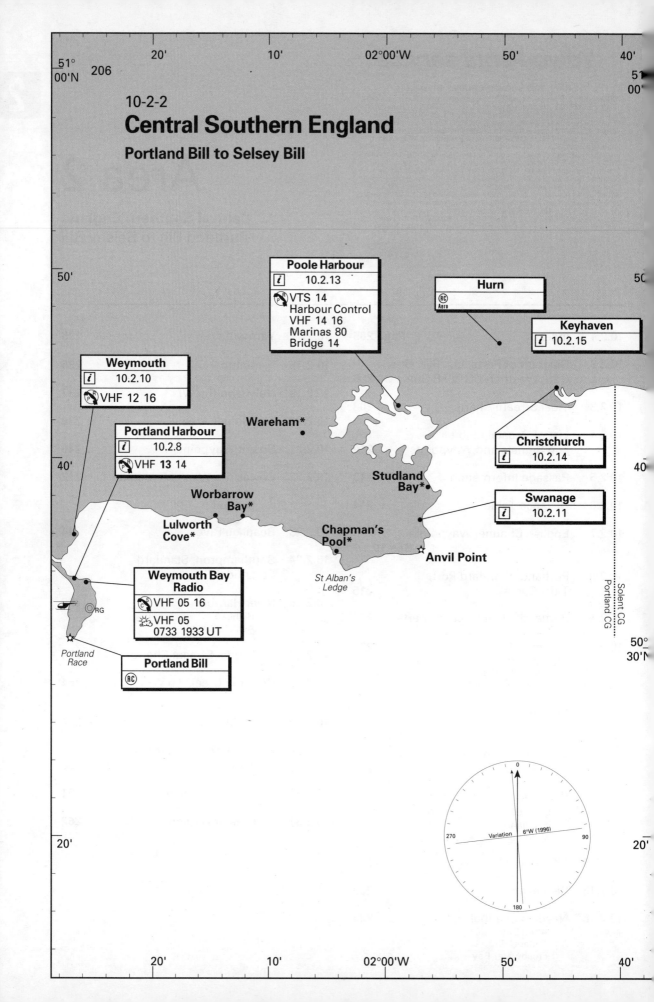

20'

10'

02°00'W

50'

40'

51°
00'

10-2-2
Central Southern England
Portland Bill to Selsey Bill

50'

Poole Harbour

i   10.2.13

VTS 14
Harbour Control
VHF 14 16
Marinas 80
Bridge 14

Hurn

RC
Aero

Keyhaven

i   10.2.15

Weymouth

i   10.2.10

VHF 12 16

Wareham*

Christchurch

i   10.2.14

Portland Harbour

i   10.2.8

VHF **13** 14

Studland
Bay*

Swanage

i   10.2.11

Worbarrow
Bay*

Lulworth
Cove*

Chapman's
Pool*

Anvil Point

RG

St Alban's
Ledge

Solent CG
Portland CG

**Weymouth Bay
Radio**

VHF 05 16

VHF 05
0733 1933 UT

50°
30'N

*Portland
Race*

Portland Bill

RC

270   Variation   6°W (1996)   90

0

180

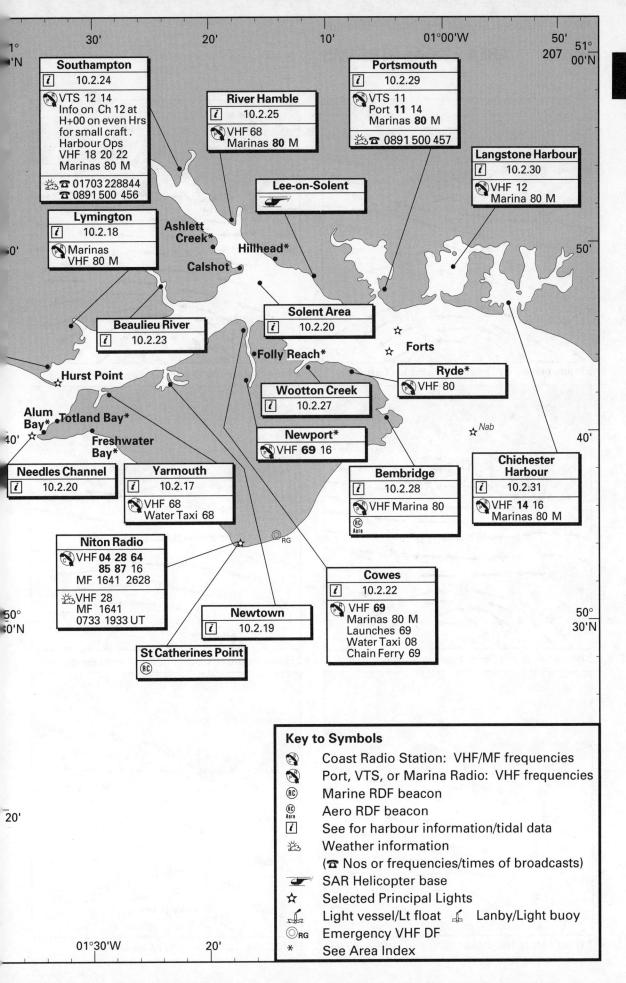

2

207

Southampton
| *i* | 10.2.24 |

VTS 12 14
Info on Ch 12 at
H+00 on even Hrs
for small craft.
Harbour Ops
VHF 18 20 22
Marinas 80 M

☎ 01703 228844
☎ 0891 500 456

River Hamble
| *i* | 10.2.25 |

VHF 68
Marinas **80** M

Portsmouth
| *i* | 10.2.29 |

VTS 11
Port **11** 14
Marinas **80** M

☎ 0891 500 457

Langstone Harbour
| *i* | 10.2.30 |

VHF 12
Marina 80 M

Lee-on-Solent

Lymington
| *i* | 10.2.18 |

Marinas
VHF 80 M

Ashlett Creek*

Calshot

Hillhead*

Beaulieu River
| *i* | 10.2.23 |

Solent Area
| *i* | 10.2.20 |

☆

☆ **Forts**

Ryde*
VHF 80

Hurst Point

Folly Reach*

Wootton Creek
| *i* | 10.2.27 |

Alum Bay*

Totland Bay*

Freshwater Bay*

Newport*
VHF **69** 16

☆ *Nab*

Needles Channel
| *i* | 10.2.20 |

Yarmouth
| *i* | 10.2.17 |

VHF 68
Water Taxi 68

Bembridge
| *i* | 10.2.28 |

VHF Marina 80

RC Aero

Chichester Harbour
| *i* | 10.2.31 |

VHF **14** 16
Marinas **80** M

Niton Radio
VHF **04 28 64**
    85 87 16
MF 1641 2628

VHF 28
MF 1641
0733 1933 UT

☆

RG

Cowes
| *i* | 10.2.22 |

VHF **69**
Marinas 80 M
Launches 69
Water Taxi 08
Chain Ferry 69

Newtown
| *i* | 10.2.19 |

St Catherines Point
RC

Key to Symbols
- Coast Radio Station: VHF/MF frequencies
- Port, VTS, or Marina Radio: VHF frequencies
- RC   Marine RDF beacon
- RC Aero   Aero RDF beacon
- *i*   See for harbour information/tidal data
- Weather information
  (☎ Nos or frequencies/times of broadcasts)
- SAR Helicopter base
- ☆   Selected Principal Lights
- Light vessel/Lt float   Lanby/Light buoy
- ©RG   Emergency VHF DF
- *   See Area Index

10-2-3   AREA 2 TIDAL STREAMS

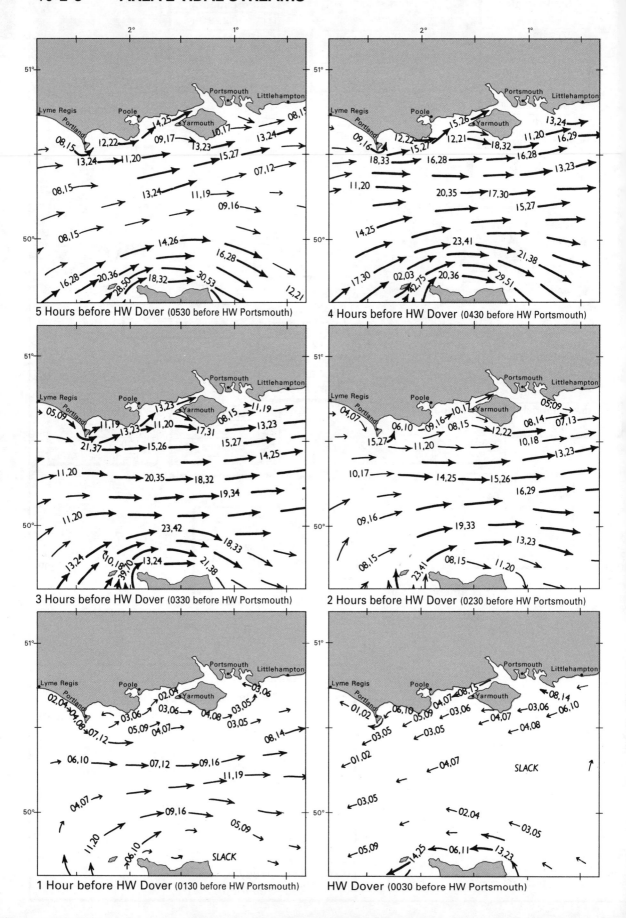

5 Hours before HW Dover (0530 before HW Portsmouth)

4 Hours before HW Dover (0430 before HW Portsmouth)

3 Hours before HW Dover (0330 before HW Portsmouth)

2 Hours before HW Dover (0230 before HW Portsmouth)

1 Hour before HW Dover (0130 before HW Portsmouth)

HW Dover (0030 before HW Portsmouth)

Westward 10.1.3   Portland 10.2.9   Isle of Wight 10.2.26   Eastward 10.3.3   Southward 10.15.3   Channel Islands 10.14.3

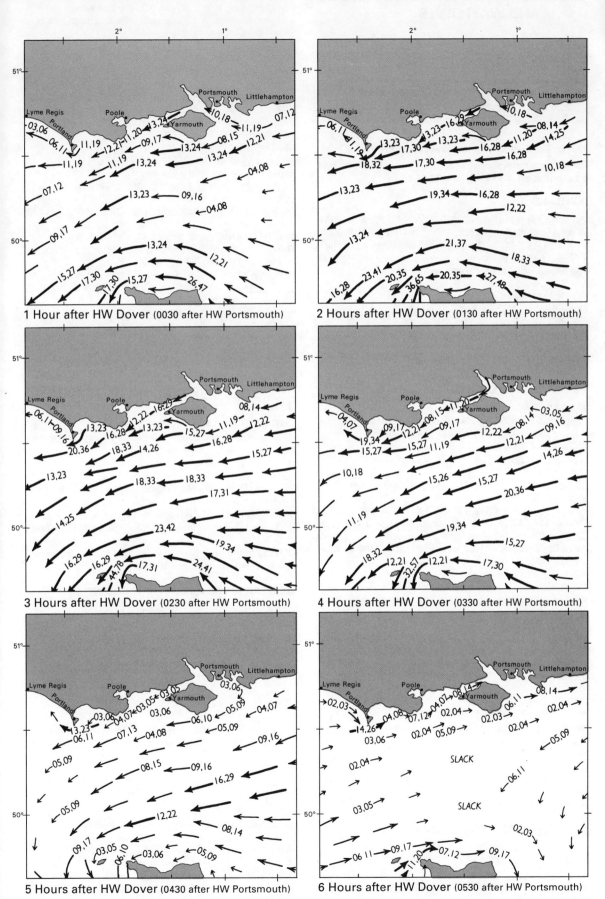

1 Hour after HW Dover (0030 after HW Portsmouth)

2 Hours after HW Dover (0130 after HW Portsmouth)

3 Hours after HW Dover (0230 after HW Portsmouth)

4 Hours after HW Dover (0330 after HW Portsmouth)

5 Hours after HW Dover (0430 after HW Portsmouth)

6 Hours after HW Dover (0530 after HW Portsmouth)

10.2.4 COASTAL LIGHTS, FOG SIGNALS AND WAYPOINTS

Abbreviations used below are given in 1.4.1. Principal lights are in **bold** print, places in CAPITALS, and light-vessels, light floats and Lanbys in *CAPITAL ITALICS*. Unless otherwise stated lights are white. m – elevation in metres; M – nominal range in miles. Fog signals are in *italics*. Useful waypoints are underlined – use those on land with care. All geographical positions should be assumed to be approximate. See 4.4.1.

NOTE: For English Channel Waypoints see 10.1.7.

For other offshore aids, near the Channel Islands and adjacent coast of France, see 10.14.4.

PORTLAND

Portland Bill 50°30'·82N 02°27'·32W Fl (4) 20s 43m **25M**; W ● Tr, R band. Changes from 1 flash to 4 flashes 221°-244°, 4 flashes 244°-117°, changes from 4 flashes to 1 flash 117°-141°; RC; FR 19m 13M (same Tr) vis 271°-291° over The Shambles; *Dia 30s max power 005°-085°*.

PORTLAND HARBOUR

Outer Bkwtr (S end) Oc R 30s 12m 5M.
Outer Bkwtr (N end) QR 14m 5M; vis 013°-268°.
NE Bkwtr (A Hd) 50°35'·12N 02°24'·99W Fl 10s 22m **20M**; W Tr.
NE Bkwtr (B Hd) 50°35'·62N 02°25'·80W Oc R 15s 11m 5M.

PORTLAND TO ISLE OF WIGHT

WEYMOUTH
S Pier Hd 50°36'·50N 02°26'·40W Q 10m 9M; tfc sigs.
Ldg Lts 239·8° both FR 5/7m 4M; R ◆ on W post.
N Pier Hd 2 FG (vert) 9m 6M. *Bell* (when vessels expected).
W Shambles Lt By 50°29'·75N 02°24'·33W Q (9) 15s; WCM; *Bell*.
E Shambles Lt By 50°30'·75N 02°20'·00W Q (3) 10s; ECM; *Whis*.
Lulworth Cove ent, E Point 50°36'·97N 02°14'·69W.
Bindon Hill 50°37'·3N 02°13'·6W and St Alban's Hd 50°34'·8N 02°03'·4W Iso R 2s (when firing taking place).
Anvil Pt 50°35'·48N 01°57'·52W Fl 10s 45m **24M**; W ● Tr; vis 237°-076°; (H24).

SWANAGE
Pier Hd 50°36'·52N 01°56'·88W 2 FR (vert) 6m 3M.
Peveril Ledge By 50°36'·38N 01°56'·02W; PHM.

POOLE
Poole Fairway Lt By 50°38'·95N 01°54'·78W L Fl 10s; SWM.
Poole Bar (No. 1) Lt By 50°39·31N 01°55'·10W QG; SHM; *Bell*
(Historic wreck) 50°39'·68N 01°54'·80W Fl Y 5s; SPM.

SWASH CHANNEL
No. 2 Lt By 50°39'·17N 01°55'·13W Fl R 2s; PHM.
Swash Chan marked by PHM and SHM, unlit except for:
Training Bank Lt By 50°39'·77N 01°55'·72W QR (T).
No. 10 Lt By 50°40'·11N 01°55'·82W Fl R 4s; PHM.
No. 9 Lt By 50°40'·16N 01°55'·72W Fl G 5s; SHM.
No. 11 (Hook Sands) Lt By 50°40'·40N 01°55'·99W Fl G 3s; SHM.
No. 12 (Channel) Lt By 50°40'·37N 01°56'·11W Fl R 2s; PHM.
No. 14 Lt By 50°40'·76N 01°56'·73W Fl R 4s; PHM.
No. 13 Lt By 50°40'·84N 01°56'·62W Fl G 5s; SHM.

EAST LOOE CHANNEL
E Looe No. 16A Lt By 50°41'·02N 01°56'·03W QR; PHM.
East Hook By 50°40'·55W 01°55'·13W; PHM.

S Haven Pt, ferry landing 2 FR (vert) 5m on either side of ramp.
Ferry landing, E side 2 FG (vert) 3m, either side of ramp.
S Deep. Marked by Lt Bns and unlit Bns from ent S of Brownsea Castle to Furzey Is.

BROWNSEA ROADS
No.18 Lt By 50°41'·02N 01°57'·32W Fl R 5s; PHM.
N Haven Pt Bn 50°41'·12N 01°57'·10W Q (9) 15s 5m; WCM.
Brownsea (No. 42) Lt By 50°41'·13N 01°57'·33W Q (3) 10s; ECM.
RMYC Pier Hds 50°41'·31N 01°56'·73W 2 FG (vert) 2M.

MIDDLE SHIP CHANNEL
No. 20 Lt By 50°41'·35N 01°57'·02W Q (6) + L Fl 15s; *Bell* SCM.
Marked by PHM and SHM Lt Bys.
Aunt Betty (No. 50) Lt By 50°41'·93N 01°57'·31W Q (3) 10s; ECM.
Diver (No.51) Lt By 50°42'·24N 01°58'·26W Q (9) 15s; WCM.

NORTH CHANNEL
The chan to Poole Hbr YC Marina and Poole Quay is marked by PHM and SHM's, mostly lit.
Bullpit Bn 50°41'·69N 01°56'·62W Q (9) 15s 7m 4M; WCM.
Salterns Marina Outer Bkwtr Hd 50°42'·20N 01°57'·01W 2 FR (vert) 2M; Tfc sigs.
Inner Bkwtr Hd 2 FG (vert) 3M.

Parkstone YC platform 50°42'·33N 01°58'·00W Q 8m 1M; hut on dolphin.
Stakes No. 55 Lt By 50°42'·39N 01°58'·93W Q (6) + L Fl 15s; SCM.
Little Chan, E side, Oyster Bank Bn 50°42'·59N 01°59'·05W Fl (2) G 5s; SHM.

WAREHAM CHANNEL
Wareham Chan marked by PHM and SHM's initially, and then by stakes.

BOURNEMOUTH
Pier Hd 2 FR (vert) 9m 1M; W Col. *Reed (2) 120s* when vessel expected.
Boscombe Pier Hd 2 FR (vert) 7m 1M; R Col.
Hengistbury Hd, groyne, Bn 50°42'·63N 01°44'·85W (unlit).

NOTE: For waypoints of navigational buoys and racing marks in Solent area, see 10.2.21.

WESTERN APPROACHES TO THE SOLENT

Needles Fairway Lt By 50°38'·20N 01°38'·90W L Fl 10s; SWM; *Whis*.
Needles Lt 50°39'·70N 01°35'·43W Oc (2) WRG 20s 24m **W17M**, **R17M**, R14M G14M; ●Tr, R band and lantern; vis Rshore -300°, W300°-083°; R(unintens) 083°-212°, W212°-217°, G217°-224°. *Horn (2) 30s*.

NEEDLES CHANNEL.
SW Shingles Lt By 50°39'·37N 01°37'·25W Fl R 2·5s; PHM.
Bridge Lt By 50°39'·59N 01°36'·80W VQ (9) 10s; Racon (T); WCM.
Shingles Elbow Lt By 50°40'·31N 01°35'·92W Fl (2) R 5s; PHM.
Mid Shingles Lt By 50°41'·18N 01°34'·58W; Fl (3) R 10s; PHM.
Totland Bay Pier Hd 2 FG (vert) 6m 2M.
Warden Lt By 50°41'·45N 01°33'·47W Fl G 2.5s; SHM; Bell.

NORTH CHANNEL
N Hd Lt By 50°42'·65N 01°35'·43W Fl (3) G 10s; SHM.
NE Shingles Lt By 50°41'·93N 01°33'·32W Q (3) 10s; ECM.
Hurst Pt Ldg Lts 042°. Front 50°42'·36N 01°33'·05W Iso 4s 15m 14M; R ■ Tr; vis 029°-053°. Rear 215m from front Iso WR 6s 23m W14/13M, R11M; W ● Tr; vis W(unintens) 080°-104°, W234°-244°, R244°-250°, W250°-053°.

2

THE WEST SOLENT

Sconce Lt By 50°42'·50N 01°31'·35W Q; NCM; *Bell*.
Black Rock By 50°42'·55N 01°30'·55W; SHM.
Fort Victoria Pier Hd 50°42'·42N 01°31'·08W 2 FG (vert) 4M.

YARMOUTH
Pier Hd, centre, 50°42'·48N 01°29'·88W 2 FR (vert) 2M;
G col. High intensity FW (occas).

LYMINGTON
Jack in the Basket 50°44'·25N 01°30'·50W Fl R 2s 9m.
Ldg Lts 319·5°. Front 50°45'·16N 01°31'·57W FR 12m 8M;
vis 309·5°-329·5°. Rear, 363m from front, FR 17m 8M; vis as
front.
Cross Boom No. 2 50°44'·33N 01°30'·50W Fl R 2s 4m 3M;
R □ on pile.
No. 1 50°44'·38N 01°30'·39W Fl G 2s 2m 3M; G △ on pile.

Durn's Pt obstn, S end, 50°45'·37N 01°26'·95W QR; dolphin.
Hampstead Ledge Lt By 50°43'·83N 01°26'10W Fl (2) G 5s; SHM.
W Lepe Lt By 50°45'20N 01°24'·00W Fl R 5s; PHM.
Salt Mead Lt By 50°44'·48N 01°22'·95W Fl (3) G 10s; SHM.
Gurnard Ledge Lt By 50°45'·48N 01°20'·50W Fl G 4s; SHM.
E Lepe Lt By 50°46'·09N 01°20'·81W Fl (2) R 5s; PHM; *Bell*.
Gurnard Lt By 50°46'·18N 01°18'·76W Q; NCM.

BEAULIEU RIVER
Beaulieu Spit, E end 50°46'·83N 01°21'·67W Fl R 5s 3M;
R dolphin; vis 277°-037°.
Ent Chan Bn Nos. 5, 9, 19, 21 Fl G 4s; Bn Nos 12, 20 Fl R 4s.

Off Stansore Pt. 50°46'·73N 01°20'·72W, 50°46'·81N
01°20'·49W, 50°46'·89N 01°20'·34W. In each of these posns
is a QR Lt 4m 1M; R ◆, W band, on R pile, marking cables.
NE Gurnard Lt By 50°47'·03N 01°19'·34W Fl (3) R 10s; PHM.
W Bramble Lt By 50°47'·17N 01°18'·57W VQ (9) 10s; WCM;
Bell 15s; Racon (T).
Thorn Knoll Lt By 50°47'·47N 01°18'·35W Fl G 5s; SHM.
Bourne Gap Lt By 50°47'·80N 01°18'·25W Fl R 3s; PHM.
N Thorn Lt By 50°47'·88N 01°17'·75W QG; SHM.
W Knoll By 50°47'·52N 01°17'·67W; SHM.
Outfall 50°48'·25N 01°18'·73W Iso R 10s 6m 5M; col on ■
structure; Ra refl; FR Lt on each corner; *Horn 20s*.

CALSHOT SPIT Lt F   50°48'·32N 01°17'·55W Fl 5s 12m
11M; R hull, Lt Tr amidships; *Horn (2) 60s*.
E Knoll By 50°47'·93N 01°16'·75W; SHM.
Castle Pt Lt By 50°48'·67N 01°17'·60W IQR 10s; PHM.
Reach Lt By 50°49'·02N 01°17'·57W Fl (3) G 10s; SHM.

SOUTHAMPTON WATER
Coronation Lt By 50°49'·52N 01°17'·53W Fl Y 5s; SPM.
Hook Lt By 50°49'·49N 01°18'·21W QG 15s; SHM; *Horn*.
Fawley Chan No. 2 Lt Bn 50°49'·45N 01°18'·75W Fl R 3s; PHM.

ASHLETT CREEK
Fawley Lt By 50°49'·97N 01°19'·38W QR; PHM.

Bald Head By 50°49'·86N 01°18'·16W; SHM.
Hamble Pt Lt By 50°50'·12N 01°18'·58W Q (6) + L Fl 15s; SCM.

RIVER HAMBLE
Ldg Lts 345·5°. Front No. 6 pile 50°50'·58N 01°18'·74W
Oc (2) R 12s 4m 2M. Rear 820m from front, QR 12m; W mast;
vis 341·5°-349·5°.
No. 1 pile 50°50'·31N 01°18'·57W Fl G 3s 3M; SHM.
No. 2 pile 50°50'·36N 01°18'·68W Q (3) 10s 3M; ECM.
Ldg Lts 026·1°, Warsash Shore. Front 50°50'·98N 01°18'·32W
QG; vis 010°-040°. Rear, Sailing Club, Iso G 6s; vis 022°-030°.
Esso Marine terminal, SE end 50°50'·05N 01°19'·33W 2 FR
(vert) 9m 10M; *Whis (2) 20s*.

BP Hamble Jetty 50°50'·90N 01°19'·50W 2 FG (vert) 5/3m
2M (on each side of the 4 dolphins).
Greenland Lt By 50°51'·08N 01°20'·33W IQ G 10s; SHM.
Cadland Lt By 50°50'·98N 01°20'·45W Fl R 3s; PHM.
Lains Lake Lt By 50°51'·55N 01°21'·57W Fl (2) R 4s; PHM.
Hound Lt By 50°51'·65N 01°21'·43W Fl (3) G 10s; SHM.
Netley Lt By 50°51'·98N 01°21'·72W Fl G 3s; SHM.
NW Netley Lt By 50°52'·28N 01°22'·65W Fl G 7s; SHM.
Deans Elbow Lt By 50°52'·13N 01°22'·68W Oc R 4s; PHM.
Weston Shelf Lt By 50°52'·68N 01°23'·17W Fl (3) G 15s; SHM.

HYTHE
Hythe Knock Lt By 50°52'·80N 01°23'·73W Fl R 3s; PHM.
Hythe Pier Hd 50°52'·45N 01°23'·52W 2 FR (vert) 12/5m 5M.
Marina Village Lt Bn 50°52'·23N 01°23'·48W Q (3) 10s; ECM.
Lock ent 50°52'·52N 01°23'·88W 2 FG (vert); G △ and 2 FR
(vert); R □.

SOUTHAMPTON/RIVER ITCHEN
Swinging Gd No. 1 Lt By 50°52'·97N 01°23'·35W Oc G 4s;
SHM.
E side. No. 1 dolphin 50°53'·12N 01°23'·32W QG; SHM.
No. 2 Dn 50°53'·27N 01°23'·28W Fl G 5s 2M; SHM.
No. 3 Dn 50°53'·45N 01°23'·18W Fl G 7s; SHM.
No. 4 pile 50°53'·58N 01°23'·07W QG 4m 2M; SHM.
Itchen Bridge. FW on bridge span each side marks main chan.
2 FG (vert) 2M each side on E pier. 2 FR (vert) 2M each side
on W pier.
Crosshouse Lt Bn 50°54'·01N 01°23'·10W Oc R 5s 5m 2M;
PHM.
Chapel Lt Bn 50°54'·12N 01°23'·13W Fl G 3s 5m 3M; SHM.
Shamrock Quay SW end 50°54'·45N 01°22'·83W 2 FR (vert)
4m, and NE end 2 FR (vert) 4m.
No. 5 Lt Bn 50°54'·47N 01°22'·68W Fl G 3s.
No. 6 Lt Bn 50°54'·57N 01°22'·55W Fl R 3s.
No. 7 Lt Bn 50°54'·57N 01°22'·40W Fl (2) G 5s.
No. 9 Lt Bn 50°54'·70N 01°22'·38W Fl (4) G 10s.
Kemps Marina Jetty Hd 50°54'·80N 01°22'·57W 2 FG (vert)
5m 1M

SOUTHAMPTON/RIVER TEST
Town Quay Marina Ent 50°53'·62N 01°24'·15W 2 FG (vert).
Gymp Lt By 50°53'·15N 01°24'·22W QR; PHM.
Queen Elizabeth II terminal, S end 50°52'·97N 01°23'·64W
4 FG (vert) 16m 3M.
Lower Foul Gd Lt Bn 50°53'·23N 01°24'·47W Fl (2) R 10s; PHM.
Upper Foul Gd Lt Bn 50°53'·50N 01°24'·80W Fl (2) R 10s; PHM.
Town Quay Ldg Lts 329°, both FY 12/22m 3/2M (occas).
Gymp Elbow Lt By 50°53'·48N 01°24'·53W Oc R 4s; PHM.
Pier Hd Lt By 50°53'·63N 01°24'·57W QG; SHM.
Dibden Bay Lt By 50°53'·66N 01°24'·84W Q; NCM.
Swinging Gd No. 2 Lt By 50°53'·78N 01°25'·03W Fl (2) R 10s;
PHM.
Cracknore Lt By 50°53'·91N 01°25'·12W Oc R 8s; PHM.
Millbrook Lt By 50°54'·08N 01°26'·73W QR; PHM.
Bury Lt By 50°54'·10N 01°27'·03W Fl R 5s; PHM.
Eling Lt By 50°54'·45N 01°27'·75W Fl R 5s; PHM.

THE EAST SOLENT

NORTH CHANNEL/HILLHEAD
Calshot Lt By 50°48'·40N 01°16'·95W VQ; NCM; *Bell 30s*.
Hillhead Lt By 50°48'·03N 01°15'·91W Fl R 2·5s; PHM.
E Bramble Lt By 50°47'·20N 01°13'·56W VQ (3) 5s; ECM; *Bell*.
Hillhead S Bkwtr Hd Bn 50°49'·01N 01°14'·44W; PHM.

COWES
No. 4 Lt By 50°46'·04N 01°17'·78W QR; PHM.
No. 3 Lt By 50°46'·04N 01°17'·95W Fl G 3s; SHM.
Ldg Lts 164°. Front 50°45'·87N 01°17'·76W Iso 2s 3m 6M.
Rear, 290m from front, Iso R 2s 5m 3M; vis 120°-240°.

E Bkwtr Hd 50°45'·84N 01°17'·43W Fl R 3s 3M.
W Cowes Marina N end 50°45'·69N 01°17'·62W 2 FG (vert) 6m.
E Cowes Marina N end 50°45'·15N 01°17'·44W 2 FR (vert).

Prince Consort Lt By 50°46'·38N 01°17'·47W VQ; NCM.
W Ryde Mid Lt By 50°46'·45N 01°15'·70W Q (9) 15s; WCM.
Norris Lt By 50°45'·92N 01°15'·40W Fl (3) R 10s; PHM.
N Ryde Mid Lt By 50°46'·58N 01°14'·28W Fl (4) R 20s; PHM.
S Ryde Mid Lt By 50°46'·10N 01°14'·08W Fl G 5s; SHM.
Peel Bank Lt By 50°45'·57N 01°13'·25W Fl (2) R 5s; PHM.
SE Ryde Mid Lt By 50°45'·90N 01°12'·00W VQ (6) + L Fl 10s; SCM.
NE Ryde Mid Lt By 50°46'·18N 01°11'·80W Fl (2) R 10s; PHM.

WOOTTON
Lt Bn 50°44'·51N 01°12'·05W Q 1M; NCM.
No. 1 Lt Bn 50°44'·37N 01°12'·26W Fl (2) G 5s.
No. 2 Lt Bn 50°44'·22N 01°12'·38W Fl R 5s.

Mother Bank Lt By 50°45'·45N 01°11'·13W Fl R 3s; PHM.
Browndown Lt By 50°46'·54N 01°10'·87W Fl G 15s; SHM.
Stokes Bay Wk By 50°46'·67N 01°10'·58W; SHM.

RYDE
Pier, NW corner, N and E corner marked by 2 FR (vert). In fog FY from N corner, vis 045°-165°, 200°-320°.
Leisure Hbr E side 50°43'·95N 01°09'·20W 2 FR (vert) 7m 1M. FY 6m shown when depth of water in Hbr greater than 1m; 2 FY when depth exceeds 1·5m.
Hbr W side 50°43'·93N 01°09'·23W 2 FG (vert) 7m 1M.

Ft Gilkicker 50°46'·40N 01°08'·38W Oc G 10s 7M.
N Sturbridge Lt By 50°45'·31N 01°08'·15W VQ; NCM.
NE Mining Gnd Lt By 50°44'·71N 01°06'·30W Fl Y 10s; SPM.

PORTSMOUTH AND APPROACHES
Horse Sand Ft 50°44'·97N 01°04'·25W Iso G 2s 21m 8M; large ● stone structure.
Saddle Lt By 50°45'·18N 01°04'·79W VQ (3) G 10s; SHM.
Horse Sand Lt By 50°45'·48N 01°05'·17W Fl G 2·5s; SHM.
Outer Spit Lt By 50°45'·55N 01°05'·41W Q (6) + L Fl 15s; SCM.
Boyne Lt By 50°46'·12N 01°05'·17W Fl G 5s; SHM.
Spit Refuge Lt By 50°46'·12N 01°05'·37W Fl R 5s; PHM.
Spit Sand Ft, N side 50°46'·20N 01°05'·85W Fl R 5s 18m 7M; large ● stone structure.
Castle Lt By 50°46'·43N 01°05'·30W Fl (2) G 6s; SHM.
Southsea Castle N corner 50°46'·66N 01°05'·25W Iso 2s 16m 11M, W stone Tr, B band; vis 339°-066°.
Dir Lt 001·5° Dir WRG 11m W13M, R5M, G5M; same structure FG 351·5°-357·5°, Al WG 357·5°-000° (W phase incr with brg), FW 000°-003°, Al WR 003°-005·5° (R phase incr with brg), FR 005·5°-011·5°.
Ridge Lt By 50°46'·42N 01°05'·57W Fl (2) R 6s; PHM.
No. 1 Lt By 50°46'·73N 01°05'·72W Fl (3) G 10s; SHM.
No. 2 Lt By 50°46'·66N 01°05'·88W Fl R 10s; PHM.
No. 3 Lt By 50°47'·04N 01°06'·17W QG; SHM.
No. 4 Lt By 50°46'·98N 01°06'·27W QR; PHM.
Ft Blockhouse 50°47'·34N 01°06'·65W Dir Lt 320°; Dir WRG 6m W13M, R5M, G5M; Oc G 310°-316°, Al WG 316°-318·5° (W phase incr with brg), Oc 318·5°-321·5°, Al WR 321·5°-324° (R phase incr with brg), Oc R 324°-330°. 2 FR (vert) 20m E.
Victoria Pile 50°47'·31N 01°06'·40W Oc G 15s 1M; SHM.
Dn, close E of C&N Marina, 50°47'·82N 01°06'·89W, Hbr Ent Dir Lt (Fuel Jetty) WRG 2m 1M; vis Iso G 2s 322·5°-330°, Al WG 330°-332·5°, Iso 2s 332·5°-335° (main chan), Al WR 335°-337·5°, Iso R 2s 337·5°-345° (Small Boat Chan).
Ballast Lt By 50°47'·59N 01°06'·76W Fl R 2·5s; PHM.
The Point 50°47'·54N 01°06'·48W QG 2M; SHM.
Port Solent Lock ent 50°50'·58N 01°06'·25W Fl (4) G 10s.

No Man's Land Ft 50°44'·37N 01°05'·60W Iso R 2s 21m 8M; large ● stone structure.
Horse Elbow Wk By 50°44'·40N 01°03'·35W; SHM.
Horse Elbow Lt By 50°44'·23N 01°03'·80W QG; SHM.
Warner Lt By 50°43'·84N 01°03'·93W QR; PHM; Whis.
Dean Elbow Lt By 50°43'·66N 01°01'·78W Fl G 5s; SHM.
St Helens Lt By 50°43'·33N 01°02'·32W Fl (3) R 15s; PHM.
Horse Tail Lt By 50°43'·20N 01°00'·14W Fl (2) G 10s; SHM.
Dean Tail Lt By 50°42'·95N 00°59'·08W Fl G 5s; SHM.
Nab East Lt By 50°42'·82N 01°00'·70W Fl (2) R 10s; PHM.
Dean Tail South Lt By 50°43'·10N 00°59'·49W Q (6) + L Fl 10s; SCM.
Nab End Lt By 50°42'·60N 00°59'·38W Fl R 5s; PHM.
New Grounds Lt By 50°41'·97N 00°58'·53W VQ (3) 5s; ECM.

BEMBRIDGE
St Helen's Ft (IOW) 50°42'·27N 01°04'·95W Fl (3) 10s 16m 8M; large ● stone structure.
Bembridge Tide Gauge 50°42'·43N 01°04'·93W Fl Y 2s 1M; SPM.

LANGSTONE AND APPROACHES
Winner By 50°45'·07N 01°00'·01W; SCM.
Roway Wk Bn 50°46'·08N 01°02'·20W Fl (2) 5s; IDM.
Langstone Fairway Lt By 50°46'·28N 01°01'·27W L Fl 10s; SWM.
Eastney Pt Lt Bn 50°47'·20N 01°01'·58W QR 2m 2M.
Eastney Gunnery Range Lt 50°47'·16N 01°02'·12W FR, Oc (2) Y 10s, and Y Lts (occas) when firing taking place.
S Lake 50°49'·45N 00°59'·80W Fl G 3s 3m 2M; SHM.
Binness 50°49'·60N 00°59'·85W Fl R 3s 3m 2M; PHM.

CHICHESTER ENTRANCE
Bar Lt Bn 50°45'·88N 00°56'·38W Fl WR 5s 14m W7M, R5M; vis W322°-080°, R080°-322°; Tide Gauge. Same structure, Fl (2) R 10s 7m 2M; vis 020°-080°.
Eastoke Lt Bn 50°46'·62N 00°56'·08W QR 2m; R □ on pile.
W Winner Lt Bn 50°46'·83N 00°55'·89W QG; G △ on pile.

EMSWORTH CHANNEL
Verner Lt Bn 50°48'·27N 00°56'·57W Fl R 10s; PHM.
Marker Pt 50°48'·87N 00°56'·65W Fl (2) G 10s 8m; SHM.
NE Hayling Lt Bn 50°49'·60N 00°56'·77W Fl (2) R 10s 8m; PHM.
Emsworth Lt Bn 50°49'·63N 00°56'·70W Q (6) + L Fl 15s; SCM, tide gauge.

CHICHESTER CHANNEL
East Hd Lt Bn 50°47'·32N 00°54'·67W Fl (4) G 10s; G △ on pile; SHM; tide gauge.
Camber Lt Bn 50°47'·83N 00°53'·93W Q (6) + L Fl 15s; SCM.
Chalkdock Lt Bn 50°48'·46N 00°53'·27W Fl (2) G 10s; G △ on pile, SHM.
Itchenor Jetty 50°48'·43N 00°51'·90W 2 FG (vert); tide gauge.
Birdham Lt Bn 50°48'·33N 00°50'·18W Fl (4) G 10s; pile, SHM, depth gauge.
Chichester Yacht Basin Lt Bn 50°48'·42N 00°49'·87W Fl G 5s 6m; SHM; tide gauge.

St Catherine's Pt 50°34'·52N 01°17'·80W Fl 5s 41m **27M**; vis 257°-117°; RC. FR 35m **17M** (same Tr) vis 099°-116°.
Ventnor Pier 50°35'·45N 01°12'·25W 2 FR (vert) 10m 3M.
Sandown Pier Hd 50°39'·04N 01°09'·10W 2 FR (vert) 7m 2M.
W Princessa Lt By 50°40'·12N 01°03'·57W Q (9) 15s; WCM.
Bembridge Ledge Lt By 50°41'·12N 01°02'·72W Q (3) 10s; ECM.

Nab Tr. 50°40'·05N 00°57'·07W Fl 10s 27m **16M**; Horn (2) 30s; Racon (T); vis 300°-120°.

10.2.5 PASSAGE INFORMATION

Reference books include: Admiralty *Channel Pilot*; *South Coast Cruising* (YM/Fishwick); *Shell Channel Pilot* (Imray/Cunliffe); *The Solent* (Imray/Bowskill); and *Creeks and Harbours of the Solent* (Adlard Coles). See 10.0.5 for distances across the Channel, and 10.3.5 for notes on cross-Channel passages.

THE PORTLAND RACE (chart 2255)

South of the Bill lies the Portland Race which can give severe and dangerous sea states. Even in settled weather it should be carefully avoided by small craft, although at neaps it may be barely perceptible.

The Race occurs at the confluence of two strong S-going tidal streams which run down each side of Portland for almost 10 hours out of 12 at springs. These streams meet the main E-W stream of the Channel, producing large eddies on either side of Portland and a highly confused sea state with heavy overfalls in the Race. The irregular contours of the sea-bed, which shoals abruptly from depths of over 100m some 2M south of the Bill to as little as 9m on Portland Ledge 1M further N, greatly contribute to the violence of the Race. Portland Ledge strongly deflects the flow of water upwards, so that on the flood the Race lies SE of the Bill and vice versa on the ebb. Conditions deteriorate with wind-against-tide, especially at springs; in an E gale against the flood stream the Race may spread eastward to The Shambles. The Race normally extends about 2M S of the Bill, but further S in bad weather.

The Tidal Stream chartlets at 10.2.9 show the approx hourly positions of the Race. They are referenced to HW Portland, for the convenience of those leaving or making for Portland/Weymouth; and to HW Dover for those on passage S of the Bill. The smaller scale chartlets at 10.2.3 show the English Chan streams referenced to HW at Dover and Portsmouth.

Small craft may avoid the Race either by passing clear to seaward of it, between 3 and 5M S of the Bill; or by using the inshore passage if conditions suit. This passage is a stretch of relatively smooth water between 2½ca and 5ca off the Bill (depending on wind), which should not however be used at springs nor at night; beware lobster pots. Timing is important to catch "slackish" water around the Bill, i.e:

> **Westbound** = from HW Dover – 1 to HW + 2
> (HW Portland + 4 to HW – 6).
> **Eastbound** = from HW Dover + 5 to HW – 4
> (HW Portland – 3 to HW + 1).

From either direction, close Portland at least 2M N of the Bill to utilise the S-going stream; once round the Bill, the N-going stream will set a yacht away from the Race area.

PORTLAND TO CHRISTCHURCH BAY (chart 2615)

The Shambles bank is about 3M E of Portland Bill, and should be avoided at all times. In bad weather the sea breaks heavily on it. It is marked by buoys on its E side and at SW end. E of Weymouth are rky ledges extending 3ca offshore as far as Lulworth Cove, which provides a reasonable anch in fine, settled weather and offshore winds; as do Worbarrow B and Chapman's Pool (10.2.10).

A firing range extends 5M offshore between Lulworth and St Alban's Hd. Yachts must pass through this area as quickly as possible, when the range is in use, see 10.2.10. Beware Kimmeridge Ledges, which extend over 5ca seaward.

St Alban's Hd (107m and conspic) is steep-to and has a dangerous race off it which may extend 3M seaward. The race lies to the E on the flood and to the W on the ebb; the latter is the more dangerous. An inshore passage, at most 5ca wide, avoids the worst of the overfalls. There is an eddy on W side of St Alban's, where the stream runs almost continuously SE. 1M S of St Alban's the ESE stream begins at HW Portsmouth + 0520, and the WNW stream at HW – 0030, with sp rates of 4·75kn.

There is deep water quite close inshore between St Alban's Hd and Anvil Pt (lt). 1M NE of Durlston Hd, Peveril Ledge runs 2½ca seaward, causing quite a bad race which extends nearly 1M eastwards, particularly on W-going stream against a SW wind. Proceeding towards the excellent shelter of Poole Harbour (10.2.13), overfalls may be met off Ballard Pt and Old Harry on the W-going stream. Studland Bay (10.2.13 and chart *2172*) is a good anch except in NE to SE winds. Anch about 4ca WNW of Handfast Pt. Avoid foul areas on chart.

Poole Bay offers good sailing in waters sheltered from W and N winds, and with no dangers to worry the average yacht. Tidal streams are weak N of a line between Handfast Pt and Hengistbury Hd. The latter is a dark headland, S of Christchurch hbr (10.2.14), with a groyne extending 1ca S and Beerpan Rks a further 100m offshore. Beware lobster pots in this area. Christchurch Ledge extends 2·75M SE from Hengistbury Hd. The tide runs hard over the ledge at sp, and there may be overfalls. Within Christchurch B the streams are weak.

WESTERN APPROACHES TO SOLENT (charts *2219*, 2050)

The Needles are distinctive rks at the W end of the Isle of Wight. The adjacent chalk cliffs of High Down are conspic from afar; the lt ho may not be seen by day until relatively close. There are drying rocks 5ca WNW of the lt ho, with remains of wreck close SW of these rocks. The NW side of Needles Chan is defined by the Shingles bank, parts of which dry and on which the sea breaks violently in the least swell. The SE side of the bank is fairly steep-to, the NW side shelves more gradually. See 10.2.16.

On the ebb the stream sets very strongly (3·4kn) WSW across the Shingles. In bad weather broken water and overfalls extend along The Bridge, a reef which runs 8ca W of the lt ho with extremity marked by WCM lt buoy. S to W gales against the ebb raise very dangerous seas in the Needles Chan. (In such conditions the E approach to the Solent, via Nab Tr and the Forts, should be used or shelter found at Poole or Studland). Even a SW F4 over the ebb will cause breaking seas near Bridge and SW Shingles buoys.

In strong winds the North Channel, N of the Shingles, is preferable to the Needles Channel. The two join S of Hurst Pt, where overfalls and tide rips may be met. Beware The Trap, a shoal spit 150m SE of Hurst Castle.

In E winds Alum B, close NE of the Needles, is an attractive daytime anch with its coloured cliffs, but beware Long Rk (dries) in middle of B, and Five Fingers Rk 1½ca SW of Hatherwood Pt on N side. Totland Bay is good anch in settled weather, but avoid Warden Ledge.

THE SOLENT (charts 2040, *394*)

Within the Solent there are few dangers in mid-chan. The most significant is Bramble bank (dries) between Cowes and Calshot. The main shipping chan (buoyed) passes S and W of the Brambles, but yachts can use the North Chan to the NE of the Brambles at any state of tide. Tidal streams are strong at sp, but principally follow the direction of the main chan.

An Area of Concern between Cowes and Calshot provides added safety for larger ships; see 10.2.20 for details.

Several inshore spits, banks, rocks and ledges, which a yachtsman should know, include: Pennington and Lymington Spits on the N shore; Black Rk 4ca W of entrance to Yarmouth (10.2.17); Hamstead Ledge 8ca W of entrance to Newtown River (10.2.19) and Saltmead Ledge 1·5M to E; Gurnard Ledge 1·5M W of Cowes; Lepe

Middle and Beaulieu Spit, S and W of the ent to Beaulieu R. (10.2.23); the shoals off Stone Pt, where three bns mark cable area; Shrape Mud, which extends N from the breakwater of Cowes hbr (10.2.22) and along to Old Castle Pt; the shoals and isolated rks which fringe the island shore from Old Castle Pt to Ryde, including either side of the ent to Wootton Creek (10.2.27); and Calshot Spit which extends almost to the lt F which marks the turn of chan into Southampton Water.

Southampton Water is a busy commercial waterway with large tankers, containerships, lesser craft and ferries. Yachts should monitor VHF Ch 12 to ascertain shipping movements. Between the Esso jetty off Fawley and the BP jetty on the E side the channel is narrow for large vessels; yachts can easily stay clear by seeking shoal water. N of this area there is adequate water for yachts close outboard of the main buoyed channel; the banks are of gently shelving soft mud, apart from foul ground between Hythe and Marchwood. Unlit marks and large mooring buoys may however be hard to see against the many shore lights. Except in strong N'lies, Southampton Water and the R Test and Itchen provide sheltered sailing. The R Hamble is convenient, but somewhat crowded.

Depending on the wind direction, there are many good anchs: For example, in W winds there is anch on E side of Hurst, as close inshore as depth permits, NE of High lt. In S winds, or in good weather, anch W of Yarmouth hbr ent, as near shore as possible; reasonably close to town, see 10.2.17.

In winds between W and N there is good anch in Stanswood Bay, about 1M NE of Stansore Pt. Just N of Calshot Spit there is shelter from SW and W. Osborne Bay, 2M E of Cowes, is sheltered from winds between S and W. In E winds Gurnard B, the other side of Cowes is preferable. In N winds anch in Stokes B. At E end of IOW there is good anch off Bembridge in winds from S, SW or W; but clear out if wind goes into E. There are also places which a shoal-draught boat can explore at the top of the tide, such as Ashlett Creek (10.2.25) between Fawley and Calshot, Eling up the R. Test, and the upper reaches of the R. Medina (10.2.22).

ISLE OF WIGHT – SOUTH COAST (chart *2045*)

From the Needles eastward to Freshwater B the cliffs can be approached to within 1ca, but beyond the E end of chalk cliffs there are ledges off Brook and Atherfield which require at least 5ca offing. The E-going stream sets towards these dangers. 4M SSW of the Needles the stream turns E x N at HW Portsmouth + 0530, and W at HW – 0030, sp rate 2kn.

St Catherine's lt ho (lt, RC) is conspic. It is safe to pass 2ca off, but a race occurs off the Point and can be very dangerous at or near sp with a strong opposing wind; particularly SE of the Pt on a W-going stream in a W gale, when St Catherine's should be given a berth of at least 2M. 1·25M SE of the Pt the stream turns E x N at HW Portsmouth + 0520, and W x S at HW – 0055, sp rate 3·75kn.

Rks extend about 2½ca either side of Dunnose where a race occurs. In Sandown B anch off Shanklin or Sandown where the streams are weak inshore. Off the centre of the B they turn NE x E at HW Portsmouth + 0500, and SW x W at HW – 0100, sp rates 2 kn. The Yarborough Monument is conspic above Culver Cliff. Whitecliff B provides an anch in winds between W and N. From here to Foreland (Bembridge Pt) the coast is fringed by a ledge of rks (dry) extending up to 3ca offshore, and it is advisable to keep to seaward (E) of Bembridge Ledge ECM lt buoy.

EASTERN APPROACHES TO SOLENT (charts 2050, *2045*)

4·5M E of Foreland is Nab Tr (lt, fog sig), a conspic steel and concrete structure (28m), marking Nab Shoal for larger vessels and of no direct significance to yachtsmen. NW of Nab Tr, the E approach to the Solent via Spithead, presents few problems and is far safer in SW/W gales than the Needles Chan.

The main chan is well buoyed and easy to follow, but there is plenty of water for the normal yacht to the S of it when approaching No Man's Land Fort and Horse Sand Fort, between which craft must pass. Submerged barriers lie SW of the former and N of the latter. Ryde Sand dries extensively and is a trap for the unwary; so too is Hamilton Bank on the W side of the chan to Portsmouth (10.2.29).

Nab Tr is also a most useful landmark when approaching the E end of Isle of Wight, or when making for the hbrs of Langstone (10.2.30) or Chichester (10.2.31). Both these hbrs, with offlying sands, are on a dangerous lee shore in strong S'ly winds. East and West Winner flank the ent to Langstone Hbr. Similarly, E and W Pole Sands, drying 1m, lie either side of the ent chan from Chichester Bar bn. SE from Chichester Bar the whole of Bracklesham Bay is shallow, with a pronounced inshore set at certain states of the tide; yachts should keep at least 2M offshore. Further along a low-lying coast, is Selsey Bill with extensive offshore rocks and shoals. Either pass these to seaward of the Owers lt Float, or via the Looe Chan (see 10.3.5) in suitable conditions. Boulder SHM lt buoy is at the W ent to this chan, about 6M SE of Chichester Bar bn. Medmery Bank, 3·7m, is 1M WNW of Boulder.

10.2.6   DISTANCE TABLE

Approximate distances in nautical miles are by the most direct route, whilst avoiding dangers and allowing for Traffic Separation Schemes. Places in *italics* are in adjoining areas; places in **bold** are also in 10.0.5, Cross-Channel Distances.

		1	2	3	4	5	6	7	8	9	10	11	12	13	14	15	16	17	18	19	20
1.	*Exmouth*	1																			
2.	*Lyme Regis*	21	2																		
3.	Portland Bill	36	22	3																	
4.	**Weymouth**	46	32	8	4																
5.	Swanage	58	44	22	22	5															
6.	**Poole Hbr ent**	65	51	28	26	6	6														
7.	**Needles Lt Ho**	73	58	35	34	14	14	7													
8.	Lymington	79	64	42	40	20	24	6	8												
9.	Yarmouth (IOW)	77	63	40	39	18	22	4	2	9											
10.	Beaulieu R. ent	84	69	46	45	25	29	11	7	7	10										
11.	Cowes	86	71	49	46	28	27	14	10	9	2	11									
12.	Southampton	93	78	55	54	34	34	20	16	16	9	9	12								
13.	R. Hamble (ent)	90	75	53	51	32	34	18	12	13	6	6	5	13							
14.	Portsmouth	96	81	58	57	37	35	23	19	19	12	10	18	13	14						
15.	Langstone Hbr	98	84	61	59	39	39	25	21	21	14	12	21	18	5	15					
16.	Chichester Bar	101	86	63	62	42	42	28	23	24	17	15	23	18	8	5	16				
17.	Bembridge	97	81	59	58	38	39	24	18	19	13	10	18	15	5	6	8	17			
18.	**Nab Tower**	102	86	64	63	43	44	29	23	24	18	15	24	19	10	7	6	6	18		
19.	St Catherine's Pt	82	68	45	44	25	25	12	19	21	27	15	36	29	20	20	19	17	15	19	
20.	*Littlehampton*	117	102	79	79	60	61	46	44	45	38	36	45	42	31	28	25	28	22	35	20

PORTLAND HARBOUR   10-2-8

Dorset 50°35'·11N 02°24'·90W (E Ship Chan)

CHARTS
AC 2268, 2255, *2610*; Imray C4, C5; Stanfords 12; OS 194
TIDES
–0430 Dover; ML 1·0; Zone 0 (UT)

Standard Port PORTLAND (→)

Times				Height (metres)			
High Water		Low Water		MHWS	MHWN	MLWN	MLWS
0100	0700	0100	0700	2·1	1·4	0·8	0·1
1300	1900	1300	1900				

LULWORTH COVE and MUPE BAY (Worbarrow Bay)

+0005	+0015	–0005	0000	+0·1	+0·1	+0·2	+0·1

NOTE: Portland is a Standard Port; predictions for each day of the year are given below. Double LWs (known locally as the Gulder) occur over a 4hr period. Predictions are for the first LW.

SHELTER
Poor, due to lack of wind breaks. ‡ N of the moorings off Castletown (best in S/SW winds) or off Castle Cove. East Fleet is only suitable for small craft with lowering masts.
Note: Low flying helicopters often operate for long periods, H24, over S part of hbr.
In April 1995 the sale was announced of Portland Harbour and HM Naval Base to Portland Port Ltd. HM Ships ceased training at the Base at the end of July 1995; the Naval Base is due to close in April 1996. A QHM is likely to remain in office until the new Harbour Authority is established. Future plans are said to include a commercial port, Ro-Ro ferry service, fishing hbr and small marina. Implementation of some of these projects may await the closure of the helicopter base in 1999. Further information will be published in the Supplements as available. Meanwhile Weymouth (new marina under consideration) remains the best option for yachtsmen, unless in emergency.

NAVIGATION
WPT 50°35'·07N 02°24'·00W, 090°/270° from/to E Ship Chan, Fort Hd, 0·50M. The S Chan is permanently closed. Speed limit in the hbr is 12kn. Beware rky reef extending 1ca off Sandsfoot Cas, shoal areas E of Small Mouth and hydrofoils from Weymouth. At night beware unlit buoys, lighters and rafts. Portland Race (see 10.2.5 and 10.2.9 Portland Tidal Streams) is extremely dangerous.

LIGHTS AND MARKS
Bill of Portland (S end) Fl (4) 20s 43m 25M; W tr, R band; gradually changes from 1 flash to 4 flashes 221°-244°, 4 flashes 244°-117°, gradually changes from 4 flashes to 1 flash 117°-141°. FR 19m 13M, same tr, vis 271°-291° (20°) over The Shambles, Dia 30s. Ldg lts 288° into E Fleet: Front QG 3m 2M; rear Iso G 4s 5m 2M.

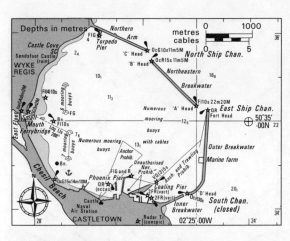

RADIO TELEPHONE
The former Portland Naval Base operated VHF Ch 13 14; subsequent changes are not known, but will be published in Supplements to this Almanac. Note: Portland CG offers radio coverage of the Casquets TSS on Ch **69** 16.
TELEPHONE (01305)
QHM 820311; MRSC 760439; ⌗ (01752) 220661; Marinecall 0891 500457; Police 63011; Dr 820311 (Emergency).
FACILITIES
Castle Cove SC ☎ 783708, M, L, FW; **Services:** Slip, M, L, FW, ME, Sh, C, CH, El (mobile workshop).
Town ⊠, Ⓑ, ⇌ (bus to Weymouth), ✈ (Bournemouth).

There is no set of the sea in Portland Race: no run and sway: no regular assault. It is a chaos of pyramidical waters leaping up suddenly without calculation, or rule of advance. It is not a charge, but a scrimmage; a wrestling bout; but a wrestling bout of a thousand against one. It purposely raises a clamour to shake its adversary's soul, wherein it most resembles a gigantic pack of fighting dogs, for it snarls, howls, yells, and all this most terrifically. Its purpose is to kill, and to kill with a savage pride.
And all these things you find out if you get mixed up in it on a very small boat.

The Cruise of the Nona: Hilaire Belloc. Pimlico (Publishers). Reprinted by permission of the Peters Fraser & Dunlop Group Ltd.

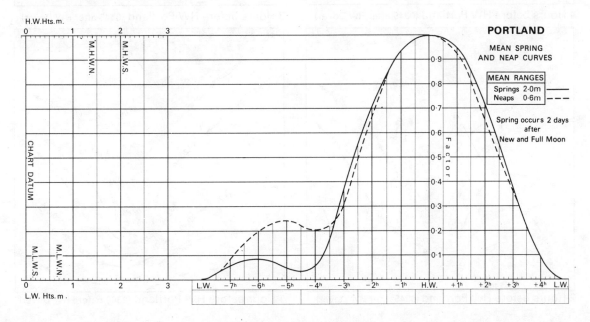

PORTLAND TIDAL STREAMS 10-2-9

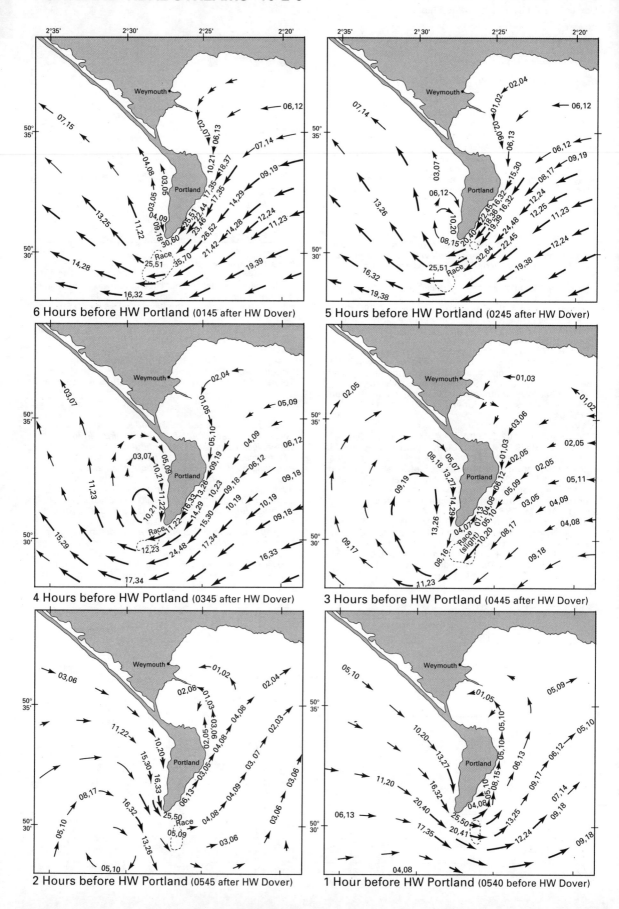

6 Hours before HW Portland (0145 after HW Dover)

5 Hours before HW Portland (0245 after HW Dover)

4 Hours before HW Portland (0345 after HW Dover)

3 Hours before HW Portland (0445 after HW Dover)

2 Hours before HW Portland (0545 after HW Dover)

1 Hour before HW Portland (0540 before HW Dover)

General Area 2   10.2.3

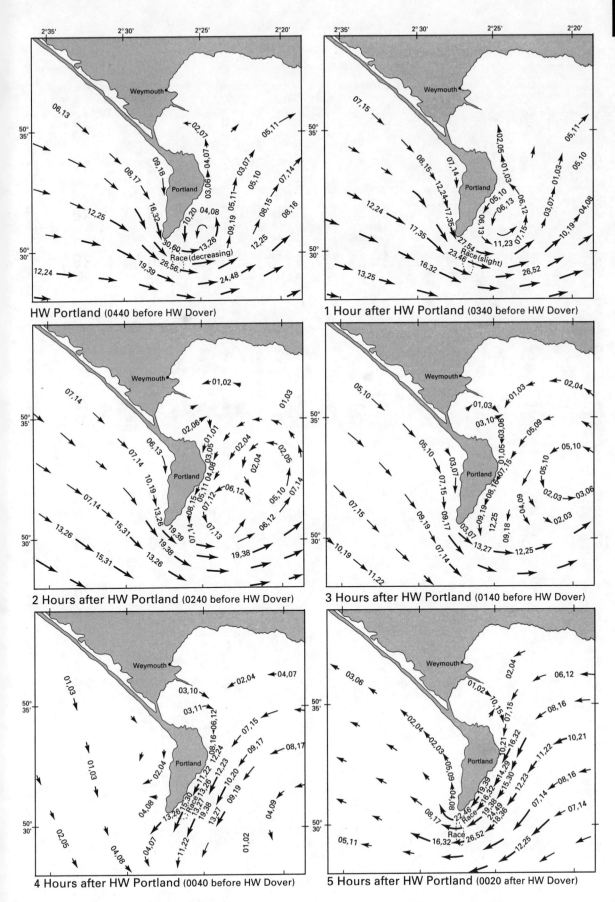

HW Portland (0440 before HW Dover)

1 Hour after HW Portland (0340 before HW Dover)

2 Hours after HW Portland (0240 before HW Dover)

3 Hours after HW Portland (0140 before HW Dover)

4 Hours after HW Portland (0040 before HW Dover)

5 Hours after HW Portland (0020 after HW Dover)

ENGLAND – PORTLAND

LAT 50°34′N   LONG 2°26′W

TIMES AND HEIGHTS OF HIGH AND LOW WATERS

YEAR **1996**

TIME ZONE (UT)
For Summer Time add ONE hour in non-shaded areas

JANUARY

Date	Day	Time	m	Time	m	Time	m	Time	m
1	M	0249	1.5	0803	0.8	1511	1.5	2028	0.6
2	TU	0350	1.6	0906	0.7	1611	1.5	2120	0.5
3	W	0440	1.7	0955	0.6	1702	1.6	2207	0.5
4	TH	0524	1.8	1039	0.5	1748	1.7	2251	0.4
5 O	F	0605	1.9	1121	0.4	1831	1.8	2334	0.3
6	SA	0643		1202	0.4	1910	1.8		
7	SU	0014	0.3	0720	2.0	1241	0.3	1947	1.8
8	M	0052	0.3	0755	2.0	1315	0.3	2022	1.8
9	TU	0124	0.3	0829	2.0	1343	0.3	2054	1.8
10	W	0151	0.3	0859	1.9	1408	0.3	2123	1.7
11	TH	0217	0.4	0926	1.8	1435	0.3	2150	1.6
12	F	0246	0.4	0955	1.7	1508	0.4	2222	1.5
13	SA	0321	0.5	1031	1.6	1551	0.4	2306	1.4
14	SU	0410	0.6	1120	1.5	1652	0.5		
15	M	0008	1.4	0524	0.8	1228	1.4	1813	0.6
16	TU	0134	1.5	0655	0.7	1357	1.5	1937	0.5
17	W	0305	1.6	0820	0.6	1530	1.6	2051	0.5
18	TH	0419	1.8	0931	0.5	1647	1.7	2155	0.3
19	F	0522	2.0	1030	0.3	1752	1.9	2251	0.2
20 ●	SA	0619	2.2	1122	0.2	1849	2.1	2341	0.1
21	SU	0712	2.3	1211	0.1	1941	2.2		
22	M	0029	0.1	0759	2.4	1258	0.0	2026	2.2
23	TU	0114	0.0	0843	2.4	1342	0.0	2108	2.1
24	W	0155	0.1	0923	2.3	1424	0.1	2145	2.0
25	TH	0236	0.2	1000	2.1	1506	0.2	2220	1.8
26	F	0315	0.3	1034	1.9	1547	0.3	2252	1.7
27	SA	0355	0.5	1106	1.7	1631	0.5	2326	1.5
28	SU	0442	0.6	1144	1.5	1723	0.6		
29	M	0012	1.4	0545	0.8	1236	1.3	1828	0.7
30	TU	0117	1.4	0710	0.8	1353	1.3	1943	0.7
31	W	0250	1.4	0835	0.8	1530	1.3	2049	0.6

FEBRUARY

Date	Day	Time	m	Time	m	Time	m	Time	m
1	TH	0403	1.5	0933	0.7	1635	1.5	2143	0.5
2	F	0455	1.7	1019	0.5	1726	1.6	2229	0.4
3	SA	0542	1.8	1101	0.4	1813	1.7	2313	0.3
4 O	SU	0626	2.0	1141	0.3	1856	1.8	2354	0.2
5	M	0707	2.0	1219	0.2	1935	1.9		
6	TU	0032	0.2	0745	2.1	1255	0.2	2011	1.9
7	W	0107	0.1	0820	2.1	1325	0.1	2043	1.9
8	TH	0137	0.1	0851	2.1	1353	0.2	2111	1.8
9	F	0205	0.2	0918	1.9	1421	0.2	2135	1.7
10	SA	0234	0.3	0945	1.7	1452	0.2	2203	1.6
11	SU	0305	0.3	1017	1.6	1527	0.3	2239	1.5
12	M	0345	0.4	1058	1.5	1617	0.4	2330	1.4
13	TU	0446	0.6	1157	1.4	1734	0.5		
14	W	0044	1.4	0622	0.7	1321	1.4	1912	0.6
15	TH	0225	1.5	0805	0.6	1507	1.5	2039	0.5
16	F	0357	1.7	0924	0.5	1635	1.6	2146	0.4
17	SA	0508	1.9	1022	0.3	1742	1.8	2241	0.2
18 ●	SU	0606	2.1	1113	0.1	1838	2.0	2330	0.1
19	M	0658	2.3	1159	0.0	1927	2.2		
20	TU	0015	0.0	0744	2.4	1243	-0.1	2009	2.2
21	W	0057	-0.1	0826	2.4	1324	-0.1	2048	2.2
22	TH	0136	0.0	0903	2.3	1403	0.0	2121	2.1
23	F	0213	0.2	0936	2.1	1439	0.1	2150	1.9
24	SA	0248	0.2	1003	1.8	1514	0.2	2215	1.7
25	SU	0322	0.4	1030	1.6	1546	0.4	2242	1.5
26	M	0356	0.5	1102	1.4	1620	0.6	2319	1.4
27	TU	0440	0.7	1147	1.3	1714	0.7		
28	W	0014	1.3	0616	0.8	1255	1.2	1853	0.8
29	TH	0133	1.3	0801	0.7	1439	1.2	2016	0.7

MARCH

Date	Day	Time	m	Time	m	Time	m	Time	m
1	F	0312	1.4	0909	0.6	1608	1.4	2116	0.6
2	SA	0422	1.6	0955	0.5	1703	1.5	2204	0.4
3	SU	0515	1.8	1036	0.3	1751	1.7	2248	0.3
4	M	0602	1.9	1115	0.2	1835	1.8	2329	0.2
5 O	TU	0647	2.0	1153	0.1	1916	1.9		
6	W	0007	0.1	0727	2.1	1229	0.1	1953	2.0
7	TH	0043	0.0	0803	2.1	1302	0.0	2026	2.0
8	F	0116	0.0	0836	2.0	1333	0.0	2055	1.9
9	SA	0148	0.1	0904	1.9	1405	0.1	2119	1.8
10	SU	0219	0.1	0932	1.8	1437	0.2	2147	1.7
11	M	0252	0.2	1004	1.7	1512	0.3	2221	1.6
12	TU	0332	0.4	1045	1.5	1558	0.4	2309	1.5
13	W	0432	0.5	1142	1.4	1714	0.6		
14	TH	0019	1.4	0610	0.6	1307	1.4	1858	0.6
15	F	0201	1.5	0757	0.6	1457	1.4	2028	0.6
16	SA	0339	1.6	0914	0.4	1624	1.6	2134	0.4
17	SU	0450	1.9	1009	0.3	1727	1.8	2226	0.3
18	M	0548	2.1	1057	0.1	1820	2.0	2313	0.1
19 ●	TU	0639	2.2	1141	0.0	1906	2.1	2356	0.0
20	W	0724	2.3	1223	-0.1	1948	2.2		
21	TH	0036	-0.1	0804	2.3	1302	-0.1	2024	2.2
22	F	0115	0.0	0839	2.2	1339	-0.1	2055	2.1
23	SA	0150	0.2	0909	2.0	1412	0.1	2120	1.9
24	SU	0224	0.2	0934	1.8	1443	0.2	2142	1.7
25	M	0254	0.3	0959	1.6	1508	0.4	2206	1.6
26	TU	0321	0.5	1029	1.4	1528	0.6	2237	1.4
27	W	0352	0.6	1110	1.2	1559	0.7	2323	1.3
28	TH	0459	0.7	1216	1.2	1730	0.8		
29	F	0037	1.3	0718	0.7	1352	1.2	1936	0.8
30	SA	0212	1.4	0833	0.6	1531	1.3	2043	0.6
31	SU	0337	1.5	0923	0.5	1631	1.5	2133	0.5

APRIL

Date	Day	Time	m	Time	m	Time	m	Time	m
1	M	0438	1.7	1004	0.3	1720	1.7	2217	0.3
2	TU	0531	1.9	1043	0.2	1806	1.9	2258	0.2
3	W	0618	2.0	1121	0.1	1849	2.0	2337	0.1
4 O	TH	0702	2.1	1158	0.0	1928	2.1		
5	F	0015	0.0	0741	2.1	1235	0.0	2004	2.1
6	SA	0052	0.0	0817	2.1	1311	0.0	2036	2.0
7	SU	0128	0.0	0849	2.0	1347	0.1	2105	2.0
8	M	0204	0.1	0920	1.9	1424	0.2	2135	1.8
9	TU	0243	0.2	0956	1.7	1504	0.3	2212	1.7
10	W	0329	0.4	1040	1.6	1555	0.5	2300	1.6
11	TH	0433	0.6	1140	1.5	1710	0.6		
12	F	0010	1.5	0602	0.7	1307	1.4	1843	0.7
13	SA	0147	1.5	0741	0.6	1447	1.5	2010	0.6
14	SU	0317	1.7	0854	0.5	1604	1.7	2114	0.5
15	M	0426	1.8	0948	0.3	1704	1.9	2206	0.4
16	TU	0524	2.0	1035	0.1	1755	2.0	2252	0.2
17 ●	W	0614	2.1	1118	0.0	1841	2.1	2334	0.1
18	TH	0700	2.2	1159	0.0	1922	2.2		
19	F	0014	0.1	0740	2.2	1238	0.0	1958	2.2
20	SA	0052	0.1	0815	2.1	1314	0.1	2028	2.1
21	SU	0128	0.1	0843	1.9	1348	0.2	2052	1.9
22	M	0202	0.2	0908	1.8	1417	0.3	2113	1.8
23	TU	0232	0.3	0934	1.6	1440	0.4	2138	1.6
24	W	0257	0.4	1004	1.4	1458	0.6	2205	1.5
25	TH	0324	0.6	1043	1.3	1529	0.7	2241	1.4
26	F	0412	0.6	1142	1.2	1629	0.8	2344	1.3
27	SA	0559	0.7	1308	1.2	1838	0.8		
28	SU	0115	1.4	0741	0.6	1439	1.3	2000	0.7
29	M	0244	1.5	0838	0.5	1548	1.5	2055	0.6
30	TU	0354	1.6	0923	0.4	1642	1.7	2142	0.4

Chart Datum: 0·93 metres below Ordnance Datum (Newlyn)

ENGLAND – PORTLAND

LAT 50°34'N   LONG 2°26'W

TIMES AND HEIGHTS OF HIGH AND LOW WATERS   YEAR **1996**

TIME ZONE (UT)
For Summer Time add ONE hour in non-shaded areas

MAY

Day	Time	m	Day	Time	m
1 W	0453 / 1005 / 1731 / 2224	1.8 / 0.2 / 1.9 / 0.3	**16** TH	0547 / 1052 / 1813 / 2311	1.9 / 0.2 / 2.0 / 0.3
2 TH	0545 / 1046 / 1817 / 2306	1.9 / 0.1 / 2.0 / 0.2	**17** F	0634 / 1133 / 1855 / 2351 ●	2.0 / 0.2 / 2.1 / 0.2
3 F O	0633 / 1127 / 1901 / 2347	2.0 / 0.1 / 2.1 / 0.1	**18** SA	0716 / 1213 / 1931	2.0 / 0.2 / 2.1
4 SA	0718 / 1208 / 1941	2.1 / 0.1 / 2.2	**19** SU	0031 / 0751 / 1251 / 2002	0.2 / 2.0 / 0.2 / 2.0
5 SU	0028 / 0758 / 1250 / 2018	0.1 / 2.1 / 0.1 / 2.1	**20** M	0109 / 0821 / 1327 / 2027	0.2 / 1.9 / 0.3 / 2.0
6 M	0110 / 0837 / 1332 / 2055	0.1 / 2.0 / 0.1 / 2.1	**21** TU	0144 / 0848 / 1358 / 2052	0.3 / 1.8 / 0.4 / 1.8
7 TU	0152 / 0915 / 1415 / 2131	0.1 / 1.9 / 0.2 / 2.0	**22** W	0215 / 0916 / 1424 / 2119	0.3 / 1.6 / 0.4 / 1.7
8 W	0237 / 0955 / 1501 / 2212	0.2 / 1.8 / 0.4 / 1.8	**23** TH	0240 / 0947 / 1444 / 2146	0.4 / 1.5 / 0.5 / 1.6
9 TH	0328 / 1043 / 1554 / 2303	0.4 / 1.7 / 0.5 / 1.7	**24** F	0305 / 1023 / 1513 / 2216	0.5 / 1.4 / 0.6 / 1.5
10 F	0430 / 1144 / 1701	0.5 / 1.6 / 0.6	**25** SA	0343 / 1111 / 1559 / 2302	0.5 / 1.3 / 0.7 / 1.4
11 SA	0008 / 0546 / 1302 / 1820	1.6 / 0.5 / 1.5 / 0.7	**26** SU	0442 / 1220 / 1716	0.6 / 1.3 / 0.8
12 SU	0131 / 0710 / 1424 / 1941	1.6 / 0.5 / 1.6 / 0.7	**27** M	0014 / 0607 / 1343 / 1852	1.4 / 0.6 / 1.3 / 0.7
13 M	0249 / 0824 / 1535 / 2048	1.7 / 0.5 / 1.7 / 0.6	**28** TU	0145 / 0730 / 1458 / 2005	1.4 / 0.5 / 1.5 / 0.6
14 TU	0356 / 0920 / 1634 / 2141	1.7 / 0.4 / 1.8 / 0.5	**29** W	0305 / 0831 / 1600 / 2100	1.5 / 0.4 / 1.7 / 0.5
15 W	0455 / 1008 / 1726 / 2228	1.9 / 0.3 / 1.9 / 0.4	**30** TH	0412 / 0923 / 1655 / 2149	1.7 / 0.3 / 1.8 / 0.4
			31 F	0511 / 1012 / 1746 / 2237	1.8 / 0.2 / 2.0 / 0.3

JUNE

Day	Time	m	Day	Time	m
1 SA O	0605 / 1100 / 1834 / 2324	2.0 / 0.2 / 2.1 / 0.2	**16** SU ●	0652 / 1150 / 1907	1.8 / 0.3 / 2.0
2 SU	0656 / 1147 / 1921	2.1 / 0.1 / 2.2	**17** M	0011 / 0730 / 1231 / 1939	0.3 / 1.9 / 0.3 / 2.0
3 M	0010 / 0743 / 1234 / 2005	0.1 / 2.1 / 0.1 / 2.2	**18** TU	0051 / 0802 / 1309 / 2009	0.1 / 1.8 / 0.3 / 2.0
4 TU	0057 / 0829 / 1321 / 2048	0.1 / 2.1 / 0.1 / 2.2	**19** W	0128 / 0832 / 1344 / 2038	0.1 / 1.8 / 0.3 / 1.9
5 W	0144 / 0913 / 1407 / 2131	0.1 / 2.0 / 0.2 / 2.1	**20** TH	0201 / 0903 / 1412 / 2107	0.3 / 1.7 / 0.4 / 1.8
6 TH	0232 / 0958 / 1455 / 2215	0.2 / 1.9 / 0.3 / 2.0	**21** F	0226 / 0934 / 1435 / 2135	0.3 / 1.6 / 0.5 / 1.7
7 F	0322 / 1045 / 1546 / 2303	0.3 / 1.8 / 0.4 / 1.9	**22** SA	0249 / 1005 / 1500 / 2203	0.4 / 1.5 / 0.5 / 1.6
8 SA	0418 / 1138 / 1642 / 2358	0.4 / 1.7 / 0.6 / 1.7	**23** SU	0319 / 1041 / 1536 / 2237	0.4 / 1.4 / 0.6 / 1.5
9 SU	0520 / 1240 / 1747	0.5 / 1.6 / 0.7	**24** M	0402 / 1129 / 1628 / 2327	0.5 / 1.4 / 0.6 / 1.4
10 M	0103 / 0630 / 1350 / 1900	1.6 / 0.5 / 1.6 / 0.7	**25** TU	0503 / 1237 / 1742	0.5 / 1.4 / 0.7
11 TU	0214 / 0743 / 1500 / 2013	1.6 / 0.5 / 1.6 / 0.7	**26** W	0037 / 0619 / 1359 / 1904	1.4 / 0.5 / 1.4 / 0.7
12 W	0323 / 0847 / 1602 / 2113	1.6 / 0.5 / 1.7 / 0.6	**27** TH	0206 / 0757 / 1515 / 2017	1.5 / 0.5 / 1.6 / 0.6
13 TH	0425 / 0940 / 1656 / 2204	1.7 / 0.4 / 1.8 / 0.5	**28** F	0329 / 0845 / 1620 / 2119	1.6 / 0.4 / 1.7 / 0.5
14 F	0519 / 1026 / 1745 / 2248	1.7 / 0.4 / 1.9 / 0.5	**29** SA	0439 / 0946 / 1718 / 2215	1.7 / 0.3 / 1.9 / 0.4
15 SA	0609 / 1109 / 1828 / 2330	1.8 / 0.3 / 2.0 / 0.4	**30** SU	0541 / 1041 / 1813 / 2308	1.9 / 0.2 / 2.1 / 0.2

JULY

Day	Time	m	Day	Time	m
1 M O	0639 / 1133 / 1906 / 2359	2.0 / 0.1 / 2.2 / 0.1	**16** TU	0710 / 1209 / 1921	1.8 / 0.3 / 2.0
2 TU	0732 / 1223 / 1955	2.1 / 0.1 / 2.3	**17** W	0031 / 0745 / 1249 / 1954	0.3 / 1.8 / 0.2 / 2.0
3 W	0047 / 0821 / 1311 / 2041	0.1 / 2.2 / 0.1 / 2.3	**18** TH	0109 / 0818 / 1325 / 2026	0.2 / 1.8 / 0.2 / 2.0
4 TH	0135 / 0907 / 1357 / 2125	0.1 / 2.1 / 0.1 / 2.3	**19** F	0142 / 0849 / 1356 / 2056	0.2 / 1.8 / 0.3 / 1.9
5 F	0222 / 0950 / 1443 / 2208	0.1 / 2.1 / 0.2 / 2.1	**20** SA	0208 / 0919 / 1421 / 2124	0.3 / 1.7 / 0.3 / 1.8
6 SA	0309 / 1033 / 1528 / 2250	0.2 / 1.9 / 0.3 / 2.0	**21** SU	0232 / 0946 / 1445 / 2150	0.3 / 1.6 / 0.4 / 1.7
7 SU	0357 / 1116 / 1617 / 2334	0.3 / 1.8 / 0.5 / 1.8	**22** M	0258 / 1014 / 1513 / 2218	0.3 / 1.5 / 0.4 / 1.6
8 M	0449 / 1205 / 1711	0.4 / 1.6 / 0.6	**23** TU	0333 / 1049 / 1553 / 2257	0.4 / 1.5 / 0.5 / 1.5
9 TU	0025 / 0548 / 1305 / 1815	1.6 / 0.5 / 1.5 / 0.7	**24** W	0420 / 1140 / 1652 / 2351	0.5 / 1.4 / 0.6 / 1.4
10 W	0128 / 0657 / 1417 / 1931	1.5 / 0.6 / 1.5 / 0.8	**25** TH	0529 / 1253 / 1815	0.5 / 1.4 / 0.7
11 TH	0244 / 0810 / 1528 / 2045	1.5 / 0.6 / 1.6 / .0.7	**26** F	0109 / 0655 / 1427 / 1944	1.4 / 0.6 / 1.5 / 0.6
12 F	0354 / 0912 / 1627 / 2142	1.5 / 0.6 / 1.7 / 0.7	**27** SA	0248 / 0820 / 1549 / 2101	1.5 / 0.5 / 1.7 / 0.5
13 SA	0453 / 1002 / 1718 / 2227	1.6 / 0.5 / 1.8 / 0.6	**28** SU	0414 / 0930 / 1657 / 2203	1.6 / 0.4 / 1.9 / 0.4
14 SU	0544 / 1046 / 1803 / 2310	1.6 / 0.4 / 1.9 / 0.4	**29** M	0525 / 1029 / 1757 / 2258	1.8 / 0.3 / 2.1 / 0.2
15 M ●	0629 / 1128 / 1844 / 2351	1.7 / 0.4 / 1.9 / 0.3	**30** TU O	0626 / 1122 / 1852 / 2349	2.0 / 0.1 / 2.3 / 0.1
			31 W	0720 / 1211 / 1942	2.1 / 0.0 / 2.4

AUGUST

Day	Time	m	Day	Time	m
1 TH	0036 / 0808 / 1258 / 2028	0.0 / 2.2 / 0.0 / 2.4	**16** F	0044 / 0758 / 1301 / 2009	0.2 / 1.9 / 0.2 / 2.0
2 F	0122 / 0852 / 1342 / 2110	0.0 / 2.2 / 0.0 / 2.4	**17** SA	0117 / 0830 / 1333 / 2040	0.2 / 1.9 / 0.2 / 2.0
3 SA	0206 / 0932 / 1424 / 2149	0.0 / 2.1 / 0.1 / 2.2	**18** SU	0145 / 0859 / 1400 / 2108	0.2 / 1.8 / 0.2 / 1.9
4 SU	0249 / 1010 / 1505 / 2226	0.1 / 2.0 / 0.2 / 2.0	**19** M	0211 / 0924 / 1425 / 2133	0.2 / 1.7 / 0.3 / 1.8
5 M	0331 / 1045 / 1547 / 2302	0.3 / 1.8 / 0.4 / 1.8	**20** TU	0237 / 0948 / 1452 / 2200	0.3 / 1.6 / 0.4 / 1.6
6 TU	0415 / 1122 / 1634 / 2340	0.4 / 1.6 / 0.6 / 1.6	**21** W	0307 / 1020 / 1525 / 2234	0.4 / 1.6 / 0.5 / 1.5
7 W	0505 / 1207 / 1732	0.6 / 1.5 / 0.7	**22** TH	0347 / 1104 / 1617 / 2323	0.5 / 1.5 / 0.6 / 1.4
8 TH	0028 / 0608 / 1313 / 1849	1.4 / 0.7 / 1.4 / 0.8	**23** F	0451 / 1209 / 1745	0.6 / 1.4 / 0.7
9 F	0148 / 0728 / 1450 / 2019	1.3 / 0.7 / 1.4 / 0.8	**24** SA	0037 / 0631 / 1345 / 1928	1.4 / 0.7 / 1.5 / 0.7
10 SA	0326 / 0844 / 1600 / 2122	1.3 / 0.7 / 1.5 / 0.7	**25** SU	0224 / 0808 / 1526 / 2052	1.4 / 0.6 / 1.6 / 0.6
11 SU	0429 / 0937 / 1652 / 2206	1.4 / 0.6 / 1.7 / 0.6	**26** M	0401 / 0921 / 1640 / 2154	1.6 / 0.5 / 1.9 / 0.4
12 M	0520 / 1021 / 1737 / 2247	1.6 / 0.5 / 1.8 / 0.5	**27** TU	0512 / 1018 / 1741 / 2247	1.8 / 0.3 / 2.1 / 0.2
13 TU	0605 / 1103 / 1819 / 2327	1.7 / 0.4 / 1.9 / 0.3	**28** W O	0611 / 1108 / 1835 / 2335	2.0 / 0.1 / 2.3 / 0.1
14 W ●	0646 / 1144 / 1858	1.8 / 0.3 / 2.0	**29** TH	0703 / 1155 / 1924	2.2 / 0.0 / 2.4
15 TH	0007 / 0724 / 1224 / 1934	0.2 / 1.9 / 0.2 / 2.1	**30** F	0020 / 0748 / 1239 / 2007	0.0 / 2.3 / 0.0 / 2.5
			31 SA	0104 / 0830 / 1321 / 2048	-0.1 / 2.3 / 0.0 / 2.4

Chart Datum: 0·93 metres below Ordnance Datum (Newlyn)

ENGLAND – PORTLAND

LAT 50°34′N   LONG 2°26′W

TIMES AND HEIGHTS OF HIGH AND LOW WATERS   YEAR **1996**

TIME ZONE (UT)
For Summer Time add ONE hour in non-shaded areas

SEPTEMBER

Day	Time	m	Time	m	Time	m	Time	m
1 SU	0145	0.0	0907	2.2	1401	0.1	2124	2.2
16 M	0117	0.2	0836	2.0	1334	0.2	2047	2.0
2 M	0223	0.1	0940	2.0	1439	0.2	2157	2.0
17 TU	0146	0.2	0901	1.9	1403	0.3	2113	1.8
3 TU	0301	0.3	1009	1.8	1516	0.4	2226	1.7
18 W	0215	0.3	0926	1.8	1432	0.4	2142	1.7
4 W	0338	0.5	1037	1.6	1557	0.6	2256	1.5
19 TH	0245	0.4	0957	1.7	1507	0.5	2218	1.6
5 TH	0417	0.6	1112	1.5	1649	0.8	2336	1.3
20 F	0324	0.5	1040	1.6	1600	0.6	2308	1.5
6 F	0513	0.8	1203	1.4	1810	0.9		
21 SA	0428	0.7	1143	1.5	1736	0.7		
7 SA	0041	1.2	0641	0.9	1326	1.4	1950	0.8
22 SU	0025	1.4	0619	0.8	1319	1.5	1922	0.7
8 SU	0301	1.3	0810	0.8	1524	1.5	2057	0.7
23 M	0219	1.5	0759	0.7	1507	1.7	2042	0.6
9 M	0408	1.4	0908	0.7	1619	1.6	2139	0.6
24 TU	0353	1.6	0909	0.6	1621	1.9	2140	0.4
10 TU	0454	1.6	0953	0.5	1705	1.8	2219	0.4
25 W	0457	1.9	1003	0.4	1720	2.1	2229	0.2
11 W	0537	1.7	1035	0.4	1748	1.9	2258	0.3
26 TH	0551	2.1	1051	0.2	1812	2.3	2315	0.1
12 TH ●	0618	1.9	1115	0.3	1829	2.0	2336	0.2
27 F ○	0640	2.2	1135	0.1	1900	2.4	2358	0.0
13 F	0657	2.0	1155	0.2	1909	2.1		
28 SA	0724	2.3	1217	0.1	1943	2.4		
14 SA	0013	0.1	0733	2.0	1231	0.2	1945	2.1
29 SU	0039	0.0	0803	2.3	1258	0.1	2022	2.3
15 SU	0047	0.1	0806	2.0	1304	0.2	2018	2.1
30 M	0118	0.0	0838	2.2	1336	0.1	2056	2.2

OCTOBER

Day	Time	m	Time	m	Time	m	Time	m
1 TU	0155	0.2	0908	2.1	1412	0.3	2125	1.9
16 W	0122	0.2	0840	2.0	1342	0.3	2056	1.9
2 W	0228	0.3	0931	1.9	1447	0.4	2150	1.7
17 TH	0156	0.3	0909	1.9	1418	0.4	2129	1.8
3 TH	0259	0.5	0954	1.7	1522	0.6	2217	1.5
18 F	0231	0.5	0942	1.8	1501	0.5	2209	1.6
4 F	0324	0.7	1024	1.5	1605	0.8	2254	1.3
19 SA	0315	0.6	1026	1.7	1602	0.6	2303	1.5
5 SA	0352	0.8	1107	1.4	1727	0.9	2356	1.2
20 SU	0425	0.8	1129	1.6	1732	0.7		
6 SU	0538	0.9	1216	1.4	1908	0.9		
21 M	0023	1.5	0606	0.8	1304	1.6	1907	0.7
7 M	0151	1.2	0725	0.9	1358	1.4	2019	0.7
22 TU	0214	1.5	0740	0.8	1445	1.7	2022	0.6
8 TU	0336	1.4	0832	0.8	1528	1.6	2105	0.6
23 W	0336	1.7	0849	0.7	1556	1.9	2118	0.4
9 W	0421	1.6	0921	0.6	1622	1.7	2145	0.5
24 TH	0435	1.9	0943	0.5	1654	2.0	2206	0.3
10 TH	0502	1.8	1003	0.5	1709	1.9	2224	0.3
25 F	0527	2.1	1030	0.4	1746	2.2	2251	0.2
11 F	0544	1.9	1043	0.4	1755	2.0	2301	0.2
26 SA ○	0614	2.2	1113	0.3	1834	2.3	2333	0.1
12 SA ●	0625	2.1	1122	0.3	1838	2.1	2338	0.2
27 SU	0657	2.3	1206	0.2	1917	2.3		
13 SU	0704	2.1	1158	0.2	1918	2.1		
28 M	0013	0.1	0735	2.3	1234	0.2	1956	2.2
14 M	0013	0.1	0739	2.2	1234	0.2	1954	2.1
29 TU	0051	0.2	0809	2.2	1312	0.3	2028	2.0
15 TU	0048	0.2	0812	2.1	1308	0.2	2026	2.0
30 W	0127	0.3	0848	2.1	1348	0.3	2055	1.9
31 TH	0159	0.4	0857	1.9	1422	0.5	2119	1.7

NOVEMBER

Day	Time	m	Time	m	Time	m	Time	m
1 F	0226	0.6	0920	1.8	1454	0.6	2147	1.5
16 SA	0226	0.5	0939	2.0	1500	0.5	2208	1.7
2 SA	0245	0.7	0947	1.6	1525	0.7	2223	1.4
17 SU	0316	0.6	1025	1.8	1600	0.6	2303	1.6
3 SU	0306	0.8	1020	1.5	1617	0.8	2317	1.3
18 M	0419	0.7	1125	1.7	1716	0.6		
4 M	0354	0.9	1117	1.4	1810	0.9		
19 TU	0018	1.6	0540	0.8	1247	1.7	1837	0.6
5 TU	0042	1.3	0625	1.0	1247	1.4	1928	0.8
20 W	0149	1.6	0707	0.8	1415	1.7	1950	0.6
6 W	0226	1.4	0749	0.9	1421	1.5	2022	0.6
21 TH	0306	1.7	0820	0.7	1526	1.8	2049	0.5
7 TH	0334	1.6	0844	0.7	1532	1.7	2105	0.5
22 F	0407	1.9	0918	0.6	1626	1.9	2140	0.4
8 F	0422	1.8	0928	0.6	1628	1.8	2145	0.4
23 SA	0459	2.0	1007	0.5	1720	2.0	2225	0.3
9 SA	0508	1.9	1009	0.5	1719	1.9	2223	0.3
24 SU	0547	2.1	1051	0.4	1809	2.1	2308	0.3
10 SU	0552	2.1	1048	0.4	1806	2.0	2302	0.2
25 M ○	0630	2.2	1133	0.4	1853	2.1	2348	0.3
11 M ●	0634	2.2	1127	0.3	1851	2.1	2342	0.2
26 TU	0709	2.2	1212	0.3	1932	2.0		
12 TU	0714	2.2	1206	0.3	1932	2.1		
27 W	0027	0.3	0742	2.2	1252	0.3	2004	1.9
13 W	0022	0.2	0751	2.2	1246	0.3	2010	2.1
28 TH	0104	0.3	0809	2.1	1329	0.4	2032	1.8
14 TH	0102	0.2	0826	2.2	1327	0.3	2046	2.0
29 F	0138	0.4	0834	2.0	1404	0.4	2058	1.7
15 F	0143	0.3	0901	2.1	1410	0.4	2124	1.9
30 SA	0206	0.5	0900	1.9	1434	0.5	2127	1.6

DECEMBER

Day	Time	m	Time	m	Time	m	Time	m
1 SU	0227	0.6	0927	1.7	1458	0.6	2201	1.5
16 M	0310	0.5	1027	1.9	1548	0.4	2258	1.7
2 M	0249	0.7	0956	1.6	1528	0.7	2244	1.4
17 TU	0404	0.6	1118	1.8	1649	0.5	2356	1.6
3 TU	0325	0.8	1037	1.5	1621	0.7	2347	1.3
18 W	0508	0.7	1220	1.7	1757	0.6		
4 W	0431	0.9	1142	1.4	1754	0.7		
19 TH	0107	1.6	0621	0.8	1335	1.6	1908	0.6
5 TH	0112	1.3	0627	0.9	1314	1.4	1916	0.7
20 F	0224	1.6	0740	0.8	1450	1.6	2014	0.6
6 F	0234	1.5	0750	0.8	1438	1.5	2012	0.6
21 SA	0333	1.7	0849	0.7	1557	1.7	2111	0.5
7 SA	0338	1.7	0844	0.7	1546	1.7	2100	0.5
22 SU	0431	1.8	0944	0.6	1654	1.8	2201	0.5
8 SU	0431	1.8	0931	0.5	1644	1.8	2146	0.4
23 M	0521	1.9	1031	0.5	1745	1.8	2245	0.4
9 M	0520	2.0	1016	0.4	1738	1.9	2232	0.3
24 TU ○	0606	2.0	1113	0.5	1831	1.9	2327	0.4
10 TU ●	0608	2.1	1100	0.3	1828	2.0	2318	0.2
25 W	0647	2.1	1154	0.4	1912	1.9		
11 W	0653	2.2	1145	0.3	1915	2.1		
26 TH	0007	0.3	0721	2.1	1234	0.3	1946	1.9
12 TH	0004	0.2	0736	2.3	1231	0.2	2000	2.1
27 F	0046	0.3	0752	2.1	1312	0.3	2016	1.8
13 F	0050	0.2	0819	2.3	1317	0.2	2043	2.0
28 SA	0122	0.3	0820	2.0	1348	0.3	2045	1.8
14 SA	0135	0.3	0900	2.2	1404	0.3	2125	2.0
29 SU	0154	0.4	0849	1.9	1417	0.4	2115	1.7
15 SU	0222	0.4	0942	2.1	1454	0.3	2209	1.9
30 M	0218	0.5	0918	1.8	1438	0.4	2145	1.6
31 TU	0238	0.5	0946	1.7	1501	0.5	2217	1.5

Chart Datum: 0·93 metres below Ordnance Datum (Newlyn)

WEYMOUTH 　　10-2-10

Dorset 50°36'·54N 02°26'·50W

CHARTS
AC *2172*, 2268, 2255, *2610*; Imray C4, C5; Stanfords 12; OS 194

TIDES
–0438 Dover; ML 1·1; Zone 0 (UT)

Standard Port PORTLAND (←)

Predictions for Weymouth are as for Portland. Mean ranges are small: 0·6m at np and 2·0m at sp.
NOTE: Double LWs occur; predictions are for first LW. At sp there is a LW stand lasting about 4 hrs; 1 hr at nps. Due to an eddy, the tidal stream in Weymouth Roads is W-going at all times except HW –0510 to HW –0310.

SHELTER
Good, but swell enters hbr in strong E wind. Berth in The Cove on pontoon S side or on the N side (Custom House Quay) opposite RDYC; in season rafting-up is the rule. The quays between The Cove and the lifting bridge are reserved for FVs. Hbr speed limit is 'Dead Slow'.
It is feasible to ‡ in Weymouth B, NE of hbr ent in about 3m, but necessarily some way offshore due to the drying sands. See also 10.2.9 for possible ‡ in Portland Harbour.
Nota Bene: A 237 berth marina (2·5m) is **provisionally** due to open in Spring/Summer 1996, subject to the usual statutory planning approval/public enquiry. It will be located as shown on the chartlet, ie beyond the Town Bridge and pontoons of the existing municipal marina. The new marina will have all the usual facilities, including visitors' berths. Further details will be published in the Supplements to this almanac, as they become known.

NAVIGATION
WPT 50°36'·68N, 02°26'·10W 060°/240° from/to front ldg lt, 0·50M. The hbr ent lies deep in the NW corner of Weymouth Bay; it could in some conditions be confused with the N ent to Portland Hbr. Fishing factory ships are often at ‡ in the NE part of Weymouth Bay.
Caution: ferries/fast catamarans entering/leaving; comply with IPTS.
Bridge lifts 0900, 1100, 1300 and 1500LT summer, or on request (2 hrs notice); clearance when down is 2·7–3·8m at HW, 4·6–5·2m at LW.
NOTE: If heading E, check Lulworth firing programme; see overleaf and Supplements for current dates.

LIGHTS AND MARKS
Conspic ch spire, 6ca NNW of hbr ent, is a useful day mark to help find the ent when approaching from SE past the Portland bkwtrs or from the E.
Portland 'A' Head lt ho, Fl 10s 22m 20M, is 1·7M SE of hbr ent and provides the best initial guidance at night. Pierhd lts are hard to see against shore lts. Ldg lts 240°, 2 FR (H24), are 500m inside the pierheads, daymarks are R open ◊s on W poles; they are not visible until the harbour entrance is opened.
IPTS must be obeyed. They are shown from a RW mast near the root of the S pier. There is one additional signal:
　2 Ⓡ over 1 Ⓖ = Ent and dep prohib (ent obstructed).
If no sigs are shown, vessels are clear to enter or leave with caution. Sigs are not too easy to see, by day/night.

RADIO TELEPHONE
VHF Ch 12 16 (0800-2000 summer and when vessel due).

TELEPHONE (01305)
Hr Mr 206278/206423; MRSC 760439; Marinecall 0891 500457; ⌗ (01752) 220661; Police 251212; Ⓗ 772211.

FACILITIES
Marina (see under SHELTER) 237 berths, usual facilities; **Hbr and The Cove** AB £9 - £12 (£4 for <4 hrs), M; **Custom House Quay** FW, AB, showers;
Royal Dorset YC ☎ 786258, M, Bar; **Weymouth SC** ☎ 785481, M, Bar;
Services: CH, Sh, ACA, Gaz, Rigging, D (pontoon), Slip, ME, Ⓔ, El, CH. D (only) from road tanker daily 0700-1900, min quantity 25ltrs; ☎ 775465 or mobile 0860 912401 or call *Raybar* VHF Ch 06.
Town EC Wed; P & D (cans), FW, V, R, Bar, ✉, Ⓑ, ⇌, ✈ (Bournemouth).

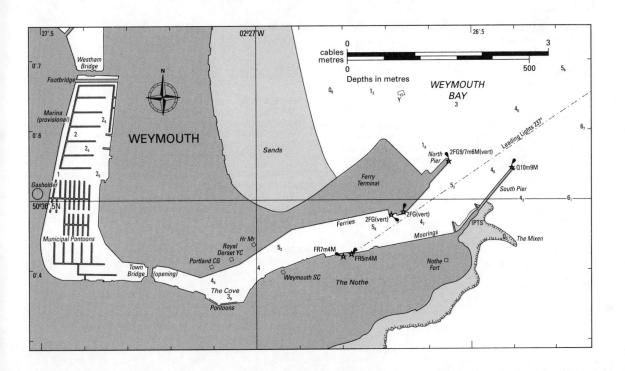

ANCHORAGES AND RANGES EAST OF WEYMOUTH

LULWORTH COVE, Dorset, 50°36′.97N 02°14′.74W. AC *2172*. HW −0449 on Dover, see 10.2.8 Tides; ML 1·2m. Good shelter in fair weather and offshore winds, but heavy swell enters the cove in S and SW winds; if strong the ⚓ becomes untenable. Enter the cove slightly E of centre. There is a YB buoy for the range safety launch in the middle of the cove in about 4m CD. ⚓ in NE part in 2·5m. Holding is poor. 8kn speed limit. Local moorings, village and slip are on W side. Facilities: EC Wed/Sat; FW at tap in car park, Bar, ⊠, R, Slip.

LULWORTH FIRING RANGES. There are 2 danger areas along the coast from Lulworth Cove to Kimmeridge Bay, thence to a position 0·5M SW of St Alban's Head: The Inner area extends 5·5M offshore and is used by the army as shown below. The Outer area extends to 12M and is never active at night and rarely at weekends. Warships may use the inner and outer ranges, firing Eastward from Adamant Shoal (approx 02°19′W) at the 3 DZ target buoys, (up to 3M SW of St Alban's Hd) which should be avoided by at least 1M. Warships fly R flags and other vessels/helicopters may patrol the area.
Firing on the Inner range occurs most weekdays from 0930-1700 (1200 on Fri), often on Tues and Thurs nights for 3-4 hrs and up to six weekends per year. There is NO firing in August. When firing is in progress R flags (Fl R lts at night) are flown from St Alban's Hd and Bindon Hill. However, further inland, some R flags fly whether or not firing is taking place; these mark the boundary of the range Land Area. VHF Ch 08 is monitored by Range Control and the Range safety boats.
Times of firing are published locally, sent to Hr Mrs and YCs and can be obtained from the Range Officer ☎ (01929) 462721 ext. 4819/4859 during office hours and at other times from the guardroom ext 4824. Firing details are broadcast by Radio Solent (221m/1359kHz, 300m/999kHz or 96·1 MHz VHF) daily (see 10·2·18) and 2 Counties Radio (362m/828kHz and 97.2MHz) and can be obtained from Portland CG (Ch 67), Portland Naval Base (Ch 13 14), or Range Safety Boats (Ch 08). The annual firing weekends and No Firing periods are published in the Supplements to this Almanac.
All the Land Area and the Inner Sea Danger Area (D026 Inner) are subject to the regulations laid down in *The Lulworth Ranges Byelaws 1978 operative from 10 Nov 1978 - Statutory Instruments 1978 No 1663.* A copy may be obtained from HMSO. A key passage states: *The Byelaws shall not apply to any vessel in the ordinary course of navigation, not being used for fishing, in the Sea Area and remaining in the Sea Area no longer than is reasonably necessary to pass through the Sea Area.* Nevertheless yachts should make every reasonable effort to keep clear when firing is in progress. If on passage between Weymouth and Anvil Pt, a track via 50°30′N 02°10′W will clear the S boundary of the Inner range and St Alban's Race, and is only 3·3M longer than a direct trk.

WORBARROW BAY, Dorset, 50°37′.00N 02°12′.00W. AC *2172*. Tides as Lulworth Cove/Mupe Bay, see 10.2.8. Worbarrow is a 1½M wide bay, close E of Lulworth Cove. It is easily identified from seaward by the V-shaped gap in the hills at Arish Mell, centre of bay just E of Bindon Hill. Bindon Hill also has a conspic white chalk scar due to cliff falls. Caution: Mupe Rks at W end and other rks 1ca off NW side. ⚓s in about 3m sheltered from W or E winds at appropriate end. The bay lies within Lulworth Ranges (see above); landing prohib at Arish Mell. No lights/facilities.

CHAPMAN'S POOL, Dorset, 50°35′.50N 02°03′.85W. AC *2172*. Tidal data is approx that for Swanage (10. 2.11). Chapman's Pool, like Worbarrow Bay, Brandy Bay and Kimmeridge Bay, is picturesque and convenient when the wind is off-shore. ⚓ in depths of about 3m in centre of bay to avoid tidal swirl, but beware large unlit B buoy (for Range Safety boat). From here to St Alban's Hd the stream runs SSE almost continuously due to a back eddy. There are no lights and no facilities.

SWANAGE   10-2-11
Dorset 50°36′.42N 01°56′.97W

CHARTS
AC *2172, 2610*, 2175; Imray C4; Stanfords 12, 15; OS 195

TIDES
HW Sp −0235 & +0125, Np −0515 & +0120 on Dover; ML 1·5

Standard Port PORTSMOUTH (→)

Times				Height (metres)			
High Water		Low Water		MHWS	MHWN	MLWN	MLWS
0000	0600	0500	1100	4·7	3·8	1·9	0·8
1200	1800	1700	2300				
Differences SWANAGE							
−0250	+0105	−0105	−0105	−2·7	−2·2	−0·7	−0·3
POOLE HARBOUR ENTRANCE							
−0240	+0105	−0100	−0030	−2·7	−2·2	−0·7	−0·3

NOTE: Double HWs occur except at nps and predictions are for the higher HW. Near nps there is a stand, and the predictions shown are for the middle of the stand. See 10·2·12.

SHELTER
Good ⚓ in winds from SW to N, but bad in E/SE winds >F4 due to swell which may persist for 6 hrs after a blow. >F6 holding gets very difficult. Pier (open Apr-Oct) is under repair and may provide landing. Nearest safe haven is Poole.

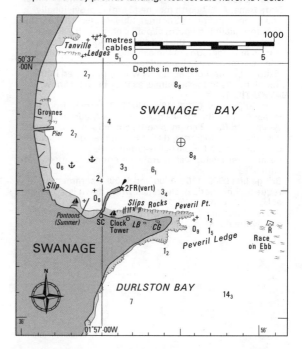

NAVIGATION
WPT 50°36′.70N 01°56′.50W, 054°/234° from/to pier hd, 0·30M. Coming from S beware Peveril Ledge and its Race which can be vicious with a SW wind against the main ebb. It is best to keep 1M seaward of Durlston Hd and Peveril Pt. On the W side of Swanage B, keep clear of Tanville and Phippards Ledges, approx 300m off the beach. On the S side of the pier are the ruins of an old pier.

LIGHTS AND MARKS
The only lts are 2 FR (vert) on the pier; difficult to see due to confusing street lts. Peveril Ledge By, PHM unlit, hard to pick out at night due to Anvil Pt lt; keep 0·5M clear to E.

RADIO TELEPHONE
None.

TELEPHONE (01929)
MRSC (01305) 760439; ⌗ (01703) 827350; Marinecall 0891 500457; Police 422004; Dr 422231; Ⓗ 422282.

FACILITIES
Pier, L, AB (HW only); **Swanage SC** ☎ 422987, Slip, L, FW, Bar; **Boat Park** (Peveril Pt), Slip, FW, L;
Services: Diving, Salvage, Towing.
Town P & D (cans), FW, V, R, Bar, ⊠, Ⓑ, ⇌ (bus to Wareham), ✈ (Bournemouth).

SPECIAL TIDAL PROBLEMS BETWEEN SWANAGE AND SELSEY 10-2-12

Due to the complex tidal variations between Portland and Portsmouth, time and height differences for harbours on this coast will give only approximate predictions. A more accurate result is achieved by using the curves which are given and discussed below.

Special curves, as shown on the following two pages, are given for individual ports owing to their rapidly changing tidal characteristics and the distorted tidal curves in this area. Since their low water (LW) points are more sharply defined than high water (HW), the times on these curves are referenced to LW, but otherwise they are used as described in 9·4. Box 17 of the tidal prediction form (NP204, shown in the RH column) should be amended to read 'Time of LW'.

Ports between Swanage and Yarmouth: Height differences, as shown for each secondary port, always refer to the higher HW (that which reaches a factor of 1·0 on the curves). The higher HW should be used to obtain the range at the Secondary Port. The time differences, which are not needed for this calculation, also refer to the higher HW.

Since the curves at these ports change considerably in shape and duration between Springs and Neaps, the tide cannot adequately be defined by only two curves. A third, "critical" curve, is therefore shown for the range at Portsmouth (indicated on the right of the graph) at which the two high waters are equal at the port concerned. Interpolation should be between this critical curve and either the spring or neap curve, as appropriate.

Note that, whilst the critical curve extends throughout the tidal cycle, the spring and neap curves stop at the higher HW. Thus for a range at Portsmouth of 3·9m, the factor for 7hrs after LW Poole (Town Quay) should be referenced to the following LW; whereas if the range at Portsmouth had been 1·9m it should be referenced to the preceding LW.

The procedure is shown step-by-step in the following example using the **Differences SWANAGE** below and the special curves for Swanage, Poole (Ent) and Bournemouth printed for convenience at the foot of this page.

Example: Find the height of tide at Swanage at 0200 on a day when the tidal predictions for Portsmouth are:

19 0100 4·6
   0613 1·1
M 1314 4·5
   1833 0·8

Standard Port PORTSMOUTH (⟶)

Times				Height (metres)			
High Water		Low Water		MHWS	MHWN	MLWN	MLWS
0000	0600	0500	1100	4·7	3·8	1·9	0·8
1200	1800	1700	2300				
Differences SWANAGE							
−0250	+0105	−0105	−0105	−2·7	−2·2	−0·7	−0·3

(1) Complete the top part of the tidal prediction form (next Col), omitting the HW time column (boxes 1, 5 & 9).
(2) On the left of the Swanage tidal curve diagram, plot the Secondary Port HW and LW heights (1·9 and 0·6m from (1) above), and join the points by a sloping line.

Tidal prediction form   Time or height required 0200

	TIME		HEIGHT	
	HW	LW	HW	LW
Standard Port *Portsmouth*	1	2 0613	3 4·6	4 1·1
Differences	5	6 −0105	7 −2·7	8 −0·5
Secondary Port *Swanage*	9	10 0508	11 1·9	12 0·6
Duration (or time from HW to LW)	13	9–10 or 10–9	Range Stand. Port 14 3·5	3–4
			Range Secdy. Port 15 1·3	11–12

*Springs/Neaps/Interpolate

Start height at given time 10	Time reqd.	16	0200	17 + 18
	Time of ~~HW~~ LW	17	0508	10
17 – 16	Interval	18	−0308	Date..19th Nov
	Factor	19	0·84	Time zone .0 (GMT)
19 x 15	Rise above LW	20	1·1	22 – 21
12	Height of LW	21	0·6	12 Start: time for given height
20 + 21	Height reqd.	22	1·7	

*Delete as necessary

(3) The time required (0200) is 3hr 8min before the time of LW at the Secondary Port, so from this point draw a line vertically up towards the curves.
(4) It is necessary to interpolate for the day's range at Portsmouth (3·5m), which is about mid-way between the spring curve (3·9m) and the critical curve (2·8m). This should give a point level with a factor of 0·84.
(5) From this point draw a horizontal line to meet the sloping line constructed in (2) above.
(6) From the point where the horizontal line meets the sloping line, proceed vertically to the height scale at the top, and read off the height required, 1·7m.

The Factor method of doing the calculation, instead of the graphical method just described, is shown in the completed lower part of the tidal prediction form above. The procedure follows that given in 9·4·3. Note that box 17 is amended to read 'Time of LW'.

Fig 10A is reproduced at the end of this section from earlier editions of Admiralty Tide Tables. It shows tabular data which provide a less accurate but quicker method of finding intermediate heights for certain places. It is useful to note that the area enclosed by the dotted lines represents the period during which the tide stands and in which a second HW may occur.
To use this table, note that the upper of the three height figures given is for mean spring tides, the middle for average and the lower for mean neap tides:
Determine whether the time required is nearer to HW or LW at Portsmouth and work out the interval (between time required and the nearest HW or LW at Portsmouth). Extract the height of the corresponding predicted HW (left hand column) or LW (right hand column). By interpolation between the heights of HW or LW, read off the height of tide under the appropriate column (hrs before/after HW or hrs before/after LW).

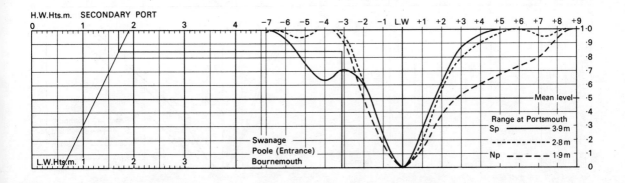

TIDAL CURVES – SWANAGE TO SELSEY

Tidal curves for places between Swanage and Selsey are given below, and their use is explained above. In this area the times of LW are defined more sharply than the times of HW, and the curves are therefore drawn with their times related to LW instead of HW.

Apart from referencing the times to LW, the procedure for obtaining intermediate heights with these curves is the same as that used for normal Secondary Ports (see 9.4.2). For most places a third curve is shown, for the range at Portsmouth at which the two HWs are equal at the port concerned; for interpolation between the curves see the previous page.

Note 1.* Due to the constriction of the R Medina, Newport requires special treatment since the hbr dries out at 1·4m. The calculation should be made using the LW time and height differences for Cowes, and the HW height differences for Newport. Any calculated heights which fall below 1·4m should be treated as 1·4m.

Note 2.* Wareham and Tuckton LWs do not fall below 0·7m except under very low river flow conditions.

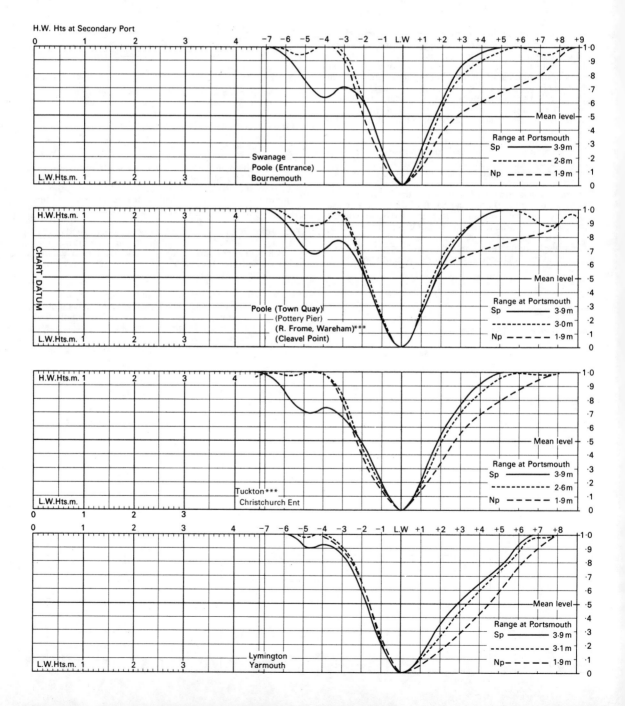

TIDAL CURVES *continued*

H.W. Hts at Secondary Port

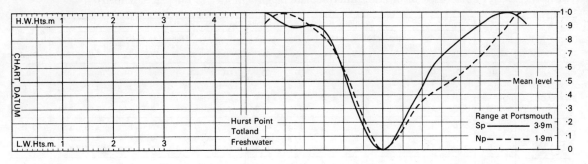

Hurst Point
Totland
Freshwater

Range at Portsmouth
Sp ——— 3·9m
Np – – – 1·9m

Mean level

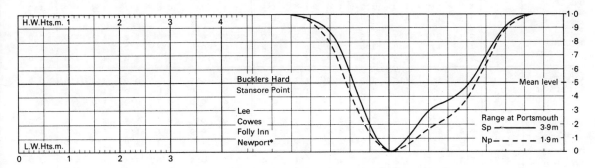

Bucklers Hard
Stansore Point

Lee
Cowes
Folly Inn
Newport*

Range at Portsmouth
Sp ——— 3·9m
Np – – – 1·9m

Mean level

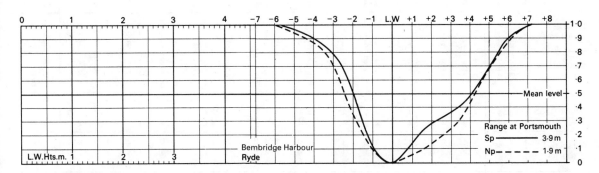

Bembridge Harbour
Ryde

Range at Portsmouth
Sp ——— 3·9m
Np – – – 1·9m

Mean level

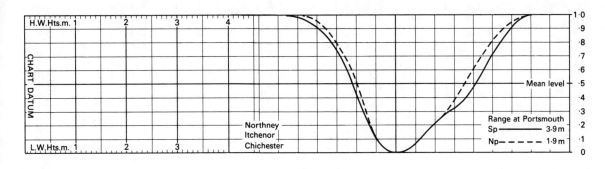

Northney
Itchenor
Chichester

Range at Portsmouth
Sp ——— 3·9m
Np – – – 1·9m

Mean level

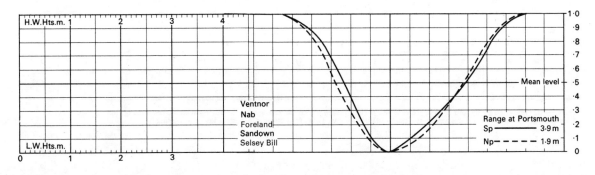

Ventnor
Nab
Foreland
Sandown
Selsey Bill

Range at Portsmouth
Sp ——— 3·9m
Np – – – 1·9m

Mean level

SWANAGE TO NAB TOWER

FIG 10A   (To be used for finding intermediate heights in metres for places named)

Place	Height of H.W. at Portsmouth m.	HOURLY HEIGHTS ABOVE CHART DATUM AT THE PLACE — Hours before or after HIGH WATER AT PORTSMOUTH							Hours before or after LOW WATER AT PORTSMOUTH						Height of L.W. at Portsmouth m.
		3b.	2b.	1b.	H.W.	1a.	2a.	3a.	2b.	1b.	L.W.	1a.	2a.	3a.	
		m.	m.	m.	m.	m.	m.	m.	m.	m.	m.	m.	m.	m.	m.
SWANAGE	4·7	1·9	1·8	1·5	1·3	1·4	1·2	0·8	0·6	0·3	0·8	1·3	1·7	1·8	0·6
	4·3	1·6	1·6	1·5	1·5	1·2	1·4	1·1	0·9	0·8	1·0	1·3	1·5	1·6	1·2
	3·8	1·5	1·5	1·5	1·5	1·6	1·5	1·3	1·2	1·1	1·2	1·3	1·4	1·4	1·8
POOLE ENTRANCE	4·7	2·0	1·9	1·6	1·4	1·5	1·4	0·9	0·7	0·3	0·8	1·3	1·6	1·9	0·6
	4·3	1·6	1·6	1·5	1·5	1·5	1·5	1·1	1·0	0·8	0·9	1·2	1·5	1·6	1·2
	3·8	1·4	1·5	1·5	1·5	1·6	1·5	1·3	1·2	1·1	1·1	1·2	1·3	1·4	1·8
POOLE BRIDGE	4·7	2·2	2·2	1·9	1·6	1·6	1·7	1·3	1·1	0·6	0·5	1·0	1·6	1·9	0·6
	4·3	1·8	1·7	1·6	1·7	1·8	1·8	1·5	1·4	1·0	0·8	1·1	1·5	1·7	1·2
	3·8	1·5	1·5	1·6	1·7	1·8	1·8	1·5	1·5	1·3	1·2	1·3	1·5	1·5	1·8
BOURNE-MOUTH	4·7	2·1	2·0	1·7	1·5	1·5	1·5	0·9	0·7	0·3	0·6	1·2	1·7	1·9	0·6
	4·3	1·6	1·7	1·6	1·6	1·6	1·5	1·2	1·0	0·8	0·8	1·2	1·4	1·5	1·2
	3·8	1·5	1·5	1·5	1·5	1·6	1·5	1·4	1·3	1·1	1·1	1·2	1·3	1·4	1·8
CHRIST- † CHURCH HARBOUR	4·7	1·8	1·8	1·5	1·3	1·5	1·1	0·7	0·7	0·5	0·4	0·9	1·3	1·6	0·6
	4·3	1·5	1·5	1·4	1·5	1·5	1·2	0·9	0·8	0·6	0·6	1·0	1·2	1·4	1·2
	3·8	1·2	1·2	1·3	1·4	1·4	1·1	0·9	0·8	0·6	0·7	0·9	1·0	1·1	1·8
FRESHWATER BAY	4·7	2·4	2·5	2·4	2·2	2·2	1·9	1·1	0·9	0·5	0·8	1·5	2·0	2·2	0·6
	4·3	2·2	2·3	2·2	2·2	2·2	1·9	1·4	1·2	0·9	1·1	1·5	1·8	2·0	1·2
	3·8	1·9	2·0	2·2	2·2	2·2	2·0	1·6	1·6	1·3	1·3	1·6	1·7	1·8	1·8
TOTLAND BAY	4·7	2·3	2·5	2·4	2·3	2·3	2·1	1·4	1·1	0·5	0·8	1·4	1·8	2·1	0·6
	4·3	2·1	2·3	2·3	2·3	2·2	2·1	1·6	1·4	0·9	1·1	1·4	1·7	1·9	1·2
	3·8	2·0	2·1	2·3	2·3	2·2	2·1	1·8	1·7	1·4	1·4	1·6	1·8	1·8	1·8
HURST-POINT	4·7	2·3	2·6	2·7	2·5	2·5	2·3	1·6	1·2	0·5	0·7	1·3	1·7	2·0	0·6
	4·3	2·0	2·3	2·5	2·5	2·4	2·3	1·7	1·5	1·1	1·0	1·4	1·7	1·9	1·2
	3·8	1·9	2·1	2·3	2·3	2·3	2·2	1·8	1·7	1·4	1·3	1·5	1·7	1·9	1·8
YARMOUTH I.O.W.	4·7	2·4	2·8	3·0	2·8	2·8	2·7	1·8	1·5	0·7	0·8	1·4	1·8	1·8	0·6
	4·3	2·2	2·5	2·7	2·7	2·7	2·6	1·9	1·6	1·1	1·2	1·6	1·8	2·0	1·2
	3·8	2·0	2·3	2·5	2·5	2·5	2·3	1·9	1·7	1·5	1·5	1·6	1·7	1·8	1·8
LYMINGTON	4·7	2·2	2·6	3·0	2·8	2·9	2·8	2·1	1·7	0·7	0·5	1·1	1·6	1·9	0·6
	4·3	2·0	2·3	2·7	2·7	2·7	2·6	2·1	1·8	1·1	1·0	1·3	1·6	1·7	1·2
	3·8	1·9	2·2	2·4	2·5	2·5	2·4	2·0	1·8	1·5	1·4	1·5	1·6	1·7	1·8
SOLENT BANKS	4·7	2·4	2·9	3·4	3·3	3·2	3·0	2·2	1·8	0·7	0·6	1·2	1·8	2·0	0·6
	4·3	2·2	2·6	3·0	3·1	3·0	2·9	2·2	1·9	1·2	1·1	1·4	1·6	1·9	1·2
	3·8	2·1	2·3	2·6	2·7	2·7	2·6	2·2	2·0	1·6	1·5	1·7	1·9	2·0	1·8
COWES ROAD	4·7	2·5	3·4	4·1	4·2	4·1	3·8	3·0	2·5	1·1	0·6	1·2	1·8	2·1	0·6
	4·3	2·4	3·1	3·7	3·8	3·7	3·5	2·8	2·6	1·5	1·2	1·5	1·8	2·1	1·2
	3·8	2·5	3·0	3·3	3·4	3·4	3·2	2·7	2·5	2·0	1·7	1·9	2·0	2·2	1·8
CALSHOT CASTLE	4·7	2·6	3·6	4·3	4·4	4·3	4·1	3·2	2·6	1·2	0·7	1·3	1·9	2·2	0·6
	4·3	2·6	3·3	3·8	4·0	4·0	3·7	3·0	2·6	1·6	1·2	1·6	2·0	2·2	1·2
	3·8	2·7	3·2	3·5	3·6	3·6	3·4	2·8	2·6	2·0	1·9	2·0	2·2	2·3	1·8
LEE-ON-SOLENT	4·7	2·7	3·6	4·4	4·5	4·4	4·2	3·1	2·5	1·1	0·6	1·2	1·8	2·1	0·6
	4·3	2·7	3·4	3·9	4·1	4·0	3·7	2·9	2·5	1·4	1·2	1·6	2·0	2·2	1·2
	3·8	2·7	3·2	3·6	3·7	3·6	3·3	2·8	2·6	2·1	1·9	2·0	2·2	2·4	1·8
RYDE	4·7	2·7	3·7	4·3	4·5	4·3	4·0	2·9	2·4	1·1	0·7	1·2	1·8	2·1	0·6
	4·3	2·7	3·4	4·0	4·1	4·0	3·7	2·9	2·6	1·6	1·3	1·6	1·9	2·2	1·2
	3·8	2·7	3·2	3·6	3·7	3·6	3·4	2·9	2·7	2·1	1·9	2·0	2·2	2·4	1·8
NAB TOWER	4·7	2·9	3·8	4·4	4·5	4·3	3·6	2·4	2·0	0·9	0·6	1·0	1·5	2·1	0·6
	4·3	2·9	3·6	4·1	4·2	4·0	3·4	2·5	2·2	1·4	1·2	1·4	1·8	2·2	1·2
	3·8	2·9	3·3	3·7	3·7	3·6	3·1	2·6	2·3	1·9	1·7	1·8	2·1	2·4	1·8
SANDOWN	4·7	2·6	3·3	3·8	4·0	3·8	3·3	2·1	1·7	0·8	0·6	1·0	1·5	1·9	0·6
	4·3	2·6	3·0	3·5	3·6	3·5	3·1	2·2	1·9	1·3	1·1	1·4	1·7	2·0	1·2
	3·8	2·6	2·9	3·2	3·3	3·1	2·8	2·3	2·1	1·8	1·6	1·7	1·9	2·2	1·8
VENTNOR	4·7	2·8	3·3	3·7	3·8	3·5	2·9	2·0	1·7	1·0	0·9	1·3	1·7	2·1	0·6
	4·3	2·6	3·1	3·4	3·4	3·2	2·8	2·1	1·9	1·4	1·3	1·6	1·9	2·2	1·2
	3·8	2·5	2·8	3·1	3·1	3·0	2·8	2·3	2·2	1·8	1·7	1·9	2·1	2·3	1·8

Note.—Area enclosed by pecked lines represents the period during which the tide stands, or during which a second high water may occur.
† Heights at Christchurch are for inside the bar; outside the bar, L.W. falls about 0·6 metres lower at Springs.

POOLE HARBOUR   10-2-13

Dorset 50°40'·90N 01°56'·88W (Ent)

CHARTS
AC *2611*, 2175; Imray C4, Y23; Stanfords 12, 15, 7; OS 195
TIDES
Town Quay –0141, +0114 Dover; ML 1·5; Zone 0 (UT)

POOLE (TOWN QUAY) (→)

Times			Height (metres)			
High Water	Low Water		MHWS	MHWN	MLWN	MLWS
–	–	0500 1100	2·1	1·6	1·2	0·6
		1700 2300				

Differences POTTERY PIER

–	–	+0005 +0005	–0·1	+0·1	+0·1	+0·2

CLEAVEL POINT

–	–	–0010 –0010	0·0	–0·1	0·0	–0·1

WAREHAM (River Frome)

–	–	+0125 +0040	+0·1	+0·1	0·0	+0·3

Differences POOLE HBR ENT are given under 10.2.11 with reference to the Standard Port of Portsmouth.

NOTE: LW predictions and heights of HW for each day of the year are given below. See also 10·2·12. Double HWs occur, except at nps, and predicted heights are for the higher HW; the height of the 2nd HW is always about 1·8m. HW occurs between LW +5 and next LW –3. Near nps there is a stand; predictions shown are for the middle of the stand. Strong and continuous winds from E to SW may raise sea levels by 0·2m, whilst W to NE winds may lower sea levels by 0·1m.

SHELTER
An excellent hbr with narrow ent; access in all conditions except very strong E/SE winds. ⚓s wherever sheltered from the wind and clear of chans, moorings and shellfish beds; especially in South Deep, off W end of Brownsea Is and off Shipstal Pt. The S half of the hbr is designated as a Quiet Area (see chartlet) with speed limit of 6kn. A 6kn limit also covers from Stakes SCM By, past Poole Quay and Poole Bridge up to Cobbs Quay in Holes Bay.
A 10kn speed limit applies to the rest of the hbr, ie West from the seaward app chans (defined by an arc of radius 1400m centred on S Haven Pt, 50°40'·78N 01°56'·91W) to the junction of R Frome with R Trent at 02°04'·60W (see chartlet). Note: From 1 Oct to 31 Mar the 10kn limit does not apply in the North, Middle Ship and Wareham Chans.
NAVIGATION
WPT Poole Bar (No 1 SHM) By, QG, 50°39'·32N 01°55'·10W, 148°/328° from/to Haven Hotel, 1·95M. In strong SE-S winds the Bar is dangerous especially on the ebb. Beware lobster pots around Studland Bay and close to training bank. From Poole Bar to Shell Bay a recreational **Boat Chan**, suitable for craft < 3m draught, parallels the W side of the Swash Channel. Caution: The **E Looe Chan** (buoyed) is liable to shift and may have less water than charted. 1ca ENE of E Looe PHM buoy there is only 1m. Within the hbr there are 2 chans up to Poole. Both are clearly marked by lateral buoys, mostly lit, with divisions marked by cardinal buoys. Outside the marked chans there are extensive shoal or drying areas.
The **Middle Ship Chan** is dredged to 6·0m for traffic to the ferry terminal at Hamworthy, and is mostly only 80m wide. Recreational craft must keep out of the Middle Ship Chan, by using the **Boat Chan**; this parallels S of the dredged chan between the PHM buoys and, further outboard, stakes with PHM topmarks marking the edge of the bank. Depth in this chan is 2·0m below CD, except close to the stakes where it reduces to 1·5m.
The **North Channel** is the other option: This is little used by ships and is advised for yachts/pleasure craft; deeper water is on the outside of chan bends.
Yachts departing W should check Lulworth gunnery range (see 10·2·10). Info is shown in the Hr Mr's office, broadcast on Radio Solent at times given in 10·2·20 and printed in the Supplements to this almanac.
LIGHTS AND MARKS
See chartlet and 10.2.4 for main buoys, beacons and lts.
Sandbanks Chain Ferry shows a Fl W lt (rotating) and a B ● above the leading Control cabin by D/N to indicate which way it is going. In fog it sounds 1 long and 2 short blasts every 2 mins. When stationary at Night it shows a FW lt; in fog it rings a bell for 5 sec every minute. Note: the chains of the new ferry are close to the surface for a greater distance astern than its predecessor.

Poole Bridge (Lights shown from bridge tr)
Ⓡ   = Do not approach bridge;
Fl Ⓖ = Bridge lifting, proceed with caution; Ⓖ= Proceed. Bridge lifts routinely for small craft at: Mon-Fri 0930, 1030, 1230, 1430, 1630, 1830, 2130; Sat, Sun & Bank hols = as Mon-Fri, plus 0730; at 2345 daily bridge will also lift if any vessels are waiting. Each lift only permits one cycle of traffic in each direction. Pleasure craft may pass when the bridge lifts on request for a commercial vessel; monitor Ch 14. Bridge will not usually lift during weekday road traffic Rush Hours 0730-0930 and 1630-1830.
RADIO TELEPHONE
Call: *Poole Hbr Control* VHF Ch 14 16 (H24). Salterns Marina Ch M 80; Parkstone Haven Ch M; Poole YC Haven, call *Pike* Ch M; Poole Bridge, call *PB* Ch 14. Cobbs Quay, call *CQ Base* Ch 80.
TELEPHONE (01202)
Hr Mr 440200; Hbr Control 440330; Pilots 666401; Bridge 674115; MRSC (01305) 760439; ⌗ (01703) 827350; Met (01703) 228844; Marinecall 0891 500457; Police 22099; Ⓗ 675100.
FACILITIES The following are some of the many facilities:
Marinas (from seaward)
Salterns Marina (300, few visitors) ☎ 709971, Fax 700398, £23, max draft 2·5m, AC, FW, P, D, ME, EI, Ⓔ, Sh, CH, Gas, Gaz, C (5 ton), BH (45 ton), Bar, R, ☒. Appr from No 31 SHM buoy.
Parkstone Haven, (Parkstone YC's new marina ☎ 743610), some ♥ berths, £12; dredged 2m. Access from North Chan near No 35 SHM buoy, Fl G 5s. Appr chan, dredged 2·5m, is marked by SHM buoy (Fl G 3s), 1 PHM and 3 SHM unlit buoys. Ldg lts 006°, both QY. 2 FG and 2FR (vert) on bkwtr hds.
Poole Quay (AB £9, Sh, FW) is close to town & facilities. Berthing Office on the quay is open 0800-2200, Apr-Sept. Hbr Office at New Quay Rd, Hamworthy (HO).
Sunseeker International Marina (50) ☎ 685335, AC, Sh, D, BH (30 ton), C (36 ton), FW, ME, EI, CH, V, R, Bar;
Cobbs Quay Marina (750, some visitors) ☎ 674299, Fax 665217, £18, Slip, P, D, Gas, ☒, SM, FW, AC, ME, EI, Ⓔ, Sh, C (10 ton), CH, R, Bar;
Dorset Yacht Co (M: 120+12 visitors) ☎ 674531, Fax 677518, Slip, P, D, Gas, Gaz, FW, ME, EI, Sh, C (5 ton), Bar, AC;
Public Landing Places: On Poole Quay, in Holes Bay and by ferry hards at Sandbanks.
Fuel Poole Bay Fuels barge (May-Sep 0900-1800; moored near Aunt Betty buoy, No 50) P, D, Gas, Gaz, V, Off licence.
Corrals (S side of Poole Quay adjacent bridge) P & D;
Salterns marina P & D.
Yacht Clubs
Royal Motor YC ☎ 707227, M, Bar, R; **Poole Hbr YC** (Salterns) ☎ 707321; **Parkstone YC** ☎ 743610 (Parkstone Haven); **Poole YC** ☎ 672687; **Cobb's Quay YC** ☎ 673690.
Services
A complete range of marine services is available; consult marina/Hr Mr for exact locations: M, L, FW, AB, ME, EI, Sh, CH, Slip, CH, SM, D, P, C (18 ton), ACA, Ⓔ, Safety Equipment and Inflatables. **Town** EC Wed; ✉, Ⓑ, ⇌, ✈. Ferry to Cherbourg (all year) and St Malo (summer).

ADJACENT HARBOUR AND ANCHORAGE

WAREHAM, Dorset, 50°41'·00N 02°06'·48W. AC *2611*. HW –0030 (Np), +0320 (Sp) on Dover (see 10·2·12 & ·13). Shelter very good, appr narrow and winding up R Frome but well marked by buoys and posts at ent. Beware prohib ⚓s (salmon holes) marked on the chart; also many moored boats. Passage is unlit; keep to the outside of all bends. Max draft 1·2m to Wareham Quay.
Facilities: **Ridge Wharf Yacht Centre** (180+6 visitors) (½M upstream of R Frome ent) ☎ (01929) 552650, Access HW±2 approx AB, M, FW, P, D, ME, EI, Gas, AC, BH (20 ton), Slip, Sh, CH; **Redclyffe YC** ☎ 551227 (½M below bridge); **Wareham Quay** AB, FW, R. **Town** EC Wed, P & D (cans), V, Gas, R, Bar, ✉, Ⓑ, ⇌, Dr ☎ 3444.

STUDLAND BAY, Dorset, 50°38'·70N 01°55'·82W. AC *2172*, 2175. Tides approx as for Swanage (10·2·11). Shelter is good except in N/ E winds. Beware Redend Rks off S shore. Best ⚓ in about 3m, 3ca NW of The Yards (three strange projections on the chalk cliffs near Handfast Pt). **Village:** EC Thurs; FW, V, R, ✉, hotel, P & D (cans), No marine facilities. A Historic Wreck (see 10.0.3g) is at 50°39'·67N 01°54'·79W, 4 ½ca NNE of Poole Bar buoy.

POOLE HARBOUR *continued*

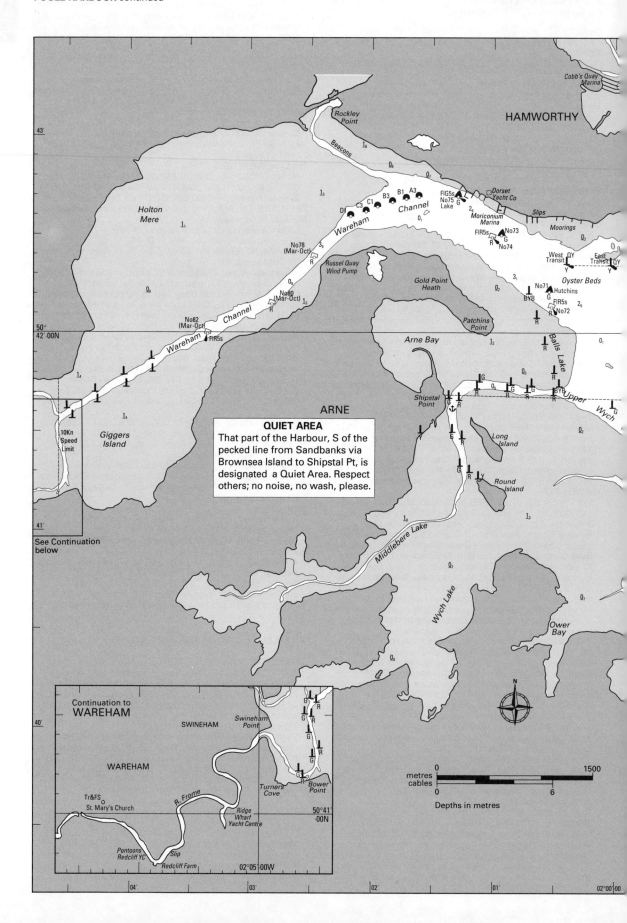

QUIET AREA
That part of the Harbour, S of the pecked line from Sandbanks via Brownsea Island to Shipstal Pt, is designated a Quiet Area. Respect others; no noise, no wash, please.

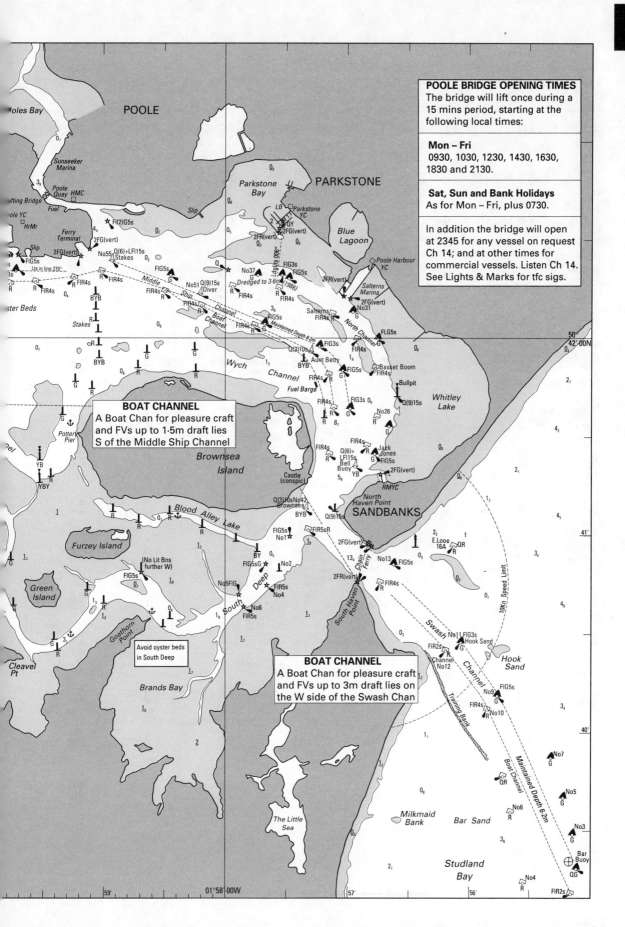

POOLE BRIDGE OPENING TIMES
The bridge will lift once during a 15 mins period, starting at the following local times:

Mon – Fri
0930, 1030, 1230, 1430, 1630, 1830 and 2130.

Sat, Sun and Bank Holidays
As for Mon – Fri, plus 0730.

In addition the bridge will open at 2345 for any vessel on request Ch 14; and at other times for commercial vessels. Listen Ch 14. See Lights & Marks for tfc sigs.

BOAT CHANNEL
A Boat Chan for pleasure craft and FVs up to 1·5m draft lies S of the Middle Ship Channel

BOAT CHANNEL
A Boat Chan for pleasure craft and FVs up to 3m draft lies on the W side of the Swash Chan

POOLE

PARKSTONE

Parkstone Bay

Blue Lagoon

Sunseeker Marina

Poole Quay

Ferry Terminal

Salterns Marina

North Channel

Middle Ship Channel

Boat Channel

Wych Channel

Whitley Lake

Brownsea Island

Basket Boom

Bullpit

Potlery Pier

Fuel Barge

Jack Jones

Castle (conspic)

Brownsea

North Haven Point

RMYC

SANDBANKS

Blood Alley Lake

Furzey Island

Deep

South

Green Island

Goathorn Point

South Haven Point

Chain Ferry

E.Looe

Cleavel Pt

Avoid oyster beds in South Deep

Brands Bay

Swash

Hook Sand

Hook Sand

Channel

Training Bank

Maintained Depth 6·2m

Boat Channel

10Kn Speed Limit

The Little Sea

Milkmaid Bank

Bar Sand

Studland Bay

Bar Buoy

ENGLAND – POOLE (TOWN QUAY)

LAT 50°43′N   LONG 1°59′W

TIMES AND HEIGHTS OF HIGH AND LOW WATERS

YEAR **1996**

TIME ZONE (UT)
For Summer Time add ONE hour in non-shaded areas

JANUARY

Day	Time	m	Day	Time	m
1 M	0044 1324	1.1 1.8 1.1 1.7	16 TU	1223	1.8 1.1 1.7
2 TU	0143 1416	1.1 1.9 1.0 1.8	17 W	0049 1334	1.0 1.9 0.9 1.9
3 W	0233 1500	1.0 1.9 0.9 1.9	18 TH	0156 1433	0.9 2.0 0.8 2.0
4 TH	0316 1541	0.9 1.9 0.8 1.9	19 F	0254 1526	0.8 2.2 0.6 2.1
5 F ○	0355 1618	0.9 2.0 0.7 1.9	20 SA ●	0347 1617	0.7 2.2 0.5 2.2
6 SA	0431 1654	0.8 2.0 0.7 2.0	21 SU	0437 1707	0.5 2.3 0.4
7 SU	0507 1728	0.8 2.0 0.7	22 M	0526 1755	2.3 0.5 2.3 0.3
8 M	0541 1800	2.0 0.8 2.0 0.7	23 TU	0614 1841	2.3 0.5 2.2 0.4
9 TU	0611 1829	2.0 0.8 2.0 0.7	24 W	0700 1925	2.3 0.5 2.2 0.4
10 W	0642 1859	2.0 0.9 1.9 0.8	25 TH	0745 2008	2.2 0.6 2.0 0.6
11 TH	0716 1936	2.0 0.9 1.9 0.8	26 F	0830 2052	2.1 0.8 1.9 0.8
12 F	0756 2018	1.9 1.0 1.8 0.9	27 SA	0919 2142	1.9 0.9 1.8 1.0
13 SA	0846 2110	1.9 1.0 1.8 1.0	28 SU	1019 2245	1.8 1.1 1.7 1.1
14 SU	0948 2216	1.8 1.7 1.1	29 M	1133	1.7 1.2 1.5
15 M	1105 2333	1.8 1.1 1.7 1.1	30 TU	0000 1248	1.3 1.7 1.2 1.5
			31 W	0112 1349	1.2 1.7 1.1 1.7

FEBRUARY

Day	Time	m	Day	Time	m
1 TH	0210 1437	1.1 1.8 1.0 1.8	16 F	0149 1423	0.9 1.9 0.8 1.9
2 F	0256 1519	1.0 1.9 0.9 1.9	17 SA	0248 1517	0.8 2.0 0.6 2.1
3 SA	0336 1558	0.9 1.9 0.7 1.9	18 SU ●	0339 1606	0.6 2.2 0.4 2.2
4 SU ○	0413 1633	0.8 1.9 0.7 2.0	19 M	0427 1652	0.5 2.2 0.3 2.3
5 M	0447 1709	0.7 2.0 0.6	20 TU	0513 1739	0.4 2.2 0.3
6 TU	0521 1740	2.0 0.7 2.0 0.6	21 W	0556 1821	2.3 0.4 2.2 0.3
7 W	0552 1809	2.0 0.7 2.0 0.6	22 TH	0638 1859	2.3 0.4 2.2 0.4
8 TH	0622 1839	2.0 0.7 2.0 0.6	23 F	0717 1938	0.5 2.0 0.5
9 F	0654 1913	2.0 0.7 1.9 0.7	24 SA	0754 2016	2.1 0.7 1.9 0.8
10 SA	0731 1953	2.0 0.8 1.9 0.8	25 SU	0834 2058	1.9 0.9 1.8 0.9
11 SU	0817 2041	1.9 1.8 0.9	26 M	0923 2153	1.8 1.7 1.1
12 M	0913 2143	1.8 1.7 1.0	27 TU	1032 2314	1.7 1.2 1.5 1.3
13 TU	1028 2306	1.8 1.1 1.7 1.1	28 W	1203	1.5 1.3 1.5
14 W	1159	1.7 1.1 1.7	29 TH	0038 1316	1.3 1.2 1.6
15 TH	0034 1320	1.1 1.8 1.0 1.5			

MARCH

Day	Time	m	Day	Time	m
1 F	0144 1409	1.2 1.7 1.0 1.7	16 SA	0141 1410	0.9 1.7 0.8 1.9
2 SA	0233 1453	1.0 1.8 0.9 1.9	17 SU	0238 1503	0.8 2.0 0.6 2.1
3 SU	0314 1531	0.9 1.8 0.8 1.9	18 M	0327 1550	0.5 2.1 0.4 2.2
4 M	0350 1608	0.8 1.9 0.7 2.0	19 TU ●	0412 1633	0.4 2.2 0.4 2.2
5 TU ○	0425 1643	0.7 1.9 0.5 2.0	20 W	0453 1716	0.4 2.2 0.3
6 W	0457 1717	0.6 2.0 0.5	21 TH	0535 1755	2.2 0.4 2.2 0.4
7 TH	0529 1748	2.0 0.5 2.0 0.5	22 F	0612 1833	2.2 0.4 2.1 0.4
8 F	0601 1820	2.0 0.5 2.0 0.5	23 SA	0648 1908	2.0 0.5 2.0 0.6
9 SA	0635 1854	2.0 0.5 2.0 0.6	24 SU	0722 1943	2.0 0.7 1.9 0.8
10 SU	0712 1935	2.0 0.6 1.9 0.7	25 M	0757 2022	1.9 0.8 1.8 0.9
11 M	0756 2022	1.9 0.7 1.9 1.0	26 TU	0838 2111	1.8 1.0 1.7 1.1
12 TU	0851 2126	1.8 0.9 1.8 1.0	27 W	0933 2225	1.6 1.1 1.3
13 W	1006 2253	1.7 1.0 1.7 1.1	28 TH	1106 2357	1.5 1.3 1.3
14 TH	1141	1.7 1.1 1.7	29 F	1233	1.4 1.3 1.5
15 F	0025 1307	1.1 1.7 0.9 1.8	30 SA	0109 1334	1.3 1.5 1.1 1.7
			31 SU	0202 1419	1.1 1.7 0.9 1.8

APRIL

Day	Time	m	Day	Time	m
1 M	0243 1500	0.9 1.8 0.8 1.9	16 TU	0309 1528	0.6 2.0 0.5 2.2
2 TU	0321 1537	0.8 1.9 0.7 2.0	17 W ●	0352 1610	0.5 2.1 0.4 2.2
3 W	0357 1613	0.7 1.9 0.6 2.0	18 TH	0432 1650	0.4 2.1 0.4 2.2
4 TH ○	0431 1648	0.5 2.0 0.5 2.0	19 F ●	0512 1729	0.4 2.1 0.5
5 F	0505 1724	0.5 2.0 0.5	20 SA	0548 1805	2.1 0.5 2.0 0.5
6 SA	0541 1801	2.1 0.5 2.0 0.5	21 SU	0623 1840	2.1 0.5 2.0 0.7
7 SU	0618 1840	2.1 0.5 2.0 0.5	22 M	0655 1915	2.0 0.7 1.9 0.8
8 M	0658 1923	0.5 2.0 0.7	23 TU	0728 1952	1.9 0.8 1.8 0.9
9 TU	0745 2015	1.9 0.7 1.9 0.8	24 W	0806 2038	1.8 0.9 1.8 1.1
10 W	0842 2119	1.8 0.8 1.8 1.0	25 TH	0853 2137	1.7 1.1 1.7 1.3
11 TH	0956 2243	1.7 0.9 1.7 1.0	26 F	1001 2302	1.5 1.2 1.6 1.3
12 F	1125	1.7 1.0 1.7	27 SA	1134	1.5 1.3 1.6
13 SA	0010 1247	1.0 1.7 0.9 1.8	28 SU	0020 1245	1.3 1.5 1.1 1.7
14 SU	0124 1351	0.9 1.8 0.8 1.9	29 M	0119 1336	1.1 1.6 1.0 1.8
15 M	0220 1442	0.8 1.9 0.7 2.0	30 TU	0205 1420	1.0 1.7 0.9 1.9

Chart Datum: 1·40 metres below Ordnance Datum (Newlyn)

2

ENGLAND – POOLE (TOWN QUAY)

LAT 50°43′N LONG 1°59′W

TIMES AND HEIGHTS OF HIGH AND LOW WATERS

YEAR **1996**

TIME ZONE (UT)
For Summer Time add ONE hour in non-shaded areas

MAY

	Time	m		Time	m
1 W	0244 1500	0.8 1.8 0.7 2.0	**16** TH	0328 1546	0.6 2.0 0.6 2.1
2 TH	0323 1540	0.7 1.9 0.7 2.0	**17** F ●	0409 1625	0.5 2.0 0.6 2.1
3 F O	0402 1619	0.6 2.0 0.5 2.1	**18** SA	0448 1704	0.5 2.0 0.6
4 SA	0440 1701	0.5 2.1 0.5	**19** SU	0525 1740	2.0 0.5 2.0 0.7
5 SU	0521 1744	2.1 0.4 2.1 0.5	**20** M	0600 1815	2.0 0.6 2.0 0.7
6 M	0605 1829	2.1 0.4 2.1 0.5	**21** TU	0633 1850	2.0 0.7 1.9 0.8
7 TU	0651 1916	2.1 0.5 2.0 0.6	**22** W	0706 1926	1.9 0.8 1.9 0.9
8 W	0742 2011	2.0 0.6 2.0 0.7	**23** TH	0741 2007	1.8 0.9 1.8 1.0
9 TH	0839 2112	1.9 0.7 1.9 0.9	**24** F	0821 2054	1.8 1.0 1.8 1.1
10 F	0946 2226	1.8 0.8 1.8 1.0	**25** SA	0912 2154	1.7 1.1 1.7 1.3
11 SA	1103 2343	1.7 0.9 1.8 1.0	**26** SU	1019 2310	1.6 1.1 1.7 1.3
12 SU	1218	1.7 0.9 1.9	**27** M	1135	1.6 1.1 1.7
13 M	0055 1323	0.9 1.8 0.8 1.9	**28** TU	0019 1240	1.2 1.6 1.1 1.8
14 TU	0155 1416	0.8 1.9 0.7 2.0	**29** W	0116 1334	1.0 1.7 0.9 1.9
15 W	0244 1503	0.7 1.9 0.7 2.0	**30** TH	0204 1421	0.9 1.8 0.8 2.0
			31 F	0249 1507	0.8 1.9 0.7 2.0

JUNE

	Time	m		Time	m
1 SA O	0334 1553	0.6 2.0 0.6 2.1	**16** SU ●	0427 1640	0.7 1.9 0.7 2.0
2 SU	0420 1639	0.5 2.1 0.5 2.2	**17** M	0505 1718	0.7 1.9 0.7
3 M	0507 1729	0.4 2.2 0.5	**18** TU	0540 1754	2.0 0.7 1.9 0.8
4 TU	0556 1819	2.2 0.4 2.2 0.5	**19** W	0613 1829	2.0 0.7 1.9 0.8
5 W	0645 1909	2.2 0.4 2.2 0.5	**20** TH	0644 1901	1.9 0.8 1.9 0.9
6 TH	0737 2001	2.1 0.5 2.1 0.7	**21** F	0716 1937	1.9 0.8 1.9 0.9
7 F	0830 2059	2.0 0.6 2.0 0.8	**22** SA	0751 2017	1.8 0.9 1.8 1.0
8 SA	0929 2201	1.9 0.8 1.9 0.9	**23** SU	0834 2105	1.8 1.0 1.8 1.1
9 SU	1034 2311	1.8 0.9 1.9 0.9	**24** M	0927 2204	1.7 1.0 1.8 1.1
10 M	1142	1.7 0.9 1.9	**25** TU	1031 2314	1.7 1.1 1.8 1.1
11 TU	0021 1250	1.0 1.7 0.9 1.9	**26** W	1140	1.7 1.1 1.8
12 W	0124 1348	0.9 1.8 0.9 1.9	**27** TH	0024 1248	1.1 1.7 1.0 1.9
13 TH	0218 1437	0.8 1.8 0.8 2.0	**28** F	0127 1347	1.0 1.8 0.9 2.0
14 F	0305 1521	0.8 1.9 0.8 2.0	**29** SA	0221 1441	0.8 1.9 0.8 2.1
15 SA	0347 1602	0.7 1.9 0.7 2.0	**30** SU	0314 1534	0.7 2.0 0.7 2.2

JULY

	Time	m		Time	m
1 M O	0404 1625	0.5 2.1 0.5 2.2	**16** TU	0442 1656	0.7 1.9 0.8 2.0
2 TU	0454 1717	0.4 2.2 0.5	**17** W	0519 1734	0.7 2.0 0.8
3 W	0545 1807	0.4 2.2 0.5	**18** TH	0552 1806	2.0 0.7 2.0 0.8
4 TH	0635 1856	2.2 0.4 2.2 0.5	**19** F	0623 1837	1.9 0.7 2.0 0.8
5 F	0724 1947	2.2 0.4 2.2 0.5	**20** SA	0651 1909	1.9 0.8 1.9 0.8
6 SA	0814 2038	2.1 0.5 2.1 0.7	**21** SU	0723 1945	1.9 0.8 1.9 0.9
7 SU	0905 2133	2.0 0.7 2.0 0.8	**22** M	0801 2028	1.8 0.9 1.9 1.0
8 M	1001 2234	1.8 0.8 1.9 0.9	**23** TU	0848 2121	1.8 1.0 1.8 1.0
9 TU	1105 2342	1.7 1.0 1.8 1.0	**24** W	0946 2228	1.7 1.0 1.8 1.1
10 W	1213	1.7 1.0 1.8	**25** TH	1059 2344	1.7 1.1 1.8 1.1
11 TH	0051 1318	1.0 1.7 1.0 1.8	**26** F	1215	1.0 1.7 1.1 1.8
12 F	0152 1413	1.0 1.8 1.0 1.9	**27** SA	0100 1327	1.0 1.8 1.0 1.9
13 SA	0242 1500	0.9 1.8 0.9 1.9	**28** SU	0204 1427	0.8 1.9 0.8 2.0
14 SU	0325 1542	0.8 1.9 0.9 1.9	**29** M	0300 1521	0.7 2.0 0.7 2.2
15 M ●	0405 1620	0.7 1.9 0.8 1.9	**30** TU O	0352 1613	0.5 2.2 0.5 2.3
			31 W	0441 1704	0.4 2.2 0.5

AUGUST

	Time	m		Time	m
1 TH	0530 1752	2.2 0.3 2.3 0.4	**16** F	0527 1742	2.0 0.6 2.0 0.7
2 F	0619 1840	2.2 0.3 2.3 0.4	**17** SA	0558 1812	2.0 0.7 2.0 0.7
3 SA	0705 1925	2.2 0.4 2.2 0.5	**18** SU	0626 1842	2.0 0.7 2.0 0.7
4 SU	0750 2011	2.1 0.5 2.2 0.6	**19** M	0656 1917	1.9 0.7 2.0 0.8
5 M	0835 2059	2.0 0.7 2.0 0.8	**20** TU	0732 1957	1.9 0.8 1.9 0.9
6 TU	0925 2153	1.9 0.9 1.9 1.0	**21** W	0816 2048	1.8 0.9 1.9 1.0
7 W	1023 2301	1.7 1.0 1.8 1.1	**22** TH	0912 2154	1.8 1.0 1.8 1.1
8 TH	1135	1.6 1.2 1.7	**23** F	1028 2319	1.7 1.1 1.7 1.1
9 F	0016 1250	1.1 1.6 1.2 1.7	**24** SA	1157	1.7 1.1 1.8
10 SA 1352	0125	1.1 1.7 1.1 1.8	**25** SU 1317	0044	1.0 1.8 1.0 1.9
11 SU 1440	0219	1.0 1.8 1.0 1.8	**26** M 1418	0153	0.9 1.9 0.9 2.0
12 M 1521	0303	0.9 1.9 0.9 1.9	**27** TU 1512	0248	0.7 2.1 0.7 2.2
13 TU 1559	0342	0.8 1.9 0.8 1.9	**28** W O 1601	0338	0.5 2.2 0.5 2.2
14 W ● 1634	0419	0.7 2.0 0.7 2.2	**29** TH 1647	0426	0.4 2.3 0.4 2.3
15 TH 1710	0454	0.6 2.0 0.7	**30** F 1734	0513	0.3 2.3 0.4
			31 SA 1818	0557	2.3 0.3 2.3 0.4

Chart Datum: 1.40 metres below Ordnance Datum (Newlyn)

ENGLAND – POOLE (TOWN QUAY)

LAT 50°43′N   LONG   1°59′W

TIMES AND HEIGHTS OF HIGH AND LOW WATERS

YEAR **1996**

TIME ZONE (UT)
For Summer Time add ONE hour in non-shaded areas

SEPTEMBER

Day	Time	m	Day	Time	m
1 SU	0640 / 1859	2.2 0.4 / 2.2 0.5	16 M	0601 / 1818	2.0 0.7 / 2.0 0.7
2 M	0721 / 1941	2.2 0.5 / 2.2 0.6	17 TU	0633 / 1853	2.0 0.7 / 2.0 0.7
3 TU	0801 / 2022	2.0 0.7 / 2.0 0.8	18 W	0710 / 1933	2.0 0.8 / 1.9 0.8
4 W	0846 / 2110	1.9 0.9 / 1.9 1.0	19 TH	0753 / 2024	1.9 0.9 / 1.9 0.9
5 TH	0941 / 2214	1.7 1.1 / 1.7 1.1	20 F	0851 / 2132	1.8 1.0 / 1.8 1.1
6 F	1057 / 2337	1.6 1.3 / 1.6 1.3	21 SA	1013 / 2302	1.7 1.2 / 1.7 1.1
7 SA	1218	1.5 1.3 / 1.5	22 SU	1147	1.7 1.2 / 1.7
8 SU	0054 / 1327	1.2 1.7 / 1.3 1.7	23 M	0030 / 1307	1.0 1.8 / 1.0 1.9
9 M	0152 / 1416	1.1 1.8 / 1.1 1.8	24 TU	0139 / 1406	0.9 1.9 / 0.9 2.0
10 TU	0236 / 1457	0.9 1.9 / 0.9 1.9	25 W	0234 / 1457	0.7 2.1 / 0.7 2.2
11 W	0316 / 1534	0.8 2.0 / 0.8 1.9	26 TH	0321 / 1544	0.5 2.2 / 0.5 2.2
12 TH ●	0353 / 1609	0.7 2.0 / 0.7 2.0	27 F O	0406 / 1628	0.4 2.3 / 0.4 2.3
13 F	0428 / 1643	0.6 2.0 / 0.7 2.0	28 SA	0450 / 1711	0.4 2.3 / 0.4
14 SA	0501 / 1716	0.6 2.0 / 0.7	29 SU	0533 / 1753	2.2 0.4 / 2.3 0.4
15 SU	0532 / 1746	2.0 0.6 / 2.0 0.7	30 M	0612 / 1832	2.2 0.5 / 2.2 0.5

OCTOBER

Day	Time	m	Day	Time	m
1 TU	0651 / 1910	2.1 0.6 / 2.1 0.7	16 W	0613 / 1835	2.1 0.7 / 2.0 0.7
2 W	0729 / 1948	2.0 0.8 / 2.0 0.8	17 TH	0654 / 1918	2.0 0.8 / 2.0 0.8
3 TH	0811 / 2031	1.9 0.9 / 1.8 1.0	18 F	0742 / 2012	1.9 0.9 / 1.9 0.9
4 F	0901 / 2127	1.8 1.1 / 1.7 1.2	19 SA	0843 / 2119	1.9 1.0 / 1.8 1.0
5 SA	1013 / 2250	1.7 1.3 / 1.6 1.3	20 SU	1002 / 2246	1.8 1.1 / 1.7 1.1
6 SU	1139	1.5 1.4 / 1.5	21 M	1132	1.7 1.1 / 1.7
7 M	0014 / 1252	1.3 1.7 / 1.3 1.6	22 TU	0010 / 1249	1.0 1.8 / 1.0 1.8
8 TU	0117 / 1345	1.1 1.8 / 1.1 1.7	23 W	0119 / 1349	0.9 2.0 / 0.9 2.0
9 W	0205 / 1427	1.0 1.9 / 1.0 1.8	24 TH	0214 / 1438	0.7 2.1 / 0.7 2.1
10 TH	0244 / 1505	0.9 2.0 / 0.9 1.9	25 F	0301 / 1524	0.6 2.2 / 0.6 2.2
11 F	0322 / 1540	0.8 2.0 / 0.8 2.0	26 SA O	0345 / 1607	0.5 2.3 / 0.5 2.2
12 SA ●	0358 / 1614	0.7 2.1 / 0.7 2.0	27 SU	0427 / 1648	0.5 2.3 / 0.5 2.2
13 SU	0431 / 1647	0.6 2.1 / 0.7 2.1	28 M	0507 / 1728	0.5 2.2 / 0.5
14 M	0504 / 1721	0.6 2.0 / 0.6	29 TU	0546 / 1806	2.2 0.5 / 2.2 0.6
15 TU	0538 / 1756	2.1 0.6 / 2.1	30 W	0624 / 1843	2.1 0.7 / 2.0 0.7
			31 TH	0700 / 1919	2.0 0.8 / 2.0 0.8

NOVEMBER

Day	Time	m	Day	Time	m
1 F	0740 / 1958	1.9 1.0 / 1.9 1.0	16 SA	0737 / 2006	2.0 0.8 / 1.9 0.8
2 SA	0826 / 2046	1.8 1.1 / 1.7 1.1	17 SU	0837 / 2109	1.9 0.9 / 1.9 0.9
3 SU	0926 / 2151	1.7 1.3 / 1.6 1.3	18 M	0948 / 2223	1.9 1.0 / 1.8 1.0
4 M	1048 / 2317	1.7 1.4 / 1.5 1.3	19 TU	1108 / 2339	1.8 1.1 / 1.8 1.0
5 TU	1204	1.7 1.4 / 1.5	20 W	1222	1.9 1.0 / 1.8
6 W	0028 / 1304	1.3 1.7 / 1.3 1.7	21 TH	0050 / 1325	0.9 2.0 / 0.9 1.9
7 TH	0123 / 1350	1.1 1.8 / 1.1 1.8	22 F	0149 / 1417	0.8 2.0 / 0.8 2.0
8 F	0206 / 1430	1.0 1.9 / 0.9 1.9	23 SA	0238 / 1504	0.7 2.2 / 0.7 2.0
9 SA	0246 / 1507	0.9 2.0 / 0.8 2.0	24 SU	0323 / 1547	0.7 2.2 / 0.7 2.1
10 SU	0323 / 1544	0.8 2.0 / 0.7 2.0	25 M O	0404 / 1629	0.7 2.2 / 0.6 2.1
11 M ●	0401 / 1620	0.7 2.1 / 0.7 2.1	26 TU	0443 / 1708	0.7 2.2 / 0.6 2.1
12 TU	0437 / 1658	0.7 2.2 / 0.6 2.2	27 W	0522 / 1746	2.1 0.7 / 2.1 0.7
13 W	0517 / 1740	2.2 0.6 / 2.2 0.6	28 TH	0600 / 1821	2.0 0.8 / 2.0 0.7
14 TH	0559 / 1824	2.2 0.7 / 2.1 0.6	29 F	0636 / 1855	2.0 0.9 / 2.0 0.8
15 F	0645 / 1912	2.1 0.7 / 2.0 0.7	30 SA	0713 / 1930	1.9 1.0 / 1.9 0.9

DECEMBER

Day	Time	m	Day	Time	m
1 SU	0752 / 2010	1.9 1.1 / 1.8 1.0	16 M	0825 / 2054	2.0 0.8 / 1.9 0.8
2 M	0839 / 2057	1.8 1.2 / 1.7 1.1	17 TU	0927 / 2156	2.0 0.9 / 1.8 0.9
3 TU	0938 / 2159	1.8 1.3 / 1.7 1.3	18 W	1037 / 2306	1.9 1.0 / 1.8 1.0
4 W	1054 / 2316	1.7 1.4 / 1.6 1.3	19 TH	1148	1.9 1.0 / 1.8
5 TH	1206	1.7 1.3 / 1.6	20 F	0016 / 1257	1.0 1.9 / 1.0 1.8
6 F	0024 / 1304	1.2 1.8 / 1.2 1.7	21 SA	0121 / 1355	1.0 1.9 / 0.9 1.9
7 SA	0120 / 1350	1.1 1.9 / 1.0 1.8	22 SU	0216 / 1445	0.9 2.0 / 0.8 1.9
8 SU	0206 / 1433	1.0 2.0 / 0.9 1.9	23 M	0303 / 1530	0.8 2.0 / 0.8 2.0
9 M	0249 / 1516	0.8 2.1 / 0.8 2.0	24 TU O	0346 / 1611	0.8 2.1 / 0.7 2.0
10 TU ●	0332 / 1559	0.7 2.2 / 0.7 2.1	25 W	0425 / 1649	0.8 2.0 / 0.7 2.0
11 W	0416 / 1642	0.7 2.2 / 0.5 2.2	26 TH	0503 / 1727	0.8 2.0 / 0.7
12 TH	0502 / 1729	0.6 2.2 / 0.5	27 F	0540 / 1802	2.0 0.8 / 2.0 0.7
13 F	0549 / 1816	0.6 2.2 / 0.5	28 SA	0614 / 1834	2.0 0.8 / 2.0 0.8
14 SA	0638 / 1906	2.2 0.7 / 2.1 0.5	29 SU	0648 / 1906	2.0 0.9 / 1.9 0.8
15 SU	0729 / 1957	2.2 0.7 / 2.0 0.7	30 M	0721 / 1938	1.9 1.0 / 1.9 0.9
			31 TU	0757 / 2015	1.9 1.1 / 1.8 1.0

Chart Datum: 1·40 metres below Ordnance Datum (Newlyn)

2

CHRISTCHURCH   10-2-14

Dorset 50°43'·50N 01°44'·25W

CHARTS
AC *2172, 2219*; Imray C4; Stanfords 7, 12; OS 195
TIDES
HW Sp –0210, Np, –0140 Dover; ML 1·2; Zone 0 (UT)

Standard Port PORTSMOUTH (→)

Times				Height (metres)			
High Water		Low Water		MHWS	MHWN	MLWN	MLWS
0000	0600	0500	1100	4·7	3·8	1·9	0·8
1200	1800	1700	2300				
Differences CHRISTCHURCH (Ent)							
–0230	+0030	–0035	–0035	–2·9	–2·4	–1·2	–0·2
CHRISTCHURCH (Tuckton)							
–0205	+0110	+0110	+0105	–3·0	–2·5	–1·0	+0·1
BOURNEMOUTH							
–0240	+0055	–0050	–0030	–2·7	–2·2	–0·8	–0·3

NOTE: Double HWs occur, except near nps; predictions are for the higher HW. Near nps there is a stand, when predictions are for mid-stand. Tidal levels are for inside the bar. Outside the bar the tide is about 0·6m lower at sp. Floods (or drought) in the two rivers cause considerable variations from predicted hts. See 10·2·12.

SHELTER
Good in lee of Hengistbury Hd, elsewhere exposed to SW winds. R Stour, navigable at HW up to Tuckton, and the R Avon up to the first bridge, give good shelter in all winds. Most ⚓s in the hbr dry. No ⚓ in chan. No berthing at ferry jetty by Mudeford sandbank. CSC has limited pontoon AB and moorings for monohulls <9m. Hbr speed limit 4kn.
NAVIGATION
WPT 50°43'·50N 01°43'·50W, 090°/270° from/to NE end of Mudeford Quay 0·5M. The bar/chan is liable to shift. The ent is difficult on the ebb which reaches 4-5kn in 'The Run'. Chan inside hbr is narrow and mostly shallow (approx 0·3m) soft mud; mean ranges are 1·2m sp and 0·7m nps.

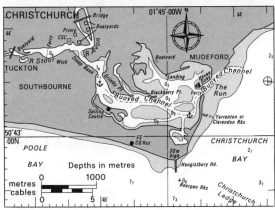

Recommended ent/dep at HW/stand. Beware groynes S of Hengistbury Hd, Beerpan and Yarranton Rks.
LIGHTS AND MARKS
2 FG (vert) at NE end of Mudeford Quay. Unlit chan buoys in hbr and apps are locally laid April-Oct inc; info from ☎ 483250.
RADIO TELEPHONE
None.
TELEPHONE (01202)
Quay & Moorings Supt (01425) 274933; MRSC (01305) 760439; ⌗ (01590) 674584; Marinecall 0891 500457; Police 486333; Ⓗ 303626; Casualty 704167.
FACILITIES
Mudeford Quay (Apl-Sept), Slip, AB, M, L, P (cans, ½M), FW, C (mobile), V; **Christchurch SC (CSC)** ☎ 483150, AB £7, M, Bar.
Services: Slip, M, D at Rossiter's BY (R Avon), FW, ME, EI, Sh, CH, ACA, C (8 ton).
Town ✉, Ⓑ, ⇌, ✈ (Bournemouth).

KEYHAVEN   10-2-15

Hampshire 50°42'·82N 01·33'·18W

CHARTS
AC *2021, 2219, 2040*; Imray C4, C3, Y20; Stanfords 7, 11, 12; OS 196
TIDES
–0020, +0105 Dover; ML 2·0; Zone 0 (UT)

Standard Port PORTSMOUTH (→)

Times				Height (metres)			
High Water		Low Water		MHWS	MHWN	MLWN	MLWS
0000	0600	0500	1100	4·7	3·8	1·9	0·8
1200	1800	1700	2300				
Differences HURST POINT							
–0115	–0005	–0030	–0025	–2·0	–1·5	–0·5	–0·1

NOTE: Double HWs occur at or near sp, when predictions are for the first HW. Off springs there is a stand of about 2 hrs; predictions are then for the middle of the stand. See 10·2·12.

SHELTER
Good, but the river gets extremely congested. Access HW ±4½. Ent difficult on ebb. All moorings and ⚓s are exposed to winds across the marshland. River is administered by New Forest DC aided by the Keyhaven Consultative Committee.
NAVIGATION
WPT 50°42'·70N 01°32'·50W, 115°/295° from/to chan ent, 0·40M. Ent should not be attempted in strong E winds. Bar is constantly changing. Leave chan SHM buoys well to stbd. Beware lobster pots. Approaching from the W, beware The Shingles bank over which seas break and which partly dries. At Hurst Narrows give 'The Trap' a wide berth.

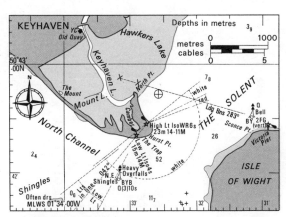

LIGHTS AND MARKS
When E of Hurst High lt, two ldg bns ('X' topmarks) lead 283° to ent of buoyed chan; the R & G ent buoys are more visible.
RADIO TELEPHONE
None.
TELEPHONE (01590)
R. Warden 645695; MRSC (01705) 552100; ⌗ (01590) 674584; Marinecall 0891 500457; Police 615101; Dr 643022; Ⓗ 677011.
FACILITIES
Quay Slip, L; **Keyhaven YC** ☎ 642165, C, M, L (on beach), FW, Bar; **New Forest District Council** ☎ (01703) 285000, Slip, M; **Milford-on-Sea** P, D, FW, CH, V, R, Bar; **Hurst Castle SC** M, L, FW;
Services: Slip, ME, EI, Sh, C (9 ton), CH.
Village EC (Milford-on-Sea) Wed; R, Bar, CH, V, ✉ and Ⓑ (Milford-on-Sea), ⇌ (bus to New Milton), ✈ (Hurn).

NEEDLES CHANNEL   10-2-16

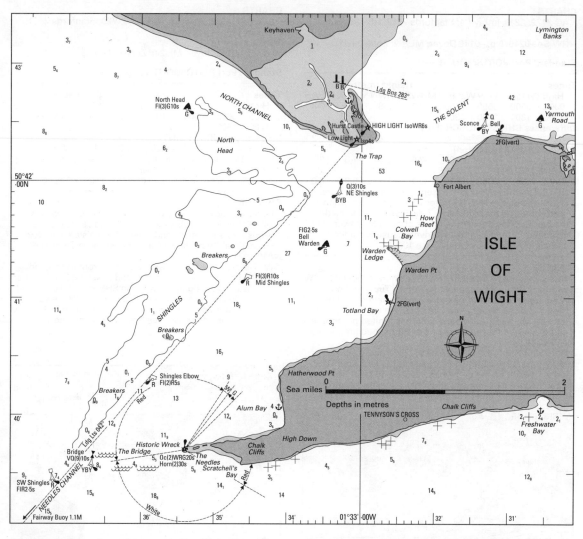

Some of the features and hazards of the Needles Channel, North Channel and Hurst Narrows are described below:

The Needles are distinctive rks at the W end of the Isle of Wight. The adjacent chalk cliffs of High Down are conspic from afar; the lt ho may not be seen by day until relatively close. There are drying rocks ½ca WNW of the lt ho, with remains of wreck close SW of these rocks. The NW side of the Needles Chan is defined by the Shingles bank, parts of which dry and on which the sea breaks violently in the least swell. The SE side of the bank is fairly steep-to, the NW side shelves more gradually. On the ebb the stream sets very strongly (3·4kn) WSW across the Shingles. The Needles Chan is well lit and buoyed and in fair weather presents no significant problems. Note: The Hurst Castle ldg lts lead 042° between SW Shingles and Bridge buoys; but further NE the ldg line is outside the buoyed chan and very adjacent to the Shingles.

In bad weather broken water and overfalls extend along The Bridge, a reef which runs 8ca W of the lt ho with extremity marked by Bridge WCM lt buoy. S to W gales against the ebb raise very dangerous seas in the Needles Chan. (In such conditions the E approach to the Solent, via Nab Tower and the Forts, should be used or shelter found at Poole or Studland.) Even a SW Force 4 against the ebb will raise breaking seas near Bridge and SW Shingles Bys. In strong winds the North Chan, N of the Shingles, is preferable to the Needles Chan. The two join S of Hurst Point where overfalls and tide rips may be met. Beware The Trap, a shoal spit extending 150m SE of Hurst Castle.

ANCHORAGES BETWEEN THE NEEDLES AND YARMOUTH

ALUM BAY, 50°40'·07N 01°34'·25W. *AC 2021.* Tides as for Totland B. Very good shelter in E and S winds, but squally in gales. Distinctive W cliffs to S and multi-coloured cliffs and chairlift to E. Appr from due W of chairlift to clear Five Fingers Rk, dries 0·6m, to the N and Long Rk, a reef drying 0·9m at its E end, to the S. ⚓ in about 4m off the new pier. A Historic Wreck (see 10.0.3g) is at 50°39'·7N 01°35'·45W.

TOTLAND BAY, 50°40'·95N 01°32'·78W. *AC 2219.* Tides, see 10.2.17 and 10.2.12; ML 1·9m. Good shelter in E'lies in wide shelving bay between Warden Ledge (rks 4ca offshore) to the N and Hatherwood Pt to the SW. Appr W of Warden SHM buoy Fl G 2·5s to ⚓ out of the tide in 2m between pier (2FG vert) and old LB house; good holding. Colwell Bay, to the N between Warden Pt and Fort Albert, is generally rky and shallow.

ANCHORAGE EAST OF THE NEEDLES, SOUTH IOW

FRESHWATER BAY, 50°40'·04N 01°30'·53W. AC *2021.* Tides see 10.2.15 and 10.2.12; ML 1·6m. Well sheltered from the N, open to the S. The bay is 3·2M E of Needles lt ho and 1·2M E of Tennyson's Cross. Redoubt Fort is conspic on W side of B, a hotel on N side and Stag, Arch and Mermaid Rks to the E. The B is shallow, with rky drying ledges ¾ca either side and a rk drying 0·1m almost in the centre. Best to ⚓ in about 2m just outside bay. Facilities: V, R, Bar, ✉.

YARMOUTH   10-2-17

Isle of Wight 50°42'·39N 01°29'·97W

CHARTS

AC *2021, 2040*; Imray C3, Y20; Stanfords 11, 18; OS 196

TIDES

Sp –0050, +0150 Np +0020 Dover; ML 2·0; Zone 0 (UT)

Standard Port PORTSMOUTH (→)

Times				Height (metres)			
High Water		Low Water		MHWS	MHWN	MLWN	MLWS
0000	0600	0500	1100	4·7	3·8	1·9	0·8
1200	1800	1700	2300				
Differences YARMOUTH							
–0105	+0005	–0025	–0030	–1·6	–1·3	–0·4	0·0
TOTLAND BAY							
–0130	–0045	–0040	–0040	–2·0	–1·5	–0·5	–0·1
FRESHWATER BAY							
–0210	+0025	–0040	–0020	–2·1	–1·5	–0·4	0·0

NOTE: Double HWs occur at or near sp; at other times there is a stand lasting about two hrs. Predictions refer to the first HW when there are two; otherwise to the middle of the stand. See 10·2·12.

SHELTER

Good from all directions of wind and sea, but swell enters if wind strong from N/NE. Hbr dredged 2m from ent to bridge; access H24. Moor fore-and-aft on piles in 5 rows, A to E; on the Town Quay, or on pontoon if <9m LOA. Boats over 15m LOA, 4m beam or 2·4m draft should give notice of arrival. Berthing on S Quay is normally only for fuel, C, FW, or to load people/cargo. Hbr gets very full, and may be closed to visitors. 12 Y ⚓s outside (see chartlet) and ⚓ further to the N or S.

NAVIGATION

WPT 50°42'·55N 01°29'·93W, 008°/188° from/to abeam car ferry terminal, 2ca. Dangers on appr are Black Rock and shoal water to the N of the E/Wbkwtr. Beware ferries.

Caution: strong ebb in the ent at sp. Speed limit 4kn in hbr apprs from abeam pierhead, in the hbr and up-river. ⚓ prohib in hbr and beyond R Yar road bridge. This swing bridge opens for access to the moorings and BYs up-river at Saltern Quay: (May-Sept) 0800, 0900, 1000, 1200, 1400, 1600, 1730, 1830, 2000LT; and on request (Oct-May). The river is navigable by dinghy at HW almost up to Freshwater.

A **Historic Wreck** (see 10.0.3g) is at 50°42'·52N 01°29'·59W, 2ca ExN from end of pier; marked by Y SPM buoy.

LIGHTS AND MARKS

Ldg bns (2 W ◊ on B/W masts) and ldg lts (FG 5/9m 2M), on quay, 188°. When hbr is closed to visitors (eg when full in summer or at week-ends) a R flag is flown at the pier head and an illuminated board 'Harbour Full' is displayed at the ent, plus an extra ®. In fog a high intensity Ⓦ lt is shown from the pier hd and from the inner E pier, together with a Ⓨ.

RADIO TELEPHONE

Hr Mr and Water Taxi VHF Ch 68.

TELEPHONE (01983 = IOW code)

Hr Mr 760321, Fax 761192; MRSC (01705) 552100; ⌗ (01703) 827350; Marinecall 0891 500457; Police 582000; Dr 760434.

FACILITIES

Hbr £8.20 on piles, Town Quay or pontoon; Slip, P, D, L, M, Gaz, FW, C (5 ton), Ice;
Yarmouth SC ☎ 760270, Bar, L;
Royal Solent YC ☎ 760256, Bar, R, L, M, Slip;
Services Note: Most marine services/BYs are located near Salterns Quay, 500m up-river above the bridge, or ½M by road. BY, Slip, M, ME, El, Sh, CH, Gas, Gaz, SM (☎ 754773 for emergency repairs H24), C, Divers.
Town EC Wed; V, R, Bar, ✉, Ⓑ (May-Sept 1000-1445, Sept-May a.m. only), ⇌ (Lymington), ✈ (Bournemouth/Southampton).

12 Orange Buoys for Visitors
Small Craft Anchorage
YARMOUTH ROAD
Depths in Metres
Black Rock
Norton
Norton Spit
Bathing Area (buoyed)
Sand Hard
Breakwater
Scrubbing Berths
R. Yar
Dredged to 2·0m
Pontoon
Tide Gauge
Fuel South Quay
FW
DIY Crane
Swing Bridge 2.5m
Salterns Quay 400m
Yarmouth SC
Car Ferry Terminal
Town Quay
Castle
HrMr
Royal Solent YC
Tr&FS
Slips
WC
Pier
Small Craft Moorings
Pontoons
Wk Obstn
Pontoon jetty
BY

LYMINGTON   10-2-18

Hampshire 50°45'·10N 01·31'·32W

CHARTS
AC *2021, 2040, 2045*; Imray C3, Y20, Y30; Stanfords 11, 18; OS 196

TIDES
Sp −0040, +0100, Np +0020 Dover; ML 2·0; Zone 0 (UT)

Standard Port PORTSMOUTH (→)

Times				Height (metres)			
High Water		Low Water		MHWS	MHWN	MLWN	MLWS
0000	0600	0500	1100	4·7	3·8	1·9	0·8
1200	1800	1700	2300				

Differences LYMINGTON
−0110	+0005	−0020	−0020	−1·7	−1·2	−0·5	−0·1

NOTE: Double HWs occur at or near sp and on other occasions there is a stand lasting about 2hrs. Predictions refer to the first HW when there are two. At other times they refer to the middle of the stand. See 10·2·12.

FACILITIES
Marinas:
Lymington Yacht Haven (475+100 visitors), 2m depth, all tides access, ☎ 677071, Fax 678186, £16.60, P, D, AC, FW, BY, ME, EI, Sh, C (10 ton), BH (40 ton), CH, Gas, Gaz, ▣;
Lymington Marina (300+100 visitors), ☎ 673312, Fax 676353, £14.10, Slip, P, AC, D, FW, ME, EI, Sh, CH, BH (100 ton), C, (37, 80 ton), Gas, Gaz, ▣;
Town Quay AB £6.50, M, FW, Slip (see Hr Mr); **Bath Road** public pontoon, FW.
Clubs: Royal Lymington YC ☎ 672677, R, Bar; **Lymington Town SC** ☎ 674514, AB, R, Bar.
Services: M, FW, ME, EI, Sh, C (16 ton), CH, Ⓔ, SM, ACA.
Town EC Wed; every facility including ✉, Ⓑ, ⇌, ✈ (Bournemouth or Southampton).

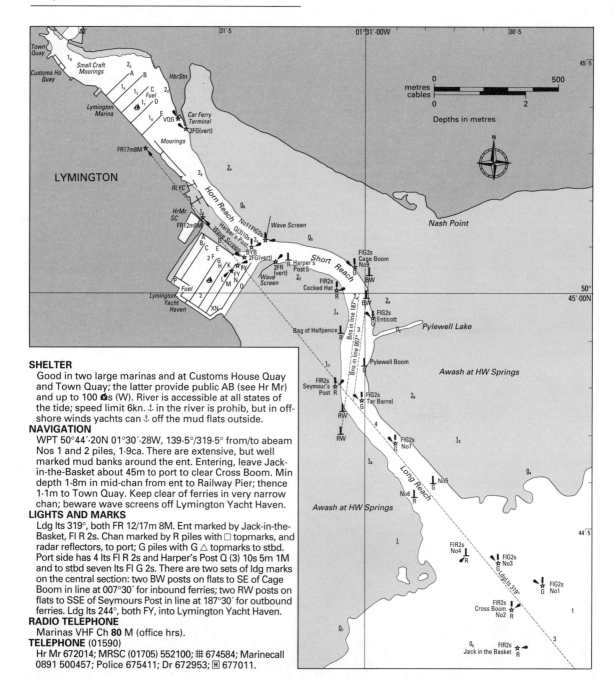

SHELTER
Good in two large marinas and at Customs House Quay and Town Quay; the latter provide public AB (see Hr Mr) and up to 100 ⚓s (W). River is accessible at all states of the tide; speed limit 6kn. ⚓ in the river is prohib, but in offshore winds yachts can ⚓ off the mud flats outside.

NAVIGATION
WPT 50°44'·20N 01°30'·28W, 139·5°/319·5° from/to abeam Nos 1 and 2 piles, 1·9ca. There are extensive, but well marked mud banks around the ent. Entering, leave Jack-in-the-Basket about 45m to port to clear Cross Boom. Min depth 1·8m in mid-chan from ent to Railway Pier; thence 1·1m to Town Quay. Keep clear of ferries in very narrow chan; beware wave screens off Lymington Yacht Haven.

LIGHTS AND MARKS
Ldg lts 319°, both FR 12/17m 8M. Ent marked by Jack-in-the-Basket, Fl R 2s. Chan marked by R piles with □ topmarks, and radar reflectors, to port; G piles with G △ topmarks to stbd. Port side has 4 lts Fl R 2s and Harper's Post Q (3) 10s 5m 1M and to stbd seven lts Fl G 2s. There are two sets of ldg marks on the central section: two BW posts on flats to SE of Cage Boom in line at 007°30' for inbound ferries; two RW posts on flats to SSE of Seymours Post in line at 187°30' for outbound ferries. Ldg lts 244°, both FY, into Lymington Yacht Haven.

RADIO TELEPHONE
Marinas VHF Ch **80** M (office hrs).

TELEPHONE (01590)
Hr Mr 672014; MRSC (01705) 552100; ⌗ 674584; Marinecall 0891 500457; Police 675411; Dr 672953; Ⓗ 677011.

NEWTOWN

10-2-19

Isle of Wight 50°43'·42N 01°24'·58W

CHARTS

AC *2021, 2040, 1905*; Imray C3, Y20; Stanfords 11, 18; OS 196

TIDES

Sp –0108, Np +0058, Dover; ML 2·3; Zone 0 (UT)

Standard Port PORTSMOUTH (→)

Times				Height (metres)			
High Water		Low Water		MHWS	MHWN	MLWN	MLWS
0000	0600	0500	1100	4·7	3·8	1·9	0·8
1200	1800	1700	2300				
Differences SOLENT BANK							
–0100	0000	–0015	–0020	–1·3	–1·0	–0·3	–0·1

NOTE: Double HWs occur at or near springs; at other times there is a stand which lasts about 2hrs. Predictions refer to the first HW when there are two. At other times they refer to the middle of the stand. See 10·2·12.

SHELTER

3½M E of Yarmouth, Newtown gives good shelter, but is exposed to N winds. There are 6 ⚓s (R/W) in Clamerkin Lake and 16 (R/W) in the main arm leading to Shalfleet, all are numbered; check with Hr Mr. Do not ⚓ above boards showing "Anchorage Limit" on account of oyster beds. Fin keel boats can stay afloat from ent to Hamstead landing or to Clamerkin Limit Boards. Public landing on E side of river N of quay. The whole peninsula ending in Fishhouse Pt is a nature reserve; yachtsmen are asked not to land there. 5kn speed limit in hbr is strictly enforced.

If no room in river, good ⚓ in 3-5m W of ent, but beware rky ledges E of Hamstead Ledge SHM By, Fl (2) G 5s, and piles with dolphin.

NAVIGATION

WPT 50°43'·80N 01°25'·10W, 310°/130° from/to ldg bn, 0·46M. From W, make good Hamstead Ledge SHM By, thence E to pick up ldg marks.

From E, keep N of Newtown gravel banks where W/SW winds over a sp ebb can raise steep breaking seas; leave R spherical bar buoy to port.

Best ent is from about HW –4, on the flood but while the mud flats are still visible. Ent lies between two shingle spits and can be rough in N winds especially near HW. There is only about 0·9m over the bar.

Inside the ent so many perches mark the mud banks that confusion may result. Near junction to Causeway Lake depth is only 0·9m and beyond this water quickly shoals. Clamerkin Lake is deeper (1·2m); chan is marked by occas perches. Keep to E to avoid gravel spit off W shore, marked by three perches. Beware many oyster beds. There is a rifle range at top of Clamerkin Lake and in Spur Lake. R flags flown during firing. High voltage power line across Clamerkin at 50°42'·78N 01°22'·58W has clearance of 9m - no shore markings.

LIGHTS AND MARKS

Conspic TV mast (152m) bearing about 150° (3·3M from hbr ent) provides initial approach track. In season a forest of masts inside the hbr are likely to be evident. The ldg bns, 130°, are off Fishhouse Pt in mud on NE side of ent: front bn, RW bands with Y-shaped topmark; rear bn, W with W disc in B circle. There are no lights.

RADIO TELEPHONE

None.

TELEPHONE (01983)

Hr Mr 531424; MRSC (01705) 552100; ⌗ (01703) 827350; Marinecall 0891 500457; Police 528000; Dr 760434.

FACILITIES

Newtown Quay M £8.50, L, FW; **Shalfleet Quay** Slip, M, L, AB; **Lower Hamstead Landing** L, FW; **R. Seabroke** ☎ 531213, Sh; **Shalfleet Village** V, Bar, P & D (cans; in emergency from garage).
Newtown EC Thurs; ✉, Ⓑ (Yarmouth or Newport), ⇌ (bus to Yarmouth, ferry to Lymington), ✈ (Bournemouth or Southampton).

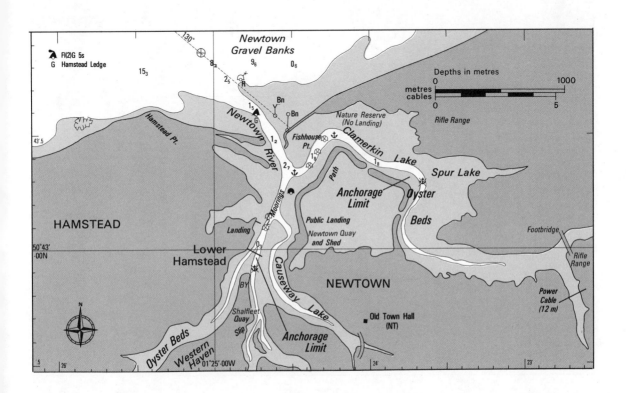

SOLENT AREA   10-2-20

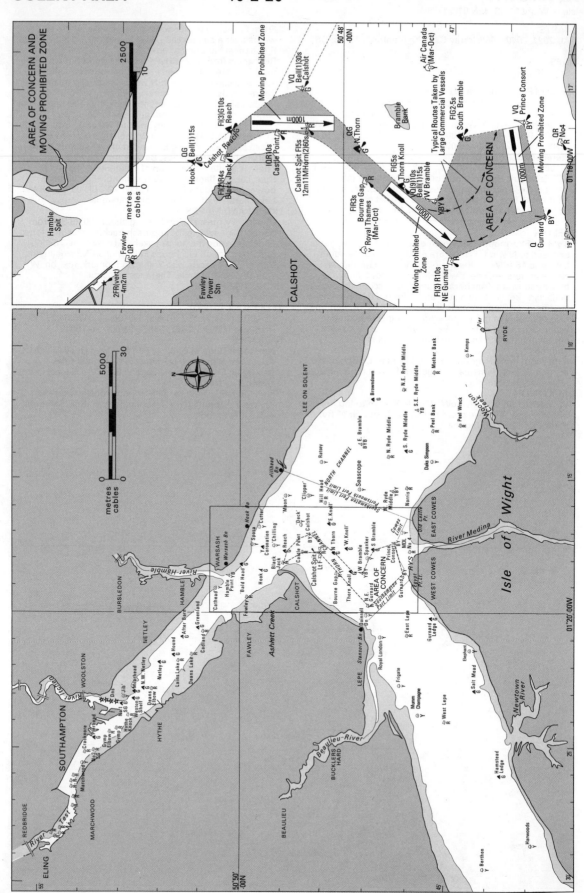

SOLENT AREA *continued*

The following paragraphs highlight some of the potential problems in the central Solent area and provide more general information applicable throughout the Solent.

Vessel Traffic Service (VTS)

A VTS, operated by Southampton on VHF Ch 12 14, controls shipping in the Solent between the Needles and Nab Tower including Southampton Water. Portsmouth Hbr and its appr's N of a line from Gilkicker Pt to Outer Spit By are controlled on Ch 11 by QHM Portsmouth.

The VTS is primarily intended to monitor and co-ordinate the safe passage of commercial ships which must make contact at designated reporting points. The VTS includes compulsory pilotage and a radar service on request, together with berthing instructions and tug assistance.

It follows that pleasure craft, particularly at night or in poor visibility, can be forewarned of shipping movements (and likely avoiding action), simply by listening on VHF Ch 12, or Ch 11 for QHM Portsmouth. Traffic information is routinely broadcast by Southampton VTS on VHF Ch 12 every H from 0600 to 2200LT, Fri-Sun and Bank Hols from Easter to last weekend in Oct. From 1 June to 30 Sept broadcasts are daily at the same times.

Pleasure Craft and Commercial Shipping

In the interests of safety it is important that good co-operation between pleasure craft and commercial shipping be maintained. Yachtsmen should always bear in mind the restricted field of vision from large ships at close quarters, their limited ability to manoeuvre at slow speeds, and the constraints of navigating through narrow and shallow channels.

An **Area of Concern** (AOC) has been designated at one of the busiest parts of the Solent to provide greater safety for large vessels. The AOC (see chartlet opposite) covers the Western Approach Channel and the Thorn Channel; it is delineated by the following lt buoys, clockwise fom Prince Consort NCM: Gurnard NCM, NE Gurnard PHM, Bourne Gap PHM, Calshot lt Float, Castle Point PHM, Black Jack PHM, Reach PHM, Calshot NCM, N Thorn SHM, Thorn Knoll SHM, W Bramble WCM and S Bramble SHM.

The AOC, which is criss-crossed by many pleasure craft, has also to be negotiated by large commercial vessels bound to/from Southampton normally via the E Solent. Such vessels, when inbound, usually pass Prince Consort NCM and turn first to the southward toward Gurnard NCM, before starting their critical stbd turn into the Thorn Chan. They turn port around Calshot to clear the AOC. Typical tracks are depicted opposite.

To minimise the risk of collision with small craft, any large vessel >150m LOA, on entering the AOC, is enclosed by a **Moving Prohibited Zone** (MPZ) which extends 1000m ahead of the vessel and 100m on either beam. *Small craft <20m LOA must remain outside this MPZ, using seamanlike anticipation of likely turns.*

The large vessel, displaying a B cylinder by day or 3 all-round Ⓡ lts (vert) by night, will normally be preceded by a Hbr patrol launch showing a Fl Bu lt and working VHF Ch 12 (callsign *SP*).

VHF Ch 12, in addition to providing VTS, will identify large vessels and approx timings of MPZ as part of the hourly broadcasts (see above). All pleasure craft in the vicinity are strongly advised to monitor Ch 12 in order to create a mental picture. Be particularly alert when in, or approaching, the triangle defined by E.Lepe, Hook and W Ryde Middle buoys.

VHF Radio Telephone

The proliferation of VHF radios in yachts and, it must be said, often poor R/T procedures cause problems for legitimate users and can seriously hamper emergency situations. Yachtsmen are reminded that Ch 16 is a DISTRESS, SAFETY and CALLING Ch. If another calling Ch is available use it in preference to Ch 16; otherwise, use Ch 16 as briefly as possible to make contact before shifting to a working Ch. Note also that initial contact with Solent CG should be on Ch 67, NOT Ch 16 (see next column). For ship-to-ship messages the recognised VHF channels include 06, 08, 72 and 77. **Yachts in the Solent should listen on Ch 12 and on Ch 11 for Portsmouth.** Other Ch's are listed under each port entry.

Local Signals

Outward bound vessels normally hoist the following flag signals during daylight hours.

Signal	Meaning
International 'E' Flag over Answering Pendant	} I am bound East (Nab Tower)
Answering Pendant Over International 'W' Flag	} I am bound West (The Needles)

Southampton patrol launches have HARBOUR MASTER painted on their after cabin in B lettering on Y background. At night a Fl Bu all-round lt is shown above the W masthead lt.

Reference

Much useful information is given in the *Solent Year Book,* published by the Solent Cruising and Racing Association (SCRA); also in a free booklet *The Yachtsman's Guide to Southampton Water* and a leaflet *Enjoy the Solent.* *Solent Hazards* by Peter Bruce, published by Boldre Marine, goes closer inshore than other Pilot books.

Weather and Navigation Broadcasts

Sailing information from BBC Radio Solent: 999 kHz (300m) and 96·1 MHz VHF. 1359 kHz (221m) in Bournemouth area.

A	Local weather forecast.
A*	Live forecast from Southampton Weather Centre.
B	Shipping forecast for Channel sea areas, with general synopsis and Coastal Station reports.
C	Coastguard Stn reports.
D	Tidal details.
E	Shipping movements.
F	Gunnery range firing times.

Daily Broadcasts (LT)

0504	A (Mon-Fri)	1104	A
0533	A, B, C, D, E, F (M-F)	1204	A
0604	A	1304	A* Sat; A on Sun
0633	A, B, C, D, E, F	1308	A (Mon-Fri)
0709	A	1328	A* (Mon-Fri)
0733	A*	1404	A (Not Sun)
0745	B, C, D, F	1504	A. A* on Sun
0745	E (Sat, Sun only)	1604	A (Mon-Fri)
0809	A	1709	A (Mon-Fri)
0833	A* (Mon-Sat)	1733	A*, D, F (Mon-Fri)
0850	E (Mon-Fri)	1758	A* (Sat only)
0904	A. (A* on Sun)	1804	A (Mon-Sat)
1000	A (Sun only)	2204	A (Mon-Fri)
1004	A (Mon-Fri)	2300	A* (2302 on Sun)

Recorded forecasts for this area can be obtained on ☎ (0891) 500 457. Southampton Weather Centre is ☎ (01703) 228844. Solent CG broadcasts on Ch 67 local strong wind warnings on receipt; and local forecasts every 4 hours from 0400LT, but every 2 hours if strong wind warnings are in force.

Solent Coastguard

The Maritime Rescue Sub Centre (MRSC) at Lee-on-Solent ☎ (01705) 552100 coordinates all SAR activities in Solent District, which is bounded by a line from Highcliffe south to the EC1 buoy; E to the Greenwich Lt V; thence N to Beachy Head. It is the busiest CG District in the UK, by virtue of the huge concentration of pleasure craft within its bounds.

It is manned H24, year round by at least 3 CG Officers who can call on the RNLI, Solent Safety rescue boats and the CG Rescue helicopter based at Lee. Sector and Auxiliary CGs are based on the IOW, Calshot, Eastney, Hayling, Littlehampton, Shoreham, Newhaven and elsewhere.

Solent CG keeps watch on VHF Ch 67 and 16. Uniquely, your initial call to *Solent Coastguard* should be made on Ch 67, the working channel; this is because Ch 16 is often very busy especially in the summer. Ch 67 is also heavily loaded and is only for essential traffic. Listen out before transmitting; be brief, to the point and use correct R/T procedures.

Save valuable R/T time by telephoning Solent CG before sailing; they will be glad to advise you. In general terms, they will always stress: Up-to-date forecasts; awareness of tidal streams; sound knowledge of "Rule of the Road" and local Notices to Mariners; adequate fuel, plus reserves, for your passage, and a sharp lookout at all times. Bon voyage!

SOLENT AREA WAYPOINTS   10.2.21

Waypoints marked with an asterisk (*) are special (yellow) racing marks, which may be removed in winter. Racing buoys marked with a bullet (•) against the longitude are only laid during Cowes week. Other waypoints are navigational buoys, unless otherwise stated.

After Barn	50°51'·50N 01°20'·73W
***Air Canada**	50°47'·30N 01°16'·75W
***Alpha** (Cowes)	50°46'·24N 01°18'·11W•
***Ashlett**	50°49'·95N 01°19'·67W
Bald Head	50°49'·86N 01°18'·16W
Bank Lt Bn	50°53'·58N 01°23'·24W
***Bay**	50°46'·02N 00°57'·81W
***Beken** (ex Keel)	50°45'·75N 01°19'·67W
Bembridge Ledge	50°41'·12N 01°02'·72W
Bembridge Tide Gauge	50°42'·43N 01°04'·93W
***Berthon**	50°44'·18N 01°29'·13W
***Beta** (Cowes)	50°46'·25N 01°17'·53W•
***Beta** (Portsmouth)	50°46'·80N 01°07'·25W
Black Jack	50°49'·10N 01°17'·98W
Black Rock	50°42'·55N 01°30'·55W
***Bob Kemp**	50°45'·15N 01°09'·55W
Boulder (Looe Chan)	50°41'·53N 00°49'·00W
Bourne Gap	50°47'·80N 01°18'·25W
***Bowring**	50°47'·28N 01°12'·00W
Boyne	50°46'·12N 01°05'·17W
Bramble Bn	50°47'·38N 01°17'·05W
Bridge	50°39'·59N 01°36'·80W
***Brookes & Gatehouse** (ex Alpha)	50°46'·40N 01°07'·80W
Browndown	50°46'·54N 01°10'·87W
Bury	50°54'·10N 01°27'·03W
Cadland	50°50'·98N 01°20'·45W
Calshot	50°48'·40N 01°16'·95W
Calshot Spit Lt F	50°48'·32N 01°17'·55W
***Camper & Nicholsons**	50°47'·05N 01°06'·68W
Castle (NB)	50°46'·43N 01°05'·30W
Castle Point	50°48'·67N 01°17'·60W
***Cathead**	50°50'·58N 01°19'·15W
***Champagne Mumm**	50°45'·60N 01°23'·03W
Chi	50°45'·48N 00°56'·91W
Chichester Bar Bn	50°45'·88N 00°56'·38W
***Chilling**	50°49'·23N 01°17'·42W
Chi Spit	50°45'·68N 00°56'·48W
***Clipper**	50°48'·26N 01°15'·38W
Coronation	50°49'·52N 01°17'·53W
Cowes Breakwater Lt	50°45'·84N 01°17'·43W
Cowes No.3	50°46'·04N 01°17'·95W
Cowes No.4	50°46'·04N 01°17'·78W
Cracknore	50°53'·92N 01°25'·12W
Crosshouse Lt Bn	50°54'·01N 01°23'·10W
***Cutter**	50°49'·47N 01°16'·81W

***Daks-Simpson**	50°45'·50N 01°14'·30W
***DB Marine**	50°46'·13N 01°13'·00W
Dean Elbow	50°43'·66N 01°01'·78W
Deans Elbow	50°52'·13N 01°22'·68W
Deans Lake	50°51'·35N 01°21'·52W
Dean Tail	50°42'·95N 00°59'·08W
Dean Tail South	50°43'·10N 00°59'·49W
***Deck**	50°48'·00N 01°16'·70W
Dibden Bay	50°53'·66N 01°24'·84W
***Durns**	50°45'·40N 01°25'·80W•
Durns Pt obstn (S end)	50°45'·37N 01°26'·95W
East Bramble	50°47'·20N 01°13'·55W
East Knoll	50°47'·93N 01°16'·75W
East Lepe	50°46'·09N 01°20'·81W
***Echo**	50°46'·05N 01°05'·66W
***Elephant**	50°44'·60N 01°21'·80W
Eling	50°54'·45N 01°27'·75W
Fairway (Needles)	50°38'·20N 01°38'·90W
Fawley	50°49'·97N 01°19'·38W
***Frigate**	50°46'·10N 01°22'·10W
Greenland	50°51'·08N 01°20'·33W
Gurnard	50°46'·18N 01°18'·76W
Gurnard Ledge	50°45'·48N 01°20'·50W
Gymp	50°53'·15N 01°24'·22W
Gymp Elbow	50°53'·48N 01°24'·53W
Hamble Point	50°50'·12N 01°18'·58W
Hamstead Ledge	50°43'·83N 01°26'·10W
***Hard**	50°44'·92N 00°57'·81W
***Harwoods**	50°42'·81N 01°28'·75W
Hillhead	50°48'·03N 01°15'·91W
Hook	50°49'·48N 01°18'·22W
Horse Elbow	50°44'·23N 01°03'·80W
Horse Sand	50°45'·48N 01°05'·17W
Horse Sand Fort Lt	50°44'·97N 01°04'·25W
Horse Tail	50°43'·20N 01°00'·14W
Hound	50°51'·65N 01°21'·43W
***Hurst**	50°42'·87N 01°32'·46W
Hythe Knock	50°52'·80N 01°23'·73W
Jack in Basket	50°44'·25N 01°30'·50W
***Jacksons**	50°44'·30N 01°28'·16W
***Jardines**	50°48'·10N 01°14'·55W
***Jib**	50°52'·93N 01°22'·97W
***Kelvin Hughes**	50°47'·30N 01°14'·50W•
Lains Lake	50°51'·55N 01°21'·57W
***Lambeth**	50°41'·50N 01°41'·60W

Langstone Fairway	50°46'·28N 01°01'·27W
Lee Pt Bn	50°47'·40N 01°11'·85W
*Lucas	50°46'·24N 01°08'·67W
Main Passage	50°45'·98N 01°04'·02W
Marchwood	50°53'·95N 01°25'·50W
*Marina Developments	50°46'·12N 01°16'·55W
*Mark	50°49'·53N 01°18'·87W
*Meon	50°49'·12N 01°15'·62W
Mid Shingles	50°41'·19N 01°34'·59W
Milbrook	50°54'·08N 01°26'·73W
Mixon Bn	50°42'·35N 00°46'·21W
Moorhead	50°52'·52N 01°22'·82W
*Moreton	50°42'·02N 01°03'·14W
*Morse (ex Delta)	50°46'·12N 01°06'·33W
Mother Bank	50°45'·45N 01°11'·13W
Nab 1	50°41'·23N 00°56'·43W
Nab 2	50°41'·70N 00°56'·71W
Nab 3	50°42'·17N 00°57'·05W
Nab East	50°42'·82N 01°00'·70W
Nab End	50°42'·60N 00°59'·38W
Nab Tower	50°40'·05N 00°57'·07W
NE Gurnard	50°47'·03N 01°19'·34W
NE Mining Ground	50°44'·70N 01°06'·30W
NE Ryde Middle	50°46'·18N 01°11'·80W
NE Shingles	50°41'·93N 01°33'·32W
Needles Fairway	50°38'·20N 01°38'·90W
Netley	50°51'·98N 01°21'·72W
New Grounds	50°41'·97N 00°58'·53W
*Newtown	50°44'·15N 01°23'·70W•
Newtown G By	50°43'·57N 01°24'·70W
No Mans Land Fort Lt	50°44'·37N 01°05'·61W
Norris	50°45'·92N 01°15'·40W
North Head	50°42'·65N 01°35'·43W
North Ryde Middle	50°46'·58N 01°14'·30W
North Sturbridge	50°45'·31N 01°08'·15W
North Thorn	50°47'·88N 01°17'·75W
NW Netley	50°52'·28N 01°22'·65W
*ODM (Lymington)	50°44'·18N 01°30'·10W
Outer Nab	50°41'·00N 00°56'·56W
Outer Spit	50°45'·55N 01°05'·41W
*Oxey	50°43'·84N 01°30'·86W
Peel Bank	50°45'·57N 01°13'·25W
Peel Wreck	50°44'·88N 01°13'·34W
*Pennington	50°43'·38N 01°31'·54W
Pier Head	50°53'·63N 01°24'·57W
Poole Fairway	50°38'·97N 01°54'·80W
Portsmouth No. 3 Bar	50°47'·04N 01°06'·17W
Portsmouth No. 4	50°46'·98N 01°06'·27W
Prince Consort	50°46'·38N 01°17'·47W
*Pylewell	50°44'·58N 01°29'·43W

*Quinnell	50°47'·02N 01°19'·48W
*Ratsey	50°47'·63N 01°13'·56W
Reach	50°49'·02N 01°17'·57W
Ridge	50°46'·42N 01°05'·57W
Roway Wk	50°46'·08N 01°02'·20W
*Royal Albert (exGamma)	50°46'·48N 01°05'·87W
*Royal London	50°46'·55N 01°21'·37W
*Royal Thames	50°47'·47N 01°19'·10W
*Ruthven	50°42'·67N 01°03'·45W
Ryde Pier Hd	50°44'·35N 01°09'·51W
*RYS flagstaff	50°45'·97N 01°17'·97W
Saddle	50°45'·18N 01°04'·79W
Salt Mead	50°44'·48N 01°22'·95W
Sconce	50°42'·50N 01°31'·35W
*Seascope	50°47'·38N 01°15'·82W
SE Ryde Middle	50°45'·90N 01°12'·00W
Shingles Elbow	50°40'·31N 01°35'·92W
*Short	50°49'·73N 01°19'·32W
*Snowden (ex Trap)	50°46'·17N 01°17'·51W
South Bramble	50°46'·95N 01°17'·65W
South Ryde Middle	50°46'·10N 01°14'·08W
*Spanker	50°47'·05N 01°17'·57W
Spit Refuge	50°46'·12N 01°05'·37W
Spit Sand Fort Lt	50°46'·20N 01°05'·85W
*Sposa	50°49'·70N 01°17'·63W
St Helens	50°43'·33N 01°02'·32W
Stokes Bay	50°46'·97N 01°09'·00W
Stokes Bay Wreck	50°46'·67N 01°10'·58W
Street	50°41'·65N 00°48'·80W
*Sunsail	50°46'·40N 01°15'·00W
Swinging Ground No. 1	50°52'·97N 01°23'·35W
Swinging Ground No. 2	50°53'·78N 01°25'·03W
SW Mining Ground	50°44'·63N 01°07'·95W
SW Shingles	50°39'·37N 01°37'·25W
*Tanners	50°44'·80N 01°28'·47W
*Tesco	50°45'·08N 01°27'·25W
Thorn Knoll	50°47'·47N 01°18'·35W
Trinity House (Cowes)	50°46'·10N 01°17'·15W
Warden	50°41'·45N 01°33'·47W
Warner	50°43'·84N 01°03'·93W
West Bramble	50°47'·17N 01°18'·57W
*W – E	50°45'·48N 00°58'·70W
West Knoll	50°47'·52N 01°17'·67W
West Lepe	50°45'·20N 01°24'·00W
Weston Shelf	50°52'·68N 01°23'·17W
West Princessa	50°40'·12N 01°03'·58W
West Ryde Middle	50°46'·45N 01°15'·70W
Winner	50°45'·07N 01°00'·01W
*Woolwich	50°43'·00N 01°38'·00W
Wootton Bn	50°44'·51N 01°12'·05W

2

COWES/RIVER MEDINA   10-2-22

Isle of Wight 50°45'·86N 01°17'·72W

CHARTS
AC *2793, 2040, 394*; Imray C3, Y20; Stanfords 11, 18; OS 196

TIDES
+0029 Dover; ML 2·7; Zone 0 (UT)

Standard Port PORTSMOUTH (→)

Times				Height (metres)			
High Water		Low Water		MHWS	MHWN	MLWN	MLWS
0000	0600	0500	1100	4·7	3·8	1·9	0·8
1200	1800	1700	2300				
Differences COWES							
−0015	+0015	0000	−0020	−0.5	−0.3	−0.1	0.0
FOLLY INN							
−0015	+0015	0000	−0020	−0.6	−0.4	−0.1	+0.2
NEWPORT							
No data		No data		−0.6	−0.4	+0.1	+0.8

NOTE: Double HWs occur at or near sp. On other occasions a stand occurs lasting up to 2hrs; times given represent the middle of the stand. See 10·2·12, especially for Newport.

SHELTER
Good at Cowes Yacht Haven and above the chain ferry, but outer hbr exposed to N and NE winds. ‡ prohib in hbr. Visitors may pick up any mooring so labelled: 4 large Øs N of front ldg lt (off The Parade); piles S of Cowes Yacht Haven; Thetis Pontoon (short stay/overnight only, dredged 2·5m); piles S of the chain ferry (W Cowes); 'E' Pontoon off E Cowes SC. See opposite for pontoons in Folly Reach; Island Harbour marina on E bank beyond Folly Inn and in Newport (dries). Good ‡ in Osborne Bay, 2M E, sheltered from SE to W; no landing.

NAVIGATION
WPT 50°46'·20N 01°17'·90W, 344°/164° from/to front ldg lt, 0·35M. Bramble Bank, 1·1m, lying 1M N of Prince Consort buoy, is a magnet to the keels of many yachts. From N, to clear it to the W keep the 2 conspic power stn chimneys at E Cowes open of each other.
On the E side of the ent, the Shrape (mud flats) extends to Old Castle Pt. Yachts must use the main chan near W shore and are advised to motor. Caution: strong tidal streams; do not sail through or ‡ in the mooring area. Speed limit 6kn in hbr. Beware high-speed catamarans/hydrofoils at W Cowes; car ferries at E Cowes, commercial shipping and the chain ferry which shows all round Fl W lt at fore-end, and gives way to all tfc; it runs Mon-Sat: 0435-0025, Sun 0635-0015LT. R Medina is navigable to Newport, but the upper reaches dry.

LIGHTS AND MARKS
Ldg lts 164°: Front Iso 2s 3m 6M, post by Customs Ho; rear, 290m from front, Iso R 2s 5m 3M, vis 120°-240°. Chan ent is marked by No.3 SHM buoy, Fl G 3s, and No.4 PHM buoy, QR. E bkwtr hd Fl R 3s 3M. Jetties and some dolphins show 2FR (vert) on E side of hbr, and 2FG (vert) on W side.

RADIO TELEPHONE
Cowes Hbr Radio and Hbr launches VHF Ch **69**, which all yachts are advised to monitor. Yachts >30m LOA should advise their arr/dep, and call *Chain Ferry* Ch 69 before passing. Casualties: (Ch 16/67) for ambulance at Fountain pontoon. Marinas Ch 80. *Cowes Water Taxi* Ch 08.

TELEPHONE (01983 for all IOW ☎s)
Hr Mr 293952; MRSC (01705) 552100; ⌗ (01703) 827350; Customs 293132; Folly Reach Hbr Office 295722; Weather Centre (01703) 228844; Marinecall 0891 500457; Police 528000; Ⓗ 524081; Dr 295251; Cowes Yachting 280770.

FACILITIES
Marinas: Cowes Yacht Haven (CYH) (35+165 Ⓥ, £13.50 to £17.10) ☎ 299975, Fax 200332, D (H24), FW, AC, Gas, Gaz, El, ME, Sh, SM, Ⓔ, C (1·5 ton), BH (40 ton), R, Ice, Ⓞ;
Cowes Marina, E Cowes (150+150 Ⓥ, £10.50 to £12.60) ☎ 293983, Fax 299276, AC, FW, BH (7.5 ton), ME, El, Sh, Gas, V, R.
Shepards Wharf (up to 75 berths, £9) ☎ 297821, ME, El, Ⓔ, BH (20 ton), C (6 ton), BY, SM, Sh, CH;
UK Sailing Centre (10 Ⓥ, £12), ☎ 294941, FW, Bar.
Yacht Clubs
Royal Yacht Squadron ☎ 292191; **Royal Corinthian YC** ☎ 292608; **Royal London YC** ☎ 299727; **Island SC** ☎ 296621; **Royal Ocean Racing Club** ☎ 295144 (manned only for Cowes events); **Cowes Corinthian YC** ☎ 296333; **E Cowes SC** ☎ 294394; **Cowes Combined Clubs** ☎ 295744.

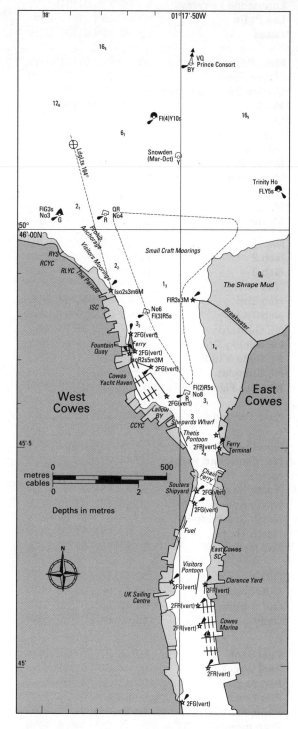

Note: Cowes Week is first week in Aug; when a free ferry runs from Island SC pontoon, call *Tenacity* Ch 06 M.
Ferries
Red Funnel ☎ 292101, all to Southampton: Car/pax from E Cowes; Hydrofoil/Catamaran (foot pax) from W Cowes.
Chain ferry ☎ 293041; **Water Taxi** ☎ 0831 325928 and VHF Ch 08 on request.
Services
A comprehensive range of marine services is available. Full details in Port Handbook & Directory, free from Hr Mr, hbr launches, marinas and Cowes Yachting.
FW from marinas, Old Town Quay, Whitegates public pontoon, Thetis pontoon and Folly Inn pontoon.
Fuel: CYH, D only H24; Lallows BY; MSB pontoon off Souters BY.
Town EC Wed; P, D, Bar, Ⓞ, Slip, ✉, Ⓑ, Gas, Gaz.

RIVER MEDINA, FOLLY REACH TO NEWPORT

FOLLY REACH, 50°44'·00N 01°16'·90W. Above Medham
ECM bn, VQ (3) 5s, there are depths of 1m to S Folly bn,
QG. There are **Ⓥ** pontoons along W bank, S of local ones.
Hr Mr ☎ 295722 and Ch 69 *Folly Launch*. **Folly Inn** ☎ 297171,
AB, L, M, Slip.
Island Harbour Marina (5ca S of Folly Inn), (150 + 100 **Ⓥ**
berths, £11.40; 2·5m), ☎ 526020, Fax 526001, AC, BH (12
ton), CH, D, El, FW, Gas, Ⓓ, ME, Sh, Slip, V, Bar. VHF Ch
80. Excellent shelter; appr via marked, dredged chan with
waiting pontoon to stbd, withies to port. Access HW ±4 to
lock (HO; H24 by arrangement) with R/G tfc lts. *Ryde
Queen* paddle steamer is conspic.

NEWPORT, 50°42'·18N 01°17'·35W. Tides see 10·2·12 and
facing page. Above Island Hbr marina the 1·2M chan to
Newport dries, but from HW Portsmouth –1½ to HW +2 it
carries 2m or more. S from Folly Inn, the hbr authority is
IoW Council. Speed limit 6kn up to Seaclose, S of
Newport Rowing Club (NRC); thence 4kn to Newport. The
chan, which is buoyed and partially lit, favours the W
bank; night appr not recommended. Power lines have
33m clearance. Ldg marks/lts are 192°, W ◇ bns 7/11m,
on the E bank, both lit 2FR (hor). In Newport, visitors'
pontoons on the E/SE sides of the basin have 1·4m HW
±2. Bilge keelers lie alongside pontoons on soft mud; fin
keelers against quay wall on firm, level bottom. Fender
boards can be supplied.
Newport Yacht Hbr (40 visitors, £7), Hr Mr ☎ 525994,
VHF Ch 69 16 (HO or as arranged), AC, FW, BY, C (10 ton).
Town EC Thurs; ME, P & D (cans), El, Sh, Slip, SM, Gas,
Ⓑ, Bar, Dr, Ⓗ, ✉, R, V.

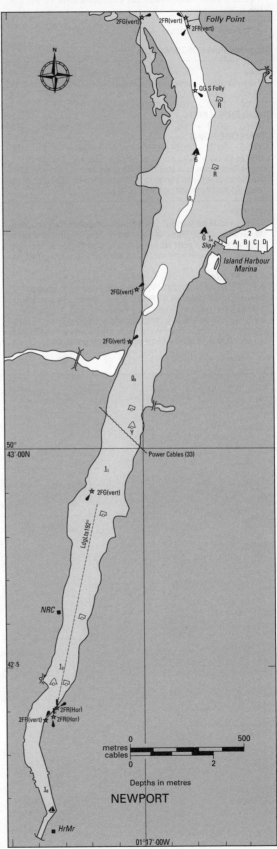

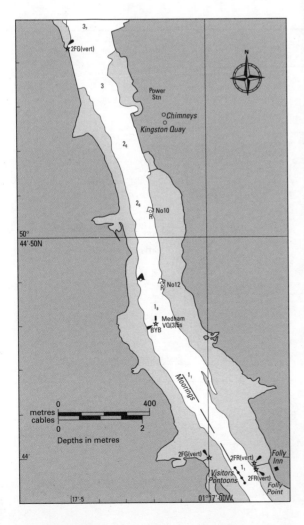

NEWPORT

BEAULIEU RIVER   10-2-23

Hampshire 50°47′·00N 01°21′·76W (Ent)

CHARTS
AC *2021, 2040, 1905*; Imray C3; Y20; Stanfords 11, 18; OS 196

TIDES
−0100 and +0140 Dover; ML 2·4; Zone 0 (UT)

Standard Port PORTSMOUTH (→)

Times				Height (metres)			
High Water		Low Water		MHWS	MHWN	MLWN	MLWS
0000	0600	0500	1100	4·7	3·8	1·9	0·8
1200	1800	1700	2300				
BUCKLER'S HARD							
−0040	−0010	+0010	−0010	−1·0	−0·8	−0·2	−0·3
STANSORE POINT							
−0050	−0010	−0005	−0010	−0·9	−0·6	−0·2	0·0

NOTE: Double HWs occur at or near springs; on other occasions there is a stand which lasts about two hrs. The predictions refer to the first HW when there are two, or to the middle of the stand. See 10.2.12.

SHELTER
Very good in all winds. ⚓ possible in reach between Lepe Ho and Beaulieu River SC, but preferable to proceed up to Buckler's Hard Yacht Hbr (pontoons and Ⓥ pile moorings).
Rabies: Craft with animals from abroad are prohibited in the river.

NAVIGATION
WPT 50°46′·50N 01°21′·45W, 159°/339° from/to abeam Beaulieu Spit dolphin (Fl R 5s), 3½ca. There are patches drying 0·3m approx 100m S of Beaulieu Spit. 1ca further SSE, almost on the ldg line, are shoal depths 0·1m. Ent dangerous LW±2. The swatchway off Beaulieu River SC is closed. A speed limit of 5kn applies to the whole river.

LIGHTS AND MARKS
Ldg bns at ent 339°, but leave marks open to E for best water. Both bns are R with Or dayglow topmarks, △ shape above □. The front is No. 2 bn, the rear is Lepe bn on shore; No 4 bn is almost in transit between these two. Beaulieu Spit, R dolphin with W band, Fl R 5s 3M vis 277°-037°; ra refl, should be left approx 40m to port. The river is clearly marked by R and G bns and perches. SHM bns 5, 9, 19 and 21 are all Fl G 4s; PHM bns 12 and 20 are Fl R 4s. Marina pontoons A, C and E have 2FR (vert).

RADIO TELEPHONE
None.

TELEPHONE (01590)
Hr Mr 616200 & 616234, mobile (0860) 919196; MRSC (01705) 552100; ⌗ (01590) 674584; Marinecall 0891 500457; Police (01703) 845511; Dr 612451 or (01703) 845955; Ⓗ 77011.

FACILITIES
Buckler's Hard Yacht Hbr £19 (110+20 visitors) ☎ 616200, Fax 616211, Slip, M, P, D, AC, FW, ME, El, Sh, C (1 ton), BH (26 ton), SM, Gas, Gaz, CH, Ⓔ, V, R, Bar.
Village V (Stores ☎ 616293), R, Bar, ✉ (Beaulieu), Ⓑ (Mon, Wed, Fri AM or Hythe), ⇌ (bus to Brockenhurst), ✈ (Bournemouth or Southampton).

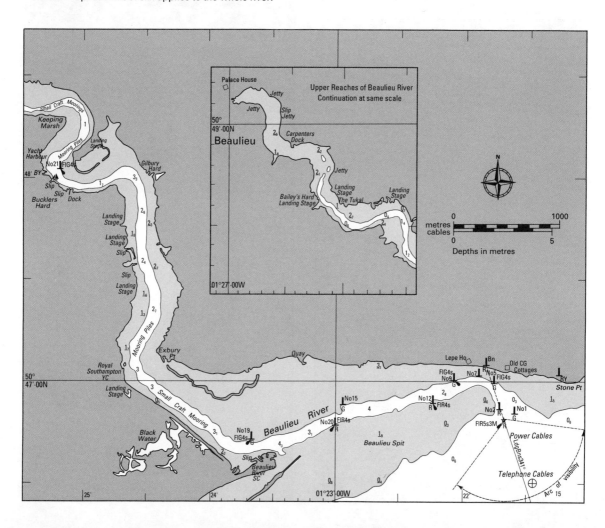

ENGLAND – SOUTHAMPTON

LAT 50°54′N   LONG 1°24′W

TIMES AND HEIGHTS OF HIGH AND LOW WATERS

YEAR **1996**

TIME ZONE (UT)
For Summer Time add ONE hour in non-shaded areas

JANUARY

Day	Time	m	Day	Time	m
1 M	0039 / 0722 / 1318 / 1956	1.7 / 4.0 / 1.6 / 3.9	**16** TU	0610 / 1213 / 1846	4.1 / 1.6 / 3.9
2 TU	0140 / 0819 / 1413 / 2052	1.6 / 4.1 / 1.4 / 4.0	**17** W	0046 / 0722 / 1328 / 2000	1.5 / 4.2 / 1.3 / 4.1
3 W	0232 / 0907 / 1500 / 2137	1.4 / 4.2 / 1.2 / 4.2	**18** TH	0157 / 0827 / 1433 / 2102	1.2 / 4.4 / 0.9 / 4.3
4 TH	0316 / 0948 / 1542 / 2215	1.2 / 4.3 / 1.0 / 4.3	**19** F	0258 / 0924 / 1531 / 2157	0.9 / 4.6 / 0.6 / 4.6
5 F ○	0357 / 1024 / 1620 / 2249	1.0 / 4.4 / 0.8 / 4.3	**20** SA ●	0353 / 1016 / 1623 / 2247	0.6 / 4.7 / 0.3 / 4.7
6 SA	0436 / 1057 / 1657 / 2321	0.9 / 4.4 / 0.7 / 4.4	**21** SU	0444 / 1104 / 1713 / 2335	0.5 / 4.8 / 0.1 / 4.8
7 SU	0513 / 1131 / 1732 / 2354	0.9 / 4.4 / 0.7 / 4.4	**22** M	0533 / 1150 / 1759	0.2 / 4.9 / 0.0
8 M	0547 / 1205 / 1804	0.9 / 4.4 / 0.8	**23** TU	0021 / 0619 / 1237 / 1842	4.8 / 0.2 / 4.8 / 0.1
9 TU	0028 / 0618 / 1240 / 1833	4.4 / 0.9 / 4.3 / 0.8	**24** W	0107 / 0703 / 1322 / 1924	4.8 / 0.4 / 4.7 / 0.3
10 W	0103 / 0649 / 1315 / 1903	4.3 / 1.0 / 4.3 / 1.0	**25** TH	0152 / 0745 / 1406 / 2004	4.6 / 0.6 / 4.6 / 0.6
11 TH	0140 / 0722 / 1352 / 1936	4.3 / 1.1 / 4.2 / 1.1	**26** F	0238 / 0828 / 1452 / 2046	4.4 / 0.9 / 4.2 / 0.9
12 F	0219 / 0759 / 1431 / 2016	4.2 / 1.3 / 4.1 / 1.3	**27** SA	0325 / 0913 / 1542 / 2132	4.2 / 1.2 / 4.0 / 1.3
13 SA	0302 / 0845 / 1517 / 2105	4.2 / 1.4 / 4.0 / 1.4	**28** SU	0418 / 1008 / 1642 / 2232	4.0 / 1.6 / 3.7 / 1.7
14 SU	0354 / 0942 / 1614 / 2208	4.1 / 1.6 / 3.9 / 1.6	**29** M	0521 / 1119 / 1758 / 2351	3.8 / 1.8 / 3.6 / 1.9
15 M	0457 / 1053 / 1726 / 2326	4.0 / 1.6 / 3.8 / 1.6	**30** TU	0637 / 1238 / 1924	3.7 / 1.8 / 3.6
			31 W	0109 / 0749 / 1346 / 2031	1.8 / 3.8 / 1.6 / 3.8

FEBRUARY

Day	Time	m	Day	Time	m
1 TH	0210 / 0846 / 1438 / 2120	1.6 / 4.0 / 1.3 / 4.0	**16** F	0144 / 0814 / 1421 / 2051	1.3 / 4.2 / 1.0 / 4.2
2 F	0258 / 0930 / 1521 / 2159	1.4 / 4.2 / 1.1 / 4.2	**17** SA	0248 / 0913 / 1520 / 2146	0.9 / 4.4 / 0.6 / 4.5
3 SA	0339 / 1007 / 1600 / 2232	1.1 / 4.3 / 0.8 / 4.3	**18** SU ●	0343 / 1004 / 1611 / 2234	0.6 / 4.6 / 0.2 / 4.7
4 SU ○	0417 / 1040 / 1638 / 2303	0.9 / 4.4 / 0.7 / 4.3	**19** M	0433 / 1050 / 1659 / 2319	0.3 / 4.8 / 0.0 / 4.8
5 M	0454 / 1112 / 1713 / 2333	0.7 / 4.4 / 0.6 / 4.4	**20** TU	0519 / 1134 / 1743	0.1 / 4.8 / -0.1
6 TU	0528 / 1144 / 1746	0.7 / 4.4 / 0.6	**21** W	0002 / 0602 / 1217 / 1823	4.8 / 0.1 / 4.8 / -0.1
7 W	0005 / 0559 / 1218 / 1815	4.4 / 0.7 / 4.4 / 0.6	**22** TH	0044 / 0642 / 1258 / 1901	4.7 / 0.2 / 4.6 / 0.1
8 TH	0039 / 0629 / 1252 / 1844	4.4 / 0.7 / 4.4 / 0.7	**23** F	0125 / 0719 / 1338 / 1936	4.6 / 0.4 / 4.5 / 0.5
9 F	0113 / 0700 / 1327 / 1915	4.4 / 0.8 / 4.3 / 0.8	**24** SA	0205 / 0755 / 1419 / 2011	4.4 / 0.7 / 4.2 / 0.8
10 SA	0150 / 0735 / 1405 / 1952	4.3 / 0.9 / 4.2 / 1.0	**25** SU	0246 / 0832 / 1503 / 2049	4.2 / 1.1 / 4.0 / 1.3
11 SU	0230 / 0816 / 1447 / 2036	4.2 / 1.1 / 4.1 / 1.2	**26** M	0330 / 0916 / 1554 / 2139	3.9 / 1.5 / 3.7 / 1.7
12 M	0317 / 0907 / 1541 / 2134	4.1 / 1.3 / 3.9 / 1.4	**27** TU	0426 / 1019 / 1705 / 2258	3.7 / 1.8 / 3.5 / 2.0
13 TU	0418 / 1015 / 1652 / 2252	4.0 / 1.5 / 3.8 / 1.6	**28** W	0543 / 1149 / 1841	3.5 / 1.9 / 3.5
14 W	0536 / 1143 / 1820	3.9 / 1.6 / 3.8	**29** TH	0034 / 0712 / 1312 / 2003	2.0 / 3.6 / 1.8 / 3.7
15 TH	0024 / 0700 / 1310 / 1944	1.6 / 4.0 / 1.4 / 4.0			

MARCH

Day	Time	m	Day	Time	m
1 F	0145 / 0820 / 1411 / 2056	1.8 / 3.8 / 1.5 / 3.9	**16** SA	0132 / 0802 / 1407 / 2039	1.3 / 4.1 / 1.0 / 4.2
2 SA	0235 / 0907 / 1456 / 2136	1.5 / 4.0 / 1.2 / 4.1	**17** SU	0236 / 0901 / 1504 / 2131	0.9 / 4.3 / 0.6 / 4.5
3 SU	0316 / 0945 / 1536 / 2209	1.2 / 4.2 / 0.9 / 4.3	**18** M	0329 / 0950 / 1554 / 2217	0.6 / 4.5 / 0.3 / 4.6
4 M	0354 / 1017 / 1613 / 2239	0.9 / 4.3 / 0.6 / 4.3	**19** TU ●	0416 / 1033 / 1639 / 2300	0.3 / 4.6 / 0.1 / 4.7
5 TU ○	0430 / 1048 / 1649 / 2308	0.7 / 4.4 / 0.5 / 4.4	**20** W	0500 / 1114 / 1721 / 2340	0.1 / 4.7 / 0.0 / 4.7
6 W	0505 / 1120 / 1723 / 2340	0.5 / 4.4 / 0.4 / 4.4	**21** TH	0541 / 1154 / 1800	0.1 / 4.7 / 0.0
7 TH	0537 / 1153 / 1755	0.5 / 4.5 / 0.4	**22** F	0019 / 0618 / 1233 / 1836	4.7 / 0.2 / 4.6 / 0.2
8 F	0013 / 0608 / 1228 / 1825	4.5 / 0.5 / 4.5 / 0.5	**23** SA	0057 / 0653 / 1311 / 1909	4.5 / 0.4 / 4.4 / 0.5
9 SA	0048 / 0640 / 1304 / 1857	4.5 / 0.5 / 4.4 / 0.6	**24** SU	0134 / 0725 / 1350 / 1940	4.4 / 0.7 / 4.2 / 0.9
10 SU	0125 / 0715 / 1343 / 1934	4.4 / 0.7 / 4.3 / 0.8	**25** M	0211 / 0757 / 1430 / 2014	4.1 / 1.0 / 4.0 / 1.3
11 M	0206 / 0755 / 1427 / 2018	4.3 / 0.9 / 4.2 / 1.1	**26** TU	0251 / 0835 / 1517 / 2057	3.9 / 1.4 / 3.8 / 1.7
12 TU	0254 / 0845 / 1522 / 2115	4.1 / 1.2 / 4.0 / 1.4	**27** W	0340 / 0926 / 1619 / 2205	3.7 / 1.7 / 3.6 / 2.0
13 W	0355 / 0953 / 1635 / 2236	3.9 / 1.4 / 3.8 / 1.6	**28** TH	0447 / 1048 / 1747 / 2345	3.5 / 1.9 / 3.5 / 2.1
14 TH	0516 / 1124 / 1807	3.8 / 1.5 / 3.8	**29** F	0618 / 1222 / 1918	3.5 / 1.9 / 3.6
15 F	0011 / 0646 / 1256 / 1933	1.6 / 3.8 / 1.4 / 3.9	**30** SA	0106 / 0738 / 1331 / 2018	1.9 / 3.6 / 1.6 / 3.9
			31 SU	0201 / 0832 / 1420 / 2100	1.6 / 3.9 / 1.3 / 4.1

APRIL

Day	Time	m	Day	Time	m
1 M	0244 / 0912 / 1503 / 2135	1.3 / 4.1 / 1.0 / 4.2	**16** TU	0308 / 0931 / 1530 / 2157	0.7 / 4.4 / 0.5 / 4.6
2 TU	0324 / 0947 / 1542 / 2207	0.9 / 4.2 / 0.7 / 4.4	**17** W ●	0354 / 1014 / 1614 / 2238	0.4 / 4.5 / 0.3 / 4.6
3 W	0401 / 1020 / 1620 / 2239	0.7 / 4.4 / 0.5 / 4.5	**18** TH	0437 / 1053 / 1656 / 2316	0.3 / 4.5 / 0.2 / 4.6
4 TH ○	0437 / 1053 / 1656 / 2313	0.5 / 4.5 / 0.4 / 4.5	**19** F	0517 / 1131 / 1735 / 2353	0.2 / 4.5 / 0.3 / 4.5
5 F	0513 / 1129 / 1731 / 2348	0.4 / 4.5 / 0.4 / 4.6	**20** SA	0554 / 1209 / 1810	0.3 / 4.4 / 0.4
6 SA	0548 / 1206 / 1806	0.3 / 4.6 / 0.4	**21** SU	0029 / 0627 / 1246 / 1843	4.4 / 0.5 / 4.4 / 0.7
7 SU	0026 / 0623 / 1246 / 1842	4.5 / 0.4 / 4.5 / 0.6	**22** M	0105 / 0658 / 1324 / 1914	4.3 / 0.7 / 4.2 / 1.0
8 M	0106 / 0701 / 1329 / 1922	4.5 / 0.5 / 4.4 / 0.8	**23** TU	0142 / 0729 / 1404 / 1947	4.2 / 1.0 / 4.1 / 1.3
9 TU	0150 / 0744 / 1417 / 2010	4.3 / 0.8 / 4.2 / 1.0	**24** W	0221 / 0804 / 1449 / 2027	4.0 / 1.3 / 3.9 / 1.6
10 W	0241 / 0836 / 1516 / 2110	4.1 / 1.1 / 4.0 / 1.3	**25** TH	0305 / 0848 / 1543 / 2124	3.8 / 1.6 / 3.7 / 1.9
11 TH	0345 / 0944 / 1631 / 2230	3.9 / 1.4 / 3.9 / 1.5	**26** F	0401 / 0951 / 1653 / 2245	3.6 / 1.8 / 3.6 / 2.1
12 F	0506 / 1111 / 1758 / 2358	3.8 / 1.5 / 3.9 / 1.5	**27** SA	0515 / 1116 / 1814	3.5 / 1.9 / 3.7
13 SA	0633 / 1236 / 1918	3.8 / 1.3 / 4.0	**28** SU	0009 / 0635 / 1234 / 1922	2.0 / 3.6 / 1.8 / 3.9
14 SU	0115 / 0746 / 1345 / 2021	1.3 / 4.0 / 1.1 / 4.3	**29** M	0112 / 0740 / 1332 / 2013	1.8 / 3.8 / 1.5 / 4.1
15 M	0216 / 0843 / 1441 / 2112	1.0 / 4.3 / 0.7 / 4.5	**30** TU	0202 / 0829 / 1420 / 2054	1.4 / 4.0 / 1.2 / 4.3

Chart Datum: 2·74 metres below Ordnance Datum (Newlyn)

ENGLAND – SOUTHAMPTON

LAT 50°54′N   LONG   1°24′W

TIMES AND HEIGHTS OF HIGH AND LOW WATERS

YEAR **1996**

TIME ZONE (UT)
For Summer Time add ONE hour in non-shaded areas

Chart Datum: 2·74 metres below Ordnance Datum (Newlyn)

MAY

	Time	m		Time	m
1 W	0246 0910 1504 2132	1.1 4.2 0.9 4.4	**16** TH	0329 0954 1547 2215	0.7 4.3 0.7 4.5
2 TH	0327 0948 1546 2209	0.8 4.4 0.7 4.5	**17** F	0412 1034 1629 2253 ●	0.6 4.4 0.6 4.5
3 F O	0408 1027 1627 2247	0.5 4.5 0.5 4.6	**18** SA	0452 1111 1709 2329	0.6 4.4 0.6 4.4
4 SA	0448 1107 1708 2326	0.4 4.6 0.4 4.7	**19** SU	0530 1148 1746	0.5 4.3 0.7
5 SU	0529 1149 1749	0.3 4.6 0.4	**20** M	0004 0604 1225 1820	4.4 0.6 4.3 0.9
6 M	0008 0609 1233 1830	4.6 0.3 4.6 0.6	**21** TU	0041 0636 1303 1853	4.3 0.8 4.2 1.1
7 TU	0053 0652 1321 1916	4.6 0.5 4.5 0.8	**22** W	0118 0707 1342 1926	4.2 1.0 4.2 1.3
8 W	0141 0739 1413 2007	4.4 0.7 4.3 1.0	**23** TH	0156 0740 1424 2004	4.1 1.2 4.1 1.6
9 TH	0236 0833 1514 2108	1.0 4.2 1.3	**24** F	0237 0819 1511 2050	3.9 1.4 3.9 1.8
10 F	0340 0938 1625 2220	4.0 1.2 4.1 1.4	**25** SA	0324 0908 1606 2150	3.8 1.7 3.9 2.0
11 SA	0454 1053 1742 2337	3.9 1.4 4.1 1.5	**26** SU	0421 1012 1711 2302	3.7 1.8 3.8 2.0
12 SU	0612 1209 1855	3.9 1.3 4.2	**27** M	0529 1126 1818	3.7 1.8 3.9
13 M	0049 0721 1316 1956	1.3 4.0 1.2 4.4	**28** TU	0011 0638 1234 1918	1.8 3.8 1.6 4.1
14 TU	0150 0820 1413 2048	1.1 4.2 1.0 4.4	**29** W	0111 0739 1332 2010	1.6 3.9 1.4 4.3
15 W	0242 0910 1502 2134	0.9 4.3 0.8 4.5	**30** TH	0204 0831 1424 2056	1.3 4.1 1.1 4.4
			31 F	0253 0918 1513 2140	1.0 4.3 0.9 4.6

JUNE

	Time	m		Time	m
1 SA O	0340 1003 1601 2224	0.7 4.5 0.7 4.7	**16** SU ●	0429 1054 1646 2309	0.8 4.3 0.9 4.4
2 SU	0427 1048 1647 2309	0.5 4.6 0.5 4.7	**17** M	0507 1130 1725 2344	0.8 4.3 0.9 4.3
3 M	0513 1135 1734 2355	0.3 4.7 0.5 4.7	**18** TU	0544 1205 1801	0.8 4.3 1.0
4 TU	0559 1223 1822	0.3 4.7 0.6	**19** W	0019 0616 1242 1835	4.3 0.9 4.3 1.1
5 W	0043 0646 1314 1910	4.7 0.4 4.6 0.7	**20** TH	0056 0648 1319 1907	4.2 1.0 4.2 1.2
6 TH	0134 0735 1408 2002	4.6 0.6 4.5 0.9	**21** F	0133 0719 1358 1941	4.2 1.2 4.2 1.4
7 F	0228 0826 1506 2058	4.4 0.8 4.4 1.1	**22** SA	0211 0801 1439 2019	4.1 1.3 4.1 1.6
8 SA	0328 0923 1609 2201	4.2 1.1 4.3 1.3	**23** SU	0251 0833 1524 2106	4.0 1.5 4.1 1.7
9 SU	0433 1027 1716 2308	4.1 1.3 4.2 1.4	**24** M	0338 0923 1617 2203	3.9 1.6 4.0 1.8
10 M	0542 1135 1824	4.0 1.4 4.2	**25** TU	0434 1025 1718 2310	3.8 1.7 4.0 1.8
11 TU	0016 0651 1242 1927	1.5 4.0 1.4 4.2	**26** W	0540 1136 1824	3.8 1.7 4.1
12 W	0120 0754 1342 2023	1.4 4.0 1.3 4.3	**27** TH	0019 0829 1246 1926	1.7 3.9 1.6 4.2
13 TH	0215 0848 1435 2111	1.2 4.1 1.2 4.4	**28** F	0124 0754 1349 2024	1.4 4.1 1.3 4.4
14 F	0304 0936 1522 2154	1.0 4.3 1.1 4.4	**29** SA	0223 0851 1446 2116	1.1 4.3 1.1 4.6
15 SA	0348 1017 1605 2233	0.9 4.3 1.0 4.4	**30** SU	0317 0943 1540 2206	0.8 4.5 0.8 4.7

JULY

	Time	m		Time	m
1 M O	0409 1034 1632 2254	0.5 4.6 0.6 4.8	**16** TU	0446 1112 1705 2325	0.9 4.3 1.0 4.3
2 TU	0500 1123 1723 2343	0.4 4.7 0.5 4.8	**17** W	0523 1145 1742 2358	0.8 4.3 1.0 4.3
3 W	0549 1213 1813	0.3 4.8 0.5	**18** TH	0558 1218 1815	0.9 4.3 1.0
4 TH	0032 0637 1303 1901	4.8 0.3 4.7 0.6	**19** F	0032 0628 1253 1846	4.3 1.0 4.3 1.1
5 F	0122 0725 1354 1950	4.7 0.4 4.7 0.7	**20** SA	0107 0657 1328 1916	4.3 1.1 4.3 1.2
6 SA	0213 0812 1447 2040	4.5 0.7 4.5 1.0	**21** SU	0143 0727 1405 1948	4.2 1.2 4.2 1.4
7 SU	0306 0901 1542 2133	4.3 0.9 4.4 1.2	**22** M	0219 0802 1445 2028	4.1 1.4 4.2 1.5
8 M	0403 0955 1642 2232	4.2 1.3 4.2 1.5	**23** TU	0300 0845 1531 2116	4.1 1.5 4.1 1.7
9 TU	0506 1057 1746 2339	4.0 1.5 4.1 1.6	**24** W	0350 0939 1627 2218	4.0 1.7 4.0 1.8
10 W	0616 1205 1854	3.9 1.7 4.1	**25** TH	0453 1048 1736 2334	3.9 1.8 4.0 1.8
11 TH	0047 0726 1314 1957	1.6 3.9 1.7 4.1	**26** F	0609 1208 1850	3.9 1.7 4.1
12 F	0149 0829 1412 2052	1.5 4.0 1.6 4.2	**27** SA	0051 0724 1323 1959	1.6 4.0 1.5 4.3
13 SA	0241 0920 1502 2137	1.3 4.1 1.4 4.3	**28** SU	0201 0831 1429 2058	1.3 4.3 1.2 4.5
14 SU	0326 1003 1546 2216	1.2 4.3 1.2 4.3	**29** M	0301 0928 1527 2151	0.9 4.5 0.9 4.7
15 M ●	0408 1039 1627 2251	1.0 4.3 1.1 4.4	**30** TU O	0357 1020 1621 2241	0.6 4.7 0.6 4.8
			31 W	0448 1110 1712 2329	0.3 4.8 0.4 4.9

AUGUST

	Time	m		Time	m
1 TH	0537 1158 1800	0.2 4.9 0.3	**16** F	0535 1151 1752	0.8 4.4 0.9
2 F	0016 0623 1246 1846	4.9 0.2 4.8 0.4	**17** SA	0006 0606 1224 1821	4.4 0.9 4.4 0.9
3 SA	0103 0708 1333 1930	4.8 0.3 4.7 0.6	**18** SU	0040 0634 1257 1849	4.4 1.0 4.4 1.0
4 SU	0150 0750 1416 2014	4.6 0.6 4.6 0.8	**19** M	0113 0702 1332 1920	4.3 1.1 4.3 1.1
5 M	0238 0833 1509 2059	4.4 0.9 4.4 1.2	**20** TU	0149 0735 1410 1956	4.3 1.2 4.3 1.3
6 TU	0328 0919 1601 2151	4.2 1.3 4.2 1.5	**21** W	0228 0814 1453 2041	4.2 1.4 4.2 1.5
7 W	0426 1015 1703 2256	3.9 1.7 3.9 1.8	**22** TH	0316 0905 1548 2141	4.1 1.6 4.1 1.7
8 TH	0536 1127 1817	3.8 1.9 3.9	**23** F	0420 1015 1701 2302	3.9 1.8 4.0 1.8
9 F	0013 0658 1247 1931	1.9 3.8 2.0 3.9	**24** SA	0541 1143 1825	3.9 1.8 4.0
10 SA	0125 0810 1354 2033	1.8 3.9 1.8 4.1	**25** SU	0031 0706 1308 1942	1.7 4.0 1.6 4.2
11 SU	0221 0904 1445 2120	1.4 4.1 1.6 4.2	**26** M	0147 0817 1418 2044	1.4 4.3 1.3 4.4
12 M	0306 0946 1527 2158	1.3 4.2 1.3 4.3	**27** TU	0249 0915 1516 2138	1.0 4.5 0.9 4.7
13 TU	0346 1021 1606 2232	1.1 4.3 1.1 4.4	**28** W O	0344 1006 1608 2226	0.6 4.7 0.6 4.8
14 W ●	0424 1051 1644 2303	0.9 4.4 0.9 4.4	**29** TH	0433 1053 1657 2311	0.3 4.9 0.3 4.9
15 TH	0501 1121 1719 2334	0.8 4.4 0.9 4.4	**30** F	0520 1138 1743 2355	0.1 4.9 0.3
			31 SA	0604 1222 1826	0.1 4.9 0.3

2

ENGLAND – SOUTHAMPTON

LAT 50°54′N   LONG   1°24′W

TIMES AND HEIGHTS OF HIGH AND LOW WATERS   YEAR **1996**

TIME ZONE (UT)
For Summer Time add ONE hour in non-shaded areas

SEPTEMBER

Time	m	Time	m
1 SU 0039 0645 1306 1906	4.8 0.3 4.8 0.5	**16** M 0011 0609 1229 1825	4.5 0.8 4.5 0.8
2 M 0123 0724 1349 1945	4.7 0.6 4.6 0.8	**17** TU 0046 0639 1304 1856	4.5 1.0 4.5 1.0
3 TU 0206 0801 1432 2024	4.4 0.9 4.4 1.1	**18** W 0123 0712 1343 1933	4.4 1.1 4.4 1.2
4 W 0252 0841 1519 2108	4.2 1.4 4.1 1.5	**19** TH 0204 0753 1427 2018	4.3 1.3 4.2 1.4
5 TH 0345 0930 1616 2208	3.9 1.8 3.9 1.9	**20** F 0254 0845 1524 2119	4.1 1.6 4.1 1.7
6 F 0453 1042 1731 2332	3.7 2.1 3.7 2.1	**21** SA 0402 0956 1640 2244	4.0 1.8 3.9 1.8
7 SA 0623 1216 1858	3.7 2.2 3.8	**22** SU 0527 1130 1809	3.9 1.8 4.0
8 SU 0055 0744 1330 2007	2.0 3.8 2.0 3.9	**23** M 0018 0654 1257 1928	1.7 4.1 1.6 4.2
9 M 0156 0840 1422 2056	1.7 4.1 1.7 4.1	**24** TU 0134 0804 1405 2030	1.4 4.3 1.3 4.4
10 TU 0241 0921 1503 2134	1.4 4.2 1.4 4.3	**25** W 0234 0900 1501 2122	1.0 4.6 0.9 4.7
11 W 0321 0955 1541 2207	1.2 4.4 1.2 4.4	**26** TH 0326 0949 1551 2208	0.6 4.8 0.6 4.8
12 TH 0358 1025 1617 ● 2236	0.9 4.4 0.9 4.5	**27** F 0414 1034 1638 O 2251	0.3 4.9 0.4 4.9
13 F 0434 1053 1652 2306	0.8 4.5 0.8 4.5	**28** SA 0458 1116 1722 2333	0.2 4.9 0.3 4.8
14 SA 0508 1123 1725 2338	0.8 4.5 0.8 4.5	**29** SU 0540 1157 1803	0.2 4.9 0.3
15 SU 0540 1154 1756	0.8 4.5 0.8	**30** M 0014 0619 1238 1840	4.8 0.4 4.7 0.5

OCTOBER

Time	m	Time	m
1 TU 0055 0655 1318 1915	4.6 0.6 4.6 0.8	**16** W 0024 0619 1243 1839	4.6 0.8 4.6 0.8
2 W 0136 0729 1358 1950	4.4 1.0 4.4 1.1	**17** TH 0105 0657 1324 1919	4.5 1.0 4.4 1.0
3 TH 0218 0805 1440 2029	4.2 1.4 4.1 1.5	**18** F 0150 0741 1412 2008	4.4 1.2 4.3 1.3
4 F 0307 0848 1530 2119	3.9 1.8 3.9 1.9	**19** SA 0245 0848 1511 2110	4.2 1.5 4.1 1.5
5 SA 0409 0952 1636 2238	3.7 2.2 3.7 2.1	**20** SU 0354 0949 1627 2233	4.0 1.7 4.0 1.7
6 SU 0533 1128 1805	3.7 2.3 3.7	**21** M 0517 1118 1753	3.7 1.8 4.0
7 M 0010 0701 1251 1924	2.1 3.8 2.2 3.8	**22** TU 0001 0639 1240 1910	1.6 4.2 1.6 4.2
8 TU 0117 0802 1347 2019	1.9 4.0 1.9 4.0	**23** W 0114 0747 1345 2012	1.3 4.4 1.3 4.4
9 W 0206 0846 1431 2100	1.6 4.2 1.6 4.2	**24** TH 0213 0842 1441 2103	1.0 4.6 0.9 4.6
10 TH 0248 0929 1510 2134	1.3 4.4 1.2 4.4	**25** F 0303 0929 1530 2148	0.7 4.8 0.7 4.7
11 F 0326 0952 1547 2206	1.0 4.5 1.0 4.5	**26** SA 0350 1013 1615 O 2230	0.5 4.8 0.5 4.7
12 SA 0403 1022 1622 ● 2238	0.8 4.6 0.8 4.6	**27** SU 0433 1053 1658 2311	0.4 4.8 0.4 4.7
13 SU 0438 1054 1657 2311	0.7 4.6 0.7 4.6	**28** M 0514 1133 1738 2350	0.4 4.8 0.5 4.6
14 M 0512 1128 1730 2346	0.7 4.7 0.7 4.6	**29** TU 0552 1211 1815	0.5 4.7 0.6
15 TU 0546 1204 1804	0.7 4.6 0.7	**30** W 0029 0627 1249 1848	4.5 0.8 4.5 0.8
		31 TH 0109 0701 1327 1921	4.4 1.1 4.4 1.1

NOVEMBER

Time	m	Time	m
1 F 0150 0735 1407 1956	4.2 1.4 4.2 1.4	**16** SA 0143 0735 1404 2003	4.5 1.1 4.4 1.1
2 SA 0235 0815 1451 2039	4.0 1.7 4.0 1.7	**17** SU 0240 0831 1503 2103	4.3 1.3 4.2 1.3
3 SU 0329 0908 1546 2139	3.9 2.0 3.8 2.0	**18** M 0346 0939 1612 2216	4.2 1.5 4.1 1.5
4 M 0437 1025 1658 2303	3.8 2.2 3.7 2.1	**19** TU 0501 1057 1730 2334	4.1 1.6 4.1 1.5
5 TU 0556 1151 1819	3.8 2.2 3.7	**20** W 0616 1213 1845	4.2 1.5 4.1
6 W 0021 0706 1258 1926	2.0 4.0 2.0 3.9	**21** TH 0045 0722 1320 1949	1.4 4.4 1.3 4.3
7 TH 0119 0758 1348 2017	1.7 4.2 1.7 4.1	**22** F 0145 0819 1416 2043	1.2 4.5 1.1 4.4
8 F 0207 0840 1432 2057	1.4 4.4 1.4 4.3	**23** SA 0237 0908 1507 2130	0.9 4.6 0.9 4.5
9 SA 0249 0917 1512 2134	1.2 4.5 1.1 4.4	**24** SU 0325 0952 1552 2213	0.8 4.7 0.7 4.5
10 SU 0329 0952 1551 2211	0.9 4.6 0.8 4.6	**25** M 0408 1032 1635 2253	0.7 4.7 0.6 4.5
11 M 0408 1027 1630 ● 2248	0.8 4.7 0.7 4.6	**26** TU 0449 1110 1714 2331	0.6 4.6 0.6 4.5
12 TU 0446 1105 1708 2327	0.7 4.8 0.6 4.7	**27** W 0528 1147 1751	0.7 4.6 0.7
13 W 0525 1145 1747	0.7 4.8 0.6	**28** TH 0008 0604 1224 1824	4.5 0.8 4.4 0.8
14 TH 0009 0604 1227 1828	4.7 0.7 4.7 0.7	**29** F 0047 0638 1302 1856	4.4 1.0 4.4 1.0
15 F 0054 0647 1313 1912	4.6 0.9 4.6 0.8	**30** SA 0126 0712 1340 1929	4.3 1.3 4.2 1.2

DECEMBER

Time	m	Time	m
1 SU 0208 0748 1420 2006	4.2 1.5 4.1 1.5	**16** M 0230 0822 1449 2049	4.5 1.0 4.4 1.0
2 M 0254 0831 1506 2052	4.1 1.8 3.9 1.7	**17** TU 0329 0921 1551 2150	4.3 1.3 4.2 1.2
3 TU 0346 0927 1600 2152	4.0 2.0 3.8 1.9	**18** W 0434 1028 1659 2259	4.2 1.4 4.0 1.4
4 W 0449 1038 1707 2306	3.9 2.1 3.7 1.9	**19** TH 0543 1140 1812	4.2 1.5 4.0
5 TH 0556 1152 1820	3.9 2.0 3.8	**20** F 0009 0651 1249 1922	1.5 4.2 1.4 4.0
6 F 0018 0659 1256 1924	1.8 4.1 1.8 3.9	**21** SA 0115 0753 1351 2024	1.4 4.3 1.3 4.1
7 SA 0118 0753 1349 2018	1.6 4.2 1.5 4.1	**22** SU 0213 0847 1444 2115	1.2 4.4 1.1 4.2
8 SU 0209 0840 1437 2104	1.3 4.4 1.2 4.3	**23** M 0302 0934 1531 2200	1.1 4.5 0.9 4.3
9 M 0256 0922 1523 2147	1.1 4.6 0.9 4.5	**24** TU 0347 1015 1614 O 2240	0.9 4.5 0.7 4.4
10 TU 0341 1004 1607 ● 2230	0.8 4.7 0.7 4.6	**25** W 0429 1053 1653 2316	0.8 4.5 0.7 4.4
11 W 0425 1046 1651 2313	0.7 4.8 0.5 4.7	**26** TH 0508 1128 1730 2352	0.8 4.5 0.6 4.4
12 TH 0509 1130 1735 2358	0.6 4.8 0.4 4.7	**27** F 0545 1203 1805	0.8 4.4 0.7
13 F 0554 1215 1820	0.6 4.8 0.4	**28** SA 0027 0619 1239 1836	4.4 0.9 4.4 0.8
14 SA 0045 0640 1303 1906	4.7 0.7 4.7 0.5	**29** SU 0104 0652 1316 1906	4.3 1.1 4.3 1.0
15 SU 0136 0729 1354 1955	4.6 0.8 4.5 0.7	**30** M 0141 0724 1353 1938	4.3 1.3 4.2 1.2
		31 TU 0221 0759 1432 2014	4.2 1.5 4.1 1.4

Chart Datum: 2·74 metres below Ordnance Datum (Newlyn)

SOUTHAMPTON   10-2-24

Hampshire 50°52'·90N 01°23'·40W

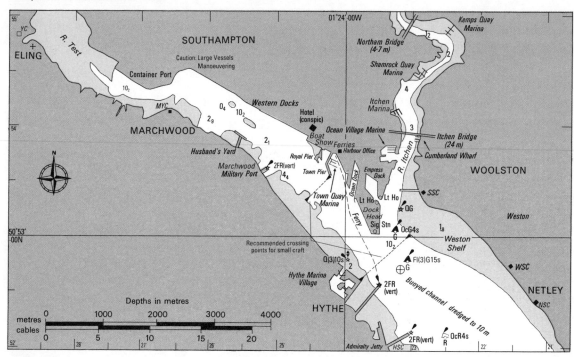

CHARTS

AC *2041, 1905, 394, 2045*; Imray C3; Stanfords 11, 18; OS 196

TIDES

HW (1st) –0001 Dover; ML 2·9; Zone 0 (UT)

Standard Port SOUTHAMPTON (←)

Times				Height (metres)			
High Water		Low Water		MHWS	MHWN	MLWN	MLWS
0400	1100	0000	0600	4·5	3·7	1·8	0·5
1600	2300	1200	1800				

Differences REDBRIDGE

–0020	+0005	0000	–0005	–0·1	–0·1	–0·1	–0·1

Southampton is a Standard Port and tidal predictions for each day of the year are given above. At sp there are two separate HWs about two hrs apart; at nps there is a long stand. Predictions are for the first HW when there are two, otherwise for the middle of the stand. See 10·2·12. NE gales combined with high barometer may lower sea level by 0·6m.

SHELTER

Good in most winds, although a heavy chop develops in SE winds >F4, when it may be best to shelter in marinas. Ⓥ berths available in Hythe Marina (with lock ent), Town Quay marina (ent to R Test), and on R Itchen at Ocean Village, Itchen, Shamrock Quay and Kemp's Marinas. There are no specific yacht ⚓s but temp ⚓ is permitted (subject to Hr Mr) off club moorings at Netley, Hythe, Weston and Marchwood in about 2m. Keep clear of main or secondary chans and Hythe Pier. Public moorings for larger yachts opposite Royal Pier near Gymp Elbow PHM buoy in 4m (contact Hr Mr); nearest landing is at Town Quay Marina.

NAVIGATION

WPT Weston Shelf SHM buoy, Fl (3) G 15s, 50°52'·68N 01°23'·16W, 138°/318° from/to Port Sig Stn, 0·40M. Main chans are well marked. Yachts should keep just outside the buoyed lit fairway and are recommended to cross it at 90° abeam Fawley chy, at Cadland/Greenland buoys, abeam Hythe and abeam Town Quay. Caution: several large unlit buoys off Hythe, both sides of the main chan, and elsewhere. It is essential to keep clear of very large tankers operating from Fawley and passenger and container ships from Southampton. See also 10·2·20 for the Area of Concern between Cowes and Calshot. .

R Test There is foul ground at Marchwood and Royal Pier; extensive container port beyond. Eling Chan dries.

R Itchen Care is necessary, particularly at night. Above Itchen Bridge the chan bends sharply to port and favours the W side. There are unlit moorings in the centre of the river. Navigation above Northam Bridge (4·7m clearance) is not advisable.

There is a speed limit of 6kn in both rivers above the line Hythe Pier to Weston Shelf.

LIGHTS AND MARKS

Main lts are on the chartlet and in 10.2.4. Fawley chimney (198m, R lts) is conspic day/night. Note also:
(1) Hythe Marina Village, close NW of Hythe Pier: appr chan marked by Q (3) 10s, ECM bn and Fl (2) R 5s PHM bn. Lock ent, N side 2 FG (vert); S side 2 FR (vert).
(2) Southampton Water divides at Dock Head which is easily identified by conspic silos and a high lattice mast showing traffic sigs which are mandatory for commercial vessels, but may be disregarded by yachts outside the main chans. Beware large ships manoeuvering off Dock Head, and craft leaving Rivers Itchen and Test.
(3) Dock Hd, W side (Queen Elizabeth II Terminal, S end) 4 FG (vert) 3M; framework tr; marks ent to R Test. Town Quay Marina has 2 FR and 2 FG (vert) on wavebreaks.
(4) Ent to R Itchen marked by SHM Oc G 4s, beyond which piles with G lts mark E side of chan ldg to Itchen bridge (24·4m); a FW lt at bridge centre marks the main chan. Ent to Ocean Village is facing Vosper Thorneycroft sheds, conspic on E bank.
(5) Above Itchen Bridge, marked by 2 FR (vert) and 2 FG (vert), the principal marks are: Crosshouse bn Oc R 5s; Chapel bn Fl G 3s. **Caution:** 8 large unlit mooring buoys in middle of river. Shamrock Quay pontoons 2 FR (vert) at SW and NE ends; No 5 bn Fl G 3s; No 7 bn Fl (2) G 5s; Millstone Pt jetty 2 FR (vert); No 9 bn Fl (4) G 10s and Kemps Quay Marina 2 FG (vert). Northam Bridge, FR/FG, has 4·7m clearance.

RADIO TELEPHONE

Vessel Traffic Services (VTS) Centre. Call: *Southampton VTS* Ch **12** 14 16 (H24).
Traffic info for small craft broadcast on Ch 12 on the hour 0600-2200 Fri-Sun and Bank Holiday Mons from Easter to last weekend in Oct. From 1 June to 30 Sept broadcasts are every day at the same times (see 10.2.20).
Southampton Hbr Patrol Call: *Southampton Patrol* VHF Ch **12** 16, 01-28, 60-88 (H24). Marinas VHF Ch **80** M.
Fuel barges in R Itchen, call *Mr Diesel* or *Wyefuel* Ch 08.

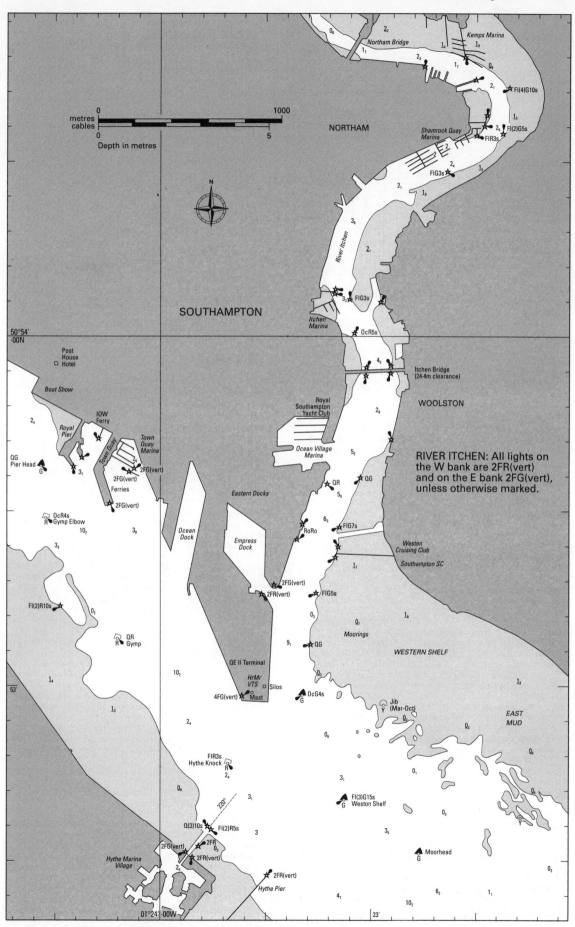

2

metres
cables

0   1000

0   5

Depth in metres

N

NORTHAM

Northam Bridge

Kemps Marina

Fl(4)G10s

Shamrock Quay
Marina

Fl(2)G5s

FlR3s

FlG3s

River Itchen

SOUTHAMPTON

FlG3s

Itchen
Marina

OcR5s

50°54'
·00N

Post
House
Hotel

Itchen Bridge
(24·4m clearance)

WOOLSTON

Boat Show

IOW
Ferry

Royal
Pier

Town
Quay
Marina

QG
Pier Head
G

2FG(vert)

2FG(vert)

Ferries

2FG(vert)

Royal
Southampton
Yacht Club

Ocean Village
Marina

RIVER ITCHEN: All lights on
the W bank are 2FR(vert)
and on the E bank 2FG(vert),
unless otherwise marked.

QR

QG

Eastern Docks

OcR4s
R Gymp Elbow

Ocean
Dock

Empress
Dock

RoRo

FlG7s

Weston
Cruising Club

Southampton SC

Fl(2)R10s

QR
R Gymp

2FG(vert)

2FR(vert)

FlG5s

Moorings

WESTERN SHELF

QG

QE II Terminal

HrMr
VTS   Silos

4FG(vert)   Mast

OcG4s
G

Jib
(Mar-Oct)
Y

EAST
MUD

53'

FlR3s
Hythe Knock
R

220°

Q(3)10s

Fl(2)R5s

Fl(3)G15s
G Weston Shelf

2FG(vert)

2FR
O₃

2FR(vert)

Hythe Marina
Village

Moorhead
G

2FR(vert)

Hythe Pier

01°24'·00W

23'

SOUTHAMPTON continued

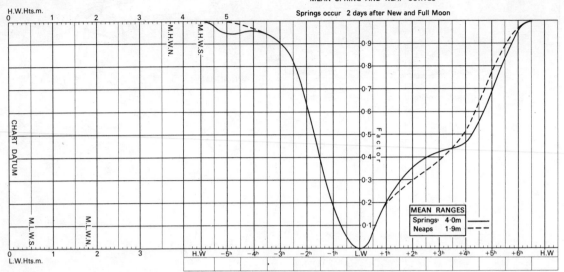

SOUTHAMPTON
MEAN SPRING AND NEAP CURVES
Springs occur 2 days after New and Full Moon

TELEPHONE (01703)

Hr Mr ABP & VTS 330022, 339733 outside HO; Fax 232991; ☎ 827350; MRSC (01705) 552100; Weather Centre 228844; Marinecall 0891 500457; Police 581111; Dr 226631 (Port Health); Ⓗ 777222.

FACILITIES

Marinas

Hythe Marina (220+50 visitors; 2·5m), Pre-call VHF Ch 80. ☎ 207073, Fax 842424, £12.98, access H24; BH (30 ton), C (12 ton), AC, P, D, El, ME, Sh, CH, FW, V, R, Bar, SM. Tfc lts (vert) at lock: 3 Ⓡ = Wait; 3 Fl R = Stop; 2 Ⓖ over Ⓦ = proceed, free-flow. Waiting pontoon outside lock, S side. Ferries from Hythe pier to Town Quay and Ocean Village.

Ocean Village Marina (450; visitors welcome). Pre-call Ch 80, ☎ 229385, Fax 233515, £16.13, FW, V, R, Bar, CH, Slip, Gas, Gaz, Kos, ME, Sh, Ⓘ, P, D, AC, (Access H24);

Itchen Marina (50) ☎ 631500, D, BY, FW, AC, C (40 ton); No Ⓥ berths, but will not refuse a vessel in difficulty.

Shamrock Quay Marina (220+40 visitors) ☎ 229461, Fax 333384, £12.83, access H24, BH (62 ton), C (12 ton), ME, El, Sh, SM, Ⓘ, R, Bar, AC, CH, FW, Gas, Gaz, Kos, V;

Kemp's Quay Marina (220; visitors welcome) ☎ 632323, £10.57, access HW±3½, AC, C (5 ton), D, FW, Gas, ME;

Town Quay Marina (136) ☎ 234397, Fax 235302, £10.70, access H24 (2·6m), AC, FW, CH, Ⓘ, R, Bar; marina ent is a dogleg between two floating wavebreaks (lit by 2 FR and 2 FG) which appear continuous from seaward. Beware adjacent fast ferries. Craft >20m LOA must get clearance from Southampton VTS to ent/dep Town Quay marina. Note: At Calshot Activities Centre there is a 40 berth pontoon, BH and a 200 boat hardstanding.

Yacht Clubs

Royal Southampton YC ☎ 223352, Bar, R, M, FW, L, Ⓘ; **Hythe SC** ☎ 846563; **Marchwood YC** ☎ 864641, Bar, M, C (10 ton), FW, L; **Netley SC** ☎ 454272; **Southampton SC** ☎ 446575; **Weston SC** ☎ 452527; **Eling SC** ☎ 863987.

Services

CH, ACA, Sh, Rigging, Spars, SM, ME, El, Ⓔ. Fuel barges in R Itchen, E side close down-river from Ocean Village.

Hards

at Hythe, Crackmore, Eling, Mayflower Park (Test), Northam (Itchen). Public landings at Cross House hard, Cross House slip, Block House hard (Itchen), Carnation public hard & Cowporters public hard.

City

V, R, Bar, Ⓑ, ✉, ⇌, ✈, Ferries/Hydrofoil to IOW, ☎ 333042; ferry Town Quay, ☎ 840722, to Hythe. Stena Sealink to Cherbourg; see 10.0.4.

Reference

ABP publish a *Yachtsman's Guide to Southampton Water* obtainable from VTS Centre, Berth 37, Eastern Docks, Southampton SO1 1GG.

RIVER HAMBLE   10-2-25

Hampshire 50°50'·90N 01°18'·41W

CHARTS

AC *2022, 1905*; Imray C3; Stanfords 11, 18; OS 196

TIDES

+0020, –0010 Dover; ML 2·9; Zone 0 (UT)

Standard Port SOUTHAMPTON (←—)

Times				Height (metres)			
High Water		Low Water		MHWS	MHWN	MLWN	MLWS
0400	1100	0000	0600	4·5	3·7	1·8	0·5
1600	2300	1200	1800				
Differences WARSASH							
+0020	+0010	+0010	0000	0·0	+0·1	+0·1	+0·3
BURSLEDON							
+0020	+0020	+0010	+0010	+0·1	+0·1	+0·2	+0·2
CALSHOT CASTLE							
0000	+0025	0000	0000	0·0	0·0	+0·2	+0·3

NOTE: Double HWs occur at or near sp; at other times there is a stand of about two hrs. Predictions are for the first HW if there are two or for the middle of the stand. See 10·2·12. NE gales can decrease depths by 0·6m.

SHELTER

Excellent, with visitors berths at 4 major marinas, many YCs, SCs, BYs and on some Hbr Authority pile moorings.

NAVIGATION

WPT Hamble Pt SCM buoy, Q (6) + L Fl 15s, 50°50'·12N 01°18'·58W, 166°/346° from/to front ldg lt, 0·48M. Unlit piles and buoys are a danger at night. River is extremely crowded; ⚓ prohib. Yachts with aux engines may not use spinnakers above Warsash jetty.

Bridge clearances: Road 4·0m; Rly 6·0m; M27 4·3m. The site of a Historic Wreck (*Grace Dieu*) is 3ca up-river of the M27 bridge, at 50°53'·51N 01°17'·24W, (see 10.0.3g).

LIGHTS AND MARKS

Ldg lts 345°: Front Oc (2) R 12s 4m 2M, No 6 pile bn; rear, 820m from front, QR 12m, W mast on shore; vis 341°-349°. No 1 pile Fl G 3s 3M, SHM. No 2 pile Q (3) 10s 3M, ECM. No 3 pile Fl (2) G 5s, SHM. No 5 pile Fl (3) G 10s, SHM. Ldg lts 026° on E shore: front QG, W mast; rear Iso G 6s. No 7 pile Fl G 3s, SHM. No 8 pile Fl R 3s, PHM. No 9 pile Fl (2) G 5s, SHM. No 10 pile Fl (2) R 5s, PHM.

In mid-stream between Warsash and Hamble Pt Marina there are Ⓥ pile moorings between 2 pontoons end-to-end, aligned N/S. The most S'ly end is lit Fl R 2s and the most N'ly end Fl (2) R 5s.

Above Warsash, jetties and pontoons on the E side are marked by 2FG (vert) lts, and those on the W side by 2FR (vert) lts. Lateral piles are Fl G 2s or Fl R 2s (see chartlet).

RIVER HAMBLE *continued*

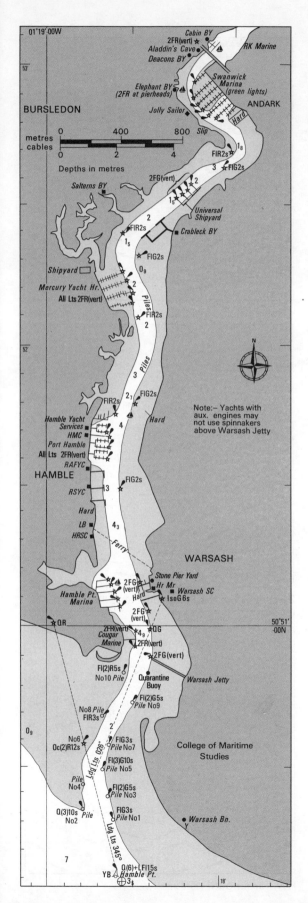

RADIO TELEPHONE
Call: *Hamble Hbr Radio* Ch **68** 16 (Mon-Fri 0830-1700; Sat & Sun April-Oct 0900-1830 Nov-Mar 0900-1300). Marinas Ch **80** M. See also 10.2.22.

TELEPHONE (01703) on Hamble side of river. See Note Hr Mr 576387; MRSC (01705) 552100; ⧫ (01703) 827350; Southampton Weather Centre 228844; Marinecall 0891 500457; Police 581111; Dr 573110.

Note: On the E side of river, Locks Heath (01489) tel nos all begin 57, 58 or 88.

FACILITIES
Marinas:

Hamble Pt Marina (220+10 ⓥ) ☎ 452464, Fax 456440, £14.81, AC, Bar, CH, D, BH (40+ ton), C (8 ton), Ⓔ, El, FW, Gas, Gaz, ME, Sh, V, YC, (Access H24);

Port Hamble Marina (340+ ⓥ) ☎ 452741, Fax 455206, £13.74, AC, ▨, Bar, BH (100 ton), C (7 ton), CH, D, Ⓔ, FW, Gas, Gaz, ME, P, Sh, El, SM, Slip, V, (Access H24);

Mercury Yacht Hbr (346+ ⓥ) ☎ 455994, Fax 457369, £10.58, AC, Bar, BH (20 ton), El, Slip, CH, D, Ⓔ, FW, Gas, Gaz, ME, P, Sh, SM, V, (Access H24);

Swanwick Marina (380+ ⓥ) ☎ 885000 (after 1700, 885262), Fax 885509, £12, AC, BH (60 ton), C (12 ton), CH, D, Ⓔ, FW, Gas, Gaz, ⌗, ▨, ME, P, ✉, Sh, SM, V, (Access H24).

The Hbr Authority jetty in front of the conspic B/W Hr Mr's Office at Warsash has limited AB (£13 for 24hrs); also ⓥ pile moorings in mid-stream. More ⓥ pile moorings are opposite Port Hamble marina.

Yacht Clubs:
Hamble River SC ☎ 452070; **RAFYC** ☎ 452208, Bar, R, L; **Royal Southern YC** ☎ 453271; **Warsash SC** ☎ 583575.

Services:
A very wide range of marine services is available; consult marina/Hr Mr for locations. CH, Ⓔ, BY, AB, C (12 ton), Ⓔ, FW, Gas, Gaz, M, ME, R, Sh, Slip, SM; Riggers, BH (25 ton), ACA, Divers. **Piper Marine Services** ☎ 454563, (or call *Piper Fuel* Ch M), D, P.

Hards. At Warsash, Hamble and Swanwick.
Slips at Warsash, Hamble, Bursledon and Lower Swanwick.
✉ (Hamble, Bursledon, Warsash and Lower Swanwick); Ⓑ (Hamble, Bursledon, Sarisbury Green, Swanwick, Warsash); ⇌ (Hamble and Bursledon); ✈ (Southampton). *Hamble River Guide* available from Hr Mr.

ADJACENT HARBOURS

ASHLETT CREEK, Hants, 50°49'·98N 01°19'·40W. AC *2022, 1905*. Tides approx as Calshot Castle (above). Small drying (2·1m) inlet across from R Hamble; best for shoal-draft vessels. Appr at HW via Fawley PHM buoy, QR, close to Esso Marine Terminal. Unlit chan, marked by 3 PHM buoys, 1 SHM buoy and 2 PHM bns, has four 90° bends. Ldg bns are hard to find; local knowledge desirable. Berth at drying quay. Facilities: AB, M, FW, Slip, Hard, Pub. **Esso SC.**

HILLHEAD, Hants, 50°49'·05N 01°14'·45W. AC *2022, 1905*. HW +0030 on Dover; see 10.2.28 for LEE diffs. Short term ⚓ for small craft at mouth of R Meon. Bar dries ¼M offshore. Ent dries 1·2m at MLWS. Appr on 030° towards Hillhead SC ho (W, conspic), bns mark chan, ● topmarks to port, ▲ ones to stbd. Small hbr to W inside ent where yachts can lie in soft mud alongside bank. Facilities: **Hillhead SC** ☎ (01329) 664843. **Hillhead village** EC Thurs; ✉, CH, V, P & D (cans).

10-2-26   ISLE OF WIGHT TIDAL STREAMS

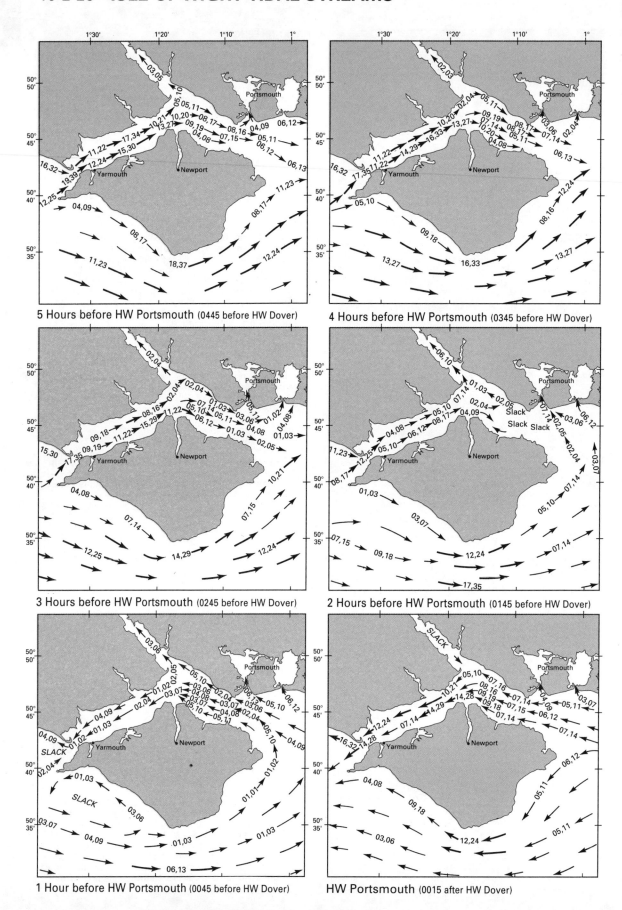

5 Hours before HW Portsmouth (0445 before HW Dover)

4 Hours before HW Portsmouth (0345 before HW Dover)

3 Hours before HW Portsmouth (0245 before HW Dover)

2 Hours before HW Portsmouth (0145 before HW Dover)

1 Hour before HW Portsmouth (0045 before HW Dover)

HW Portsmouth (0015 after HW Dover)

General Area 2: 10.2.3

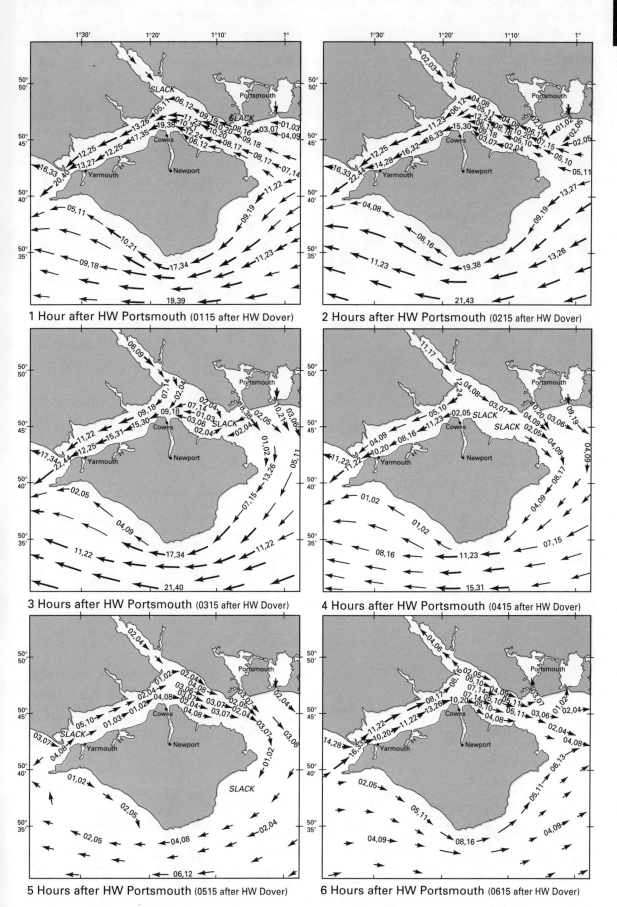

1 Hour after HW Portsmouth (0115 after HW Dover)

2 Hours after HW Portsmouth (0215 after HW Dover)

3 Hours after HW Portsmouth (0315 after HW Dover)

4 Hours after HW Portsmouth (0415 after HW Dover)

5 Hours after HW Portsmouth (0515 after HW Dover)

6 Hours after HW Portsmouth (0615 after HW Dover)

WOOTTON CREEK 10-2-27

Isle of Wight 50°44'·06N 01°12'·68W

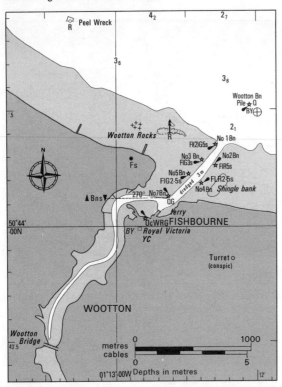

CHARTS
AC 2022, 394; Imray C3, Y20; Stanfords 11, 18; OS 196
TIDES
+0023 Dover; ML 2·8; Zone 0 (UT). Use RYDE differences 10.2.28; see also 10.2.12.
SHELTER
Good except in stormy N or E winds. Above the ferry, the creek dries. Moor to piles or ⚓s off RVYC, or AB in 2m off Fishbourne Quay. No ⚓ in the fairway. Speed limit 5kn.
NAVIGATION
WPT Wootton NCM Bn, Q, 50°44'·51N 01°12'·04W, 044°/224° from/to ferry slip, 0·64M. Beware large ferries, leaving astern and turning at Wootton Bn. It is difficult to beat in on the ebb.
LIGHTS AND MARKS
Ent to creek due S of SE Ryde Middle SCM and 1·75M W of Ryde Pier. Once in chan follow 4 lit SHM bns and 2 PHMs. Keep in W sector of Dir lt, Oc WRG 10s, G221°-224°, W224°-225½°, R225½°-230½°. By ferry terminal, turn onto ldg marks on W shore △ ▽, which form a ◇ when in transit 270°.
RADIO TELEPHONE
None.
TELEPHONE (01983)
Royal Victoria YC 882325; MRSC (01705) 552100; Fairways Association 882763; ⌗ (01703) 827350; Marinecall 0891 500457; Police 528000; Dr 882424.
FACILITIES
Royal Victoria YC ☎ 882325, Slip, M, FW, R, Bar; **Fishbourne Quay BY** ☎ 882200, £10, C (40 ton), D (cans), El, Ⓔ, ME, Sh, SM. **Village** EC = Thurs, Wootton Bridge = Wed; ✉ (Wootton Bridge, Ryde), Ⓑ (Ryde), ⟱ (ferry to Portsmouth), ✈ (Southampton).

ADJACENT HARBOUR

RYDE, Isle of Wight 50°43'·95N 01°09'·22W. AC 394. HW +0022 on Dover; ML 2·8m; see 10.2.12 and 10.2.28. Small hbr 300m E of Ryde Pier; dries approx 1·7m. Access for shoal draft approx HW−2½ to +2. Appr 197° across drying Ryde Sands, via chan marked by 3 unlit SHM/PHM buoys. Ent lts 2 F R/G (vert). Depth at ent shown by 2 Ⓨ (vert) lts focused on appr chan: 1 Ⓨ = >1·0m; 2 Ⓨ = >1·5m. Hbr has W floodlt. Beware hovercraft operating between pier and hbr. VHF Ch 80. Hr Mr ☎ (01983) 613879, Fax 812034. Facilities: **Marina** (75+70 visitors) £7.50, FW. **Town** EC Thurs; all facilities adjacent, P & D (cans).

BEMBRIDGE 10-2-28

Isle of Wight 50°41'·59N 01°06'·31W
CHARTS
AC 2022, 2050, 2045; Imray C3, C9; Stanfords 18; OS 196
TIDES
+0020 Dover; Zone 0 (UT). See 10.2.12

Standard Port PORTSMOUTH (→)

Times				Height (metres)			
High Water		Low Water		MHWS	MHWN	MLWN	MLWS
0000	0600	0500	1100	4·7	3·8	1·9	0·8
1200	1800	1700	2300				
Differences BEMBRIDGE HARBOUR							
−0010	+0005	+0020	0000	−1·6	−1·5	−1·4	−0·6
RYDE							
−0010	+0010	−0005	−0010	−0·2	−0·1	0·0	+0·1
FORELAND (LB Slip)							
−0005	0000	+0005	+0010	−0·1	−0·1	0·0	+0·1
VENTNOR							
−0025	−0030	−0025	−0030	−0·8	−0·6	−0·2	+0·2
SANDOWN							
0000	+0005	+0010	+0025	−0·6	−0·5	−0·2	0·0

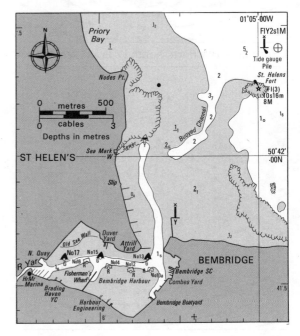

SHELTER
Good, but difficult ent in NNE gales. No access LW ±2½ for 1·5m draft; carefully check tide gauge which indicates depth over the bar. Speed limit 6kn. Visitors' berths at marina, Fisherman's Wharf and afloat on pontoon between Nos 15 & 17 SHM buoys. No ⚓ in chan and hbr, but Priory Bay is sheltered ⚓ in winds from S to WNW.
NAVIGATION
WPT tide gauge, Fl Y 2s, 50°42'·43N 01°04'·93W, approx 2ca E of ent to well-buoyed, but unlit chan. The bar, between Nos 6 and 8 buoys, almost dries. Avoid the gravel banks between St. Helen's Fort, Nodes Pt and N to Seaview, by keeping to ent times above.
LIGHTS AND MARKS
St Helens Fort Fl (3) 10s 16m 8M; no ⚓ within 1ca radius of Fort. Conspic W seamark on shore where chan turns S.
RADIO TELEPHONE
Call Bembridge Marina VHF Ch **80**; Hbr Launch Ch M.
TELEPHONE (01983)
Hr Mr 872828; MRSC (01705) 552100; ⌗ (01703) 827350; Marinecall 0891 500457; Police 528000; Dr 872614.
FACILITIES
Marina (40+100 visitors) ☎ 872828, Fax 872922, £12, FW, ME, El, AC, ⚡, V, R, Bar; **St Helen's Quay** FW, CH; **Brading Haven YC** ☎ 872289, Bar, R, FW; **Bembridge SC** ☎ 872686; **Services:** M, Slip, BY, P & D (cans), ME, El, Sh, Gas. **Town** EC Thurs; V, R, Bar, ✉, Ⓑ, ⟱ (Ryde), ✈ (So'ton).

ENGLAND – PORTSMOUTH

LAT 50°48′N   LONG 1°07′W

TIMES AND HEIGHTS OF HIGH AND LOW WATERS

YEAR **1996**

JANUARY

Time	m		Time	m
1 0052	1.8	**16** 0647	4.2
0753	4.2	1230	1.7
M 1333	1.7	TU 1922	4.0
2032	4.0		
2 0153	1.7	**17** 0057	1.6
0852	4.3	0759	4.4
TU 1427	1.5	W 1343	1.4
2127	4.1	2034	4.3
3 0244	1.6	**18** 0206	1.4
0939	4.4	0901	4.6
W 1512	1.3	TH 1444	1.1
2212	4.3	2135	4.5
4 0328	1.4	**19** 0306	1.1
1019	4.4	0956	4.8
TH 1554	1.2	F 1539	0.8
2250	4.4	2230	4.7
5 0408	1.3	**20** 0400	0.9
1054	4.5	1049	4.9
F 1632	1.0	SA 1631	0.6
O 2323	4.4	● 2323	4.9
6 0446	1.2	**21** 0452	0.7
1127	4.5	1140	5.0
SA 1709	1.0	SU 1721	0.4
2355	4.5		
7 0521	1.1	**22** 0013	5.0
1201	4.5	0540	0.6
SU 1742	0.9	M 1230	5.0
		1808	0.3
8 0028	4.5	**23** 0102	5.0
0554	1.1	0627	0.6
M 1235	4.5	TU 1318	4.9
1813	1.0	1853	0.4
9 0102	4.5	**24** 0149	5.0
0624	1.2	0712	0.6
TU 1310	4.5	W 1405	4.8
1841	1.0	1936	0.5
10 0137	4.5	**25** 0233	4.9
0654	1.3	0755	0.8
W 1346	4.4	TH 1450	4.6
1911	1.1	2017	0.8
11 0213	4.5	**26** 0316	4.7
0727	1.4	0839	1.1
TH 1422	4.3	F 1534	4.4
1946	1.2	2100	1.1
12 0251	4.4	**27** 0400	4.4
0806	1.5	0927	1.4
F 1502	4.2	SA 1619	4.1
2027	1.3	2149	1.5
13 0334	4.3	**28** 0447	4.2
0854	1.6	1025	1.7
SA 1549	4.1	SU 1712	3.9
2118	1.5	2250	1.8
14 0426	4.2	**29** 0544	4.0
0955	1.8	1139	1.9
SU 1647	4.0	M 1825	3.7
2222	1.7		
15 0531	4.2	**30** 0007	2.0
1110	1.8	0700	3.9
M 1800	3.9	TU 1256	1.9
2339	1.7	1957	3.7
		31 0121	1.9
		0818	3.9
		W 1359	1.7
		2104	3.9

FEBRUARY

Time	m		Time	m
1 0221	1.8	**16** 0159	1.4
0915	4.1	0845	4.4
TH 1449	1.5	F 1434	1.1
2152	4.1	2124	4.4
2 0308	1.5	**17** 0300	1.1
0958	4.3	0943	4.6
F 1532	1.3	SA 1529	0.8
2231	4.3	2219	4.7
3 0349	1.3	**18** 0352	0.8
1035	4.4	1036	4.8
SA 1611	1.0	SU 1620	0.5
2305	4.4	● 2310	4.9
4 0427	1.1	**19** 0441	0.6
1109	4.4	1126	4.9
SU 1648	0.9	M 1707	0.3
O 2337	4.5	2357	5.0
5 0502	1.0	**20** 0527	0.4
1143	4.5	1214	4.9
M 1723	0.8	TU 1752	0.3
6 0010	4.5	**21** 0042	5.0
0535	1.0	0609	0.4
TU 1218	4.5	W 1300	4.9
1753	0.8	1833	0.3
7 0042	4.6	**22** 0126	5.0
0605	0.9	0650	0.5
W 1253	4.5	TH 1343	4.8
1822	0.8	1911	0.5
8 0115	4.6	**23** 0206	4.8
0634	1.0	0728	0.7
TH 1328	4.5	F 1424	4.6
1851	0.8	1948	0.7
9 0148	4.6	**24** 0243	4.7
0706	1.0	0804	0.9
F 1403	4.4	SA 1503	4.4
1924	0.9	2025	1.1
10 0224	4.5	**25** 0321	4.4
0742	1.1	0843	1.3
SA 1441	4.3	SU 1543	4.2
2003	1.1	2106	1.4
11 0303	4.4	**26** 0400	4.1
0826	1.3	0930	1.6
SU 1524	4.2	M 1629	3.9
2049	1.3	2200	1.8
12 0351	4.2	**27** 0449	3.9
0921	1.5	1038	1.9
M 1606	4.0	TU 1730	3.7
2150	1.6	2320	2.1
13 0452	4.1	**28** 0557	3.7
1034	1.7	1210	2.0
TU 1732	3.9	W 1907	3.6
2311	1.8		
14 0612	4.0	**29** 0046	2.1
1206	1.7	0732	3.7
W 1900	3.9	TH 1325	1.9
		2033	3.8
15 0042	1.7		
0735	4.1		
TH 1329	1.5		
2019	4.1		

MARCH

Time	m		Time	m
1 0154	1.9	**16** 0151	1.4
0846	3.9	0832	4.2
F 1420	1.6	SA 1421	1.1
2125	4.0	2111	4.4
2 0244	1.6	**17** 0250	1.1
0934	4.1	0931	4.5
SA 1505	1.3	SU 1515	0.8
2205	4.3	2204	4.7
3 0326	1.3	**18** 0340	0.7
1012	4.2	1022	4.7
SU 1544	1.1	M 1603	0.6
2241	4.4	2252	4.8
4 0403	1.1	**19** 0426	0.5
1047	4.4	1110	4.8
M 1622	0.9	TU 1648	0.4
2314	4.5	● 2337	4.9
5 0439	0.9	**20** 0508	0.4
1122	4.4	1155	4.8
TU 1658	0.7	W 1730	0.3
O 2347	4.5		
6 0512	0.8	**21** 0020	4.9
1158	4.5	0548	0.4
W 1731	0.7	TH 1239	4.8
		1808	0.4
7 0019	4.6	**22** 0100	4.9
0543	0.7	0625	0.5
TH 1234	4.5	F 1319	4.7
1801	0.7	1845	0.5
8 0052	4.6	**23** 0136	4.8
0614	0.7	0700	0.6
F 1309	4.6	SA 1357	4.6
1832	0.7	1919	0.8
9 0125	4.6	**24** 0211	4.6
0647	0.7	0733	0.9
SA 1346	4.5	SU 1434	4.4
1906	0.8	1953	1.1
10 0200	4.5	**25** 0246	4.4
0723	0.8	0807	1.2
SU 1425	4.4	M 1512	4.2
1945	1.0	2031	1.4
11 0240	4.4	**26** 0322	4.1
0806	1.0	0846	1.5
M 1508	4.3	TU 1556	4.0
2031	1.2	2119	1.8
12 0326	4.2	**27** 0406	3.8
0859	1.3	0940	1.8
TU 1603	4.1	W 1650	3.7
2133	1.5	2231	2.1
13 0427	4.0	**28** 0506	3.6
1013	1.6	1111	2.0
W 1716	3.9	TH 1807	3.6
2258	1.8		
14 0548	3.9	**29** 0004	2.1
1148	1.7	0629	3.5
TH 1845	3.9	F 1241	2.0
		1942	3.7
15 0033	1.7	**30** 0118	2.0
0718	4.0	0759	3.7
F 1315	1.4	SA 1343	1.7
2007	4.1	2044	4.0
		31 0212	1.7
		0857	3.9
		SU 1430	1.4
		2129	4.2

APRIL

Time	m		Time	m
1 0255	1.4	**16** 0321	0.8
0939	4.1	1005	4.6
M 1512	1.2	TU 1541	0.6
2207	4.4	2231	4.8
2 0334	1.1	**17** 0405	0.6
1018	4.3	1051	4.7
TU 1550	0.9	W 1624	0.5
2243	4.5	● 2315	4.8
3 0410	0.9	**18** 0447	0.5
1056	4.4	1135	4.7
W 1627	0.8	TH 1705	0.5
2318	4.6	2355	4.8
4 0445	0.7	**19** 0526	0.5
1134	4.5	1216	4.7
TH 1703	0.7	F 1743	0.6
O 2353	4.6		
5 0519	0.6	**20** 0033	4.7
1212	4.6	0601	0.6
F 1738	0.6	SA 1255	4.6
		1818	0.7
6 0028	4.7	**21** 0108	4.7
0554	0.6	0635	0.7
SA 1251	4.6	SU 1331	4.5
1814	0.6	1852	0.9
7 0105	4.7	**22** 0141	4.5
0630	0.6	0707	0.9
SU 1330	4.6	M 1407	4.4
1852	0.7	1926	1.1
8 0143	4.6	**23** 0215	4.3
0710	0.7	0739	1.2
M 1413	4.5	TU 1445	4.2
1934	0.9	2002	1.4
9 0224	4.4	**24** 0251	4.1
0755	0.9	0815	1.4
TU 1500	4.4	W 1527	4.1
2024	1.2	2046	1.7
10 0313	4.2	**25** 0332	3.9
0850	1.2	0901	1.7
W 1556	4.2	TH 1616	3.9
2127	1.5	2144	2.0
11 0414	4.0	**26** 0425	3.7
1003	1.4	1008	1.9
TH 1707	4.0	F 1719	3.8
2248	1.6	2307	2.1
12 0533	3.9	**27** 0533	3.6
1131	1.5	1140	2.0
F 1832	4.0	SA 1836	3.8
13 0017	1.6	**28** 0027	2.0
0702	3.9	0652	3.6
SA 1255	1.4	SU 1253	1.8
1950	4.2	1946	3.9
14 0133	1.4	**29** 0128	1.8
0816	4.2	0802	3.8
SU 1401	1.1	M 1346	1.6
2053	4.4	2041	4.1
15 0231	1.1	**30** 0215	1.5
0914	4.4	0855	4.0
M 1454	0.9	TU 1431	1.3
2145	4.6	2126	4.3

Chart Datum: 2·73 metres below Ordnance Datum (Newlyn)

ENGLAND – PORTSMOUTH

LAT 50°48′N   LONG   1°07′W

TIMES AND HEIGHTS OF HIGH AND LOW WATERS   YEAR **1996**

TIME ZONE (UT)
For Summer Time add ONE hour in non-shaded areas

Chart Datum: 2·73 metres below Ordnance Datum (Newlyn)

MAY

Day	Time	m	Time	m	Time	m	Time	m
1 W	0256	1.2	0941	4.2	1512	1.0	2207	4.5
16 TH	0341	0.8	1031	4.5	1559	0.8	2251	4.7
2 TH	0336	1.0	1024	4.4	1553	0.9	2247	4.6
17 F ●	0423	0.7	1115	4.5	1639	0.8	2331	4.7
3 F O	0415	0.8	1107	4.5	1633	0.7	2326	4.7
18 SA	0503	0.7	1154	4.5	1718	0.8		
4 SA	0455	0.6	1150	4.7	1715	0.6		
19 SU	0006	4.6	0539	0.7	1232	4.5	1753	0.9
5 SU	0006	4.7	0535	0.5	1233	4.7	1757	0.6
20 M	0040	4.6	0613	0.8	1307	4.5	1828	1.0
6 M	0048	4.7	0618	0.5	1317	4.7	1841	0.7
21 TU	0113	4.5	0645	1.0	1342	4.4	1902	1.2
7 TU	0130	4.7	0703	0.6	1404	4.6	1927	0.8
22 W	0147	4.4	0717	1.2	1420	4.3	1937	1.4
8 W	0216	4.5	0752	0.8	1455	4.5	2020	1.0
23 TH	0224	4.2	0751	1.3	1500	4.2	2016	1.6
9 TH	0307	4.3	0847	1.0	1552	4.3	2120	1.3
24 F	0303	4.1	0830	1.5	1544	4.1	2102	1.8
10 F	0408	4.1	0953	1.2	1658	4.2	2232	1.5
25 SA	0349	3.9	0920	1.7	1636	4.0	2201	2.0
11 SA	0520	4.0	1108	1.4	1813	4.2	2350	1.5
26 SU	0445	3.8	1025	1.8	1737	3.9	2315	2.0
12 SU	0641	4.0	1225	1.4	1926	4.3		
27 M	0551	3.8	1141	1.8	1845	4.0		
13 M	0103	1.4	0753	4.1	1332	1.2	2028	4.4
28 TU	0026	1.9	0703	3.8	1248	1.7	1947	4.1
14 TU	0205	1.2	0852	4.4	1427	1.0	2121	4.6
29 W	0125	1.6	0807	4.0	1343	1.4	2041	4.3
15 W	0256	1.0	0944	4.4	1515	0.9	2208	4.6
30 TH	0214	1.3	0902	4.2	1432	1.2	2130	4.5
31 F	0301	1.1	0952	4.4	1519	1.0	2216	4.6

JUNE

Day	Time	m	Time	m	Time	m	Time	m
1 SA O	0347	0.8	1041	4.6	1606	0.8	2301	4.7
16 SU ●	0441	0.9	1134	4.4	1655	1.0	2342	4.5
2 SU	0434	0.6	1129	4.7	1654	0.7	2347	4.8
17 M	0519	0.9	1210	4.4	1732	1.0		
3 M	0521	0.5	1217	4.8	1743	0.6		
18 TU	0014	4.5	0553	0.9	1244	4.4	1807	1.1
4 TU	0033	4.8	0609	0.5	1306	4.8	1831	0.6
19 W	0048	4.5	0626	1.0	1319	4.4	1841	1.2
5 W	0121	4.8	0657	0.5	1356	4.8	1920	0.7
20 TH	0123	4.4	0656	1.1	1355	4.4	1913	1.3
6 TH	0210	4.7	0747	0.6	1448	4.7	2011	0.9
21 F	0159	4.3	0727	1.2	1432	4.3	1947	1.4
7 F	0302	4.5	0839	0.8	1543	4.5	2107	1.1
22 SA	0236	4.2	0801	1.4	1512	4.2	2026	1.6
8 SA	0358	4.3	0936	1.1	1642	4.4	2208	1.3
23 SU	0317	4.1	0843	1.5	1556	4.2	2113	1.7
9 SU	0501	4.2	1040	1.3	1745	4.3	2317	1.4
24 M	0404	4.0	0934	1.6	1646	4.1	2211	1.8
10 M	0611	4.0	1149	1.4	1853	4.3		
25 TU	0501	3.9	1037	1.7	1747	4.1	2320	1.8
11 TU	0028	1.5	0723	4.0	1258	1.4	1957	4.3
26 W	0610	3.9	1147	1.7	1855	4.2		
12 W	0133	1.4	0828	4.1	1358	1.3	2055	4.4
27 TH	0032	1.7	0723	4.0	1256	1.6	2000	4.3
13 TH	0229	1.2	0924	4.2	1449	1.2	2145	4.5
28 F	0136	1.5	0828	4.2	1357	1.3	2057	4.5
14 F	0317	1.1	1012	4.3	1534	1.1	2228	4.5
29 SA	0232	1.2	0926	4.4	1453	1.1	2150	4.7
15 SA	0400	1.0	1056	4.4	1616	1.0	2307	4.5
30 SU	0326	0.9	1020	4.6	1547	0.9	2240	4.8

JULY

Day	Time	m	Time	m	Time	m	Time	m
1 M O	0418	0.7	1112	4.7	1639	0.7	2330	4.9
16 TU	0457	0.9	1149	4.4	1711	1.1	2351	4.5
2 TU	0509	0.5	1203	4.9	1731	0.6		
17 W	0533	0.9	1222	4.5	1747	1.1		
3 W	0019	4.9	0558	0.4	1255	4.9	1820	0.6
18 TH	0024	4.5	0605	0.9	1256	4.5	1819	1.1
4 TH	0109	4.9	0647	0.4	1345	4.9	1908	0.6
19 F	0059	4.4	0635	1.0	1330	4.5	1849	1.1
5 F	0159	4.8	0735	0.5	1435	4.8	1957	0.7
20 SA	0135	4.4	0703	1.1	1404	4.4	1920	1.2
6 SA	0249	4.7	0823	0.7	1525	4.7	2046	0.9
21 SU	0210	4.3	0734	1.2	1440	4.4	1955	1.3
7 SU	0340	4.5	0913	0.9	1615	4.5	2140	1.2
22 M	0248	4.2	0811	1.3	1518	4.3	2037	1.5
8 M	0434	4.2	1008	1.2	1710	4.3	2240	1.4
23 TU	0330	4.1	0856	1.5	1602	4.2	2129	1.6
9 TU	0535	4.0	1110	1.5	1812	4.2	2349	1.6
24 W	0422	4.0	0953	1.6	1658	4.1	2234	1.8
10 W	0647	3.9	1220	1.6	1922	4.1		
25 TH	0529	3.9	1104	1.8	1808	4.1	2351	1.7
11 TH	0059	1.6	0801	3.9	1327	1.6	2027	4.2
26 F	0649	4.0	1222	1.7	1925	4.2		
12 F	0202	1.5	0904	4.1	1424	1.5	2122	4.3
27 SA	0108	1.5	0804	4.2	1336	1.5	2032	4.4
13 SA	0254	1.3	0955	4.2	1512	1.4	2207	4.3
28 SU	0214	1.2	0908	4.4	1438	1.2	2129	4.6
14 SU	0338	1.2	1038	4.3	1555	1.3	2245	4.4
29 M	0312	0.9	1004	4.6	1534	1.0	2222	4.8
15 M ●	0419	1.0	1116	4.4	1634	1.1	2319	4.4
30 TU O	0405	0.6	1057	4.8	1627	0.7	2313	4.9
31 W	0456	0.4	1149	4.9	1718	0.6		

AUGUST

Day	Time	m	Time	m	Time	m	Time	m
1 TH	0004	4.9	0544	0.3	1239	5.0	1805	0.5
16 F	0002	4.5	0541	0.8	1231	4.5	1755	1.0
2 F	0054	4.9	0631	0.3	1328	5.0	1852	0.5
17 SA	0037	4.5	0611	0.9	1303	4.6	1825	1.0
3 SA	0142	4.9	0716	0.4	1414	4.9	1936	0.6
18 SU	0111	4.5	0638	0.9	1336	4.5	1854	1.0
4 SU	0229	4.7	0800	0.6	1459	4.4	2020	0.8
19 M	0146	4.4	0708	1.0	1409	4.5	1928	1.1
5 M	0315	4.5	0844	0.9	1543	4.6	2107	1.1
20 TU	0221	4.4	0743	1.2	1445	4.4	2007	1.3
6 TU	0401	4.3	0932	1.3	1629	4.3	2200	1.5
21 W	0301	4.2	0825	1.4	1527	4.3	2056	1.5
7 W	0454	4.0	1029	1.6	1724	4.1	2306	1.7
22 TH	0351	4.1	0920	1.6	1620	4.1	2201	1.7
8 TH	0604	3.8	1141	1.9	1836	3.9		
23 F	0459	3.9	1034	1.8	1732	4.0	2325	1.8
9 F	0023	1.8	0732	3.8	1258	1.9	1957	3.9
24 SA	0625	3.9	1204	1.8	1858	4.1		
10 SA	0134	1.7	0844	4.0	1402	1.8	2100	4.1
25 SU	0052	1.6	0747	4.1	1326	1.6	2013	4.3
11 SU	0230	1.5	0937	4.2	1452	1.6	2147	4.2
26 M	0203	1.3	0854	4.4	1429	1.3	2114	4.6
12 M	0315	1.3	1019	4.3	1534	1.4	2224	4.3
27 TU	0300	0.9	0950	4.7	1524	1.0	2207	4.8
13 TU	0355	1.1	1055	4.4	1612	1.2	2257	4.4
28 W O	0351	0.6	1042	4.9	1614	0.7	2257	4.9
14 W ●	0433	0.9	1127	4.5	1649	1.0	2329	4.5
29 TH	0440	0.4	1131	5.0	1702	0.5	2346	5.0
15 TH	0509	0.8	1159	4.5	1724	1.0		
30 F	0527	0.3	1219	5.0	1747	0.4		
31 SA	0033	5.0	0610	0.3	1304	5.0	1830	0.5

ENGLAND – PORTSMOUTH

LAT 50°48′N   LONG 1°07′W

TIMES AND HEIGHTS OF HIGH AND LOW WATERS

YEAR 1996

TIME ZONE (UT)
For Summer Time add ONE hour in non-shaded areas

SEPTEMBER

Day	Time	m	Day	Time	m
1 SU	0119 / 0652 / 1348 / 1911	4.9 / 0.4 / 4.9 / 0.6	**16** M	0047 / 0614 / 1308 / 1830	4.6 / 0.9 / 4.6 / 0.9
2 M	0203 / 0732 / 1428 / 1951	4.8 / 0.7 / 4.8 / 0.8	**17** TU	0122 / 0645 / 1342 / 1905	4.6 / 0.9 / 4.6 / 1.0
3 TU	0245 / 0811 / 1508 / 2031	4.6 / 1.0 / 4.5 / 1.2	**18** W	0159 / 0721 / 1418 / 1944	4.5 / 1.1 / 4.4 / 1.2
4 W	0327 / 0854 / 1549 / 2118	4.3 / 1.4 / 4.3 / 1.5	**19** TH	0240 / 0803 / 1500 / 2033	4.3 / 1.3 / 4.3 / 1.4
5 TH	0415 / 0948 / 1636 / 2220	4.0 / 1.8 / 4.0 / 1.8	**20** F	0331 / 0859 / 1555 / 2139	4.1 / 1.6 / 4.1 / 1.7
6 F	0517 / 1102 / 1741 / 2343	3.8 / 2.0 / 3.8 / 2.0	**21** SA	0440 / 1019 / 1708 / 2307	4.0 / 1.9 / 4.0 / 1.8
7 SA	0654 / 1225 / 1920	3.7 / 2.1 / 3.7	**22** SU	0607 / 1154 / 1838	3.9 / 1.9 / 4.0
8 SU	0102 / 0818 / 1336 / 2034	1.9 / 3.9 / 2.0 / 3.9	**23** M	0038 / 0733 / 1315 / 1958	1.6 / 4.1 / 1.6 / 4.3
9 M	0202 / 0912 / 1427 / 2123	1.7 / 4.1 / 1.7 / 4.1	**24** TU	0149 / 0840 / 1417 / 2059	1.3 / 4.4 / 1.3 / 4.5
10 TU	0248 / 0953 / 1509 / 2200	1.4 / 4.3 / 1.4 / 4.3	**25** W	0245 / 0935 / 1509 / 2152	0.9 / 4.7 / 0.9 / 4.8
11 W	0328 / 1028 / 1547 / 2233	1.1 / 4.5 / 1.2 / 4.4	**26** TH	0334 / 1024 / 1557 / 2240	0.6 / 4.9 / 0.7 / 4.9
12 TH ●	0406 / 1101 / 1623 / 2305	0.9 / 4.5 / 1.0 / 4.5	**27** F O	0420 / 1110 / 1642 / 2326	0.4 / 5.0 / 0.5 / 5.0
13 F	0442 / 1132 / 1658 / 2338	0.8 / 4.6 / 0.9 / 4.6	**28** SA	0505 / 1155 / 1725	0.4 / 5.0 / 0.5
14 SA	0515 / 1204 / 1730	0.8 / 4.6 / 0.9	**29** SU	0011 / 0546 / 1239 / 1806	4.9 / 0.4 / 5.0 / 0.5
15 SU	0012 / 0545 / 1236 / 1759	4.6 / 0.8 / 4.6 / 0.9	**30** M	0055 / 0625 / 1319 / 1844	4.9 / 0.6 / 4.9 / 0.7

OCTOBER

Day	Time	m	Day	Time	m
1 TU	0136 / 0703 / 1357 / 1921	4.7 / 0.8 / 4.7 / 0.9	**16** W	0103 / 0626 / 1320 / 1847	4.7 / 0.9 / 4.6 / 0.9
2 W	0215 / 0740 / 1434 / 1958	4.6 / 1.1 / 4.5 / 1.2	**17** TH	0142 / 0706 / 1359 / 1929	4.6 / 1.1 / 4.5 / 1.1
3 TH	0255 / 0820 / 1512 / 2040	4.3 / 1.4 / 4.2 / 1.5	**18** F	0227 / 0752 / 1444 / 2021	4.4 / 1.3 / 4.3 / 1.3
4 F	0340 / 0909 / 1555 / 2134	4.1 / 1.8 / 4.0 / 1.9	**19** SA	0320 / 0851 / 1541 / 2127	4.3 / 1.6 / 4.1 / 1.6
5 SA	0435 / 1019 / 1652 / 2255	3.9 / 2.1 / 3.8 / 2.1	**20** SU	0428 / 1009 / 1653 / 2251	4.1 / 1.8 / 4.0 / 1.7
6 SU	0556 / 1146 / 1816	3.7 / 2.2 / 3.7	**21** M	0552 / 1138 / 1821	4.0 / 1.8 / 4.0
7 M	0021 / 0733 / 1300 / 1952	2.1 / 3.9 / 2.1 / 3.8	**22** TU	0017 / 0715 / 1257 / 1941	1.6 / 4.2 / 1.6 / 4.2
8 TU	0126 / 0833 / 1355 / 2047	1.8 / 4.1 / 1.8 / 4.0	**23** W	0128 / 0821 / 1359 / 2043	1.3 / 4.5 / 1.3 / 4.5
9 W	0215 / 0917 / 1438 / 2127	1.6 / 4.3 / 1.5 / 4.2	**24** TH	0225 / 0915 / 1450 / 2135	1.0 / 4.7 / 1.0 / 4.7
10 TH	0256 / 0953 / 1517 / 2202	1.3 / 4.5 / 1.3 / 4.4	**25** F	0313 / 1003 / 1537 / 2222	0.8 / 4.9 / 0.8 / 4.8
11 F	0335 / 1028 / 1553 / 2237	1.1 / 4.6 / 1.1 / 4.5	**26** SA O	0358 / 1048 / 1621 / 2307	0.6 / 5.0 / 0.7 / 4.8
12 SA ●	0411 / 1102 / 1628 / 2312	0.9 / 4.6 / 0.9 / 4.6	**27** SU	0441 / 1132 / 1703 / 2350	0.6 / 5.0 / 0.6 / 4.9
13 SU	0445 / 1135 / 1702 / 2348	0.8 / 4.7 / 0.9 / 4.7	**28** M	0521 / 1212 / 1742	0.6 / 4.9 / 0.7
14 M	0518 / 1209 / 1735	0.8 / 4.7 / 0.8	**29** TU	0031 / 0559 / 1251 / 1819	4.8 / 0.7 / 4.8 / 0.8
15 TU	0025 / 0551 / 1244 / 1809	4.7 / 0.8 / 4.7 / 0.8	**30** W	0110 / 0636 / 1327 / 1855	4.7 / 0.9 / 4.6 / 1.0
			31 TH	0148 / 0712 / 1403 / 1930	4.5 / 1.2 / 4.5 / 1.2

NOVEMBER

Day	Time	m	Day	Time	m
1 F	0226 / 0750 / 1439 / 2008	4.4 / 1.5 / 4.3 / 1.5	**16** SA	0220 / 0747 / 1437 / 2015	4.6 / 1.2 / 4.4 / 1.1
2 SA	0309 / 0835 / 1521 / 2054	4.2 / 1.8 / 4.1 / 1.8	**17** SU	0314 / 0845 / 1533 / 2117	4.4 / 1.4 / 4.3 / 1.4
3 SU	0359 / 0933 / 1611 / 2158	4.0 / 2.1 / 3.8 / 2.0	**18** M	0418 / 0955 / 1640 / 2229	4.3 / 1.6 / 4.1 / 1.5
4 M	0501 / 1053 / 1715 / 2323	3.9 / 2.2 / 3.7 / 2.1	**19** TU	0532 / 1113 / 1759 / 2346	4.2 / 1.7 / 4.1 / 1.5
5 TU	0620 / 1211 / 1835	3.9 / 2.2 / 3.7	**20** W	0649 / 1229 / 1917	4.3 / 1.6 / 4.2
6 W	0036 / 0733 / 1312 / 1948	2.0 / 4.0 / 2.0 / 3.9	**21** TH	0058 / 0756 / 1334 / 2021	1.4 / 4.5 / 1.4 / 4.4
7 TH	0132 / 0828 / 1400 / 2041	1.8 / 4.2 / 1.7 / 4.1	**22** F	0159 / 0852 / 1428 / 2116	1.2 / 4.6 / 1.2 / 4.5
8 F	0217 / 0911 / 1441 / 2125	1.5 / 4.4 / 1.4 / 4.3	**23** SA	0250 / 0942 / 1516 / 2205	1.0 / 4.8 / 1.0 / 4.6
9 SA	0258 / 0951 / 1519 / 2205	1.3 / 4.5 / 1.2 / 4.5	**24** SU	0336 / 1027 / 1600 / 2251	0.9 / 4.8 / 0.9 / 4.7
10 SU	0336 / 1029 / 1557 / 2245	1.1 / 4.6 / 1.0 / 4.6	**25** M O	0418 / 1109 / 1643 / 2332	0.9 / 4.8 / 0.8 / 4.7
11 M ●	0414 / 1107 / 1634 / 2325	0.9 / 4.7 / 0.9 / 4.7	**26** TU	0458 / 1148 / 1722	0.9 / 4.8 / 0.8
12 TU	0452 / 1145 / 1713 / 2350	0.9 / 4.8 / 0.8 / 4.9	**27** W	0011 / 0536 / 1225 / 1759	4.7 / 0.9 / 4.7 / 0.9
13 W	0005 / 0531 / 1224 / 1753	4.8 / 0.8 / 4.8 / 0.8	**28** TH	0048 / 0613 / 1300 / 1833	4.6 / 1.1 / 4.6 / 1.0
14 TH	0048 / 0612 / 1305 / 1836	4.8 / 0.9 / 4.7 / 0.8	**29** F	0124 / 0648 / 1335 / 1907	4.5 / 1.3 / 4.5 / 1.2
15 F	0132 / 0657 / 1348 / 1923	4.7 / 1.0 / 4.6 / 0.9	**30** SA	0201 / 0740 / 1411 / 1941	4.4 / 1.5 / 4.3 / 1.4

DECEMBER

Day	Time	m	Day	Time	m
1 SU	0241 / 0802 / 1450 / 2019	4.3 / 1.7 / 4.1 / 1.6	**16** M	0306 / 0834 / 1524 / 2102	4.6 / 1.2 / 4.4 / 1.1
2 M	0325 / 0847 / 1534 / 2105	4.2 / 1.9 / 4.0 / 1.8	**17** TU	0403 / 0934 / 1623 / 2203	4.5 / 1.4 / 4.2 / 1.3
3 TU	0416 / 0945 / 1626 / 2206	4.1 / 2.1 / 3.9 / 2.0	**18** W	0506 / 1043 / 1730 / 2311	4.4 / 1.5 / 4.1 / 1.5
4 W	0516 / 1059 / 1728 / 2322	4.0 / 2.2 / 3.8 / 2.0	**19** TH	0615 / 1155 / 1845	4.3 / 1.6 / 4.1
5 TH	0624 / 1213 / 1840	4.0 / 2.1 / 3.8	**20** F	0023 / 0724 / 1305 / 1956	1.5 / 4.3 / 1.5 / 4.1
6 F	0032 / 0729 / 1312 / 1948	1.9 / 4.2 / 1.9 / 4.0	**21** SA	0130 / 0826 / 1405 / 2059	1.5 / 4.4 / 1.4 / 4.3
7 SA	0129 / 0825 / 1400 / 2044	1.7 / 4.3 / 1.6 / 4.2	**22** SU	0227 / 0921 / 1457 / 2151	1.3 / 4.6 / 1.2 / 4.4
8 SU	0217 / 0913 / 1444 / 2134	1.5 / 4.5 / 1.3 / 4.4	**23** M	0315 / 1008 / 1543 / 2238	1.2 / 4.6 / 1.1 / 4.5
9 M	0301 / 0957 / 1528 / 2220	1.2 / 4.7 / 1.1 / 4.6	**24** TU O	0359 / 1050 / 1625 / 2318	1.1 / 4.7 / 1.0 / 4.5
10 TU ●	0345 / 1040 / 1612 / 2305	1.0 / 4.8 / 0.9 / 4.7	**25** W	0439 / 1127 / 1704 / 2355	1.1 / 4.6 / 0.9 / 4.6
11 W	0430 / 1123 / 1657 / 2350	0.9 / 4.8 / 0.7 / 4.8	**26** TH	0517 / 1202 / 1741	1.1 / 4.6 / 0.9
12 TH	0516 / 1207 / 1743	0.8 / 4.8 / 0.6	**27** F	0029 / 0553 / 1236 / 1815	4.6 / 1.1 / 4.5 / 1.0
13 F	0036 / 0602 / 1253 / 1829	4.9 / 0.8 / 4.8 / 0.6	**28** SA	0103 / 0627 / 1311 / 1846	4.5 / 1.2 / 4.5 / 1.1
14 SA	0124 / 0650 / 1340 / 1917	4.8 / 0.9 / 4.7 / 0.7	**29** SU	0138 / 0700 / 1346 / 1917	4.5 / 1.3 / 4.4 / 1.2
15 SU	0213 / 0740 / 1430 / 2007	4.8 / 1.0 / 4.6 / 0.9	**30** M	0215 / 0732 / 1423 / 1948	4.4 / 1.5 / 4.3 / 1.4
			31 TU	0253 / 0807 / 1502 / 2024	4.3 / 1.7 / 4.1 / 1.5

Chart Datum: 2·73 metres below Ordnance Datum (Newlyn)

PORTSMOUTH   10-2-29

Hampshire 50°47'·35N 01°06'·58W (Entrance)

CHARTS

AC 2628, 2629, 2625, *2631, 394, 2050, 2045*; Imray C3, C9; Stanfords 11, 18; OS 197

TIDES

+0029 Dover; ML 2·8; Zone 0 (UT)

Standard Port PORTSMOUTH (←)

Times				Height (metres)			
High Water		Low Water		MHWS	MHWN	MLWN	MLWS
0500	1000	0000	0600	4·7	3·8	1·9	0·8
1700	2200	1200	1800				
Differences LEE-ON-SOLENT							
−0005	+0005	−0015	−0010	−0·2	−0·1	+0·1	+0·2

Portsmouth is a Standard Port; daily predictions are given above. See also 10·2·12. Strong winds from NE to SE, coupled with a high barometer, may lower levels by 1m and delay times of HW and LW by 1hr; the opposite may occur in strong W'lies with low pressure.

SHELTER

Excellent. This very large hbr affords shelter in some area for any wind. There are two marinas on the Gosport side, two at Fareham and one at the N end of Portchester Lake, plus several yacht pontoons/jetties and many moorings (see Facilities). Good shelter in The Camber, but this is a busy little commercial dock and often full; beware the Isle of Wight car ferry docking near the ent. Portsmouth is a major naval base and Dockyard Port; all vessels come under the QHM's authority. If > 20m LOA, ask QHM's permission (VHF Ch 11) to enter, leave or move in hbr, especially in fog. Fishing and ⚓ in chans are prohib.

NAVIGATION

WPT No 4 Bar buoy, QR, 50°46'·75N 01°06'·27W, 150°/330° from/to hbr ent (W side), 4½ca. Beware very strong tides in hbr ent, commercial shipping and ferries, Gosport ferry and HM Ships.

Speed limit is 10kn within hbr and within 1000 yds of the shore in any part of the Dockyard Port; speed = speed through the water. Outside the hbr ent, the Dockyard Port limits embrace the Solent from Hillhead and Old Castle Pt (close NE of Cowes) eastward to Eastney and Shanklin (IOW), thence almost out to Nab Tr (see AC 394 & 2050).

Historic Wrecks (see 10.0.3g) are at: 50°45'·8N 01°06'·2W (site of *Mary Rose*), marked by SPM buoys; 5ca SSW of Spit Sand Ft. *Invincible* lies at 50°44'·34N 01°02'·23W, 117° Horse Sand Fort 1·45M, marked by SPM buoy.

Approaches: From the W, yachts can use the Swashway Chan (to NW of Spit Sand Fort) which carries about 2m; keep War Memorial and RH edge of block of flats on at 049°. The Inner Swashway Chan (Round Tr on 029°. NB: rear transit, diving tank, has been demolished) carries only 0·1m; local knowledge required.

Approaching inshore from E, the submerged barrier, which extends from Southsea to Horse Sand Fort, should only be crossed via the unlit Inshore Boat passage (0·9m) 1ca off the beach, marked by R & G piles; or via the Main Passage (min depth 1·2m) 7ca further S, marked by G pile and dolphin, QR.

A Small Boat Channel for craft < 20m LOA lies at the hbr ent, parallel to and outboard of the W edge of the main dredged chan; it runs from abeam No 4 Bar buoy, QR (off Clarence Pier) to Ballast buoy, Fl R 2·5s, and extends about 50m off Fort Blockhouse. A depth gauge is on pile BC4. Yachts should enter by the Small Boat Chan; they may also enter on the E side of the main chan, but clear of it and close inshore. All yachts must leave via the Small Boat Chan. Yachts may only cross the main chan N of Ballast buoy or S of No 4 Bar buoy. Yachts must motor (if so fitted) between No 4 Bar and Ballast buoys; winds at the ent may be fickle or gusty and tides run hard.

FIRING RANGE

Tipner Rifle Range as shown on chartlet; danger area extends 2,500 metres from firing range. When firing is in progress, R flag or Ⓡ lt on Tipner Range FS indicates yachts should clear the range danger area or transit it as quickly as possible.

LIGHTS AND MARKS

From E of the IOW, Nab Tower, Fl 10s 27m 16M, is conspic about 10M SE of the hbr ent. In the inner appr's there are 3 conspic forts: Horse Sand Fort, Iso G 2s; No Man's Land Fort, Iso R 2s, and Spit Sand Fort, Fl R 5s.

Ldg marks/lts: St Jude's ✠ spire and Southsea Castle lt ho in transit 003° lead between Outer Spit SCM buoy, Q (6) + L Fl 15s, and Horse Sand SHM buoy, Fl G 2·5s. At night keep in the W sector (000°-003°) between the Al WG and Al WR sectors of the Dir lt (H24) on Southsea Castle, which also shows an Iso 2s lt, vis 339°-066°.

The Small Boat Chan is covered, until close to the hbr ent, by the Oc R sector (324°-330°) of the Dir WRG lt on Fort Blockhouse (W side of hbr ent). Thereafter the Iso R 2s sector (337·5°-345°) of the Dir WRG lt 2m 1M (on dolphin E of Gosport Marina) leads 341° through the ent and close abeam Ballast Bank PHM buoy, Fl R 2·5s.

RADIO TELEPHONE

Yachts should monitor Ch **11** (H24) for traffic/nav info. For the Camber call *Portsmouth Hbr Radio* (Commercial Port) Ch 11 14 (H24).

Haslar Marina and *Port Solent* Ch **80** M (H24). *Gosport Marina* call Ch **80** M (HO). Fareham Marina Ch M (summer 0900-1730). Wicor Marina Ch 80 (0900-1730, Mon-Sat). Naval activities to the S/SE of Portsmouth and IOW may be advised by Solent CG Ch 67 or ☎ (01705) 552100; or Naval Ops ☎ 722008. Naval vessels use Ch 13. The positions and times of naval firings and underwater explosions are broadcast daily at 0800 and 1400LT Ch 06; preceded by a Securité call on Ch 16. Warnings of underwater explosions will also be broadcast on Ch 16 at 1 hour, at 30 mins and just before the detonation.

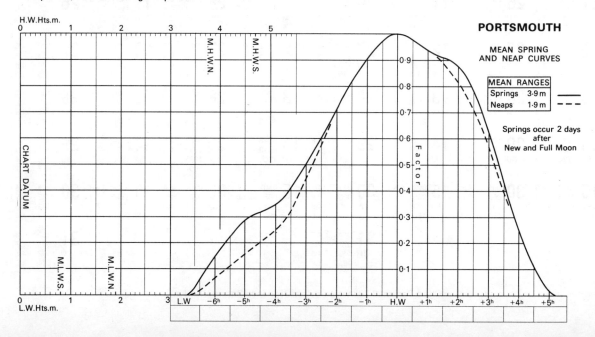

PORTSMOUTH

MEAN SPRING
AND NEAP CURVES

MEAN RANGES	
Springs	3·9 m ———
Neaps	1·9 m - - -

Springs occur 2 days
after
New and Full Moon

PORTSMOUTH *continued*

2

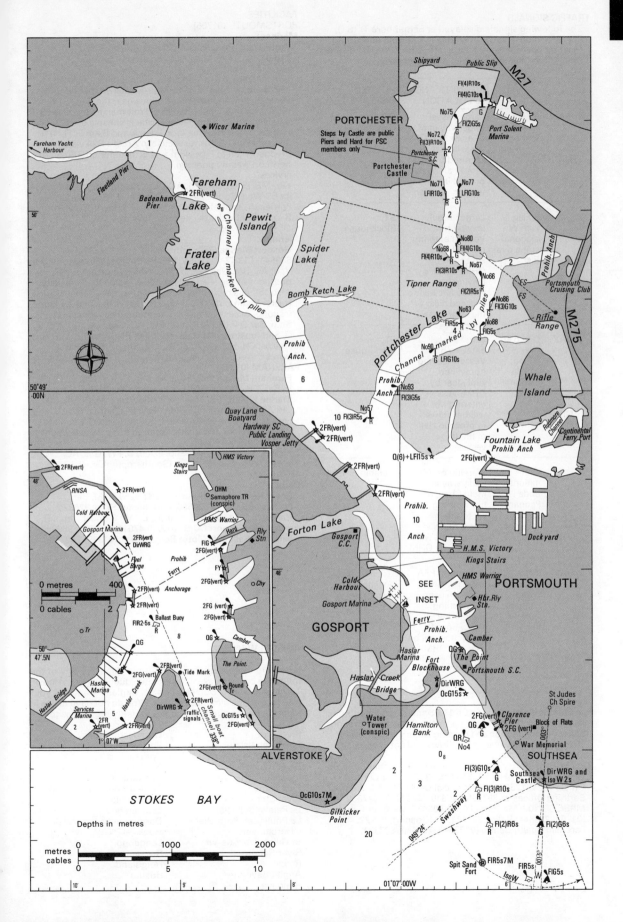

PORTCHESTER

Steps by Castle are public
Piers and Hard for PSC
members only

Shipyard
Public Slip
M27

Fl(4)R10s
Fl(4)G10s
No75
Fl(2)G5s
G
Port Solent
Marina

No72
Fl(3)R10s
R
G

No71
LFlR10s
R
No77
LFlG10s
G

Portchester
S.C.

Portchester
Castle

No80
No68 Fl(4)G10s
Fl(4)R10s R G
No67
No66
Fl(3)R10s R
Fl(2)R5s R

Tipner Range

No86
No63 Fl(3)G10s
Fl(5s R G
No88
Portchester Lake
Fl(5s
4 *marked by piles*
Channel marked by piles

No90
LFlG10s
G

*Rifle
Range*
M275

*Whale
Island*

*Portsmouth
Cruising Club*
ES
ES

Prohib. Anch.

No93
*Prohib.
Anch.*
Fl(3)G5s

*Fareham Yacht
Harbour*

Fleetland Pier

Wicor Marine

1

*Fareham
Lake*
2FR(vert)
3 6

*Bedenham
Pier*

*Pewit
Island*

*Frater
Lake*

*Channel
4 marked by piles*

*Spider
Lake*

6

Bomb Ketch Lake
2 1

*Prohib.
Anch.*

6

*Quay Lane
Boatyard*
Hardway SC
Public Landing
Vosper Jetty

10 Fl(3)R5s
No57
R

2FR(vert)
2FR(vert)

2FR(vert)

Q(6)+LFl15s

*Ridmore
Channel*
*Continental
Ferry Port*

Fountain Lake
Prohib Anch
2FG(vert)

2FR(vert)

*Prohib.
10
Anch*

Dockyard

HMS Victory
Kings
Stairs

QHM
Semaphore TR
(conspic)

HMS Warrior
Hard
Rly
Stn

Forton Lake

*Gosport
C.C.*

H.M.S. Victory
Kings Stairs

HMS Warrior

PORTSMOUTH

Hbr.Rly
Sta.

FIG
2FG(vert)

FY
2FG(vert)

Chy

Prohib
Ferry

2FR(vert)
2FR(vert)
DirWRG
Fuel
Barge

2FR(vert)

2FR(vert)

Anchorage

2FG (vert)
2FG(vert)

FlR2·5s
R
Ballast Buoy

8
QG QG

Camber

*Cold
Harbour*

Gosport Marina

GOSPORT

Camber

QG
The Point
Portsmouth S.C.

*Haslar
Marina*
*Fort
Blockhouse*

DirWRG
OcG15s

2FG(vert) Clarence
QG Pier
G 2FG(vert)
G

St Judes
Ch Spire

Block of Flats

War Memorial

SOUTHSEA

Fl(3)G10s
G
Southsea
Castle DirWRG and
IsoW 2s

Fl(3)R10s
R

Fl(2)R6s
R
Fl(2)G6s
G

FlR5s7M
Spit Sand
Fort
FlR5s
IsoW
W
FlG5s

*Hamilton
Bank*

QR
No4

*Haslar
Marina*

*Haslar Creek
Bridge*

*Water
Tower
(conspic)*

2
0 8

3

2

4 *Swashway*

20

ALVERSTOKE

2FR(vert)
RNSA
48'

2FR(vert)

Cold Harbour

Gosport Marina
2FR(vert)
DirWRG

*Fuel
Barge*

0 metres 400

0 cables 2

2FR(vert)

2FR(vert)

FlR2·5s
R

Tr

QG

50°
47'.5N

2FR(vert)
2FR(vert)

*Haslar
Marina*

*Services
Marina*

2FR
(vert)

2FR(vert)

1° 07'W

SEE
INSET

Ballast Buoy

8

QG

Tide Mark
DirWRG
2FG(vert)
2FR(vert)

The Point.

2FG(vert)
Round
Tr

2FR(vert)
Traffic
signals
OcG15s
2FG(vert)

*small boat
channel 338°*

3

*Haslar
Bridge*

5

Haslar Creek

2

Ferry
*Prohib.
Anch.*

Swashway
049°24'

STOKES BAY

Depths in metres

metres
cables

0 1000 2000

0 5 10

OcG10s7M
Gilkicker
Point

003°

01°07'·00W

10' 9' 8' 7'

PORTSMOUTH *continued*

TRAFFIC SIGNALS

The following signals displayed at Semaphore Tr (ST), Fort Blockhouse and sometimes in HM Ship concerned must be obeyed; except that craft <20m LOA may use the Small Boat Chan H24 despite displayed tfc sigs.

	SIGNAL	MEANING AND APPLICATION	HOISTED/ DISPLAYED BY
1. DAY NIGHT	R Flag, W diagonal stripe. Ⓡ Ⓖ Ⓖ	Large vessel underway in Main Chan or hbr. Other vessels may be required by QHM to wait alongside or hold in a waiting position.	ST, Blockhouse.
2. DAY NIGHT	R Flag with W diagonal stripe over B ● Ⓦ Ⓖ	Large vessel leaving hbr. Vessels entering hbr will be kept clear by QHM. Vessels leaving hbr will be allowed to proceed clear of the large vessel.	ST, Blockhouse.
3. DAY NIGHT	One B ● over R Flag with W diagonal stripe. Ⓖ Ⓦ	Large vessel entering hbr. Vessels leaving hbr will be kept clear by QHM. Vessels entering hbr will be allowed to proceed clear of the large vessel.	ST, Blockhouse.
4. DAY	International Code Pennant superior to Pennant Zero.	Warship or RFA underway in Main Chan, or hbr warning sig to other ships. Specific instructions will be given by QHM.	Warship or RFA
5. DAY NIGHT	International Code Pennant superior to Pennant NINE. Ⓖ Ⓖ Ⓖ	Warship or RFA underway in Main Chan, or hbr warning sig to other ships. Specific instruction will be given by QHM.	ST, Blockhouse.

Fog Routine is broadcast on Ch 11, 13 and 73, when it comes into force. Yachts may continue at the skipper's discretion, but with great caution and keeping well clear of the main chan; they are however strongly advised not to proceed. Monitor VHF Ch 11.

TELEPHONE (Portsmouth/Gosport 01705; Fareham 01329) QHM 723124; AQHM 723344/Fax 837715; Hbr Control Officer (H24) 723694; Commercial Docks 297395; Camber Berthing Offices ☎ 297395 Ext 310; ⌗ (01703) 827350; MRSC 552100; Marinecall 0891 500457; Weather Centre (01703) 228844; Police 321111; Dr (Gosport) 80922; Fareham Health Centre (01329) 282911; Ⓗ 822331.

FACILITIES
PORTSMOUTH (01705)
Marinas
Port Solent, Portchester, (900) ☎ 210765, Fax 324241, £16.04, P, D, FW, ME, El, Ⓔ, Sh, BH (40 ton), CH, V, AC, R, Bar, Gas, Gaz, Ⓞ.
Portchester Lake is marked by lit/unlit piles; unusually, PHMs are numbered 57 to 74 (from seaward), and SHMs 95 to 75. Beware unlit naval buoys near the S end. Do not delay crossing Tipner Range, S limit marked by piles 63/87 and N by 70/78. Portchester Castle is conspic 5ca SSW of marina. 140m W of the lock, Piles A and B are lit Fl (4) R 10s and Fl (4) G 10s respectively. Access H24 via chan dredged 1·5m to lock (43m x 12·5m); enter on 3 Ⓖ (vert) or berth on waiting pontoon.
Services
FW, ME, El, Ⓔ, Sh, SM, ACA, CH; **Hbr** Moorings ☎ 832484.
City EC Wed (Southsea Sat); ✉, Ⓑ, ⇌, ✈ (Southampton). Ferries to Ouistreham, Cherbourg, Le Havre, St Malo, Bilbao, Santander (winter) and IoW (see 10.0.4).
GOSPORT (01705)
Marinas
Gosport Marina (350, some visitors) ☎ 524811, Fax 589541, £13.47, P, D, FW, ME, El, Sh, BH (150, 40 ton), CH, V, R, AC, Bar, Gas, Gaz, SM, Ⓞ. Note: There are RNSA pontoons at the N end of Cold Hbr, inside the Fuel Jetty. Also 150 pile moorings (some dry); contact Haslar Marina **Haslar Marina**, ☎ 601201, Fax 602201, £10.47, (600+ some visitors), Access H24; Ⓥ at L pontoon, near conspic Lt Ship, Bar & R (RN & RAYC); FW, AC, Gas, Gaz, CH, ME, Ⓔ, Ⓞ, Slip (upstream of Haslar bridge). RNSA berths at S end.
Services: CH, P, D, ACA, El, Ⓔ, ME, Sh, BY, SM, Slip, C.
Town EC Wed; ✉, Ⓑ, ⇌ (Portsmouth), ✈ (Southampton).
FAREHAM (01329)
Fareham Marina ☎ 822445, M, Slip, D, FW, ME, El, Ⓔ, Sh, V, Bar, CH; (Access HW±3); **Fareham Yacht Hbr; Wicor Marine** (200) ☎ 237112, Fax 825660, Slip, M, D, ME, Sh, CH, AC, BH (10 ton), C (7 ton), FW, El, Ⓔ, Gas, Gaz. Fareham Lake is well marked, but only partially lit up to Bedenham Pier and unlit thereafter. Chan dries 0·9m in final 5ca to Town Quay.
Services: M, Sh, CH, ME, Slip, El, Ⓔ, D, FW, Gas, AC, SM.
Town EC Wed; ✉, Ⓑ, ⇌, ✈ (Southampton).

Clubs
Royal Naval & Royal Albert YC ☎ 825924, M, Bar; **Portsmouth SC** ☎ 820596; **Portchester SC** ☎ 376375; **Hardway SC** ☎ 581875, Slip, M, L, FW, C (mast stepping only), AB; **Gosport CC** ☎ (01329) 47014 or (0860) 966390; **Fareham Sailing & Motor Boat Club** ☎ (01329) 280738.

AGENTS WANTED

If you are interested in becoming our agent for any of the following ports, please write to: The Editor, Edington House, Trent, Sherborne, Dorset DT9 4SR, England – and get your free copy of the almanac annually. You do not have to live in a port to be the agent, but at least a fairly regular visitor.

River Exe	Grandcamp-Maisy
Port Ellen (Islay)	Port-en-Bessin
Glandore/Union Hall	Courseulles
River Rance/Dinan	Boulogne
Lampaul	Dunkerque
Port Tudy	Terneuzen/Westerschelde
River Etel	Oudeschild
Le Palais (Belle Ile)	Lauwersoog
Le Pouliguen/Pornichet	Dornumer-Accumersiel
L'Herbaudière	Hooksiel
St Gilles-Croix-de-Vie	Langeoog
River Seudre	Bremerhaven
Royan	Helgoland
Anglet/Bayonne	Büsum
Hendaye	

LANGSTONE HARBOUR   10-2-30

Hampshire 50°47'·20N 01°01'·45W (Ent)

CHARTS

AC *3418, 2045*; Imray C3, Y33; Stanfords 10, 11; OS 196, 197

TIDES

+0022 Dover; Zone 0 (UT)

Standard Port PORTSMOUTH (←)

Times				Height (metres)			
High Water		Low Water		MHWS	MHWN	MLWN	MLWS
0500	1000	0000	0600	4·7	3·8	1·9	0·8
1700	2200	1200	1800				
Differences LANGSTONE							
0000	0000	+0010	+0010	+0·1	+0·1	0·0	0·0
NAB TOWER							
+0015	0000	+0015	+0015	–0·2	0·0	+0·2	0·0

SHELTER

Very good in marina (2·4m) to W inside ent, access HW±3 over sill 1·6m CD; waiting pontoon. Ent is 7m wide. 6 Y ⚓s at W side of hbr ent, 6 more on E side; max LOA 9m. Or ⚓ out of the fairway in Russell's Lake and Langstone Chan (water ski area); or see Hr Mr (E side of ent). Hbr speed limit 10kn.

NAVIGATION

WPT Langstone Fairway SWM buoy , L Fl 10s, 50°46'·28N 01°01'·27W, 168°/348° from/to QR lt at ent, 0·94M. Bar has about 1·8m. Ent chan lies between E & W Winner drying banks, which afford some protection. Appr is easy in fair weather, best from HW –3 to +1, but avoid entry against the ebb, esp at sp and in onshore winds. In strong S/SE winds do not attempt entry.

Fraser Range, Eastney, in use Mon to Fri 0800-1800, or as notified. Details from (01705) 722351 ext 6420 or Radio Solent (see 10.2.20). Range area is a circle 1M radius centred on 50°47'·30N 01°01'·90W, with sector 120°-155° out to 9M. Live firing does not take place, but 30 mins before use, 2 R flags are flown at range site; FR, Oc (2) Y 10s and Y lts on same lattice tr are shown when in use.

LIGHTS AND MARKS

Ldg marks (concrete dolphins), or Fairway buoy on with conspic chy, lead 344° just clear of E Winner. The ent itself deepens and favours the W side. The narrow appr chan to Langstone Marina is marked by 7 SHM piles, only the first of which is lit, Fl G. There are 9 PHM piles; the 4th, 6th and 9th are Fl R. The lock has R/G ent sigs, as it is too narrow for 2 boats to pass; outbound have priority.

RADIO TELEPHONE

VHF Ch 12 16 (Summer 0830-1700. Winter: Mon-Fri 0830-1700; Sat-Sun 0830-1300 LT). Marina Ch **80** M (H24).

TELEPHONE (01705)

Hr Mr 463419; MRSC 552100; ⌗ (01703) 827350; Marinecall 0891 500457; Police 321111; Dr 465721.

FACILITIES

Langstone Marina (300) ☎ 822719, Fax 822220, £10.81, CH, BH (20 ton), D, Gaz, C, AC, FW, Access HW±3; **Hayling Pontoon** (E side of ent), AB, P, D, FW, L, Slip; **Langstone SC** ☎ 484577, Slip, M, L, FW, Bar; **Eastney Cruising Ass'n** (ECA) ☎ 734103, 6 ⚓s; **Solatron SC; Locks SC** ☎ 829833; **Tudor SC** (Hilsea) ☎ 662002, Slip, M, FW, Bar. **Towns**: EC Havant Wed; ✉ (Eastney, Hayling), Ⓑ (Havant, Hayling, Emsworth), ⇌ (bus to Havant), ✈ (Southampton).

We left behind the painted buoy
  That tosses at the harbour-mouth;
  And madly danced our hearts with joy,
  As fast we fleeted to the South:
How fresh was every sight and sound
On open main or winding shore!
We knew the merry world was round,
And we might sail for evermore.

The Voyage: Alfred, Lord Tennyson

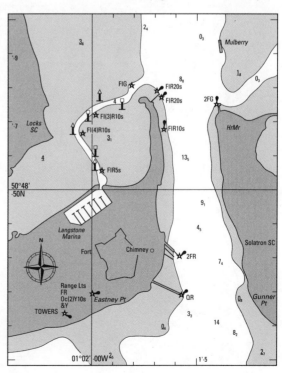

CHICHESTER HARBOUR   10-2-31

W. Sussex 50°46'.83N 00°55'.97W

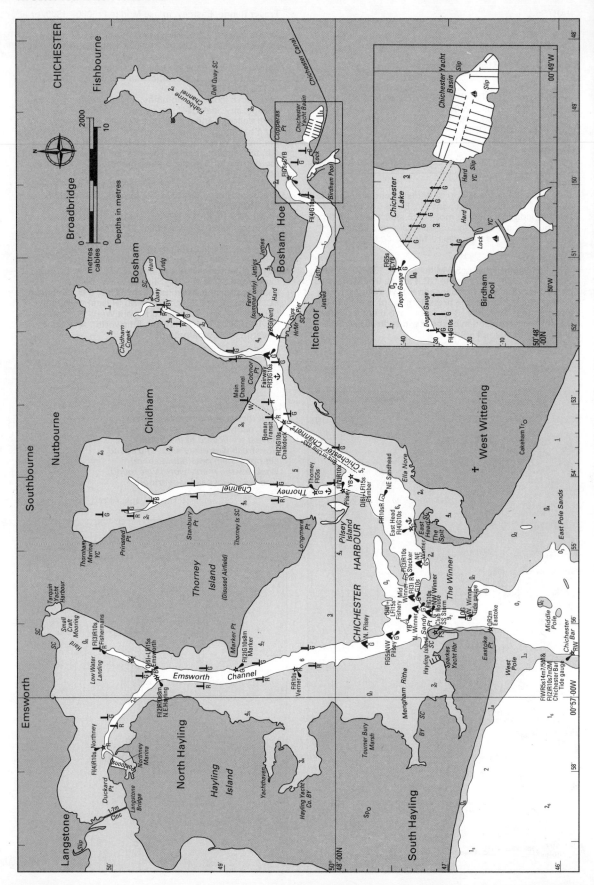

CHICHESTER HARBOUR *continued*

CHARTS
AC *3418, 2045*; Imray C4, C9, Y33; Stanfords 10, 11; OS 197
TIDES
+0027 Dover; ML 2·8; Zone 0 (UT); see curves on 10·2·12

Standard Port PORTSMOUTH (←—)

Times				Height (metres)			
High Water		Low Water		MHWS	MHWN	MLWN	MLWS
0500	1000	0000	0600	4·7	3·8	1·9	0·8
1700	2200	1800	1800				
Differences HARBOUR ENTRANCE							
–0010	+0005	+0015	+0020	+0·2	+0·2	0·0	+0·1
NORTHNEY							
+0010	+0015	+0015	+0025	+0·2	0·0	–0·2	–0·3
ITCHENOR							
–0005	+0005	+0005	+0025	+0·1	0·0	–0·2	–0·2
BOSHAM							
0000	+0010	No data		+0·2	+0·1	No data	
DELL QUAY							
+0005	+0015	No data		+0·2	+0·1	No data	
SELSEY BILL							
–0005	–0005	+0035	+0035	+0·6	+0·6	0·0	0·0

SHELTER
Excellent in all 5 main chans: Emsworth, Thorney, Chichester, Bosham, Itchenor Reach and Fishbourne. There are six yacht hbrs and marinas (see FACILITIES); also about 50 ⚓s at Emsworth and Itchenor. Recognised ⚓s in Thorney Chan off Pilsey Is; off E Head (uncomfortable in NE winds); and in the Chichester Chan off Chalkdock Pt. Hbr speed limit of 8kn is rigidly enforced.
NAVIGATION
WPT 50°45'·50N 00°56'·50W, 193°/013° from/to Bar Bn, 0·40M. Best entry is HW –3 to +1, to avoid confused seas during the ebb, esp in onshore winds >F 5. Do not attempt entry in S'ly gales. Bar is dredged 1·5m, but depths may vary ±0·75m after gales. Leave Bar Bn (depth gauge) close to port.
APPROACHES: From the W, the astern transit 255° of No Man's Land Fort and Ryde ✠ spire (hard to see) leads to the Bar Bn. Closer in, transit 064° of Target NCM Bn with Cakeham Tr leads 6ca S of Bar Bn; thence alter 013° as Eastoke Pt opens to E of Bar Bn. CHI SPIT unlit PHM buoy (some 2ca SxW of Bar Bn, Apr-Nov) must be rounded to clear W Pole spit, dries 0·2m.
From the E/SE (Looe Chan) keep W for 2M, then NW; pick up an astern brg 184° of Nab Tr, toward the Bar Bn, so as to clear the shoals of Bracklesham Bay. The former Owers LANBY is now a SCM buoy, Q (6) + L Fl 15s, Whis, Racon. Note: An Historic Wreck (*Hazardous*) lies at 50°45'·10N 00°51'·47W, brg 105°/3·2M from Bar Bn; see 10.0.3g.
ENTRANCE: Pass between Eastoke bn QR and W Winner bn QG (tide gauge). Three SHM lt buoys mark the edge of The Winner shoal, dries, to stbd of the ent. At Fishery SCM buoy, Q (6) + L Fl 15s, chan divides: N to Emsworth and ENE toward Chichester. Stocker's Sand, dries 2·4m, is marked by 3 PHM lt buoys. East Head bn, Fl (4) G 10s, (tide gauge) marks start of anchorage.
EMSWORTH CHANNEL: Chan is straight, broad, deep and well marked/lit in the 2·5M reach to Emsworth SCM bn, Q (6) + L Fl 15s, where Sweare Deep forks NW to Northney. Good ⚓s especially N of Sandy Pt near ent to chan. Here an unlit ECM bn marks chan to Sparkes Yacht Hbr.
THORNEY CHANNEL: Strangers should go up at half-flood. Ent is at Camber SCM bn, Q (6) + L Fl 15s; pass between Pilsey and Thorney Lt bns, thereafter chan is marked by perches. Above Stanbury Pt chan splits, Prinsted Chan to port (full of moorings) and Nutbourne Chan to stbd; both dry at N ends. There is plenty of room to ⚓ in Thorney Chan, well protected from E and SE winds.
CHICHESTER CHANNEL: This runs up to Itchenor Reach and Bosham Chan. From NE Sandhead PHM by, Fl R 10s, transit 033° of Roman Transit bn on with Main Chan Bn and distant clump of trees leads to Chalkdock Bn, Fl (2) G 10s. Here alter 082° to Fairway buoy, Fl (3) G 10s; on this reach a measured half-mile is marked by Y perches. At Deep End SCM bn turn N into Bosham Chan, or ESE into Itchenor Reach, for Birdham Pool and Chichester Marina. ⚓ prohib in Itchenor Reach and Bosham Chan.

LIGHTS AND MARKS
Bar Bn, wooden twr + R can topmark, Fl WR 5s 14m 7/5M, vis W 322°-080°, R080°-322°; and same tr, Fl (2) R 10s 7m 2M, 020°-080°; also tide gauge. 3 SHM Bys: NW Winner Fl G 10s; N Winner Fl (2) G10s; Mid Winner Fl (3) G 10s. Fishery SCM Q (6)+L Fl 15s. All chans well marked.
RADIO TELEPHONE
Hr Mr, call *Chichester* VHF Ch **14** 16 (Patrol craft *Regnum* on Ch14). (Apl-Sept: 0900-1300, 1400-1730. Oct-Mar: Mon-Fri 0900-1300, 1400-1730. Sat 0900-1300). Tarquin Yacht Hbr and Northney Marina Ch **80** M. Chichester Marina Ch M.
TELEPHONE (01243)
Chichester Hbr Conservancy Office 512301; ⌗ (01703) 827350; MRSC (01705) 552100; Weather info (01705) 8091; Marinecall 0891 500457; Police 536733; Ⓗ 787970.
FACILITIES
EMSWORTH CHANNEL
Tarquin Yacht Harbour (200+20 visitors) ☎ 375211, Fax 378498, £11; access HW±2 over 2·4m sill which maintains 1·5m inside, Slip, Gas, ME, El, AC, Sh, P, D, FW, BH (60 ton), C (20 ton);
Slips at South St, Kings St, and Slipper Mill; contact the Warden ☎ 376422.
Services: ME, Sh, CH, El, ACA; Emsworth EC Wed.
HAYLING ISLAND (01705)
Sparkes Yacht Hbr (140) ☎ 463572, mobile 0370-365610, Fax 461325, £12.50, access all tides via chan dredged 2m; pontoons have 1·6m. Slip, ME, El, FW, P, D, Gas, Gaz, ▣, Sh, C (20 ton), CH. From close N of Sandy Pt, appr on transit 277° of two x bns; thence alter S, past 3 PHM bns to marina.
Northney Marina (260+27 visitors) ☎ 466321, Fax 461467, £8.50; access all tides via chan 1m, D, BH (35 ton), Bar, FW, AC, El, Sh, R, CH, ME;
Services: ME, El, Slip, BH (8 ton), P, FW, Sh, CH. EC Wed.
THORNEY CHANNEL
Thornham Marina (77+6 visitors) ☎ 375335, Fax 371522, £7.00, appr via drying chan, P & D (cans), FW, Sh, ME, C (10 ton), BH (12 ton), Slip, R, Bar. **Services:** CH, BY.
CHICHESTER CHANNEL/ITCHENOR REACH
Hard available at all stages of the tide. There are 6 ⚓s off Itchenor jetty and a 90ft pontoon. For moorings apply Hr Mr. **Services:** Slip, P & D (cans), CH, Sh, FW, M, El, Ⓔ, ME. Itchenor EC Thurs.
BOSHAM CHANNEL
For moorings (200+) contact the Quaymaster ☎ 573336. ⚓ prohib in chan which mostly dries, access HW±2.
Bosham Quay Hard, L, FW, AB; **Services:** SM. EC Wed.
CHICHESTER LAKE
Birdham Pool: (230+10 visitors) ☎ 512310, £14, enter chan at Birdham SHM bn, Fl (4) G 10s, with depth gauge; access HW ±3 via lock. **Services:** Slip, P, D, FW, El, Ⓔ, AC, Sh, CH, Gas, ME, SM, C (3 ton).
Chichester Marina: (1000+50 visitors) ☎ 512731, Fax 513472, £13.00, enter chan at CYB SHM pile, Fl G 5s, with depth gauge; 6kn speed limit. Well marked chan has approx 0·5m below CD; no access LW ±1½; waiting pontoon outside the lock.
Traffic sigs:
   Q Ⓡ (S of tr) = <1m water in chan.
   Q Ⓨ (top of tr) = both gates open (free flow).
Lock sigs: Ⓡ = Wait; Ⓖ = Enter.
From Easter to 30 Sep, lock is manned Mon-Thur 0700-2100; Fri 0700 -2359; Sat, Sun, Bank Hols 0600-2359; all LT. 1 Oct to Easter: Contact ☎ 512731 or call VHF Ch M.
Services: Slip, P, D, FW, ME, El, Sh, AC, Gas, Gaz, CH, BY, BH (20 ton), V, R, Bar, ▣, ACA, SM.
FISHBOURNE CHANNEL
Dell Quay: Possible drying berth alongside the Quay, public slip. **Services:** Sh, Slip, BH, M, L.

Clubs
Birdham YC; Bosham SC ☎ 572341; **Chichester YC** ☎ 512918, R, Bar, ▣; **Chichester Cruiser and Racing Club** ☎ 371731; **Dell Quay SC** ☎ 785080; **Emsworth SC** ☎ 373065; **Emsworth Slipper SC** ☎ 372523; **Hayling Island SC** ☎ (01705) 463768; **Itchenor SC** ☎ 512400; **Mengham Rithe SC** ☎ (01705) 463337; **Thorney Island SC; W Wittering SC.**

REQUIRING EXPERT HELP?
Look in The Pink

and make your call with confidence

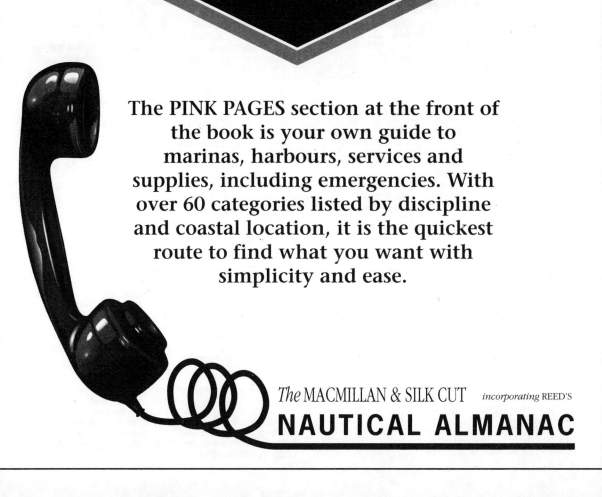

The PINK PAGES section at the front of the book is your own guide to marinas, harbours, services and supplies, including emergencies. With over 60 categories listed by discipline and coastal location, it is the quickest route to find what you want with simplicity and ease.

The MACMILLAN & SILK CUT   *incorporating* REED'S
NAUTICAL ALMANAC

3

Area 3

South-East England
Selsey Bill to North Foreland

South-East England

Gravesend*
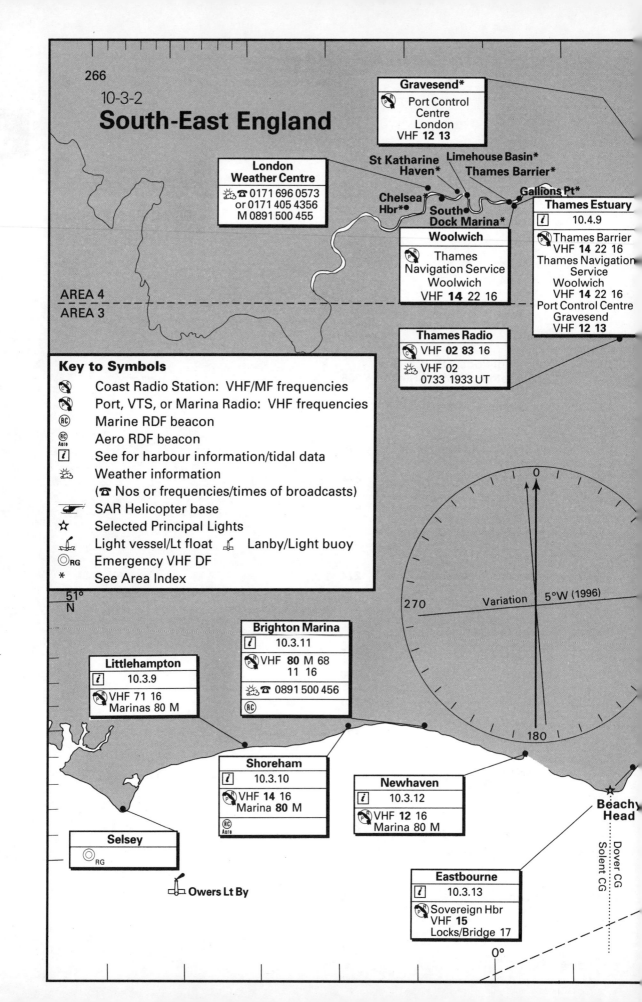
Port Control
Centre
London
VHF **12 13**

**London
Weather Centre**
☁ ☎ 0171 696 0573
or 0171 405 4356
M 0891 500 455

St Katharine
Haven*

Limehouse Basin*
Thames Barrier*

Chelsea
Hbr*●

Gallions Pt*

South
Dock Marina*

Thames Estuary
ⓘ   10.4.9

Thames Barrier
VHF **14** 22 16
Thames Navigation
Service
Woolwich
VHF **14** 22 16
Port Control Centre
Gravesend
VHF **12 13**

Woolwich
Thames
Navigation Service
Woolwich
VHF **14** 22 16

AREA 4
AREA 3

Thames Radio
VHF **02 83** 16
☁ VHF 02
0733 1933 UT

Key to Symbols

Coast Radio Station: VHF/MF frequencies

Port, VTS, or Marina Radio: VHF frequencies

ⓇⒸ Marine RDF beacon

ⓇⒸ Aero RDF beacon
Aero

ⓘ See for harbour information/tidal data

☁ Weather information
(☎ Nos or frequencies/times of broadcasts)

SAR Helicopter base

☆ Selected Principal Lights

Light vessel/Lt float   Lanby/Light buoy

ⓄRG Emergency VHF DF

* See Area Index

51°
N

0

270   Variation   5°W (1996)

180

Brighton Marina
ⓘ   10.3.11
VHF **80** M 68
11 16
☁ ☎ 0891 500 456
ⓇⒸ

Littlehampton
ⓘ   10.3.9
VHF 71 16
Marinas 80 M

Shoreham
ⓘ   10.3.10
VHF **14** 16
Marina **80** M
ⓇⒸ
Aero

Newhaven
ⓘ   10.3.12
VHF **12** 16
Marina 80 M

Selsey
ⓄRG

Beachy
Head

Dover CG
Solent CG

Owers Lt By

Eastbourne
ⓘ   10.3.13
Sovereign Hbr
VHF **15**
Locks/Bridge 17

0°

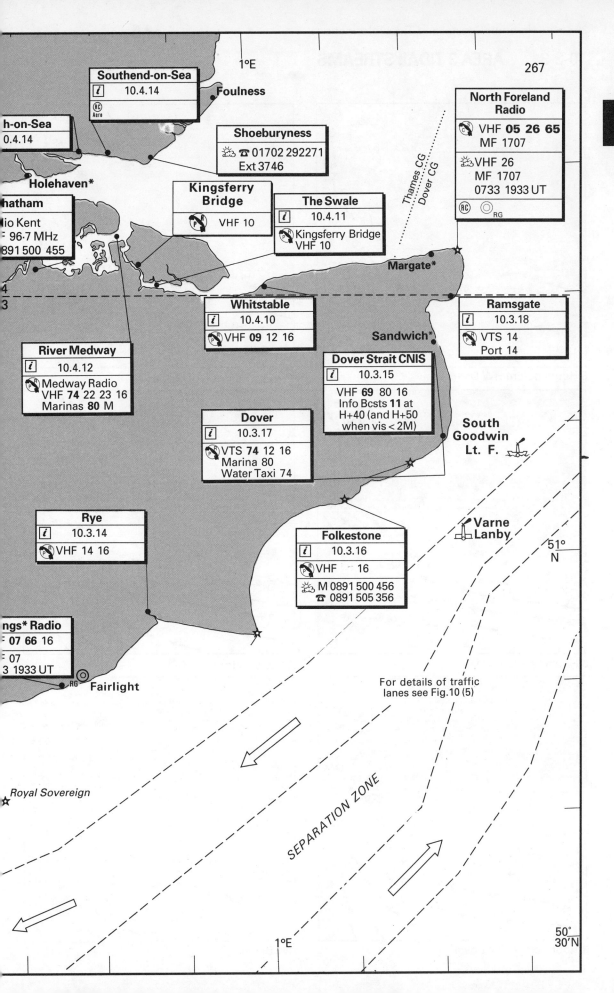

3

Southend-on-Sea
i 10.4.14
RC Aero

Foulness

h-on-Sea
0.4.14

Holehaven*

Shoeburyness
☎ 01702 292271
Ext 3746

hatham
io Kent
F 96·7 MHz
891 500 455

Kingsferry Bridge
P VHF 10

The Swale
i 10.4.11
P Kingsferry Bridge VHF 10

North Foreland Radio
VHF **05 26 65**
MF 1707
VHF 26
MF 1707
0733 1933 UT
RC ◎ RG

Thames CG
Dover CG

Margate*

Whitstable
i 10.4.10
P VHF **09** 12 16

Sandwich*

Ramsgate
i 10.3.18
P VTS 14
Port 14

River Medway
i 10.4.12
P Medway Radio
VHF **74** 22 23 16
Marinas **80** M

Dover Strait CNIS
i 10.3.15
VHF **69** 80 16
Info Bcsts **11** at
H+40 (and H+50
when vis < 2M)

South Goodwin Lt. F.

Dover
i 10.3.17
P VTS **74** 12 16
Marina 80
Water Taxi 74

Rye
i 10.3.14
P VHF 14 16

Folkestone
i 10.3.16
P VHF 16
M 0891 500 456
☎ 0891 505 356

Varne Lanby

51°
N

For details of traffic
lanes see Fig.10 (5)

ngs* Radio
F **07 66** 16
F 07
3 1933 UT
RG **Fairlight**

Royal Sovereign

SEPARATION ZONE

50°
30'N

1°E

1°E

10-3-3   AREA 3 TIDAL STREAMS

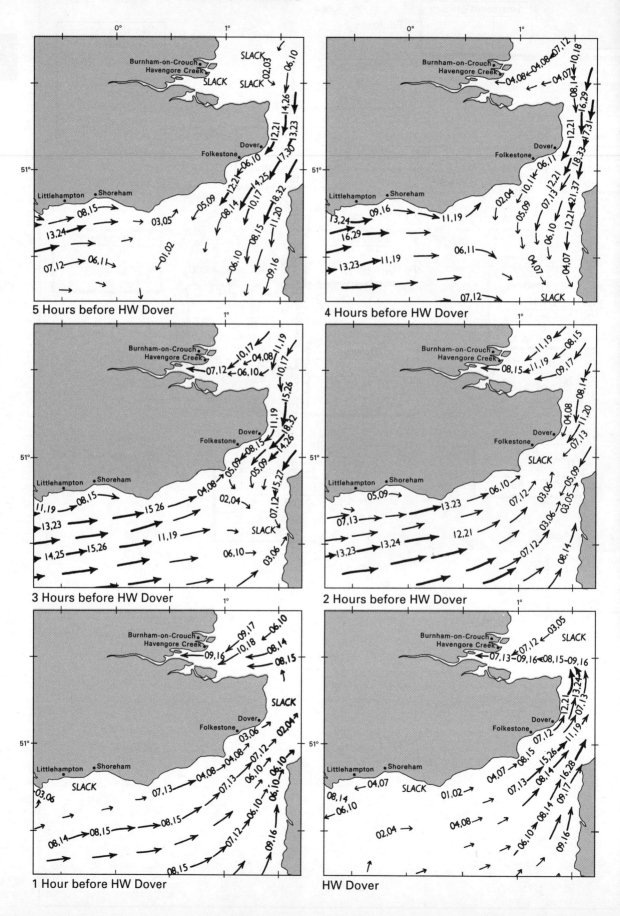

5 Hours before HW Dover

4 Hours before HW Dover

3 Hours before HW Dover

2 Hours before HW Dover

1 Hour before HW Dover

HW Dover

Westward 10.2.3   Southward 10.19.3   Northward 10.4.3   Thames Estuary 10.4.8   Eastward 10.20.3

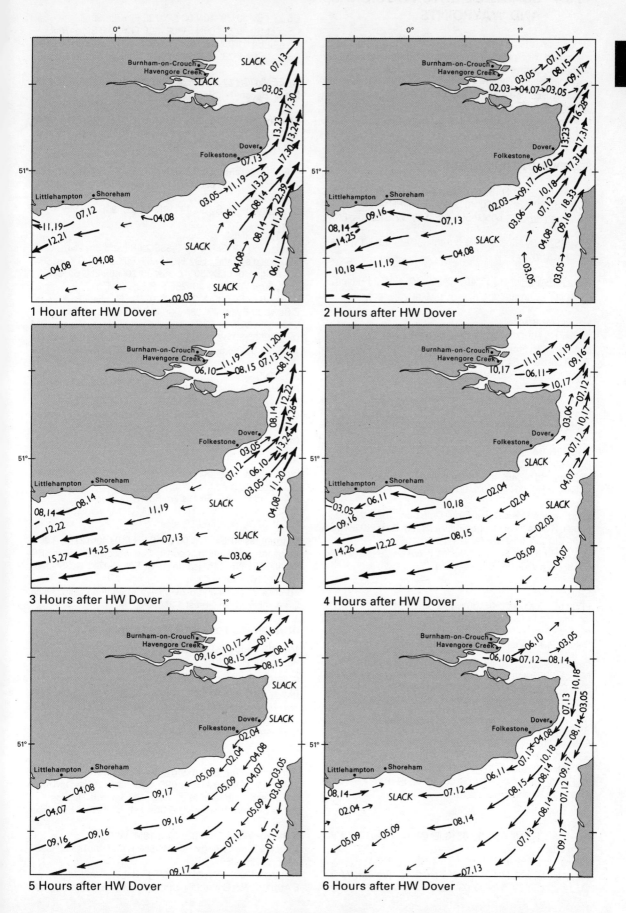

1 Hour after HW Dover

2 Hours after HW Dover

3 Hours after HW Dover

4 Hours after HW Dover

5 Hours after HW Dover

6 Hours after HW Dover

10.3.4 COASTAL LIGHTS, FOG SIGNALS AND WAYPOINTS

Abbreviations used below are given in 1.4.1. Principal lights are in **bold** print, places in CAPITALS, and light-vessels, light floats and Lanbys in *CAPITAL ITALICS*. Unless otherwise stated lights are white. m – elevation in metres; M – nominal range in miles. Fog signals are in *italics*. Useful waypoints are underlined – use those on land with care. All geographical positions should be assumed to be approximate. See 4.4.1.

SELSEY BILL TO DUNGENESS

Boulder Lt By 50°41'·53N 00°49'·00W Fl G 2·5s; SHM.
Mixon Bn 50°42'·35N 00°46'·21W (unlit); PHM.
E Borough Hd Lt By 50°41'·50N 00°39'·00W Q (3) 10s; ECM.

OWERS Lt By 50°37'·27N 00°40'·60W Q (6) + L Fl 15s; Racon (O) *Whis*

Bognor Regis Pier Hd 50°46'·70N 00°40'·42W 2 FR (vert).
Outfall Lt By 50°46'·20N 00°30'·45W Fl Y 5s; SPM.

LITTLEHAMPTON
W Pier Hd 50°47'·85N 00°32'·37W 2 FR (vert) 7m 6M.
Ldg Lts 346°. Front E Pier Hd 59°48'·1N 00°32'·4W FG 6m 7M; B col. Rear, 64m from front, Oc WY 7·5s 9m 10M; W Tr; vis W290°-356°, Y356°-042°.

WORTHING
Pier Hd 2 FR (vert) 6m 1M.
Outfall Lt By 50°48'·45N 00°19'·40W Fl (2) R 10s; PHM.

SHOREHAM
Lt By 50°47'·00N 00°15'·20W Fl Y 5s; SPM.
W Bkwtr Hd 50°49'·45N 00°14'·78W Fl R 5s 7m 7M.
E Bkwtr Hd 50°49'·50N 00°14'·70W Fl G 5s 7m 8M; *Siren 120s.*
Ldg Lts 355°. Middle Pier Front Oc 5s 8m 10M; W watch-house, R base; tidal Lts; tfc sigs; *Horn 20s.* **Rear**, 192m from front, Fl 10s 13m **15M**; Gy Tr vis 283°-103°.
W Pier Hd 50°49'·54N 00°14'·81W F WR 6m; R to seaward.
E Pier Hd F WG 7m; G to seaward.

BRIGHTON
Lt By 50°46'·00N 00°08'·30W Fl Y 3s; SPM.
W Pier Hd Fl R 10s 13m 2M; *Bell (1) 13s* (when vessel expected).
Marine Palace Pier Hd 2 FR (vert) 10m 2M.

Lowenbrau Lt By 50°48'·4N 00°06'·4W Fl Y 4s; SPM.
Mercantile Credit Lt By 50°48'·9N 00°08'·4W Fl Y 6s; SPM.
BMYC 'B' Lt By 50°46'·1N 00°08'·1W Fl Y 3s; SPM.
Saft Lt By 50°46'·2N 00°04'·5W Fl Y 2s; SPM.

BRIGHTON MARINA
E Bkwtr 50°48'·53N 00°06'·27W Fl (4) WR 20s 16m W10M, R8M; W pillar, G bands; vis R260°-295°, W295°-100°.
E Bkwtr Hd QG 8m 7M.
W Bkwtr Hd 50°48'·47N 00°06'·30W QR 10m 7M; W ● structure, R bands; *Horn (2) 30s.*

NEWHAVEN
Bkwtr Hd 50°46'·52N 00°03'·60E Oc (2) 10s 17m 12M; *Horn 30s.*
W Pier Hd 2 FR (vert).
E Pier Hd 50°46'·77N 00°03'·68E Iso G 5s 12m 6M; W Tr.
CS 1 Lt By 50°33'·67N 00°03'·83W Fl Y 2·5s; SPM; *Whis.*

NOTE: For English Channel Waypoints see 10.1.7.

CS 2 Lt By 50°39'·10N 00°32'·70E Fl Y 5s; SPM.
CS 3 Lt By 50°52'·00N 01°02'·30E Fl Y 10s; SPM; *Bell.*
CS 4 Lt By 51°08'·58N 01°34'·03E Fl (4) Y 15s; SPM; *Whis.*
CS 5 Lt By 51°23'·00N 01°50'·00E Fl (4) Y 15s; SPM.

GREENWICH Lt V 50°24'·50N 00°00'·00 Fl 5s 12m **21M**; R hull; Racon (M); Ra refl; *Horn 30s.*

Beachy Hd 50°44'·00N 00°14'·60E Fl (2) 20s 31m **25M**; W ● Tr, R band and lantern; vis 248°-101°; (H24); *Horn 30s.* Fog Det Lt vis 085·5°-265·5°.

Royal Sovereign 50°43'·42N 00°26'·18E Fl 20s 28m 12M; W Tr, R band on W cabin on concrete col; helicopter platform; *Horn (2) 30s.*
Royal Sovereign By 50°44'·18N 00°25'·93E; PHM.

EASTBOURNE
Pier Hd 50°45'·88N 00°17'·85E 2 FR (vert) 8m 2M.
St Leonard's Outfall Lt By 50°49'·27N 00°32'·00E Fl Y 5s; SPM.
Sovereign Hbr Lt By 50°47'·38N 00°20'·45E Fl G 5s; SHM.
Lt By 50°47'·29N 00°20'·25E Fl R 5s; PHM.
W Bkwtr Lt By 50°47'·27N 00°20'·10E Fl R 5s; PHM.
E Bkwtr Lt By 50°47'·28N 00°20'·02E Fl G 5s; SHM.
Sovereign Marina. 50°47'·18N 00°19'·87E Fl (3) 15s 12m 7M.
Dir Lt 258° 50°47'·23N 00°19'·70E Dir Fl WRG 3s 4m 1M; vis G252·5°-256·5°, W256·5°-259·5°, R259·5°-262·5°.

HASTINGS
Pier Hd 2 FR (vert) 8m 5M; W hut.
W Bkwtr Hd 50°51'·13N 00°35'·70E Fl R 2·5s 5m 4M.
Ldg Lts 356·3°. Front FR 14m 4M. Rear West Hill, 357m from front, FR 55m 4M; W Tr.
Groyne No. 3 Fl G 5s 2m.

RYE
Rye Fairway Lt By 50°54'·00N 00°48'·13E L Fl 10s; SWM.
W Groyne Hd 50°55'·55N 00°46'·65E Fl R 5s 7m 6M; Ra refl.
E Arm Hd No. 1 Q (9) 15s 7m 5M; G △; *Horn 7s.*
E Bank No. 11 Oc WG 4s W7M, G6M; vis W326°-331°, G331°-326°; Tidal and Tfc sigs.

Dungeness 50°54'·77N 00°58'·67E Fl 10s 40m **27M**; B ● Tr, W bands and lantern, floodlit; Part obsc 078°-shore; RC; (H24). F RG 37m 11M (same Tr); vis R057°-073°, G073°-078°, R196°-216°; *Horn (3) 60s.*
FR Lts shown 2·4 and 5·2M WNW when firing taking place.
QR and FR on radio mast 1·2M NW;

DUNGENESS TO NORTH FORELAND

VARNE Lanby 51°01'·25N 01°24'·00E Fl R 20s 12m **19M**; Racon (T); *Horn 30s*; .

FOLKESTONE
Bkwtr Hd 51°04'·53N 01°11'·79E Fl (2) 10s 14m **22M**; *Dia (4) 60s.* In fog Fl 2s; vis 246°-306°, intens 271·5°-280·5°.
Outer Hbr E Pier Hd QG 16m 1M.
Shakespeare Cliff E end Fl R 5s.

DOVER
Admiralty Pier Extension Hd 51°06'·65N 01°19'·77E Fl 7·5s 21m **20M**; W Tr; vis 096°-090°, obsc in The Downs by S Foreland inshore of 226°; *Horn 10s*; Int Port Tfc sigs.
Prince of Wales Pier Hd VQ G 14m 4M; W Tr; Fl Y 1·5s (intens, occas).
S Bkwtr, W Hd Oc R 30s 21m **18M**; W Tr.
Knuckle Fl (4) WR 10s 15m **W15M**, R13M; W Tr; vis R059°-239°, W239°-059°.
N Head 51°07'·17N 01°20'·72E Fl R 2·5s 11m 5M.
E Arm Hd, Port Control Sig Stn; Fl G 5s 12m 5M; *Horn (2) 30s.*

3

S GOODWIN Lt F 51°07'·95N 01°28'·60E Fl (2) 30s 12m **21M**; R hull with Lt Tr amidships; *Horn (2) 60s.*
SW Goodwin Lt By 51°08'·57N 01°28'·80E Q (6) + L Fl 15s; SCM.
S Goodwin Lt By 51°10'·57N 01°32'·37E Fl (4) R 15s; PHM.
SE Goodwin Lt By 51°12'·95N 01°34'·55E Fl (3) R 10s; PHM.

E GOODWIN Lt F 51°13'·05N 01°36'·31E Fl 15s 12m **21M**; R hull with Lt Tr amidships; Racon; *Horn 30s.*
E Goodwin Lt By 51°16'·00N 01°35'·60E Q (3) 10s; ECM.
NE Goodwin Lt By 51°20'·28N 01°34'·27E Q (3) 10s; ECM; Racon.

DEAL
Pier Hd 51°13'·40N 01°24'·65E 2 FR (vert) 7m 5M.
Outfall 51°14'·5N 01°24'·6E Fl R 2·5s; Ra refl.

THE DOWNS
Deal Bank Lt By 51°12'·90N 01°25'·67E; QR; PHM.
Goodwin Fork Lt By 51°13'·25N 01°27'·13E Q (6) + L Fl 15s; SCM; *Bell.*
Downs Lt By 51°14'·32N 01°26'·92E Fl (2) R 5s; PHM.

GULL STREAM
W Goodwin Lt By 51°15'·28N 01°27'·32E Fl G 5s; SHM.
S Brake Lt By 51°15'·40N 01°27'·00E Fl (3) R 10s; PHM.
NW Goodwin Lt By 51°16'·78N 01°28'·76E Q (9) 15s; WCM *Bell* .
Brake Lt By 51°16'·90N 01°28'·40E Fl (4) R 15s; PHM; *Bell.*
N Goodwin Lt By 51°17'·88N 01°30'·55E Fl G 2·5s; SHM.
Gull Stream Lt By 51°18'·10N 01°30'·02E QR; PHM.
Gull Lt By 51°19'·55N 01°31'·40E VQ (3) 5s; ECM.
Goodwin Knoll Lt By 51°19'·55N 01°32'·30E Fl (2) G 5s; SHM.

RAMSGATE CHANNEL
B1 By 51°15'·75N 01°25'·60E; SHM.
B2 By 51°18'·03N 01°24'·20E; SHM.
Sandwich Fairway Lt By 51°19'·11N 01°24'·62E L Fl 10s; SWM.

RAMSGATE
RA Lt By 51°19'·57N 01°30'·23E Q(6) + L Fl 15s; SCM.
E Brake Lt By 51°19'40N 01°29'·05E Fl R 5s; PHM; Ra refl.
No. 1 Lt By 51°19'·52N 01°27'·40E Fl G 5s; SHM.
No. 2 Lt By 51°19'·43N 01°27'·40E Fl (4) R 10s; PHM.
No. 3 Lt By 51°19'·52N 01°26'·71E Fl G 2·5s; SHM.
No. 4 Lt By 51°19'·43N 01°28'·67E QR; PHM.
No. 5 Lt By 51°19'·52N 01°26'·02E Q(6) + L Fl 15s; SCM.
No. 6 Lt By 51°19'·43N 01°26'·02E Fl (2) R 5s; PHM.
W Pier Hd FR or G 12m 7M; tfc sigs; *Horn 60s.*
N Quern Lt By 51°19'·38N 01°26'·25E Q; NCM.
W Quern Lt By 51°18'·95N 01°25'·50E Q (9) 15s; WCM.
S Bkwtr Hd VQ R 10m 5M; W pillar, R bands.
N Bkwtr Hd Q G 10m 5M; W pillar, G bands.
W Marine terminal Dir Lt 270°, Dir Oc WRG 10s 10m 5M; B △, Or stripe; vis G259°-269°, W269°-271°, R271°-281°. Rear 493m from front Oc 5s 17m 5M; B ▽, Or stripe; vis 263°-278°.

RIVER STOUR
Chan marked by PHM & SHM Bys and Bns.
Pegwell Bay, Sandwich app 51°18'·72N 01°23'·05E Fl R 10s 3m 4M; framework Tr; moved to meet changes in chan.

BROADSTAIRS
Broadstairs Knoll Lt By 51°20'·85N 01°29'·58E Fl R 2·5s; PHM.
Pier SE end 51°21'·46N 01° 26'·83E 2 FR (vert) 7m 4M.

N Foreland 51°22'·47N 01°26'·80E Fl (5) WR 20s 57m **W19M, R16M, R15M**; W 8-sided Tr; vis W shore-150°, R(16M)150°-181°, R(15M) 181°-200°, W200°-011°; RC.

F1 Lt By 51°11'·20N 01°45'·03E; Fl (4) Y 15s; SPM.
Inter Bank Lt By 51°16'·45N 01°52'·33E Fl Y 5s; Racon; SPM.
Mid Falls Lt By 51°18'·60N 01°47'·10E Fl (3) R 10s; PHM; *Bell.*
F2 Lt By 51°20'·38N 01°56'·30E Fl (4) Y 15s; SPM; *Bell.*

10.3.5   PASSAGE INFORMATION

Reference books include: Admiralty *Channel Pilot*; *Shell Channel Pilot* (Imray/Cunliffe); and *South Coast Cruising* (YM/ Fishwick). See 10.0.5 for cross-Channel distances.

THE EASTERN CHANNEL

This area embraces the greatest concentration of commercial shipping in the world. In such waters the greatest danger to a small yacht is being run down by a larger vessel, especially in poor visibility. In addition to the many ships plying up and down the traffic lanes, there are fast ferries, hovercraft and hydrofoils passing to and fro between English and Continental harbours; warships and submarines on exercises; fishing vessels operating both inshore and offshore; many other yachts; and static dangers such as lobster pots and fishing nets which are concentrated in certain places.

Even for coastal cruising it is essential to know about the TSS and ITZ, see Fig.10 (5); eg, note that the SW-bound TSS lane from the Dover Strait passes only 4M off Dungeness. Radar surveillance of the Dover Strait (10.3.15) is maintained at all times by the Channel Navigation Information Service (CNIS).

In this area the weather has a big effect on tidal streams, and on the range of tides. The rates of tidal streams vary with the locality, and are greatest in the narrower parts of the Chan and off major headlands. In the Dover Strait sp rates can reach 4kn, but elsewhere in open water they seldom exceed 2kn. Also N winds, which give smooth water and pleasant sailing off the shores of England, can cause rough seas on the French coast; and vice versa. With strong S'lies the English coast between Isle of Wight and Dover is very exposed, and shelter is hard to find. The Dover Strait has a funnelling effect and in strong winds can become very rough.

SELSEY BILL AND THE OWERS (chart *1652*)

Selsey Bill is a low headland, and off it lie the Owers – groups of rks and shoals extending 3M to the S, and 5M to the SE. Just W and SW of the Bill, The Streets (awash) extend 1·25M seaward. 1·25M SSW of the Bill are The Grounds (or Malt Owers) and The Dries (dry). 1M E of The Dries, and about 1·25M S of the lifeboat house on E side of Selsey Bill is a group of rks called The Mixon, marked by bn at E end.

Immediately S of dangers above is the Looe chan, which runs E/W about 0·75M S of Mixon bn, and is marked by buoys at W end, where it is narrowest between Brake (or Cross) Ledge on N side and Boulder Bank to the S. In daylight and in good vis and moderate weather, the Looe chan is an easy and useful short cut. The E-going stream begins at HW Portsmouth + 0430, and the W-going at HW Portsmouth – 0135, sp rates 2·5 kn. Beware lobster pots in this area.

In poor vis or in bad weather (and always in darkness) keep S of the Owers Lanby, moored 7M SE of Selsey Bill, marking SE end of Owers. Over much of Owers there is less than 3m, and large parts virtually dry: so a combination of tidal stream and strong wind produces heavy breaking seas and overfalls over a large area.

OWERS TO BEACHY HEAD (charts *1652, 536*)

The coast from Selsey Bill to Brighton is low, faced by a shingle beach, and with few offlying dangers, Bognor Rks (dry in places) extend 1·75M E from a point 1M W of the pier, and Bognor Spit extends E and S from the end of them. Middleton ledge are rks running 0·8M offshore, about 1·5M E of Bognor pier, with depths of less than 1m. Shelley Rks lie 5ca S of Middleton ledge, with depths of less than 1m.

Winter Knoll, about 2·5M SSW of Littlehampton (10.3.9) has depths of 2·1m. Kingston Rks, depth 2m, lie about 3·25M ESE of Littlehampton. An unlit outfall bn is 3ca off Goring -on- sea (2M W of Worthing pier). Grass Banks, an extensive shoal with 2m depth at W end, lie about 1M S of Worthing pier. Elbow shoal, with depth of 3·1m, lies E of Grass Banks.

Off Shoreham (10.3.10) Church Rks, with depth of 0·3m, lie 1·5M W of the hbr ent and 2½ca offshore. Jenny Rks, with depth 0·9m, are 1·25M E of the ent, 3ca offshore.

At Brighton (10.3.11) the S Downs form the coastline, and high chalk cliffs are conspic from here to Beachy Hd. There are no dangers more than 3ca offshore, until Birling Gap, where a rky ledge begins, on which is built Beachy Hd lt ho (fog sig). Head Ledge (dries) extends about 4ca S. 2M S of Beachy Hd the W-going stream begins at HW Dover + 0030, and the E-going at HW Dover – 0520, sp rates 2·25kn. In bad weather there are overfalls off the Head, which should then be given a berth of 2M.

BEACHY HEAD TO DUNGENESS

Royal Sovereign lt tr (fog sig) is 7·4M E of Beachy Head. The extensive Royal Sovereign shoals lie from 3M NW of the tr to 1·5M N of it, and have a minimum depth of 3·5m. There are strong eddies over the shoals at sp, and the sea breaks on them in bad weather.

On the direct course from Royal Sovereign lt tr to clear Dungeness there are no dangers. Along the coast in Pevensey B and Rye B there are drying rky ledges or shoals extending 5ca offshore in places. These include Boulder Bank near Wish tr, S of Eastbourne (10.3.13); Oyster Reef off Cooden; Bexhill Reef off Bexhill-on-Sea; Bopeep Rks off St Leonards; and the shoals at the mouth of R Rother, at entrance to Rye (10.3.14). There are also banks 2-3M offshore, on which the sea builds in bad weather. Avoid the firing range danger area between Rye and Dungeness (lt, fog sig, RC). The nuclear power station is conspic at SE extremity of the low-lying spit. The Pt is steep-to on SE side. Good anch close NE of Dungeness.

DUNGENESS TO NORTH FORELAND (charts *1892, 1828*)

From Dungeness to Folkestone (10.3.16) the coast forms a bay. Beware Roar bank, depth 2·7m, E of New Romney: otherwise there are no offlying dangers, apart from Hythe firing range. Good anch off Sandgate in offshore winds. Off Folkestone the E-going stream starts at HW Dover – 0155, sp rate 2kn; the W-going at HW Dover + 0320, sp rate 1·5kn.

Passing Dover (10.3.17) and S Foreland keep 1M offshore. Do not pass too close to Dover, because ferries/jetfoils leave at speed, and there can be considerable backwash and lumpy seas off the breakwaters. 8M S of Dover in the TSS is the Varne, a shoal 7M long with least depth 3·3m and heavy seas in bad weather, marked by Lanby and 3 buoys. Between S and N Foreland the N-going stream begins at about HW Dover – 0150, and the S-going at about HW Dover + 0415.

The Goodwin Sands are drying, shifting shoals, extending about 10M from S to N, and 5M from W to E at their widest part. The E side is relatively steep-to; large areas dry up to 2·7m. The sands are well marked by lt Fs and buoys. Kellett Gut is an unmarked chan about 5ca wide, running SW/NE through the middle of the sands, but it is not regularly surveyed and is liable to change. The Gull Stream (buoyed) leads from The Downs, inside Goodwin Sands and outside Brake Sands to the S of Ramsgate (10.3.18). The Ramsgate chan leads inside the Brake Sands and Cross Ledge.

CROSS-CHANNEL PASSAGES

Factors which need to be considered when planning passages between England and the Continent or Channel Islands, and vice versa, include the following:

a. Selection of points of departure and landfalls so that passage time and time out of sight of identifiable marks is minimised. This can considerably reduce anxiety and fatigue (which can soon become apparent in a family crew). The risk of navigational errors, particularly those due to leeway and tidal streams, is also reduced. Bear in mind the importance of taking back bearings on the departure mark.

b. Careful prior study of the meteorological situation, so that windows of opportunity may be predicted, ie high pressure; and periods of bad weather may best be avoided.

c. Prevailing winds and the forecast wind direction, so that the probability of obtaining a good slant can be improved. The prevailing winds are from the S and W, except in the spring (March, April, May) when the frequency of winds from the NE and E is about the same as from SW/ W.

d. The direction and rate of tidal streams during any coastal passage before taking departure across Channel; equally streams during (and after) the crossing, so as to lay off the drift angle required to make good the desired track.

e. The legal requirement to head at right angles across the TSS (10.0.9), and the possible use of the engine in order to expedite such crossing.

f. The probable meteorological visibility and thus the range at which daymarks may be seen. Bear in mind the additional range provided by lights when a landfall is made at night or dawn/dusk. Statistically the probability of fog is about 5% in the summer months and a meteorological visibility greater than 6M can be expected 50% of the time.

g. The availability of additional navigational information such as clearly identifiable radar targets if equipped with radar; soundings, for example when crossing the distinctive contours of the Hurd Bank; the rising or dipping ranges of major lights and the sighting of TSS buoys and lt Floats (but keep 2M clear of EC1, EC2 and EC3 buoys).

h. Finally, in this electronic age, a firm resolve should be made to keep a dead reckoning plot. This is both a safeguard, and a source of pride (when proven accurate); it also tends to ensure a higher degree of navigational awareness.

If proceeding from Brighton to St Malo, for example, it might pay to cruise coastwise to take departure from St Catherines Point, the Needles, Anvil Point or Portland Bill when crossing towards Barfleur, Cherbourg, Cap de la Hague or Alderney. The advantages of getting well to windward and working the tides to advantage cannot be overemphasised. The times and areas of races and overfalls should also be included in the passage plan.

Passages from Brighton, Newhaven or Eastbourne to Dieppe are relatively short and direct. The route crosses the Dover Strait TSS whose SW-bound lane lies only 7M S of Beachy Hd. A departure from close W of CS2 buoy will satisfy the 90° crossing rule and minimise the time spent in the TSS. During the 19M crossing of the W-bound and E-bound lanes, it is worth listening to the VHF broadcasts of navigational and traffic information made by CNIS. These include details of vessels which appear to be contravening Rule 10.

Dover to Calais or Boulogne is about 25M (see 10.3.17). Keep a very sharp lookout; listen to CNIS and to the relevant hbr VHF channel; do not attempt it in fog or poor visibility.

10.3.6   DISTANCE TABLE

Approximate distances in nautical miles are by the most direct route, whilst avoiding dangers and allowing for Traffic Separation Schemes. Places in *italics* are in adjoining areas; places in **bold** are in 10.0.5, Cross-Channel Distances; places underlined are in 10.0.7, Distances across the North Sea.

	1	2	3	4	5	6	7	8	9	10	11	12	13	14	15	16	17	18	19	20
1. *Portland Bill Lt*	**1**																			
2. **Nab Tower**	60	**2**																		
3. Boulder Buoy	65	5	**3**																	
4. Owers Lanby	69	11	8	**4**																
5. **Littlehampton**	78	19	13	12	**5**															
6. **Shoreham**	90	32	24	21	13	**6**														
7. **Brighton**	93	35	28	24	17	5	**7**													
8. **Newhaven**	97	40	34	29	24	12	7	**8**												
9. Beachy Head Lt	104	46	41	36	30	20	14	8	**9**											
10. **Eastbourne**	111	51	45	40	34	24	19	12	7	**10**										
11. **Rye**	129	72	67	62	56	46	41	34	25	23	**11**									
12. Dungeness Lt	134	76	71	66	60	50	44	38	30	26	9	**12**								
13. **Folkestone**	152	92	84	81	76	65	60	53	43	40	23	13	**13**							
14. **Dover**	157	97	89	86	81	70	65	58	48	45	28	18	5	**14**						
15. <u>Ramsgate</u>	172	112	104	101	96	85	80	73	63	60	43	33	20	15	**15**					
16. N Foreland Lt	175	115	107	104	99	88	83	76	66	63	46	36	23	18	3	**16**				
17. <u>*Sheerness*</u>	206	146	139	135	132	119	114	107	97	96	79	67	54	49	34	31	**17**			
18. <u>*London Bridge*</u>	248	188	184	177	177	161	156	149	139	141	124	109	96	91	76	73	45	**18**		
19. <u>*Burnham-on-Crouch*</u>	216	156	148	145	140	129	124	117	107	104	87	75	64	59	44	41	34	76	**19**	
20. <u>*Harwich*</u>	212	152	144	141	136	125	120	113	103	100	83	73	60	55	40	37	50	83	31	**20**

S.E. ENGLAND
WAYPOINTS   10-3-8

Selected waypoints for use in Areas 3 and 4 are listed in
alphabetical order below. Further tabulated waypoint listings
for use in coastal waters are given in sections 10.2.21, 10.4.7,
and 10.9.15. Selected waypoints for use in English Channel
crossings are given in 10.1.7.

AREA 3

Boulder By	50°41'·53N 00°49'·00W
Brake Lt By	51°16'·90N 01°28'·40E
Brighton Marina Hd	50°48'·45N 00°06'·30W
Broadstairs Knoll Lt By	51°20'·85N 01°29'·58E
Bullock Bank Lt By	50°46'·90N 01°07'·70E
Colbart N Lt By	50°57'·44N 01°23'·40E
Colbart SW Lt By	50°48'·82N 01°16'·40E
CS 1 Lt By	50°33'·67N 00°03'·83W
CS 2 Lt By	50°39'·10N 00°32'·70E
CS 3 Lt By	50°52'·00N 01°02'·30E
CS 4 Lt By	51°08'·58N 01°34'·03E
Deal Bank Lt By	51°12'·90N 01°25'·67E
Downs Lt By	51°14'·32N 01°26'·92E
Dungeness Lt	50°54'·77N 00°58'·67E
Dungeness Lt By	50°54'·43N 00°58'·33E
East Brake Lt By	51°19'·40N 01°29'·05E
East Borough Hd Lt By	50°41'·50N 00°39'·00W
East Goodwin Lt F	51°13'·05N 01°36'·31E
East Goodwin Lt By	51°16'·00N 01°35'·60E
East Varne Lt By	50°58'·20N 01°21'·00E
F1 Lt By	51°11'·20N 01°45'·03E
F2 Lt By	51°20'·38N 01°56'·30E
Faversham Spit By	51°20'·74N 00°54'·31E
Goodwin Fork Lt By	51°13'·25N 01°27'·13E
Goodwin Knoll Lt By	51°19'·55N 01°32'·30E
Greenwich Lt V	50°24'·50N 00°00'·00
Gull Lt By	51°19'·55N 01°31'·40E
Gull Stream Lt By	51°18'·10N 01°30'·02E
Inter Bank Lt By	51°16'·45N 01°52'·33E
Mid Falls Lt By	51°18'·60N 01°47'·10E
Mid Varne Lt By	50°58'·90N 01°20'·00E
MPC Lt By	51°06'·09N 01°38'·36E
Newhaven Bkwtr Hd	50°46'·52N 00°03'·60E
NE Goodwin Lt By	51°20'·28N 01°34'·27E
North Goodwin Lt By	51°17'·88N 01°30'·55E
NW Goodwin Lt By	51°16'·78N 01°28'·76E
Outer Owers By	50°38'·75N 00°41'·30W
Owers Lt By	50°37'·27N 00°40'·60W
Pullar By	50°40'·45N 00°50'·00W
Ramsgate Chan B.1 By	51°15'·75N 01°25'·60E
Ramsgate Chanl B.2 By	51°18'·03N 01°24'·20E
Royal Sovereign Lt	50°43'·42N 00°26'·18E
Rye Fairway Lt By	50°54'·00N 00°48'·13E
Sandwich Fairway Lt By	51°19'·11N 01°24'·62E
Sandettié Lt F	51°09'·40N 01°47'·20E
Shoreham Lt By	50°47'·00N 00°15'·20W
South Brake Lt By	51°15'·40N 01°27'·00E
SE Goodwin Lt By	51°12'·95N 01°34'·55E

South Falls Lt By	51°13'·80N 00°44'·03E
South Goodwin Lt By	51°10'·57N 01°32'·37E
South Goodwin Lt F	51°07'·95N 01°28'·60E
S Inner Gabbard Lt By	51°51'·20N 01°52'·40E
South Varne Lt By	50°55'·60N 01°17'·40E
SW Goodwin Lt By	51°08'·57N 01°28'·80E
SW Sandettié Lt By	51°09'·72N 01°45'·73E
Street By	50°41'·65N 00°48'·80W
Varne Lanby	51°01'·25N 01°24'·00E
West Goodwin Lt By	51°15'·28N 01°27'·32E
West Quern Lt By	51°18'·95N 91°25'·00E
WSW Sandettié Lt By	51°12'·32N 01°51'·23E

AREA 4

Blacktail E Bn	51°31'·75N 00°56'·60E
Blacktail W Bn	51°31'·43N 00°55'·30E
Columbine By	51°24'·23N 01°01'·45E
Columbine Spit By	51°23'·83N 01°00'·13E
CS 5 Lt By	51°23'·00N 01°50'·00E
Drill Stone Lt By	51°25'·80N 01°43'·00E
East Cant Lt By	51°28'·50N 00°55'·70E
East Last Lt By	51°24'·00N 01°12'·28E
East Margate Lt By	51°27'·00N 01°26'·50E
East Redsand Lt By	51°29'·38N 01°04'·15E
East Tongue Lt By	51°28'·72N 01°18'·72E
Edinburgh Lt By	51°31'·35N 01°21'·14E
Elbow Lt By	51°23'·20N 01°31'·70E
F3 Lt By	51°23'·82N 02°00'·62E
Falls Hd Lt By	51°28'·20N 01°50'·00E
Girdler Lt By	51°29'·15N 01°06'·50E
Hook Spit By	51°24'·05N 01°12'·65E
Margate Hook Bn	51°24'·12N 01°14'·41E
Medway Lt By	51°28'·80N 00°52'·92E
Mid Shingles Lt By	51°31'·93N 01°12'·08E
North Redsand Trs Lt By	51°28'·70N 00°59'·42E
North Shingles Lt By	51°32'·63N 01°14'·35E
North Tongue Lt By	51°28'·78N 01°13'·18E
NE Knob Lt By	51°32'·00N 01°10'·10E
NE Spit Lt By	51°27'·90N 01°30'·00E
NE Tongue Sand Tr Lt By	51°29'·65N 01°22'·13E
NW Shingles Lt By	51°31'·23N 01°09'·83E
Outer Tongue Lt By	51°30'·70N 01°26'·50E
Pollard Spit Lt By	51°22'·95N 00°58'·67E
Shingles Patch Lt By	51°32'·98N 01°15'·47E
Shoebury Lt Bn	51°30'·28N 00°49'·38E
SE Girdler Lt By	51°29'·47N 01°10'·00E
SE Margate Lt By	51°24'·10N 01°20'·50E
South Margate Lt By	51°23'·88N 01°16'·75E
South Oaze Lt By	51°30'·00N 01°00'·80E
S Redsand Towers Lt By	51°28'·57N 00°59'·77E
South Shingles Lt By	51°29'·20N 01°16'·12E
SW Oaze Lt By	51°29'·03N 00°57'·03E
SW Tongue Tr Lt By	51°29'·40N 01°22'·13E
Spaniard Lt By	51°26'·20N 01°04'·10E
Spile Lt By	51°26'·40N 00°55'·80E
Tizard Lt By	51°32'·90N 01°13'·00E
West Girdler Lt By	51°29'·58N 01°06'·82E
Whitstable St Lt By	51°23'·83N 01°01'·70E

LITTLEHAMPTON   10-3-9
W. Sussex 50°47'·84N 00°32'·33W

3

CHARTS
AC 1991, 1652; Imray C9; Stanfords 9; OS 197
TIDES
+0015 Dover; ML 2·8; Zone 0 (UT)

Standard Port SHOREHAM (→)

Times				Height (metres)			
High Water		Low Water		MHWS	MHWN	MLWN	MLWS
0500	1000	0000	0600	6·3	4·8	1·9	0·6
1700	2200	1200	1800				
Differences LITTLEHAMPTON (ENT)							
+0010	0000	−0005	−0010	−0·4	−0·4	−0·2	−0·2
LITTLEHAMPTON (NORFOLK WHARF)							
+0015	+0005	0000	+0045	−0·7	−0·7	−0·3	+0·2
ARUNDEL							
No data	+0120	No data		−3·1	−2·8	No data	
PAGHAM							
+0015	0000	−0015	−0025	−0·7	−0·5	−0·1	−0·1
BOGNOR REGIS							
+0010	−0005	−0005	−0020	−0·6	−0·5	−0·2	−0·1

NOTE: Tidal hts in hbr are affected by flow down R Arun. Tide seldom falls lower than 0·7m above CD.

SHELTER
Good. Ent dangerous in strong SE winds which cause swell up the hbr. The bar (0·4 to 0·7m) is rough in SW'lies. Visitors berth initially at County Wharf and contact Hr Mr.
NAVIGATION
WPT 50°47'·50N 00°32'·20W, 166°/346° from/to front ldg lt, 0·60M. Bar ½M offshore. Hbr accessible from HW−3 to HW+2½ for approx 1·5m draft. The ebb runs so fast (4 – 6 kn) at sp that yachts may have difficulty entering. From HW−1 to HW+4 a strong W-going tidal stream sets across the ent; keep to E side. Speed limit 6½kn.
On E side of ent chan a training wall which covers at half-tide is marked by 7 poles and unlit bn at S end. The W pier is a long, prominent structure of wood piles; tide gauge on end shows ht of tide above CD. To calculate depth on the bar deduct 0·7m from indicated depth.

River Arun. A retractable footbridge (3·6m clearance MHWS; 9·4m above CD) 3ca above County Wharf gives access for masted craft to Littlehampton marina. It is opened by request to Hr Mr before 1630 previous day. The River Arun is navigable on the tide by small, unmasted craft for 24M via Ford, Arundel and beyond; consult Hr Mr.
LIGHTS AND MARKS
High-rise bldg (38m) is conspic 0·4M NNE of hbr ent. Ldg lts 346°: Front FG on B column; Rear, lt ho Oc WY 7·5s at root of E bkwtr, W 290°-356°, Y 356°-042°. The Fl G 3s lt at Norfolk Wharf indicates that you have overshot! When Pilot boat with P at the bow displays the Pilot flag 'H' (WR vert halves) or Ⓦ over Ⓡ lts, all boats keep clear of ent; large ship moving.
Footbridge sigs, from high mast to port:
Fl G lt = open; Fl R = closed.
Bridge's retractable centre section (22m wide) has 2 FR (vert) to port and 2 FG (vert) to stbd on each side.
RADIO TELEPHONE
Port VHF Ch 71 16 (0900-1799LT); Pilots Ch 71 16 when vessel due. Marinas Ch 80 M (office hrs).
TELEPHONE (01903)
Hr Mr 721215; MRSC (01705) 552100; ⌗ (01703) 827350; Marinecall 0891 500456; Police 731733; Dr 714113.
FACILITIES
County Wharf AB £10, FW, C (5 ton), ME, Sh;
Services: BY, M, Sh (Wood), ACA.
Littlehampton Sailing & Motor Club ☎ 715859, M, FW, Bar;
Arun YC (90+10 visitors) ☎ 714533, (dries; access HW±3), M, AC, FW, Bar, Slip;
Littlehampton Marina (120+30 visitors) ☎ 713553, Slip, BH (16 ton), CH, P, D, V, R, Bar, FW, AC, Sh, ME;
Ship and Anchor Marina, about 2M up-river at Ford, (182, some visitors) ☎ (01243) 551262, (access HW±4), Slip, FW, ME, Sh, CH, V, R, Bar.
Town EC Wed; P, D, V, R, Bar, ✉, Ⓑ, ⇌, ✈ (Shoreham).

Littlehampton chart

SHOREHAM 10-3-10

W. Sussex 50°49'·50N 00°14'·76W

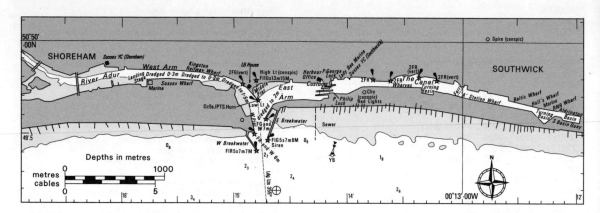

CHARTS

AC 2044, *1652*; Imray C9; Stanfords 9; OS 197/8

TIDES

+0009 Dover; ML 3·3; Duration 0605; Zone 0 (UT)

Standard Port SHOREHAM (→)

Times				Height (metres)			
High Water		Low Water		MHWS	MHWN	MLWN	MLWS
0500	1000	0000	0600	6·3	4·8	1·9	0·6
1700	2200	1200	1800				
Differences WORTHING							
+0010	0000	−0005	−0010	−0·1	−0·2	0·0	0·0

NOTE: Shoreham is a Standard Port and tidal predictions for the year are given below.

SHELTER

Excellent, once through the lock and into Southwick Canal (alias The Canal). The shallow water (dredged 2·5m) at the ent can be very rough in strong on-shore winds; do not attempt ent in onshore gales. Lady Bee and Aldrington (E end of The Canal) marinas both welcome visitors.

NAVIGATION

WPT 50°49'·20N 00°14'·72W, 175°/355° from/to front ldg lt, 0·52M. From E, beware Jenny Rks (0·9m) and from the W, Church Rks (0·3m). Yachtsmen are advised not to use the drying W arm if possible. Speed limit = 4kn. Prince George Lock, the N'ly of two, opens on request for yachts; ent 6m wide, pontoon inside on S wall. Outside, there may be waiting space on S side jetties. Prince Philip Lock is for commercial ships; yachts should keep clear.

LIGHTS AND MARKS

Conspic, light-coloured chy (109m), 0.6M ENE of hbr ent, is visible from 20M offshore. Radio mast, R lts, is conspic 170m N of High lt.
Ldg lts 355°: front Oc 5s 8m 10M; rear High lt Fl 10s 13m 15M.
Traffic Sigs IPTS (Sigs 2 and 5, Oc) are shown from Middle Pier. Note : (Y) exemption lt is also shown.
Oc R 3s (from LB ho, directed at E or W Arms) = No exit.
Lock Sigs (Comply strictly to avoid turbulence):
3 (R) (vert) = do not approach lock.
(G)(W) G (vert) = clear to approach lock.

RADIO TELEPHONE

VHF Ch **14** 16 (H24) Hr Mr and lock. Lady Bee Marina Ch **80** M.

TELEPHONE (01273)

Hr Mr 592613; Locks 592366; MRSC (01705) 552100; ∭ (01703) 827350; Marinecall 0891 500456; Police 454521; Ⓗ 455622; Dr 461101 (Health Centre).

FACILITIES

Lady Bee Marina (110+10 visitors) ☎ 593801, Fax 870349, £5 (best to pre-arrange), Slip, P, D, FW, ME, El, Sh, SM, AC, R, V, CH; Access HW±3½.
Sussex YC ☎ 464868, ½ tide pontoon (limited visitors' berths), R, Bar; **Sussex Motor YC** ☎ 453078, M, L, Bar; **Surry BY** ☎ 461491, Slip, M, FW, AB, Access HW ±2½;
Services: ACA.
Town EC Wed; Ⓞ, ✉, Ⓑ, ⇌, ✈.

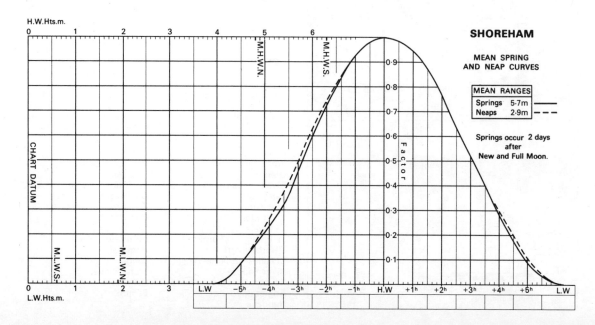

SHOREHAM

MEAN SPRING AND NEAP CURVES

MEAN RANGES	
Springs	5·7m
Neaps	2·9m

Springs occur 2 days after New and Full Moon.

ENGLAND – SHOREHAM

LAT 50°50′N   LONG 0°15′W

TIMES AND HEIGHTS OF HIGH AND LOW WATERS

YEAR 1996

TIME ZONE (UT)
For Summer Time add ONE hour in non-shaded areas

3

JANUARY

Day	Time	m	Time	m	Time	m	Time	m
1 M	0135	1.7	0746	5.2	1411	1.6	2028	5.1
16 TU	0014	1.7	0636	5.2	1303	1.6	1917	5.1
2 TU	0233	1.6	0852	5.4	1504	1.4	2125	5.3
17 W	0134	1.5	0755	5.4	1415	1.3	2033	5.4
3 W	0324	1.4	0941	5.6	1550	1.2	2210	5.5
18 TH	0243	1.2	0900	5.8	1516	0.9	2134	5.8
4 TH	0408	1.2	1022	5.7	1631	1.0	2248	5.7
19 F	0342	0.9	0957	6.2	1610	0.6	2229	6.2
5 F O	0448	1.1	1056	5.9	1710	0.9	2322	5.9
20 SA ●	0434	0.6	1049	6.4	1701	0.3	2320	6.5
6 SA	0525	1.0	1127	5.9	1747	0.8	2353	5.9
21 SU	0523	0.4	1140	6.6	1750	0.2		
7 SU	0601	1.0	1158	5.9	1822	0.8		
22 M	0009	6.7	0611	0.3	1229	6.7	1837	0.1
8 M	0023	6.0	0634	1.0	1229	5.9	1855	0.9
23 TU	0057	6.7	0659	0.3	1315	6.6	1924	0.2
9 TU	0052	5.9	0707	1.0	1259	5.9	1927	0.9
24 W	0141	6.6	0745	0.4	1400	6.4	2009	0.4
10 W	0122	5.9	0737	1.1	1332	5.8	1956	1.0
25 TH	0225	6.4	0831	0.6	1443	6.1	2053	0.6
11 TH	0154	5.8	0809	1.2	1407	5.7	2028	1.1
26 F	0307	6.1	0916	0.9	1527	5.8	2137	1.0
12 F	0231	5.7	0847	1.3	1447	5.5	2107	1.2
27 SA	0352	5.7	1003	1.3	1615	5.4	2224	1.4
13 SA	0314	5.6	0934	1.4	1535	5.3	2156	1.4
28 SU	0441	5.3	1057	1.6	1710	5.0	2321	1.8
14 SU	0406	5.4	1033	1.6	1632	5.1	2257	1.6
29 M	0539	5.0	1213	1.9	1813	4.7		
15 M	0512	5.2	1145	1.7	1746	5.0		
30 TU	0047	2.0	0644	4.8	1339	1.9	1931	4.7
31 W	0206	1.9	0805	4.9	1440	1.7	2057	5.0

FEBRUARY

Day	Time	m	Time	m	Time	m	Time	m
1 TH	0303	1.7	0916	5.2	1529	1.4	2148	5.3
16 F	0231	1.3	0848	5.5	1503	1.0	2124	5.7
2 F	0349	1.4	1000	5.5	1611	1.1	2227	5.6
17 SA	0331	0.9	0948	6.0	1558	0.6	2219	6.2
3 SA	0429	1.1	1034	5.7	1650	0.9	2300	5.8
18 SU ●	0423	0.6	1040	6.3	1647	0.3	2309	6.5
4 SU O	0506	1.0	1106	5.9	1726	0.7	2330	5.9
19 M	0511	0.3	1129	6.6	1734	0.1	2356	6.7
5 M	0541	0.9	1136	6.0	1802	0.7		
20 TU	0557	0.2	1215	6.7	1820	0.1		
6 TU	0000	6.0	0614	0.8	1208	6.0	1835	0.7
21 W	0040	6.8	0640	0.2	1259	6.7	1903	0.1
7 W	0030	6.0	0646	0.8	1240	6.0	1905	0.7
22 TH	0121	6.7	0723	0.3	1340	6.5	1944	0.3
8 TH	0100	6.1	0714	0.8	1312	6.0	1932	0.8
23 F	0200	6.5	0803	0.5	1419	6.2	2022	0.6
9 F	0133	6.0	0744	0.8	1347	6.0	2003	0.8
24 SA	0237	6.1	0844	0.8	1456	5.9	2100	0.9
10 SA	0208	6.0	0820	0.9	1424	5.8	2041	0.9
25 SU	0314	5.7	0920	1.2	1538	5.4	2141	1.3
11 SU	0247	5.8	0903	1.1	1508	5.6	2127	1.2
26 M	0358	5.3	1005	1.6	1629	5.0	2230	1.8
12 M	0335	5.5	0958	1.3	1602	5.3	2225	1.4
27 TU	0455	4.8	1111	1.9	1732	4.6	2335	2.1
13 TU	0436	5.2	1109	1.6	1712	5.0	2342	1.7
28 W	0601	4.6	1234	2.1	1842	4.5		
14 W	0600	5.0	1235	1.6	1851	4.9		
29 TH	0129	2.1	0713	4.6	1410	1.9	2005	4.7
15 TH	0114	1.6	0734	5.1	1358	1.4	2018	5.2

MARCH

Day	Time	m	Time	m	Time	m	Time	m
1 F	0237	1.9	0835	4.9	1503	1.6	2116	5.1
16 SA	0219	1.3	0838	5.4	1449	1.0	2112	5.7
2 SA	0325	1.5	0930	5.2	1546	1.2	2157	5.5
17 SU	0317	0.9	0937	5.9	1542	0.6	2205	6.1
3 SU	0405	1.2	1006	5.6	1624	1.0	2230	5.8
18 M	0407	0.6	1027	6.2	1630	0.4	2253	6.5
4 M	0441	1.0	1039	5.8	1700	0.8	2302	6.0
19 TU ●	0454	0.3	1114	6.5	1715	0.3	2337	6.6
5 TU O	0516	0.8	1111	6.0	1736	0.7	2333	6.1
20 W	0537	0.2	1158	6.6	1758	0.2		
6 W	0550	0.7	1144	6.1	1809	0.6		
21 TH	0019	6.7	0619	0.2	1239	6.6	1839	0.2
7 TH	0005	6.2	0620	0.6	1219	6.1	1839	0.6
22 F	0058	6.6	0658	0.3	1318	6.4	1916	0.4
8 F	0038	6.2	0650	0.6	1253	6.2	1908	0.6
23 SA	0134	6.4	0734	0.5	1353	6.2	1952	0.6
9 SA	0112	6.2	0723	0.6	1328	6.1	1942	0.6
24 SU	0206	6.1	0809	0.8	1427	5.9	2027	0.9
10 SU	0147	6.1	0800	0.7	1406	6.0	2021	0.8
25 M	0237	5.7	0845	1.1	1503	5.5	2106	1.3
11 M	0227	5.9	0844	0.9	1450	5.7	2108	1.1
26 TU	0312	5.2	0927	1.4	1550	5.1	2152	1.7
12 TU	0313	5.5	0938	1.2	1543	5.3	2207	1.4
27 W	0405	4.8	1021	1.8	1655	4.7	2253	2.0
13 W	0415	5.1	1049	1.5	1656	5.0	2327	1.7
28 TH	0522	4.5	1130	2.1	1804	4.5		
14 TH	0541	4.9	1218	1.6	1836	4.9		
29 F	0012	2.2	0632	4.4	1316	2.0	1913	4.7
15 F	0102	1.6	0720	5.0	1344	1.4	2006	5.2
30 SA	0158	2.0	0741	4.7	1426	1.7	2019	5.0
31 SU	0251	1.6	0842	5.1	1512	1.4	2111	5.4

APRIL

Day	Time	m	Time	m	Time	m	Time	m
1 M	0333	1.3	0927	5.4	1551	1.1	2151	5.7
16 TU	0348	0.6	1009	6.1	1609	0.5	2232	6.3
2 TU	0410	1.0	1006	5.7	1628	0.9	2228	6.0
17 W ●	0433	0.4	1055	6.3	1653	0.4	2316	6.4
3 W	0445	0.8	1043	6.0	1704	0.7	2304	6.1
18 TH	0515	0.3	1137	6.4	1735	0.4	2356	6.5
4 TH O	0519	0.6	1120	6.1	1738	0.6	2339	6.2
19 F	0556	0.4	1217	6.4	1814	0.4		
5 F	0553	0.5	1157	6.2	1812	0.5		
20 SA	0033	6.4	0633	0.4	1255	6.2	1850	0.6
6 SA	0015	6.3	0628	0.5	1235	6.3	1847	0.5
21 SU	0107	6.2	0708	0.6	1329	6.1	1925	0.7
7 SU	0052	6.3	0706	0.5	1313	6.2	1926	0.5
22 M	0137	5.9	0742	0.8	1401	5.8	2000	1.0
8 M	0131	6.2	0747	0.6	1354	6.0	2009	0.7
23 TU	0205	5.6	0818	1.0	1434	5.5	2038	1.2
9 TU	0213	5.9	0834	0.8	1440	5.8	2059	1.0
24 W	0236	5.3	0859	1.3	1514	5.2	2122	1.6
10 W	0303	5.6	0930	1.1	1537	5.4	2200	1.3
25 TH	0316	4.9	0947	1.6	1613	4.9	2217	1.9
11 TH	0407	5.2	1040	1.4	1651	5.1	2319	1.6
26 F	0430	4.6	1048	1.9	1724	4.7	2324	2.1
12 F	0530	4.9	1206	1.5	1823	5.0		
27 SA	0550	4.5	1200	2.0	1830	4.7		
13 SA	0048	1.5	0705	5.0	1326	1.3	1948	5.3
28 SU	0041	2.0	0656	4.6	1321	1.8	1930	5.0
14 SU	0201	1.3	0821	5.3	1429	1.0	2053	5.7
29 M	0157	1.7	0756	4.9	1423	1.5	2024	5.3
15 M	0258	0.9	0920	5.7	1522	0.7	2146	6.1
30 TU	0249	1.4	0847	5.3	1509	1.2	2111	5.6

Chart Datum: 3·27 metres below Ordnance Datum (Newlyn)

ENGLAND – SHOREHAM

LAT 50°50'N   LONG 0°15'W

TIMES AND HEIGHTS OF HIGH AND LOW WATERS   YEAR 1996

TIME ZONE (UT)
For Summer Time add ONE hour in non-shaded areas

MAY

Day	Time	m		Day	Time	m
1 W	0330	1.1		16 TH	0410	0.6
	0932	5.6			1034	6.0
	1549	1.0			1630	0.7
	2153	5.9			2252	6.2
2 TH	0409	0.8		17 F ●	0453	0.6
	1014	5.9			1116	6.1
	1628	0.8			1712	0.7
	2234	6.1			2332	6.2
3 F O	0448	0.6		18 SA	0534	0.6
	1055	6.1			1156	6.1
	1707	0.6			1751	0.7
	2314	6.3				
4 SA	0527	0.4		19 SU	0008	6.1
	1137	6.3			0611	0.6
	1747	0.5			1232	6.0
	2355	6.4			1828	0.7
5 SU	0609	0.4		20 M	0041	6.0
	1219	6.3			0646	0.7
	1830	0.5			1306	5.9
					1903	0.8
6 M	0036	6.3		21 TU	0112	5.8
	0652	0.3			0721	0.8
	1302	6.3			1338	5.8
	1914	0.5			1938	1.0
7 TU	0119	6.2		22 W	0140	5.6
	0739	0.4			0757	1.0
	1347	6.1			1410	5.6
	2001	0.6			2015	1.2
8 W	0206	6.0		23 TH	0210	5.4
	0829	0.6			0835	1.2
	1438	5.9			1443	5.4
	2054	0.9			2056	1.4
9 TH	0259	5.7		24 F	0246	5.1
	0925	0.9			0918	1.4
	1536	5.6			1524	5.1
	2155	1.2			2144	1.6
10 F	0402	5.3		25 SA	0333	4.9
	1032	1.2			1009	1.7
	1645	5.3			1623	5.0
	2309	1.4			2241	1.8
11 SA	0516	5.1		26 SU	0442	4.7
	1149	1.3			1109	1.8
	1802	5.3			1737	4.9
					2344	1.9
12 SU	0028	1.4		27 M	0605	4.7
	0640	5.1			1215	1.8
	1303	1.3			1842	5.0
	1921	5.4				
13 M	0137	1.2		28 TU	0050	1.7
	0757	5.3			0709	4.9
	1404	1.1			1321	1.6
	2027	5.6			1939	5.2
14 TU	0235	1.0		29 W	0152	1.5
	0857	5.6			0806	5.2
	1458	0.9			1419	1.4
	2122	5.9			2032	5.6
15 W	0325	0.8		30 TH	0246	1.2
	0948	5.8			0858	5.5
	1546	0.8			1509	1.1
	2209	6.1			2120	5.9
				31 F	0334	0.9
					0946	5.8
					1556	0.8
					2207	6.1

JUNE

Day	Time	m		Day	Time	m
1 SA O	0420	0.6		16 SU ●	0513	0.8
	1033	6.1			1135	5.9
	1642	0.6			1732	0.9
	2252	6.3			2344	5.9
2 SU	0505	0.4		17 M	0552	0.7
	1120	6.3			1210	5.9
	1728	0.5			1809	0.9
	2338	6.4				
3 M	0552	0.3		18 TU	0017	5.9
	1207	6.4			0627	0.8
	1815	0.4			1244	5.9
					1844	0.9
4 TU	0024	6.4		19 W	0048	5.8
	0640	0.3			0702	0.8
	1255	6.4			1316	5.8
	1903	0.4			1919	1.0
5 W	0112	6.3		20 TH	0117	5.7
	0729	0.3			0737	0.9
	1344	6.3			1345	5.7
	1953	0.6			1954	1.1
6 TH	0201	6.1		21 F	0147	5.5
	0821	0.5			0812	1.1
	1435	6.1			1415	5.6
	2046	0.7			2030	1.2
7 F	0254	5.9		22 SA	0220	5.4
	0916	0.7			0849	1.2
	1530	5.9			1449	5.5
	2144	1.0			2110	1.4
8 SA	0352	5.6		23 SU	0300	5.2
	1017	1.0			0929	1.4
	1628	5.7			1532	5.3
	2249	1.2			2156	1.5
9 SU	0454	5.3		24 M	0348	5.0
	1124	1.2			1018	1.6
	1731	5.5			1625	5.1
	2359	1.3			2252	1.6
10 M	0604	5.2		25 TU	0449	4.9
	1233	1.3			1117	1.7
	1841	5.4			1732	5.1
					2356	1.7
11 TU	0108	1.3		26 W	0607	4.9
	0722	5.2			1225	1.7
	1336	1.3			1848	5.2
	1953	5.4				
12 W	0209	1.2		27 TH	0103	1.5
	0829	5.3			0723	5.1
	1433	1.2			1335	1.5
	2054	5.6			1953	5.4
13 TH	0301	1.1		28 F	0208	1.3
	0925	5.5			0827	5.4
	1523	1.1			1437	1.2
	2145	5.7			2051	5.7
14 F	0349	0.9		29 SA	0305	0.9
	1013	5.7			0923	5.7
	1609	1.0			1532	0.9
	2229	5.8			2144	6.0
15 SA	0433	0.8		30 SU	0358	0.6
	1056	5.8			1016	6.1
	1652	0.9			1623	0.7
	2309	5.9			2235	6.3

JULY

Day	Time	m		Day	Time	m
1 M O	0448	0.4		16 TU	0532	0.8
	1107	6.3			1150	5.9
	1713	0.5			1750	0.9
	2325	6.4			2354	5.8
2 TU	0538	0.2		17 W	0608	0.8
	1157	6.5			1221	5.9
	1802	0.4			1826	0.9
3 W	0015	6.5		18 TH	0024	5.8
	0627	0.2			0643	0.8
	1247	6.5			1251	5.9
	1851	0.4			1859	0.9
4 TH	0105	6.3		19 F	0053	5.8
	0717	0.2			0716	0.9
	1336	6.5			1318	5.8
	1941	0.4			1931	1.0
5 F	0154	6.3		20 SA	0123	5.7
	0807	0.3			0747	1.0
	1425	6.4			1347	5.8
	2032	0.6			2002	1.1
6 SA	0243	6.1		21 SU	0155	5.6
	0859	0.5			0817	1.1
	1514	6.2			1420	5.7
	2124	0.8			2035	1.2
7 SU	0334	5.8		22 M	0231	5.5
	0952	0.8			0852	1.2
	1604	5.9			1458	5.6
	2220	1.1			2115	1.3
8 M	0427	5.5		23 TU	0314	5.4
	1050	1.1			0935	1.4
	1657	5.6			1544	5.4
	2322	1.3			2206	1.5
9 TU	0525	5.2		24 W	0406	5.1
	1156	1.4			1030	1.6
	1755	5.3			1641	5.2
					2309	1.6
10 W	0034	1.5		25 TH	0511	5.0
	0633	5.0			1139	1.7
	1306	1.6			1755	5.1
	1903	5.1				
11 TH	0141	1.5		26 F	0023	1.6
	0757	5.0			0640	5.0
	1409	1.5			1300	1.6
	2021	5.2			1919	5.2
12 F	0239	1.4		27 SA	0139	1.4
	0902	5.2			0802	5.2
	1503	1.4			1414	1.4
	2121	5.4			2029	5.5
13 SA	0329	1.2		28 SU	0246	1.0
	0954	5.4			0906	5.6
	1551	1.2			1522	1.0
	2208	5.6			2129	5.9
14 SU	0414	1.0		29 M	0342	0.7
	1038	5.6			1003	6.0
	1634	1.1			1610	0.7
	2248	5.7			2223	6.2
15 M ●	0454	0.9		30 TU O	0434	0.4
	1116	5.8			1055	6.4
	1713	1.0			1700	0.5
	2323	5.8			2314	6.5
				31 W	0523	0.2
					1146	6.6
					1749	0.3

AUGUST

Day	Time	m		Day	Time	m
1 TH	0004	6.6		16 F	0620	0.8
	0611	0.1			1222	6.0
	1235	6.7			1836	0.9
	1836	0.3				
2 F	0053	6.6		17 SA	0027	5.9
	0659	0.1			0651	0.8
	1322	6.7			1250	6.0
	1924	0.3			1906	0.9
3 SA	0139	6.5		18 SU	0059	5.9
	0747	0.3			0719	0.9
	1407	6.6			1320	6.0
	2011	0.5			1934	0.9
4 SU	0224	6.3		19 M	0131	5.9
	0834	0.5			0747	0.9
	1451	6.3			1353	5.9
	2057	0.7			2005	1.0
5 M	0309	5.9		20 TU	0205	5.8
	0920	0.8			0821	1.1
	1535	6.0			1429	5.8
	2144	1.1			2044	1.1
6 TU	0357	5.5		21 W	0245	5.6
	1009	1.2			0904	1.3
	1623	5.5			1513	5.5
	2236	1.4			2132	1.3
7 W	0449	5.1		22 TH	0334	5.3
	1106	1.6			0958	1.5
	1716	5.2			1607	5.2
	2342	1.7			2235	1.6
8 TH	0551	4.8		23 F	0438	5.0
	1226	1.9			1109	1.7
	1818	4.9			1721	5.0
					2353	1.7
9 F	0111	1.8		24 SA	0612	4.9
	0708	4.7			1238	1.8
	1345	1.9			1857	5.1
	1936	4.9				
10 SA	0217	1.7		25 SU	0119	1.5
	0840	4.9			0746	5.1
	1444	1.7			1401	1.5
	2059	5.1			2015	5.4
11 SU	0310	1.4		26 M	0232	1.2
	0935	5.3			0854	5.6
	1532	1.4			1504	1.1
	2149	5.4			2117	5.9
12 M	0354	1.2		27 TU	0329	0.7
	1018	5.6			0951	6.1
	1614	1.2			1557	0.7
	2228	5.6			2212	6.2
13 TU	0433	1.0		28 W O	0419	0.4
	1054	5.8			1042	6.5
	1652	1.0			1646	0.4
	2300	5.8			2302	6.5
14 W ●	0510	0.8		29 TH	0507	0.2
	1126	5.9			1131	6.7
	1728	0.9			1732	0.3
	2329	5.9			2350	6.7
15 TH	0546	0.8		30 F	0553	0.1
	1155	6.0			1217	6.8
	1803	0.9			1818	0.2
	2358	5.9				
				31 SA	0036	6.7
					0638	0.2
					1302	6.8
					1902	0.3

Chart Datum: 3·27 metres below Ordnance Datum (Newlyn)

ENGLAND – SHOREHAM

LAT 50°50′N   LONG 0°15′W

TIMES AND HEIGHTS OF HIGH AND LOW WATERS

YEAR **1996**

3

TIME ZONE (UT)
For Summer Time add ONE hour in non-shaded areas

SEPTEMBER

Day	Time	m	Day	Time	m
1 SU	0120 / 0722 / 1343 / 1945	6.6 / 0.3 / 6.6 / 0.5	**16** M	0035 / 0650 / 1254 / 1907	6.1 / 0.8 / 6.1 / 0.8
2 M	0201 / 0804 / 1424 / 2026	6.3 / 0.6 / 6.3 / 0.7	**17** TU	0108 / 0721 / 1328 / 1941	6.0 / 0.9 / 6.0 / 0.9
3 TU	0242 / 0846 / 1504 / 2106	6.0 / 0.9 / 5.9 / 1.1	**18** W	0143 / 0758 / 1405 / 2021	5.9 / 1.0 / 5.9 / 1.0
4 W	0325 / 0928 / 1547 / 2151	5.6 / 1.3 / 5.5 / 1.5	**19** TH	0223 / 0842 / 1448 / 2111	5.7 / 1.2 / 5.6 / 1.3
5 TH	0415 / 1018 / 1640 / 2246	5.1 / 1.7 / 5.0 / 1.9	**20** F	0313 / 0938 / 1544 / 2215	5.4 / 1.5 / 5.2 / 1.6
6 F	0515 / 1125 / 1742	4.8 / 2.1 / 4.7	**21** SA	0419 / 1052 / 1702 / 2335	5.0 / 1.8 / 4.9 / 1.7
7 SA	0014 / 0625 / 1316 / 1852	2.1 / 4.6 / 2.2 / 4.7	**22** SU	0600 / 1225 / 1843	4.9 / 1.8 / 5.0
8 SU	0151 / 0805 / 1421 / 2029	2.0 / 4.8 / 1.9 / 4.9	**23** M	0105 / 0733 / 1348 / 2003	1.6 / 5.2 / 1.5 / 5.4
9 M	0245 / 0909 / 1510 / 2123	1.6 / 5.2 / 1.6 / 5.3	**24** TU	0218 / 0841 / 1450 / 2106	1.2 / 5.7 / 1.1 / 5.8
10 TU	0330 / 0950 / 1551 / 2200	1.3 / 5.6 / 1.3 / 5.6	**25** W	0314 / 0937 / 1541 / 2158	0.8 / 6.1 / 0.7 / 6.2
11 W	0408 / 1024 / 1627 / 2231	1.0 / 5.8 / 1.0 / 5.8	**26** TH	0402 / 1026 / 1628 / 2247	0.5 / 6.5 / 0.4 / 6.5
12 TH	0444 / 1054 / 1703 / ●2300	0.9 / 5.8 / 0.9 / 6.0	**27** F	0448 / 1112 / 1713 / O2332	0.3 / 6.7 / 0.3 / 6.7
13 F	0519 / 1123 / 1737 / 2330	0.8 / 6.1 / 0.8 / 6.0	**28** SA	0532 / 1156 / 1757	0.2 / 6.8 / 0.3
14 SA	0552 / 1151 / 1809	0.7 / 6.1 / 0.8	**29** SU	0016 / 0615 / 1238 / 1838	6.7 / 0.3 / 6.7 / 0.4
15 SU	0002 / 0622 / 1222 / 1838	6.1 / 0.8 / 6.1 / 0.8	**30** M	0057 / 0656 / 1317 / 1917	6.5 / 0.6 / 6.5 / 0.5

OCTOBER

Day	Time	m	Day	Time	m
1 TU	0136 / 0735 / 1354 / 1955	6.3 / 0.7 / 6.2 / 0.8	**16** W	0049 / 0701 / 1308 / 1924	6.2 / 0.8 / 6.1 / 0.8
2 W	0213 / 0813 / 1431 / 2033	6.0 / 1.0 / 5.8 / 1.1	**17** TH	0127 / 0742 / 1348 / 2008	6.0 / 0.9 / 5.9 / 1.0
3 TH	0252 / 0853 / 1511 / 2114	5.6 / 1.4 / 5.4 / 1.5	**18** F	0210 / 0829 / 1434 / 2059	5.8 / 1.2 / 5.6 / 1.2
4 F	0340 / 0941 / 1603 / 2206	5.2 / 1.8 / 5.0 / 1.9	**19** SA	0302 / 0928 / 1532 / 2203	5.5 / 1.5 / 5.3 / 1.5
5 SA	0441 / 1041 / 1707 / 2311	4.8 / 2.1 / 4.7 / 2.1	**20** SU	0412 / 1043 / 1652 / 2322	5.1 / 1.7 / 5.0 / 1.6
6 SU	0548 / 1206 / 1815	4.7 / 2.3 / 4.6	**21** M	0546 / 1212 / 1826.	5.0 / 1.7 / 5.0
7 M	0104 / 0701 / 1347 / 1928	2.1 / 4.8 / 2.1 / 4.8	**22** TU	0048 / 0714 / 1330 / 1947	1.6 / 5.3 / 1.5 / 5.3
8 TU	0211 / 0818 / 1439 / 2036	1.8 / 5.1 / 1.7 / 5.1	**23** W	0158 / 0823 / 1431 / 2049	1.2 / 5.7 / 1.1 / 5.8
9 W	0258 / 0907 / 1520 / 2119	1.5 / 5.5 / 1.4 / 5.5	**24** TH	0254 / 0918 / 1522 / 2141	0.9 / 6.1 / 0.8 / 6.1
10 TH	0337 / 0943 / 1557 / 2155	1.2 / 5.8 / 1.1 / 5.8	**25** F	0342 / 1006 / 1608 / 2229	0.6 / 6.4 / 0.5 / 6.4
11 F	0413 / 1016 / 1633 / 2229	1.0 / 6.0 / 0.9 / 6.0	**26** SA	0427 / 1051 / 1652 / O2313	0.4 / 6.6 / 0.4 / 6.5
12 SA	0448 / 1049 / 1707 / ●2303	0.8 / 6.2 / 0.8 / 6.1	**27** SU	0511 / 1133 / 1735 / 2355	0.4 / 6.6 / 0.4 / 6.5
13 SU	0521 / 1122 / 1740 / 2338	0.8 / 6.2 / 0.8 / 6.2	**28** M	0552 / 1213 / 1815	0.5 / 6.6 / 0.5
14 M	0553 / 1156 / 1812	0.7 / 6.3 / 0.7	**29** TU	0034 / 0631 / 1251 / 1853	6.4 / 0.6 / 6.4 / 0.6
15 TU	0013 / 0625 / 1232 / 1846	6.2 / 0.7 / 6.2 / 0.7	**30** W	0112 / 0708 / 1325 / 1929	6.2 / 0.8 / 6.1 / 0.9
			31 TH	0147 / 0745 / 1359 / 2005	6.0 / 1.1 / 5.8 / 1.1

NOVEMBER

Day	Time	m	Day	Time	m
1 F	0223 / 0824 / 1434 / 2046	5.7 / 1.4 / 5.4 / 1.4	**16** SA	0204 / 0822 / 1427 / 2053	6.0 / 1.1 / 5.8 / 1.0
2 SA	0305 / 0910 / 1519 / 2133	5.3 / 1.7 / 5.1 / 1.7	**17** SU	0258 / 0921 / 1526 / 2154	5.7 / 1.3 / 5.5 / 1.3
3 SU	0402 / 1005 / 1625 / 2231	5.0 / 2.0 / 4.7 / 2.0	**18** M	0405 / 1033 / 1638 / 2306	5.4 / 1.5 / 5.2 / 1.4
4 M	0509 / 1111 / 1735 / 2340	4.8 / 2.2 / 4.6 / 2.1	**19** TU	0524 / 1151 / 1800	5.3 / 1.6 / 5.2
5 TU	0615 / 1232 / 1840	4.8 / 2.2 / 4.7	**20** W	0023 / 0645 / 1305 / 1921	1.5 / 5.4 / 1.4 / 5.3
6 W	0105 / 0717 / 1351 / 1941	2.0 / 5.0 / 1.9 / 5.0	**21** TH	0132 / 0757 / 1407 / 2027	1.3 / 5.6 / 1.2 / 5.6
7 TH	0211 / 0812 / 1440 / 2033	1.7 / 5.4 / 1.6 / 5.3	**22** F	0230 / 0854 / 1500 / 2121	1.1 / 5.9 / 0.9 / 5.9
8 F	0257 / 0858 / 1521 / 2117	1.4 / 5.7 / 1.3 / 5.7	**23** SA	0321 / 0944 / 1548 / 2210	0.9 / 6.2 / 0.7 / 6.1
9 SA	0337 / 0938 / 1558 / 2158	1.2 / 6.0 / 1.0 / 5.9	**24** SU	0407 / 1030 / 1633 / 2254	0.7 / 6.3 / 0.6 / 6.2
10 SU	0413 / 1017 / 1635 / 2237	1.0 / 6.2 / 0.8 / 6.1	**25** M	0451 / 1112 / 1715 / O2336	0.7 / 6.4 / 0.6 / 6.3
11 M	0450 / 1055 / 1711 / ●2316	0.8 / 6.3 / 0.7 / 6.3	**26** TU	0532 / 1150 / 1755	0.7 / 6.3 / 0.6
12 TU	0526 / 1133 / 1750 / 2355	0.7 / 6.4 / 0.6 / 6.3	**27** W	0014 / 0610 / 1227 / 1833	6.2 / 0.8 / 6.2 / 0.7
13 W	0605 / 1212 / 1830	0.7 / 6.4 / 0.6	**28** TH	0050 / 0647 / 1300 / 1908	6.1 / 0.9 / 6.0 / 0.9
14 TH	0035 / 0646 / 1253 / 1913	6.3 / 0.7 / 6.3 / 0.7	**29** F	0124 / 0723 / 1332 / 1944	6.0 / 1.1 / 5.8 / 1.0
15 F	0118 / 0732 / 1337 / 2000	6.2 / 0.8 / 6.1 / 0.8	**30** SA	0157 / 0801 / 1403 / 2022	5.8 / 1.3 / 5.5 / 1.3

DECEMBER

Day	Time	m	Day	Time	m
1 SU	0231 / 0843 / 1437 / 2105	5.5 / 1.5 / 5.3 / 1.5	**16** M	0252 / 0911 / 1516 / 2140	6.0 / 1.0 / 5.8 / 1.0
2 M	0310 / 0930 / 1521 / 2153	5.3 / 1.8 / 5.0 / 1.7	**17** TU	0350 / 1014 / 1617 / 2242	5.8 / 1.2 / 5.5 / 1.2
3 TU	0406 / 1026 / 1628 / 2250	5.0 / 2.0 / 4.8 / 1.9	**18** W	0454 / 1123 / 1725 / 2352	5.5 / 1.4 / 5.3 / 1.4
4 W	0520 / 1129 / 1746 / 2353	4.9 / 2.1 / 4.7 / 2.0	**19** TH	0604 / 1235 / 1842	5.4 / 1.4 / 5.2
5 TH	0626 / 1235 / 1852	5.0 / 2.0 / 4.8	**20** F	0102 / 0720 / 1340 / 1958	1.4 / 5.4 / 1.4 / 5.3
6 F	0100 / 0724 / 1340 / 1949	1.9 / 5.2 / 1.8 / 5.1	**21** SA	0205 / 0828 / 1438 / 2100	1.3 / 5.6 / 1.2 / 5.5
7 SA	0203 / 0816 / 1435 / 2041	1.7 / 5.5 / 1.5 / 5.4	**22** SU	0300 / 0923 / 1529 / 2152	1.2 / 5.8 / 1.0 / 5.7
8 SU	0255 / 0904 / 1522 / 2128	1.4 / 5.8 / 1.1 / 5.8	**23** M	0349 / 1011 / 1615 / 2238	1.0 / 6.0 / 0.9 / 5.9
9 M	0340 / 0948 / 1605 / 2213	1.1 / 6.1 / 0.9 / 6.0	**24** TU	0434 / 1053 / 1658 / O2320	0.9 / 6.1 / 0.8 / 6.0
10 TU	0423 / 1031 / 1648 / ●2257	0.9 / 6.3 / 0.7 / 6.2	**25** W	0516 / 1131 / 1739 / 2357	0.9 / 6.1 / 0.7 / 6.1
11 W	0506 / 1114 / 1732 / 2341	0.7 / 6.4 / 0.5 / 6.4	**26** TH	0554 / 1206 / 1816	0.9 / 6.1 / 0.8
12 TH	0550 / 1158 / 1817	0.6 / 6.5 / 0.4	**27** F	0031 / 0630 / 1238 / 1851	6.1 / 0.9 / 6.0 / 0.8
13 F	0026 / 0635 / 1244 / 1903	6.4 / 0.6 / 6.4 / 0.4	**28** SA	0103 / 0705 / 1308 / 1926	6.0 / 1.0 / 5.9 / 0.9
14 SA	0112 / 0723 / 1331 / 1952	6.4 / 0.7 / 6.3 / 0.5	**29** SU	0133 / 0740 / 1337 / 2001	5.9 / 1.1 / 5.7 / 1.0
15 SU	0200 / 0815 / 1421 / 2044	6.2 / 0.8 / 6.0 / 0.7	**30** M	0200 / 0816 / 1407 / 2036	5.7 / 1.3 / 5.5 / 1.2
			31 TU	0230 / 0855 / 1442 / 2114	5.6 / 1.5 / 5.3 / 1.4

Chart Datum: 3.27 metres below Ordnance Datum (Newlyn)

BRIGHTON   10-3-11

E. Sussex 50°48'·50N 00°06'·28W

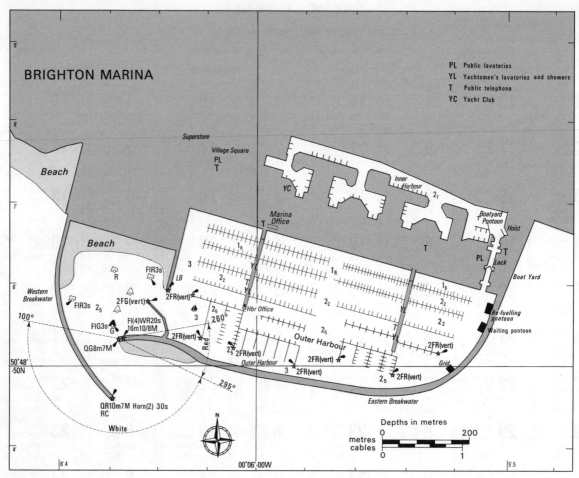

CHARTS
AC *1991, 1652*; Imray C9; Stanfords 9; OS 198
TIDES
+0004 Dover; ML 3·5; Duration 0605; Zone 0 (UT)

Standard Port SHOREHAM (←)

Times				Height (metres)			
High Water		Low Water		MHWS	MHWN	MLWN	MLWS
0500	1000	0000	0600	6·3	4·8	1·9	0·6
1700	2200	1200	1800				
Differences BRIGHTON							
−0010	−0005	−0005	−0005	+0·3	+0·1	0·0	−0·1

SHELTER
Good in the marina under all conditions, but in strong S'ly winds confused seas can make the final appr very rough. Speed limit 5kn.
NAVIGATION
WPT 50°48'·20N 00°06'·29W, 180°/000° from/to W bkwtr lt, 0·26M. Ent chan dredged 2·5m, but after gales silting may occur especially on E side. In heavy weather, best appr is from SSE to avoid worst of the backlash from bkwtrs; beware shallow water E of ent in R sector of lt Fl (4) WR 20s. A Historic Wreck (see 10.0.3g) is at 50°48'·6N 00°06'·49W, immediately W of the marina's W bkwtr.
LIGHTS AND MARKS
The marina is at the E end of the town, where white cliffs extend eastward. Daymark: conspic white hospital block, brg 334° leads to ent. Y spar buoy is 2ca S of W bkwtr. Navigational lts may be hard to see against shore glare: E bkwtr Fl (4) WR 20s (intens) 16m 10/8M; vis R260°-295°, W295°-100°. E bkwtr hd QG 8m 7M. W bkwtr hd, tr R/W bands, QR 10m 7M; Horn (2) 30s. RC = BM 294·5 kHz, 10M. Inner Hbr lock controlled by normal R/G lts, 0800-2000 LT.

RADIO TELEPHONE
Call: *Brighton Control* VHF Ch **M** 80 16 (H24); 68 11.
TELEPHONE (01273)
Hr Mr 693636; BY 609235; MRSC (01705) 552100; ⌗ (01703) 827350; Marinecall 0891 500456; Police 606744; Ⓗ 696955; Dr 686863.
FACILITIES
Marina (1600+200 visitors) ☎ 693636, Fax 675082, £14.25, ⌗, FW, P, D, AC, Gas, Gaz, ▣, R, Bar, BY, BH (60 ton), C (35 ton); **Brighton Marina YC** ☎ 818711, Bar, R.
Services El, Ⓔ, ME, Sh, SM, CH, ACA, Divers, Riggers, Superstore.
Hbr Guides available from Hbr Office or by post.
Bus service from Marina; timetable info ☎ 674881.
Electric Railway runs from Marina to Palace Pier, Mar-Oct.
Town V, R, Bar, ✉, Ⓑ, ⇌, ✈ (Shoreham).

NEWHAVEN   10-3-12

E. Sussex 50°46'·80N 00°03'·63E

CHARTS

AC 2154, *1652*; Imray C9; Stanfords 9; OS 198

TIDES

+0004 Dover; ML 3·6; Duration 0550; Zone 0 (UT)

Standard Port SHOREHAM (←—)

Times				Height (metres)			
High Water		Low Water		MHWS	MHWN	MLWN	MLWS
0500	1000	0000	0600	6·3	4·8	1·9	0·6
1700	2200	1200	1800				
Differences NEWHAVEN							
–0015	–0010	0000	0000	+0·4	+0·2	0·0	–0·2
EASTBOURNE							
–0010	–0005	+0015	+0020	+1·1	+0·6	+0·2	+0·1

SHELTER

Good in all weathers, but there is often a dangerous sea at the ent in strong on-shore winds. Appr from the SW and pass close to bkwtr to avoid heavy breaking seas on E side of dredged chan. At marina, berth inside **Ⓥ** pontoon (1·5m), access HW±5; caution silting has been reported.

NAVIGATION

WPT 50°46'·20N 00°03'·70E, 168°/348° from/to W bkwtr lt, 0·32M. Hbr silts and dredging is continuous. Ferries and cargo vessels may warp off with hawsers across the hbr.

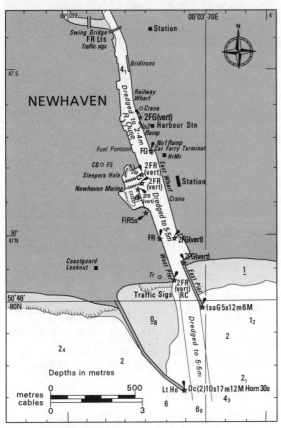

LIGHTS AND MARKS

Lt Ho on W bkwtr is conspic, as is an orange container crane opposite the marina.

Traffic sigs, displayed from tr on W side of river:

▼ over ●, or Ⓖ = only ent permitted.
● over ▼, or Ⓡ = only departure permitted.
● ▼ ● (vert) or
  ⓇⒼⓇ (vert) = No ent or departure.
● or ⒼⓇ (vert) = Entry and dep permitted with care for vessels under 15m LOA.

Swing bridge sigs:
Fl Ⓖ = Bridge opening or closing.
Ⓡ = Vessels may pass N to S.
Ⓖ = Vessels may pass S to N.

RADIO TELEPHONE

Port VHF Ch 12 16 (H24). Marina Ch **80** M (0800-1700).

TELEPHONE (01273)

Hr Mr 514131; MRSC (01705) 552100; Hbr Sig Stn 514131 ext. 247; ⌗ (01703) 827350; Marinecall 0891 500456; Police 515801; Dr 515076; Ⓗ 609411 (Casualty 696955).

FACILITIES

Marina (300+50 visitors) ☎ 513881, £15, FW, fuel pontoon 200 yds N of ent, ME, El, Sh, AC, BH (18 ton), C (10 ton), CH, Gas, Gaz, Slip, V, R, Bar, Ⓞ; **Marina YC** ☎ 513976; **Newhaven YC** ☎ 513770, AB, M, P, D, ME, El, Sh, Slip, CH; **Newhaven & Seaford SC** ☎ (01323) 890077, M, FW. **Town** EC Wed; ACA, SM, P, Ⓔ, V, R, Bar, ✉, Ⓑ, ≠, ✈ (Shoreham). Ferry to Dieppe; Stena Sealink ☎ 516699.

EASTBOURNE   10-3-13

E. Sussex 50°47'·30N 00°20'·00E

CHARTS

AC *536*; Imray C8; Stanfords 9; OS 199

TIDES

–0005 Dover; ML 3·8; Duration 0540; Zone 0 (UT)

Standard Port SHOREHAM (←—)

See Differences under 10.3.12

SHELTER

Good, but apprs exposed to NE/SE winds. Access H24 via chan dredged 2·0m and twin locks into inner basin (4m).

NAVIGATION

WPT 50°47'·20N 00°20'·75E, 078°/258° from/to hbr ent, 0·52M. There are shoals to the NE in Pevensey Bay and from 2·5M SE toward Royal Sovereign lt. From Beachy Head, keep 0·75M offshore to clear Holywell Bank.

LIGHTS AND MARKS

Beachy Hd lt, Fl (2) 20s, is 5M SW; Royal Sovereign lt, Fl 20s, is 5·5M to SE. Martello tr No 66 at root of S bkwtr has high intens Xenon lt, Fl (3) 15s 12m 7M, vis H24; but hard to see by day. From E, by day R roofs are conspic WSW of ent. Dir lt, Fl WRG 5s 4m 1M, G252·5°-256·5°, W256·5°-259·5°, R259·5°-262·5°, leads 258° into chan. A SWM Fairway buoy, Fl 10s, is about 3ca ENE of first SHM buoy Fl G 5s marking wk close N; a PHM pillar buoy Fl R 5s is close SW. Ent chan buoys are four SHM Fl G 3s, three PHM Fl R 3s, and an unlit pair. Eastbourne pier, 2 FR, is 2M S of hbr ent; an unlit PHM buoy is approx 5ca S.

RADIO TELEPHONE

Call *Sovereign Harbour* VHF Ch 15 (H24) for entry and Ch 17 for locks/bridges and berthing.

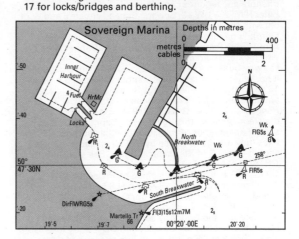

TELEPHONE (01323)

Hr Mr 470099; MRSC (01304) 210008; Marinecall 0891 500456; Police 722522; Dr 720555; Ⓗ 417400.

FACILITIES

Sovereign Marina (332 berths), ☎ 470099, Fax 470077, £13.50, FW, AC, D & P (H24), BH (50 tons), ME, Sh, CH, Ⓞ, supermarket. **Town** (2½M) all facilities, ≠, ✈ (Gatwick).

RYE   10-3-14

E. Sussex 50°55'·57N 00°46'·69E

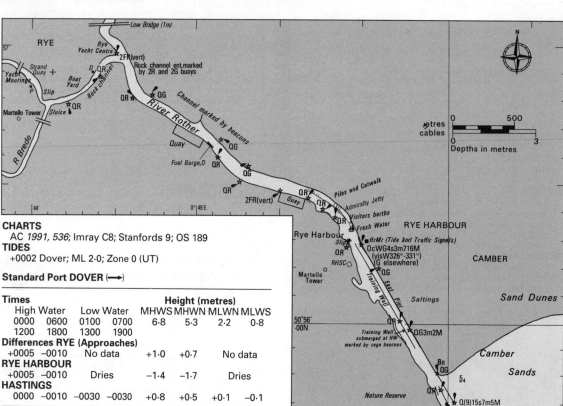

CHARTS
AC *1991, 536*; Imray C8; Stanfords 9; OS 189
TIDES
+0002 Dover; ML 2·0; Zone 0 (UT)

Standard Port DOVER (⟶)

Times				Height (metres)			
High Water		Low Water		MHWS	MHWN	MLWN	MLWS
0000	0600	0100	0700	6·8	5·3	2·2	0·8
1200	1800	1300	1900				
Differences RYE (Approaches)							
+0005	−0010	No data		+1·0	+0·7	No data	
RYE HARBOUR							
+0005	−0010	Dries		−1·4	−1·7	Dries	
HASTINGS							
0000	−0010	−0030	−0030	+0·8	+0·5	+0·1	−0·1

SHELTER
Very good in R Rother, but hbr is exposed to prevailing SW winds with little shelter in Rye Bay. Good ⚓ in lee of Dungeness (6M to E) or in N'lies ⚓ 5ca N of Fairway buoy. Rye Hbr is a small village, ¾M inside ent on W bank, used by commercial shipping. Hbr dries completely to soft mud. Berth on Admiralty Jetty; see Hr Mr for AB or M; ⚓ prohib. Speed limit 6kn. Rye town (a Cinque Port) is 2M up river; ent via Rock Chan, visitors' AB on NE side of Strand Quay.
NAVIGATION
WPT Rye Fairway SWM By, L Fl 10s, 50°54'·00N 00°48'·13E, 150°/330° from/to W Arm tripod lt, 1·81M. Ent dries to 5ca offshore and requires care when wind >F6 from SE to SW. Enter HW −2 to HW +3. Beware: Bar and shoals E and W of ent with ground swell or surf; narrow ent (42m) and chan (30m); flood runs up to 4·5kn (max HW −3 to HW −1).
Army Firing Ranges at Lydd have a Sea Danger Area which extends 3M offshore and stretches E from Rye Fairway buoy to a N/S line approx 1·5M W of Dungeness lt ho. When firing takes place, about 300 days p.a. 0830–1630LT (often to 2300), R flags/R lts are displayed ashore and a Range Safety Craft may be on station. Call *Lydd Ranges* Ch 73 13 or ☎ 01303 249541 Ext 8518/9. Vessels may legally transit through the Sea Danger Area, but should not enter or remain in it for other purposes. Radar fixes may also be obtained by VHF. If possible vessels should transit S of Stephenson Shoal. See also 10.3.15.
LIGHTS AND MARKS
Dir Oc WG 4s lt on Hr Mr's office has W sector (326°-331°) covering ent/river. W Arm lt Fl R 5s 7m 6M, wooden tripod, radar reflector. E Arm hd, Q (9) 15s 7m 5M; Horn 7s, G △. On E Pier an illuminated "Welcome to Rye" sign is considered too bright by some, but helpful by others. Rock Chan ent marked by a QR and QG lt buoy in season.
IPTS (Sigs 2 and 5 only) are shown to seaward (3M) from Hr Mr's office and up-river (1M) from Admiralty Jetty. Yachts should monitor VHF Ch 14 and keep clear of commercial ships.
Tide Signals on Hr Mr's office:
Night: ⓖ   = 2·1 - 3·0m on bar.
F Purple   = Over 3·0m on bar.
Day: 3, 2 or 1 horiz timber(s) visible on W Arm bn indicate depths of 5', 10' or 15' (1·5m, 3·0m or 4·5m) above CD.

RADIO TELEPHONE
VHF Ch 14 16 (0900-1700 LT, HW±2 or when vessel due).
TELEPHONE (01797)
Hr Mr 225225; MRCC (01304) 210008; ⌗ (01304) 202441; Marinecall 0891 500456; Police 222112; Dr 222031; Ⓗ 222109.
FACILITIES
Admiralty Jetty AB £10, Slip, M, L, FW; **Strand Quay** AB, M, P and D (50m, cans), L, FW, Shwrs; **Hbr** ME, El, C (15 ton), BY, C (3 ton), Slip (26 ton), Sh, CH, Ⓔ, ACA; **Rye Hbr SC** ☎ 223136. **Town** EC Tues; ✉, Ⓑ, ⇌, ✈ (Lydd).
Note: A Historic Wreck (*Anne*; see 10.0.3g) is about 4M WSW of Rye, close inshore at 50°53'·42N 00°41'·91E.

ADJACENT ANCHORAGE

HASTINGS, E Sussex, 50°50'·84N 00°35'·60E. AC *536*. HW −0005 on Dover; HW +0·7m on Dover; ML 3·8m; Duration 0530. See 10·3·14. Strictly a settled weather ⚓ or emergency shelter; landing places on pier. The stone bkwtr is in disrepair and serves only to protect FVs. Beware dangerous wreck 3ca SE of pier head. Ldg lts 356°, both FR 14/55m 4M: front on W metal column; rear 357m from front, on 5-sided W tr on West Hill. Pier hd 2 FR (vert) 8m 5M from white hut; W bkwtr hd Fl R 2·5s 5m 4M; Fl G 5s 2m, 30m from head of No3 Groyne (E bkwtr). A Historic Wreck (*Amsterdam*; see 10.0.3g) is about 2M W of pier, close inshore at 50°50'·7N 00°31'·65E. Facilities: EC Wed; ⌗ (01304) 202441. ACA (St Leonards). Few marine facilities; all shore needs at Hastings and St Leonards. YC ☎ (01424) 420656.

DOVER STRAIT   10-3-15

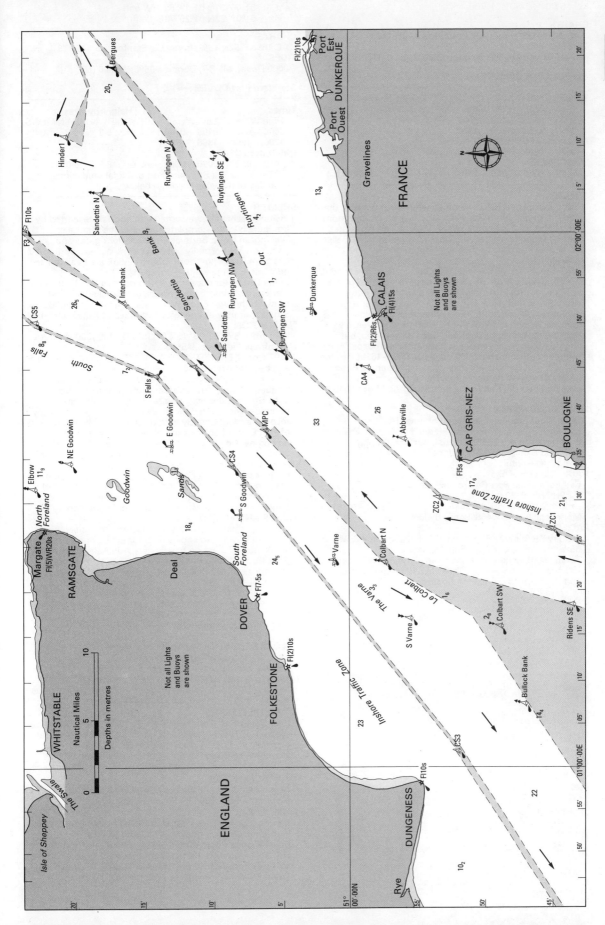

3

Bergues
20₂

Hinder1

Ruytingen N

Ruytingen SE   4₄

Ruytingen   4₂

F3 Fl10s

Sandettie N

Ruytingen NW

Out   1₇

Interbank

Bank 9₁

26₅

Sandettie   5

Sandettie N

Ruytingen SW

Dunkerque

CS5

Falls 8₈

South

7₂

S Falls

MPC

33

NE Goodwin

E Goodwin

CS4

S Goodwin

Goodwin

Sands

18₄

Elbow   11₉

North Foreland

Margate Fl(5)WR20s

RAMSGATE

Deal

South Foreland

24₅

DOVER   Fl7·5s

Varne

Colbart N

The Varne

Le Colbart   6₁

S Varne   3₅

Colbart SW

FOLKESTONE   Fl(2)10s

Inshore Traffic Zone

23

CS3

Fl10s

DUNGENESS

Rye

10₂

22

Bullock Bank

14₄

Ridens SE

2₆

ZC1

21₅

ZC2

17₆

Fl5s

CAP GRIS-NEZ

BOULOGNE

Abbeville

26

CA4   4₇

Fl(2)R6s

CALAIS   Fl(4)15s

FRANCE

Gravelines

Not all Lights and Buoys are shown

Port Ouest

Port Est   Fl(2)10s

DUNKERQUE

13₈

N

Inshore Traffic Zone

WHITSTABLE

Isle of Sheppey

The Swale

ENGLAND

Not all Lights and Buoys are shown

10

5

0

Nautical Miles

Depths in metres

02°00'·00E

01°00'·00E

51°00'·00N

20'

15'

10'

5'

00'

55'

50'

45'

20'

15'

10'

5'

00'

55'

50'

45'

FOLKESTONE   10-3-16

Kent 51°04'·56N 01°11'·78E

CHARTS
AC *1991, 1892*; Imray C8; Stanfords 9; OS 179
TIDES
−0010 Dover; ML 3·9; Duration 0500; Zone 0 (UT)

Standard Port DOVER (→)

Times				Height (metres)			
High Water		Low Water		MHWS	MHWN	MLWN	MLWS
0000	0600	0100	0700	6·8	5·3	2·2	0·8
1200	1800	1300	1900				
Differences FOLKESTONE							
−0020	−0005	−0010	−0010	+0·4	+0·4	0·0	−0·1
DUNGENESS							
−0010	−0015	−0020	−0010	+1·0	+0·6	+0·4	+0·1

SHELTER
Good except in strong E-S winds when seas break at the hbr ent. Drying Inner Hbr has many FVs, so limited room for yachts; access approx HW±2. Visitors can berth on S Quay; fender board needed. Depth gauge on hd of E Pier. Ferry area is prohib to yachts; no room to ⚓ off.
NAVIGATION
WPT 51°04'·30N 01°12'·00E, 150°/330° from/to bkwtr hd lt, 0·26M. Beware Mole Hd Rks and Copt Rks to stbd of the ent. Also ferries and pulling off wires from the jetty.
Army Firing Ranges at Hythe have a Sea Danger Area extending 2M offshore, from Hythe to Dymchurch (approx 5M and 8M WSW of Folkestone hbr). Vessels may legally transit through the Sea Danger Area, but should not enter or remain in it for other purposes. When firing takes place, about 300 days p.a. 0830–1630LT (often to 2300), R flags/R lts are displayed ashore and a Range Safety Craft may be on station. Radar fixes may also be obtained by VHF. Call *Hythe Ranges* Ch 73 13 or ☎ 01303 249541 Ext 8179. See also 10.3.14.
LIGHTS AND MARKS
Hotel block is conspic at W end of Inner Hbr.
Ldg lts 295° at ferry terminal, FR and FG (occas). QG lt at E pierhead on brg 305° leads to inner hbr. Bu flag or 3 Ⓡ (vert) at FS on S arm, ¼ hr before ferry sails = hbr closed. 3 Ⓖ (vert) = enter.
RADIO TELEPHONE
Call *Folkestone Port Control* VHF Ch 22 16.
TELEPHONE (01303)
Hr Mr 220544; MRCC (01304) 210008; ☰ (01304) 224251; Marinecall 0891 500456; Police 850055.
FACILITIES
S Quay BR Slipway Slip (free), FW; **Folkestone Y & MB Club** ☎ 251574, D, FW, L, Slip, M, Bar.
Town EC Wed (larger shops open all day); P & D (cans, 100 yds), V, R, Bar, ✉, Ⓑ, ⇶, ✈ (Lydd). Freight ferries and Hoverspeed (Seacat) to Boulogne.

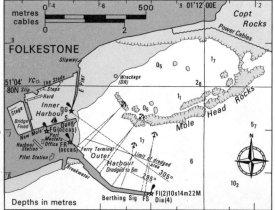

metres cables   500   ·9 01°12'·00E   Copt Rocks   Power Cables

FOLKESTONE

Slipway   Wreckage (DR)   The Stade   Steps   Hard   Inner Harbour   QG   Quay   Bridge Fixed   New Mole   FG (occas)   Port Masters Office FR (occas)   Harbour Station   Pilot Station   Ferry Terminal   Outer Harbour   Dredged to 5m   Breakwater   Limit of dredged area   Mole   Head   Rocks   305°   295°   Berthing Sig FS   Fl(2)10s14m22M Dia(4)

Depths in metres
⚠ Contact Hr Mr

DOVER   10-3-17

Kent   51°06'·71N 01°19'·83E (W ent)
       51°07'·22N 01°20'·71E (E ent)

CHARTS
AC 1698, *1828, 1892*; Imray C8; Stanfords 9; OS 179
TIDES
0000 Dover; ML 3·7; Duration 0505; Zone 0 (UT)

Standard Port DOVER (→)

Times				Height (metres)			
High Water		Low Water		MHWS	MHWN	MLWN	MLWS
0000	0600	0100	0700	6·8	5·3	2·2	0·8
1200	1800	1300	1900				
Differences DEAL							
+0010	+0020	+0010	+0005	−0·6	−0·3	0·0	0·0

NOTE: Dover is a Standard Port and tidal predictions for each day of the year are given below.

SHELTER
Visiting yachts are welcomed and normally escorted by hbr launch to the complete shelter of the Marina at Wellington Dock. Berth as directed. Dock gates and swing bridge normally open HW ±1½. Waiting pontoon has 1·5m. Three pontoons (approx 2·5m) are available in tidal hbr, E of the waiting pontoon.
In the Outer Hbr the small craft moorings (33 W ⚓s) and ⚓ are tenable in offshore winds, but exposed to winds from NE through S to SW; in gales a heavy sea builds up. Small craft may not be left unattended at ⚓ in Outer Hbr.
NAVIGATION
WPT from SW, 51°06'·15N 01°19'·77E, 180°/000° from/to Admiralty Pier lt ho, 0·5M.
WPT from NE, 51°07'·27N 01°21'·51E, 090°/270° from/to S end Eastern Arm, 0·5M.
Beware lumpy seas/overfalls outside the bkwtrs and frequent ferries, hovercraft and jetfoils through both ents. Strong tides across ents and high walls make ent under sail slow and difficult; use of engine very strongly recommended. Comply with tfc sigs and VHF instructions of Port Control and hbr patrol launch; advise if you have no engine. Do not go between NCM buoy, Q, (marking wreck inside W ent) and S bkwtr. Beware fast hovercraft/jetfoils on rounding Prince of Wales pier.
Note: A Historic Wreck (see 10.0.3g) is adjacent to the Eastern Arm bkwtr at 51°07'·6N 01°20'·8E (see chartlet). There are four more Historic Wrecks on the Goodwin Sands in positions where a yacht would hope not to be.
LIGHTS AND MARKS
Lts as on chartlet & 10.3.4. Port Control tr (conspic) is at S end of E Arm and shows IPTS for the E ent on panels; for W ent, IPTS are on panels near Admiralty Pier sig stn.
Specific permission to ent/leave via E or W ent must first be obtained from Port Control on VHF Ch 74. Clearance for small/slow craft is not normally given until within 200m of ent. If no VHF, use following Aldis Lamp sigs:
SV (··· ··−−) = I wish to enter port
SW (··· ·−−) = I wish to leave port
Port Control will reply OK (−−− −·−) or
                Wait (·−− ·− ·· −).
A Q Ⓦ lt from Port Control tr or patrol launch = keep clear of ent you are approaching.
Marina signals: In the final approach it is important, especially near LW, to stay in the W sector (324°-333°) of the F WR lt on the waiting pontoon. IPTS are shown, plus a small Fl Ⓨ lt 5 min before bridge is swung.
RADIO TELEPHONE
Call: *Dover Port Control* VHF Ch **74** 12 16. Hbr launch and Water Taxi Ch 74. *Dover Marina* Ch 80, only within tidal hbr/marina. *Dover Coastguard* Ch **69** 16 11 80, inc TSS surveillance. Chan Nav Info Service (CNIS) broadcasts nav/wx/tidal info Ch 11 at H+40; also, if vis < 2M, at H+55.
TELEPHONE (01304)
Hr Mr 240400 Ext 4540; MRCC 210008; ☰ 224251; Marinecall 0891 500456; Police 240055; Ⓗ 201624.
FACILITIES
Marina (350+300 visitors) ☎ 241663, Fax 240465, £11.70 in marina; £9.90 in tidal hbr (both inc AC), FW, C, Slip, D; **Royal Cinque Ports YC** ☎ 206262, L, M, C, FW, Bar, R; *Dover Yachtman's Manual* from marina. **Services**: D (fuel barge in hbr), ME, EI, Sh, SM, ACA, CH, Ⓔ (H24 service). **Town** EC Wed; P (cans), V, R, Bar, ✉, Ⓑ, ⇶, ✈ (Lydd).

3

DOVER *continued*

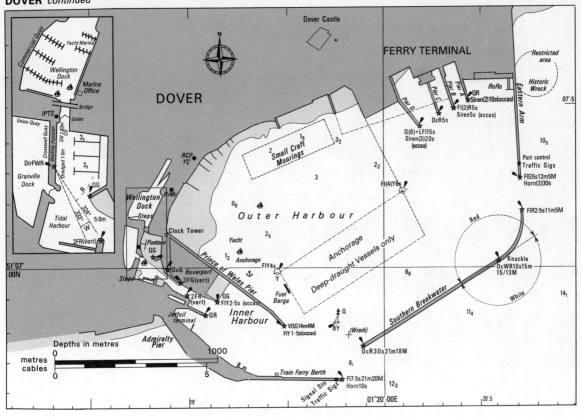

DOVER

MEAN SPRING AND NEAP CURVES

Springs occur 2 days after New and Full Moon.

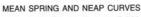

MEAN RANGES	
Springs	6·0m
Neaps	3·1m

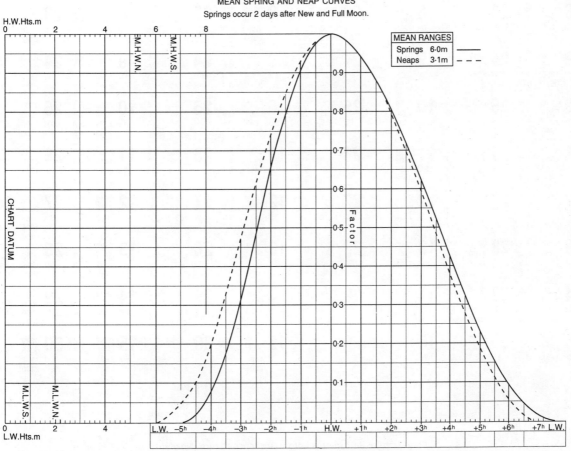

ENGLAND – DOVER

LAT 51°07′N   LONG 1°19′E

TIMES AND HEIGHTS OF HIGH AND LOW WATERS   YEAR **1996**

TIME ZONE (UT)
For Summer Time add ONE hour in non-shaded areas

JANUARY

Day	Time	m	Day	Time	m
1 M	0206 / 0734 / 1446 / 2018	2.1 / 5.7 / 1.9 / 5.6	16 TU	0100 / 0630 / 1347 / 1919	2.0 / 5.7 / 1.8 / 5.6
2 TU	0315 / 0839 / 1551 / 2113	1.9 / 5.8 / 1.7 / 5.8	17 W	0224 / 0746 / 1501 / 2024	1.9 / 5.9 / 1.5 / 5.9
3 W	0418 / 0932 / 1646 / 2158	1.7 / 6.0 / 1.4 / 6.1	18 TH	0334 / 0849 / 1608 / 2121	1.5 / 6.2 / 1.2 / 6.3
4 TH	0507 / 1016 / 1728 / 2237	1.5 / 6.2 / 1.4 / 6.3	19 F	0440 / 0945 / 1712 / 2213	1.2 / 6.5 / 1.0 / 6.6
5 F ○	0546 / 1053 / 1803 / 2313	1.3 / 6.3 / 1.3 / 6.4	20 SA ●	0543 / 1037 / 1813 / 2302	0.8 / 6.7 / 0.8 / 6.8
6 SA	0620 / 1127 / 1834 / 2346	1.2 / 6.3 / 1.3 / 6.5	21 SU	0641 / 1126 / 1909 / 2348	0.6 / 6.8 / 0.6 / 7.0
7 SU	0652 / 1159 / 1905	1.2 / 6.3 / 1.3	22 M	0734 / 1212 / 1958	0.4 / 6.9 / 0.5
8 M	0017 / 0725 / 1229 / 1937	6.5 / 1.2 / 6.3 / 1.3	23 TU	0032 / 0822 / 1257 / 2040	7.1 / 0.3 / 6.8 / 0.6
9 TU	0045 / 0759 / 1254 / 2011	6.4 / 1.2 / 6.2 / 1.3	24 W	0117 / 0905 / 1342 / 2119	7.0 / 0.4 / 6.7 / 0.7
10 W	0110 / 0834 / 1320 / 2046	6.4 / 1.3 / 6.2 / 1.3	25 TH	0201 / 0944 / 1427 / 2156	6.9 / 0.6 / 6.5 / 0.9
11 TH	0139 / 0910 / 1352 / 2121	6.4 / 1.3 / 6.2 / 1.4	26 F	0247 / 1023 / 1515 / 2234	6.6 / 0.9 / 6.2 / 1.3
12 F	0214 / 0947 / 1431 / 2200	6.3 / 1.4 / 6.1 / 1.6	27 SA	0336 / 1103 / 1608 / 2316	6.3 / 1.3 / 5.8 / 1.7
13 SA	0258 / 1028 / 1520 / 2244	6.2 / 1.5 / 5.9 / 1.8	28 SU	0430 / 1150 / 1708	5.9 / 1.7 / 5.5
14 SU	0352 / 1119 / 1622 / 2341	5.9 / 1.7 / 5.6 / 2.0	29 M	0009 / 0533 / 1250 / 1816	2.0 / 5.5 / 2.0 / 5.3
15 M	0503 / 1225 / 1751	5.7 / 1.8 / 5.5	30 TU	0118 / 0646 / 1358 / 1934	2.2 / 5.4 / 2.1 / 5.3
			31 W	0230 / 0805 / 1507 / 2045	2.2 / 5.4 / 2.0 / 5.5

FEBRUARY

Day	Time	m	Day	Time	m
1 TH	0340 / 0912 / 1609 / 2137	1.9 / 5.6 / 1.8 / 5.8	16 F	0314 / 0845 / 1553 / 2115	1.6 / 6.0 / 1.4 / 6.1
2 F	0436 / 0959 / 1659 / 2218	1.6 / 5.9 / 1.5 / 6.1	17 SA	0427 / 0944 / 1703 / 2207	1.2 / 6.3 / 1.0 / 6.5
3 SA	0521 / 1035 / 1740 / 2252	1.4 / 6.1 / 1.3 / 6.3	18 SU ●	0535 / 1035 / 1806 / 2254	0.8 / 6.6 / 0.7 / 6.8
4 SU ○	0559 / 1106 / 1815 / 2323	1.2 / 6.2 / 1.2 / 6.4	19 M	0633 / 1121 / 1858 / 2337	0.8 / 6.8 / 0.5 / 7.0
5 M	0634 / 1136 / 1849 / 2353	1.1 / 6.3 / 1.1 / 6.5	20 TU	0723 / 1202 / 1943	0.3 / 6.9 / 0.4
6 TU	0709 / 1205 / 1923	1.0 / 6.3 / 1.1	21 W	0018 / 0806 / 1241 / 2022	7.1 / 0.2 / 6.8 / 0.4
7 W	0021 / 0744 / 1232 / 1956	6.5 / 1.0 / 6.4 / 1.1	22 TH	0058 / 0845 / 1320 / 2056	7.1 / 0.3 / 6.7 / 0.6
8 TH	0048 / 0819 / 1259 / 2029	6.6 / 1.0 / 6.4 / 1.1	23 F	0138 / 0919 / 1400 / 2128	6.9 / 0.5 / 6.6 / 0.8
9 F	0117 / 0852 / 1329 / 2102	6.6 / 1.0 / 6.4 / 1.1	24 SA	0219 / 0952 / 1442 / 2159	6.7 / 0.9 / 6.3 / 1.2
10 SA	0151 / 0925 / 1406 / 2136	6.6 / 1.1 / 6.4 / 1.3	25 SU	0302 / 1025 / 1530 / 2232	6.3 / 1.3 / 5.9 / 1.6
11 SU	0231 / 1001 / 1451 / 2217	6.4 / 1.3 / 6.1 / 1.5	26 M	0351 / 1102 / 1626 / 2316	5.9 / 1.7 / 5.5 / 2.0
12 M	0320 / 1047 / 1547 / 2310	6.1 / 1.5 / 5.8 / 1.8	27 TU	0451 / 1156 / 1732	5.4 / 2.1 / 5.2
13 TU	0424 / 1148 / 1708	5.8 / 1.8 / 5.4	28 W	0026 / 0602 / 1314 / 1848	2.3 / 5.2 / 2.3 / 5.1
14 W	0023 / 0600 / 1313 / 1858	2.0 / 5.5 / 1.9 / 5.4	29 TH	0149 / 0724 / 1429 / 2009	2.3 / 5.2 / 2.2 / 5.3
15 TH	0154 / 0734 / 1439 / 2014	1.9 / 5.7 / 1.7 / 5.7			

MARCH

Day	Time	m	Day	Time	m
1 F	0301 / 0844 / 1534 / 2109	2.1 / 5.4 / 1.9 / 5.6	16 SA	0259 / 0839 / 1540 / 2103	1.6 / 5.9 / 1.4 / 6.1
2 SA	0401 / 0934 / 1628 / 2151	1.7 / 5.7 / 1.6 / 6.0	17 SU	0417 / 0937 / 1652 / 2155	1.2 / 6.3 / 1.0 / 6.5
3 SU	0451 / 1008 / 1713 / 2224	1.4 / 6.0 / 1.3 / 6.2	18 M	0523 / 1026 / 1751 / 2239	0.8 / 6.6 / 0.7 / 6.8
4 M	0533 / 1038 / 1752 / 2254	1.2 / 6.2 / 1.2 / 6.4	19 TU ●	0618 / 1107 / 1840 / 2320	0.5 / 6.7 / 0.5 / 7.0
5 TU ○	0611 / 1108 / 1828 / 2324	1.0 / 6.3 / 1.0 / 6.5	20 W	0705 / 1145 / 1921 / 2359	0.3 / 6.8 / 0.5 / 7.0
6 W	0649 / 1138 / 1903 / 2354	0.9 / 6.4 / 1.0 / 6.6	21 TH	0745 / 1220 / 1958	0.3 / 6.8 / 0.5
7 TH	0725 / 1207 / 1937	0.8 / 6.5 / 0.9	22 F	0037 / 0820 / 1257 / 2029	7.0 / 0.4 / 6.8 / 0.6
8 F	0024 / 0759 / 1237 / 2010	6.7 / 0.8 / 6.6 / 0.9	23 SA	0115 / 0851 / 1334 / 2059	6.9 / 0.7 / 6.6 / 0.9
9 SA	0055 / 0832 / 1309 / 2043	6.7 / 0.8 / 6.6 / 0.9	24 SU	0152 / 0919 / 1413 / 2125	6.6 / 1.0 / 6.3 / 1.2
10 SU	0130 / 0904 / 1347 / 2118	6.7 / 0.9 / 6.5 / 1.1	25 M	0231 / 0945 / 1456 / 2153	6.3 / 1.4 / 6.0 / 1.5
11 M	0210 / 0941 / 1432 / 2159	6.5 / 1.2 / 6.3 / 1.3	26 TU	0315 / 1014 / 1548 / 2230	5.9 / 1.7 / 5.6 / 1.9
12 TU	0259 / 1026 / 1528 / 2251	6.2 / 1.5 / 5.9 / 1.7	27 W	0413 / 1057 / 1651 / 2329	5.4 / 2.1 / 5.3 / 2.2
13 W	0404 / 1126 / 1652	5.7 / 1.8 / 5.4	28 TH	0524 / 1221 / 1803	5.1 / 2.4 / 5.1
14 TH	0004 / 0550 / 1253 / 1841	2.0 / 5.4 / 2.0 / 5.4	29 F	0103 / 0638 / 1349 / 1919	2.3 / 5.1 / 2.3 / 5.2
15 F	0136 / 0726 / 1423 / 2001	1.9 / 5.5 / 1.8 / 5.7	30 SA	0219 / 0755 / 1455 / 2024	2.1 / 5.3 / 2.0 / 5.5
			31 SU	0320 / 0850 / 1550 / 2110	1.8 / 5.6 / 1.7 / 5.8

APRIL

Day	Time	m	Day	Time	m
1 M	0412 / 0929 / 1638 / 2146	1.4 / 5.9 / 1.4 / 6.1	16 TU	0504 / 1008 / 1728 / 2220	0.8 / 6.5 / 0.9 / 6.7
2 TU	0458 / 1003 / 1721 / 2219	1.2 / 6.2 / 1.2 / 6.4	17 W ●	0556 / 1047 / 1815 / 2300	0.6 / 6.6 / 0.7 / 6.8
3 W	0542 / 1036 / 1801 / 2252	1.0 / 6.4 / 1.0 / 6.5	18 TH	0641 / 1123 / 1855 / 2339	0.5 / 6.7 / 0.7 / 6.9
4 TH	0623 / 1109 / 1839 / 2326	0.8 / 6.5 / 0.9 / 6.7	19 F	0719 / 1159 / 1931	0.6 / 6.8 / 0.7
5 F	0702 / 1142 / 1916	0.8 / 6.6 / 0.8	20 SA	0016 / 0752 / 1236 / 2002	6.8 / 0.7 / 6.7 / 0.8
6 SA	0000 / 0738 / 1216 / 1951	6.8 / 0.7 / 6.7 / 0.8	21 SU	0053 / 0821 / 1312 / 2030	6.7 / 0.9 / 6.6 / 1.0
7 SU	0035 / 0812 / 1253 / 2026	6.8 / 0.7 / 6.7 / 0.8	22 M	0129 / 0846 / 1349 / 2054	6.5 / 1.1 / 6.4 / 1.2
8 M	0114 / 0848 / 1334 / 2104	6.7 / 0.9 / 6.6 / 1.0	23 TU	0204 / 0909 / 1428 / 2122	6.2 / 1.4 / 6.1 / 1.5
9 TU	0157 / 0927 / 1423 / 2149	6.5 / 1.1 / 6.3 / 1.2	24 W	0243 / 0939 / 1512 / 2159	5.9 / 1.7 / 5.8 / 1.8
10 W	0250 / 1014 / 1524 / 2243	6.1 / 1.4 / 5.9 / 1.6	25 TH	0336 / 1020 / 1609 / 2250	5.5 / 2.0 / 5.5 / 2.0
11 TH	0404 / 1116 / 1647 / 2357	5.7 / 1.8 / 5.6 / 1.8	26 F	0444 / 1119 / 1716	5.2 / 2.3 / 5.2
12 F	0542 / 1242 / 1820	5.5 / 1.9 / 5.5	27 SA	0007 / 0554 / 1255 / 1825	2.2 / 5.1 / 2.3 / 5.2
13 SA	0122 / 0712 / 1407 / 1941	1.8 / 5.6 / 1.8 / 5.7	28 SU	0131 / 0702 / 1408 / 1929	2.1 / 5.2 / 2.1 / 5.4
14 SU	0243 / 0825 / 1522 / 2044	1.5 / 5.9 / 1.4 / 6.1	29 M	0235 / 0800 / 1506 / 2021	1.8 / 5.5 / 1.8 / 5.7
15 M	0359 / 0922 / 1631 / 2135	1.2 / 6.2 / 1.1 / 6.4	30 TU	0329 / 0846 / 1557 / 2103	1.5 / 5.8 / 1.5 / 6.1

Chart Datum: 3·67 metres below Ordnance Datum (Newlyn)

ENGLAND – DOVER

LAT 51°07′N LONG 1°19′E

TIMES AND HEIGHTS OF HIGH AND LOW WATERS

YEAR **1996**

3

TIME ZONE (UT)
For Summer Time add ONE hour in non-shaded areas

MAY

Day	Time	m	Day	Time	m
1 W	0420	1.2	**16** TH	0530	0.9
	0925	6.1		1024	6.4
	1645	1.3		1747	1.0
	2142	6.3		2239	6.6
2 TH	0508	1.0	**17** F	0615	0.9
	1003	6.4		1102	6.6
	1730	1.1		1828	0.9
	2220	6.6		● 2319	6.6
3 F	0554	0.9	**18** SA	0652	0.9
	1040	6.6		1139	6.6
	1813	0.9		1904	0.9
O	2258	6.7		2357	6.6
4 SA	0638	0.7	**19** SU	0725	1.0
	1118	6.7		1216	6.6
	1855	0.8		1936	1.0
	2337	6.8			
5 SU	0718	0.7	**20** M	0033	6.5
	1158	6.8		0752	1.1
	1935	0.7		1253	6.5
				2003	1.1
6 M	0018	6.8	**21** TU	0108	6.4
	0757	0.7		0816	1.3
	1241	6.8		1328	6.4
	2015	0.8		2030	1.3
7 TU	0103	6.7	**22** W	0141	6.2
	0838	0.8		0842	1.4
	1328	6.7		1403	6.2
	2059	0.9		2100	1.4
8 W	0152	6.5	**23** TH	0215	5.9
	0921	1.0		0915	1.6
	1421	6.4		1438	6.0
	2147	1.1		2138	1.6
9 TH	0251	6.2	**24** F	0254	5.7
	1012	1.3		0955	1.8
	1523	6.1		1521	5.7
	2244	1.4		2223	1.8
10 F	0403	5.9	**25** SA	0350	5.4
	1114	1.6		1043	2.0
	1634	5.9		1618	5.5
	2352	1.6		2320	2.0
11 SA	0524	5.7	**26** SU	0502	5.3
	1228	1.7		1146	2.2
	1751	5.7		1726	5.4
12 SU	0106	1.6	**27** M	0033	2.0
	0647	5.7		0610	5.3
	1342	1.7		1309	2.1
	1910	5.8		1832	5.5
13 M	0219	1.5	**28** TU	0145	1.9
	0800	5.8		0711	5.5
	1452	1.5		1417	1.9
	2017	6.0		1930	5.7
14 TU	0331	1.2	**29** W	0246	1.6
	0857	6.1		0803	5.8
	1600	1.3		1515	1.7
	2111	6.3		2020	6.0
15 W	0437	1.0	**30** TH	0341	1.3
	0944	6.3		0849	6.1
	1659	1.1		1608	1.4
	2157	6.5		2106	6.3
			31 F	0435	1.1
				0932	6.4
				1700	1.1
				2150	6.6

JUNE

Day	Time	m	Day	Time	m
1 SA	0526	0.9	**16** SU	0626	1.2
	1015	6.6		1120	6.5
	1749	0.9		1839	1.1
O	2235	6.7	●	2339	6.4
2 SU	0615	0.8	**17** M	0658	1.2
	1100	6.8		1157	6.5
	1837	0.8		1912	1.1
	2320	6.8			
3 M	0703	0.7	**18** TU	0015	6.4
	1145	6.9		0726	1.2
	1924	0.7		1234	6.5
				1941	1.1
4 TU	0007	6.8	**19** W	0048	6.3
	0749	0.7		0753	1.3
	1233	6.9		1307	6.4
	2011	0.7		2010	1.2
5 W	0056	6.7	**20** TH	0119	6.2
	0835	0.7		0822	1.3
	1323	6.8		1337	6.3
	2059	0.7		2043	1.3
6 TH	0148	6.6	**21** F	0147	6.0
	0922	0.9		0856	1.4
	1415	6.6		1606	6.2
	2149	0.9		2119	1.4
7 F	0246	6.3	**22** SA	0216	5.9
	1012	1.1		0933	1.6
	1512	6.4		1439	6.0
	2242	1.1		2159	1.5
8 SA	0349	6.1	**23** SU	0254	5.7
	1106	1.3		1017	1.7
	1612	6.2		1522	5.8
	2339	1.3		2244	1.7
9 SU	0456	5.9	**24** M	0345	5.6
	1206	1.5		1102	1.9
	1717	6.0		1619	5.7
				2338	1.8
10 M	0041	1.4	**25** TU	0457	5.4
	0609	5.7		1202	2.0
	1310	1.7		1729	5.6
	1829	5.9			
11 TU	0146	1.5	**26** W	0047	1.8
	0723	5.7		0616	5.5
	1415	1.7		1321	2.0
	1941	5.9		1840	5.7
12 W	0255	1.5	**27** TH	0200	1.7
	0826	5.8		0722	5.7
	1522	1.6		1432	1.8
	2043	6.0		1943	5.9
13 TH	0403	1.4	**28** F	0305	1.5
	0918	6.0		0830	6.0
	1626	1.4		1535	1.5
	2135	6.2		2038	6.2
14 F	0501	1.2	**29** SA	0405	1.2
	1002	6.2		0909	6.3
	1719	1.3		1633	1.2
	2220	6.3		2130	6.5
15 SA	0547	1.2	**30** SU	0502	1.0
	1042	6.4		0959	6.5
	1802	1.2		1729	0.9
	2301	6.4		2220	6.7

JULY

Day	Time	m	Day	Time	m
1 M	0558	0.8	**16** TU	0634	1.3
	1047	6.8		1138	6.5
	1823	0.7		1849	1.2
O	2310	6.8		2355	6.3
2 TU	0652	0.7	**17** W	0704	1.2
	1136	6.9		1212	6.5
	1917	0.6		1920	1.1
	2359	6.8			
3 W	0745	0.6	**18** TH	0026	6.3
	1224	7.0		0732	1.2
	2009	0.5		1243	6.5
				1951	1.1
4 TH	0048	6.8	**19** F	0054	6.2
	0833	0.6		0803	1.2
	1313	7.0		1310	6.4
	2057	0.5		2024	1.2
5 F	0138	6.7	**20** SA	0118	6.2
	0919	0.7		0836	1.3
	1402	6.9		1336	6.3
	2143	0.6		2059	1.2
6 SA	0230	6.5	**21** SU	0144	6.1
	1002	0.8		0911	1.4
	1453	6.7		1405	6.3
	2229	0.8		2134	1.3
7 SU	0325	6.3	**22** M	0217	6.1
	1047	1.1		0947	1.5
	1546	6.4		1443	6.2
	2316	1.1		2211	1.5
8 M	0422	6.0	**23** TU	0300	5.9
	1136	1.4		1027	1.7
	1643	6.1		1531	6.0
				2255	1.6
9 TU	0008	1.4	**24** W	0355	5.7
	0524	5.7		1116	1.9
	1232	1.7		1633	5.7
	1746	5.8		2352	1.8
10 W	0108	1.7	**25** TH	0512	5.5
	0635	5.6		1224	2.0
	1336	1.9		1755	5.6
	1859	5.7			
11 TH	0215	1.8	**26** F	0112	1.9
	0748	5.6		0646	5.6
	1444	1.9		1352	1.9
	2013	5.7		1915	5.8
12 F	0324	1.7	**27** SA	0233	1.7
	0851	5.8		0757	5.8
	1553	1.7		1506	1.6
	2115	5.9		2022	6.1
13 SA	0429	1.6	**28** SU	0341	1.4
	0942	6.0		0856	6.2
	1651	1.5		1611	1.3
	2205	6.1		2120	6.3
14 SU	0519	1.4	**29** M	0444	1.1
	1024	6.2		0949	6.5
	1738	1.3		1713	0.9
	2246	6.2		2213	6.6
15 M	0600	1.3	**30** TU	0545	0.8
	1102	6.4		1038	6.8
	1816	1.2		1814	0.7
●	2322	6.3	O	2304	6.8
			31 W	0644	0.7
				1126	7.0
				1910	0.4
				2351	6.9

AUGUST

Day	Time	m	Day	Time	m
1 TH	0737	0.5	**16** F	0711	1.2
	1211	7.1		1214	6.5
	2001	0.3		1930	1.0
2 F	0037	6.9	**17** SA	0026	6.3
	0823	0.5		0742	1.1
	1257	7.1		1241	6.5
	2046	0.3		2003	1.0
3 SA	0122	6.8	**18** SU	0050	6.3
	0904	0.5		0815	1.2
	1342	7.0		1307	6.5
	2127	0.4		2036	1.1
4 SU	0208	6.6	**19** M	0116	6.4
	0942	0.7		0847	1.2
	1428	6.8		1336	6.5
	2206	0.7		2108	1.2
5 M	0255	6.4	**20** TU	0148	6.3
	1020	1.0		0920	1.3
	1517	6.5		1412	6.4
	2246	1.1		2142	1.3
6 TU	0347	6.1	**21** W	0228	6.2
	1101	1.4		0958	1.5
	1609	6.1		1457	6.2
	2331	1.5		2222	1.6
7 W	0444	5.7	**22** TH	0319	5.9
	1152	1.8		1044	1.8
	1709	5.7		1554	5.8
				2315	1.8
8 TH	0028	1.9	**23** F	0429	5.5
	0549	5.4		1147	2.0
	1256	2.1		1722	5.5
	1818	5.5			
9 F	0136	2.1	**24** SA	0031	2.0
	0706	5.4		0624	5.4
	1409	2.1		1320	2.1
	1940	5.4		1901	5.6
10 SA	0249	2.0	**25** SU	0209	1.9
	0824	5.5		0744	5.7
	1522	1.9		1445	1.8
	2058	5.6		2014	5.9
11 SU	0356	1.8	**26** M	0324	1.5
	0922	5.8		0846	6.1
	1624	1.6		1556	1.3
	2150	5.9		2115	6.3
12 M	0451	1.6	**27** TU	0430	1.2
	1005	6.1		0939	6.5
	1713	1.4		1702	0.9
	2229	6.1		2208	6.6
13 TU	0535	1.4	**28** W	0533	0.9
	1042	6.4		1027	6.8
	1752	1.2		1803	0.6
	2301	6.3	O	2256	6.8
14 W	0610	1.3	**29** TH	0630	0.6
	1114	6.5		1112	7.1
	1826	1.1		1857	0.4
●	2330	6.3		2339	6.9
15 TH	0641	1.2	**30** F	0720	0.5
	1145	6.5		1155	7.2
	1858	1.1		1944	0.3
	2359	6.4			
			31 SA	0019	7.0
				0802	0.5
				1237	7.2
				2025	0.3

Chart Datum: 3·67 metres below Ordnance Datum (Newlyn)

ENGLAND – DOVER

LAT 51°07'N LONG 1°19'E

TIMES AND HEIGHTS OF HIGH AND LOW WATERS

YEAR **1996**

TIME ZONE (UT)
For Summer Time add ONE hour in non-shaded areas

SEPTEMBER

Day	Time	m	Time	m	Time	m	Time	m
1 SU	0100	6.9	0840	0.6	1319	7.1	2102	0.5
16 M	0022	6.5	0751	1.1	1240	6.7	2012	1.0
2 M	0141	6.7	0914	0.8	1402	6.8	2137	0.8
17 TU	0051	6.6	0824	1.1	1311	6.6	2043	1.1
3 TU	0225	6.5	0949	1.1	1447	6.5	2212	1.2
18 W	0124	6.5	0857	1.3	1347	6.5	2117	1.3
4 W	0313	6.1	1025	1.5	1537	6.1	2251	1.7
19 TH	0205	6.3	0935	1.5	1432	6.2	2158	1.6
5 TH	0409	5.7	1108	1.9	1635	5.6	2343	2.1
20 F	0256	6.0	1022	1.8	1530	5.8	2250	1.9
6 F	0512	5.4	1213	2.3	1742	5.3		
21 SA	0410	5.6	1126	2.1	1712	5.5		
7 SA	0057	2.4	0625	5.3	1334	2.3	1901	5.2
22 SU	0006	2.1	0608	5.4	1300	2.1	1851	5.4
8 SU	0215	2.3	0749	5.4	1449	2.1	2034	5.5
23 M	0151	2.0	0729	5.7	1429	1.8	2005	5.9
9 M	0323	2.0	0855	5.7	1553	1.8	2128	5.8
24 TU	0309	1.6	0832	6.1	1543	1.3	2106	6.3
10 TU	0420	1.7	0939	6.1	1642	1.5	2204	6.1
25 W	0416	1.2	0925	6.5	1649	0.9	2157	6.6
11 W	0505	1.4	1014	6.3	1723	1.2	2232	6.3
26 TH	0517	0.9	1011	6.9	1747	0.6	2241	6.8
12 TH	0542	1.3	1044	6.5	1758	1.1	● 2259	6.4
27 F	0610	0.7	1054	7.1	1837	0.5	O 2321	6.9
13 F	0614	1.2	1114	6.6	1832	1.0	2328	6.5
28 SA	0656	0.6	1135	7.2	1922	0.4	2358	7.0
14 SA	0646	1.1	1143	6.6	1906	1.0	2356	6.5
29 SU	0736	0.6	1215	7.1	2000	0.5		
15 SU	0719	1.1	1211	6.6	1940	1.0		
30 M	0036	6.9	0812	0.7	1255	7.0	2034	0.7

OCTOBER

Day	Time	m	Time	m	Time	m	Time	m
1 TU	0116	6.7	0845	0.9	1335	6.8	2105	1.0
16 W	0030	6.7	0804	1.1	1250	6.7	2023	1.1
2 W	0157	6.5	0916	1.2	1418	6.4	2135	1.4
17 TH	0108	6.6	0840	1.2	1330	6.6	2100	1.3
3 TH	0242	6.2	0946	1.6	1505	6.0	2205	1.8
18 F	0152	6.4	0921	1.4	1418	6.2	2143	1.6
4 F	0335	5.8	1023	2.0	1602	5.6	2246	2.2
19 SA	0247	6.1	1011	1.7	1523	5.8	2237	1.9
5 SA	0436	5.5	1120	2.3	1707	5.3		
20 SU	0407	5.7	1116	2.0	1706	5.6	2354	2.1
6 SU	0005	2.5	0545	5.3	1250	2.5	1819	5.2
21 M	0546	5.6	1245	2.0	1835	5.6		
7 M	0135	2.5	0702	5.3	1409	2.3	1942	5.3
22 TU	0130	2.0	0707	5.8	1410	1.8	1949	5.9
8 TU	0244	2.2	0813	5.6	1511	1.9	2045	5.7
23 W	0248	1.7	0812	6.1	1524	1.4	2049	6.2
9 W	0341	1.9	0900	6.0	1602	1.6	2122	6.0
24 TH	0356	1.3	0905	6.5	1630	1.0	2139	6.5
10 TH	0427	1.6	0935	6.2	1645	1.3	2153	6.2
25 F	0455	1.0	0952	6.8	1726	0.8	2222	6.7
11 F	0507	1.4	1007	6.5	1725	1.1	2224	6.4
26 SA	0546	0.9	1034	7.0	1814	0.7	O 2300	6.7
12 SA	0543	1.2	1038	6.6	1803	1.0	● 2255	6.5
27 SU	0630	0.8	1114	7.0	1856	0.7	2337	6.9
13 SU	0619	1.1	1110	6.7	1840	1.0	2326	6.6
28 M	0709	0.8	1154	7.0	1933	0.8		
14 M	0654	1.1	1142	6.8	1916	0.9	2357	6.7
29 TU	0014	6.8	0744	0.9	1233	6.9	2005	1.0
15 TU	0729	1.0	1215	6.8	1950	1.0		
30 W	0053	6.7	0816	1.1	1311	6.7	2034	1.2
31 TH	0132	6.5	0845	1.3	1351	6.4	2059	1.5

NOVEMBER

Day	Time	m	Time	m	Time	m	Time	m
1 F	0214	6.3	0913	1.6	1435	6.0	2126	1.8
16 SA	0147	6.5	0916	1.3	1414	6.3	2137	1.4
2 SA	0301	5.9	0947	1.9	1527	5.7	2203	2.1
17 SU	0245	6.3	1009	1.5	1522	6.0	2232	1.7
3 SU	0357	5.6	1035	2.2	1630	5.3	2256	2.4
18 M	0356	6.0	1113	1.7	1646	5.7	2343	1.9
4 M	0501	5.4	1148	2.4	1738	5.2		
19 TU	0515	5.8	1227	1.8	1809	5.7		
5 TU	0031	2.6	0610	5.3	1314	2.3	1846	5.3
20 W	0103	1.9	0635	5.9	1343	1.7	1923	5.8
6 W	0152	2.4	0716	5.5	1420	2.1	1947	5.5
21 TH	0217	1.8	0744	6.0	1456	1.5	2025	6.0
7 TH	0252	2.1	0809	5.8	1515	1.7	2034	5.8
22 F	0325	1.5	0841	6.3	1604	1.2	2117	6.3
8 F	0343	1.8	0851	6.1	1604	1.4	2113	6.1
23 SA	0428	1.3	0930	6.5	1702	1.0	2201	6.5
9 SA	0429	1.5	0927	6.4	1650	1.2	2149	6.4
24 SU	0521	1.1	1015	6.7	1751	0.9	2240	6.6
10 SU	0511	1.3	1003	6.6	1733	1.1	2224	6.6
25 M	0606	1.0	1056	6.8	1832	1.0	O 2318	6.7
11 M	0552	1.1	1040	6.7	1814	1.0	● 2259	6.7
26 TU	0645	1.0	1135	6.8	1907	1.0	2356	6.7
12 TU	0632	1.0	1117	6.8	1854	0.9	2336	6.8
27 W	0720	1.1	1214	6.7	1939	1.2		
13 W	0711	1.0	1155	6.8	1932	0.9		
28 TH	0034	6.7	0752	1.2	1251	6.5	2005	1.3
14 TH	0015	6.8	0749	1.0	1236	6.8	2009	1.0
29 F	0112	6.6	0820	1.3	1328	6.3	2030	1.5
15 F	0058	6.7	0830	1.1	1321	6.6	2050	1.2
30 SA	0149	6.4	0849	1.5	1405	6.1	2059	1.7

DECEMBER

Day	Time	m	Time	m	Time	m	Time	m
1 SU	0226	6.1	0923	1.7	1446	5.8	2136	1.9
16 M	0236	6.5	1008	1.1	1509	6.2	2227	1.4
2 M	0308	5.8	1005	1.9	1539	5.5	2221	2.1
17 TU	0335	6.3	1103	1.3	1617	5.9	2325	1.6
3 TU	0402	5.6	1057	2.1	1645	5.3	2317	2.3
18 W	0441	6.1	1203	1.5	1729	5.8		
4 W	0508	5.4	1205	2.2	1753	5.2		
19 TH	0029	1.8	0552	5.9	1309	1.6	1844	5.7
5 TH	0037	2.4	0615	5.4	1321	2.1	1855	5.4
20 F	0137	1.8	0707	5.9	1418	1.6	1953	5.8
6 F	0154	2.2	0715	5.6	1425	1.9	1948	5.6
21 SA	0247	1.8	0813	6.0	1530	1.5	2052	6.0
7 SA	0256	2.0	0806	5.9	1522	1.6	2034	6.0
22 SU	0357	1.6	0910	6.2	1636	1.4	2141	6.2
8 SU	0350	1.6	0850	6.2	1615	1.3	2116	6.3
23 M	0457	1.4	0959	6.3	1728	1.2	2224	6.4
9 M	0440	1.4	0932	6.5	1704	1.1	2157	6.5
24 TU	0544	1.2	1042	6.5	1810	1.2	O 2303	6.5
10 TU	0527	1.1	1014	6.7	1751	1.0	● 2239	6.7
25 W	0625	1.1	1121	6.5	1846	1.2	2341	6.6
11 W	0612	1.0	1057	6.8	1836	0.9	2321	6.8
26 TH	0701	1.1	1158	6.5	1917	1.2		
12 TH	0657	0.9	1141	6.9	1920	0.9		
27 F	0017	6.6	0732	1.2	1234	6.4	1943	1.3
13 F	0005	6.9	0742	0.8	1227	6.8	2003	0.9
28 SA	0053	6.2	0801	1.2	1307	6.3	2009	1.4
14 SA	0052	6.9	0829	0.8	1315	6.7	2049	1.0
29 SU	0125	6.4	0830	1.3	1337	6.1	2040	1.5
15 SU	0142	6.7	0917	1.0	1408	6.5	2136	1.2
30 M	0153	6.3	0903	1.4	1405	6.0	2114	1.6
31 TU	0221	6.1	0941	1.5	1437	5.8	2153	1.8

Chart Datum: 3·67 metres below Ordnance Datum (Newlyn)

RAMSGATE   10-3-18

Kent 51°19'·48N 01°25'·60E

CHARTS
AC 1827, *1828, 323*; Imray C1, C8; Stanfords 5, 9; OS 179

TIDES
+0030 Dover; ML 2·7; Duration 0530; Zone 0 (UT)

Standard Port DOVER (←)

Times				Height (metres)			
High Water		Low Water		MHWS	MHWN	MLWN	MLWS
0000	0600	0100	0700	6·8	5·3	2·2	0·8
1200	1800	1300	1900				
Differences RAMSGATE							
+0030	+0030	+0017	+0007	−1·6	−1·3	−0·8	−0·4
RICHBOROUGH							
+0015	+0015	+0030	+0030	−3·4	−2·6	−1·7	−0·7

HW Broadstairs = HW Dover +0037 approx.

SHELTER
Good in marina, min depth 3m. Access approx HW ±2 via flap gate and lifting bridge. Outside and close NE of the marina ent, 107 pontoon berths (2m) are accessible H24, protected by wavebreaks; (273 more berths are planned). **Anti-Rabies Byelaw:** Animals, inc dogs/cats, are totally banned ashore or afloat within the Royal Hbr limits.

NAVIGATION
WPT 51°19'·40N 01°27'·80E, 090°/270° from/to S bkwtr, 1·45M. Many ferries/jetfoils uses the well-marked main E-W chan (3·3M long, dredged 7·5m, 110m wide; as upper chartlet). Jetfoils are 'flying' at 40kn within the buoyed chan. For ent/dep yachts must use the Recommended Yacht Track parallel to, and on the S side of, the main buoyed chan.

Enter/dep under power; or advise Port Control if unable to motor. Holding area to the S of the S bkwtr must be used by yachts to keep the hbr ent clear for ferry tfc. Beware Dike Bank to the N and Quern Bank close S of the appr chan. Cross Ledge and Brake shoals are further S.

LIGHTS AND MARKS
Ldg lts 270°: front Dir Oc WRG 10s 10m 5M, G259°-269°, W269°-271°, R271°-281°; rear, Oc 5s 17m 5M.
N bkwtr hd = QG 10m 5M; S bkwtr hd = VQ R 10m 5M.
IPTS at W Pier control appr chan, outer hbr and ent to Royal Hbr. Also at W Pier, depth between piers indicated by Ⓡ = >3m; Ⓖ = <3m.
Ent to marina controlled by separate IPTS to stbd of ent. Siren sounded approx 10 mins before gate closes; non-opening indicated by R ● or Ⓡ.
Quern Bank, 0·5M SE of the hbr ent, is marked on its N side by Quern Bank NCM lt buoy, Q, and on the W by a WCM lt buoy, Fl (9) 15s.

RADIO TELEPHONE
Call *Port Control* Ch 14 (H24) to enter/cross main chan & hbr; due to frequent tfc, yachts **must** comply with any orders. Also on Ch 14, call *Dock Office* for marina berth.

TELEPHONE (01843)
Hr Mr 592277, Fax 590941; Broadstairs Hr Mr 861879; MRCC (01304) 210008; ⌗ (01304) 202441; Marinecall 0891 500456; Police 581724; Dr 852853; Ⓗ 225544.

FACILITIES
Marina (400+100 visitors) ☎ 592277, Fax 590941, AC, FW, Slip, C (20 ton), Ⓔ, ME, El, Sh, BH, CH, ACA, Gaz, SM, Ⓞ; **Outer Hbr** (107 berths), 2m, access H24, AC, FW. P & D from Fuel Barge, *Foy Boat* Ch 14 or ☎ 592662.
Royal Temple YC ☎ 591766, Bar.
Town EC Thurs; Gas, Gaz, V, R, Bar, ✉, Ⓑ, ⇌, ✈ (Manston).

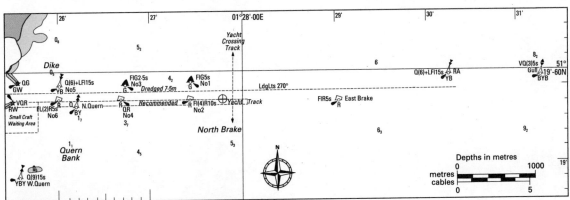

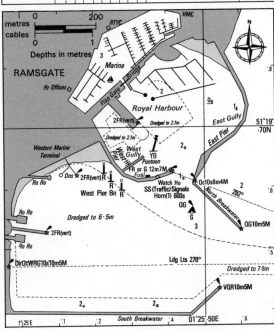

ADJACENT HARBOUR

SANDWICH, Kent, 51°16'·80N 01°21'·30E. AC *1828*. Tides above. Richborough ML 1·4m; Duration 0520. Access HW ±2 for draft 2m to reach Sandwich at sp; arrive off river ent at HW Dover. Sandwich is on the S bank of the River Stour, 3M SSE of the conspic cooling trs and chy at Richborough power stn. From Ramsgate the chy on with LH cooling tr leads approx 257° to the ent marked by SWM By, Fl 10s, 51°19'·10N 01°24'·60E. Thence past Shell Ness via bn Fl R 10s and lateral buoys, all with rotating reflective topmarks (spotlight needed, but night ent definitely not for visitors). Visitors' berths at Sandwich Town Quay ☎ (01304) 613283. Limited turning room before the swing bridge. Facilities: EC Wed; Slip; ⌗ ☎ 202441; **Marina** (50+some visitors) ☎ 613783 (max LOA 18m, 2·1m draft), BH (15 ton), Sh, Slip, FW, SM, CH, ME, Gas; D & P (cans from garage); **Sandwich Sailing and Motorboat Club** ☎ 611116 and **Sandwich Bay Sailing and Water Ski Clubs** offer some facilities. Both ports are administered by Sandwich Port & Haven Commissioners.

Volvo Penta service

Sales and service centres in area 4

KENT *John Hawkins Marine*, Ships Stores, Medway Bridge Marina, Manor Lane, Borstal, Rochester ME1 3HS Tel (01634) 840812 **ESSEX** *Volspec Ltd*, Woodrolfe Road, Tollesbury, Maldon CM9 8SE Tel (01621) 869756 *French Marine Motors Ltd*, 61/63 Waterside, Brightlingsea CO7 0AX Tel (01206) 302133 **NORFOLK** *Marinepower Engineering*, The Mill, (off Station Road), Wood Green, Salhouse, Norwich NR13 6NS Tel (01603) 720001 **NORTHAMPTONSHIRE** *CVS Pentapower*, St. Andrews Road, Northampton NN1 2LF Tel (01604) 38537/ 38409/36173 **SUFFOLK** *A. D. Truman Ltd*, Old Maltings Boatyard, Caldecott Road, Oulton Broad, Lowestoft NR32 3PH Tel (01502) 565950 *French Marine Motors Ltd*, Suffolk Yacht Harbour, Levington, Ipswich IP10 0LN Tel (01473) 659882 *Volspec Ltd*, Woolverstone Marina, Woolverstone, Ipswich IP9 1AS Tel (01473) 780144

VOLVO PENTA

Area 4 4

Thames Estuary
North Foreland to Great Yarmouth

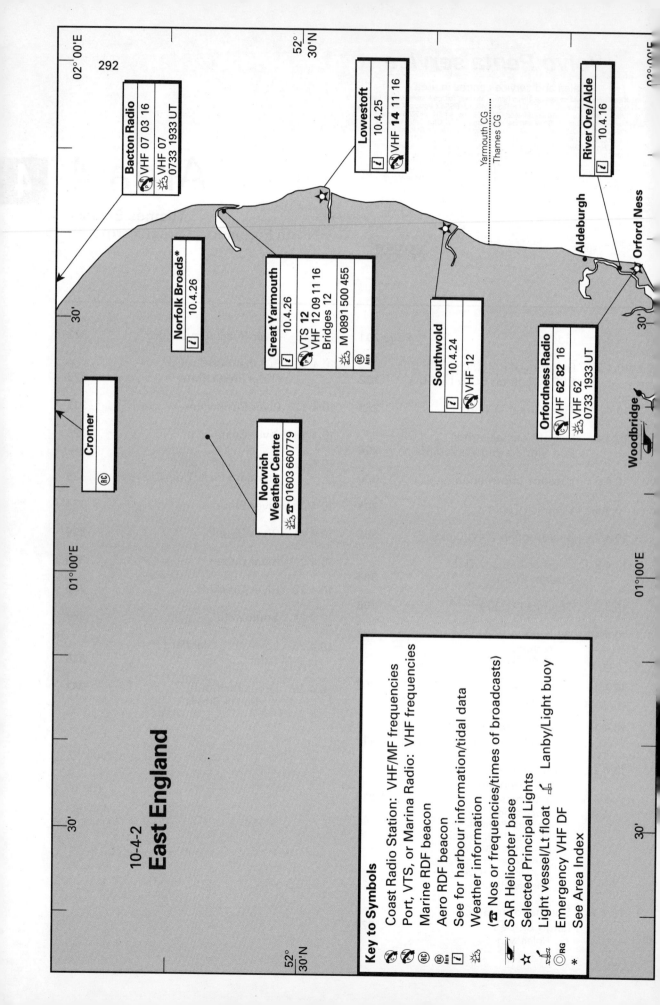

10-4-2
East England

Bacton Radio
🌊 VHF 07 03 16
☁ VHF 07
0733 1933 UT

Lowestoft
ℹ 10.4.25
🌊 VHF **14** 11 16

River Ore/Alde
ℹ 10.4.16

Norfolk Broads*
ℹ 10.4.26

Great Yarmouth
ℹ 10.4.26
🌊 VTS **12**
VHF 12 09 11 16
Bridges 12
☁ M 0891 500 455
RC Aero

Southwold
ℹ 10.4.24
🌊 VHF 12

Yarmouth CG
Thames CG

Cromer
RC

Aldeburgh

Orford Ness

Norwich
Weather Centre
☁ ☎ 01603 660779

Orfordness Radio
🌊 VHF 62 82 16
☁ VHF 62
0733 1933 UT

Woodbridge

52°
30'N

02° 00'E

30'

52°
30'N

01° 00'E

30'

01° 00'E

30'

Key to Symbols

🌊 Coast Radio Station: VHF/MF frequencies
🌊 Port, VTS, or Marina Radio: VHF frequencies
RC Marine RDF beacon
RC Aero RDF beacon
ℹ See for harbour information/tidal data
☁ Weather information
(☎ Nos or frequencies/times of broadcasts)
⛵ SAR Helicopter base
☆ Selected Principal Lights
⚓ Light vessel/Lt float ⚓ Lanby/Light buoy
◎RG Emergency VHF DF
* See Area Index

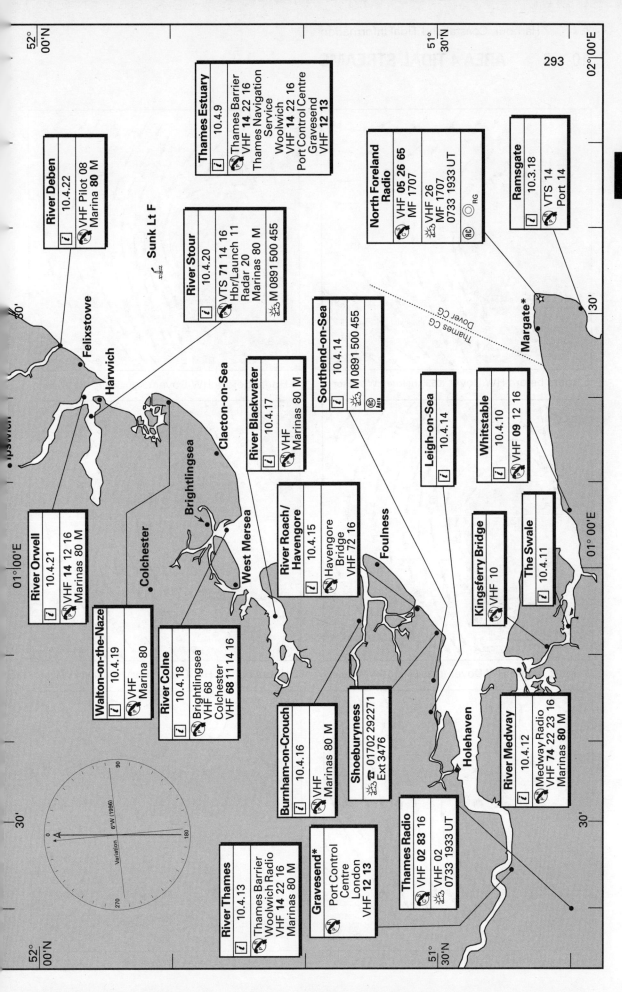

4

River Deben
10.4.22
i
VHF Pilot 08
Marina **80** M

Thames Estuary
10.4.9
i
Thames Barrier
VHF **14** 22 16
Thames Navigation
Service
Woolwich
VHF **14** 22 16
Port Control Centre
Gravesend
VHF **12 13**

North Foreland Radio
VHF **05 26 65**
MF 1707
VHF **26**
MF 1707
0733 1933 UT
RC RG

Ramsgate
10.3.18
i
VTS **14**
Port 14

Sunk Lt F

River Stour
10.4.20
i
VTS **71** 14 16
Hbr/Launch 11
Radar 20
Marinas **80** M
M 0891 500 455

Felixstowe

Harwich

Southend-on-Sea
10.4.14
i
M 0891 500 455
RC Aero

Thames CG
Dover CG

Margate*

30'

River Orwell
10.4.21
i
VHF **14** 12 16
Marinas **80** M

Ipswich

Clacton-on-Sea

River Blackwater
10.4.17
i
VHF
Marinas **80** M

Leigh-on-Sea
10.4.14
i

Whitstable
10.4.10
i
VHF **09** 12 16

Walton-on-the-Naze
10.4.19
i
VHF
Marina 80

Brightlingsea

West Mersea

Colchester

River Roach/Havengore
10.4.15
i
Havengore
Bridge
VHF **72** 16

Foulness

Kingsferry Bridge
VHF 10

The Swale
10.4.11
i

01° 00'E

River Colne
10.4.18
i
Brightlingsea
VHF 68
Colchester
VHF **68** 11 14 16

Burnham-on-Crouch
10.4.16
i
VHF
Marinas **80** M

Shoeburyness
☎ 01702 292271
Ext 3476

Holehaven

River Medway
10.4.12
i
Medway Radio
VHF **74** 22 23 16
Marinas **80** M

90

6°W (1996)

Variation

0

180

270

River Thames
10.4.13
i
Thames Barrier
Woolwich Radio
VHF **14** 22 16
Marinas **80** M

Gravesend*
i
Port Control
Centre
London
VHF **12 13**

Thames Radio
VHF **02** 83 16
VHF **02**
0733 1933 UT

30'

52°
00'N

01°00'E

52°
00'N

30'

51°
30'N

51°
30'N

02°00'E

30'

52°
00'N

10-4-3   AREA 4 TIDAL STREAMS

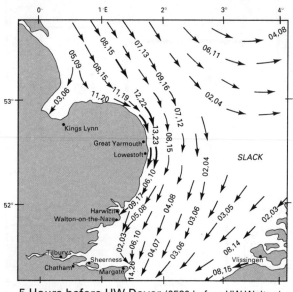

5 Hours before HW Dover (0530 before HW Walton)

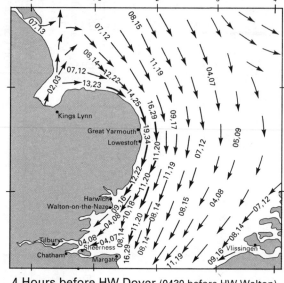

4 Hours before HW Dover (0430 before HW Walton)

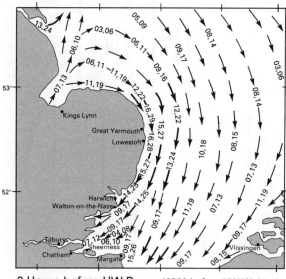

3 Hours before HW Dover (0330 before HW Walton)

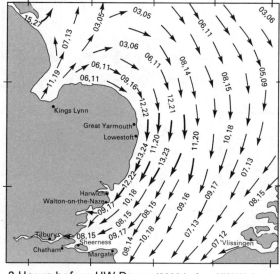

2 Hours before HW Dover (0230 before HW Walton)

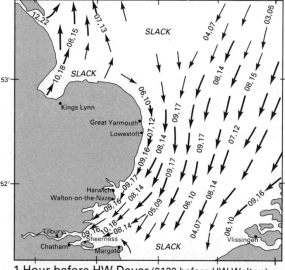

1 Hour before HW Dover (0130 before HW Walton)

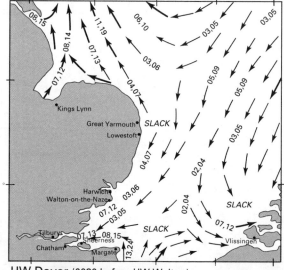

HW Dover (0030 before HW Walton)

Southward 10.3.3   Thames Estuary 10.4.8   Northward 10.5.3   Eastward 10.20.3

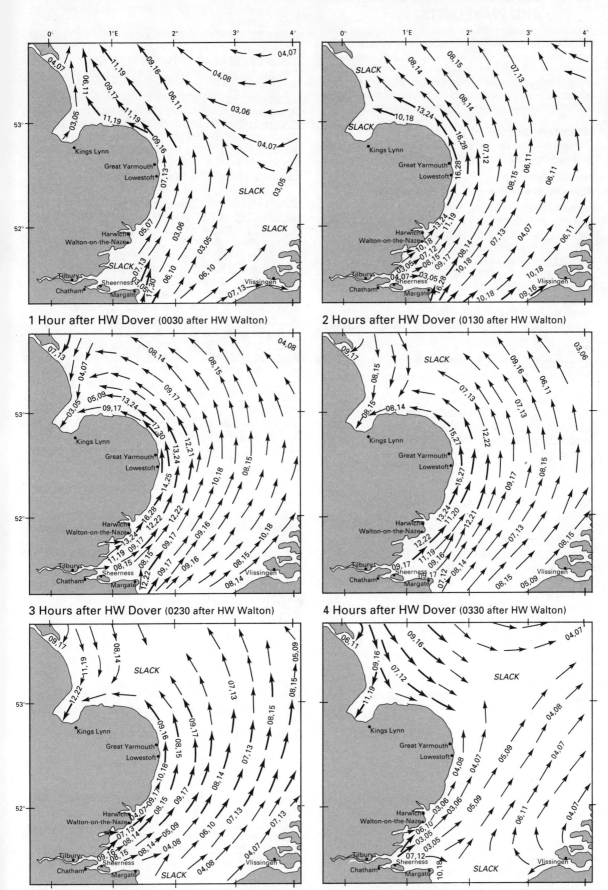

4

1 Hour after HW Dover (0030 after HW Walton)

2 Hours after HW Dover (0130 after HW Walton)

3 Hours after HW Dover (0230 after HW Walton)

4 Hours after HW Dover (0330 after HW Walton)

5 Hours after HW Dover (0430 after HW Walton)

6 Hours after HW Dover (0530 after HW Walton)

10.4.4 COASTAL LIGHTS, FOG SIGNALS AND WAYPOINTS

Abbreviations used below are given in 1.4.1. Principal lights are in **bold** print, places in CAPITALS, and light-vessels, light floats and Lanbys in *CAPITAL ITALICS*. Unless otherwise stated lights are white. m – elevation in metres; M – nominal range in miles. Fog signals are in *italics*. Useful waypoints are underlined – use those on land with care. All geographical positions should be assumed to be approximate. See 4.4.1.

IMPORTANT NOTE.
Changes are regularly made to buoyage in the Thames Estuary. Check Notices to Mariners for the latest information.

THAMES ESTUARY
(Direction of buoyage generally East to West)

APPROACHES TO THAMES ESTUARY
F3 Lt F 51°23'·82N 02°00'·62E Fl 10s 12m **22M**; Racon; *Horn 10s*.
Falls Hd Lt By 51°28'·20N 01°50'·00E Q; NCM.
Drill Stone Lt By 51°25'·80N 01°43'·00E Q (3) 10s; NCM.
NE Spit Lt By 51°27'·90N 01°30'·00E VQ (3) 5s; ECM.
Elbow Lt By 51°23'·20N 01°31'·70E Q; NCM.
Foreness Pt Outfall Lt By 51°24'·60N 01°26'·10E Fl Y 5s; SPM.
Longnose By 51°24'·12N 01°26'·18E; PHM.
Longnose Spit By 51°23'·90N 01°25'·85E; NCM.
Margate Outfall Lt By 51°24'·59N 01°26'·10E Fl R 5s; PHM.

MARGATE
Promenade Pier N Hd 51°23'·65N 01°22'·93E Fl (3) R 10s.
Stone Pier Hd FR 18m 4M. (QW marks tide gauge 385m NNW.)

GORE CHANNEL
SE Margate Lt By 51°24'·10N 01°20'·50E Q (3) 10s; ECM.
S Margate Lt By 51°23'·88N 01°16'·75E Fl G 2.5s; SHM.
Margate Hook Bn 51°24'·14N 01°14'·39E; SCM.
Hook Spit By 51°24'·05N 01°12'·65E; SHM.
E Last Lt By 51°24'·00N 01°12'·28E QR; PHM.

HERNE BAY
Pier Hd 51°22'·90N 01°07'·00E Q 8m 4M, (isolated).
Pier, near root 51°22'·36N 01°07'·30E 2 FR (vert).

WHITSTABLE
Whitstable Street Lt By 51°23'·83N 01°01'·70E Q; NCM.
Whitstable Oyster Lt By 51°22'·03N 01°01'·16E Fl (2) R 10s; PHM.
NE Arm F 15m 8M; W mast; FR 10m 5M (same structure) shown when ent/dep prohib.
W Quay Dn 51°21'·82N 01°01'·55E Fl WRG 5s 2m W5M, R3M, G3M; vis W118°-156°, G156°-178°, R178°-201°.
E Quay, N end 51°21'·80N 01°01'·65E 2 FR (vert) 4m 1M.
Ldg Lts 122·5°. Front FR 7m. Rear, 30m from front, FR 13m.

THE SWALE
Columbine By 51°24'·23N 01°01'·45E; SHM.
Columbine Spit By 51°23'·83N 01°00'·13E; SHM.
Pollard Spit Lt By 51°22'·95N 00°58'·67E QR; PHM.
Ham Gat By 51°23'·05N 00°58'·42E; SHM.
Sand End Lt By 51°21'·40N 00°56'·00E Fl G 5s; SHM.
Faversham Spit By 51°20'·74N 00°54'·31E; NCM.
Queenborough Hard S1 Lt By 51°24'·96N 00°44'·28E Fl R 3s; PHM.
Queenborough Pt Lt (S) 51°25'·31N 00°44'·13E Fl R 4s.
Queenborough Pt Lt (N) 51°25'·42N 00°44'·11E QR 3m 2M.
Queenborough Spit Lt By 51°25'·78N 00°44'·03E Q (3) 10s; ECM.

QUEENS CHANNEL/FOUR FATHOMS CHANNEL
E Margate Lt By 51°27'·00N 01°26'·50E Fl R 2.5s; PHM.
Spaniard Lt By 51°26'·20N 01°04'·10E Q (3) 10s; ECM.
Spile Lt By 51°26'·40N 00°55'·80E Fl G 2.5s; SHM.

PRINCES CHANNEL
Outer Tongue Lt By 51°30'·70N 01°26'·50E L Fl 10s; SWM; Racon (T); *Whis*.
Tongue Sand Tr 51°29'·55N 01°22'·10E (unlit) (NCM & SCM Lt Bys close N and S).
E Tongue Lt By 51°28'·72N 01°18'·72E Fl (2) R 5s; PHM.
S Shingles Lt By 51°29'·20N 01°16'·12E Q (6) + L Fl 15s; SCM; *Bell*.
N Tongue Lt By 51°28'·78N 01°13'·18E Fl (3) R 10s; PHM.
SE Girdler Lt By 51°29'·47N 01°10'·00E Fl (3) G 10s; SHM.
W Girdler Lt By 51°29'·58N 01°06'·82E Q (9)15s; WCM; *Bell*.
Girdler Lt By 51°29'·15N 01°06'·50E Fl (4) R 15s; PHM.
Shivering Sand Tr 51°29'·90N 01°04'·90E. NCM & SCM Lt Bys close N and S.
E Redsand Lt By 51°29'·38N 01°04'·15E Fl (2) R 5s; PHM.

NORTH EDINBURGH CHANNEL/KNOB CHANNEL
Edinburgh Lt By 51°31'·35N 01°21'·14E QR; PHM.
No. 1 Lt By 51°31'·44N 01°21'·67E Q (6) + L Fl 15s; SCM; *Horn (1) 10s*.
Patch Lt By 51°32'·24N 01°20'·84E Fl (2) R 10s; PHM.
SE Longsand Lt By 51°32'·24N 01°21'·22E QG; SHM.
No. 2 Lt By 51°32'·86N 01°20'·18E Fl (3) R 10s; PHM.
No. 3 Lt By 51°32'·98N 01°20'·46E Q (9) 15s; WCM.
No. 4 Lt By 51°33'·19N 01°19'·41E Fl R 2.5s; PHM; *Bell*.
No. 5 Lt By 51°33'·42N 01°19'·43E Fl G 2.5s; SHM.
No. 6 Lt By 51°33'·36N 01°18'·19E Fl R 2.5s; PHM.
No. 7 Lt By 51°33'·58N 01°18'·24E Fl G 2.5s; SHM.
No. 8 Lt By 51°33'·19N 01°16'·65E Fl (3) R 10s; PHM.
No. 9 Lt By 51°33'·46N 01°16'·70E Fl (3) G 10s; SHM; *Bell*.
Shingles Patch Lt By 51°32'·98N 01°15'·47E Q; NCM.
N Shingles Lt By 51°32'·63N 01°14'·35E Fl R 2.5s; PHM.
Tizard Lt By 51°32'·90N 01°13'·00E Q (6) + L Fl 15s; SCM.
Mid Shingles Lt By 51°31'·93N 01°12'·08E Fl (2) R 5s; PHM.
NE Knob Lt By 51°32'·00N 01°10'·10E QG; SHM.
NW Shingles Lt By 51°31'·23N 01°09'·83E VQ; NCM.
SE Knob Lt By 51°30'·86N 01°06'·51E Fl G 5s; SHM.
Knob Lt By 51°30'·66N 01°04'·38E Iso 5s; SWM; *Bell*.

OAZE DEEP
S Oaze Lt By 51°30'·00N 01°00'·80E Fl (2) G 5s; SHM.
Red Sand Tr 51°28'·60N 00°59'·50E (unlit PHM & SHM Lt Bys close NW and E).
SW Oaze Lt By 51°29'·03N 00°57'·03E Q (6) + L Fl 15s; SCM.
W Oaze Lt By 51°29'·03N 00°55'·53E Q (9) 10s; WCM.
Cant Bn 51°27'·73N 00°55'·45E (unlit).
E Cant Lt By 51°28'·50N 00°55'·70E QR; PHM.
W Cant Lt By 51°27'·19N 00°45'·61E QR; PHM.

Medway Lt By 51°28'·80N 00°52'·92E Mo (A) 6s; SWM.

MEDWAY, SHEERNESS
Grain Edge By 51°27'·58N 00°45'·57E; SHM.
Jacobs Bank Obstn Lt By 51°26'·94N 00°45'·29E VQ; NCM.
Garrison Pt Ro Ro 51°26'·91N 00°44'·92E 2 FR (vert); Dn; *Horn(3) 30s*.
Grain Hard Lt By 51°26'·94N 00°44'·27E Fl G 5s; SHM.
Isle of Grain 51°26'·6N 00°43'·5E Q WRG 20m W13M, R7M, G8M; R & W ◊ on R Tr; vis R220°-234°, G234°-241°, W241°-013°; Ra refl.
N. Kent Lt By 51°26'·10N 00°43'·57E QG; SHM.
S. Kent Lt By 51°25'·95N 00°43'·77E Fl R 5s; PHM.
Victoria Lt By 51°25'·93N 00°42'·94E Fl (3) G 10s; SHM.
Stoke No. 13 Lt By 51°25'·73N 00°39'·91E Fl G 5s; SHM.
No. 15 Lt By 51°24'·72N 00°38'·53E Fl G 10s; SHM.
Darnett No. 23 Lt By 51°24'·57N 00°35'·72E QG; SHM.
Folly No. 25 Lt By 51°24'·07N 00°35'·33E Fl (3) G 10s; SHM.
Gillingham Reach No. 27 Lt By 51°23'·88N 00°34'·82E Fl G 10s; SHM.

RIVER THAMES

SEA REACH, NORE AND YANTLET
No. 1 Lt By 51°29'·42N 00°52'·67E Fl Y 2·5s; SPM; Racon.
No. 2 Lt By 51°29'·37N 00°49'·85E Iso 5s; SWM.
No. 3 Lt By 51°29'·30N 00°46'·65E L Fl 10s; SWM.
No. 4 Lt By 51°29'·58N 00°44'·28E Fl Y 2·5s; SPM.
No. 5 Lt By 51°29'·92N 00°41'·54E Iso 5s; SWM.
No. 6 Lt By 51°30'·00N 00°39'·94E Iso 2s; SWM.
No. 7 Lt By 51°30'·07N 00°37'·15E Fl Y 2·5s; SPM; Racon.
Nore Swatch Lt By 51°28'·26N 00°45'·65E Fl (4) R 15s; PHM.
Mid Swatch Lt By 51°28'·75N 00°44'·27E Fl G 5s; SHM.
W Nore Sand Lt By 51°29'·26N 00°41'·80E Fl (3) R 10s; PHM.
East Blyth Lt By 51°29'·63N 00°37'·92E Fl (2) R 10s; PHM.
West Lee Middle Lt By 51°30'·46N 00°38'·93E QG; SHM.
Chapman Lt By 51°30'·40N 00°37'·03E Fl (3) G 10s; SHM; Bell.
Mid Blyth Lt By 51°30'·05N 00°32'·50E Q; NCM.

LEIGH-ON-SEA/SOUTHEND-ON-SEA
South Shoebury Lt By 51°30'·26N 00°51'·33E Fl G 5s; SHM.
Shoebury Lt Bn 51°30'·28N 00°49'·38E Fl (3) G 10s 5m 5M.
Inner Shoebury Bn 51°30'·15N 00°49'·05E Fl Y 2·5s.
SE Leigh Lt By 51°29'·40N 00°47'·17E Q (6) + L Fl 15s; SCM.
West Shoebury Lt By 51°30'·21N 00°45'·83E Fl G 2·5s; SHM.
Southend Pier E end 51°30'·84N 00°43'·51E 2 FG (vert) 7m; *Horn Mo (N) 30s* (TE 1986).
Pier W Hd 2 FG (vert) 13m 8M.
Leigh By 51°31'·04N 00°42'·67E; SHM.

CANVEY ISLAND/HOLEHAVEN
Canvey Jetty Hd E end 51°30'·36N 00°34'·25E 2 FG (vert); *Bell (1) 10s.*
W Hd 2 FG (vert) 13m 8M.
Lts 2 FR (vert) to port, and 2 FG (vert) to stbd, are shown from wharves etc above this Pt.

Shornmead 51°26'·97N 00°26'·63E Fl (2) WRG 10s 12m **W17M**, R13M, G13M; vis G054°-081·5°, R081·5°-086·2°, W086·2°-088·7°, G088·7°-141°, W141°-205°, R205°-213°.

GRAVESEND
Thames Navigation Service Pier 51°26'·68N 00°22'·57E FR.

Northfleet Lower 51°26'·9N 00°20'·4E Oc WR 5s 15m **W17M**, R14M; vis W164°-271°, R271°-S shore.
Northfleet Upper 51°26'·90N 00°20'·17E Oc WRG 10s 30m **W16M**, R12M, G12M; vis R126°-149°, W149°-159°, G159°-268°, W268°-279°.
Broadness 51°28'·0N 00°18'·7E Oc R 5s 12m 12M; R metal Tr.
Queen Elizabeth II Bridge NE 51°27'·95N 00°15'·72E Fl G 5s.

THAMES TIDAL BARRIER
Span E (approx centre) 51°29'·82N 00°02'·32E.

SOUTH DOCK MARINA
Greenland Pier S Hd 51°29'·64N 00°01'·80W Lt.

LIMEHOUSE BASIN MARINA/REGENT'S CANAL
Victoria Wharf W end 51°30'·52N 00°02'·14W Lt.

ST KATHARINE YACHT HAVEN.
Harrison's Wharf 51°30'·33N 00°04'·23W 2 FG (vert).

CHELSEA HARBOUR MARINA
Lock SS 51°28'·45N 00°10'·73W 2 FG (vert).

THAMES ESTUARY – NORTHERN PART

KENTISH KNOCK
Kentish Knock Lt By 51°38'·50N 01°40·50E Q (3) 10s; ECM; *Whis.*
S Knock Lt By 51°34'·73N 01°36'·10E Q (6) + L Fl 15s; SCM; *Bell.*

KNOCK JOHN CHANNEL
No. 7 Lt By 51°32'·00N 01°06'·50E Fl (4) G 15s; SHM.
No. 5 Lt By 51°32'·75N 01°08'·68E Fl (3) G 10s; SHM.
No. 4 Lt By 51°32'·60N 01°08'·82E L Fl R 10s; PHM.
No. 2 Lt By 51°33'·08N 01°09'·95E Fl (3) R 10s; PHM.
No. 3 Lt By 51°33'·20N 01°09'·80E Q (6) + L Fl 15s; SCM.
No. 1 Lt By 51°33'·72N 01°10'·82E Fl G 5s; SHM.
Knock John Lt By 51°33'·46N 01°11'·08E Fl (2) R 5s; PHM.

BLACK DEEP
No. 12 Lt By 51°33'·80N 01°13'·60E Fl (4) R 15s; PHM.
No. 11 Lt By 51°34'·30N 01°13'·50E Fl (3) G 10s; SHM.
No. 10 Lt By 51°34'·70N 01°15'·70E QR; PHM.
No. 9 Lt By 51°35'·10N 01°15'·20E Q (6) + L Fl 15s; SCM.
No. 8 Lt By 51°36'·20N 01°20'·00E Q; NCM.
No. 7 Lt By 51°37'·05N 01°17'·80E QG; SHM.
No. 6 Lt By 51°38'·49N 01°24'·51E Fl R 2·5s; PHM.
No. 5 Lt By 51°39'·50N 01°23'·10E VQ (3) 5s; ECM; *Bell.*
No. 4 Lt By 51°41'·39N 01°28'·59E Fl (2) R 5s; PHM.
No. 3 Lt By 51°41'·95N 01°26'·07E Fl (3) G 15s; SHM.
No. 1 Lt By 51°44'·00N 01°28'·20E Fl G 5s; SHM.
Sunk Head Tr Lt By 51°46'·60N 01°30'·60E Q; NCM.
No. 2 Lt By 51°45'·60N 01°32'·30E Fl (4) R 15s; WCM.
Black Deep Lt By 51°46'·60N 01°34'·05E QR; PHM.
Trinity Lt By 51°49'·00N 01°36'·50E Q (6) + L Fl 15s; SCM; *Whis.*
Long Sand Hd Lt By 51°47'·87N 01°39'·53E VQ; NCM; *Bell.*

BARROW DEEP (selected Bys)
SW Barrow Lt By 51°31'·80N 01°00'·53E Q (6) + L Fl 15s; SCM; *Bell.*
Barrow No. 11 Lt By 51°33'·73N 01°05'·85E Fl G 2·5s; SHM.
Barrow No. 9 Lt By 51°35'·31N 01°10'·40E VQ (3) 5s; ECM.
Barrow No. 6 Lt By 51°37'·27N 01°14'·79E Fl (4) R 15s; PHM.
Barrow No. 4 Lt By 51°39'·85N 01°17'·60E VQ (9) 10s; WCM.
Barrow No. 3 Lt By 51°41'·99N 01°20'·35E Q (3) 10s; ECM; Racon (M).
Barrow No. 2 Lt By 51°41'·95N 01°23'·00E Fl (2) R 5s; PHM.

WEST SWIN AND MIDDLE DEEP
Blacktail (W) Bn 51°31'·43N 00°55'·30E Iso G 10s 10m 6M.
Blacktail (E) Bn 51°31'·75N 00°56'·60E Iso G 5s 10m 6M.
Blacktail Spit Lt By 51°31'·45N 00°56'·85E Fl (3) G 10s; SHM.
SW Swin Lt By 51°32'·73N 01°01'·18E Fl (2) R 5s; PHM.
W Swin By 51°33'·82N 01°03'·30E; PHM.
Maplin Lt By 51°34'·00N 01°02'·40E Q (3) 10s; ECM; *Bell.*
Maplin Edge By 51°35'·30N 01°03'·75E; SHM.
Maplin Bank Lt By 51°35'·47N 01°04'·80E Fl (3) R 10s; PHM.

EAST SWIN (KING'S) CHANNEL
NE Maplin Lt By 51°37'·43N 01°04'·90E Fl G 5s; SHM; *Bell.*
W Hook Middle By 51°39'·15N 01°08'·07E; PHM.
S Whitaker Lt By 51°40'·20N 01°09'·15E Fl (2) G 10s; SHM.
N Middle By 51°41'·00N 01°12'·00E; NCM.
W Sunk Lt By 51°44'·30N 01°25'·90E Q (9) 15s; WCM.
Gunfleet Spit Lt By 51°45'·30N 01°21'·80E Q (6) + LFl 15s; SCM; *Bell.*
Gunfleet Old Lt Ho 51°46'·08N 01°20'·52E.

WHITAKER CHANNEL AND RIVER CROUCH
Whitaker Lt By 51°41'·40N 01°10'·61E Q (3) 10s; ECM; *Bell.*
Whitaker No. 6 Lt By 51°40'·66N 01°08'·17E Q; NCM.
Swin Spitway Lt By 51°41'·92N 01°08'·45E Iso 10s; SWM; *Bell.*
Whitaker Bn 51°39'·62N 01°06'·30E; IDM.
Swallow Tail By 51°40'·44N 01°04'·81E; SHM.
Ridge Lt By 51°40'·10N 01°05'·00E Fl R 10s; PHM.
S Buxey Lt By 51°39'·82N 01°02'·60E Fl (3) G 15s; SHM.
Sunken Buxey Lt By 51°39'·50N 01°00'·70E Q; NCM.
Buxey No. 1 Lt By 51°39'·02N 01°00'·86E VQ (6) + L Fl 10s; SCM.

Buxey No. 2 Lt By 51°38'·94W 01°00'·26E Fl R 10s; PHM.
Outer Crouch Lt By 51°38'·35N 00°58'·61E Q (6) + L Fl 15s; SCM.
Crouch Lt By 51°37'·60N 00°56'·49E Fl R 10s; PHM.
Inner Crouch Lt By 51°37'·19N 00°55'·22E L Fl 10s; SWM.
Horse Shoal Lt By 51°37'·07N 00°51'·62E Q; NCM.

RIVER ROACH/HAVENGORE
Branklet By 51°36'·95N 00°52'·24E; SPM.

BURNHAM-ON-CROUCH
Fairway No. 1 Lt By 51°37'·08N 00°51'·11E QG; SHM.
Fairway No. 5 Lt By 51°37'·16N 00°49'·67E QG; SHM.
Fairway No. 9 Lt By 51°37'·32N 00°48'·87E QG; SHM.
Fairway No. 11 Lt By 51°37'·41N 00°48'·40E QG; SHM.
Burnham Yacht Hbr Lt By 51°37'·47N 00°48'·33E L Fl 10s;
SWM.

RAY SAND CHANNEL
Buxey Bn 51°41'·13N 01°01'·38E (unlit); NCM.

GOLDMER GAT/WALLET
NE Gunfleet Lt By 51°49'·90N 01°27'·90E Q (3) 10s; ECM.
Wallet No. 2 Lt By 51°48'·85N 01°23'·10E Fl R 5s; PHM.
Wallet No. 4 Lt By 51°46'·50N 01°17'·33E Fl (4) R 10s;PHM.
Walton Pier Hd 51°50'·58N 01°16'·90E 2 FG (vert) 5m 2M.
Wallet Spitway Lt By 51°42'·83N 01°07'·42E L Fl 10s; SWM;
Bell.
Knoll Lt By 51°43'·85N 01°05'·17E Q; NCM.
Eagle Lt By 51°44'·10N 01°03'·92E QG; SHM.
NW Knoll Lt By 51°44'·32N 01°02'·27E Fl (2) R 5s; PHM.
Colne Bar Lt By 51°44'·58N 01°02'·67E Fl (2) G 5s; SHM.
Bench Head By 51°44'·66N 01°01'·20E; SHM.

RIVER BLACKWATER
The Nass Bn 51°45'·75N 00°54'·88E VQ (3) 5s 6m 2M; ECM.
Thirslet Lt By 51°43'·71N 00°50'·49E Fl (3) G 10s; SHM.
No. 1 By 51°43'·41N 00°48'·13E; SHM.
No. 2 Lt By 51°42'·78N 00°46'·58E Fl R 3s; PHM.
Osea I Pier Hd 51°43'·05N 00°46'·59E 2 FG (vert).
No. 3 By 51°42'·88N 00°46'·16E; SHM.
N Double No. 7 Lt By 51°43'·22N 00°44'·87E Fl G 3s; SHM.
No. 8 By 51°43'·91N 00°43'·35E; PHM.

RIVER COLNE/BRIGHTLINGSEA
Inner Bench Hd No. 2 Lt By 51°45'·93N 01°01'·86E Fl (2) R 5s;
PHM.
No. 9 Lt By 51°47'·33N 01°01'·17E Fl G 3s; SHM.
No. 13 Lt By 51°47'·72N 01°00'·91E Fl G; SHM.
Brightlingsea Spit Lt By 51°48'·05N 01°00'·80E Q (6) + L Fl
15s; SCM.
Brightlingsea Lt By 51°48'·19N 01°01'·18E Fl (3) G 5s; SHM.
Ldg Lts 041°. Front 51°48'·4N 01°01'·3E FR 7m 4M; W □, R
stripe on post; vis 020°-080°. Rear, 50m from front, FR 10m
4M; W ■, R stripe on post. FR Lts are shown on 7 masts
between 1·5M and 3M NW when firing occurs.
Hardway Hd 51°48'·2N 01°01'·5E 2 FR (vert) 2m.
Batemans 51°48'·3N 01°00'·8E FY 12m.
Fingringhoe Wick Pier Hd 2 FR (vert) 6m (occas).
No. 23 51°50'·6N 00°59'·0E Fl G 5s 5m.
Rowhedge Wharf FY 11m.

CLACTON-ON-SEA
Berthing arm 51°47'·00N 01°09'·60E 2 FG (vert) 5m 4M;
Reed (2) 120s (occas).

WALTON BACKWATERS
Naze Tr 51°51'·85N 01°17'·40E.
Pye End Lt By 51°55'·00N 01°18'·00E L Fl 10s; SWM.
No. 2 By 51°54'·54N 01°16'·90E; PHM; Ra refl.
No. 3 Crab Knoll By 51°54'·36N 01°16'·49E; SHM; Ra refl.

No. 4 High Hill By 51°54'·02N 01°16'·07E; PHM.
No. 5 By 51°54'·25N 01°16'·33E; SHM; Ra refl.
No. 6 By 51°53'·76N 01°15'·80E; PHM.
No. 7 By 51°53'·78N 01°15'·65E; SHM.
No. 8 By 51°53'·39N 01°15'·53E; PHM.
Island Pt By 51°53'·27N 01°15'·44E; NCM; Ra refl.
No. 10 Mussel Bk By 51°53'·31N 01°15'·49E; PHM.
No. 12 By 51°53'·26N 01°15'·51E; PHM.
No. 14 Frank Bloom By 51°53'·21N 01°15'·61E; PHM.
East Coast Sails By 51°53'·14N 01°15'·66E; SHM.
Plumtrees Stone Pt By 51°53'·01N 01°15'·73E; PHM.

HARWICH APPROACHES
(Direction of buoyage North to South.)

MEDUSA CHANNEL
Medusa Lt By 51°51'·20N 01°20'·46E Fl G 5s; SHM.
Stone Banks By 51°53'·18N 01°19'·32E; PHM.

CORK SAND /ROUGH SHOALS
S Cork By 51°51'·30N 01°24'·20E; SCM.
Roughs Tr SE Lt By 51°53'·61N 01°29'·06E Q (3) 10s; ECM; Bell.
Roughs Tr NW Lt By 51°53'·78N 01°28'·88E Q (9) 15s; WCM.
Rough Lt By 51°55'·16N 01°30'·10E VQ; NCM.
Cork Lt By 51° 55'·43N 01°24'·95E QR; PHM.
Cork Sand Lt Bn 51°55'·20N 01°25'·28E Q; NCM.

HARWICH CHANNEL
Trinity Lt By 51°49'·00N 01°36'·50E Q (6) + L Fl 15s; SCM.
SUNK Lt F 51°51'·00N 01°35'·00E Fl (2) 20s 12m **24M**; R hull
with Lt Tr; RC; Racon (T); Horn(2) 60s.
S Threshold Lt By 51°52'·44N 01°34'·16E Q (6) + L Fl 15s.
S Shipwash Lt By 51°52'·68N 01°34'·16E Q (6) + L Fl 15s; SCM.
E Fort Massac Lt By 51°53'·34N 01°32'·90E VQ (3) 5s; ECM.
Ship Head Lt By 51°53'·76N 01°34'·01E Fl R 5s; PHM.
N Threshold Lt By 51°54'·46N 01°33'·58E Fl Y 5s; SPM.
SW Shipwash Lt By 51°54'·72N 01°34'·32E Q (9)15s; WCM.
Haven Lt By 51°55'·72N 01°32'·68E Mo (A) 5s; SWM.
Shipway Lt By 51°56'·73N 01°30'·77E Iso 5s; SWM; Whis.
Cross Lt By 51°56'·20N 01°30'·58E Fl (3) Y 10s; SPM.
Harwich Chan No. 1 Lt By 51°56'·10N 01°27'·30E Fl Y 2·5s;
SPM; Racon (T).
Washington Lt By 51°56'·49N 01°26'·70E QG; SHM.
Felixstowe Ledge Lt By 51°56'·30N 01°24'·53E Fl (3) G10s;
SHM.
Wadgate Ledge Lt By 51°56'·08N 01°22'·20E Fl (4) G 15s; SHM.
Platters Lt By 51°55'·62N 01°21'·08E; Q (6) + L Fl 15s; SCM.
Rolling Ground Lt By 51°55'·51N 01°19'·86E; QG; SHM.
Beach End Lt By 51°55'·59N 01°19'·31E Fl (2) G 5s; SHM.
NW Beach Lt By 51°55'·87N 01°18'·97E Fl (3) G 10s; SHM;
Bell.
Fort Lt By 51°56'·18N 01°18'·98E Fl (4) G 15s; SHM.

EDGE OF RECOMMENDED YACHT TRACK
Cork Sand Lt By 51°55'·42N 01°24'·57E Fl (3) R 10s; PHM.
Pitching Ground Lt By 51°55'·38N 01°21'·16E Fl (4) R 15s;
PHM.
Inner Ridge Lt By 51°55'·31N 01°19'·68E QR; PHM.
Landguard Lt By 51°55'·35N 01°18'·98E Q; NCM.
Cliff Foot Lt By 51°55'·69N 01°18'·64E Fl R 5s; PHM.
S Shelf Lt By 51°56'·17N 01°18'·67E Fl (2) R 5s; PHM.
N Shelf Lt By 51°56'·65N 01°18'·70E QR; PHM.
Grisle Lt By 51°56'·87N 01°18'·43E Fl R 2·5s; PHM.
Guard Lt By 51°57'·04N 01°17'·88E Fl R 5s; PHM; Bell.

RIVER STOUR/HARWICH
Wharves, Jetties and Piers show 2 FR (vert).
Shotley Spit Lt By 51°57'·26N 01°17'·67E Q (6) + L Fl 15s;
SCM.
Shotley Marina Lock E side Dir Lt 339·5° 51°57'·43N
01°16'·71E 3m 1M (uses Moiré pattern); Or structure.

Shotley Marina Ent E side 51°57'·23N 01°16'·84E Fl (4) G 15s;
G △ on pile.
Shotley Marina W side VQ (3) 5s; ECM.
Shotley Ganges Pier E Hd 51°57'·18N 01°16'·34E 2 FG (vert)
4m 1M; G post.
Parkeston Lt By 51°57'·03N 01°14'·89E Fl (3) G 10s; SHM.
Erwarton Ness Lt Bn 51°57'·08N 01°13'·35E Q (6) + L Fl 15s
4M; SCM Bn.
Holbrook Lt Bn 51°57'·19N 01°10'·46E VQ (6) + L Fl 10s 4M;
SCM Bn.
Mistley, Baltic wharf 51°56'·69N 01°05'·31E 2 FR (vert).

ORWELL/IPSWICH
Walton Lt By 51°57'·60N 01°17'·41E Fl (3) G 10s; SHM.
Fagbury Lt By 51°57'·94N 01°16'·91E Fl G 2·5s; SHM.
Orwell Lt By 51°58'·14N 01°16'·65E Fl R 2·5s; PHM.
No. 1 Lt By 51°58'·256N 01°16'·775E Fl G 5s; SHM.
Suffolk Yacht Harbour. Ldg Lts 51°59'·77N 01°16'·22E. Front
Iso Y 1M, Rear Oc Y 4s 1M.
Woolverstone Marina 52°00'·4N 01°11'·8E 2 FR (vert).
Orwell Bridge FY 39m 3M at centre; 2 FR (vert) on Pier 9 and
2 FG (vert) on Pier 10.
No. 12 Lt By (off Fox's Marina) 52°02'·07N 01°09'·45E
Fl R 12s; PHM.
Ipswich Lock SS (Tfc) 52°02'·77N 01°09'·85E.

HARWICH TO ORFORDNESS

FELIXSTOWE/RIVER DEBEN/WOODBRIDGE HAVEN
Felixstowe Town Pier Hd 51°57'·37N 01°21'·02E 2 FG (vert) 7m.
Woodbridge Haven By 51°58'·36N 01°24'·20E; SWM.
Ldg Lts Fl or Fl Y moved as required (on request). Front W
△ on R I. Rear; R line on I.
Felixtowe Ferry, E side 51°59'·40N 01°23'·72E 2 FG (vert).
W side 2 FR (vert).
Groyne, outer end 51°59'·35N 01°23'·62E QR; (TE. 1988).

RIVER ORE/RIVER ALDE
Orford Haven By 52°01'·63N 01°27'·67E; SHM.

OFFSHORE MARKS
S Galloper Lt By 51°43'·95N 01°56'·50E Q (6) L Fl 15s; SCM;
Racon (T); *Whis.*
N Galloper Lt By 51°50'·00N 01°59'·50E Q; NCM.
S Inner Gabbard Lt By 51°51'·20N 01°52'·40E Q (6) + L Fl 15s;
SCM.
N Inner Gabbard Lt By 51°59'·10N 01°56'·10E Q; NCM.
Outer Gabbard Lt By 51°57'·80N 02°04'·30E Q (3) 10s; ECM;
Racon (O); *Whis.*
NHR-SE Lt By 51°45'·50N 02°40'·00E Fl G 5s; SHM; Racon (N).
NHR-S Lt By 51°51'·40N 02°28'·79E Fl Y 10s; SPM; *Bell.*

SHIPWASH/BAWDSEY BANK
E Shipwash Lt By 51°57'·05N 01°38'·00E VQ (3) 5s; ECM.
NW Shipwash Lt By 51°58'·33N 01°36'·33E Fl R 5s; PHM.
N Shipwash Lt By 52°01'·70N 01°38'·38E Q 7M; NCM;
Racon (M); *Bell*
S Bawdsey Lt By 51°57'·20N 01°30'·32E Q (6) + L Fl 15s;
SCM; *Whis.*
Mid Bawdsey Lt By 51°58'·85N 01°33'·70E Fl (3) G 10s; SHM.
NE Bawdsey Lt By 52°01'·70N 01°36'·20E Fl G 10s; SHM.

CUTLER/WHITING BANKS
Cutler By 51°58'·50N 01°27'·60E; SHM.
SW Whiting By 52°01'·22N 01°30'·90E; SCM.
Whiting Hook By 52°02'·95N 01°31'·93E; PHM.
NE Whiting By 52°03'·77N 01°33'·88E; ECM.

Orford Ness 52°05'·00N 01°34'·60E Fl 5s 28m **25M**; W ● Tr,
R bands. F RG 14m R14M, **G15M** (same Tr); vis R shore-210°,
R038°-047°, G047°-shore; Racon (T).

ORFORDNESS TO GREAT YARMOUTH
(Direction of buoyage South to North.)

Aldeburgh Ridge By 52°06'·82N 01°37'·60E; PHM.
Sizewell Power station, Pipeline Hds 52°12'·70N 01°37'·90E
2 FR (vert) 12/10m.
Sizewell Cooling Water intake and outfall 52°12'·90N
01°38'·15E each Fl R 5s.

SOUTHWOLD
Southwold Lt Ho 52°19'·60N 01°41'·00E Fl (4) WR 20s 37m
W17M, **R15M**, R14M; W ● Tr; vis R (intens) 204°-220°,
W220°-001°, R001°-032·3°.
N Pier Hd 52°18'·77N 01°40'·63E Fl G 1·5s 4m 4M.
S Pier Hd QR 4m 2M.

LOWESTOFT AND APPROACHES VIA STANFORD CHANNEL.
E Barnard Lt By 52°25'·11N 01°46'·50E Q (3) 10s; ECM.
Newcombe Sand Lt By 52°26'·65N 01°47'·15E QR; PHM.
S Holm Lt By 52°27'·30N 01°47'·35E VQ(6) + L Fl 10s; SCM.
Stanford Lt By 52°27'·65N 01°46'·80E Fl R 2·5s; PHM.
N Newcome Lt By 52°28'·29N 01°46'·43E Fl (4) R 15s; PHM.
SW Holm Lt By 52°28'·36N 01°47'·28E Fl (2) G 5s; SHM.
Lowestoft 52°29'·18N 01°45'·46E Fl 15s 37m **28M**; W Tr; part
obscd 347°-shore. FR 30m **18M** (same Tr); vis 184°-211·5°.
Outer Hbr S Pier Hd Oc R 5s 12m 6M; *Horn (4) 60s*; Tfc sigs.
N Pier Hd 52°28'·29N 01°45'·50E Oc G 5s 12m 8M.
Claremont Pier 52°27'·86N 01°44'·98E 2 FR (vert) 5/4m 4M.

LOWESTOFT NORTH AND CORTON ROADS
Lowestoft Ness SE Lt By 52°28'·82N 01°46'·38E Q (6) + L Fl
15s; SCM; *Bell.*
Lowestoft Ness N Lt By 52°28'·87N 01°46'·35E VQ (3) 5s;
ECM; *Bell.*
W Holm Lt By 52°29'·80N 01°47'·20E Fl (3) G 10s; SHM.
NW Holm Lt By 52°31'·90N 01°46'·80E Fl (4) G 15s; SHM.

GREAT YARMOUTH/GORLESTON APPROACHES VIA
HOLM CHANNEL
E Newcome Lt By 52°28'·48N 01°49'·32E Fl (2) R 5s; PHM.
Corton Lt By 52°31'·10N 01°51'·50E Q (3) 10s; ECM; *Whis.*
E. Holm Lt By 52°31'·33N 01°49'·42E Fl (3) R 10s; PHM.
S Corton Lt By 52°32'·19N 01°50'·00E Q (6) + L Fl 15s; SCM.
NE Holm Lt By 52°32'·27N 01°48'·31E Fl R 2·5s; PHM.
Holm Lt By 52°33'·25N 01°48'·26E Fl G 2·5s; SHM
Holm Sand Lt By 52°33'·37N 01°47'·08E Q; NCM.
W Corton Lt By 52°34'·29N 01°46'·50E Q (9) 15s; WCM.

GREAT YARMOUTH/GORLESTON
Gorleston S Pier Hd Fl R 3s 11m 11M; vis 235°-340°; *Horn (3) 60s.*
Ldg Lts 264°. Front 52°34'·30N 01°44'·07E Oc 3s 6m 10M.
Rear Brush Oc 6s 7m 10M, also FR 20m 6M; R ● Tr.
N Pier Hd 52°34'·36N 01°44'·49E QG 8m 6M; vis 176°-078°.
Haven Bridge 52°36'·38N 01°43'·47E marked by pairs of 2 FR
(vert) and 2 FG (vert) showing up and down stream.

10.4.5 PASSAGE INFORMATION

Reference books include: *East Coast Rivers* (YM/Coote) from the Swale to Southwold. The Admiralty *Dover Strait Pilot* also goes to Southwold. *North Sea Passage Pilot* (Imray/Navin) and *The East Coast* (Imray/Bowskill) cover the whole Area.

THE THAMES ESTUARY (chart *1183, 1975*)

To appreciate the geography of the Thames Estuary there is a well-known analogy between its major sandbanks and the fingers and thumb of the left hand, outstretched palm-down: With the thumb lying E over Margate Sand, the index finger covers Long Sand; the middle finger represents Sunk Sand and the third finger delineates West and East Barrow; the little finger points NE along Buxey and Gunfleet Sands.

The intervening channels are often intricate, but the main ones, in sequence from south to north, are:
a. between the Kent coast and thumb – Four Fathoms, Horse, Gore and South Chans; sometimes known as the overland route due to relatively shallow water.
b. between thumb and index finger – Queens and Princes Chans leading seaward to Knock Deep.
c. between index and middle finger – Knob Chan leading to Knock Deep via the Edinburgh Chans across Long Sand and the Shingles. Knock John Chan and Black Deep, the main shipping channels.
d. between middle and third fingers – Barrow Deep.
e. between third and little fingers – W and E Swin, Middle Deep and Whitaker Chan leading seaward to King's Chan.
f. between little finger and the Essex coast – The Wallet and Goldmer Gat.

The sandbanks shift constantly in the Thames Estuary. Up-to-date charts showing the latest buoyage changes are essential, but it is unwise to put too much faith in charted depths over the banks; a reliable echosounder is vital. The main chans carry much commercial shipping and are well buoyed and lit, but this is not so in lesser chans and swatchways which are convenient for yachtsmen, particularly when crossing the estuary from N to S, or vice versa. Unlit, unmarked minor chans (eg Fisherman's Gat or S Edinburgh Chan; in the latter there is a Historic Wreck (see 10.0.3g) at 51°31'·7N 01°14'·9E) should be used with great caution, which could indeed be the hallmark of all passage-making in the Thames Estuary. Good vis is needed to pick out buoys/marks, and to avoid shipping.

CROSSING THE THAMES ESTUARY

Study the tides carefully and understand them, so as to work the streams to best advantage and to ensure sufficient depth at the times and places where you expect to be, or might be later (see 10.4.3 and 10.4.8). In principle it is best to make most of the crossing on a rising tide, ie departing N Foreland or the vicinity of the Whitaker buoy at around LW. The stream runs 3kn at sp in places, mostly along the chans but sometimes across the intervening banks. With wind against tide a short, steep sea is raised, particularly in E or NE winds.

Making N from N Foreland to Orford Ness or beyond (or vice versa) it may be preferable to keep to seaward of the main banks, via Kentish Knock and Long Sand Head buoys, thence to N Shipwash lt buoy 14M further N.

Bound NW from N Foreland it is approximately 26M to the R Crouch, Blackwater or Colne. A safe route is through either the Princes or the North Edinburgh Chans and thence S of the Tizard, Knob and West Barrow banks to the West Swin, before turning NE into Middle Deep and the East Swin. This is just one of many routes which could be followed, depending on wind direction, tidal conditions and confidence in electronic aids in the absence of marks.

A similar, well-used route in reverse, ie to the SE, lies via the Wallet Spitway, to the Whitaker lt buoy, through Barrow Swatchway to SW Sunk bn; thence via the N Edinburgh Chan, toward the E Margate lt buoy keeping E of Tongue Sand tr. Beware shoal waters off Barrow and Sunk Sands.

Port Control London can give navigational help to yachts on VHF Ch 13; Thames CG at Walton-on-the-Naze can also assist. The Thames Navigation Service has radar coverage between the Naze and Margate out to near the Dutch coast.

NORTH FORELAND TO LONDON BRIDGE

N Foreland has a conspic lt ho, RC (chart *1828*), with buoys offshore. From HW Dover – 0120 to + 0045 the stream runs N from The Downs and W into Thames Estuary. From HWD + 0045 to + 0440 the N-going stream from The Downs meets the E-going stream from Thames Estuary, which in strong winds causes a bad sea. From HWD – 0450 to – 0120 the streams turn W into Thames Estuary and S towards The Downs. If bound for London, round N Foreland against the late ebb in order to carry a fair tide from Sheerness onward.

For vessels drawing less than 2m the most direct route from North Foreland to the Thames and Medway is via South Chan, Gore Chan, Horse Chan, Kentish Flats, Four Fathom Chan and Cant; but it is not well marked particularly over the Kentish Flats. An alternative, deeper route is East of Margate Sand and the Tongue, to set course through Princes Chan to Oaze Deep; larger vessels proceed via the North Edinburgh Chan. W-going streams begin at about HW Sheerness – 0600 and E-going at HW Sheerness + 0030.

Margate and Whitstable (10.4.10) afford little shelter for yachts. The Swale (10.4.11) provides an interesting inside route S of the Isle of Sheppey with access to Sheerness and the R Medway (10.4.12). If on passage from N Foreland to the Thames, Queenborough offers the first easily accessible, all-tide, deep-water shelter. The Medway Chan is the main appr to Sheerness from the Warp and the Medway Fairway buoy.

Close N is Sea Reach No 1 buoy and the start of Yanlet Chan and the Thames river which is buoyed up to Gravesend. See 10.4.13 for the Thames Barrier, yacht facilities in London and some PLA regulations on this busy waterway. Yachts should beware the large amount of floating debris, general turbulence and absence of bolt-holes other than listed marinas. Off Shoeburyness, Leigh Chan diverges to Southend, Leigh-on-sea (10.4.14) and Canvey Island/Benfleet.

SHOEBURYNESS TO RIVER COLNE (charts *1185, 1975*)

Maplin and Foulness Sands extend nearly 6M NE from Foulness Pt, the extremity being marked by Whitaker bn. On N side of Whitaker chan leading to R. Crouch (10.4.16 and chart *3750*) lies Buxey Sand, inshore of which is the Ray Sand chan (dries), a convenient short cut between R. Crouch and R. Blackwater with sufficient rise of tide.

To seaward of Buxey Sand and the Spitway, Gunfleet Sand extends 10M NE, marked by buoys and drying in places. A conspic disused lt tr stands on SE side of Gunfleet Sand, about 6M SSE of the Naze tr, and here the SW-going (flood) stream begins about HW Sheerness + 0600, and the NE-going stream at about HW Sheerness – 0030, sp rates 2kn.

The Rivers Blackwater (10.4.17) and Colne (10.4.18) share a common estuary which is approached from the NE via NE Gunfleet lt buoy; thence along Goldmer Gat and the Wallet towards Knoll and Eagle lt buoys. For the Colne turn NNW via Colne Bar buoy towards Inner Bench Hd buoy keeping in mid-chan. For R. Blackwater, head WNW for NW Knoll and Bench Hd buoys. From the S or SE, make for the Whitaker ECM buoy, thence through the Spitway, via Swin Spitway and Wallet Spitway buoys to reach Knoll buoy and deeper water.

RIVER COLNE TO HARWICH (chart *1975, 1593*)

4M SW of the Naze tr at Hollands Haven a conspic radar tr (67m, unlit) is an excellent daymark. From the S, approach Walton and Harwich via the Medusa chan about 1M E of Naze tr. At N end of this chan, 1M off Dovercourt, Pye End buoy marks chan SSW to Walton Backwaters (10.4.19). Harwich and Landguard Pt are close to the N. Making Harwich from the SE beware the drying Cork Sand, which lies N/S.

Sunk It Float (Fog sig, RC), 11M E of The Naze, marks the outer apprs to Harwich (10.4.20), an extensive and well sheltered hbr accessible at all times (chart *2693*). The Harwich DW channel begins 1·5M NNW of Sunk It Float and runs N between Rough and Shipwash shoals, then W past the Cork Sand PHM It buoy. It is in constant use by commercial shipping and yachts should approach via the Recommended Track for yachts. Approaching from NE and 2M off the ent to R. Deben (10.4.22), beware Cutler shoal, with least depth of 1·2m, marked by SHM buoy on E side; Wadgate Ledge and the Platters are about 1·5M ENE of Landguard Pt. S of Landguard Pt the W-going (flood) stream begins at HW Harwich + 0600, and the E-going stream at HW Harwich, sp rates about 1·5kn. Note: HW Harwich is never more than 7 mins after HW Walton; LW times are about 10 mins earlier.

HARWICH TO ORFORDNESS (chart *2052*)

Shipwash shoal, buoyed and with least depth 0·5m near its S end, runs NNE from 9M E of Felixstowe to 4M SSE of Orford Ness. Inshore of this is Shipway Chan, then Bawdsey Bank, buoyed with depths of 2m, on which the sea breaks in E'ly swell. The Sledway Chan lies between Bawdsey Bank and Whiting Bank (buoyed) which is close SW of Orford Ness, and has least depth of 1m. Hollesley Chan, about 1M wide, runs inshore W and N of this bank. In the SW part of Hollesley B is the ent to Orford Haven and the R Ore/Alde (10.4.23).

There are overfalls S of Orford Ness on both the ebb and flood streams. 2M E of Orford Ness the SW-going stream begins at HW Harwich + 0605, sp rate 2·5kn; the NE-going stream begins at HW Harwich – 0010, sp rate 3kn.

Note: The direction of local buoyage becomes S to N off Orford Ness (52°05'N).

ORFORDNESS TO GREAT YARMOUTH (chart 1543)

N of Orford Ness seas break on Aldeburgh Ridge (1.3m), but the coast is clear of offlying dangers past Aldeburgh and Southwold (10.4.24), as far as Benacre Ness, 5M S of Lowestoft. Sizewell power stn is a conspic □ bldg 1·5M N of Thorpe Ness. Keep 1·5M offshore to avoid fishing floats.

Lowestoft (10.4.25) is approached from S by the buoyed/lit Stanford chan to E of Newcome Sand and SW of Holm Sand; beware possible strong set across hbr ent. From the N, approach through Yarmouth Road and then proceed S through Gorleston, Corton and Lowestoft North Roads (buoyed). From E, approach through the Holm chan. 1M E of hbr ent, the S-going stream begins at HW Dover –0600, and the N-going at HW Dover, sp rates 2·6kn.

In the approaches to Great Yarmouth (10.4.26) from seaward the banks are continually changing; use the buoyed chans. The sea often breaks on North Scroby, Middle Scroby and Caister Shoal (all of which dry), and there are heavy tide rips over parts of Corton and South Scroby Sands, Middle and South Cross Sands, and Winterton Overfalls.

1M NE of ent to Gt Yarmouth the S-going stream begins at HW Dover –0600, and the N-going at HW Dover – 0015, sp rates 2·3kn. Breydon Water (tidal) affects streams in the Haven; after heavy rain the out-going stream at Brush Quay may exceed 5kn. For Norfolk Broads, see 10.4.26. About 12M NE of Great Yarmouth lie Newarp Banks, on which the sea breaks in bad weather.

CROSSING FROM THAMES ESTUARY TO BELGIUM OR THE NETHERLANDS (charts 1610, 1872, 3371, *1406*, 1408)

Important factors in choosing a route include the need to head at 90° across the various TSSs; to avoid areas where traffic converges; to make full use of available ITZs and to keep well clear of offshore oil/gas activities (see 10.5.5). It is best to avoid the areas westward of W Hinder It, around Nord Hinder It buoy and the Maas routes W of the Hook of Holland. For Distances across N Sea, see 10.0.7 and for further notes on North Sea crossings, see 10.20.5.

Fig. 10 (6) illustrates the strategy of crossing the N Hinder South TSS and then either crossing the W Hinder TSS eastward of W Hinder It before proceeding to Belgian ports; or proceeding on a more direct route for ports between Zeebrugge and Hook of Holland.

From Rivers Crouch, Blackwater, Colne or Harwich take departure from Long Sand Hd It buoy to S Galloper It buoy, thence to W Hinder It (see 10.20.5), crossing the TSS at right angles near Garden City It buoy; see Fig. 10 (6). Care must be taken throughout with tidal streams, which may be setting across the yacht's track. The area is relatively shallow, and in bad weather seas are steep and short.

For ports between Hook of Holland and Texel it may be best to diverge to the NE so as to cross the several Deep Water (DW) routes, and their extensions, as quickly as possible, to the N of Nord Hinder It buoy and the Maas TSS. If bound for ports NE of Texel keep well S of the TX1 It buoy and then inshore of the Off Texel-Vlieland-Terschelling-German Bight TSS (Fig. 10 (7)), which is well buoyed on its S side.

10.4.6 DISTANCE TABLE

Approximate distances in nautical miles are by the most direct route, whilst avoiding dangers and allowing for Traffic Separation Schemes. Places in *italics* are in adjoining areas; places in **bold** are in 10.0.7, Distances across the North Sea.

1. *Ramsgate*	1																			
2. Whitstable	22	2																		
3. **Sheerness**	34	14	3																	
4. Gravesend	56	36	22	4																
5. **London Bridge**	76	55	45	23	5															
6. Southend-on-Sea	35	17	6	20	43	6														
7. Havengore	33	15	12	32	55	12	7													
8. **Burnham-on-Crouch**	44	36	34	53	76	33	30	8												
9. West Mersea	43	38	29	49	72	30	29	22	9											
10. **Brightlingsea**	41	36	28	47	71	28	26	22	8	10										
11. Walton-on-the-Naze	40	40	46	59	82	39	37	25	23	23	11									
12. **Harwich**	40	40	50	65	83	40	41	31	24	24	6	12								
13. Ipswich	49	49	59	74	92	49	50	40	33	33	15	9	13							
14. River Deben (ent)	45	45	55	71	89	46	46	35	38	38	10	6	15	14						
15. River Ore (ent)	47	47	60	75	93	50	51	38	43	43	14	10	19	4	15					
16. Southwold	62	67	80	95	113	70	71	58	63	63	33	30	39	23	20	16				
17. **Lowestoft**	72	77	90	105	123	80	81	68	73	73	43	40	49	33	30	10	17			
18. Great Yarmouth	79	84	97	112	130	87	88	76	81	80	51	52	61	41	38	18	7	18		
19. *Blakeney*	123	128	141	156	174	131	132	120	125	124	95	96	105	85	82	62	51	44	19	
20. *Bridlington*	207	198	224	226	244	201	215	204	205	204	181	175	184	169	165	145	135	114	79	20

EAST ANGLIAN WAYPOINTS 10-4-7

Selected waypoints for use in the Thames Estuary are listed below. Further waypoints in adjacent waters are given in 10.3.4, 10.3.8 and 10.4.4 for the English Coast; and 10.19.4, 10.20.4 and 10.21.4 for the coasts Central NE France, Belgium, the Netherlands and Germany.

Waypoint	Latitude	Longitude
Aldeburgh Ridge By	52°06'·82N	01°37'·60E
Barrow No.3 Lt By	51°41'·99N	01°20'·35E
Barrow No.6 Lt By	51°37'·27N	01°14'·79E
Barrow No.9 Lt By	51°35'·31N	01°10'·40E
Barrow No.11 Lt By	51°33'·73N	01°05'·85E
Black Deep No. 1 Lt By	51°44'·00N	01°28'·20E
Black Deep No. 3 Lt By	51°41'·95N	01°26'·07E
Black Deep No. 5 Lt By	51°39'·50N	01°23'·10E
Black Deep No. 7 Lt By	51°37'·05N	01°17'·80E
Black Deep No. 11 Lt By	51°34'·30N	01°13'·50E
Blacktail Spit Lt By	51°31'·45N	00°56'·85E
Black Deep Lt By	51°46'·60N	01°34'·05E
Blakeney Overfalls Lt By	53°03'·00N	01°01'·50E
Boston No. 1 Lt By	52°57'·87N	00°15'·22E
Boston Roads Lt By	52°57'·67N	00°16'·23E
Burnham Flats Lt By	53°07'·50N	00°35'·00E
Buxey No. 1 Lt By	51°39'·02N	01°00'·86E
Colne Bar Lt By	51°44'·58N	01°02'·67E
Cockle Lt By	52°44'·00N	01°43'·70E
Cork Lt By	51°55'·44N	01°27'·30E
Cork Sand Lt By	51°55'·42N	01°24'·57E
Corton Lt By	52°31'·10N	01°51'·50E
Cross Sand Lt By	52°37'·00N	01°59'·25E
Crouch Lt By	51°37'·60N	00°56'·49E
Cutler Lt By	51°58'·50N	01°27'·60E
Eagle Lt By	51°44'·10N	01°03'·92E
East Barnard Lt By	52°25'·11N	01°46'·50E
East Cross Sand Lt By	52°40'·00N	01°53'·80E
East Cocking Lt By	53°09'·80N	00°50'·50E
East Hammond Knoll Lt By	52°52'·30N	01°58'·75E
East Newcome Lt By	52°28'·48N	01°49'·32E
East Sheringham Lt By	53°02'·20N	01°15'·00E
East Shipwash Lt By	51°57'·05N	01°38'·00E
F3 Lanby	51°23'·82N	02°00'·62E
Felixstowe Ledge Lt By	51°56'·30N	01°24'·56E
Foulness Lt By	51°39'·82N	01°03'·92E
Gunfleet Spit Lt By	51°45'·30N	01°21'·80E
Harwich HA Lt By	51°56'·73N	01°30'·77E
Hemsby Lt By	52°41'·84N	01°45'·00E
Horse Shoal Lt By	51°37'·07N	00°51'·62E
Inner Crouch Lt By	51°37'·19N	00°55'·22E
Kentish Knock Lt By	51°38'·50N	01°40'·50E
Knob Lt By	51°30'·66N	01°04'·38E
Knock John Lt By	51°33'·46N	01°11'·08E
Knoll Lt By	51°43'·85N	01°05'·17E
Landguard Lt By	51°55'·35N	01°18'·98E
Long Sand Hd Lt By	51°47'·87N	01°39'·53E
Lynn Knock Lt By	53°04'·40N	00°27'·31E
Maplin Bank Lt By	51°35'·47N	01°04'·80E
Medusa Lt By	51°51'·20N	01°20'·46E
Mid Bawdsey Lt By	51°58'·85N	01°33'·70E
Mid Caister Lt By	52°38'·96N	01°45'·77E
Mid Haisboro Lt By	52°54'·20N	01°41'·70E
Newcome Sand Lt By	52°26'·65N	01°47'·15E
Newarp Lt V	52°48'·35N	01°55'·80E
NHR-S Lt By	51°51'·40N	02°28'·79E
NHR-SE Lt By	51°45'·50N	02°40'·00E
North Caister Lt By	52°40'·40N	01°45'·66E
North Docking Lt By	53°14'·80N	00°41'·60E
North East Bawdsey Lt By	52°01'·70N	01°36'·20E
North East Cross Sand Lt By	52°43'·00N	01°53'·80E
North East Gunfleet Lt By	51°49'·90N	01°27'·90E
North East Maplin Lt By	51°37'·43N	01°04'·90E
North East Whiting Lt By	52°03'·77N	01°33'·88E
North Galloper Lt By	51°50'·00N	01°59'·50E
North Haisbro Lt By	53°00'·20N	01°32'·40E
North Inner Gabbard Lt By	51°59'·10N	01°56'·10E
North Newcome Lt By	52°28'·29N	01°46'·43E
North Scroby Lt By	52°42'·49N	01°44'·80E
North Shipwash Lt By	52°01'·70N	01°38'·38E
North Well Lt By	53°03'·00N	00°28'·00E
North West Scroby Lt By	52°40'·35N	01°46'·44E
Orford Haven By	52°01'·63N	01°27'·67E
Outer Crouch Lt By	51°38'·35N	00°58'·61E
Outer Gabbard Lt By	51°57'·80N	02°04'·30E
Ridge Lt By	51°40'·10N	01°05'·00E
Rough Lt By	51°55'·16N	01°31'·11E
Scott Patch Lt By	53°11'·10N	00°36'·50E
Scroby Elbow Lt By	52°37'·32N	01°46'·50E
Ship Head Lt By	51°53'·76N	01°34'·01E
Smiths Knoll Lt By	52°43'·50N	02°18'·00E
South Bawdsey Lt By	51°57'·20N	01°30'·32E
South Buxey Lt By	51°39'·82N	01°02'·60E
South Cork By	51°51'·30N	01°24'·20E
South Corton Lt By	52°32'·50N	01°49'·86E
South Holm Lt By	52°27'·41N	01°47'·34E
South Inner Gabbard Lt By	51°51'·20N	01°52'·40E
South Galloper Lt By	51°43'·95N	01°56'·50E
South Haisbro Lt By	52°50'·80N	01°48'·40E
South Race Lt By	53°08'·18N	00°56'·81E
South Shipwash Lt By	51°52'·68N	01°34'·16E
South Winterton Ridge Lt By	52°47'·20N	02°03'·60E
South Whitaker Lt By	51°40'·20N	01°09'·15E
South West Barrow Lt By	51°31'·80N	01°00'·53E
South West Holm Lt By	52°28'·36N	01°47'·28E
South West Scroby Lt By	52°35'·81N	01°46'·55E
South West Shipwash Lt By	51°54'·72N	01°34'·32E
South West Swin Lt By	51°32'·73N	01°01'·18E
South West Whiting Lt By	52°01'·22N	01°30'·90E
Stanford Lt By	52°27'·65N	01°46'·80E
Stone Banks Lt By	51°53'·18N	01°19'·32E
Sunk Lt F	51°51'·00N	01°35'·00E
Sunk Lt By (Wash- Cork Hole)	52°56'·27N	00°23'·50E
Sunk Head Tr Lt By	51°46'·60N	01°30'·60E
Sunken Buxey Lt By	51°39'·50N	01°00'·70E
Swallow Tail By	51°40'·44N	01°40'·81E
Swin Spitway Lt By	51°41'·92N	01°08'·45E
Trinity Lt By	51°49'·00N	01°36'·50E
Wallet No.2 Lt By	51°48'·85N	01°23'·10E
Wallet No.4 Lt By	51°46'·50N	01°17'·33E
Wallet Spitway Lt By	51°42'·83N	01°07'·42E
Washington Lt By	51°56'·54N	01°27'·30E
Wells Fairway Lt By	52°59'·92N	00°49'·61E
West Corton Lt By	52°34'·46N	01°46'·42E
West Holm Lt By	52°29'·80N	01°47'·20E
West Hook Middle By	51°39'·15N	01°08'·07E
West Sheringham Lt By	53°02'·93N	01°06'·87E
West Sunk Lt By	51°44'·30N	01°25'·90E
Whitaker Lt By	51°41'·40N	01°10'·61E
Whiting Hook By	52°02'·95N	01°31'·93E
Woodbridge Haven By	51°58'·36N	01°24'·20E
Woolpack Lt By	53°02'·65N	00°31'·55E

SOUTHERN NORTH SEA WAYPOINTS

AREAS 19 AND 20

A1 Lt By	51°21'·72N 02°58'·20E
A2 Lt By	51°22'·50N 03°07'·05E
A 17 Lt By	49°41'·60N 00°01'·75E
A 18 Lt By	49°42'·07N 00°02'·21E
Abbeville Lt By	50°56'·08N 01°37'·42E
Adriana Lt By	51°56'·13N 03°50'·58E
Akkaert NE Lt By	51°27'·31N 02°59'·38E
Akkaert Mid Lt By	51°24'·23N 02°53'·50E
Akkaert SW Lt By	51°22'·33N 02°46'·42E
A-Noord Lt By	51°23'·50N 02°37'·00E
A-Zuid Lt By	51°21'·50N 02°37'·00E
Bergues N Lt By	51°20'·00N 02°24'·62E
Bergues Lt By	51°17'·20N 02°18'·70E
Bergues S Lt Buoy	51°15'·16N 02°19'·50E
Binnenstroombank Lt By	51°14'·50N 02°53'·73E
Birkenfels Lt By	51°39'·05N 02°32'·05E
Bol van Heist Lt By	51°23'·15N 03°12'·05E
Bollen Lt By	51°50'·00N 03°33'·00E
BT Ratel Lt By	51°11'·62N 02°28'·00E
Buitenbank Lt By	51°51'·20N 03°25'·80E
Buitenstroombank Lt By	51°15'·20N 02°51'·80E
CA2 Lt By	51°00'·91N 01°48'·86E
CA3 Lt By	50°56'·80N 01°41'·25E
CA4 Lt By	50°58'·94N 01°45'·18E
CA6 Lt By	50°58'·30N 01°45'·70E
CP-Q-A Platform	52°35'·56N 04°31'·98E
DKA Lt By	51°02'·59N 01°57'·06E
DKB Lt By	51°03'·00N 02°09'·34E
Dunkerque Lanby	51°03'·00N 01°51'·83E
DW5 Lt By	51°02'·20N 02°01'·00E
DW23 Lt By	51°03'·60N 02°15'·25E
DW29 Lt By	51°03'·88N 02°20'·32E
Dyck E Lt By	51°05'·70N 02°05'·70E
Fairy S Lt By	51°21'·22N 02°17'·35E
Fairy W Lt By	51°23'·90N 02°09'·44E
Garden City Lt By	51°29'·20N 02°17'·90E
Goote Bank Lt By	51°27'·00N 02°52'·72E
Haut-fond de Gravelines Lt By	
	51°04'·10N 02°05'·10E
Hinder Lt By	51°54'·60N 03°55'·50E
Hinder 1	51°20'·90N 02°11'·06E
IJmuiden Lt By (IJM)	52°28'·50N 04°23'·87E
Kaloo Lt By	51°35'·60N 03°23'·30E
Kwintebank Lt By	51°21'·75N 02°43'·00E
Le Havre Lanby	49°31'·44N 00°09'·78W
LST '420' Lt By	51°15'·50N 02°40'·70E
Maas Centre Lt By	52°01'·18N 03°53'·57E
Magne Lt By	51°39'·15N 03°19'·60E
MD 3 Lt By	51°42'·55N 03°26'·65E
Middelbank Lt By	51°40'·90N 03°18'·30E

Middelkerk Bk N Lt By	51°20'·87N 02°46'·40E
Middelkerk S Lt By	51°14'·78N 02°42'·00E
Middelkerk Bk Lt By	51°18'·25N 02°42'·80E
MPC Lt By	51°06'·09N 01°38'·36E
MV Lt By	51°57'·45N 03°58'·50E
MW 1 Lt By	51°51'·25N 03°09'·40E
Nautica Ena Lt By	51°18'·12N 02°52'·85E
NHR-N	52°10'·90N 03°05'·00E
Nieuwpoort Bk Lt By	51°10'·21N 02°36'·17E
Noordhinder Lt By	52°00'·04N 02°51'·48E
Oost Dyck Lt By	51°21'·55N 02°31'·20E
Oost Dyck W Lt By	51°17'·18N 02°26'·42E
Oostendebank N Lt By	51°21'·25N 02°53'·00E
Oostendebank Oost Lt By	51°17'·36N 02°52'·00E
Oostendebank W Lt By	51°16'·25N 02°44'·85E
Ooster Lt By	51°47'·97N 03°41'·32E
Ouistreham Lt By	49°20'·48N 00°14'·73W
Petten Lt By	52°47'·38N 04°36'·80E
Rabsbank Lt By	51°38'·30N 03°10'·00E
RCE Lt By	51°02'·40N 01°53'·20E
Ruytingen SW Lt By	51°04'·99N 01°46'·90E
Ruytingen SE Lt By	51°09'·20N 02°09'·00E
Ruytingen N Lt By	51°13'·12N 02°10'·42E
Ruytingen NW Lt By	51°09'·05N 01°57'·40E
Ruytingen W Lt By	51°06'·90N 01°50'·60E
Sandettie Lt F	51°09'·40N 01°47'·20E
Sandettie N Lt By	51°18'·42N 02°04'·80E
Sandettie SW Lt By	51°09'·72N 01°45'·73E
Sandettie WSW Lt By	51°12'·32N 01°51'·23E
SBZ Lt By	51°42'·50N 03°16'·70E
Scheur 3 Lt By	51°24'·35N 03°02'·90E
Scheur 4 Lt By	51°25'·07N 03°02'·93E
Scheur-Wielingen Lt By	51°24'·26N 03°18'·00E
Scheur-Zand Lt By	51°23'·68N 03°07'·68E
Schouwenbank Lt By	51°45'·00N 03°14'·40E
SG Lt By	51°52'·00N 03°51'·50E
SM Lt By	53°19'·29N 04°55'·71E
TB Lt By	51°34'·45N 02°59'·15E
Thornton SW Lt By	51°31'·01N 02°51'·00E
Track Ferry Lt By	51°33'·80N 02°36'·50E
Trapegeer Lt By	51°08'·46N 02°34'·52E
Twin Lt By	51°32'·10N 02°22'·62E
TX 1 Lt By	52°48'·17N 04°15'·60E
TX 3 Lt By	52°58'·60N 04°22'·60E
Vergoyer SW Lt By	50°26'·90N 01°00'·10E
VL 1 Lt By	53°11'·00N 04°35'·40E
VL 11 Lt By	53°28'·12N 05°04'·00E
Wandelaar SW Lt By	51°22'·00N 03°01'·00E
Wenduinebank E Lt By	51°18'·85N 03°01'·70E
Wenduinebank N Lt By	51°21'·50N 03°02'·71E
Wenduinebank W Lt By	51°17'·28N 02°52'·87E
West Hinder Lt	51°23'·36N 02°26'·36E
Westpit Lt By	51°33'·70N 03°10'·00E
Westroombank Lt Buoy	51°11'·39N 02°43'·15E
WG Lt By	53°32'·25N 06°06'·11E
Wielingen Zand Lt By	51°22'·60N 03°10'·80E
Zand Lt By	51°22'·52N 03°10'·16E
ZSB Lt By	51°36'·80N 03°15'·00E
Zuidstroombank Lt Buoy	51°12'·33N 02°47'·50E

4

10-4-8   THAMES ESTUARY TIDAL STREAMS

Due to very strong rates of tidal streams in some areas, eddies may occur. Where possible, some indication of these is shown, but in many areas there is insufficient information or eddies are unstable.

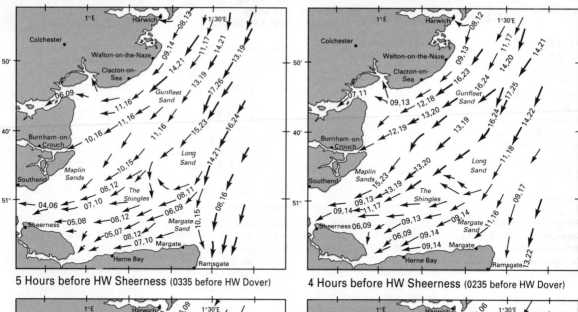

5 Hours before HW Sheerness (0335 before HW Dover)

4 Hours before HW Sheerness (0235 before HW Dover)

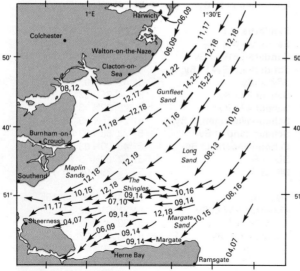

3 Hours before HW Sheerness (0135 before HW Dover)

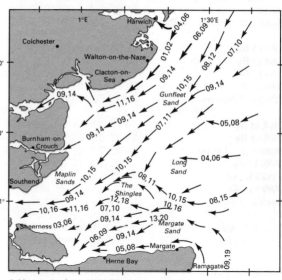

2 Hours before HW Sheerness (0035 before HW Dover)

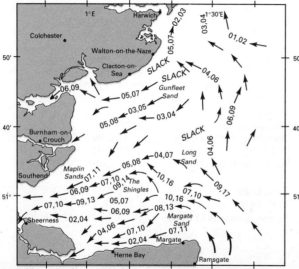

1 Hour before HW Sheerness (0025 after HW Dover)

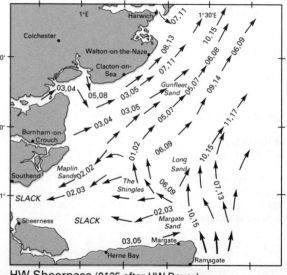

HW Sheerness (0125 after HW Dover)

Due to very strong rates of tidal streams in some areas, eddies may occur. Where possible, some indication of these is shown, but in many areas there is insufficient information or eddies are unstable.

4

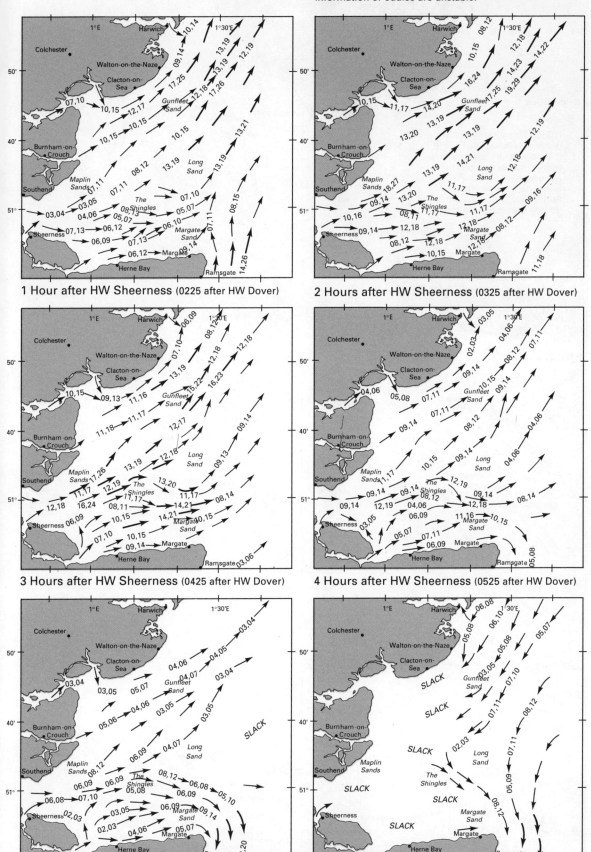

1 Hour after HW Sheerness (0225 after HW Dover)

2 Hours after HW Sheerness (0325 after HW Dover)

3 Hours after HW Sheerness (0425 after HW Dover)

4 Hours after HW Sheerness (0525 after HW Dover)

5 Hours after HW Sheerness (0600 before HW Dover)

6 Hours after HW Sheerness (0500 before HW Dover)

THAMES ESTUARY   10-4-9

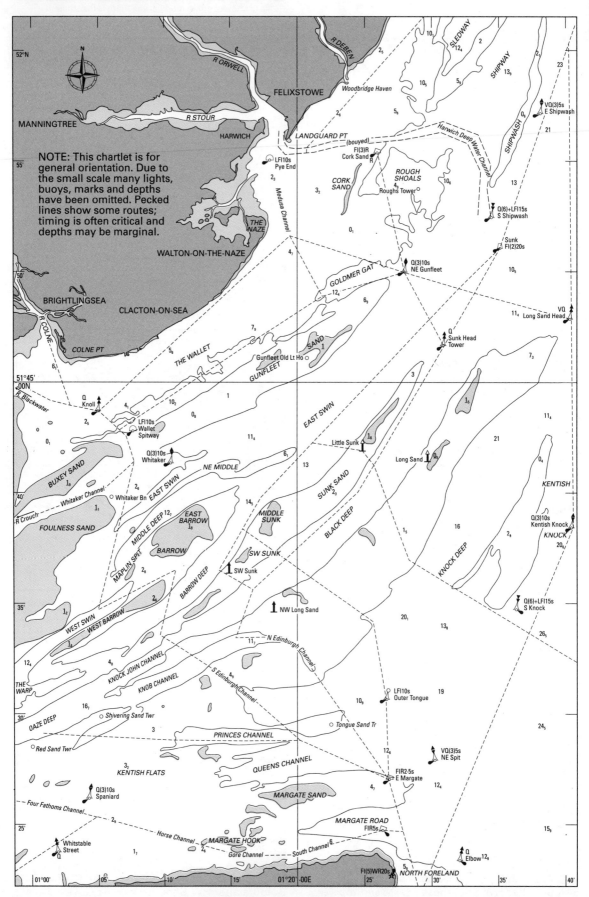

NOTE: This chartlet is for general orientation. Due to the small scale many lights, buoys, marks and depths have been omitted. Pecked lines show some routes; timing is often critical and depths may be marginal.

WHITSTABLE 10-4-10

Kent 51°21'·83N 01°01'·56E

CHARTS
AC 2571, *1607*; Imray Y14; Stanfords 5; OS 179

TIDES
+0135 Dover; ML 3·0; Duration 0605; Zone 0 (UT)

Standard Port SHEERNESS (→)

Times				Height (metres)			
High Water		Low Water		MHWS	MHWN	MLWN	MLWS
0200	0800	0200	0700	5·8	4·7	1·5	0·6
1400	2000	1400	1900				
Differences WHITSTABLE							
−0008	−0011	+0005	0000	−0·3	−0·3	0·0	−0·1
MARGATE							
−0050	−0040	−0020	−0050	−0·9	−0·9	−0·1	0·0
HERNE BAY							
−0025	−0015	0000	−0025	−0·5	−0·5	−0·1	−0·1

SHELTER
Good, except in strong winds from NNW to NE. Hbr dries. Access HW±1 for strangers. Berthing is limited to genuine refuge seekers since priority is given to commercial shipping. Fender board needed against piled quays or seek a mooring to NW of hbr, as controlled by YC.

NAVIGATION
WPT 51°22'·62N 01°01'·20E, 165°/345° from/to W Quay dolphin, 0·83M. From E keep well seaward of Whitstable Street, a hard drying sandspit, which extends 1M N from the coast; shoals a further 1M to seaward are marked by Whitstable Street NCM lt buoy. From W avoid Columbine and Pollard Spits. Appr (not before half flood) either direct in the G sector or in W sector via Whitstable Oyster PHM buoy and ldg lts. Beware shoals near approaches, which are very shallow. Oyster beds are numerous.

LIGHTS AND MARKS
Ldg lts 122°, both FR. Off head of W Quay is a dolphin, Fl WRG 5s, vis W118°-156°, G156°-178°, R178°-201°. NE arm FW 15m 8M = hbr open; FR below this lt = hbr closed.

RADIO TELEPHONE
VHF Ch **09** 12 16 (Mon-Fri: 0800-1700 LT. Other times: HW −3 to HW+1). Tidal info on request.

TELEPHONE (01227)
Hr Mr 274086; MRSC (01255) 675518; ⌗ (01304) 202441; Marinecall 0891 500455; Police 770055; Dr 263844/263033.

FACILITIES
Hbr ☎ 274086, AB £10.50, FW, D, C (15 ton); **Whitstable YC ☎** 272942, M, R, Slip, L, FW, Bar.
Services: ME, Sh, C, CH, ACA, SM, Gas, El, Ⓔ.
Town EC Wed; Ⓞ, P, V, R, Bar, ✉, Ⓑ, ⇌, ✈ Lydd/Manston.

MINOR HARBOURS WEST OF NORTH FORELAND

MARGATE, Kent, 51°23'·40N 01°22'·75E. AC 1827, 1828, 323; Imray Y7, C1; Stanfords 5; OS 179. HW+0045 on Dover; ML 2·6; Duration 0610; see 10.4.10. Small hbr drying 3m, inside bkwtr (Stone Pier) FR 18m 4M; exposed to NW'lies. Tide gauge with Q lt, 350°/170° from/to hbr ent, 0·22M. Appr's: from E, via Longnose NCM buoy, keeping about 5ca offshore; from N, via Margate PHM buoy Fl R 2·5s; from W via Gore Chan and S Chan to SE Margate ECM buoy, Q (3) 10s. Beware ruins of old pier, known as the Iron Jetty, Fl (3) R 10s, extending 2½ca N from root of Stone Pier. VHF none. Facilities: **Margate YC ☎** (01843) 292602, R, Bar. **Town** EC Thurs; D & P (cans from garage), R, V, Bar, ✉, Ⓑ, ⇌, ✈ Manston.

HERNE BAY, Kent, 51°22'·37N 01°07'·32E. AC 1607. Tides see 10.4.10. Close E of pier, a new 400m long bkwtr offers drying shelter for dayboats/dinghies. Lts: QW 8m 4M is 6ca offshore (former pier hd); bkwtr hd 2FR (vert); pier hd 2FG (vert). Reculvers conspic twrs are 3M to the E. Slip.

MINOR HARBOUR SOUTH OF SHEERNESS (See 10.4.11)

QUEENBOROUGH, Kent (Isle of Sheppey). 51°25'·01N 00°44'·29E. AC *1834*. Tides as Sheerness 10.4.12. The first deep-water refuge W of N Foreland, accessible at all tides from Garrison Pt; or from the Swale on the tide. Speed limit 8kn. Enter at Queenborough Spit ECM buoy, Q (3) 10s, via narrow chan between drying banks & moorings. An all-tide pontoon/jetty (5m) on E bank is for landing/short stay only; both sides of the jetty are foul. 4 Ⓥ berths on concrete lighter on W side or at 2 Y ⚓s (4 boats on each) close S of The Hard, a drying causeway. Lights: As chartlet. Note: Q 16m 5M lt, vis 163°-168°, on river bend covers the chan. All-tide landing 2 FR (vert). Concrete lighter Fl G 3s. Facilities: Hbr Controller (AB/⚓ £6.00) ☎ (01795) 662051, AC, FW on all-tide Landing. **Queenborough YC ☎** 663955, M, R, Bar; Water Taxi: call *Queen Base* Ch M in season. **The Creek** (dries) FW, Slip, Scrubbing berth. **Services:** BY, ME, El, Sh, CH, C (10 ton), Gas; **Town** EC Wed; V, R, Bar, ✉, Ⓑ, ⇌, ✈ (Manston).

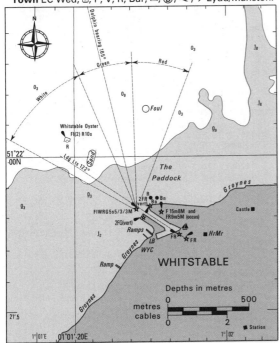

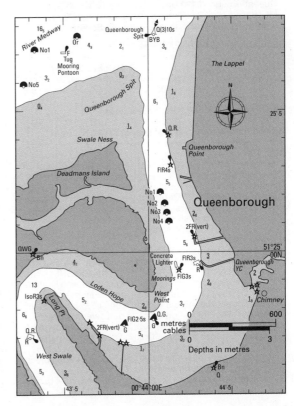

THE SWALE
Kent.

10-4-11

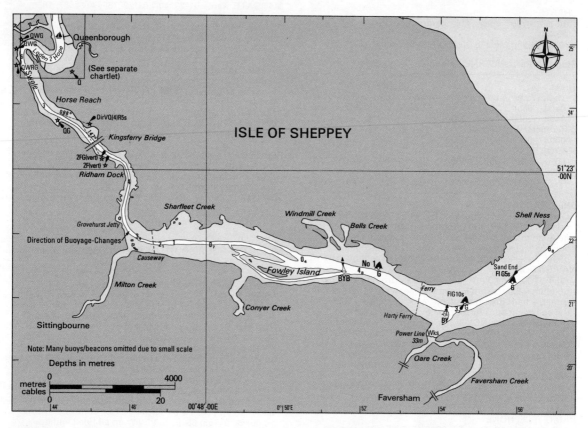

CHARTS
AC 2571, 2482, 2572, *1834*, 3683; Imray Y18, Y14;
Stanfords 5, 8; OS 178

TIDES
Queenborough +0130 Dover; Harty Ferry +0120 Dover;
ML (Harty Ferry) 3·0; Duration 0610; Zone 0 (UT). HW
differences at Faversham are –0·2m on Sheerness.

Standard Port SHEERNESS (→)

Times				Height (metres)			
High Water		Low Water		MHWS	MHWN	MLWN	MLWS
0200	0800	0200	0700	5·8	4·7	1·5	0·6
1400	2000	1400	1900				

Differences R. SWALE (Grovehurst Jetty)

–0007	0000	0000	+0016	0·0	0·0	0·0	–0·1

Grovehurst Jetty is close N of the ent to Milton Creek.

SHELTER
Excellent in the Swale, the 14M chan between the Isle of
Sheppey and the N Kent coast, from Shell Ness in the E
to Queenborough in the W. Yachts can enter the drying
creeks of Faversham, Oare, Conyer, and Milton. Beware
wrecks at ent to Faversham Creek. Many moorings line
the chan from Faversham to Conyer. See overleaf for
Queenborough, all-tide access.

NAVIGATION
E ent WPT: Columbine Spit SHM, 51°23'·84N 01°00'·13E,
050°/230° from/to ent to buoyed chan 1·3M. The first chan
buoys are Pollard Spit PHM QR and Ham Gat SHM unlit;
buoys are moved to suit the shifting chan. Speed limit 8kn.
The chan is well marked, but unlit from Faversham to
Milton Creek. The middle section from 1·5M E of Conyer
Creek to 0·5M E of Milton Creek is narrowed by drying
mudbanks and carries least depths of 0·4m. Direction of
buoyage changes at Milton Creek. There are numerous
oyster beds in the area. Kingsferry Bridge (see below)
normally opens for masted craft on request, but subject
to railway trains; temp anchs off SW bank.
The **W ent** is marked by Queenborough Spit ECM buoy,
Q (3) 10s, 1M S of Garrison Pt, at 51°25'·78N 00°44'·03E.

LIGHTS AND MARKS
No fixed lts at E ent. In W Swale the following lights are
intended for large coasters using the narrow chan:
(1) Dir ent lt Q 16m 5M; vis 163°-168°.
(2) Round Loden Hope bend: two Q WG and one Q WRG
on bns; keep in G sectors.
(3) Horse Reach ldg lts 113°: front QG 7m 5M; rear Fl G 3s
10m 6M. Dir lt 098°, VQ (4) R 5s 6m 5M.
(4) Kingsferry Bridge ldg lts 147°: front 2FG(vert) 9m 7M;
rear 2 FW (vert) 11m 10M. Lts on bridge: two x 2 FG
(vert) on SW buttresses; two x 2 FR (vert) on NE.

Kingsferry Bridge traffic sigs:

No lts	= Bridge down (3·35m MHWS).
Al Q Ⓡ/Ⓖ	= Centre span lifting.
F Ⓖ	= Bridge open (29m MHWS).
Q Ⓡ	= Centre span lowering. Keep clear.
Q Ⓨ	= Bridge out of action.

Best to request bridge opening on VHF Ch 10; or hoist a
bucket in the rigging; or sound 1 long and 4 short blasts.

RADIO TELEPHONE
Call: *Medway Radio* VHF Ch **74** 16 22 (H24); Kingsferry
Bridge Ch 10 (H24).

TELEPHONE (01795)
Hr Mr (Medway Ports Ltd) 580003; MRSC (01255) 675518;
⌗ (01304) 202441; Marinecall 0891 500455; Police 536639;
Dr or Ⓗ contact Medway Navigation Service 663025.

FACILITIES
FAVERSHAM: **Services:** BY, AB £5, M, AC, FW, Ⓔ, ME, El,
Sh, C (40 ton), SM, D, C (25 ton).
 Town EC Thurs; V, R, Bar, Gas, ✉, Ⓑ, ⇌, ✈ Gatwick.
OARE CREEK: **Services:** AB £5, M, C (8 ton), ME, El, Sh, CH;
 Hollow Shore Cruising Club ☎ 533254, Bar.
CONYER CREEK: **Swale Marina** ☎/Fax 521562, £5, BH (15
ton), ME, Sh, C (3 ton), Slip; **Conyer CC**.
 Services: CH, SM, Rigging, BY, ME, Sh, El, Ⓔ, Slip, D.
MILTON CREEK (Sittingbourne): **Crown Quay** M, FW.
 Town EC Wed; V, R, Bar, ✉, Ⓑ, ⇌, ✈ (Gatwick); also the
Dolphin Yard Sailing Barge Museum.
QUEENBOROUGH: See overleaf for details/chartlet.

ENGLAND – SHEERNESS

LAT 51°27'N　LONG　0°45'E

TIMES AND HEIGHTS OF HIGH AND LOW WATERS　　YEAR **1996**

TIME ZONE (UT)
For Summer Time add ONE hour in non-shaded areas

4

JANUARY

Day	Time (m)	Day	Time (m)
1 M	0232 1.5 / 0851 4.9 / 1515 1.3 / 2129 5.1	**16** TU	0110 1.4 / 0741 4.9 / 1413 1.1 / 2029 4.9
2 TU	0345 1.3 / 0952 5.1 / 1612 1.2 / 2224 5.2	**17** W	0242 1.4 / 0859 5.0 / 1528 1.0 / 2141 5.1
3 W	0443 1.1 / 1046 5.3 / 1700 1.1 / 2314 5.4	**18** TH	0401 1.1 / 1011 5.3 / 1635 0.8 / 2244 5.4
4 TH	0531 1.0 / 1135 5.4 / 1743 1.1 / 2357 5.5	**19** F	0510 0.8 / 1113 5.6 / 1734 0.6 / 2340 5.7
5 F O	0614 0.8 / 1218 5.5 / 1821 1.0	**20** SA ●	0611 0.4 / 1209 5.9 / 1827 0.5
6 SA	0036 5.6 / 0652 0.8 / 1257 5.5 / 1855 1.0	**21** SU	0031 6.0 / 0705 0.2 / 1301 6.1 / 1916 0.4
7 SU	0111 5.5 / 0727 0.8 / 1331 5.5 / 1925 1.0	**22** M	0120 6.0 / 0755 0.0 / 1351 6.1 / 2002 0.4
8 M	0142 5.5 / 0759 0.8 / 1404 5.5 / 1954 1.0	**23** TU	0206 6.0 / 0841 0.0 / 1438 6.1 / 2044 0.4
9 TU	0213 5.5 / 0831 0.8 / 1437 5.5 / 2023 1.0	**24** W	0251 6.0 / 0923 0.1 / 1524 6.0 / 2123 0.5
10 W	0245 5.5 / 0902 0.8 / 1513 5.5 / 2053 1.0	**25** TH	0334 5.9 / 1002 0.2 / 1608 5.8 / 2200 0.7
11 TH	0320 5.4 / 0933 0.8 / 1551 5.4 / 2125 1.0	**26** F	0416 5.7 / 1038 0.5 / 1654 5.5 / 2238 0.9
12 F	0358 5.4 / 1002 0.8 / 1634 5.3 / 2201 1.1	**27** SA	0501 5.4 / 1117 0.8 / 1741 5.2 / 2322 1.1
13 SA	0442 5.3 / 1038 0.9 / 1721 5.2 / 2246 1.2	**28** SU	0552 5.1 / 1203 1.1 / 1837 4.9
14 SU	0533 5.1 / 1131 1.0 / 1815 5.0 / 2345 1.4	**29** M	0016 1.4 / 0656 4.8 / 1301 1.3 / 1941 4.7
15 M	0632 4.9 / 1249 1.1 / 1918 4.9	**30** TU	0124 1.5 / 0810 4.7 / 1412 1.5 / 2049 4.7
		31 W	0252 1.5 / 0920 4.8 / 1532 1.4 / 2152 4.9

FEBRUARY

Day	Time (m)	Day	Time (m)
1 TH	0416 1.3 / 1021 5.0 / 1633 1.3 / 2246 5.2	**16** F	0349 1.1 / 0956 5.1 / 1621 0.9 / 2228 5.2
2 F	0511 1.0 / 1112 5.2 / 1721 1.1 / 2333 5.4	**17** SA	0503 0.7 / 1102 5.5 / 1721 0.6 / 2326 5.6
3 SA	0555 0.8 / 1157 5.4 / 1802 1.0	**18** SU ●	0602 0.3 / 1158 5.8 / 1814 0.4
4 SU O	0014 5.5 / 0634 0.7 / 1236 5.5 / 1836 0.9	**19** M	0018 5.8 / 0652 0.1 / 1249 6.0 / 1901 0.3
5 M	0052 5.5 / 0709 0.7 / 1312 5.5 / 1906 0.9	**20** TU	0106 6.0 / 0739 -0.1 / 1336 6.1 / 1945 0.2
6 TU	0125 5.5 / 0741 0.7 / 1345 5.5 / 1935 0.9	**21** W	0150 6.0 / 0821 -0.1 / 1420 6.1 / 2026 0.3
7 W	0156 5.5 / 0813 0.7 / 1417 5.5 / 2004 0.9	**22** TH	0231 6.0 / 0859 0.0 / 1501 5.9 / 2102 0.4
8 TH	0227 5.5 / 0842 0.6 / 1451 5.6 / 2033 0.8	**23** F	0309 5.9 / 0933 0.2 / 1539 5.7 / 2135 0.5
9 F	0259 5.6 / 0909 0.6 / 1527 5.6 / 2102 0.8	**24** SA	0347 5.7 / 1004 0.5 / 1617 5.5 / 2208 0.7
10 SA	0336 5.6 / 0933 0.7 / 1607 5.5 / 2134 0.8	**25** SU	0425 5.5 / 1037 0.8 / 1655 5.2 / 2245 1.0
11 SU	0417 5.5 / 1004 0.7 / 1652 5.3 / 2214 0.9	**26** M	0508 5.1 / 1118 1.1 / 1739 4.8 / 2333 1.3
12 M	0505 5.3 / 1049 0.9 / 1743 5.1 / 2306 1.1	**27** TU	0602 4.8 / 1213 1.4 / 1841 4.5
13 TU	0601 5.1 / 1156 1.1 / 1843 4.9	**28** W	0036 1.5 / 0720 4.5 / 1321 1.6 / 2003 4.4
14 W	0020 1.4 / 0709 4.8 / 1341 1.3 / 1956 4.7	**29** TH	0151 1.6 / 0845 4.5 / 1442 1.6 / 2115 4.6
15 TH	0215 1.4 / 0834 4.8 / 1509 1.2 / 2117 4.9		

MARCH

Day	Time (m)	Day	Time (m)
1 F	0334 1.4 / 0951 4.8 / 1603 1.4 / 2215 4.9	**16** SA	0341 1.1 / 0947 5.1 / 1607 1.0 / 2212 5.1
2 SA	0443 1.1 / 1045 5.1 / 1657 1.1 / 2305 5.2	**17** SU	0451 0.6 / 1051 5.5 / 1705 0.7 / 2310 5.5
3 SU	0529 0.9 / 1131 5.4 / 1738 1.0 / 2348 5.4	**18** M	0546 0.3 / 1145 5.8 / 1756 0.4
4 M	0607 0.7 / 1210 5.5 / 1813 0.9	**19** TU ●	0001 5.8 / 0633 0.1 / 1233 6.0 / 1842 0.3
5 TU O	0027 5.5 / 0643 0.6 / 1247 5.6 / 1843 0.8	**20** W	0047 5.9 / 0716 0.0 / 1317 6.0 / 1924 0.2
6 W	0103 5.6 / 0716 0.6 / 1321 5.6 / 1914 0.8	**21** TH	0129 6.0 / 0756 0.0 / 1358 6.0 / 2004 0.3
7 TH	0135 5.6 / 0749 0.6 / 1355 5.6 / 1945 0.7	**22** F	0208 6.0 / 0831 0.2 / 1435 5.8 / 2039 0.4
8 F	0207 5.6 / 0820 0.6 / 1429 5.7 / 2014 0.7	**23** SA	0244 5.9 / 0902 0.4 / 1508 5.7 / 2111 0.5
9 SA	0240 5.7 / 0846 0.6 / 1505 5.7 / 2043 0.7	**24** SU	0318 5.7 / 0931 0.6 / 1540 5.5 / 2141 0.7
10 SU	0316 5.7 / 0911 0.6 / 1544 5.6 / 2116 0.7	**25** M	0354 5.5 / 1002 0.8 / 1615 5.2 / 2214 0.8
11 M	0358 5.7 / 0944 0.7 / 1627 5.4 / 2156 0.8	**26** TU	0435 5.2 / 1040 1.1 / 1655 5.0 / 2259 1.1
12 TU	0446 5.4 / 1030 0.9 / 1717 5.1 / 2247 1.0	**27** W	0524 4.9 / 1131 1.4 / 1748 4.6
13 W	0542 5.1 / 1134 1.2 / 1817 4.8	**28** TH	0000 1.4 / 0629 4.5 / 1239 1.6 / 1906 4.4
14 TH	0001 1.3 / 0652 4.8 / 1323 1.4 / 1933 4.7	**29** F	0111 1.5 / 0800 4.5 / 1353 1.7 / 2032 4.5
15 F	0203 1.3 / 0822 4.8 / 1455 1.3 / 2059 4.8	**30** SA	0226 1.4 / 0914 4.7 / 1514 1.5 / 2138 4.8
		31 SU	0351 1.2 / 1011 5.0 / 1619 1.2 / 2231 5.1

APRIL

Day	Time (m)	Day	Time (m)
1 M	0448 0.9 / 1058 5.3 / 1703 1.0 / 2316 5.3	**16** TU	0523 0.3 / 1125 5.8 / 1734 0.5 / 2339 5.7
2 TU	0530 0.7 / 1139 5.5 / 1740 0.9 / 2357 5.5	**17** W ●	0609 0.2 / 1212 5.9 / 1820 0.4
3 W	0609 0.6 / 1218 5.7 / 1815 0.8	**18** TH	0025 5.8 / 0650 0.2 / 1255 5.9 / 1902 0.4
4 TH O	0034 5.6 / 0646 0.6 / 1255 5.7 / 1851 0.7	**19** F	0107 5.9 / 0727 0.3 / 1334 5.9 / 1942 0.4
5 F	0110 5.7 / 0722 0.5 / 1330 5.8 / 1927 0.7	**20** SA	0145 5.8 / 0801 0.4 / 1409 5.7 / 2017 0.5
6 SA	0145 5.8 / 0757 0.5 / 1407 5.8 / 2001 0.6	**21** SU	0221 5.6 / 0833 0.6 / 1440 5.6 / 2049 0.6
7 SU	0222 5.8 / 0828 0.5 / 1444 5.8 / 2033 0.6	**22** M	0254 5.7 / 0903 0.7 / 1510 5.5 / 2119 0.7
8 M	0301 5.8 / 0859 0.6 / 1525 5.7 / 2108 0.6	**23** TU	0330 5.5 / 0932 0.9 / 1544 5.3 / 2151 0.8
9 TU	0345 5.7 / 0936 0.7 / 1609 5.5 / 2150 0.7	**24** W	0409 5.3 / 1006 1.1 / 1624 5.1 / 2232 1.0
10 W	0435 5.5 / 1023 1.0 / 1700 5.2 / 2244 1.0	**25** TH	0456 5.0 / 1053 1.4 / 1713 4.8 / 2328 1.2
11 TH	0534 5.1 / 1131 1.3 / 1802 4.9	**26** F	0552 4.7 / 1156 1.6 / 1817 4.6
12 F	0006 1.2 / 0647 4.9 / 1310 1.4 / 1919 4.7	**27** SA	0034 1.4 / 0704 4.5 / 1306 1.7 / 1938 4.5
13 SA	0158 1.2 / 0814 4.9 / 1437 1.3 / 2041 4.8	**28** SU	0141 1.3 / 0823 4.6 / 1414 1.6 / 2050 4.7
14 SU	0326 0.9 / 0931 5.2 / 1547 1.0 / 2151 5.2	**29** M	0247 1.2 / 0927 4.9 / 1518 1.4 / 2148 4.9
15 M	0431 0.6 / 1033 5.5 / 1644 0.7 / 2248 5.5	**30** TU	0351 1.0 / 1018 5.2 / 1613 1.1 / 2238 5.2

Chart Datum: 2·90 metres below Ordnance Datum (Newlyn)

ENGLAND – SHEERNESS

LAT 51°27′N   LONG 0°45′E

TIMES AND HEIGHTS OF HIGH AND LOW WATERS

YEAR **1996**

TIME ZONE (UT)

For Summer Time add ONE hour in non-shaded areas

MAY

Day	Time	m	Time	m	Time	m	Time	m
1 W	0445	0.8	1104	5.5	1701	0.9	2322	5.5
2 TH	0532	0.6	1146	5.7	1745	0.8		
3 F ○	0004	5.6	0615	0.5	1227	5.8	1828	0.7
4 SA	0044	5.8	0657	0.5	1307	5.9	1911	0.6
5 SU	0125	5.9	0737	0.5	1347	5.9	1953	0.5
6 M	0207	6.0	0816	0.5	1428	5.9	2034	0.5
7 TU	0251	5.9	0854	0.6	1512	5.8	2114	0.5
8 W	0339	5.8	0935	0.7	1559	5.6	2200	0.7
9 TH	0431	5.6	1025	1.0	1651	5.3	2258	0.8
10 F	0532	5.3	1129	1.2	1754	5.1		
11 SA	0018	1.0	0642	5.1	1251	1.3	1905	5.0
12 SU	0145	1.0	0757	5.1	1410	1.3	2018	5.0
13 M	0302	0.9	0906	5.3	1520	1.1	2123	5.2
14 TU	0405	0.7	1007	5.5	1619	0.9	2222	5.4
15 W	0457	0.5	1100	5.7	1711	0.7	2314	5.6
16 TH	0542	0.5	1148	5.8	1758	0.6		
17 F ●	0002	5.7	0622	0.5	1232	5.8	1841	0.6
18 SA	0046	5.7	0700	0.6	1311	5.8	1921	0.6
19 SU	0125	5.7	0735	0.7	1346	5.7	1958	0.6
20 M	0201	5.6	0807	0.8	1416	5.6	2031	0.7
21 TU	0235	5.5	0838	0.9	1447	5.5	2102	0.7
22 W	0310	5.4	0907	1.0	1521	5.4	2134	0.8
23 TH	0348	5.3	0939	1.1	1600	5.2	2212	0.9
24 F	0431	5.1	1019	1.3	1645	5.0	2259	1.1
25 SA	0520	4.9	1113	1.4	1738	4.8	2358	1.2
26 SU	0618	4.8	1217	1.5	1841	4.7		
27 M	0100	1.2	0724	4.7	1323	1.5	1951	4.7
28 TU	0202	1.1	0832	4.9	1426	1.4	2057	4.9
29 W	0303	1.0	0933	5.1	1526	1.2	2155	5.1
30 TH	0403	0.8	1026	5.4	1624	1.0	2246	5.4
31 F	0458	0.7	1114	5.6	1718	0.8	2334	5.6

JUNE

Day	Time	m	Time	m	Time	m	Time	m
1 SA ○	0549	0.5	1200	5.8	1810	0.7		
2 SU	0021	5.8	0636	0.5	1246	5.9	1900	0.4
3 M	0108	6.0	0722	0.4	1331	6.0	1950	0.4
4 TU	0155	6.1	0807	0.5	1416	6.0	2038	0.4
5 W	0243	6.1	0851	0.5	1502	5.9	2125	0.4
6 TH	0333	5.9	0935	0.7	1551	5.7	2214	0.5
7 F	0426	5.8	1023	0.8	1643	5.5	2308	0.6
8 SA	0523	5.5	1119	1.0	1741	5.3		
9 SU	0009	0.7	0625	5.3	1224	1.2	1844	5.2
10 M	0118	0.9	0731	5.2	1335	1.3	1949	5.1
11 TU	0228	0.9	0836	5.2	1446	1.2	2054	5.2
12 W	0333	0.9	0937	5.4	1550	1.1	2154	5.3
13 TH	0427	0.8	1033	5.5	1647	1.0	2250	5.4
14 F	0514	0.8	1123	5.6	1736	0.8	2340	5.6
15 SA	0556	0.8	1209	5.7	1822	0.7		
16 SU ●	0026	5.6	0635	0.8	1250	5.7	1903	0.7
17 M	0108	5.6	0712	0.9	1326	5.6	1942	0.7
18 TU	0144	5.5	0745	0.9	1358	5.5	2016	0.7
19 W	0218	5.5	0816	0.9	1429	5.5	2048	0.8
20 TH	0251	5.4	0845	1.0	1501	5.4	2119	0.8
21 F	0327	5.4	0916	1.0	1537	5.3	2153	0.8
22 SA	0406	5.3	1003	1.1	1618	5.1	2231	0.9
23 SU	0449	5.2	1033	1.2	1703	5.1	2318	1.0
24 M	0539	5.0	1127	1.4	1755	4.9		
25 TU	0015	1.1	0634	4.9	1232	1.4	1854	4.8
26 W	0118	1.1	0738	4.9	1340	1.4	2001	4.9
27 TH	0223	1.1	0846	5.0	1447	1.3	2110	5.0
28 F	0328	0.9	0949	5.2	1552	1.1	2212	5.3
29 SA	0430	0.8	1046	5.5	1656	0.9	2309	5.6
30 SU	0527	0.6	1138	5.7	1756	0.6		

JULY

Day	Time	m	Time	m	Time	m	Time	m
1 M ○	0002	5.8	0620	0.5	1228	5.9	1852	0.4
2 TU	0053	6.0	0710	0.4	1316	6.0	1945	0.3
3 W	0144	6.1	0758	0.4	1404	6.0	2036	0.2
4 TH	0233	6.2	0843	0.4	1451	6.0	2123	0.1
5 F	0322	6.1	0928	0.5	1539	5.9	2209	0.2
6 SA	0412	5.9	1012	0.7	1627	5.8	2255	0.4
7 SU	0504	5.7	1058	0.8	1719	5.5	2342	0.6
8 M	0559	5.4	1149	1.1	1815	5.3		
9 TU	0036	0.9	0659	5.2	1250	1.3	1917	5.1
10 W	0141	1.1	0802	5.1	1401	1.4	2022	5.0
11 TH	0252	1.2	0905	5.1	1517	1.3	2127	5.1
12 F	0355	1.2	1004	5.2	1623	1.2	2226	5.2
13 SA	0448	1.1	1058	5.4	1717	1.0	2320	5.4
14 SU	0533	1.0	1146	5.5	1805	0.8		
15 M ●	0007	5.5	0614	1.0	1229	5.6	1847	0.8
16 TU	0050	5.5	0652	0.9	1307	5.6	1926	0.7
17 W	0127	5.5	0726	1.0	1340	5.5	2001	0.7
18 TH	0159	5.5	0757	1.0	1411	5.5	2032	0.7
19 F	0231	5.5	0825	1.0	1442	5.4	2101	0.8
20 SA	0304	5.5	0854	1.0	1514	5.4	2131	0.8
21 SU	0340	5.4	0925	1.0	1550	5.4	2200	0.8
22 M	0419	5.4	0959	1.1	1630	5.3	2233	0.9
23 TU	0503	5.2	1039	1.2	1716	5.2	2317	1.0
24 W	0554	5.1	1134	1.3	1810	5.0		
25 TH	0026	1.1	0653	4.9	1252	1.4	1914	4.9
26 F	0146	1.2	0802	4.9	1413	1.4	2030	4.9
27 SA	0300	1.1	0916	5.0	1528	1.2	2145	5.1
28 SU	0409	0.9	1022	5.3	1641	0.9	2250	5.5
29 M	0511	0.6	1119	5.6	1746	0.6	2348	5.8
30 TU	0606	0.5	1212	5.9	1844	0.3		
31 W ○	0040	6.0	0657	0.4	1302	6.0	1936	0.1

AUGUST

Day	Time	m	Time	m	Time	m	Time	m
1 TH	0131	6.2	0745	0.3	1349	6.1	2024	0.0
2 F	0219	6.2	0830	0.3	1435	6.1	2109	0.0
3 SA	0305	6.1	0912	0.4	1519	6.0	2150	0.1
4 SU	0351	6.0	0951	0.5	1603	5.9	2227	0.3
5 M	0437	5.7	1031	0.7	1649	5.6	2304	0.6
6 TU	0526	5.4	1113	1.0	1739	5.3	2347	1.0
7 W	0620	5.1	1204	1.3	1838	5.0		
8 TH	0041	1.3	0723	4.8	1308	1.5	1948	4.8
9 F	0154	1.5	0830	4.8	1432	1.5	2059	4.8
10 SA	0318	1.5	0934	4.9	1558	1.3	2203	5.0
11 SU	0422	1.3	1031	5.2	1657	1.1	2258	5.3
12 M	0511	1.1	1121	5.4	1745	0.9	2346	5.5
13 TU	0554	1.0	1205	5.6	1827	0.7		
14 W ●	0028	5.6	0632	0.9	1244	5.6	1904	0.7
15 TH	0104	5.6	0706	0.9	1318	5.6	1938	0.7
16 F	0137	5.6	0735	0.9	1350	5.5	2009	0.7
17 SA	0207	5.5	0802	1.0	1419	5.5	2038	0.7
18 SU	0239	5.5	0830	0.9	1450	5.5	2104	0.7
19 M	0312	5.6	0859	0.9	1523	5.5	2128	0.8
20 TU	0350	5.5	0929	1.0	1601	5.5	2153	0.8
21 W	0431	5.4	1004	1.1	1645	5.3	2230	1.0
22 TH	0519	5.2	1052	1.2	1737	5.1	2327	1.2
23 F	0616	4.9	1205	1.4	1840	4.9		
24 SA	0109	1.4	0725	4.8	1347	1.5	2000	4.8
25 SU	0238	1.3	0848	4.8	1512	1.3	2127	5.0
26 M	0352	1.1	1002	5.2	1631	0.9	2237	5.4
27 TU	0455	0.8	1102	5.5	1736	0.5	2335	5.8
28 W ○	0550	0.5	1155	5.8	1830	0.2		
29 TH	0027	6.0	0640	0.4	1244	6.0	1919	0.0
30 F	0115	6.2	0726	0.3	1330	6.1	2004	0.0
31 SA	0200	6.2	0810	0.3	1413	6.1	2045	0.0

Chart Datum: 2·90 metres below Ordnance Datum (Newlyn)

ENGLAND – SHEERNESS

LAT 51°27′N   LONG   0°45′E

TIMES AND HEIGHTS OF HIGH AND LOW WATERS

YEAR **1996**

4

TIME ZONE (UT)
For Summer Time add ONE hour in non-shaded areas

SEPTEMBER

Day	Time	m	Day	Time	m
1 SU	0243 / 0850 / 1455 / 2121	6.1 / 0.4 / 6.0 / 0.2	**16** M	0212 / 0807 / 1425 / 2036	5.7 / 0.9 / 5.6 / 0.8
2 M	0324 / 0926 / 1534 / 2153	5.9 / 0.5 / 5.9 / 0.4	**17** TU	0246 / 0836 / 1458 / 2059	5.7 / 0.9 / 5.6 / 0.8
3 TU	0404 / 1002 / 1615 / 2225	5.6 / 0.7 / 5.6 / 0.7	**18** W	0322 / 0906 / 1537 / 2126	5.6 / 0.9 / 5.6 / 0.9
4 W	0445 / 1039 / 1658 / 2303	5.3 / 1.0 / 5.3 / 1.1	**19** TH	0403 / 0941 / 1621 / 2204	5.5 / 1.0 / 5.4 / 1.0
5 TH	0531 / 1125 / 1753 / 2353	5.0 / 1.2 / 4.9 / 1.4	**20** F	0450 / 1028 / 1714 / 2300	5.2 / 1.2 / 5.2 / 1.3
6 F	0633 / 1225 / 1908	4.7 / 1.5 / 4.6	**21** SA	0546 / 1140 / 1818	4.9 / 1.4 / 4.9
7 SA	0100 / 0750 / 1339 / 2027	1.7 / 4.6 / 1.6 / 4.6	**22** SU	0039 / 0657 / 1330 / 1942	1.5 / 4.7 / 1.5 / 4.7
8 SU	0229 / 0900 / 1524 / 2135	1.7 / 4.7 / 1.5 / 4.8	**23** M	0218 / 0826 / 1501 / 2114	1.5 / 4.8 / 1.2 / 5.0
9 M	0352 / 1000 / 1629 / 2231	1.5 / 5.0 / 1.2 / 5.2	**24** TU	0335 / 0943 / 1619 / 2223	1.2 / 5.1 / 0.8 / 5.4
10 TU	0446 / 1051 / 1717 / 2319	1.2 / 5.3 / 0.9 / 5.5	**25** W	0438 / 1043 / 1719 / 2319	0.9 / 5.5 / 0.5 / 5.8
11 W	0530 / 1136 / 1758	1.0 / 5.6 / 0.7	**26** TH	0531 / 1135 / 1810	0.6 / 5.8 / 0.2
12 TH ●	0000 / 0607 / 1216 / 1834	5.6 / 0.7 / 5.6 / 0.7	**27** F O	0009 / 0619 / 1223 / 1855	6.0 / 0.4 / 6.0 / 0.1
13 F	0036 / 0639 / 1251 / 1908	5.7 / 0.9 / 5.6 / 0.7	**28** SA	0055 / 0704 / 1307 / 1937	6.1 / 0.3 / 6.1 / 0.1
14 SA	0109 / 0708 / 1324 / 1939	5.7 / 0.9 / 5.6 / 0.7	**29** SU	0137 / 0746 / 1349 / 2015	6.1 / 0.4 / 6.1 / 0.2
15 SU	0141 / 0737 / 1354 / 2009	5.6 / 0.9 / 5.6 / 0.7	**30** M	0217 / 0825 / 1428 / 2048	6.0 / 0.4 / 6.0 / 0.4

OCTOBER

Day	Time	m	Day	Time	m
1 TU	0254 / 0900 / 1505 / 2119	5.8 / 0.6 / 5.8 / 0.6	**16** W	0222 / 0819 / 1439 / 2039	5.8 / 0.8 / 5.8 / 0.8
2 W	0328 / 0934 / 1543 / 2149	5.6 / 0.7 / 5.6 / 0.9	**17** TH	0300 / 0852 / 1520 / 2111	5.7 / 0.9 / 5.7 / 0.9
3 TH	0402 / 1009 / 1623 / 2224	5.3 / 1.0 / 5.3 / 1.2	**18** F	0341 / 0930 / 1607 / 2152	5.5 / 0.9 / 5.5 / 1.1
4 F	0441 / 1052 / 1711 / 2311	5.0 / 1.2 / 4.9 / 1.5	**19** SA	0428 / 1020 / 1701 / 2249	5.3 / 1.1 / 5.2 / 1.3
5 SA	0533 / 1149 / 1817	4.7 / 1.4 / 4.6	**20** SU	0525 / 1136 / 1807	5.0 / 1.3 / 4.9
6 SU	0015 / 0656 / 1258 / 1945	1.8 / 4.5 / 1.6 / 4.5	**21** M	0019 / 0638 / 1318 / 1931	1.6 / 4.8 / 1.3 / 4.8
7 M	0133 / 0819 / 1417 / 2058	1.8 / 4.6 / 1.5 / 4.7	**22** TU	0156 / 0804 / 1446 / 2055	1.5 / 4.8 / 1.1 / 5.0
8 TU	0305 / 0923 / 1544 / 2156	1.7 / 4.9 / 1.3 / 5.1	**23** W	0313 / 0919 / 1558 / 2202	1.3 / 5.1 / 0.8 / 5.4
9 W	0411 / 1016 / 1637 / 2244	1.4 / 5.2 / 1.0 / 5.4	**24** TH	0415 / 1019 / 1656 / 2257	1.0 / 5.4 / 0.5 / 5.7
10 TH	0456 / 1101 / 1719 / 2326	1.1 / 5.4 / 0.8 / 5.6	**25** F	0509 / 1111 / 1745 / 2346	0.7 / 5.7 / 0.4 / 5.7
11 F	0532 / 1142 / 1757	1.0 / 5.6 / 0.7	**26** SA O	0557 / 1159 / 1829	0.5 / 5.9 / 0.3
12 SA ●	0003 / 0604 / 1220 / 1832	5.7 / 0.9 / 5.7 / 0.7	**27** SU	0031 / 0641 / 1244 / 1908	6.0 / 0.8 / 6.0 / 0.4
13 SU	0039 / 0637 / 1255 / 1906	5.7 / 0.9 / 5.7 / 0.7	**28** M	0113 / 0723 / 1325 / 1945	6.0 / 0.5 / 5.9 / 0.5
14 M	0113 / 0711 / 1328 / 1939	5.8 / 0.9 / 5.7 / 0.7	**29** TU	0150 / 0801 / 1404 / 2018	5.9 / 0.5 / 5.9 / 0.6
15 TU	0147 / 0746 / 1402 / 2010	5.8 / 0.8 / 5.7 / 0.8	**30** W	0224 / 0837 / 1440 / 2048	5.7 / 0.6 / 5.7 / 0.8
			31 TH	0256 / 0910 / 1517 / 2118	5.6 / 0.8 / 5.6 / 1.0

NOVEMBER

Day	Time	m	Day	Time	m
1 F	0328 / 0943 / 1555 / 2151	5.4 / 0.9 / 5.3 / 1.2	**16** SA	0327 / 0933 / 1600 / 2149	5.6 / 0.8 / 5.6 / 1.1
2 SA	0405 / 1024 / 1639 / 2233	5.2 / 1.1 / 5.1 / 1.5	**17** SU	0415 / 1026 / 1655 / 2244	5.4 / 0.9 / 5.4 / 1.3
3 SU	0452 / 1116 / 1734 / 2331	4.9 / 1.3 / 4.8 / 1.7	**18** M	0512 / 1137 / 1800 / 2359	5.1 / 1.1 / 5.1 / 1.5
4 M	0554 / 1219 / 1845	4.6 / 1.4 / 4.6	**19** TU	0622 / 1300 / 1915	4.9 / 1.1 / 5.0
5 TU	0041 / 0720 / 1325 / 2004	1.8 / 4.5 / 1.4 / 4.6	**20** W	0126 / 0739 / 1421 / 2029	1.5 / 4.9 / 1.1 / 5.1
6 W	0153 / 0834 / 1431 / 2109	1.8 / 4.7 / 1.3 / 4.9	**21** TH	0243 / 0850 / 1531 / 2134	1.3 / 5.1 / 0.9 / 5.4
7 TH	0303 / 0933 / 1535 / 2202	1.6 / 5.0 / 1.1 / 5.2	**22** F	0349 / 0952 / 1629 / 2231	1.1 / 5.4 / 0.7 / 5.6
8 F	0401 / 1022 / 1628 / 2247	1.3 / 5.2 / 0.9 / 5.5	**23** SA	0445 / 1047 / 1718 / 2321	0.9 / 5.6 / 0.6 / 5.8
9 SA	0447 / 1106 / 1713 / 2328	1.1 / 5.5 / 0.8 / 5.7	**24** SU	0534 / 1136 / 1801	0.7 / 5.7 / 0.6
10 SU	0528 / 1147 / 1755	0.9 / 5.6 / 0.7	**25** M O	0007 / 0620 / 1223 / 1841	5.9 / 0.6 / 5.8 / 0.7
11 M ●	0008 / 0608 / 1226 / 1835	5.8 / 0.8 / 5.7 / 0.7	**26** TU	0049 / 0702 / 1305 / 1917	5.8 / 0.5 / 5.8 / 0.7
12 TU	0046 / 0649 / 1305 / 1914	5.8 / 0.8 / 5.8 / 0.7	**27** W	0127 / 0741 / 1345 / 1951	5.7 / 0.6 / 5.7 / 0.7
13 W	0124 / 0730 / 1344 / 1951	5.9 / 0.7 / 5.9 / 0.7	**28** TH	0200 / 0818 / 1421 / 2023	5.6 / 0.7 / 5.6 / 0.9
14 TH	0203 / 0810 / 1426 / 2028	5.8 / 0.7 / 5.9 / 0.8	**29** F	0231 / 0851 / 1456 / 2052	5.5 / 0.8 / 5.5 / 1.0
15 F	0243 / 0850 / 1511 / 2105	5.8 / 0.7 / 5.8 / 0.8	**30** SA	0303 / 0923 / 1532 / 2123	5.4 / 0.9 / 5.4 / 1.2

DECEMBER

Day	Time	m	Day	Time	m
1 SU	0339 / 0959 / 1613 / 2158	5.3 / 1.0 / 5.2 / 1.3	**16** M	0406 / 1030 / 1646 / 2235	5.6 / 0.6 / 5.6 / 1.1
2 M	0421 / 1044 / 1659 / 2245	5.1 / 1.1 / 5.0 / 1.5	**17** TU	0500 / 1127 / 1745 / 2334	5.4 / 0.8 / 5.4 / 1.2
3 TU	0511 / 1138 / 1753 / 2347	4.8 / 1.2 / 4.8 / 1.6	**18** W	0601 / 1232 / 1850	5.2 / 0.9 / 5.2
4 W	0613 / 1238 / 1856	4.6 / 1.3 / 4.7	**19** TH	0046 / 0709 / 1344 / 1957	1.4 / 5.0 / 1.0 / 5.1
5 TH	0055 / 0725 / 1339 / 2005	1.7 / 4.6 / 1.3 / 4.8	**20** F	0205 / 0818 / 1456 / 2103	1.4 / 5.0 / 1.0 / 5.2
6 F	0201 / 0836 / 1440 / 2109	1.6 / 4.7 / 1.2 / 5.0	**21** SA	0318 / 0924 / 1558 / 2203	1.3 / 5.2 / 1.0 / 5.4
7 SA	0304 / 0936 / 1538 / 2205	1.4 / 5.0 / 1.0 / 5.3	**22** SU	0421 / 1023 / 1651 / 2257	1.1 / 5.3 / 0.9 / 5.5
8 SU	0401 / 1028 / 1633 / 2253	1.2 / 5.3 / 0.9 / 5.5	**23** M	0515 / 1116 / 1736 / 2345	0.9 / 5.5 / 0.9 / 5.6
9 M	0454 / 1115 / 1723 / 2338	1.0 / 5.5 / 0.8 / 5.7	**24** TU O	0602 / 1205 / 1817	0.7 / 5.6 / 0.9
10 TU ●	0544 / 1200 / 1810	0.8 / 5.7 / 0.7	**25** W	0029 / 0646 / 1249 / 1855	5.7 / 0.7 / 5.6 / 0.9
11 W	0022 / 0632 / 1245 / 1855	5.8 / 0.7 / 5.9 / 0.7	**26** TH	0108 / 0726 / 1329 / 1930	5.6 / 0.7 / 5.6 / 0.9
12 TH	0105 / 0721 / 1330 / 1938	5.9 / 0.6 / 6.0 / 0.7	**27** F	0142 / 0802 / 1404 / 2002	5.6 / 0.7 / 5.5 / 1.0
13 F	0148 / 0808 / 1416 / 2021	5.9 / 0.5 / 6.0 / 0.7	**28** SA	0212 / 0835 / 1437 / 2030	5.5 / 0.7 / 5.5 / 1.1
14 SA	0232 / 0854 / 1503 / 2102	5.9 / 0.5 / 5.9 / 0.8	**29** SU	0243 / 0906 / 1510 / 2058	5.4 / 0.8 / 5.4 / 1.1
15 SU	0317 / 0941 / 1553 / 2146	5.7 / 0.5 / 5.8 / 0.9	**30** M	0317 / 0937 / 1547 / 2129	5.4 / 0.8 / 5.3 / 1.1
			31 TU	0354 / 1012 / 1627 / 2204	5.3 / 0.9 / 5.2 / 1.2

Chart Datum: 2·90 metres below Ordnance Datum (Newlyn)

RIVER MEDWAY
(SHEERNESS)   10-4-12

Kent 51°27'·00N 00°44'·60E (Off Garrison Point)

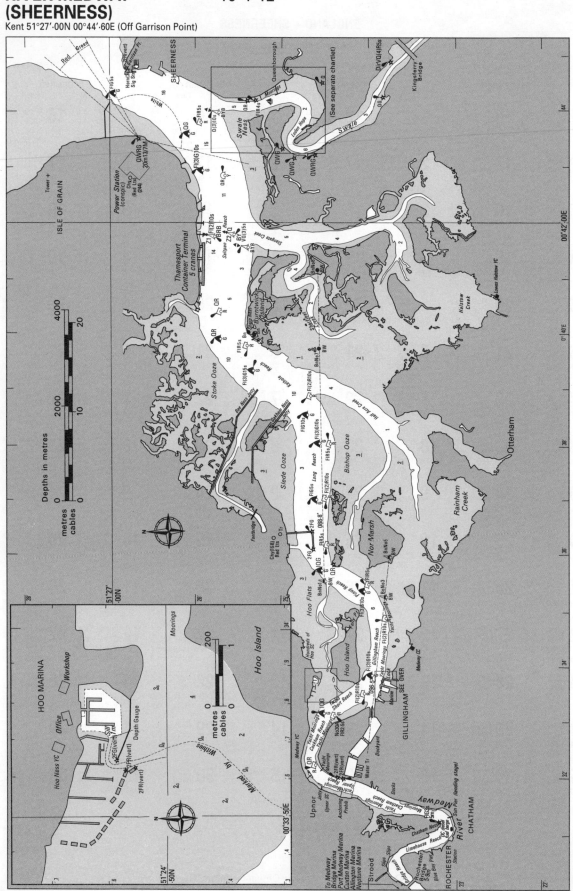

CHARTS
AC 3683, 2482, 1835, *1834, 1185*; Imray Y18; Stanfords 5, 8; OS 178

TIDES
+0130 Dover; ML 3·1; Duration 0610; Zone 0 (UT)

Standard Port SHEERNESS (⟵)

Times				Height (metres)			
High Water		Low Water		MHWS	MHWN	MLWN	MLWS
0200	0800	0200	0700	5·8	4·7	1·5	0·6
1400	2000	1400	1900				
Differences BEE NESS							
+0002	+0002	0000	+0005	+0·2	+0·1	0·0	0·0
CHATHAM (Lock Approaches)							
+0010	+0012	+0012	+0018	+0·3	+0·1	−0·1	−0·2
UPNOR							
+0015	+0015	+0015	+0025	+0·2	+0·2	−0·1	−0·1
ROCHESTER (STROOD PIER)							
+0018	+0018	+0018	+0028	+0·2	+0·2	−0·2	−0·3
ALLINGTON LOCK							
+0050	+0035	No data		−2·1	−2·2	−1·3	−0·4

NOTE: Sheerness is a Standard Port and tidal predictions for each day of the year are given above.

SHELTER
There are 4 marinas downriver of Rochester Bridge and 5 above. Sheerness is a ferry/commercial hbr with no yacht berths. Lower reaches of the Medway are exposed to strong NE winds, but Stangate and Half Acre Creeks are secure in all weathers and give access to lesser creeks. There are good ⚓s in Sharfleet Creek; from about HW−4 it is possible to go via the "back-door" into Half Acre Creek. Speed limit is 6kn W of Folly Pt (Hoo Is). See also 10.4.11 for Queenborough and access to The Swale.

NAVIGATION
WPT Medway SWM buoy, Mo(A) 6s, 51°28'·80N 00°52'·92E, 069°/249° from/to Garrison Pt, 5·5M. The wreck of the 'Richard Montgomery' lies 2M NE of river ent. The estuary offers a huge area to explore, although much of it dries out to mud. Some minor creeks are buoyed. The river is well buoyed and perched up to Rochester and tidal up to Allington Lock (21·6M). If planning to go up river, get the *Medway Ports River Byelaws 1991* from Port of Sheerness Ltd, Sheerness Docks, Kent ME12 1RX.

Bridge Clearances (MHWS):
Rochester	5·9m
Medway (M2)	29·6m
New Hythe (footbridge)	11·3m
Aylesford (Stone)	2·87m
Aylesford (Bailey)	3·26m
Maidstone Bypass (M20)	9·45m

LIGHTS AND MARKS
See 10.4.4 and chartlet for details of lts. Isle of Grain lt Q WRG 20m 13/7/8M R220°-234°, G234°-241°, W241°-013°. Power stn chy (242m) Oc and FR lts. Tfc Sigs: Powerful lt, Fl 7s, at Garrison Pt means large vessel under way: if shown up river = inbound; if to seaward = outbound. Note: not every buoy is shown due to scale limitations.

RADIO TELEPHONE
Call: *Medway Radio* VHF Ch **74** 16 11 22 73 (H24). Radar assistance on request Ch 22. Monitor Ch 74 underway and Ch 16 at ⚓. Ch **80** M for marinas: Gillingham, Hoo (H24), Medway Bridge (0900-1700 LT) and Port Medway (0800-2000LT). Link calls via Thames Radio Ch 02, 83.

TELEPHONE (01795 Sheerness; 01634 Medway)
Hr Mr (01795) 561234; MRSC (01255) 675518; ⌗ (01474) 537115; Marinecall 0891 500455; Police (01634) 811281, (01795) 661451; Dr via Medway Nav Service (01795) 663025.

FACILITIES (all 01634 code, unless otherwise stated)
Marinas (from seaward up to Rochester Bridge)
Mariners Farm BY (Rainham Creek) ☎ 233179, M, BH, Slip;
Gillingham Marina (250+12 visitors) ☎ 280022, Fax 280164, £15.03 E basin (access via lock HW±4½), W basin HW±2, P, D, AC, FW, ME, EI, Ⓔ, Sh, Gas, Gaz, CH, BH (20 ton), C (1 ton), Slip, V, Bar;
Medway Pier Marine ☎ 851113, D, FW, Slip, C (6 ton), BY, Ⓔ;
Hoo Marina (220) ☎ 250311, Fax 251761, FW, Sh, C (20 ton), ME, D (cans), SM, AC, CH, EI, Ⓔ, Gas, Gaz; access HW±1½ to W basin; HW±3 to E basin (via sill 1m above CD) ; waiting buoys in Short Reach.

Continued

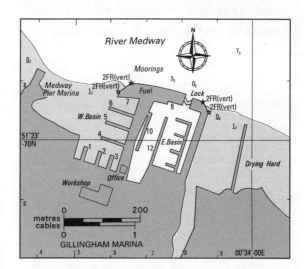

GILLINGHAM MARINA

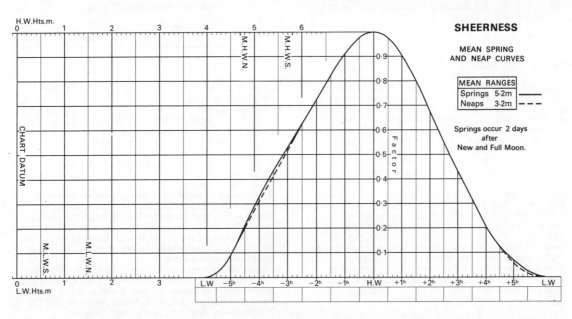

SHEERNESS

MEAN SPRING AND NEAP CURVES

MEAN RANGES	
Springs	5·2m ———
Neaps	3·2m - - - -

Springs occur 2 days after New and Full Moon.

RIVER MEDWAY continued

Marinas (above Rochester Bridge)
Medway Bridge Marina (160+15 visitors) ☎ 843576, Fax 843820, £11.75, Slip, D, P, FW, ME, El, Ⓔ, Sh, C (3 ton), BH (10 ton), Gas, Gaz, SM, AC, CH, V, R, Bar; **Port Medway Marina** (50) ☎ 720033, Fax 720315, FW, AC, BH (16 ton), C; **Cuxton Marina** (150+some visitors) ☎ 721941, Fax 290853, Slip, FW, ME, El, Ⓔ, Sh, BH (12 ton), AC, CH; **Elmhaven Marina** (60) ☎ 240489, Slip, FW, ME, El, Sh, C, AC; **Allington Marina** (120) ☎ (01622) 752057, CH, ME, El, Sh, P, D, Slip, C (10 ton), FW, Gas, Gaz; (non-tidal; lock operates HW–3 to +2, ☎ (01622) 752450).
Notes: All moorings are administered by YCs or marinas. There are landing facilities (only) at Gillingham Pier, Gillingham Dock steps, Sun Pier (Chatham), Ship Pier, Town Quay steps (Rochester) and Strood Pier. There are slips at Commodores Hard, Gillingham; Upnor Causeway opposite The Pier public house; Cuxton (HW ±3).
Clubs
Sheppey YC (Sheerness) ☎ 663052; **Lower Halstow YC** ☎ (01227) 458554; **Medway Cruising Club** (Gillingham) ☎ 856489, Bar, M, L, FW; **Hoo Ness YC** ☎ 250052, Bar, R, M, L, FW; **Hundred of Hoo SC** ☎ 250102; **Medway Motor Cruising Club** ☎ 827194; **Medway Motor YC** ☎ 389856; **Medway YC** (Upnor) ☎ 718399; **Upnor SC** ☎ 718043; **Royal Engineers YC** ☎ 844555; **RNSA** (Chatham) ☎ 823524; **Rochester CC** ☎ 841350, Bar, R, M, FW, L, Ⓞ; **Strood YC** ☎ 718261, Bar, M, C (1·5 ton), FW, L, Slip.
Services
ME, El, Sh, dry dock, SM, D, CH, ACA (Sheerness).
Refuelling Barge (Ship Pier, Rochester) ☎ 813773, D, CH, ACA.
Towns: EC Wed; all facilities R, V, Ⓞ, ⊠, ⇌, ✈ (Gatwick).

HARBOUR IN LOWER REACHES OF RIVER THAMES

GRAVESEND, Kent, 51°23'·61N 00°23'·00E. AC 1186, 2151. HW +0150 on Dover; ML 3·3m; Duration 0610. See 10·4·13 Tilbury diffs. Caution: Off the N bank, from Coalhouse Pt to 7ca E of Gravesend, 6 groynes extend approx 400m almost into the fairway; the outer ends are marked by SHM bns, Fl G 2·5s. ⚓ E of the Sea School jetty, close to S shore, but remote from town. There are ⚓s off the Club. Lock opens HW –1½ to HW on request to lock-keeper, ☎ (01474) 352392 (24hrs notice required for night tides).
Note: Boats can be left unattended in canal basin but not at ⚓s. Royal Terrace Pier hd FR. Call *Port Control London* VHF Ch 13 to seaward of Sea Reach No 4 By; Ch 12 from there to Crayford Ness. Broadcasts on Ch 12 every H+00, H+30. # 537115; Facilities: **Gravesend SC** ☎ 533974, Bar, FW, M, P & D (cans); **Services:** C (at canal ent, ask at SC), CH, Ⓔ, ME, El, Sh. **Town** EC Wed, R, V.

THAMES TIDAL BARRIER

Description: Located at Woolwich Reach, it protects London from flooding. There are 9 piers between which gates can be rotated upwards from the river bed to form a barrier. The piers are numbered 1-9 from N to S; the spans are lettered A-K from S to N (see diagram). A, H, J & K are not navigable. C-F, with depth 5·8m, are for larger vessels; B and G, with 1·25m, are for small craft/yachts, W-bound via G and E-bound via B.
Control & Communications: The Thames Barrier Navigation Centre controls all traffic in a Zone from Margaret Ness to Blackwall Pt, using callsign *Woolwich Radio* on VHF Ch 14, 22. Inbound vessels should pass their Barrier ETA to *Woolwich Radio* when abeam Crayfordness; at Margaret Ness they should obtain clearance to proceed through the Barrier. Outbound vessels should adopt the same procedure abeam Tower Bridge and Blackwall Pt. Non-VHF craft should, if possible, pre-notify Barrier Control ☎ 0181-855 0315, observe all visual signals, proceed with caution keeping clear of larger vessels and use spans B or G as

THE THAMES BARRIER 51°29'·88N 00°02'·31E (Span G)

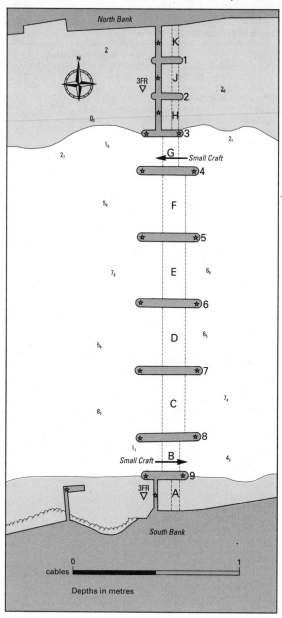

appropriate. Sailing vessels should transit the Barrier under power, not sail.
Lights and Signals: At Thamesmead & Barking Power Stn to the E, and Blackwall Stairs (N bank) and Blackwall Pt (S bank) to the W, noticeboards and lts indicate:
Fl Ⓨ = proceed with extreme caution.
Fl Ⓡ = navigation within Zone is prohibited.
Loudhailers may pass instructions and Morse K (–·–) = Barrier closed.
On the Barrier piers:
St Andrew's Cross (R lts) = barrier or span closed.
Arrows (G lts) = span indicated is open to traffic.
Spans A, H, J and K are lit with 3 Ⓡ in ▽ = No passage.
Testing: The Barrier is completely closed for testing one day per month, LW –1½ to LW +1½. Dates of testing are shown in the Supplements to this almanac. Individual spans are tested weekly.
Beware: When all spans are closed, keep 200m clear to avoid turbulence. It is dangerous to transit a closed span, as the gate may be semi-raised. Small craft should not navigate between Thames Refinery Jetty and Gulf Oil Island, unless intending to transit the Barrier.

RIVER THAMES   10-4-13
London

CHARTS
AC 3319, 2484, 3337, 2151, 1186, *1185*; Imray C2, C1;
Stanfords 5; OS 176, 177, 178. Other references include:
*Nicholsons Guide to the Thames; London Waterways
Guide* (Imray); the *Port of London River Bye Laws* and
Yachtsman's Guide to the tidal Thames, obtainable from
PLA, Devon House, 58-60 St Katherine's Way, London E1
9LB; ☎ (0171) 265 2656.

TIDES
+0252 Dover; ML 3·6; Duration 0555; Zone 0 (UT)

Standard Port LONDON BRIDGE (→)

Times				Height (metres)			
High Water		Low Water		MHWS	MHWN	MLWN	MLWS
0300	0900	0400	1100	7·1	5·9	1·3	0·5
1500	2100	1600	2300				

Differences TILBURY

−0055	−0040	−0050	−0115	−0·7	−0·5	+0·1	0·0

WOOLWICH (GALLIONS POINT)

−0020	−0020	−0035	−0045	−0·1	0·0	+0·2	0·0

ALBERT BRIDGE

+0025	+0020	+0105	+0110	−0·9	−0·8	−0·7	−0·4

HAMMERSMITH BRIDGE

+0040	+0035	+0205	+0155	−1·4	−1·3	−1·0	−0·5

KEW BRIDGE

+0055	+0050	+0255	+0235	−1·8	−1·8	−1·2	−0·5

RICHMOND LOCK

+0105	+0055	+0325	+0305	−2·2	−2·2	−1·3	−0·5

London Bridge is a Standard Port; daily predictions are
below. The river is tidal up to Richmond Footbridge where
there is a half-tide lock and a weir with overhead sluice
gates. When down, ie closed, these gates maintain at least
1·72m between Richmond and Teddington bridges; the
half-tide lock, on the Surrey bank, must then be used. At
other times (approx HW ±2) pass through the 3 central
arches. If the Thames Barrier is closed, water levels will
vary greatly from predictions.

TIDES – TIME DIFFERENCES ON LONDON BRIDGE

Place	MHWS	MHWN	MLWN	MLWS
Teddington Lock	+0106	+0056	—	—
Chiswick Bridge	+0049	+0044	+0235	+0224
Putney Bridge	+0032	+0030	+0138	+0137
Battersea Bridge	+0023	+0020	+0109	+0110
Westminster Bridge	+0012	+0011	+0031	+0035
London Bridge	0000	0000	0000	0000
Surrey Dock Greenland Ent	−0010	−0008	−0013	−0015
Millwall Dock Ent	−0010	−0008	−0014	−0016
Deptford Creek	−0012	−0011	−0018	−0021
Greenwich Pier	−0014	−0012	−0020	−0023
India & Millwall Dock Ent	−0018	−0015	−0026	−0029
Royal Victoria Dock Ent	−0021	−0018	−0031	−0025
Woolwich Ferry	−0028	−0024	−0042	−0047
Royal Albert Dock Ent	−0029	−0024	−0043	−0050
Coldharbour Point	−0037	−0030	−0053	−0103
Stoneness Lt Ho	−0048	−0037	−0059	−0114
Broadness Lt Ho	−0052	−0040	−0101	−0119
Gravesend Town Pier	−0059	−0044	−0106	−0125

SHELTER
Very good shelter in many places above the Thames
Barrier: in Bow Creek (Bugsby's Reach), Deptford Creek
(HW±2), S Dock Marina*, St Katharine's Yacht Haven*,
Lambeth Pier (PLA), Chelsea Harbour Marina*, Chelsea
Yacht & Boat Co (Cheyne Walk), Cadogan Pier (PLA),
Hurlingham YC, Chas Newens (BY, Putney), Alan See
(Hammersmith), Hammersmith Pier, Chiswick Quay
Marina, Auto Marine Services (Chiswick), Grand Union
Canal ent (Brentford), Howlett's BY (Twickenham) and
Tough's BY (Teddington); and in many PLA Draw Docks.
*See separate entries on following page.

PIERS WHERE LANDING CAN BE MADE BY ARRANGEMENT

Hampton Court Pier	)	PLA Central booking
Richmond Landing Stage	)	Service
Kew Pier	)	0171-265 2666
Putney Pier	)	Fax 0171-265 2699
Cadogan Pier	)	
Festival Pier	)	
Hammersmith Pier		0181-748 5405
Chelsea Hbr Pier		0171-351 4433

Lambeth Pier	)	PLA Central booking
Westminster Pier*	)	Service
Charing Cross Pier*	)	0171-265 2666
London Bridge City Pier	)	Fax 0171-265 2699
Greenwich Pier	)	* Only bookable in
Tower Pier*	)	off-peak hrs
Swan Lane Pier		0171-987 1185/730 4812
Greenland Pier	)	
Great Eastern Pier	)	0171-512 3000
London City Airport Pier		0171-474 5555
Thames Barrier Pier		0171-854 5555

NAVIGATION
The tidal Thames is divided by the PLA into a lower
section = from the sea to Crayfordness (2M above QE II
bridge); and an upper section = from Crayfordness to
Teddington.

Some general points: Going up or down river, keep as far
to stbd as is safe and seamanlike. Boats approaching a
bridge against the tide give way to those approaching
with the tide; but pleasure craft should always keep clear
of commercial vessels, especially tug/barge tows. Above
Cherry Garden Pier (Wapping), vessels over 40m always
have priority. Speed should be such as to minimise wash,
but an 8kn speed limit applies inshore off Southend, off
Shellhaven and Coryton, and above Wandsworth Bridge.
Some of the potential hazards are outlined below:

Lower section. In Sea Reach, keep well S of the main chan
to clear tankers turning abeam Canvey Is and Shellhaven.
In Lower Hope hold the NW bank until Ovens SHM buoy;
long groynes extend from the N bank for the next 2M. The
Tilbury landing stage is used by the Gravesend ferry and
cruise liners. In Northfleet Hope beware ships/tugs turning
into Tilbury Docks; container berths and a grain terminal
are close up-river. Long Reach has Ro-Ro berths on both
banks up/down stream of QE II bridge. Tankers berth at
Purfleet (N bank).

Upper section. Avoid unhandy tug/lighter tows en route
to Erith. Thames Police and harbour launches are very
helpful to yachtsmen, especially in emergency (*Thames
Patrol* Ch 14); state position relative to landmarks, rather
than lat/long. Expect frequent passenger launches from/
to Greenwich, The Tower and Westminster. Passage by
night is not advised. See below for bridge warning lights.

BRIDGES

Name of Bridge	Distance from London Bridge Nautical Miles	Clearance below centre span MHWS (m)
Richmond	13·97	5·3
Richmond Railway	13·67	5·3
Twickenham	13·64	5·9
Richmond Footbridge	13·49	4·8
Kew	11·33	5·3
Kew Railway	10·98	5·6
Chiswick	10·22	6·9
Barnes Railway	9·55	5·4
Hammersmith	7·97	3·7
Putney	6·45	5·5
Fulham Railway	6·31	6·9
Wandsworth	5·46	5·8
Battersea Railway	4·83	6·1
Battersea	4·27	5·5
Albert	4·04	4·9
Chelsea	3·40	6·6
Victoria Railway	3·31	6·0
Vauxhall	2·46	5·6
Lambeth	2·02	6·5
Westminster	1·64	5·4
Charing Cross Rly	1·32	7·0
Waterloo	1·12	8·5
Blackfriars	0·63	7·1
Blackfriars Rly	0·62	7·0
Southwark	0·24	7·4
Cannon St. Rly	0·16	7·1
London Bridge	0·00	8·9
Tower	below 0·49	8·6
Dartford (QEII)	below 17·68	54·1

LIGHTS AND MARKS
Glare from the many shore lts inhibits night navigation.
Margaret Ness Fl (2) 5s 11m 8M. Tower Bridge sounds
horn 20s or gong 30s when bascules open for shipping.
Iso W lts on both sides of certain bridges warn of an
approaching large vessel or tug, (which has switched on
the Iso lts electronically); other craft should keep clear.
A ▽ of R discs (Ⓡ lts) below a bridge = this arch closed.

4

RADIO TELEPHONE

Pleasure craft are encouraged to participate in the Thames Navigation Service by monitoring:

Port Control London   Ch 13   Sea to Sea Reach No 4 buoy;
                                        Ch 12   No 4 buoy to Crayfordness.
Woolwich Radio   Ch 14   Up-river from Crayfordness.

Craft >20m LOA must have VHF radio. Smaller craft without VHF should advise ☎ 0181-855 0315 before and after passage. Routine broadcasts of traffic, weather, tidal and navigational info are made at H and H +30 on Ch 12 by *Port Control London* and at H +15 and H +45 on Ch 14 by *Woolwich Radio*. For individual marinas the VHF Ch(s) are shown overleaf.

TELEPHONE (0171/0181)

PLA, Chief Hr Mr (01474) 562200; Hr Mr (Upper Section) 0171-265 2656; Hr Mr (Lower Section) (01474) 562212; Duty Officer Woolwich 0181-855 0315; Port Controller Gravesend & London Port Control Centre (01474) 560311; PLA Enquiries 0171-265 2656, Fax 265 2699; Port Health Authority (Tilbury) 01375-842663 (H24); MRSC (01255) 675518; River Police (Waterloo) 0171-321 7278, (Wapping) 0171-488 5291; London Weather Centre 0171-831 5968; Tower Bridge 0171-407 0922; ⌗ (01474) 537115; Richmond Lock 0181-940 0634; **Marinecall** 0891 500455; Ⓗ 0171-9877011.

FACILITIES (Letters in brackets appear on chartlets)

TEDDINGTON (0181)
  (A), BY, CH, AC, ME, M, Gas, C (6 ton), Sh, El, FW; **(B)**, D, M, ME, El, Sh, FW, Gas, Slip, AB, C (30 ton), CH.
RICHMOND (0181)
  (C), BY, CH, D, Gas, M, FW, ME, El, Sh, M.
BRENTFORD (0181)
  Thames Locks (No 101) ☎ 560 8942, Ent to Grand Union Canal, M, AB. **Brentford Dock Marina (D)** (80+10 visitors) ☎ 568 0287 (VHF Ch M), AC, Bar, CH, El, FW, ME, R, V, Sh, Access HW±2½;
KEW (0181)
  (F), CH, D, P, Gas, SM; **Kew Marina** ☎ 940 8364, M; **Dove Marina** ☎ 748 9474, M, FW.
CHISWICK (0181)
  Chiswick Quay Marina (50) ☎ 994 8743, Access HW±2, M, FW, BY, M, ME, El, Sh.
WANDSWORTH (0181)
  Hurlingham YC ☎ 788 5547, M; **Services:** CH, ME, FW, El, Sh.
CHELSEA (0171)
  Chelsea Hbr (G) (see right); **Chelsea Yacht & Boat Co (H)** ☎ 352 1427, M, Gas; **Cadogan Pier (I)** ☎ 352 4604, M, L.
WESTMINSTER BRIDGE (S side)
  Westminster Petroleum Ltd (Fuel barge Thames Refueller) ☎ 0831 110681, Gas, CH, D, L.
POOL OF LONDON (0171)
  St Katharine Haven (J) ☎ 488 2400 (see right); **Westminster Petroleum Ltd (K)** ☎ 481 1774, (Fuel barge Burgan), D, Gas; **Services:** CH, ACA.
LIMEHOUSE REACH (0171)
  See opp for **S Dock Marina (M)** and **Limehouse Basin Marina**.
GREENWICH (0181)
  Greenwich YC ☎ 8587339; **Services: (L)** ME, P, D, CH, BY.

ADMIRALTY CHART AGENTS (Central London)

Brown & Perring, 36/44 Tabernacle St   ☎ 0171-253 4517
Kelvin Hughes, 145 Minories   709 9076
Ocean Leisure, 13/14 Northumberland Ave   930 5050
Capt. O.M.Watts, 7 Dover St   493 4633
London Yacht Centre, 13 Artillery Lane   247 0521
Telesonic Marine, 60/62 Brunswick Centre   837 4106
Stanfords, 12/14 Long Acre   836 1321

HARBOURS ON THE THAMES (Woolwich to Chelsea)

GALLIONS POINT MARINA, London, 51°30'·27N 00°04'·73E at entry basin for Royal Albert Dock. AC 2151, 2484. Tides as for Gallions Pt (10.4.13). Marina ☎ 0171-476 7054 (H24). VHF Ch 68, when vessel expected. Access HW±2 (nps), HW±5 (Sp); deep water in basin. AB approx £9.40. DLR to W end, until 0030. Woolwich ferry & tunnel 15 mins walk.

SOUTH DOCK MARINA, London, 51°29'·64N 00°01'·80W. AC 3337, 2484. Tides as for Surrey Dock Greenland Ent (10.4.13). 1·1M above Greenwich, 2·5M below Tower Bridge. Marina ☎ 0171-252 2244, Fax 702 2252, (372 + visitors £11). VHF Ch M 80. Waiting pontoon at Greenland Pier. Approx access via lock HW±2 for 2m draft; HW±4 for 1m draft. Facilities: AC, ME, Sh, El, FW, CH, (20 ton), Bar, R, V, Ⓒ, SDYC; Dr ☎ 237 1078; Ⓗ ☎ 955 5000; Police ☎ 252 2836. ⇌, Surrey Quays Tube stn, ✈ City Airport.

LIMEHOUSE BASIN, London, 51°30'·55N 00°02'·16W. Access HW±4½ via bridge and lock, 0800-1700LT daily; waiting pontoon. VHF Ch 80. Facilities: (90 berths £10.57) FW, AC, entry to Regents Canal and R Lea, ⇌, DLR. BWB lock ☎ 0171-308 9930. Marina is managed by The Cruising Association, HQ at: 1 Northey St, Limehouse Basin, E14 8BT, ☎ 0171-537 2828, Fax 537 2266.

ST KATHARINE HAVEN, London, 51°30'·30N 00°04'·26W. AC 3337, 3319. HW +0245 on Dover. Tides as London Bridge (10·4·13). Good shelter under all conditions. Lock (42·7m x 9·1m with 2 lifting bridges), access HW −2 to HW +1½, summer 0600-2030, winter 0800-1800, (lock shut Tues and Wed, Nov to Feb). Six Y waiting buoys are downstream of ent. Ferry Pier, 30m upstream of ent, has limited berthing/shore access; berth on inboard side, only for shoal draft. Call *St Katharine* VHF Ch 80. **St Katherine Haven** (100+50 visitors) ☎ 0171-481 8350, Fax 702 2252, £13, CH, M, ME, El, Sh, AC, Bar, YC, FW, Gas, R, V, ⌗, Ⓒ.

CHELSEA HARBOUR, London, 51°28'·00N 00°11'·00W. AC 3319. Tides: see 10·4·13. Good shelter under all conditions. Basin ent (5·5m beam x 2·0m draft) with bascule bridge. Lock opens when 2·5m over sill; tide gauge outside, access HW ±1½. Waiting berths on Chelsea Hbr Pier close upriver. Call *Chelsea Hbr* VHF Ch 80 14. **Marina** (50+10 visitors, £11.75). ☎ 0171-351 9680, Hr Mr ☎ (pager) 0459-117143, Fax 352 4534, £11.75, AC, FW, Bar, R, YC, Ⓑ, V.

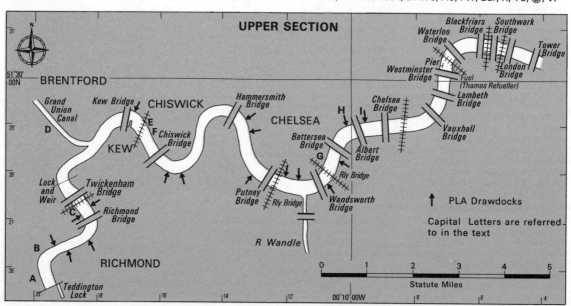

RIVER THAMES continued

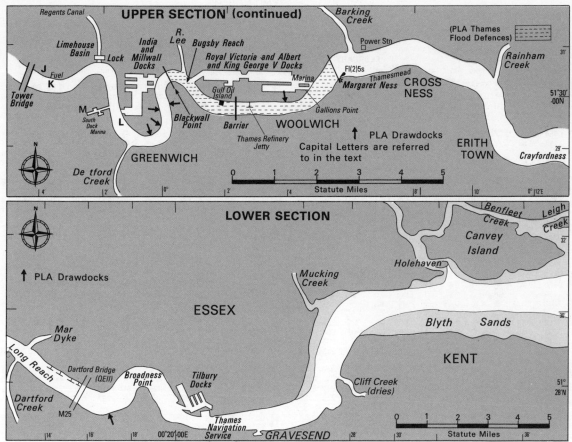

UPPER SECTION (continued)

LOWER SECTION

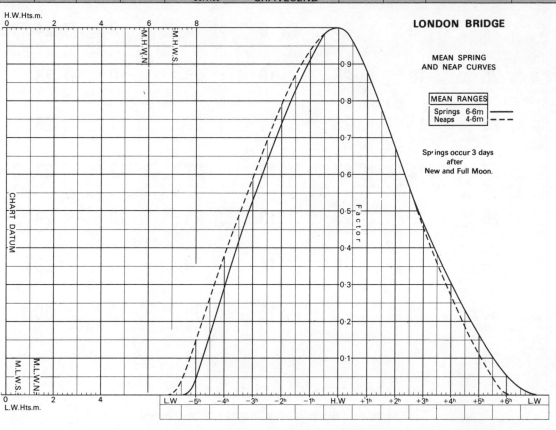

LONDON BRIDGE

MEAN SPRING
AND NEAP CURVES

MEAN RANGES
Springs 6·6m ———
Neaps 4·6m – – –

Springs occur 3 days
after
New and Full Moon.

ENGLAND – LONDON BRIDGE

LAT 51°30′N   LONG   0°05′W

TIMES AND HEIGHTS OF HIGH AND LOW WATERS

YEAR **1996**

TIME ZONE (UT)
For Summer Time add ONE hour in non-shaded areas

Chart Datum: 3·20 metres below Ordnance Datum (Newlyn)

JANUARY

Day	Time	m	Day	Time	m
1 M	0328 / 1013 / 1625 / 2245	1.3 / 6.3 / 1.0 / 6.5	**16** TU	0218 / 0901 / 1526 / 2150	1.3 / 6.1 / 1.1 / 6.3
2 TU	0454 / 1114 / 1738 / 2342	1.2 / 6.5 / 0.9 / 6.6	**17** W	0405 / 1020 / 1703 / 2302	1.4 / 6.2 / 1.0 / 6.5
3 W	0610 / 1209 / 1834	1.0 / 6.7 / 0.9	**18** TH	0538 / 1132 / 1815	1.1 / 6.5 / 0.8
4 TH	0033 / 0704 / 1257 / 1921	6.7 / 0.9 / 6.7 / 0.9	**19** F	0005 / 0650 / 1234 / 1915	6.8 / 0.8 / 6.9 / 0.6
5 F ○	0117 / 0750 / 1339 / 2002	6.6 / 0.8 / 6.6 / 1.0	**20** SA ●	0101 / 0751 / 1328 / 2010	7.0 / 0.4 / 7.2 / 0.4
6 SA	0153 / 0831 / 1417 / 2038	6.6 / 0.8 / 6.6 / 1.1	**21** SU	0151 / 0847 / 1420 / 2101	7.2 / 0.2 / 7.4 / 0.3
7 SU	0226 / 0909 / 1452 / 2108	6.6 / 0.8 / 6.6 / 1.1	**22** M	0240 / 0937 / 1509 / 2148	7.3 / −0.1 / 7.5 / 0.3
8 M	0257 / 0942 / 1526 / 2132	6.6 / 0.8 / 6.7 / 1.0	**23** TU	0326 / 1023 / 1557 / 2230	7.4 / −0.2 / 7.6 / 0.3
9 TU	0331 / 1010 / 1601 / 2200	6.7 / 0.8 / 6.7 / 1.0	**24** W	0410 / 1103 / 1641 / 2307	7.3 / −0.1 / 7.5 / 0.4
10 W	0406 / 1034 / 1637 / 2231	6.6 / 0.8 / 6.7 / 0.9	**25** TH	0451 / 1138 / 1723 / 2340	7.2 / 0.1 / 7.2 / 0.6
11 TH	0440 / 1101 / 1714 / 2303	6.6 / 0.8 / 6.7 / 0.9	**26** F	0529 / 1209 / 1804	7.0 / 0.3 / 6.9
12 F	0516 / 1131 / 1754 / 2338	6.5 / 0.8 / 6.6 / 0.9	**27** SA	0011 / 0607 / 1242 / 1846	0.7 / 6.8 / 0.5 / 6.6
13 SA	0556 / 1207 / 1839	6.4 / 0.8 / 6.5	**28** SU	0046 / 0652 / 1323 / 1937	0.9 / 6.4 / 0.8 / 6.2
14 SU	0018 / 0644 / 1253 / 1932	0.9 / 6.3 / 0.9 / 6.3	**29** M	0134 / 0759 / 1418 / 2052	1.1 / 6.0 / 1.1 / 6.0
15 M	0110 / 0746 / 1355 / 2037	1.1 / 6.2 / 1.0 / 6.2	**30** TU	0237 / 0935 / 1523 / 2209	1.4 / 5.9 / 1.3 / 5.9
			31 W	0347 / 1047 / 1638 / 2312	1.5 / 6.0 / 1.4 / 6.1

FEBRUARY

Day	Time	m	Day	Time	m
1 TH	0518 / 1146 / 1758	1.4 / 6.2 / 1.3	**16** F	0529 / 1118 / 1801 / 2348	1.2 / 6.3 / 0.9 / 6.5
2 F	0007 / 0641 / 1236 / 1854	6.3 / 1.2 / 6.4 / 1.2	**17** SA	0643 / 1222 / 1903	0.7 / 6.8 / 0.6
3 SA	0054 / 0729 / 1320 / 1937	6.4 / 1.0 / 6.5 / 1.1	**18** SU ●	0045 / 0741 / 1316 / 1956	6.8 / 0.3 / 7.1 / 0.4
4 SU ○	0133 / 0810 / 1357 / 2015	6.5 / 0.9 / 6.5 / 1.1	**19** M	0136 / 0833 / 1405 / 2046	7.1 / 0.0 / 7.4 / 0.2
5 M	0207 / 0849 / 1432 / 2049	6.5 / 0.8 / 6.6 / 1.0	**20** TU	0222 / 0921 / 1452 / 2131	7.3 / −0.2 / 7.5 / 0.1
6 TU	0241 / 0926 / 1506 / 2121	6.7 / 0.7 / 6.8 / 0.9	**21** W	0306 / 1004 / 1536 / 2213	7.4 / −0.3 / 7.6 / 0.1
7 W	0315 / 0958 / 1542 / 2152	6.7 / 0.6 / 6.9 / 0.8	**22** TH	0348 / 1042 / 1617 / 2249	7.4 / −0.2 / 7.5 / 0.2
8 TH	0350 / 1026 / 1618 / 2222	6.8 / 0.6 / 6.9 / 0.8	**23** F	0426 / 1115 / 1655 / 2321	7.4 / 0.0 / 7.3 / 0.4
9 F	0423 / 1050 / 1654 / 2252	6.8 / 0.7 / 6.8 / 0.8	**24** SA	0503 / 1143 / 1730 / 2348	7.2 / 0.2 / 7.0 / 0.6
10 SA	0457 / 1115 / 1731 / 2322	6.7 / 0.7 / 6.7 / 0.8	**25** SU	0538 / 1210 / 1805	6.9 / 0.5 / 6.7
11 SU	0535 / 1146 / 1813 / 2357	6.6 / 0.7 / 6.5 / 0.8	**26** M	0015 / 0616 / 1244 / 1844	0.8 / 6.5 / 0.8 / 6.3
12 M	0620 / 1226 / 1902	6.4 / 0.8 / 6.3	**27** TU	0053 / 0705 / 1332 / 1935	1.0 / 6.0 / 1.2 / 5.8
13 TU	0041 / 0716 / 1320 / 2001	1.0 / 6.2 / 1.1 / 6.1	**28** W	0152 / 0819 / 1436 / 2101	1.4 / 5.6 / 1.5 / 5.5
14 W	0142 / 0829 / 1440 / 2118	1.3 / 5.9 / 1.3 / 6.0	**29** TH	0303 / 1014 / 1546 / 2235	1.6 / 5.6 / 1.6 / 5.6
15 TH	0324 / 0957 / 1642 / 2240	1.5 / 6.0 / 1.3 / 6.2			

MARCH

Day	Time	m	Day	Time	m
1 F	0414 / 1118 / 1659 / 2335	1.6 / 5.8 / 1.6 / 5.9	**16** SA	0518 / 1106 / 1744 / 2330	1.1 / 6.3 / 1.0 / 6.4
2 SA	0557 / 1209 / 1815	1.4 / 6.1 / 1.4	**17** SU	0627 / 1208 / 1844	0.5 / 6.8 / 0.5
3 SU	0024 / 0658 / 1254 / 1905	6.2 / 1.1 / 6.3 / 1.2	**18** M	0027 / 0722 / 1301 / 1936	6.8 / 0.1 / 7.2 / 0.3
4 M	0106 / 0742 / 1331 / 1946	6.4 / 0.9 / 6.5 / 1.1	**19** TU ●	0117 / 0811 / 1347 / 2024	7.1 / −0.1 / 7.4 / 0.1
5 TU ○	0143 / 0822 / 1407 / 2025	6.5 / 0.8 / 6.7 / 0.9	**20** W	0201 / 0856 / 1431 / 2109	7.2 / −0.2 / 7.5 / 0.1
6 W	0219 / 0901 / 1443 / 2104	6.7 / 0.6 / 6.9 / 0.8	**21** TH	0244 / 0938 / 1512 / 2150	7.3 / −0.2 / 7.5 / 0.0
7 TH	0255 / 0939 / 1519 / 2141	6.9 / 0.5 / 7.0 / 0.6	**22** F	0324 / 1015 / 1551 / 2227	7.4 / −0.1 / 7.4 / 0.1
8 F	0331 / 1011 / 1557 / 2214	7.0 / 0.5 / 7.0 / 0.6	**23** SA	0402 / 1048 / 1626 / 2300	7.4 / 0.1 / 7.2 / 0.3
9 SA	0407 / 1038 / 1633 / 2243	6.9 / 0.6 / 6.9 / 0.6	**24** SU	0438 / 1116 / 1658 / 2326	7.2 / 0.3 / 7.0 / 0.5
10 SU	0442 / 1102 / 1710 / 2309	6.9 / 0.7 / 6.8 / 0.7	**25** M	0513 / 1140 / 1731 / 2348	6.9 / 0.6 / 6.7 / 0.7
11 M	0520 / 1129 / 1750 / 2340	6.7 / 0.7 / 6.5 / 0.7	**26** TU	0550 / 1204 / 1808	6.5 / 0.9 / 6.3
12 TU	0603 / 1206 / 1835	6.4 / 1.0 / 6.2	**27** W	0017 / 0633 / 1243 / 1853	1.0 / 6.1 / 1.3 / 5.9
13 W	0022 / 0656 / 1258 / 1931	1.0 / 6.1 / 1.2 / 5.9	**28** TH	0108 / 0729 / 1347 / 1951	1.3 / 5.6 / 1.6 / 5.5
14 TH	0121 / 0808 / 1415 / 2051	1.3 / 5.8 / 1.5 / 5.8	**29** F	0224 / 0901 / 1501 / 2125	1.5 / 5.3 / 1.8 / 5.4
15 F	0301 / 0944 / 1622 / 2220	1.5 / 5.9 / 1.4 / 6.0	**30** SA	0335 / 1037 / 1610 / 2250	1.5 / 5.6 / 1.7 / 5.6
			31 SU	0444 / 1133 / 1717 / 2345	1.4 / 5.9 / 1.5 / 6.0

APRIL

Day	Time	m	Day	Time	m
1 M	0559 / 1218 / 1817	1.1 / 6.2 / 1.3	**16** TU	0004 / 0654 / 1240 / 1910	6.9 / 0.0 / 7.3 / 0.2
2 TU	0030 / 0658 / 1259 / 1907	6.3 / 0.9 / 6.5 / 1.0	**17** W ●	0054 / 0743 / 1326 / 1959	7.1 / −0.1 / 7.4 / 0.1
3 W	0111 / 0744 / 1337 / 1953	6.5 / 0.7 / 6.8 / 0.8	**18** TH	0139 / 0828 / 1408 / 2044	7.2 / −0.1 / 7.4 / 0.1
4 TH ○	0150 / 0829 / 1415 / 2039	6.8 / 0.5 / 7.0 / 0.6	**19** F	0221 / 0909 / 1448 / 2126	7.2 / 0.0 / 7.3 / 0.1
5 F	0229 / 0911 / 1455 / 2123	7.0 / 0.4 / 7.1 / 0.5	**20** SA	0301 / 0947 / 1524 / 2204	7.2 / 0.1 / 7.2 / 0.1
6 SA	0310 / 0950 / 1535 / 2203	7.1 / 0.3 / 7.2 / 0.4	**21** SU	0340 / 1021 / 1558 / 2237	7.2 / 0.3 / 7.1 / 0.3
7 SU	0350 / 1023 / 1614 / 2237	7.1 / 0.5 / 7.0 / 0.5	**22** M	0416 / 1049 / 1630 / 2305	7.1 / 0.5 / 6.9 / 0.5
8 M	0430 / 1052 / 1653 / 2305	7.0 / 0.7 / 6.8 / 0.7	**23** TU	0452 / 1111 / 1703 / 2325	6.8 / 0.8 / 6.7 / 0.7
9 TU	0511 / 1120 / 1733 / 2335	6.8 / 0.9 / 6.5 / 0.8	**24** W	0529 • / 1131 / 1740 / 2349	6.5 / 1.0 / 6.4 / 0.9
10 W	0555 / 1156 / 1816	6.5 / 1.1 / 6.2	**25** TH	0610 / 1203 / 1823	6.1 / 1.3 / 6.0
11 TH	0015 / 0648 / 1253 / 1911	1.0 / 6.1 / 1.3 / 5.9	**26** F	0028 / 0658 / 1253 / 1914	1.1 / 5.8 / 1.6 / 5.7
12 F	0115 / 0801 / 1402 / 2033	1.2 / 5.9 / 1.5 / 5.8	**27** SA	0137 / 0759 / 1408 / 2020	1.4 / 5.6 / 1.8 / 5.6
13 SA	0255 / 0932 / 1555 / 2159	1.3 / 6.0 / 1.4 / 6.0	**28** SU	0253 / 0920 / 1523 / 2142	1.4 / 5.6 / 1.7 / 5.6
14 SU	0454 / 1046 / 1717 / 2307	0.9 / 6.5 / 0.9 / 6.5	**29** M	0401 / 1037 / 1630 / 2252	1.2 / 5.9 / 1.5 / 5.9
15 M	0601 / 1147 / 1818	0.4 / 7.0 / 0.5	**30** TU	0507 / 1132 / 1732 / 2346	1.0 / 6.2 / 1.2 / 6.3

ENGLAND – LONDON BRIDGE

LAT 51°30′N   LONG 0°05′W

TIMES AND HEIGHTS OF HIGH AND LOW WATERS

YEAR **1996**

4

TIME ZONE (UT)
For Summer Time add ONE hour in non-shaded areas

MAY

Day		Time	m	Time	m	Time	m	Time	m
1	W	0610	0.8	1220	6.6	1829	1.0		
2	TH	0033	6.6	0704	0.6	1304	6.9	1921	0.7
3	F O	0118	6.9	0754	0.4	1347	7.1	2012	0.5
4	SA	0203	7.1	0842	0.3	1430	7.2	2102	0.3
5	SU	0248	7.3	0927	0.2	1514	7.2	2148	0.3
6	M	0334	7.3	1008	0.3	1558	7.1	2231	0.3
7	TU	0420	7.2	1044	0.5	1640	6.9	2308	0.5
8	W	0505	6.9	1118	0.8	1722	6.5	2343	0.7
9	TH	0552	6.6	1155	1.1	1807	6.3		
10	F	0023	0.9	0646	6.3	1244	1.3	1901	6.0
11	SA	0120	1.0	0755	6.2	1350	1.4	2018	6.0
12	SU	0240	1.0	0912	6.3	1517	1.3	2134	6.2
13	M	0417	0.8	1020	6.7	1641	0.9	2240	6.6
14	TU	0527	0.4	1120	7.0	1747	0.5	2338	6.9
15	W	0623	0.1	1214	7.3	1843	0.3		
16	TH	0030	7.1	0713	0.0	1303	7.3	1932	0.2
17	F ●	0118	7.1	0758	0.1	1346	7.2	2018	0.2
18	SA	0201	7.1	0840	0.2	1425	7.1	2101	0.3
19	SU	0242	7.0	0920	0.4	1501	7.0	2141	0.3
20	M	0320	7.0	0955	0.5	1533	6.9	2216	0.4
21	TU	0357	6.9	1024	0.7	1605	6.8	2245	0.6
22	W	0433	6.7	1045	0.9	1639	6.6	2306	0.8
23	TH	0509	6.5	1105	1.0	1716	6.4	2328	0.9
24	F	0549	6.3	1136	1.2	1757	6.2		
25	SA	0002	1.0	0632	6.1	1217	1.3	1843	6.0
26	SU	0050	1.1	0724	5.9	1312	1.5	1940	5.8
27	M	0200	1.1	0826	5.9	1426	1.5	2047	5.9
28	TU	0314	1.1	0935	6.0	1543	1.4	2156	6.0
29	W	0424	0.9	1042	6.3	1651	1.2	2300	6.3
30	TH	0531	0.7	1140	6.6	1754	1.0	2356	6.6
31	F	0631	0.5	1231	6.9	1853	0.7		

JUNE

Day		Time	m	Time	m	Time	m	Time	m
1	SA O	0048	6.9	0725	0.3	1320	7.2	1949	0.5
2	SU	0139	7.4	0817	0.2	1408	7.3	2043	0.3
3	M	0229	7.4	0907	0.2	1456	7.3	2136	0.2
4	TU	0319	7.4	0954	0.2	1543	7.2	2224	0.1
5	W	0409	7.4	1037	0.4	1629	7.0	2308	0.3
6	TH	0457	7.2	1116	0.6	1713	6.8	2348	0.4
7	F	0546	6.9	1154	0.8	1758	6.6		
8	SA	0027	0.6	0637	6.7	1237	1.0	1849	6.4
9	SU	0114	0.7	0737	6.5	1330	1.1	1954	6.3
10	M	0213	0.8	0844	6.5	1437	1.1	2105	6.4
11	TU	0327	0.7	0950	6.6	1554	1.0	2211	6.6
12	W	0445	0.6	1052	6.9	1711	0.8	2312	6.8
13	TH	0549	0.4	1148	7.0	1814	0.5		
14	F	0007	6.9	0643	0.3	1240	7.1	1907	0.4
15	SA	0058	6.9	0731	0.4	1325	7.0	1955	0.4
16	SU ●	0143	6.9	0814	0.5	1405	6.9	2039	0.5
17	M	0224	6.8	0855	0.6	1441	6.8	2120	0.5
18	TU	0303	6.8	0931	0.7	1513	6.7	2156	0.6
19	W	0339	6.7	1002	0.8	1545	6.7	2227	0.7
20	TH	0414	6.7	1023	0.9	1619	6.6	2250	0.8
21	F	0450	6.6	1046	1.0	1646	6.5	2311	0.8
22	SA	0527	6.5	1116	1.0	1733	6.3	2341	0.8
23	SU	0608	6.3	1152	1.1	1815	6.2		
24	M	0019	0.8	0653	6.2	1236	1.1	1904	6.1
25	TU	0109	0.9	0748	6.2	1333	1.3	2005	6.1
26	W	0217	0.9	0950	6.6	1449	1.4	2112	6.2
27	TH	0339	0.9	0959	6.3	1612	1.3	2221	6.3
28	F	0457	0.8	1105	6.6	1725	1.0	2325	6.6
29	SA	0604	0.6	1204	6.9	1831	0.8		
30	SU	0024	6.9	0703	0.4	1258	7.1	1932	0.5

JULY

Day		Time	m	Time	m	Time	m	Time	m
1	M O	0119	7.2	0759	0.2	1348	7.3	2031	0.3
2	TU	0212	7.4	0852	0.2	1438	7.3	2125	0.1
3	W	0304	7.5	0942	0.1	1527	7.4	2216	0.0
4	TH	0355	7.5	1028	0.3	1614	7.3	2301	0.0
5	F	0443	7.4	1109	0.3	1658	7.1	2341	0.1
6	SA	0530	7.2	1146	0.5	1741	6.9		
7	SU	0017	0.3	0617	6.9	1224	0.7	1826	6.7
8	M	0055	0.5	0709	6.6	1306	0.9	1920	6.5
9	TU	0140	0.6	0810	6.4	1359	1.0	2029	6.4
10	W	0238	0.8	0917	6.4	1503	1.1	2140	6.4
11	TH	0350	0.9	1021	6.5	1620	1.1	2246	6.5
12	F	0509	0.8	1121	6.7	1743	0.9	2345	6.7
13	SA	0613	0.7	1216	6.8	1845	0.7		
14	SU	0038	6.7	0705	0.7	1304	6.8	1934	0.7
15	M ●	0125	6.7	0750	0.7	1346	6.7	2019	0.7
16	TU	0207	6.7	0832	0.8	1422	6.7	2100	0.7
17	W	0244	6.8	0910	0.8	1454	6.7	2138	0.7
18	TH	0319	6.7	0942	0.8	1527	6.7	2210	0.7
19	F	0353	6.8	1007	0.9	1601	6.7	2235	0.7
20	SA	0428	6.7	1030	0.9	1635	6.6	2255	0.7
21	SU	0504	6.7	1059	0.9	1710	6.5	2320	0.7
22	M	0541	6.6	1131	0.9	1747	6.4	2352	0.7
23	TU	0623	6.4	1208	1.0	1830	6.3		
24	W	0032	0.8	0712	6.3	1254	1.1	1926	6.2
25	TH	0127	0.9	0812	6.2	1357	1.3	2033	6.1
26	F	0247	1.1	0922	6.2	1534	1.4	2147	6.2
27	SA	0427	1.0	1035	6.4	1703	1.2	2300	6.4
28	SU	0544	0.8	1141	6.7	1818	0.8		
29	M	0005	6.8	0647	0.6	1239	7.0	1922	0.5
30	TU O	0103	7.1	0745	0.3	1331	7.2	2020	0.2
31	W	0157	7.4	0838	0.2	1420	7.3	2114	0.0

AUGUST

Day		Time	m	Time	m	Time	m	Time	m
1	TH	0248	7.5	0928	0.1	1508	7.4	2202	-0.2
2	F	0337	7.6	1014	0.1	1553	7.4	2245	-0.2
3	SA	0423	7.6	1054	0.1	1636	7.4	2323	-0.1
4	SU	0507	7.4	1131	0.3	1716	7.2	2356	0.2
5	M	0549	7.1	1204	0.5	1756	6.9		
6	TU	0027	0.4	0632	6.7	1239	0.8	1840	6.6
7	W	0105	0.7	0723	6.3	1323	1.0	1940	6.2
8	TH	0155	1.0	0833	6.1	1421	1.2	2105	6.0
9	F	0259	1.2	0948	6.1	1530	1.3	2220	6.1
10	SA	0414	1.3	1053	6.2	1657	1.3	2322	6.3
11	SU	0538	1.1	1150	6.5	1821	1.0		
12	M	0017	6.5	0639	1.0	1241	6.6	1913	0.8
13	TU	0104	6.6	0727	0.9	1323	6.6	1957	0.7
14	W ●	0145	6.7	0809	0.9	1400	6.7	2038	0.7
15	TH	0221	6.7	0847	0.8	1433	6.7	2116	0.7
16	F	0255	6.8	0922	0.8	1506	6.8	2150	0.6
17	SA	0329	6.9	0951	0.8	1540	6.8	2217	0.7
18	SU	0404	6.9	1017	0.8	1613	6.7	2237	0.7
19	M	0439	6.8	1044	0.8	1646	6.6	2259	0.7
20	TU	0514	6.7	1112	0.9	1721	6.5	2326	0.8
21	W	0553	6.5	1143	0.9	1802	6.4		
22	TH	0001	0.8	0637	6.3	1223	1.1	1853	6.2
23	F	0048	1.0	0733	6.1	1318	1.3	1959	6.0
24	SA	0157	1.3	0845	5.9	1455	1.5	2118	6.0
25	SU	0400	1.4	1007	6.1	1648	1.3	2241	6.2
26	M	0528	1.0	1120	6.4	1809	0.8	2351	6.7
27	TU	0633	0.6	1220	6.8	1911	0.3		
28	W O	0048	7.1	0729	0.3	1312	7.1	2005	0.0
29	TH	0140	7.4	0821	0.1	1359	7.3	2055	-0.1
30	F	0228	7.6	0910	0.0	1445	7.5	2141	-0.2
31	SA	0314	7.6	0954	0.0	1528	7.5	2223	-0.2

Chart Datum: 3·20 metres below Ordnance Datum (Newlyn)

ENGLAND – LONDON BRIDGE

LAT 51°30'N   LONG   0°05'W

TIMES AND HEIGHTS OF HIGH AND LOW WATERS

YEAR **1996**

TIME ZONE (UT)
For Summer Time add ONE hour in non-shaded areas

SEPTEMBER

Day	Time	m	Time	m	Time	m	Time	m
1 SU	0358	7.6	1034	0.0	1610	7.5	2259	−0.1
16 M	0337	7.0	1001	0.7	1550	6.9	2216	0.7
2 M	0439	7.4	1110	0.2	1649	7.3	2330	0.2
17 TU	0413	7.0	1029	0.7	1624	6.8	2238	0.7
3 TU	0517	7.1	1141	0.5	1726	7.0	2357	0.5
18 W	0448	6.8	1056	0.9	1700	6.6	2304	0.9
4 W	0552	6.7	1211	0.7	1804	6.6		
19 TH	0525	6.5	1123	1.0	1741	6.4	2337	1.0
5 TH	0027	0.8	0629	6.3	1249	1.0	1850	6.2
20 F	0607	6.3	1200	1.1	1830	6.2		
6 F	0111	1.2	0718	5.9	1343	1.3	2006	5.8
21 SA	0021	1.2	0658	6.0	1252	1.4	1933	5.9
7 SA	0214	1.5	0901	5.7	1450	1.5	2149	5.7
22 SU	0125	1.5	0810	5.8	1425	1.6	2057	5.9
8 SU	0326	1.6	1020	5.8	1603	1.5	2255	6.0
23 M	0332	1.6	0943	5.9	1638	1.3	2225	6.2
9 M	0447	1.5	1120	6.1	1746	1.2	2350	6.3
24 TU	0509	1.2	1059	6.3	1754	0.7	2335	6.7
10 TU	0606	1.2	1211	6.4	1844	0.9		
25 W	0614	0.7	1159	6.8	1852	0.2		
11 W	0037	6.5	0657	1.0	1254	6.6	1927	0.8
26 TH	0031	7.2	0708	0.3	1251	7.2	1943	−0.1
12 TH	0118	6.7	0740	0.9	1332	6.7	●2008	0.7
27 F	0121	7.4	0759	0.1	1337	7.4	○2031	−0.2
13 F	0153	6.8	0818	0.8	1406	6.8	2046	0.6
28 SA	0206	7.6	0846	0.0	1420	7.5	2115	−0.1
14 SA	0227	6.9	0854	0.7	1440	6.9	2122	0.6
29 SU	0249	7.6	0930	0.0	1502	7.5	2155	−0.1
15 SU	0302	7.0	0929	0.7	1515	6.9	2153	0.6
30 M	0330	7.5	1011	0.0	1543	7.5	2231	0.1

OCTOBER

Day	Time	m	Time	m	Time	m	Time	m
1 TU	0409	7.4	1047	0.2	1622	7.3	2301	0.4
16 W	0350	7.0	1016	0.6	1607	7.0	2223	0.8
2 W	0443	7.1	1118	0.5	1659	7.0	2326	0.7
17 TH	0427	6.8	1046	0.8	1647	6.8	2250	1.0
3 TH	0515	6.8	1145	0.8	1736	6.6	2349	1.0
18 F	0505	6.5	1115	1.0	1729	6.5	2323	1.1
4 F	0549	6.4	1216	1.0	1818	6.2		
19 SA	0545	6.2	1150	1.2	1818	6.2		
5 SA	0023	1.3	0630	6.0	1305	1.3	1911	5.7
20 SU	0007	1.3	0633	6.0	1242	1.4	1919	6.0
6 SU	0122	1.7	0727	5.6	1413	1.5	2054	5.5
21 M	0109	1.6	0742	5.8	1413	1.5	2043	5.9
7 M	0240	1.9	0930	5.5	1523	1.5	2217	5.7
22 TU	0255	1.7	0920	5.9	1616	1.1	2206	6.3
8 TU	0353	1.8	1040	5.8	1636	1.3	2314	6.1
23 W	0441	1.2	1035	6.4	1728	0.6	2312	6.8
9 W	0507	1.5	1134	6.2	1755	1.1		
24 TH	0548	0.7	1135	6.8	1825	0.2		
10 TH	0002	6.4	0610	1.3	1219	6.4	1845	0.8
25 F	0009	7.2	0643	0.3	1228	7.2	○1916	0.0
11 F	0043	6.6	0657	1.0	1258	6.6	1928	0.7
26 SA	0058	7.5	0733	0.1	1314	7.3	○2003	0.0
12 SA	0120	6.8	0739	0.8	1335	6.8	●2008	0.6
27 SU	0143	7.5	0821	0.1	1358	7.4	2046	0.1
13 SU	0156	7.0	0820	0.7	1411	7.0	2047	0.6
28 M	0225	7.4	0905	0.1	1440	7.4	2126	0.2
14 M	0233	7.1	0901	0.6	1449	7.1	2123	0.6
29 TU	0304	7.3	0946	0.1	1520	7.3	2203	0.4
15 TU	0311	7.1	0941	0.6	1528	7.1	2155	0.6
30 W	0340	7.2	1023	0.3	1559	7.2	2234	0.6
31 TH	0413	7.0	1056	0.5	1636	7.0	2257	0.8

NOVEMBER

Day	Time	m	Time	m	Time	m	Time	m
1 F	0445	6.8	1122	0.8	1713	6.6	2315	1.1
16 SA	0452	6.6	1120	0.9	1723	6.7	2321	1.1
2 SA	0519	6.5	1148	1.1	1753	6.3	2343	1.3
17 SU	0533	6.3	1156	1.1	1812	6.4		
3 SU	0559	6.1	1226	1.3	1840	5.9		
18 M	0003	1.3	0619	6.1	1246	1.2	1911	6.2
4 M	0027	1.6	0647	5.8	1329	1.5	1938	5.6
19 TU	0100	1.5	0725	6.0	1400	1.5	2026	6.2
5 TU	0136	1.8	0754	5.5	1440	1.5	2101	5.6
20 W	0220	1.5	0855	6.1	1540	1.0	2141	6.4
6 W	0258	1.9	0932	5.6	1546	1.4	2218	5.8
21 TH	0401	1.2	1008	6.4	1656	0.6	2246	6.8
7 TH	0408	1.7	1042	5.9	1651	1.2	2314	6.2
22 F	0516	0.8	1110	6.8	1755	0.3	2344	7.2
8 F	0511	1.4	1134	6.2	1751	0.9		
23 SA	0616	0.4	1204	7.1	1848	0.2		
9 SA	0001	6.5	0607	1.2	1219	6.5	1842	0.8
24 SU	0035	7.3	0708	0.3	1254	7.2	1935	0.2
10 SU	0044	6.8	0658	0.9	1301	6.8	1928	0.6
25 M	0121	7.3	0757	0.2	1339	7.2	○2019	0.3
11 M	0124	7.0	0746	0.7	1342	7.0	●2013	0.5
26 TU	0203	7.2	0842	0.3	1421	7.2	2100	0.5
12 TU	0206	7.2	0835	0.5	1424	7.2	2056	0.5
27 W	0241	7.1	0924	0.3	1502	7.1	2138	0.6
13 W	0248	7.2	0922	0.4	1509	7.3	2137	0.6
28 TH	0316	7.0	1003	0.4	1540	7.0	2210	0.8
14 TH	0330	7.1	1006	0.5	1554	7.2	2214	0.7
29 F	0348	6.9	1036	0.6	1617	6.9	2232	1.0
15 F	0412	6.9	1045	0.7	1638	7.0	2247	0.6
30 SA	0420	6.7	1103	0.8	1653	6.6	2249	1.1

DECEMBER

Day	Time	m	Time	m	Time	m	Time	m
1 SU	0455	6.5	1125	1.0	1731	6.4	2316	1.2
16 M	0526	6.6	1203	0.7	1804	6.7		
2 M	0534	6.3	1153	1.1	1813	6.2	2353	1.3
17 TU	0002	1.1	0610	6.4	1245	0.9	1857	6.5
3 TU	0617	6.0	1236	1.3	1901	6.0		
18 W	0049	1.2	0705	6.3	1338	0.9	2001	6.4
4 W	0040	1.5	0710	5.8	1339	1.4	1958	5.9
19 TH	0149	1.3	0823	6.2	1448	0.9	2111	6.4
5 TH	0145	1.7	0817	5.7	1452	1.3	2105	5.9
20 F	0306	1.2	0938	6.4	1612	0.8	2218	6.6
6 F	0307	1.7	0933	5.8	1559	1.2	2214	6.1
21 SA	0435	1.1	1044	6.6	1722	0.6	2318	6.9
7 SA	0420	1.5	1040	6.1	1704	1.0	2315	6.4
22 SU	0548	0.8	1143	6.9	1820	0.5		
8 SU	0525	1.2	1137	6.4	1803	0.8		
23 M	0013	7.0	0646	0.5	1236	7.0	1910	0.5
9 M	0007	6.7	0624	1.0	1228	6.8	1856	0.6
24 TU	0102	7.0	0737	0.4	1323	7.0	○1956	0.6
10 TU	0055	7.0	0719	0.7	1316	7.0	●1946	0.5
25 W	0145	6.9	0823	0.5	1407	6.9	2038	0.7
11 W	0142	7.2	0814	0.5	1404	7.3	2036	0.5
26 TH	0224	6.8	0906	0.5	1447	6.9	2117	0.8
12 TH	0228	7.3	0907	0.4	1453	7.4	2124	0.5
27 F	0258	6.8	0945	0.6	1524	6.8	2151	0.9
13 F	0314	7.2	0958	0.3	1542	7.4	2208	0.6
28 SA	0329	6.7	1020	0.7	1559	6.8	2213	1.0
14 SA	0400	7.1	1044	0.4	1629	7.2	2248	0.7
29 SU	0401	6.7	1047	0.8	1634	6.7	2230	1.1
15 SU	0443	6.9	1125	0.6	1716	7.0	2324	0.9
30 M	0435	6.6	1105	0.9	1709	6.6	2256	1.1
31 TU	0512	6.4	1128	0.9	1747	6.4	2329	1.1

Chart Datum: 3·20 metres below Ordnance Datum (Newlyn)

SOUTHEND-ON-SEA/
LEIGH-ON-SEA   10-4-14
Essex (Lat/Long as for Waypoint)

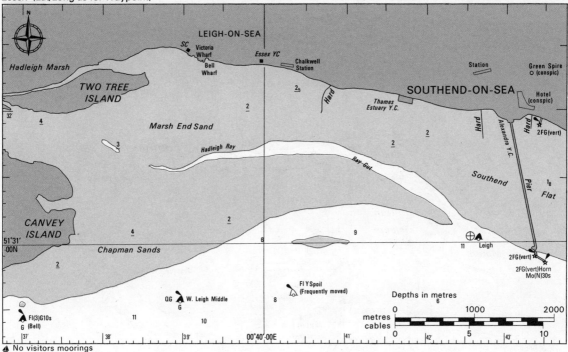

▲ No visitors moorings

CHARTS
AC *1185, 1183*; Imray C2, Y6; Stanfords 5, 8; OS 178
TIDES
+0125 Dover; ML 3·0; Duration 0610; Zone 0 (UT)

Standard Port SHEERNESS (←—)

Times				Height (metres)			
High Water		Low Water		MHWS	MHWN	MLWN	MLWS
0200	0800	0200	0700	5·8	4·7	1·5	0·6
1400	2000	1400	1900				
Differences SOUTHEND-ON-SEA							
−0005	−0005	−0005	−0005	0·0	0·0	−0·1	−0·1
CORYTON							
+0010	+0010	0000	+0010	+0·5	+0·4	−0·1	−0·1

SHELTER
The whole area dries soon after half ebb, except Ray Gut
(0·4 - 4·8m) which leads to Leigh Creek and Hadleigh Ray,
either side of Two Tree Island, thence to Benfleet Creek; all
are buoyed, but echo-sounder is invaluable. At Leigh-on-Sea
some drying moorings are available; or yachts can take the
ground alongside Bell Wharf or Victoria Wharf. It is also
possible to secure at the end of Southend Pier to collect
stores, FW. NOTE: Southend-on-Sea and Leigh-on-Sea are
both part of the lower PLA Area and an 8kn speed limit is
enforced in inshore areas. Southend BC launches *Alec
White II* , *Sidney Bates II* or *Low Way* patrol area (VHF Ch
12 16), Apr-Oct.
NAVIGATION
WPT Leigh SHM buoy, 51°31′·04N 00°42′·67E, at ent to
Ray Gut; this SHM buoy can be left close to port on
entering Ray Gut, since there is now more water NE of it
than to the SW. Appr from Shoeburyness, keep outside
the W Shoebury (SHM buoy Fl G 2·5s). Beware some 3000
small boat moorings 1M either side of Southend Pier.
Speed limit in Canvey Island/Hadleigh Ray areas is 8kn.
LIGHTS AND MARKS
Pier lts as on chartlet.
RADIO TELEPHONE
Thames Navigation Service: *Port Control London* VHF Ch 12.
TELEPHONE (01702)
Hr Mr 611889, Fax 355110; Hr Mr Leigh-on-Sea 710561;
MRSC (01255) 675518; Essex Police Marine Section
(01268) 775533; ‡‡ (01474) 537115; Marinecall 0891 500455;
Police 341212; Dr 49451; Ⓗ 348911.

FACILITIES
SOUTHEND-ON-SEA: **Southend Pier** ☎ 355620, AB £5.50, M, L,
FW, Bar; **Alexandra YC** ☎ 340363, Bar, FW; **Thorpe Bay YC**
☎ 587563, Bar, L, Slip, R, FW; **Thames Estuary YC** ☎ 345967;
Halfway YC ☎ 582025;
Services: CH, ACA, Ⓔ. **Town** EC Wed. V, R, Bar, ✉, Ⓑ, ⇌, ✈.
LEIGH-ON-SEA: **Essex YC** ☎ 78404, FW, Bar; **Leigh on Sea SC**
☎ 76788, FW, Bar; **Bell Wharf**, AB (first 24hrs free, then
£4.75; **Victoria Wharf** AB, SM, Slip;
Services: Slip, D (cans), L, FW, ME, El, Sh, C, CH, SM; EC Wed.
CANVEY ISLAND: **Services:** Slip, M, D, FW, ME, El, Sh, C, Gas,
CH, Access HW±2; **Island YC** ☎ 683729.
BENFLEET: **Benfleet YC** ☎ (01268) 792278, Slip, FW, Bar;
Services: Access HW±2½, M, Slip, D, FW, ME, El, Sh, C, .

ADJACENT HARBOUR

HOLEHAVEN, Essex, 51°30′·55N 00°33′·50E. AC 2484, 1186.
HW +0140 on Dover; see 10·4·14 Tides (use differences for
CORYTON); ML 3·0m; Duration 0610. Shelter is good, but
beware swell from passing traffic. Note: There is an 8kn
speed limit in the river off Coryton and Shellhaven. See
Piermaster for 4 Y ⚓s on extreme W of ent with 12m at
MLWS. Keep to Canvey Is side on ent. ⚓ on W edge of
chan as long stone groynes extend from E side. 0·5M N
of ent an overhead oil pipe crosses chan with 11m
clearance, plus 2 FY lts (horiz). VHF Ch 12 *Canvey Patrol*.
Lts Coryton Refinery Jetty No 4 2 FG (vert). **Piermaster** ☎
(01268) 683041; Facilities: FW at pier in office hours (also
from 'The Lobster Smack' yard), P & D from Canvey
Village (1M); EC Thurs; all other facilities on Canvey Is.

RIVER ROACH/HAVENGORE

Essex 51°36'·95N 00°52'·24E (Branklet SPM buoy); 51°33'·59N 00°50'·62E (Havengore Bridge)

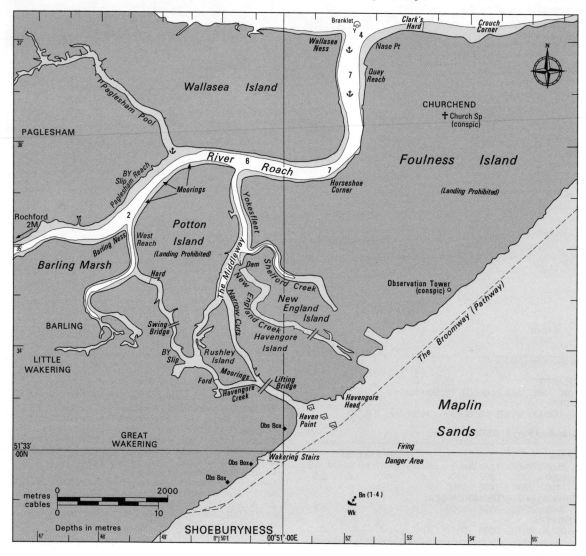

CHARTS
AC *3750, 1185*; Imray C1, Y17; Stanfords 4, 5; OS 178

TIDES
+0110 Dover; ML 2·7; Duration 0615; Zone 0 (UT)

Standard Port WALTON-ON-THE-NAZE (→)

Times				Height (metres)			
High Water		Low Water		MHWS	MHWN	MLWN	MLWS
0000	0600	0500	1100	4·2	3·4	1·1	0·4
1200	1800	1700	2300				
Differences ROCHFORD							
+0050	+0040	Dries		−0·8	−1·1	Dries	

SHELTER
Good. The Roach gives sheltered sailing and access to a network of secluded creeks, including Havengore (the "backdoor" from the Crouch to the Thames Estuary). ‡s behind sea-walls can be found for all winds at: Quay Reach (often more protected than the Crouch), Paglesham Reach (possible moorings from BY at East End), West Reach, Barling Reach and Yokes Fleet. An ‡ light is essential due to freighters H24. Speed limit 8kn. Crouch Hbr Authority controls R Roach and Crouch, out to Foulness Pt.

NAVIGATION
Normal access H24 to the Roach is from R Crouch (see 10.4.16 for WPT from seaward); the ent between Branklet SPM buoy and Nase Pt is narrowed by mudbanks. Unlit buoys up-river to Barling Ness, above which few boats go.

To exit at Havengore Creek, appr via Middleway and Narrow Cuts to reach the bridge before HW.
Entry via Havengore Creek is possible in good weather, with great care and adequate rise of tide (max draft 1·5m at HW sp). Shoeburyness Range is usually active Mon-Fri 0600-1700LT; give 24hrs notice to Range Officer by ☎. Subsequent clearance on VHF by Havengore lifting bridge (☎ HW±2, HJ); no passage unless bridge raised. Least water is over the shifting bar, just inside creek ent. From the S, cross Maplin Sands at HW −1 from S Shoebury SHM buoy, Fl G 5s (51°30'·26N 00°51'·33E), leaving Pisces wreck (conspic, 1M from ent) to port.

LIGHTS AND MARKS
None.

RADIO TELEPHONE
Range Officer (*Shoe Base*) Ch 72 16 office hrs. Bridge keeper (*Shoe Bridge*) Ch 72 16 HW±2 (HJ). *Port Control London* broadcasts nav/met info Ch 12 every H and H+30.

TELEPHONE (01702= Southend)
Range Officer 292271 Ext 3211; Havengore Bridge Ext 3436; Police 431212; Dr 218678; ⌗ (01473) 219481; MRSC (01255) 675518; Marinecall 0891 500455.

FACILITIES
Paglesham (East End) M £5, FW, D, slip, El, ME (from BY), Sh, Bar; **Gt Wakering:** Slip, P, D, FW, ME, El, Sh, C, CH (from BY); @ Rochford **Wakering YC** ☎ 530926, M, L, Bar; **Towns** EC Wed Gt Wakering & Rochford; V, R, Bar, ✉ (Great Wakering and Barling); most facilities, Ⓑ and ⇌ in Rochford and Shoeburyness, ✈ (Southend).

BURNHAM-ON-CROUCH   10-4-16

Essex 51°37'·47N 00°48'·33E (Yacht Hbr)

CHARTS
AC 3750, 1975, 1183; Imray Y17; Stanfords 4, 5; OS 168

TIDES
+0115 Dover; ML 2·5; Duration 0610; Zone 0 (UT). Full daily predictions for Burnham are on following pages. Ranges: Sp = 5·0m; Np = 3·2m. Use Walton Tidal Curves (10.4.19)

Standard Port WALTON-ON-THE-NAZE (⟶)

Times				Height (metres)			
High Water		Low Water		MHWS	MHWN	MLWN	MLWS
0000	0600	0500	1100	4·2	3·4	1·1	0·4
1200	1800	1700	2300				

Differences WHITAKER BEACON

+0022	+0024	+0033	+0027	+0·6	+0·5	+0·2	+0·1

HOLLIWELL POINT

+0034	+0037	+0100	+0037	+1·1	+0·9	+0·3	+0·1

BURNHAM-ON-CROUCH (but see also full predictions)

+0050	+0035	+0115	+0050	+1·0	+0·8	−0·1	−0·2

NORTH FAMBRIDGE

+0115	+0050	+0130	+0100	+1·1	+0·8	0·0	−0·1

HULLBRIDGE

+0115	+0050	+0135	+0105	+1·1	+0·8	0·0	−0·1

BATTLESBRIDGE

+0120	+0110	Dries	Dries	−1·8	−2·0	Dries	Dries

SHELTER
River is exposed to most winds. There are 6 marinas or yacht hbrs. ⚓ prohib in fairway but possible just above or below the moorings. Cliff Reach is sheltered from SW winds. Speed limit in river is 8kn.

NAVIGATION
WPT Outer Crouch SCM, Q (6) + L Fl 15s, 51°38'·35N 00°58'·61E. The main appr from the Swin or the Spitway is via the Whitaker Chan. The drying Ray Sand Chan is usable by shoal draft boats on the tide as a short cut from the River Blackwater.

There are few landmarks to assist entering. A 'Firing Danger Area' lies E and S of Foulness Pt. The Crouch is navigable up to Battlesbridge, 15M from Foulness. Landing on Bridgemarsh Is (up river) is prohib.

LIGHTS AND MARKS
The Whitaker Chan and R Crouch are lit as far W as No 15 Fairway SHM buoy, QG. From Sunken Buxey NCM, Q, St Mary's ✠ spire leads 233° to Outer Crouch SCM, Q (6) + L Fl 15s, (⊕); thence 240° leads into river via Crouch PHM buoy, Fl R 10s and Inner Crouch SWM buoy, L Fl 10s.

RADIO TELEPHONE
Essex Marina VHF Ch 80 (0900-1700 LT). W Wick Marina Ch 80 M (1000-1700 LT). Burnham Yacht Harbour Ch 80.

TELEPHONE (Maldon = 0621)
Hr Mr 783602; MRSC (0255) 675518; ⌗ (0473) 219481; Marinecall 0891 500455; Police 782121; Dr 2782054.

FACILITIES
BURNHAM
Burnham Yacht Hbr (350) ☎ 782150, Fax 785848, Access H24, £8, AC, FW, ME, EI, Sh, BH (30 ton), CH, ▣, R, Slip;
Royal Corinthian YC ☎ 782105, AB, FW, M, L, R, Bar;
Royal Burnham YC ☎ 782044, FW, L, R, Bar;
Crouch YC ☎ 782252, L, FW, R, Bar;
Services: AB, BY, C (15 ton), D, FW, L, ME, EI, Sh, M, Slip, CH, ACA, Gas, Gaz, SM, P, Rigging.
Town EC Wed; V, R, Bar, ✉, Ⓑ, ⇌, ✈ (Southend).
WALLASEA
Essex Marina (400) ☎ (01702) 258531, Fax 258227, BY, Gas, Bar, C (13 ton), BH (40 ton), CH, D, EI, FW, L, M, ME, P, R, Sh, Slip, V, YC; **Essex YC; Services:** ACA.
FAMBRIDGE
N Fambridge Yacht Stn (150) ☎ 740370, Access HW±5, L, CH, Sh, M, ME, BY, C (5 ton), EI, FW, Slip, Gas, Gaz;
W Wick Marina (Stow Creek) (180) ☎ 741268, Access HW±5, Gas, Gaz, CH, EI, Slip, FW, D, C (5 ton), YC, Bar;
Brandy Hole Yacht Stn (120) ☎ (0702) 230248, L, M, ME, Sh, Slip, Gas, Gaz, Bar, BY, D, FW, Access HW±4.
ALTHORNE
Bridge Marsh Marina (125+6 visitors) ☎ 740414, Fax 742216, Access HW±4, FW, Sh, ▣, ME, EI, C (8 ton), Slip.

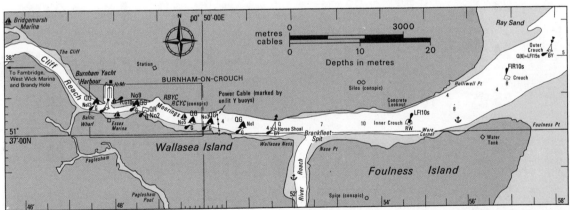

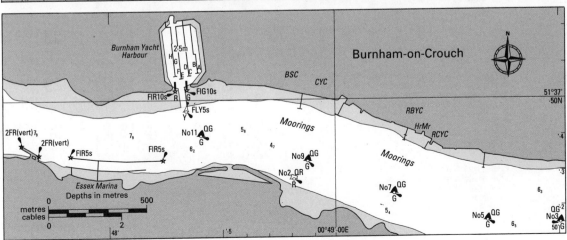

ENGLAND – BURNHAM–ON–CROUCH

LAT 51°37'N   LONG   0°48'E

TIMES AND HEIGHTS OF HIGH AND LOW WATERS

YEAR 1996

TIME ZONE (UT)
For Summer Time add ONE hour in non-shaded areas

JANUARY

Day	Time	m	Time	m	Time	m	Time	m
1 M	0247	1.0	0842	4.5	1531	0.8	2120	4.5
16 TU	0127	1.0	0735	4.3	1427	0.8	2018	4.3
2 TU	0357	0.9	0946	4.6	1628	0.8	2216	4.7
17 W	0250	0.9	0852	4.5	1541	0.7	2130	4.6
3 W	0455	0.8	1041	4.7	1716	0.7	2306	4.8
18 TH	0408	0.7	1003	4.7	1648	0.5	2235	4.8
4 TH	0546	0.5	1130	4.8	1759	0.7	2352	5.0
19 F	0517	0.4	1105	5.1	1746	0.3	2333	5.1
5 F O	0630	0.4	1215	5.0	1836	0.7		
20 SA •	0619	0.2	1202	5.3	1836	0.2		
6 SA	0031	5.0	0705	0.4	1254	5.0	1907	0.7
21 SU	0026	5.2	0708	0.0	1256	5.5	1920	0.2
7 SU	0106	5.0	0737	0.4	1327	5.0	1937	0.7
22 M	0114	5.3	0753	-0.3	1343	5.6	2001	0.2
8 M	0136	5.0	0807	0.3	1357	5.0	2007	0.7
23 TU	0158	5.5	0836	-0.3	1426	5.6	2042	0.2
9 TU	0205	5.0	0835	0.3	1427	5.0	2037	0.7
24 W	0239	5.5	0918	-0.3	1509	5.5	2122	0.3
10 W	0236	5.0	0907	0.3	1500	5.0	2109	0.7
25 TH	0320	5.3	1000	-0.1	1551	5.5	2202	0.4
11 TH	0309	5.0	0941	0.3	1538	5.0	2144	0.7
26 F	0401	5.2	1042	0.1	1633	5.0	2243	0.7
12 F	0347	4.8	1019	0.4	1619	4.8	2223	0.8
27 SA	0444	4.8	1126	0.3	1720	4.6	2329	0.8
13 SA	0428	4.7	1102	0.5	1706	4.6	2309	0.9
28 SU	0534	4.6	1219	0.7	1813	4.3		
14 SU	0518	4.6	1155	0.7	1800	4.5		
29 M	0029	1.0	0636	4.2	1325	0.9	1923	4.1
15 M	0008	1.0	0619	4.3	1308	0.8	1904	4.3
30 TU	0148	1.1	0759	4.2	1439	1.0	2038	4.2
31 W	0318	1.0	0915	4.3	1549	1.0	2145	4.3

FEBRUARY

Day	Time	m	Time	m	Time	m	Time	m
1 TH	0429	0.9	1017	4.5	1648	0.9	2240	4.6
16 F	0353	0.7	0947	4.6	1632	0.5	2217	4.7
2 F	0525	0.7	1110	4.7	1736	0.8	2328	4.8
17 SA	0509	0.3	1053	5.0	1731	0.4	2318	5.0
3 SA	0613	0.4	1155	5.0	1818	0.7		
18 SU •	0610	0.1	1152	5.2	1823	0.2		
4 SU O	0011	5.0	0650	0.4	1236	5.0	1850	0.7
19 M	0012	5.2	0657	-0.1	1244	5.5	1905	0.2
5 M	0048	5.0	0721	0.3	1308	5.0	1921	0.5
20 TU	0101	5.3	0739	-0.3	1329	5.6	1946	0.1
6 TU	0119	5.0	0751	0.3	1338	5.0	1950	0.5
21 W	0143	5.5	0820	-0.3	1410	5.6	2024	0.1
7 W	0149	5.0	0819	0.2	1408	5.1	2020	0.5
22 TH	0222	5.5	0857	-0.3	1449	5.5	2102	0.2
8 TH	0219	5.0	0847	0.2	1440	5.1	2050	0.4
23 F	0259	5.3	0934	-0.1	1526	5.2	2138	0.3
9 F	0251	5.1	0918	0.2	1515	5.1	2123	0.4
24 SA	0335	5.2	1010	0.1	1602	5.0	2214	0.4
10 SA	0325	5.0	0951	0.3	1554	5.0	2200	0.5
25 SU	0413	5.0	1047	0.4	1639	4.7	2253	0.7
11 SU	0403	4.8	1031	0.4	1637	4.7	2242	0.7
26 M	0455	4.6	1131	0.8	1721	4.3	2340	0.9
12 M	0449	4.7	1117	0.5	1728	4.5	2334	0.8
27 TU	0547	4.2	1228	1.0	1813	4.1		
13 TU	0546	4.5	1223	0.8	1828	4.3		
28 W	0048	1.0	0702	4.0	1340	1.1	1942	4.0
14 W	0048	0.9	0701	4.3	1351	0.9	1946	4.2
29 TH	0219	1.1	0838	4.1	1501	1.1	2106	4.1
15 TH	0219	0.9	0829	4.3	1517	0.8	2106	4.3

MARCH

Day	Time	m	Time	m	Time	m	Time	m
1 F	0354	0.9	0950	4.3	1613	1.0	2209	4.5
16 SA	0344	0.5	0937	4.6	1616	0.7	2201	4.6
2 SA	0456	0.7	1045	4.6	1708	0.8	2301	4.7
17 SU	0456	0.2	1042	5.0	1714	0.4	2301	5.0
3 SU	0545	0.5	1131	4.8	1752	0.7	2345	5.0
18 M	0554	0.0	1138	5.3	1805	0.3	2354	5.2
4 M	0625	0.3	1212	5.1	1829	0.5		
19 TU •	0640	-0.1	1227	5.5	1848	0.2		
5 TU O	0023	5.0	0658	0.3	1246	5.1	1900	0.5
20 W	0043	5.3	0720	-0.3	1311	5.5	1928	0.1
6 W	0057	5.1	0728	0.2	1317	5.1	1930	0.4
21 TH	0124	5.3	0758	-0.1	1351	5.5	2005	0.1
7 TH	0129	5.1	0757	0.2	1348	5.1	2000	0.4
22 F	0202	5.3	0833	0.0	1427	5.3	2041	0.2
8 F	0200	5.1	0825	0.2	1419	5.1	2031	0.3
23 SA	0237	5.3	0906	0.1	1500	5.2	2114	0.2
9 SA	0233	5.1	0855	0.2	1455	5.1	2105	0.3
24 SU	0311	5.2	0938	0.3	1532	5.0	2147	0.3
10 SU	0307	5.1	0928	0.3	1532	5.0	2141	0.4
25 M	0347	5.0	1012	0.5	1604	4.7	2221	0.5
11 M	0346	5.0	1005	0.4	1615	4.8	2223	0.7
26 TU	0424	4.7	1051	0.8	1640	4.5	2303	0.7
12 TU	0431	4.8	1053	0.7	1704	4.5	2315	0.7
27 W	0509	4.3	1142	1.0	1726	4.2		
13 W	0529	4.5	1156	0.9	1805	4.2		
28 TH	0002	0.9	0608	4.1	1252	1.2	1829	4.0
14 TH	0026	0.8	0644	4.2	1327	1.0	1923	4.1
29 F	0122	1.0	0743	4.0	1410	1.2	2009	4.0
15 F	0204	0.8	0816	4.3	1500	0.9	2047	4.3
30 SA	0256	1.0	0910	4.2	1528	1.1	2126	4.2
31 SU	0413	0.8	1011	4.6	1630	0.9	2222	4.6

APRIL

Day	Time	m	Time	m	Time	m	Time	m
1 M	0506	0.5	1059	4.8	1717	0.7	2308	4.8
16 TU	0531	0.0	1117	5.3	1743	0.5	2332	5.1
2 TU	0549	0.3	1140	5.1	1758	0.5	2350	5.0
17 W •	0619	0.0	1206	5.3	1828	0.2		
3 W	0627	0.3	1216	5.1	1834	0.4		
18 TH	0020	5.2	0657	0.2	1250	5.3	1908	0.2
4 TH O	0028	5.1	0701	0.2	1252	5.2	1906	0.4
19 F	0104	5.2	0733	0.1	1329	5.2	1946	0.2
5 F	0105	5.2	0732	0.2	1326	5.2	1939	0.3
20 SA	0141	5.2	0807	0.2	1404	5.1	2021	0.2
6 SA	0140	5.2	0803	0.2	1400	5.2	2013	0.2
21 SU	0216	5.2	0838	0.3	1436	5.0	2052	0.2
7 SU	0216	5.2	0835	0.2	1436	5.1	2049	0.2
22 M	0249	5.1	0909	0.4	1504	4.8	2123	0.4
8 M	0254	5.2	0909	0.3	1516	5.0	2128	0.2
23 TU	0323	5.0	0940	0.7	1535	4.7	2156	0.4
9 TU	0335	5.1	0950	0.4	1559	4.8	2213	0.3
24 W	0359	4.7	1017	0.8	1611	4.6	2236	0.5
10 W	0424	4.8	1038	0.7	1649	4.6	2307	0.5
25 TH	0441	4.5	1103	1.0	1655	4.3	2329	
11 TH	0524	4.6	1143	0.9	1751	4.3		
26 F	0533	4.2	1206	1.2	1752	4.1		
12 F	0020	0.7	0637	4.3	1312	1.0	1908	4.2
27 SA	0038	0.9	0657	4.1	1320	1.2	1904	4.1
13 SA	0159	0.7	0804	4.5	1442	0.9	2029	4.3
28 SU	0156	0.9	0807	4.1	1434	1.2	2026	4.2
14 SU	0329	0.4	0920	4.7	1555	0.7	2139	4.6
29 M	0313	0.8	0920	4.5	1541	1.0	2131	4.5
15 M	0437	0.2	1023	5.1	1653	0.4	2239	5.0
30 TU	0417	0.5	1014	4.7	1635	0.8	2224	4.7

Chart Datum: 2·35 metres below Ordnance Datum (Newlyn)

ENGLAND – BURNHAM–ON–CROUCH

LAT 51°37′N   LONG   0°48′E

TIMES AND HEIGHTS OF HIGH AND LOW WATERS

YEAR **1996**

TIME ZONE (UT)
For Summer Time add ONE hour in non-shaded areas

4

MAY

Day	Time	m	Time	m	Time	m	Time	m
1 W	0507	0.4	1100	5.0	1721	0.7	2311	5.0
16 TH	0553	0.1	1141	5.2	1809	0.3	2356	5.1
2 TH	0553	0.3	1142	5.1	1804	0.4	2356	5.1
17 F ●	0634	0.2	1226	5.2	1850	0.3		
3 F O	0632	0.2	1223	5.2	1843	0.3		
18 SA	0041	5.1	0709	0.3	1306	5.1	1928	0.3
4 SA	0039	5.2	0708	0.2	1304	5.2	1921	0.2
19 SU	0120	5.1	0742	0.4	1342	5.0	2002	0.3
5 SU	0120	5.3	0744	0.2	1343	5.2	2000	0.2
20 M	0157	5.0	0813	0.5	1414	4.8	2034	0.3
6 M	0200	5.3	0820	0.2	1422	5.2	2039	0.1
21 TU	0229	5.0	0843	0.5	1442	4.8	2103	0.3
7 TU	0242	5.3	0857	0.3	1503	5.1	2122	0.1
22 W	0302	4.8	0913	0.7	1513	4.7	2136	0.4
8 W	0329	5.2	0940	0.4	1550	4.8	2209	0.2
23 TH	0337	4.7	0948	0.8	1549	4.7	2213	0.4
9 TH	0419	5.0	1031	0.7	1640	4.7	2305	0.3
24 F	0417	4.6	1028	0.9	1631	4.5	2300	0.5
10 F	0518	4.7	1132	0.8	1741	4.5		
25 SA	0503	4.5	1120	1.0	1723	4.3	2355	0.7
11 SA	0017	0.4	0626	4.6	1252	0.9	1850	4.3
26 SU	0558	4.3	1226	1.1	1821	4.2		
12 SU	0144	0.4	0742	4.6	1415	0.9	2004	4.5
27 M	0106	0.8	0702	4.2	1339	1.2	1930	4.2
13 M	0305	0.3	0854	4.8	1528	0.7	2112	4.7
28 TU	0218	0.7	0815	4.3	1447	1.1	2037	4.3
14 TU	0412	0.2	0956	5.0	1628	0.5	2212	4.8
29 W	0326	0.5	0921	4.6	1549	0.9	2138	4.6
15 W	0506	0.1	1051	5.2	1721	0.3	2306	5.0
30 TH	0425	0.4	1017	4.8	1643	0.7	2233	4.8
31 F	0517	0.3	1107	5.0	1734	0.5	2324	5.1

JUNE

Day	Time	m	Time	m	Time	m	Time	m
1 SA O	0605	0.2	1156	5.1	1823	0.3		
16 SU ●	0020	5.0	0648	0.4	1245	5.0	1914	0.3
2 SU	0014	5.2	0648	0.2	1243	5.2	1906	0.2
17 M	0102	5.2	0720	0.5	1323	5.0	1948	0.3
3 M	0102	5.3	0728	0.2	1327	5.2	1950	0.1
18 TU	0138	4.8	0751	0.5	1355	4.8	2019	0.3
4 TU	0147	5.3	0808	0.2	1410	5.0	2034	0.0
19 W	0211	4.8	0821	0.7	1424	4.8	2047	0.3
5 W	0233	5.3	0849	0.2	1454	5.2	2119	0.0
20 TH	0242	4.8	0851	0.7	1454	4.8	2118	0.3
6 TH	0320	5.3	0933	0.3	1540	5.1	2207	0.0
21 F	0316	4.8	0933	0.7	1528	4.7	2152	0.3
7 F	0411	5.2	1020	0.5	1630	5.0	2301	0.1
22 SA	0353	4.7	1000	0.8	1607	4.7	2232	0.4
8 SA	0505	5.0	1115	0.7	1725	4.7		
23 SU	0434	4.7	1042	0.9	1652	4.6	2317	0.5
9 SU	0002	0.2	0606	4.7	1223	0.9	1826	4.6
24 M	0524	4.5	1133	1.0	1743	4.5		
10 M	0116	0.3	0713	4.7	1341	0.9	1934	4.6
25 TU	0015	0.5	0618	4.5	1240	1.1	1841	4.3
11 TU	0234	0.3	0821	4.7	1457	0.8	2041	4.6
26 W	0125	0.7	0723	4.3	1354	1.1	1948	4.3
12 W	0342	0.3	0926	4.8	1603	0.7	2144	4.7
27 TH	0236	0.7	0832	4.5	1503	1.0	2056	4.5
13 TH	0439	0.3	1023	5.0	1659	0.5	2241	4.8
28 F	0344	0.5	0938	4.7	1609	0.8	2159	4.7
14 F	0527	0.3	1114	5.0	1749	0.4	2332	5.0
29 SA	0445	0.4	1036	4.8	1710	0.5	2257	5.0
15 SA	0612	0.4	1201	5.1	1835	0.4		
30 SU	0541	0.3	1131	5.1	1808	0.3	2353	5.2

JULY

Day	Time	m	Time	m	Time	m	Time	m
1 M O	0631	0.2	1223	5.2	1857	0.1		
16 TU	0045	5.0	0702	0.5	1304	5.0	1934	0.4
2 TU	0047	5.3	0715	0.1	1312	5.3	1944	0.0
17 W	0121	5.0	0732	0.7	1337	5.0	2004	0.4
3 W	0134	5.5	0757	0.1	1358	5.3	2028	-0.1
18 TH	0153	4.8	0801	0.5	1406	4.8	2031	0.3
4 TH	0221	5.5	0838	0.2	1441	5.3	2112	-0.3
19 F	0222	4.8	0831	0.5	1435	4.8	2058	0.3
5 F	0308	5.5	0921	0.2	1527	5.3	2157	-0.1
20 SA	0253	4.8	0901	0.7	1505	4.8	2129	0.3
6 SA	0355	5.3	1005	0.4	1612	5.2	2245	0.0
21 SU	0327	4.8	0935	0.7	1541	4.8	2203	0.3
7 SU	0445	5.1	1054	0.5	1701	5.0	2336	0.2
22 M	0406	4.8	1012	0.8	1619	4.7	2241	0.4
8 M	0539	4.8	1148	0.8	1756	4.7		
23 TU	0450	4.7	1055	0.9	1705	4.6	2327	0.5
9 TU	0038	0.4	0637	4.6	1300	0.9	1858	4.6
24 W	0541	4.6	1149	1.0	1759	4.5		
10 W	0151	0.5	0745	4.5	1419	1.0	2008	4.5
25 TH	0031	0.7	0639	4.3	1304	1.1	1905	4.3
11 TH	0304	0.7	0853	4.6	1535	0.9	2116	4.5
26 F	0149	0.8	0751	4.3	1424	1.0	2019	4.3
12 F	0408	0.7	0954	4.7	1638	0.7	2217	4.7
27 SA	0307	0.7	0904	4.6	1541	0.9	2131	4.6
13 SA	0500	0.7	1049	4.8	1732	0.5	2312	4.8
28 SU	0419	0.7	1011	4.8	1653	0.5	2237	4.8
14 SU	0547	0.5	1140	5.0	1820	0.4		
29 M	0521	0.4	1110	5.1	1756	0.3	2338	5.1
15 M ●	0001	4.8	0628	0.5	1224	5.0	1859	0.4
30 TU O	0615	0.2	1207	5.2	1848	0.1		
31 W	0032	5.3	0700	0.2	1258	5.5	1933	-0.1

AUGUST

Day	Time	m	Time	m	Time	m	Time	m
1 TH	0122	5.6	0742	0.1	1343	5.6	2016	-0.3
16 F	0133	5.0	0740	0.5	1345	5.0	2009	0.3
2 F	0208	5.6	0824	0.1	1426	5.6	2057	-0.3
17 SA	0159	5.0	0809	0.5	1413	5.0	2035	0.3
3 SA	0252	5.6	0904	0.2	1508	5.5	2138	-0.3
18 SU	0229	5.0	0839	0.5	1442	5.0	2103	0.3
4 SU	0335	5.5	0946	0.3	1550	5.3	2220	0.0
19 M	0300	5.1	0911	0.5	1514	5.0	2134	0.3
5 M	0419	5.2	1029	0.5	1633	5.1	2304	0.2
20 TU	0337	5.0	0947	0.7	1550	4.8	2208	0.4
6 TU	0506	4.8	1117	0.8	1723	4.8	2352	0.5
21 W	0418	4.8	1028	0.8	1631	4.7	2250	0.5
7 W	0559	4.6	1217	1.0	1820	4.5		
22 TH	0506	4.6	1117	0.9	1724	4.5	2343	0.8
8 TH	0057	0.7	0703	4.3	1336	1.1	1932	4.3
23 F	0605	4.5	1226	1.0	1829	4.3		
9 F	0213	1.0	0816	4.3	1501	1.0	2047	4.3
24 SA	0107	0.9	0716	4.3	1354	1.0	1952	4.3
10 SA	0328	1.0	0925	4.5	1613	0.9	2155	4.5
25 SU	0236	0.9	0837	4.5	1523	0.9	2114	4.5
11 SU	0430	0.9	1024	4.7	1711	0.7	2252	4.7
26 M	0356	0.8	0950	4.7	1641	0.5	2223	4.8
12 M	0522	0.8	1115	5.0	1800	0.5	2342	4.8
27 TU	0501	0.5	1052	5.1	1743	0.2	2324	5.2
13 TU	0605	0.7	1201	5.1	1839	0.4		
28 W O	0556	0.3	1149	5.3	1835	0.0		
14 W ●	0024	5.0	0640	0.7	1242	5.1	1913	0.4
29 TH	0019	5.5	0643	0.2	1240	5.5	1918	-0.1
15 TH	0102	5.0	0711	0.7	1315	5.1	1942	0.3
30 F	0107	5.6	0724	0.2	1326	5.6	1959	-0.3
31 SA	0152	5.6	0805	0.2	1407	5.6	2037	-0.3

Chart Datum: 2·35 metres below Ordnance Datum (Newlyn)

ENGLAND – BURNHAM–ON–CROUCH

LAT 51°37′N   LONG   0°48′E

TIMES AND HEIGHTS OF HIGH AND LOW WATERS

YEAR **1996**

TIME ZONE (UT)
For Summer Time add ONE hour in non-shaded areas

SEPTEMBER

Date	Time	m		Date	Time	m
1 SU	0232 / 0845 / 1446 / 2114	5.6 / 0.2 / 5.6 / -0.1		16 M	0204 / 0817 / 1419 / 2037	5.2 / 0.5 / 5.1 / 0.3
2 M	0311 / 0923 / 1525 / 2151	5.5 / 0.3 / 5.3 / 0.1		17 TU	0236 / 0850 / 1451 / 2108	5.1 / 0.5 / 5.1 / 0.4
3 TU	0351 / 1004 / 1604 / 2229	5.2 / 0.4 / 5.1 / 0.4		18 W	0312 / 0925 / 1527 / 2142	5.1 / 0.7 / 5.0 / 0.5
4 W	0431 / 1047 / 1647 / 2311	4.8 / 0.7 / 4.8 / 0.7		19 TH	0352 / 1006 / 1609 / 2223	5.0 / 0.8 / 4.8 / 0.7
5 TH	0515 / 1137 / 1739	4.6 / 0.9 / 4.5		20 F	0438 / 1057 / 1701 / 2316	4.7 / 0.9 / 4.6 / 0.9
6 F	0003 / 0612 / 1248 / 1850	1.0 / 4.2 / 1.1 / 4.1		21 SA	0536 / 1204 / 1809	4.5 / 1.0 / 4.3
7 SA	0113 / 0733 / 1418 / 2016	1.2 / 4.1 / 1.1 / 4.1		22 SU	0037 / 0650 / 1336 / 1938	1.0 / 4.3 / 1.0 / 4.3
8 SU	0236 / 0851 / 1540 / 2129	1.2 / 4.2 / 1.0 / 4.3		23 M	0213 / 0816 / 1511 / 2101	1.0 / 4.5 / 0.8 / 4.6
9 M	0353 / 0954 / 1641 / 2227	1.1 / 4.6 / 0.8 / 4.6		24 TU	0337 / 0930 / 1626 / 2210	0.9 / 4.7 / 0.4 / 5.0
10 TU	0450 / 1046 / 1731 / 2317	1.0 / 4.8 / 0.5 / 5.0		25 W	0441 / 1033 / 1725 / 2308	0.7 / 5.1 / 0.2 / 5.2
11 W	0536 / 1132 / 1813 / 2358	0.8 / 5.1 / 0.4 / 5.1		26 TH	0534 / 1128 / 1816	0.4 / 5.3 / 0.0
12 TH ●	0614 / 1213 / 1845	0.7 / 5.2 / 0.4		27 F O	0000 / 0617 / 1218 / 1857	5.5 / 0.3 / 5.5 / -0.1
13 F	0036 / 0646 / 1248 / 1915	5.1 / 0.7 / 5.2 / 0.3		28 SA	0049 / 0705 / 1304 / 1936	5.6 / 0.2 / 5.6 / 0.0
14 SA	0106 / 0715 / 1319 / 1942	5.1 / 0.5 / 5.1 / 0.3		29 SU	0131 / 0745 / 1345 / 2013	5.6 / 0.2 / 5.6 / 0.0
15 SU	0134 / 0746 / 1349 / 2010	5.1 / 0.5 / 5.1 / 0.3		30 M	0210 / 0824 / 1423 / 2047	5.5 / 0.3 / 5.5 / 0.2

OCTOBER

Date	Time	m		Date	Time	m
1 TU	0246 / 0901 / 1500 / 2121	5.3 / 0.3 / 5.3 / 0.3		16 W	0215 / 0832 / 1433 / 2046	5.2 / 0.5 / 5.2 / 0.4
2 W	0320 / 0938 / 1536 / 2154	5.1 / 0.5 / 5.1 / 0.5		17 TH	0251 / 0909 / 1511 / 2123	5.1 / 0.5 / 5.1 / 0.5
3 TH	0353 / 1017 / 1614 / 2231	4.8 / 0.7 / 4.7 / 0.9		18 F	0331 / 0953 / 1556 / 2205	5.0 / 0.7 / 4.8 / 0.8
4 F	0429 / 1102 / 1658 / 2317	4.6 / 0.9 / 4.5 / 1.1		19 SA	0417 / 1046 / 1651 / 2301	4.7 / 0.8 / 4.6 / 1.0
5 SA	0514 / 1202 / 1758	4.3 / 1.1 / 4.1		20 SU	0516 / 1152 / 1800	4.5 / 0.9 / 4.3
6 SU	0021 / 0622 / 1323 / 1930	1.3 / 4.1 / 1.1 / 4.0		21 M	0017 / 0629 / 1324 / 1923	1.1 / 4.3 / 0.8 / 4.3
7 M	0140 / 0801 / 1450 / 2052	1.5 / 4.1 / 1.1 / 4.2		22 TU	0151 / 0756 / 1453 / 2043	1.1 / 4.5 / 0.7 / 4.6
8 TU	0302 / 0914 / 1559 / 2153	1.3 / 4.5 / 0.9 / 4.6		23 W	0313 / 0908 / 1605 / 2150	0.9 / 4.7 / 0.4 / 5.0
9 W	0409 / 1009 / 1651 / 2242	1.1 / 4.7 / 0.7 / 4.8		24 TH	0418 / 1010 / 1701 / 2247	0.7 / 5.1 / 0.2 / 5.2
10 TH	0458 / 1056 / 1733 / 2325	0.9 / 5.0 / 0.5 / 5.1		25 F	0512 / 1105 / 1752 / 2339	0.4 / 5.2 / 0.1 / 5.5
11 F	0540 / 1136 / 1812	0.8 / 5.2 / 0.4		26 SA O	0602 / 1155 / 1835	0.3 / 5.3 / 0.1
12 SA ●	0002 / 0617 / 1214 / 1844	5.2 / 0.7 / 5.2 / 0.4		27 SU	0025 / 0645 / 1242 / 1912	5.5 / 0.3 / 5.5 / 0.2
13 SU	0036 / 0650 / 1250 / 1915	5.2 / 0.5 / 5.2 / 0.4		28 M	0107 / 0725 / 1323 / 1947	5.5 / 0.3 / 5.3 / 0.3
14 M	0107 / 0722 / 1324 / 1944	5.2 / 0.5 / 5.2 / 0.4		29 TU	0146 / 0803 / 1400 / 2021	5.4 / 0.3 / 5.3 / 0.4
15 TU	0141 / 0756 / 1358 / 2014	5.2 / 0.5 / 5.2 / 0.5		30 W	0219 / 0840 / 1436 / 2052	5.2 / 0.4 / 5.2 / 0.5
				31 TH	0251 / 0915 / 1510 / 2123	5.0 / 0.4 / 5.0 / 0.8

NOVEMBER

Date	Time	m		Date	Time	m
1 F	0320 / 0951 / 1546 / 2156	4.8 / 0.7 / 4.8 / 0.9		16 SA	0317 / 0946 / 1549 / 2155	5.0 / 0.4 / 5.0 / 0.8
2 SA	0353 / 1032 / 1626 / 2237	4.7 / 0.8 / 4.6 / 1.1		17 SU	0404 / 1039 / 1642 / 2249	4.8 / 0.5 / 4.7 / 0.9
3 SU	0432 / 1124 / 1715 / 2333	4.7 / 0.9 / 4.3 / 1.3		18 M	0500 / 1143 / 1748 / 2356	4.6 / 0.5 / 4.6 / 1.0
4 M	0527 / 1231 / 1818	4.2 / 1.0 / 4.1		19 TU	0610 / 1306 / 1901	4.5 / 0.7 / 4.5
5 TU	0047 / 0641 / 1345 / 1948	1.5 / 4.1 / 1.0 / 4.1		20 W	0122 / 0729 / 1428 / 2017	1.1 / 4.5 / 0.5 / 4.7
6 W	0202 / 0812 / 1459 / 2103	1.5 / 4.2 / 0.9 / 4.3		21 TH	0244 / 0841 / 1538 / 2123	1.0 / 4.7 / 0.4 / 4.8
7 TH	0314 / 0919 / 1559 / 2157	1.2 / 4.6 / 0.8 / 4.7		22 F	0352 / 0944 / 1637 / 2221	0.8 / 5.0 / 0.3 / 5.1
8 F	0412 / 1011 / 1650 / 2243	1.0 / 4.8 / 0.5 / 5.0		23 SA	0450 / 1040 / 1727 / 2312	0.5 / 5.1 / 0.2 / 5.2
9 SA	0500 / 1057 / 1733 / 2324	0.8 / 5.1 / 0.4 / 5.1		24 SU	0541 / 1131 / 1812	0.4 / 5.2 / 0.3
10 SU	0543 / 1139 / 1814	0.7 / 5.2 / 0.4		25 M O	0000 / 0628 / 1219 / 1850	5.2 / 0.3 / 5.2 / 0.4
11 M ●	0004 / 0624 / 1220 / 1850	5.2 / 0.5 / 5.2 / 0.4		26 TU	0045 / 0709 / 1302 / 1925	5.2 / 0.3 / 5.2 / 0.4
12 TU	0042 / 0702 / 1301 / 1923	5.3 / 0.4 / 5.3 / 0.4		27 W	0122 / 0747 / 1340 / 1957	5.1 / 0.3 / 5.1 / 0.5
13 W	0119 / 0739 / 1339 / 1957	5.3 / 0.4 / 5.3 / 0.4		28 TH	0157 / 0823 / 1416 / 2027	5.0 / 0.4 / 5.1 / 0.7
14 TH	0158 / 0819 / 1418 / 2033	5.2 / 0.3 / 5.2 / 0.4		29 F	0226 / 0856 / 1448 / 2057	5.0 / 0.4 / 5.0 / 0.8
15 F	0236 / 0900 / 1501 / 2111	5.1 / 0.3 / 5.1 / 0.5		30 SA	0254 / 0928 / 1522 / 2129	4.8 / 0.5 / 4.8 / 0.9

DECEMBER

Date	Time	m		Date	Time	m
1 SU	0326 / 1005 / 1558 / 2205	4.8 / 0.5 / 4.7 / 1.0		16 M	0353 / 1032 / 1630 / 2236	5.0 / 0.2 / 5.0 / 0.8
2 M	0405 / 1050 / 1641 / 2250	4.7 / 0.7 / 4.5 / 1.1		17 TU	0444 / 1129 / 1726 / 2333	4.8 / 0.3 / 4.7 / 0.9
3 TU	0452 / 1143 / 1731 / 2349	4.5 / 0.8 / 4.3 / 1.2		18 W	0545 / 1237 / 1830	4.6 / 0.5 / 4.6
4 W	0549 / 1249 / 1830	4.3 / 0.9 / 4.2		19 TH	0047 / 0654 / 1354 / 1943	1.0 / 4.5 / 0.5 / 4.6
5 TH	0103 / 0659 / 1358 / 1945	1.3 / 4.2 / 0.9 / 4.2		20 F	0208 / 0809 / 1506 / 2052	1.0 / 4.6 / 0.5 / 4.7
6 F	0215 / 0815 / 1504 / 2058	1.2 / 4.3 / 0.8 / 4.5		21 SA	0324 / 0917 / 1609 / 2153	0.9 / 4.7 / 0.4 / 4.8
7 SA	0322 / 0920 / 1604 / 2155	1.1 / 4.6 / 0.7 / 4.7		22 SU	0428 / 1017 / 1702 / 2247	0.7 / 4.8 / 0.4 / 4.7
8 SU	0420 / 1015 / 1656 / 2245	0.9 / 4.8 / 0.5 / 5.0		23 M	0524 / 1111 / 1750 / 2338	0.5 / 5.0 / 0.4 / 4.7
9 M	0511 / 1105 / 1744 / 2332	0.7 / 5.1 / 0.4 / 5.1		24 TU O	0615 / 1200 / 1832	0.4 / 5.1 / 0.5
10 TU ●	0601 / 1153 / 1828	0.5 / 5.2 / 0.4		25 W	0023 / 0657 / 1245 / 1906	5.1 / 0.3 / 5.1 / 0.7
11 W	0018 / 0646 / 1240 / 1906	5.2 / 0.4 / 5.3 / 0.3		26 TH	0103 / 0734 / 1324 / 1938	5.0 / 0.3 / 5.0 / 0.7
12 TH	0102 / 0729 / 1324 / 1945	5.3 / 0.2 / 5.3 / 0.3		27 F	0137 / 0810 / 1358 / 2008	5.0 / 0.3 / 5.0 / 0.7
13 F	0143 / 0812 / 1407 / 2024	5.3 / 0.2 / 5.3 / 0.4		28 SA	0207 / 0840 / 1429 / 2037	4.8 / 0.3 / 5.0 / 0.7
14 SA	0224 / 0855 / 1452 / 2104	5.2 / 0.1 / 5.3 / 0.4		29 SU	0235 / 0909 / 1500 / 2107	4.8 / 0.3 / 4.8 / 0.7
15 SU	0306 / 0941 / 1539 / 2148	5.1 / 0.1 / 5.2 / 0.5		30 M	0304 / 0941 / 1533 / 2140	4.8 / 0.4 / 4.8 / 0.8
				31 TU	0340 / 1019 / 1612 / 2218	4.8 / 0.4 / 4.7 / 0.9

Chart Datum: 2·35 metres below Ordnance Datum (Newlyn)

RIVER BLACKWATER   10-4-17

Essex 51°41'·30N 00°55'·00E (½ca S of Nass bn)

CHARTS
AC *3741, 1975, 1183*; Imray, Y17; OS 168

TIDES
Maldon +0130 Dover; ML 2·8; Duration 0620; Zone 0 (UT)

Standard Port WALTON-ON-THE-NAZE (→)

Times				Height (metres)			
High Water		Low Water		MHWS	MHWN	MLWN	MLWS
0000	0600	0500	1100	4·2	3·4	1·1	0·4
1200	1800	1700	2300				
Differences SUNK HEAD							
0000	+0002	–0002	+0002	–0.3	–0.3	–0.1	–0.1
CLACTON-ON-SEA							
+0012	+0010	+0025	+0008	+0.3	+0.1	0.0	0.0
WEST MERSEA							
+0035	+0015	+0055	+0010	+0.9	+0.4	+0.1	+0.1
BRADWELL							
+0035	+0023	+0047	+0004	+1.1	+0.8	+0.2	+0.1
OSEA ISLAND							
+0057	+0045	+0050	+0007	+1.1	+0.9	+0.1	0.0
MALDON							
+0107	+0055	No data		–1.3	–1.1		No data

SHELTER
Good, as appropriate to wind. Marinas at Tollesbury, Bradwell and Maylandsea. ⚓ restricted by oyster beds and many moorings. At W Mersea there is a pontoon for landing (limited waiting); also pile moorings in Ray Chan or ⚓ in Mersea Quarters, access approx HW±1½. Berths at Heybridge Basin, access via lock approx HW –1 to HW, thence to Chelmer & Blackwater Canal (not navigable).

NAVIGATION
WPT Knoll NCM, Q, 51°43'·85N 01°05'·17E, 107°/287° from/to Nass bn, ECM VQ (3) 5s, 6·7M. Speed limit 8kn W of Osea Is.
WEST MERSEA: Beware oyster beds between Cobmarsh Is and Packing Marsh Is and in Salcott Chan.
BRADWELL: No dangers, but only suitable for small craft and area gets very crowded; see below under Lts & Marks.
TOLLESBURY FLEET: Proceeding via S Chan up Woodrolfe Creek, a tide gauge shows depth over marina ent sill (approx 3m at MHWS and 2m at MHWN). Speed limits: Woodrolfe Creek 4kn upper reaches; Tollesbury Fleet S Chan 8kn.

LIGHTS AND MARKS
Bradwell Creek ent has bn QR with tide gauge showing depth in ft in Creek; this bn must be left to STBD on entry. 4 PHM buoys, 3 SHM withies and 2 B/W △ ldg bns mark the chan which doglegs past a SHM buoy to marina ent. Power stn is conspic 7ca NNE.
MALDON: From S of Osea Is, 'The Doctor', No 3 SHM buoy on with Blackwater SC lt, Iso G 5s, lead 300° approx up the chan; or No 3 and No 8 buoys in line at 305°. Beyond No 8 buoy, the chan which shifts and carries 0·2m, is buoyed up to Maldon. Access near HW; pontoons dry to soft mud.

TELEPHONE (01621 Maldon; 01206 Colchester/W Mersea)
Hr Mr 856726; R. Bailiff (Maldon Quay) 856487, Office 875837, Mobile 0860 456802; Canal lockmaster 853506; MRSC (01255) 675518; ⌗ (01473) 219481; Marinecall 0891 500455; Police (Colchester) 762212, (W Mersea) 382930; Dr 854118, or W Mersea 382015.

FACILITIES
WEST MERSEA (01206)
W Mersea YC ☎ 382947, M , R, Bar, scrubbing posts.
Services: Slip (+ dock), M, L (at HW), FW, ME, El, C (10 ton), CH, D, BY, C (mobile), Sh, SM;
Town EC Wed; P, D, FW, ME, El, CH, V, R, Bar, ✉, Ⓑ, ≠ (bus to Colchester, Ⓗ ☎ 0206-853535), ✈ (Southend/ Stansted).
TOLLESBURY (01621)
Tollesbury Marina (240+20 visitors) ☎ 868471, Fax 868489, Slip, D, AC, BH (10 ton), Gas, Gaz, FW, ME, El, Sh, C (5 ton), CH, V, R, Bar, ▢, Access HW±1½;
Tollesbury Cruising Club ☎ 869561, Bar, R, M, C (20 ton), D, CH, FW, L, Slip, AC, ME, El, Sh;
Services: Slip access HW±2 , FW, ME, El, Sh, CH.
Village EC Wed; P, V, R, Bar, ✉, Ⓑ (Tues, Thurs 1000-1430), ≠ (bus to Witham), ✈ (Southend or Cambridge).
BRADWELL (01621)
Bradwell Marina (280, some Ⓥ) ☎ 776235, Fax 776393, £9.75, Slip, AC, Gas, Gaz, D, P, FW, ME, El, Sh, BH (16 ton), CH, R, Bar, Access HW±4½, approx 2m; **Bradwell Quay YC** ☎ 776539, M, FW, Bar, L, Slip. **Town** ✉, ≠ (bus/ taxi to Southminster), ✈ (Southend).
MAYLANDSEA (01621)
Blackwater Marina (230) ☎ 740264, Fax 742122, £6, Slip, D, Sh, CH, R, Bar; Access HW±2. 150 moorings in chan. Taxi to Southminster ≠.
MALDON (01621)
Maldon Quay Slip, M, P, D, FW, AB; **Maldon Little Ship Club** ☎ 854139, Bar;
Services: Slip, D, Sh, CH, M, ACA, SM, ME, El, Ⓔ.
Town EC Wed; ✉, Ⓑ, ≠ (bus to Chelmsford, Ⓗ ☎ (01245) 440761), ✈ (Southend, Cambridge or Stansted).
HEYBRIDGE BASIN (01621)
Blackwater SC ☎ 853923, L, FW; **Services:** Slip, D, L, M, FW, CH, ME, El, SH, C. Bus to Heybridge/Maldon.

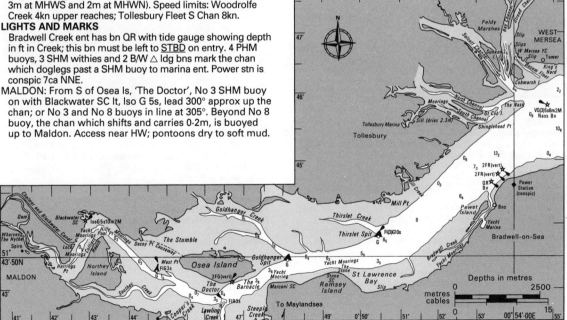

RADIO TELEPHONE
Bradwell and Tollesbury Marinas VHF Ch **80** M (HO).
Blackwater Marina VHF Ch M, 0900-2300.

RIVER COLNE   10-4-18

Essex 51°47'·95N 01°00'·70E (Brightlingsea)

CHARTS
AC 3741, 1975, 1183; Imray, Y17; Stanfords 4, 5; OS 168
TIDES
+0050 Dover; ML 2·5; Duration 0615; Zone 0 (UT)

Standard Port WALTON-ON-THE-NAZE (→)

Times				Height (metres)			
High Water		Low Water		MHWS	MHWN	MLWN	MLWS
0000	0600	0500	1100	4·2	3·4	1·1	0·4
1200	1800	1700	2300				

Differences BRIGHTLINGSEA

+0025	+0021	+0046	+0004	+0·8	+0·4	+0·1	0·0

COLCHESTER

+0035	+0025	Dries out		0·0	−0·3	Dries out	

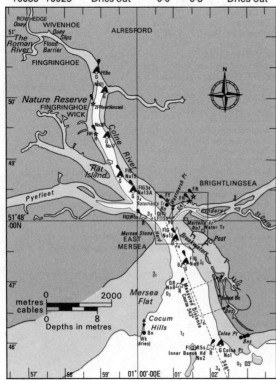

LIGHTS AND MARKS
Well buoyed/lit up to Wivenhoe. Ldg lts/marks 041° for Brightlingsea: both FR 7/10m 4M; dayglo W □, orange stripe on posts; adjusted to suit the chan. Then Spit SCM buoy, Q (6) + L Fl 15s, and chan buoys Fl (3) G 5s and Fl R 5s, plus NCM bn Q where chan is divided by Cindery Is. Bateman's Tr (conspic) by Westmarsh Pt has a FY sodium lt 12m. Pyefleet Chan and other creeks are unlit.
The flood barrier is marked by 2FR/FG (vert) on both sides and there are bns, QR/QG, up/downstream on the river banks. To facilitate the passage of large vessels, Dir lts above and below the barrier are as follows: for up-stream tfc 305°, Oc WRG 5s 5/3M, vis G300°-304·7°, W304·7°-305·3°, R305·3°-310°; and for down-stream tfc 125°, Oc WRG 5s 5/3M, vis G120°-124.8, W°124.8°-125.2°, R125.2°-130°. Daymarks are W ▽ with Or vert stripe.
RADIO TELEPHONE
Brightlingsea Port Radio VHF Ch 68. Colchester Ch **68** 11 14 16 (Office hrs and HW−2 to HW+1).
TELEPHONE (01206 Brightlingsea and Colchester)
Hr Mr (Brightlingsea) 302200; Hr Mr (Colchester) 827316; MRSC (01255) 675518; ⌗ (01473) 219481; Marinecall 0891 500455; Police (01255) 221312; Dr 303875.

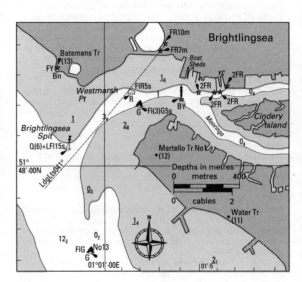

SHELTER
Suitable shelter can be found for most winds, but outer hbr is exposed to W'lies. Some pile moorings for visitors in the creek S of Cindery Is; none to the N. ⚓s to the NW of Mersea Stone Pt and in Pyefleet Chan, E of Pewit Is. R Colne is navigable for 4·5m draft to Wivenhoe, where the river dries; and to The Hythe, Colchester (3m draft).
NAVIGATION
WPT Colne Bar By, SHM Fl (2) G 5s, 51°44'·58N 01°02'·66E, 160°/340° from/to Mersea Stone, 3·6M. See also 10·4·17.
Extensive mud and sand banks flank the ent chan. Much traffic in the Colne; large coasters use the Brightlingsea chans. The ent to Brightlingsea Creek is very narrow at LW and carries about 1m.
A flood barrier 2ca below Wivenhoe church is normally open (30m wide) allowing unrestricted passage; keep to stbd, max speed 5kn. Tfc lts on N pier are 3FR (vert), vis up/downstream. When lit, they indicate either the barrier gates are shut or a large vessel is passing through; other traffic must keep clear. (See LIGHTS AND MARKS).
Speed limits in the approaches and up-river:
No 13 buoy to Fingringhoe (No 24 buoy) = 8kn; but Nos 12 to 16 buoys = 5kn;
No 24 buoy to Colchester = 4kn;
Brightlingsea Harbour = 4kn.

FACILITIES
BRIGHTLINGSEA
Town Hard ☎ 303535, L, FW, Pile moorings £5; **Colne YC** ☎ 302594, L, FW, R, Bar; **Brightlingsea SC** Slip, Bar; **Services:** M, L, FW, ME, El, Ⓔ, Sh, CH, ACA, P & D (cans), Gas, SM, BY, C, Slip.
Town P & D (cans), FW, ME, El, Sh, C (mobile), CH, V, R, Bar, ✉, Ⓑ, ⇌ (bus to Wivenhoe or Colchester), ✈ (Southend or Stansted).
WIVENHOE: **Colne Marine Yacht** ☎ 822417, L, ME, El, Sh, C; **Wivenhoe SC**.
Village P, V, Bar, ✉, Ⓑ (AM only), ⇌.

WALTON BACKWATERS   10-4-19

Essex 51°54'·54N 01°16'·90E (No 2 PHM buoy)

CHARTS
AC 2695, *2052*; Imray, Y16; Stanfords 5, 6; OS 169

TIDES
+0030 Dover; ML 2·2; Duration 0615; Zone 0 (UT). Walton is a Standard Port. Predictions are for Walton Pier, ie to seaward. Differences for Bramble Creek (N of Hamford Water) are +10, –7, –5, +10 mins; heights are all +0·3m.

SHELTER
Good in all weather, but ent not advised if a big sea is running from the NE. Berth HW±5 in Titchmarsh Marina, ent dredged 1·3m; or on adjacent pontoons in the Twizzle. Good ⚓s in Hamford Water (keep clear of Oakley Creek) and in N end of Walton Chan, 2ca S of Stone Pt on E side. Walton Yacht Basin more suited for long stay; appr dries.

NAVIGATION
WPT Pye End SWM buoy, L Fl 10s, 51°55'·00N 01°18'·00E, 054°/234° from/to buoyed chan ent, 1·0M. NB this stretch carries only 0·9m. From S, appr via Medusa Chan; from N and E via the Harwich recomended yacht track. At narrow ent to Walton Chan leave No. 9 NCM buoy to stbd, and 3 PHM buoys close to port; after a fourth PHM off Stone Pt stay mid-chan. Beware lobster pots off the Naze and Pye Sands and oyster beds in the Backwaters.

LIGHTS AND MARKS
Naze Tr (49m) is conspic 3M S of Pye End By. 2M NNE at Felixstowe, cranes and Y flood lts are conspic D/N. Chan buoys inward from Pye End are unlit.

RADIO TELEPHONE
Titchmarsh marina Ch 80, 0800-2000 in season.

TELEPHONE (01255)
Hr Mr 851887; MRSC 675518; ⌗ (01473) 219481; Marinecall 0891 500455; Police 241312; Ⓗ 502446.

FACILITIES
Titchmarsh Marina (450+visitors), ☎ 672185, Fax 851901, £9, Access HW±5 over sill 1·3m, D, FW, AC, Gas, Gaz, ME, CH, El, BH (10 ton), TraveLift (35 ton), Slip, R, Bar; **Walton Yacht Basin/Walton & Frinton YC** (60) ☎ 675526, AB (long stay), FW, AC, R, Bar; **Services:** Slip, M, D, C (½ ton), El. **Town** EC Wed; P, SM, V, R, Bar, ✉, Ⓑ, ⇌, ✈ (Southend/Cambridge).

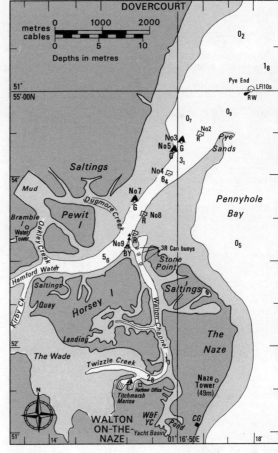

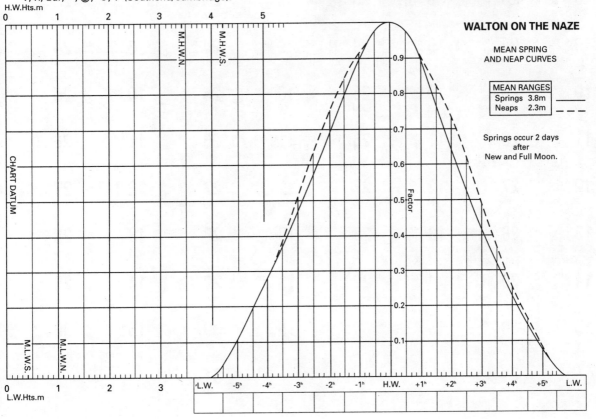

WALTON ON THE NAZE

MEAN SPRING AND NEAP CURVES

MEAN RANGES
Springs 3.8m
Neaps 2.3m

Springs occur 2 days after New and Full Moon.

ENGLAND – WALTON–ON–THE–NAZE

LAT 51°51′N   LONG 1°16′E

TIMES AND HEIGHTS OF HIGH AND LOW WATERS

YEAR 1996

TIME ZONE (UT)
For Summer Time add ONE hour in non-shaded areas

JANUARY

	Time	m		Time	m
1 M	0146 0802 1427 2038	1.1 3.6 0.9 3.6	**16** TU	0031 0657 1327 1939	1.1 3.5 0.9 3.5
2 TU	0251 0903 1520 2132	1.0 3.7 0.9 3.8	**17** W	0149 0811 1436 2048	1.0 3.6 0.8 3.7
3 W	0345 0956 1605 2220	0.9 3.8 0.8 3.9	**18** TH	0301 0919 1538 2150	0.8 3.8 0.7 3.9
4 TH	0433 1043 1645 2304	0.7 3.9 0.8 4.0	**19** F	0406 1019 1633 2246	0.6 4.1 0.5 4.1
5 F O	0516 1126 1722 2342	0.6 4.0 0.8 4.0	**20** SA ●	0504 1114 1723 2337	0.4 4.3 0.4 4.2
6 SA	0554 1204 1756	0.6 4.0 0.8	**21** SU	0557 1206 1810	0.2 4.4 0.4
7 SU	0017 0628 1238 1828	4.0 0.6 4.0 0.8	**22** M	0025 0645 1255 1854	4.3 0.0 4.5 0.4
8 M	0048 0700 1309 1900	4.0 0.5 4.0 0.8	**23** TU	0111 0732 1340 1938	4.4 0.0 4.5 0.4
9 TU	0118 0731 1341 1933	4.0 0.5 4.0 0.8	**24** W	0154 0817 1425 2021	4.4 0.0 4.4 0.5
10 W	0150 0805 1416 2007	4.0 0.5 4.0 0.8	**25** TH	0236 0902 1508 2104	4.3 0.1 4.2 0.6
11 TH	0225 0842 1455 2045	4.0 0.5 4.0 0.8	**26** F	0319 0947 1553 2148	4.2 0.3 4.0 0.8
12 F	0304 0923 1538 2127	3.9 0.6 3.9 0.9	**27** SA	0404 1034 1641 2238	3.9 0.5 3.7 0.9
13 SA	0347 1009 1627 2216	3.8 0.7 3.7 1.0	**28** SU	0456 1127 1737 2337	3.7 0.8 3.5 1.1
14 SU	0439 1105 1723 2317	3.7 0.8 3.6 1.1	**29** M	0601 1229 1846	3.4 1.0 3.3
15 M	0543 1213 1828	3.5 0.9 3.5	**30** TU	0051 0720 1338 1958	1.2 3.4 1.1 3.4
			31 W	0215 0833 1443 2102	1.1 3.5 1.1 3.5

FEBRUARY

	Time	m		Time	m
1 TH	0321 0933 1538 2155	1.0 3.6 1.0 3.7	**16** F	0247 0904 1523 2133	0.8 3.7 0.7 3.8
2 F	0413 1024 1623 2241	0.8 3.8 0.9 3.9	**17** SA	0358 1008 1619 2231	0.5 4.0 0.6 4.0
3 SA	0458 1107 1703 2322	0.6 4.0 0.8 4.0	**18** SU ●	0455 1104 1709 2323	0.3 4.2 0.4 4.2
4 SU O	0537 1146 1738 2358	0.6 4.0 0.8 4.0	**19** M	0545 1154 1754	0.1 4.4 0.4
5 M	0611 1219 1811	0.5 4.0 0.7	**20** TU	0011 0630 1240 1837	4.3 0.0 4.5 0.3
6 TU	0030 0643 1250 1842	4.0 0.5 4.0 0.7	**21** W	0055 0714 1323 1919	4.4 0.0 4.5 0.3
7 W	0101 0713 1321 1914	4.0 0.4 4.1 0.7	**22** TH	0136 0755 1404 2000	4.3 0.0 4.4 0.4
8 TH	0133 0744 1355 1947	4.0 0.4 4.1 0.6	**23** F	0214 0834 1442 2039	4.3 0.1 4.2 0.5
9 F	0206 0817 1431 2023	4.1 0.4 4.1 0.6	**24** SA	0252 0913 1520 2117	4.2 0.3 4.0 0.6
10 SA	0241 0853 1512 2102	4.0 0.5 4.0 0.7	**25** SU	0332 0953 1559 2159	4.0 0.6 3.8 0.8
11 SU	0321 0935 1557 2147	3.9 0.6 3.8 0.8	**26** M	0415 1040 1642 2249	3.7 0.8 3.5 0.8
12 M	0409 1025 1650 2243	3.8 0.7 3.6 0.9	**27** TU	0509 1136 1737 2354	3.4 1.1 3.3 1.1
13 TU	0508 1131 1753 2354	3.6 0.9 3.5 1.0	**28** W	0626 1243 1904	3.2 1.2 3.2
14 W	0625 1253 1908	3.5 1.0 3.4	**29** TH	0120 0758 1359 2025	1.2 3.3 1.2 3.3
15 TH	0120 0749 1414 2025	1.0 3.5 0.9 3.5			

MARCH

	Time	m		Time	m
1 F	0248 0907 1506 2125	1.0 3.5 1.1 3.6	**16** SA	0239 0854 1508 2117	0.7 3.7 0.8 3.7
2 SA	0346 1000 1557 2215	0.8 3.7 0.9 3.8	**17** SU	0346 0957 1603 2215	0.4 4.0 0.6 4.0
3 SU	0432 1044 1638 2257	0.7 3.9 0.8 4.0	**18** M	0440 1050 1651 2306	0.3 4.3 0.5 4.2
4 M	0511 1123 1715 2334	0.5 4.1 0.7 4.0	**19** TU ●	0527 1138 1735 2353	0.1 4.4 0.4 4.3
5 TU O	0546 1156 1748	0.5 4.1 0.7	**20** W	0610 1222 1818	0.0 4.4 0.3
6 W	0007 0618 1228 1820	4.1 0.4 4.1 0.6	**21** TH	0035 0650 1303 1858	4.3 0.1 4.4 0.3
7 TH	0040 0649 1300 1852	4.1 0.4 4.1 0.6	**22** F	0115 0728 1341 1937	4.3 0.2 4.3 0.4
8 F	0113 0720 1333 1926	4.1 0.4 4.1 0.5	**23** SA	0152 0804 1416 2013	4.3 0.3 4.2 0.4
9 SA	0147 0752 1410 2003	4.1 0.4 4.1 0.5	**24** SU	0227 0839 1449 2048	4.2 0.4 4.0 0.5
10 SU	0223 0828 1449 2042	4.1 0.5 4.0 0.5	**25** M	0304 0915 1525 2125	4.0 0.7 3.8 0.7
11 M	0303 0908 1534 2127	4.0 0.6 3.9 0.8	**26** TU	0343 0957 1600 2210	3.8 0.9 3.6 0.8
12 TU	0351 0959 1625 2223	3.9 0.8 3.6 0.8	**27** W	0430 1051 1648 2311	3.5 1.1 3.4 1.0
13 W	0451 1106 1728 2334	3.6 1.0 3.4 0.9	**28** TH	0532 1158 1754	3.3 1.3 3.2
14 TH	0609 1231 1846	3.4 1.1 3.3	**29** F	0026 0705 1311 1930	1.1 3.2 1.3 3.2
15 F	0106 0737 1358 2007	0.9 3.5 1.0 3.5	**30** SA	0154 0829 1424 2044	1.1 3.2 1.2 3.4
			31 SU	0306 0927 1522 2138	0.9 3.7 1.0 3.7

APRIL

	Time	m		Time	m
1 M	0355 1013 1606 2222	0.7 3.9 0.8 3.9	**16** TU	0419 1030 1630 2245	0.2 4.3 0.5 4.1
2 TU	0436 1052 1644 2302	0.5 4.1 0.7 4.0	**17** W ●	0504 1117 1714 2331	0.2 4.3 0.4 4.2
3 W	0513 1127 1720 2339	0.5 4.1 0.6 4.1	**18** TH	0545 1200 1757	0.2 4.3 0.4
4 TH O	0549 1202 1755	0.4 4.2 0.6	**19** F	0014 0624 1240 1837	4.2 0.3 4.3 0.4
5 F O	0015 0622 1237 1830	4.2 0.4 4.2 0.5	**20** SA	0053 0700 1317 1915	4.2 0.4 4.1 0.4
6 SA	0052 0656 1313 1907	4.2 0.4 4.2 0.4	**21** SU	0129 0734 1350 1949	4.2 0.5 4.0 0.4
7 SU	0129 0730 1351 1946	4.2 0.4 4.1 0.4	**22** M	0204 0807 1420 2023	4.1 0.6 3.9 0.5
8 M	0209 0808 1432 2028	4.2 0.5 4.0 0.4	**23** TU	0239 0841 1452 2058	4.0 0.8 3.8 0.6
9 TU	0252 0851 1517 2116	4.1 0.6 3.9 0.5	**24** W	0317 0920 1529 2141	3.8 0.9 3.7 0.7
10 W	0343 0943 1609 2214	3.9 0.8 3.7 0.7	**25** TH	0401 1010 1616 2237	3.6 1.1 3.5 0.9
11 TH	0445 1052 1714 2328	3.7 1.0 3.5 0.8	**26** F	0455 1115 1715 2345	3.4 1.3 3.3 1.0
12 F	0602 1217 1831	3.5 1.1 3.4	**27** SA	0603 1224 1828	3.3 1.3 3.3
13 SA	0101 0725 1341 1949	0.8 3.6 1.0 3.5	**28** SU	0058 0728 1334 1946	1.0 3.3 1.3 3.4
14 SU	0225 0838 1449 2056	0.6 3.8 0.8 3.7	**29** M	0210 0838 1436 2049	0.8 3.6 1.1 3.6
15 M	0328 0939 1543 2154	0.4 4.1 0.6 4.0	**30** TU	0309 0930 1526 2140	0.7 3.8 0.9 3.8

Chart Datum: 2·16 metres below Ordnance Datum (Newlyn)

ENGLAND – WALTON-ON-THE-NAZE

LAT 51°51′N   LONG 1°16′E

TIMES AND HEIGHTS OF HIGH AND LOW WATERS

YEAR **1996**

TIME ZONE (UT)
For Summer Time add ONE hour in non-shaded areas

4

MAY

	Time	m		Time	m
1 W	0356 1014 1609 2225	0.6 4.0 0.8 4.0	**16** TH	0439 1053 1654 2308	0.3 4.2 0.5 4.1
2 TH	0439 1054 1650 2308	0.5 4.1 0.6 4.1	**17** F ●	0520 1137 1737 2351	0.4 4.2 0.5 4.1
3 F O	0518 1134 1730 2349	0.4 4.2 0.5 4.2	**18** SA	0558 1217 1818	0.5 4.1 0.5
4 SA	0557 1214 1811	0.4 4.2 0.4	**19** SU	0031 0633 1254 1855	4.1 0.6 4.0 0.5
5 SU	0031 0635 1255 1852	4.3 0.4 4.2 0.4	**20** M	0109 0706 1327 1929	4.0 0.7 3.9 0.5
6 M	0113 0714 1336 1935	4.3 0.4 4.2 0.3	**21** TU	0143 0739 1357 2001	4.0 0.7 3.9 0.5
7 TU	0157 0755 1419 2021	4.3 0.5 4.1 0.3	**22** W	0218 0812 1429 2036	3.9 0.8 3.8 0.6
8 W	0245 0841 1507 2112	4.2 0.6 3.9 0.4	**23** TH	0254 0849 1506 2116	3.8 0.9 3.8 0.6
9 TH	0338 0935 1600 2212	4.0 0.8 3.8 0.5	**24** F	0336 0932 1551 2206	3.7 1.0 3.6 0.7
10 F	0439 1041 1703 2325	3.8 0.9 3.6 0.6	**25** SA	0424 1028 1644 2305	3.6 1.1 3.5 0.8
11 SA	0550 1158 1814	3.7 1.0 3.5	**26** SU	0521 1134 1745	3.5 1.2 3.4
12 SU	0047 0704 1316 1925	0.6 3.7 1.0 3.6	**27** M	0011 0626 1242 1852	0.9 3.4 1.3 3.4
13 M	0203 0813 1424 2030	0.5 3.9 0.8 3.8	**28** TU	0119 0736 1346 1957	0.8 3.5 1.2 3.5
14 TU	0305 0913 1520 2128	0.4 4.0 0.7 3.9	**29** W	0222 0839 1443 2055	0.7 3.7 1.0 3.7
15 W	0355 1006 1609 2220	0.3 4.2 0.5 4.0	**30** TH	0317 0933 1534 2148	0.6 3.9 0.8 3.9
			31 F	0406 1021 1622 2237	0.5 4.0 0.7 4.1

JUNE

	Time	m		Time	m
1 SA O	0451 1108 1709 2325	0.4 4.1 0.5 4.2	**16** SU ●	0535 1155 1803	0.6 4.0 0.5
2 SU	0535 1153 1755	0.4 4.2 0.4	**17** M	0012 0610 1234 1840	4.0 0.7 4.0 0.5
3 M	0012 0618 1238 1842	4.3 0.4 4.2 0.3	**18** TU	0050 0643 1307 1913	3.9 0.7 3.9 0.5
4 TU	0059 0701 1323 1929	4.3 0.4 4.2 0.2	**19** W	0124 0715 1338 1944	3.9 0.8 3.9 0.5
5 W	0147 0746 1409 2018	4.3 0.4 4.2 0.2	**20** TH	0157 0748 1409 2017	3.9 0.8 3.9 0.5
6 TH	0236 0833 1457 2110	4.3 0.5 4.1 0.2	**21** F	0232 0823 1444 2054	3.9 0.8 3.8 0.5
7 F	0329 0924 1549 2207	4.2 0.7 4.0 0.3	**22** SA	0310 0902 1525 2136	3.8 0.9 3.8 0.6
8 SA	0426 1023 1647 2311	4.0 0.8 3.8 0.4	**23** SU	0354 0947 1612 2225	3.8 1.0 3.7 0.7
9 SU	0529 1131 1750	3.8 1.0 3.7	**24** M	0445 1042 1705 2323	3.6 1.1 3.6 0.7
10 M	0021 0636 1244 1856	0.5 3.8 1.0 3.7	**25** TU	0542 1147 1806	3.6 1.2 3.5
11 TU	0134 0742 1355 2001	0.6 3.8 0.9 3.7	**26** W	0029 0646 1256 1910	0.8 3.5 1.2 3.5
12 W	0237 0844 1456 2101	0.5 3.9 0.8 3.8	**27** TH	0136 0752 1401 2015	0.8 3.6 1.1 3.6
13 TH	0330 0939 1549 2156	0.5 4.0 0.7 3.9	**28** F	0239 0855 1502 2115	0.7 3.8 0.9 3.8
14 F	0415 1028 1636 2245	0.5 4.0 0.6 4.0	**29** SA	0336 0951 1559 2211	0.6 3.9 0.7 4.0
15 SA	0457 1113 1721 2331	0.6 4.1 0.6 4.0	**30** SU	0428 1044 1653 2305	0.5 4.1 0.5 4.2

JULY

	Time	m		Time	m
1 M O	0517 1134 1745 2357	0.4 4.2 0.5 4.3	**16** TU	0550 1214 1825	0.7 4.0 0.6
2 TU	0604 1223 1835	0.3 4.3 0.2	**17** W	0032 0622 1249 1857	4.0 0.8 4.0 0.6
3 W	0046 0649 1310 1923	4.4 0.3 4.3 0.1	**18** TH	0105 0654 1319 1926	3.9 0.7 3.9 0.5
4 TH	0135 0734 1356 2011	4.4 0.4 4.3 0.0	**19** F	0136 0726 1349 1956	3.9 0.7 3.9 0.5
5 F	0224 0820 1443 2059	4.4 0.4 4.3 0.1	**20** SA	0208 0759 1421 2029	3.9 0.8 3.9 0.5
6 SA	0313 0908 1531 2150	4.3 0.6 4.2 0.2	**21** SU	0243 0835 1458 2105	3.9 0.8 3.8 0.5
7 SU	0405 1000 1622 2245	4.1 0.7 4.0 0.4	**22** M	0324 0915 1538 2146	3.9 0.9 3.8 0.6
8 M	0501 1058 1719 2345	3.9 0.9 3.8 0.6	**23** TU	0410 1001 1626 2235	3.8 1.0 3.7 0.7
9 TU	0602 1205 1822	3.7 1.0 3.7	**24** W	0503 1059 1722 2338	3.7 1.1 3.6 0.8
10 W	0053 0707 1320 1929	0.7 3.6 1.1 3.6	**25** TH	0604 1209 1829	3.5 1.2 3.5
11 TH	0202 0812 1430 2034	0.8 3.7 1.0 3.7	**26** F	0052 0713 1324 1940	0.9 3.5 1.1 3.5
12 F	0301 0911 1529 2133	0.8 3.8 0.8 3.8	**27** SA	0205 0823 1436 2049	0.8 3.7 1.0 3.7
13 SA	0350 1004 1620 2226	0.8 3.9 0.7 3.9	**28** SU	0311 0927 1543 2152	0.8 3.9 0.7 3.9
14 SU	0434 1052 1705 2313	0.7 4.0 0.6 3.9	**29** M	0409 1024 1642 2250	0.6 4.1 0.5 4.1
15 M ●	0514 1135 1747 2355	0.7 4.0 0.6 4.0	**30** TU O	0500 1118 1735 2343	0.4 4.2 0.3 4.3
			31 W	0548 1208 1824	0.4 4.4 0.1

AUGUST

	Time	m		Time	m
1 TH	0033 0633 1255 1910	4.5 0.3 4.5 0.0	**16** F	0044 0631 1257 1902	4.0 0.7 4.0 0.5
2 F	0121 0718 1340 1955	4.5 0.3 4.5 0.0	**17** SA	0112 0702 1326 1931	4.0 0.7 4.0 0.5
3 SA	0207 0802 1424 2039	4.5 0.4 4.4 0.0	**18** SU	0143 0735 1357 2001	4.0 0.7 4.0 0.5
4 SU	0252 0847 1507 2124	4.4 0.5 4.3 0.2	**19** M	0216 0810 1430 2034	4.1 0.7 4.0 0.5
5 M	0338 0933 1553 2211	4.2 0.7 4.1 0.4	**20** TU	0254 0848 1507 2111	4.0 0.8 3.9 0.6
6 TU	0427 1025 1644 2302	3.9 0.9 3.9 0.7	**21** W	0337 0932 1551 2156	3.9 0.9 3.8 0.7
7 W	0522 1125 1744	3.7 1.1 3.6	**22** TH	0427 1025 1645 2253	3.7 1.0 3.6 0.9
8 TH	0003 0627 1239 1854	0.9 3.5 1.2 3.5	**23** F	0528 1134 1754	3.6 1.1 3.5
9 F	0114 0737 1359 2007	1.1 3.5 1.1 3.5	**24** SA	0012 0639 1256 1914	1.0 3.5 1.1 3.5
10 SA	0224 0843 1506 2112	1.1 3.6 1.0 3.6	**25** SU	0136 0757 1419 2032	1.0 3.6 1.0 3.6
11 SU	0322 0940 1600 2207	1.0 3.8 0.8 3.8	**26** M	0250 0907 1532 2139	0.9 3.8 0.7 3.9
12 M	0410 1029 1646 2254	0.9 4.0 0.7 3.9	**27** TU	0351 1007 1630 2237	0.7 4.1 0.4 4.2
13 TU	0451 1113 1726 2335	0.8 4.1 0.6 4.0	**28** W O	0442 1101 1721 2330	0.5 4.3 0.2 4.4
14 W ●	0527 1152 1802	0.8 4.1 0.6	**29** TH	0530 1150 1808	0.4 4.4 0.1
15 TH	0012 0600 1226 1833	4.0 0.8 4.1 0.5	**30** F	0018 0614 1237 1851	4.5 0.4 4.5 0.0
			31 SA	0104 0658 1320 1933	4.5 0.4 4.5 0.0

Chart Datum: 2·16 metres below Ordnance Datum (Newlyn)

ENGLAND – WALTON–ON–THE–NAZE

LAT 51°51′N   LONG 1°16′E

TIMES AND HEIGHTS OF HIGH AND LOW WATERS   YEAR **1996**

TIME ZONE (UT)
For Summer Time add ONE hour in non-shaded areas

SEPTEMBER

Day	Time	m	Time	m	Time	m	Time	m
1 SU	0146	4.5	0741	0.4	1401	4.5	2013	0.1
2 M	0227	4.4	0823	0.5	1441	4.3	2053	0.3
3 TU	0308	4.2	0906	0.6	1522	4.1	2133	0.6
4 W	0350	3.9	0952	0.8	1607	3.9	2218	0.8
5 TH	0436	3.7	1046	1.0	1701	3.6	2312	1.1
6 F	0536	3.4	1154	1.2	1814	3.3		
7 SA	0018	1.3	0655	3.3	1319	1.2	1937	3.3
8 SU	0136	1.3	0810	3.4	1435	1.1	2047	3.5
9 M	0247	1.2	0911	3.7	1532	0.9	2143	3.7
10 TU	0340	1.1	1001	3.9	1619	0.7	2230	4.0
11 W	0423	0.9	1045	4.1	1658	0.6	2310	4.1
12 TH	0459	0.8	1124	4.2	1732	0.6	● 2346	4.1
13 F	0533	0.8	1158	4.2	1804	0.5		
14 SA	0017	4.1	0604	0.7	1230	4.1	1833	0.5
15 SU	0046	4.1	0637	0.7	1301	4.1	1903	0.5
16 M	0117	4.2	0711	0.7	1333	4.1	1933	0.5
17 TU	0151	4.1	0747	0.7	1406	4.1	2006	0.6
18 W	0228	4.1	0825	0.8	1443	4.0	2043	0.7
19 TH	0309	4.0	0909	0.9	1527	3.9	2127	0.8
20 F	0358	3.8	1003	1.0	1622	3.7	2224	1.0
21 SA	0458	3.6	1113	1.1	1733	3.5	2344	1.1
22 SU	0614	3.5	1239	1.1	1900	3.5		
23 M	0114	1.1	0737	3.6	1408	0.9	2020	3.7
24 TU	0232	1.0	0848	3.8	1518	0.6	2126	4.0
25 W	0332	0.8	0948	4.1	1613	0.4	2222	4.2
26 TH	0422	0.6	1041	4.3	1701	0.2	2312	4.4
27 F	0509	0.5	1129	4.4	1745	0.1	O 2359	4.5
28 SA	0554	0.4	1214	4.5	1827	0.2		
29 SU	0042	4.5	0636	0.4	1257	4.5	1906	0.2
30 M	0123	4.4	0718	0.5	1337	4.4	1944	0.4

OCTOBER

Day	Time	m	Time	m	Time	m	Time	m
1 TU	0201	4.3	0759	0.5	1415	4.3	2020	0.5
2 W	0236	4.1	0839	0.7	1453	4.1	2056	0.7
3 TH	0311	3.9	0920	0.8	1533	3.8	2135	1.0
4 F	0348	3.7	1009	1.0	1619	3.6	2225	1.2
5 SA	0435	3.5	1111	1.2	1721	3.3	2329	1.4
6 SU	0546	3.3	1227	1.2	1852	3.2		
7 M	0043	1.5	0722	3.3	1349	1.2	2011	3.4
8 TU	0200	1.4	0832	3.6	1453	1.0	2110	3.7
9 W	0302	1.2	0925	3.8	1541	0.7	2157	3.9
10 TH	0348	1.0	1010	4.0	1621	0.7	2238	4.1
11 F	0427	0.9	1049	4.2	1657	0.6	2314	4.2
12 SA	0502	0.8	1125	4.2	1731	0.6	● 2346	4.2
13 SU	0537	0.7	1200	4.2	1804	0.6		
14 M	0018	4.2	0612	0.7	1235	4.2	1835	0.6
15 TU	0053	4.2	0648	0.7	1310	4.2	1908	0.7
16 W	0128	4.2	0727	0.7	1347	4.2	1943	0.6
17 TH	0206	4.1	0808	0.7	1427	4.1	2022	0.7
18 F	0248	4.0	0855	0.8	1514	3.9	2108	0.9
19 SA	0336	3.8	0951	0.9	1611	3.7	2207	1.1
20 SU	0437	3.6	1102	1.0	1723	3.5	2325	1.2
21 M	0554	3.5	1228	0.9	1846	3.5		
22 TU	0053	1.2	0717	3.6	1352	0.8	2003	3.7
23 W	0210	1.0	0827	3.8	1458	0.6	2107	4.0
24 TH	0310	0.8	0926	4.1	1551	0.4	2202	4.2
25 F	0401	0.6	1019	4.2	1638	0.3	2251	4.4
26 SA	0448	0.5	1107	4.3	1721	0.5	O 2336	4.4
27 SU	0532	0.5	1152	4.4	1801	0.4		
28 M	0018	4.4	0615	0.5	1234	4.3	1839	0.5
29 TU	0058	4.3	0656	0.5	1313	4.3	1915	0.6
30 W	0133	4.2	0736	0.6	1350	4.2	1949	0.7
31 TH	0206	4.0	0814	0.6	1426	4.0	2022	0.9

NOVEMBER

Day	Time	m	Time	m	Time	m	Time	m
1 F	0236	3.9	0852	0.8	1503	3.9	2058	1.0
2 SA	0310	3.8	0936	0.9	1545	3.7	2142	1.2
3 SU	0352	3.6	1032	1.0	1636	3.5	2242	1.4
4 M	0449	3.4	1138	1.1	1742	3.3	2353	1.5
5 TU	0606	3.3	1248	1.1	1910	3.3		
6 W	0104	1.4	0733	3.4	1357	1.0	2022	3.5
7 TH	0211	1.3	0837	3.7	1453	0.9	2114	3.8
8 F	0305	1.1	0927	3.9	1540	0.7	2158	4.0
9 SA	0350	0.9	1011	4.1	1621	0.6	2237	4.1
10 SU	0430	0.8	1051	4.2	1659	0.6	2315	4.2
11 M	0510	0.7	1131	4.2	1737	0.6	● 2352	4.3
12 TU	0550	0.6	1211	4.3	1813	0.6		
13 W	0030	4.3	0630	0.6	1251	4.3	1849	0.6
14 TH	0110	4.2	0713	0.5	1332	4.2	1928	0.6
15 F	0150	4.1	0758	0.5	1417	4.2	2010	0.7
16 SA	0233	4.0	0847	0.6	1506	4.0	2057	0.9
17 SU	0322	3.9	0944	0.7	1602	3.8	2155	1.0
18 M	0421	3.7	1053	0.7	1710	3.7	2306	1.1
19 TU	0534	3.6	1211	0.8	1825	3.6		
20 W	0026	1.2	0651	3.6	1328	0.7	1938	3.8
21 TH	0143	1.1	0801	3.8	1433	0.6	2041	3.9
22 F	0246	0.9	0901	4.0	1528	0.5	2137	4.1
23 SA	0340	0.7	0955	4.1	1615	0.4	2226	4.2
24 SU	0428	0.6	1044	4.2	1657	0.6	2312	4.2
25 M	0514	0.5	1130	4.2	1738	0.6	O 2355	4.2
26 TU	0558	0.5	1212	4.2	1815	0.6		
27 W	0033	4.1	0639	0.5	1252	4.1	1849	0.7
28 TH	0109	4.0	0717	0.6	1329	4.1	1922	0.8
29 F	0140	4.0	0753	0.6	1403	4.0	1955	0.9
30 SA	0209	3.9	0828	0.7	1438	3.9	2029	1.0

DECEMBER

Day	Time	m	Time	m	Time	m	Time	m
1 SU	0242	3.9	0908	0.7	1516	3.8	2107	1.1
2 M	0323	3.8	0956	0.8	1601	3.6	2156	1.2
3 TU	0412	3.6	1053	0.9	1653	3.5	2259	1.3
4 W	0512	3.5	1155	1.0	1755	3.4		
5 TH	0008	1.4	0623	3.4	1300	1.0	1907	3.4
6 F	0116	1.3	0736	3.5	1402	0.9	2017	3.6
7 SA	0218	1.2	0838	3.7	1457	0.8	2112	3.8
8 SU	0312	1.0	0931	3.9	1546	0.7	2200	4.0
9 M	0400	0.8	1019	4.1	1631	0.6	2245	4.1
10 TU	0447	0.7	1105	4.2	1714	0.6	● 2329	4.2
11 W	0533	0.6	1150	4.3	1755	0.5		
12 TH	0012	4.3	0619	0.4	1235	4.3	1836	0.5
13 F	0055	4.3	0705	0.4	1320	4.3	1918	0.6
14 SA	0138	4.2	0752	0.3	1407	4.3	2002	0.6
15 SU	0222	4.1	0842	0.3	1456	4.2	2049	0.7
16 M	0310	4.0	0936	0.4	1549	4.0	2141	0.9
17 TU	0404	3.9	1037	0.5	1648	3.8	2242	1.0
18 W	0507	3.7	1144	0.6	1755	3.7	2353	1.1
19 TH	0618	3.6	1256	0.7	1905	3.7		
20 F	0109	1.1	0730	3.7	1404	0.7	2011	3.8
21 SA	0220	1.0	0835	3.8	1502	0.6	2110	3.9
22 SU	0320	0.8	0933	3.9	1552	0.6	2202	4.0
23 M	0412	0.7	1025	4.0	1637	0.6	2250	4.0
24 TU	0500	0.6	1112	4.1	1718	0.7	O 2334	4.1
25 W	0545	0.5	1155	4.1	1755	0.8		
26 TH	0013	4.0	0625	0.5	1235	4.0	1829	0.8
27 F	0049	4.0	0703	0.5	1310	4.0	1901	0.8
28 SA	0120	3.9	0736	0.5	1343	4.0	1933	0.9
29 SU	0149	3.9	0808	0.5	1415	3.9	2005	0.8
30 M	0220	3.9	0842	0.6	1450	3.9	2041	0.9
31 TU	0257	3.9	0922	0.6	1530	3.8	2121	1.0

Chart Datum: 2·16 metres below Ordnance Datum (Newlyn)

THIS PAGE IS INTENTIONALLY BLANK

RIVERS STOUR, ORWELL AND DEBEN   10-4-20, 21 & 22

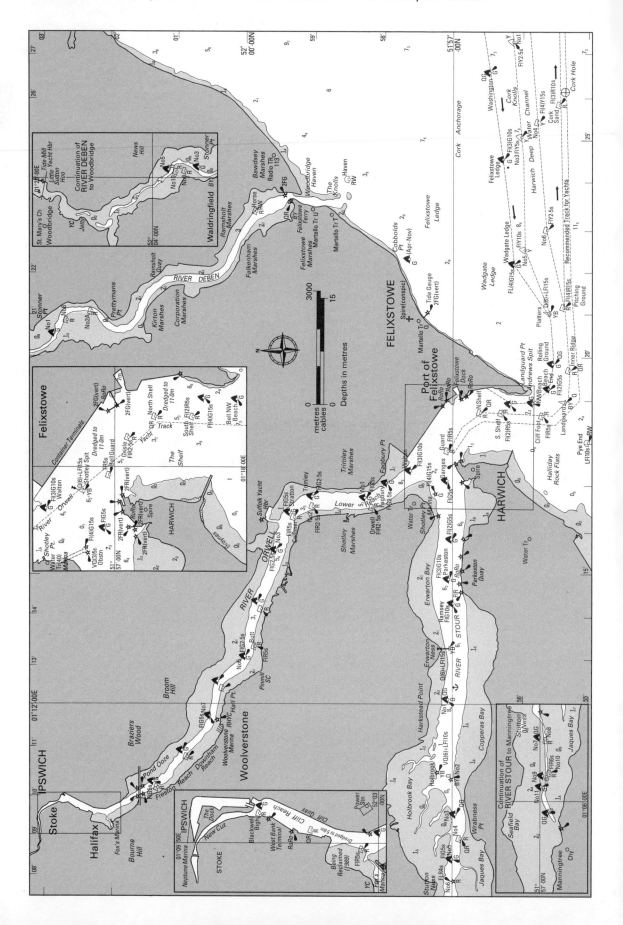

RIVER STOUR   10-4-20

Essex/Suffolk 51°57'·03N 01°17'·88E (Guard PHM buoy)

CHARTS
AC *2693*, 1594, 1491, 1593, *2052*; Imray Y16; Stanfords 5, 6; OS 169

TIDES
Harwich+0050 Dover; ML 2·1; Duration 0630; Zone 0 (UT)

Standard Port WALTON-ON-THE-NAZE (←—)

Times				Height (metres)			
High Water		Low Water		MHWS	MHWN	MLWN	MLWS
0000	0600	0500	1100	4·2	3·4	1·1	0·4
1200	1800	1700	2300				
Differences HARWICH							
+0007	+0002	–0010	–0012	–0·2	0·0	0·0	0·0
WRABNESS							
+0017	+0015	–0010	–0012	–0·1	0·0	0·0	0·0
MISTLEY							
+0032	+0027	–0010	–0012	0·0	0·0	–0·1	–0·1

Note: Although Harwich is a Standard Port, it has only two Secondary Ports referenced to it. Harwich HW and LW times differ by only 5 and 10 minutes from Walton-on-the-Naze.

SHELTER
Good at Shotley Pt Marina, access at all tides via a chan dredged 2m, outer limits lit, to lock. AB also at Harwich Pound (dries; access only near HW), Mistley, Manningtree (both dry). No yachts at Parkeston Quay. ⚓s off Erwarton Ness, Wrabness Pt, Holbrook Creek and Stutton Ness.

NAVIGATION
WPT Cork Sand PHM lt buoy, Fl (3) R 10s, 51°55'·43N 01°25'·95E, 087°/267° from/to position 7ca S of Landguard Pt, 4M. Keep clear of commercial shipping. Stay out of the DW chan by using recommended yacht track, parallel to S of it from the WPT and thence to W of it past Harwich.
Caution: Bkwtr, ESE of Blackman's Hd, covers at HW; it is marked by small inconspic unlit PHM bn, only 5ca W of main chan. The Guard shoal (0·8m), about 2ca S of Guard PHM buoy, lies close to the recommended yacht track. Outside the hbr, yachts should cross the DW chan at 90° between Rolling Ground and Platters buoys. See 10.4.5. The R Stour is well marked; speed limit 8kn. Beware 'The Horse' 4ca NE and a drying bank 1½ca NW of Wrabness Pt. From Mistley Quay local knowledge is needed for the narrow, tortuous chan to Manningtree.
Special Local Sound Signals
Commercial vessels may use these additional sigs:
Four short and rapid blasts followed by one short blast } = I am turning short around to stbd.

Four short and rapid blasts followed by two short blasts } = I am turning short around to port.
One prolonged blast = I am leaving a dock, quay or ⚓.

LIGHTS AND MARKS
The R Stour to Mistley Quay is lit. At Cattawade, 8M up river, a conspic chy leads 270° through the best water up to Harkstead Pt.
Shotley Pt Marina: a Dir lt at lock indicates the dredged chan (2·0m) by Inogen (or Moiré) visual marker lts which are square, ambered displays; a vert B line indicates on the appr centre line 339°. If off the centre line, arrows indicate the direction to steer to regain it.

RADIO TELEPHONE
Harwich Hbr Radio Ch **71** 11 14 16 (H24). Yachts should monitor Ch 71 for tfc info, but not transmit. Weather, tidal info and possibly help in poor vis may be available on request. The Hbr Patrol launch listens on Ch 11. Hbr Radar Ch 20. Shotley Pt Marina Ch **80** M (lock master).

TELEPHONE (01255)
Harwich Hr Mr 243030; Hbr Ops 243000; Marinecall 0891 500455; MRSC 675518; ⌗ 508966/502267 (H24); Police 241312; Dr 506451; Ⓗ 502446.

FACILITIES
HARWICH: **Town Pier** L, FW, AB (tidal); **Town** EC Wed; P, D, ME, SM, Gas, El, Sh, V, R, Bar, ✉, Ⓑ, ⇌, ✈ (Cambridge).
SHOTLEY: (01473) **Shotley Pt Marina** (350, visitors welcome) ☎ 788982, Fax 788868, £14, access H24 via lock; FW, AC, D, P, Ⓖ, ME, El, Ⓔ, Sh, Slip, BH (30 ton), C, V, BY, CH, SM, Bar, R; **Shotley SC** ☎ 787500, Slip, FW, Bar. WRABNESS: M, FW, V. MISTLEY and MANNINGTREE: AB, M, FW, V, P & D (cans), Gas, Bar. **Stour SC** ☎ (01206) 393924 M, Bar.

RIVER ORWELL   10-4-21

Suffolk 51°57'·03N 01°17'·88E (Guard PHM buoy)

CHARTS
AC *2693*, 1491, *2052*; Imray Y16; Stanfords 5, 6; OS 169. A *Yachting Guide to Harwich Harbour and its Rivers* has much useful info, inc Harwich tidal predictions; it can be obtained free from Harwich Haven Authority, Angel Gate, Harwich CO12 3EJ; ☎ (01255) 243000, Fax 241325.

TIDES
Pin Mill +0100 Dover; Ipswich +0115 Dover; ML 2·4; Duration 0555; Zone 0 (UT)

Standard Port WALTON-ON-THE-NAZE (←—)

Times				Height (metres)			
High Water		Low Water		MHWS	MHWN	MLWN	MLWS
0000	0600	0500	1100	4·2	3·4	1·1	0·4
1200	1800	1700	2300				
Differences IPSWICH							
+0022	+0027	0000	–0012	0·0	0·0	–0·1	–0·1
PIN MILL							
+0012	+0015	–0008	–0012	–0·1	0·0	0·0	0·0

SHELTER
Good. Ent and river well marked, but many unlit moorings off both banks. ⚓s above Shotley Pt on W side, or in Buttermans B. No yacht facilities at Felixstowe. Visitors' berths (pre-arrange) at Suffolk Yacht Hbr, Woolverstone Marina and Fox's Marina (Ipswich). Ipswich Dock opens from HW –2 to HW+¾, but mainly for commercial vessels. For entry to Ipswich Dock it is essential first to call *Ipswich Port Radio* Ch 14 before arrival, then call *Neptune Marina* also Ch 14 for alongside berth in 5m.

NAVIGATION
Appr/ent from sea as in 10.4.20. WPT Shotley Spit SCM buoy, Q (6)+L Fl 15s, 51°57'·22N 01°17'·70E, at river ent. Keep clear of the many merchant ships, ferries etc from/to Harwich, Felixstowe and Ipswich. Speed limit in the R Orwell is 6kn.

LIGHTS AND MARKS
Ent between Shotley Spit bn and Walton SHM, Fl (3) G 10s. Suffolk Yacht Hbr appr marked by four bns and ldg lts: front Iso Y; rear Oc Y 4s. Woolverstone Marina lts 2 FR (vert). A14 bridge lts: Centre FY (clearance 38m)
No 9 Pier 2 FR (vert)) shown up and
No 10 Pier 2 FG (vert)) down stream.
Ⓡ and Ⓖ tfc lts control ent to Ipswich Dock (H24). New Cut, W of Ipswich Dock: 3 FR (vert) = Cut closed, ie a water velocity control structure is raised from the river bed to just below water level; vessels must not proceed.

RADIO TELEPHONE
Call: *Ipswich Port Radio* VHF Ch **14** 16 12 (H24). Once above Shotley Pt, monitor Ch 14 continuously for tfc info. Suffolk Yacht Hbr, Woolverstone Marina, Fox's Marina: Ch 80 M. Neptune Marina: Ch M 14 (0800-1730 LT).

TELEPHONE (01473)
Orwell Navigation Service 231010 (also Ipswich Hr Mr and Port Radio); MRSC (01255) 675518; ⌗ 219481 (H24); Marinecall 0891 500455; Police 233000; Ⓗ 712233.

FACILITIES
LEVINGTON
Suffolk Yacht Hbr (500+10 visitors) ☎ 659240, Fax 659632, £10.58, Slip, P, D, FW, ME, El, Ⓔ, Sh, C (5/20 ton), BH (10/20 ton), CH, V, Gas, Gaz, AC, SM, Access H24; **Haven Ports YC** ☎ 659658, R, Bar. **Town** ✉, Ⓑ (Felixstowe), ⇌ (bus to Ipswich), ✈ (Cambridge/Norwich).
PIN MILL
Hr Mr ☎ 780276, M £4.50, L, CH, C (6 ton), SH, ME, El, FW, D (cans), Bar, R; **Pin Mill SC** ☎ 780271; Facilities at Ipswich.
WOOLVERSTONE
Woolverstone Marina (300+22 visitors) ☎ 780206, Fax 780273, £11.76, Slip, P (cans), D, FW, BY, ME, El, Sh, AC, Gas, Gaz, Ⓖ, C (25 ton mobile), CH, V; **Royal Harwich YC** ☎ 780319, R, Bar. **Town** EC Chelmondiston Wed; ✉, V.
IPSWICH
Fox's Marina (100+some visitors) ☎ 689111, Fax 601737, £10.80, FW, AC, P & D (cans), Gas, Gaz, BH (26 and 44 ton), C (7 ton), ME, El, Ⓔ, Sh, Bar, CH, ACA;
Neptune Marina (100+50 Ⓥ), ☎ 215204, Fax 780366, £11, near town centre, wet Dock (5·8m), access via lock HW –2 to HW+¾, waiting pontoon, FW, AC, D, P (cans), Sh, ME, C (14 ton), BH (40 ton), BY, El, Ⓔ, Gas, Gaz, R, Bar;
Orwell YC ☎ 602288, Slip, L, FW, Bar;
City No EC; ✉, Ⓑ, ⇌, ✈ (Cambridge/Norwich).

4

RIVER DEBEN   10-4-22

Suffolk 51°59'·35N 01°23'·69E (Felixstowe Ferry)

CHARTS
AC *2693, 2052*; Imray C28, Y15; Stanfords 3, 5, 6; OS 169
TIDES
Woodbridge Haven +0025 Dover; Woodbridge +0105
Dover; ML 1·9; Duration 0635; Zone 0 (UT)

Standard Port WALTON-ON-THE-NAZE (←—)

Times				Height (metres)			
High Water		Low Water		MHWS	MHWN	MLWN	MLWS
0100	0700	0100	0700	4·2	3·4	1·1	0·4
1300	1900	1300	1900				
Differences FELIXSTOWE PIER							
−0005	−0007	−0018	−0020	−0.5	−0.4	0.0	0.0
BAWDSEY							
−0010	−0012	−0028	−0032	−0.8	−0.7	−0.2	−0.2
WOODBRIDGE HAVEN (Ent)							
0000	−0005	−0020	−0025	−0.5	−0.5	−0.1	+0.1
WOODBRIDGE (Town)							
+0045	+0025	+0025	−0020	−0.2	−0.3	−0.2	0.0

SHELTER
Good at all times in Tide Mill Yacht Hbr at Woodbridge;
clearance over sill is 1·8m at MHWN and 2·8m MHWS.
Accurate tide gauge and waiting buoys. ⌁s up-river (clear
of moorings) above Horse Sand, at Ramsholt, Waldringfield,
Methersgate, Kyson Pt and Woodbridge (9M from ent).
NAVIGATION
WPT Woodbridge Haven unlit SWM buoy, 51°58'·36N
01°24'·20E, 306°/126° from/to Martello tower T, 0·65M. If a
pilot is required call VHF Ch 08 or dip the burgee when
passing Martello tower T. There is a shifting shingle bar
which may be crossed at HW−4 to HW depending on draft.
It is recommended to enter after half-flood, and to leave
on the flood. The ent is only 1ca wide and with strong onshore winds gets dangerously choppy; the chan is well
buoyed and marked. Keep E of Horse Sand, just up river
of the SC. No commercial tfc. Speed limit is 8kn above
Green Reach.
Note: For current sketch map of the approaches, send SAE
(plus 2 first-class stamps for the RNLI LB) to Tidemill Yacht
Hbr, Woodbridge, Suffolk IP12 1BP.
LIGHTS AND MARKS
Ldg marks (may be lit Fl W or Y), between Martello trs T
and U, are: Front W △ on R ■ background, rear R ■;
moved according to the chan. No lights other than 2 FR
(vert) on Felixstowe Ferry side, and 2 FG (vert) on E side,
marking the ferry landings. Bawdsey Radio mast (113m) is
conspic 0·6M ENE of ent.
RADIO TELEPHONE
Pilot Ch 08, call *Late Times* (pilot launch). Tide Mill Yacht
Hbr VHF Ch **80** M (some VHF dead spots down-river).
TELEPHONE (01394)
Hr Mr 385745; MRSC (01255) 675518; Marinecall 0891
500455; Pilot 270853; ⌗ (01473) 219481; Police 383377.
FACILITIES
FELIXSTOWE FERRY
   Quay Slip, M, L, FW, ME, El, Sh, CH, V, R, Bar; **Felixstowe
   Ferry SC** ☎ 283785; **Felixstowe Ferry BY** ☎ 282173, M (200),
   Gas, Slip.
RAMSHOLT **Services:** M, FW, ME, Bar.
WALDRINGFIELD
   Waldringfield SC ☎ 736633, Bar; **Services:** BY, C, Slip, D, FW,
   BH (40 ton), CH, Gas, Gaz, V.
WOODBRIDGE
   Tide Mill Yacht Hbr (150+50 visitors) ☎ 385745, Fax 380735,
   D, L, FW, ME, El, Sh, C (10 ton), AC, V, entry over sill (2·8m at
   MHWS); **Services:** CH, Slip, C, M, ACA; **Deben YC.**
   Town P, D, L (opposite Everson BY), FW, CH, V, R, Bar, ✉, Ⓑ,
   ⇌, ✈ (Cambridge or Norwich).

RIVER ORE/ALDE   10-4-23

Suffolk 52°02'·10N 01°27'·60E (Ent)

CHARTS
AC 2695, *2693*, 1543, *2052*; Imray Y15, C28; Stanfords 3, 6;
OS 169
TIDES
Ent. +0015 Dover Slaughden Quay +0155 Dover; ML1·6;
Duration 0620; Zone 0 (UT)

Standard Port WALTON-ON-THE-NAZE (←—)

Times				Height (metres)			
High Water		Low Water		MHWS	MHWN	MLWN	MLWS
0100	0700	0100	0700	4·2	3·4	1·1	0·4
1300	1900	1300	1900				
Differences ORFORD HAVEN BAR							
−0015	−0017	−0038	−0042	−1.0	−0.8	−0.2	−0.1
ORFORD QUAY							
+0040	+0040	+0055	+0055	−1.6	−1.3	+0.2	0.0
SLAUGHDEN QUAY							
+0100	+0100	+0115	+0115	−1.3	−1.0	+0.2	0.0
SNAPE							
+0200	+0200	No data		−1.3	−1.0	−0.3	+0.4

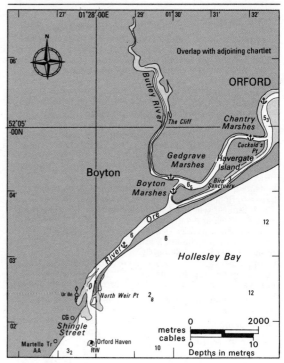

SHELTER
R Ore changes name to R Alde between Orford and
Aldeburgh (NB: overlap on chartlets), and is navigable up
to Snape. Good ⌁s as shown, also between Slaughden
Quay and Martello Tower and at Iken. Upper reaches of
river are shallow and winding, and although marked by
withies these may be damaged. Havergate Island is a
bird sanctuary; landing prohib.
NAVIGATION
WPT Orford Haven unlit SWM By, 52°01'·63N 01°27'·67E;
but this is moved depending on changes to the bar. The
bar (0·5m) shifts after onshore gales and is dangerous in
rough or confused seas. These result from tidal streams
within the shingle banks running in opposition to those
offshore. Ebb runs up to 6kn. Without local info do not
enter before half flood. Beware shoals off the Or ♦ bn on
W shore just inside ent (keep well to E side), and S to SW
of Dove Pt (the most SW point of Havergate Island).
Latest plan of ent available £1 from Alde & Ore Assoc'n,
Woodlands, Sandy Lane, Snape, Suffolk IP17 1SD or from
Aldeburgh YC.

RIVER ORE/ALDE *continued*

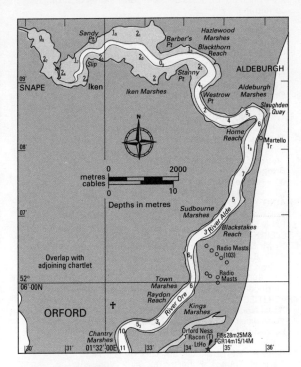

LIGHTS AND MARKS
Orfordness lt ho, W tr/R bands, Fl 5s, is 5·5M NE of Haven buoy. Shingle Street, about 2ca S of ent, is located by Martello tr 'AA', CG Stn, terrace houses and DF aerial. Haven buoy and Or ♦ bn are rarely moved; buoy does not indicate the chan. Up-river, Orford Castle (ru) is conspic, as is the Martello Tr 3ca S of Slaughden Quay.

RADIO TELEPHONE
None

TELEPHONE (01728 Aldeburgh; 01394 Orford/Shottisham)
Hr Mr Aldeburgh 452896; Hr Mr Orford 450481; Orford River Warden 450267; MRSC (01255) 675518; Contact CG Aldeburgh and Shingle Street (week ends, bad weather) through MRSC; ‖ (01473) 219481; Marinecall 0891 500455; Police 452716; Dr (01394) 450315/ 450369, (01394) 411214, and (01728) 452027.

FACILITIES
ORFORD
Orford Quay Slip, AB (1 hour free, then £10/hour); M £4 night, L, FW, D (cans), C (mobile 5 ton), CH, SH (small craft), SC, R, Bar;
Village (¼ M). EC Wed; P & D (cans), Gas, Gaz, ⊠, V, R, Bar, ≫ (occas. bus to Woodbridge).
ALDEBURGH
Slaughden Quay L, FW, Slip, BH (20 ton), CH; **Aldeburgh YC** ☎ 452562.
Services: M £3, Sh, Slip, D, ME, BY, Gas, Gaz, P, CH.
Town (¾M), EC Wed; P, V, R, Bar, ⊠, Ⓑ, ≫ (bus to Wickham Market), ✈ (Norwich).

SOUTHWOLD   10-4-24
Suffolk 52°18'·75N 01°40'·65E

CHARTS
AC 2695, 1543; Imray C28; Stanfords 3; OS 156

TIDES
–0105 Dover; ML 1·5; Duration 0620; Zone 0 (UT)

Standard Port LOWESTOFT (→)

Times				Height (metres)			
High Water		Low Water		MHWS	MHWN	MLWN	MLWS
0300	0900	0200	0800	2·4	2·1	1·0	0·5
1500	2100	1400	2000				
Differences SOUTHWOLD							
+0105	+0105	+0055	+0055	0·0	0·0	–0·1	0·0
MINSMERE							
+0110	+0110	+0110	+0110	0·0	–0·1	–0·2	–0·2
ALDEBURGH (seaward)							
+0120	+0120	+0120	+0110	+0·3	+0·4	–0·1	–0·1
ORFORD NESS							
+0135	+0135	+0135	+0125	+0·4	+0·6	–0·1	0·0

SHELTER
Good, but the ent is dangerous in strong winds from N through E to S. Visitors berth on a staging (max 16 boats, rafted 4 deep) 6ca from the ent, on N bank near to the Hbr Inn. If rafted, shore lines are essential due to current.

NAVIGATION
WPT 52°18'·06N 01°41'·80E, 135°/315° from/to N Pier lt, 1M. Enter on the flood since the ebb runs up to 6kn. Some shoals are unpredictable; a sand and shingle bar, extent/depth variable, lies off the hbr ent. Obtain details of appr chans from Hr Mr before entering (Ch 12 or ☎ 724712). Enter between piers in midstream. When chan widens, at The Knuckle (2 FG vert), turn *immediately* to stbd; keep within 10m of quay wall until it ends, when resume midstream. Unlit low footbridge ¾M upstream of ent. Note: A Historic Wreck (see 10.0.3g) is 3·6M S of the hbr ent on Dunwich Bank at 52°15'·14N 01°38'·53E.

LIGHTS AND MARKS
Ldg lines as chartlet. In addition: Walberswick ✠ on with N Pier lt = 268°. Hbr ent opens on 300°. 3 FR (vert) at N pier = port closed. Lt ho, W ○ tr, is in Southwold town, 0·86M NNE of hbr ent, Fl (4) WR 20s 37m 18/17/14M; vis R (intens) 204°-220°, W220°-001°, R001°-032°.

RADIO TELEPHONE
Southwold Port Radio Ch 12 16 09 (0800-1800LT).

TELEPHONE (01502)
Hr Mr 724712; MRCC (01493) 851338; ‖ (01473) 219481; Marinecall 0891 500455; Weather (01603) 660779; Police 722666; Dr 722326; Ⓗ 723333; Pilot 724712.

FACILITIES
Hbr AB £8.75, FW, Sh, Slip; **Southwold SC;**
Services: D, CH, ME, Sh, Slip, BH (20 ton), SM.
Town (¾M), EC Wed (Southwold & Walberswick); Gas, Gaz, Kos, P (cans, 1M), R, V, ⊠, Ⓑ, ≫ (bus to Brampton/Darsham), ✈ (Norwich).

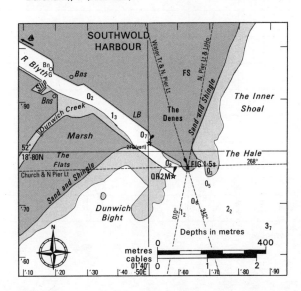

LOWESTOFT   10-4-25

Suffolk 52°28'·28N 01°45'·50E

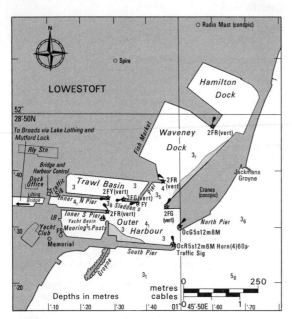

CHARTS
AC 1536, 1543; Imray C28; Stanfords 3; OS 156/134

TIDES
–0133 Dover; ML 1·6; Duration 0620; Zone 0 (UT)
Lowestoft is a Standard port and tidal predictions for each day of the year are given below

SHELTER
Good, except in E winds; hbr accessible H24. Fairway dredged 4·7m. Speed limit 4kn. Yacht Basin in SW corner of Outer Hbr is controlled by RN & S YC; yachts lie on the N side in 1·5m CD. Mooring on N side of S Pier is prohib. Bridge to Inner Hbr (and Lake Lothing) lifts at the following local times (20 mins notice required):
Mon-Fri   0700, 0930, 1100, 1600, 1900, 2100
Sat/Sun, Bank Hols 0745, 0930, 1100, 1400, 1730, 1900, 2100
and also, by prior arrangement, when ships transit. Small craft may pass under the bridge (clearance 2·2m) at any time but VHF Ch 14 contact advisable.

NAVIGATION
Sands are continually shifting. Beware shallows and drying areas, and do not cross banks in bad weather or strong tidal conditions.
From S, WPT is E Barnard ECM buoy, Q (3) 10s, 52°25'·11N 01°46'·50E; thence via Stanford Chan E of Newcome Sand QR, Stanford Fl R 2.5s and N Newcome Fl (4) R 15s, all PHM buoys. S Holm SCM, VQ (6)+L Fl 10s, and SW Holm SHM, Fl (2) G 5s, buoys mark the seaward side of this chan.
From E, WPT is Corton ECM buoy, Q (3) 10s Whis, 52°31'·10N 01°51'·50E; then via Holm Chan (buoyed) into Corton Road. Or approach direct to S Holm SCM buoy for Stanford Chan.
From N, appr via Yarmouth, Gorleston and Corton Roads.

LIGHTS AND MARKS
N Newcome PHM lt buoy bears 086°/5·5ca from hbr ent.
Tfc Sigs: Comply with IPTS (only Nos 2 & 5 are shown) on S pierhead when entering and leaving; also get clearance on VHF Ch 14 due restricted vis in appr and ent.
Bridge Sigs (on N side of bridge):
Ⓨ = bridge operating, keep 150m clear.
Ⓖ = vessels may enter/leave Inner Hbr.

RADIO TELEPHONE
Lowestoft Hbr Control VHF Ch **14** 16 11 (H24). Pilot Ch 14. RN & SYC Ch M 14.

TELEPHONE (01502)
Hr Mr & Bridge Control 572286; Mutford Bridge and Lock 531778 (+Ansafone, checked daily at 0830, 1300 & 1730); Oulton Broad Yacht Stn 574946; MRCC (01493) 851338; Pilot 560277; ⊞ (01473) 219481; Weather (01603) 660779; Marinecall 0891 500455; Police 562121; Ⓗ 600611.

FACILITIES
Royal Norfolk & Suffolk YC ☎ 566726, Fax 517981, £12.50 inc YC facilities, M, D, L, FW, C (2 ton), Slip, R, Bar;
Lowestoft Cruising Club ☎ 574376 (occas), AB £5 (no club facilities), M, L, FW, Slip;
Services: ME, El, Sh, CH, SM, Gas, Gaz, Ⓔ, ACA.
Town EC Thurs; V, R, Bar, ⌧, Ⓑ, ⇌, ✈ (Norwich).

Entry to the Broads: Passage to Oulton Broad, from Lake Lothing via two bridges and Mutford Lock (openings are coordinated; fee £5), is available 7 days/wk in working hrs HJ as pre-arranged with Mutford Br/Lock ☎ (01502) 531778/523003 or VHF Ch 09 14(occas), who will also advise visitors drawing >1·7m. Mutford Control operates in response to bookings and daily 0800-1100 and 1300-1600LT. Oulton Broad Yacht Station ☎ (01502) 574946. From Oulton Broad, access into the R. Waveney is via Oulton Dyke. New Cut is a short cut from the R. Waveney to the R Yare for air draft <7·3m. See 10.4.26 for Broads.

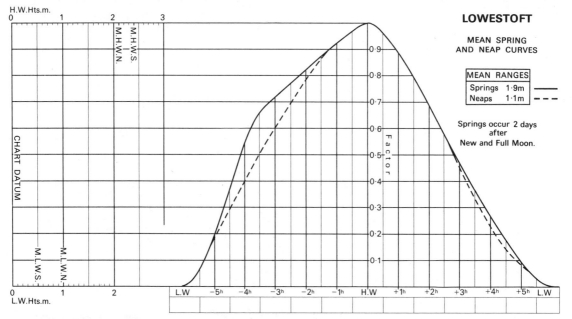

LOWESTOFT

MEAN SPRING AND NEAP CURVES

MEAN RANGES	
Springs	1·9m
Neaps	1·1m

Springs occur 2 days after New and Full Moon.

4

ENGLAND – LOWESTOFT

LAT 52°28′N   LONG 1°45′E

TIMES AND HEIGHTS OF HIGH AND LOW WATERS

YEAR **1996**

TIME ZONE (UT)
For Summer Time add ONE hour in non-shaded areas

JANUARY

	Time	m		Time	m
1 M	0556 1229 1841	2.2 0.9 2.2	**16** TU	0427 1128 1742 2356	2.2 0.8 2.2 1.1
2 TU	0101 0657 1324 1926	1.1 2.3 0.9 2.3	**17** W	0547 1231 1842	2.3 0.8 2.3
3 W	0152 0751 1409 2005	0.9 2.3 0.9 2.4	**18** TH	0104 0700 1329 1933	0.9 2.3 0.7 2.4
4 TH	0236 0837 1446 2041	0.8 2.3 1.0 2.4	**19** F	0203 0802 1423 2022	0.7 2.4 0.7 2.5
5 F O	0316 0916 1514 2116	0.8 2.3 1.0 2.5	**20** SA ●	0258 0900 1514 2111	0.4 2.5 0.6 2.6
6 SA	0350 0953 1533 2152	0.7 2.3 1.0 2.5	**21** SU	0349 0954 1601 2159	0.3 2.5 0.6 2.7
7 SU	0419 1030 1600 2228	0.7 2.3 1.0 2.5	**22** M	0438 1045 1646 2245	0.1 2.5 0.6 2.7
8 M	0447 1108 1632 2300	0.7 2.3 0.9 2.5	**23** TU	0524 1133 1726 2330	0.1 2.5 0.6 2.7
9 TU	0518 1144 1706 2331	0.6 2.3 0.9 2.5	**24** W	0608 1219 1804	0.1 2.4 0.7
10 W	0552 1218 1741	0.6 2.2 0.9	**25** TH	0013 0651 1308 1842	2.7 0.3 2.3 0.8
11 TH	0005 0626 1251 1819	2.5 0.7 2.2 1.0	**26** F	0057 0736 1401 1923	2.5 0.4 2.2 0.9
12 F	0047 0706 1330 1903	2.5 0.7 2.2 1.0	**27** SA	0145 0825 1505 2015	2.4 0.6 2.1 1.0
13 SA	0134 0752 1418 1953	2.4 0.8 2.1 1.1	**28** SU	0248 0918 1609 2118	2.2 0.8 2.0 1.1
14 SU	0225 0850 1514 2052	2.3 0.8 2.1 1.2	**29** M	0413 1015 1708 2227	2.1 1.0 2.1 1.1
15 M	0322 1015 1624 2209	2.3 0.9 2.1 1.2	**30** TU	0533 1121 1804	2.1 1.0 2.1
			31 W	0036 0641 1258 1854	1.1 2.1 1.1 2.2

FEBRUARY

	Time	m		Time	m
1 TH	0134 0738 1348 1937	0.9 2.2 1.1 2.3	**16** F	0051 0653 1317 1910	0.8 2.2 0.8 2.3
2 F	0219 0824 1427 2016	0.8 2.2 1.0 2.4	**17** SA	0153 0758 1412 2003	0.5 2.3 0.7 2.5
3 SA	0258 0900 1455 2054	0.8 2.3 1.0 2.4	**18** SU ●	0246 0853 1502 2053	0.3 2.4 0.6 2.6
4 SU O	0332 0934 1514 2132	0.7 2.3 1.0 2.5	**19** M	0335 0943 1547 2141	0.1 2.5 0.6 2.7
5 M	0401 1011 1541 2208	0.6 2.3 0.9 2.5	**20** TU	0421 1029 1631 2227	0.1 2.5 0.5 2.7
6 TU	0428 1047 1613 2240	0.6 2.3 0.9 2.5	**21** W	0505 1112 1710 2310	0.0 2.4 0.6 2.7
7 W	0458 1121 1646 2311	0.6 2.3 0.8 2.5	**22** TH	0546 1153 1746 2351	0.1 2.3 0.6 2.6
8 TH	0529 1149 1722 2346	0.5 2.3 0.8 2.5	**23** F	0625 1231 1820	0.3 2.2 0.6
9 F	0602 1219 1759	0.5 2.3 0.8	**24** SA	0031 0704 1309 1857	2.5 0.5 2.1 0.7
10 SA	0026 0638 1257 1840	2.5 0.6 2.2 0.8	**25** SU	0114 0748 1353 1945	2.3 0.7 2.0 0.9
11 SU	0112 0720 1342 1926	2.4 0.7 2.1 0.9	**26** M	0209 0838 1458 2046	2.2 0.9 2.0 1.0
12 M	0202 0810 1434 2022	2.3 0.8 2.1 1.0	**27** TU	0329 0934 1613 2152	2.1 1.0 2.0 1.0
13 TU	0259 0914 1533 2131	2.2 0.9 2.1 1.0	**28** W	0504 1032 1717 2303	2.0 1.1 2.0 1.0
14 W	0405 1052 1648 2333	2.2 0.9 2.1 1.0	**29** TH	0619 1137 1814	2.1 1.2 2.1
15 TH	0532 1211 1809	2.2 0.9 2.2			

MARCH

	Time	m		Time	m
1 F	0105 0716 1320 1904	1.0 2.1 1.1 2.2	**16** SA	0039 0652 1307 1849	0.7 2.2 0.9 2.3
2 SA	0151 0800 1401 1948	0.8 2.2 1.1 2.3	**17** SU	0138 0751 1400 1944	0.4 2.3 0.8 2.4
3 SU	0229 0833 1432 2029	0.7 2.3 1.0 2.4	**18** M	0229 0840 1447 2035	0.2 2.4 0.6 2.5
4 M	0302 0908 1456 2108	0.7 2.3 0.9 2.4	**19** TU ●	0316 0925 1531 2122	0.1 2.4 0.5 2.6
5 TU O	0333 0945 1523 2144	0.6 2.3 0.8 2.5	**20** W	0400 1007 1612 2208	0.1 2.4 0.5 2.6
6 W	0403 1021 1554 2217	0.5 2.3 0.8 2.5	**21** TH	0442 1046 1650 2250	0.1 2.4 0.4 2.6
7 TH	0434 1052 1628 2250	0.5 2.3 0.7 2.5	**22** F	0521 1122 1726 2330	0.2 2.3 0.5 2.5
8 F	0506 1120 1704 2327	0.5 2.3 0.6 2.5	**23** SA	0557 1154 1759	0.4 2.2 0.5
9 SA	0540 1152 1742	0.5 2.3 0.6	**24** SU	0009 0632 1228 1834	2.4 0.5 2.2 0.6
10 SU	0008 0616 1231 1822	2.5 0.5 2.3 0.6	**25** M	0051 0711 1307 1919	2.3 0.8 2.1 0.7
11 M	0054 0657 1314 1908	2.4 0.7 2.2 0.7	**26** TU	0143 0800 1400 2018	2.1 1.0 2.0 0.9
12 TU	0144 0746 1404 2004	2.3 0.8 2.1 0.8	**27** W	0256 0858 1516 2125	2.0 1.1 2.0 0.9
13 W	0243 0847 1502 2113	2.2 1.0 2.1 0.9	**28** TH	0421 0959 1627 2231	2.0 1.2 2.0 1.0
14 TH	0357 1017 1614 2318	2.1 1.0 2.1 0.9	**29** F	0537 1101 1730 2342	2.1 1.2 2.1 0.9
15 F	0534 1159 1743	2.1 1.0 2.1	**30** SA	0637 1211 1826	2.1 1.2 2.1
			31 SU	0058 0721 1316 1914	0.8 2.2 1.1 2.3

APRIL

	Time	m		Time	m
1 M	0144 0759 1356 1958	0.7 2.3 1.0 2.3	**16** TU	0209 0820 1429 2016	0.3 2.4 0.6 2.4
2 TU	0223 0837 1429 2037	0.7 2.3 0.9 2.4	**17** W ●	0255 0902 1512 2104	0.2 2.4 0.5 2.5
3 W	0258 0915 1501 2115	0.6 2.4 0.8 2.4	**18** TH	0338 0942 1553 2149	0.2 2.4 0.5 2.5
4 TH O	0333 0951 1535 2151	0.5 2.4 0.6 2.5	**19** F	0418 1019 1631 2231	0.3 2.4 0.4 2.4
5 F	0408 1023 1611 2230	0.5 2.4 0.6 2.5	**20** SA	0455 1052 1706 2311	0.4 2.3 0.4 2.4
6 SA	0443 1055 1649 2310	0.4 2.4 0.5 2.5	**21** SU	0528 1125 1739 2350	0.5 2.3 0.5 2.3
7 SU	0520 1130 1729 2353	0.5 2.4 0.5 2.5	**22** M	0601 1159 1814	0.7 2.3 0.6
8 M	0559 1209 1812	0.6 2.3 0.5	**23** TU	0032 0635 1238 1856	2.2 0.8 2.2 0.7
9 TU	0040 0641 1253 1859	2.4 0.7 2.2 0.6	**24** W	0124 0718 1322 1951	2.1 1.0 2.1 0.8
10 W	0132 0731 1342 1956	2.3 0.9 2.2 0.7	**25** TH	0231 0816 1428 2056	2.0 1.2 2.1 0.9
11 TH	0237 0830 1440 2108	2.2 1.0 2.1 0.8	**26** F	0343 0921 1544 2200	2.0 1.2 2.1 0.9
12 F	0407 0950 1557 2306	2.1 1.1 2.1 0.7	**27** SA	0447 1024 1646 2302	2.1 1.3 2.1 0.9
13 SA	0533 1145 1724	2.2 1.1 2.1	**28** SU	0546 1126 1742	2.1 1.2 2.1
14 SU	0021 0640 1251 1829	0.6 2.3 0.9 2.2	**29** M	0001 0638 1226 1834	0.8 2.2 1.1 2.2
15 M	0119 0733 1342 1925	0.4 2.3 0.8 2.3	**30** TU	0055 0724 1315 1920	0.7 2.3 1.0 2.3

Chart Datum: 1·50 metres below Ordnance Datum (Newlyn)

ENGLAND – LOWESTOFT

LAT 52°28′N   LONG 1°45′E

TIMES AND HEIGHTS OF HIGH AND LOW WATERS

YEAR **1996**

TIME ZONE (UT)
For Summer Time add ONE hour in non-shaded areas

MAY

Day	Time	m	Day	Time	m
1 W	0142 / 0806 / 1357 / 2003	0.6 / 2.3 / 0.9 / 2.3	**16** TH	0233 / 0837 / 1453 / 2047	0.4 / 2.4 / 0.6 / 2.4
2 TH	0223 / 0845 / 1436 / 2044	0.5 / 2.4 / 0.8 / 2.4	**17** F ●	0315 / 0917 / 1535 / 2133	0.4 / 2.4 / 0.5 / 2.4
3 F ○	0303 / 0921 / 1516 / 2127	0.5 / 2.4 / 0.6 / 2.5	**18** SA	0354 / 0953 / 1614 / 2216	0.5 / 2.4 / 0.5 / 2.3
4 SA	0343 / 0957 / 1557 / 2211	0.4 / 2.4 / 0.5 / 2.5	**19** SU	0429 / 1027 / 1649 / 2256	0.6 / 2.4 / 0.5 / 2.3
5 SU	0422 / 1034 / 1639 / 2256	0.4 / 2.5 / 0.4 / 2.5	**20** M	0459 / 1102 / 1723 / 2334	0.7 / 2.4 / 0.5 / 2.3
6 M	0503 / 1113 / 1722 / 2342	0.5 / 2.5 / 0.4 / 2.5	**21** TU	0528 / 1138 / 1757	0.8 / 2.4 / 0.6
7 TU	0545 / 1154 / 1808	0.6 / 2.4 / 0.4	**22** W	0016 / 0600 / 1215 / 1835	2.2 / 0.9 / 2.3 / 0.6
8 W	0031 / 0628 / 1238 / 1857	2.4 / 0.7 / 2.4 / 0.5	**23** TH	0104 / 0636 / 1252 / 1923	2.1 / 1.0 / 2.3 / 0.7
9 TH	0128 / 0717 / 1327 / 1956	2.3 / 0.9 / 2.3 / 0.6	**24** F	0203 / 0719 / 1333 / 2022	2.1 / 1.1 / 2.2 / 0.8
10 F	0242 / 0814 / 1427 / 2111	2.2 / 1.0 / 2.2 / 0.6	**25** SA	0308 / 0819 / 1426 / 2125	2.1 / 1.2 / 2.2 / 0.8
11 SA	0404 / 0924 / 1549 / 2245	2.2 / 1.1 / 2.2 / 0.6	**26** SU	0408 / 0932 / 1545 / 2223	2.1 / 1.3 / 2.1 / 0.8
12 SU	0515 / 1115 / 1704 / 2357	2.2 / 1.1 / 2.2 / 0.5	**27** M	0505 / 1038 / 1647 / 2319	2.1 / 1.3 / 2.1 / 0.8
13 M	0617 / 1226 / 1808	2.3 / 1.0 / 2.2	**28** TU	0559 / 1139 / 1745	2.2 / 1.2 / 2.2
14 TU	0055 / 0709 / 1321 / 1906	0.4 / 2.3 / 0.8 / 2.3	**29** W	0013 / 0649 / 1235 / 1837	0.7 / 2.2 / 1.1 / 2.2
15 W	0147 / 0755 / 1409 / 1958	0.4 / 2.4 / 0.7 / 2.3	**30** TH	0104 / 0734 / 1325 / 1927	0.6 / 2.3 / 0.9 / 2.3
			31 F	0151 / 0814 / 1412 / 2016	0.6 / 2.4 / 0.8 / 2.4

JUNE

Day	Time	m	Day	Time	m
1 SA ○	0236 / 0854 / 1459 / 2105	0.5 / 2.5 / 0.6 / 2.5	**16** SU ●	0333 / 0930 / 1600 / 2204	0.7 / 2.4 / 0.6 / 2.3
2 SU	0320 / 0934 / 1546 / 2155	0.5 / 2.5 / 0.5 / 2.5	**17** M	0404 / 1006 / 1636 / 2243	0.8 / 2.5 / 0.6 / 2.3
3 M	0404 / 1016 / 1632 / 2244	0.5 / 2.6 / 0.4 / 2.5	**18** TU	0429 / 1043 / 1708 / 2320	0.8 / 2.5 / 0.6 / 2.2
4 TU	0448 / 1059 / 1719 / 2334	0.5 / 2.6 / 0.3 / 2.5	**19** W	0457 / 1119 / 1739 / 2359	0.9 / 2.5 / 0.6 / 2.2
5 W	0532 / 1143 / 1807	0.6 / 2.6 / 0.3	**20** TH	0529 / 1153 / 1814	0.9 / 2.5 / 0.6
6 TH	0026 / 0616 / 1228 / 1857	2.4 / 0.7 / 2.5 / 0.3	**21** F	0040 / 0601 / 1225 / 1852	2.2 / 1.0 / 2.4 / 0.7
7 F	0125 / 0703 / 1317 / 1954	2.3 / 0.8 / 2.4 / 0.4	**22** SA	0128 / 0637 / 1300 / 1939	2.1 / 1.0 / 2.3 / 0.7
8 SA	0234 / 0755 / 1417 / 2100	2.3 / 1.0 / 2.3 / 0.5	**23** SU	0224 / 0719 / 1343 / 2037	2.1 / 1.1 / 2.3 / 0.8
9 SU	0344 / 0856 / 1530 / 2213	2.2 / 1.1 / 2.3 / 0.6	**24** M	0325 / 0831 / 1433 / 2140	2.1 / 1.2 / 2.2 / 0.8
10 M	0449 / 1016 / 1641 / 2326	2.2 / 1.1 / 2.2 / 0.6	**25** TU	0423 / 0928 / 1528 / 2239	2.1 / 1.3 / 2.2 / 0.8
11 TU	0548 / 1155 / 1746	2.2 / 1.1 / 2.2	**26** W	0519 / 1052 / 1629 / 2335	2.1 / 1.2 / 2.2 / 0.7
12 W	0030 / 0642 / 1259 / 1847	0.6 / 2.3 / 0.9 / 2.3	**27** TH	0613 / 1158 / 1749	2.2 / 1.1 / 2.2
13 TH	0125 / 0730 / 1350 / 1942	0.6 / 2.3 / 0.8 / 2.3	**28** F	0030 / 0701 / 1257 / 1855	0.7 / 2.3 / 1.0 / 2.3
14 F	0212 / 0813 / 1437 / 2033	0.6 / 2.4 / 0.7 / 2.3	**29** SA	0123 / 0745 / 1352 / 1953	0.6 / 2.4 / 0.8 / 2.4
15 SA	0255 / 0853 / 1520 / 2121	0.7 / 2.4 / 0.6 / 2.3	**30** SU	0213 / 0828 / 1445 / 2048	0.6 / 2.5 / 0.6 / 2.4

JULY

Day	Time	m	Day	Time	m
1 M ○	0302 / 0913 / 1537 / 2142	0.5 / 2.6 / 0.5 / 2.5	**16** TU	0342 / 0946 / 1621 / 2225	0.9 / 2.5 / 0.6 / 2.3
2 TU	0350 / 0959 / 1627 / 2234	0.5 / 2.7 / 0.3 / 2.5	**17** W	0401 / 1022 / 1650 / 2300	0.9 / 2.5 / 0.6 / 2.3
3 W	0436 / 1045 / 1715 / 2325	0.5 / 2.7 / 0.2 / 2.5	**18** TH	0429 / 1058 / 1718 / 2336	0.9 / 2.6 / 0.6 / 2.3
4 TH	0520 / 1130 / 1802	0.6 / 2.7 / 0.2	**19** F	0501 / 1129 / 1748	0.9 / 2.5 / 0.6
5 F	0016 / 0603 / 1216 / 1849	2.5 / 0.6 / 2.7 / 0.2	**20** SA	0011 / 0533 / 1159 / 1820	2.3 / 0.9 / 2.5 / 0.6
6 SA	0110 / 0647 / 1303 / 1939	2.4 / 0.7 / 2.6 / 0.3	**21** SU	0043 / 0608 / 1234 / 1854	2.2 / 0.9 / 2.5 / 0.7
7 SU	0211 / 0734 / 1356 / 2034	2.3 / 0.9 / 2.5 / 0.5	**22** M	0117 / 0647 / 1316 / 1935	2.2 / 1.0 / 2.4 / 0.7
8 M	0317 / 0828 / 1504 / 2135	2.3 / 1.0 / 2.3 / 0.6	**23** TU	0200 / 0734 / 1404 / 2031	2.1 / 1.1 / 2.3 / 0.8
9 TU	0419 / 0931 / 1617 / 2243	2.2 / 1.1 / 2.3 / 0.7	**24** W	0254 / 0831 / 1458 / 2153	2.1 / 1.2 / 2.3 / 0.8
10 W	0518 / 1055 / 1725	2.2 / 1.1 / 2.2	**25** TH	0410 / 0952 / 1557 / 2300	2.1 / 1.2 / 2.2 / 0.8
11 TH	0000 / 0613 / 1236 / 1830	0.8 / 2.2 / 1.0 / 2.2	**26** F	0527 / 1126 / 1710	2.2 / 1.1 / 2.2
12 F	0103 / 0703 / 1333 / 1929	0.8 / 2.3 / 0.9 / 2.2	**27** SA	0001 / 0625 / 1235 / 1832	0.8 / 2.3 / 1.0 / 2.3
13 SA	0154 / 0748 / 1422 / 2021	0.8 / 2.4 / 0.8 / 2.3	**28** SU	0100 / 0716 / 1336 / 1939	0.7 / 2.4 / 0.8 / 2.4
14 SU	0238 / 0829 / 1506 / 2108	0.9 / 2.4 / 0.7 / 2.3	**29** M	0155 / 0804 / 1433 / 2037	0.7 / 2.5 / 0.6 / 2.4
15 M ●	0315 / 0908 / 1546 / 2149	0.9 / 2.5 / 0.7 / 2.3	**30** TU	0248 / 0852 / 1526 / 2132	0.6 / 2.6 / 0.4 / 2.5
			31 W ○	0337 / 0940 / 1615 / 2223	0.6 / 2.7 / 0.2 / 2.6

AUGUST

Day	Time	m	Day	Time	m
1 TH	0423 / 1027 / 1702 / 2311	0.5 / 2.8 / 0.1 / 2.6	**16** F	0405 / 1033 / 1651 / 2308	0.9 / 2.6 / 0.6 / 2.4
2 F	0507 / 1112 / 1747 / 2357	0.5 / 2.8 / 0.1 / 2.5	**17** SA	0436 / 1103 / 1719 / 2337	0.8 / 2.6 / 0.6 / 2.4
3 SA	0548 / 1157 / 1831	0.6 / 2.8 / 0.2	**18** SU	0509 / 1134 / 1749	0.8 / 2.6 / 0.6
4 SU	0045 / 0628 / 1241 / 1915	2.4 / 0.7 / 2.7 / 0.3	**19** M	0003 / 0544 / 1211 / 1820	2.3 / 0.8 / 2.5 / 0.6
5 M	0137 / 0711 / 1329 / 2003	2.3 / 0.8 / 2.5 / 0.5	**20** TU	0038 / 0623 / 1253 / 1857	2.3 / 0.9 / 2.5 / 0.7
6 TU	0240 / 0800 / 1430 / 2056	2.2 / 0.9 / 2.3 / 0.7	**21** W	0121 / 0707 / 1340 / 1944	2.3 / 0.9 / 2.4 / 0.8
7 W	0345 / 0859 / 1552 / 2153	2.1 / 1.0 / 2.2 / 0.9	**22** TH	0211 / 0800 / 1434 / 2046	2.2 / 1.0 / 2.3 / 0.9
8 TH	0446 / 1006 / 1706 / 2258	2.1 / 1.1 / 2.2 / 1.0	**23** F	0308 / 0910 / 1534 / 2224	2.2 / 1.1 / 2.2 / 1.0
9 F	0543 / 1208 / 1815	2.2 / 1.1 / 2.2	**24** SA	0418 / 1100 / 1650 / 2338	2.2 / 1.1 / 2.2 / 1.0
10 SA	0041 / 0635 / 1315 / 1915	1.0 / 2.3 / 1.0 / 2.2	**25** SU	0546 / 1218 / 1825	2.3 / 0.9 / 2.3
11 SU	0136 / 0722 / 1404 / 2007	1.0 / 2.4 / 0.8 / 2.3	**26** M	0043 / 0648 / 1323 / 1934	0.9 / 2.4 / 0.7 / 2.4
12 M	0219 / 0804 / 1447 / 2051	1.0 / 2.4 / 0.8 / 2.3	**27** TU	0142 / 0741 / 1411 / 2029	0.8 / 2.5 / 0.5 / 2.5
13 TU	0255 / 0844 / 1525 / 2127	1.0 / 2.5 / 0.7 / 2.3	**28** W ○	0235 / 0831 / 1510 / 2119	0.7 / 2.7 / 0.3 / 2.5
14 W ●	0320 / 0921 / 1558 / 2201	1.0 / 2.6 / 0.7 / 2.4	**29** TH	0323 / 0919 / 1558 / 2206	0.6 / 2.8 / 0.1 / 2.6
15 TH	0337 / 0958 / 1624 / 2235	0.9 / 2.6 / 0.6 / 2.4	**30** F	0408 / 1006 / 1643 / 2250	0.5 / 2.8 / 0.1 / 2.6
			31 SA	0449 / 1051 / 1725 / 2332	0.5 / 2.8 / 0.1 / 2.5

Chart Datum: 1·50 metres below Ordnance Datum (Newlyn)

ENGLAND – LOWESTOFT

LAT 52°28′N   LONG   1°45′E

TIMES AND HEIGHTS OF HIGH AND LOW WATERS   YEAR **1996**

TIME ZONE (UT)
For Summer Time add ONE hour in non-shaded areas

4

SEPTEMBER

Day	Time	m		Day	Time	m
1 SU	0529 / 1134 / 1806	0.5 / 2.8 / 0.2		**16** M	0447 / 1110 / 1721 / 2333	0.7 / 2.6 / 0.6 / 2.4
2 M	0013 / 0607 / 1217 / 1847	2.4 / 0.6 / 2.6 / 0.4		**17** TU	0524 / 1149 / 1754	0.7 / 2.6 / 0.6
3 TU	0053 / 0647 / 1259 / 1930	2.3 / 0.7 / 2.5 / 0.7		**18** W	0009 / 0603 / 1232 / 1831	2.4 / 0.8 / 2.5 / 0.7
4 W	0138 / 0734 / 1351 / 2019	2.2 / 0.9 / 2.3 / 0.9		**19** TH	0052 / 0648 / 1320 / 1916	2.4 / 0.9 / 2.4 / 0.9
5 TH	0254 / 0832 / 1522 / 2114	2.1 / 1.0 / 2.2 / 1.1		**20** F	0140 / 0741 / 1414 / 2014	2.3 / 1.0 / 2.3 / 1.0
6 F	0407 / 0937 / 1647 / 2213	2.1 / 1.1 / 2.1 / 1.2		**21** SA	0236 / 0850 / 1518 / 2136	2.2 / 1.0 / 2.2 / 1.1
7 SA	0507 / 1048 / 1755 / 2319	2.2 / 1.1 / 2.2 / 1.2		**22** SU	0341 / 1043 / 1650 / 2318	2.2 / 1.0 / 2.2 / 1.1
8 SU	0602 / 1248 / 1856	2.3 / 1.0 / 2.2		**23** M	0509 / 1204 / 1826	2.3 / 0.8 / 2.3
9 M	0108 / 0651 / 1337 / 1945	1.2 / 2.4 / 0.9 / 2.3		**24** TU	0030 / 0623 / 1308 / 1927	1.0 / 2.4 / 0.6 / 2.4
10 TU	0151 / 0735 / 1418 / 2025	1.1 / 2.5 / 0.8 / 2.4		**25** W	0128 / 0719 / 1402 / 2016	0.9 / 2.5 / 0.4 / 2.5
11 W	0225 / 0815 / 1453 / 2058	1.1 / 2.5 / 0.7 / 2.4		**26** TH	0219 / 0810 / 1451 / 2102	0.8 / 2.7 / 0.3 / 2.5
12 TH	0249 / 0853 / 1523 / ●2131	1.0 / 2.6 / 0.7 / 2.4		**27** F	0305 / 0858 / 1536 / O2145	0.6 / 2.7 / 0.2 / 2.6
13 F	0312 / 0930 / 1551 / 2205	0.9 / 2.6 / 0.7 / 2.5		**28** SA	0348 / 0945 / 1620 / 2225	0.6 / 2.8 / 0.2 / 2.5
14 SA	0341 / 1004 / 1620 / 2237	0.9 / 2.6 / 0.6 / 2.5		**29** SU	0430 / 1029 / 1701 / 2303	0.5 / 2.7 / 0.2 / 2.5
15 SU	0413 / 1036 / 1650 / 2304	0.8 / 2.6 / 0.6 / 2.5		**30** M	0509 / 1112 / 1739 / 2338	0.5 / 2.7 / 0.4 / 2.4

OCTOBER

Day	Time	m		Day	Time	m
1 TU	0546 / 1152 / 1817	0.6 / 2.6 / 0.6		**16** W	0508 / 1131 / 1734 / 2346	0.7 / 2.6 / 0.7 / 2.5
2 W	0011 / 0624 / 1234 / 1855	2.4 / 0.7 / 2.4 / 0.8		**17** TH	0550 / 1215 / 1813	0.7 / 2.5 / 0.8
3 TH	0048 / 0709 / 1322 / 1941	2.3 / 0.8 / 2.3 / 1.0		**18** F	0028 / 0636 / 1304 / 1858	2.4 / 0.8 / 2.4 / 0.9
4 F	0136 / 0806 / 1440 / 2037	2.2 / 0.9 / 2.1 / 1.2		**19** SA	0116 / 0731 / 1359 / 1953	2.4 / 0.9 / 2.2 / 1.1
5 SA	0302 / 0911 / 1619 / 2138	2.2 / 1.0 / 2.1 / 1.3		**20** SU	0211 / 0841 / 1511 / 2103	2.3 / 0.9 / 2.2 / 1.2
6 SU	0421 / 1018 / 1726 / 2240	2.2 / 1.1 / 2.1 / 1.3		**21** M	0316 / 1028 / 1658 / 2254	2.3 / 0.9 / 2.2 / 1.2
7 M	0520 / 1134 / 1825 / 2348	2.3 / 1.0 / 2.2 / 1.3		**22** TU	0445 / 1147 / 1813	2.3 / 0.7 / 2.3
8 TU	0614 / 1251 / 1913	2.4 / 0.9 / 2.3		**23** W	0012 / 0559 / 1249 / 1909	1.1 / 2.4 / 0.6 / 2.4
9 W	0059 / 0700 / 1334 / 1950	1.2 / 2.4 / 0.8 / 2.4		**24** TH	0110 / 0658 / 1341 / 1956	1.0 / 2.5 / 0.7 / 2.5
10 TH	0140 / 0742 / 1410 / 2024	1.1 / 2.5 / 0.8 / 2.4		**25** F	0200 / 0750 / 1429 / 2039	0.8 / 2.6 / 0.3 / 2.5
11 F	0213 / 0821 / 1443 / 2059	1.0 / 2.6 / 0.7 / 2.5		**26** SA	0245 / 0838 / 1514 / O2120	0.6 / 2.6 / 0.3 / 2.5
12 SA	0244 / 0858 / 1516 / ●2134	0.9 / 2.6 / 0.7 / 2.5		**27** SU	0329 / 0925 / 1556 / 2159	0.6 / 2.6 / 0.4 / 2.5
13 SU	0317 / 0934 / 1549 / 2206	0.8 / 2.6 / 0.6 / 2.5		**28** M	0410 / 1010 / 1636 / 2235	0.6 / 2.6 / 0.4 / 2.5
14 M	0352 / 1010 / 1623 / 2235	0.8 / 2.6 / 0.6 / 2.5		**29** TU	0449 / 1052 / 1712 / 2308	0.6 / 2.6 / 0.6 / 2.5
15 TU	0429 / 1049 / 1657 / 2308	0.7 / 2.6 / 0.6 / 2.5		**30** W	0527 / 1132 / 1746 / 2341	0.6 / 2.5 / 0.7 / 2.4
				31 TH	0604 / 1213 / 1820	0.7 / 2.3 / 0.9

NOVEMBER

Day	Time	m		Day	Time	m
1 F	0017 / 0646 / 1300 / 1857	2.4 / 0.8 / 2.2 / 1.1		**16** SA	0011 / 0631 / 1253 / 1844	2.5 / 0.7 / 2.4 / 0.9
2 SA	0100 / 0739 / 1404 / 1949	2.3 / 0.9 / 2.1 / 1.2		**17** SU	0058 / 0726 / 1352 / 1936	2.5 / 0.7 / 2.3 / 1.1
3 SU	0201 / 0843 / 1527 / 2056	2.3 / 1.0 / 2.1 / 1.4		**18** M	0151 / 0835 / 1514 / 2037	2.4 / 0.8 / 2.2 / 1.2
4 M	0324 / 0946 / 1636 / 2200	2.3 / 1.0 / 2.1 / 1.4		**19** TU	0257 / 1006 / 1640 / 2207	2.3 / 0.8 / 2.2 / 1.2
5 TU	0429 / 1047 / 1735 / 2303	2.3 / 1.0 / 2.2 / 1.4		**20** W	0423 / 1122 / 1748 / 2346	2.3 / 0.7 / 2.3 / 1.2
6 W	0527 / 1145 / 1826	2.3 / 0.9 / 2.3		**21** TH	0537 / 1225 / 1844	2.4 / 0.6 / 2.3
7 TH	0002 / 0618 / 1239 / 1909	1.3 / 2.4 / 0.9 / 2.3		**22** F	0048 / 0638 / 1319 / 1932	1.0 / 2.4 / 0.5 / 2.4
8 F	0054 / 0704 / 1324 / 1949	1.2 / 2.4 / 0.8 / 2.4		**23** SA	0140 / 0732 / 1408 / 2015	0.9 / 2.5 / 0.5 / 2.4
9 SA	0137 / 0746 / 1405 / 2027	1.1 / 2.5 / 0.7 / 2.5		**24** SU	0227 / 0822 / 1452 / 2056	0.7 / 2.5 / 0.5 / 2.5
10 SU	0216 / 0826 / 1443 / 2104	0.9 / 2.5 / 0.7 / 2.5		**25** M	0311 / 0910 / 1534 / O2134	0.7 / 2.5 / 0.6 / 2.5
11 M	0255 / 0906 / 1521 / ●2138	0.8 / 2.6 / 0.6 / 2.5		**26** TU	0354 / 0956 / 1612 / 2209	0.6 / 2.5 / 0.7 / 2.5
12 TU	0334 / 0948 / 1559 / 2212	0.7 / 2.6 / 0.6 / 2.6		**27** W	0433 / 1038 / 1646 / 2243	0.6 / 2.4 / 0.9 / 2.5
13 W	0416 / 1032 / 1638 / 2249	0.7 / 2.6 / 0.6 / 2.5		**28** TH	0511 / 1117 / 1716 / 2318	0.6 / 2.4 / 0.9 / 2.5
14 TH	0459 / 1116 / 1718 / 2329	0.6 / 2.6 / 0.7 / 2.6		**29** F	0547 / 1156 / 1743 / 2354	0.6 / 2.3 / 1.0 / 2.5
15 F	0544 / 1203 / 1759	0.6 / 2.5 / 0.8		**30** SA	0625 / 1240 / 1814	0.7 / 2.2 / 1.1

DECEMBER

Day	Time	m		Day	Time	m
1 SU	0032 / 0710 / 1333 / 1849	2.4 / 0.8 / 2.1 / 1.2		**16** M	0044 / 0720 / 1345 / 1918	2.6 / 0.5 / 2.3 / 1.0
2 M	0114 / 0806 / 1437 / 1937	2.4 / 0.9 / 2.1 / 1.3		**17** TU	0135 / 0822 / 1458 / 2012	2.5 / 0.6 / 2.2 / 1.1
3 TU	0210 / 0908 / 1541 / 2058	2.3 / 0.9 / 2.1 / 1.4		**18** W	0236 / 0934 / 1612 / 2118	2.4 / 0.7 / 2.2 / 1.2
4 W	0328 / 1006 / 1640 / 2214	2.3 / 0.9 / 2.1 / 1.4		**19** TH	0359 / 1049 / 1717 / 2305	2.3 / 0.7 / 2.2 / 1.2
5 TH	0431 / 1101 / 1737 / 2316	2.3 / 0.9 / 2.2 / 1.3		**20** F	0514 / 1158 / 1815	2.3 / 0.7 / 2.3
6 F	0528 / 1154 / 1829	2.3 / 0.9 / 2.3		**21** SA	0025 / 0619 / 1258 / 1906	1.1 / 2.3 / 0.7 / 2.3
7 SA	0013 / 0620 / 1244 / 1914	1.2 / 2.3 / 0.8 / 2.4		**22** SU	0123 / 0718 / 1349 / 1951	0.9 / 2.4 / 0.7 / 2.4
8 SU	0104 / 0709 / 1330 / 1956	1.1 / 2.4 / 0.7 / 2.4		**23** M	0213 / 0811 / 1434 / 2033	0.8 / 2.4 / 0.7 / 2.4
9 M	0150 / 0756 / 1414 / 2034	0.9 / 2.5 / 0.7 / 2.5		**24** TU	0258 / 0901 / 1516 / O2112	0.7 / 2.4 / 0.8 / 2.5
10 TU	0236 / 0842 / 1457 / ●2112	0.8 / 2.5 / 0.7 / 2.6		**25** W	0341 / 0947 / 1553 / 2148	0.6 / 2.4 / 0.8 / 2.5
11 W	0321 / 0930 / 1540 / 2151	0.6 / 2.5 / 0.6 / 2.6		**26** TH	0421 / 1029 / 1623 / 2223	0.6 / 2.3 / 0.9 / 2.5
12 TH	0408 / 1019 / 1622 / 2233	0.6 / 2.6 / 0.6 / 2.6		**27** F	0458 / 1105 / 1646 / 2258	0.6 / 2.3 / 0.9 / 2.5
13 F	0454 / 1107 / 1705 / 2315	0.5 / 2.6 / 0.7 / 2.7		**28** SA	0530 / 1140 / 1711 / 2333	0.6 / 2.3 / 1.0 / 2.5
14 SA	0541 / 1155 / 1747 / 2359	0.5 / 2.5 / 0.8 / 2.6		**29** SU	0602 / 1218 / 1741	0.6 / 2.2 / 1.0
15 SU	0629 / 1246 / 1831	0.5 / 2.4 / 0.9		**30** M	0007 / 0637 / 1301 / 1812	2.5 / 0.7 / 2.2 / 1.1
				31 TU	0042 / 0719 / 1350 / 1850	2.4 / 0.8 / 2.1 / 1.1

Chart Datum: 1·50 metres below Ordnance Datum (Newlyn)

GREAT YARMOUTH   10-4-26

Norfolk 52°34'·33N 01°44'·50E

CHARTS

AC 1536, 1543; Imray C28; Stanfords 3; OS 134

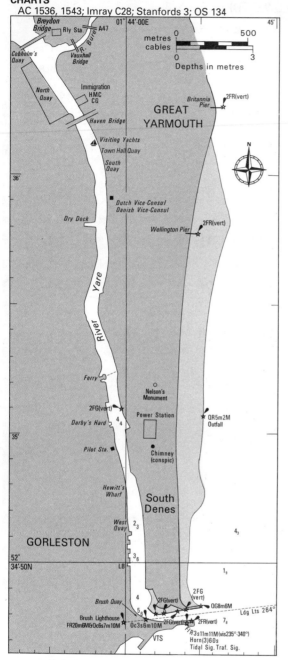

SHELTER

Excellent on Town Hall Quay, close S of Haven Bridge; ⚓ prohib in hbr which is a busy commercial port.

NAVIGATION

WPT 52°34'·40N 01°45'·67E, 084°/264° from/to front ldg lt, 1·0M. Access is H24, subject to clearance, but small craft must not attempt ent in strong SE winds which cause dangerous seas, especially on the ebb. Except at local slack water, which occurs at HW+1½ and LW+1¾, tidal streams at the ent are strong. On the flood, the stream eddies NW past S pier, thence up-river; beware being set onto N pier; a QY tidal lt on S pier warns of this D/N. Temp shoaling may occur in the ent during strong E'lies, with depths 1m less than those charted. Beware strong tidal streams that sweep through the Haven Bridge.

LIGHTS AND MARKS

Main lt Fl R 3s 11m 11M, vis 235°-340°, Horn (3) 60s. (Note: Tfc Sigs and the tidal QY are co-located with the Main lt on a R brick bldg, W lower half floodlit, at S pier). Ldg lts 264°: front Oc 3s 6m 10M; rear Oc 6s 7m 10M, (below the FR 20m 6M on Brush lt ho). N pier lt, QG 8m 6M, vis 176°-078° (262°). Lesser lts as on chartlet.

TRAFFIC SIGNALS

Tfc sigs and VTS instructions (Ch 12) must be obeyed at all times. S pier: 3 Ⓡ (vert), vis 235°-295° = Ent prohib. VTS office: 3 Ⓡ (vert) = no vessel to go down-river S of the LB shed.
Haven and Breydon bridges: 3 Ⓡ (vert) = passage prohib.

RADIO TELEPHONE

Call: Yarmouth Ch 12 (both H24) 09. Both bridges Ch 12.

TELEPHONE (01493)

Hr Mr 855151; VTS (H24) 855153; MRCC 851338; ⌗ (01473) 219481; Police 336200; Breydon Bridge 651275; Broads Navigation Authority (01603) 610734.

FACILITIES

Town Hall Quay (50m stretch) AB £10, may be limited to only 2 nights in season.
Burgh Castle Marina (on Breydon Water) (90+10 visitors) ☎ 780263, Slip, D, FW, ME, El, Sh, C (6 ton), ▣, Gas, Gaz, CH, V, R, Bar, Access HW ±4; Services: BY, P & D, ME, El, FW, Slip, Diving, AB, L, M, Sh, SM, ACA.
Town EC Thurs; P, D, CH, V, R, Bar, ✉, Ⓑ, ⇌, ✈ (Norwich).

Entry to the Broads: Pass up R Yare at slack LW, under Haven Bridge (2·3m MHWS) thence to Breydon Water via Breydon Bridge (4·0m) or to R Bure. Both bridges lift in co-ordination to pass small craft in groups. They are manned 0800-1700 Mon-Thurs, 0800-1600 Fri, but do not open 0800-0900 or 1700-1800. Call the Bridge Officer on VHF Ch 12. R Bure has two fixed bridges (2·3m MHWS).

NORFOLK BROADS: The Broads comprise about 120 miles of navigable rivers and lakes in Norfolk and Suffolk. The main rivers (Bure, Yare and Waveney) are tidal, flowing into the sea at Great Yarmouth. The N Broads have a 2·3m headroom limit. Unlimited headroom restricts cruising to R Yare (Great Yarmouth to Norwich) and R Waveney (Lowestoft to Beccles). The Broads may be entered from sea at Great Yarmouth (as above) or Lowestoft (10.4.25).
Tidal data on the rivers and Broads is based on the time of LW at Yarmouth Yacht Stn (mouth of R Bure), which is LW Gorleston +0100 (see TIDES). Add the differences below to time of LW Yarmouth Yacht Stn to get local LW times:

R Bure		R Waveney	
Acle Bridge	+0230	Burney Arms	+0100
Horning	+0300	St Olaves	+0115
Potter Heigham	+0400	Oulton Broad	+0300
R Yare		Beccles	+0320
Reedham	+0115		
Cantley	+0200		
Norwich	+0430		

LW at Breydon (mouth of R Yare) is LW Yarmouth Yacht Stn +0100. Tide starts to flood on Breydon Water whilst still ebbing from R Bure. Max draft is 1·8m; 2m with care. Tidal range varies from 0·6m to 1·8m.
Licences are compulsory; get temp one from The Broads Authority, 18 Colegate, Norwich NR3 1BQ, ☎ 01603-610734; from Mutford Lock or from River Inspectors. Hamilton's Guide to the Broads is recommended.

TIDES

–0210 Dover; ML 1·5; Duration 0620; Zone 0 (UT)

Standard Port LOWESTOFT (←)

Times				Height (metres)			
High Water		Low Water		MHWS	MHWN	MLWN	MLWS
0300	0900	0200	0800	2·4	2·1	1·0	0·5
1500	2100	1400	2000				

Differences GORLESTON (To be used for Great Yarmouth)

–0035	–0035	–0030	–0030	0·0	–0·1	0·0	0·0

CAISTER-ON-SEA

–0130	–0130	–0100	–0100	0·0	–0·1	0·0	0·0

WINTERTON-ON-SEA

–0225	–0215	–0135	–0135	+0·8	+0·5	+0·2	+0·1

Rise of tide occurs mainly during 3½ hours after LW. From HW Lowestoft –3 until HW the level is usually within 0·3m of predicted HW. Flood tide runs until about HW +1½ and Ebb until about LW +2½. See also under NAVIGATION.

Volvo Penta service

Sales and service centres in area 5
YORKSHIRE Auto Unit Repairs (Leeds) Ltd, Henshaw Works, Henshaw Lane, Yeadon, Leeds LS19 7XY Tel (01132) 501222 Anglo Dansk Engineering Co Ltd, Robinson Lane, Fish Docks, Grimsby DN31 3SF Tel (01472) 351457/8/9
NOTTINGHAM Newark Marina Ltd, 26 Farndon Road, Newark NG24 4SD Tel (01636) 704022 **TYNE & WEAR** Royston Engineering Group Ltd, 40 Bell Street, Fish Quay, North Shields NE30 1HF Tel 0191-259 5935/6797

Area 5

East England
Blakeney to Berwick-on-Tweed

5

VOLVO PENTA

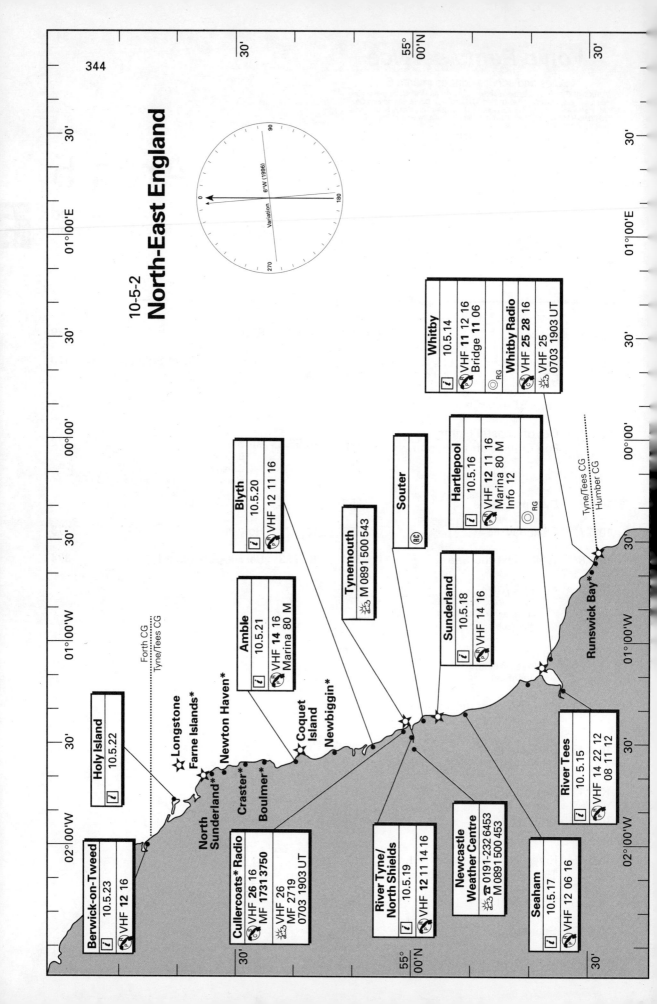

10-5-2
North-East England

Variation
6°W (1996)

Forth CG
Tyne/Tees CG

Berwick-on-Tweed
10.5.23
VHF 12 16

Holy Island
10.5.22

☆ Longstone
Farne Islands*
North Sunderland*
Newton Haven*
Craster*
Boulmer*

Cullercoats* Radio
VHF 26 16
MF 1731 3750
MF 2719
0703 1903 UT

Amble
10.5.21
VHF 14 16
Marina 80 M

☆ Coquet
Island
Newbiggin*

Blyth
10.5.20
VHF 12 11 16

Tynemouth
M 0891 500 543

Souter
RC

**River Tyne/
North Shields**
10.5.19
VHF 12 11 14 16

**Newcastle
Weather Centre**
☎ 0191-232 6453
M 0891 500 453

Sunderland
10.5.18
VHF 14 16

Hartlepool
10.5.16
VHF 12 11 16
Marina 80 M
Info 12
RG

Seaham
10.5.17
VHF 12 06 16

River Tees
10.5.15
VHF 14 22 12
08 11 12

Whitby
10.5.14
VHF 11 12 16
Bridge 11 06
RG

Whitby Radio
VHF 25 28 16
VHF 25
0703 1903 UT

Tyne/Tees CG
Humber CG

Runswick Bay*

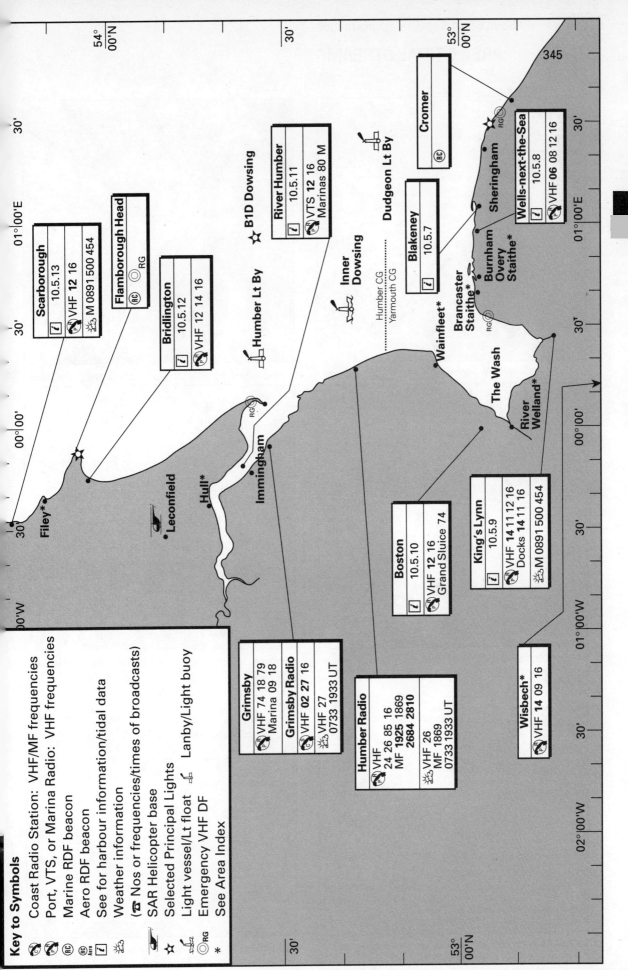

Key to Symbols

🎙️	Coast Radio Station: VHF/MF frequencies
🎙️	Port, VTS, or Marina Radio: VHF frequencies
⊙RC	Marine RDF beacon
⊙	Aero RDF beacon
i	See for harbour information/tidal data
📻	Weather information (☎ Nos or frequencies/times of broadcasts)
✪	Selected Principal Lights
🚁	SAR Helicopter base
🚢	Light vessel/Lt float
⊙RG	Emergency VHF DF
*	See Area Index
⬗	Lanby/Light buoy

5

345

Scarborough
10.5.13
i | 🎙️ VHF **12** 16
📻 M 0891 500 454

Flamborough Head ⊙RG

Bridlington
10.5.12
i | 🎙️ VHF 12 14 16

✪ **Humber Lt By**

☆ **B1D Dowsing**

River Humber
10.5.11
i | 🎙️ VTS **12** 16
Marinas 80 M

🚢 **Inner Dowsing**

Dudgeon Lt By

Humber CG .... Yarmouth CG

Cromer
⊙RC

⊙RG

Sheringham

Blakeney
10.5.7
i

Burnham Overy Staithe *

Brancaster Staithe *
⊙RG

Wells-next-the-Sea
10.5.8
i | 🎙️ VHF **06** 08 12 16

Wainfleet *

The Wash

River Welland *

Filey *

🚢 **Leconfield**

Hull *

Immingham

Boston
10.5.10
i | 🎙️ VHF **12** 16
Grand Sluice 74

King's Lynn
10.5.9
i | 🎙️ VHF **14** 11 12 16
Docks **14** 11 16
📻 M 0891 500 454

Grimsby
🎙️ VHF 74 18 79
Marina 09 18

Grimsby Radio
🎙️ VHF **02 27** 16
📻 VHF 27
0733 1933 UT

Humber Radio
🎙️ VHF
24 26 85 16
MF **1925** 1869
2684 2810
📻 VHF 26
MF 1869
0733 1933 UT

Wisbech *
🎙️ VHF **14** 09 16

54° 00'N

30'

01°00'E

30'

00'00'

30'

00'W

02°00'W

30'

01°00'W

30'

00°00'

30'

01°00'E

30'

53° 00'N

53° 00'N

30'

10-5-3   AREA 5 TIDAL STREAMS

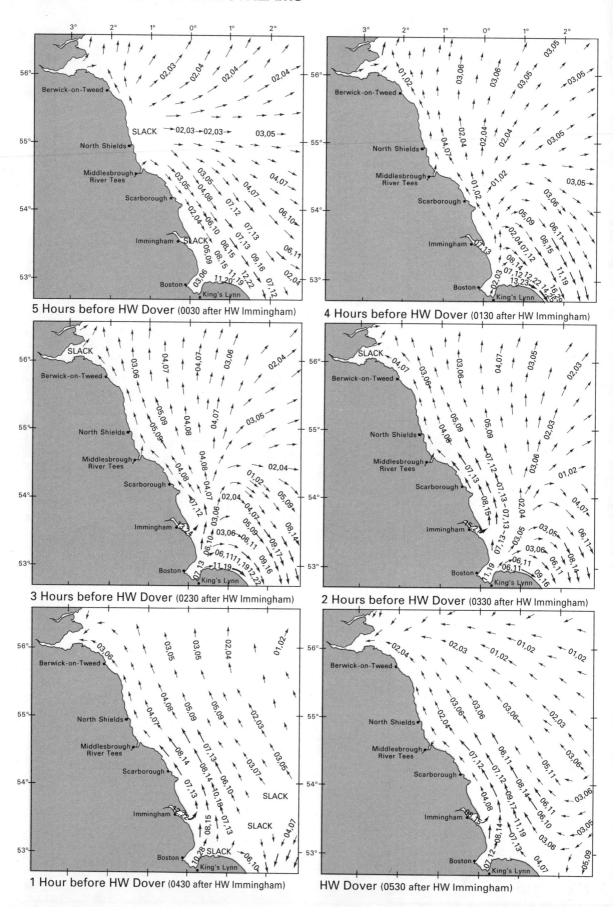

5 Hours before HW Dover (0030 after HW Immingham)

4 Hours before HW Dover (0130 after HW Immingham)

3 Hours before HW Dover (0230 after HW Immingham)

2 Hours before HW Dover (0330 after HW Immingham)

1 Hour before HW Dover (0430 after HW Immingham)

HW Dover (0530 after HW Immingham)

Northward 10.6.3   Southward 10.4.3

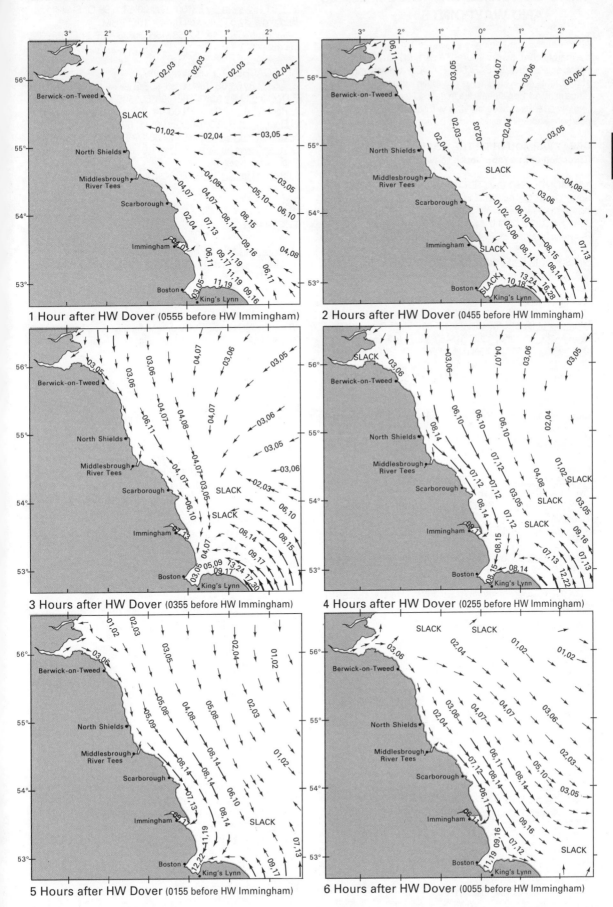

1 Hour after HW Dover (0555 before HW Immingham)

2 Hours after HW Dover (0455 before HW Immingham)

3 Hours after HW Dover (0355 before HW Immingham)

4 Hours after HW Dover (0255 before HW Immingham)

5 Hours after HW Dover (0155 before HW Immingham)

6 Hours after HW Dover (0055 before HW Immingham)

10.5.4 COASTAL LIGHTS, FOG SIGNALS AND WAYPOINTS

Abbreviations used below are given in 1.4.1. Principal lights are in **bold** print, places in CAPITALS, and light-vessels, light floats and Lanbys in *CAPITAL ITALICS*. Unless otherwise stated lights are white. m – elevation in metres; M – nominal range in miles. Fog signals are in *italics*. Useful waypoints are underlined – use those on land with care. All geographical positions should be assumed to be approximate. See 4.4.1.

GREAT YARMOUTH TO THE WASH
(Direction of buoyage South to North)

YARMOUTH AND CAISTER ROADS/COCKLE GATWAY
South Denes Outfall 52°35'·10N 01°44'·50E QR 5m 2M; R △.
Wellington Pier Hd 52°35'·92N 01°44'·42E 2 FR (vert) 8m 3M.
Jetty Hd 52°36'·10N 01°44'·48E 2 FR(vert) 7m 2M.
Britannia Pier Hd 52°36'·47N 01°44'·57E 2 FR (vert) 11m 4M; W col.
SW Scroby Lt By 52°35'·81N 01°46'·55E Fl G 2·5s; SHM.
Scroby Elbow Lt By 52°37'·70N 01°46'·50E Fl (2) G 5s; SHM; *Bell.*
Mid Caister Lt By 52°38'·96N 01°45'·77E Fl (2) R 5s; PHM; *Bell.*
NW Scroby Lt By 52°40'·35N 01°46'·44E Fl (3) G 10s; SHM.
N Caister Lt By 52°40'·40N 01°45'·66E Fl (3) R 10s; PHM.
Hemsby Lt By 52°41'·84N 01°45'·00E Fl R 2·5s; PHM.
N Scroby Lt By 52°42'·49N 01°44'·80E VQ; NCM; *Whis.*
Cockle Lt By 52°44'·00N 01°43'·70E VQ (3) 5s; ECM; *Bell.*
Winterton Old Lt Ho 52°42'·75N 01°41'·80E Racon (T).

OFFSHORE ROUTE
Cross Sand Lt By 52°37'·00N 01°59'·25E L Fl 10s 6m 5M; SWM; Racon (T).
E. Cross Sand Lt By 52°40'·00N 01° 53'·80E Fl (4) R 15s; PHM.
NE Cross Sand Lt By 52°43'·00N 01° 53'·80E VQ (3) 5s; ECM.
Smith's Knoll Lt By 52°43'·50N 02°18'·00E Q (6) + L Fl 15s 7M; SCM; Racon (T); *Whis.*
S Winterton Ridge Lt By 52°47'·20N 02°03'·60E Q (6) + L Fl 15s; SCM.
E Hammond Knoll Lt By 52°52'·30N 01°58'·75E Q (3) 10s; ECM.
Hammond Knoll Lt By 52°49'·72N 01°57'·70E Q (9) 15s; WCM.
NEWARP Lt F 52°48'·35N 01°55'·80E Fl 10s 12m **21M** (H24); Racon (O); *Horn 20s* (continuous).
S Haisbro Lt By 52°50'·80N 01°48'·40E Q (6) + L Fl 15s; SCM; *Bell.*

(Direction of buoyage East to West)

Mid Haisbro Lt By 52°54'·20N 01°41'·70E Fl (2) G 5s; SHM.
N Haisbro Lt By 53°00'·20N 01°32'·40E Q; NCM; Racon (T); *Bell.*
Happisburgh Lt Ho 52°49'·20N 01°32'·30E Fl (3) 30s 41m 14M; W Tr, 3 R bands.

CROMER
Cromer 52°55'·45N 01°19'·12E Fl 5s 84m **23M**; W 8-sided Tr; RC; vis 102°-307°; Racon (C).
Lifeboat Ho 52°56'·00N 01°18'·20E 2 FR (vert) 8m 5M.

Tayjack Wk Lt By 52°57'·70N 01°15'·40E VQ; NCM.
E Sheringham Lt By 53°02'·20N 01°15'·00E Q (3) 10s; ECM.
W Sheringham Lt By 53°02'·93N 01°06'·87E Q (9) 15s; WCM.
Blakeney Overfalls Lt By 53°03'·00N 01°01'·50E Fl (2) R 5s; PHM; *Bell.*

BLAKENEY
Fairway By 52°59'·17N 00°57'·38E; SPM.
Hjordis Wk By 52°58'·97N 00°58'·20E; PHM.
Bar Lt By 52°59'·11N 00°58'·23E QY; SPM.

WELLS-NEXT-THE-SEA/BRANCASTER STAITHE
Wells Fairway Lt By 53°00'·17N 00°51'·15E Q; SWM.
Bridgirdle By 53°01'·72N 00°44'·10E; PHM.
Brancaster Club Ho 52°58'·45N 00°38'·25E Fl 5s 8m 3M; vis 080°-270°.

APPROACHES TO THE WASH
S Race Lt By 53°08'·18N 00°56'·80E Q (6) + L Fl 15s; SCM; *Bell.*
E Docking Lt By 53°09'·80N 00°50'·50E Fl R 2·5s; PHM.
N Race Lt By 53°14'·97N 00°44'·00E Fl G 5s; SHM; *Bell.*
N Docking Lt By 53°14'·80N 00°41'·60E Q; NCM.
Scott Patch Lt By 53°11'·10N 00°36'·50E VQ (3) 5s; ECM.
S Inner Dowsing Lt By 53°12'·10N 00°33'·80E Q (6) + L Fl 15s; SCM; *Bell.*
Burnham Flats Lt By 53°07'·50N 00°35'·00E Q (9) 15s; WCM; *Bell.*

THE WASH

Lynn Knock Lt By 53°04'·40N 00°27'·31E QG; SHM.
North Well Lt By 53°03'·00N 00°28'·00E L Fl 10s; SWM; *Whis*; Racon (T).
Woolpack Lt By 53°02'·65N 00°31'·55E Fl R 10s; PHM.

ROARING MIDDLE Lt F 52°58'·50N 00°21'·00E Q 5m 8M; NCM; *Bell.* Replaced May-June annually by B&Y pillar and Bell By Q.

CORK HOLE/KING'S LYNN
Sunk Lt By 52°56'·27N 00°23'·50E Q (9) 15s; WCM.
No 1 Lt By 52°55'·70N 00°22'·10E VQ; NCM; *Bell* .
No 3 Lt By 52°54'·42N 00°24'·51E Q (3) 10s; ECM.
No 3A Lt By 52°53'·70N 00°23'·96E Fl G 5s; SHM.
(Buoyage from Cork Hole to Lynn Cut subject to change.)
W Stones Lt Bn 52°49'·71N 00°21'·22E Q 3m 2M; NCM.
Bn B 52°49'·10N 00°21'·22E Fl Y 2s 3m 2M; △ on B post.
Bn E 52°48'·18N 00°21'·52E Fl Y 6s 3m 2M; △ on B post.
West Bank Lt Bn 52°47'·4N 00°22'·1E Fl Y 2s 3m 4M; R pile.
King's Lynn W Bk Ferry 52°45'·35N 00°23'·46E Fl Y 2s 5m 2M (when tide is falling) and 2 FG (vert).

WISBECH CHANNEL/RIVER NENE
(Note: Bns are moved as required.)
Bar Flat Lt By 52°55'·25N 00°16'·64E Q (3) 10s; ECM.
Big Tom 52°49'·57N 00°13'·17E Fl (2) R 10s; R Bn.
West End 52°49'·5N 00°13'·0E Fl G 5s 3M; B mast, Ra refl.
Marsh 52°49'·0N 00°13'·0E QR.
Scottish Sluice West Bk 52°48'·5N 00°12'·7E FG 9m; Mast; Stakes on W side of River Nene to Wisbech carry QW Lts and those on E side QR Lts.

FREEMAN CHANNEL
Boston Roads Lt By 52°57'·67N 00°16'·23E L Fl 10s; SWM.
Boston No. 1 Lt By 52°57'·87N 00°15'·22E Fl G 3s; SHM.
No. 3 Lt By 52°58'·10N 00°14'·15E Fl G 6s; SHM.
No. 5 Lt By 52°58'·52N 00°12'·78E Fl G 3s; SHM.
Freeman Inner Lt By 52°58'·45N 00°11'·43E Q (9) 15s; WCM.
Delta Lt By 52°58'·34N 00°11'·26E Fl R 6s; PHM.

BOSTON LOWER ROAD
Boston No. 7 Lt By 52°58'·57N 00°10'·00E Fl G 3s; SHM.
Boston No. 9 Lt By 52° 57'·58N 00°08'·45E Fl G 3s; SHM.
Boston No. 11 Lt By 52°56'·51N 00°07'·64E Fl G 6s; SHM.
Boston No. 13 Lt By 52°56'·22N 00°07'·13E Fl G 3s; SHM.
Boston No.15 Lt By 52°56'·29N 00°05'·70E Fl (2) G 6s; SHM.

Welland Lt Bn 52°56'·06N 00°05'·37E QR 5m; R ☐ on Bn.
Tabs Hd 52°55'·99N 00°05'·01E Q WG 4m 1M; R ☐ on W mast; vis W shore-251°, G251°-shore; Ra refl.

BOSTON, NEW CUT AND RIVER WITHAM
Ent N side, Dollypeg Lt Bn 52°56'·10N 00°05'·15E QG 4m
1M; B △ on Bn; Ra refl.
Tabs Hd Q WG wm 1M; vis shore-251°, G251°-shore.
New Cut 52°55'·97N 00°04'·79E Fl G 3s; △ on pile.
New Cut Ldg Lts 240°. Front, No. 1 52°55'·82N 00°04'·49E
F 5m 5M. Rear, 90m from front, F 8m 5M.
Boston Ldg Lts 324°. Front, No. 10 52°58'·02N 00°00'·49W
F. Rear, No. 10A 150m from front, F.

WELLAND CUT/RIVER WELLAND
SE side Iso R 2s; NW side Iso G 2s. Lts QR (to port) and
QG (to stbd) mark the chan upstream.
Fosdyke Bridge 52°52'·26N 00°02'·45W FY.

(Direction of buoyage North to South)

BOSTON DEEP/WAINFLEET ROADS
Wainfleet Range UQ R, with FR on Trs SW & NE.
Scullridge By 52°59'·68N 00°14'·00E; SHM.
Friskney By 53°00'·48N 00°16'·68E; SHM.
Long Sand By 53°01'·10N 00°18'·30E; SHM.
Pompey By 53°02'·20N 00°19'·37E; SHM.
Swatchway By 53°03'·76N 00°19'·80E; SHM.
Inner Knock By 53°04'·85N 00°20'·50E; PHM.
Wainfleet Roads By 53°06'·20N 00°21'·40E; PHM.
Skegness S By 53°06'·70N 00°23'·35E; SHM.
Skegness By 53°08'·42N 00°23'·80E; SHM.

WASH TO THE RIVER HUMBER
(Direction of buoyage South to North)

Dudgeon Lt By 53°16'·60N 01°17'·00E Q (9) 15s 7M; WCM;
Racon (O); *Whis*.
E Dudgeon Lt By 53°19'·70N 00°58'·80E Q (3) 10s; ECM; *Bell*.
Mid Outer Dowsing Lt By 53°24'·80N 01°07'·90E Fl (3) G 10s;
SHM; *Bell*.
N Outer Dowsing Lt By 53°33'·50N 00°59'·70E Q; NCM.
B.1D Platform Dowsing 53°33'·71N 00°52'·72E Fl (2) 10s
28m **22M**; Morse (U) R 15s 28m 3M; *Horn (2) 60s*; Racon (T).

RIVER HUMBER APPROACHES
W Ridge Lt By 53°19'·05N 00°44'·60E Q (9) 15s; WCM.
Inner Dowsing Lt F 53°19'·50N 00°33'·96E Fl 10s 12m **15M**;
Racon (T); *Horn 60s*.
Protector Lt By 53°24'·83N 00°25'·25E Fl R 2·5s; PHM.
DZ No. 4 Lt By 53°27'·12N 00°19'·17E Fl Y 5s; SPM.
DZ No. 3 Lt By 53°29'·17N 00°19'·19E Fl Y 2·5s; SPM.
Rosse Spit Lt By 53°30'·40N 00°17'·04E Fl (2) R 5s; PHM.
Haile Sand No. 2 Lt By 53°32'·14N 00°12'·80E Fl (3) R 10s;
PHM.
Humber Lt By 53°36'·72N 00°21'·60E L Fl 10s; SWM; *Whis*;
Racon (T).
N Binks Lt By 53°36'·22N 00°18'·70E Fl Y 2·5s; SPM.
Outer Haile Lt By 53°34'·80N 00°18'·70E Fl (4) 15s; SPM.
S Binks Lt By 53°34'·72N 00°16'·65E Fl Y 5s; SPM.
SPURN Lt F 53°33'·54N 00°14'·33E Q (3) 10s 10m 8M; ECM;
Horn 20s; Racon (M).
SE CHEQUER Lt F 53°33'·37N 00°12'·65E VQ (6) + L Fl 10s
6m 6M; SCM; Ra refl; *Horn 30s*.
No. 3 Chequer Lt By 53°33'·05N 00°10'·70E Q (6) + L Fl 15s;
SCM.
Tetney Monobuoy 53°32'·34N 00°06'·85E 2 VQ Y (vert); Y
SBM; *Horn Mo (A) 60s*; QY on 290m floating hose.

RIVER HUMBER/GRIMSBY/HULL
Spurn Pt Lt Bn 53°34'·36N 00°06'·59E Fl G 3s 11m 5M; G △.
Spurn Hd Military Pier Hd and Pilot Jetty each show 2 FG
(vert) Lts 6m 2M.
BULL Lt F 53°33'·78N 00°05'·65E VQ 8m 6M; NCM;
Horn (2) 20s.

Bull Sand Fort 53°33'·69N 00°04'·14E Fl (2) 5s 20m 4M;
Horn 30s.
Haile Sand Fort 53°32'·05N 00°02'·14E Fl R 5s 21m 3M.
Haile Chan No. 4 Lt By 53°33'·63N 00°02'·94E Fl R 4s; PHM.
Middle No. 7 Lt F VQ (6) + L Fl 10s; SCM; *Horn 20s*.
Grimsby Royal Dock ent E side 53°35'·06N 00°03'·93W Fl (2)
R 6s 10m 8M; Dn.
Killingholme Lts in line 292°. Front 53°38'·78N 00°12'·87W
Iso R 2s 10m 14M. Rear, 189m from front, Oc R 4s 21m 14M.
Immingham Oil Terminal SE end 53°37'·68N 00°09'·32W
2 QR (vert) 8m 5M; *Horn Mo (N) 30s*.
Clay Huts No. 13 Lt F 53°38'·52N 00°11'·28W Iso 2s 5m 9M;
SWM.
Sand End No. 16 Lt F 53°42'·52N 00°14'·47W Fl R 4s 5m 3M;
PHM.
Hebbles No. 21 Lt By 53°44'·03N 00°15'·88W Fl G 1·5s; SHM.
Lower W Middle No. 24 Lt By 53°44'·26N 00°18'·24W
Fl R 4s; PHM.
Hull Marina, Humber Dk Basin, E ent 53°44'·22N 00°20'·05W
2 FG (vert).

RIVER HUMBER TO WHITBY

Canada & Giorgios Wk Lt By 53°42'·33N 00°07'·22E
VQ (3) 5s; ECM.
Hornsea Sewer Outfall Lt By 53°55'·00N 00°01'·70E
Fl Y 20s; SPM.
Atwick Sewer Outfall Lt By 53°57'·10N 00°10'·20W
Fl Y 10s; SPM.

BRIDLINGTON
SW Smithic Lt By 54°02'·40N 00°09'·10W Q (9) 15s; WCM.
N Pier Hd 54°04'·77N 00°11'·08W Fl 2s 12m 9M; *Horn 60s*.
S Pier FR or G R 8/12m, R4M, G3M, (Tidal Lts).
N Smithic Lt By 54°06'·20N 00°03'·80W Q; NCM; *Bell*.

Flamborough Hd 54°06'·97N 00°04'·87W Fl (4) 15s 65m
24M; W ● Tr; RC; Horn *(2) 90s*.

FILEY/SCARBOROUGH/WHITBY
Filey on cliff above CG Stn FR 31m 1M; vis 272°-308°.
Filey Brigg Lt By 54°12'·73N 00°14'·48W Q (3) 10s; ECM;
Bell.
Scarborough E Pier Hd 54°16'·87N 00°23'·27W QG 8m 3M.
Scarborough Lt Ho Pier Iso 5s 17m 9M; W ● Tr; vis 219°-039°
and FY 8m; vis 233°-030°; (tide sigs); *Dia 60s*.
Scalby Ness Diffusers Lt By 54°18'·60N 00°23'·25W Fl R 5s;
PHM.
Whitby Lt By 54°30'·32N 00°36'·48W Q; NCM; *Bell*.
High Lt Ling Hill 54°28'·60N 00°34'·00W Iso RW 10s 73m
18M, R16M; W 8-sided Tr and dwellings; vis R128°-143°,
W143°-319°.
Whitby E Pier Hd FR 14m 3M; R Tr.
Whitby W Pier Hd 53°29'·64N 00°36'·69W FG (occas) 14m
3M; G Tr; *Horn 30s*.

WHITBY TO RIVER TYNE

RUNSWICK/REDCAR
Runswick Bay Pier 54°31'·99N 00°44'·90W 2 FY (occas).
Boulby Outfall Lt By 54°34'·51N 00°48'·15W Fl (4) Y 10s;
SPM.
Outfall Lt By 54°36'·63N 01°00'·30W Fl Y 10s; SPM.
Salt Scar Lt By 54°38'·10N 01°00'·00W Q; NCM; *Horn(1) 15s*;
Bell.
Luff Way Ldg Lts 197°. Front, on Esplanade, FR 8m 7M; vis
182°-212°. Rear, 115m from front, FR 12m 7M; vis 182°-212°.
High Stone. Lade Way Ldg Lts 247°. Front 54°37'·15N
01°03'·81W Oc R 2·5s 9m 7M. Rear, 43m from front, Oc R
2·5s 11m 7M; vis 232°-262°.

TEES APPROACHES/HARTLEPOOL

Tees Fairway Lt By 54°40'·93N 01°06'·38W Iso 4s 9m 8M; SWM; Racon (B); *Horn 5s.*

Tees N (Fairway) Lt By 54°40'·28N 01°06'·95W Fl G 5s;SHM.

Tees S (Fairway) Lt By 54°40'·18N 01°06'·95W Fl R 5s; PHM.

Bkwtr Hd **S Gare** 54°38'·83N 01°08'·15W Fl WR 12s 16m **W20M, R17M**; W ● Tr; vis W020°-274°, R274°-357°; *Sig Stn; Horn 30s.*

Ldg Lts 210·1° Front 54°37'·22N 01°10'·08W. Both FR 18/20m 13/10M.

Longscar Lt By 54°40'·85N 01°09'·80W Q(3) 10s; ECM; *Bell.*

The Heugh 54°41'·78N 01°10'·47W Fl (2) 10s 19m **19M** (H24); W Tr.

Hartlepool Old Pier Hd 54°41'·59N 01°10'·99W QG 13m 7M; B Tr.

W Hbr N Pier Hd 54°41'·31N 01°11'·47W Oc G 5s 12m 2M. Harlepool Yacht Haven Lock Dir Lt 308° 54°41'·43N 01°11'·82W Dir Fl WRG 2s 6m 3M; vis G305·5°-307°, W307°-309°, R309°-310·5°.

N Sands, Pipe Jetty Hd 54°42'·80N 01°12'·40W 2 FR (vert) 1M; *Bell 15s.*

SEAHAM/SUNDERLAND

Seaham N Pier Hd 54°50'·25N 01°19'·15W Fl G 10s 12m 5M; W col, B bands; Di*a 30s.*

Sunderland Roker Pier Hd 54°55'·27N 01°21'·05W Fl 5s 25m **23M**; W ● Tr, 3 R bands and cupola: vis 211°-357°; S*iren 20s.*

Old N Pier Hd 54°55'·12N 01°21'·52W QG 12m 8M; Y Tr; *Horn 10s.*

Whitburn Steel By 54°56'·30N 01°20'·80W; PHM.

Whitburn Firing Range 54°57'·2N 01°21'·3W and 54°57'·7N 01°21'·2W both FR when firing is taking place.

DZ Lt Bys 54°57'·04N 01°18'·81W and 54°58'·58N 01°19'·80W, both Fl Y 2·5s; SPM.

TYNE ENTRANCE/NORTH SHIELDS

Oslo Fjord/Eugenia Chandris Lt By 55°00'·26N 01°23'·58W; Fl (3) R 10s; PHM.

Ent N Pier Hd 55°00'·87N 01°24'·08W Fl (3) 10s 26m **26M**; Gy ● Tr, W lantern; *Horn 10s.*

S Pier Hd 55°00'·67N 01°23'·97W Oc WRG 10s 15m W13M, R9M, G8M; Gy ● Tr, R&W lantern; vis W075°-161°, G161°-179° over Bellhues rk, W179°-255°, R255°-075°; *Bell (1) 10s* (TD 1988).

Fish Quay Ldg Lts 258°. **Front** 55°00'·54N 01°25'·98W F 25m **20M**; W ■ Tr. **Rear**, 220m from front, F 39m **20M**; W ■ Tr.

Herd Groyne Hd 55°00'·48N 01°25'·34W Oc WR 10s 13m W13M, R11M, R1M; R pile structure, R&W lantern; vis R (unintens) 080°-224°, W224°-255°, R255°-277°; *Bell (1) 5s (TD 1988).*

Saint Peter's Marina ent 54°57'·93N 01°34'·25E (unmarked).

RIVER TYNE TO BERWICK-ON-TWEED

CULLERCOATS/BLYTH/NEWBIGGIN

Cullercoats Ldg Lts 256°. Front 55°02'·05N 01°25'·77W FR 27m 3M. Rear, 38m from front, FR 35m 3M.

Blyth Ldg Lts 324°. Front 55°07'·42N 01°29'·72W F Bu 11m 10M. Rear, 180m from front, F Bu 17m 10M. Both Or ◇ on Tr.

Blyth Fairway Lt By 55°06'·58N 01°28'·50W Fl G 3s; SHM; *Bell.*

Blyth E Pier Hd 55°06'·98N 01°29'·11W Fl (4) 10s 19m **21M**; W Tr. FR 13m 13M (same Tr); vis 152°-249°; *Horn (3) 30s.*

Blyth W Pier Hd 55°06'·98N 01°29'·27W 2 FR (vert) 7m 8M; W Tr.

Newbiggin Bkwtr Hd 55°11'·00N 01°30'·22W Fl G 10s 4M.

Lynemouth Lt By 55°12'·50N 01°30'·70W Fl R 10s; PHM.

COQUET ISLAND/WARKWORTH AND AMBLE

Coquet 55°20'·03N 01°32'·28W Fl (3) WR 30s 25m **W23M, R19M**; W ■ Tr, turreted parapet, lower half Gy; vis R330°-140°, W140°-163°, R163°-180°, W180°-330°; sector boundaries are indeterminate and may appear as Alt WR; *Horn 30s.*

Outfall Lt By 55°20'·32N 01°33'·63W Fl R 10s; PHM; *Bell.*

Amble S Pier Hd 55°20'·38N 01°34'·14W Fl R 5s 9m 5M; W ● Tr, R bands, W base.

N Pier Hd 55°20'·38N 01°34'·15W Fl G 6s 12m 6M; W pylon.

BOULMER/CRASTER/NEWTON HAVEN/BEADNELL BAY

Boulmer Haven Bn 55°24'·75N 01°34'·40W; SHM.

Craster Hbr 55°28'·37N 01°35'·45W (unmarked).

Newton Rk By 55°32'·17N 01°35'·75W; PHM.

N SUNDERLAND (SEAHOUSES)/BAMBURGH/FARNE ISLANDS

The Falls By 55°34'·62N 01°37'·02W; PHM.

N Sunderland NW Pier Hd 55°35'·03N 01°38'.84W FG 11m 3M; W Tr; vis 159°-294°; Tfc Sigs; *Siren 90s* (occas).

N. Sunderland Bkwtr Hd 55°35'·05N 01°38'·79W Fl R 2·5s 6m. (TE 1989)

Shoreston Outcars By 55°35'·88N 01°39'·22W; PHM.

Black Rocks Pt **Bamburgh**   55°37'·00N 01°43'·35W Oc (2) WRG 15s 12m **W17M**, R13M, G13M; W bldg; vis G122°-165°, W165°-175°, R175°-191°, W191°-238°, R238°-275°, W275°-289°, G289°-300°.

Inner Farne 55°36'·93N 01°39'·25W Fl (2) WR 15s 27m W8M, R6M; W ● Tr; vis R119°-280°, W280°-119°.

Longstone W side 55°38'·63N 01°36'·55W Fl 20s 23m **24M**; R Tr, W band; *Horn (2) 60s.*

Swedman By 55°37'·65N 01°41'·52W; SHM.

HOLY ISLAND

Goldstone By 55°40'·12N 01°43'·45W; SHM.

Ridge By 55°39'·70N 01°45'·87W; ECM.

Triton Shoal By 55°39'·62N 01°46'·65W; SHM.

Old Law E Bn 55°39'·49N 01°47'·50W Oc RG 6s 9m 4M; Vis G170°-260°, R260°-020°.

Heugh 55°40'·09N 01°47'·89W Oc RG 6s 24m 5M; R △ on Tr; vis G135°-310°, R310°-125°.

Plough Seat By 55°40'·37N 01°44'·87W; PHM.

BERWICK-ON-TWEED

Bkwtr Hd 55°45'·88N 01°58'·95W Fl 5s 15m 10M; W ● Tr, R cupola and base; vis E of Seal Carr ledges-shore. FG (same Tr) 8m 1M; vis 010°-154°; *Reed 60s* (occas).

10.5.5 PASSAGE INFORMATION

For directions and pilotage refer to: *The East Coast* (Imray/ Bowskill) as far as The Wash; *Tidal Havens of the Wash and Humber* (Imray/Irving) carefully documents the hbrs of this little-frequented cruising ground. N from R. Humber see the Royal Northumberland YC's *Sailing Directions, Humber to Rattray Head*. The Admiralty Pilot *North Sea (West)* covers the whole coast. *North Sea Passage Pilot* (Imray/Navin) goes as far N as Cromer and across to Den Helder.

NORTH NORFOLK COAST (charts 106, 108)

The coast of N Norfolk is unfriendly in bad weather, with no hbr accessible when there is any N in the wind. The hbrs all dry, and seas soon build up in the entrances or over the bars, some of which are dangerous even in a moderate breeze and an ebb tide. But in settled weather and moderate offshore winds it is a peaceful area to explore, particularly for boats which can take the ground. At Blakeney and Wells (see 10.5.7 and 10.5.8) chans shift almost every year, so local knowledge is essential and may best be acquired in advance from the Hr Mr; or in the event by following a friendly FV of suitable draft.

Haisborough Sand (buoyed) lies parallel to and 8M off the Norfolk coast at Happisburgh lt ho, with depths of less than 1m in many places, and drying 0·3m near the mid-point. The shoal is steep-to, on its NE side in particular, and there are tidal eddies. Even a moderate sea or swell breaks on the shallower parts. There are dangerous wks near the S end. Haisborough Tail and Hammond Knoll (with wk depth 1m) lie to the E of S end of Haisborough Sand. Newarp lt F is 5M SE. Similar banks lie parallel to and up to 60M off the coast.

The streams follow the generally NW/SE direction of the coast and offshore chans. But in the outer chans the stream is somewhat rotatory: when changing from SE-going to NW-going it sets SW, and when changing from NW-going to SE-going it sets NE, across the shoals. Close S of Haisborough Sand the SE-going stream begins at HW Immingham –0030; the NW-going at HW Immingham +0515, sp rates up to 2·5kn. It is possible to carry a fair tide from Gt Yarmouth to the Wash.

If proceeding direct from Cromer to the Humber, pass S of Sheringham Shoal (buoyed) where the ESE-going stream begins at HW Immingham – 0225, and the WNW-going at + 0430. Proceed to NE of Blakeney Overfalls and Docking Shoal, and to SW of Race Bank, so as to fetch Inner Dowsing lt tr (lt, fog sig). Thence pass E of Protector Overfalls, and steer for Rosse Spit buoy at SE ent to R Humber (10.5.11).

THE WASH (charts 108, 1200)

The Wash is formed by the estuaries of the rivers Great Ouse, Nene, Welland and Witham; it is an area of shifting sands, most of which dry. Important features are the strong tidal streams, the low-lying shore, and the often poor vis. Keep a careful watch on the echo sounder, because buoys may (or may not) have been moved to accommodate changes in the chan. Near North Well, the in-going stream begins at HW Immingham – 0430, and the out-going at HW Immingham + 0130, sp rates about 2kn. The in-going stream is usually stronger than the out-going, but its duration is less. Prolonged NE winds cause an in-going current, which can increase the rate and duration of the in-going stream and raise the water level at the head of the estuary. Do not attempt entry to the rivers too early on the flood, which runs hard in the rivers.

North Well SWM lt buoy and Roaring Middle lt F are the keys to entering the Wash from N or E. But from the E it is also possible to appr via a shallow route N of Stiffkey Overfalls and

Bridgirdle PHM buoy; thence via Sledway and Woolpack PHM lt buoy to North Well and into Lynn Deeps. Near north end of Lynn Deeps there are overfalls over Lynn Knock at sp tides. For King's Lynn (10.5.9) and R Nene (Wisbech) follow the buoyed/lit Cork Hole and Wisbech Chans. Boston (10.5.10) and R Welland are reached via Freeman Chan, westward from Roaring Middle; or via Boston Deep, all lit.

The NW shore of The Wash is fronted by mudflats extending 2–3M offshore and drying more than 4m; a bombing range is marked by Y bns and buoys. Wainfleet Swatchway should only be used in good vis; the buoyed chan shifts constantly, and several shoals (charted depths unreliable) off Gibraltar Pt obstruct access to Boston Deep. For Wainfleet, see 10.5.10.

THE WASH TO THE RIVER HUMBER (charts 108, 107)

Inner Dowsing is a narrow N/S sandbank with a least depth of 1·2m, 8M offshore between Skegness and Mablethorpe. There are overfalls off the W side of the bank at the N end. Inner Dowsing lt vessel (fog sig) is 1M NE of the bank.

In the outer approaches to The Wash and R. Humber there are many offlying banks, but few of them are of direct danger to yachts. The sea however breaks on some of them in bad weather, when they should be avoided. Fishing vessels may be encountered, and there are many oil/gas installations offshore (see below).

RIVER HUMBER (charts 109, 1188, 3497)

R. Humber is formed by R. Ouse and R. Trent, which meet 13M above Kingston-upon-Hull. It is commercially important and gives access to these rivers and inland waterways; it also drains most of Yorkshire and the Midlands. Where the Humber estuary reaches the sea between Northcoates Pt and Spurn Hd it is 4M wide. A VTS scheme is in operation to regulate commercial shipping in the Humber, Ouse and Trent and provide full radar surveillance. Yachts are advised to listen out on the Humber VTS frequency.

Approaching from the S, a yacht should make good Rosse Spit and then Haile Sand No 2, both PHM lt buoys, before altering westward to intercept the buoyed appr chan, which leads SW from the Humber fairway lt buoy to Spurn lt float.

If bound to/from the N, avoid The Binks, a shoal (dries 0·4m in places) extending 3M E from Spurn Hd, with a rough sea when wind is against tide. Depths offshore are irregular and subject to frequent change; it would be best to round the Outer Binks ECM buoy, unless in calm conditions and with local knowledge.

Haile Sand and Bull Sand Forts are both conspic to the SW of Spurn Head; beyond them it is advisable to follow one of the buoyed chans, since shoals are liable to change. Hawke Chan (later Sunk) is the main dredged chan to the N. Haile Chan favours the S side and Grimsby. Bull Chan takes a middle course before merging with Haile Chan. There are good yachting facilities at Grimsby and Hull (10.5.11).

Streams are strong, even fierce at sp; local info suggests that they are stronger than shown in 10.5.3, which is based upon NP 251 (Admiralty Tidal Stream Atlas). 5ca S of Spurn Hd the flood sets NW from about HW Immingham – 0520, sp rate 3·5kn; the ebb sets SE from about HW Immingham, sp rate 4kn. The worst seas are experienced in NW gales against a strong flood tide. 10M E of Spurn Hd the tidal streams are not affected by the river; relative to HW Immingham, the S-going stream begins at – 0455, and the N-going at + 0130. Nearer the entrance the direction of the S-going stream becomes more W'ly, and that of the N-going stream more E'ly.

Flamborough Head (lt, fog sig, RC) is a steep, W cliff with conspic lt ho on summit. The lt may be obsc by cliffs when close inshore. An old lt ho, also conspic, is 2½ca WNW. Tides run hard around the Hd which, in strong winds against a sp tide, is best avoided by 2M. From here the coast runs NW, with no offshore dangers until Filey Brigg where rky ledges extend 5ca ESE, marked by an ECM lt buoy. There is anch in Filey B (10.5.12) in N or offshore winds. NW of Filey Brigg beware Old Horse Rks and foul ground 5ca offshore; maintain this offing past Scarborough (10.5.13) to Whitby High lt. Off Whitby (10.5.14) beware Whitby Rk and The Scar (dry in places) to E of hbr, and Upgang Rks (dry in places) 1M to WNW; swell breaks heavily on all these rocks.

From Whitby to Hartlepool (10.5.16) there are no dangers more than 1M offshore. Runswick B (10.5.14 and chart 1612), 5M NW of Whitby, provides anch in winds from S and W but is dangerous in onshore winds. The little hbr of Staithes is only suitable for yachts which can take the ground, and only in good weather and offshore winds.

Redcliff, dark red and 205m high is a conspic feature of this coast which, along to Hunt Cliff, is prone to landslides and is fringed with rky ledges which dry for about 3ca off. There is a conspic radio mast 4ca SSE of Redcliff. Off Redcar and Coatham beware W Scar and Salt Scar, detached rky ledges (dry) lying 1 – 8ca offshore. Other ledges lie close SW and S of Salt Scar which has NCM lt buoy. Between R. Tees (10.5.15) and Hartlepool (10.5.16) beware Long Scar, detached rky ledge (dries 2m) with extremity marked by ECM lt buoy. Tees and Hartlepool Bays are exposed to strong E/SE winds.

HARTLEPOOL TO COQUET ISLAND (charts 134, 152, 156)

From The Heugh an offing of 1M clears all dangers until past Seaham (10.5.17) and approaching Sunderland (10.5.18), where White Stones, rky shoals with depth 2·6m, lie 1·75M SSE of Roker Pier lt ho, and Hendon Rk, depth 0·9m, lies 1·25M SE of the lt ho. 1M N of Sunderland is Whitburn Steel, a rky ledge with less than 2m over it; a dangerous wreck (buoyed) lies 1ca SE of it. A firing range at Souter Pt is marked by R flags (R lts) when active. Along this stretch of coast industrial smoke haze may reduce vis and obscure lights.

The coast N of Tynemouth (10.5.19) is foul, and on passage to Blyth (10.5.20) it should be given an offing of 1M. 3·5M N of Tynemouth is St Mary's Island (with disused lt ho), joined to mainland by causeway. The small, drying hbr of Seaton Sluice, 1M NW of St Mary's Island, is accessible only in offshore winds via a narrow ent.

Proceeding N from Blyth, keep well seaward of The Sow and Pigs rks, and set course to clear Newbiggin Pt and Beacon Pt by about 1M. There are conspic measured mile bns here. Near Beacon Pt are conspic chys of aluminium smelter and power stn. 2M NNW of Beacon Pt is Snab Pt where rks extend 3ca seaward. Further offshore Cresswell Skeres, rky patches with depth 3m, lie about 1·5M NNE of Snab Pt.

COQUET ISLAND TO FARNE ISLANDS (chart 156)

Coquet Is (lt, fog sig) lies about 5ca offshore at SE end of Alnmouth B, and nearly 1M NNE of Hauxley Pt, off which dangerous rks extend 6ca offshore, drying 1·9m. On passage, normally pass 1M E of Coquet Is in the W sector of the lt. Coquet chan may be used in good vis by day; but it is only 2ca wide, not buoyed, has least depth of 0·3m near the centre; and the stream runs strongly: S-going from HW Tyne – 0515 and N-going from HW Tyne + 0045. In S or W winds, there are good anchs in Coquet Road, W and NW of the Island.

Amble (Warkworth) hbr ent (10.5.21) is about 1M W of Coquet Is, and 1·5M SE of Warkworth Castle (conspic). 4ca NE and ENE of ent is Pan Bush, rky shoal with least depth of 0·3m on which dangerous seas can build in any swell. The bar has varying depths, down to less than 1m. The entrance is dangerous in strong winds from N/E when broken water may extend to Coquet Is. Once inside, the hbr is safe.

Between Coquet Is and the Farne Is, 19M to N, keep at least 1M offshore to avoid various dangers. To seaward, Craster Skeres lie 5M E of Castle Pt, and Dicky Shad and Newton Skere lie 1·75M and 4·5M E of Beadnell Pt; these are three rky banks on which the sea breaks heavily in bad weather. For Newton Haven and N Sunderland (Seahouses), see 10.5.21.

FARNE ISLANDS (charts 111, 160)

The coast between N Sunderland Pt (Snook) and Holy Island, 8M NW, has fine hill (Cheviots) scenery fronted by dunes and sandy beaches. The Farne Is and offlying shoals extend 4·5M offshore, and are a mini-cruising ground well worth visiting in good weather. The islands are a bird sanctuary, owned and operated by the National Trust, with large colonies of sea birds and grey seals. AC 111 is essential.

Inner Sound separates the islands from the mainland; in good conditions it is a better N/S route than keeping outside the whole group; but the stream runs at 3kn at sp, and with strong wind against tide there is rough water. If course is set outside Farne Is, pass 1M E of Longstone (lt, fog sig) to clear Crumstone Rk 1M to S, and Knivestone (dries 3·6m) and Whirl Rks (depth 0·6m) respectively 5 and 6ca NE of Longstone lt ho. The sea breaks on these rks.

The islands, rks and shoals are divided by Staple Sound, running NW/SE, into an inner and outer group. The former comprises Inner Farne, W and E Wideopens and Knock's Reef. Inner Farne (lt) is the innermost Is; close NE there is anch called The Kettle, sheltered except from NW, but anch out of stream close to The Bridges connecting Knock's Reef and W Wideopen. 1M NW of Inner Farne Is and separated by Farne Sound, which runs NE/SW, lies the Megstone, a rk 5m high. Beware Swedman reef (dries 0·5m), marked by SHM buoy 4ca WSW of Megstone.

The outer group of Islands comprises Staple and Brownsman Islands, N and S Wamses, the Harcars and Longstone. There is occas anch between Staple and Brownsman Is. Piper Gut and Crafords Gut may be negotiated in calm weather and near HW, stemming the S-going stream.

HOLY ISLAND TO BERWICK (charts 1612, 111, 160)

Near the Farne Is and Holy Is the SE-going stream begins at HW Tyne – 0430, and the NW-going at HW Tyne + 0130. Sp rates are about 2.5kn in Inner Sound, 4kn in Staple Sound and about 3·5kn 1M NE of Longstone, decreasing to seaward. There is an eddy S of Longstone on NW-going stream.

Holy Is (or Lindisfarne; 10.5.22) lies 6M WNW of Longstone, and is linked to mainland by a causeway covered at HW. There is a good anch on S side (chart 1612) with conspic daymarks and dir lts. The castle and a W obelisk at Emanuel Head are also conspic. The stream runs strongly in and out of hbr, W-going from HW Tyne + 0510, and E-going from HW Tyne – 0045. E of Holy Is, Goldstone chan runs N/S between Goldstone Rk (dries) SHM buoy on E side and Plough Seat Reef and Plough Rk (both dry) on W side, with PHM buoy.

Berwick Bay has some offlying shoals. Berwick-upon-Tweed (10.5.23) is easily visible against the low shoreline, which rises again to high cliffs further north. The hbr entrance is restricted by a shallow bar, dangerous in onshore winds.

NORTH SEA PASSAGES

See 10.0.7 for Distances across the North Sea. There are also further passage Notes in 10.4.5 for the Southern North Sea TSS; in 10.6.5 for crossing to Norway and the Baltic; in 10.20.5 for crossings from Belgium and the Netherlands; and in 10.21.5 for crossings from the Frisian Is and German Bight.

HARTLEPOOL TO SOUTHERN NETHERLANDS
(charts 2182A, 1191, *1190*, 1503, 1408, 1610, 3371, 110)

From abeam Whitby the passage can, theoretically, be made on one direct course, but this would conflict with oil/gas activities and platforms including Rough and Amethyst fields off Humber, Hewett off Cromer and very extensive fields further offshore. Commercial, oil-rig support and fishing vessels may be met S of Flamborough Hd and particularly off NE Norfolk where it is advisable to follow an inshore track.

After passing Flamborough Hd, Dowsing B1D, Dudgeon It buoy and Newarp It F, either:
Proceed SxE'ly to take departure from the Outer Gabbard; thence cross N Hinder South TSS (Fig. 10(6)) at right angles before heading for Roompotsluis via Middelbank and subsequent buoyed chan.
Or set course ESE from the vicinity of Cross Sand It buoy and Smith's Knoll, so as to cross the N/S deep-water traffic routes to the E (see 10.20.5). Thence alter SE toward Hoek van Holland, keeping N of Maas Approaches TSS, Figs 10 (6) & (7).

HARTLEPOOL TO THE GERMAN BIGHT
(charts 2182A, 1191, 266, 1405)

Taking departure eastward from abeam Whitby High It, skirt the SW Patch off Dogger Bank, keeping clear S of Gordon Gas Field and then N of German Bight W Approach TSS (Fig. 10(7)). Thence head for the Elbe or Helgoland; the latter may also serve as a convenient haven in order to adjust the passage for Elbe tides and streams (10.21.5), without greatly increasing passage distance. Tidal streams are less than 1kn away from the coast and run E/W along much of the route.

OIL AND GAS INSTALLATIONS

Any yacht going offshore in the N Sea is likely to encounter oil or gas installations. These are shown on Admiralty charts, where scale permits; the position of mobile rigs is updated in weekly NMs. Safety zones of radius 500m are established round all permanent platforms, mobile exploration rigs, and tanker loading moorings, as described in the Annual Summary of Admiralty Notices to Mariners No 20. Some of these platforms are close together or inter-linked. Unauthorised vessels, including yachts, must not enter these zones except in emergency or due to stress of weather.

Platforms show a main It, Fl Mo (U) 15s 15M. In addition secondary Its, Fl Mo (U) R 15s 2M, synchronised with the main It, may mark projections at each corner of the platform if not marked by a W It. The fog signal is Horn Mo (U) 30s. See the Admiralty List of Lights and Fog Signals, Vol A.

5

10.5.6   DISTANCE TABLE

Approximate distances in nautical miles are by the most direct route, whilst avoiding dangers and allowing for Traffic Separation Schemes. Places in *italics* are in adjoining areas; places in **bold** are in 10.0.7, Distances across the North Sea.

		1	2	3	4	5	6	7	8	9	10	11	12	13	14	15	16	17	18	19	20
1.	*Great Yarmouth*	1																			
2.	Blakeney	44	2																		
3.	**King's Lynn**	85	42	3																	
4.	Boston	83	39	34	4																
5.	Humber Lt Buoy	82	45	55	54	5															
6.	**Grimsby**	99	54	61	58	17	6														
7.	Hull	113	68	75	72	31	14	7													
8.	Bridlington	114	79	87	83	35	44	58	8												
9.	Scarborough	130	96	105	98	50	59	81	20	9											
10.	Whitby	143	101	121	114	66	75	97	35	16	10										
11.	River Tees (ent)	166	122	138	135	87	96	118	56	37	21	11									
12.	**Hartlepool**	169	126	140	137	89	98	122	58	39	24	4	12								
13.	Seaham	175	137	151	145	100	106	133	66	47	33	15	11	13							
14.	Sunderland	180	142	156	149	105	110	138	70	51	36	20	16	5	14						
15.	Tynemouth	183	149	163	154	112	115	145	75	56	41	27	23	12	7	15					
16.	Blyth	190	156	171	162	120	123	153	83	64	49	35	31	20	15	8	16				
17.	Amble	203	170	185	176	126	143	157	102	81	65	46	42	32	27	21	14	17			
18.	Holy Island	225	191	196	198	148	166	180	126	104	88	68	65	54	50	44	37	22	18		
19.	**Berwick-on-Tweed**	232	200	205	205	157	166	189	126	107	91	82	78	67	61	55	47	31	9	19	
20.	*Eyemouth*	240	208	213	213	165	174	197	134	115	99	90	86	75	69	63	55	39	17	8	20

BLAKENEY   10-5-7
Norfolk 52°59'·10N 00°58'·35E

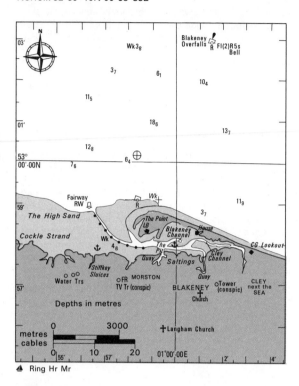

⚓ Ring Hr Mr

CHARTS
AC 108, 1190; Imray C28; Stanfords 19; OS 133
TIDES
–0445 Dover; ML Cromer 2·8; Duration 0530; Zone 0 (UT)

Standard Port IMMINGHAM (⟶)

Times				Height (metres)			
High Water		Low Water		MHWS	MHWN	MLWN	MLWS
0100	0700	0100	0700	7·3	5·8	2·6	0·9
1300	1900	1300	1900				
Differences BLAKENEY							
+0115	+0055	No data		–3·9	–3·8	No data	
BLAKENEY BAR							
+0035	+0025	+0030	+0040	–1·6	–1·3	No data	
CROMER							
+0050	+0030	+0050	+0130	–2·1	–1·7	–0·5	–0·1

SHELTER
Very good, but hbr inaccessible with fresh on-shore winds when conditions in the ent deteriorate very quickly, especially on the ebb. Entry, sp HW ±2½, nps HW ±1. Moorings in The Pit or at Stiffkey Sluices. Speed limit 8kn.
NAVIGATION
WPT 53°00'·00N 00°58'·20E, approx 045°/225° 1M from/to Fairway RW buoy (52°59'·17N 00°56'·38E , April-Oct) at ent to chan. Large dangerous wk, approx 1·5M E of ent, is marked by unlit R PHM buoy. The bar is shallow and shifts often. The chan is marked by 15 unlit G SHM buoys. Beware mussel lays, drying, off Blakeney Spit.
LIGHTS AND MARKS
Y ldg bns on dunes at Blakeney Pt are erected only when the chan ent moves adjacent to the Pt. Conspic marks are: Blakeney and Langham churches; a chy on the house on Blakeney Pt neck; TV mast (R lts) approx 2M S of ent.
RADIO TELEPHONE
None.
TELEPHONE (01263)
Hr Mr 740362; MRCC (01493) 851338; ✠ (01473) 219481; Marinecall 0891 500455; Dr 740314; Pilot 740362.
FACILITIES
Quay AB (Free), Slip, M, D, FW, EI, C (15 ton), CH; **Services:** Pilot (☎ 740362), AB, BY, M, P & D (cans), FW, ME, EI, Sh, SM, Gas, Gaz, AC. **Village** EC Wed; V, R, Bar, ✉, Ⓑ, ⇌ (Sherringham), ✈ (Norwich).

WELLS-NEXT-THE-SEA   10-5-8
Norfolk 52°59'·30N 00°49'·75E (ent shifts)

CHARTS
AC 108, 1190; Imray C28, Y9; OS 132
TIDES
–0445 Dover; ML 1·2 Duration 0540; Zone 0 (UT)

Standard Port IMMINGHAM (⟶)

Times				Height (metres)			
High Water		Low Water		MHWS	MHWN	MLWN	MLWS
0100	0700	0100	0700	7·3	5·8	2·6	0·9
1300	1900	1300	1900				
Differences WELLS-NEXT-THE-SEA							
+0035	+0045	+0340	+0310	–3·8	–3·8	Not below CD	
WELLS BAR							
+0020	+0020	+0020	+0020	–1·3	–1·0	No data	
BURNHAM OVERY STAITHE							
+0045	+0055	No data		–5·0	–4·9	No data	

Note: LW time differences at Wells are for the end of a LW stand which lasts about 4 hrs at sp and about 5 hrs at nps.

SHELTER
Good, except in strong N winds when swell renders entry impossible for small craft. Max draft 3m at sp. Access from HW –1½ to HW +1, but recommended on the flood.
NAVIGATION
WPT Fairway SWM buoy, 52°59'·92N 00°49'·61E, 020°/200° from/to chan ent, 0·7M. The bar and ent vary in depth and position; buoys are altered to suit. Keep to port side of chan from No 12 to quay. Best to follow FV or take a pilot.

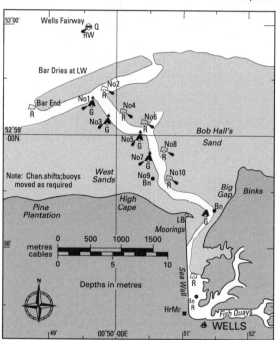

LIGHTS AND MARKS
Fairway buoy SWM, Q. Chan is marked by SHM buoys, four of which are Fl 3s, and two Fl G 3s PHM buoys; plus unlit buoys. Temp buoys may be laid when chan changes. A white LB ho with R roof is conspic at hbr ent. A pine plantation is visible close W of ent.
RADIO TELEPHONE
Wells Hbr Radio VHF Ch 12 16 (when vessel due, HW–2).
TELEPHONE (01328 Fakenham)
Hr Mr 711744; Pilot 710550; MRCC (01493) 851338; ✠ (01473) 219481; Marinecall 0891 500455; Police 710212; Ⓗ 710218.
FACILITIES
Main Quay M (see Hr Mr), AB (£9), FW, ME, EI, Sh, C (5 ton mobile), CH, V, R, Bar; **E Quay** Slip, M, L; **Wells SC** ☎ 711320, Slip, Bar; **Services:** M, ME, EI, Ⓔ, Sh, CH, ACA. **Town** EC Thurs; P & D (bowser on quay; up to 500 galls), Gas, V, R, Bar, ✉, Ⓑ, ⇌ (bus to Norwich/King's Lynn), ✈ (Norwich).

KING'S LYNN   10-5-9

Norfolk 52°49'·72N 00°21'·30E (West Stones bn)

CHARTS
AC 1200, 108, *1190*; Imray Y9; OS 132

TIDES
–0443 Dover; ML 3·6; Duration 0340 Sp, 0515 Np;
Zone 0 (UT)

Standard Port IMMINGHAM (→)

Times				Height (metres)			
High Water		Low Water		MHWS	MHWN	MLWN	MLWS
0100	0700	0100	0700	7·3	5·8	2·6	0·9
1300	1900	1300	1900				
Differences KING'S LYNN							
+0030	+0030	+0305	+0140	–0·5	–0·8	–0·8	+0·1
HUNSTANTON							
+0010	+0020	+0105	+0025	+0·1	–0·2	–0·1	0·0
WEST STONES							
+0025	+0025	+0115	+0040	–0·3	–0·4	–0·3	+0·2
WISBECH CUT							
+0020	+0025	+0200	+0030	–0·3	–0·7	–0·4	No data

SHELTER
Hbr is well sheltered 1½M up river. Entry recommended HW±3. The Alexandra dock is open from about HW –1½ to HW and yachts can be left there with the Dockmaster's permission. Drying moorings at S Quay, S side of Boal Quay or at Friars Fleet; keep clear of FV moorings.

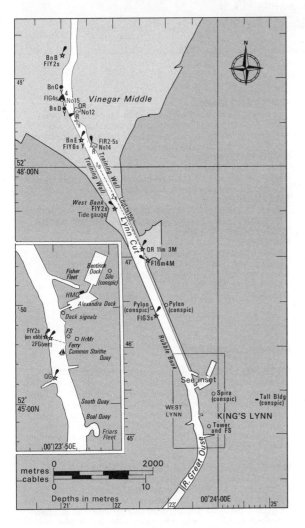

NAVIGATION
WPT Roaring Middle lt float NCM, Q 5m 8M, 52°58'·50N 00°21'·00E, 347°/167° from/to No 1 NCM buoy, 2·9M. NB: Roaring Middle lt float (WPT) is replaced temporarily every May/Jun by a NCM pillar buoy, Q, for maintenance. Extensive shifting sand banks extend several miles into the Wash. The best and safest appr is via the Cork Hole route, marked by lt buoys. Chans are subject to frequent changes particularly between No 7 lt buoy and Lynn Cut. S of W Stones bn the deeper water is on E side of chan. Advice may be obtained from Pilot launches which are often in vicinity of 52°56'·3N 00°22'·2E (boarding point); or follow them in to harbour.

LIGHTS AND MARKS
Conspic white Lt Ho (disused, 18m) on Hunstanton cliffs. West Stones bn NCM, Q 3m 2M. Lynn Cut ldg lts 155°: front QR 11m 3M; rear FW 16m 4M, both on masts. Entry sigs for Alexandra Dock:
Bu flag or Ⓡ = Vessels can enter;
R flag or Ⓖ = Vessels leaving dock.

RADIO TELEPHONE
Call *KLCB* VHF Ch 14 16 11 12 (Mon-Fri: 0800-1730 LT). Other times: HW –4 to HW+1.
King's Lynn Docks (ABP) Ch 14 16 11 (HW–2½ to HW+1).

TELEPHONE (01553)
Hr Mr 773411; Dock 691555; MRCC (01493) 851338; ⌗ (01473) 219481; Marinecall 0891 500455; Dr via Hr Mr.

FACILITIES
A commercial port with virtually no facilities for yachts.
Docks ☎ 691555, AB £12 if available, M, FW, C (32 ton); **Services:** CH, Sh, ME, El, Ⓔ, D.
Town EC Wed; P, D, V, R, Bar, ✉, Ⓑ, ⇌, ✈ (Humberside or Norwich).
Note: 24M up the Great Ouse river, Ely Marina ☎ (01353) 664622, Slip, M, P, D, FW, ME, El, Sh, C (10 ton), CH. Lock half-way at Denver Sluice ☎ (01366) 382340/VHF Ch 73, and low bridges beyond.

ADJACENT HARBOURS

BURNHAM OVERY STAITHE, Norfolk, 52°59'·00N 00°46'·50E. AC 108, *1190*. HW –0420 on Dover. See 10·5·8. Small drying hbr; ent chan has 0·3m MLWS. ⚓ off the Staithe only suitable in good weather. No lts. Scolt Hd is conspic to W and Gun Hill to E; Scolt Hd Island is a conspic 3M long sandbank which affords some shelter. Chan varies constantly and buoys are moved to suit. Local knowledge advisable. Facilities: (01328) **Burnham Overy Staithe SC** ☎ 738348, M, L; **Services:** CH, M, ME, Sh, Slip, FW; **Burnham Market** EC Wed; Bar, P and D (cans), R, V.

BRANCASTER STAITHE, Norfolk, 52°59'·00N 00°38'·50E. AC 108, *1190*. HW –0425 on Dover; See 10.5.8. Small drying hbr; dangerous to enter except by day in settled weather. Speed limit 6kn. Appr from due N. Conspic golf club house with lt, Fl 5s 8m 3M, is 0·5M S of chan ent and Fairway buoy. Beware wk shown on chart. Sandbanks vary constantly and buoys changed to suit. Scolt Hd conspic to E. Local knowledge or Pilot advised. ⚓s available occasionally in The Hole. Hr Mr ☎ (01485) 210638, . Facilities: **Brancaster Staithe SC** ☎ 210249, R, Bar; **Scolt Hd NT Warden** ☎ 210330 (Access HW ±3); **Services:** BY, CH, El, FW, P & D (cans), ME, R, Sh, Bar, V.

WISBECH, Cambridgeshire, 52°40'·00N 00°09'·65E. AC 1200, *1190*. HW –0450 on Dover; ML 3·5m; Duration 0520. See 10·5·9. Excellent shelter. Vessels of 4·8m draft can reach Wisbech at sp (3·4m at nps). Ent to R Nene and inland waterways. Landing at W Nene tr; moorings at Sutton Port (W bank 0·5M downstream from Sutton Bridge) or at Wisbech town quay. Ent well marked with lit buoys and bns from RAF No 6 ECM buoy to Nene trs. Best ent HW –3. Big Tom bn to Sutton br is 3½M, thence to Wisbech 6M, with F & Fl 5s lts to stbd. Call on VHF Ch 16 09 14 or ☎ (01945) 582125, HW –3 to HW. Take care when ships entering or leaving the berthing area. Hr Mr ☎ (01406) 351530 at Sutton Bridge, not H24.
Town P & D (cans), Bar, R, V, Gas.

BOSTON   10-5-10

Lincs 52°56'·00N 00°05'·00E (Tabs Head bn)

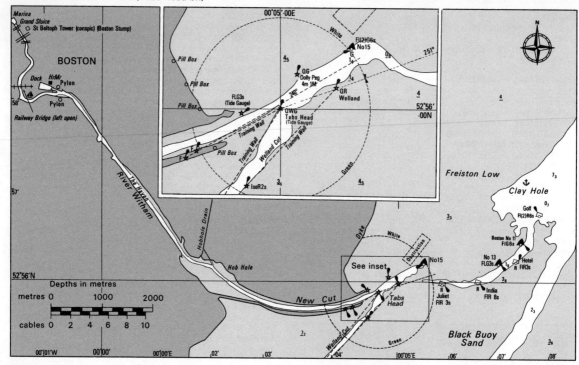

CHARTS
AC 1200, 108; Imray Y9; OS 131
TIDES
–0415 Dover; ML 3·3; Duration Flood 0500, Ebb 0700;
Zone 0 (UT)

Standard Port IMMINGHAM (→)

Times				Height (metres)			
High Water		Low Water		MHWS	MHWN	MLWN	MLWS
0100	0700	0100	0700	7·3	5·8	2·6	0·9
1300	1900	1300	1900				
Differences BOSTON							
0000	+0010	+0140	+0050	–0·5	–1·0	–0·9	–0·5
TABS HEAD (WELLAND RIVER)							
0000	+0005	+0125	+0020	+0·2	–0·2	–0·2	–0·2
SKEGNESS							
+0010	+0015	+0030	+0020	–0·4	–0·5	–0·1	0·0
INNER DOWSING LIGHT TOWER							
0000	0000	+0010	+0010	–0·9	–0·7	–0·1	+0·3

SHELTER
Very good, but berthing in the Dock is prohib except in
emergency. Yachts secure just above Dock ent and see
Hr Mr. The port is administered by Port of Boston Ltd.
Moorings may be possible (on S side) below first fixed
bridge.
Yachts which can lower masts should pass the Grand
Sluice lock into fresh water (24 hrs notice required); the
lock is 22·7m x 4·6m and opens approx HW±2. It leads
into the R Witham Navigation which goes 31M to
Lincoln. Marina is to stbd immediately beyond the sluice.
British Waterways have 50 moorings, with FW and AC,
beyond Grand Sluice.
NAVIGATION
WPT Boston Rds SWM lt buoy, L Fl 10s, 52°57'·53N
00°16'·23E, 100°/280° from/to Freeman Chan ent, 0·70M.
The chan is liable to change but is well marked. Tabs
Head marks the ent to the river, and should be passed
not earlier than HW–3 to enable the Grand Sluice to be
reached before the start of the ebb. On reaching Boston
Dock, masts should be lowered to negotiate swing bridge
(cannot always be opened) and three fixed bridges. Chan
through town is narrow and un-navigable at LW.

LIGHTS AND MARKS
St Boltoph's ch tr, (the Boston Stump) is conspic from
afar. New Cut and R Witham are marked by bns with
topmarks. FW lts mark ldg lines: six pairs going upstream
and six pairs going downstream.
RADIO TELEPHONE
Call: *Boston Dock* VHF Ch 12 11 16 (Mon-Fri 0700-1700LT
and HW –2½ to HW +1½). All boats between Golf buoy and
Grand Sluice must listen Ch 12. Call: *Grand Sluice* Ch 74.
TELEPHONE (01205)
Hr Mr 362328; MRCC (01493) 851338; Port Sig Stn 362328;
⌗ 363070; Lock Keeper 364864; Marinecall 0891 500455;
Police 366222; Ⓗ 364801.
FACILITIES
Boston Marina (50 + some visitors) ☎ 364420, £3.00, D
(cans), ACA, FW, CH, C in dock, see Hr Mr (emergency
only) Access HW±2; **Port of Boston** ☎ 366566, ME;
Services: El, ME, Sh, Gas.
Town EC Thurs; V, R, Bar, ⊠, Ⓑ, ⇌, ✈ (Humberside).

ADJACENT HARBOURS

RIVER WELLAND, Lincolnshire, 52°56'·00N 00°05'·00E
(Tabs Head bn). AC 1200, 1190. At Welland Cut HW –0440
on Dover; ML 0·3m; Duration 0520. See 10.5.10. At Tabs
Head bn HW ±3, ent Welland Cut which is defined by
training walls and lt bns. Beware sp flood of up to 5kn.
Berth 6M up, at Fosdyke on small quay 300m NE of
bridge on stbd side. Recommended for short stay only.
Very limited facilities.

WAINFLEET, Lincolnshire, 53°04'·77N 00°20'·00E (chan
ent). AC 108. Skegness HW +0500 on Dover. See 10.5.10
(Skegness). ML 4·0m; Duration 0600. Shelter good, but
emergency only. Drying chan starts close WSW of Inner
Knock PHM buoy. Swatchway buoyed but not lit; chan
through saltings marked by posts with radar reflectors
and lateral topmarks. Enter HW ±1½. No lts. Facilities: M,
AB (larger boats at fishing jetties, smaller at YC), FW at
Field Study Centre on stbd side of ent. All shore facilities
at Skegness (3½ miles), EC Thurs.

ENGLAND – IMMINGHAM

LAT 53°38′N   LONG   0°11′W

TIMES AND HEIGHTS OF HIGH AND LOW WATERS

YEAR **1996**

TIME ZONE (UT)
For Summer Time add ONE hour in non-shaded areas

5

JANUARY

	Time	m		Time	m
1 M	0206 0836 1447 2106	6.1 2.3 6.0 2.5	**16** TU	0043 0731 1349 2000	6.1 2.2 6.0 2.4
2 TU	0310 0933 1541 2203	6.2 2.2 6.3 2.2	**17** W	0213 0847 1500 2117	6.2 2.0 6.4 2.0
3 W	0405 1022 1628 2251	6.3 2.0 6.5 1.9	**18** TH	0327 0952 1558 2223	6.6 1.7 6.8 1.5
4 TH	0452 1105 1709 2334	6.5 1.9 6.7 1.6	**19** F	0429 1049 1650 2321	6.9 1.3 7.2 1.0
5 F O	0533 1145 1745	6.7 1.7 6.9	**20** SA	0524 1142 1738 ●	7.2 1.1 7.5
6 SA	0014 0610 1221 1818	1.4 6.7 1.7 7.0	**21** SU	0014 0614 1232 1824	0.6 7.5 0.9 7.7
7 SU	0051 0645 1254 1852	1.4 6.8 1.6 7.1	**22** M	0104 0703 1318 1909	0.4 7.5 0.8 7.8
8 M	0126 0720 1324 1925	1.4 6.8 1.6 7.1	**23** TU	0151 0750 1403 1954	0.3 7.5 0.9 7.8
9 TU	0159 0754 1353 1956	1.4 6.8 1.7 7.0	**24** W	0236 0835 1445 2038	0.4 7.3 1.1 7.6
10 W	0230 0827 1423 2026	1.5 6.7 1.7 6.9	**25** TH	0318 0920 1525 2122	0.7 7.0 1.4 7.2
11 TH	0259 0900 1457 2100	1.6 6.5 1.8 6.8	**26** F	0359 1005 1604 2208	1.1 6.6 1.7 6.8
12 F	0332 0937 1535 2140	1.7 6.4 1.9 6.7	**27** SA	0438 1053 1646 2300	1.6 6.2 2.1 6.3
13 SA	0413 1020 1621 2228	1.8 6.2 2.2 6.4	**28** SU	0522 1150 1736	2.1 5.9 2.5
14 SU	0505 1113 1717 2327	2.0 6.0 2.4 6.2	**29** M	0008 0615 1259 1840	5.9 2.5 5.7 2.8
15 M	0611 1222 1833	2.2 5.9 2.5	**30** TU	0128 0729 1406 2020	5.7 2.7 5.7 2.8
			31 W	0241 0856 1507 2139	5.8 2.6 6.0 2.5

FEBRUARY

	Time	m		Time	m
1 TH	0343 0955 1600 2230	6.0 2.4 6.3 2.1	**16** F	0321 0935 1541 2211	6.3 1.9 6.6 1.5
2 F	0433 1042 1644 2314	6.3 2.1 6.6 1.7	**17** SA	0425 1035 1636 2309	6.8 1.5 7.1 1.0
3 SA	0514 1123 1722 2355	6.5 1.8 6.8 1.5	**18** SU ●	0519 1128 1725	7.2 1.1 7.4
4 SU O	0550 1201 1757	6.7 1.7 7.0	**19** M	0001 0605 1217 1810	0.5 7.4 0.8 7.7
5 M	0033 0624 1236 1832	1.3 6.8 1.6 7.1	**20** TU	0049 0650 1302 1853	0.3 7.5 0.7 7.8
6 TU	0110 0659 1307 1905	1.2 6.9 1.5 7.1	**21** W	0133 0731 1345 1935	0.2 7.5 0.7 7.8
7 W	0143 0732 1336 1936	1.2 6.9 1.5 7.1	**22** TH	0214 0811 1424 2016	0.4 7.3 1.0 7.6
8 TH	0212 0803 1406 2006	1.3 6.9 1.5 7.1	**23** F	0252 0849 1500 2055	0.7 7.0 1.2 7.2
9 F	0239 0835 1439 2039	1.3 6.8 1.5 7.1	**24** SA	0326 0921 1534 2134	1.1 6.7 1.5 6.8
10 SA	0310 0909 1515 2117	1.4 6.7 1.6 6.9	**25** SU	0359 1000 1610 2216	1.6 6.3 1.9 6.3
11 SU	0346 0949 1556 2201	1.6 6.5 1.8 6.7	**26** M	0436 1044 1654 2312	2.1 5.9 2.4 5.8
12 M	0431 1037 1647 2257	1.9 6.2 2.1 6.3	**27** TU	0525 1152 1754	2.6 5.6 2.7
13 TU	0532 1139 1758	2.2 6.0 2.4	**28** W	0044 0629 1310 1910	5.5 2.9 5.5 2.8
14 W	0010 0655 1309 1932	6.0 2.4 5.9 2.4	**29** TH	0211 0754 1431 2107	5.5 2.9 5.7 2.6
15 TH	0156 0824 1436 2100	6.0 2.3 6.2 2.1			

MARCH

	Time	m		Time	m
1 F	0318 0923 1530 2204	5.8 2.6 6.1 2.2	**16** SA	0315 0921 1524 2158	6.3 2.0 6.5 1.4
2 SA	0410 1015 1616 2248	6.1 2.2 6.4 1.8	**17** SU	0417 1020 1620 2254	6.7 1.5 7.0 0.9
3 SU	0451 1058 1655 2329	6.4 1.9 6.7 1.4	**18** M	0507 1111 1708 2343	7.1 1.1 7.3 0.5
4 M	0526 1137 1732	6.7 1.7 7.0	**19** TU ●	0551 1158 1752	7.3 0.8 7.5
5 TU O	0008 0559 1213 1806	1.2 6.8 1.5 7.1	**20** W	0028 0630 1243 1834	0.4 7.4 0.7 7.6
6 W	0045 0633 1246 1840	1.1 6.9 1.4 7.2	**21** TH	0110 0708 1324 1915	0.4 7.4 0.7 7.6
7 TH	0119 0706 1316 1912	1.1 7.0 1.3 7.2	**22** F	0148 0743 1401 1953	0.5 7.2 0.8 7.4
8 F	0149 0738 1348 1945	1.1 7.0 1.2 7.3	**23** SA	0223 0816 1435 2030	0.8 7.0 1.1 7.1
9 SA	0218 0809 1423 2020	1.1 7.0 1.2 7.2	**24** SU	0254 0847 1507 2105	1.2 6.7 1.4 6.7
10 SU	0250 0845 1459 2059	1.2 6.9 1.4 7.0	**25** M	0324 0918 1541 2142	1.6 6.4 1.7 6.2
11 M	0326 0925 1540 2144	1.5 6.7 1.6 6.7	**26** TU	0359 0955 1623 2230	2.1 6.0 2.2 5.8
12 TU	0411 1012 1631 2241	1.8 6.3 1.9 6.3	**27** W	0445 1049 1720 2351	2.5 5.7 2.5 5.4
13 W	0510 1113 1743 2358	2.2 6.0 2.2 5.9	**28** TH	0548 1224 1832	2.9 5.4 2.7
14 TH	0634 1243 1918	2.5 5.9 2.3	**29** F	0132 0705 1349 1958	5.4 3.0 5.6 2.6
15 F	0154 0807 1416 2049	5.9 2.4 6.1 2.0	**30** SA	0244 0824 1452 2121	5.6 2.8 5.9 2.2
			31 SU	0338 0936 1541 2211	6.0 2.4 6.3 1.8

APRIL

	Time	m		Time	m
1 M	0420 1024 1623 2255	6.4 2.0 6.6 1.5	**16** TU	0447 1051 1647 2320	7.0 1.2 7.1 0.7
2 TU	0456 1105 1701 2336	6.7 1.7 6.9 1.2	**17** W ●	0528 1137 1733	7.2 0.9 7.3
3 W	0531 1143 1737	6.9 1.5 7.1	**18** TH	0004 0606 1221 1815	0.6 7.2 0.8 7.3
4 TH O	0014 0605 1220 1813	1.0 7.0 1.3 7.2	**19** F	0045 0642 1302 1855	0.7 7.2 0.8 7.3
5 F	0050 0638 1255 1848	1.0 7.1 1.1 7.3	**20** SA	0122 0716 1339 1933	0.8 7.1 0.9 7.1
6 SA	0124 0712 1332 1925	0.9 7.2 1.0 7.3	**21** SU	0155 0747 1412 2008	1.1 7.0 1.1 6.9
7 SU	0158 0747 1410 2004	1.0 7.1 1.0 7.2	**22** M	0225 0817 1444 2042	1.3 6.8 1.3 6.6
8 M	0234 0825 1450 2048	1.1 7.0 1.2 7.0	**23** TU	0256 0848 1518 2118	1.7 6.5 1.6 6.2
9 TU	0314 0908 1535 2137	1.4 6.8 1.4 6.7	**24** W	0329 0924 1559 2202	2.0 6.2 2.0 5.8
10 W	0401 0957 1630 2237	1.8 6.4 1.7 6.2	**25** TH	0411 1010 1651 2305	2.4 5.8 2.3 5.5
11 TH	0501 1101 1741	2.2 6.1 2.0	**26** F	0507 1122 1758	2.8 5.5 2.5
12 F	0003 0621 1229 1908	5.9 2.6 6.0 2.0	**27** SA	0036 0620 1254 1911	5.4 2.9 5.5 2.5
13 SA	0147 0750 1356 2034	6.0 2.4 6.1 1.7	**28** SU	0154 0736 1402 2023	5.5 2.8 5.7 2.2
14 SU	0259 0901 1502 2138	6.3 2.0 6.5 1.3	**29** M	0253 0844 1457 2124	5.9 2.5 6.1 1.9
15 M	0358 0959 1558 2232	6.7 1.6 6.8 1.0	**30** TU	0340 0939 1543 2214	6.2 2.1 6.4 1.5

Chart Datum: 3·90 metres below Ordnance Datum (Newlyn)

ENGLAND – IMMINGHAM

LAT 53°38′N   LONG 0°11′W

TIMES AND HEIGHTS OF HIGH AND LOW WATERS

YEAR 1996

TIME ZONE (UT)
For Summer Time add ONE hour in non-shaded areas

MAY

Day	Time	m	Time	m	Time	m	Time	m
1 W	0420	6.6	1027	1.8	1625	6.7	2259	1.2
16 TH	0502	6.9	1116	1.2	1713	7.0	2339	1.0
2 TH	0459	6.8	1111	1.5	1706	7.0	2341	1.0
17 F ●	0541	7.0	1200	1.0	1756	7.0		
3 F ○	0536	7.1	1153	1.2	1746	7.2		
18 SA	0020	1.1	0618	7.0	1241	1.0	1837	7.0
4 SA	0021	0.9	0612	7.2	1235	1.0	1827	7.3
19 SU	0057	1.2	0652	7.0	1319	1.0	1915	6.9
5 SU	0101	0.9	0650	7.3	1317	0.9	1909	7.4
20 M	0130	1.3	0724	6.9	1353	1.2	1950	6.7
6 M	0141	0.9	0729	7.3	1400	0.9	1954	7.3
21 TU	0201	1.5	0755	6.8	1426	1.3	2024	6.5
7 TU	0222	1.1	0812	7.2	1446	0.9	2043	7.0
22 W	0233	1.7	0828	6.6	1501	1.5	2100	6.3
8 W	0306	1.3	0858	6.9	1535	1.2	2136	6.7
23 TH	0305	1.9	0903	6.3	1539	1.8	2140	6.0
9 TH	0356	1.7	0950	6.6	1631	1.4	2239	6.3
24 F	0342	2.2	0943	6.1	1625	2.0	2229	5.8
10 F	0454	2.0	1054	6.3	1737	1.7		
25 SA	0429	2.5	1034	5.8	1721	2.2	2333	5.6
11 SA	0003	6.1	0605	2.3	1213	6.2	1853	1.7
26 SU	0529	2.7	1144	5.7	1826	2.3		
12 SU	0125	6.1	0724	2.3	1331	6.2	2009	1.6
27 M	0049	5.6	0640	2.8	1301	5.7	1932	2.2
13 M	0232	6.3	0835	2.0	1436	6.4	2112	1.4
28 TU	0157	5.8	0750	2.6	1404	6.0	2034	2.0
14 TU	0330	6.5	0935	1.7	1534	6.6	2206	1.2
29 W	0253	6.1	0852	2.3	1500	6.3	2131	1.6
15 W	0419	6.8	1027	1.4	1626	6.8	2255	1.1
30 TH	0342	6.5	0948	1.9	1550	6.6	2222	1.4
31 F	0426	6.8	1040	1.5	1637	6.9	2310	1.1

JUNE

Day	Time	m	Time	m	Time	m	Time	m
1 SA ○	0508	7.1	1129	1.2	1724	7.2	2356	0.9
16 SU ●	0555	6.9	1223	1.2	1820	6.7		
2 SU	0550	7.3	1217	0.9	1811	7.3		
17 M	0035	1.4	0631	6.9	1302	1.2	1857	6.7
3 M	0041	0.8	0632	7.4	1305	0.7	1858	7.4
18 TU	0110	1.5	0704	6.9	1338	1.2	1932	6.7
4 TU	0126	0.8	0716	7.5	1353	0.6	1947	7.3
19 W	0142	1.5	0738	6.8	1412	1.3	2006	6.6
5 W	0212	0.9	0802	7.4	1442	0.7	2039	7.1
20 TH	0214	1.6	0811	6.7	1447	1.5	2041	6.4
6 TH	0258	1.1	0850	7.2	1532	0.8	2133	6.9
21 F	0245	1.8	0844	6.6	1521	1.6	2117	6.3
7 F	0348	1.4	0943	6.9	1625	1.1	2235	6.6
22 SA	0317	2.0	0920	6.4	1558	1.8	2157	6.1
8 SA	0442	1.8	1043	6.6	1723	1.3	2345	6.3
23 SU	0355	2.2	1000	6.2	1640	2.0	2244	5.9
9 SU	0542	2.1	1149	6.4	1828	1.6		
24 M	0442	2.4	1049	6.0	1734	2.1	2342	5.8
10 M	0054	6.2	0651	2.2	1302	6.3	1938	1.7
25 TU	0542	2.5	1151	5.9	1839	2.2		
11 TU	0158	6.2	0803	2.2	1408	6.3	2042	1.7
26 W	0054	5.8	0654	2.6	1305	6.0	1947	2.1
12 W	0256	6.3	0908	2.0	1509	6.4	2139	1.6
27 TH	0205	6.0	0806	2.4	1417	6.2	2052	1.8
13 TH	0349	6.5	1004	1.7	1605	6.5	2229	1.5
28 F	0305	6.3	0913	2.0	1520	6.5	2151	1.5
14 F	0436	6.6	1055	1.5	1654	6.6	2315	1.3
29 SA	0357	6.6	1014	1.6	1616	6.8	2245	1.2
15 SA	0517	6.8	1141	1.3	1739	6.7	2357	1.4
30 SU	0446	7.1	1110	1.2	1710	7.1	2336	1.0

JULY

Day	Time	m	Time	m	Time	m	Time	m
1 M ○	0532	7.4	1203	0.8	1801	7.3		
16 TU	0015	1.6	0609	6.9	1245	1.3	1838	6.7
2 TU	0025	0.8	0618	7.6	1255	0.6	1850	7.4
17 W	0051	1.5	0644	7.0	1322	1.3	1912	6.7
3 W	0114	0.7	0704	7.7	1345	0.4	1940	7.4
18 TH	0125	1.5	0719	7.0	1357	1.3	1945	6.7
4 TH	0200	0.8	0751	7.6	1433	0.4	2031	7.3
19 F	0155	1.6	0752	6.9	1430	1.4	2019	6.7
5 F	0247	0.9	0839	7.5	1521	0.6	2122	7.1
20 SA	0224	1.6	0824	6.8	1500	1.5	2052	6.6
6 SA	0333	1.2	0929	7.2	1610	0.8	2216	6.8
21 SU	0254	1.7	0856	6.7	1529	1.6	2126	6.4
7 SU	0421	1.5	1023	6.9	1659	1.2	2315	6.5
22 M	0327	1.9	0931	6.5	1601	1.8	2205	6.3
8 M	0512	1.9	1123	6.5	1754	1.6		
23 TU	0407	2.1	1013	6.4	1644	2.0	2253	6.1
9 TU	0017	6.2	0610	2.2	1230	6.2	1857	2.0
24 W	0458	2.3	1107	6.2	1744	2.1	2355	5.9
10 W	0120	6.0	0722	2.4	1338	6.1	2008	2.1
25 TH	0605	2.5	1216	6.0	1901	2.2		
11 TH	0221	6.0	0839	2.3	1444	6.1	2111	2.1
26 F	0117	6.0	0727	2.4	1342	6.1	2019	2.1
12 F	0318	6.2	0943	2.1	1544	6.2	2206	2.0
27 SA	0233	6.2	0846	2.2	1501	6.3	2127	1.8
13 SA	0409	6.4	1036	1.8	1637	6.4	2253	1.8
28 SU	0335	6.6	0955	1.7	1605	6.7	2226	1.4
14 SU	0453	6.6	1123	1.6	1722	6.5	2336	1.7
29 M	0428	7.0	1057	1.2	1702	7.1	2320	1.1
15 M ●	0533	6.8	1206	1.4	1802	6.6		
30 TU ○	0517	7.4	1152	0.7	1754	7.4		
31 W	0011	0.8	0604	7.7	1243	0.4	1842	7.5

AUGUST

Day	Time	m	Time	m	Time	m	Time	m
1 TH	0059	0.7	0650	7.8	1332	0.2	1929	7.6
16 F	0104	1.5	0656	7.1	1336	1.2	1921	6.9
2 F	0146	0.6	0736	7.8	1418	0.2	2016	7.4
17 SA	0134	1.5	0729	7.1	1408	1.3	1953	6.9
3 SA	0230	0.8	0823	7.7	1503	0.4	2101	7.2
18 SU	0202	1.5	0800	7.0	1435	1.4	2024	6.8
4 SU	0313	1.0	0909	7.4	1545	0.8	2148	6.9
19 M	0230	1.6	0831	6.9	1500	1.5	2056	6.7
5 M	0355	1.4	0957	7.0	1628	1.3	2237	6.5
20 TU	0303	1.7	0905	6.8	1529	1.6	2132	6.5
6 TU	0438	1.8	1050	6.6	1712	1.9	2333	6.1
21 W	0341	1.8	0946	6.6	1608	1.9	2217	6.3
7 W	0527	2.3	1154	6.1	1804	2.3		
22 TH	0428	2.1	1036	6.3	1702	2.2	2314	6.0
8 TH	0038	5.9	0628	2.6	1308	5.8	1918	2.6
23 F	0532	2.4	1145	6.0	1822	2.4		
9 F	0144	5.8	0805	2.7	1419	5.8	2043	2.6
24 SA	0036	5.9	0659	2.5	1323	5.9	1954	2.4
10 SA	0247	6.0	0923	2.4	1523	6.0	2143	2.4
25 SU	0209	6.1	0827	2.2	1453	6.2	2109	2.0
11 SU	0342	6.3	1017	2.1	1618	6.2	2232	2.1
26 M	0317	6.6	0943	1.7	1600	6.7	2211	1.6
12 M	0429	6.6	1103	1.7	1703	6.3	2315	1.8
27 TU	0413	7.0	1044	1.1	1655	7.1	2305	1.2
13 TU	0509	6.8	1145	1.4	1740	6.7	2354	1.6
28 W ○	0502	7.5	1138	0.7	1744	7.4	2355	0.8
14 W ●	0546	7.0	1227	1.3	1815	6.8		
29 TH	0549	7.8	1227	0.3	1829	7.6		
15 TH	0030	1.5	0621	7.1	1301	1.2	1848	6.9
30 F	0042	0.6	0633	7.9	1313	0.2	1911	7.6
31 SA	0127	0.6	0717	7.9	1357	0.3	1953	7.5

Chart Datum: 3·90 metres below Ordnance Datum (Newlyn)

ENGLAND – IMMINGHAM

LAT 53°38′N   LONG 0°11′W

TIMES AND HEIGHTS OF HIGH AND LOW WATERS

YEAR **1996**

TIME ZONE (UT)
For Summer Time add ONE hour in non-shaded areas

SEPTEMBER

Day	Time	m	Time	m	Time	m	Time	m
1 SU	0209	0.7	0801	7.7	1437	0.6	2033	7.2
16 M	0138	1.4	0734	7.2	1407	1.3	1955	7.0
2 M	0249	1.0	0844	7.4	1515	1.0	2112	6.9
17 TU	0208	1.4	0807	7.1	1434	1.4	2027	6.9
3 TU	0326	1.4	0928	7.0	1551	1.5	2152	6.5
18 W	0242	1.5	0843	7.0	1506	1.6	2104	6.7
4 W	0404	1.8	1015	6.5	1628	2.0	2239	6.1
19 TH	0321	1.7	0925	6.7	1545	1.9	2149	6.4
5 TH	0447	2.3	1114	6.0	1713	2.5	2346	5.8
20 F	0409	2.0	1018	6.3	1638	2.3	2245	6.1
6 F	0543	2.7	1234	5.6	1816	2.9		
21 SA	0514	2.3	1130	6.0	1757	2.6		
7 SA	0105	5.7	0700	2.8	1352	5.6	1957	3.0
22 SU	0008	5.9	0643	2.4	1319	5.9	1935	2.6
8 SU	0214	5.8	0858	2.6	1458	5.8	2116	2.7
23 M	0148	6.1	0815	2.2	1445	6.3	2052	2.2
9 M	0313	6.2	0953	2.2	1554	6.2	2206	2.3
24 TU	0258	6.6	0929	1.6	1549	6.7	2154	1.7
10 TU	0402	6.5	1037	1.8	1631	6.5	2249	1.9
25 W	0355	7.0	1028	1.1	1641	7.1	2247	1.2
11 W	0442	6.8	1117	1.5	1714	6.7	2328	1.7
26 TH	0444	7.4	1119	0.7	1727	7.4	2335	0.9
12 TH ●	0519	7.1	1156	1.3	1748	6.9		
27 F ○	0530	7.7	1206	0.5	1809	7.5		
13 F	0004	1.5	0554	7.2	1234	1.2	1820	7.0
28 SA	0021	0.7	0613	7.8	1250	0.4	1848	7.6
14 SA	0038	1.4	0629	7.2	1309	1.2	1853	7.0
29 SU	0105	0.6	0656	7.8	1331	0.5	1925	7.4
15 SU	0109	1.4	0702	7.2	1340	1.2	1924	7.0
30 M	0145	0.8	0738	7.6	1409	0.8	2002	7.2

OCTOBER

Day	Time	m	Time	m	Time	m	Time	m
1 TU	0223	1.0	0819	7.3	1443	1.2	2036	6.9
16 W	0150	1.3	0747	7.2	1413	1.4	2004	7.1
2 W	0258	1.4	0859	6.9	1514	1.7	2110	6.6
17 TH	0228	1.4	0827	7.0	1449	1.6	2044	6.9
3 TH	0332	1.8	0941	6.4	1547	2.1	2148	6.2
18 F	0310	1.6	0914	6.7	1531	1.9	2130	6.6
4 F	0413	2.2	1034	5.9	1628	2.6	2244	5.8
19 SA	0401	1.9	1025	6.3	1625	2.3	2228	6.3
5 SA	0506	2.6	1151	5.6	1728	3.0		
20 SU	0508	2.2	1125	6.0	1741	2.6	2348	6.1
6 SU	0014	5.6	0617	2.8	1316	5.5	1849	3.1
21 M	0631	2.2	1309	6.0	1913	2.6		
7 M	0135	5.7	0757	2.7	1425	5.7	2026	2.9
22 TU	0123	6.2	0758	2.0	1426	6.2	2030	2.3
8 TU	0238	6.0	0914	2.3	1521	6.1	2129	2.5
23 W	0234	6.5	0909	1.6	1528	6.7	2132	1.8
9 W	0328	6.4	1000	1.9	1606	6.4	2214	2.1
24 TH	0332	6.9	1006	1.2	1620	7.0	2225	1.4
10 TH	0410	6.8	1042	1.6	1643	6.7	2254	1.8
25 F	0422	7.3	1056	0.9	1704	7.3	2314	1.1
11 F	0448	7.0	1122	1.3	1717	6.9	2332	1.5
26 SA ○	0509	7.5	1142	0.7	1745	7.4	2359	0.9
12 SA ●	0524	7.2	1200	1.2	1751	7.1		
27 SU	0553	7.6	1206	0.7	1823	7.4		
13 SU	0007	1.4	0559	7.3	1237	1.2	1824	7.2
28 M	0042	0.8	0635	7.5	1305	0.9	1859	7.3
14 M	0041	1.3	0635	7.3	1309	1.2	1856	7.2
29 TU	0122	0.9	0716	7.4	1341	1.1	1933	7.2
15 TU	0115	1.3	0710	7.3	1340	1.2	1929	7.2
30 W	0159	1.1	0756	7.1	1413	1.4	2005	7.0
31 TH	0232	1.4	0834	6.8	1442	1.7	2037	6.7

NOVEMBER

Day	Time	m	Time	m	Time	m	Time	m
1 F	0306	1.7	0913	6.4	1513	2.1	2112	6.4
16 SA	0306	1.4	0909	6.8	1523	1.8	2119	6.8
2 SA	0345	2.0	0959	6.0	1551	2.5	2157	6.0
17 SU	0359	1.6	1007	6.5	1617	2.1	2216	6.6
3 SU	0435	2.4	1100	5.7	1643	2.9	2308	5.7
18 M	0501	1.8	1119	6.2	1723	2.4	2329	6.3
4 M	0540	2.6	1221	5.5	1755	3.1		
19 TU	0614	2.0	1245	6.1	1844	2.5		
5 TU	0036	5.7	0653	2.7	1336	5.6	1916	3.0
20 W	0053	6.3	0733	1.9	1357	6.3	2000	2.3
6 W	0148	5.9	0808	2.4	1436	5.9	2029	2.7
21 TH	0205	6.5	0842	1.7	1458	6.5	2106	2.0
7 TH	0244	6.2	0909	2.1	1525	6.3	2127	2.4
22 F	0306	6.7	0939	1.4	1552	6.8	2202	1.6
8 F	0331	6.5	0959	1.8	1607	6.6	2214	2.0
23 SA	0400	7.0	1030	1.3	1639	7.0	2252	1.3
9 SA	0412	6.8	1043	1.5	1644	6.9	2256	1.7
24 SU	0449	7.2	1117	1.2	1720	7.1	2339	1.1
10 SU	0452	7.1	1125	1.3	1720	7.1	2336	1.4
25 M ○	0535	7.2	1200	1.1	1759	7.2		
11 M ●	0531	7.2	1203	1.2	1756	7.2		
26 TU	0022	1.0	0618	7.2	1240	1.2	1835	7.2
12 TU	0015	1.3	0610	7.3	1241	1.1	1831	7.3
27 W	0102	1.1	0658	7.1	1315	1.4	1909	7.1
13 W	0055	1.1	0650	7.4	1318	1.2	1908	7.3
28 TH	0139	1.2	0737	7.0	1347	1.5	1941	7.0
14 TH	0136	1.1	0732	7.3	1356	1.3	1947	7.3
29 F	0212	1.4	0813	6.7	1416	1.7	2013	6.8
15 F	0219	1.2	0818	7.1	1437	1.5	2030	7.1
30 SA	0246	1.6	0850	6.5	1447	2.0	2047	6.6

DECEMBER

Day	Time	m	Time	m	Time	m	Time	m
1 SU	0323	1.8	0929	6.2	1521	2.2	2125	6.3
16 M	0352	1.2	0958	6.7	1604	1.8	2203	6.9
2 M	0406	2.1	1016	5.9	1602	2.5	2213	6.1
17 TU	0447	1.5	1101	6.5	1701	2.1	2306	6.6
3 TU	0500	2.4	1115	5.7	1656	2.8	2319	5.8
18 W	0548	1.7	1212	6.3	1807	2.4		
4 W	0603	2.5	1226	5.6	1809	3.0		
19 TH	0019	6.4	0658	1.9	1320	6.2	1923	2.4
5 TH	0038	5.8	0710	2.5	1335	5.8	1925	2.9
20 F	0133	6.4	0809	1.9	1423	6.3	2036	2.3
6 F	0147	6.0	0814	2.3	1434	6.0	2031	2.6
21 SA	0239	6.4	0911	1.8	1521	6.4	2138	2.0
7 SA	0244	6.2	0912	2.0	1525	6.4	2129	2.2
22 SU	0339	6.6	1006	1.7	1612	6.6	2232	1.7
8 SU	0334	6.6	1003	1.7	1610	6.7	2220	1.9
23 M	0432	6.7	1054	1.6	1658	6.8	2321	1.4
9 M	0421	6.9	1049	1.4	1651	7.0	2308	1.5
24 TU ○	0520	6.9	1139	1.5	1738	7.0		
10 TU ●	0506	7.1	1134	1.2	1731	7.3	2354	1.2
25 W	0005	1.3	0603	6.9	1219	1.5	1815	7.1
11 W	0551	7.3	1217	1.1	1811	7.4		
26 TH	0046	1.2	0642	6.9	1255	1.5	1850	7.1
12 TH	0039	1.0	0636	7.4	1300	1.1	1852	7.5
27 F	0123	1.2	0719	6.9	1327	1.6	1923	7.1
13 F	0126	0.9	0722	7.4	1344	1.1	1935	7.5
28 SA	0157	1.3	0754	6.8	1357	1.7	1955	7.0
14 SA	0213	0.9	0811	7.2	1428	1.3	2020	7.4
29 SU	0230	1.4	0827	6.6	1426	1.8	2027	6.8
15 SU	0301	1.0	0902	7.0	1514	1.5	2109	7.2
30 M	0303	1.6	0902	6.4	1456	2.0	2100	6.6
31 TU	0338	1.8	0939	6.2	1529	2.2	2135	6.4

Chart Datum: 3·90 metres below Ordnance Datum (Newlyn)

5

RIVER HUMBER   10-5-11

Humberside 53°35'·10N 00°03'·87W (Grimsby)
53°44'·22N 00°20'·60W (Hull marina)

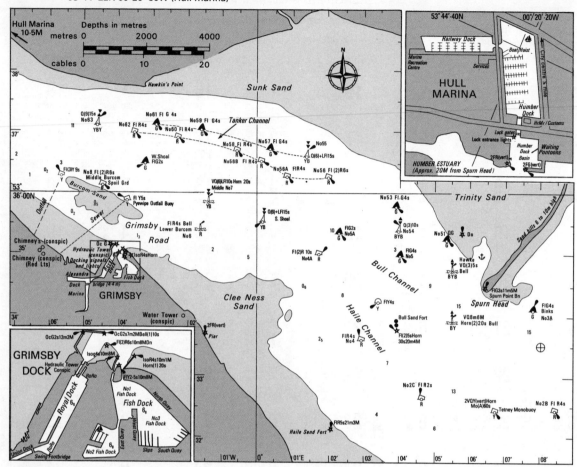

CHARTS

AC *109*, 3497, 1188, *1190*; Imray C29; OS 107; ABP (local)

TIDES

−0510 Immingham, −0452 Hull, Dover; ML 4·1; Duration
0555; Zone 0 (UT)

Standard Port IMMINGHAM (←)

Times				Height (metres)			
High Water		Low Water		MHWS	MHWN	MLWN	MLWS
0100	0700	0100	0700	7·3	5·8	2·6	0·9
1300	1900	1300	1900				
Differences BULL SAND FORT							
−0020	−0030	−0035	−0015	−0·4	−0·3	+0·1	+0·2
GRIMSBY							
−0003	−0011	−0015	−0002	−0·3	−0·2	0·0	+0·1
HULL (ALBERT DOCK)							
+0019	+0019	+0033	+0027	+0·3	+0·1	−0·1	−0·2
HUMBER BRIDGE							
+0024	+0022	+0047	+0036	−0·1	−0·4	−0·7	−0·7
BURTON STATHER (R. Trent)*							
+0105	+0045	+0335	+0305	−2·1	−2·3	−2·3	Dries
KEADBY (R. Trent)*							
+0135	+0120	+0425	+0410	−2·5	−2·8	Dries	Dries
BLACKTOFT (R. Ouse)†							
+0100	+0055	+0325	+0255	−1·6	−1·8	−2·2	−1·1
GOOLE (R. Ouse)†							
+0130	+0115	+0355	+0350	−1·6	−2·1	−1·9	−0·6

NOTE: Daily predictions for Immingham are given above.

---

* Normal river level at Burton Stather is about 0·1m below
  CD, and at Keadby 0·1m to 0·2m below CD.

† Heights of LW can increase by up to 0·3m at Blacktoft
  and 0·6m at Goole when river in spate. HW heights are
  little affected.

SHELTER

R Humber is the estuary of R Ouse and R Trent. Yachts
can ‡ inside Spurn Hd, except in strong SW/NW winds.
ABP is the Authority for the Humber and owns the ports
of Hull, Grimsby, Immingham and Goole. Immingham
should be used by yachts only in emergency. If unable to
reach Hull on the tide, in S to W winds there is a good ‡
off the SW bank 8ca above Killingholme Oil jetty, well
clear of main chan

The **marinas** at Grimsby, Hull, S Ferriby and the docks at
Goole are all entered by lock, access HW±3. S Ferriby
should not be attempted without up-to-date ABP charts
which cover the ever-changing buoyed chan above Hull.
Entry to Winteringham (HW±½) and Brough Havens
(HW±1) should not be attempted without first contacting
Humber Yawl Club for up-to-date appr chan details and
mooring availability. Bad silting has been reported at
Winteringham; both havens dry to soft mud.

NAVIGATION

WPT 53°33'·50N 00°08'·00E, 095°/275° from/to Bull Sand
Fort, 2·3M. From the S, make for Rosse Spit PHM buoy,
then keep N of the Haile Sand buoys via Haile Chan.

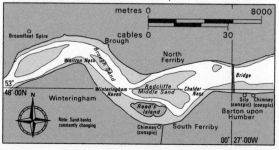

RIVER HUMBER *continued*

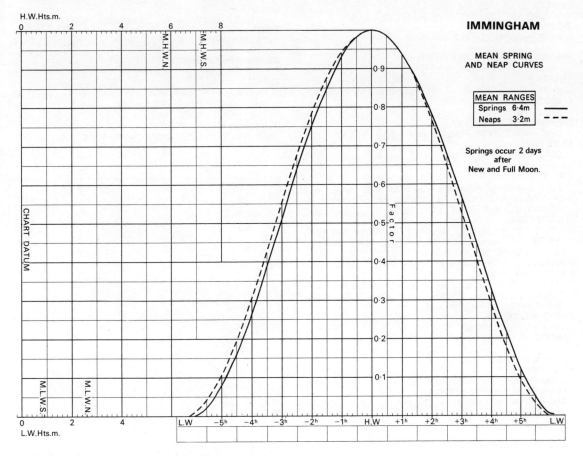

H.W.Hts.m.

IMMINGHAM

MEAN SPRING
AND NEAP CURVES

MEAN RANGES	
Springs 6·4m	——
Neaps 3·2m	- - -

Springs occur 2 days
after
New and Full Moon.

5

CHART DATUM

M.H.W.N.   M.H.W.S.

M.L.W.S.   M.L.W.N.

Factor

L.W.   −5ʰ   −4ʰ   −3ʰ   −2ʰ   −1ʰ   H.W.   +1ʰ   +2ʰ   +3ʰ   +4ʰ   +5ʰ   L.W.

L.W.Hts.m.

From the N, make good Spurn Lt Float to keep clear of the Binks; then enter the estuary to the S of the Chequers buoys and Spurn Head for Hawke or Bull Chans.
The Humber is a busy commercial waterway best entered at LW. Sp tides are fierce; 4·4kn ebb off Spurn Head and Immingham. Off R Hull there is a tidal eddy and streams can be rotatory, ie the flood makes W up Hull Roads for ¾hr whilst the ebb is already running down-river over Skitter Sand on the opposite bank (reaches 2½kn at springs). Humber bridge has 30m clearance.

LIGHTS AND MARKS
The Humber is well buoyed/lit for its whole length. At Grimsby a conspic tr (94m) marks ent to Royal Dock. IPTS control entry to Grimsby (shown W of ent to Royal Dock), Immingham, Killingholme, Hull and Goole.

RADIO TELEPHONE
Keep listening watch on Ch **12** 16 *VTS Humber* (located at Queen Elizabeth Dock, Hull ☎ (01482) 701787) for tfc movements, nav, wx and safety info; also tidal data on request. The VTS covers the R Humber, Ouse and Trent. VTS broadcasts weather (inc vis reports), nav and tidal info every odd H+03 on Ch 12.
Other VHF stns or destinations:
Grimsby Docks Radio Ch 74 (H24) 18 79. Marina Ch 09 18.
Immingham Docks Radio Ch 19 68 (H24).
R Hull Port Ops Service call *Drypool Radio* Ch 22 11 (Ch 22: Mon-Fri HW−2 to HW+1; Sat 0900-1100 LT).
Hull Marina, Ch M 80 (0700-2200); Albert Dock Ch 09.
S Ferriby Marina and Humber YC, Ch 80 (0930-1700).
Goole Docks Radio Ch 14 (H24) 09 19. Boothferry Bridge Ch 09 (H24). Selby Railway and Toll Bridges Ch 09.

TELEPHONE (Grimsby 01472; Hull 01482)
GRIMSBY Port Mgr 359181; ⌗ (01469) 574748; MRSC (01262) 672317; Marinecall 0891 500454; Police 59171; Ⓗ 74111.
HULL Hr Mr 783538; Lock 215357; MRSC (01262) 672317; ⌗ 782107; Marinecall 0891 500454; Police 26111; Dr contact Humber VTS 701787.

FACILITIES
GRIMSBY
Grimsby Marina (150+25 visitors) ☎ 360404, D, P (cans), FW, ME, AC, Gas, Gaz, El, Sh, BH (30 ton), R, CH, Bar, (access HW±3 via Royal Dock and Union Dock, but fixed bridge clearance is only 4·45m; marina is just off the SW corner of chartlet).
The **Fish Docks** are entered by lock 300m E of conspic tr. Access is HW±3, with R/G tfc lts, but yachts should enter HW±2, "on the level", after being cleared in by *Fish Dock Island* Ch 74.
No 2 Fish Dock: marina,100 berths + 20 visitors on pontoon along the W quay, £8 inc AC. Contact Humber Cruising Association ☎ (01472) 268424; usual facilities.
Grimsby and Cleethorpes YC ☎ 356678, Bar, R, M, FW, Ⓞ; **Town** EC Thurs; all facilities, ACA.
HULL
Hull Marina, ent at 53°44'·22N 00°20'·07W, (310 + 20 visitors) ☎ 593451; £12, access HW±3 via lock, (waiting pontoon to be installed); (open 0800-1800 LT weekdays; 0700-2200 LT Fri, Sat, Sun); P, D, FW, AC, CH, BH (50 ton), C (2 ton), Gas, ⌗, ME, El, Sh, Slip, Ⓞ, SM, ACA.
SOUTH FERRIBY
Marina (100+20 visitors) ☎ (01652) 635620; access HW±3, £8 inc lock fee, D, P (cans), FW, ME, El, Sh, C (30 ton), CH, Gas, Gaz. **Village** V, Bar.
WINTERINGHAM HAVEN (belongs to Humber Yawl Club) ☎ (01724) 734452, ✉.
BROUGH HAVEN
Humber Yawl Club ☎ (01482) 667224, Slip, FW, Bar, limited AB; contact club.
NABURN (R Ouse, 4M S of York and 80M above Spurn Pt).
Naburn Marina (450+50 visitors) ☎ (01904) 621021; £5.00; VHF Ch **80** M; CH, P, D, FW, AC, Sh, ME, BH (16 ton), R.

BRIDLINGTON   10-5-12

Humberside 54°04'·77N 00°11'·12W

CHARTS
AC 1882, 121, 129, 1191, *1190*; Imray C29; OS 101
TIDES
+0553 Dover; ML 3·6; Duration 0610; Zone 0 (UT)

Standard Port RIVER TEES ENT. (→)

Times				Height (metres)			
High Water		Low Water		MHWS	MHWN	MLWN	MLWS
0000	0600	0000	0600	5·5	4·3	2·0	0·9
1200	1800	1200	1800				
Differences BRIDLINGTON							
+0100	+0050	+0055	+0050	+0·6	+0·4	+0·3	+0·2
FILEY BAY							
+0042	+0042	+0047	+0034	+0·3	+0·6	+0·4	+0·1

SHELTER
Good, except in E, SE and S winds. Hbr dries, available from HW±3 (for draft of 2·7m). Visitors normally berth on S pier or near Hr Mr's Office.
NAVIGATION
WPT SW Smithic WCM, Q (9) 15s, 54°02'·41N 00°09'·10W, 153°/333° from/to ent, 2·6M. Close-in appr is with N pier hd lt on brg 002° to keep W of drying patch (The Canch). Beware bar, 1m at MLWN, could dry out at MLWS.
LIGHTS AND MARKS
Hbr is 4M WSW of Flamborough Hd lt, Fl (4) 15s 65m 24M. Tidal sigs from S pier: FG (No sig by day) = < 2·7m in hbr; FR (R flag by day) = >2·7m in hbr.
RADIO TELEPHONE
VHF Ch **12** 16 14 (occas).
TELEPHONE (01262)
Hr Mr 670148; CG 672317; MRSC 672317; ⌘ (01947) 602074; Marinecall 0891 500454; Police 672222; Ⓗ 673451.
FACILITIES
S Pier FW, C (5 ton), C, Slip; See Hr Mr for M, AB £8.23 to £9.96; **Royal Yorks YC** ☎ 672041, L, FW, R, Bar;
Town EC Thurs; P & D (cans), CH, ME, El, V, R, Bar, ✉, Ⓑ, ⇌, ✈ (Humberside).

ADJACENT ANCHORAGE

FILEY, N Yorkshire, 54°12'·80N 00°16'·10W, AC 1882, 129. HW +0532 on Dover; ML 3·5m; Duration 0605. See 10.5.12. Good ⚓ in winds from S to NNE in 4 – 5m on hard sand. Lt on cliff above CG Stn, G metal column, FR 31m 1M vis 272°-308°. The natural bkwtr, Filey Brigg marked by ECM buoy, Q(3)10s, Bell. Beware Horse Rk, N of Filey Brigg, foul ground extending ½M from shore. Facilities EC Wed; V, R, Bar, L, Ⓗ ☎ (01723) 68111, ✉, Ⓑ, ⇌.

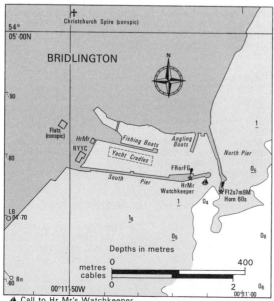

▲ Call to Hr Mr's Watchkeeper

SCARBOROUGH   10-5-13

N. Yorkshire 54°16'·87N 00°23'·28W

CHARTS
AC 1612, 129, 1191; Imray C29; OS 101
TIDES
+0527 Dover; ML 3·5; Duration 0615; Zone 0 (UT)

Standard Port RIVER TEES ENT. (→)

Times				Height (metres)			
High Water		Low Water		MHWS	MHWN	MLWN	MLWS
0000	0600	0000	0600	5·5	4·3	2·0	0·9
1200	1800	1200	1800				
Differences SCARBOROUGH							
+0040	+0040	+0030	+0030	+0·2	+0·3	+0·3	0·0

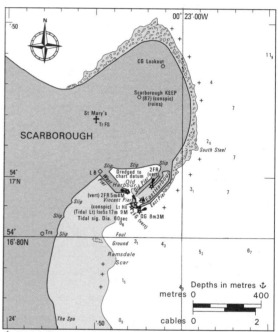

▲ Contact Watchman on duty at Lt Ho

SHELTER
Good in E hbr, access HW±3 via narrow ent by E pier, but not in strong E/SE winds. Ⓥ drying berths on Old Pier just N of Lt Ho, by the bridge. The Old Hbr is strictly for FVs.
NAVIGATION
WPT 54°16'·50N 00°22'·00W, 122°/302° from/to E pier lt, 0·83M. Beware rks SW of E pier running out for approx 20m. Appr from the E to avoid Ramsdale Scar, rky patch 0·9m. Keep careful watch for salmon nets E & SE of ent.
LIGHTS AND MARKS
Lt ho (conspic), Iso 5s 17m 9M, on Old Pier. No ldg lts/marks.
Tidal sigs on Old Pier:
Ⓨ = 1·8 - 3·7m depth;
Iso 5s or B ● = >3·7m.
At W pier: 2FR (vert) 5m 4M = >1·8m.
These depths are for Old Hbr; E hbr ent has approx 1·5m less.
RADIO TELEPHONE
Call *Scarborough Lt Ho* VHF Ch **12** 16 (H24). Watchkeeper will offer guidance to approaching visitors and help moor.
TELEPHONE (01723)
Hr Mr (HO) 373530 and Fax, 360684 (OT); CG 372323; MRSC (01262) 672317; ⌘ (01947) 602074; Marinecall 0891 500454; Police 500300; Ⓗ 368111.
FACILITIES
Harbour AB £5.73, M (Long waiting list – some visitors berths available), FW, C (3 ton), Slip, D; **Scarborough YC** ☎ 373821, Slip, M*, L, FW, ME, El, AB;
Services: ME, El, Sh, CH, P & D (cans), Ⓔ.
Town EC Wed; P, D, V, R, Bar, ✉, Ⓑ, ⇌, ✈ (Humberside).

WHITBY
10-5-14

N. Yorkshire 54°29'·64N 00°36'·68W

CHARTS
AC 1612, 134, 129; Imray C29; OS 94
TIDES
+0500 Dover; ML 3·3; Duration 0605; Zone 0 (UT)

Standard Port RIVER TEES ENT. (→)

Times				Height (metres)			
High Water		Low Water		MHWS	MHWN	MLWN	MLWS
0000	0600	0000	0600	5·5	4·3	2·0	0·9
1200	1800	1200	1800				
Differences WHITBY							
+0015	+0030	+0020	+0005	+0·1	0·0	−0·1	−0·1

SHELTER
Good except in lower hbr in strong NW to NE winds. Hbr available from HW±4 for drafts of approx 2m. In strong winds from NW through N to SE the sea breaks a long way out and ent is difficult. Marina (dredged approx 2m) is 2ca beyond swing bridge, which opens on request at ½ hour intervals HW±2; extra openings at weekends by arrangement with WYC. FG lts = open; FR lts = shut.
NAVIGATION
WPT 54°30'·20N 00°36'·86W, 349°/169° from/to ent, 0·57M. Hbr can be apprd safely from any direction except SE. From SE beware Whitby Rk; leave Whitby NCM buoy, Q, to port. Beware strong set to E when appr piers from HW −2 to HW. Vessels >37m LOA must embark pilot; arrange via Hr Mr.
LIGHTS AND MARKS
Whitby High lt ho, Iso RW 10s 73m 18/16M, (R128°-143°, W143°-319°), is 2M ESE of hbr ent. Ldg lines:
(1) Chapel spire in line 176° with E lt ho.
(2) FR lt or 2 bns, seen between E and W pier extension, lts (FR and FG), lead 169° into hbr. Continue on this line until bns (W △ and W ○ with B stripe) on E pier (two FY lts) are abeam.
(3) On course 209° keep these same bns in line astern.

RADIO TELEPHONE
VHF Ch **11** 16 12 (H24). Whitby Bridge Ch **11** 16 06 (listens on Ch 16 HW–2 to HW+2).
TELEPHONE (01947)
Hr Mr 602354; MRSC (01262) 672317; ⌗ 602074; Marinecall 0891 500454/453; Police 603443; Dr 820888.
FACILITIES
Whitby Marina (200+10 visitors) ☎ 600165, £13, AC, D, FW, P (cans), Slip, ME, El, Sh, C, CH; **Fish Quay** M, D, L, FW, C (1 ton), CH, AB, R, Bar; **Whitby YC** ☎ 603623, M, L, Bar; **Services:** ME, El, Sh, CH, BH, ACA, SM, Gas, Gaz. **Town** EC Wed; usual amenities, ⊠, Ⓑ, ⇌, ✈ (Teesside).

ADJACENT ANCHORAGE

RUNSWICK BAY, N. Yorkshire, 54°32'·10N 00°44'·10W. AC 1612. HW +0505 on Dover: +0010 on R Tees Ent; HW −0·1m on R Tees Ent; ML 3·1m; Duration 0605. Good shelter in all winds from NW by W to SSE. Enter bay at 225° keeping clear of many rks at base of cliffs. Two W posts (2FY by night when required by lifeboat) 18m apart are ldg marks 270° to LB ho and can be used to lead into ⚓. Good holding in 6m to 9m in middle of bay. Facilities: **Runswick Bay Rescue Boat Station** ☎ (01947) 840965; **Village** Bar, R, V.

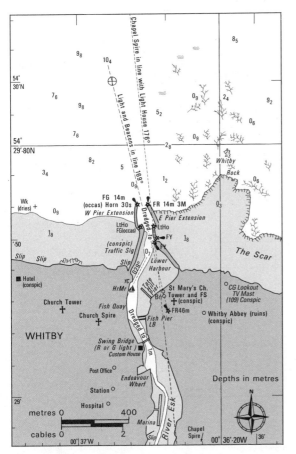

RIVER TEES
MIDDLESBROUGH
10-5-15

Cleveland 54°38'·93N 01°08'·38W

CHARTS
AC 2566, 2567, 152; Imray C29; OS 93
TIDES
+0450 Dover; ML 3·1; Duration 0605; Zone 0 (UT)

Standard Port RIVER TEES ENT. (→)

Times				Height (metres)			
High Water		Low Water		MHWS	MHWN	MLWN	MLWS
0000	0600	0000	0600	5·5	4·3	2·0	0·9
1200	1800	1200	1800				
Differences MIDDLESBROUGH (Dock Ent)							
0000	+0002	0000	−0003	+0·1	+0·2	+0·1	−0·1

NOTE: River Tees Entrance is a Standard Port and daily tidal predictions are given below.

SHELTER
Entry is not recommended for small craft in heavy weather especially with strong winds from NE to SE. Small craft berths are not readily available, but may be arranged at Paddy's Hole (Bran Sands), at Stockton Castlegate Marine Club approx 10M from S. Gare or by Hr Mr; see also under Facilities.
NAVIGATION
WPT Tees Fairway SWM, Iso 4s, Horn 5s, Racon, 54°40'·94N 01°06'·39W, 030°/210° from/to S Gare bkwtr, 2·4M. Beware Saltscar, Eastscar and Longscar Rks on appr. Bridges up river have following clearances at MHWS:
(1) ½M above Middlesbrough Dock, transporter br, 48m;
(2) 2M from there, Newport br, 6·4m;
(3) ½M from there, A19 road br, 18·0m;
(4) ½M from there, new bridge, 5·0m; but transit the barrage via lock 25m x 6m (see R/T);
(5) 1½M from there, Teesdale road br, 5·5m;
(6) ½M from there, Stockton-Victoria br, 5·4m.

5

RIVER TEES/MIDDLESBROUGH *continued*

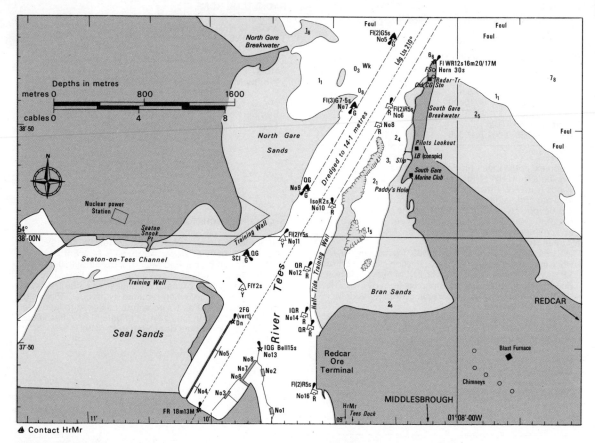

⚓ Contact HrMr

LIGHTS AND MARKS

Q lt, or 3 Ⓡ (vert) at Old CG stn, means no entry without approval of Hr Mr. Ldg lts 210°, FR on framework trs. Chan well marked to beyond Middlesbrough.

RADIO TELEPHONE

Call: *Tees Hbr Radio* VHF Ch **14** 22 16 12 (H24). Monitor Ch 14; also info Ch 14 22. *Tees Barrage Radio* Ch M (37).

TELEPHONE (01642)

Hr Mr 468127 (HO)/ 452541 (H24); MRSC (0191) 257 2691; ⌗ 440111; Marinecall 0891 500454; Police 248184; Ⓗ (N Tees) 672122, Ⓗ (S Tees) 850850.

FACILITIES

Limited berthing on R. Tees for small pleasure craft; visitors would be advised to go to Hartlepool (4M). Or make prior arrangements with Club Secretaries or Hr Mr. **S Gare Marine Club** ☎ 491039 Slip, M (check with Secretary), L, FW, Bar; **Castlegate Marine Club** ☎ 583299 Slip, M, FW, ME, EI, Sh, CH, L, V; **Tees Motor Boat Club** M (check with Secretary); **Services:** EI, ME, Ⓔ, ACA.
Town EC Wed; ⊠, Ⓑ, ⇌, ✈.

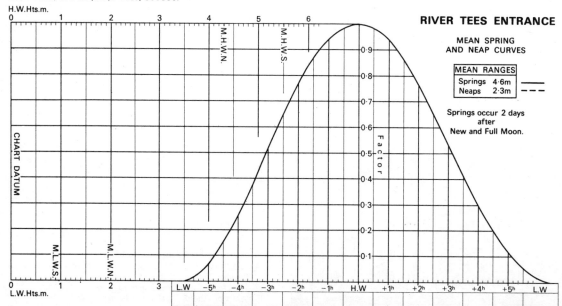

RIVER TEES ENTRANCE

MEAN SPRING AND NEAP CURVES

MEAN RANGES	
Springs 4·6m	——
Neaps 2·3m	- - -

Springs occur 2 days after New and Full Moon.

ENGLAND – RIVER TEES ENTRANCE

LAT 54°38'N   LONG 1°09'W

TIMES AND HEIGHTS OF HIGH AND LOW WATERS

YEAR **1996**

TIME ZONE (UT)
For Summer Time add ONE hour in non-shaded areas

Chart Datum: 2·85 metres below Ordnance Datum (Newlyn)

JANUARY

Day	Time	m	Day	Time	m
1 M	0628 / 1236 / 1857	1.7 / 4.5 / 1.9	**16** TU	0527 / 1136 / 1802	1.8 / 4.4 / 1.9
2 TU	0051 / 0727 / 1335 / 1952	4.5 / 1.7 / 4.6 / 1.7	**17** W	0008 / 0640 / 1245 / 1912	4.6 / 1.6 / 4.7 / 1.6
3 W	0148 / 0815 / 1421 / 2038	4.6 / 1.6 / 4.7 / 1.5	**18** TH	0117 / 0744 / 1346 / 2014	4.8 / 1.3 / 5.0 / 1.2
4 TH	0235 / 0856 / 1500 / 2117	4.7 / 1.5 / 4.9 / 1.3	**19** F	0217 / 0840 / 1439 / 2107	5.2 / 1.0 / 5.3 / 0.8
5 F	0315 / 0931 / 1535 / 2153	4.8 / 1.4 / 5.0 / 1.1	**20** SA ●	0310 / 0929 / 1527 / 2156	5.5 / 0.8 / 5.6 / 0.4
6 SA	0353 / 1002 / 1607 / 2226	4.9 / 1.3 / 5.1 / 1.0	**21** SU	0359 / 1016 / 1613 / 2242	5.6 / 0.7 / 5.8 / 0.3
7 SU	0428 / 1032 / 1639 / 2259	4.9 / 1.3 / 5.1 / 0.9	**22** M	0446 / 1101 / 1658 / 2328	5.7 / 0.6 / 5.8 / 0.2
8 M	0502 / 1104 / 1712 / 2333	4.9 / 1.2 / 5.1 / 0.9	**23** TU	0533 / 1145 / 1744	5.6 / 0.7 / 5.8
9 TU	0538 / 1138 / 1747	4.9 / 1.2 / 5.1	**24** W	0013 / 0620 / 1230 / 1830	0.3 / 5.5 / 0.9 / 5.6
10 W	0008 / 0615 / 1215 / 1824	0.9 / 4.9 / 1.3 / 5.1	**25** TH	0058 / 0708 / 1314 / 1918	0.5 / 5.2 / 1.1 / 5.4
11 TH	0045 / 0655 / 1252 / 1903	1.0 / 4.8 / 1.4 / 4.9	**26** F	0145 / 0758 / 1400 / 2009	0.9 / 4.9 / 1.4 / 5.1
12 F	0123 / 0739 / 1332 / 1946	1.2 / 4.6 / 1.6 / 4.8	**27** SA	0233 / 0850 / 1451 / 2105	1.2 / 4.7 / 1.7 / 4.7
13 SA	0207 / 0827 / 1418 / 2037	1.4 / 4.5 / 1.8 / 4.6	**28** SU	0327 / 0946 / 1550 / 2205	1.6 / 4.4 / 2.0 / 4.5
14 SU	0259 / 0923 / 1519 / 2140	1.6 / 4.4 / 2.0 / 4.5	**29** M	0430 / 1048 / 1701 / 2310	1.9 / 4.2 / 2.1 / 4.3
15 M	0408 / 1027 / 1641 / 2253	1.7 / 4.3 / 2.1 / 4.4	**30** TU	0546 / 1154 / 1823	2.0 / 4.2 / 2.1
			31 W	0018 / 0658 / 1302 / 1929	4.2 / 2.0 / 4.3 / 1.9

FEBRUARY

Day	Time	m	Day	Time	m
1 TH	0123 / 0753 / 1357 / 2019	4.3 / 1.9 / 4.5 / 1.6	**16** F	0102 / 0728 / 1328 / 2001	4.7 / 1.5 / 4.8 / 1.1
2 F	0215 / 0836 / 1440 / 2100	4.3 / 1.7 / 4.7 / 1.4	**17** SA	0206 / 0826 / 1424 / 2055	5.0 / 1.1 / 5.2 / 0.7
3 SA	0258 / 0913 / 1516 / 2136	4.6 / 1.5 / 4.9 / 1.1	**18** SU ●	0258 / 0915 / 1513 / 2143	5.4 / 0.8 / 5.5 / 0.4
4 SU	0335 / 0944 / 1549 / 2209	4.8 / 1.3 / 5.0 / 1.0	**19** M	0344 / 1000 / 1557 / 2227	5.6 / 0.6 / 5.8 / 0.2
5 M	0409 / 1014 / 1619 / 2241	5.0 / 1.2 / 5.1 / 0.8	**20** TU	0427 / 1042 / 1639 / 2309	5.7 / 0.5 / 5.8 / 0.1
6 TU	0441 / 1046 / 1651 / 2314	5.0 / 1.1 / 5.2 / 0.7	**21** W	0510 / 1123 / 1721 / 2350	5.6 / 0.6 / 5.7 / 0.3
7 W	0515 / 1120 / 1725 / 2347	5.0 / 1.0 / 5.2 / 0.7	**22** TH	0553 / 1204 / 1804	5.5 / 0.7 / 5.6
8 TH	0551 / 1155 / 1801	5.0 / 1.0 / 5.2	**23** F	0031 / 0636 / 1245 / 1848	0.5 / 5.2 / 1.0 / 5.4
9 F	0022 / 0629 / 1232 / 1838	0.8 / 4.9 / 1.1 / 5.1	**24** SA	0112 / 0721 / 1325 / 1935	0.9 / 4.9 / 1.3 / 5.0
10 SA	0059 / 0710 / 1309 / 1918	0.9 / 4.8 / 1.3 / 4.9	**25** SU	0154 / 0808 / 1409 / 2026	1.3 / 4.6 / 1.6 / 4.7
11 SU	0139 / 0754 / 1351 / 2005	1.1 / 4.6 / 1.5 / 4.7	**26** M	0239 / 0901 / 1500 / 2124	1.7 / 4.3 / 1.9 / 4.3
12 M	0227 / 0846 / 1443 / 2106	1.4 / 4.4 / 1.7 / 4.3	**27** TU	0335 / 1001 / 1605 / 2230	2.1 / 4.1 / 2.2 / 4.1
13 TU	0329 / 0950 / 1557 / 2222	1.7 / 4.3 / 1.9 / 4.3	**28** W	0445 / 1109 / 1728 / 2341	2.2 / 4.1 / 2.2 / 4.0
14 W	0453 / 1103 / 1729 / 2345	1.8 / 4.3 / 1.9 / 4.4	**29** TH	0616 / 1219 / 1855	2.3 / 4.1 / 2.0
15 TH	0617 / 1219 / 1853	1.7 / 4.5 / 1.6			

MARCH

Day	Time	m	Day	Time	m
1 F	0050 / 0721 / 1321 / 1950	4.2 / 2.1 / 4.3 / 1.8	**16** SA	0045 / 0708 / 1307 / 1943	4.6 / 1.6 / 4.7 / 1.1
2 SA	0147 / 0808 / 1409 / 2032	4.4 / 1.8 / 4.6 / 1.5	**17** SU	0150 / 0807 / 1405 / 2038	4.9 / 1.2 / 5.1 / 0.7
3 SU	0231 / 0845 / 1447 / 2108	4.6 / 1.6 / 4.8 / 1.2	**18** M	0241 / 0856 / 1454 / 2124	5.3 / 0.9 / 5.4 / 0.4
4 M	0308 / 0917 / 1521 / 2142	4.8 / 1.3 / 5.0 / 0.9	**19** TU ●	0324 / 0940 / 1536 / 2206	5.5 / 0.7 / 5.6 / 0.3
5 TU	0342 / 0949 / 1552 / 2215	5.0 / 1.1 / 5.1 / 0.8	**20** W	0405 / 1021 / 1617 / 2245	5.6 / 0.6 / 5.7 / 0.3
6 W	0414 / 1023 / 1625 / 2249	5.1 / 1.0 / 5.2 / 0.6	**21** TH	0444 / 1100 / 1656 / 2324	5.6 / 0.6 / 5.7 / 0.4
7 TH	0448 / 1058 / 1700 / 2323	5.2 / 0.9 / 5.3 / 0.6	**22** F	0523 / 1138 / 1737	5.4 / 0.7 / 5.5
8 F	0525 / 1134 / 1737 / 2359	5.2 / 0.9 / 5.3 / 0.7	**23** SA	0001 / 0602 / 1215 / 1818	0.7 / 5.2 / 0.9 / 5.3
9 SA	0603 / 1211 / 1817	5.1 / 0.9 / 5.2	**24** SU	0037 / 0643 / 1252 / 1902	1.0 / 5.0 / 1.2 / 4.9
10 SU	0037 / 0644 / 1250 / 1859	0.8 / 5.0 / 1.1 / 5.0	**25** M	0113 / 0726 / 1332 / 1949	1.4 / 4.7 / 1.5 / 4.6
11 M	0118 / 0728 / 1332 / 1948	1.1 / 4.8 / 1.3 / 4.8	**26** TU	0152 / 0814 / 1418 / 2043	1.8 / 4.4 / 1.8 / 4.3
12 TU	0205 / 0819 / 1424 / 2048	1.4 / 4.6 / 1.5 / 4.5	**27** W	0240 / 0911 / 1518 / 2146	2.1 / 4.2 / 2.1 / 4.1
13 W	0305 / 0921 / 1534 / 2204	1.7 / 4.4 / 1.7 / 4.4	**28** TH	0347 / 1018 / 1631 / 2257	2.4 / 4.1 / 2.2 / 4.0
14 TH	0430 / 1036 / 1705 / 2326	1.7 / 4.3 / 1.7 / 4.4	**29** F	0506 / 1129 / 1750	2.4 / 4.1 / 2.1
15 F	0555 / 1155 / 1832	1.8 / 4.4 / 1.5	**30** SA	0008 / 0624 / 1234 / 1859	4.1 / 2.3 / 4.3 / 1.9
			31 SU	0108 / 0721 / 1326 / 1948	4.3 / 2.0 / 4.5 / 1.6

APRIL

Day	Time	m	Day	Time	m
1 M	0154 / 0803 / 1408 / 2028	4.6 / 1.7 / 4.8 / 1.3	**16** TU	0218 / 0833 / 1430 / 2100	5.1 / 1.1 / 5.3 / 0.6
2 TU	0233 / 0841 / 1445 / 2106	4.9 / 1.4 / 5.0 / 1.0	**17** W ●	0302 / 0917 / 1513 / 2141	5.3 / 0.9 / 5.5 / 0.5
3 W	0307 / 0918 / 1520 / 2143	5.1 / 1.2 / 5.2 / 0.8	**18** TH	0340 / 0957 / 1553 / 2220	5.4 / 0.8 / 5.5 / 0.6
4 TH	0342 / 0956 / 1556 / 2220	5.2 / 1.0 / 5.3 / 0.7	**19** F	0417 / 1035 / 1632 / 2256	5.4 / 0.7 / 5.4 / 0.7
5 F	0419 / 1034 / 1635 / 2258	5.3 / 0.9 / 5.3 / 0.7	**20** SA	0454 / 1112 / 1712 / 2330	5.3 / 0.8 / 5.3 / 0.9
6 SA	0458 / 1113 / 1716 / 2337	5.3 / 0.8 / 5.3 / 0.7	**21** SU	0531 / 1147 / 1752	5.2 / 1.0 / 5.1
7 SU	0539 / 1153 / 1800	5.2 / 0.9 / 5.2	**22** M	0003 / 0609 / 1224 / 1834	1.2 / 5.0 / 1.2 / 4.9
8 M	0018 / 0622 / 1236 / 1847	0.9 / 5.1 / 1.0 / 5.1	**23** TU	0037 / 0650 / 1303 / 1919	1.5 / 4.8 / 1.4 / 4.6
9 TU	0102 / 0709 / 1322 / 1940	1.1 / 4.9 / 1.1 / 4.9	**24** W	0113 / 0735 / 1347 / 2008	1.8 / 4.6 / 1.7 / 4.4
10 W	0152 / 0801 / 1416 / 2042	1.4 / 4.7 / 1.3 / 4.7	**25** TH	0157 / 0826 / 1441 / 2104	2.1 / 4.4 / 1.9 / 4.2
11 TH	0255 / 0904 / 1526 / 2153	1.7 / 4.5 / 1.5 / 4.5	**26** F	0257 / 0927 / 1547 / 2208	2.3 / 4.2 / 2.0 / 4.1
12 F	0414 / 1017 / 1648 / 2308	1.9 / 4.5 / 1.5 / 4.5	**27** SA	0414 / 1035 / 1655 / 2316	2.4 / 4.2 / 2.0 / 4.2
13 SA	0532 / 1132 / 1808	1.9 / 4.5 / 1.4	**28** SU	0525 / 1140 / 1758	2.3 / 4.3 / 1.8
14 SU	0022 / 0643 / 1242 / 1918	4.6 / 1.7 / 4.8 / 1.1	**29** M	0018 / 0626 / 1237 / 1854	4.4 / 2.1 / 4.5 / 1.6
15 M	0127 / 0743 / 1341 / 2014	4.9 / 1.4 / 5.1 / 0.8	**30** TU	0109 / 0718 / 1324 / 1943	4.6 / 1.8 / 4.8 / 1.3

5

ENGLAND – RIVER TEES ENTRANCE

LAT 54°38′N   LONG   1°09′W

TIMES AND HEIGHTS OF HIGH AND LOW WATERS

YEAR **1996**

TIME ZONE (UT)
For Summer Time add ONE hour in non-shaded areas

MAY

	Time	m		Time	m
1 W	0153 0804 1407 2028	4.9 1.5 5.0 1.1	**16** TH	0238 0854 1451 2116	5.1 1.1 5.2 0.9
2 TH	0232 0848 1448 2110	5.1 1.2 5.2 0.9	**17** F	0317 0935 1532 2154 ●	5.2 1.0 5.2 0.9
3 F O	0312 0930 1530 2153	5.3 1.0 5.3 0.8	**18** SA	0354 1013 1612 2230	5.2 0.9 5.2 1.0
4 SA	0352 1012 1614 2235	5.4 0.9 5.4 0.8	**19** SU	0430 1050 1651 2303	5.2 0.9 5.1 1.2
5 SU	0435 1056 1701 2319	5.4 0.8 5.4 0.8	**20** M	0506 1125 1731 2335	5.1 1.0 5.0 1.3
6 M	0520 1140 1750	5.4 0.8 5.3	**21** TU	0543 1202 1812	5.0 1.1 4.8
7 TU	0004 0606 1227 1842	1.0 5.3 0.9 5.2	**22** W	0008 0622 1241 1854	1.5 4.9 1.3 4.6
8 W	0052 0656 1318 1937	1.2 5.1 1.0 5.0	**23** TH	0045 0705 1323 1939	1.7 4.8 1.5 4.5
9 TH	0146 0751 1415 2037	1.4 5.0 1.1 4.8	**24** F	0127 0752 1410 2028	1.9 4.6 1.6 4.4
10 F	0248 0853 1521 2142	1.6 4.8 1.3 4.7	**25** SA	0218 0845 1507 2124	2.1 4.5 1.8 4.3
11 SA	0357 1000 1631 2248	1.8 4.7 1.3 4.6	**26** SU	0325 0945 1609 2224	2.2 4.4 1.8 4.3
12 SU	0507 1108 1741 2356	1.8 4.7 1.3 4.7	**27** M	0437 1047 1712 2325	2.2 4.4 1.8 4.4
13 M	0614 1214 1848	1.7 4.8 1.2	**28** TU	0541 1148 1810	2.1 4.5 1.6
14 TU	0059 0715 1314 1945	4.8 1.5 5.0 1.1	**29** W	0022 0639 1244 1904	4.6 1.9 4.7 1.4
15 W	0153 0808 1406 2034	5.0 1.3 5.1 1.0	**30** TH	0114 0731 1335 1954	4.9 1.6 5.0 1.2
			31 F	0201 0821 1423 2043	5.1 1.3 5.2 1.0

JUNE

	Time	m		Time	m
1 SA O	0246 0908 1510 2130	5.3 1.0 5.3 0.9	**16** SU ●	0336 0956 1556 2208	5.0 1.1 4.9 1.3
2 SU	0331 0955 1559 2217	5.4 0.8 5.4 0.8	**17** M	0412 1033 1635 2240	5.1 1.0 4.9 1.3
3 M	0417 1043 1649 2305	5.5 0.7 5.4 0.9	**18** TU	0447 1108 1713 2312	5.1 1.0 4.9 1.3
4 TU	0504 1131 1741 2353	5.5 0.7 5.4 0.9	**19** W	0522 1144 1751 2347	5.0 1.0 4.8 1.4
5 W	0554 1221 1835	5.5 0.7 5.3	**20** TH	0559 1221 1830	5.0 1.1 4.7
6 TH	0043 0646 1313 1929	1.1 5.5 0.7 5.2	**21** F	0023 0639 1300 1911	1.5 4.9 1.2 4.6
7 F	0137 0741 1409 2026	1.3 5.2 0.9 5.0	**22** SA	0103 0721 1341 1955	1.6 4.8 1.4 4.5
8 SA	0234 0840 1508 2124	1.5 5.0 1.0 4.8	**23** SU	0147 0808 1428 2045	1.7 4.7 1.5 4.4
9 SU	0335 0941 1610 2225	1.6 4.9 1.2 4.7	**24** M	0239 0901 1523 2140	2.0 4.5 1.6 4.4
10 M	0439 1044 1713 2327	1.7 4.8 1.3 4.7	**25** TU	0346 1001 1627 2239	2.1 4.4 1.7 4.4
11 TU	0544 1147 1818	1.7 4.8 1.3	**26** W	0458 1105 1731 2341	2.1 4.5 1.7 4.5
12 W	0029 0647 1248 1917	4.7 1.6 4.8 1.3	**27** TH	0604 1209 1832	1.9 4.6 1.5
13 TH	0127 0744 1344 2009	4.8 1.5 4.9 1.3	**28** F	0040 0703 1309 1929	4.7 1.6 4.8 1.3
14 F	0216 0834 1432 2054	4.9 1.3 4.9 1.2	**29** SA	0135 0757 1404 2022	5.0 1.3 5.1 1.1
15 SA	0258 0917 1516 2133	5.0 1.2 4.9 1.2	**30** SU ●	0226 0852 1456 2113	5.3 1.0 5.3 0.9

JULY

	Time	m		Time	m
1 M O	0314 0942 1547 2203	5.5 0.7 5.5 0.8	**16** TU	0356 1016 1618 2221	5.0 1.0 4.8 1.3
2 TU	0402 1031 1637 2252	5.6 0.5 5.5 0.8	**17** W	0429 1050 1653 2252	5.1 0.9 4.9 1.2
3 W	0450 1120 1728 2340	5.7 0.4 5.5 0.8	**18** TH	0501 1124 1728 2326	5.1 0.9 4.9 1.2
4 TH	0540 1210 1820	5.6 0.4 5.5	**19** F	0535 1159 1803	5.1 0.9 4.8
5 F	0029 0630 1300 1911	0.9 5.6 0.5 5.3	**20** SA	0001 0612 1235 1841	1.3 5.0 1.0 4.8
6 SA	0119 0723 1351 2005	1.1 5.4 0.7 5.1	**21** SU	0039 0651 1312 1923	1.4 4.9 1.1 4.7
7 SU	0212 0819 1445 2100	1.3 5.2 0.9 4.9	**22** M	0118 0733 1352 2009	1.5 4.8 1.3 4.6
8 M	0307 0917 1543 2157	1.5 5.0 1.2 4.7	**23** TU	0202 0821 1440 2100	1.7 4.6 1.5 4.4
9 TU	0408 1018 1644 2257	1.7 4.8 1.4 4.6	**24** W	0256 0918 1541 2159	1.9 4.5 1.7 4.4
10 W	0514 1121 1749	1.8 4.6 1.6	**25** TH	0410 1027 1655 2304	2.0 4.4 1.8 4.4
11 TH	0000 0622 1225 1852	4.5 1.8 4.6 1.6	**26** F	0530 1140 1806	1.9 4.5 1.7
12 F	0103 0725 1325 1948	4.6 1.7 4.6 1.6	**27** SA	0011 0640 1250 1910	4.6 1.7 4.6 1.5
13 SA	0157 0817 1417 2035	4.7 1.5 4.7 1.5	**28** SU	0114 0743 1351 2007	4.9 1.3 5.0 1.2
14 SU	0243 0902 1502 2114	4.8 1.3 4.8 1.4	**29** M	0210 0839 1445 2100	5.2 0.9 5.3 0.9
15 M ●	0321 0941 1542 2113	4.9 1.1 4.8 0.9	**30** TU O	0300 0930 1534 2149	5.5 0.6 5.6 0.6
			31 W	0347 1018 1622 2236	5.7 0.3 5.7 0.6

AUGUST

	Time	m		Time	m
1 TH	0434 1105 1709 2322	5.8 0.2 5.7 0.7	**16** F	0436 1100 1700 2303	5.2 0.8 5.0 1.1
2 F	0521 1151 1757	5.8 0.2 5.6	**17** SA	0509 1133 1734 2337	5.2 0.8 5.0 1.1
3 SA	0008 0608 1238 1845	0.8 5.7 0.4 5.4	**18** SU	0544 1206 1812	5.1 0.8 4.9
4 SU	0054 0657 1325 1935	1.0 5.5 0.7 5.1	**19** M	0013 0621 1242 1851	1.2 5.0 1.0 4.8
5 M	0142 0750 1415 2027	1.2 5.2 1.0 4.9	**20** TU	0050 0700 1321 1934	1.3 4.9 1.2 4.7
6 TU	0234 0846 1509 2123	1.5 4.9 1.4 4.6	**21** W	0131 0745 1405 2023	1.5 4.7 1.4 4.5
7 W	0332 0947 1610 2224	1.8 4.6 1.7 4.4	**22** TH	0220 0842 1502 2121	1.7 4.5 1.7 4.3
8 TH	0440 1053 1719 2330	1.9 4.4 1.9 4.3	**23** F	0328 0956 1622 2231	1.9 4.4 1.9 4.3
9 F	0557 1202 1830	2.0 4.3 1.9	**24** SA	0500 1117 1745 2345	1.9 4.3 1.8 4.4
10 SA	0037 0706 1308 1928	4.4 1.8 4.4 1.8	**25** SU	0621 1235 1855	1.7 4.6 1.6
11 SU	0137 0800 1401 2015	4.5 1.6 4.5 1.7	**26** M	0055 0729 1340 1953	4.8 1.3 5.0 1.3
12 M	0224 0844 1445 2054	4.7 1.3 4.7 1.5	**27** TU	0155 0826 1432 2045	5.2 0.8 5.3 0.9
13 TU	0302 0921 1523 2128	4.9 1.1 4.8 1.4	**28** W O	0245 0915 1519 2132	5.5 0.4 5.6 0.7
14 W ●	0336 0955 1557 2159	5.0 1.0 4.9 1.2	**29** TH	0330 1000 1603 2216	5.8 0.2 5.8 0.5
15 TH	0406 1027 1629 2230	5.1 0.8 5.0 1.1	**30** F	0414 1044 1646 2259	5.9 0.1 5.8 0.5
			31 SA	0457 1127 1729 2342	5.9 0.2 5.6 0.7

Chart Datum: 2·85 metres below Ordnance Datum (Newlyn)

ENGLAND – RIVER TEES ENTRANCE

LAT 54°38′N   LONG 1°09′W

TIMES AND HEIGHTS OF HIGH AND LOW WATERS

YEAR **1996**

TIME ZONE (UT)
For Summer Time add ONE hour in non-shaded areas

5

SEPTEMBER

	Time	m		Time	m
1 SU	0541 1210 1813	5.7 0.4 5.4	**16** M	0516 1138 1742 2348	5.2 0.8 5.1 1.1
2 M	0025 0627 1254 1859	0.9 5.5 0.8 5.1	**17** TU	0554 1214 1822	5.1 1.0 5.0
3 TU	0109 0716 1338 1948	1.2 5.2 1.2 4.8	**18** W	0026 0635 1254 1903	1.2 5.0 1.2 4.8
4 W	0155 0810 1427 2042	1.5 4.8 1.6 4.5	**19** TH	0107 0722 1338 1951	1.4 4.8 1.5 4.6
5 TH	0250 0911 1526 2143	1.9 4.5 2.0 4.3	**20** F	0156 0820 1434 2050	1.6 4.5 1.8 4.4
6 F	0400 1020 1641 2252	2.1 4.2 2.2 4.2	**21** SA	0302 0934 1557 2203	1.8 4.3 2.0 4.3
7 SA	0527 1135 1803	2.1 4.2 2.2	**22** SU	0436 1058 1725 2321	1.9 4.3 2.0 4.4
8 SU	0005 0642 1244 1904	4.3 2.0 4.3 2.1	**23** M	0603 1218 1838	1.6 4.6 1.7
9 M	0108 0735 1338 1950	4.4 1.7 4.5 1.9	**24** TU	0035 0713 1325 1937	4.7 1.2 5.0 1.4
10 TU	0156 0817 1421 2028	4.7 1.4 4.7 1.6	**25** W	0136 0809 1417 2027	5.1 0.8 5.3 1.0
11 W	0234 0853 1457 2101	4.9 1.2 4.9 1.4	**26** TH	0226 0857 1501 2112	5.5 0.5 5.6 0.7
12 TH ●	0307 0927 1529 2132	5.1 1.0 5.0 1.2	**27** F ○	0310 0940 1541 2155	5.8 0.3 5.8 0.6
13 F	0337 0959 1559 2204	5.2 0.8 5.1 1.1	**28** SA	0352 1021 1621 2236	5.9 0.2 5.8 0.6
14 SA	0407 1031 1630 2238	5.2 0.7 5.2 1.0	**29** SU	0432 1101 1700 2316	5.9 0.3 5.6 0.7
15 SU	0440 1104 1705 2312	5.3 0.7 5.2 1.0	**30** M	0514 1141 1740 2355	5.7 0.6 5.4 0.9

OCTOBER

	Time	m		Time	m
1 TU	0557 1219 1822	5.4 1.0 5.2	**16** W	0534 1152 1757	5.2 1.0 5.2
2 W	0035 0643 1259 1907	1.2 5.1 1.4 4.8	**17** TH	0008 0619 1234 1840	1.1 5.1 1.2 5.0
3 TH	0117 0710 1340 1956	1.5 4.7 1.8 4.5	**18** F	0052 0710 1321 1930	1.3 4.9 1.5 4.8
4 F	0206 0831 1432 2055	1.9 4.4 2.2 4.3	**19** SA	0143 0810 1418 2029	1.5 4.6 1.8 4.6
5 SA	0311 0939 1544 2205	2.1 4.1 2.5 4.2	**20** SU	0250 0921 1538 2140	1.7 4.5 2.0 4.5
6 SU	0435 1055 1715 2319	2.2 4.1 2.5 4.2	**21** M	0417 1039 1703 2257	1.7 4.4 2.0 4.5
7 M	0601 1207 1827	2.1 4.2 2.3	**22** TU	0541 1157 1816	1.5 4.6 1.8
8 TU	0025 0658 1304 1916	4.4 1.9 4.4 2.1	**23** W	0010 0651 1305 1916	4.8 1.2 4.9 1.5
9 W	0117 0741 1357 1954	4.6 1.6 4.7 1.8	**24** TH	0114 0748 1357 2007	5.1 0.9 5.2 1.2
10 TH	0158 0819 1425 2029	4.9 1.3 4.9 1.5	**25** F	0206 0836 1441 2052	5.4 0.6 5.5 0.9
11 F	0233 0853 1458 2103	5.1 1.1 5.1 1.3	**26** SA ○	0251 0919 1520 2134	5.6 0.5 5.6 0.7
12 SA ●	0305 0927 1528 2137	5.2 0.9 5.2 1.1	**27** SU	0331 0959 1558 2214	5.7 0.5 5.6 0.7
13 SU	0338 1002 1601 2213	5.3 0.8 5.3 1.0	**28** M	0411 1037 1634 2252	5.7 0.6 5.6 0.8
14 M	0414 1037 1637 2250	5.4 0.8 5.3 1.0	**29** TU	0451 1113 1712 2330	5.5 0.9 5.4 0.9
15 TU	0453 1114 1716 2328	5.3 0.8 5.3 1.0	**30** W	0533 1148 1751	5.3 1.2 5.2
			31 TH	0007 0616 1223 1832	1.2 5.0 1.5 4.9

NOVEMBER

	Time	m		Time	m
1 F	0047 0702 1259 1917	1.5 4.7 1.9 4.7	**16** SA	0045 0705 1311 1916	1.1 5.0 1.5 5.0
2 SA	0131 0754 1341 2008	1.8 4.4 2.2 4.5	**17** SU	0139 0804 1409 2015	1.2 4.8 1.7 4.9
3 SU	0226 0853 1440 2110	2.0 4.2 2.5 4.3	**18** M	0243 0908 1519 2122	1.4 4.7 1.9 4.7
4 M	0336 1003 1601 2221	2.2 4.1 2.6 4.3	**19** TU	0358 1017 1635 2233	1.5 4.6 2.0 4.7
5 TU	0452 1114 1722 2330	2.2 4.1 2.5 4.3	**20** W	0514 1129 1747 2343	1.4 4.6 1.9 4.8
6 W	0601 1217 1825	2.0 4.4 2.2	**21** TH	0625 1238 1852	1.3 4.8 1.6
7 TH	0028 0654 1308 1913	4.5 1.7 4.6 1.9	**22** F	0048 0725 1335 1947	5.0 1.1 5.0 1.4
8 F	0116 0738 1349 1954	4.8 1.5 4.9 1.6	**23** SA	0145 0816 1422 2034	5.2 0.9 5.2 1.1
9 SA	0157 0818 1424 2034	5.0 1.2 5.1 1.4	**24** SU	0233 0900 1503 2117	5.3 0.8 5.4 1.0
10 SU	0235 0857 1459 2113	5.2 1.0 5.3 1.1	**25** M ○	0315 0940 1539 2157	5.4 0.8 5.4 0.9
11 M ●	0313 0935 1536 2152	5.3 0.9 5.4 1.0	**26** TU	0355 1016 1615 2235	5.4 0.9 5.4 0.9
12 TU	0353 1014 1615 2232	5.4 0.9 5.5 0.9	**27** W	0434 1051 1650 2311	5.3 1.1 5.3 1.0
13 W	0436 1055 1656 2314	5.4 0.9 5.4 0.9	**28** TH	0514 1123 1727 2347	5.1 1.3 5.2 1.1
14 TH	0522 1137 1740 2358	5.3 1.0 5.3 0.9	**29** F	0555 1155 1806	4.9 1.5 5.0
15 F	0612 1222 1826	5.2 1.2 5.2	**30** SA	0024 0637 1230 1846	1.3 4.7 1.7 4.9

DECEMBER

	Time	m		Time	m
1 SU	0105 0721 1308 1931	1.5 4.5 2.0 4.7	**16** M	0133 0752 1357 2001	0.9 5.0 1.5 5.1
2 M	0150 0811 1354 2022	1.7 4.3 2.2 4.5	**17** TU	0231 0850 1457 2102	1.1 4.8 1.7 4.9
3 TU	0244 0907 1456 2122	1.9 4.2 2.4 4.4	**18** W	0334 0952 1604 2207	1.3 4.7 1.8 4.8
4 W	0350 1010 1613 2227	2.0 4.2 2.4 4.3	**19** TH	0443 1058 1714 2314	1.4 4.6 1.9 4.7
5 TH	0458 1116 1725 2332	2.0 4.3 2.3 4.4	**20** F	0555 1206 1825	1.4 4.6 1.8
6 F	0601 1216 1827	1.9 4.5 2.1	**21** SA	0022 0701 1311 1927	4.8 1.4 4.7 1.6
7 SA	0030 0656 1307 1920	4.6 1.6 4.7 1.8	**22** SU	0125 0757 1405 2019	4.9 1.3 4.9 1.3
8 SU	0121 0745 1352 2007	4.9 1.4 5.0 1.5	**23** M	0219 0844 1449 2104	5.0 1.2 5.0 1.1
9 M	0208 0831 1434 2052	5.1 1.2 5.2 1.2	**24** TU ○	0304 0925 1527 2145	5.1 1.1 5.1 1.0
10 TU	0253 0914 1515 2136	5.3 1.0 5.4 1.0	**25** W	0344 1001 1601 2222	5.1 1.1 5.2 0.9
11 W	0338 0958 1558 2220	5.4 0.9 5.5 0.8	**26** TH	0422 1034 1635 2257	5.1 1.2 5.2 0.9
12 TH	0425 1042 1642 2305	5.5 0.9 5.6 0.7	**27** F	0459 1105 1709 2331	5.0 1.3 5.2 1.0
13 F	0514 1127 1727 2352	5.4 0.9 5.5 0.7	**28** SA	0536 1135 1744	4.9 1.3 5.1
14 SA	0605 1214 1815	5.3 1.1 5.4	**29** SU	0005 0613 1208 1821	1.1 4.8 1.5 5.0
15 SU	0041 0657 1303 1906	0.8 5.2 1.2 5.3	**30** M	0042 0652 1244 1900	1.2 4.7 1.6 4.9
			31 TU	0120 0734 1323 1944	1.4 4.5 1.8 4.7

Chart Datum: 2·85 metres below Ordnance Datum (Newlyn)

HARTLEPOOL   10-5-16

Cleveland 54°41'·30N 01°11'·49W (West Hbr ent)

CHARTS
AC 2566, 2567, 152; Imray C29; OS 93
TIDES
+0437 Dover; ML 3·0; Duration 0600; Zone 0 (UT)

Standard Port RIVER TEES ENT. (←—)

Times				Height (metres)			
High Water		Low Water		MHWS	MHWN	MLWN	MLWS
0000	0600	0000	0600	5·5	4·3	2·0	0·9
1200	1800	1200	1800				
Differences HARTLEPOOL							
−0004	−0004	−0006	−0006	−0·1	−0·1	−0·2	−0·1

SHELTER
Excellent in marina (5m), access HW±4½ via chan dredged 0·8m and lock (ent 9m wide; pontoon on S side). Speed limit 4kn in W Hbr and marina. Strong E'lies cause swell, making ent chan hazardous, but possible. In such conditions, call VHF Ch M to shelter in the lock, awaiting tide; or call Victoria Hbr (commercial dock not normally for yachts) Ch 12 for short-stay berth, access H24.
NAVIGATION
WPT Longscar ECM buoy, Q (3) 10s, Bell, 54°40'·85N 01°09'·79W, 115°/295° from/to W Hbr ent 1·06M; (or, for Victoria Hbr, 128°/308° from/to Nos 1/2 buoys, 0·65M). From S, beware Longscar Rks, only 0·4M WSW of WPT. Note: Tees Fairway SWM buoy, Iso 4s 8M, (54°40'·93N 01°06'·38W) is 2M E of Longscar ECM buoy and may assist the initial landfall.
LIGHTS AND MARKS
The Heugh lt ho Fl (2) 10s 19m 19M, H24. Dir lt Fl WRG 2s 6m 3M leads 308° to W Hbr/marina lock; vis G305·5°-307°, W307°-309°, R309°-310·5°. W Hbr outer piers, Oc R/G 5s 12m 2M; bright street lts on S pier. Inner piers, FR/FG 7m 2M.
Lock sigs: Ⓖ = Enter; Ⓡ = Wait; 2Ⓡ = Lock closed.
Dir lt Iso WRG 3s 42m, W324·4°-325·4°, leads 325° via lit buoyed chan to Victoria Hbr. 2 FG (vert) on Kafiga pontoons.
RADIO TELEPHONE
Marina VHF Ch **M** 80. Call: *Hartlepool Dock Radio* VHF Ch **12** 16 11 (HJ and at HW). Info service (HJ) on Ch 12.
TELEPHONE (01429)
Marina 865744; Hr Mr 266127; MRSC (0191) 257 2691; Tees & Hartlepool Port Authority 276771; ⌗ 861390; Marinecall 0891 500453; Police 221151; Dr 272679.
FACILITIES
Hartlepool Marina (262 + visitors) ☎ 865744, £10.47, FW, AC, D, P (cans), BY, El, Sh, Ⓞ, BH (40 tons), C (15 ton), Gas, Gaz; **Hartlepool YC** ☎ 274931, Bar; **Tees SC** ☎ 267151, Bar;
Services: CH, ME, EL, Sh, C (Mobile 15+30 ton).
Town EC Wed; P (cans), V, R, Bar, ✉, Ⓑ, ⇌, ✈ (Teesside).

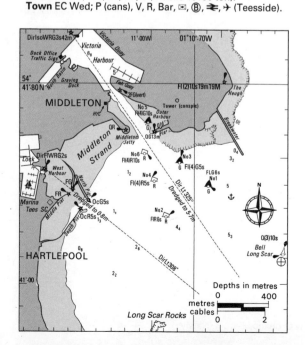

SEAHAM   10-5-17

Durham 54°50'·23N 01°19'·17W

CHARTS
AC 1627, 152; Imray C29; OS 88
TIDES
+0435 Dover; ML 3·0; Duration 0600; Zone 0 (UT)

Standard Port RIVER TEES ENT. (←—)

Times				Height (metres)			
High Water		Low Water		MHWS	MHWN	MLWN	MLWS
0000	0600	0000	0600	5·5	4·3	2·0	0·9
1200	1800	1200	1800				
Differences SEAHAM							
−0015	−0015	−0015	−0015	−0·3	−0·2	0·0	0·2

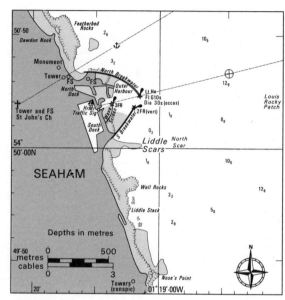

Depths in metres

SHELTER
Small boats normally berth in N Dock where shelter is excellent, but it dries. Larger boats may lock into S Dock; gates open from HW −2 to HW+1. Speed limit 5kn. Or ⚓ 0.25M off shore with clock tr in transit 240° with St John's church tr.
NAVIGATION
WPT 54°50'·35N 01°18'·50W, 076°/256° from/to N bkwtr lt ho, 0·40M. Shoals and rks to S of S bkwtr (Liddle Scars). Ent should not be attempted in strong on-shore winds.
LIGHTS AND MARKS
No ldg lts, but hbr is easily identified by lt ho (W with B bands) on N pier, Fl G 10s 12m 5M (often shows FG in bad weather), Dia 30s (sounded HW−2½ to +1½). FS at NE corner of S dock on with N lt ho leads in 256° clear of Tangle Rks. 3FR lts on wave screen are in form of a △.
Traffic sigs at S Dock:
Ⓡ = Vessels enter
Ⓖ = Vessels leave
RADIO TELEPHONE
VHF Ch **12** 16 06 (HW−2½ to HW+1½ between 0800-1800 LT Mon-Fri).
TELEPHONE (0191)
Hr Mr 581 3246; Hbr Ops Office 581 3877; MRSC 257 2691; ⌗ 5130385; Marinecall 0891 500453; Police 581 2255; Dr 581 2332.
FACILITIES
S Dock ☎ 5813877, L, FW, C (40 ton), AB; **N Dock** M.
Town (½M) EC Wed; P, D, FW, ME, El, CH (5M), V, R, Bar, ✉, Ⓑ, ⇌, ✈ (Teesside or Newcastle).

SUNDERLAND   10-5-18

Tyne and Wear 54°55'·22N 01°21'·05W

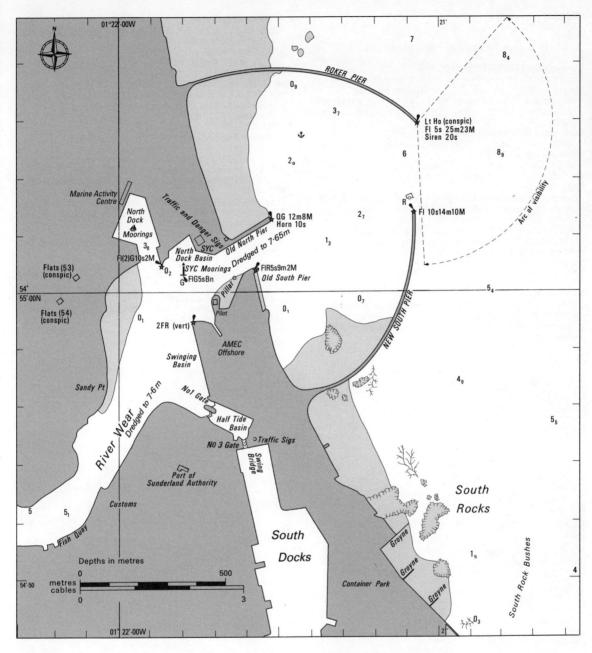

CHARTS
AC 1627, 152; Imray C29; OS 88

TIDES
+0430 Dover; ML 2·9; Duration 0600; Zone 0 (UT)

Standard Port RIVER TEES ENT. (←)

Times				Height (metres)			
High Water		Low Water		MHWS	MHWN	MLWN	MLWS
0000	0600	0000	0600	5·5	4·3	2·0	0·9
1200	1800	1200	1800				
Differences SUNDERLAND							
–0017	–0017	–0016	–0016	–0·3	–0·1	0·0	–0·1

SHELTER
Very good, but strong E'lies cause heavy swell in ent and outer hbr. There are fore-and-aft ⚓s in N Dock Marina (3·8m); pontoons are due to be installed winter 1996. App to marina ent is marked by SHM dolphin, Fl G 5s, and E jetty, Fl (2) G 10s.

NAVIGATION
WPT 54°55'·20N 01°20'·00W, 098°/278° from/to Roker Pier lt, 0·61M. Beware wreck at Whitburn Steel about 1M N of ent, and Hendon Rk (0·9m), 1·2M SE of hbr ent.

LIGHTS AND MARKS
3 FL ⓡ lts from Pilot Stn on Old N Pier = danger in hbr; no ent/dep.

RADIO TELEPHONE
N Dock Marina Ch M. Port VHF Ch 14 16 (H24); tide and visibility reports on request.

TELEPHONE (0191)
Hr Mr 514 0411 (HO), 567 2626 (OT); Marina 514 4721; MRSC 257 2691; ⌗ 5130385; Marinecall 0891 500453; Police 5102020; Ⓗ 565 6256.

FACILITIES
North Dock Marina (130 moorings) ☎ 514 4721, M £5.88, Slip, FW; **Sunderland YC** ☎ 567 5133, Slip (Dinghy), FW, AB, Bar; **Wear Boating Association** ☎ 567 5313, AB.
Town EC Wed; P & D (cans), Gas, Gaz, CH, El, ME, SM, V, R, Bar, ✉, Ⓞ, Ⓑ, ⇌, ✈ (Newcastle).

RIVER TYNE/NORTH SHIELDS

Tyne and Wear 55°00'·78N 01°24'·00W   **10-5-19**

CHARTS
AC 1934, 152; Imray C29; OS 88

TIDES
+0430 Dover; ML 3·0; Duration 0604; Zone 0 (UT)

Standard Port RIVER TEES ENT. (⟵)

Times				Height (metres)			
High Water		Low Water		MHWS	MHWN	MLWN	MLWS
0000	0600	0000	0600	5·5	4·3	2·0	0·9
1200	1800	1200	1800				
Differences NORTH SHIELDS							
−0016	−0018	−0017	−0022	−0·5	−0·4	−0·2	−0·2
NEWCASTLE-UPON-TYNE							
−0013	−0015	−0009	−0014	−0·2	−0·2	−0·1	−0·1

SHELTER
Good in all weathers. Access H24, but in strong E and NE winds appr is difficult for small craft. Limited berthing for yachts which are charged a conservancy fee £6.50, as well as any private berthing dues. Prior arrangements must be made with Club Secretaries or Hr Mr. Yachts may use Albert Edward Dock giving excellent shelter and protection from heavy river traffic; obtain permission from Hr Mr by VHF or ☎. Ent is on N bank, 1M up river from No 1 Groyne, Fl G 5s.

NAVIGATION
WPT 55°01'·00N 01°22'·22W, 078°/258° from/to front ldg lt, 2·2M. From S, no dangers. From N, beware Bellhues Rk (approx 1M N of hbr and ¾M off shore); give old N pier a wide berth. Dredged chan in Lower Hbr is buoyed.

LIGHTS AND MARKS
Ldg lts 258°, FW 25/39m 20M, two W trs. Castle conspic on cliff 26m high, N of hbr.

RADIO TELEPHONE
Call: *Tyne Hbr Radio* VHF Ch **12** 16 11 14 (H24).

TELEPHONE (0191)
Hr Mr 257 0407; MRSC 257 2691; ⌗ 257 9441; Marinecall 0891 500453; Met 2326453; Police 232 3451; Dr via Tyne Hbr Radio 257 2080; Ⓗ (Tynemouth) 259 6660; Ⓗ (Newcastle) 273 8811.

FACILITIES
St Peter's Basin Marina (140 + 20 visitors) ☎ 265 4472, approx 7·8M above hbr ent; max draft is 2·8m, access HW±4, AC, FW, D, P; **Hebburn Marina** (50) ☎ 483 2876, FW, Slip; **Friars Goose Marina** (50) ☎ 469 2545, FW, ME, El, CH, Slip; **Tynemouth SC** ☎ 2529157; **South Shields SC** ☎ 4565821.
Services: Slip, M, L, FW, ME, El, Sh, C, CH, AB, ACA, Ⓔ.
Town EC Wed; P & D (cans), V, R, Bar, ✉, Ⓑ, ⇌ (Tynemouth or S Shields), ✈ (Newcastle).

ADJACENT HARBOUR

CULLERCOATS, Tyne and Wear, 55°02'·07N 01°25'·71W. AC 1191. +0430 Dover. Tides as 10.5.19. Small drying hbr 1·6M N of R Tyne ent. Appr on ldg line 256°, two bns (FR lts), between drying rks. An occas fair weather ⚓ or dry against S pier. Facilities at Tynemouth.

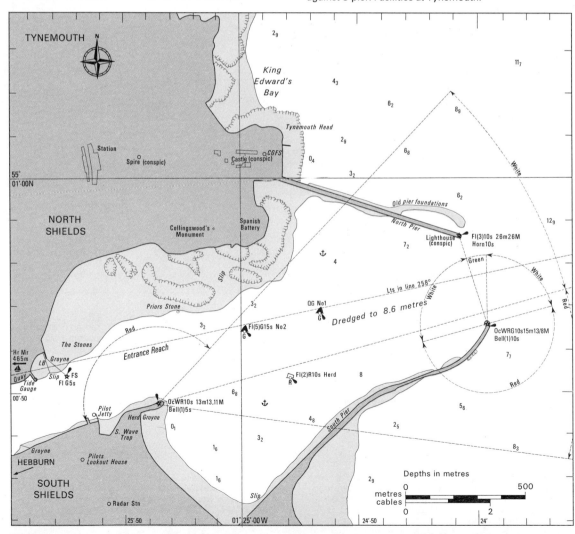

BLYTH 10-5-20

Northumberland 55°06'·98N 01° 29'·17W

CHARTS
AC 1626, 152, 156; Imray C29; OS 81, 88

TIDES
+0430 Dover; ML 2·8; Duration 0558; Zone 0 (UT)

Standard Port RIVER TEES ENT. (←)

Times				Height (metres)			
High Water		Low Water		MHWS	MHWN	MLWN	MLWS
0000	0600	0000	0600	5·5	4·3	2·0	0·9
1200	1800	1200	1800				
Differences BLYTH							
−0011	−0025	−0018	+0013	−0·5	−0·4	−0·3	−0·1

SHELTER
Very good; access H24. Visitors normally pick up RNYC mooring in S Hbr, E section or berth on Middle Jetty and see Hr Mr. At LW in strong SE winds, seas break across ent.

NAVIGATION
WPT Fairway SHM buoy, Fl G 3s, Bell, 55°06'·58N 01°28'·50W, 140°/320° from/to E pier lt, 0·53M. From N, beware The Pigs, The Sow and Seaton Sea Rks. No dangers from S.

LIGHTS AND MARKS
There are 8 conspic wind turbines on the E pier (shown on chartlet as X) and 1 on shore. Outer ldg lts 324°, F Bu 11/17m 10M, Or ◇ on framework trs. Inner ldg lts 338°, F Bu 5/11m 10M, front W 6-sided tr; rear W △ on mast.

RADIO TELEPHONE
Call: Blyth Hbr Control VHF Ch 12 11 16 (H24).

TELEPHONE (01670)
Hr Mr 352678; MRSC (0191) 257 2691; ⌗ 361521; Marinecall 0891 500453; Police (01661) 72555; Dr 353226.

FACILITIES
R Northumberland YC ☎ 353636, M £8, FW, C (1½ ton), Bar; South Hbr ☎ 352678, AB, M, FW, C (30 ton); Services: Slip, ME, El, Sh, Gas, Gaz. Town EC Wed; P & D (cans), V, R, Bar, ✉, Ⓑ, bus to Newcastle ⇌ ✈.

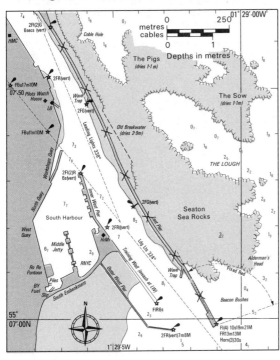

A Cautionary Tale; or the Perils of making a landfall in Fog.

We were weary after our slow passage of four days from Aberdeen, so I said to the crew "Let us not stay out here and wait for the bad weather to overtake us. Let us rather try to find our way into port". So we started the engine and we steamed to the south'ard through the fog.

Presently we heard the explosive signal on Coquet Island; and we continued slowly on our way until, by a rough bearing of the sound (in which we placed no confidence other than as a rough guide, for it is well known that sounds travel by odd and devious ways in fog), we estimated that the light house was abeam. We then set a careful compass course, and every seven minutes (the period of the fog signal being seven minutes and a half) we slowed down the motor, so that we could hear clearly and again judge the approximate direction of the sound. We had our patent log streamed, and we carefully noted the distance run from the time the light was abeam. In this way, when the sound bore about forty five degrees on our starboard quarter, we obtained an approximate four point bearing, by sound, of the light house; from which we put down, very roughly, our estimated position on the chart. And from this area (for we were not so foolish as to consider it a point) we laid our course for the bell buoy off the entrance to Blyth. We read the log, allowed carefully for the tide, and steamed slowly on.

All went well until we were within some three miles, according to our estimate, from the buoy. We then noticed that the seas were suddenly becoming steeper, for no apparent reason. We next saw that their backs were flecked with foam. Then we heard a mighty thundering of surf. At that moment, for an instant the fog thinned slightly and showed us, to our horror, a mass of ugly black rocks **right under our bows**! We rose on the back of one huge swell, and the next sea **was actually breaking on the shore**.

To put the helm hard over and head away from the land was the work of an instant, but it had been a close call. A glance at the chart showed not only that we were a good way inshore of where we had thought, but that we had nearly ended our voyage on Newbiggin Point. Why had we not heard the roar of the breakers sooner? I cannot tell, save that our engine was running, and may have partly drowned the noise. But I think a more likely explanation is that we must have run into a curious dead pocket in the fog, where sounds did not travel. It is well known that such phenomena occur.

Our position thus established, we made a direct course for the bell buoy, and picked it up without difficulty, whence to steer into the harbour, making allowance for the tide across the entrance, was a simple matter. The noise of trains ashore was an added guide. Nevertheless we saw nothing of the land until the two piers loomed up through the fog, one on each side of us. We were thankful to be in. Half an hour after we had berthed the fog cleared, and there followed a perfect sunny day.

The Yachtman's England: Frank G.G. Carr, 1937, Seeley Service.

ADJACENT ANCHORAGE

NEWBIGGIN, Northumberland, 55°10'·75N 01°30'·00W. AC 156. Tides approx as for Blyth, 3·5M to the S. Temp, fair weather ⚓ in about 4m in centre of Bay, sheltered from SW to N winds. Caution: offlying rky ledges to N and S. Two pairs of framework trs (marking a measured mile) bracket the bay. Conspic church on N side of bay; bkwtr lt Fl G 10s 4M. Facilities: SC (dinghies). Town V, R, Bar.

AMBLE   10-5-21

Northumberland 55°20'·37N 01°34'·15W

CHARTS
AC 1627, 156; Imray C29; OS 81

TIDES
+0412 Dover; ML 3·1; Duration 0606; Zone 0 (UT)

Standard Port RIVER TEES ENT. (←)

Times				Height (metres)			
High Water		Low Water		MHWS	MHWN	MLWN	MLWS
0000	0600	0000	0600	5·5	4·3	2·0	0·9
1200	1800	1200	1800				
Differences AMBLE							
−0039	−0033	−0040	−0036	−0·5	−0·2	0·0	−0·1
COQUET ISLAND							
−0023	−0028	−0037	−0042	−0·4	−0·1	−0·2	−0·1

SHELTER
The hbr (also known as Warkworth Hbr) is safe in all weathers, but ent is dangerous in strong N to E winds or in swell which causes heavy breakers on Pan Bush shoal and on the bar at the hbr ent. Once inside the N bkwtr, beware drying banks to stbd, ie on S side of ruined N jetty; chan favours the S quays. Visitors should go to Amble marina on S bank of R Coquet, approx 5ca from ent, access HW±4 via sill (0·75m above CD); the sill is marked by PHM and ECM buoys, both unlit. 4kn speed limit in hbr.

NAVIGATION
WPT 55°21'·00N 01°33'·00W, 045°/225° from/to hbr ent, 0·9M. Ent recommended from NE, passing N and W of Pan Bush. A wreck, 1·7m, lies 1·5ca ENE of N pier hd. The S-going stream sets strongly across ent. In NE'ly gales, when broken water can extend to Coquet Island, keep E of island and go to Blyth where app/ent may be safer. Coquet Chan (min depth 0·3m) is not buoyed and should only be used with local knowledge, by day, in fair weather and with adequate rise of tide.

LIGHTS AND MARKS
Coquet Island lt ho, (conspic) W □ tr, turreted parapet, lower half grey; Fl (3) WR 30s 25m 23/19M R330°-140°, W140°-163°, R163°-180°, W180°-330°. Sector boundaries are indeterminate and may appear as Al WR. Horn 30s. The Fl R 5s lt on S pier is only shown when the bar has >3m water and is not dangerous.

RADIO TELEPHONE
Call Amble Marina Ch 80 (H24). Amble Hbr VHF Ch 14 16 (Mon-Fri 0900-1700 LT). Coquet YC Ch M (occas).

TELEPHONE (01665)
Hr Mr 710306 (part-time); MRSC (0191) 257 9441; ⌗ (01670) 361521; Marinecall 0891 500453; Ⓗ (01670) 521212.

FACILITIES
Amble Marina (210+40 visitors) ☎ 712168 AC, BY, C, Gas, FW, D, P, R, Gaz, Slip, BH (20 ton), ME, El, Sh, Ⓔ, SM, Bar; V, CH, Ⓞ; **Hbr** D, AB; **Coquet YC** ☎ 711179 Slip, Bar, M, FW, L; **Services:** ME, Slip, CH, El, Sh, SM, Ⓔ.
Town EC Wed; V, R, Bar, ✉, ⇌ (Alnmouth), ✈ (Newcastle).

HARBOURS AND ANCHORAGES BETWEEN AMBLE AND HOLY ISLAND

BOULMER, Northumberland, 55°25'·00N 01°33'·80W. AC 156. Tides approx as for Amble, 4·5M to the S. A small haven almost enclosed by N and S Rheins, rky ledges either side of the narrow (30m) ent, Marmouth; only advised in settled offshore weather. 2 unlit bns lead approx 262° through the ent, leaving close to stbd a bn on N Rheins. ⌘ just inside in about 1·5m or dry out on sand at the N end. Few facilities: Pub, ✉ in village. Alnwick is 4M inland.

CRASTER, Northumberland, 55°28'·40N 01°35'·20W. AC 156. Tidal differences: interpolate between Amble (10.5.21) and N Sunderland (10.5.22). Strictly a fair weather ⌘ in offshore winds, 1M S of the conspic Dunstanburgh Castle (ru). The ent, 40m wide, is N of Muckle Carr and S of Little Carr which partly covers and has a bn on its S end. ⌘ in about 3·5m just inshore of these 2 rky outcrops; or berth at the E pier on rk/sand inside the tiny drying hbr. Facilities: V, R, Bar.

NEWTON HAVEN and BEADNELL BAY, Northumberland, 55°30'·90N 01° 36'·60W. AC 156. HW +0342 on Dover, −0102 on R Tees Ent; HW ht −0·7m on R Tees Ent; ML 2·6m; Duration 0625. A safe ⌘ in winds from NNW to SE via S but susceptible to swell. Ent to S of Newton PHM buoy and Newton Pt. Beware Fills Rks. ⌘ between Fills Rks and Low Newton by the Sea in 4/5m. A very attractive ⌘ with no lts, marks or facilities except a pub. Further ⌘ S of Beadnell Pt (1M N of Newton Pt) in 4-6m; small, private hbr; Beadnell SC. Village 0·5M.

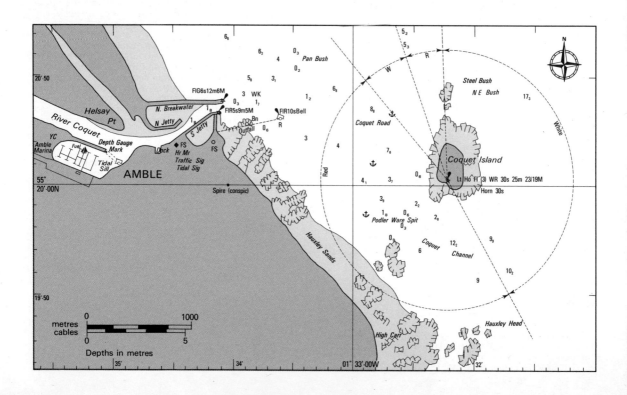

Continued

NORTH SUNDERLAND (Seahouses), Northumberland, 55°35´.04N 01°38´.81W. AC 1612. HW +0340 on Dover; ML 2·7m; Duration 0618. See 10.5.22. Good shelter except in on-shore winds when swell makes outer hbr berths (0·7m) very uncomfortable and dangerous. Access HW±3. Inner hbr has excellent berths but usually full of FVs. Beware The Tumblers (rks) to the W of ent and rks protruding NE from bkwtr hd Fl R 2·5s 6m; NW pier hd FG 11m 3M; vis 159°-294°, on W tr; traffic sigs; Siren 90s when vessels expected. When it is dangerous to enter a ⓇR is shown over the FG lt (or R flag over a Bu flag) on NW pier hd. Facilities: EC Wed; Gas; all facilities available.

FARNE ISLANDS, Northumberland, 55°37´.00N 01°39´.00W. AC 111, 156, 160. HW +0345 on Dover; ML 2·6m; Duration 0630. See 10.5.22. The islands are a NT nature reserve in a beautiful area; they should only be attempted in good weather. Landing is only allowed on Farne Island, Staple Is and Longstone. In the inner group, ‡ in The Kettle on the NE side of Inner Farne; near the Bridges (which connect Knocks Reef to West Wideopen); or to the S of West Wideopen. In the outer group, ‡ in Pinnacle Haven (between Staple Is and Brownsman). Beware turbulence over Knivestone and Whirl Rks and eddy S of Longstone during NW tidal streams. Lts and marks: Black Rocks Pt, Oc (2) WRG 15s 12m 17/13M; G122°-165°, W165°-175°, R175°-191°, W191°-238°, R238°-275°, W275°-289°, G289°-300°. Bamburgh Castle is conspic 6ca to the SE. Farne Is lt ho at SW Pt, Fl (2) WR 15s 27m 8/6M; W ○ tr; R119°-280°, W280°-119°. Longstone Fl 20s 23m 24M, R tr with W band (conspic), RC, horn (2) 60s. Caution: reefs extend about 7ca seaward. No facilities.

HOLY ISLAND   10-5-22

Northumberland 55°40´.00N 01°48´.00W

CHARTS
AC 1612, 111; Imray C24; OS 75
TIDES
+0344 Dover; ML 2·6; Duration 0630; Zone 0 (UT)

Standard Port RIVER TEES ENT. (←)

Times				Height (metres)			
High Water		Low Water		MHWS	MHWN	MLWN	MLWS
0000	0600	0000	0600	5·5	4·3	2·0	0·9
1200	1800	1200	1800				
Differences HOLY ISLAND							
–0059	–0057	–0122	–0132	–0·7	–0·6	–0·5	–0·3
NORTH SUNDERLAND (Seahouses)							
–0104	–0102	–0115	–0124	–0·7	–0·6	–0·4	–0·2

SHELTER
Good S of The Heugh in 3-6m, but ‡ is uncomfortable in fresh W/SW winds esp at sp flood. Better shelter in The Ouse on sand/mud if able to dry out; but not in S/SE winds.
NAVIGATION
WPT 55°39´.76N 01°44´.78W, 080°/260° from/to Old Law E bn 1·55M. From N identify Emanuel Hd, conspic W △ bn, then appr via Goldstone Chan leaving Plough Seat PHM buoy to stbd. From S, clear Farne Is thence to WPT. Outer ldg bns lead 260° close past Ridge End ECM and Triton Shoal SHM buoys. Possible overfalls in chan across bar (2·1m) with sp ebb up to 4kn. Inner ldg marks lead 310° to ‡. Alternative route, rounding Castle Pt via Hole Mouth and The Yares, may be more sheltered, but is not advised for strangers.

LIGHTS AND MARKS
Outer ldg marks/lts are Old Law bns (conspic), 2 white obelisks 21/25m on 260°; E bn has sectored lt, Oc RG 6s 9m 4M, G170°-260°, R260°-020°. Inner ldg marks/lts are The Heugh tr, R △, on with St Mary's ch belfry 310°. The Heugh has sectored lt, Oc RG 6s 24m 5M, G135°-310°, R310°-125°. Sector lts Oc RG are aligned on 260° and 310° respectively.
RADIO TELEPHONE
None.
TELEPHONE (01289)
Hr Mr 89217; MRSC 0191-257 2691.
FACILITIES
Limited. FW on village green, R, Bar, limited V, P & D from Beal (5M); bus (occas) to Berwick. Note Lindisfarne is ancient name; Benedictine Abbey (ruins) and Castle (NT) are worth visiting. Causeway to mainland covers at HW. It is usable by vehicles HW+3½ to HW–2; less in adverse wx.

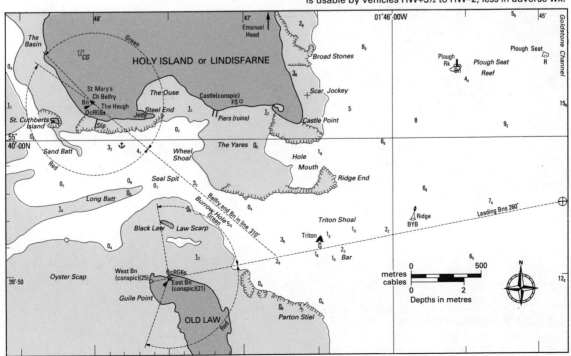

BERWICK-ON-TWEED   10-5-23

Northumberland 55°45'·87N 01°58'·95W

CHARTS
AC 1612, 111, 160; OS 75

TIDES
+0348 Dover; ML 2·5; Duration 0620; Zone 0 (UT)

Standard Port RIVER TEES ENT. (←)

Times				Height (metres)			
High Water		Low Water		MHWS	MHWN	MLWN	MLWS
0000	0600	0000	0600	5·5	4·3	2·0	0·9
1200	1800	1200	1800				
Differences BERWICK							
–0109	–0111	–0126	–0131	–0·8	–0·5	–0·7	–0·3

SHELTER
Good shelter or ⚓ except in strong E/SE winds. Yachts lie in Tweed dock (the dock gates have been removed; 0·6m in ent, approx 1·2m inside at MLWS) or temporarily at W end of Fish Jetty (1·2m).

NAVIGATION
WPT 55°45'·65N 01°58'·00W, 114°/294° from/to bkwtr lt ho, 0·58M. On-shore winds and ebb tides cause very confused state over the bar (0·6m). Access HW ±4 at sp. From HW–2 to HW+1 strong flood tide sets across the ent; keep well up to bkwtr. The sands at the mouth of the Tweed shift so often that local knowledge is essential. The Berwick bridge (first and lowest) has about 3m clearance.

LIGHTS AND MARKS
Town hall clock tr and lt ho in line at 294°. When past Crabwater Rk, keep bns at Spittal in line at 207°. Bns are B and W with △ top marks (both FR).

RADIO TELEPHONE
Hr Mr VHF Ch 12 16 (HO).

TELEPHONE (01289)
Hr Mr 307404; MRSC 01333 450666; ☒ 307547; Marinecall 0891 500453/452; Police 307111; Dr 307484.

FACILITIES
Tweed Dock ☎ 307404, AB £3.50, M, P, D, FW, ME, El, Sh, C (Mobile 3 ton), Slip, SM.
Town EC Thurs; P, V, R, Bar, ☒, Ⓑ, ⇌ and ✈ (Newcastle or Edinburgh).

AGENTS WANTED

If you are interested in becoming our agent for any of the following ports, please write to: The Editor, Edington House, Trent, Sherborne, Dorset DT9 4SR, England – and get your free copy of the almanac annually. You do not have to live in a port to be the agent, but at least a fairly regular visitor.

River Exe
Port Ellen (Islay)
Glandore/Union Hall
River Rance/Dinan
Lampaul
Port Tudy
River Etel
Le Palais (Belle Ile)
Le Pouliguen/Pornichet
L'Herbaudière
St Gilles-Croix-de-Vie
River Seudre
Royan
Anglet/Bayonne
Hendaye

Grandcamp-Maisy
Port-en-Bessin
Courseulles
Boulogne
Dunkerque
Terneuzen/Westerschelde
Oudeschild
Lauwersoog
Dornumer-Accumersiel
Hooksiel
Langeoog
Bremerhaven
Helgoland
Büsum

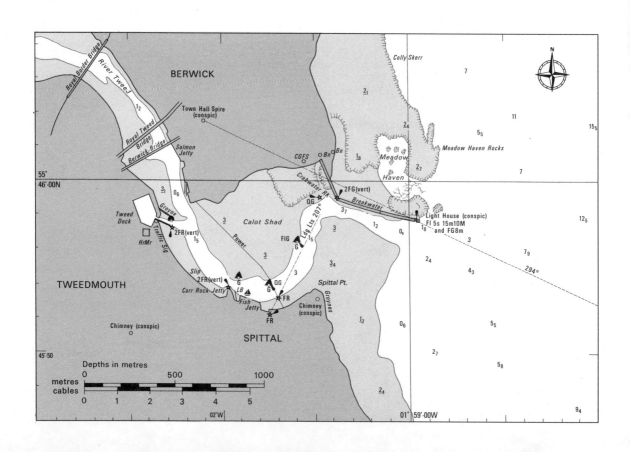

Volvo Penta service

Sales and service centres in area 6
LOTHIAN *Port Edgar Marine Services Ltd*, Port Edgar Marina, South
Queensferry, Nr. Edinburgh EH30 9SQ Tel 0131-331 1233

Area 6

South-East Scotland
Eyemouth to Rattray Head

VOLVO PENTA

6

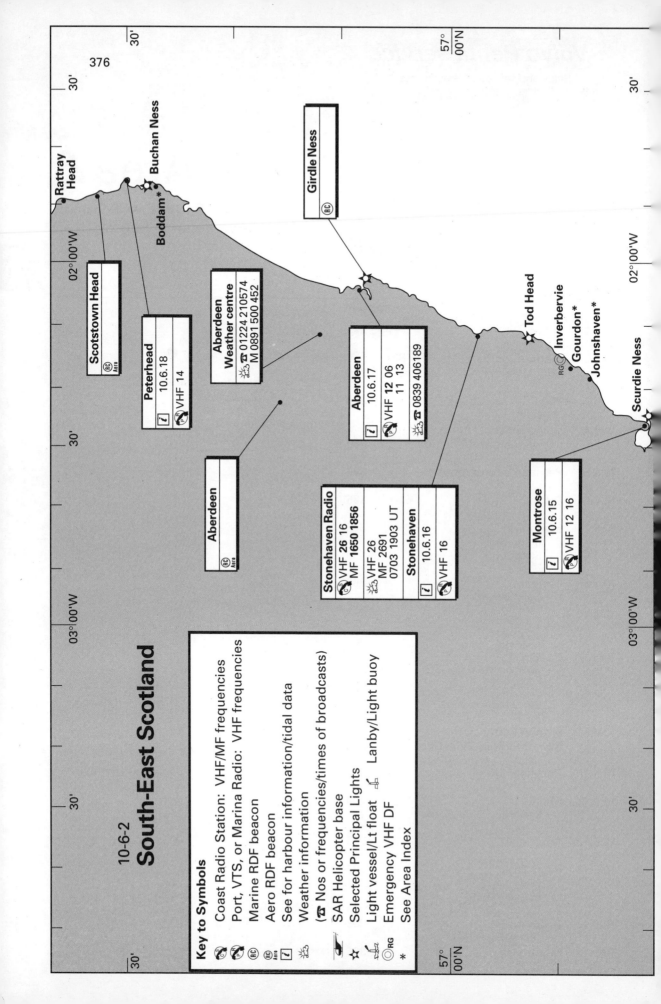

10·6·2
South-East Scotland

Key to Symbols

🎧🎧	Coast Radio Station: VHF/MF frequencies
🎧🎧	Port, VTS, or Marina Radio: VHF frequencies
(RC)	Marine RDF beacon
(RC) Aero	Aero RDF beacon
i	See for harbour information/tidal data
🎧	Weather information (☎ Nos or frequencies/times of broadcasts)
🚁	SAR Helicopter base
☆	Selected Principal Lights
⌓	Light vessel/Lt float ⌓ Lanby/Light buoy
⊙RG	Emergency VHF DF
*	See Area Index

Rattray Head

Buchan Ness

Boddam*

Scotstown Head

(RC) Aero

Peterhead

i	10.6.18
🎧	VHF 14

Aberdeen Weather centre

☎ 01224 210574
M 0891 500 452

Aberdeen

(RC) Aero

Girdle Ness

(RC)

Tod Head

Inverbervie

Gourdon*

Johnshaven*

Scurdie Ness

Aberdeen

i	10.6.17
🎧	VHF **12** 06 11 13
🎧	☎ 0839 406189

RG⊙

Stonehaven Radio

🎧	VHF **26** 16 MF **1650 1856**
🎧	VHF 26 MF 2691 0703 1903 UT

Stonehaven

i	10.6.16
🎧	VHF 16

Montrose

i	10.6.15
🎧	VHF 12 16

57° 00'N

57° 00'N

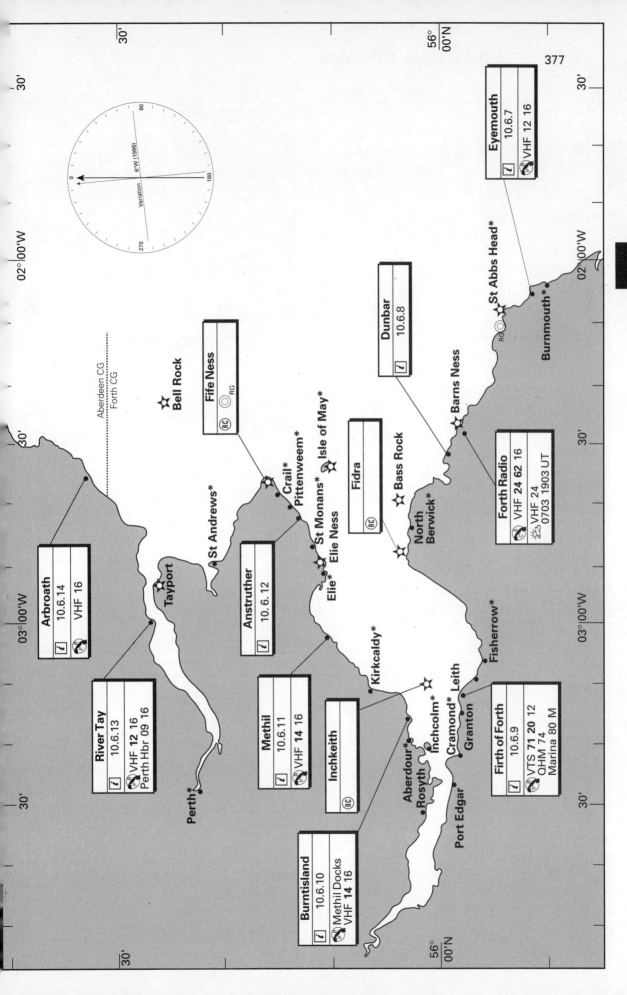

6

Eyemouth
10.6.7
VHF 12 16

Dunbar
10.6.8

St Abbs Head*

Burnmouth*

Fife Ness
RG

Bell Rock

Aberdeen CG
Forth CG

Variation
6°W (1996)
0
90
180
270

02°00'W

03°00'W

02°00'W

30'

30'

30'

56°
00'N

56°
00'N

Crail*
Pittenweem*
St Monans*
Isle of May*
Elie Ness
Elie*

St Andrews*

Tayport

Anstruther
10.6.12

Fidra
RG

Bass Rock

North
Berwick*

Barns Ness

Forth Radio
VHF 24 62 16
VHF 24
0703 1903 UT

Arbroath
10.6.14
VHF 16

River Tay
10.6.13
VHF **12** 16
Perth Hbr 09 16

Perth*

Methil
10.6.11
VHF **14** 16

Inchkeith
RG

Kirkcaldy*

Inchcolm*

Cramond* Leith
Granton

Aberdour*
Rosyth

Port Edgar

Fisherrow*

Firth of Forth
10.6.9
VTS 71 20 12
QHM 74
Marina 80 M

Burntisland
10.6.10
Methil Docks
VHF **14** 16

10-6-3   AREA 6 TIDAL STREAMS

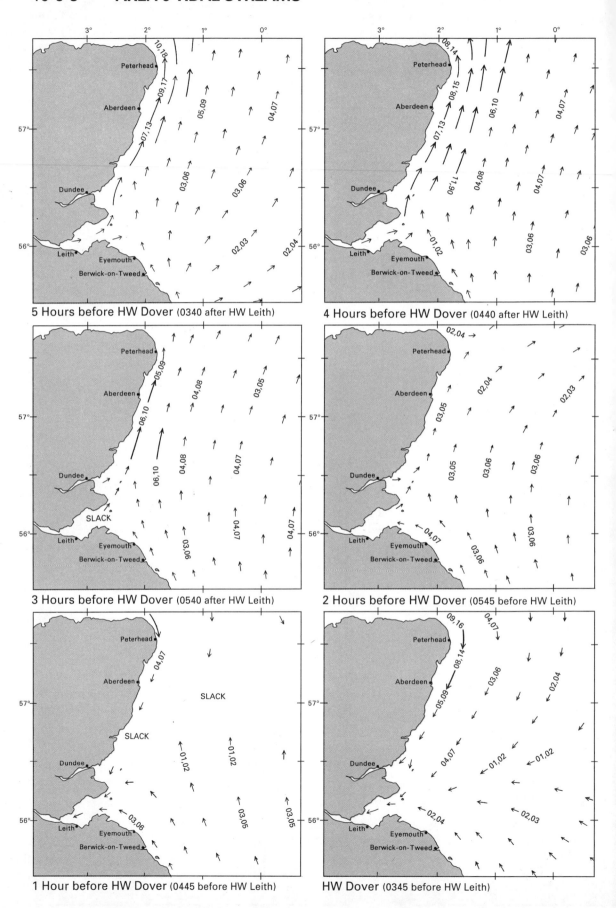

5 Hours before HW Dover (0340 after HW Leith)

4 Hours before HW Dover (0440 after HW Leith)

3 Hours before HW Dover (0540 after HW Leith)

2 Hours before HW Dover (0545 before HW Leith)

1 Hour before HW Dover (0445 before HW Leith)

HW Dover (0345 before HW Leith)

Northward 10.7.3   Southward 10.5.3

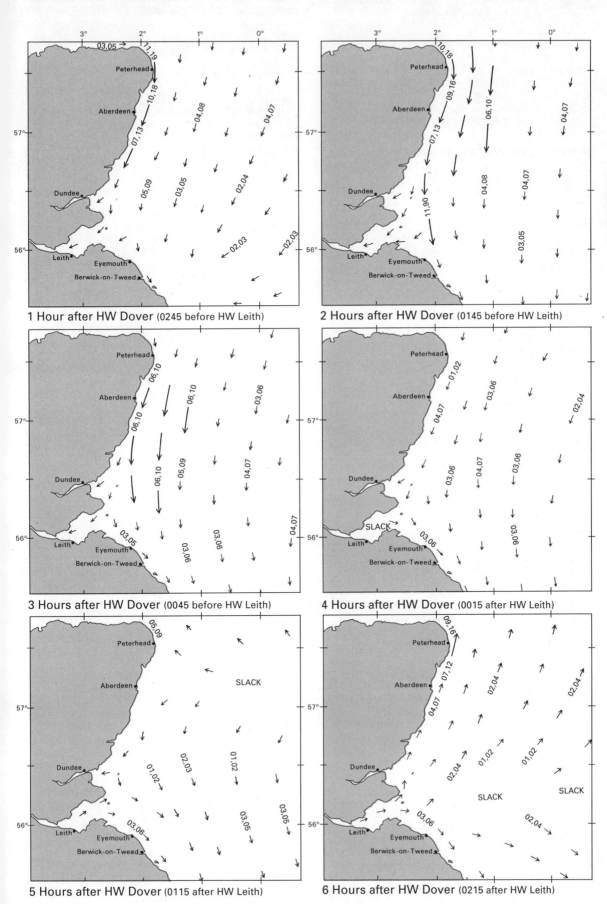

1 Hour after HW Dover (0245 before HW Leith)

2 Hours after HW Dover (0145 before HW Leith)

3 Hours after HW Dover (0045 before HW Leith)

4 Hours after HW Dover (0015 after HW Leith)

5 Hours after HW Dover (0115 after HW Leith)

6 Hours after HW Dover (0215 after HW Leith)

10.6.4   COASTAL LIGHTS, FOG SIGNALS AND WAYPOINTS

Abbreviations used below are given in 1.4.1. Principal lights are in **bold** print, places in CAPITALS, and light-vessels, light floats and Lanbys in *CAPITAL ITALICS*. Unless otherwise stated lights are white. m – elevation in metres; M – nominal range in miles. Fog signals are in *italics*. Useful waypoints are underlined – use those on land with care. All geographical positions should be assumed to be approximate. See 4.4.1.

BERWICK-UPON-TWEED TO BASS ROCK

BURNMOUTH
Ldg Lts 274°. Front 55°50'·55N 02°04'·12W FR 29m 4M. Rear, 45m from front, FR 35m 4M. Both on W posts.

EYEMOUTH
Ldg Lts 174°. Front, W Bkwtr Hd, 55°52'·47N 02°05'·18W FG 7m 5M. Rear, elbow 55m from front, FG 10m 4M.
E Bkwtr Hd 55°52'·51N 02°05'·18W Iso R 2s 8m 8M; *Siren 30s.*

ST ABB'S
Hd of inside Jetty 55°53'·95N 02°07'·60W FR 4m 1M.
St Abb's Hd 55°54'·97N 02°08'·20W Fl 10s 68m **26M**; W Tr; Racon (T).
Torness Power Station Pier Hd 55°58'·40N 02°24'·32W Fl R 5s 10m 5M.
Barns Ness Lt Bn Tr 55°59'·21N 02°26'·68W Iso 4s 36m 10M; W ● Tr.

DUNBAR
Bayswell Hill Ldg Lts 198°. Front 56°00'·26N 02°31'·08W Oc G 6s 15m 3M; W ▲ on Or col; intens 188°-208°. Rear, Oc G 6s 22m 3M; ▼ on Or col; synch with front, intens 188°-208°.
Victoria Hbr, Middle Quay, 56°00'·32N 02°30'·80W QR 6m 3M; vis through cliffs at hbr ent.

Bellhaven Bay Outfall By 56°00'·98N 02°33'·00W; SPM.
S Carr Bn (12) 56°03'·44N 02°37'·60W.
Bass Rock, S side, 56°04'·60N 02°38'·37W Fl (3) 20s 46m 10M; W Tr; vis 241°-107°.

FIRTH OF FORTH AND SOUTH SHORE
(Direction of buoyage East to West)

NORTH BERWICK
Outfall Lt By 56°04'·27N 02°40'·78W Fl Y 5s; SPM.
N Pier Hd 56°03'·73N 02°42'·92W F WR 7m 3M; vis R seaward, W over hbr. Not lit if ent closed by weather.

Fidra, near summit 56°04'·40N 02°47'·00W Fl (4) 30s 34m **24M**; W Tr; RC; obsc by Bass Rk, Craig Leith and Lamb Is.
Wreck Lt By 56°04'·40N 02°52'·30W Fl (2) R 10s; PHM.

PORT SETON/COCKENZIE/FISHERROW/SOUTH CHANNEL
Port Seton, E Pier Hd, 55°58'·40N 02°57'·10W Iso WR 4s 10m W9M, R6M; R shore-105°, W105°-225°, R225°-shore; *Bell* (occas).
Cockenzie Power Station, Jetty Hd 55°58'·25N 02°58'·32W QR 6m 1M.
Fisherrow E Pier Hd 55°58'·80N 03°04'·03W Oc W 6s 5m 6M; framework Tr.
South Chan Appr Lt By 56°01'·42N 03°02'·15W L Fl 10s; SWM.
Narrow Deep Lt By 56°01'·47N 03°04'·50W Fl (2) R 10s; PHM.
Herwit Lt By 56°01'·05N 03°06'·43W Fl (3) G 10s; SHM; *Bell.*
North Craig By 56°00'·75N 03°03'·80W; SHM.
Craigh Waugh Lt By 56°00'·27N 03°04'·38W Q; NCM.
Diffuser Hds By (Outer) 55°59'·81N 03°07'·75W; NCM.

Diffuser Hds By (Inner) 55°59'·38N 03°07'·94W; SCM
Leith Approach Lt By 55°59'·95N 03°11'·42W Fl R 3s; PHM.

LEITH
East Bkwtr Hd 55°59'·48N 03°10'·85W Iso R 4s 7m 9M; *Horn (3) 30s.*
W Bkwtr Hd L Fl G 6s.

GRANTON
E Pier Hd 55°59'·28N 03°13'·17W Fl R 2s 5m 6M; W ■ Bldg.

CRAMOND
Church Tr 55°58'·67N 03°17'·92W.

NORTH CHANNEL/MIDDLE BANK
Inchkeith Fairway Lt By 56°03'·50N 03°00'·00W Iso 2s; SWM; Racon (T).
No. 1 Lt By 56°03'·23N 03°03'·63W Fl G 9s; SHM.
No. 2 Lt By 56°02'·90N 03°03'·63W Fl R 9s; PHM.
No. 3 Lt By 56°03'·23N 03°06'·00W Fl G 6s; SHM.
No. 4 Lt By 56°02'·90N 03°06'·00W Fl R 6s; PHM.
No. 5 Lt By 56°03'·18N 03°07'·80W Fl G 3s; SHM.
No. 6 Lt By 56°03'·05N 03°08'·35W Fl R 3s; PHM.
No. 8 Lt By 56°02'·95N 03°09'·54W Fl R 9s; PHM.
Inchkeith, summit 56°02'·01N 03°08'·09W Fl 15s 67m **22M**; stone Tr; RC.
E Stell Pt *Horn 15s.*
Pallas Rock Lt By 56°01'·50N 03°09'·22W VQ (9) 10s; WCM.
East Gunnet Lt By 56°01'·42N 03°10'·30W Q (3) 10s; ECM.
West Gunnet Lt By 56°01'·35N 03°10'·97W Q (9) 15s; WCM.
No. 7 Lt By 56°02'·80N 03°10'·87W QG; *Bell*; Racon (T).
No. 9 Lt By 56°02'·37N 03°13'·38W Fl G 6s; SHM.
No. 10 Lt By 56°02'·05N 03°13'·30W Fl R 6s; PHM.
No. 11 Lt By 56°02'·08N 03°15'·15W Fl G 3s; SHM.
No. 12 Lt By 56°01'·77N 03°15'·05W Fl R 3s; PHM.
No. 13 Lt By 56°01'·77N 03°16'·94W Fl G 9s; SHM.
No. 14 Lt By 56°01'·52N 03°16'·82W Fl R 9s; PHM.
Oxcars Lt Bn Tr 56°01'·36N 03°16'·74W Fl (2) WR 7s 16m W13M, R12M; W Tr, R band; vis W072°-087°, R087°-196°, W196°-313°, R313°-072°; Ra refl.
Inchcolm E Pt 56°01'·73N 03°17'·75W Fl (3) 15s 20m 10M; Gy Tr; part obsc 075°-145°; *Horn (3) 45s.*
No. 15 Lt By 56°01'·43N 03°18'·70W Fl G 6s; SHM.

MORTIMER'S DEEP.
Hawkcraig Pt Ldg Lts 292°. Front 56°03'·04N 03°16'·98W Iso 5s 12m 14M; W Tr; vis 282°-302°. Rear, 96m from front, Iso 5s 16m 14M; W Tr; vis 282°-302°.
No. 1 Lt By 56°02'·68N 03°15'·19W QG; SHM.
No. 2 Lt By 56°02'·70N 03°15'·76W QR; PHM.
No. 3 Lt By 56°02'·51N 03°17'·44W Fl (2) G 5s; SHM.
No. 4 Lt By 56°02'·38N 03°17'·35W Fl (2) R 5s; PHM.
No. 5 Lt By 56°02'·37N 03°17'·86W Fl G 4s; SHM.
No. 6 Lt By 56°02'·28N 03°17'·78W Fl R 4s; PHM.
No. 7 Lt By 56°01'·94N 03°18'·92W Fl (2) G 5s; SHM.
No. 8 Lt By 56°02'·10N 03°18'·17W Fl R 2s; PHM.
No. 9 Lt By 56°01'·69N 03°19'·08W QG; SHM.
No. 10 Lt By 56°01'·83N 03°18'·48W Fl (2) R 5s; PHM.
No. 14 Lt By 56°01'·56N 03°18'·96W Q (9) 15s; WCM.
Inchcolm S Lts in line 066°. Front, 84m from rear, Q 7m 7M; W Tr; vis 062·5°-082·5°. Common Rear 56°01'·80N 03°18'·13W Iso 5s 11m 7M; W Tr; vis 062°-082°.
N Lts in line 076·7°. Front, 80m from rear, Q 7m 7M; W Tr; vis 062·5°-082·5°.

APPROACHES TO FORTH BRIDGES
No. 16 Lt By 56°00'·75N 03°19'·81W Fl R 3s; PHM.
No. 17 Lt By 56°01'·17N 03°20'·12W Fl G 3s; SHM.
No. 19 Lt By 56°00'·72N 03°22'·40W Fl G 9s; SHM.
Hound Pt Terminal NE Dn 56°00'·48N 03°21'·14W 2 FR 7m 5M; *Siren (3) 90s.*

Centre Pier 2 Aero FR 47m 5M.

Hound Pt SW Dn 56°00'·28N 03°21'·83W FR 7m 5M.

Inch Garvie, NW end 56°00'·01N 03°23'·29W L Fl 5s 9m 11M; B ● Bn, W lantern.

N Queensferry. Oc 5s and QR or QG tfc signals.

Forth Rail Bridge. Centres of spans have W Lts and ends of cantilevers R Lts, defining N and S chans.

Forth Road Bridge. N suspension Tr Iso G 4s 7m 6M on E and W sides; 2 Aero FR 155m 11M and 2 FR 109m 7M on same Tr. Main span, N part QG 50m 6M on E and W sides. Main span, centre Iso 4s 52m 8M on E and W sides. Main span, S part QR 50m 6M on E and W sides. S suspension Tr Iso R 4s 7m 6M on E and W sides; 2 Aero FR 155m and 2 Fr 109m 7M on same Tr.

PORT EDGAR

Dir Lt 244°. W Bkwtr Hd 55°59'·85N 03°24'·69W Dir Fl R 4s 4m 8M; W blockhouse; 4 QY mark floating bkwtr.

3 x 2 FR (vert) mark N ends of Marina pontoons inside hbr.

Beamer Rk Lt Bn Tr 56°02'·28N 03°24'·66W Fl 3s 6m 9M; W Tr, R top; *Horn 20s.*

FIRTH OF FORTH – NORTH SHORE (INWARD)

BURNTISLAND

W Pier outer Hd 56°03'·2N 03°22'·2W Fl (2) R 6s 7m; W Tr.

E Pier outer Hd 56°03'·23N 03°14'·08W Fl (2) G 6s 6m 5M.

ABERDOUR/BRAEFOOT BAY/INCHCOLM

Hawkcraig Pt (see MORTIMER'S DEEP above)

Aberdour Bay Outfall Bn 56°02'·97N 03°17'·62W; Y Bn.

Braefoot Bay Terminal, W Jetty. Ldg Lts 247·25°. **Front** 56°02'·15N 03°18'·63W Fl 3s 6m **15M**; W ▲ on E dolphin; vis 237·2°-257·2°; four dolphins marked by 2 FG (vert). **Rear**, 88m from front, Fl 3s 12m **15M**; W ▼ on appr gangway; vis 237·2°-257·2°; synch with front.

Inchcolm Abbey Tr 56°01'·81N 03°18'·02W.

INVERKEITHING BAY

St Davids Dir Lt Bn 56°01'·37N 03°22'·20W Dir 098° Fl G 5s 3m 7M; Or □, on pile.

Channel Lt By 56°01'·43N 03°22'·94W QG; SHM.

Channel Lt By 56°01'·44N 03°23'·30W QR; PHM.

HM NAVAL BASE, ROSYTH

Main Chan Dir Lt 323·5°. Bn A 56°01'·19N 03°25'·53W Dir Oc WRG 7m 4M; R ■ on W post with R bands, on B&W diagonal ■ on W Bn; vis G318°-321°, W321°-326°, R326°-328° (H24).

Dir Lt 115°, Bn C 56°00'·61N 03°24'·17W Dir Oc WRG 6s 7m 4M; W ▼ on W Bn; vis R110°-113°, W113°-116·5°, G116·5°-120°.

Dir Lt 295°, Bn E 56°01'·30N 03°26'·83W Dir Oc 6s 11m 4M; vis 293·5°-296·5°.

No. 1 Lt By 56°00'·54N 03°24'·48W Fl (2) G 10s; SHM.

Whale Bank No. 2 Lt By 56°00'·70N 03°25'·10W Q (3) 10s; ECM.

No. 3 Lt By 56°00'·87N 03°24'·98W Fl G 5s; SHM.

No. 4 Lt By 56°00'·82N 03°25'·18W Fl R 3s; PHM.

No. 5 Lt By 56°01'·08N 03°25'·80W QG; SHM.

No. 6 Lt By 56°01'·01N 03°25'·94W QR; PHM.

S Arm Jetty Hd 56°01'·08N 03°26'·48W L Fl (2) WR 12s 5m W9M; R6M; vis W010°-280°, R280°-010°; *Siren 20s (occas).*

RIVER FORTH

ROSYTH TO GRANGEMOUTH

Dhu Craig Lt By 56°00'·76N 03°27'·15W Fl G 5s; SHM.

Blackness Lt By 56°01'·07N 03°30'·22W QR; PHM.

Charlestown. Lts in line. Front 56°02'·20N 03°30'·60W FG 4m 10M; Y ▲ on Y pile; vis 017°-037°; marks line of HP gas main. Rear FG 6m 10M; Y ▼ on Y pile; vis 017°-037°.

Crombie Jetty, downstream dolphin 56°01'·94N 03°31'·76W 2 FG (vert) 8m 4M; *Horn (2) 60s.*

Crombie Jetty, upstream dolphin 56°02'·00N 03°32'·03W 2 FG (Vert) 8m 4M.

Tancred Bank Lt By 56°01'·59N 03°31'·83W Fl (2) R 10s; PHM.

Dods Bank Lt By 56°02'·03N 03°33'·99W Fl R 3s; PHM.

Bo'ness Lt By 56°02'·23N 03°35'·31W Fl R 10s; PHM.

Bo'ness. Carriden outfall 56°01'·32N 03°33'·62W Fl Y 5s 3M; Y ■ on Y Bn.

Torry 56°02'·47N 03°35'·20W Fl G 10s 5m 7M; G ● structure.

Bo'ness Platform 56°01'·84N 03°36'·13W QR 3m 2M; R pile Bn.

GRANGEMOUTH

Grangemouth App No. 1 pile 56°02'·13N 03°38'·01W Fl (3) R 20s 4m 6M.

Hen & Chickens Lt By 56°02'·37N 03°38'·00W Fl (3) G 20s; SHM.

No. 2 pile 56°02'·35N 03°39'·13W Fl G 5s 4m 6M; G ■ on pile.

No. 3 pile 56°02'·26N 03°39'·13W Fl R 5s 4m 6M.

No. 4 pile 56°02'·39N 03°39'·83W Fl G 2s 4m 5M.

No. 5 pile 56°02'·25N 03°39'·82W Fl R 2s 4m 5M.

Grangemouth W Lt By 56°02'·38N 03°40'·50W QG; SHM.

Dock entrance, E Jetty; *Horn 30s;* docking signals.

Longannet Power Station, intake L Fl G 10s 5m 6M.

Inch Brake By 56°03'·62N 03°43'·19W; SHM.

KINCARDINE

Swing bridge 56°03'·9N 03°43'·5W FW at centre of each span; FR Lts mark each side of openings.

FIRTH OF FORTH – NORTH SHORE (OUTWARD)

KIRKCALDY

East Pier Hd 56°06'·78N 03°08'·81W Fl WG 10s 12m 8M; vis G156°-336°, W336°-156°.

S Pier Hd 56°06'·81N 03°08'·88W 2 FR (vert) 7m 5M.

W Rockheads By 56°07'·00N 03°06'·90W; SHM.

E Rockheads By 56°07'·15N 03°06'·33W; SHM.

Kirkcaldy Wreck Lt By 56°07'·26N 03°05'·20W Fl (3) G 18s; SHM.

METHIL

Outer Pier Hd 56°10'·77N 03°00'·39W Oc G 6s 8m 5M; W Tr; vis 280°-100°.

ELIE

Thill Rk By 56°10'·88N 02°49'·60W; PHM.

Elie Ness 56°11'·05N 02°48'·65W Fl 6s 15m **18M**; W Tr.

ST MONANCE

Bkwtr Hd 56°12'·20N 02°45'·80W Oc WRG 6s 5m W7M, R4M, G4M; vis G282°-355°, W355°-026°, R026°-038°.

E Pier Hd 2 FG(vert) 6m 4M; Or tripod; *Bell* (occas).

W Pier near Hd, 2 FR (vert) 6m 4M.

PITTENWEEM

Ldg Lts 037° Middle Pier Hd. Front FR 4m 5M. Rear FR 8m 5M. Both Gy Cols, Or stripes.

E Bkwtr Hd 56°12'·36N 02°43'·36W Fl (2) RG 5s 9m R9M; G6M; vis R265°-345°, G345°-055°.

Beacon Rk Lt Bn QR 3m 2M.

W Pier Elbow, *Horn 90s* (occas).

ANSTRUTHER EASTER
Ldg Lts 019°. Front 56°13'·29N 02°41'·68W FG 7m 4M.
Rear, 38m from front, FG 11m 4M, (both W masts)
W Pier Hd 2 FR (vert) 5m 4M; Gy mast; *Horn (3) 60s (occas)*.
E Pier Hd 56°13'·15N 02°41'·72W Fl G 3s 6m 4M.

MAY ISLAND
Isle of May, Summit 56°11'·13N 02°33'·30W Fl (2) 15s 73m
22M; ■ Tr on stone dwelling.

CRAIL
Ldg Lts 295°. Front 56°15'·48N 02°37'·70W FR 24m 6M (not
lit when hbr closed). Rear, 30m from front, FR 30m 6M.

Fife Ness Lt 56°16'·73N 02°35'·10W Iso WR 10s 12m
W21M, R20M; W bldg; vis W143°-197°, R197°-217°, W217°-
023°; RC.

FIFE NESS TO MONTROSE

N Carr Lt By 56°18'·07N 02°32'·85W Q (3) 10s; ECM.
Bell Rk Lt Tr 56°26'·05N 02°23'·07W Fl 5s 28m **18M**; W ●
Tr; Racon (M).

RIVER TAY/TAYPORT/DUNDEE/PERTH
Tay Fairway Lt By 56°28'·92N 02°37'·42W L Fl 10s; SWM;
Bell.
Middle Green Lt By (N) 56°28'·33N 02°38'·83W Fl (3) G 18s; SHM.
Middle Red Lt By (S) 56°28'·17N 02°38'·50W Fl (2) R 12s;
PHM.
Abertay N Lt By 56°27'·41N 02°40'·66W Q (3) 10s; ECM;
Racon (T).
Abertay S (Elbow) Lt By 56°27'·17N 02°40'·33W Fl R 6s; PHM.
High Lt Ho Dir Lt 269°, 56°27'·17N 02°53'·85W Dir Iso WRG
3s 24m **W22M, R17M, G16M**; W Tr; vis G267°-268°, W268°-
270°, R270°-271°.
Inner Lt Buoy 56°27'·10N 02°44'·23W Fl (2) R 12s; PHM.
N Lady Lt By 56°27'·43N 02°46'·56W Fl (3) G 18s; SHM.
S Lady Lt By 56°27'·20N 02°46'·76W Fl (3) R 18s; PHM.
Pool Lt By 56°27'·15N 02°48'·50W Fl R 6s; PHM.
Tentsmuir Pt 56°26'·6N 02°49'·5W Fl Y 5s; Y Bn; vis 198°-
208°; marks gas pipeline.
Monifieth 56°28'·9N 02°47'·8W Fl Y 5s; Y Bn; vis 018°-028°;
marks gas pipeline.
Horse Shoe Lt By 56°27'·28N 02°50'·11W VQ (6) + L Fl 15s; SCM.
Larick Scalp Lt By 56°27'·19N 02°51'·50W Fl (2) R 12s; PHM;
Bell.
Broughty Castle 56°27'·76N 02°52'·10W 2 FG (vert) 10m 4M;
Gy col; FR is shown at foot of old Lt Ho at Buddon Ness, 4M
to E, and at other places on firing range when practice is
taking place.
Craig Lt By 56°27'·48N 02°52'·94W QR; PHM.
Newcombe Shoal Lt By 56°27'·73N 02°53'·50W Fl R 6s; PHM.
Dundee Tidal Basin E Ent 56°27'·92N 02°55'·92W 2 FG (vert).
E Deep Lt By 56°27'·35N 02°55'·62W QR; PHM.
Middle Bank Lt By 56°27'·40N 02°56'·39W Q (3) 10s; ECM.
West Deep Lt By 56°27'·15W 02°56'·15W Fl R 3s; PHM.
Tay Road Bridge N navigation span, centre 56°27'·03N
02°56'·44W 2 x VQ 27m.
Tay Road Bridge S navigation span, centre 56°27'·01N
02°56'·38W 2 x VQ 28m.
Tay Railway Bridge navigation 56°26'·28N 02°59'·20W 2 x 2
F (vert) 23m.
Jock's Hole 56°21'·75N 03°12'·10W QR 8m 2M.
Cairnie Pier 56°21'·50N 03°17'·80W.
Pipeline S by Elcho Castle 56°22'·50N 03°20'·80W Iso R 4s
4m 4M.

ARBROATH
Outfall Lt By 56°32'·64N 02°34'·97W Fl Y 3s; SPM.
Ldg Lts 299·2°. Front 56°33'·30N 02°35'·07W FR 7m 5M; W
col. Rear, 50m from front, FR 13m 5M; W col.
W Bkwtr E end, VQ (2) 6s 6m 4M; W post.
E Pier S Elbow 56°33'·26N 02°34'·89W Fl G 3s 8m 5M; W Tr;
shows FR when hbr closed; *Siren (3) 60s (occas)*.

MONTROSE
Scurdie Ness 56°42'·12N 02°26'·15W Fl (3) 20s 38m **23M**;
W Tr; Racon (T).
Ldg Lts 271·5°. Front FR 11m 5M; W twin pillars, R bands.
Rear, 272m from front, FR 18m 5M; W Tr, R cupola.
Scurdie Rks Lt By 56°42'·15N 02°25'·42W QR; PHM.
Annat Lt By 56°42'·24N 02°25'·85W Fl G 3s; SHM.
Annat Shoal Lt By 56°42'·38N 02°25'·50W QG; SHM.

MONTROSE TO RATTRAY HEAD

JOHNSHAVEN
Ldg Lts 316°. Front 56°47'·65N 02°20'·05W FR 5m; R
structure. Rear, 85m from front, FG 20m; G structure; shows
R when unsafe to enter hbr.

GOURDON HARBOUR
Ldg Lts 358°. Front 56°49'·70N 02°17'·10W FR 5m 5M; W Tr;
shows G when unsafe to enter; *Siren (2) 60s (occas)*. Rear,
120m from front, FR 30m 5M; W Tr.
W Pier Hd 56°49'·62N 02°17'·15W Fl WRG 3s 5m W9M,
R7M, G7M; vis G180°-344°, W344°-354°, R354°-180°.
E Bkwtr Hd Q 3m 7M.

Todhead 56°53'·00N 02°12'·85W Fl (4) 30s 41m **29M**; W Tr.

STONEHAVEN
Outer Pier Hd 56°57'·59N 02°11'·89W Iso WRG 4s 7m W11M,
R7M, G8M; vis G214°-246°, W246°-268°, R268°-280°.

Girdle Ness 57°08'·35N 02°02'·82W Fl (2) 20s 56m **22M**; W
● Tr; obsc by Greg Ness when brg more than about 020°; RC;
Racon (G).

ABERDEEN
Fairway Lt By 57°09'·33N 02°01'·85W Q; SWM; Racon (T).
Ldg Lts 235·7°. Front 57°08'·39N 02°04'·41W FR or G 14m
5M; W Tr; R when ent safe, FG when dangerous to navigation;
vis 195°-279°. Rear, 205m from front, FR 19m 5M; W Tr;
vis 195°-279°.
S Bkwtr Hd 57°08'·70N 02°03'·23W Fl (3) R 8s 23m 7M.
N Pier Hd 57°08'·75N 02°03'·58W Oc WR 6s 11m 9M; W Tr;
vis W145°-055°, R055°-145°. In fog FY 10m (same Tr) vis
136°-336°; *Bell (3) 12s*.

Buchan Ness 57°28'·23N 01°46'·37W Fl 5s 40m **28M**; W Tr,
R bands; Racon (O); *Horn (3) 60s*.
Cruden Scaurs Lt By 57°23'·25N 01°50'·00W Fl R 10s; PHM; *Bell*.

PETERHEAD
Kirktown Ldg Lts 314°. Front 57°30'·23N 01°47'·10W FR
13m 8M; R mast, W ▲ on Or mast. Rear, 91m from front,
R 17m 8M; W ▼ on Or mast.
S Bkwtr Hd 57°29'·81N 01°46'·43W Fl (2) R 12s 24m 7M; W
●Tr with B base.
N Bkwtr Hd 57°29'·85N 01°46'·22W Iso RG 6s 19m 11M; W
tripod; vis R165°-230°, G230°-165°; *Horn 30s*.
Marina Bkwtr Hd 57°29'·82N 01°47'·33W Fl R 3s 6m 2M.

Rattray Hd. Ron Rk 57°36'·62N 01°48'·90W Fl (3) 30s 28m
24M; W Tr; Racon (M); *Horn (2) 45s*.

10.6.5   PASSAGE INFORMATION

For these waters refer to the Admiralty *North Sea (West) Pilot*; R Northumberland YC's *Sailing Directions Humber to Rattray Head*, and the *Forth Yacht Clubs Association Pilot Handbook*, which covers the Firth of Forth in detail.

BERWICK-UPON-TWEED TO BASS ROCK (charts 160, 175)

From Berwick-upon-Tweed to the Firth of Forth there is no good hbr which can be approached with safety in strong onshore winds. So, if on passage with strong winds from N or E, plan accordingly and keep well to seaward. In late spring and early summer fog (haar) is likely in onshore winds.

The coast N from Berwick is rky with cliffs rising in height to Burnmouth, then diminishing gradually to Eyemouth (10.6.7). Keep 5ca offshore to clear outlying rks. Burnmouth, although small, has more alongside space than Eyemouth, which is a crowded fishing hbr. 2M NW is St Abb's Hbr (10.6.7), with temp anch in offshore winds in Coldingham B close to the S.

St Abb's Hd (lt) is a bold, steep headland, 92m high, with no offlying dangers. The stream runs strongly round the Hd, causing turbulence with wind against tide; this can be largely avoided by keeping close inshore. The ESE-going stream begins at HW Leith – 0345, and the WNW-going at HW Leith + 0240. There is a good anch in Pettico Wick, on NW side of Hd, in S winds, but dangerous if the wind shifts onshore. There are no off-lying dangers between St Abb's Hd and Fast Castle Hd, 3M WNW. Between Fast Castle Hd and Barns Ness, about 8M NW, is the attractive little hbr of Cove; but it dries and should only be approached in ideal conditions.

Torness Power Station (conspic; lt on bkwtr) is 1·75M SE of Barns Ness (lt) which lies 2·5M ESE of Dunbar (10.6.8) and is fringed with rks; tidal streams as for St Abb's Hd. Conspic chys are 7½ca WSW inland of Barns Ness. Between here and Dunbar keep at least 2½ca offshore to clear rky patches. Sicar Rk (7·9m depth) lies about 1·25M ENE of Dunbar, and sea breaks on it in onshore gales.

The direct course from Dunbar to Bass Rk (lt) is clear of all dangers; inshore of this line beware Wildfire Rks (dry) on NW side of Bellhaven B. In offshore winds there is anch in Scoughall Road. Great Car is ledge of rks, nearly covering at HW, 1M ESE of Gin Hd, with Car bn (stone tr surmounted by cross) at its N end. Drying ledges of rks extend 1M SE of Great Car, up to 3ca offshore. Keep at least 5ca off Car bn in strong onshore winds. Tantallon Castle (ruins) is on cliff edge 1M W of Great Car. Bass Rk (lt) lies 1·25M NNE of Gin Hd, and is a sheer, conspic rk (115m) with no offlying dangers; landing difficult due to swell.

FIRTH OF FORTH, SOUTH SHORE (chart 734, 735)

Westward of Bass Rk, Craigleith (51m), Lamb Is (24m) and Fidra (31m) lie 5ca or more offshore, while the coast is generally foul. Craigleith is steep-to, and temporary anchorage can be found on SE and SW sides; if passing inshore of it keep well to N side of chan. N Berwick hbr (dries) lies S of Craigleith, but is unsafe in onshore winds. Between Craigleith and Lamb Is, beware drying rks up to 3ca from land. Lamb Is is 1·5M WNW of N Berwick (10.6.8) and has a rky ledge extending 2½ca SW. Fidra Is (lt, RC) is a bird reserve, nearly connected to the shore by rky ledges, and should be passed to the N; passage and anch on S side are tricky. Anchor on E or W sides, depending on wind, in good weather.

In the B between Fidra and Edinburgh some shelter can be found in SE winds in Aberlady B and Gosford B. The best anch is SW of Craigielaw Pt. Port Seton is a drying fishing hbr 7½ca E of the conspic chys of Cockenzie Power Station; the E side of the hbr can be entered HW ±3, but not advisable in strong onshore wind or sea. Cockenzie (dries) is close to power station; beware Corsik Rk 400m to E. Access HW ± 2·5, but no attractions except boatyard. For Fisherrow, see 10.6.8.

There are no dangers on the direct course from Fidra to Inchkeith (lt, RC), which stands between the buoyed deep water chans. Rks extend 7½ca SE from Inchkeith, and 5ca off the W side where there is a small hbr below the lt ho; landing is forbidden without permission. N Craig and Craig Waugh (least depth 0·6m) are buoyed shoals 2·5M SE from Inchkeith lt ho. For Cramond and Inchcolm, see 10.6.8.

In N Chan, close to Inchkeith the W-going (flood) stream begins about HW Leith – 0530, and the E-going at HW Leith + 0030, sp rates about 1kn. The streams gather strength towards the Forth bridges, where they reach 2·25kn and there may be turbulence.

Leith is wholly commercial; Granton has yacht moorings in the E hbr; Port Edgar (10.6.9) is a major yacht hbr close W of Forth road bridge. Hound Point oil terminal is an artificial 'island-jetty' almost in mid-stream, connected to the shore by underwater pipeline (no ⚓). Yachts may pass the terminal on either side at least 30m off and well clear of tankers berthing.

RIVER FORTH TO KINCARDINE (charts 736, 737, 738)

The main shipping chan under the N span of the rail bridge is busy with commercial traffic for Grangemouth and warships to/from Rosyth dockyard. In the latter case a Protected Chan may be activated; see 10.6.9 for details. W of Beamer Rk the Firth widens as far as Bo'ness (small drying hbr) on the S shore where the chan narrows between drying mudbanks. Charlestown (N bank) dries, but is a secure hbr. Grangemouth is industrially conspic. Caution: gas carriers, tankers, cargo vessels; no yacht facilities. Few yachts go beyond Kincardine swing bridge, clearance 9m, which is no longer opened.

FIRTH OF FORTH, NORTH SHORE (charts 734, 190)

From Burntisland (10.6.10) the N shore of Firth of Forth leads E to Kinghorn Ness. 1M SSW of Kinghorn Ness Blae Rk (SHM lt buoy) has least depth of 4·1m, and seas break on it in E gales. Rost Bank lies halfway between Kinghorn Ness and Inchkeith, with tide rips at sp tides or in strong winds.

From Kinghorn Ness to Kirkcaldy, drying rks lie up to 3ca offshore. Kirkcaldy hbr (10.6.8) is effectively closed, but yachts can enter inner dock near HW by arrangement; ent is dangerous in strong E'lies, when seas break a long way out.

Between Kirkcaldy and Methil (10.6.11) the only dangers more than 2ca offshore are The Rockheads, extending 4ca SE of Dysart, and marked by 2 SHM buoys. Largo B is anch, well sheltered from N and E, but avoid gaspipes near E side. Close SW of Elie, beware W Vows (dries) and E Vows (dries, bn). There is anch close W of Elie Ness (10.6.8). Ox Rk (dries 2m) lies 5ca ENE of Elie Ness, and 2½ca offshore; otherwise there are no dangers more than 2ca offshore past St Monans, Pittenweem (10.6.8) and Anstruther (10.6.12), but in bad weather the sea breaks on Shield Rk 4ca off Pittenweem. From Anstruther to Crail (10.6.8) and on to Fife Ness keep 3ca offshore to clear Caiplie Rk and other dangers. May Island (lt) (10.6.8) lies about 5M S of Fife Ness; its shores are bold except at NW end where rks extend 1ca off. Anch near N end at E or W Tarbert, on lee side according to winds; in good weather it is possible to land. lt ho boats use Kirkhaven, close SE of lt ho

FIFE NESS TO MONTROSE (chart 190)

Fife Ness is fringed by rky ledges, and a reef extends 1M NE to N Carr Rk (dries 1·4m, marked by bn). In strong onshore winds keep to seaward of N Carr ECM lt buoy. From here keep 5ca offshore to clear dangers entering St Andrews B, where there is anch; the little hbr (10.6.13) dries, and should not be approached in onshore winds.

Northward from Firth of Forth to Rattray Hd the coast is mostly rky and steep-to, and there are no out-lying dangers within 2M of the coast except those off R. Tay and Bell Rk. But in an onshore blow there are few safe havens; both yachts and crews need to be prepared for offshore cruising rather than coast-crawling.

R. Tay (10.6.13 and chart 1481) is approached from the NE via Fairway buoy; it is dangerous to cut corners from the S. The Bar, NE of Abertay lt buoy, is dangerous in heavy weather, particularly in strong onshore wind or swell. Abertay Sands extend nearly 4M E of Tentsmuir Pt on S side of chan (buoyed); Elbow is a shoal extension eastward. Gaa Sands running 1·75M E from Buddon Ness, are marked by Abertay lt buoy (Racon) on N side of chan. Passage across Abertay and Gaa Sands is very dangerous. The estuary is shallow, with many shifting sandbanks; Tayport is a good passage stop and best yacht hbr (dries) in the Tay. S of Buddon Ness the W-going (flood) stream begins about HW Aberdeen – 0400, and the E-going at about HW Aberdeen + 0230, sp rates 2kn.

Bell Rk (lt, Racon) lies about 11·5M E of Buddon Ness. 2M E of Bell Rk the S-going stream begins HW Aberdeen – 0220, and the N-going at HW Aberdeen + 0405, sp rates 1kn. W of Bell Rk the streams begin earlier.

N from Buddon Ness the coast is sandy. 1·25M SW of Arbroath (10.6.14) beware Elliot Horses, rky patches with depth 1·9m, which extend about 5ca offshore. Between Whiting Ness and Scurdie Ness, 9·5M NNE, the coast is clear of out-lying dangers, but is mostly fringed with drying rks up to 1ca off. In offshore winds there is temp anch in SW of Lunan B, off Ethie Haven.

Scurdie Ness (lt, Racon) is conspic on S side of ent to Montrose (10.6.15). Scurdie Rks (dry) extend 2ca E of the Ness. On N side of chan Annat Bank dries up to about 5ca E of the shore, opposite Scurdie Ness (chart 1438). The in-going stream begins at HW Aberdeen – 0500, and the outgoing at HW Aberdeen + 0115; both streams are very strong, up to 7kn at sp, and there is turbulence off the ent on the ebb. The ent is dangerous in strong onshore winds, with breaking seas extending to Scurdie Ness on the ebb. In marginal conditions the last quarter of the flood is best time to enter.

MONTROSE TO ABERDEEN (chart 210)

N from Montrose the coast is sandy for 5M to Milton Ness, where there is anch on S side in N winds. Johnshaven (10.6.16), 2M NE, is a small hbr (dries) with tight entrance, which should not be approached with onshore wind or swell. 5ca NE, off Brotherton Cas, drying rks extend 4ca offshore. Gourdon (10.6.16) has a small hbr (mostly dries) approached on ldg line between rky ledges; inner hbr has storm gates. Outside the hbr rks extend both sides of entrance, and the sea breaks heavily in strong E winds. Keep a sharp lookout for lobster pot dan buoys between Montrose and Stonehaven.

North to Inverbervie the coast is fringed with rky ledges up to 2ca offshore. Just N of Todhead Pt (lt) is Catterline, a small B which forms a natural anch in W winds, but open to E. Downie Pt, SE of Stonehaven (10.6.16) should be

rounded 1ca off. The Bay is encumbered by rky ledges up to 2ca from shore and exposed to the E; anch 6ca E of Bay Hotel or berth afloat in outer hbr.

From Garron Pt to Girdle Ness the coast is mostly steep-to. Fishing nets may be met off headlands during fishing season. Craigmaroinn and Seal Craig (dry) are parts of reef 3ca offshore SE of Portlethen, a fishing village with landing sheltered by rks. Cove B has a very small fishing hbr, off which there is anch in good weather; Mutton Rk (dries 2·1m) lie 1½ca offshore. From Cove to Girdle Ness keep 5ca offshore, avoiding Hasman Rks (dries 3·4m) 1ca off Altens .

Greg Ness and Girdle Ness (lt, RC, Racon), at SE corner of Aberdeen B (10.6.17), are fringed by rks. Girdlestone is a rky patch, depth less than 2m, 2ca ENE of lt ho. A drying patch lies 2ca SE of lt ho. Off Girdle Ness the S-going stream begins at HW Aberdeen – 0430, and the N-going at HW Aberdeen + 0130, sp rates 2·5kn. A race forms on S-going stream.

ABERDEEN TO RATTRAY HEAD (chart 213)

From Aberdeen there are few offshore dangers to Buchan Ness. R. Ythan, 1·75M SSW of Hackley Hd, is navigable by small craft, but chan shifts constantly. 3M North is the very small hbr of Collieston (mostly dries), only accessible in fine weather. 4·75M NNE of Hackley Head lie The Skares, rks (marked by PHM lt buoy) extending 3½ca from S point of Cruden B, where there is anch in offshore winds. On N side of Cruden B is Port Erroll (dries 2·5m).

Buchan Ness (lt, fog sig, Racon) is a rky peninsula. 2ca N is Meikle Mackie islet, close W of which is the small hbr of Boddam (dries) (10.6.18). 3ca NE of Meikle Mackie is The Skerry, a rk 6m high on S side of Sandford B; rks on which the sea breaks extend 2ca NNE. The chan between The Skerry and the coast is foul with rks and not advised. Peterhead (10.6.18) is easy to enter in almost all conditions and is an excellent passage port with marina at SW corner of the Bay.

Rattray Hd (with lt, fog sig on The Ron, rk 2ca E of Hd) has rky foreshore, drying for 2ca off. Rattray Briggs is a detached reef, depth 0·2m, 2ca E of lt ho. Rattray Hard is a rky patch, depth 10·7m, 1·5M ENE of lt ho, which raises a dangerous sea during onshore gales. Off Rattray Hd the S-going stream begins at HW Aberdeen – 0420, and the N-going at HW Aberdeen + 0110, sp rates 3kn. In normal conditions keep about 1M E of Rattray Hd, but pass 5M off in bad weather, preferably at slack water. Conspic radio masts with R lts lie 2·5M WNW and 2·2M W of lt ho.

For notes on offshore oil/gas installations, see 10.5.5.

NORTH SEA PASSAGE

For distances across the N Sea, see 10.0.7.

FORTH TO NORWAY AND BALTIC (charts 2182B, 2182C)

Heading ENE'ly from Forth the main hazards result from offshore industrial activities and the associated traffic. In summer particularly, oil/gas exploration, movement of drilling rigs, pipe laying etc create situations which could endanger other vessels. Rig movements and many of the more intense activities are published in Notices to Mariners, but even so it is wise to avoid the gas and oil fields where possible and never to approach within 500m of installations (see 10.5.5). There are TSS to be avoided off the S and SW coast of Norway. Strong currents and steep seas may be experienced in the approaches to the Skagerrak..

10.6.6   DISTANCE TABLE

Approximate distances in nautical miles are by the most direct route, whilst avoiding dangers and allowing for Traffic Separation Schemes. Places in *italics* are in adjoining areas; places in **bold** are in 10.0.7, Distances across the North Sea.

1. *Great Yarmouth*	**1**																			
2. ***Berwick-on-Tweed***	232	**2**																		
3. Eyemouth	240	10	**3**																	
4. Dunbar	257	26	17	**4**																
5. North Berwick	266	35	25	9	**5**															
6. Granton	285	54	44	27	19	**6**														
7. **Port Edgar**	290	58	50	34	26	7	**7**													
8. Burntisland	283	53	43	26	18	5	8	**8**												
9. Methil	276	45	36	20	13	14	20	12	**9**											
10. Anstruther	269	38	29	14	10	23	29	22	11	**10**										
11. Fife Ness	269	38	29	17	14	28	34	27	16	5	**11**									
12. Bell Rock	276	43	36	27	25	40	47	39	28	17	12	**12**								
13. **Dundee**	289	58	49	37	34	48	54	47	36	25	20	20	**13**							
14. Arbroath	284	51	44	34	31	45	51	44	33	22	17	10	15	**14**						
15. Montrose	291	59	51	43	41	55	61	54	43	32	27	17	27	12	**15**					
16. Stonehaven	300	72	66	60	58	72	78	71	60	49	44	32	45	30	20	**16**				
17. **Aberdeen**	308	82	78	73	70	84	90	83	72	61	56	44	57	42	32	13	**17**			
18. Peterhead	318	105	98	93	95	106	108	105	94	83	78	68	80	64	54	35	25	**18**		
19. *Fraserburgh*	334	121	114	109	108	122	128	121	110	99	94	83	96	79	68	51	39	16	**19**	
20. *Wick*	391	178	171	166	165	179	185	178	167	156	151	140	153	136	125	108	96	72	57	**20**

EYEMOUTH   10-6-7

Berwick 55°32'·51N 02°05'·19W

CHARTS
AC 1612, 160; OS 67

TIDES
+0330 Dover; ML No data; Duration 0610; Zone 0 (UT)

Standard Port LEITH (⟶)

Times				Height (metres)			
High Water		Low Water		MHWS	MHWN	MLWN	MLWS
0300	0900	0300	0900	5·6	4·5	2·1	0·8
1500	2100	1500	2100				
Differences EYEMOUTH							
−0015	−0025	−0014	−0004	−0·9	−0·8	No data	

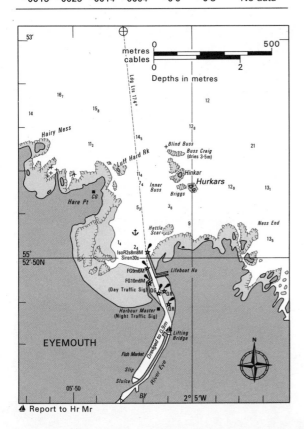

▲ Report to Hr Mr

SHELTER
Good in all weathers but entry should not be attempted in strong N/E winds. Busy fishing hbr, but yachts are welcome; expect to berth at E quay knuckle, near lifting bridge in about 2m; or ⚓ in bay only in off-shore winds. Note: WIP '95/'96 to build new basin for FVs and dredge ent to 3m; giving more space for yachts in old hbr.

NAVIGATION
WPT 55°53'·00N 02°05'·28W, 354°/174° from/to E bkwtr lt, 0·50M. Appr can be made N or S of Hurkar Rks but there are no ldg marks to the S; keep in mid-chan. To the N, beware Blind Buss. Ent and basin dredged to 0·9m.

LIGHTS AND MARKS
St. Abbs Hd lt ho Fl 10s 68m 26M is 3M NW. Ldg lts 174° (orange column) both FG 9/10m 6M on W pier. Ⓡ or R flag = unsafe to enter.

RADIO TELEPHONE
VHF Ch 16 12 (No regular watch).

TELEPHONE (018907)
Hr Mr 50223; MRSC (01333) 450666; ⌗ (0131) 469 7400; Marinecall 0891 500452; Police 50217; Dr 50599.

FACILITIES
Jetty AB £2.35, FW, D (by delivery), P (cans), Slip;
Services: BH, ME, Sh, El, C (12 ton mobile), CH, Gas, Ⓔ.
Town EC Wed; LB, P, D, CH, V, R, Bar, ✉, Ⓓ, Gas, Gaz, Ⓑ, ⇌ (bus to Berwick-on-Tweed), ✈ (Edinburgh).

ADJACENT HARBOURS

BURNMOUTH, Berwick, 55°50'·60N 02°04'·00W. AC 160. HW +0315 on Dover, −0025 on Leith; Duration 0615. Use Eyemouth tides 10.6.7. From S beware Quarry Shoal Rks; from N beware E and W Carrs. 2 W bns (FR 29/35m 4M), 45m apart, lead 274° towards the hbr mouth until ent opens and 2FG (vert) come in line with outer hbr ent. Min depth at ent at LWS is 0·6m. Good shelter especially in inner hbr (dries). With on-shore winds, swell makes outer hbr uncomfortable. Hr Mr (018907) 81283. Facilities: AB £4, FW, limited stores, Bar at top of valley.

ST ABBS, Berwick, 55°54'·100N 02°07'·65W. AC 175. HW +0330 on Dover, −0017 on Leith; HW −0·6m on Leith; Duration 0605. Ldg line (about 228°) S face of Maw Carr on village hall (conspic R roof) leads SW until the hbr ent opens to port and the 2nd ldg line (about 167°) can be seen 2FR 4/8m 1M, or Y LB ho visible thru' ent. On E side of ent chan, beware Hog's Nose and on W side the Maw Carr. Shelter good. In strong on-shore winds outer hbr suffers from waves breaking over E pier. Inner hbr is best but often full of FVs and dries. Access HW±3. Hr Mr will direct visitors. Hr Mr (018907) 71323. Facilities: AB £6, FW on quay, R, V, more facilities & bar at Coldingham (5M).

DUNBAR   10-6-8

East Lothian 56°00'·39N 02°31'·00W

CHARTS
AC 734, 175; Imray 27; OS 67
TIDES
+0330 Dover; ML 3·0; Duration 0600; Zone 0 (UT)

Standard Port LEITH (→)

Times				Height (metres)			
High Water		Low Water		MHWS	MHWN	MLWN	MLWS
0300	0900	0300	0900	5·6	4·5	2·1	0·8
1500	2100	1500	2100				
Differences DUNBAR							
−0005	−0010	+0010	+0017	−0·4	−0·3	−0·1	−0·1
FIDRA							
+0006	+0006	−0006	−0006	−0·2	−0·2	0·0	0·0

SHELTER
Outer (Victoria) Hbr is subject to surge in strong NW to NE winds; N side dries, but pool 1·25m at LWS in SW corner. Inner (Old or Cromwell) Hbr (dries) is safe at all times: ent through a bridge, opened on request to Hr Mr.
NAVIGATION
WPT 56°00'·70N 02°30'·80W, 018°/198° from/to front ldg lt 198°, 0·50M. Min depth at ent 0·9m. Ent is unsafe in heavy on-shore swell. Beware Outer Bush Rk (0·6m). Keep to port on entry to avoid rockfall off castle.
LIGHTS AND MARKS
Church and Castle ruin both conspic. From NE, ldg lts, Oc G 6s 15/22m 3M, synch, intens 188°-208°, 2 W △ on Or cols, lead 198° through Dunbar Steeples to the Roads; thence narrow hbr ent opens with QR vis brg 132°. From NW, appr on brg 132° between bns on Wallaces Hd and Half Ebb Rk.
RADIO TELEPHONE
None.

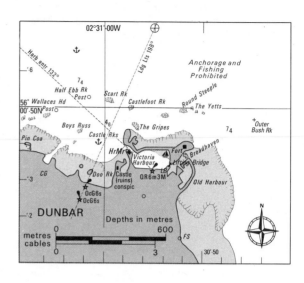

TELEPHONE (01368)
Hr Mr 863206; MRSC (01333) 450666; ⌗ (0131) 4697400; Police 862718; Marinecall 0891 500452; Dr 862327; Ⓗ (031) 2292477.
FACILITIES
Quay AB £4, Slip, FW, D (delivery), P (cans); **N Wall** M, AB; **Inner Hbr** Slip, AB; **Services** ME, Gas, Gaz.
Town EC Wed; LB, P, ▣, V, R, Bar, ✉, Ⓑ, ⇌, ✈ Edinburgh.

HARBOURS AND ANCHORAGES ON THE SOUTH BANK OF THE FIRTH OF FORTH

NORTH BERWICK, East Lothian, 56°03'·74N 02°42'·95W. AC 734. Fidra HW +0344 on Dover; ML 3·0m; Duration 0625. See 10.6.8 Fidra. Shelter good with winds from S to W but dangerous with on-shore winds. Ent is 8m wide. Hbr dries. From E or W, from position 0·25M S of Craigleith, steer S for Plattock Rks, thence SSW 40m off bkwtr before turning 180° port into hbr. Bkwtr lt F WR 7m 3M, R to seaward, W over hbr; not lit when bad weather closes hbr. Beware Maiden Rks (bn) 100m NW of this lt. Facilities: AB £5.70, P & D (cans), FW on pier, CH. **East Lothian YC** ☎ (01620) 2698 Bar.
Town EC Thurs; V, Gas, Ⓑ, ✉, ⇌ and bus Edinburgh.

FISHERROW, Midlothian, 55°56'·79N 03°04'·00W. AC 735, 734. HW +0345 on Dover, −0005 on Leith; HW −0·1m on Leith; ML 3·0m; Duration 0620. Shelter good except in NW winds. Mainly a pleasure craft hbr, dries 5ca offshore. Appr dangerous in on-shore winds. Access HW±2. High-rise block (38m) is conspic 9ca W of hbr. E pier lt, Oc 6s 5m 6M on metal framework tr. Berth on E pier. Hr Mr ☎ (0131) 665 5900; **Fisherrow YC** FW.
Town EC Wed; V, P & D from garage, R, Bar, Ⓑ, ✉, SM.

CRAMOND, Midlothian, 55°59'·80N 03°17'·40W. AC 736. Tides as Leith (see 10.6.9). Cramond Island, approx 1M offshore, is connected to the S shore of the Firth by a drying causeway. A chan, marked by 7 SHM posts, leads W of Cramond Island to Cramond hbr at the mouth of R Almond, conspic white houses. Access HW±2; AB free or ⌕ off the Is. Seek local advice from: **Cramond Boat Club** ☎ (0131) 336 1356, FW, M, Bar. **Village** V, R, Pub, Bus.

HARBOURS AND ANCHORAGES ON THE NORTH SHORE OF THE FIRTH OF FORTH

INCHCOLM, Fife, 56°01'·85N, 03°17'·80W. AC 736. Tides see 10.6.10. Best ⚓ in 4m, N of abbey (conspic); appr from NW or ESE, to land at pier close E (small fee). Meadulse Rks (dry) on N side. Ends of island foul. At SE end, lt Fl (3) 15s, obsc 075°-145°, horn (3) 45s. No facilities. ☎ 0131-244 3101. Keep clear of large ships under way in Mortimer's Deep.

ABERDOUR, Fife, 56°03'·00N 03°17'·40W. AC 735, 736. HW +0345 on Dover; +0005 on Leith; HW 0·5m on Leith; ML 3·3m; Duration 0630. See 10.6.10. Good shelter except in SE winds when a swell occurs. The ⚓ between The Little Craigs and the disused pier is good but exposed to winds from E to SW. Temp berths £2 are available in hbr (dries) alongside the quay wall. Beware Little Craigs (dries 2·2m) and outfall 2ca N marked by bn. There are no lts/ marks. Hr Mr ☎ (01383) 860452. Facilities: FW (tap on pier), P, R, V, Bar in village, EC Wed; **Aberdour BC** ☎ (01592) 202827.

BURNTISLAND: See 10.6.10
KIRKCALDY: See 10.6.11
METHIL: See 10.6.11

ELIE, Fife, 56°11'·20N 02°49'·20W. AC 734. HW +0325 on Dover, –0015 on Leith; HW –0·1m on Leith; ML 3·0m; Duration 0620; Elie B provides good shelter from N winds for small craft but local knowledge is needed. Hbr dries; 3 short term waiting buoys available. Beware ledge off end of pier which dries. From E beware Ox Rk (dries 1m) 5M ENE of Elie Ness; from W beware rks off Chapel Ness, W Vows, E Vows (surmounted by cage bn) and Thill Rk, marked by PHM buoy. Lt: Elie Ness Fl 6s 15m 18M, W tr. Hr Mr (01333) 330502; AB (3) drying £5, M, AC, FW, CH, SC, Slip. Police 310333. Dr ☎ 330302; **Services:** P & D (tanker), Gas, Gaz. El. In Elie & Earlsferry: R, V, Bar, ✉, Ⓑ.

ST MONANS, Fife, 56°12'·25N 02°45'·85W. AC 734. HW +0335 on Dover, –0020 on Leith; HW –0·1m on Leith; ML 3·0m; Duration 0620. Shelter good except in strong SE to SW winds when scend occurs in the hbr (dries). Berth alongside E pier until contact with Hr Mr. From NE keep at least 2½ca from coast. Bkwtr hd Oc WRG 6s 5m 7/4M;

E pier hd 2 FG (vert) 6m 4M. W pier hd 2 FR (vert) 6m 4M. Facilities: Hr Mr ☎ (01333) 730428; AB £5.10, FW, AC, El. **Services:** Gas, P & D (tanker), AC. **Village** R, Bar, V, ✉, Ⓑ.

PITTENWEEM, Fife, 56°12'·60N 02°43'·70W. AC 734. HW +0325 Dover; –0015 and –0·1m on Leith; ML 3m. Duration 0620. Busy fishing hbr, dredged 1-2m, access all tides, but not in onshore winds. Yachts not encouraged; contact Hr Mr for berth at W end of inner hbr, but only for emergency use. Outer hbr dries to rock; is only suitable for temp stop in calm weather. Appr 037° on ldg marks/lts, Gy cols/Y stripe, both FR 3/8m 5M. Rks to port marked by bn, QR 3m 2M, and 3 unlit bns. E bkwtr lt Fl (2) RG 5s 9m 9/6M, R265°-345°, G345°-055°. No VHF. Hr Mr ☎ (01333) 312591. Facilities: FW, CH, D & P (tanker), Gas, V, Bar.

ANSTRUTHER: See 10.6.12

CRAIL, Fife, 56°15'·35N 02°37'·20W. AC 175. HW +0320 on Dover, –0020 on Leith; HW –0·2m on Leith; ML 3·0m; Duration 0615. Good shelter but only for boats able to take the ground alongside. Appr between S pier and bn on rks to S following ldg line 295°, two W concrete pillars with FR lts, 24/30m 6M. Turn 150° to stbd for ent. Call Forth CG on VHF Ch 16 before entering. Hr Mr ☎ (01333) 450820. Facilities: AB £5.10, El, FW, AC, Slip, P. **Village** EC Wed; Bar, R, V, ✉, Ⓑ.

ISLE OF MAY, Fife, 56°11'·40N 02°33'·60W. AC 734. HW +0325 on Dover, –0025 on Leith. In settled weather only, and depending on the wind, ⚓ at E or W Tarbert in 4m; landing at Altarstanes. Near the SE tip there is a tiny hbr at Kirkhaven, with narrow, rky ent; yachts can moor fore-and-aft to rings in rks, in about 1-1·5m. SDs are needed. Beware Norman Rk to N of Island, and Maiden Hair Rk to S. At the summit, a ☐ tr on stone ho, Fl (2) 15s 73m 22M. A SPM buoy, Fl Y 3s, is 1M WSW. The island is a bird sanctuary, owned by Scottish Natural Heritage ☎ (01334) 654038. Avoid the breeding season, mid-Mar to end Jul. Landing only at Altarstanes or Kirkhaven, 1000-1700; not on Tues, April to July inc.

6

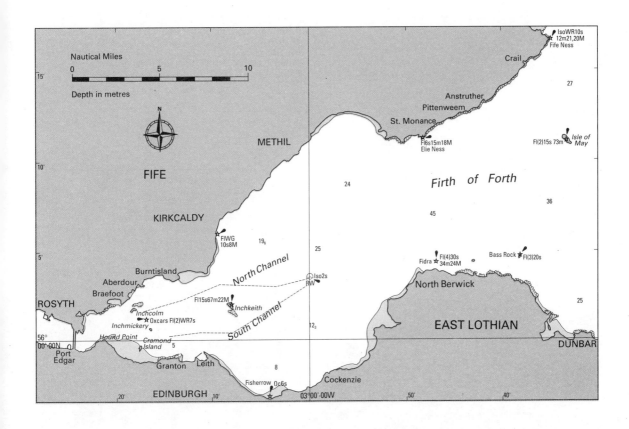

FIRTH OF FORTH   10-6-9
Lothian/Fife

CHARTS
AC 734, 735, 736; Imray C27; OS 66, 59

TIDES
+0350 (Granton) Dover; ML 3·3; Duration 0620; Zone 0 (UT)

Standard Port LEITH (→)

Times				Height (metres)			
High Water		Low Water		MHWS	MHWN	MLWN	MLWS
0300	0900	0300	0900	5·6	4·5	2·1	0·8
1500	2100	1500	2100				

Differences COCKENZIE

–0007	–0015	–0013	–0005	–0·2	0·0	No data

GRANTON: Same as LEITH

Kincardine: Time difference Leith +0030.
Alloa: Time difference Leith +0048.
Leith is a Standard Port and tidal predictions for each day of the year are given below.

SHELTER
Granton mostly dries and is open to swell in N'lies. Some berths on E side of Middle pier in about 1·2m; Pilot boats berth at seaward end. W side is mainly for FVs. Good shelter in Port Edgar marina (South Queensferry). Leith is wholly commercial. Rosyth Naval Dockyard is not for yachts except in emergency.

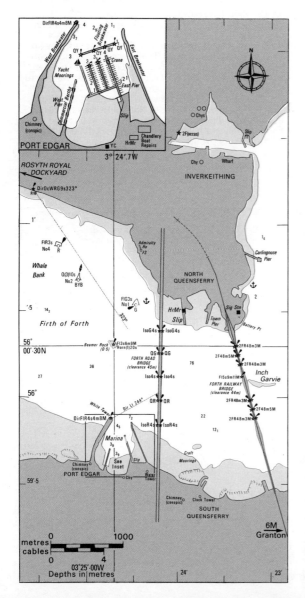

NAVIGATION
WPT Granton 56°00'·00N 03°13'·22W, 000°/180° from/to ent, 0·72M.
WPT Port Edgar 56°N 03°24'·2W, 064°/244° from/to Dir Lt, Fl R 4s, on W bkwtr, 3ca. Beware Hound Pt terminal; Forth railway and road bridges; H.M. Ships entering and leaving Rosyth Dockyard. On N shore, no vessel may enter Mortimer's Deep (Braefoot gas terminal) without prior approval from Forth Navigation Service. 12kn speed limit W of Forth Rly Bridge.
Note: Forth Ports Authority controls the Forth Estuary, all commercial impounded docks and Granton Hbr.
A Protected Chan 150m wide extends from Nos 13 and 14 lt buoys (NNW of Oxcars) under the bridges (N of Inch Garvie and Beamer Rk), to the ent of Rosyth Dockyard. When the Protected Chan is in operation an Oc 5s lt and a QR lt are shown from N Queensferry Naval sig stn, and all other vessels must clear the chan for naval traffic.

LIGHTS AND MARKS
Granton: R flag with W diagonal cross (or Ⓖ lt) on signal mast at middle pier hd = Entry prohib.
Port Edgar: On W pier Dir lt Fl R 4s 4m 8M 244°; 4 QY lts mark floating bkwtr; 3 x 2 FR (vert) mark N ends of marina pontoons.

RADIO TELEPHONE
Call *Forth Navigation* (at Leith) Ch **71** (H24) 16; **20** 12 (use 71 within area for calling and for short messages).
N Queensferry Naval Sig Stn at Battery Pt, call: *Queensferry* VHF Ch **74** 71 16 (H24).
Rosyth Naval Base, call *QHM* Ch 74 73 (Mon-Fri: 0730-1700).
Grangemouth Docks Ch 14 (H24). Leith Docks Ch 12.
Port Edgar Marina Ch M **80** (Apl-Sept 0900-1930; Oct-Mar 0900-1630LT).

TELEPHONE (0131)
Hr Mr Leith 554 3661; MRSC (01333) 450666; ☷ (0131) 469 7400; Forth Yacht Clubs Assn 552 3452; Weather (0141) 248 3451; Marinecall 0891 500452; Police (S. Queensferry) 331 1798; Ⓗ Edinburgh Royal Infirmary 229-2477; Maritime HQ, Pitreavie (01383) 412161, ask for Naval Ops room, for Naval activities on N and E coasts of Scotland.

FACILITIES
GRANTON
Hr Mr ☎ 552 3385, AB £11.50, FW, Slip; **Royal Forth YC** ☎ 552 3006, Fax 552 8560, Slip, M, L, FW, C (5 ton), D, ME, El, Sh, Bar; **Forth Corinthian YC** ☎ 552 5939, Slip, M, L, Bar; Access HW±3½.
Services: Gas, Gaz, Sh, CH, ME.
Town D, P, V, R, Bar, ☒, Ⓑ, ⇌, ✈ (Buses to Edinburgh).
SOUTH QUEENSFERRY
Port Edgar Marina (300+8 visitors) ☎ 331 3330, Fax 331 4878, £10.20, Access H24, M, Slip, AC, CH, D, El, Ⓔ, ME, Sh, SM, Gas, Gaz, FW, R, C (5 ton); Port Edgar YC.
Town EC Wed; P, V, R, Bar, ☒, Ⓑ, ⇌ (Dalmeny), ✈ Edinburgh.
EDINBURGH: ACA.

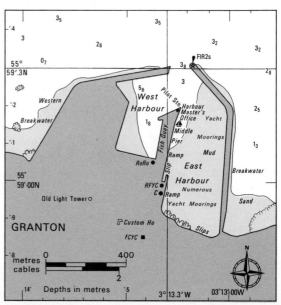

SCOTLAND – LEITH

LAT 55°59′N   LONG 3°10′W

TIMES AND HEIGHTS OF HIGH AND LOW WATERS

YEAR **1996**

TIME ZONE (UT)
For Summer Time add ONE hour in non-shaded areas

JANUARY

Day	Time	m	Day	Time	m
1 M	0519	1.9	**16** TU	0404	1.7
	1119	4.7		1012	4.7
	1746	1.9		1632	1.9
	2343	4.8		2245	4.8
2 TU	0612	1.8	**17** W	0508	1.6
	1215	4.9		1122	4.9
	1838	1.7		1739	1.6
				2355	5.0
3 W	0036	4.8	**18** TH	0608	1.3
	0654	1.7		1226	5.2
	1305	5.0		1842	1.2
	1920	1.5			
4 TH	0125	5.0	**19** F	0057	5.4
	0730	1.6		0706	1.0
	1348	5.2		1324	5.5
	1956	1.3		1942	0.8
5 F O	0206	5.1	**20** SA	0153	5.6
	0759	1.5		0801	0.8
	1425	5.3		1415	5.8
	2028	1.2	●	2036	0.4
6 SA	0243	5.1	**21** SU	0244	5.8
	0825	1.4		0850	0.6
	1458	5.4		1504	6.0
	2058	1.1		2123	0.2
7 SU	0317	5.2	**22** M	0332	5.9
	0853	1.3		0936	0.5
	1531	5.4		1550	6.0
	2129	1.0		2206	0.2
8 M	0351	5.2	**23** TU	0420	5.8
	0922	1.3		1018	0.6
	1604	5.4		1636	5.9
	2159	1.0		2247	0.3
9 TU	0428	5.2	**24** W	0508	5.7
	0950	1.3		1058	0.8
	1641	5.3		1725	5.7
	2227	1.1		2326	0.5
10 W	0507	5.1	**25** TH	0558	5.4
	1015	1.4		1138	1.1
	1720	5.2		1815	5.5
	2250	1.2			
11 TH	0548	5.1	**26** F	0005	0.9
	1044	1.5		0648	5.1
	1802	5.1		1218	1.4
	2317	1.3		1907	5.2
12 F	0632	5.0	**27** SA	0045	1.3
	1118	1.6		0741	4.8
	1846	4.9		1304	1.7
	2353	1.5		2003	4.8
13 SA	0717	4.8	**28** SU	0132	1.7
	1200	1.8		0837	4.6
	1934	4.8		1400	2.0
				2104	4.6
14 SU	0041	1.6	**29** M	0233	2.0
	0807	4.7		0937	4.4
	1255	1.9		1518	2.2
	2028	4.7		2209	4.4
15 M	0244	1.8	**30** TU	0435	2.2
	0904	4.7		1041	4.4
	1505	2.1		1727	2.1
	2132	4.7		2313	4.4
			31 W	0554	2.1
				1142	4.6
				1826	1.8

FEBRUARY

Day	Time	m	Day	Time	m
1 TH	0011	4.6	**16** F	0556	1.4
	0640	1.9		1205	5.0
	1237	4.8		1837	1.1
	1910	1.6			
2 F	0102	4.7	**17** SA	0044	5.2
	0717	1.7		0655	1.1
	1324	5.0		1307	5.3
	1946	1.3		1936	0.7
3 SA	0145	4.9	**18** SU	0141	5.5
	0747	1.5		0749	0.8
	1404	5.2	●	1401	5.7
	2017	1.1		2026	0.3
4 SU O	0222	5.1	**19** M	0231	5.7
	0810	1.3		0836	0.5
	1439	5.3		1449	5.9
	2043	0.9		2109	0.1
5 M	0256	5.2	**20** TU	0317	5.8
	0837	1.1		0919	0.4
	1513	5.4		1534	6.0
	2111	0.8		2148	0.0
6 TU	0330	5.2	**21** W	0400	5.8
	0906	1.0		0959	0.4
	1546	5.4		1617	5.9
	2139	0.8		2224	0.2
7 W	0406	5.3	**22** TH	0444	5.6
	0934	1.0		1036	0.5
	1621	5.4		1701	5.8
	2205	0.8		2258	0.5
8 TH	0443	5.3	**23** F	0529	5.4
	0959	1.1		1112	0.8
	1659	5.3		1747	5.5
	2227	0.9		2330	0.9
9 F	0523	5.2	**24** SA	0614	5.1
	1025	1.1		1147	1.2
	1739	5.2		1834	5.1
	2252	1.0			
10 SA	0605	5.1	**25** SU	0003	1.3
	1056	1.2		0702	4.8
	1821	5.1		1227	1.5
	2325	1.2		1925	4.8
11 SU	0650	4.9	**26** M	0045	1.7
	1135	1.4		0754	4.5
	1908	4.9		1318	1.9
				2024	4.5
12 M	0008	1.4	**27** TU	0142	2.1
	0737	4.8		0854	4.3
	1224	1.6		1426	2.2
	2000	4.7		2133	4.2
13 TU	0107	1.7	**28** W	0258	2.4
	0832	4.6		1002	4.2
	1329	1.9		1653	2.2
	2103	4.6		2241	4.2
14 W	0337	1.8	**29** TH	0533	2.3
	0938	4.6		1108	4.4
	1611	1.9		1805	1.9
	2218	4.6		2343	4.4
15 TH	0451	1.7			
	1054	4.7			
	1728	1.5			
	2336	4.8			

MARCH

Day	Time	m	Day	Time	m
1 F	0622	2.0	**16** SA	0543	1.5
	1206	4.6		1148	4.9
	1849	1.6		1826	1.0
2 SA	0036	4.6	**17** SU	0033	5.1
	0659	1.7		0641	1.1
	1256	4.8		1251	5.2
	1925	1.3		1922	0.6
3 SU	0120	4.8	**18** M	0129	5.4
	0727	1.5		0732	0.8
	1338	5.0		1345	5.5
	1954	1.0		2008	0.3
4 M	0157	5.0	**19** TU	0216	5.6
	0747	1.2		0817	0.5
	1415	5.2		1432	5.7
	2019	0.8	●	2049	0.2
5 TU O	0231	5.2	**20** W	0258	5.7
	0814	1.0		0859	0.4
	1449	5.3		1516	5.8
	2046	0.7		2125	0.2
6 W	0305	5.3	**21** TH	0338	5.7
	0845	0.8		0937	0.4
	1524	5.4		1557	5.8
	2114	0.6		2159	0.3
7 TH	0341	5.4	**22** F	0418	5.6
	0915	0.8		1012	0.5
	1559	5.5		1638	5.6
	2141	0.6		2230	0.6
8 F	0418	5.4	**23** SA	0457	5.4
	0941	0.8		1047	0.7
	1637	5.4		1719	5.4
	2205	0.7		2259	1.0
9 SA	0457	5.3	**24** SU	0538	5.1
	1007	0.8		1121	1.1
	1717	5.3		1801	5.1
	2231	0.8		2329	1.4
10 SU	0539	5.2	**25** M	0619	4.8
	1038	1.0		1158	1.4
	1800	5.2		1847	4.8
	2305	1.1			
11 M	0625	5.0	**26** TU	0004	1.8
	1117	1.2		0705	4.6
	1848	5.0		1246	1.8
	2348	1.4		1940	4.4
12 TU	0714	4.8	**27** W	0058	2.2
	1206	1.4		0802	4.3
	1942	4.8		1351	2.1
				2050	4.2
13 W	0048	1.7	**28** TH	0215	2.4
	0809	4.6		0918	4.2
	1315	1.7		1508	2.2
	2045	4.5		2204	4.1
14 TH	0319	1.9	**29** F	0343	2.4
	0916	4.5		1029	4.2
	1558	1.7		1720	2.0
	2202	4.6		2309	4.3
15 F	0437	1.8	**30** SA	0549	2.2
	1033	4.6		1129	4.4
	1718	1.4		1811	1.7
	2325	4.8			
			31 SU	0002	4.5
				0624	1.8
				1221	4.7
				1846	1.4

APRIL

Day	Time	m	Day	Time	m
1 M	0047	4.8	**16** TU	0112	5.3
	0644	1.5		0711	0.9
	1305	4.9		1325	5.4
	1914	1.1		1945	0.5
2 TU	0126	5.0	**17** W	0158	5.5
	0710	1.2		0755	0.7
	1344	5.2		1413	5.6
	1942	0.8	●	2025	0.5
3 W	0202	5.2	**18** TH	0239	5.5
	0744	0.9		0836	0.5
	1421	5.3		1456	5.6
	2015	0.6		2100	0.5
4 TH	0238	5.4	**19** F	0316	5.5
	0820	0.7		0914	0.5
	1459	5.5		1536	5.6
O	2048	0.5	O	2133	0.6
5 F	0315	5.5	**20** SA	0352	5.5
	0854	0.6		0949	0.6
	1537	5.6		1615	5.5
	2119	0.5		2203	0.8
6 SA	0354	5.5	**21** SU	0428	5.3
	0925	0.6		1023	0.6
	1616	5.6		1653	5.3
	2148	0.6		2231	1.1
7 SU	0434	5.4	**22** M	0504	5.1
	0954	0.7		1059	1.1
	1659	5.5		1732	5.1
	2217	0.8		2259	1.4
8 M	0517	5.3	**23** TU	0541	4.9
	1027	0.8		1134	1.4
	1744	5.3		1813	4.8
	2253	1.1		2327	1.8
9 TU	0604	5.1	**24** W	0623	4.7
	1108	1.0		1218	1.7
	1834	5.1		1859	4.5
	2340	1.4			
10 W	0656	4.9	**25** TH	0005	2.1
	1203	1.3		0711	4.5
	1930	4.8		1319	1.9
				1954	4.2
11 TH	0105	1.8	**26** F	0130	2.3
	0754	4.7		0813	4.3
	1410	1.6		1428	2.0
	2035	4.6		2110	4.2
12 F	0302	1.9	**27** SA	0252	2.4
	0902	4.6		0936	4.2
	1546	1.5		1540	2.0
	2153	4.6		2221	4.3
13 SA	0420	1.8	**28** SU	0407	2.3
	1019	4.7		1043	4.4
	1704	1.3		1647	1.8
	2313	4.8		2319	4.5
14 SU	0526	1.5	**29** M	0507	2.0
	1130	4.9		1138	4.6
	1808	1.0		1740	1.5
15 M	0018	5.1	**30** TU	0007	4.7
	0621	1.2		0551	1.6
	1231	5.2		1226	4.8
	1900	0.7		1822	1.2

Chart Datum: 2·90 metres below Ordnance Datum (Newlyn)

SCOTLAND – LEITH

LAT 55°59′N   LONG 3°10′W

TIMES AND HEIGHTS OF HIGH AND LOW WATERS   YEAR **1996**

TIME ZONE (UT)
For Summer Time add ONE hour in non-shaded areas

Chart Datum: 2·90 metres below Ordnance Datum (Newlyn)

MAY

Day	Time	m	Day	Time	m
1 W	0050 / 0632 / 1309 / 1903	5.0 / 1.3 / 5.1 / 0.9	**16** TH	0138 / 0734 / 1352 / 2001	5.3 / 0.9 / 5.3 / 0.8
2 TH	0131 / 0713 / 1352 / 1943	5.2 / 1.0 / 5.4 / 0.7	**17** F ●	0220 / 0815 / 1437 / 2037	5.4 / 0.8 / 5.4 / 0.9
3 F ○	0211 / 0755 / 1433 / 2024	5.5 / 0.7 / 5.5 / 0.5	**18** SA	0257 / 0853 / 1517 / 2109	5.4 / 0.8 / 5.4 / 0.9
4 SA	0251 / 0835 / 1515 / 2102	5.6 / 0.6 / 5.7 / 0.5	**19** SU	0331 / 0929 / 1555 / 2139	5.4 / 0.8 / 5.3 / 1.1
5 SU	0332 / 0915 / 1558 / 2139	5.6 / 0.5 / 5.7 / 0.6	**20** M	0404 / 1003 / 1631 / 2207	5.3 / 0.9 / 5.2 / 1.2
6 M	0415 / 0952 / 1644 / 2215	5.6 / 0.6 / 5.6 / 0.8	**21** TU	0438 / 1037 / 1708 / 2234	5.2 / 1.1 / 5.0 / 1.5
7 TU	0500 / 1031 / 1732 / 2256	5.5 / 0.7 / 5.4 / 1.1	**22** W	0514 / 1114 / 1747 / 2300	5.0 / 1.3 / 4.9 / 1.7
8 W	0549 / 1119 / 1825 / 2351	5.3 / 0.9 / 5.2 / 1.4	**23** TH	0555 / 1153 / 1829 / 2328	4.9 / 1.5 / 4.7 / 1.9
9 TH	0644 / 1238 / 1923	5.1 / 1.2 / 5.0	**24** F	0641 / 1244 / 1916	4.7 / 1.7 / 4.6
10 F	0117 / 0744 / 1407 / 2027	1.7 / 4.9 / 1.3 / 4.8	**25** SA	0015 / 0731 / 1347 / 2009	2.1 / 4.5 / 1.8 / 4.4
11 SA	0239 / 0851 / 1527 / 2140	1.8 / 4.8 / 1.4 / 4.7	**26** SU	0155 / 0830 / 1452 / 2113	2.3 / 4.4 / 1.9 / 4.4
12 SU	0355 / 1002 / 1641 / 2251	1.8 / 4.8 / 1.3 / 4.8	**27** M	0312 / 0939 / 1554 / 2222	2.2 / 4.4 / 1.8 / 4.5
13 M	0502 / 1108 / 1744 / 2354	1.6 / 4.9 / 1.1 / 5.0	**28** TU	0416 / 1045 / 1651 / 2320	2.1 / 4.6 / 1.6 / 4.7
14 TU	0600 / 1208 / 1837	1.3 / 5.1 / 1.0	**29** W	0510 / 1142 / 1742	1.8 / 4.8 / 1.3
15 W	0049 / 0649 / 1303 / 1921	5.2 / 1.1 / 5.2 / 0.9	**30** TH	0012 / 0558 / 1233 / 1830	4.9 / 1.4 / 5.1 / 1.1
			31 F	0100 / 0646 / 1322 / 1917	5.2 / 1.1 / 5.3 / 0.8

JUNE

Day	Time	m	Day	Time	m
1 SA ○	0146 / 0734 / 1410 / 2005	5.5 / 0.8 / 5.6 / 0.6	**16** SU ●	0239 / 0837 / 1459 / 2050	5.3 / 1.0 / 5.2 / 1.2
2 SU	0230 / 0823 / 1457 / 2051	5.6 / 0.6 / 5.7 / 0.6	**17** M	0313 / 0912 / 1535 / 2119	5.3 / 0.9 / 5.2 / 1.2
3 M	0315 / 0911 / 1543 / 2135	5.7 / 0.5 / 5.8 / 0.6	**18** TU	0345 / 0946 / 1610 / 2147	5.3 / 1.0 / 5.1 / 1.3
4 TU	0359 / 0959 / 1631 / 2219	5.8 / 0.4 / 5.8 / 0.7	**19** W	0418 / 1019 / 1645 / 2214	5.2 / 1.0 / 5.1 / 1.4
5 W	0447 / 1048 / 1721 / 2306	5.7 / 0.5 / 5.6 / 0.9	**20** TH	0453 / 1053 / 1723 / 2239	5.2 / 1.2 / 5.0 / 1.5
6 TH	0538 / 1142 / 1815 / 2359	5.5 / 0.7 / 5.4 / 1.2	**21** F	0533 / 1126 / 1804 / 2304	5.0 / 1.3 / 4.9 / 1.7
7 F	0633 / 1242 / 1913	5.3 / 0.9 / 5.2	**22** SA	0616 / 1159 / 1847 / 2338	4.9 / 1.5 / 4.8 / 1.8
8 SA	0100 / 0733 / 1347 / 2013	1.5 / 5.1 / 1.1 / 5.0	**23** SU	0702 / 1241 / 1933	4.8 / 1.6 / 4.7
9 SU	0208 / 0835 / 1457 / 2117	1.7 / 5.0 / 1.3 / 4.8	**24** M	0022 / 0750 / 1355 / 2023	2.0 / 4.7 / 1.7 / 4.6
10 M	0321 / 0939 / 1611 / 2222	1.8 / 4.9 / 1.4 / 4.8	**25** TU	0141 / 0845 / 1507 / 2122	2.1 / 4.6 / 1.9 / 4.5
11 TU	0434 / 1042 / 1718 / 2325	1.7 / 4.9 / 1.4 / 4.9	**26** W	0328 / 0948 / 1611 / 2229	2.1 / 4.6 / 1.7 / 4.6
12 W	0537 / 1142 / 1813	1.6 / 5.0 / 1.3	**27** TH	0433 / 1056 / 1709 / 2332	1.9 / 4.7 / 1.5 / 4.8
13 TH	0022 / 0631 / 1239 / 1900	5.0 / 1.4 / 5.1 / 1.3	**28** F	0531 / 1159 / 1804	1.6 / 5.0 / 1.2
14 F	0115 / 0718 / 1332 / 1940	5.1 / 1.2 / 5.1 / 1.2	**29** SA	0029 / 0626 / 1256 / 1858	5.1 / 1.2 / 5.3 / 1.0
15 SA	0200 / 0800 / 1418 / 2017	5.2 / 1.1 / 5.2 / 1.2	**30** SU	0122 / 0721 / 1350 / 1951	5.4 / 0.9 / 5.6 / 0.7

JULY

Day	Time	m	Day	Time	m
1 M ○	0212 / 0817 / 1440 / 2041	5.7 / 0.6 / 5.8 / 0.6	**16** TU	0254 / 0858 / 1514 / 2102	5.3 / 1.0 / 5.2 / 1.2
2 TU	0259 / 0909 / 1529 / 2129	5.8 / 0.3 / 5.9 / 0.5	**17** W	0326 / 0929 / 1547 / 2129	5.3 / 0.9 / 5.2 / 1.2
3 W	0345 / 0957 / 1618 / 2214	5.9 / 0.2 / 5.9 / 0.6	**18** TH	0358 / 0959 / 1621 / 2155	5.3 / 0.9 / 5.2 / 1.2
4 TH	0433 / 1045 / 1708 / 2259	5.9 / 0.3 / 5.8 / 0.7	**19** F	0432 / 1029 / 1658 / 2218	5.3 / 1.0 / 5.1 / 1.3
5 F	0524 / 1133 / 1800 / 2346	5.7 / 0.4 / 5.6 / 1.0	**20** SA	0509 / 1055 / 1737 / 2241	5.2 / 1.1 / 5.1 / 1.4
6 SA	0618 / 1222 / 1854	5.6 / 0.7 / 5.3	**21** SU	0550 / 1116 / 1818 / 2310	5.1 / 1.2 / 5.0 / 1.5
7 SU	0035 / 0714 / 1315 / 1950	1.3 / 5.3 / 1.0 / 5.1	**22** M	0633 / 1143 / 1902 / 2346	5.0 / 1.4 / 4.9 / 1.7
8 M	0130 / 0811 / 1413 / 2048	1.6 / 5.1 / 1.3 / 4.9	**23** TU	0718 / 1223 / 1948	4.8 / 1.6 / 4.7
9 TU	0235 / 0912 / 1527 / 2149	1.8 / 4.9 / 1.6 / 4.7	**24** W	0032 / 0807 / 1324 / 2039	1.9 / 4.7 / 1.8 / 4.6
10 W	0358 / 1014 / 1650 / 2252	1.9 / 4.8 / 1.7 / 4.7	**25** TH	0142 / 0906 / 1530 / 2142	2.0 / 4.6 / 1.7 / 4.6
11 TH	0518 / 1117 / 1754 / 2353	1.8 / 4.8 / 1.7 / 4.8	**26** F	0403 / 1016 / 1644 / 2254	2.0 / 4.7 / 1.7 / 4.7
12 F	0619 / 1216 / 1843	1.6 / 4.8 / 1.6	**27** SA	0511 / 1129 / 1745	1.7 / 4.9 / 1.4
13 SA	0049 / 0707 / 1312 / 1925	4.9 / 1.4 / 4.9 / 1.5	**28** SU	0001 / 0613 / 1235 / 1843	5.0 / 1.3 / 5.2 / 1.1
14 SU	0139 / 0749 / 1359 / 2001	5.1 / 1.2 / 5.0 / 1.4	**29** M	0101 / 0714 / 1332 / 1939	5.3 / 0.9 / 5.5 / 0.8
15 M ●	0219 / 0825 / 1439 / 2034	5.2 / 1.1 / 5.1 / 1.3	**30** TU ○	0154 / 0811 / 1425 / 2030	5.7 / 0.5 / 5.8 / 0.6
			31 W	0243 / 0901 / 1514 / 2117	5.9 / 0.2 / 6.0 / 0.4

AUGUST

Day	Time	m	Day	Time	m
1 TH	0330 / 0947 / 1601 / 2201	6.0 / 0.0 / 6.0 / 0.4	**16** F	0334 / 0933 / 1554 / 2131	5.4 / 0.8 / 5.3 / 1.1
2 F	0416 / 1030 / 1649 / 2243	6.0 / 0.1 / 5.9 / 0.5	**17** SA	0407 / 0959 / 1630 / 2155	5.4 / 0.8 / 5.3 / 1.1
3 SA	0505 / 1112 / 1738 / 2324	5.9 / 0.3 / 5.7 / 0.8	**18** SU	0444 / 1022 / 1708 / 2218	5.3 / 0.9 / 5.3 / 1.2
4 SU	0555 / 1153 / 1829	5.7 / 0.6 / 5.4	**19** M	0523 / 1043 / 1749 / 2244	5.2 / 1.1 / 5.2 / 1.3
5 M	0006 / 0647 / 1235 / 1920	1.1 / 5.4 / 1.0 / 5.1	**20** TU	0604 / 1111 / 1831 / 2318	5.1 / 1.2 / 5.0 / 1.5
6 TU	0053 / 0742 / 1322 / 2015	1.5 / 5.1 / 1.5 / 4.8	**21** W	0649 / 1148 / 1916	5.0 / 1.5 / 4.9
7 W	0147 / 0841 / 1421 / 2115	1.8 / 4.8 / 1.9 / 4.6	**22** TH	0002 / 0737 / 1239 / 2007	1.7 / 4.8 / 1.7 / 4.7
8 TH	0304 / 0945 / 1614 / 2219	2.0 / 4.6 / 2.1 / 4.5	**23** F	0101 / 0835 / 1509 / 2107	1.9 / 4.7 / 1.9 / 4.6
9 F	0501 / 1051 / 1737 / 2323	2.0 / 4.5 / 2.0 / 4.6	**24** SA	0342 / 0946 / 1624 / 2222	2.0 / 4.6 / 1.8 / 4.7
10 SA	0607 / 1154 / 1828	1.8 / 4.6 / 1.9	**25** SU	0456 / 1107 / 1729 / 2337	1.7 / 4.8 / 1.6 / 4.9
11 SU	0022 / 0655 / 1251 / 1909	4.8 / 1.5 / 4.8 / 1.7	**26** M	0603 / 1218 / 1829	1.5 / 5.2 / 1.2
12 M	0113 / 0735 / 1338 / 1945	5.0 / 1.3 / 5.0 / 1.5	**27** TU	0040 / 0704 / 1317 / 1924	5.3 / 0.8 / 5.5 / 0.9
13 TU	0155 / 0809 / 1416 / 2015	5.2 / 1.1 / 5.1 / 1.3	**28** W ○	0135 / 0759 / 1409 / 2014	5.7 / 0.4 / 5.8 / 0.6
14 W ●	0230 / 0839 / 1449 / 2040	5.3 / 0.9 / 5.2 / 1.2	**29** TH	0224 / 0846 / 1456 / 2059	5.9 / 0.1 / 6.0 / 0.4
15 TH	0302 / 0906 / 1521 / 2105	5.4 / 0.8 / 5.2 / 1.1	**30** F	0310 / 0928 / 1541 / 2141	6.1 / 0.0 / 6.0 / 0.3
			31 SA	0355 / 1008 / 1625 / 2221	6.1 / 0.1 / 5.9 / 0.5

SCOTLAND – LEITH

LAT 55°59′N   LONG 3°10′W

TIMES AND HEIGHTS OF HIGH AND LOW WATERS   YEAR **1996**

TIME ZONE (UT)
For Summer Time add ONE hour in non-shaded areas

6

SEPTEMBER

	Time	m		Time	m
1 SU	0440 1045 1710 2259	6.0 0.3 5.7 0.7	**16** M	0418 0951 1640 2154	5.5 0.8 5.4 1.0
2 M	0527 1120 1757 2338	5.7 0.7 5.4 1.1	**17** TU	0457 1015 1720 2222	5.4 1.0 5.3 1.2
3 TU	0617 1156 1846	5.4 1.2 5.1	**18** W	0539 1045 1803 2257	5.3 1.2 5.2 1.4
4 W	0019 0709 1237 1939	1.5 5.0 1.7 4.8	**19** TH	0624 1124 1850 2341	5.1 1.5 5.0 1.6
5 TH	0110 0808 1331 2038	1.8 4.7 2.1 4.5	**20** F	0715 1217 1942	4.9 1.8 4.8
6 F	0217 0914 1447 2145	2.1 4.4 2.4 4.4	**21** SA	0044 0814 1450 2043	1.9 4.7 2.0 4.6
7 SA	0435 1023 1715 2252	2.2 4.4 2.3 4.5	**22** SU	0328 0927 1606 2159	1.9 4.7 1.9 4.7
8 SU	0546 1128 1807 2351	1.9 4.5 2.1 4.7	**23** M	0443 1052 1713 2318	1.6 4.8 1.6 5.0
9 M	0632 1223 1848	1.6 4.7 1.8	**24** TU	0550 1204 1812	1.2 5.2 1.3
10 TU	0042 0710 1310 1921	4.9 1.3 4.9 1.6	**25** W	0021 0648 1302 1905	5.3 0.8 5.5 0.9
11 W	0125 0743 1347 1948	5.1 1.1 5.1 1.3	**26** TH	0116 0740 1351 1954	5.7 0.5 5.8 0.7
12 TH ●	0201 0810 1420 2008	5.3 0.9 5.3 1.2	**27** F ○	0204 0825 1436 2038	5.9 0.3 5.9 0.5
13 F	0234 0833 1452 2034	5.4 0.8 5.4 1.0	**28** SA	0249 0905 1518 2118	6.0 0.2 6.0 0.4
14 SA	0307 0900 1526 2103	5.5 0.7 5.5 0.9	**29** SU	0332 0942 1559 2157	6.0 0.3 5.9 0.5
15 SU	0341 0926 1602 2129	5.5 0.7 5.5 1.0	**30** M	0415 1016 1641 2233	5.9 0.6 5.7 0.8

OCTOBER

	Time	m		Time	m
1 TU	0459 1048 1723 2309	5.6 0.9 5.4 1.1	**16** W	0435 0955 1655 2206	5.6 1.0 5.5 1.1
2 W	0544 1120 1808 2349	5.3 1.4 5.1 1.5	**17** TH	0518 1028 1739 2243	5.4 1.2 5.3 1.3
3 TH	0633 1158 1857	5.0 1.8 4.8	**18** F	0606 1111 1828 2333	5.2 1.5 5.1 1.5
4 F	0038 0730 1250 1955	1.9 4.6 2.2 4.5	**19** SA	0700 1214 1923	5.0 1.9 4.9
5 SA	0141 0837 1400 2106	2.1 4.4 2.5 4.4	**20** SU	0143 0800 1431 2027	1.8 4.8 2.0 4.7
6 SU	0300 0948 1632 2215	2.3 4.3 2.6 4.4	**21** M	0313 0914 1546 2143	1.7 4.7 1.9 4.8
7 M	0507 1053 1735 2315	2.1 4.4 2.3 4.6	**22** TU	0426 1036 1653 2259	1.5 4.9 1.7 5.0
8 TU	0556 1148 1815	1.8 4.7 2.0	**23** W	0531 1146 1751	1.2 5.2 1.4
9 W	0006 0634 1235 1845	4.8 1.5 4.9 1.7	**24** TH	0001 0627 1243 1843	5.3 0.9 5.5 1.1
10 TH	0050 0703 1313 1903	5.1 1.3 5.1 1.4	**25** F	0055 0717 1331 1931	5.6 0.7 5.7 0.9
11 F	0128 0725 1348 1928	5.3 1.0 5.3 1.2	**26** SA ○	0144 0800 1415 2015	5.8 0.6 5.8 1.0
12 SA ●	0204 0753 1423 2000	5.4 0.8 5.5 1.0	**27** SU	0228 0840 1456 2055	5.9 0.6 5.8 0.7
13 SU	0239 0825 1458 2034	5.6 0.7 5.6 0.9	**28** M	0311 0915 1534 2133	5.8 0.7 5.7 0.7
14 M	0316 0857 1535 2105	5.6 0.7 5.6 0.9	**29** TU	0351 0948 1612 2208	5.7 0.9 5.6 0.9
15 TU	0354 0926 1614 2134	5.6 0.8 5.6 0.9	**30** W	0432 1018 1650 2243	5.5 1.2 5.4 1.2
			31 TH	0513 1048 1728 2322	5.3 1.5 5.1 1.5

NOVEMBER

	Time	m		Time	m
1 F	0556 1121 1809	5.0 1.9 4.9	**16** SA	0553 1111 1812 2345	5.4 1.5 5.2 1.4
2 SA	0008 0644 1206 1857	1.8 4.7 2.2 4.7	**17** SU	0649 1236 1909	5.1 1.8 5.0
3 SU	0106 0742 1314 2003	2.1 4.5 2.5 4.5	**18** M	0134 0750 1405 2013	1.5 4.9 1.9 4.9
4 M	0213 0855 1431 2124	2.2 4.3 2.6 4.4	**19** TU	0251 0900 1519 2125	1.6 4.8 1.9 4.9
5 TU	0325 1005 1550 2230	2.2 4.4 2.5 4.5	**20** W	0402 1014 1628 2236	1.5 4.9 1.8 5.0
6 W	0436 1103 1659 2324	2.0 4.6 2.2 4.7	**21** TH	0507 1121 1729 2338	1.3 5.1 1.6 5.2
7 TH	0526 1153 1739	1.7 4.8 1.9	**22** F	0604 1218 1823	1.2 5.3 1.3
8 F	0011 0603 1236 1815	5.0 1.4 5.1 1.6	**23** SA	0033 0653 1310 1911	5.4 1.1 5.4 1.1
9 SA	0053 0640 1315 1852	5.3 1.2 5.3 1.3	**24** SU	0124 0737 1355 1955	5.5 1.0 5.6 1.0
10 SU	0133 0717 1350 1931	5.4 1.0 5.4 1.1	**25** M ○	0210 0816 1436 2036	5.6 1.0 5.6 0.9
11 M ●	0213 0756 1433 2010	5.6 0.8 5.7 0.9	**26** TU	0252 0851 1513 2112	5.6 1.1 5.6 0.9
12 TU	0253 0834 1512 2048	5.7 0.8 5.7 0.8	**27** W	0331 0923 1548 2147	5.5 1.2 5.5 1.0
13 W	0334 0910 1534 2124	5.8 0.8 5.7 0.8	**28** TH	0409 0952 1622 2222	5.4 1.3 5.4 1.2
14 TH	0417 0945 1635 2201	5.7 1.0 5.6 1.0	**29** F	0447 1020 1657 2258	5.3 1.5 5.2 1.2
15 F	0503 1023 1721 2244	5.6 1.2 5.4 1.1	**30** SA	0526 1050 1735 2338	5.0 1.8 5.1 1.6

DECEMBER

	Time	m		Time	m
1 SU	0608 1120 1818	4.9 2.0 4.9	**16** M	0004 0636 1223 1855	1.0 5.3 1.5 5.2
2 M	0028 0654 1202 1907	1.8 4.7 2.2 4.7	**17** TU	0110 0735 1331 1956	1.2 5.1 1.7 5.1
3 TU	0128 0747 1328 2005	2.0 4.5 2.4 4.5	**18** W	0217 0838 1441 2102	1.4 4.9 1.9 4.9
4 W	0231 0850 1447 2118	2.1 4.5 2.4 4.5	**19** TH	0328 0944 1555 2209	1.5 4.8 1.9 4.9
5 TH	0332 1001 1553 2229	2.0 4.5 2.3 4.6	**20** F	0439 1050 1708 2312	1.5 4.9 1.8 5.0
6 F	0429 1102 1650 2326	1.8 4.7 2.1 4.8	**21** SA	0541 1151 1806	1.5 5.0 1.6
7 SA	0519 1155 1738	1.6 4.9 1.8	**22** SU	0011 0634 1247 1858	5.1 1.4 5.2 1.4
8 SU	0016 0605 1242 1823	5.0 1.3 5.2 1.4	**23** M	0106 0718 1336 1943	5.2 1.4 5.3 1.2
9 M	0104 0649 1327 1909	5.3 1.1 5.4 1.2	**24** TU ○	0154 0758 1419 2023	5.2 1.3 5.4 1.1
10 TU	0149 0734 1411 1955	5.5 0.9 5.7 0.9	**25** W	0236 0833 1456 2059	5.3 1.3 5.4 1.0
11 W	0233 0820 1453 2041	5.7 0.8 5.8 0.9	**26** TH	0314 0904 1530 2132	5.3 1.3 5.4 1.0
12 TH	0318 0904 1536 2127	5.8 0.8 5.8 0.7	**27** F	0350 0932 1602 2204	5.2 1.3 5.4 1.1
13 F	0403 0948 1620 2214	5.8 0.9 5.8 0.7	**28** SA	0424 1000 1634 2236	5.2 1.4 5.3 1.2
14 SA	0450 1032 1707 2304	5.7 1.0 5.6 0.8	**29** SU	0501 1026 1711 2310	5.1 1.5 5.2 1.3
15 SU	0541 1122 1758	5.5 1.3 5.5	**30** M	0540 1050 1751 2342	5.0 1.7 5.0 1.5
			31 TU	0623 1117 1836	4.9 1.9 4.9

Chart Datum: 2·90 metres below Ordnance Datum (Newlyn)

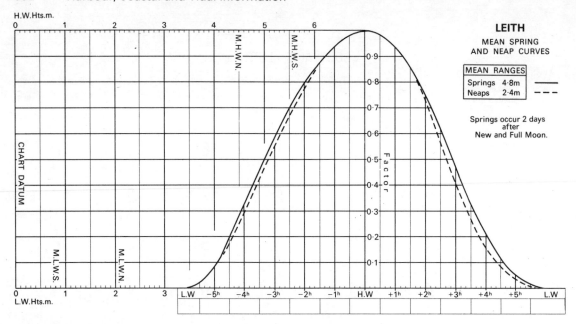

H.W.Hts.m.

LEITH
MEAN SPRING
AND NEAP CURVES

MEAN RANGES	
Springs	4·8m
Neaps	2·4m

Springs occur 2 days
after
New and Full Moon.

CHART DATUM

Factor

L.W.Hts.m.

BURNTISLAND 10-6-10

Fife 56°03'·23N 03°14'·12W

CHARTS
AC 733, 739, 735; Imray C27; OS 66
TIDES
+0340 Dover; ML 3·3; Duration 0625; Zone 0 (UT)

Standard Port LEITH (←—)

Times				Height (metres)			
High Water		Low Water		MHWS	MHWN	MLWN	MLWS
0300	0900	0300	0900	5·6	4·5	2·1	0·8
1500	2100	1500	2100				
Differences BURNTISLAND							
+0002	−0002	+0002	−0003	0·0	0·0	+0·1	+0·1

SHELTER
Good in the industrial docks but only fair in the outer hbr; unsuitable for yachts in strong winds. E dock can be entered from HW−3 to HW; not recommended unless in emergency.

NAVIGATION
WPT 56°03'·00N 03°14'·00W, 163°/343° from/to ent, 0·23M. To the E, beware Black Rks (off chartlet) and to the W, Familars Rks. Keep clear of ships using DG ranges SW of port. Commercial barge operations can cause delays.
LIGHTS AND MARKS
As chartlet. Conspic marks: Radio mast 1·1M N of hbr ent; Shed to NW; Radar tr on E pier. Tfc Sigs for E dock only.
RADIO TELEPHONE
Forth Navigation Ch **71** 16 12 20 (H24), for ent to E Dock.
TELEPHONE (01592)
Hr Mr (01333) 426725; MRSC (01333) 450666; ⌗ (0131) 4697400; Marinecall 0891 500452; Police 204444; Dr 872761.
FACILITIES
Dock ☎ 872236, AB (limited) £19.97, FW, C (10 ton); **Outer Hbr** Slip, FW, AB (limited); **Burntisland YC** M or AB for small fee, if room in Boat Shelter; FW; **Services:** D, ME, El, Ⓔ, Sh, BY, C (30 ton), CH, Gas, Gaz. **Town** EC Wed; P, D, ME, El, C, V, R, Bar, ✉, Ⓑ, ⇌, Ⓗ Kirkcaldy, ✈ Edinburgh.

KIRKCALDY, 4·7M to NE, is officially closed; see Methil.

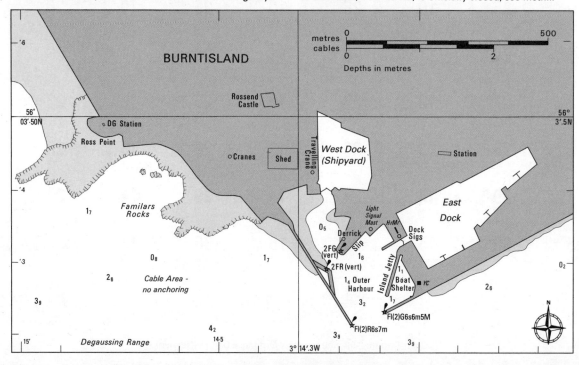

BURNTISLAND

metres
cables
Depths in metres

Rossend
Castle

DG Station

Ross Point

Cranes

Shed

Travelling Crane

West Dock
(Shipyard)

Station

Familars
Rocks

East
Dock

Light
Signal
Mast

HrMr

Derrick

Dock
Sigs

2FG
(vert)

Slip

2FR (vert)

Island Jetty

Boat
Shelter

YC

Cable Area -
no anchoring

Fl(2)G6s6m5M

Fl(2)R6s7m

Degaussing Range

METHIL   10-6-11

Fife 56°10'·76N 03°00'·45W

CHARTS
AC 739, 734; Imray C27; OS 59
TIDES
+0330 Dover; ML 3·0; Duration 0615; Zone 0 (UT)

Standard Port LEITH (←)

Times				Height (metres)			
High Water		Low Water		MHWS	MHWN	MLWN	MLWS
0300	0900	0300	0900	5·6	4·5	2·1	0·8
1500	2100	1500	2100				
Differences METHIL							
+0007	+0007	−0007	−0007	0·0	0·0	+0·1	+0·1
KIRKCALDY							
+0009	+0009	−0009	−0009	−0·3	−0·3	−0·2	−0·2

SHELTER
Commercial port, but good emergency shelter in No 2 dock.
NAVIGATION
WPT 56°10'·50N 03°00'·00W, 140°/320° from/to pier hd lt, 0·34M. Beware silting. A sand bar forms rapidly to seaward of the lt ho and dredged depth is not always maintained.
LIGHTS AND MARKS
By day and night (vert lts):
ⓇⒼ = Dangerous to enter; Bring up in roads.

ⓇⓌ = Clear to enter No 2 dock.

Ⓡ = Remain in roads until another signal is made.
RADIO TELEPHONE
VHF Ch 14 16 (HW–3 to HW+1).
TELEPHONE (01592)
Hr Mr (Port Manager) (01333) 426725; MRSC (01333) 450666; ⌗ (0131) 469 7400; Marinecall 0891 500452; Police 712881; Dr (01333) 426913.
FACILITIES
Hbr No 2 Dock £19.97, FW, C (7 ton);
Town EC Thurs; P, D, Gas, Gaz, V, R, Bar, ✉, Ⓑ, ⇌ (bus to Markinch or Kirkcaldy), Ⓗ Kirkcaldy, ✈ (Edinburgh).

ADJACENT HARBOUR, 6M to SW.

KIRKCALDY, Fife, 56°06'·81N 03°08'·86W. AC 739. HW +0345 on Dover, −0005 on Leith; HW −0·1m on Leith; ML 3·2m; Duration 0620. See 10.6.11. Shelter good except in strong E winds; an emergency refuge. Officially the hbr is closed (no commercial tfc) and unmanned; depths may be less than charted due to silting. Small craft should contact Forth Ports Authority ☎ (01333) 426725, or call *Methil Docks Radio* Ch 16 14 for advice.

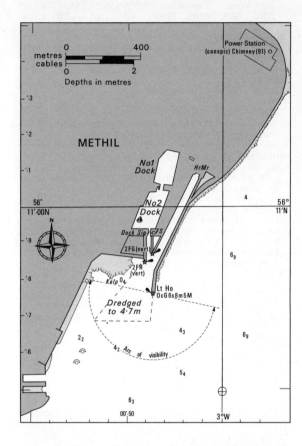

6

ANSTRUTHER 10-6-12

Fife 56°13'·16N 02°41'·72W

CHARTS
AC 734, 175; Imray C27; OS 59
TIDES
+0315 Dover; ML 3·1; Duration 0620; Zone 0 (UT)

Standard Port LEITH (←)

Times				Height (metres)			
High Water		Low Water		MHWS	MHWN	MLWN	MLWS
0300	0900	0300	0900	5·6	4·5	2·1	0·8
1500	2100	1500	2100				
Differences ANSTRUTHER EASTER							
−0010	−0035	−0020	−0020	−0·1	−0·1	−0·1	−0·1

SHELTER
Good, but do not enter in strong E and S winds. Hbr dries; access approx HW±2. Caution: ledge at base of W pier. No ⚓ to W of hbr; do not go N of W Pier lt due to rocks.
NAVIGATION
WPT 56°12'·60N 02°42'·10W, 199°/019° from/to ent, 0·60M. Beware lobster pots and FVs.
LIGHTS AND MARKS
Conspic tr on W pier. Ldg lts 019°, both FG 7/11m 4M. Pier lts as chartlet. Horn (3) 60s in tr.
RADIO TELEPHONE
Forth Navigation Service. See 10.6.9.

TELEPHONE (01333)
Hr Mr 310836; MRSC (01333) 450666; ⌗ (0131) 469 7400; Marinecall 0891 500452; Police 310333; Dr 310352.
FACILITIES
Hbr AB £5.99, Slip, FW, LB, AC, Shwrs;
Services: D (tanker), CH, ACA, ME, Gas, Gaz, El, Ⓔ, Ⓞ.
Town EC Wed; P, V, R, Bar, ✉, Ⓑ, ⇌ (bus Cupar or Leuchars), Ⓗ St Andrews, ✈ Edinburgh/Dundee.

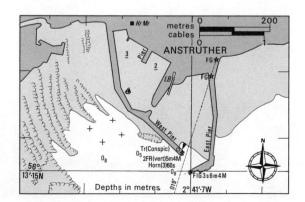

RIVER TAY   10-6-13

Fife/Angus 56°27'·11N 02°52'·78W (Tayport)

CHARTS
AC 1481, 190; OS 54, 59

TIDES
+0401 (Dundee) Dover; ML 3·1; Duration 0610; Zone 0 (UT)

Standard Port ABERDEEN (→)

Times				Height (metres)			
High Water		Low Water		MHWS	MHWN	MLWN	MLWS
0000	0600	0100	0700	4·3	3·4	1·6	0·6
1200	1800	1300	1900				
Differences BAR							
+0100	+0100	+0050	+0110	+0·9	+0·8	+0·3	+0·1
DUNDEE							
+0140	+0120	+0055	+0145	+1·1	+0·9	+0·3	+0·1
NEWBURGH							
+0215	+0200	+0250	+0335	−0·2	−0·4	−1·1	−0·5
PERTH							
+0220	+0225	+0510	+0530	−0·9	−1·4	−1·2	−0·3

NOTE: At Perth LW time differences give the start of the rise, following a LW stand of about 4 hours.

SHELTER
Good in the Tay estuary, but ent is dangerous in strong E/SE winds or in an on-shore swell. Tayport is best place for yachts on passage, access HW±4. Hbr partly dries except W side of NE pier; S side is full of yacht moorings. Gates at Dundee (Camperdown) commercial docks open HW−2 to HW (Fl R lt = no entry/exit). Possible moorings off Royal Tay YC. ⚓s as on chartlet: the ⚓ off the city is exposed and landing difficult. Off S bank good shelter at Woodhaven and ⚓s from Wormit BC. There are ⚓s up river at Balmerino, Newburgh and Inchyra.

NAVIGATION
WPT Tay Fairway SWM buoy, L Fl 10s, Bell, 56°28'·92N 02°37'·42W, 045°/225° from/to the Middle Bar buoys, 9½ca. Do not try to cross Abertay or Gaa Sands as charted depths are unreliable. Chan is well buoyed, minimum depth 5·2m. Beware strong tidal streams.

LIGHTS AND MARKS
Tayport High lt Dir 269° Iso WRG 3s, W sector 268°-270°. The HFP "Abertay" ECM buoy, Q (3) 10s (Racon), at E end of Gaa Sands is a clear visual mark. Keep N of Larick, a conspic disused lt bn.

RADIO TELEPHONE
Dundee Hbr Radio VHF Ch **12** 16 (H24); local nav warnings, weather, vis and tides on request. Royal Tay YC, Ch M.

TELEPHONE (01382)
Hr Mr (Dundee) 224121/Fax 200834; Hr Mr (Perth) (01738) 624056; MRSC (01333) 450666; ⌗ (0131) 469 7400; Tayport Boatowners' Ass'n 553679; Marinecall 0891 500452; Police (Tayport) 552222, (Dundee) 223200; Dr 221953; Ⓗ 223125.

FACILITIES
N BANK: **Camperdown Dock**, AB £13.30, FW, ME, EI, C (8 ton); **Victoria Dock** FW, ME, C (8 ton), AB; **Royal Tay YC** (Broughty Ferry) ☎ 477516, M, L, R, Bar;
Services: CH, M, L, ME, EI, Sh, C (2 ton), ACA.
Dundee City EC Wed; P, D, CH, V, R, Bar, ✉, Ⓑ, ⇌, ✈.
S BANK: **Tayport Hbr** ☎ 553679 AB £7.00, Slip, L, FW, AC;
Wormit Boating Club ☎ 541400 M, Slip, L, FW, V.

ADJACENT HARBOURS

PERTH, Perthshire, 56°22'·90N 03°25'·65W. AC 1481; OS 53, 58. Tides, see 10.6.13. FYCA Pilot Handbook is needed. Leave Tay rly bridge at about HW Dundee −2 to carry a fair tide the 16·5M to Perth. The buoyed/lit chan favours the S bank for 9M to Newburgh. Here care is needed due to mudbanks in mid-stream; keep S of Mugdrum Is. Up-river, power cables have clearance of 33m and Friarton bridge 26m. Keep S of Willow Is, past the gasworks to hbr on the W bank. Hbr has approx 1·5m; keep clear of coasters. See Hr Mr, ☎ (01738) 624056, for berth. VHF Ch 09 16. FW, D & P (cans), usual city amenities, ⇌, ✈.

ST ANDREWS, Fife, 56°20'·33N 02°46'·70W. AC 190. HW −0015 Leith. Small drying hbr 7M S of Tay Estuary and 8M NW of Fife Ness. In strong onshore winds breaking seas render appr/ent impossible. Appr at HW±2 on 270°; N bkwtr bn in transit with conspic cathedral tr; no lights. Keep about 10m S of the bkwtr for best water. Berth on W side of inner hbr (drying 2·5m). 8m wide ent has lock gates, usually open, and retractable footbridge. Facilities: FW, SC. EC Thurs; All amenities of university town, inc golf course.

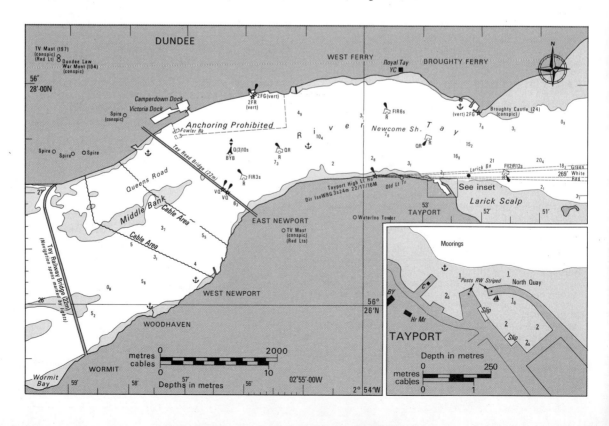

ARBROATH   10-6-14

Angus 56°33'·24N 02°34'·88W

CHARTS
AC 1438, 190; OS 54

TIDES
+0317 Dover; ML 2·9; Duration 0620; Zone 0 (UT)

Standard Port ABERDEEN (→)

Times				Height (metres)			
High Water		Low Water		MHWS	MHWN	MLWN	MLWS
0000	0600	0100	0700	4·3	3·4	1·6	0·6
1200	1800	1300	1900				
Differences ARBROATH							
+0056	+0037	+0034	+0055	+0·7	+0·7	+0·2	+0·1

SHELTER
Good, especially in Wet Dock, but ent can be dangerous in moderate SE swell. Dock gates normally remain open, but will be closed on request. Entry should not be attempted LW±2½.

NAVIGATION
WPT 56°33'·00N 02°34'·10W, 119°/299° from/to ent, 0·50M. Beware Knuckle rks to stbd and Cheek Bush rks to port on entering. Arbroath is a very busy fishing hbr so beware heavy traffic.

LIGHTS AND MARKS
Ldg lts 299°, both FR 7/13m 5M; or twin trs of St Thomas' ✠ visible between N pier lt ho and W bkwtr bn.
Entry sigs: Fl Ⓖ= Entry safe
                   Ⓡ   = Entry dangerous

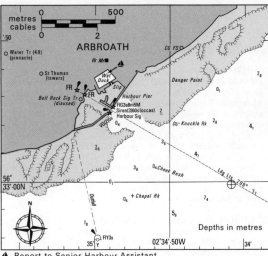

⚓ Report to Senior Harbour Assistant

RADIO TELEPHONE
Contact AFA (Arbroath Fishermen's Ass'n) VHF Ch 16.
TELEPHONE (01241)
Hr Mr 872166; MRSC (01224) 592334; ⌗ (0131) 469 7400; Marinecall 0891 500452; Police 722222; Dr 876836.
FACILITIES
Pier Slip, D, L, FW, AB; **Services:** BY, Slip, L, ME, El, Sh, C (8 ton) Ⓔ, M, Gas, CH.
Town EC Wed; P, D, V, R, Bar, ✉, Ⓑ, ⇌, ✈ (Dundee).

MONTROSE   10-6-15

Angus 56°42'·21N 02°26'·49W

CHARTS
AC 1438, 190; OS 54

TIDES
+0320 Dover; ML 2·9; Duration 0645; Zone 0 (UT)

Standard Port ABERDEEN (→)

Times				Height (metres)			
High Water		Low Water		MHWS	MHWN	MLWN	MLWS
0000	0600	0100	0700	4·3	3·4	1·6	0·6
1200	1800	1300	1900				
Differences MONTROSE							
+0055	+0055	+0030	+0040	+0·5	+0·4	+0·2	0·0

SHELTER
Good; yachts are welcome in this busy commercial port. Contact Hr Mr for AB, usually available, but beware wash from other traffic. Double mooring lines advised due to strong tidal streams (up to 6kn).

NAVIGATION
WPT 56°42'·20N 02°25'·00W, 091°/271° from/to front ldg lt, 1·25M. Beware Annat Bank to N and Scurdie Rks to S of ent chan. In quiet weather best access is LW to LW+1, but in strong onshore winds only safe access would be from HW −2 to HW. Ent is dangerous with strong onshore winds against ebb tide as heavy overfalls develop.

LIGHTS AND MARKS
Scurdie Ness lt ho Fl (3) 20s 38m 23M (conspic). Two sets of ldg lts: Outer 271·5°, both FR 11/18m 5M. Inner 265°, both FG 21/33m 5M, Orange △ front and ▽ rear.
RADIO TELEPHONE
VHF Ch 12 16 (H24).
TELEPHONE (01674)
Hr Mr 672302/673153; MRCC (01224) 592334; ⌗ (0131) 469 7400; Marinecall 0891 500452; Police 672222; Dr 673400.
FACILITIES
N Quay ☎ 672302, AB £7.05, D (by tanker via Hr Mr), FW, ME, El, C (1½ to 40 ton), CH, Gas.
Town EC Wed; V, R, P, Bar, ✉, Ⓑ, ⇌, ✈ (Aberdeen).

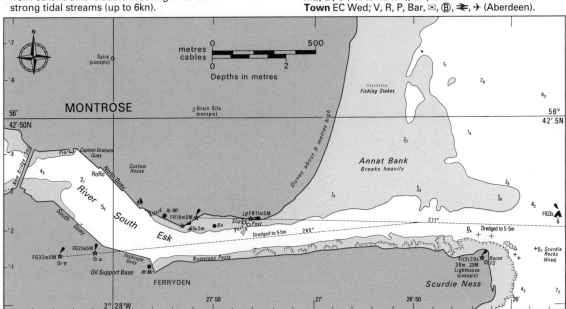

HARBOURS SOUTH OF STONEHAVEN

JOHNSHAVEN, Angus, 56°47'·61N 02°19'·96W. AC 210.
HW +0245 on Dover; +0025 and +0·4m on Aberdeen; ML
2·7m; Duration 0626. Very small drying hbr 6·5M N of
Montrose. Ent impossible in strong onshore winds;
strictly a fair weather visit. Appr from 5ca SE at HW±2½.
Conspic W shed at N end of hbr. Ldg marks/lts on 316°:
front, R structure with FR 5m; rear is G structure, 20m up
the hill and 85m from front, with FG (FR when entry
unsafe). Transit leads between rky ledges to very narrow
(20m) ent. Turn 90° port into Inner Basin (dries 2·5m) and
berth on outer wall. Hr Mr ☎ (01561) 362262 (home).
Facilities: Slip, AB, AC, C (5 ton), FW, V, R, ME, Bar, ✉.
Bus to Montrose and Aberdeen.

GOURDON, Kincardine, 56°49'·50N 02°17'·10W. AC 210.
HW +0240 on Dover; +0020 on Aberdeen; HW +0·4m on
Aberdeen; ML 2·7m; Duration 0620. Shelter good in inner
W hbr (drys about 2m; protected by storm gates); access
from about mid-flood. E (or Gutty) hbr is rky, with
difficult access. Beware rky ledges marked by bn and
extending 200m S from W pier end. A dangerous rk dries
on the ldg line about 1½ca S of pier heads. Ldg marks/lts
358°, both FR 5/30m 5M, 2 W trs; front lt shows G when
not safe to enter. W pier hd Fl WRG 3s 5m 9/7M, vis
G180°-344°, W344°-354° (10°), R354°-180°. E bkwtr hd Q
3m 7M. Hr Mr ☎ (01569) 762741 (part-time, same as
10.6.16). Facilities: Slip, FW from standpipe, D, ME, AC,
M, V, R, Bar. Fish market held Mon-Fri 1130 and 1530.

STONEHAVEN   10-6-16

Kincardine 56°57'·58N 02°11'·91W

CHARTS
AC 1438, 210; OS 45

TIDES
+0235 Dover; ML 2·6; Duration 0620; Zone 0 (UT)

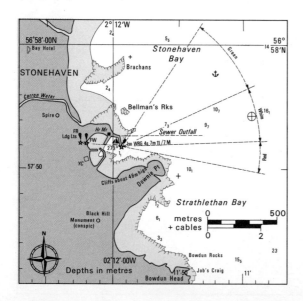

Standard Port ABERDEEN (→)

Times				Height (metres)			
High Water		Low Water		MHWS	MHWN	MLWN	MLWS
0000	0600	0100	0700	4·3	3·4	1·6	0·6
1200	1800	1300	1900				
Differences STONEHAVEN							
+0013	+0008	+0013	+0009	+0·2	+0·2	+0·1	0·0

SHELTER
Good, especially from offshore winds. Berth in outer hbr
(0·4m) on bkwtr or N wall; sandbank forms in middle to
W side. Or ⚓ outside in fair weather. Hbr speed limit 3kn.
Inner hbr dries 3·4m and in bad weather storm gates are
shut. Do not go S of ldg line, to clear rks E of inner hbr wall.

NAVIGATION
WPT 56°57'·70N 02°11'·00W, 078°/258° from/to bkwtr lt,
0·50M. Give Downie Pt a wide berth. Do not enter in
strong on-shore winds. Radar assistance on Ch 16 in fog.

LIGHTS AND MARKS
N pier Iso WRG 4s 7m 11/7M; appr in W sector, 246°-268°.
Inner hbr ldg lts 273°, only visible within outer hbr: front
FW 6m 5M; rear FR 8m 6M, but FG = storm gates closed.

RADIO TELEPHONE
Maritime Rescue International VHF Ch 16; ☎ 764065.

TELEPHONE (01569)
Hr Mr (part-time) 762741; MRCC (01224) 592334; ◫ (0131)
469 7400; Marinecall 0891 500452; Police 762963;
Dr 762945.

FACILITIES
Hbr AB £7.50 for 7 days, M, L, FW, AC, Slip, C (1·5 ton), LB;
Aberdeen and Stonehaven YC Slip, Bar.
Town EC Wed; V, R, Bar, ✉, Ⓑ, ⇌, ✈ (Aberdeen).

ABERDEEN   10-6-17

Aberdeen 57°08'·72N 02°03'·48W

CHARTS
AC 1446, 210; OS 38

TIDES
+0231 Dover; ML 2·5; Duration 0620; Zone 0 (UT)
Note: Aberdeen is a Standard Port and tidal predictions for each day of the year are given below.

SHELTER
Good in hbr; open at all tides, but do not enter in strong NE/ESE winds. For berthing instructions call Hr Mr on VHF or berth at Pocra Quay first. Yachts usually lie in Upper Dock or on N side of Albert Basin alongside floating linkspan, but are not encouraged in this busy commercial port. ⚓ in Aberdeen Bay gives some shelter from S and W winds.

NAVIGATION
WPT Fairway SWM, Q, Racon, 57°09'·32N 02°01'·83W, 056°/236° from/to ent 1·05M. Give Girdle Ness a berth of at least ¼M (more in bad weather) and do not pass close round pier hds. Strong tidal streams and, with river in spate, possible overfalls. Chan dredged to 6m on ldg line.

LIGHTS AND MARKS
Ldg lts 236° (FR = port open; FG = port closed).
Traffic sigs at root of N pier:
Ⓖ	=	Entry prohib
Ⓡ	=	Dep prohib
Ⓡ & Ⓖ	=	Port closed

RADIO TELEPHONE
VHF Ch 06 11 **12** 13 16 (H24).

TELEPHONE (01224)
Hr Mr 592571; MRCC 592334; ⌗ (0131) 469 7400; Weather 722334; Marinecall 0891 500452/0839 406189; Police 639111.

FACILITIES
Services: AB £14, El, Ⓔ, CH, ME, ACA.
City EC Wed/Sat; all amenities, ⇌, ✈.

6

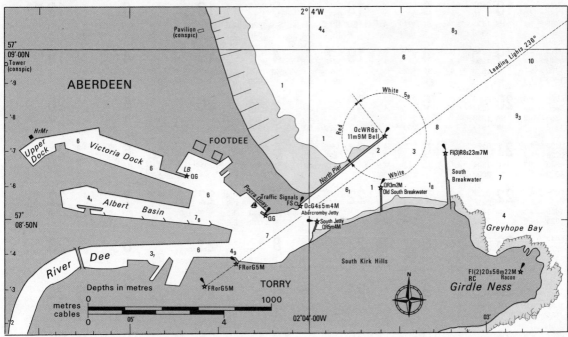

▲ After berthing at Pocra Quay report to HrMr

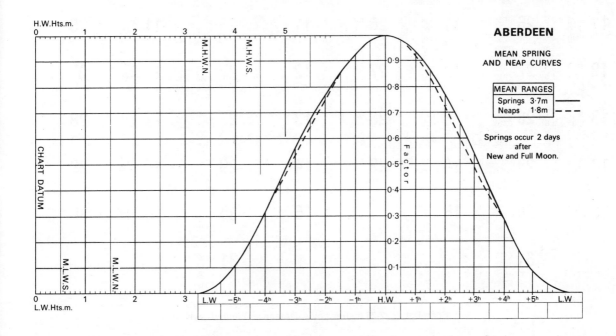

ABERDEEN
MEAN SPRING
AND NEAP CURVES

MEAN RANGES	
Springs	3·7m
Neaps	1·8m

Springs occur 2 days after
New and Full Moon.

SCOTLAND – ABERDEEN

LAT 57°09′N   LONG   2°05′W

TIMES AND HEIGHTS OF HIGH AND LOW WATERS

YEAR **1996**

TIME ZONE (UT)
For Summer Time add ONE hour in non-shaded areas

Chart Datum: 2·25 metres below Ordnance Datum (Newlyn)

JANUARY

No	Day	Time	m	Time	m	Time	m	Time	m	No	Day	Time	m	Time	m	Time	m	Time	m
1	M	0345	1.6	1019	3.7	1615	1.7	2239	3.8	16	TU	0245	1.5	0906	3.7	1515	1.7	2134	3.8
2	TU	0443	1.6	1108	3.9	1711	1.6	2330	3.9	17	W	0358	1.4	1014	3.8	1629	1.4	2245	4.0
3	W	0531	1.5	1151	4.0	1758	1.4			18	TH	0503	1.2	1115	4.1	1733	1.1	2348	4.2
4	TH	0014	4.0	0613	1.4	1229	4.1	1840	1.2	19	F	0558	1.0	1208	4.3	1828	0.8		
5	F O	0054	4.0	0652	1.4	1306	4.2	1918	1.1	20	SA ●	0043	4.4	0646	0.8	1258	4.5	1917	0.5
6	SA	0131	4.1	0726	1.3	1343	4.3	1953	1.0	21	SU	0134	4.5	0732	0.7	1344	4.7	2003	0.3
7	SU	0208	4.1	0757	1.3	1419	4.3	2025	1.0	22	M	0222	4.5	0816	0.6	1428	4.7	2047	0.3
8	M	0244	4.1	0827	1.2	1454	4.3	2058	0.9	23	TU	0308	4.5	0859	0.7	1511	4.7	2131	0.3
9	TU	0320	4.0	0859	1.3	1527	4.2	2133	1.0	24	W	0353	4.4	0943	0.8	1555	4.5	2216	0.5
10	W	0357	4.0	0934	1.3	1601	4.1	2210	1.0	25	TH	0437	4.2	1028	1.0	1640	4.4	2303	0.8
11	TH	0436	3.9	1010	1.4	1640	4.0	2250	1.1	26	F	0524	4.0	1116	1.3	1730	4.1	2353	1.1
12	F	0519	3.8	1049	1.5	1725	3.9	2335	1.3	27	SA	0615	3.7	1210	1.5	1825	3.9		
13	SA	0607	3.7	1135	1.6	1819	3.8			28	SU	0048	1.4	0720	3.6	1315	1.8	1932	3.6
14	SU	0030	1.4	0700	3.6	1237	1.7	1919	3.7	29	M	0153	1.7	0838	3.5	1427	1.9	2103	3.5
15	M	0134	1.5	0759	3.6	1353	1.8	2024	3.7	30	TU	0304	1.8	0941	3.6	1541	1.8	2212	3.6
										31	W	0412	1.8	1037	3.7	1647	1.7	2308	3.7

FEBRUARY

No	Day	Time	m	Time	m	Time	m	Time	m	No	Day	Time	m	Time	m	Time	m	Time	m
1	TH	0508	1.7	1126	3.8	1740	1.5	2355	3.8	16	F	0448	1.3	1055	3.9	1726	1.0	2337	4.0
2	F	0555	1.6	1209	4.0	1823	1.3			17	SA	0545	1.1	1151	4.2	1821	0.7		
3	SA	0036	3.9	0634	1.4	1249	4.2	1901	1.1	18	SU ●	0031	4.3	0634	0.8	1241	4.4	1907	0.4
4	SU O	0114	4.0	0708	1.3	1326	4.2	1934	1.0	19	M	0120	4.4	0718	0.6	1326	4.6	1949	0.2
5	M	0149	4.1	0738	1.2	1401	4.3	2005	0.9	20	TU	0204	4.5	0759	0.5	1408	4.7	2029	0.2
6	TU	0223	4.1	0807	1.1	1434	4.3	2035	0.8	21	W	0246	4.4	0839	0.5	1449	4.6	2108	0.3
7	W	0257	4.1	0839	1.0	1505	4.3	2108	0.8	22	TH	0325	4.3	0919	0.6	1530	4.5	2148	0.5
8	TH	0331	4.1	0911	1.0	1537	4.2	2143	0.8	23	F	0405	4.2	1000	0.8	1613	4.3	2230	0.8
9	F	0408	4.0	0945	1.1	1614	4.1	2219	0.9	24	SA	0446	4.0	1043	1.1	1658	4.1	2315	1.1
10	SA	0449	3.9	1021	1.2	1657	4.0	2259	1.1	25	SU	0530	3.7	1130	1.4	1748	3.8		
11	SU	0534	3.8	1103	1.3	1749	3.9	2349	1.3	26	M	0004	1.5	0620	3.5	1228	1.6	1847	3.5
12	M	0625	3.7	1157	1.5	1850	3.7			27	TU	0104	1.8	0735	3.4	1343	1.8	2022	3.4
13	TU	0054	1.5	0724	3.6	1313	1.6	1957	3.6	28	W	0221	2.0	0900	3.4	1506	1.9	2142	3.4
14	W	0213	1.6	0833	3.6	1447	1.6	2113	3.6	29	TH	0339	2.0	1003	3.5	1619	1.7	2242	3.5
15	TH	0337	1.5	0949	3.7	1615	1.4	2231	3.8										

MARCH

No	Day	Time	m	Time	m	Time	m	Time	m	No	Day	Time	m	Time	m	Time	m	Time	m
1	F	0442	1.8	1057	3.7	1715	1.5	2331	3.7	16	SA	0435	1.3	1037	3.8	1718	0.9	2328	3.9
2	SA	0532	1.5	1144	3.9	1759	1.3			17	SU	0533	1.1	1135	4.1	1809	0.6		
3	SU	0013	3.8	0611	1.4	1226	4.0	1836	1.1	18	M	0020	4.1	0620	0.8	1224	4.3	1852	0.3
4	M	0051	4.0	0644	1.2	1303	4.2	1909	0.9	19	TU ●	0105	4.3	0702	0.6	1307	4.4	1931	0.2
5	TU O	0125	4.1	0715	1.1	1338	4.3	1940	0.7	20	W	0144	4.3	0740	0.5	1347	4.5	2006	0.2
6	W	0158	4.1	0745	0.9	1409	4.3	2011	0.6	21	TH	0221	4.3	0817	0.5	1427	4.5	2042	0.3
7	TH	0231	4.2	0817	0.8	1440	4.3	2043	0.6	22	F	0257	4.2	0855	0.5	1507	4.4	2119	0.5
8	F	0305	4.2	0848	0.8	1515	4.3	2116	0.7	23	SA	0333	4.1	0934	0.7	1548	4.2	2158	0.8
9	SA	0342	4.1	0922	0.8	1553	4.2	2152	0.8	24	SU	0412	3.9	1015	0.9	1631	3.9	2239	1.1
10	SU	0421	4.0	0959	0.9	1638	4.0	2232	1.0	25	M	0453	3.7	1059	1.2	1718	3.7	2324	1.5
11	M	0506	3.8	1043	1.1	1730	3.9	2322	1.2	26	TU	0539	3.5	1152	1.5	1811	3.4		
12	TU	0557	3.7	1137	1.3	1832	3.7			27	W	0018	1.8	0636	3.4	1300	1.7	1930	3.2
13	W	0029	1.5	0658	3.5	1255	1.5	1943	3.5	28	TH	0129	2.0	0811	3.3	1423	1.7	2106	3.2
14	TH	0153	1.6	0812	3.5	1433	1.4	2103	3.5	29	F	0258	2.0	0923	3.4	1541	1.6	2209	3.4
15	F	0321	1.6	0929	3.6	1608	1.2	2224	3.7	30	SA	0407	1.8	1022	3.5	1640	1.4	2300	3.5
										31	SU	0459	1.6	1112	3.7	1726	1.2	2343	3.7

APRIL

No	Day	Time	m	Time	m	Time	m	Time	m	No	Day	Time	m	Time	m	Time	m	Time	m
1	M	0540	1.4	1155	3.9	1804	1.0			16	TU	0005	4.0	0603	0.8	1206	4.1	1832	0.4
2	TU	0021	3.9	0615	1.2	1234	4.0	1838	0.8	17	W ●	0047	4.1	0643	0.7	1248	4.2	1908	0.4
3	W	0056	4.0	0648	1.0	1308	4.2	1912	0.6	18	TH	0122	4.2	0720	0.5	1327	4.3	1941	0.4
4	TH O	0130	4.1	0721	0.8	1342	4.3	1945	0.5	19	F	0155	4.2	0756	0.5	1406	4.2	2016	0.5
5	F	0204	4.2	0754	0.7	1417	4.3	2018	0.5	20	SA	0229	4.1	0833	0.5	1446	4.1	2052	0.7
6	SA	0240	4.2	0828	0.6	1456	4.3	2053	0.6	21	SU	0305	4.0	0912	0.7	1526	4.0	2129	0.9
7	SU	0318	4.1	0904	0.6	1538	4.2	2132	0.7	22	M	0343	3.9	0952	0.8	1608	3.8	2208	1.2
8	M	0359	4.1	0945	0.7	1626	4.0	2216	0.9	23	TU	0423	3.7	1035	1.0	1653	3.6	2250	1.4
9	TU	0445	3.9	1033	0.9	1721	3.8	2310	1.2	24	W	0507	3.6	1124	1.3	1743	3.4	2339	1.7
10	W	0538	3.7	1133	1.1	1825	3.6			25	TH	0559	3.4	1222	1.5	1844	3.2		
11	TH	0018	1.4	0643	3.5	1253	1.2	1936	3.5	26	F	0040	1.9	0707	3.3	1332	1.6	2011	3.2
12	F	0138	1.6	0758	3.5	1422	1.2	2056	3.3	27	SA	0157	1.9	0831	3.3	1447	1.5	2124	3.3
13	SA	0303	1.5	0911	3.6	1555	1.1	2214	3.7	28	SU	0315	1.8	0936	3.4	1552	1.4	2219	3.4
14	SU	0417	1.3	1018	3.7	1701	0.8	2316	3.9	29	M	0413	1.7	1030	3.5	1643	1.2	2305	3.6
15	M	0516	1.1	1117	3.9	1751	0.6			30	TU	0500	1.4	1116	3.7	1726	1.0	2345	3.8

SCOTLAND – ABERDEEN

LAT 57°09′N　LONG 2°05′W

TIMES AND HEIGHTS OF HIGH AND LOW WATERS　　　　YEAR **1996**

TIME ZONE (UT)
For Summer Time add ONE hour in non-shaded areas

Chart Datum: 2·25 metres below Ordnance Datum (Newlyn)

MAY

Day	Time	m	Time	m
1 W	0541 / 1157 / 1805	1.2 / 3.9 / 0.8	**16** TH 0023 / 0623 / 1231 / 1844	4.0 / 0.8 / 4.0 / 0.7
2 TH	0022 / 0619 / 1236 / 1842	4.0 / 0.9 / 4.1 / 0.6	**17** F 0058 / 0701 / 1310 ● / 1918	4.0 / 0.7 / 4.1 / 0.7
3 F O	0100 / 0657 / 1316 / 1920	4.1 / 0.7 / 4.2 / 0.5	**18** SA 0131 / 0738 / 1349 / 1953	4.0 / 0.6 / 4.0 / 0.8
4 SA	0139 / 0734 / 1357 / 1957	4.2 / 0.6 / 4.3 / 0.5	**19** SU 0206 / 0815 / 1428 / 2028	4.0 / 0.6 / 4.0 / 0.9
5 SU	0218 / 0813 / 1441 / 2037	4.2 / 0.5 / 4.3 / 0.5	**20** M 0243 / 0853 / 1508 / 2104	4.0 / 0.7 / 3.9 / 1.0
6 M	0259 / 0854 / 1528 / 2120	4.2 / 0.5 / 4.2 / 0.7	**21** TU 0321 / 0932 / 1550 / 2142	3.9 / 0.8 / 3.7 / 1.2
7 TU	0343 / 0940 / 1620 / 2208	4.1 / 0.5 / 4.0 / 0.9	**22** W 0400 / 1013 / 1632 / 2221	3.8 / 0.9 / 3.6 / 1.3
8 W	0431 / 1033 / 1716 / 2304	3.9 / 0.7 / 3.9 / 1.1	**23** TH 0442 / 1057 / 1718 / 2305	3.7 / 1.1 / 3.4 / 1.5
9 TH	0527 / 1135 / 1818	3.8 / 0.9 / 3.7	**24** F 0529 / 1146 / 1809 / 2356	3.5 / 1.2 / 3.3 / 1.7
10 F	0007 / 0631 / 1245 / 1927	1.3 / 3.6 / 1.0 / 3.6	**25** SA 0623 / 1242 / 1906	3.4 / 1.4 / 3.3
11 SA	0119 / 0740 / 1401 / 2042	1.5 / 3.6 / 1.1 / 3.6	**26** SU 0057 / 0725 / 1343 / 2011	1.8 / 3.3 / 1.4 / 3.3
12 SU	0236 / 0849 / 1528 / 2153	1.5 / 3.6 / 1.0 / 3.6	**27** M 0205 / 0830 / 1447 / 2118	1.8 / 3.4 / 1.4 / 3.4
13 M	0350 / 0956 / 1635 / 2253	1.3 / 3.7 / 0.9 / 3.8	**28** TU 0313 / 0931 / 1549 / 2214	1.7 / 3.5 / 1.2 / 3.5
14 TU	0451 / 1056 / 1726 / 2342	1.2 / 3.8 / 0.7 / 3.9	**29** W 0412 / 1027 / 1643 / 2303	1.5 / 3.6 / 1.1 / 3.7
15 W	0541 / 1147 / 1808	1.0 / 4.0 / 0.7	**30** TH 0503 / 1117 / 1730 / 2348	1.2 / 3.8 / 0.9 / 3.9
			31 F 0550 / 1205 / 1815	1.0 / 4.0 / 0.7

JUNE

Day	Time	m	Time	m
1 SA O	0031 / 0634 / 1253 / 1858	4.1 / 0.7 / 4.2 / 0.6	**16** SU 0111 / 0723 / 1334 / 1934 ●	4.0 / 0.8 / 3.9 / 1.0
2 SU	0116 / 0718 / 1341 / 1941	4.2 / 0.5 / 4.3 / 0.5	**17** M 0147 / 0800 / 1413 / 2009	4.0 / 0.8 / 3.9 / 1.0
3 M	0159 / 0803 / 1429 / 2025	4.3 / 0.4 / 4.3 / 0.5	**18** TU 0225 / 0836 / 1452 / 2043	4.0 / 0.7 / 3.9 / 1.1
4 TU	0244 / 0849 / 1519 / 2111	4.3 / 0.3 / 4.2 / 0.6	**19** W 0303 / 0912 / 1531 / 2118	4.0 / 0.8 / 3.8 / 1.1
5 W	0330 / 0938 / 1611 / 2200	4.2 / 0.4 / 4.1 / 0.8	**20** TH 0341 / 0949 / 1611 / 2155	3.9 / 0.8 / 3.7 / 1.2
6 TH	0419 / 1030 / 1705 / 2252	4.1 / 0.6 / 4.0 / 1.0	**21** F 0419 / 1039 / 1652 / 2235	3.8 / 0.9 / 3.6 / 1.4
7 F	0513 / 1126 / 1804 / 2350	4.0 / 0.6 / 3.8 / 1.2	**22** SA 0500 / 1112 / 1737 / 2319	3.7 / 1.1 / 3.5 / 1.5
8 SA	0613 / 1226 / 1909	3.8 / 0.8 / 3.7	**23** SU 0546 / 1200 / 1826	3.6 / 1.2 / 3.4
9 SU	0053 / 0716 / 1332 / 2018	1.4 / 3.7 / 1.0 / 3.6	**24** M 0009 / 0638 / 1253 / 1919	1.6 / 3.5 / 1.3 / 3.4
10 M	0202 / 0824 / 1446 / 2124	1.4 / 3.7 / 1.1 / 3.6	**25** TU 0109 / 0736 / 1352 / 2017	1.7 / 3.5 / 1.3 / 3.4
11 TU	0313 / 0932 / 1559 / 2222	1.4 / 3.7 / 1.1 / 3.7	**26** W 0216 / 0837 / 1455 / 2120	1.7 / 3.5 / 1.3 / 3.5
12 W	0420 / 1034 / 1656 / 2314	1.3 / 3.7 / 1.1 / 3.8	**27** TH 0324 / 0940 / 1558 / 2221	1.5 / 3.6 / 1.2 / 3.7
13 TH	0516 / 1128 / 1742 / 2358	1.2 / 3.8 / 1.0 / 3.9	**28** F 0427 / 1042 / 1659 / 2316	1.3 / 3.8 / 1.0 / 3.9
14 F	0603 / 1214 / 1821	1.0 / 3.9 / 1.0	**29** SA 0525 / 1141 / 1752	1.0 / 4.0 / 0.8
15 SA	0035 / 0644 / 1255 / 1858	3.9 / 0.9 / 3.9 / 1.0	**30** SU 0007 / 0616 / 1235 / 1840	4.1 / 0.7 / 4.2 / 0.7

JULY

Day	Time	m	Time	m
1 M O	0055 / 0706 / 1326 / 1927	4.3 / 0.5 / 4.3 / 0.5	**16** TU 0130 / 0743 / 1355 / 1950	4.1 / 0.8 / 4.0 / 1.1
2 TU	0142 / 0753 / 1416 / 2012	4.4 / 0.3 / 4.4 / 0.5	**17** W 0207 / 0817 / 1432 / 2021	4.1 / 0.8 / 4.0 / 1.1
3 W	0228 / 0840 / 1505 / 2058	4.4 / 0.2 / 4.4 / 0.5	**18** TH 0244 / 0849 / 1509 / 2054	4.1 / 0.8 / 3.9 / 1.1
4 TH	0314 / 0928 / 1555 / 2145	4.4 / 0.2 / 4.3 / 0.6	**19** F 0319 / 0923 / 1546 / 2129	4.1 / 0.8 / 3.9 / 1.1
5 F	0402 / 1016 / 1646 / 2234	4.3 / 0.3 / 4.1 / 0.8	**20** SA 0353 / 1000 / 1624 / 2206	4.0 / 0.8 / 3.8 / 1.2
6 SA	0452 / 1107 / 1740 / 2326	4.2 / 0.5 / 4.0 / 1.0	**21** SU 0429 / 1039 / 1704 / 2245	3.9 / 0.9 / 3.7 / 1.3
7 SU	0546 / 1201 / 1840	4.0 / 0.8 / 3.8	**22** M 0510 / 1121 / 1750 / 2327	3.8 / 1.1 / 3.6 / 1.4
8 M	0023 / 0645 / 1300 / 1945	1.3 / 3.8 / 1.0 / 3.6	**23** TU 0600 / 1210 / 1840	3.7 / 1.2 / 3.5
9 TU	0128 / 0753 / 1405 / 2050	1.4 / 3.7 / 1.2 / 3.6	**24** W 0020 / 0656 / 1309 / 1935	1.6 / 3.6 / 1.3 / 3.5
10 W	0237 / 0906 / 1517 / 2150	1.5 / 3.6 / 1.4 / 3.6	**25** TH 0131 / 0758 / 1416 / 2038	1.6 / 3.6 / 1.4 / 3.5
11 TH	0348 / 1012 / 1623 / 2245	1.5 / 3.6 / 1.4 / 3.7	**26** F 0248 / 0906 / 1528 / 2146	1.6 / 3.6 / 1.4 / 3.7
12 F	0452 / 1108 / 1716 / 2332	1.4 / 3.7 / 1.4 / 3.8	**27** SA 0401 / 1017 / 1635 / 2250	1.4 / 3.7 / 1.4 / 3.9
13 SA	0544 / 1157 / 1801	1.2 / 3.8 / 1.3	**28** SU 0507 / 1123 / 1733 / 2345	1.1 / 4.0 / 1.0 / 4.1
14 SU	0013 / 0628 / 1239 / 1840	3.9 / 1.1 / 3.9 / 1.2	**29** M 0604 / 1219 / 1825	0.7 / 4.2 / 0.7
15 M	0052 / 0707 / 1318 / 1917 ●	4.0 / 0.9 / 3.9 / 1.2	**30** TU 0036 / 0655 / 1311 / 1911 O	4.3 / 0.4 / 4.4 / 0.6
			31 W 0124 / 0741 / 1400 / 1956	4.5 / 0.2 / 4.5 / 0.5

AUGUST

Day	Time	m	Time	m
1 TH	0209 / 0826 / 1448 / 2041	4.6 / 0.1 / 4.5 / 0.5	**16** F 0221 / 0824 / 1444 / 2030	4.2 / 0.7 / 4.1 / 1.0
2 F	0254 / 0910 / 1534 / 2125	4.6 / 0.1 / 4.4 / 0.5	**17** SA 0254 / 0856 / 1518 / 2103	4.2 / 0.7 / 4.1 / 1.0
3 SA	0338 / 0955 / 1620 / 2211	4.5 / 0.2 / 4.2 / 0.7	**18** SU 0325 / 0931 / 1554 / 2137	4.1 / 0.8 / 4.0 / 1.1
4 SU	0425 / 1042 / 1708 / 2259	4.3 / 0.5 / 4.0 / 1.0	**19** M 0359 / 1006 / 1633 / 2212	4.0 / 0.9 / 3.9 / 1.2
5 M	0514 / 1131 / 1800 / 2352	4.1 / 0.8 / 3.8 / 1.2	**20** TU 0440 / 1044 / 1716 / 2250	3.9 / 1.0 / 3.8 / 1.3
6 TU	0609 / 1225 / 1903	3.9 / 1.2 / 3.6	**21** W 0529 / 1129 / 1805 / 2339	3.8 / 1.2 / 3.7 / 1.5
7 W	0053 / 0717 / 1327 / 2013	1.5 / 3.6 / 1.5 / 3.5	**22** TH 0626 / 1230 / 1901	3.7 / 1.4 / 3.6
8 TH	0203 / 0839 / 1438 / 2117	1.6 / 3.5 / 1.7 / 3.5	**23** F 0053 / 0730 / 1347 / 2006	1.6 / 3.6 / 1.5 / 3.5
9 F	0317 / 0949 / 1551 / 2215	1.7 / 3.5 / 1.7 / 3.6	**24** SA 0224 / 0843 / 1506 / 2120	1.6 / 3.6 / 1.5 / 3.6
10 SA	0428 / 1048 / 1651 / 2306	1.6 / 3.6 / 1.6 / 3.7	**25** SU 0345 / 1002 / 1618 / 2228	1.4 / 3.7 / 1.3 / 3.9
11 SU	0524 / 1138 / 1740 / 2351	1.4 / 3.7 / 1.5 / 3.9	**26** M 0456 / 1110 / 1718 / 2326	1.0 / 3.9 / 1.1 / 4.1
12 M	0609 / 1220 / 1821	1.2 / 3.8 / 1.4	**27** TU 0554 / 1206 / 1809	0.7 / 4.2 / 0.8
13 TU	0031 / 0647 / 1258 / 1856	4.0 / 1.0 / 3.9 / 1.2	**28** W 0017 / 0642 / 1256 / 1855 O	4.4 / 0.4 / 4.4 / 0.6
14 W	0110 / 0722 / 1334 / 1928 ●	4.1 / 0.9 / 4.0 / 1.1	**29** TH 0104 / 0726 / 1342 / 1938	4.6 / 0.2 / 4.5 / 0.5
15 TH	0147 / 0753 / 1410 / 1958	4.2 / 0.8 / 4.1 / 1.0	**30** F 0148 / 0807 / 1426 / 2020	4.7 / 0.1 / 4.5 / 0.5
			31 SA 0230 / 0848 / 1508 / 2101	4.7 / 0.1 / 4.4 / 0.5

6

SCOTLAND – ABERDEEN

LAT 57°09′N   LONG 2°05′W

TIMES AND HEIGHTS OF HIGH AND LOW WATERS

YEAR 1996

TIME ZONE (UT)
For Summer Time add ONE hour in non-shaded areas

SEPTEMBER

Day	Time	m	Day	Time	m
1 SU	0313 / 0929 / 1549 / 2144	4.6 / 0.3 / 4.3 / 0.7	16 M	0258 / 0901 / 1525 / 2110	4.2 / 0.7 / 4.1 / 1.0
2 M	0356 / 1012 / 1631 / 2230	4.4 / 0.6 / 4.1 / 0.9	17 TU	0334 / 0934 / 1603 / 2144	4.2 / 0.9 / 4.0 / 1.1
3 TU	0442 / 1058 / 1716 / 2320	4.1 / 1.0 / 3.8 / 1.2	18 W	0416 / 1009 / 1646 / 2223	4.0 / 1.0 / 3.9 / 1.2
4 W	0533 / 1148 / 1809	3.8 / 1.3 / 3.6	19 TH	0507 / 1054 / 1736 / 2314	3.9 / 1.3 / 3.7 / 1.4
5 TH	0018 / 0636 / 1248 / 1925	1.5 / 3.6 / 1.7 / 3.5	20 F	0606 / 1159 / 1834	3.7 / 1.5 / 3.6
6 F	0129 / 0808 / 1401 / 2040	1.7 / 3.4 / 1.9 / 3.5	21 SA	0034 / 0713 / 1325 / 1942	1.5 / 3.6 / 1.7 / 3.6
7 SA	0246 / 0922 / 1518 / 2142	1.8 / 3.4 / 1.9 / 3.6	22 SU	0208 / 0830 / 1448 / 2059	1.5 / 3.6 / 1.6 / 3.6
8 SU	0400 / 1023 / 1623 / 2237	1.6 / 3.5 / 1.8 / 3.7	23 M	0334 / 0952 / 1603 / 2208	1.3 / 3.7 / 1.4 / 3.9
9 M	0458 / 1113 / 1715 / 2325	1.5 / 3.7 / 1.6 / 3.9	24 TU	0446 / 1058 / 1703 / 2307	1.0 / 4.0 / 1.2 / 4.1
10 TU	0543 / 1156 / 1756	1.2 / 3.8 / 1.4	25 W	0541 / 1152 / 1753 / 2358	0.7 / 4.2 / 0.9 / 4.3
11 W	0007 / 0620 / 1234 / 1830	4.1 / 1.0 / 4.0 / 1.3	26 TH	0627 / 1239 / 1837	0.4 / 4.4 / 0.7
12 TH ●	0046 / 0654 / 1310 / 1902	4.2 / 0.9 / 4.1 / 1.1	27 F O	0044 / 0707 / 1322 / 1917	4.5 / 0.3 / 4.5 / 0.5
13 F	0122 / 0726 / 1344 / 1933	4.3 / 0.8 / 4.2 / 1.0	28 SA	0126 / 0744 / 1401 / 1957	4.6 / 0.2 / 4.5 / 0.5
14 SA	0155 / 0757 / 1416 / 2005	4.3 / 0.7 / 4.2 / 0.9	29 SU	0207 / 0821 / 1439 / 2037	4.6 / 0.3 / 4.4 / 0.6
15 SU	0226 / 0829 / 1449 / 2037	4.3 / 0.7 / 4.2 / 0.9	30 M	0248 / 0900 / 1516 / 2118	4.5 / 0.5 / 4.3 / 0.7

OCTOBER

Day	Time	m	Day	Time	m
1 TU	0330 / 0941 / 1555 / 2202	4.3 / 0.8 / 4.1 / 0.9	16 W	0316 / 0907 / 1538 / 2124	4.2 / 0.9 / 4.2 / 0.9
2 W	0414 / 1023 / 1637 / 2250	4.1 / 1.1 / 3.9 / 1.2	17 TH	0401 / 0947 / 1621 / 2208	4.1 / 1.1 / 4.0 / 1.1
3 TH	0502 / 1111 / 1724 / 2346	3.8 / 1.5 / 3.7 / 1.5	18 F	0454 / 1036 / 1711 / 2305	3.9 / 1.3 / 3.8 / 1.3
4 F	0558 / 1206 / 1825	3.5 / 1.8 / 3.5	19 SA	0554 / 1144 / 1812	3.7 / 1.6 / 3.7
5 SA	0054 / 0726 / 1319 / 1955	1.7 / 3.3 / 2.0 / 3.5	20 SU	0026 / 0702 / 1306 / 1923	1.4 / 3.6 / 1.7 / 3.6
6 SU	0210 / 0848 / 1440 / 2104	1.8 / 3.4 / 2.1 / 3.5	21 M	0152 / 0820 / 1428 / 2037	1.4 / 3.6 / 1.7 / 3.7
7 M	0323 / 0951 / 1549 / 2203	1.7 / 3.5 / 1.9 / 3.7	22 TU	0317 / 0939 / 1543 / 2146	1.2 / 3.7 / 1.5 / 3.9
8 TU	0422 / 1043 / 1642 / 2254	1.5 / 3.7 / 1.7 / 3.9	23 W	0428 / 1043 / 1644 / 2247	1.0 / 4.0 / 1.3 / 4.1
9 W	0509 / 1126 / 1724 / 2338	1.3 / 3.8 / 1.5 / 4.0	24 TH	0522 / 1134 / 1734 / 2339	0.8 / 4.2 / 1.0 / 4.3
10 TH	0549 / 1205 / 1800	1.1 / 4.0 / 1.3	25 F	0606 / 1220 / 1818	0.6 / 4.3 / 0.8
11 F	0018 / 0623 / 1241 / 1834	4.2 / 0.9 / 4.2 / 1.1	26 SA O	0025 / 0645 / 1300 / 1857	4.4 / 0.5 / 4.4 / 0.7
12 SA ●	0055 / 0657 / 1315 / 1907	4.3 / 0.8 / 4.3 / 1.0	27 SU	0107 / 0720 / 1336 / 1935	4.5 / 0.5 / 4.5 / 0.6
13 SU	0127 / 0729 / 1348 / 1940	4.3 / 0.7 / 4.3 / 0.9	28 M	0147 / 0756 / 1411 / 2014	4.5 / 0.6 / 4.4 / 0.6
14 M	0200 / 0801 / 1422 / 2013	4.3 / 0.7 / 4.3 / 0.8	29 TU	0227 / 0833 / 1447 / 2055	4.4 / 0.8 / 4.3 / 0.8
15 TU	0236 / 0833 / 1459 / 2046	4.3 / 0.8 / 4.3 / 0.9	30 W	0307 / 0912 / 1525 / 2138	4.2 / 1.0 / 4.2 / 0.9
			31 TH	0350 / 0952 / 1605 / 2224	4.0 / 1.3 / 4.0 / 1.2

NOVEMBER

Day	Time	m	Day	Time	m
1 F	0436 / 1035 / 1650 / 2316	3.8 / 1.6 / 3.8 / 1.4	16 SA	0445 / 1028 / 1653 / 2304	4.0 / 1.3 / 4.0 / 1.1
2 SA	0526 / 1124 / 1741	3.6 / 1.8 / 3.6	17 SU	0543 / 1131 / 1754	3.9 / 1.5 / 3.9
3 SU	0017 / 0628 / 1229 / 1850	1.6 / 3.4 / 2.0 / 3.5	18 M	0013 / 0648 / 1243 / 1901	1.2 / 3.7 / 1.7 / 3.8
4 M	0125 / 0758 / 1348 / 2014	1.7 / 3.4 / 2.1 / 3.5	19 TU	0127 / 0802 / 1359 / 2012	1.3 / 3.7 / 1.7 / 3.8
5 TU	0235 / 0908 / 1501 / 2120	1.7 / 3.4 / 2.0 / 3.6	20 W	0246 / 0917 / 1513 / 2122	1.2 / 3.8 / 1.6 / 3.8
6 W	0337 / 1004 / 1559 / 2216	1.6 / 3.6 / 1.9 / 3.7	21 TH	0400 / 1020 / 1618 / 2226	1.1 / 3.9 / 1.4 / 4.0
7 TH	0429 / 1051 / 1646 / 2304	1.4 / 3.8 / 1.7 / 3.9	22 F	0457 / 1114 / 1712 / 2322	1.0 / 4.1 / 1.2 / 4.1
8 F	0512 / 1132 / 1726 / 2346	1.2 / 4.0 / 1.4 / 4.1	23 SA	0543 / 1159 / 1758	0.9 / 4.2 / 1.0
9 SA	0551 / 1209 / 1804	1.1 / 4.1 / 1.2	24 SU	0009 / 0622 / 1238 / 1839	4.2 / 0.8 / 4.3 / 0.9
10 SU	0023 / 0627 / 1245 / 1841	4.2 / 0.9 / 4.3 / 1.0	25 M O	0051 / 0658 / 1313 / 1918	4.3 / 0.9 / 4.3 / 0.8
11 M ●	0100 / 0703 / 1321 / 1918	4.3 / 0.8 / 4.4 / 0.9	26 TU	0131 / 0734 / 1348 / 1957	4.3 / 0.9 / 4.3 / 0.8
12 TU	0138 / 0738 / 1358 / 1954	4.4 / 0.8 / 4.4 / 0.8	27 W	0211 / 0811 / 1424 / 2037	4.2 / 1.0 / 4.3 / 0.8
13 W	0219 / 0814 / 1437 / 2032	4.4 / 0.8 / 4.4 / 0.8	28 TH	0250 / 0848 / 1502 / 2118	4.1 / 1.2 / 4.2 / 0.9
14 TH	0303 / 0852 / 1518 / 2114	4.3 / 0.9 / 4.3 / 0.8	29 F	0331 / 0924 / 1541 / 2200	4.0 / 1.3 / 4.1 / 1.1
15 F	0351 / 0936 / 1603 / 2204	4.2 / 1.1 / 4.2 / 0.9	30 SA	0414 / 1002 / 1623 / 2245	3.8 / 1.5 / 4.0 / 1.3

DECEMBER

Day	Time	m	Day	Time	m
1 SU	0459 / 1043 / 1709 / 2335	3.7 / 1.7 / 3.8 / 1.4	16 M	0527 / 1113 / 1733 / 2353	4.0 / 1.3 / 4.1 / 1.0
2 M	0548 / 1132 / 1801	3.6 / 1.9 / 3.7	17 TU	0626 / 1215 / 1834	3.9 / 1.5 / 3.9
3 TU	0031 / 0643 / 1235 / 1901	1.6 / 3.5 / 2.0 / 3.6	18 W	0057 / 0734 / 1323 / 1941	1.2 / 3.8 / 1.7 / 3.8
4 W	0133 / 0749 / 1348 / 2009	1.6 / 3.5 / 2.1 / 3.6	19 TH	0207 / 0847 / 1436 / 2054	1.3 / 3.8 / 1.7 / 3.8
5 TH	0237 / 0903 / 1459 / 2117	1.6 / 3.5 / 2.0 / 3.6	20 F	0321 / 0952 / 1546 / 2205	1.3 / 3.8 / 1.6 / 3.9
6 F	0337 / 1002 / 1558 / 2216	1.5 / 3.7 / 1.8 / 3.8	21 SA	0427 / 1048 / 1649 / 2305	1.3 / 3.9 / 1.4 / 4.0
7 SA	0429 / 1050 / 1648 / 2306	1.4 / 3.9 / 1.6 / 3.9	22 SU	0519 / 1137 / 1741 / 2356	1.2 / 4.0 / 1.3 / 4.1
8 SU	0515 / 1133 / 1734 / 2351	1.2 / 4.1 / 1.3 / 4.1	23 M	0602 / 1218 / 1826	1.2 / 4.1 / 1.1
9 M	0558 / 1215 / 1817	1.1 / 4.2 / 1.1	24 TU O	0039 / 0641 / 1255 / 1906	4.1 / 1.2 / 4.2 / 1.0
10 TU ●	0035 / 0639 / 1257 / 1859	4.3 / 1.0 / 4.4 / 0.9	25 W	0119 / 0718 / 1330 / 1944	4.2 / 1.2 / 4.3 / 0.9
11 W	0120 / 0719 / 1338 / 1941	4.4 / 0.9 / 4.5 / 0.7	26 TH	0157 / 0754 / 1407 / 2022	4.1 / 1.2 / 4.3 / 0.9
12 TH	0206 / 0801 / 1420 / 2025	4.4 / 0.8 / 4.5 / 0.6	27 F	0235 / 0828 / 1444 / 2059	4.1 / 1.2 / 4.3 / 0.9
13 F	0252 / 0843 / 1502 / 2110	4.4 / 0.9 / 4.5 / 0.6	28 SA	0313 / 0900 / 1522 / 2136	4.2 / 1.3 / 4.2 / 1.0
14 SA	0341 / 0929 / 1548 / 2200	4.3 / 1.0 / 4.4 / 0.7	29 SU	0352 / 0934 / 1600 / 2213	3.9 / 1.4 / 4.1 / 1.1
15 SU	0432 / 1018 / 1637 / 2254	4.2 / 1.2 / 4.3 / 0.8	30 M	0432 / 1010 / 1639 / 2254	3.8 / 1.5 / 4.0 / 1.2
			31 TU	0514 / 1050 / 1723 / 2338	3.7 / 1.6 / 3.8 / 1.4

Chart Datum: 2·25 metres below Ordnance Datum (Newlyn)

PETERHEAD
10-6-18
Aberdeen 57°29'·83N 01°46'·31W

CHARTS
AC 1438, 213; OS 30
TIDES
+0140 Dover; ML 2·3; Duration 0620; Zone 0 (UT)

Standard Port ABERDEEN (←)

Times				Height (metres)			
High Water		Low Water		MHWS	MHWN	MLWN	MLWS
0000	0600	0100	0700	4·3	3·4	1·6	0·6
1200	1800	1300	1900				
Differences PETERHEAD							
–0035	–0045	–0035	–0040	–0·5	–0·3	–0·1	–0·1

SHELTER
Good in marina (2·3m). A useful passage hbr, also a major fishing and oil/gas industry port. Access any weather/tide.
NAVIGATION
WPT 57°29'·46N 01°45'·64W, 134°/314° from/to ent, 0·5M. No dangers. 5kn speed limit in Bay; 4kn in marina. Chan between marina bkwtr and ECM lt buoy is <30m wide.
LIGHTS AND MARKS
Power stn chy (183m) is conspic 1·25M S of ent. Ldg lts 314°, both FR 13/17m 8M (H24); front △, rear ▽ on Y cols. Marina bkwtr has Fl R 3s 6m 2M on 2·5m high ⚓ symbol.

Unless already cleared on VHF, the following tfc sigs (all Hor) from Control tr above Hr Mr office must be obeyed:
3 Fl Ⓡ = No entry to Bay Hbr from sea.
2 Fl Ⓡ = No exit Bay Hbr to sea.
4 Fl Ⓡ = Bay Hbr closed; no traffic movement.
3F Ⓡ = No entry to fishing hbr from Bay Hbr.
2F Ⓡ = No exit from fishing hbr to Bay Hbr.
RADIO TELEPHONE
Call *Peterhead Hbr Radio* VHF Ch **14** 9 16 for ent/dep.
TELEPHONE (01779)
Hr Mr (Hbr Trust) 474281; Hr Mr (Bay Authority) 474020; MRCC (01224) 592334; ⌖ (0131) 469 7400; Marinecall 0891 500452; Police 472571; Dr 474841; Ⓗ 472316.
FACILITIES
Marina ☎ via 474020 (HO)/Fax 475712, 90 berths, access all tides, 2·3m at ent, AC, FW, V and Ⓒ at caravan site; **Peterhead SC** ☎ (011358) 751340 (Sec'y).
Services: D available in S Hbr, Slip, ME, El, Ⓔ, Sh, C, Gas.
Town EC Wed; P, D, V, R, ✉, bus to Aberdeen for ⇌ & ✈.

ADJACENT HARBOUR

BODDAM, Aberdeen, 57°28'·38N 01°46'·30W. AC 213. HW +0145 on Dover; Tides as 10.6.18. Good shelter, in the lee of Meikle Mackie, the island just N of Buchan Ness, Fl 5s 40m 28M Horn (3) 60s. Hbr dries/unlit. Beware rks around Meikle Mackie and to the SW of it. Appr from 1½ca NW of The Skerry. Yachts lie along N wall. All facilities at Peterhead, 4 miles N.

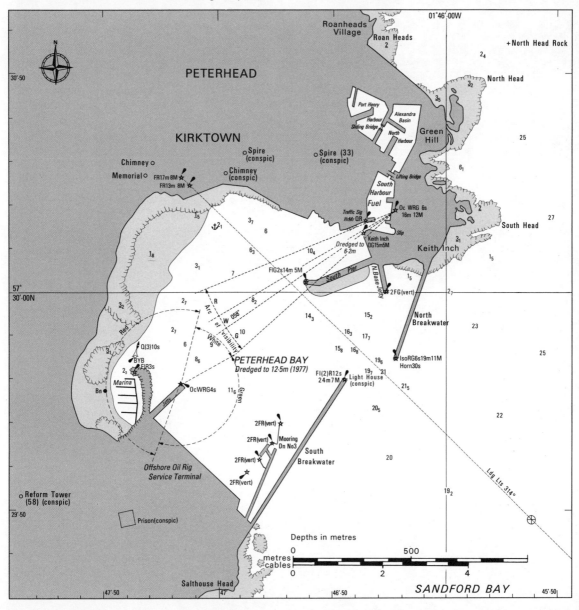

Volvo Penta service

Sales and service centres in area 7
HIGHLANDS AND ISLANDS Caley Marina, Canal Road, Muirtown, Inverness
1V3 6NF Tel (01463) 236539

Area 7

North-East Scotland
Rattray Head to Cape Wrath
including Orkney and Shetland Islands

7

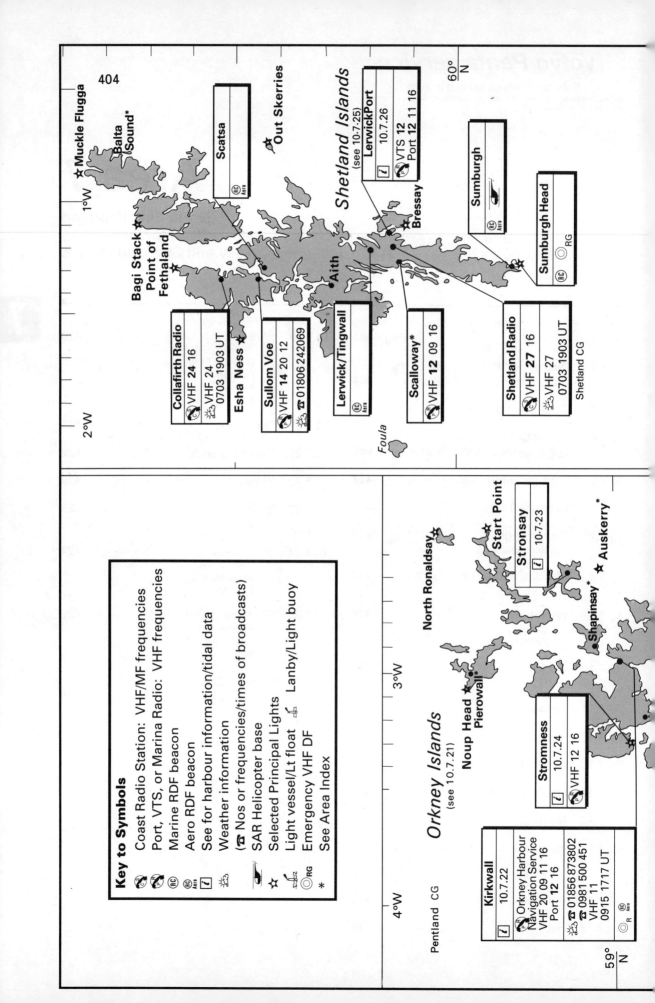

Key to Symbols

📻 Coast Radio Station: VHF/MF frequencies
📻 Port, VTS, or Marina Radio: VHF frequencies
Ⓡ Marine RDF beacon
Ⓡ Aero RDF beacon
ℹ See for harbour information/tidal data
📡 Weather information
(☎ Nos or frequencies/times of broadcasts)
✈ SAR Helicopter base
★ Selected Principal Lights
⛴ Light vessel/Lt float   Lanby/Light buoy
◎RG Emergency VHF DF
✶ See Area Index

★ Muckle Flugga

Balta Sound*

1°W

Scatsa

Ⓡ Aero

✶ Out Skerries

Shetland Islands
(see 10·7·25)

60°
N

LerwickPort   10.7.26
| ℹ | 📻 VTS **12** |
| | Port **12** 11 16 |

Bagi Stack ★
Point of
Fethaland ★

2°W

Esha Ness ★

Aith ★

★ Bressay

Sumburgh

Ⓡ Aero

Collafirth Radio
| 📻 VHF **24** 16 |
| 📡 VHF 24 |
| 0703 1903 UT |

Sumburgh Head

◎RG

Ⓡ Aero

Sullom Voe
| 📻 VHF **14** 20 12 |
| 📡 ☎ 01806 242069 |

Lerwick/Tingwall

Ⓡ Aero

Scalloway*
| 📻 VHF **12** 09 16 |

Shetland Radio
| 📻 VHF **27** 16 |
| 📡 VHF 27 |
| 0703 1903 UT |
| Shetland CG |

Foula

North Ronaldsay ★

Start Point

Stronsay   10.7.23
| ℹ |

★ Auskerry*

Shapinsay*

Orkney Islands
(see 10.7.21)

Noup Head ★
Pierowall*

3°W

Stromness   10.7.24
| ℹ | 📻 VHF **12** 16 |

Kirkwall   10.7.22
| ℹ |
| 📻 Orkney Harbour |
| Navigation Service |
| VHF 20 09 11 16 |
| Port **12** 16 |
| 📡 ☎ 01856 873802 |
| ☎ 0981 500 451 |
| VHF 11 |
| 0915 1717 UT |

◎R

Ⓡ Aero

Pentland CG

4°W

59°
N

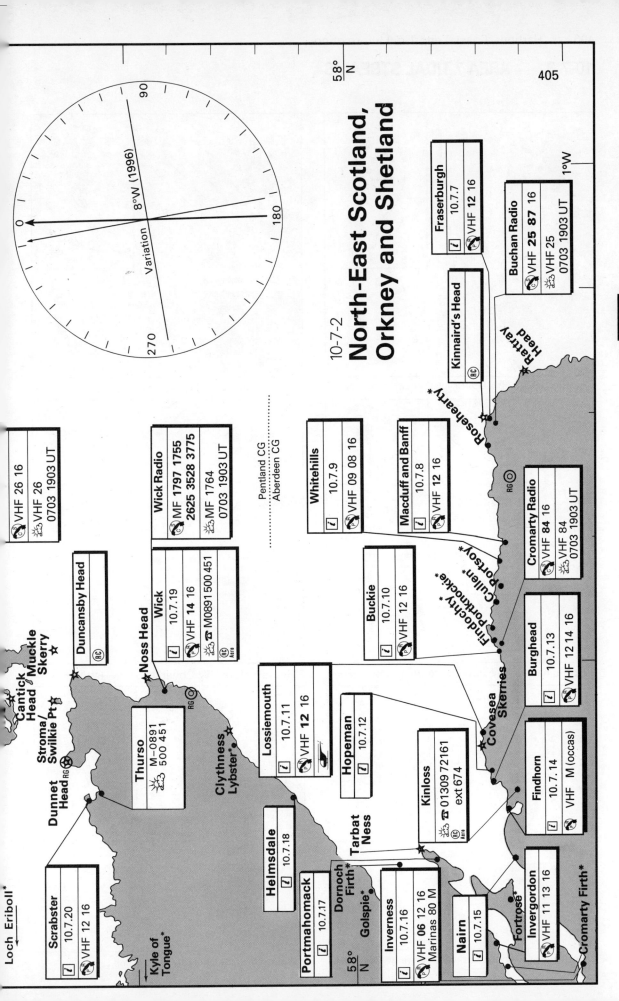

10-7-2
North-East Scotland, Orkney and Shetland

58°N

1°W

Fraserburgh
ℹ 10.7.7
📻 VHF 12 16

Buchan Radio
📻 VHF **25 87** 16
🌦 VHF 25
0703 1903 UT

Kinnaird's Head
Ⓡⓒ

Rattray Head

Rosehearty*

Whitehills
ℹ 10.7.9
📻 VHF 09 08 16

Macduff and Banff
ℹ 10.7.8
📻 VHF 12 16

Wick Radio
📻 MF 1797 1755
2625 3528 3775
🌦 MF 1764
0703 1903 UT

Pentland CG
Aberdeen CG

Duncansby Head
Ⓡⓒ

Wick
ℹ 10.7.19
📻 VHF 14 16
☎ M0891 500 451
Ⓡⓒ Auto

Noss Head

Buckie
ℹ 10.7.10
📻 VHF 12 16

Portsoy*
Cullen*
Findochty*
Portknockie*

Cromarty Radio
📻 VHF **84** 16
🌦 VHF 84
0703 1903 UT

RG ◎

VHF 26 16
🌦 VHF 26
0703 1903 UT

Cantick
Head / Muckle
Skerry ☆

Stroma /
Swilkie Pt ☆

Dunnet
Head RG

Thurso
☎ M–0891
500 451

Clythness
Lybster*

Lossiemouth
ℹ 10.7.11
📻 VHF **12** 16

Hopeman
ℹ 10.7.12

Covesea
Skerries

Burghead
ℹ 10.7.13
📻 VHF 12 14 16

Loch Eriboll*

Scrabster
ℹ 10.7.20
📻 VHF 12 16

Kyle of
Tongue*

Helmsdale
ℹ 10.7.18

Tarbat
Ness

Kinloss
☎ 01309 72161
ext 674
🌦 Ⓡⓒ Auto

Findhorn
ℹ 10.7.14
🌦 VHF M (occas)

58°N

Portmahomack
ℹ 10.7.17

Dornoch
Firth*

Golspie*

Inverness
ℹ 10.7.16
📻 VHF **06** 12 16
Marinas 80 M

Nairn
ℹ 10.7.15

Fortrose*

Invergordon
📻 VHF 11 13 16

Cromarty Firth*

8°W (1996)

Variation

90

180

270

0

10-7-3   AREA 7 TIDAL STREAMS

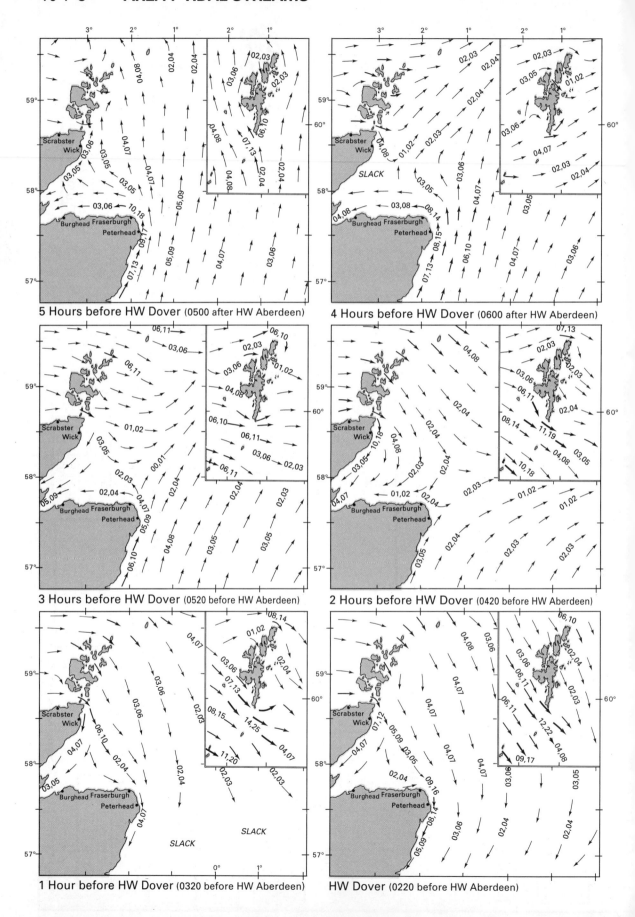

5 Hours before HW Dover (0500 after HW Aberdeen)

4 Hours before HW Dover (0600 after HW Aberdeen)

3 Hours before HW Dover (0520 before HW Aberdeen)

2 Hours before HW Dover (0420 before HW Aberdeen)

1 Hour before HW Dover (0320 before HW Aberdeen)

HW Dover (0220 before HW Aberdeen)

Southward 10.6.3   Westward 10.8.3

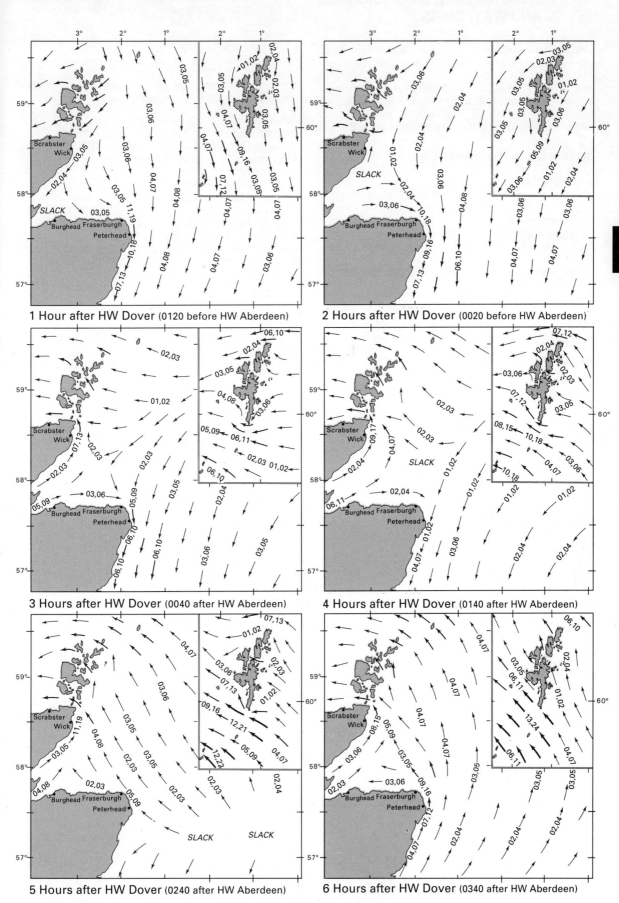

1 Hour after HW Dover (0120 before HW Aberdeen)

2 Hours after HW Dover (0020 before HW Aberdeen)

3 Hours after HW Dover (0040 after HW Aberdeen)

4 Hours after HW Dover (0140 after HW Aberdeen)

5 Hours after HW Dover (0240 after HW Aberdeen)

6 Hours after HW Dover (0340 after HW Aberdeen)

10.7.4 COASTAL LIGHTS, FOG SIGNALS AND WAYPOINTS

Abbreviations used below are given in 1.4.1. Principal lights are in **bold** print, places in CAPITALS, and light-vessels, light floats and Lanbys in *CAPITAL ITALICS*. Unless otherwise stated lights are white. m – elevation in metres; M – nominal range in miles. Fog signals are in *italics*. Useful waypoints are underlined – use those on land with care. All geographical positions should be assumed to be approximate. See 4.4.1.

RATTRAY HEAD TO INVERNESS

FRASERBURGH
Cairnbulg Briggs 57°41'·12N 01°56'·35W Fl (2) 10s 6M; Bn.
Ldg Lt 291°. 57°41'·58N 02°00'·03W QR 12m 5M. Rear, 75 from front, Oc R 6s 17m 5M.
Balaclava Bkwtr Hd 57°41'·53N 01°59'·63W Fl (2) G 8s 26m 6M; dome on W Tr; vis 178°-326°; *Siren 20s* (fishing).

Kinnaird Hd 57°41'·87N 02°00'·15W Fl 5s 25m **22M**; vis 092°-297°; W Tr; RC.
Bombing range Lt By 57°43'·80N 02°00'·75W Fl Y 5s; SPM.
Target float 57°42'·00N 02°10'·00W Fl Y 10s; bombing target; Ra refl.
Traget float 57°43'·33N 02°07'·25W Fl Y 3s.

MACDUFF/BANFF/WHITEHILLS
Macduff Lt Ho Pier Hd 57°40'·26N 02°29'·90W Fl (2) WRG 6s 12m W9M, R7M; W Tr; vis G shore-115°, W115°-174°, R174°-210°; *Horn (2) 20s* .
Macduff W Pier Hd 57°40'·23N 02°29'·88W QG 4m 5M.
Whitehills Pier Hd 57°40'·82N 02°34'·75W Fl WR 3s 7m W9M, R6M; W Tr; vis R132°-212°, W212°-245°.

PORTSOY
Pier Ldg Lts 160°. Front 57°41'·18N 02°41'·30W F 12m 5M; Tr. Rear FR 17m 5M; mast.

BUCKIE
West Muck 57°41'·07N 02°57'·93W QR 5m 7M; tripod.
NW Pier Hd 57°40'·85N 02°57'·62W 2 FR (vert) 7m 11M; R col. (3 FR when Hbr closed).
Ldg Lts 125°. **Front** 57°40'·85N 02°57'·56W Oc R 10s 15m **15M**; W Tr; *Siren (2) 60s*. **Rear**, 365m from front, Iso WG 2s 30m **W16M**, G12M; vis G090°-110°, W110°-225°.
W Pier, NW corner 2 FG (vert) 4m 9M; G col.

LOSSIEMOUTH
S Pier Hd 57°43'·44N 03°16'·59W Fl R 6s 11m 5M; *Siren 60s*.

Covesea Skerries 57°43'·50N 03°20'·30W Fl WR 20s 49m **W24M, R20M**; W Tr; vis W076°-267°, R267°-282°.

HOPEMAN
W Pier Hd 57°42'·71N 03°26'·20W Oc G 4s 8m 4M shown 1/8-30/4.
Ldg Lts 081°. Front 57°42'·73N 03°26'·09W FR 3m. Rear, 10m from front, FR 4m. Shown 1/8-30/4.

BURGHEAD/FINDHORN
Burghead N Bkwtr Hd 57°42'·10N 03°29'·94W Oc 8s 7m 5M.
Burghead Spur 57°42'·11N 03°29'·94W Hd QR 3m 5M; vis from SW only.
Findhorn By 57°40'·40N 03°37'·65W; SWM.

NAIRN
W Pier Hd 57°35'·62N 03°51'·56W QG 5m 1M; Gy post.
E Pier Hd Oc WRG 4s 6m 5M; 8-sided Tr; vis G shore-100°, W100°-207°, R207°-shore.

Whiteness Hd, McDermott Base Dir Lt 142·5° 57°35'·88N 04°00'·15W Dir Iso WRG 4s 6m 10M; vis G138°-141°, W141°-144°, R144°-147°. (TE 1990).

INVERNESS FIRTH
Riff Bank E Lt By 57°38'·40N 03°58'·07W Fl Y 10s; SPM.
Navity Bank Lt By 57°38'·18N 04°01'·10W Fl (3) G 15s; SHM.
Riff Bank N Lt By 57°37'·25N 04°02'·65W Fl (2) R 12s; PHM.
Riff Bank W Lt By 57°35'·80N 04°03'·95W Fl Y 5s; SPM.

South Channel
Riff Bank S Lt By 57°36'·75N 04°00'·87W Q (6) + LFl 15s; SCM.
Craigmee Lt By 57°35'·32N 04°04'·90W Fl R 6s; PHM.
Chanonry 57°34'·46N 04°05'·48W Oc 6s 12m **15M**; W Tr; vis 148°-073°.
Avoch 57°34'·04N 04°09'·82W 2 FR (vert) 7/5m 5M; (occas).
Munlochy Lt By 57°32'·93N 04°07'·55W L Fl 10s; SWM.
Meikle Mee Lt By 57°30'·27N 04°11'·94W Fl G 3s; SHM.
Longman Pt 57°30'·02N 04°13'·22W Fl WR 2s 7m W5M, R4M; R ▲ Bn; vis W078°-258°, R258°-078°.
Craigton Pt 57°30'·07N 04°14'·01W Fl WRG 4s 6m W11M, R7M, G7M; vis W312°-048°, R048°-064°, W064°-085°, G085°-shore.
Kessock Bridge. N Trs Oc G 6s 28m 5M and QG 3m 3M; S Trs Oc R 6s 28m 5M and QR 3m 3M.

INVERNESS
R. Ness Outer Bn 57°29'·84N 04°13'·85W QR 3m 4M.
Inner Bn 57°29'·73N 04°14'·02W QR 3m 4M.
Embankment Hd Fl G 2s 8m 4M; G framework Tr.
E side Fl R 3s 7m 6M.

CALEDONIAN CANAL
Clachnaharry, S training wall Hd 57°29'·44N 04°15'·78W Iso G 4s 5m 2M; W △ on W mast; tfc signals.
N Training Wall Hd QR 5m 2M.

INVERNESS TO DUNCANSBY HEAD

CROMARTY FIRTH/INVERGORDON
Fairway Lt By 57°39'·98N 03°54'·10W L Fl 10s; SWM; Racon.
Cromarty Bank Lt By 57°40'·68N 03°56'·69W Fl (2) G 10s; SHM.
Buss Bank Lt By 57°41'·00N 03°59'·45W Fl R 3s; PHM.
The Ness 57°40'·99N 04°02'·10W Oc WR 10s 18m **W15M**, R11M; W Tr; vis R079°-088°, W088°-275°, obsc by N Sutor when brg less than 253°.
Nigg Ferry Jetty, SE corner, 2 FG (vert) 6m 2M.
SW corner 2 FG (vert) 6m 2M.
Nigg Oil Terminal Pier Hd 57°41'·57N 04°02'·51W Oc G 5s 31m 5M; Gy Tr, floodlit.
E and W ends marked by 2 FG (vert) 9 4M.
Nigg Sands E Lt By 57°41'·62N 04°04'·25W Fl (2) G 10s; SHM.
Nigg Sands W Lt By 57°41'·29N 04°07'·15W Fl G 3s; SHM.
British Alcan Pier Hd 57°41'·30N 04°08'·27W QG 17m 5M.
Dockyard Pier Hd 57°41'·17N 04°09'·64W Fl (3) G 10s 15m 4M.
Supply Base SE corner Iso G 4s 9m 6M; Gy mast.
Quay, W end Oc G 8s 9m 6M; Gy mast.
Queen's Dock W Arm Iso G 2s 9m 6M.
Three Kings Lt By 57°43'·75N 03°54'·17W Q (3) 10s; ECM.
Tarbat Ledge/Culloden Rk By 57°52'·45N 03°45'·45W; PHM.
Lt By 57°53'·00N 03°47'·00W Fl Y 5s; SPM.

DORNOCH FIRTH/TAIN
Tarbat Ness 57°51'·92N 03°46'·52W Fl (4) 30s 53m **24M**; W Tr, R bands; Racon.
Firing range 57°49'·45N 03°57'·50W Fl R 5s, when firing occurs.
Target float 57°51'·59N 03°52'·46W Fl Y 5s.

HELMSDALE/LYBSTER

Ben-a-chielt 58°19'·80N 03°22'·20W Aero 5 FR (vert) 448-265m; radio mast.

Lybster, S Pier Hd 58°17'·80N 03°17'·25W Oc R 6s 10m 3M; W Tr; occas.

Clythness 58°18'·70N 03°12'·50W Fl (2) 30s 45m **16M**; W Tr, R band.

WICK

S Pier Hd 58°26'·36N 03°04'·65W Fl WRG 3s 12m W5M, R3M, G3M; W 8-sided Tr; vis G253°-269°, W269°-286°, R286°-329°; *Bell (2) 10s* (occas).

Dir Lt 288·5° 58°26'·56N 03°05'·26W Dir F WRG 9m W10M, R7M, G7M; col on N end of bridge; vis G283·5°-287·2°, W287·2°-291·7°, R289·7°-293·5°.

Noss Hd 58°28'·75N 03°02'·90W Fl WR 20s 53m **W25M, R 21M**; W Tr; vis R shore-191°, W191°-shore.

DUNCANSBY HEAD TO CAPE WRATH

Duncansby Hd 58°38'·62N 03°01'·44W Fl 12s 67m **24M**; W Tr; RC; Racon (T).

Pentland Skerries 58°41'·43N 02°55'·39W Fl (3) 30s 52m **23M**; W Tr; *Horn 45s.*

Lother Rock 58°43'·80N 02°58'·58W Q 11m 6M; Racon.

S Ronaldsay, Burwick Bkwtr Hd 2 FR (vert) 8m 5M.

Swona, near SW end 58°44'·28N 03°04'·13W Fl 8s 17m 9M; W col; vis 261°-210°.

Swona N Hd 58°45'·13N 03°03'·00W Fl (3) 10s 16m 10M.

Stroma, Swilkie Pt 58°41'·78N 03°06'·92W Fl (2) 20s 32m **26M**; W Tr; *Horn (2) 60s* .

Inner sound, John O'Groats, Pier Hd 58°38'·73N 03°04'·12W Fl R 3s 4m 2M; W post; Ra refl.

Dunnet Hd 58°40'·31N 03°22'·48W Fl (4) 30s 105m **23M**; W Tr; RG.

THURSO/SCRABSTER

Holburn (Little) Hd 58°36'·90N 03°32'·28W Fl WR 10s 23m **W15M**, R11M; W Tr; vis W198°-358°, R358°-shore.

Thurso Bkwtr Hd 58°35'·97N 03°30'·63W QG 5m 4M; G post; shown 1/9-30/4.

Thurso Ldg Lts 195°. Front 58°35'·98N 03°30'·65W FG 5m 4M; Gy post. Rear FG 6m 4M; Gy mast.

Scrabster Outer Pier Hd 58°36'·63N 03°32'·48W QG 6m 4M.

Strathy Pt 58°36'·10N 04°01'·00W Fl 20s 45m **27M**; W Tr on W dwelling.

Sule Skerry 59°05'·10N 04°24'·30W Fl (2) 15s 34m **21M**; W Tr; Racon (T).

North Rona 59°07'·30N 05°48'·80W Fl (3) 20s 114m **24M**; W Tr.

Sula Sgeir 59°05'·65N 06°09'·50W Fl 15s 74m 11M; ■ structure.

Loch Eriboll, White Hd 58°31'·10N 04°38'·80W Fl WR 3s 18m W13M, R12M; W Tr and bldg; vis W030°-172°, R172°-191°, W191°-212°.

Cape Wrath 58°37'·55N 04°59'·87W Fl (4) 30s 122m **24M**; W Tr; *Horn (3) 45s.*

ORKNEY ISLANDS

Tor Ness 58°46'·71N 03°17'·70W Fl 3s 21m 10M; W Tr.

S Walls, SE end, **Cantick Hd** 58°47'·25N 03°07'·76W Fl 20s 35m **18M**; W Tr.

SCAPA FLOW AND APPROACHES

Ruff Reef, off Cantick Hd 58°47'·48N 03°07'·68W Fl (2) 10s 10m 6M; B Bn.

Long Hope, S Ness Pier Hd, 58°48'·08N 03°12'·22W Fl WRG 3s 6m W7M, R5M, G5M; vis G082°-242°, W242°-252°, R252°-082°.

Hoxa Hd 58°49'·35N 03°01'·93W Fl WR 3s 15m W9M, R6M; W Tr; vis W026°-163°, R163°-201°, W201°-215°.

Stanger Hd 58°48'·98N 03°04'·60W Fl R 5s 25m 8M.

Roan Hd 58°50'·75N 03°03'·81W Fl (2) R 6s 12m 7M.

Nevi Skerry 58°50'·70N 03°02'·60W Fl (2) 6s 7m 6M; IDM.

Calf of Flotta 58°51'·30N 03°03'·90W QR 8m 4M.

Flotta Terminal. N end of E Jetty. 2 FR (vert) 10m 3M.

West Jetty 2 FR (vert) 10m 3M; *Bell (1)10s.*

Mooring dolphins, E and W, both QR 8m 3M.

SPM Tr No. 1 58°52'·20N 03°07'·37W Fl Y 5s 12m 3M; *Horn Mo(A) 60s.*

SPM Tr No. 2 58°52'·27N 03°05'·82W Fl (4) Y 15s 12m 3M; *Horn Mo(N) 60s.*

Gibraltar Pier 58°50'·29N 03°07'·77W 2 FG (vert) 7m 3M.

Golden Wharf N end 58°50'·16N 03°11'·36W 2 FR (vert) 7m 3M.

Lyness Wharf S end 58°50'·04N 03°11'·31W 2 FR (vert) 7m 3M.

St Margaret's Hope, Needle Pt Reef 58°50'·12N 02°57'·38W Fl G 3s 6m 3M; ◆ on post.

Pier Hd 2 FG (vert) 6m 2M.

Ldg Lts 196°, both FR 7/11m.

Rose Ness 58°52'·36N 02°49'·80W Fl 6s 24m 8M; W Tr.

Scapa Pier W end 58°57'·44N 02°58'·32W Fl G 3s 6m 8M; W mast.

Barrel of Butter 58 53'·45N 03°07'·47W Fl (2) 10s 6m 7M; Gy platform on ● Tr.

Cava Lt Tr 58°53'·26N 03°10'·58W Fl WR 3s 11m W10M, R8M; W ● Tr; vis W351°-143°, R143°-196°, W196°-251°, R251°- 271°, W271°-298°.

Houton Bay Ldg Lts 316°. Front 58°55'·00N 03°11'·46W Fl G 3s 8m. Rear, 200m from front, FG 16m both R ▲ on W pole, B bands, vis 312°-320°.

Ro-Ro terminal, S end Iso R 4s 7m 5M.

CLESTRAN SOUND

Peter Skerry Lt By 58°55'·28N 03°13'·42W Fl G 6s; SHM.

Riddock Shoal Lt By 58°55'·88N 03°15'·07W Fl (2) R 12s; PHM.

HOY SOUND

Ebbing Eddy Rks Lt By 58°56'·62N 03°16'·90W Q; NCM.

Graemsay Is Ldg Lts 104°. **Front** 58°56'·46N 03°18'·50W Iso 3s 17m **15M**; W Tr; vis 070°-255°. **Rear**, 1·2M from front, Oc WR 8s 35m **W20M, R16M**; W Tr; vis R097°-112°, W112°-163°, R163°-178°, W178°-332°; obsc on Ldg line within 0·5M.

Skerry of Ness 58°56'·98N 03°17'·73W Fl WG 4s 7m W7M, G4M; vis W shore-090°, G090°-shore.

STROMNESS

Stromness Can Lt By 58°57'·27N 03°17'·52W QR; PHM.

Stromness Conical Lt By 58°57'·43N 03°17'·55W Fl G 3s; SHM.

Ldg Lts 317°. Front 58°57'·64N 03°18'·06W FR 29m 11M; post on W Tr. Rear, 55m from front FR 39m 11M; both vis 307°-327°.

N Pier Hd 58°57'·78N 03°17'·62W Fl R 3s 8m 5M.

AUSKERRY.

Copinsay 58°53'·82N 02°40'·25W Fl (5) 30s 79m **21M**; W Tr; *Horn (4) 60s.* Fog Det Lt UQ, vis 192°.

Auskerry 59°01'·58N 02°34'·25W Fl 20s 34m **18M**; W Tr.

Helliar Holm S end 59°01'·17N 02°53'·95W Fl WRG 10s 18m W14M, R10M; W Tr; vis G256°-276°, W276°-292°, R292°-098°, W098°-116°, G116°-154°.

Balfour Pier, Shapinsay 59°01'·89N 02°54'·40W Q WRG 5m W3M, R2M, G2M; vis G270°-010°, W010°-020°, R020°-090°.

KIRKWALL
Scargun Shoal By 59°00'·83N 02°58'·57W; SHM.
Pier N end 58°59'·32N 02°57'·62W Iso WRG 5s 8m **W15M**, R13M, G13M; W Tr; vis G153°-183°, W183°-192°, R192°-210°.

WIDE FIRTH
Linga Skerry Lt By 59°02'·44N 02°57'·45W Q (3) 10s; ECM.
Boray Skerries Lt By 59°03'·68N 02°57'·55W Q (6) + L Fl 15s; SCM.
Skertours Lt By 59°04'·15N 02°56'·61W Q; NCM.
Galt Skerry Lt By 59°05'·25N 02°54'·10W Q; NCM.
Brough of Birsay 59°08'·25N 03°20'·30W Fl (3) 25s 52m **18M**; W castellated Tr and Bldg.
Papa Stronsay NE end, The Ness 59°09'·38N 02°34'·80W Iso 4s 8m 9M; W Tr.

STRONSAY, PAPA SOUND
Quiabow Lt By 59°09'·85N 02°36'·20W Fl (2) G 12s; SHM.
No. 1 Lt By (off Jacks Reef) 59°09'·20N 02°36'·40W Fl G 5s; SHM.
No. 2 Lt By 59°08'·95N 02°36'·50W Fl R 5s; PHM.
No. 3 Lt By 59°08'·73N 02°36'·08W Fl (2) G 5s; SHM.
No. 4 Lt By 59°08'·80N 02°36'·37W Fl (2) R 5s; PHM.
Whitehall Pier 50°08'·61N 02°35'·79W 2 FG (vert) 8m 4M.

SANDAY ISLAND/NORTH RONALDSAY
Start Pt 59°16'·70N 02°22'·50W Fl (2) 20s 24m **19M**; W Tr, B stripes.
Kettletoft Pier Hd 59°13'·90N 02°35'·72W Fl WRG 3s 7m W7M, R5M, G5M; W Tr; vis W351°-011°, R011°-180°, G180°-351°.
N Ronaldsay NE end, 59°23'·40N 02°22'·80W Fl 10s 43m **19M**; R Tr, W bands; Racon; Horn 60s.
Nouster Pier Hd 59°21'·32N 02°26'·35W QR 5m.

EDAY/EGILSAY
Calf Sound 59°14'·30N 02°45'·70W Iso WRG 5s 8m W8M, R7M, G6M; W Tr; vis R shore-216°, W216°-223°, G223°-302°, W302°-307°.
Backaland Pier 59°09'·45N 02°44'·75W Fl R 3s 5m 4M; vis 192°-250°.
Egilsay Pier S end 59°09'·32N 02°56'·65W Fl G 3s 4m 4M.

WESTRAY/PIEROWALL.
Noup Hd 59°19'·90N 03°04'·10W Fl 30s 79m **22M**, W Tr; vis 335°-242°, 248°-282°; obsc on E bearings within 0·8M, part obsc 240°-275°.
Pierowall E Pier Hd 59°19'·39N 02°58'·41W Fl WRG 3s 7m W11M, R7M, G7M; vis G254°-276°, W276°-291°, R291°-308°, G308°-215°.
Papa Westray, Moclett Bay Pier Hd 59°19'·65N 02°53'·40W Fl WRG 5s 7m W5M, R3M, G3M; vis G306°-341°, W341°-040°, R040°-074°.

SHETLAND ISLES

FAIR ISLE
Skadan S end 59°30'·85N 01°39'·08W Fl (4) 30s 32m **24M**; W Tr; vis 260°-146°, obsc inshore 260°-282°; Horn(2) 60s.
Skroo N end 59°33'·16N 01°36'·49W Fl (2) 30s 80m **22M**; W Tr; vis 086·7°-358°; Horn (3) 45s.

MAINLAND, SOUTH
Sumburgh Hd 59°51'·30N 01°16'·37W Fl (3) 30s 91m **23M**; W Tr; RC.
Pool of Virkie, Marina E Bkwtr Hd 59°53'·05N 01°17'·00W 2 FG (vert) 6m 5M.
Mousa, Perie Bard, 59°59'·85N 01°09'·40W Fl 3s 20m 10M; W Tr.
Aithsvoe 60°02'·30N 01°12'·83W Fl R 3s 3m 2M.

BRESSAY/LERWICK
Kirkabister Ness 60°07'·25N 01°07'·18W Fl (2) 20s 32m **23M**; W Tr; FR Lts on radio masts 0·95M NE.
Cro of Ham 60°08'·20N 01°07'·40W Fl 3s 3M.
Twageos Pt 60°08'·95N 01°07'·83W L Fl 6s 8m 6M; W Bn.
Maryfield, Ferry Terminal 60°09'·47N 01°07'·32W Oc WRG 6s 5m 5M; vis W008°-013°, R013°-111°, G111°-008°.
Bkwtr N Hd 60°09'·27N 01°08'·29W 2 FR (vert) 5m 4M.
N Ness 60°09'·60N 01°08'·66W Iso WG 4s 4m 5M; vis G158°-216°, W216°-158°.
Loofa Baa 60°09'·75N 01°08'·67W Q (6) + L Fl 15s 4m 5M; SCM.
Soldian Rk Lt By 60°12'·54N 01°04'·61W VQ(6) + L Fl 10s; SCM.
N ent Dir Lt 215°. 60°10'·49N 01°09'·40W Dir Oc WRG 6s 27m 8M; Y ▲, Or stripe; vis R211°-214°, W214°-216°, G216°-221°.
Gremista Marina S Bkwtr Hd 60°10'·23N 01°09'·49W Iso R 4s 3m 2M.
Greenhead 60°10'·87N 01°08'·98W Q (4) R 10s 4m 3M.
Rova Hd 60°11'·45N 01°08'·45W Fl (3) WRG 18s 10m W8M, R7M, G6M; W Tr; vis R shore-180°, W180°-194°, G194°-213°, R213°-241°, W241°-261·5°, G261·5°-009°, W009°-shore.
The Brethren Rk Lt By 60°12'·38N 01°08'·12W Q (9) 15s; WCM.
The Unicorn Rk Lt By 60°13'·54N 01°08'·35W VQ (3) 5s; ECM
Dales Voe 60°11'·82N 01°11'·10W Fl (2) WRG 8s 5m W4M, R3M, G3M; vis G220°-227°, W227°-233°, R233°-240°.
Dales Voe Quay 60°11'·60N 01°10'·48W 2 FR (vert) 9m 3M.
Laxfirth Pier Hd 60°12'·77N 01°12'·01W 2 FG (vert) 4m 2M.
Hoo Stack 60°14'·99N 01°05'·25W Fl (4) WRG 12s 40m W7M, R5M, G5M; W pylon; vis R169°-180°, W180°-184°, G184°-193°, W193°-169°. Dir Lt 182°. Dir Fl (4) WRG 12s 33m W9M, R6M, G6M; same structure; vis R177°-180°, W180°-184°, G184°-187°; synch with upper Lt.
Mull (Moul) of Eswick 60°15'·80N 01°05'·80W Fl WRG 3s 50m W9M, R6M, G6M; W Tr; vis R 028°-200°, W200°-207°, G207°-018°, W018°-028°.

WHALSAY/SKERRIES
Symbister Ness 60°20'·46N 01°02'·15W Fl (2) WG 12s 11m W8M, G6M; W Tr; vis W shore-203°, G203°-shore.
Symbister Bay S Bkwtr Hd 60°20'·60N 01°01'·50W QG 4m 2M.
N Bkwtr Hd 60°20'·67N 01°01'·60W Oc G 7s 3m 3M.
E Bkwtr Hd Oc R 7s 3m 3M.
Marina N pontoon 60°20'·50N 01°01'·40W 2 FG (vert) 2m 3M.
Skate of Marrister 60°21'·42N 01°01'·25W Fl G 6s 4m 4M; G mast with platform.
Suther Ness 60°22'·15N 01°00'·05W Fl WRG 3s 8m W10M, R8M, G7M; vis W shore-038°, R038°-173°, W173°-206°, G206°-shore.
Mainland. Laxo Voe ferry terminal 60°21'·1N 01°10'·0W 2 FG (vert) 4m 2M.
Bound Skerry 60°25'·50N 00°43'·50W Fl 20s 44m **20M**; W Tr.
South Mouth. Ldg Lts 014°. Front 60°25'·37N 00°44'·89W FY 3m 2M. Rear, FY 12m 2M.
Bruray Bn D Fl (3) G 6s 3m 3M.
Bruray Bn B VQ G 3m 3M.
Housay Bn A VQ R 3m 3M.
Bruray ferry berth 60°25'·4N 00°45'·10W 2 FG (vert) 6m 4M.
Muckle Skerry 60°26'·40N 00°51'·70W Fl (2) WRG 10s 13m W7M, R5M, G5M; W Tr; vis W046°-192°, R192°-272°, G272°-348°, W348°-353°, R353°-046°.

YELL SOUND
S ent, Lunna Holm 60°27'·38N 01°02'·39W Fl (3) WRG 15s 19m W10M, R7M, G7M; W ● Tr; vis R shore-090°, W090°-094°, G094°-209°, W209°-275°, R275°-shore.
Firths Voe, N shore 60°27'·24N 01°10'·50W Oc WRG 8s 9m **W15M**, R10M, G10M; W Tr; vis W189°-194°, G194°-257°, W257°-263°, R263°-339°, W339°-066°.

Linga Is. Dir Lt 60°26'·83N 01°09'·00W Dir Q (4) WRG 8s 10m W9M, R9M, G9M; concrete col; vis R145°-148°, W148°-152°, G152°-155°. Q (4) WRG 8s 10m W7M, R4M, G4M; same structure; vis R052°-146°, G154°-196°, W196°-312°; synch with Dir Lt.

The Rumble Bn 60°28'·20N 01°07'·12W R Bn; Racon (O).

Yell, Ulsta Ferry Terminal Bkwtr Hd 60°29'·78N 01°09'·40W Oc RG 4s 7m R5M, G5M; vis G shore-354°, R044°-shore. Oc WRG 4s 5m W8M, R5M, G5M; same structure; vis G shore-008°, W008°-036°, R036°-shore.

Toft ferry terminal 60°28'·06N 01°12'·26W 2 FR (vert) 5m 2M.

Ness of Sound, W side, 60°31'·38N 01°11'·15W Iso WRG 5s 18m W9M, R6M, G6M; vis G shore-345°, W345°-350°, R350°-160°, W160°-165°, G165°-shore.

Brother Is Dir Lt 329°, 60°30'·99N 01°13'·99W Dir Fl (4) WRG 8s 16m W10M, R7M, G7M; vis G323·5°-328°, W328°-330°, R330°-333·5°.

Mio Ness 60°29'·70N 01°13'·55W Q (2) WR 10s 12m W7M, R4M; W ● Tr; W282°-238°, R238°-282°.

Tinga Skerry 60°30'·52N 01°14'·73W Q (2) G 10s 9m 5M; W ● Tr.

YELL SOUND, NORTH ENTRANCE

Bagi Stack 60°43'·55N 01°07'·40W Fl (4) 20s 45m 10M; W Tr.

Gruney Is 60°39'·20N 01°18'·03W Fl WR 5s 53m W8M, R6M; W Tr; vis R064°-180°, W180°-012°; Racon (T).

Point of Fethaland 60°38'·09N 01°18'·58W Fl (3) WR 15s 65m **W24M, R20M**; W Tr; vis R080°-103°, W103°-160°, R160°-206°, W206°-340°.

Muckle Holm 60°34'·85N 01°15'·90W Fl (2) 10s 32m 10M; W Tr.

Little Holm 60°33'·46N 01°15'·75W Iso 4s 12m 6M; W Tr.

Outer Skerry 60°33'·08N 01°18'·20W Fl 6s 12m 8M; W col, B bands.

Quey Firth 60°31'·48N 01°19'·46W Oc WRG 6s 22m W12M, R8M, G8M; W Tr; vis W shore (through S and W)-290°, G290°-327°, W327°-334°, R334°-shore.

Lamba, S side, 60°30'·76N 01°17'·70W Fl WRG 3s 30m W8M, R5M, G5M; W Tr; vis G shore-288°, W288°-293°, R293°-327°, W327°-044°, R044°-140°, W140°-shore. Dir Lt 290·5° Dir Fl WRG 3s 24m W10M, R7M, G7M; vis 285·5°-288°, W288°-293°, R293°-295·5°.

SULLOM VOE

Gluss Is Ldg Lts 194·7° (H24). **Front** 60°29'·81N 01°19'·31W F 39m **19M**; ■ on Gy Tr. **Rear**, 0·75M from front, F 69m **19M**; ■ on Gy Tr. Both Lts 9M by day.

Little Roe 60°30'·05N 01°16'·35W Fl (3) WR 10s 16m W5M, R4M; Y and W structure; vis R036°-095·5°, W095·5°-036°.

Skaw Taing 60°29'·13N 01°16'·72W Fl (2) WRG 5s 21m W8M, R5M, G5M; Or and W structure; vis W049°-078°, G078°-147°, W147°-154°, R154°-169°, W169°-288°.

Ness of Bardister 60°28'·22N 01°19'·50W Oc WRG 8s 20m W9M, R6M, G6M; Or and W structure; vis W180·5°-240°, R240°-310·5°, W310·5°-314·5°, G314·5°-030·5°.

Vats Houllands 60°27'·97N 01°17'·48W Oc WRGY 3s 73m 6M; Gy Tr; vis W343·5°-029·5°, Y029·5°-049°, G049°-074·5°, R074·5°-098·5°, G098·5°-123·5°, Y123·5°-148°, W148°-163·5°.

Fugla Ness. Lts in line 212·3°. Rear 60°27'·3N 01°19'·7W Iso 4s 45m 14M. Common front 60°27'·48N 01°19'·43W Iso 4s 27m 14M; synch with rear Lts. Lts in line 203°. Rear 60°27'·3N 01°19'·6W Iso 4s 45m 14M.

Sella Ness. Upper Lt 60°26'·92N 01°16'·52W Q WRG 14m 7M; Gy Tr; vis G084·5°-098·7°, W098·7°-099·7°, W126°-128·5°, R128·5°-174·5°; by day F WRG 2M (occas). Lower Lt. Q WRG 10m 7M; vis: G084·5°-106·5°, W106·5°-115°, R115°-174·5°; by day F WRG 2M (occas).

Tug Jetty finger, Pier Hd 60°26'·79N 01°16'·25W Iso G 4s 4m 3M.

Garth Pier N arm Hd 60°26'·72N 01°16'·22W Fl (2) G 5s 4m 3M.

Scatsa Ness Upper Lt 60°26'·52N 01°18'·13W Oc WRG 5s 14m 7M; Gy Tr; vis G161·5°-187·2°, W187·2°-188·2°, W207·2°-208·2°, R208·2°-251·5°; by day F WRG 2M (occas). Lower Lt Oc WRG 5s 10m 7M; vis G161·5°-197·2°, W197·2°-202·2°, R202·2°-251·5°; by day F WRG 2M (occas).

Ungam Is 60°27'·27N 01°18'·50W VQ (2) 5s 2m 2M; W col; Ra refl.

EAST YELL /UNST/BALTA SOUND

Whitehill 60°34'·85N 01°00'·01W Fl WR 3s 24m W9M, R6M; vis W shore-163°, R163°-211°, W211°-349°, R349°-shore.

Uyea Sound 60°41'·19N 00°55'·37W Fl (2) 8s 8m 7M; R & W Tr.

Balta Sound 60°44'·47N 00°47'·56W Fl WR 10s 17m 10M, R7M; vis W249°-010°, R010°-060°, W060°-154°; Q Lt (occas) marks Unst Aero RC 0·7M W.

Balta Marina Bkwtr Hd 60°45'·60N 00°50'·20W Fl R 6s 2m 2M.

Holme of Skaw 60°49'·92N 00°46'·19W Fl 5s 8m 8M.

Muckle Flugga 60°51'·33N 00°53'·00W Fl (2) 20s 66m **22M**; W Tr.

Yell. Cullivoe Bkwtr Hd 60°41'·91N 00°59'·66W Oc R 7s 5m 2M; Gy col.

MAINLAND, WEST

Esha Ness 60°29'·35N 01°37'·55W Fl 12s 61m **25M**; W ■ Tr.

Hillswick, S end of Ness 60°27'·20N 01°29'·70W Fl (4) WR 15s 34m W9M, R6M; W house: vis W217°-093°, R093°-114°.

Muckle Roe, Swarbacks Minn, 60°21'·05N 01°26'·90W Fl WR 3s 30m W9M, R6M; vis W314°-041°, R041°-075°, W075°-137°.

W Burra Firth Outer Lt 60°17'·84N 01°33'·47W Oc WRG 8s 27m W9M, R7M, G7M; vis G 136°-142°, W142°-150°, R150°-156°.

W Burra Firth Inner Lt 60°17'·84N 01°32'·03W F WRG 9m W15M, R9M, G9M; vis G095°-098°, W098°-102°, W098°-102°, R102°-105°.

Aith Bkwtr. RNLI berth 60°17'·20N 01°22'·30W QG 5m 3M.

W Burra Firth Transport Pier Hd 60°17'·75N 01°32'·30W Iso G 4s 4m 4M.

Ve Skerries 60°22'·40N 01°48'·67W Fl (2) 20s 17m 11M; W Tr; Racon (T).

Rams Hd 60°12'·00N 01°33'·40W Fl WG 8s 16m W9m, G6M, R6M; W house; vis G265°-355°, W355°-012°, R012°-090°, W090°-136°, obsc by Vaila I when brg more than 030°.

Vaila Pier 60°13'·47N 01°34'·00W 2 FR (vert) 4m.

Skelda Voe. Skeld Pier Hd 60°11'·20N 01°26'·10W 2 FR (vert) 4m 3M.

North Havra 60°09'·88N 01°20'·17W Fl WRG 12s 24m W7M, R5M, G5M; W Tr; vis G 001°-053·5°, W053·5°-060·5°, G274°-334°, W334°-337·5°, R337·5°-001°.

SCALLOWAY

Pt of the Pund 60°08'·02N 01°18'·20W Fl WRG 5s 20m W7M, R5M, G5M; W Tr; vis R350°-090°, G090°-111°, R111°-135°, W135°-140°, G140°-177°, W267°-350°.

Whaleback Skerry Lt By 60°07'·98N 01°18'·79W Q; NCM.

Moores slipway Jetty Hd 60°08'·21N 01°16'·72W 2 FR (vert) 4m 1M.

Centre Pier 60°08'·11N 01°16'·38W Oc WRG 10s 7m W14M, G11M, R11M; vis G045·7°-056·8°, W056·8°-058·8°, R058·8°-069·9°.

Fugla Ness 60°06'·40N 01°20'·75W Fl (2) WRG 10s 20m W10M, R7M, G7M; W Tr; vis G014°-032°, W032°-082°, R082°-134°, W134°-shore.

FOULA

60°06'·78N 02°03'·72W Fl (3) 15s 36m **18M**; W Tr. Obscured 123°-221°.

10.7.5 PASSAGE INFORMATION

Refer to the *N Coast of Scotland Pilot*; the CCC's SDs (3 vols) for *N and NE coasts of Scotland*; *Orkney*; and *Shetland*.

MORAY FIRTH: SOUTH COAST (charts 115, 222, 223)

Crossing the Moray Firth from Rattray Hd (lt, fog sig) to Duncansby Hd (lt,RC, Racon) heavy seas may be met in strong W winds. Most hbrs in the Firth are exposed to NE-E winds. For oil installations, see 10.5.5; the Beatrice Field is 20M S of Wick. Tidal streams attain 3kn at sp close off Rattray Hd, but 5M NE of the Head the NE-going stream begins at HW Aberdeen + 0140, and the SE-going stream at HW Aberdeen – 0440, sp rates 2kn. Streams are weak elsewhere in the Moray Firth, except in the inner part. In late spring/early summer fog (haar) is likely in onshore winds.

In strong winds the sea breaks over Steratan Rk in the E approach to Fraserburgh (10.7.7), and over Colonel Rk 1·75M E of Kinnairds Hd (lt). Rosehearty firing range is 3M NW of Fraserburgh. Banff B is shallow; N of Macduff (10.7.8) beware Collie Rks. Banff hbr dries, and should not be approached in fresh NE-E winds, when seas break well offshore; Macduff would then be a feasible alternative.

From Meavie Pt to Scar Nose dangers extend up to 3ca from shore in places. Beware Caple Rk (depth 0·2m) 7½ca W of Logie Hd. Spey B is clear of dangers more than 7½ca from shore; anch here, but only in offshore winds. Beware E Muck (dries) 5ca SW of Craigenroan, an above-water rky patch 5ca SW of Craig Hd, and Middle Muck and W Muck in approach to Buckie (10.7.10); Findochty & Portknockie are 2 and 3.5M ENE. Halliman Skerries (dry; bn) lie 1·5M WNW of Lossiemouth (10.7.11). Covesea Skerries (dry) lie 5ca NW of their lt ho.

Inverness Firth is approached between Nairn (10.7.15) and S Sutor. In heavy weather there is a confused sea with overfalls on Guillam Bank, 9M S of Tarbat Ness. The sea also breaks on Riff Bank (S of S Sutor) which dries in places. Chans run both N and S of Riff Bank. Off Fort George, on E side of ent to Inverness Firth (chart 1078), the SW-going stream begins HW Aberdeen + 0605, sp rate 2·5kn; the NE-going stream begins at HW Aberdeen – 0105, sp rate 3·5kn. There are eddies and turbulence between Fort George and Chanonry Pt when stream is running hard. Much of Inverness Firth is shallow, but a direct course from Chanonry Pt to Kessock Bridge, via Munlochy SWM and Meikle Mee SHM lt buoys, carries a least depth of 2·1m. Meikle Mee bank dries 0·2m. For Fortrose and Avoch, see 10.7.16.

MORAY FIRTH: NORTH WEST COAST (chart 115)

Cromarty Firth (charts 1889, 1890) is entered between N Sutor and S Sutor, both fringed by rks, some of which dry. Off the entrance the in-going stream begins at HW Aberdeen + 0605, and the out-going at HW Aberdeen – 0105, sp rates 1·5 kn. Good sheltered anchs within the firth, see 10.7.19.

The coast NE to Tarbat Ness (lt) is fringed with rks. Beware Three Kings (dries) about 3M NE of N Sutor. Culloden Rk, a shoal with depth of 1·8m, extends 2½ca NE of Tarbat Ness, where stream is weak. Beware salmon nets between Tarbat Ness and Portmahomack (10.7.17). Dornoch Firth (10.7.19) is shallow, with shifting banks, and in strong E winds the sea breaks heavily on the bar E of Dornoch Pt.

At Lothbeg Pt, 5M SW of Helmsdale (10.7.18), a rky ledge extends 5ca offshore. Near Berriedale, 7M NE of Helmsdale, is The Pinnacle, a detached rk 61m high, standing close offshore. The Beatrice oil field lies on Smith Bank, 28M NE of Tarbat Ness, and 11M off Caithness coast. Between Dunbeath (10.7.18) and Lybster (10.7.18) there are no dangers more than 2ca offshore. Clyth Ness (lt) is fringed by detached and drying rks. From here to Wick (10.7.19) the only dangers are close inshore. There is anch in Sinclair's B in good weather, but Freswick B further N is to await the tide in Pentland Firth (beware wreck in centre of bay). Stacks of Duncansby and Baxter Rk (depth 2·7m) lie 1M and 4ca S of Duncansby Hd.

PENTLAND FIRTH (charts 2162, 2581)

This potentially dangerous chan should only be attempted with moderate winds (less than F4), good vis, no swell and a fair np tide; when it presents few problems. A safe passage depends on a clear understanding of tidal streams and correct timing. The Admiralty Tidal Stream Atlas for Orkney and Shetland (NP 209) gives large scale vectors and is essential. Even in ideal conditions the races off Duncansby Hd, Swilkie Pt (N end of Stroma), and Rks of Mey (Merry Men of Mey) must be avoided as they are always dangerous to small craft. Also avoid the Pentland Skerries, Muckle Skerry, Old Head, Lother Rock (S Ronaldsay), and Dunnet Hd on E-going flood. For passages across the Firth see CCC *SDs for Orkney*.

At E end the Firth is entered between Duncansby Hd and Old Hd (S Ronaldsay), between which lie Muckle Skerry and the Pentland Skerries. Near the centre of Firth are the Islands of Swona (N side) and Stroma (S side). Outer Sound (main chan, 2·5M wide) runs between Swona and Stroma; Inner Sound (1·5M wide) between Stroma and the mainland. Rks of Mey extend about 2ca N of St John's Pt. The W end of the Firth is between Dunnet Hd and Tor Ness (Hoy).

Tidal streams reach 8-9kn at sp in the Outer Sound, and 9-12kn between Pentland Skerries and Duncansby Hd. The resultant dangerous seas, very strong eddies and violent races should be avoided by yachts at all costs. Broadly the E-going stream begins at HW Aberdeen + 0500, and the W-going at HW Aberdeen – 0105. **Duncansby Race** extends ENE towards Muckle Skerry on the SE-going stream, but by HW Aberdeen – 0440 it extends NW from Duncansby Hd. Note: HW at Muckle Skerry is the same time as HW Dover. A persistent race off **Swilkie Pt** at N end of Stroma, is very dangerous with a strong W'ly wind over a W-going stream. The most dangerous and extensive race in the Firth is **Merry Men of Mey**, which forms off St John's Pt on W-going stream at HW Aberdeen – 0150 and for a while extends right across to Tor Ness with heavy breaking seas even in fine weather.

Passage Westward: This is the more difficult direction due to prevailing W winds. Freswick B, 3·5M S of Duncansby Hd, is a good waiting anch; here an eddy runs N for 9 hrs. Round Duncansby Hd close in at HW Aberdeen –0220, as the ebb starts to run W. Take a mid-course through the Inner Sound to appr the Rks of Mey from close inshore. Gills Bay is a temp anch if early; do not pass Rks of Mey until ebb has run for at least 2 hrs. Pass 100m N of the Rks (awash).

Passage Eastward: With a fair wind and tide, no race forms and the passage is easier. Leave Scrabster at local LW+1 so as to be close off Dunnet Hd at HW Aberdeen +0240 as the E-going flood starts to make. If late, give the Hd a wide berth. Having rounded the Rks of Mey, steer S initially to avoid being set onto the rky S tip of Stroma, marked by unlit SCM bn. Then keep mid-chan through the Inner Sound and maintain this offing to give Duncansby Hd a wide berth.

PENTLAND FIRTH TO CAPE WRATH (chart 1954)

Dunnet B, S of Dunnet Hd (lt) gives temp anch in E or S winds, but dangerous seas enter in NW'lies. On W side of Thurso B is Scrabster (10.7.20) sheltered from S and W. Between Holborn Hd and Strathy Pt the E-going stream begins at HW Ullapool – 0150, and the W-going at HW Ullapool + 0420, sp rates 1·8kn. Close to Brims Ness off Ushat Hd the sp rate is 3kn, and there is often turbulence.
SW of Ushat Hd the Dounreay poer stn is conspic, near shore. Dangers extend 2½ca seaward off this coast.

Along E side of Strathy Pt (lt) an eddy gives almost continuous N-going stream, but there is usually turbulence off the Pt where this eddy meets the main E or W stream. Several small B's along this coast give temp anch in offshore winds, but must not be used or approached with wind in a N quarter.

Kyle of Tongue (10.7.19) is entered from E through Caol Raineach, S of Eilean nan Ron, or from N between Eilean Iosal and Cnoc Glass. There is no chan into the kyle W of Rabbit Is, to which a drying spit extends 0·5M NNE from the mainland shore. Further S there is a bar across entrance to inner part of kyle. There are anchs on SE side of Eilean nan Ron, SE side of Rabbit Is, off Skullomie, or S of Eilean Creagach off Talmine. Approach to the latter runs close W of Rabbit Islands, but beware rks to N and NW of them.

Loch Eriboll, (chart 2076 and 10.7.19), provides secure anchs, but in strong winds violent squalls blow down from mountains. Eilean Cluimhrig lies on W side of entrance; the E shore is fringed with rks up to 2ca offshore. At White Hd (lt) the loch narrows to 6ca. There are chans W and E of Eilean Choraidh. Best anchs in Camas an Duin (S of Ard Neackie) or in Rispond B close to entrance (but not in E winds, and beware Rispond Rk which dries).

The coast to C. Wrath (10.8.5) is indented, with dangers extending 3ca off the shore and offlying rks and Is. Once a yacht has left Loch Eriboll she is committed to a long and exposed passage until reaching Loch Inchard. The Kyle of Durness is dangerous if the wind or sea is onshore. Give Cape Wrath a wide berth when wind-against-tide which raises a severe sea. A firing exercise area extends 8M E of C. Wrath, and 4M offshore. When in use, R flags or pairs of R lts (vert) are shown from E and W limits, and yachts should keep clear.

ORKNEY ISLANDS (10.7.21 and charts 2249, 2250)

The Islands are mostly indented and rky, but with sandy beaches especially on NE sides. Pilotage is easy in good vis, but in other conditions great care is needed since tides run strongly. For details refer to Clyde Cruising Club's *Orkney Sailing Directions* and the Admiralty Tidal Atlas NP 209.

When cruising in Orkney it is essential to understand and use the tidal streams to the best advantage, avoiding the various tide races and overfalls, particularly near sp. A good engine is needed since, for example, there are many places where it is dangerous to get becalmed. Swell from the Atlantic or North Sea can contribute to dangerous sea conditions, or penetrate to some of the anchorages. During summer months winds are not normally unduly strong, and can be expected to be Force 7 or more on about two days a month. But in winter the wind reaches this strength for 10-15 days per month, and gales can be very severe in late winter and early spring. Cruising conditions are best near midsummer, when of course the hours of daylight are much extended.

Stronsay Firth and Westray Firth run SE/NW through the group. The many good anchs, include: Deer Sound (W of Deer Ness); B of Firth, B of Isbister, and off Balfour in Elwick B (all leading from Wide Firth); Rysa Sound, B of Houton, Hunda Sound (in Scapa Flow); Rousay Sound; and Pierowall Road (Westray). Plans for some of these are on chart 2622. For Auskerry, see 10.7.23. For Houton Bay Shapinsay and Pierowall, see 10.7.24. There is a major oil terminal and prohibited area at Flotta, on the S side of Scapa Flow.

Tide races or dangerous seas occur at the entrances to most of the firths or sounds when the stream is against strong winds. This applies particularly to Hoy Sound, Eynhallow Sound, Papa Sound (Westray), Lashy Sound, and North Ronaldsay Firth. Also off Mull Head, over Dowie Sand, between Muckle Green Holm and War Ness (where violent turbulence may extend right across the firth), between Faraclett Head and Wart Holm, and off Sacquoy Hd. Off War Ness the SE-going stream begins at HW Aberdeen + 0435, and the NW-going at HW Aberdeen – 0200, sp rates 7kn.

7

SHETLAND ISLANDS (10.7.25 and charts 3281, 3282, 3283)

These Islands mostly have bold cliffs and are relatively high, separated by narrow sounds through which the tide runs strongly, so that in poor vis great care is needed. Avoid sp tides, swell and wind against tide conditions. Although there are many secluded and attractive anchs, remember that the weather can change very quickly, with sudden shifts of wind. Also beware salmon fisheries and mussel rafts (unlit) in many Voes, Sounds and hbrs. Lerwick (10.7.26) is the busy main port and capital; for Scalloway and Balta Sound see 10.7.24. Refer to the Clyde Cruising Club's *Shetland Sailing Directions*.

Coming from the S, beware a most violent and dangerous race (roost) off Sumburgh Hd (at S end of Mainland) on both streams. Other dangerous areas include between Ve Skerries and Papa Stour; the mouth of Yell Sound with strong wind against N-going stream; and off Holm of Skaw (N end of Unst). Tidal streams run mainly NW/SE and are not strong except off headlands and in the major sounds; the Admiralty Tidal Atlas NP 209 gives detail. The sp range is about 2m.

The 50M passage from Orkney can conveniently be broken by a stop at Fair Isle (North Haven). Note that races form off both ends of the Is, especially S (Roost of Keels); see 10.7.24. Lerwick to Bergen, Norway is about 210M.

10.7.6   DISTANCE TABLE

Approximate distances in nautical miles are by the most direct route, whilst avoiding dangers and allowing for Traffic Separation Schemes. Places in *italics* are in adjoining areas; places in **bold** are in 10.0.7, Distances across the North Sea.

	1	2	3	4	5	6	7	8	9	10	11	12	13	14	15	16	17	18	19	20
1. *Peterhead*	1																			
2. **Fraserburgh**	16	2																		
3. Banff/Macduff	33	18	3																	
4. Buckie	46	31	15	4																
5. Lossiemouth	56	41	25	11	5															
6. Findhorn	69	54	38	24	13	6														
7. Nairn	79	64	48	34	23	10	7													
8. **Inverness**	90	75	59	45	34	23	13	8												
9. Tarbat Ness	72	57	41	27	18	14	17	27	9											
10. Helmsdale	74	59	44	33	26	28	32	43	16	10										
11. **Wick**	72	57	50	46	44	51	58	69	42	29	11									
12. Duncansby Head	82	67	62	58	57	64	71	81	54	41	13	12								
13. Scrabster	100	85	80	76	75	82	89	99	72	59	31	18	13							
14. **Kirkwall**	115	100	95	91	90	97	104	114	87	74	46	34	50	14						
15. Stromness	104	89	84	80	79	85	92	103	76	63	35	22	25	32	15					
16. Fair Isle	122	111	116	118	120	130	137	148	121	108	79	68	85	55	77	16				
17. **Lerwick**	160	150	156	160	162	172	170	190	162	148	120	109	124	95	110	42	17			
18. Loch Eriboll (ent)	137	122	117	113	112	119	126	136	109	96	68	55	37	80	50	110	150	18		
19. Cape Wrath	145	130	125	121	120	127	126	144	117	104	76	63	47	79	58	120	155	13	19	
20. *Ullapool*	198	183	178	174	173	180	179	197	170	157	129	116	100	132	111	173	208	66	53	20

FRASERBURGH   10-7-7

Aberdeen 57°41'·52N 01°59'·70W

CHARTS
AC 1462, 222,115; OS 30
TIDES
+0120 Dover; ML 2·3; Duration 0615; Zone 0 (UT)

Standard Port ABERDEEN (←)

Times				Height (metres)			
High Water		Low Water		MHWS	MHWN	MLWN	MLWS
0000	0600	0100	0700	4·3	3·4	1·6	0·6
1200	1800	1300	1900				
Differences FRASERBURGH							
−0105	−0115	−0120	−0110	−0·6	−0·5	−0·2	0·0

SHELTER
A safe refuge/passage stop, but does not cater for yachts. Ent is dangerous in NE/SE gales. Berth as directed by Hr Mr.
NAVIGATION
WPT 57°41'·32N 01°58'·71W, 111°/291° from/to ent, 0·57M. This is a very busy fishing port and FVs come and go H24. Good lookout on entering/leaving. Yachts can enter under radar control in poor visibility. Hbr is dredged 3·4m.
LIGHTS AND MARKS
Kinnairds Hd lt ho, Fl 5s 25m 22M, is 0·45M NNW of ent. Cairnbulg Briggs bn, Fl (2) 10s 9m 6M, is 1·8M ESE of ent. Ldg lts 291°: front QR 12m 5M; rear Oc R 6s 17m 5M.
Entry sigs at W Pier: 2 B ●s or 2 FR (vert) = No entry. R flag or one FR = Hbr open, but special care needed.
RADIO TELEPHONE
Call on approach VHF Ch 12 16 (H24).
TELEPHONE (01346)
Hr Mr 516069; Watch Tr 515926; Port Office 515858; MRCC (01224) 592334; ⌗ (0131) 469 7400; Marinecall 0891 500 451; Police 513151; Dr 518088.
FACILITIES
Port ☎ 515858, AB £5 (in S Hbr), Slip, P (cans), D, FW, CH, ME, EI, Sh, C (70 ton mobile), V, R, Bar; **Services:** C (30 ton), SM. **Town** EC Wed; ✉, Ⓑ, ⇌, ✈ (bus to Aberdeen).

ADJACENT HARBOURS

ROSEHEARTY, Aberdeen, 57°42'·10N 02°06'·78W. AC 222, 213. HW Aberdeen −1. E pier and inner hbr dry, but end of W pier is accessible at all states of tide. Ent exposed in N/E winds; in E/SE winds hbr can be uncomfortable. Ldg marks B/W on approx 220°; rks E of ldg line. When 30m from pier, steer midway between ldg marks and W pier. Port Rae, close to E, has unmarked rks; local knowledge. Hr Mr ☎ (01346) 571292 (home), AB £4. **Town** V, R, Bar, ✉.
Pennan Cove, 5M to the W, has council ⚓s (10 tons max) at approx 57°40'·95N 02°15'·60W. There are similar ⚓s at **Gardenstown** (Gamrie Bay), approx 57°40'·90N 02°19'·50W.

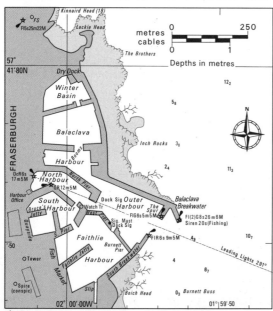

⚓ Apply harbour office if not previously directed.

MACDUFF/BANFF   10-7-8

Banff   Macduff 57°40'·27N 02°29'·94W
         Banff   57°40'·24N 02°31'·18W

CHARTS
AC 1462, 222, 115; OS 29
TIDES
+ 0055 Dover; ML 2·0; Duration 0615; Zone 0 (UT)

Standard Port ABERDEEN (←)

Times				Height (metres)			
High Water		Low Water		MHWS	MHWN	MLWN	MLWS
0200	0900	0400	0900	4·3	3·4	1·6	0·6
1400	2100	1600	2100				
Differences BANFF							
−0100	−0150	−0150	−0050	−0·8	−0·6	−0·5	−0·2

SHELTER
Macduff: Reasonably good, but ent not advised in strong NW/N winds. Slight/moderate surge in outer hbr with N/NE gales. Hbr ent is 17m wide with 3 basins; approx 2·6m in outer hbr and 2m inner hbr. A busy cargo/fishing port with limited space for yachts.
Banff: Popular hbr (dries); access HW±4. Y waiting ⚓s. When Macduff ent is very rough in strong NW/N winds, Banff can be a safe refuge; berth in outside basin and contact Hr Mr. In strong N/ENE winds Banff is unusable.
NAVIGATION
WPT 57°40'·50N 02°30'·50W, 307°/127° from/to Macduff ent, 0·4M. Same WPT 056°/236° from/to Banff ent, 0·44M. Beware Feachie Craig, Collie Rks and rky coast N and S of hbr ent.
LIGHTS AND MARKS
Macduff: Ldg lts/marks 127° both FR 44/55m 3M, orange △s. Pier hd lt, Fl (2) WRG 6s 12m 9/7M, W tr; W115°-174°. Banff: W bn (unlit) at end of N pier.

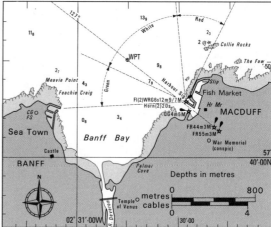

⚓ Apply to harbour office if not previously directed

RADIO TELEPHONE
VHF Ch 12 16 (H24).
TELEPHONE (01261)
Hr Mr (Macduff) 832236; Hr Mr (Banff) 815093 (home, part-time); MRCC (01224) 592334; ⌗ (0131) 469 7400; Marinecall 0891 500 451; Police 812555; Dr Banff 812027.
FACILITIES
MACDUFF: **Hbr** Slip, P (cans), D, FW, ME, EI, Sh, CH. **Town** EC Wed; V, R, Bar, ✉, ⇌ (bus to Keith).
BANFF: **Hbr** £6, FW, AC, Slip; **Banff SC**. **Town**, P, D, V, R, Bar, ⇌, Ⓑ, ✈ (Aberdeen).

ADJACENT HARBOUR (3·5M W of WHITEHILLS)

PORTSOY, Banff, 57°41'·36N 02°41'·50W. AC 222. HW+0047 on Dover; −0132 and Ht −0·3m on Aberdeen. Small drying hbr; ent exposed to NW/NE winds. New hbr to port of ent partially dries; inner hbr dries to clean sand. Ldg lts 160°, front FW 12m 5M on twr; rear FR 17m 5M. Hr Mr ☎ (01261) 815093 (home). Facilities: limited. AB, Slip, FW, V, R, Bar, ✉.
Sandend Bay, 1·7M W (57°41'N 02°44'·5W). There are Y ⚓s.

WHITEHILLS   10-7-9

Banff 57°40'·82N 02°34'·78W

CHARTS
AC 222, 115; OS 29

TIDES
+0050 Dover; ML 2·4; Duration 0610; Zone 0 (UT)

Standard Port ABERDEEN (←)

Times				Height (metres)			
High Water		Low Water		MHWS	MHWN	MLWN	MLWS
0200	0900	0400	0900	4·3	3·4	1·6	0·6
1400	2100	1600	2100				
Differences WHITEHILLS							
−0122	−0137	−0117	−0127	−0·4	−0·3	+0·1	+0·1

SHELTER
Safe. In strong NW/N winds beware surge in the narrow ent and outer hbr (2·4m), when ent is best not attempted. See Hr Mr for vacant pontoon berth (1·2m), or berth on N or E walls of inner hbr (1·8m) as space permits.

NAVIGATION
WPT 57°42'·00N 02°34'·80W, 000°/180° from/to bkwtr lt, 1·2M. Reefs on S side of chan marked by 2 rusty/white SHM bns. Beware fishing floats.

LIGHTS AND MARKS
Fl WR 25s (timing is unreliable) on pier hd, vis R132°–212°, W212°–245°; appr in R sector.

RADIO TELEPHONE
Whitehills Hbr Radio VHF Ch 09 08 16.

TELEPHONE (01261)
Hr Mr 861291; MRCC (01224) 592334; ⌗ (0131) 469 7400; Marinecall 0891 500451; Police (01542) 32222; Dr 812027.

FACILITIES
Harbour AB £5, P, D, FW, ME, EI, CH.
Town V, R, Bar, ✉, Ⓑ (AM only), ⇌ (bus to Keith), ✈ (Aberdeen).

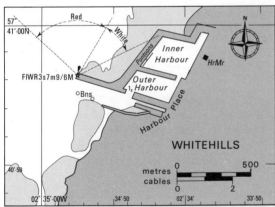

⚠ Apply to harbour office if not previously directed

ADJACENT HARBOURS

CULLEN, Banff, 57°41'·65N 02°49'·20W. AC 222. HW +0045 on Dover, −0135 on Aberdeen; HW ht −0·3m Aberdeen; ML 2·4m; Duration 0555. Shelter good, but ent hazardous in strong W/N winds. There are council ⚓s (10 tons max). Small hbr, dries, access approx HW ±2. Moor S of Inner jetty if < 1m draft. Beware local moorings across inner basin ent. W bn on N pier; no lts. Best suited to shoal draft and bilge keelers. Hr Mr ☎ (01261) 842477 (home, part-time), £5. **Town** V, R, Bar, ✉. Note: 8ca ENE are Y ⚓s.

PORTKNOCKIE, Banff, 57°42'·30N 02°51'·70W. AC 222. HW +0045 on Dover, −0135 and ht −0·3m on Aberdeen; ML 2·3m; Duration 0555; access at all states of tide at ent. Good shelter in one of the safest hbrs on S side of Moray Firth, but care needed entering in strong N'ly winds. Scend is often experienced. Ldg lts, conspic FW, approx 148°, to ent. W mark on S pier hd. Orange street lts surround the hbr. Most of inner hbr dries, so berth at W or N jetties on firm sand. Hr Mr ☎ (01542) 840833; Facilities: Slip, AB £5, FW, Sh; Dr ☎ 840272. **Town** EC Wed; Ⓑ, P & D, ✉, V, Bar.

BUCKIE   10-7-10

Banff 57°40'·84N 02°57'·63W

CHARTS
AC 1462, 222, 115; OS 28

TIDES
+0040 Dover; ML 2·4; Duration 0550; Zone 0 (UT)

Standard Port ABERDEEN (←)

Times				Height (metres)			
High Water		Low Water		MHWS	MHWN	MLWN	MLWS
0200	0900	0400	0900	4·3	3·4	1·6	0·6
1400	2100	1600	2100				
Differences BUCKIE							
−0130	−0145	−0125	−0140	−0·2	−0·2	0·0	+0·1

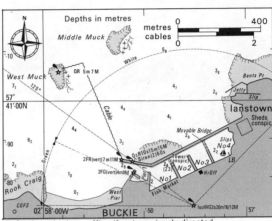

⚠ Apply to harbour office if not previously directed

SHELTER
Good in all weathers, but in strong NNW to NE winds there is a dangerous swell over the bar at hbr ent; access H24. Berth in No 4 basin; see Hr Mr if drawbridge closed.

NAVIGATION
WPT 57°41'·32N 02°58'·80W, 306°/126° from/to ent, 0·80M. Beware W Muck (QR 5m tripod, 7M), Middle Muck and E Muck Rks, 3ca off shore.

LIGHTS AND MARKS
Ldg lts lead 125° clear of W Muck; front Oc R 10s 15m 15M, W tr; rear Iso WG 2s 20m 16/12M, W tr, R top. NB: This line does not lead into hbr ent; but 2FG (vert) on W pier in transit with same Iso WG 2s do lead 119° to ent (24m wide). White tr of ice plant on pier 2 is conspic. Entry sigs on N pier:
3 Ⓡ lts = hbr closed. Traffic is controlled by VHF.

RADIO TELEPHONE
VHF Ch 12 16 (H24)

TELEPHONE (01542)
Hr Mr 831700; MRCC (01224) 592334; ⌗ (01343) 552861; Marinecall 0891 500 451; Police 832222; Dr 831555.

FACILITIES
No 4 Basin AB £6, FW; **Services:** D & P (delivery), BY, ME, EI, Sh, CH, ACA, SM, BH, Slip, C (15 ton), Gas.
Town EC Wed; V, Bar, Ⓑ, ✉, ⇌ (bus to Elgin), ✈ (Aberdeen or Inverness).

ADJACENT HARBOUR (2M ENE of BUCKIE)

FINDOCHTY, Banff, 57°41'·96N 02°54'·20W. AC 222. HW +0045 on Dover, −0140 on Aberdeen; HW ht −0·2m on Aberdeen; ML 2·3m; Duration 0550. Ent is approx 2ca W of conspic church/belfry. 1ca N of ent, leave Beacon Rk (3m high) to stbd. Ldg lts, FW, lead approx 166° into Outer Basin which dries and has many rky outcrops. Ent faces N and is 20m wide; unlit white bn at hd of W pier. Good shelter in inner basin which has 3 pontoons for 100 yachts; AB £10. Access (1·5m draft) HW ± 4. Hr Mr ☎ (01542) 831466 (home, part-time). **Town** V, R, Bar, ✉, Ⓑ.

7

LOSSIEMOUTH   10-7-11

Moray 57°43'·43N 03°16'·54W

CHARTS
AC 1462, 223; OS 28
TIDES
+0040 Dover; ML 2·3; Duration 0605; Zone 0 (UT)

Standard Port ABERDEEN (←—)

Times				Height (metres)			
High Water		Low Water		MHWS	MHWN	MLWN	MLWS
0200	0900	0400	0900	4·3	3·4	1·6	0·6
1400	2100	1600	2100				
Differences LOSSIEMOUTH							
–0125	–0200	–0130	–0130	–0·2	–0·2	0·0	0·0

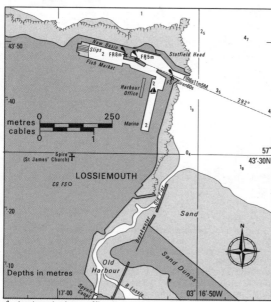

▲ Apply to harbour office if not previously directed

SHELTER
Very good in winds from SSE to NW. In strong N to SE winds appr to ent can be dangerous, with swell in outer hbr. Turn hard port for marina in S Basin, dredged 2m; access HW±4. But chan and Basin are prone to silting; a vessel drawing 2m would have little clearance at LWS ±1. West (or New) Basin is for commercial and FVs.
NAVIGATION
WPT 57°43'·40N 03°16'·00W, 097°/277° from/to ent, 0·30M. Rks to N and S of hbr ent; appr from E. Near ent, beware current from R Lossie setting in N'ly direction and causing confused water in N to SE winds at sp.
LIGHTS AND MARKS
Ldg lts 292°, both FR 5/8m; S pier hd Fl R 6s 11m 5M. Traffic sigs:
B ● at S pier (Ⓡ over Fl R 6s) = hbr closed.
RADIO TELEPHONE
VHF Ch 12 16 HO. Call before ent/dep due to restricted visibility in entrance.
TELEPHONE (01343)
Hr Mr 813066/HN 814696; MRCC (01224) 592334; ⌗ (0131) 4697400 or (01343) 552861; Marinecall 0891 500451; Police 812022; Dr 812277.
FACILITIES
Marina (43), ☎ 813066, £11.28 inc AC, FW; Hbr ME, EI, Sh, C, SM (see Hr Mr); Lossiemouth SC ☎ 812928; Hbr Service Stn ☎ 813001, Mon-Fri 0800-2030, Sat 0800-1800, Sun 0930-1730, P & D cans, Gas. Services: CH, Slip. Town EC Thurs; V, R, Bar, ✉, Ⓑ, ⇌ (bus to Elgin), ✈ (Inverness).

HOPEMAN   10-7-12

Moray 57°42'·72N 03°26'·22W

CHARTS
AC 1462, 223; OS 28
TIDES
+0050 Dover; ML 2·4; Duration 0610; Zone 0 (UT)

Standard Port ABERDEEN (←—)

Times				Height (metres)			
High Water		Low Water		MHWS	MHWN	MLWN	MLWS
0200	0900	0400	0900	4·3	3·4	1·6	0·6
1400	2100	1600	2100				
Differences HOPEMAN							
–0120	–0150	–0135	–0120	–0·2	–0·2	0·0	0·0

SHELTER
Once in SW basin, shelter good from all winds; but hbr dries, access HW ± 2 (for 1·5m draft). Ent is difficult in winds from NE to SE. A popular yachting hbr with AB and good facilities; run by Grampian Regional Council.
NAVIGATION
WPT 57°42'·68N, 03°26'·50W, 263°/083° from/to ent, 0·17M. Dangerous rks lie off hbr ent. Do not attempt entry in heavy weather. Beware salmon stake nets E and W of hbr (Mar to Aug) and lobster pot floats.
LIGHTS AND MARKS
Ldg lts 081°, FR 3/4m; S pier hd FG 4s 8m 4M. All lit only 1 Aug – 30 Apr.
RADIO TELEPHONE
None.
TELEPHONE (01343)
Hr Mr 830650 (home, part-time); MRCC (01224) 592334; ⌗ 552745; Marinecall 0891 500 451; Police 830222; Dr 543141.
FACILITIES
Hbr AB £10, D, FW, Slip.
Services: CH, ME, Gas, Sh, EI, P (cans).
Town EC Wed; V, R, Bar, ✉, Ⓑ, ⇌ (bus to Elgin), ✈ (Inverness).

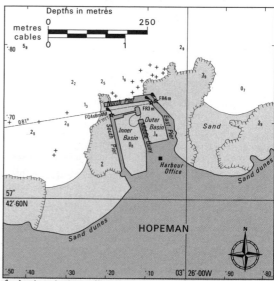

▲ Apply to harbour office if not previously directed

BURGHEAD
10-7-13

Moray 57°42'·08N 03°29'·93W

CHARTS
AC 1462, 223; OS 28

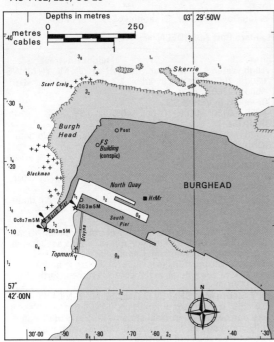

⚓ Apply to harbour office if not previously directed

TIDES
+0035 Dover; ML 2·4; Duration 0610; Zone 0 (UT)

Standard Port ABERDEEN (←—)

Times				Height (metres)			
High Water		Low Water		MHWS	MHWN	MLWN	MLWS
0200	0900	0400	0900	4·3	3·4	1·6	0·6
1400	2100	1600	2100				
Differences BURGHEAD							
−0120	−0150	−0135	−0120	−0·2	−0·2	0·0	0·0

SHELTER
One of the few Moray Firth hbrs open in strong E winds. Go alongside where available and contact Hr Mr. Can become very congested with FVs.

NAVIGATION
WPT 57°42'·30N 03°30'·30W, 317°/137° from/to N pier lt QR, 0·28M. Chan is variable due to sand movement. Appr from SW. Access HW ±4.

LIGHTS AND MARKS
No ldg lts but night ent is safe after identifying the N pier lts: QR 3m 5M and Oc 8s 7m 5M. S pier hd QG 3m 5M.

RADIO TELEPHONE
Hr Mr VHF Ch 12 14 16 (HO and when vessel due).

TELEPHONE (01343)
Hr Mr 835337; MRCC (01224) 592334; ☷ 552745; Marinecall 0891 500 451; Dr 812277.

FACILITIES
Hbr £10, D, FW, AB, C (50 ton mobile), L, Slip, BY, Sh.
Town EC Thurs; Bar, ☒, V, P (cans), Ⓑ, ⇌ (bus to Elgin), ✈ (Inverness).

FINDHORN
10-7-14

Moray 57°39'·66N 03°37'·38W

CHARTS
AC 223; OS 27

TIDES
+0110 Dover; ML 2·5; Duration 0615; Zone 0 (UT)

Standard Port ABERDEEN (←—)

Times				Height (metres)			
High Water		Low Water		MHWS	MHWN	MLWN	MLWS
0200	0900	0400	0900	4·3	3·4	1·6	0·6
1400	2100	1600	2100				
Differences FINDHORN							
−0120	−0150	−0135	−0130	0·0	−0·1	0·0	+0·1

SHELTER
⚓ off N pier or dry out alongside, inside piers and ask at YC. Do not attempt entry in strong NW/NE winds or with big swell running.
THE OLD BAR. The original mouth of Findhorn River 4M SW of Findhorn gives excellent shelter in all weathers. Chan changes; local knowledge needed.

NAVIGATION
WPT 57°40'·31N 03°38'·55W, SWM spar buoy, 313°/133° from/to Ee Point, 0·85M. From WPT, proceed SSE to the buoys marking the gap in the sand bar; thence ESE via SHM buoy to 3 poles with PHM topmarks to be left a boat's length to port. Once past The Ee, turn port inside G buoys.

LIGHTS AND MARKS
Unlit. There is a windsock on FS by The Ee.

RADIO TELEPHONE
VHF Ch M *Chadwick Base* (when racing in progress).

TELEPHONE (01309)
MRCC (01224) 592334; ☷ (01343) 552745; G.Mackenzie (Findhorn Pilot) 690546; Marinecall 0891 500 451; Police 672224; Dr 672221.

FACILITIES
Royal Findhorn YC ☎ 690247, M, FW, Bar;
Services: BY, L, M, AC, FW, Slip, C (16 ton), P & D (cans), El, ME, CH, ACA, Gas, Sh.
Town V, R, Bar, ☒, Ⓑ, ⇌ (Forres), ✈ (Inverness).

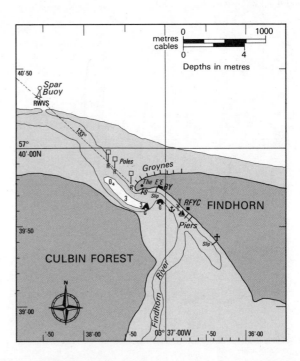

NAIRN   10-7-15

Nairn 57°35'·63N 03°51'·56W

CHARTS
AC 1462, 223; OS 27
TIDES
+0110 Dover; ML 2·2; Duration 0615; Zone 0 (UT)

Standard Port ABERDEEN (←—)

Times				Height (metres)			
High Water		Low Water		MHWS	MHWN	MLWN	MLWS
0200	0900	0400	0900	4·3	3·4	1·6	0·6
1400	2100	1600	2100				
Differences NAIRN							
−0120	−0150	−0135	−0130	0·0	−0·1	0·0	+0·1

SHELTER
Good, but entry difficult in fresh NNE'ly. Pontoons in hbr with ♥ berths. Best entry HW ± 1½. No commercial ships.
NAVIGATION
WPT 57°35'·90N 03°51'·80W, 335°/155° from/to ent, 0·3M. The approach dries to 100m off the pierheads. Inside, the best water is to the E side of the river chan.
LIGHTS AND MARKS
Lt ho on E pier hd, Oc WRG 4s 6m 5M, vis G shore-100°, W100°-207°, R207°-shore. Keep in W sector. McDermott Base, 4·5M to the W, has a large conspic cream-coloured building; also useful if making for Inverness Firth.
RADIO TELEPHONE
None. Ch M (weekends only).
TELEPHONE (01667)
Hr Mr 454704; MRCC (01224) 592334; ⌗ (01343) 552745; Clinic 455092; Marinecall 0891 500 451; Police 452222; Dr 453421.
FACILITIES
Nairn Basin AB £10, FW (standpipes), Slip, AC (110 volts), P, D; **Nairn SC** ☎ 453897, Bar.
Town EC Wed; V, R, Bar, ⊠, Ⓑ, ⇌, ✈ (Inverness).

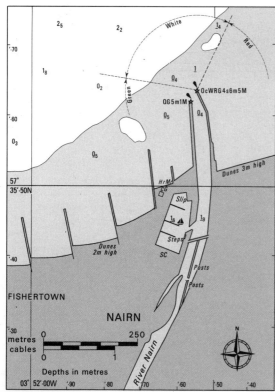

NAIRN

⚓ Nairn, apply to SC

INVERNESS   10-7-16

Inverness 57°29'·75N 04°14'·08W

CHARTS
AC 1078, 1077, 223; OS 26/27
TIDES
+0100 Dover; ML 2·7; Duration 0620; Zone 0 (UT)

Standard Port ABERDEEN (←—)

Times				Height (metres)			
High Water		Low Water		MHWS	MHWN	MLWN	MLWS
0300	1000	0000	0700	4·3	3·4	1·6	0·6
1500	2200	1200	1900				
Differences INVERNESS							
−0050	−0150	−0200	−0150	+0·5	+0·3	+0·2	+0·1
FORTROSE							
−0125	−0125	−0125	−0125	0·0	0·0	No data	
CROMARTY							
−0120	−0155	−0155	−0120	0·0	0·0	+0·1	+0·2
INVERGORDON							
−0105	−0200	−0200	−0110	+0·1	+0·1	+0·1	+0·1
DINGWALL							
−0045	−0145	No data		+0·1	+0·2	No data	

SHELTER
Good in all weathers. Berth in R Ness at Longman Yacht Haven (3m at LW) or alongside quays; or, via sea lock, at two marinas in Caledonian Canal, ent to which can be difficult in strong tides (see 10.8.15). Fortrose and Avoch (see below) are safe ⚓s at the ent to Inverness Firth.
NAVIGATION
WPT Meikle Mee SHM By Fl G 3s, 57°30'·28N 04°11'·93W, 070°/250° from/to Longman Pt bn, 0·74M. Ent to R Ness is very narrow but deep. Tidal streams strong S of Craigton Pt (E-going stream at sp exceeds 5kn). Beware marine farms S of Avoch (off chartlet).
LIGHTS AND MARKS
Longman Pt bn Fl WR 2s 7m 5/4M, vis W078°-258°, R258°-078°. Craigton Pt lt, Fl WRG 4s 6m 11/7M vis W312°-048°, R048°-064°, W064°-085°, G085°-shore. Ent to Canal marked by QR and Iso G 4s on ends of training walls.
RADIO TELEPHONE
Call: *Inverness Hbr Office* VHF Ch 06 12 16 (Mon-Fri: 0900-1700 LT). Inverness Boat Centre Ch 80 M (0900-1800 LT). Caley Marina Ch 80 M.
Ch 74 is used by all stns on the Canal. Call: *Clachnaharry Sea Lock*; or for office: *Caledonian Canal* .
TELEPHONE (01463)
Hr Mr 715715; Clachnaharry Sea Lock 713896; Canal Office 233140; MRCC (01224) 592334; ⌗ (0141) 887 9369; Marinecall 0891 500 451; Police 239191; Dr 234151.
FACILITIES
Longman Yacht Haven (15+5 visitors) ☎ 715715 AC, D, ME, FW, access H24 (3m at LW);
Citadel and Shore Street Quays (R Ness) ☎ 715715, AB, P, D, L, FW, ME, EI;
Seaport Marina, (20 + 20 visitors) ☎ 239475, Fax 710942, £10, AC, D, FW, Gas, Gaz, C (40 ton), access HW±4;
Caley Marina (25 + 25 visitors) ☎ 236539, £10, ACA, AC, C (20 ton), CH, D, ME, EI, Sh, FW;
Services: Slip, M, ME, EI, C (100 ton), CH, FW, P, SM, Gas.
Town EC Wed; V, R, Bar, ⊠, Ⓑ, ⇌, ✈.

MINOR HARBOURS IN INVERNESS FIRTH

FORTROSE, Ross and Cromarty, 57°34'·73N 04°07'·95W. AC 1078. HW +0055 on Dover; ML 2·5m; Duration 0620. See 10.7.16. Small drying unlit hbr, well protected by Chanonry Ness to E; access HW±2, limited space. Follow ldg line 296°, Broomhill Ho (conspic on hill to NW) in line with school spire until abeam SPM buoy; then turn W to avoid Craig an Roan rks (1·8m) ESE of ent. Chanonry Pt lt, Oc 6s 12m 15M, obscd 073°-shore. Hr Mr ☎ (01381) 620861; Dr ☎ 620909. Facilities: EC Thurs; AB £3, L, M, P, D, Slip, Gas, R, V, ⊠, Ⓑ; **Chanonry SC** (near pier) ☎ 621010.

AVOCH, Ross & Cromarty, 57°34'·05N 04°09'·85W. AC 1078. Tides as Fortrose (1·25M to the ENE). Hbr dries, mostly on the N side, but is bigger than Fortrose; access HW±2. Small craft may stay afloat at nps against the S pier, which has 2FR (vert) at E-facing ent. Hr Mr ☎ (01381) 620378, AB, FW. Village: ⊠, V, R, Bar, P & D (cans), ME.

INVERNESS *continued*

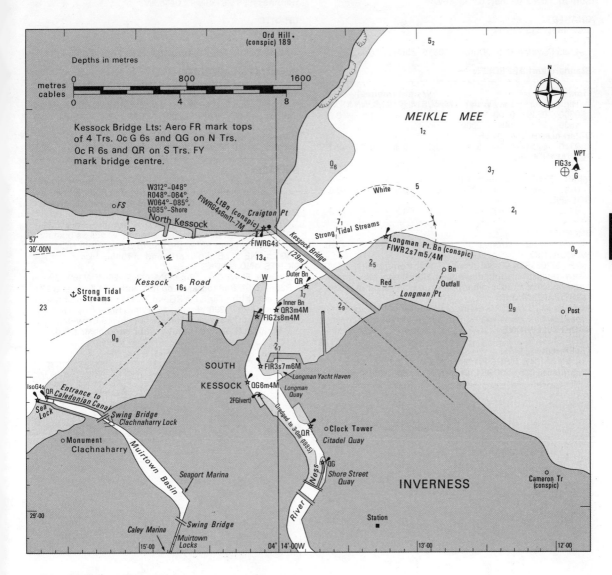

Ord Hill.
(conspic) 189

Depths in metres

metres
cables

0   800   1600
0   4   8

Kessock Bridge Lts: Aero FR mark tops
of 4 Trs. Oc G 6s and QG on N Trs.
Oc R 6s and QR on S Trs. FY
mark bridge centre.

MEIKLE MEE

W312°–048°,
R048°–064°,
W064°–085°,
G085°–Shore

LtBn (conspic) Craigton Pt
FlWRG4s6m11-7M

FlG3s   WPT
G

White

Strong Tidal Streams

North Kessock
FS
G
57°
30'·00N
FlWRG4s
Kessock Bridge (29m)
FlWR2s7m5/4M
Longman Pt. Bn (conspic)
13₄
Outer Bn
QR
W
Kessock   Road
16₅
Inner Bn
QR3m4M
FlG2s8m4M
Red
Longman Pt
Bn
Outfall
23
Strong Tidal
Streams
R
0₉
2₇
FlR3s7m6M
SOUTH
KESSOCK
Longman Yacht Haven
QG6m4M
Longman
Quay
2FG(vert)
IsoG4s
QR
Entrance to
Caledonian Canal
Sea
Lock
Swing Bridge
Clachnaharry Lock
Dredged to 3·0m (085°)
QR
Clock Tower
Citadel Quay
Monument
Clachnaharry
Muirtown Basin
QG
Shore Street
Quay
INVERNESS
Cameron Tr
(conspic)
Seaport Marina
River Ness
29'·00
Caley Marina
Swing Bridge
Muirtown
Locks
Station
15'·00
04' 14'·00W
13'·00
12'·00

5₂

1₂

O₆

5

3₇

2₁

O₉

7₁

2₅

O₉

Post

2₉

1₇

PORTMAHOMACK   10-7-17

Ross and Cromarty 57°50'·30N 03°49'·70W

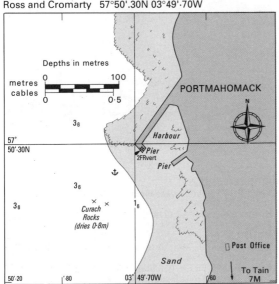

Depths in metres

metres
cables

0   100
0   0·5

PORTMAHOMACK

3₆

Harbour

57°
50'·30N

Pier
2FRvert

Pier

3₆

3₆

1₆

Curach
Rocks
(dries 0·8m)

Post Office

Sand

50'·20   '·80   03' 49'·70W   '·60   To Tain
7M

CHARTS
AC 223, 115; OS 21
TIDES
+0035 Dover; ML 2·5; Duration 0600; Zone 0 (UT); See
10.7.18 for Differences
SHELTER
Good, but uncomfortable in SW/NW winds. Access to hbr
at HW only. Hbr dries but good ⚓ close SW of pier.
NAVIGATION
WPT SPM buoy, FlY 5s, 57°53'·03N 03°47'·02W, 346°/166°
from/to Tarbat Ness lt, 1·13M. Beware Curach Rks which
lie from 2ca SW of pier to the shore. Rks extend N and W
of the pier. Beware lobster pot floats and salmon nets N
of hbr. Tain Range activity shown by R flags or R lts.
LIGHTS AND MARKS
Tarbert Ness lt ho Fl (4) 30s 53m 24M, W twr R bands, is
2·6M to NE of hbr. Pier hd 2 FR (vert) 7m 5M.
RADIO TELEPHONE
None.
TELEPHONE (01862)
Hr Mr 871441; MRCC (01224) 592334; ☰ (01463) 222787;
Marinecall 0891 500 451; Dr 892759.
FACILITIES
Hbr, M, L, FW, AB. **Town** EC Wed; R, V, Bar, ✉, ⇌ (bus to
Tain), ✈ (Inverness).

HELMSDALE   10-7-18

Sutherland 58°06'.85N 03°38'.80W

CHARTS
AC 1462, 115; OS 17
TIDES
+0035 Dover; ML 2·2; Duration 0615; Zone 0 (UT)

Standard Port ABERDEEN (←)

Times				Height (metres)			
High Water		Low Water		MHWS	MHWN	MLWN	MLWS
0300	0800	0200	0800	4·3	3·4	1·6	0·6
1500	2000	1400	2000				
Differences HELMSDALE							
−0140	−0200	−0150	−0135	−0.5	−0.4	−0.1	−0.1
PORTMAHOMACK							
−0120	−0210	−0140	−0110	−0.2	−0.1	+0.1	+0.1
MEIKLE FERRY (Dornoch Firth)							
−0100	−0140	−0120	−0055	+0.1	0.0	−0.1	0.0
GOLSPIE							
−0130	−0215	−0155	−0130	−0.3	−0.3	−0.1	0.0

SHELTER
Good, except in strong E/SE'lies. AB on NW pier, approx 1m.
NAVIGATION
WPT 58°06'.61N 03°38'.3W, 133°/313° from/to ent, 0·35M.
Beware spate coming down river after heavy rain. Shoal
both sides of chan and bar builds up when river in spate.
LIGHTS AND MARKS
Ldg lts 313°. Front FG (= hbr open) or FR (= hbr closed);
rear FG; both on W masts. By day Or disc on each mast.
RADIO TELEPHONE
VHF Ch 12 16.
TELEPHONE (01431)
Hr Mr 821347; MRCC (01224) 592334; ⌗ (01955) 3650;
Marinecall 0891 500 451; Dr 821221, or 821225 (Home).

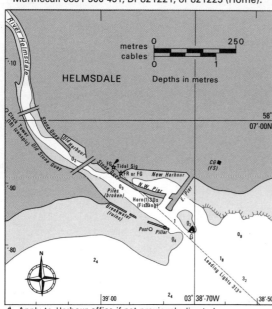

⚓ Apply to Harbour office if not previously directed

FACILITIES
Hbr AB £13.80, M (See Hr Mr), FW, Slip.
Town EC Wed; P, D, Gas, V, R, Bar, ✉, Ⓑ (Brora), ⇌ (Wick).

ADJACENT HARBOUR

LYBSTER, Caithness, 58°17'·75N 03°17'·30W. AC 115. HW
+0020 on Dover; −0150 sp, −0215 np on Aberdeen; HW ht
−0.6m on Aberdeen; ML 2·1m; Duration 0620. Excellent
shelter in basin (SW corner of inner hbr); AB on W side of
pier in about 1·2m. Most of hbr dries to sand/mud and is
much used by FVs; no bollards on N wall. Appr on about
350°. Beware rks close on E side of ent; narrow (10m) ent
is difficult in strong E to S winds. Min depth 2·5m in ent.
S pier hd, Oc R 6s 10m 3M, occas in fishing season.
Facilities: FW on W quay. Town EC Thurs; Bar, D, P, R, V.

WICK   10-7-19

Caithness 58°26'·38N 03°04'·63W

CHARTS
AC 1462, 115; OS 12
TIDES
+0010 Dover; ML 2·0; Duration 0625; Zone 0 (UT)

Standard Port ABERDEEN

Times				Height (metres)			
High Water		Low Water		MHWS	MHWN	MLWN	MLWS
0300	0800	0200	0800	4·3	3·4	1·6	0·6
1500	2000	1400	2000				
Differences WICK							
−0155	−0220	−0210	−0220	−0.9	−0.7	−0.2	−0.1

SHELTER
Good, except in strong NNE to SSE winds. Berth where
directed in the Inner Hbr, 2·4m. NB: The River Hbr is
leased and must *not* be entered without prior approval.
NAVIGATION
WPT 58°26'·20N 03°·30W, 104°/284° from/to S pier lt,
0·72M. Hbr ent dangerous in strong E winds as boats
have to turn port 90° at the end of S pier. Unlit NCM bn,
300m ENE of LB slip, marks end of ruined bkwtr.
LIGHTS AND MARKS
S pier lt, Fl WRG 3s 12m 5/3M, G253°-269°, W269°-286°,
R286°-329°, Bell (occas). Ldg lts , both FR 5/8m, lead 234°
into outer hbr. Dir lt FWRG 9m 10/7M on N end of bridge,
W sector 287°-290°, leads 288·5° into River Hbr. Tfc sigs:
B ● (Ⓖ) at CG stn on S Head = hbr closed by weather.
B ● (Ⓡ) at S pier hd = caution; hbr temp obstructed.

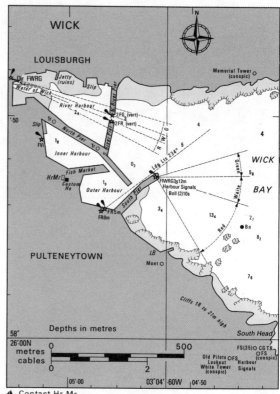

⚓ Contact Hr Mr

RADIO TELEPHONE
VHF Ch 14 16 (when vessel expected).
TELEPHONE (01955)
Hr Mr 602030; MRSC (01856) 873268; ⌗ (0141) 887 9369;
Police 603551; Ⓗ 602434, 602261.
FACILITIES
Inner Hbr Slip, L, ME, AB (see Hr Mr), V; Outer Hbr L, ME;
Fish Jetty D, L, FW, CH;
Services: ME, EI, Sh, CH, Slip, Gas, C (15 to 100 ton).
Town EC Wed; P, V, R, Bar, ✉, Ⓑ, ⇌, ✈.

OTHER HARBOURS ON THE NORTH WEST SIDE OF THE MORAY FIRTH

CROMARTY FIRTH, Ross and Cromarty, 57°41'·20N 04°02'·00W. AC 1889, 1890. HW +0100 on Dover; ML 2·5m; Duration 0625. See 10.7.16. Excellent hbr extending 7·5M W, past Invergordon, then 9M SW. Good shelter always available, depending on wind direction. Beware rks and reefs round N and S Sutor at the ent; many unlit oil rig mooring buoys and fish cages within the firth. Cromarty Village Hbr (partly dries) is formed by 2 piers, but congested with small craft and probably foul ground; ⚓ 2ca W of S pier hd in approx 6m. Hr Mr ☎ (01381) 600502. Cromarty lt ho, on the Ness, Oc WR 10s 18m 15/11M, R079°–088°, W088°–275°, obsc by N Sutor when brg < 253°. *Cromarty Firth Port Control* VHF Ch 11 16 13 (H24) ☎ (01349) 852308; ⌧ (0141) 887 9369. **Invergordon Boating Club**. Facilities: AB, Bar, C (3 ton), D, FW, ✉, P, R, V, Gas, L; EC Wed. Ferry: Local to Nigg; also Invergordon-Kirkwall.

DORNOCH FIRTH, Ross and Cromarty/Sutherland. 57°51'·30N 03°59'·30W. AC 223, 115. HW +0115 on Dover; ML 2·5m; Duration 0605. See 10.7.17. Excellent shelter but difficult ent. There are many shifting sandbanks, especially near the ent, between N edge of Whiteness Sands and S edge of Gizzen Briggs. ⚓s in 7m ¾M ESE of Dornoch Pt (sheltered from NE swell by Gizzen Briggs); in 7m 2ca SSE of Ard na Cailc; in 3·3m 1M below Bonar Bridge. Firth extends 15M inland, but AC coverage ceases ¼M E of Ferry Pt. The A9 road bridge, 3·3M W of Dornoch Pt, with 11m clearance, has 3 spans lit on both sides; span centres show Iso 4s, N bank pier Iso G 4s, S bank pier Iso R 4s and 2 midstream piers QY. Tarbat Ness lt ho Fl (4) 30s 53m 24M. Fl R 5s lt shown when Tain firing range active. Very limited facilities at Ferrytown and Bonar Bridge. CG ☎ (01862) 810016.
Dornoch: EC Thur; V, P, ✉, Dr, Ⓑ, R, Bar.

GOLSPIE, Sutherland, 57°58'·73N 03°56'·70W. AC 223. HW +0045 on Dover; ML 2·3m; Duration 0610. See 10.7.18. Golspie pier projects 60m SE across foreshore with arm projecting SW at the hd, giving shelter during NE winds. Beware The Bridge, a bank (0·3m to 1·8m) running parallel to the shore ¼M to seaward of pier hd. Seas break heavily over The Bridge in NE winds. There are no lts. To enter, keep Duke of Sutherlands Memorial in line 316° with boathouse SW of pier, until church spire in village is in line 006° with hd of pier, then keep on those marks. Hbr gets very congested; good ⚓ off pier.
Town EC Wed; Bar, D, Dr, Ⓗ, L, M, P, Gas, ✉, R, ⇶, V, Ⓑ.

ANCHORAGES BETWEEN SCRABSTER AND CAPE WRATH

KYLE OF TONGUE, Sutherland, 58°32'·00N 04°22'·60W (ent). +0050 on Ullapool; HW ht –0·4m on Ullapool. The Kyle runs about 7M inland. Entry (see 10.7.5) should not be attempted in strong N winds. ⚓ at Talmine (W of Rabbit Is) protected from all but NE winds; at Skullomie Hr, protected from E winds; off Mol na Coinnle, a small bay on SE side of Eilean nan Ron, protected from W and N winds; off S of Rabbit Is, protected from W to N winds. No ldg lts/marks. Facilities: Limited supplies at Talmine (½M from slip) or at Coldbachie (1½M from Skullomie).

LOCH ERIBOLL, Sutherland, 58°32'·60N 04°37'·40W. AC 2076. HW –0345 on Dover; ML 2·7m; Duration 0610. See 10.8.7. Enter between Whiten Hd and Klourig Is in W sector of White Hd lt, Fl WR 3s, vis W030°–172°, R172°–191°, W191°–212°.In SW winds fierce squalls funnel down the loch. Yachts can enter Rispond Hbr, access approx HW ± 3, and dry out alongside; no lts/marks and very limited facilities. Good ⚓s: at Rispond Bay on W side of loch, ent good in all but E winds, in approx 5m; off Portnancon in 5·5m; at the head of the loch; at Camus an Duin and in bays to N and S of peninsula at Heilam on E side of loch.

SCRABSTER   10-7-20
Caithness 58°36'·63N 03°32'·52W

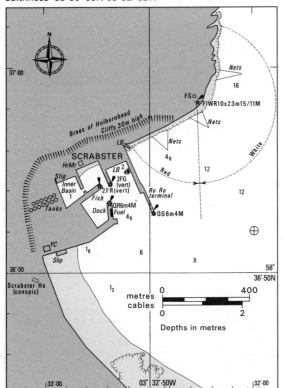

CHARTS
AC 1462, 2162, 1954; OS 12
TIDES
-0240 Dover; ML 3·2; Duration 0615; Zone 0 (UT)

Standard Port ABERDEEN (←—)

Times				Height (metres)			
High Water		Low Water		MHWS	MHWN	MLWN	MLWS
0300	1000	0100	0800	4·3	3·4	1·6	0·6
1500	2200	1300	2000				
Differences SCRABSTER							
–0455	–0510	–0500	–0445	+0·7	+0·3	+0·5	+0·2
STROMA							
–0320	–0320	–0320	–0320	–1·2	–1·1	–0·3	–0·1
DUNCANSBY HEAD							
–0320	–0320	–0320	–0320	–1·2	–1·0		No data

SHELTER
Very good except for swell in NW winds. ⚓ is not recommended. Secure alongside NE wall and contact Hr Mr. Yachts normally use Inner Basin.
NAVIGATION
WPT 58°36'·60N 03°32'·00W, 098°/278° from/to E pier lt, 0·25M. Can be entered at all tides in all weathers. Do not confuse hbr lts with those of Thurso. Beware FVs, merchant ships and the Orkney ferries.
LIGHTS AND MARKS
There are no ldg marks/lts. Entry is simple once the pier lt, QG 6m 4M, has been located.
RADIO TELEPHONE
VHF Ch 12 16 (0800-2200LT).
TELEPHONE (01847)
Hr Mr 892779; MRSC (01856) 873268; ⌧ (01955) 603650; Marinecall 0891 500 451; Police 893222; Dr 893154.
FACILITIES
Hbr Slip, D, P (cans), L, FW, ME, El, C (30 ton mobile), CH, AB, R, Bar; **Pentland Firth YC** M, R, Bar. **Thurso** EC Thurs; V, R, Bar, ✉, Ⓑ, ⇶, ✈ (Wick). Ferry to Stromness.

ORKNEY ISLANDS   10-7-21

The Orkney Islands number about 70, of which some 24 are inhabited. They extend from Duncansby Hd 5 to 50M NNE, and are mostly low-lying, but Hoy in the SW of the group reaches 475m (1560ft). Coasts are generally rky and much indented, but there are many sandy beaches. A passage with least width of about 3M runs NW/SE through the group. The islands are separated from Scotland by Pentland Firth, a very dangerous stretch of water (see 10.7.5). The principal island is Mainland (or Pomona) on which stands Kirkwall, the capital. Severe gales blow in winter and early spring (see 10.7.5). The climate is mild but windy, and very few trees grow. There are LBs at Longhope, Stromness and Kirkwall. There is a CG MRSC at Kirkwall, ☎ (01856) 873268, with Auxiliary (Watch & Rescue) Stns at Longhope (S Walls), Brough Ness (S Ronaldsay), Stromness and Deerness (both Mainland), Westray, Papa Westray, N Ronaldsay, Sanday, and all inhabited isles except Egilsay and Wyre.

CHARTS
AC 2249, 2250 and 2162 at medium scale. For larger scale charts, see under individual hbrs. OS sheets 5 and 6.

TIDES
Aberdeen (10.6.17) is the Standard Port. Tidal streams are strong, particularly in Pentland Firth and in the firths and sounds among the islands (see 10.7.5).

SHELTER
There are piers (fender board advised) at all the main islands. Yachts can pay 4 or 14 day hbr dues (£8.71 or £17.94 in 1995) to berth on any pier in Orkney except St Margaret's Hope. Some of the many ⚓s are listed below:

Mainland
SCAPA BAY: good except in S winds. No yacht berths alongside pier due to heavy hbr traffic. Only ents to Scapa Flow are via Hoy Snd, Hoxa Snd or W of Flotta.
ST MARYS (known as Holm, pronounced Ham): N side of Kirk Sound; ⚓ in B of Ayre or berth E side of pier HW±4. P & D (cans), ✉, Bar, R, Bus to Kirkwall & Burwick Ferry.
KIRK SOUND (E ent): ⚓ N of Lamb Holt; beware fish cages.
DEER SOUND: ⚓ in Pool of Mirkady or off pier on NW side of sound; very good shelter, no facilities.

Burray
E WEDDEL SOUND: ⚓ to E of pier in E'lies, sheltered by No 4 Churchill Barrier; pier is exposed in strong W'lies. P & D (cans), BY, Slip, V, ✉, Bar, R, Bus to Kirkwall.
HUNDA SOUND: good ⚓ in all winds.

S Ronaldsay
ST MARGARET'S HOPE: ⚓ in centre of bay; beware Flotta ferries at the pier, AB £5.87. Hr Mr ☎ 831454; Dr 831206. FW, P & D (cans), V, R, Bar, ✉, Bus Kirkwall.
WIDEWALL B: ⚓ sheltered from all but SW winds

Flotta
Berth on Sutherland Pier, SW of oil terminal. Hr Mr ☎ 701411. P & D (cans), V, ✉.

Hoy
LONG HOPE: ⚓ E of S Ness pier, used by steamers, or berth on pier (safest at slack water) ☎ 701273; Dr 701209. Facilities: FW, P & D (cans), ✉, V, Bar.
LYNESS: berth on pier; keep clear of disused piles. Also ⚓ in Ore Bay. Hr Mr ☎ 791228. FW, P & D (cans), Bar, ✉.
PEGAL B: good ⚓ except in strong W winds.

Rousay
WYRE SOUND: ⚓ E of Rousay pier, or berth on it. ✉, V, R.

Eday
FERSNESS B: good holding, sheltered from S winds.
BACKALAND B: berth on pier clear of ferry or ⚓ to NW. Beware cross tides. FW, P & D, V, ✉.
CALF SND: ⚓ in Carrick B; good shelter from SW-NW'lies.

Westray
RAPNESS: Berth on pier, clear of Ro-Ro. Open to SSW.
B OF MOCLETT (Papa Westray): Good ⚓ but open to S.
S WICK (Papa Wray): ⚓ off the old pier or ESE of pier off Holm of Papa.

Sanday
LOTH B: berth on pier, clear of ferry. Beware strong tides.
KETTLETOFT B: ⚓ in bay or berth on pier; very exposed to SE'lies. Hr Mr ☎ 600227. P & D (cans), ✉, Ⓑ, V, hotel.
NORTH BAY: on NW side of island, exposed to NW.
OTTERSWICK: good ⚓ except in N or E winds.

N Ronaldsay
SOUTH B: ⚓ in middle of bay or berth on pier; open to S and W, and subject to swell. V, ✉.
LINKLET B: ⚓ off jetty at N of bay, open to E.

OTHER HARBOURS AND ⚓s. Auskerry see facing page. For Houton Bay, Shapinsay and Pierowall, see after 10.7.24 .

NAVIGATION
Navigation is easy in clear weather, apart from the strong tidal streams in all the firths and sounds. The associated races and overfalls are off Brough of Birsay (Mainland), Noup Head (Westray) and Dennis Head (N Ronaldsay); see 10.7.5. Beware many lobster pots (creels).

LIGHTS AND MARKS
The main hbrs and sounds are well lit; for details see 10.7.4. Powerful lts are shown from Cantick Hd, Graemsay Island, Copinsay, Auskerry, Kirkwall, Brough of Birsay, Sanday Island, N Ronaldsay and Noup Hd.

RADIO TELEPHONE
Orkney Hbrs Navigation Service (call: *Orkney Hbr Radio*, Ch 11 16 (H24)) covers Scapa Flow, Wide Firth and Shapinsay Sound. Forecasts are broadcast on Ch 11 at 0915 and 1715. For other local stations see individual hbrs. The local Coast Radio Station is Orkney Radio; call Ch 26 (H24), unreliably controlled from Wick Radio.

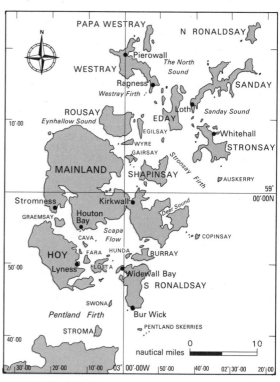

TELEPHONE Area Code for islands SW of Stronsay and Westray Firths is 01856; islands to the NE are 01857.

MEDICAL SERVICES
Doctors are available at Kirkwall, Stromness, Rousay, Hoy, Shapinsay, Eday, S and N Ronaldsay, Stronsay, Sanday and Westray (Pierowall); Papa Westray is looked after by Westray. The only hospital (and dentist) are at Kirkwall. Serious cases are flown to Aberdeen (1 hour).

SALMON CAGES
Beware salmon cages (may be marked by Y buoys/lts) at:

Rysa Sound	Pegal Bay (Hoy)
Lyrawa Bay	Hunda Sound
Ore Bay (Hoy)	Kirk Sound
Widewall Bay (S Ronaldsay)	Carness Bay
St Margaret's Hope	Bay of Ham

OYSTERS AND LONGLINES
Beware oysters and longlines at:

Widewall Bay	Bay of Firth
Swandister Bay	Damsay Sound
Water Sound	Millburn Bay (Gairsay)
Hunda Sound	Pierowall
Deer Sound	Bay of Skaill (Westray)
Inganess Bay	Longhope

KIRKWALL   10-7-22

Orkney Islands, Mainland 58°59'·33N 02°57'·60W

CHARTS
AC 1553, 2584, 2249, 2250; OS 6
TIDES
–0045 Dover; ML 1·7; Duration 0620; Zone 0 (UT)

Standard Port ABERDEEN (←)

Times				Height (metres)			
High Water		Low Water		MHWS	MHWN	MLWN	MLWS
0300	1100	0200	0900	4·3	3·4	1·6	0·6
1500	2300	1400	2100				
Differences KIRKWALL							
–0237	–0302	–0252	–0301	–1·3	–1·0	–0·3	–0·1
DEER SOUND							
–0245	–0245	–0245	–0245	–1·1	–0·9	–0·3	0·0
TINGWALL							
–0355	–0345	–0355	–0340	–1·2	–1·0	–0·3	–0·1

SHELTER
Good except in N winds or W gales when there is a surge at the ent. At SW end of main pier, enter inner hbr (very full in Jun/Jul); or safe ⚓ between pier and Crow Ness Pt.
NAVIGATION
WPT 59°01'·40N 02°57'·00W, 008°/188° from/to pier hd lt, 2·2M. Appr in W sector of pier hd lt. Bay is shoal to SW.

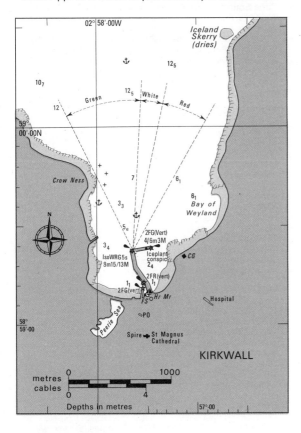

LIGHTS AND MARKS
Appr with St Magnus Cathedral (very conspic) brg 190°.
RADIO TELEPHONE
VHF Ch 12 16 (0900-1700LT). Orkney Hbrs Navigation Service, call: Orkney Hbr Radio Ch 11 16 (H24). Local weather on Ch 11 at 0915 and 1715LT.
TELEPHONE (01856)
Hr Mr 872292; Port Office 873636; Fuel 873105; MRSC 873268; ⌗ 872108 and (0141) 887 9369; Weather 873802; Marinecall 0891 500451; Police 872241; Dr 872763/873201.
FACILITIES
Pier P, D, FW, CH, C (mobile, 25 ton); N and E Quays M; Orkney SC ☎ 872331, M, L, C, AB, Slip.
Town EC Wed; P, D, ME, El, Sh, CH, V, Gas, R, Bar, ✉, Ⓑ, ▣, ⇌ (Ferry to Scrabster, bus to Thurso), ✈.

STRONSAY   10-7-23

Orkney Islands, Stronsay 59°08'·60N 02°35'·90W

CHARTS
AC 2622, 2250; OS 6
TIDES
–0140 Dover; ML 1·7; Duration 0620; Zone 0 (UT)

Standard Port ABERDEEN (←)

Times				Height (metres)			
High Water		Low Water		MHWS	MHWN	MLWN	MLWS
0300	1100	0200	0900	4·3	3·4	1·6	0·6
1500	2300	1400	2100				
Differences LOTH (Sanday)							
–0257	–0257	–0308	–0308	–1·0	–0·9	–0·2	+0·2
KETTLETOFT PIER (Sanday)							
–0230	–0230	–0225	–0225	–1·1	–0·9	–0·3	0·0
RAPNESS (Westray)							
–0410	–0410	–0410	–0410	–0·5	–0·6	0·0	0·0
PIEROWALL (Westray)							
–0355	–0355	–0350	–0350	–0·6	–0·6	–0·2	–0·1

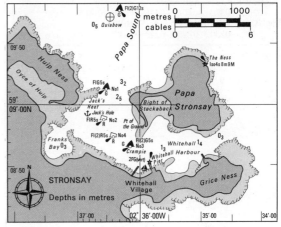

SHELTER
Good from all winds. Good ⚓ between seaward end of piers, or berth on outer end of either pier and contact Hr Mr. Many other sheltered ⚓s around the bay.
NAVIGATION
WPT 59°09'·85N 02°36'·20W, Quiabow SHM By, Fl (2) G 12s, 009°/189° from/to No 1 lt buoy, 6·5ca. 800m NE of Huip Ness is Quiabow, a submerged rk. Jack's Reef extends 400m E from Huip Ness, and is marked by No 1 SHM buoy Fl G 5. A bank extends 350m SW from Papa Stronsay. Crampie Shoal is in mid-chan, marked by No 3 buoy. The buoyed chan to Whitehall pier is dredged 3·5m. Spit to E of Whitehall pier extends 400m N. The E ent is narrow, shallow and should not be attempted.
LIGHTS AND MARKS
As chartlet. Pier hd lts, 2FG (vert).
RADIO TELEPHONE
See Kirkwall.
TELEPHONE (01857)
Hr Mr 616257; MRSC (01856) 873268; ⌗ (01856) 872108; Marinecall 0891 500451; Police (01856) 872241; Dr 616321.
FACILITIES
W Pier M, L, AB; Main Pier M, L, FW, AB.
Village (Whitehall) EC Thurs; P, D, V, Bar, ✉, Ⓑ, ⇌ (ferry to Scrabster, bus to Thurso), ✈.

ADJACENT HARBOUR

AUSKERRY, Orkney Islands, 59°02'·05N 02°34'·55W. AC 2250. HW –0010 on Dover, –0315 on Aberdeen, HW ht –1m on Aberdeen. Small island at ent to Stronsay Firth with small hbr on W side. Safe ent and good shelter except in SW winds. Ent has 3·5m; at pier 1·2m alongside pier. Yachts can lie secured between ringbolts at ent and the pier. Auskerry Sound and Stronsay Firth are dangerous with wind over tide. Auskerry lt at S end, Fl 20s 34m 18M, W tr. No facilities.

STROMNESS   10-7-24

Orkney Islands, Mainland 58°57'·81N 03°17'·62W

CHARTS
AC 2568, 2249; OS 6
TIDES
-0145 Dover; ML 2·0; Duration 0620; Zone 0 (UT)

Standard Port ABERDEEN (←)

Times				Height (metres)			
High Water		Low Water		MHWS	MHWN	MLWN	MLWS
0300	1100	0200	0900	4·3	3·4	1·6	0·6
1500	2300	1400	2100				
Differences STROMNESS							
−0430	−0355	−0415	−0420	−0·7	−0·8	−0·1	−0·1
ST MARY'S (Scapa Flow)							
−0345	−0345	−0345	−0345	−0·1	−0·1	−0·2	−0·2
BURRAY NESS (Burray)							
−0200	−0200	−0155	−0155	−1·0	−0·9	−0·3	0·0
WIDEWALL BAY (S Ronaldsay)							
−0400	−0400	−0355	−0355	−0·7	−0·7	−0·3	−0·2
BUR WICK (S Ronaldsay)							
−0255	−0320	−0400	−0410	−0·8	−0·6	0·0	0·0
MUCKLE SKERRY (Pentland Firth)							
−0230	−0230	−0225	−0225	−1·7	−1·4	−0·6	−0·2

SHELTER
Very good. Northern Lights Board have sole use of pier near to ldg lts. ‡ in hbr or berth at ferry piers further N.

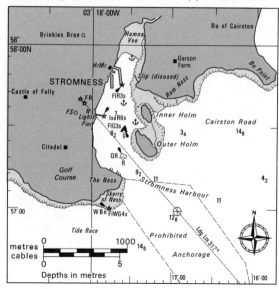

NAVIGATION
WPT 58°57'·00N 03°16'·90W, 137°/317° from/to front ldg lt, 0·88M. Tides in Hoy Sound are very strong (>7kn sp); if entering against the ebb, stand on to avoid being swept onto Skerry of Ness. Ent should not be attempted in bad weather or with strong wind against tide. No tidal stream in hbr.
LIGHTS AND MARKS
For Hoy Sound, ldg lts 104° on Graemsay Is: front Iso 3s 17m 15M, W tr; rear Oc WR 8s 35m 20/16M, ldg sector is R097°-112°. Skerry of Ness, Fl WG 4s 7m 7/4M; W shore-090°, G090°-shore.
Hbr ldg lts 317°, both FR 29/39m 11M (H24), W trs, vis 307°-327°.
RADIO TELEPHONE
VHF Ch 12 16 (0900-1700LT). (See also Kirkwall).
TELEPHONE (01856)
Hr Mr 850744; Fuel 851286; MRSC 873268; ⌗ 872108; Marinecall 0891 500 451; Police 850222; Dr 850205.
FACILITIES
Services: Sh, El, Ⓔ, ME, C (mobile, 30 ton), Slip.
Town EC Thurs; FW, D, V, R, Bar, Gas, ⊠, ▣, Ⓑ, ⇌ (ferry to Scrabster, bus to Thurso), ✈ (Kirkwall).
Note: Yachtsmen may contact for help: **J. Stout** ☎ 850100, **S. Mowat** ☎ 850624 or **W.Burgon** ☎ 850215.

OTHER HARBOURS IN THE ORKNEY ISLANDS

HOUTON BAY, Mainland, 58°54'·88N 03°11'·23W. AC 2568, 35. HW −0140 on Dover, −0400 on Aberdeen; HW ht +0·3m on Kirkwall; ML 1·8m; Duration 0615. ‡ in the bay in approx 5·5m at centre, sheltered from all winds. The ent is to the E of the island Holm of Houton; ent chan dredged 3·5m for 15m each side of ldg line. Keep clear of merchant vessels/ferries plying to Flotta.
Ldg lts 316°: front Fl G 3s 8m, rear FG 16m; both R △ on W pole, B bands. Ro Ro terminal in NE corner marked by Iso R 4s. Bus to Kirkwall; Slip close E of piers. Yachtsmen may contact **M. Grainger** ☎ 811356 for help.

SHAPINSAY, Orkney Islands, 59°02'·00N 02°54'·00W. AC 2584, 2249. HW −0015 on Dover, −0330 on Aberdeen; HW ht −1·0m on Aberdeen. Good shelter in Elwick Bay off Balfour on SW end of island in 2·5-3m. Enter bay passing W of Helliar Holm which has lt Fl WRG 10s on S end. Keep mid-chan. Balfour Pier lt Q WRG 5m 3/2M; vis G270°-010°, W010°-020°, R020°-090°. Tides in The String reach 5kn at sp. Facilities: ⊠, P & D (cans), shop, Bar.

PIEROWALL, Westray, 59°19'·35N 02°58'·41W. AC 2622, 2250. HW −0135 on Dover; ML 2·2m; Duration 0620. See 10.7.23. The bay is a good ‡ in 2-7m and well protected. Deep water AB at Gill Pt piers may be available; see Hr Mr. From S, beware Skelwick Skerry rks, and from the N the rks extending approx 1ca off Vest Ness. The N ent via Papa Sound needs local knowledge; tide race on the ebb. A dangerous tide race runs off Mull Hd at the N of Papa Westray. Lights: E pier hd Fl WRG 3s 7m 11/7M, G254°-276°, W276°-291°, R291°-308°, G308°-215°. W pier hd 2 FR (vert) 4/6m 3M. VHF Ch 16. Hr Mr ☎ (01857) 677273. Facilities: FW (at Gill Pier), P & D (cans), Bar, ⊠, Ⓑ, R, V.

OTHER HARBOURS IN THE SHETLAND ISLANDS

FAIR ISLE, Shetland Islands, 59°32'·40N 01°36'·10W (North Haven). AC 2622. HW −0030 on Dover; ML 1·4m; Duration 0620. See 10.7.26 Good shelter in N Haven, but uncomfortable in NE winds. Lie alongside pier or ‡ in approx 2m. Beware cross-tides in the apprs and rks all round the island, particularly in S Haven and South Hbr which are not recommended. Ldg marks 199° into N Haven: Stack of N Haven on with top of Sheep Craig. Dir lt, 209° into N Haven, Oc WRG 8s 10m 6M, vis G204°-208°, W208°- 211°, R211°-221°. Other lts: In the S, Skadan Fl (4) 30s 32m **24**M, vis 260°-146°, but obscd close inshore from 260°-282°, Horn (2) 60s. In the N, Skroo Fl (2) 30s 80m **22**M, vis 086·7°-358°, Horn (3) 45s. Facilities: V, ⊠ at N Shriva, and a bi-weekly ferry to Shetland.

SCALLOWAY, Mainland, 60°07'·80N 01°16'·60W. AC 3294. HW −0200 on Dover; ML 0·9m; Duration 0620. See 10.7.26. A well sheltered ‡ in all weathers, but care is needed passing through the islands in strong SW winds. The N Chan is easier and safer than the S Chan. ‡ off Scalloway 6 -10m or in Hamna Voe (W Burra). Lts: Fugla Ness Fl (2) WRG 10s 20m 10/7M, W Tr; W sector, 032°-082° covers the S Chan. Dir Oc 058°, WRG 10s 7m 14/11M, on hbr quay (at 60°08'·11N 01°16'·39W), vis G045·7°-056·8°, W056·8°-058·8°, R058·8°-069·9°. Hbr: Moores Slipway jetty hd 2 FR (vert) 4/3m 1M. Blacksness W pier hd 2 FG (vert) 6/4m 3M; E pier hd Oc R 7s 5m 3M. VHF Ch 16; 09 12 (Mon–Fri 0600–1800LT; Sat 0600–1230LT). Hr Mr/Port Control ☎ (01595) 880574 (H24). Facilities: **Scalloway Boating Club** ☎ 880409; **Town** EC Thurs; AB, M, Slip, P, D, FW, SM, BY, CH, C, El, ME, Sh, ⊠, R, V, Bar.

BALTA SOUND, Unst, 60°44'·35N 00°48'·00W. AC 3293. HW −0105 on Dover; ML 1·3; Duration 0640. See 10.7.26. Balta Sound is a large almost landlocked inlet with good shelter from all winds. Beware bad holding on kelp. Safest entry is via S Chan between Huney Is and Balta Is; inner chan marked by an unlit SPM buoy and two lit PHM buoys. N Chan is deep but narrow; keep to Unst shore. ‡ off Sandisons Wharf (2FG vert) in approx 6m or enter marina close W (one visitor's berth); jetty has Fl R 6s 2m 2M. S end of Balta Is, Fl WR 10s 17m 10/7M, W249°-010°, R010°-060°, W060°-154°. VHF Ch 16; 20 (HO). Facilities: BY, FW, D, El, ME, Sh; Hotel by pier. **Baltasound village**, Bar, R, V, ⊠.

SHETLAND ISLANDS   10-7-25

The Shetland Islands consist of approx 100 islands, holms and rks of which fewer than 20 are inhabited. They lie 90 to 150M NNE of the Scottish mainland. By far the biggest island is Mainland with Lerwick (10.7.26), the capital, on the E side and Scalloway (facing page), the only other town and old capital, on the W side. At the very S is Sumburgh airport and there are airstrips at Baltasound, Scalsta and Tingwall. Two islands of the Shetland group not shown on the chartlet are Fair Isle (see facing page), 20M SSW of Sumburgh Hd and owned by the NT for Scotland, and Foula (see below) 12M WSW of Mainland. There are LBs at Lerwick and Aith. The CG MRSC is at Lerwick ☎ (01595) 692976, with a Sector Base at Sella Ness (Sullom Voe) and an Auxiliary Station (Watch & Rescue) at Fair Isle.

CHARTS
AC: Med scale 3281, 3282, 3283; larger scale 3290, 3291, 3292, 3293, 3294, 3295, 3297, 3298; OS sheets 1-4.

TIDES
Lerwick is the Standard Port. Tidal streams run mostly N/ S or NW/SE and in open waters to the E and W are mostly weak. But rates >6kn can cause dangerous disturbances at the N and S extremities of the islands and in the two main sounds (Yell Snd and Bluemull/ Colgrave Snds). Keep 3M off Sumburgh Head to clear a dangerous race (roost) or pass close inshore.

SHELTER
Weather conditions are bad in winter; yachts should only visit Apr – Sept. Around mid-summer it is day light H24. Some 11 small, non-commercial "marinas" are asterisked below; they are mostly full of local boats but supposedly each reserves 1 berth for visitors. Of the many ⚓s, the following are safe to enter in most weathers:

Mainland (anti-clockwise from Sumburgh Head)
GRUTNESS VOE*: 1·5M N of Sumburgh Hd, a convenient passage ⚓, open to NE. Beware 2 rks awash in mid-ent.
CAT FIRTH: excellent shelter, ⚓ in approx 6m. Facilities: ✉ (Skellister), FW, V (both at Lax Firth).
GRUNNA VOE: off S side of Dury Voe, good shelter and holding, ⚓ in 5-10m; beware prohib ⚓ areas. Facilities: V, FW, ✉ (Lax Firth).
WHALSAY*: Small FV hbr at Symbister. FW, D, V, ✉.
OUT SKERRIES*: Quay and ⚓ at Bruray. FW, D, V, ✉.
S OF YELL SOUND*: Tides –0025 on Lerwick. W of Lunna Ness, well-protected ⚓s with good holding include: Boatsroom Voe, W Lunna Voe (small hotel, FW), Colla Firth* (excellent pier) and Dales Voe. Facilities: none.
SULLOM VOE: tides –0130 on Lerwick. 6·5M long deep water voe, partly taken over by the oil industry. ⚓ S of the narrows. Facilities at Brae: FW, V, ✉, D, ME, El, Sh, Bar.
HAMNA VOE: Tides –0200 on Lerwick; very good shelter. Ldg line 153° old house on S shore with prominent rk on pt of W shore 3ca within ent. Almost land-locked; ⚓ in 6m approx, but bottom foul with old moorings. Facilities: ✉ (0·5M), Vs, D (1·5M), L (at pier).
URA FIRTH: NE of St Magnus Bay, ⚓ off Hills Wick on W side or in Hamar Voe on E side, which has excellent shelter in all weathers and good holding, but no facilities. Facilities: Hills Wick FW, ✉, D, ME, El, Sh, V, R, Bar.
OLNA FIRTH: NE of Swarbacks Minn, beware rk 1ca off S shore which dries. ⚓ in firth, 4-8m or in Gon Firth or go alongside pier at Voe. Facilities: (Voe) FW, V, D, ✉, Bar.
SWARBACKS MINN*: a large complex of voes and isles SE of St Magnus Bay. Best ⚓ Uyea Sound or Aith Voe*, both well sheltered and good holding. Facilities: former none; Aith FW, ✉, V, Bar, LB.
VAILA SOUND: on SW of Mainland, ent via Easter Sound (do not attempt Wester Sound); very good shelter, ⚓ N of Salt Ness in 4-5m in mud. Facilities: FW, V, ✉.
GRUTING VOE*: tides –0150 on Lerwick, ⚓ in main voe or in Seli, Scutta or Browland* voes. Facilities: V and ✉ at Bridge of Walls (hd of Browland Voe).

Yell
MID YELL VOE: tides –0040 on Lerwick, enter through S Sd or Hascosay Sd, good ⚓ in wide part of voe 2·5– 10m. Facilities: ✉, FW at pier on S side, D, V, ME, Sh, El.
BASTA VOE: good ⚓ above shingle bank in 5-15m; good holding in places. Facilities: FW, V, Hotel, ✉.
BLUE MULL SND*: ⚓ at Cullivoe, pier and slip. D, FW, V.
Foula: Ham Voe on E side has tiny hbr/pier, unsafe in E'ly; berth clear of mailboat. Avoid Hoevdi Grund, 2M ESE.

NAVIGATION
A careful lookout must be kept for salmon farming cages, mostly marked by Y buoys and combinations of Y lts. The Clyde Cruising Club's *Shetland Sailing Directions and Anchorages* are essential for visitors. For general passage information see 10.7.5. Weather forecasting and the avoidance of wind-over-tide conditions assume yet more significance than elsewhere in the UK. Local magnetic anomalies may be experienced.

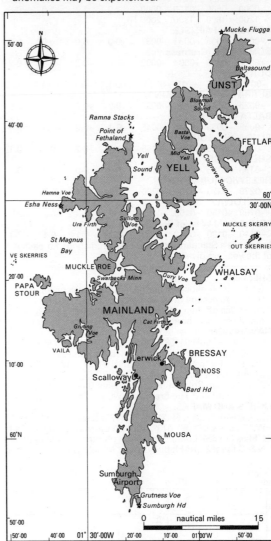

Note: There are two Historic Wrecks (*Kennemerland* and *Wrangels Palais*) on Out Skerries at 60°25'·2N 00°45'·0W and 60°25'·5N 00°43'·27W (see 10.0.3g).

LIGHTS AND MARKS
See 10.7.4. Powerful lights show offshore from Fair Isle, Sumburgh Head, Kirkabister Ness, Bound Skerry, Muckle Flugga, Pt of Fethaland, Esha Ness and Foula.

RADIO TELEPHONE
For Port Radio services see 10.7.26. Local Coast Radio Stns are Shetland Radio (Ch 27 16), and Collafirth Radio (Ch 24 16). Weather messages are broadcast by Shetland Radio (Ch 27) and Collafirth Radio (Ch 24) at 0703 and 1903 UT. Gale warnings after next silence period and at 0303 0903 1503 2103 UT.

TELEPHONE (01595)
MRSC 692976; Sullom Voe Port Control 242551; Weather 692239; Forecaster 242069; Sumburgh Airport 460654.

FACILITIES
See Shelter above. All stores can be obtained in Lerwick and to a lesser extent in Scalloway. Elsewhere in Shetland there is little available.

LERWICK
10-7-26

Shetland Islands, Mainland 60°09'·29N 01°08'·30W

CHARTS
AC 3290, 3291, 3283; OS 4
TIDES
–0001 Dover; ML 1·4; Duration 0620; Zone 0 (UT)

Standard Port LERWICK (→)

Times				Height (metres)			
High Water		Low Water		MHWS	MHWN	MLWN	MLWS
0000	0600	0100	0800	2·2	1·7	1·0	0·6
1200	1800	1300	2000				
Differences FAIR ISLE							
–0006	–0015	–0031	–0037	0·0	0·0	0·0	0·0
SUMBURGH (Grutness Voe)							
+0006	+0008	+0004	–0002	–0·4	–0·3	–0·3	–0·2
DURY VOE							
–0015	–0015	–0010	–0010	–0·1	–0·1	–0·1	–0·3
BURRA VOE (YELL SOUND)							
–0025	–0025	–0025	–0025	+0·2	+0·2	0·0	0·0
BALTA SOUND							
–0055	–0055	–0045	–0045	+0·1	+0·2	–0·1	–0·1
BLUE MULL SOUND							
–0135	–0135	–0155	0155	+0·4	+0·2	0·0	–0·1
SULLOM VOE							
–0135	–0125	–0135	–0120	0·0	0·0	–0·2	–0·2
HILLSWICK (URA FIRTH)							
–0220	–0220	–0200	–0200	0·0	–0·4	–0·4	–0·1
SCALLOWAY							
–0150	–0150	–0150	–0150	–0·6	–0·3	–0·3	0·0
FOULA (23M West of Scalloway)							
–0140	–0140	–0140	–0120	–0·2	–0·1	–0·1	–0·1

Lerwick is a Standard Port and tidal predictions for each day of the year are given below.

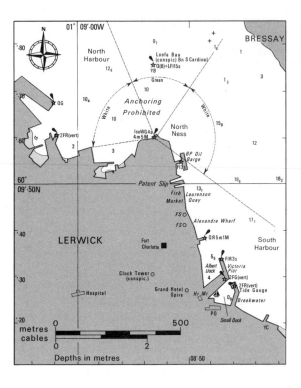

SHELTER
Good. Hr Mr allocates berths in Small Dock or Albert Dock. FVs occupy most alongside space. ⚓ prohib for about 2ca off the waterfront. Gremista marina in N hbr, is mainly for local boats, and is about 1M from the town.
NAVIGATION
WPT 60°06'·00N 01°08'·50W, 190°/010° from/to Maryfield lt, 3·5M, in W sector. From S, Bressay Sound is clear of dangers. From N, WPT 60°11'·60N 01°07'·88W, 035°/215° from/to N ent Dir lt, 1·34M; lt Oc WRG 6s, W sector 214°-216°. Beware Soldian Rk (dries), Nive Baa (0·6m), Green Holm (10m) and The Brethren (two rks 2m and 1·5m).
LIGHTS AND MARKS
Kirkabister Ness lt Fl (2) 20s 32m 23M; Maryfield lt Oc WRG 6s, vis W 008°-013°; both on Bressay. Twageos Pt lt L Fl 6s 8m 6M. Loofa Baa SCM lt bn marks shoal between N & S hbrs. 2 SHM lt buoys mark Middle Ground in N hbr.

RADIO TELEPHONE
VHF Ch **12** 11 16 (H24).
Other stns: Sullom Voe Ch **14** 12 20 16 (H24). Traffic info and local forecasts broadcast on request Ch 14 or 16. Scalloway Ch **12** 09 16 (Mon-Fri: 0800-1700; Sat: 0800-1200LT). Balta Sound Ch 16 20 (occas).
TELEPHONE (01595)
Hr Mr 692991; MRSC 692976; ⌗ (0131) 469 7400; Weather 692239; Police 692110; Dr 693201.
FACILITIES
Hbr Slip, M, P, D, L, FW, ME, Sh, Gas; **Lerwick Hbr Trust** ☎ 692991, M, FW, D, P, AB; **Lerwick Boating Club** ☎ 692407, L, C, Bar, 🚽;
Services: ME, EI, Ⓔ, Sh, Slip, BY, CH, SM, Gas, ACA.
Town EC Wed (all day); V, R, Bar, ✉, Ⓑ, ⇌, (ferry to Aberdeen), ✈.

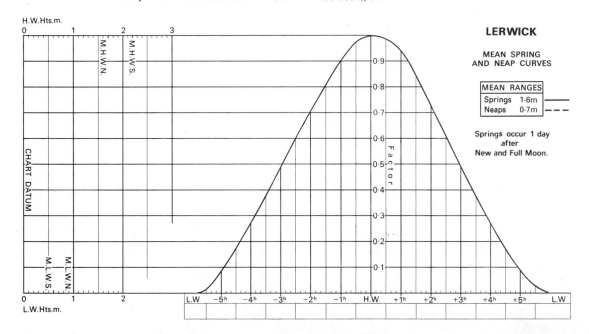

SCOTLAND – LERWICK

LAT 60°09′N   LONG   1°08′W

TIMES AND HEIGHTS OF HIGH AND LOW WATERS

YEAR **1996**

TIME ZONE (UT)
For Summer Time add ONE hour in non-shaded areas

7

JANUARY

Time	m	Time	m
1 M 0137 0754 1404 2018	1.1 2.0 1.1 2.0	**16** TU 0014 0638 1259 1916	1.1 2.1 1.2 2.1
2 TU 0226 0845 1452 2108	1.1 2.1 1.0 2.0	**17** W 0133 0748 1412 2025	1.0 2.2 1.0 2.2
3 W 0308 0928 1534 2151	1.1 2.2 0.9 2.1	**18** TH 0233 0848 1507 2124	1.0 2.3 0.8 2.3
4 TH 0346 1006 1612 2228	1.0 2.2 0.9 2.1	**19** F 0325 0941 1557 2216	0.9 2.5 0.7 2.4
5 F 0420 1040 1647 2302 O	1.0 2.3 0.8 2.2	**20** SA 0412 1030 1645 2305 ●	0.8 2.6 0.5 2.5
6 SA 0454 1112 1722 2335	1.0 2.3 0.8 2.2	**21** SU 0458 1153 1731 2352	0.7 2.7 0.5 2.5
7 SU 0528 1143 1756	0.9 2.3 0.8	**22** M 0543 1202 1817	0.7 2.7 0.5
8 M 0008 0601 1216 1830	2.2 0.9 2.3 0.8	**23** TU 0038 0627 1247 1902	2.5 0.7 2.6 0.5
9 TU 0043 0634 1248 1905	2.2 1.0 2.3 0.8	**24** W 0123 0711 1332 1948	2.4 0.8 2.6 0.6
10 W 0118 0708 1322 1941	2.2 1.0 2.3 0.8	**25** TH 0208 0757 1417 2036	2.3 0.9 2.4 0.8
11 TH 0156 0744 1400 2021	2.1 1.0 2.2 0.9	**26** F 0253 0845 1505 2127	2.2 1.0 2.3 1.0
12 F 0237 0826 1442 2106	2.1 1.1 2.2 0.9	**27** SA 0342 0940 1558 2233	2.1 1.1 2.1 1.1
13 SA 0323 0914 1532 2157	2.0 1.2 2.1 1.0	**28** SU 0437 1108 1701	2.0 1.2 2.0
14 SU 0417 1013 1634 2259	2.0 1.2 2.1 1.1	**29** M 0001 0544 1239 1825	1.2 2.0 1.2 1.9
15 M 0523 1126 1753	2.0 1.2 2.0	**30** TU 0110 0711 1343 1952	1.3 2.0 1.2 1.9
		31 W 0204 0818 1435 2049	1.2 2.0 1.1 2.0

FEBRUARY

Time	m	Time	m
1 TH 0250 0906 1518 2133	1.2 2.1 1.0 2.1	**16** F 0222 0833 1458 2115	1.0 2.2 0.8 2.3
2 F 0329 0947 1555 2211	1.1 2.2 0.9 2.1	**17** SA 0313 0928 1546 2206	0.9 2.4 0.6 2.4
3 SA 0403 1021 1629 2244	1.0 2.3 0.8 2.2	**18** SU 0359 1017 1631 2252 ●	0.8 2.5 0.5 2.4
4 SU 0436 1053 1702 2315 O	1.0 2.3 0.8 2.2	**19** M 0442 1103 1714 2336	0.7 2.6 0.4 2.5
5 M 0509 1123 1735 2346	0.9 2.4 0.7 2.3	**20** TU 0525 1146 1757	0.6 2.6 0.4
6 TU 0541 1153 1807	0.9 2.4 0.7	**21** W 0018 0606 1229 1838	2.5 0.6 2.6 0.5
7 W 0018 0612 1225 1840	2.3 0.9 2.4 0.7	**22** TH 0059 0647 1311 1919	2.4 0.7 2.5 0.5
8 TH 0052 0645 1300 1915	2.2 0.9 2.4 0.7	**23** F 0139 0729 1352 2000	2.3 0.8 2.4 0.8
9 F 0128 0720 1338 1953	2.2 0.9 2.3 0.8	**24** SA 0220 0811 1436 2041	2.2 0.9 2.2 1.0
10 SA 0207 0801 1419 2036	2.2 1.0 2.3 0.9	**25** SU 0302 0857 1523 2125	2.1 1.0 2.1 1.1
11 SU 0250 0848 1507 2125	2.1 1.1 2.2 1.0	**26** M 0350 0956 1619 2233	2.0 1.2 1.9 1.3
12 M 0340 0944 1604 2224	2.1 1.1 2.1 1.1	**27** TU 0448 1204 1731	1.9 1.2 1.8
13 TU 0439 1054 1721 2338	2.0 1.2 2.0 1.2	**28** W 0038 0605 1317 1913	1.3 1.8 1.2 1.9
14 W 0558 1237 1858	2.0 1.1 2.0	**29** TH 0140 0738 1411 2024	1.3 1.9 1.1 1.8
15 TH 0115 0724 1402 2015	1.1 2.1 1.0 2.1		

MARCH

Time	m	Time	m
1 F 0227 0838 1454 2109	1.2 2.0 1.0 1.9	**16** SA 0209 0820 1445 2104	0.9 2.1 0.6 2.1
2 SA 0306 0920 1530 2146	1.1 2.1 0.9 2.0	**17** SU 0258 0915 1531 2152	0.8 2.2 0.5 2.2
3 SU 0340 0955 1603 2218	1.0 2.2 0.8 2.1	**18** M 0342 1002 1613 2235	0.7 2.4 0.4 2.3
4 M 0413 1027 1635 2249	0.9 2.2 0.7 2.1	**19** TU 0424 1047 1654 2317 ●	0.6 2.4 0.4 2.3
5 TU 0445 1058 1708 2320 O	0.8 2.3 0.6 2.2	**20** W 0504 1129 1733 2356	0.5 2.4 0.4 2.3
6 W 0517 1129 1740 2352	0.7 2.3 0.6 2.3	**21** TH 0544 1209 1811	0.5 2.4 0.4
7 TH 0549 1202 1814	0.7 2.4 0.6	**22** F 0033 0623 1248 1848	2.3 0.5 2.3 0.6
8 F 0026 0622 1239 1849	2.3 0.7 2.3 0.6	**23** SA 0111 0702 1328 1924	2.2 0.6 2.2 0.7
9 SA 0103 0659 1318 1928	2.2 0.7 2.3 0.7	**24** SU 0148 0742 1409 2001	2.1 0.7 2.1 0.9
10 SU 0142 0741 1402 2011	2.2 0.8 2.2 0.8	**25** M 0227 0825 1454 2041	2.0 0.8 1.9 1.0
11 M 0225 0828 1450 2100	2.1 0.9 2.1 0.9	**26** TU 0312 0915 1546 2129	1.9 1.0 1.7 1.1
12 TU 0314 0925 1548 2159	2.0 1.0 2.0 1.0	**27** W 0406 1036 1652 2337	1.8 1.0 1.6 1.2
13 W 0411 1036 1705 2316	1.9 1.0 1.9 1.1	**28** TH 0515 1239 1812	1.7 1.0 1.6
14 TH 0529 1232 1850	1.9 1.0 1.9	**29** F 0105 0636 1336 1935	1.1 1.8 0.9 1.6
15 F 0104 0707 1352 2007	1.1 2.0 0.8 2.0	**30** SA 0156 0749 1419 2029	1.0 1.7 0.8 1.7
		31 SU 0235 0839 1455 2108	0.9 1.8 0.7 1.8

APRIL

Time	m	Time	m
1 M 0309 0919 1529 2144	0.8 1.9 0.6 1.9	**16** TU 0323 0945 1551 2215	0.5 2.1 0.3 2.1
2 TU 0343 0955 1603 2218	0.7 2.0 0.5 2.0	**17** W 0404 1028 1630 2255 ●	0.5 2.2 0.3 2.1
3 W 0417 1029 1637 2251	0.6 2.1 0.4 2.1	**18** TH 0444 1109 1707 2332	0.4 2.2 0.2 2.1
4 TH 0450 1104 1712 2326	0.5 2.2 0.4 2.1	**19** F 0523 1148 1743	0.4 2.1 0.4
5 F 0525 1141 1747	0.5 2.2 0.4	**20** SA 0008 0600 1227 1818	2.1 0.4 2.1 0.5
6 SA 0002 0601 1221 1825	2.2 0.5 2.2 0.5	**21** SU 0043 0638 1305 1853	2.0 0.5 2.0 0.6
7 SU 0041 0642 1303 1906	2.1 0.5 2.2 0.5	**22** M 0119 0717 1345 1929	2.0 0.5 1.8 0.7
8 M 0122 0726 1349 1951	2.1 0.5 2.1 0.7	**23** TU 0158 0800 1429 2009	1.9 0.6 1.7 0.8
9 TU 0207 0816 1441 2042	2.0 0.6 1.9 0.8	**24** W 0240 0847 1518 2055	1.7 0.7 1.6 0.9
10 W 0256 0914 1541 2142	1.9 0.7 1.8 0.9	**25** TH 0329 0945 1617 2155	1.6 0.8 1.5 1.0
11 TH 0355 1030 1700 2304	1.8 0.7 1.7 0.9	**26** F 0430 1114 1724 2353	1.6 0.8 1.5 1.0
12 F 0511 1220 1841	1.8 0.7 1.7	**27** SA 0542 1237 1833	1.5 0.8 1.5
13 SA 0047 0650 1332 1953	0.9 1.8 0.6 1.8	**28** SU 0105 0650 1329 1933	0.9 1.6 0.7 1.6
14 SU 0150 0802 1425 2046	0.8 1.9 0.5 1.9	**29** M 0151 0748 1411 2022	0.8 1.6 0.6 1.7
15 M 0240 0857 1510 2133	0.7 2.0 0.4 2.0	**30** TU 0231 0836 1450 2105	0.7 1.7 0.5 1.8

Chart Datum: 1·22 metres below Ordnance Datum (Local)

SCOTLAND – LERWICK

LAT 60°09′N   LONG 1°08′W

TIMES AND HEIGHTS OF HIGH AND LOW WATERS

YEAR 1996

TIME ZONE (UT)
For Summer Time add ONE hour in non-shaded areas

MAY

Day	Time	m	Time	m	Day	Time	m	Time	m
1 W	0309	0.6	0919	1.9	16 TH	0346	0.4	1009	1.9
	1528	0.4	2144	1.9		1607	0.4	2232	1.9
2 TH	0346	0.5	1000	2.0	17 F	0426	0.4	1051	1.9
	1606	0.3	2222	2.0	●	1643	0.4	2309	2.0
3 F	0424	0.4	1041	2.0	18 SA	0504	0.3	1129	1.9
O	1644	0.3	2301	2.0		1718	0.5	2344	2.0
4 SA	0503	0.3	1123	2.1	19 SU	0542	0.3	1206	1.9
	1724	0.3	2341	2.1		1752	0.5		
5 SU	0545	0.3	1206	2.1	20 M	0018	1.9	0619	0.4
	1805	0.3				1244	1.8	1827	0.6
6 M	0022	2.1	0629	0.3	21 TU	0054	1.9	0658	0.4
	1253	2.0	1849	0.4		1323	1.7	1904	0.6
7 TU	0107	2.0	0717	0.3	22 W	0131	1.8	0738	0.5
	1342	1.9	1936	0.5		1405	1.6	1944	0.7
8 W	0153	2.0	0809	0.4	23 TH	0211	1.7	0822	0.5
	1435	1.8	2028	0.6		1451	1.6	2027	0.8
9 TH	0245	1.9	0909	0.4	24 F	0254	1.6	0911	0.6
	1536	1.7	2129	0.7		1542	1.5	2118	0.8
10 F	0343	1.8	1024	0.5	25 SA	0344	1.5	1007	0.6
	1650	1.6	2249	0.8		1639	1.4	2221	0.9
11 SA	0455	1.7	1154	0.5	26 SU	0446	1.5	1114	0.6
	1817	1.6				1740	1.5	2343	0.9
12 SU	0019	0.8	0624	1.7	27 M	0553	1.5	1222	0.6
	1305	0.5	1928	1.6		1841	1.5		
13 M	0125	0.7	0738	1.7	28 TU	0054	0.8	0656	1.6
	1400	0.4	2023	1.7		1320	0.6	1935	1.6
14 TU	0218	0.6	0835	1.8	29 W	0147	0.7	0753	1.7
	1446	0.4	2110	1.8		1408	0.5	2025	1.7
15 W	0304	0.5	0925	1.9	30 TH	0234	0.6	0845	1.8
	1528	0.4	2152	1.9		1453	0.4	2111	1.8
					31 F	0318	0.5	0933	1.9
						1537	0.4	2155	1.9

JUNE

Day	Time	m	Time	m	Day	Time	m	Time	m
1 SA	0401	0.3	1020	2.0	16 SU	0449	0.4	1112	1.8
O	1620	0.2	2238	2.0	●	1657	0.6	2323	2.0
2 SU	0446	0.2	1107	2.0	17 M	0526	0.4	1148	1.8
	1704	0.3	2322	2.1		1731	0.6	2356	1.9
3 M	0532	0.2	1155	2.0	18 TU	0602	0.4	1223	1.8
	1749	0.3				1807	0.6		
4 TU	0007	2.1	0619	0.2	19 W	0030	1.9	0639	0.4
	1243	2.0	1835	0.4		1300	1.8	1843	0.6
5 W	0054	2.1	0708	0.2	20 TH	0106	1.9	0717	0.4
	1334	1.9	1924	0.5		1339	1.7	1921	0.7
6 TH	0142	2.0	0801	0.2	21 F	0142	1.8	0757	0.5
	1426	1.8	2015	0.5		1419	1.7	2001	0.7
7 F	0233	1.9	0859	0.3	22 SA	0219	1.7	0839	0.5
	1523	1.7	2113	0.6		1503	1.6	2044	0.8
8 SA	0329	1.8	1004	0.4	23 SU	0301	1.7	0924	0.6
	1627	1.6	2223	0.7		1551	1.6	2133	0.8
9 SU	0433	1.7	1120	0.5	24 M	0350	1.6	1016	0.6
	1741	1.6	2345	0.7		1645	1.5	2231	0.9
10 M	0551	1.7	1232	0.5	25 TU	0452	1.6	1116	0.7
	1853	1.6				1746	1.6	2343	0.9
11 TU	0057	0.7	0708	1.7	26 W	0603	1.6	1223	0.7
	1332	0.5	1954	1.7		1848	1.6		
12 W	0156	0.6	0812	1.7	27 TH	0059	0.8	0712	1.7
	1422	0.5	2044	1.7		1326	0.7	1947	1.7
13 TH	0246	0.6	0905	1.7	28 F	0201	0.7	0815	1.8
	1506	0.5	2130	1.8		1423	0.6	2041	1.9
14 F	0330	0.5	0951	1.8	29 SA	0254	0.5	0911	1.9
	1546	0.6	2211	1.9		1513	0.5	2131	2.0
15 SA	0411	0.5	1033	1.8	30 SU	0344	0.4	1004	2.0
	1622	0.6	2248	1.9		1601	0.4	2219	2.1

JULY

Day	Time	m	Time	m	Day	Time	m	Time	m
1 M	0432	0.3	1054	2.1	16 TU	0508	0.5	1129	1.9
O	1647	0.4	2307	2.2		1713	0.6	2335	2.0
2 TU	0520	0.2	1143	2.1	17 W	0542	0.4	1201	1.9
	1734	0.4	2353	2.3		1747	0.6		
3 W	0608	0.1	1231	2.1	18 TH	0007	2.2	0617	0.4
	1821	0.4				1235	1.9	1822	0.6
4 TH	0040	2.3	0656	0.1	19 F	0039	2.0	0652	0.4
	1320	2.0	1908	0.5		1309	1.9	1857	0.7
5 F	0128	2.2	0746	0.2	20 SA	0112	2.0	0728	0.5
	1410	2.0	1957	0.5		1345	1.8	1933	0.7
6 SA	0217	2.1	0838	0.3	21 SU	0148	1.9	0806	0.5
	1501	1.9	2050	0.6		1424	1.8	2011	0.8
7 SU	0309	2.0	0935	0.5	22 M	0227	1.9	0848	0.6
	1556	1.8	2151	0.7		1506	1.8	2056	0.9
8 M	0406	1.9	1042	0.6	23 TU	0312	1.8	0934	0.7
	1658	1.7	2307	0.8		1554	1.7	2148	0.9
9 TU	0513	1.7	1157	0.7	24 W	0407	1.8	1029	0.8
	1809	1.7				1652	1.7	2253	0.9
10 W	0029	0.8	0634	1.7	25 TH	0516	1.7	1135	0.8
	1304	0.7	1920	1.7		1801	1.7		
11 TH	0135	0.8	0748	1.7	26 F	0015	0.9	0638	1.8
	1400	0.8	2019	1.8		1252	0.8	1912	1.8
12 F	0230	0.7	0847	1.7	27 SA	0137	0.8	0752	1.8
	1447	0.8	2109	1.8		1400	0.7	2016	1.9
13 SA	0316	0.7	0935	1.8	28 SU	0238	0.6	0855	2.0
	1528	0.8	2152	1.9		1455	0.7	2112	2.1
14 SU	0357	0.6	1018	1.8	29 M	0330	0.5	0950	2.1
	1605	0.7	2230	2.0		1545	0.6	2203	2.2
15 M	0434	0.5	1055	1.8	30 TU	0418	0.3	1041	2.2
●	1639	0.7	2304	2.0	O	1632	0.5	2252	2.3
					31 W	0505	0.2	1129	2.2
						1717	0.4	2338	2.4

AUGUST

Day	Time	m	Time	m	Day	Time	m	Time	m
1 TH	0551	0.2	1215	2.2	16 F	0551	0.5	1205	2.0
	1803	0.4				1758	0.7		
2 F	0024	2.4	0637	0.2	17 SA	0011	2.1	0624	0.5
	1301	2.2	1848	0.5		1238	2.0	1831	0.7
3 SA	0110	2.4	0723	0.3	18 SU	0044	2.1	0659	0.5
	1346	2.1	1934	0.6		1312	2.0	1905	0.7
4 SU	0156	2.2	0811	0.4	19 M	0120	2.1	0735	0.6
	1433	2.0	2022	0.7		1349	2.0	1943	0.8
5 M	0244	2.1	0901	0.6	20 TU	0159	2.0	0815	0.7
	1521	1.9	2116	0.8		1430	1.9	2026	0.9
6 TU	0336	1.9	0958	0.8	21 W	0244	2.0	0900	0.8
	1614	1.8	2225	0.9		1516	1.9	2117	0.9
7 W	0436	1.8	1116	0.9	22 TH	0337	1.9	0954	0.9
	1718	1.7				1611	1.8	2221	1.0
8 TH	0001	1.0	0555	1.7	23 F	0444	1.8	1100	1.0
	1237	1.0	1840	1.7		1720	1.8	2347	1.0
9 F	0115	0.9	0726	1.7	24 SA	0615	1.8	1227	1.0
	1338	1.0	1954	1.8		1844	1.9		
10 SA	0212	0.9	0830	1.7	25 SU	0124	0.8	0740	1.9
	1428	1.0	2048	1.9		1346	0.9	1958	2.0
11 SU	0259	0.8	0919	1.8	26 M	0227	0.7	0844	2.0
	1510	0.9	2132	2.0		1442	0.8	2057	2.2
12 M	0338	0.7	0959	1.9	27 TU	0317	0.5	0938	2.1
	1546	0.8	2210	2.0		1530	0.6	2149	2.3
13 TU	0413	0.6	1035	1.9	28 W	0403	0.3	1026	2.2
	1619	0.8	2242	2.1	O	1615	0.5	2236	2.4
14 W	0445	0.5	1105	2.0	29 TH	0447	0.2	1111	2.3
●	1652	0.7	2311	2.1		1659	0.5	2321	2.5
15 TH	0518	0.5	1135	2.0	30 F	0531	0.2	1155	2.3
	1725	0.7	2340	2.1		1742	0.4		
					31 SA	0005	2.5	0613	0.3
						1238	2.3	1825	0.5

Chart Datum: 1·22 metres below Ordnance Datum (Local)

SCOTLAND – LERWICK

LAT 60°09′N   LONG 1°08′W

TIMES AND HEIGHTS OF HIGH AND LOW WATERS   YEAR **1996**

TIME ZONE (UT)
For Summer Time add ONE hour in non-shaded areas

7

SEPTEMBER

Day	Time	m	Day	Time	m
1 SU	0049	2.4	**16** M	0018	2.2
	0656	0.4		0630	0.5
	1319	2.2		1242	2.1
	1908	0.6		1840	0.7
2 M	0132	2.3	**17** TU	0056	2.2
	0739	0.5		0706	0.6
	1401	2.1		1320	2.1
	1953	0.7		1919	0.7
3 TU	0217	2.1	**18** W	0138	2.1
	0823	0.7		0747	0.7
	1445	2.0		1401	2.0
	2041	0.8		2003	0.8
4 W	0306	2.0	**19** TH	0224	2.0
	0911	0.9		0833	0.8
	1533	1.9		1447	1.9
	2141	1.0		2056	0.9
5 TH	0402	1.8	**20** F	0318	1.9
	1016	1.1		0927	0.9
	1631	1.8		1541	1.9
	2328	1.0		2201	0.9
6 F	0515	1.7	**21** SA	0427	1.8
	1206	1.1		1036	1.0
	1748	1.7		1650	1.8
				2335	0.9
7 SA	0051	1.0	**22** SU	0604	1.8
	0658	1.6		1214	1.0
	1315	1.1		1823	1.9
	1921	1.8			
8 SU	0149	0.9	**23** M	0113	0.8
	0809	1.7		0732	1.9
	1406	1.0		1333	0.9
	2022	1.8		1943	2.0
9 M	0235	0.8	**24** TU	0213	0.6
	0856	1.8		0833	2.0
	1447	1.0		1427	0.8
	2107	1.9		2043	2.1
10 TU	0313	0.7	**25** W	0301	0.5
	0934	1.9		0924	2.1
	1522	0.9		1513	0.6
	2143	2.0		2133	2.3
11 W	0345	0.6	**26** TH	0345	0.4
	1007	2.0		1009	2.2
	1555	0.8		1557	0.5
	2214	2.1		2220	2.4
12 TH	0417	0.6	**27** F	0427	0.3
	1036	2.0		1052	2.3
●	1628	0.7	O	1639	0.5
	2243	2.1		2303	2.4
13 F	0450	0.5	**28** SA	0508	0.3
	1105	2.1		1133	2.3
	1701	0.6		1721	0.4
	2313	2.2		2345	2.4
14 SA	0523	0.5	**29** SU	0549	0.4
	1135	2.1		1212	2.3
	1733	0.6		1803	0.5
	2344	2.2			
15 SU	0556	0.5	**30** M	0027	2.3
	1207	2.1		0628	0.5
	1806	0.6		1251	2.2
				1844	0.5

OCTOBER

Day	Time	m	Day	Time	m
1 TU	0109	2.2	**16** W	0038	2.2
	0707	0.6		0642	0.6
	1330	2.1		1257	2.2
	1926	0.7		1902	0.6
2 W	0151	2.1	**17** TH	0122	2.1
	0746	0.8		0725	0.7
	1411	2.1		1340	2.1
	2011	0.8		1949	0.7
3 TH	0238	1.9	**18** F	0211	2.0
	0828	1.0		0812	0.8
	1456	1.9		1427	2.0
	2103	0.9		2043	0.8
4 F	0331	1.8	**19** SA	0307	1.9
	0916	1.1		0908	1.0
	1551	1.8		1522	1.9
	2233	1.0		2151	0.8
5 SA	0437	1.6	**20** SU	0418	1.8
	1115	1.2		1018	1.0
	1700	1.7		1631	1.9
				2328	0.8
6 SU	0016	1.0	**21** M	0555	1.8
	0603	1.6		1200	1.0
	1242	1.2		1804	1.9
	1824	1.7			
7 M	0117	0.9	**22** TU	0056	0.7
	0730	1.7		0718	1.8
	1336	1.1		1316	1.0
	1939	1.8		1926	2.0
8 TU	0203	0.8	**23** W	0154	0.6
	0820	1.8		0817	2.0
	1418	1.0		1409	0.8
	2028	1.9		2026	2.1
9 W	0240	0.7	**24** TH	0242	0.5
	0858	1.9		0905	2.1
	1453	0.9		1456	0.7
	2106	2.0		2116	2.2
10 TH	0313	0.7	**25** F	0325	0.4
	0931	2.0		0949	2.2
	1527	0.8		1539	0.6
	2140	2.1		2202	2.3
11 F	0346	0.6	**26** SA	0406	0.4
	1002	2.0		1031	2.3
	1601	0.7		1621	0.5
	2213	2.1	O	2245	2.3
12 SA	0420	0.5	**27** SU	0446	0.4
	1034	2.1		1110	2.3
●	1635	0.6		1702	0.5
	2246	2.2		2327	2.3
13 SU	0455	0.5	**28** M	0525	0.5
	1107	2.2		1148	2.3
	1709	0.6		1743	0.5
	2321	2.2			
14 M	0529	0.5	**29** TU	0007	2.3
	1141	2.2		0602	0.6
	1743	0.6		1225	2.2
	2358	2.2		1822	0.6
15 TU	0604	0.5	**30** W	0047	2.2
	1217	2.2		0638	0.7
	1821	0.6		1302	2.2
				1903	0.6
			31 TH	0128	2.0
				0715	0.8
				1341	2.1
				1946	0.8

NOVEMBER

Day	Time	m	Day	Time	m
1 F	0212	1.9	**16** SA	0203	2.1
	0754	1.0		0758	0.8
	1424	1.9		1414	2.1
	2033	0.9		2036	0.7
2 SA	0301	1.8	**17** SU	0300	1.9
	0838	1.1		0853	1.0
	1513	1.8		1509	2.0
	2133	1.0		2142	0.8
3 SU	0400	1.7	**18** M	0407	1.8
	0937	1.2		1002	1.0
	1615	1.8		1615	2.0
	2309	1.0		2309	0.8
4 M	0508	1.6	**19** TU	0532	1.8
	1142	1.2		1134	1.0
	1726	1.7		1739	1.9
5 TU	0026	1.0	**20** W	0030	0.7
	0619	1.7		0653	1.9
	1252	1.1		1252	1.0
	1836	1.7		1903	2.0
6 W	0118	0.9	**21** TH	0132	0.7
	0721	1.7		0754	2.0
	1339	1.0		1350	0.9
	1935	1.8		2006	2.1
7 TH	0159	0.8	**22** F	0222	0.7
	0809	1.8		0845	2.1
	1419	0.9		1439	0.8
	2022	1.9		2059	2.2
8 F	0237	0.7	**23** SA	0306	0.6
	0850	1.9		0929	2.2
	1457	0.8		1524	0.7
	2104	2.0		2146	2.2
9 SA	0315	0.7	**24** SU	0347	0.6
	0928	2.1		1011	2.2
	1534	0.7		1607	0.6
	2143	2.1		2229	2.3
10 SU	0351	0.6	**25** M	0427	0.7
	1004	2.2		1050	2.3
	1610	0.7		1648	0.6
	2222	2.2	O	2310	2.2
11 M	0428	0.6	**26** TU	0504	0.7
	1041	2.2		1127	2.3
	1647	0.6		1728	0.6
●	2301	2.3		2349	2.2
12 TU	0505	0.6	**27** W	0540	0.8
	1119	2.3		1202	2.3
	1726	0.6		1806	0.5
	2342	2.3			
13 W	0544	0.6	**28** TH	0027	2.1
	1158	2.3		0614	0.8
	1807	0.5		1238	2.2
				1845	0.7
14 TH	0026	2.2	**29** F	0106	2.1
	0624	0.7		0650	0.9
	1240	2.3		1315	2.2
	1851	0.6		1924	0.8
15 F	0113	2.2	**30** SA	0147	2.0
	0709	0.7		0728	1.0
	1325	2.2		1355	2.1
	1940	0.6		2007	0.8

DECEMBER

Day	Time	m	Day	Time	m
1 SU	0232	1.9	**16** M	0247	2.1
	0809	1.1		0839	0.9
	1438	2.0		1455	2.2
	2054	0.9		2126	0.7
2 M	0322	1.8	**17** TU	0347	2.0
	0857	1.1		0941	1.0
	1528	1.9		1555	2.1
	2150	1.0		2239	0.8
3 TU	0418	1.7	**18** W	0457	1.9
	0958	1.2		1100	1.1
	1629	1.8		1708	2.1
	2300	1.0		2359	0.9
4 W	0521	1.7	**19** TH	0617	1.9
	1131	1.2		1224	1.1
	1737	1.8		1833	2.0
5 TH	0014	1.0	**20** F	0106	0.9
	0622	1.8		0727	2.0
	1247	1.2		1331	1.0
	1841	1.8		1945	2.1
6 F	0112	0.9	**21** SA	0202	0.9
	0719	1.9		0822	2.1
	1340	1.1		1425	0.9
	1938	1.9		2043	2.1
7 SA	0200	0.9	**22** SU	0249	0.9
	0809	2.0		0910	2.2
	1425	1.0		1513	0.9
	2029	2.0		2132	2.2
8 SU	0243	0.8	**23** M	0332	0.9
	0855	2.1		0954	2.3
	1507	0.9		1557	0.8
	2116	2.2		2216	2.2
9 M	0325	0.8	**24** TU	0412	0.9
	0937	2.2		1033	2.3
	1549	0.8		1638	0.8
	2201	2.3	O	2257	2.2
10 TU	0405	0.7	**25** W	0449	0.9
	1019	2.3		1110	2.3
	1630	0.7		1716	0.7
●	2245	2.3		2334	2.2
11 W	0446	0.7	**26** TH	0523	0.9
	1100	2.4		1144	2.4
	1713	0.6		1752	0.7
	2330	2.4			
12 TH	0528	0.7	**27** F	0009	2.2
	1143	2.4		0556	0.9
	1757	0.5		1218	2.3
				1827	0.7
13 F	0016	2.4	**28** SA	0045	2.2
	0611	0.7		0630	0.9
	1227	2.5		1252	2.3
	1843	0.5		1903	0.8
14 SA	0104	2.2	**29** SU	0122	2.1
	0657	0.8		0706	1.0
	1313	2.4		1328	2.2
	1932	0.6		1941	0.8
15 SU	0154	2.2	**30** M	0201	2.0
	0745	0.9		0744	1.1
	1402	2.3		1405	2.1
	2026	0.6		2021	0.9
			31 TU	0242	2.0
				0824	1.1
				1444	2.1
				2104	1.0

Chart Datum: 1·22 metres below Ordnance Datum (Local)

Volvo Penta service

Sales and service centres in area 8
ARGYLL Crinan Boats Ltd, Crinan, PA31 8SP Tel 0154 683 232

VOLVO PENTA

Area 8

North-West Scotland
Cape Wrath to Crinan Canal

8

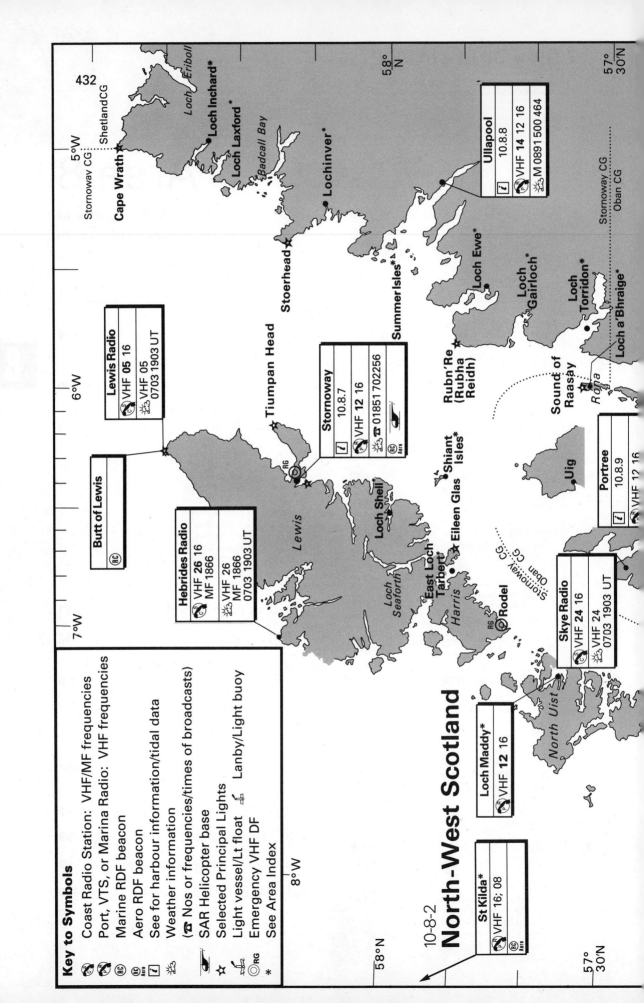

Key to Symbols

📻🐟 Coast Radio Station: VHF/MF frequencies
📻⚓ Port, VTS, or Marina Radio: VHF frequencies
(RC) Marine RDF beacon
(RC)Aero Aero RDF beacon
ℹ️ See for harbour information/tidal data
🌦️ Weather information
(☎ Nos or frequencies/times of broadcasts)
🚁 SAR Helicopter base
☆ Selected Principal Lights
Light vessel/Lt float ⚓ Lanby/Light buoy
(RG) Emergency VHF DF
* See Area Index

10-8-2
North-West Scotland

432

St Kilda*
| ℹ️📻⚓ | VHF 16; 08 |
| (RC)Aero | |

Loch Maddy*
| 📻⚓ | VHF 12 16 |

Skye Radio
| 📻🐟 | VHF 24 16 |
| 🌦️ | VHF 24 0703 1903 UT |

Portree
10.8.9
| ℹ️ | |
| 📻⚓ | VHF 12 16 |

North Uist
Uig
Sound of Raasay
Rona
Loch a'Bhraige*
Loch Torridon*
Loch Gairloch*
Rubn'Re (Rubha Reidh)
Loch Ewe*

Hebrides Radio
| 📻🐟 | VHF 26 16 MF 1866 |
| 🌦️ | VHF 26 MF 1866 0703 1903 UT |

Butt of Lewis
| (RC) | |

Harris
Rodel (RG)
East Loch Tarbert*
☆ Eileen Glas*
Shiant Isles*
Loch Seaforth
Loch Shell*
Lewis

Stornoway
10.8.7
ℹ️	
📻⚓	VHF 12 16
☎	01851 702256
(RC)Aero	

RG
☆ Tiumpan Head
Stornoway CG

Lewis Radio
| 📻🐟 | VHF 05 16 |
| 🌦️ | VHF 05 0703 1903 UT |

☆ Stoerhead
Summer Isles*▲

Ullapool
10.8.8
ℹ️	
📻⚓	VHF 14 12 16
🌦️	M 0891 500 464

● Lochinver*
Badcall Bay
Loch Laxford*
● Loch Inchard*
Loch Eriboll
☆ Cape Wrath
Shetland CG
Stornoway CG

Stornoway CG
Oban CG

58°N
57° 30'N
8°W
7°W
6°W
5°W
58° N
57° 30'N

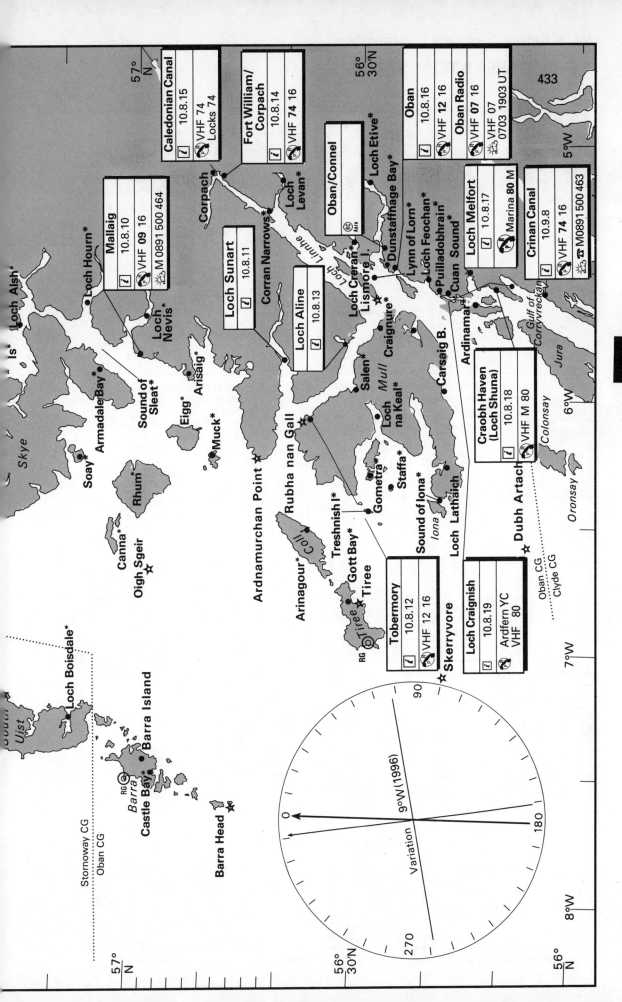

433

10-8-3 AREA 8 TIDAL STREAMS

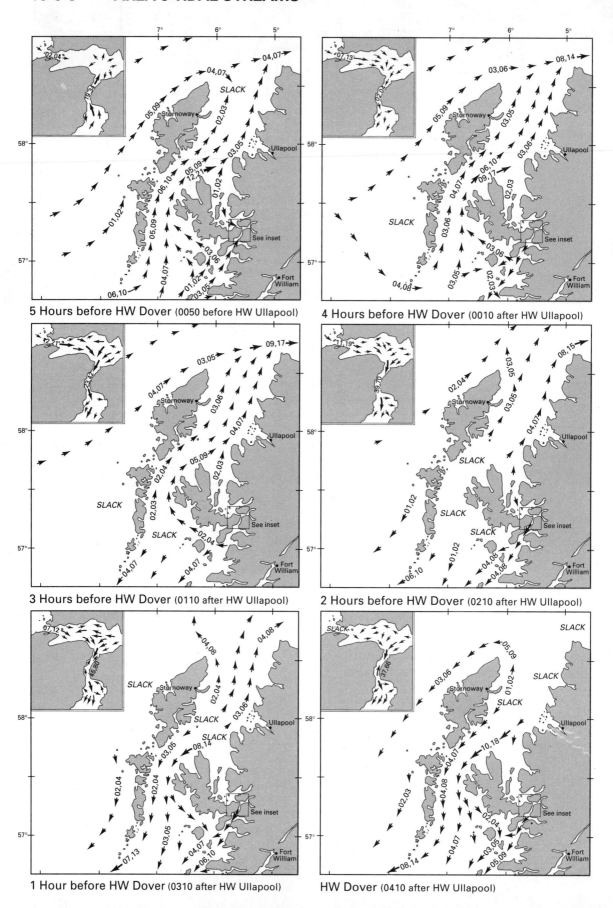

5 Hours before HW Dover (0050 before HW Ullapool)

4 Hours before HW Dover (0010 after HW Ullapool)

3 Hours before HW Dover (0110 after HW Ullapool)

2 Hours before HW Dover (0210 after HW Ullapool)

1 Hour before HW Dover (0310 after HW Ullapool)

HW Dover (0410 after HW Ullapool)

Eastward 10.7.3   Southward 10.9.3

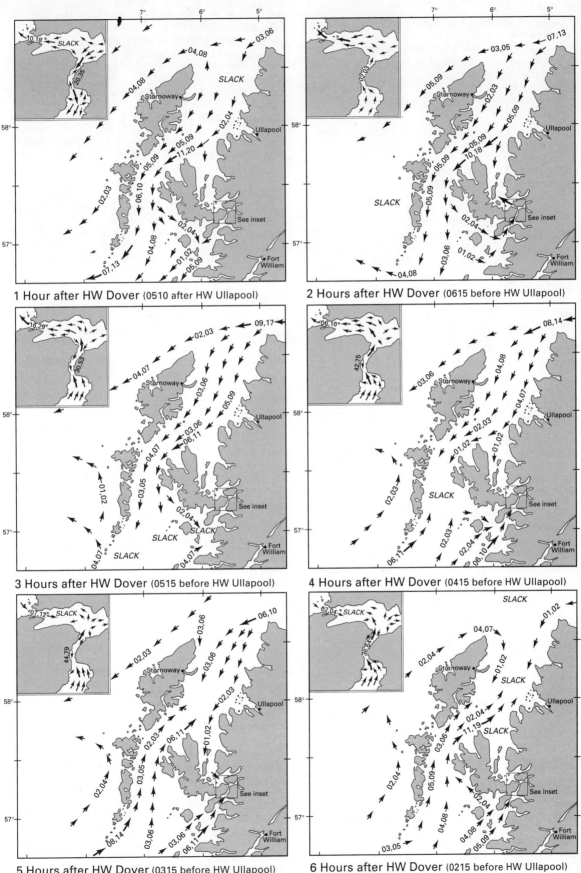

1 Hour after HW Dover (0510 after HW Ullapool)

2 Hours after HW Dover (0615 before HW Ullapool)

3 Hours after HW Dover (0515 before HW Ullapool)

4 Hours after HW Dover (0415 before HW Ullapool)

5 Hours after HW Dover (0315 before HW Ullapool)

6 Hours after HW Dover (0215 before HW Ullapool)

8

10.8.4 COASTAL LIGHTS, FOG SIGNALS AND WAYPOINTS

Abbreviations used below are given in 1.4.1. Principal lights are in **bold** print, places in CAPITALS, and light-vessels, light floats and Lanbys in *CAPITAL ITALICS*. Unless otherwise stated lights are white. m – elevation in metres; M – nominal range in miles. Fog signals are in *italics*. Useful waypoints are underlined – use those on land with care. All geographical positions should be assumed to be approximate. See 4.4.1.

Rockall 57°35'·8N 13°41'·3W Fl 15s 19m 13M (unreliable). Extinguised (T) 1993.

CAPE WRATH TO LOCH TORRIDON
Cape Wrath 58°37'·55N 04°59'·87W Fl (4) 30s 122m **24M**; W Tr; *Horn (3) 45s.*

LOCH INCHARD/LOCH LAXFORD
Rubha na Leacaig 58°27'·43N 05°04'·51W Fl (2) 10s 30m 8M. Kinlochbervie Ldg Lts 327°. Front 58°27'·52N 05°03'·01W Oc G 8s 16m 9M W□, Or △ on Gy Tr. Rear, 330m from front, Oc G 8s 26m 9M; W □, Or ▽ on Gy Tr.
Stoer Hd 58°14'·43N 05°24'·08W Fl 15s 59m **24M**; W Tr.

LOCH INVER
Soyea I 58°08'·58N 05°19'·59W Fl (2) 10s 34m 6M; Y post. Glas Leac 58°08'·70N 05°16'·27W Fl WRG 3s 7m; Gy col; vis W071°-080°, R080°-090°, G090°-103°, W103°-111°, R111°-243°, W243°-251°, G251°-071°.

The Perch (off Aird Ghlas) 58°08'·91N 05°15'·02W QG 3m 1M; B col, W bands; TE 1991.
Culag Hbr Pier Hd 58°08'·93N 05°14'·61W 2 FG (vert) 6m.

SUMMER ISLES
Old Dornie, new Pier Hd 58°02'·59N 05°25'·31W Fl G 3s 5m.

Rubha Cadail 57°55'·53N 05°13'·30W Fl WRG 6s 11m W9M, R6M, G6M; W Tr; vis G311°-320°, W320°-325°, R325°-103°, W103°-111°, G111°-118°, W118°-127°, R127°-157°, W157°-199°.

ULLAPOOL
Ullapool Pt Lt By 57°53'·43N 05°10'·35W QR; PHM.
Ullapool Pt 57°53'·62N 05°09'·67W Iso R 4s 8m 6M.
Cailleach Hd 57°55'·83N 05°24'·15W Fl (2) 12s 60m 9M; W Tr; vis 015°-236°.

LOCH EWE/LOCH GAIRLOCH
Fairway Lt By 57°52'·00N 05°40'·02W L Fl 10s; SWM.
NATO Jetty, NW corner Fl G 4s 5m 3M.
Rubha Reidh 57°51'·55N 05°48'·61W Fl (4) 15s 37m **24M**.
Glas Eilean 57°42'·82N 05°42'·36W Fl WRG 6s 9m W6M, R4M; vis W080°-102°, R102°-296°, W296°-333°, G333°-080°.

OUTER HEBRIDES – EAST SIDE
LEWIS
Butt of Lewis 58°30'·93N 06°15'·72W Fl 5s 52m **25M**; R Tr; vis 056°-320°; RC.
Tiumpan Hd 58°15'·6N 06°08'·3W Fl (2) 15s 55m **25M**; W Tr.

STORNOWAY
Arnish Pt 58°11'·50N 06°22'·17W Fl WR 10s 17m **W19M**, **R15M**; W ● Tr; vis W088°-198°, R198°-302°, W302°-013°.

Sandwick Bay, NW side Oc WRG 6s 10m 9M; vis G334°-341°, W341°-347°, R347°-354°.
Eitshal 58°10'·7N 06°35'·0W 4 FR (vert) on radio mast.

LOCH ERISORT/LOCH SHELL/EAST LOCH TARBERT
Tabhaidh Bheag 58° 07'·22N 06°23'·15W Fl 3s 13m 3M.
Eilean Chalabrigh 58°06'·81N 06°26'·62W QG 5m 3M.
Gob na Milaid Pt 58°01'·0N 06°21'·8W Fl 15s 14m 10M.
Rubh' Uisenis 57°56'·2N 06°28'·2W Fl 5s 24m 11M; W Tr.
Sgeir Inoe Lt By 57°50'·95N 06°33'·90W Fl G 6s; SHM.
Shiants Lt By 57°54'·60N 06°25'·60W QG; SHM.
Scalpay, **Eilean Glas** 57°51'·43N 06°38'·45W Fl (3) 20s 43m **23M**; W Tr, R bands; Racon (T).
Scalpay N Hbr Lt By 57°52'·58N 06°42'·16W Fl G 2s;SHM.
Dun Cor Mòr Fl R 5s 10m 5M.
Sgeir Graidach Lt By 57°50'·38N 06°41'·31W Q (6) + L Fl 15s; SCM.
Sgeir Ghlas 57°52'·38N 06°45'·18W Iso WRG 4s 9m W9M, R6M, G6M; W ● Tr; vis G282°-319°, W319°-329°, R329°-153°, W153°-164°, G164°-171°.

SOUND OF HARRIS/LEVERBURGH
Dubh Sgeir 57°45'·54N 07°02'·56W Q (2) 5s 9m 6M; R Tr, B bands.
Ldg Lts 014·7°. Front, 57°46'·25N 07°01'·98W Q 10m 4M. Rear Oc 3s 12m 4M.
Jane's Tr 57°45'·79N 07°02'·05W Q (2) G 5s 6m 4M; obsc 273°-318°.
Leverburgh Pier Hd 57°46'·04N 07°01'·56W Oc WRG 8s 5m 2M; Gy col; vis G305°-059°, W059°-066°, R066°-125°.

BERNERAY
W side, **Barra Hd** 57°47'·13N 07°39'·18W Fl 15s 208m **18M**; W Tr; obsc by islands to NE.
Berneray Bkwtr Hd 57°42'·9N 07°10'·0W Iso R 4s 6m 4M.
Drowning Rock Q (2) G 8s 2m 2M; G pillar.
Reef Chan No. 1 QG 2m 4M.
Reef Chan No. 2 Iso G 4s 2m 4M.

NORTH UIST
Eilean Fuam 57°41'·9N 07°10'·6W Q 6m 2M; W col.
Newton Jetty Root 57°41'·5N 07°11'·5W 2 FG (vert) 9m 4M.
Griminish Hbr Ldg Lts 183°. Front, 57°39'·4xN 07°26'·6xW QG 6m 4M. Rear, 110m from front, QG 7m 4M.
Pier Hd 57°39'·3N 07°26'·3W 2 FG (vert) 6m 4M; Gy col (shown Mar-Oct).

LOCH MADDY
Weaver's Pt 5 7°36'·51N 07°05'·95W Fl 3s 21m 7M; W hut.
Glas Eilean Mòr 57°35'·97N 07°06'·64W Fl G 4s 8m 5M.
Rubna Nam Pleàc 57°35'·78N 07°06'·70W Fl R 4s 7m 5M.
Ruigh Liath E Islet 57°35'·74N 07°08'·36W QG 6m 5M.

Vallaquie I 57°35'·52N 07°09'·34W Fl (3) WRG 8s 11m W7M, R5M, G5M; W pillar; vis G shore-205°, W205°-210°, R210°-240°, G240°-254°, W254°-257°, R257°-shore (P).

Lochmaddy Ldg Lts 298°. Front, Ro-Ro Pier 57°35'·79N 07°09'·29W 2 FG (vert) 8m 4M. Rear, 110m from front, Oc G 8s 10m 4M; vis 284°-304°.

GRIMSAY
Kallin Hbr Bkwtr NE corner 57°28'·90N 07°12'·25W 2 FR (vert) 6m 5M; Gy col.

SOUTH UIST, LOCH CARNAN
Landfall Lt By 57°22'·30N 07°11'·45W L Fl 10s; SWM.
No. 2 Lt By 57°22'·41N 07°14'·87W Fl R 2s; PHM.
No. 3 Lt By 57°22'·33N 07°15'·54W Fl R 5s; PHM.
No. 4 Lt By 57°22'·27N 07°15'·82W QR; PHM.
Ldg Lts 222°. Front 57°22'·02N 07°16'·28W Fl R 2s 7m 5M; W ◊ on post. Rear, 58m from front, Iso R 10s 11m 5M; W ◊ on post.
Ushenish (S Uist) 57°17'·91N 07°11'·50W Fl WR 20s 54m **W19M**, **R15M**; W Tr; vis W193°-356°, R356°-013°.

LOCH BOISDALE

Calvay E End 57°08'·55N 07°15'·32W Fl (2) WRG 10s 16m W7M, R4M, G4M; W Tr; vis W111°-190°, G190°-202°, W202°-286°, R286°-111°, .

N side 57°08'·99N 07°16'·98W Fl G 6s 3m 3M.

Gasay I Fl WR 5s 10m W7M, R4M; W Tr; vis W120°-284°, R284°-120°, .

Channel Lt By 57°09'·04N 07°17'·38W QG; SHM.

Sgeir Rk Lt By 57°09'·11N 07°17'·70W Fl G 3s; SHM.

Ro-Ro Jetty Hd 57°09'·15N 07°18'·17W Iso RG 4s 8m 2M; vis G shore-283°, R283°-shore; 2 FG (vert) 8m 3M on dn 84m W.

LUDAIG

Ludaig Dir Lt 297° 57°06'·2N 07°19'·7W Dir Oc WRG 6s 8m W7M, R4M, G4M; vis G287°-296°, W296°-298°, R298°-307°.

Stag Rk 57°05'·88N 07°18'·31W Fl (2) 8s 7m 4M.

The Witches Lt By 57°05'·75N 07°20'·77W Fl R 5s; PHM.

Ludaig Pier 2 FG (vert) 5m 3M.

ERISKAY

Bank Rk 57°05'·60N 07°17'·51W Q (2) 4s 5m 4M.

Haun Dir Lt 236° Dir Oc WRG 3s 9m W7M, R4M, G4M; vis G226°-234.5°, W234·5°-237·5°, R237·5°-246°.

Pier 2 FG(vert) 5m 5M.

Acairseid Mhor Ldg Lts 285°. Front 57°03'·92N 07°17'·18W Oc R 6s 9m 4M. Rear, 24m from front, Oc R 6s 10m 4M.

BARRA/CASTLEBAY, VATERSAY SOUND

Drover Rks Lt By 57°04'·18N 07°23'·58W Fl (2) 10s; IDM.

Curachan Lt By 56°58'·58N 07°20'·45W Q (3) 10s; ECM.

Ardveenish 57°00'·23N 07°24'·37W Oc WRG 6m 9/6M; vis G300°-304°, W304°-306°, R306°-310°.

Bo Vich Chuan Lt By 56°56'·17N 07°23'·27W Q (6) + L Fl 15s; SCM; Racon.

Sgeir Dubh 56°56'·42N 07°28'·87W Q (3) WG 6s 6m W6M, G4M; vis W280°-180°, G180°-280°. In line 283° with Sgeir Leadh (Liath) below.

Sgeir Leadh (Liath) 56°56'·65N 07°30'·72W Fl 3s 7m 8M.

Castlebay 56°57'·23N 07°29'·22W Fl R 5s 2m 3M.

Rubha Glas. Ldg Lts 295°. Front 56°56'·78N 07°30'·59W FG 9m 11M; Or △ on W Tr. Rear, 457m from front, FG 15m 11M; Or ▽ on W Tr.

OUTER HEBRIDES – WEST SIDE

Flannan I, Eilean Mór 58°17'·32N 07°35'·23W Fl (2) 30s 101m **20M**; W Tr; obsc in places by Is to W of Eilean Mór.

EAST LOCH ROAG

Aird Laimishader Carloway 58°17'·06N 06°49'·50W L Fl 12s 61m 8M; W hut; obsc on some brgs.

Ardvanich Pt 58°13'·48N 06°47'·68W Fl G 3s 4m 2M.

Tidal Rk 58°13'·45N 06°47'·57W Fl R 3s 2m 2M (synch with Ardvanich Pt above).

Gt Bernera Kirkibost Jetty 2 FG (vert) 7m 2M.

Grèinam 58°13'·30N 06°46'·16W Fl WR 6s 8m W8M, R7M; W Bn; vis R143°-169°, W169°-143°.

Rudha Arspaig Jetty Hd 2 FR (vert) 10m 4M.

NORTH UIST/SOUTH UIST

Vallay I 57°39'·70N 07°26'·10W Fl WRG 3s 8M; vis W206°-085°, G085°-140°, W140°-145°, R145°-206°.

Falconet Tr 57°21'·5N 07°23'·6W FR 25m 8M (3M by day); shown 1h before firing, changes to Iso R 2s 15 min before firing until completion.

ST KILDA

Ldg Lts 270°. Front 57°48'·36N 08°34'·27W Oc 5s 26m 3M. Rear, 100m from front, Oc 5s 38m 3M; synch.

SKYE

Eilean Trodday 57°43'·65N 06°17'·87W Fl (2) WRG 10s 49m W12M, R9M, G9M; W Bn; vis W062°-088°, R088°-130°, W130°-322°, G322°-062°.

RONA/LOCH A'BHRAIGE

NE Point 57°34'·71N 05°57'·48W Fl 12s 69m **19M**; W Tr; vis 050°-358°.

Sgeir Shuas 57°35'·04N 05°58'·54W Fl R 2s 6m 3M; vis 070°-199°.

Jetty, NE end 57°34'·68N 05°57'·86W 2FR (vert).

Rock 57°34'·62N 05°57'·94W Fl R 5s 4m 3M.

Ldg Lts 136·5° Front No. 9 Bn 57°34'·43N 05°58'·02W Q WRG 3m W4M, R3M; W and Or Bn; vis W135°-138°, R138°-318°, G318°-135°. Rear No. 10 Iso 6s 28m 5M; W Bn.

No. 1 Bn Fl G 3s 91m 3M, Or Bn.

Rubha Chùiltairbh Fl 3s 6m 5M; W Bn.

No. 11 Bn QY 6m 4M; Or Bn.

No. 3 Bn Fl (2) 10s 9m 4M; W Bn and Or stripes.

No. 12 Bn QR 5m 3M; Or Bn.

Garbh Eilean SE Pt No. 8 Bn Fl 3s 8m 5M; W Bn.

INNER SOUND

Ru Na Lachan 57°29'·04N 05°52'·07W Oc WR 8s 21m 10M; Tr; vis W337°-022°, R022°-117°, W117°-162°.

SOUND OF RAASAY, PORTREE

Portree Pier Hd 57°24'·66N 06°11'·34W 2 FR (vert) 6m 4M; occas.

CROWLIN ISLANDS

Eilean Beag 57°21'·23N 05°51'·33W Fl 6s 32m 6M; W Bn.

RAASAY/LOCH SLIGACHAN

Suisnish 2 FG (vert) 8m 2M.

Eyre Pt 57°20'·03N 06°01'·22W Fl WR 3s 5m W9M, R6M; W Tr; vis W215°-266°, R266°-288°, W288°-063°.

Sconser Ferry Terminal 57°18'·9N 06°06'·6W QR 8m 3M.

McMillan's Rk Lt By 57°21'·13N 06°06'·24W Fl (2) G 12s; SHM.

LOCH CARRON

No. 1 Lt By 57°21'·43N 05°38'·82W Fl G 3s; SHM.

Old Lt Ho 57°20'·97N 05°38'·81W (unlit).

KYLE AKIN AND KYLE OF LOCH ALSH

Kyle Akin Lt Ho 57°16'·68N 05°44'·48W (unlit)

Carragh Rk Lt By 57°17'·20N 05°45'·30W Fl (2) G 12s; SHM; Racon (T).

Bow Rk Lt By 57°16'·78N 05°45'·85W Fl (2) R 12s; PHM.

Fork Rks Lt By 57°16'·86N 05°44'·87W Fl G 6s; SHM.

Black Eye Rk Lt By 57°16'·73N 05°45'·24W Fl R 6s; PHM.

Eileanan Dubha 57°16'·58N 05°42'·25W Fl (2) 10s 9m 8M; vis obscured 104°-146°.

String Rk Lt By 57°16'·51N 05°42'·82W Fl R 6s; PHM.

Allt-an-Avaig Jetty 2 FR (vert) 10m; vis 075°-270°.

S shore, ferry slipway QR 6m (vis in Kyle of Loch Alsh).

Mooring dolphin 57°16'·38N 05°43'·36W Q 5m 3M.

Ferry Pier, W and E sides, 2 FG (vert) 6/5m 5/4M.

Butec Jetty W end N corner 57°16'·77N 05°42'·36W Oc G 6s 5m 3M each end, synch.

Sgeir-na-Caillich 57°15'·63N 05°38'·83W Fl (2) R 6s 3m 4M.

SOUND OF SLEAT

Kyle Rhea 57°14'·24N 05°39'·85W Fl WRG 3s 7m W11M, R9M, G8M; W Bn; vis R shore-219°, W219-228°, G228°-338°, W338°-346°, R346°-shore.

Sandaig I, NW point Fl 6s 12m 8M; W 8-sided Tr.

Ornsay, N end 57°09'·10N 05°46'·5W Fl R 6s 8m 4M; W Tr.

Ornsay, SE end 57°08'·60N 05°46'·80W Oc 8s 18m **15M**; W Tr; vis 157°-030°.

Eilean Iarmain, off Pier Hd 2 FR (vert) 3m 2M.

Armadale Bay Pier Centre Oc R 6s 6m 6M.
Pt of Sleat 57°01'·11N 06°01'·00W Fl 3s 20m 9M; W Tr.

MALLAIG, ENTRANCE TO LOCH NEVIS
Northern Pier E end 57°00'·48N 05°49'·43W Iso WRG 4s 6m
W9M, R6M, G6M; Gy Tr; vis G181°-185°, W185°-197°,
R197°-201°. Fl G 3s 14m 6M; same structure.
Sgeir Dhearg 57°00'·64N 05°49'·53W Fl (2) WG 8s 6m 5M;
Gy Bn; vis G190°-055°, W055°-190°.

NW SKYE, UIG/LOCH DUNVEGAN/LOCH HARPORT
Uig Edward Pier Hd 57°35'·14N 06°22'·22W Iso WRG 4s 9m
W7M, R4M, G4M; vis W180°-008°, G008°-052°, W052°-075°,
R075°-180°.
Waternish Pt 57°36'·5N 06°38'·0W Fl 20s 21m 8M; W Tr.
Loch Dunvegan Uiginish Pt 57°26'·8N 06°36'·5W Fl WG
3s 14m W7M, G5M; W hut; vis G040°-128°, W128°-306°,
obsc by Fiadhairt Pt when brg more than 148°.
Neist Pt 57°25'·4N 06°47'·2W Fl 5s 43m **16M**; W Tr.
Loch Harport Ardtreck Pt 57°20'·4N 06°25'·8W Iso 4s 17m
9M; small W Tr.

SMALL ISLES AND WEST OF MULL

CANNA, RHUM
E end Sanday Is 57°02'·84N 06°27'·92W Fl 6s 32m 9M; W Tr;
vis 152°-061°

ÒIGH SGEIR/EIGG/ARISAIG
Humla Lt By 57°00'·43N 06°37'·40W Fl G 6s; SHM.
S end, **Hyskeir** 56°58'·13N 06°40'·80W Fl (3) 30s 41m **24M**;
W Tr. N end Horn 30s.
SE point of Eigg (Eilean Chathastail) 56°52'·25N 06°07'·20W
Fl 6s 24m 8M; W Tr; vis 181°-shore.

Bo Faskadale Lt By 56°48'·18N 06°06'·35W Fl (3) G 18s; SHM.
Ardnamurchan 56°43'·64N 06°13'·46W Fl (2) 20s 55m **24M**;
Gy Tr; vis 002°-217°; Horn (2) 20s.
Cairns of Coll, Suil Ghorm 56°42'·27N 06°26'·70W Fl 12s 23m
10M; W Tr.

COLL/ARINAGOUR
Loch Eatharna, Bogha Mor Lt By 56°36'·67N 06°30'·90W
Fl G 6s; SHM.
Arinagour Pier 2 FR (vert) 12m.

TIREE
Roan Bogha Lt By 56°32'·25N 06°40'·10W Q (6) + L Fl 15s; SCM.
Placaid Bogha Lt By 56°33'·24N 06°43'·93W Fl G 4s; SHM.
Scarinish, S side of ent 56°30'·02N 06°48'·20W Fl 3s 11m
16M; W ■ Tr; vis 210°-030°.
Gott Bay Ldg Lts 286·5°. Front 56°30'·63N 06°47'·75W FR
8m (when vessel expected). Rear 30m from front FR 11m.
Skerryvore 56°19'·40N 07°06'·75W Fl 10s 46m **23M**; Gy Tr;
Racon (M); Horn 60s.

LOCH NA LÀTHAICH (LOCH LATHAICH)
Eileanan na Liathanaich, SE end 56°20'·58N 06°16'·30W
Fl WR 6s 12m W8M, R6M; vis R088°-108°, W108°-088°.
Dubh Artach 56°07'·95N 06°37'·95W Fl (2) 30s 44m **20M**;
Gy Tr, R band; Horn 45s.

SOUND OF MULL

LOCH SUNART/TOBERMORY/LOCH ALINE
Ardmore Pt 56°39'·39N 06°07'·62W Fl (2) 10s 17m 8M.
New Rks Lt By 56°39'·07N 06°03'·22W Fl G 6s; SHM.
Rubha nan Gall 56°38'·33N 06°03'·91W Fl 3s 17m **15M**,
W Tr.
Bogha Bhuilg By 56°36'·15N 05°59'·07W; SHM.
Hispania Wk Lt By 56°34'·70N 05°59'·30W Fl (2) R 10s; PHM.
Bo Rks By 56°31'·54N 05°55'·47W; SHM.
Eileanan Glasa, Green I (Dearg Sgeir) 56°32'·27N 05°54'·72W
Fl 6s 7m 8M; W ● Tr.

Fuinary Spit Lt By 56°32'·66N 05°53'·09W Fl G 6s; SHM.
Avon Rk By 56°30'·80N 05°46'·72W; PHM.
Lochaline Lt By 56°32'·99N 05°46'·41W QR; PHM.
Lochaline Ldg Lts 356°. Front 56°32'·40N 05°46'·40W F 2M.
Rear, 88m from front, F 4M; H24.
Ardtornish Pt 56°31'·10N 05°45'·15W Fl (2) WRG 10s 7m W8M,
R5M, G5M; W Tr; vis G shore-302°, W302°-310°, R310°-342°,
W342°-057°, R057°-095°, W095°-108°, G108°-shore.
Yule Rk By 56°30'·03N 05°43'·88W; PHM.
Glas Eileanan Gy Rks 56°29'·78N 05°42'·76W Fl 3s 11m 6M;
W ● Tr on W base.
Craignure Ldg Lts 240·9°. Front 56°28'·30N 05°42'·21W FR 10m.
Rear, 150m from front, FR 12m; vis 225·8°-255·8° (on req).

MULL TO CALEDONIAN CANAL AND OBAN

Lismore SW end 56°27'·35N 05°36'·38W Fl 10s 31m **19M**;
W Tr; vis 237°-208°.
Lady's Rk 56°26'·91N 05°36'·98W Fl 6s 12m 5M; R ● on W Bn.

Duart Pt 56°26'·85N 05°38'·69W Fl (3) WR 18s 14m W5M,
R3M; vis W162°-261°, R261°-275°, W275°-353°, R353°-shore.

LOCH LINNHE
Ent W side, Corran Pt 56°43'·27N 05°14'·47W Iso WRG 4s
12m W10M, R7M; W Tr; vis R shore-195°, W195°-215°,
G215°-305°, W305°-030°, R030°-shore.
Corran Narrows NE 56°43'·62N 05°13'·83W Fl 5s 4m 4M;
W Tr; vis S shore-214°.
Jetty 56°43'·42N 05°14'·56W Fl R 5s 7m 3M; Gy mast.

FORT WILLIAM/CALEDONIAN CANAL
Corpach, Caledonian Canal Lock ent Iso WRG 4s 6m 5M;
W Tr; vis G287°-310°, W310°-335°, R335°-030°.

LYNN OF LORN
Sgeir Bhuidhe Appin 56°33'·65N 05°24'·57W Fl (2) WR 7s 7m
9M; W Bn; vis R184°-220°, W220°-184°.
Off Airds Pt 56°32'·22N 05°25'·13W Fl WRG 2s 2m W3M,
R1M, G1M; R col; vis R196°-246°, W246°-258°, G258°-041°,
W041°-058°, R058°-093°, W093°-139°.
Eriska NE Pt, QG 2m 2M; G col; vis 128°-329°.

DUNSTAFFNAGE BAY
Pier Hd, NE end 56°27'·22N 05°26'·10W 2 FG (vert) 4m 2M.

OBAN
N spit of Kerrera 56°25'·50N 05°29'·50W Fl R 3s 9m 5M;
W col, R bands.
Dunollie 56°25'·39N 05°28'·98W Fl (2) WRG 6s 7m W5M,
G4M, R4M; vis G351°-009°, W009°-047°, R047°-120°, W120°-
138°, G138°-143°.
Rubbh'a' Chruidh 56°25'·33N 05°29'·22W QR 3m 2M.

OBAN TO LOCH CRAIGNISH

Kerrera Sound, Dubh Sgeir 56°22'·82N 05°32'·20W Fl (2) 12s
7m 5M; W ● Tr.

Fladda 56°14'·90N 05°40'·75W Fl (2) WRG 9s 13m W11M,
R9M, G9M; W Tr; vis R169°-186°, W186°-337°, G337°-344°.
W344°-356°, R356°-026°.
Dubh Sgeir (Luing) 56°14'·78N 05°40'·12W Fl WRG 6s 9m
W6M, R4M. G4M; W Tr; vis W000°-010°, R010°-025°, W025°-
199°, G199°-000°; Racon.
The Garvellachs, Eileach an Naoimh, SW end 56°13'·05N
05°48'·97W Fl 6s 21m 9M; W Bn; vis 240°-215°.

LOCH MELFORT/CRAOBH HAVEN
Fearnach Bay Pier 56°16'·15N 05°30'·11W 2 FR (vert) 6/5m
3M; (Private shown 1/4 to 31/10). TE 1993.

For Colonsay, and Sounds of Jura and Islay see 10.9.4.

10.8.5   PASSAGE INFORMATION

It is essential to carry large scale charts, and pilotage information as in *W Coast of Scotland Pilot*; Clyde Cruising Club's *Sailing Directions, Pt 2 Kintyre to Ardnamurchan* and *Pt 3 Ardnamurchan to Cape Wrath*; and the *Yachtsman's Pilot to W Coast of Scotland* (3 Vols) by Martin Lawrence. See 10.9.5 for some of the more relevant terms in Gaelic.

The West coast of Scotland provides splendid, if sometimes boisterous, sailing and unmatched scenery. In summer the long hours of daylight and warmth of the Gulf Stream compensate for the lower air temperatures and higher wind speeds experienced when depressions run typically north of Scotland. Inshore the wind is often unpredictable, due to the geographical effects of lochs, mountains and islands offshore; calms and squalls can alternate rapidly. Local magnetic anomalies occur in Kilbrannan Sound, Passage of Tiree, Sound of Mull, Canna, and East Loch Roag. A yacht must rely on good anchors. HIE and public ⚓s are listed, but it should not be assumed that these will always be available. Particularly in N of area, facilities are very dispersed. Beware ever more fish farms in many inlets. Submarines exercise throughout these waters: see 10.8.20 for info on active areas (Subfacts).

CAPE WRATH TO ULLAPOOL (charts 1785, 1794)

C. Wrath (lt, fog sig) is a steep headland (110m). To N of it the E-going stream begins at HW Ullapool – 0350, and W- going at HW Ullapool + 0235, sp rates 3kn. Eddies close inshore cause almost continuous W-going stream E of Cape, and N-going stream SW of it. Where they meet is turbulence, with dangerous seas in bad weather. Duslic Rk, 7ca NE of lt ho, dries 3·4m. 6M SW of C. Wrath is Islet of Am Balg (45m), foul for 2ca around.

There are anchs in Loch Inchard (chart 2503), the best shelter being in Loch Bervie on N shore; also good anchs among Is along S shore of Loch Laxford, entered between Ardmore Pt and Rubha Ruadh (see 10.8.7). Handa Is to WSW is bird sanctuary. Handa Sound is navigable with care, but beware Bogha Morair in mid-chan and associated overfalls. Tide turns 2hrs earlier in the Sound than offshore.

Strong winds against tide raise a bad sea off Pt of Stoer. The best shelter is 8M S at Loch Inver (10.8.8 and chart 2504), with good anch off hotel near head of loch. S lies Enard B.

ULLAPOOL TO LOCH TORRIDON (charts 1794, 2210)

The Summer Isles (chart 2501), 12M NW of the major fishing port of Ullapool (10.8.8), offer some sheltered anchs and tight approaches. The best include the B on E side of Tanera Mor; off NE of Tanera Beg (W of Eilean Fada Mor); and in Caolas Eilean Ristol, between the Is and mainland.

Loch Ewe (10.8.7 and chart 3146) provides good shelter and easy access. Best anchs are in Poolewe B (beware Boor Rks off W shore) and in SW corner of Loch Thuirnaig (entering, keep close to S shore to avoid rks extending from N side).

Off Rubha Reidh (lt) seas can be dangerous. The NE-going stream begins at HW Ullapool – 0335; the SW-going at HW Ullapool + 0305. Sp rates 3kn, but slacker to SW of point.

Longa Is lies N of ent to Loch Gairloch (10.8.7 and chart 2528). The chan N of it is navigable but narrow at E end. Outer loch is free of dangers, but exposed to swell. Best anch is on S side of loch in Caolas Bad a' Chrotha, W of Eilean Horrisdale.

Loch Torridon (chart 2210) has few dangers. Streams are weak except where they run 2-3 kn in narrows between Loch Shieldaig and Upper Loch Torridon. Entering Loch Torridon from S or W beware Murchadh Breac (dries 1·5m) 3ca NNW of Rubha na Fearna. Best anchs are SW of Eilean Mor (to W of Ardheslaig); in Loch a 'Chracaich, 7ca further SE; E of Shieldaig Is; and near head of Upper Loch Torridon.

OUTER HEBRIDES (charts 1785, 1794, 1795)

The E sides of these Is have many good, sheltered anchs, but W coasts give little shelter. The Clyde Cruising Club's *Outer Hebrides Sailing Directions* are advised. The Minches and Sea of the Hebrides can be very rough, particularly in the Little Minch between Skye and Harris, and around Shiant Is where tide runs locally 4kn at sp, and heavy overfalls can be met. The NE-going stream begins at HW Ullapool – 0335; the SW-going stream at HW Ullapool + 0250, sp rates 2·5kn.

From N to S, the better hbrs in Outer Hebrides include: *Lewis*. Stornoway (10.8.7); Loch Grimshader (beware Sgeir a'Chaolais, dries in entrance); Loch Erisort; Loch Odhairn; Loch Shell (10.8.7). Proceeding S from here, or to E Loch Tarbert beware Sgeir Inoe (dries 2·3m) 3M ESE of Eilean Glas lt ho at SE end of Scalpay.

Harris. E Loch Tarbert; Loch Scadaby; Loch Stockinish; Loch Finsby; W Loch Tarbert; L Rodel (HIE ⚓)
N Uist. Loch Maddy (HIE ⚓); Loch Eport, Kallin Hbr (HIE ⚓).
S Uist. Loch Skiport; Loch Eynort; Loch Boisdale (HIE ⚓); L Carnan (HIE ⚓).
Barra. Castlebay (HIE ⚓), see 10.8.7, and Berneray, on N side, E of Shelter Rk.

Range activity at the Army Artillery Range, Benbecula is broadcast at 1000LT (1 Apr - 30 Oct) on VHF Ch 12 (Ch 73 emergency only) and on MF 2660 kHz.

SKYE TO ARDNAMURCHAN PT (charts 1795, 2210, 2209, 2208, 2207)

Skye and the Is around it provide many good and attractive anchs, of which the most secure are: Acairseid Mhor on the W side of Rona; Portree (10.8.9); Isleornsay; Portnalong, near the ent to Loch Harport, and Carbost at the head; L. Dunvegan; and Uig B in Loch Snizort. HIE ⚓s at Stein (L. Dunvegan), Portree, Acairseid Mhor (Rona), Churchton B (Raasay) and Armadale Bay (S tip).

Tides are strong off Rubha Hunish at N end of Skye, and heavy overfalls occur with weather-going tide against fresh or strong winds. Anch behind Fladday Is near the N end of Raasay can be squally and uncomfortable except in settled weather; and Loch Scavaig (S. Skye, beneath the Cuillins) more so, though the latter is so spectacular as to warrant a visit in fair weather. Soay Is has a small, safe hbr on its N side, but the bar at ent almost dries at LW sp.

Between N. Skye and the mainland there is the choice of Sound of Raasay or Inner Sound. **The direction of buoyage in both Sounds is Northward.** In the former, coming S from Portree, beware Sgeir Chnapach (3m) and Ebbing Rk (dries 2·9m), both NNW of Oskaig Pt. At the Narrows (chart 2534) the SE- going stream begins at HW Ullapool – 0605, and the NW-going at HW Ullapool + 0040; sp rate 1·4kn in mid-chan, but more near shoals each side. Beware McMillan's Rk (0·4m depth) in mid-chan, marked by SHM lt buoy.

The chan between Scalpay and Skye narrows to 2½ca with drying reefs each side and least depth 0·1m. Here the E-going stream begins at HW Ullapool + 0550, and W-going at HW Ullapool – 0010, sp rate 1kn.

Inner Sound, which is a Submarine exercise area, is wider and easier than Sound of Raasay; the two are connected by Caol Rona and Caol Mor, respectively N and S of Raasay. Dangers extend about 1M N of Rona, and Cow Is lies off the mainland 8M to S; otherwise approach from N is clear to Crowlin Is, which should be passed to W. There is a good anch between Eilean Mor and Eilean Meadhonach, see 10.8.9.

A torpedo range in the Inner Sound does not normally restrict passage, but vessels may be requested to keep to the E side of the Sound if the range is active. Range activity is broadcast at 0800 and 1600LT on VHF Ch 08, 16 and is indicated by R Flags and International Code NE4 flown at the range building at Applecross, by all range vessels and at the naval pier at Kyle of Lochalsh (10.8.11).

Approaching Kyle Akin (chart 2540) from W, beware dangerous rks to N, off Bleat Is (at S side of entrance to Loch Carron); on S side of chan, Bogha Beag (dries 0·6m) and Black Eye Rk (depth 3·8m), respectively 6ca and 4ca W of bridge. For Plockton (Loch Carron), see 10.8.9. Pass at least 100m N or S of Eileanan Dubha in Kyle Akin. On S side of chan String Rk (dries) is marked by PHM lt buoy. For Loch Alsh, see 10.8.9.

Kyle Rhea connects Loch Alsh with NE end of Sound of Sleat. The tidal streams are very strong: N-going stream begins HW Ullapool + 0600, sp rate 6-7kn; S-going stream begins at HW Ullapool, sp rate 8kn. Eddies form both sides of the Kyle and there are dangerous overfalls off S end in fresh S'ly winds on S-going stream. Temp anch in Sandaig Bay, 3M to SW.

The Sound of Sleat widens to 4M off Pt of Sleat and is exposed to SW winds until Eigg and Muck give a lee . Mallaig (10.8.10) is a busy fishing and ferry hbr, convenient for supplies. Further S the lochs require intricate pilotage. 6M NE of Ardnamurchan Pt (lt, fog sig) are Bo Faskadale rks, drying 0·5m and marked by SHM lt buoy, and Elizabeth Rk with depth of 0·7m. Ardnamurchan Pt is an exposed headland onto which the ebb sets. With onshore winds, very heavy seas extend 2M offshore and it should be given a wide berth. Here the N-going stream begins at HW Oban – 0525, and the S-going at HW Oban + 0100, sp rates 1·5kn.

THE SMALL ISLES (charts 2207, 2208)

These consist of Canna, Rhum, Eigg (10.8.10) and Muck. Dangers extend SSW from Canna: at 1M Jemina Rk (depth 1·5m) and Belle Rk (depth 3·6m); at 2M Humla Rk (5m high), marked by buoy and with offlying shoals close W of it; at 5M Oigh Sgeir (lt, fog sig), the largest of a group of small Is; and at 7M Mill Rks (with depths of 1·8m).

The tide runs hard here, and in bad weather the sea breaks heavily up to 15M SW of Canna. Between Skerryvore and Neist Pt the stream runs generally N and S, starting N-going at HW Ullapool + 0550, and S-going at HW Ullapool – 0010. It rarely exceeds 1kn, except near Skerryvore, around headlands of The Small Is, and over rks and shoals.

1M off the N side of Muck are Godag Rks, some above water but with submerged dangers extending 2ca further N. Most other dangers around the Small Isles are closer inshore, but there are banks on which the sea breaks heavily in bad weather. A local magnetic anomaly exists about 2M E of Muck. The hbrs at Eigg (SE end), Rhum (Loch Scresort) and Canna (between Canna and Sanday) are all exposed to E'lies; Canna has best shelter and is useful for the Outer Hebrides.

ARDNAMURCHAN TO CRINAN (charts 2171, 2169)

S of Ardnamurchan the route lies either W of Mull via Passage of Tiree (where headlands need to be treated with respect in bad weather); or via the more sheltered Sound of Mull and Firth of Lorne. The former permits a visit to Coll and Tiree, where best anchs are at Arinagour (HIE ⚓s) and Gott B respectively. Beware Cairns of Coll, off the N tip.

The W coast of Mull is rewarding in settled weather, but careful pilotage is needed. Beware tide rip off Caliach Pt (NW corner) and Torran Rks off SW end of Mull (large scale chart 2617 required). Apart from the attractions of Iona and of Staffa (Fingal's Cave), the remote Treshnish Is are worth visiting. The best anchs in this area are at Ulva, Gometra, Bull Hole and Tinker's Hole in Iona Sound. The usual passage through Iona Sound avoids overfalls W of Iona, but heed shoal patches. Loch Lathaich on the N side of Ross of Mull is 5M to the E; a good base with anch and boatyard at Bunessan.

The Sound of Mull gives access to Tobermory (10.8.12, HIE ⚓), Dunstaffnage Bay, Oban (10.8.16), and up Loch Linnhe through Corran Narrows (where tide runs strongly) to Fort William (10.8.14) and to Corpach for the Caledonian Canal (10.8.15). But, apart from these places, there are dozens of lovely anchs in the sheltered lochs inside Mull, as for example in Loch Sunart (10.8.11) with HIE ⚓s at Kilchoan; also at Craignure and Salen Bays on Sound of Mull. For Loch Aline see 10.8.13.

On the mainland shore Puilladobhrain is a sheltered anch. Cuan Sound (see 10.8.16 for details) is a useful short cut to Loch Melfort, (10.8.17) and Craobh Haven (10.8.118). Good shelter, draft permitting, in Ardinamar B, SW of Torsa.

Sound of Luing (chart 2326) between Fladda (lt), Lunga and Scarba on the W side, and Luing and Dubh Sgeir (lt) on the E side, is the normal chan to or from Sound of Jura, despite dangers at the N end and strong tidal streams. The N and W-going flood begins at HW Oban + 0430; the S and E-going ebb at HW Oban –0155. Sp rates are 2·5kn at S end of Sound, increasing to 6kn or more in Islands off N entrance, where there are eddies, races and overfalls.

At N end of Sound of Jura (chart 2326) is Loch Craignish (10.8.19). From the N, beware very strong streams, eddies and whirlpools in Dorus Mor, off Craignish Pt. The W and N-going stream begins at HW Oban + 0330, and the E and S-going at HW Oban – 0215, sp rates 8kn.

For Gulf of Corryvreckan, Colonsay, Islay, Loch Crinan and passage south through the Sound of Jura, see 10.9.5.

10.8.6   DISTANCE TABLE

Approximate distances in nautical miles are by the most direct route, keeping East of Skye and Mull where appropriate, and avoiding dangers. Places in *italics* are in adjoining areas.

		1	2	3	4	5	6	7	8	9	10	11	12	13	14	15	16	17	18	19	20
1.	*Cape Wrath*	**1**																			
2.	Ullapool	54	**2**																		
3.	Stornoway	53	45	**3**																	
4.	East Loch Tarbert	75	56	33	**4**																
5.	Portree	83	57	53	42	**5**															
6.	Loch Harport	110	82	65	45	66	**6**														
7.	Kyle of Lochalsh	91	63	62	63	21	53	**7**													
8.	Mallaig	112	82	83	84	42	33	21	**8**												
9.	Eigg	123	98	97	75	54	34	35	14	**9**											
10.	Castlebay (Barra)	133	105	92	69	97	43	76	59	46	**10**										
11.	Tobermory	144	114	115	87	74	52	53	32	20	53	**11**									
12.	Loch Aline	157	127	128	100	87	65	66	45	33	66	13	**12**								
13.	Fort William	198	161	162	134	121	99	98	75	63	96	43	34	**13**							
14.	Oban	169	138	139	111	100	76	77	56	44	77	24	13	29	**14**						
15.	Loch Lathaich	160	130	124	98	91	62	67	49	35	56	31	53	77	48	**15**					
16.	Loch Melfort	184	154	155	117	114	92	93	69	61	92	40	27	45	18	45	**16**				
17.	Craobh Haven	184	155	155	117	114	93	92	70	60	93	40	27	50	21	43	5	**17**			
18.	Loch Craignish	188	158	159	131	118	95	96	76	64	98	44	31	55	26	46	17	14	**18**		
19.	*Crinan*	187	157	158	129	112	95	95	74	63	97	42	30	54	25	45	14	9	6	**19**	
20.	*Mull of Kintyre*	232	203	189	175	159	133	143	121	105	120	89	87	98	72	78	62	57	54	51	**20**

STORNOWAY   10-8-7
Lewis (Outer Hebrides) 58°11'·60N 06°21'·75W

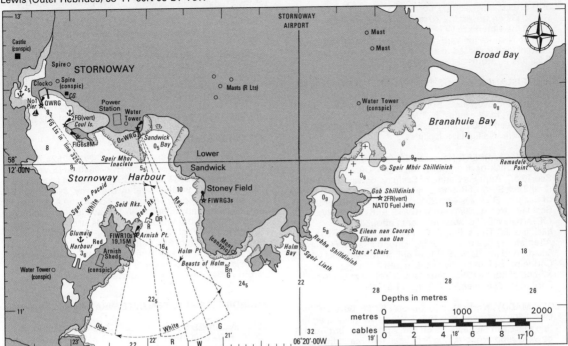

CHARTS
AC 2529, 1794; OS 8

TIDES
–0428 Dover; ML 2·8; Duration 0610; Zone 0 (UT)

Standard Port ULLAPOOL (⟶)

Times				Height (metres)			
High Water		Low Water		MHWS	MHWN	MLWN	MLWS
0100	0700	0300	0900	5·2	3·9	2·1	0·7
1300	1900	1500	2100				
Differences STORNOWAY							
–0010	–0010	–0010	–0010	–0.4	–0.2	–0.1	0.0
LOCH ERIBOLL (Portnancon) (See 10.7.20)							
+0055	+0105	+0055	+0100	0.0	+0.1	+0.1	+0.2
KYLE OF DURNESS (See 10.7.20)							
+0030	+0030	+0050	+0050	–0.6	–0.4	–0.3	–0.1
LOCH SHELL (Harris)							
–0023	–0010	–0010	–0027	–0.4	–0.3	–0.2	0.0
EAST LOCH TARBERT (Harris)							
–0035	–0020	–0020	–0030	–0.2	–0.2	0.0	+0.1
LEVERBURGH (Sound of Harris)							
–0051	–0030	–0025	–0035	–0.6	–0.4	–0.2	–0.1
LOCH MADDY (N.Uist)							
–0054	–0024	–0026	–0040	–0.4	–0.3	–0.2	0.0
LOCH CARNAN (S.Uist)							
–0100	–0020	–0030	–0050	–0.7	–0.7	–0.2	–0.1
LOCH SKIPORT (S.Uist)							
–0110	–0035	–0034	–0034	–0.6	–0.6	–0.4	–0.2
LOCH BOISDALE (S.Uist)							
–0105	–0040	–0030	–0050	–1.1	–0.9	–0.4	–0.2
BARRA (North Bay)							
–0113	–0041	–0044	–0058	–1.0	–0.7	–0.3	–0.1
CASTLEBAY (Barra)							
–0125	–0050	–0055	–0110	–0.9	–0.8	–0.4	–0.1
BARRA HEAD (Berneray)							
–0125	–0050	–0055	–0105	–1.2	–0.9	–0.3	+0.1
WEST LOCH TARBERT (W.Harris)							
–0025	–0025	–0056	–0056	–1.5	–1.1	–0.6	0.0
LITTLE BERNERA (W.Lewis)							
–0031	–0021	–0027	–0037	–0.9	–0.8	–0.5	–0.2
CARLOWAY (W.Lewis)							
–0050	+0010	–0045	–0025	–1.0	–0.7	–0.5	–0.1
BALIVANICH (W.Benbecula)							
–0113	–0027	–0041	–0055	–1.1	–0.8	–0.6	–0.2
SCOLPAIG (W North Uist)							
–0043	–0043	–0050	–0050	–1.4	–1.1	–0.6	0.0
SHILLAY (Monach Islands)							
–0113	–0053	–0057	–0117	–1.0	–0.9	–0.8	–0.3

Standard Port ULLAPOOL (⟶)

Times				Height (metres)			
High Water		Low Water		MHWS	MHWN	MLWN	MLWS
0000	0600	0300	0900	5·2	3·9	2·1	0·7
1200	1800	1500	2100				
VILLAGE BAY (St Kilda)							
–0050	–0050	–0055	–0055	–1.8	–1.4	–0.9	–0.3
FLANNAN ISLES							
–0036	–0026	–0026	–0036	–1.3	–0.9	–0.7	–0.2
ROCKALL							
–0105	–0105	–0115	–0115	–2.2	–1.7	–1.0	–0.2

SHELTER
Good, but S swells make the ⚓ uncomfortable. ⚓s at: Poll nam Portan opposite commercial quays, clear of LB moorings; Glumaig Hbr in W sector is best ⚓, but oil works may preclude this; in bay NW of Coul Is; or yachts can go alongside Cromwell St Quay. It is possible to lie alongside FVs in the inner hbr. Visitors land at steps N of FG ldg lts and report to Hr Mr. Ullapool ferries use the hbr.

NAVIGATION
WPT 58°10'·00N 06°20'·80W, 163°/343° from/to Oc WRG lt, 2·3M. Reef Rks, W side of ent marked by PHM buoy, QR. An unlit G bn marks the rky patch off Holm Pt, on which is a conspic memorial. A local magnetic anomaly exists over a small area in mid-hbr, 1·75ca N of Seid Rks.

LIGHTS AND MARKS
Arnish sheds are conspic 3ca SW of Arnish Pt lt, Fl WR 10s 17m 19/15M, W tr; W sector 302°-013° covers ent. Then in turn follow W sectors of: Sandwick Bay lt, NW side (close E of 3 conspic power stn chys and water tr) Oc WRG 6s 10m 9M, W341°-347°; then Stoney Field Fl WRG 3s 8m 11M, vis W102°-109° across hbr; and finally No 1 Pier, Q WRG 5m 11M, W335°-352°. Ldg lts 325° to Ro Ro jetty, both FG.

RADIO TELEPHONE
VHF Ch 12 16 (H24).

TELEPHONE (01851)
Hr Mr 702688; MRSC 702013; ☰ (0141) 887 9369; Marinecall 0891 500464; Police 702222; Dr 703145.

FACILITIES
Pier N end of Bay FW, C (10 ton), CH, AB; **W Pier** Slip, P, FW; **Steamer Pier** FW; **Services:** ACA, ME, El, Sh. **Town** EC Wed; P (cans), D, El, V, R, Bar, Gas, ✉, Ⓑ, ⇌ (ferry to Ullapool, bus to Garve), ✈.

HARBOURS AND ANCHORAGES ON THE EAST SIDE OF THE OUTER HEBRIDES

LOCH SHELL, Harris, 58°00´·00N 06°25´·00W. AC 1794.
HW −0437 on Dover; ML 2·7m. See 10.8.7. Pass S of Eilean
Iuvard; beware rks to W of Is. ⚓ in Tob Eishken, 2½M up
loch on N shore (beware rk awash on E side of ent), or at
head of loch (exposed to E winds; dries some distance).
Facilities: ✉/Stores at Lemreway.

SHIANT ISLANDS, Lewis, 58°53´·70N 06°21´·30W. AC 1794,
1795. Tides as Loch Shell 10.8.7. Beware strong tidal
streams and overfalls in Sound of Shiant. Strictly a fair
weather ⚓; in W winds ⚓ E of Mol Mor, isthmus between
Garbh Eileen (160m) and Eileen an Tighe. In E winds ⚓ W
of Mol Mor. No lights or facilities.

EAST LOCH TARBERT, Harris, 57°50´·00N 06°41´·00W.
AC 2905. HW −0446 on Dover; ML 3·0m; Duration 0605.
See 10.8.7. Appr via Sound of Scalpay; beware Elliot Rk
(2m) 2½ca SSW of Rubha Crago. Eilean Glas lt ho at E end
of Scalpay, Fl (3) 20s 43m 23M; W tr, R bands. In Sound of
Scalpay, stream sets W from HW +3, and E from HW −3. ⚓
off Tarbert WSW of steamer pier in about 2·5m.
Facilities: EC Thurs; Bar, D, Dr, FW, P, ✉, R, V, ferry to Uig.
Alternatively Scalpay N Hbr gives good shelter. Beware rk
5ca off Alrd an Aiseig, E side of ent. SHM By marks wk off
Coddem; 5ca E of the By is a rk, depth 1·1m. Fish pier at
SE end of hbr has 2FG (vert) lts; ⚓ 7ca N, in about 3m.
Facilities: FW at pier, ✉, V, ferry to Harris.

LOCH MADDY, North Uist, 57°36´·00N 07°06´·00W. AC 2825
HW −0500 on Dover. See 10.8.7. With strong wind against
tide there can be bad seas off ent. Appr clear, but from S
beware submerged rk ½ca N of Leacnam Madadh. Lts:
Weaver's Pt Fl 3s 21m 7M; Glas Eilean Mor Fl (2) G 4s 8m
5M; Rubna Nam Pleac Fl R 4s 7m 5M. Inside loch: Ruigh
Liath QG 6m 5M; Vallaquie Is Fl (3) WRG 8s. Ferry pier
ldg lts 298°: front 2FG(vert) 4M; rear Oc G 8s 10m 4M, vis
284°-304°. 2 HIE ⚓s in Bagh Aird nam Madadh; 5 HIE ⚓s
SW of pier ☎ (01870) 602425; 2 HIE ⚓s E of Oronsay. ⚓s
off Steamer Pier; in Charles Hbr; Oronsay, berth on
private pier, but ⚓ not recommended due to moorings;
Sponish Hbr; Loch Portain; Vallaquie. VHF Ch 12 16. Port
Manager ☎ (01876) 5003337 (day), 5003226 (night).
Facilities: Lochmaddy, EC Wed; Shop, Ⓑ, Gas, ✉, P, D,
FW; Loch Portain ✉, Shop.

LOCH SKIPPORT, South Uist, 57°20´·00N 07°13´·60W. AC
2825, 2904. HW −0602 on Dover; see 10.8.7. Easy ent 3M
NNE of Hecla (604m). No lights, but 2¼M SSE is Usinish
lt ho Fl WR 20s 54m 19/15M. ⚓s at: Wizard Pool in 7m;
beware Float Rk, dries 2·3m; Caolas Mor in 7m on N side;
Bagh Charmaig in 5m. Linne Arm has narrow ent, many
fish farms and poor holding. No facilities.

LOCH BOISDALE, South Uist, 57°08´·80N 07°16´·00W.
AC 2770. HW −0455 on Dover; ML 2·4m; Duration 0600.
See 10.8.7. Good shelter except in SE gales when swell
runs right up the M loch. Safest appr from N is between
Rubha na Cruibe and Calvay Is; ldg line 245°, pier (ru) on
with Hollisgeir. From S beware Clan Ewan Rk, dries 1m,
and McKenzie Rk, marked by PHM lt buoy Fl (3) R 15s.
Chan up to Boisdale Hbr is N of Gasay Is; beware rks off
E end. ⚓ off pier in approx 4m, or SW of Gasay Is in
approx 9m. 4 HIE ⚓s NE of pier ☎ (01870) 602425. There
are fish cages W of Rubha Bhuailt. Lts: E end of Calvay Is
Fl (2) WRG 10s 16m 7/4M. Gasay Is Fl WR 5s 10m 7/4M. N
side of loch, opp Gasay Is, Fl G 6s. Ro Ro terminal Iso RG
4s 8m 2M. See 10.8.4. Linkspan 2FG (vert). Facilities: EC
Tues; Bar, FW (tap on pier), P, ✉, R, V, ferry to mainland.

CASTLEBAY, Barra, 56°56´·80N 07°29´·60W. AC 2769.
HW −0525 on Dover; ML 2·3m; Duration 0600. See 10.8.7.
Very good shelter and holding ground. Best ⚓ NW of
Kiessimul Castle (on an Island) in approx 8m; NE of
castle are rks. There are 8 HIE ⚓s to W of pier ☎ (01870)
602425. Or ⚓ in Vatersay Bay in approx 9m. Vatersay
Sound has been closed by a causeway across its W end.
Beware rks NNW of Dubh Sgeir; Dubh Sgeir lt Fl (2) WG
6s 6m 7/5M, vis W280°-180°, G180°-280°. Sgeir Liath Fl
3s 7m 8M. Ldg lts 295°: front on Rubha Glas, FG 9m 4M,
Or stripe on W framework tr; rear, 550m from front, FG
15m 4M, Or stripe on W framework tr. Facilities: Bar, D,
FW, P, ✉, R, V, Ferry to mainland.

HIE ⚓s are also located in the Outer Hebrides at:
L Rodel, Harris. AC 2642. 3 ⚓s at 57°44´·2N 06°57´·4W in
Poll an Tigh-mhàil; enter from SW past jetties. No lts. ☎
(01851) 703773.
Kallin, Grimsay. AC 2904. 1 ⚓ at 57°28´·9N 07°12´·2W,
NE of hbr. 3 chan lt buoys and 2 FR (vert) on hbr bkwtr.
☎ (01870) 602425.
L Carnan, S Uist. AC 2825. 2 ⚓s at 57°22´·15N 07°16´·4W
☎ (01870) 602425. App chan has lt buoys and ldg lts 222°
to Sandwick quay; front Fl R 2s, rear Iso R 10s, both 5M,
W ◇s on posts.
Acairseid Mhór, Eriskay. AC 2770. 3 ⚓s at 57°04´·0N
07°17´·4W on S side of inlet, opp pier, 2 FG (vert). Ldg
lts 285°, both Oc R 6s 9/10m 4M. ☎ (01870) 602425.

ATLANTIC ISLAND

ST KILDA, 57°48´·30N 08°33´·00W. AC 2721, 2524. Tidal
figures for Village Bay, Hirta; HW −0510 on Dover; ML
1·9m; Duration 0615. See 10.8.7. A group of four Is and
three stacks now taken over by the Army. ⚓ in Village Bay,
SE-facing, in approx 5m about 1·5ca off the Army pier. If
wind is between NE and SSW big swells enter the bay;
good holding, but untenable if winds strong. Levenish Is
(55m) is 1·5M E of Hirta with offlying rks. Ldg lts 270°,
both Oc 5s 26/38m 3M. Call *Kilda Radar* VHF Ch 16 08 (HJ)
for permission to land. Alternative ⚓ at Glen Bay on N
side is only satisfactory in S and E winds. Facilities: FW
from wells near landings (courtesy of the Army), ☎.

ANCHORAGES BETWEEN CAPE WRATH AND ULLAPOOL

LOCH INCHARD, Sutherland, 58°27´·33N 05°05´·00W. AC
2503. HW −0400 on Dover. ML 2·70m. See 10.8.8 (Loch
Bervie). The most N'ly shelter before/after Cape Wrath,
12M to the N. Foinaven, conspic mountain 899m, brg 110°
leads to ent abeam Rubha na Leacaig, Fl (2) 10s 30m 8M.
4ca ESE of this lt, beware rk (3m depth) almost in mid-
chan. Kinlochbervie on N shore is a busy FV port, but has
yacht pontoon in NNE corner. Ldg lts 327°, Oc G 8s 9M,
and 3 lt bns. Close NW is ⚓ at Loch Clash, open to W;
other ⚓s at Camus Blair, 5ca SW of L. Bervie; and up the
loch at L. Sheigra, Achriesgill B and Rhiconich. Facilities:
FW, D at quay, P (cans), CH, Sh, ME, ✉, Bar, V, R.

LOCH LAXFORD, Sutherland, 58°24´·80N 05°07´·10W.
AC 2503. HW −0410 on Dover. ML 2·7m. See 10.8.8. Ent
between Rubha Ruadh and Ardmore Pt, 1M ENE, clearly
identified by 3 isolated mountains Ben Stack, Ben Arkle
and Foinaven inland. The many ⚓s in the loch include:
Loch a'Chadh-fi, on N/NE sides of islet (John Ridgeway's
Adventure School on Pt on W side of narrows has
moorings); Bagh nah-Airde Beag, next bay to E, (beware
rk 5ca off SE shore which covers at MHWS); Weaver's
Bay on SW shore, 3M from ent (beware drying rk off NW
Pt of ent); Bagh na Fionndalach Mor on SW shore (4-6m);
Fanagmore Bay on SW shore (beware head of bay foul
with old moorings). Beware many fish farming cages.
Facilities: none, nearest stores at Scourie (5M).

LOCH INVER, Sutherland, 58°09´·00N 05°14´·70W. AC 2504. HW
−0433 on Dover; ML 3·0m. See 10.8.8. Good shelter in all wx;
busy fishing hbr. Ent N or S of Soyea Is, Fl (2) 10s 34m 6M, in
W sectors of Glas Leac lt, Fl WRG 3s 7m, W071°-080°, R080°-
090°, G090°-103°, W103°-111°, R111°-243°, W243°-251°,
G251°-071°. Beware drying rk about 50m off Kirkaig Pt. Pass
N or S of Glas Leac. New Aird Ghlas pier has QG lt; Middle
pier has 2FG (vert). ⚓ at top of loch in 6m off old E pier, or
inshore of the LB, or as Hr Mr directs. VHF Ch 09 16. Facilities:
Gas, FW, P, D, V, ✉, Hotel. Marina (20 berth) planned near LB.

SUMMER ISLES, Ross & Cromarty. 58°01´N 05°25´W. AC
2501, 2509. HW −0425 Dover; ML −; See 10.8.8 for Tanera
Mor; streams are weak and irregular. In the N apps to
Loch Broom some 30 islands and rks, the main ones being
Eilean Mullagrach, Isle Ristol, Glas-leac Mor, Tanera Beg,
Eilean a' Char, Eilean Fada Mor. ⚓s: Isle Ristol, ⚓ to the S
of drying causeway; close to slip is lt Fl G 3s. Tanera Beg,
⚓ in the chan to the E inside Eilean Fada Mor (beware bys,
nets and drying rks). Tanera Mor on E side, ⚓ in bay (the
"Cabbage Patch"); new pier but many moorings; or in
NW, ⚓ close E of Eilean na Saille, but N of drying rk. Temp
⚓ at Badentarbat B for Achiltibuie on mainland. Facilities:
V, R, Gas, FW, D (emerg) ☎ (01854) 622261.

ULLAPOOL 10-8-8

Ross and Cromarty 57°53'·72N 05°09'·30W

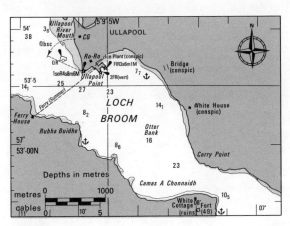

CHARTS
AC 2500, 2501, 2509, 1791; OS 19

TIDES
–0415 Dover; ML 3·0; Duration 0610; Zone 0 (UT)

Standard Port ULLAPOOL (⟶)

Times				Height (metres)			
High Water		Low Water		MHWS	MHWN	MLWN	MLWS
0000	0600	0300	0900	5·2	3·9	2·1	0·7
1200	1800	1500	2100				
Differences LOCH BERVIE							
+0030	+0010	+0010	+0020	–0·3	–0·3	–0·2	0·0
LOCH LAXFORD							
+0015	+0015	+0005	+0005	–0·3	–0·4	–0·2	0·0
BADCALL BAY							
+0005	+0005	+0005	+0005	–0·7	–0·5	–0·5	+0·2
LOCH NEDD							
0000	0000	0000	0000	–0·3	–0·2	–0·2	0·0
LOCH INVER							
–0005	–0005	–0005	–0005	–0·2	0·0	0·0	+0·1
SUMMER ISLES (Tanera Mor)							
–0005	–0005	–0005	–0005	–0·1	+0·1	0·0	+0·1
LOCH EWE (Mellon Charles)							
–0010	–0010	–0010	–0010	–0·1	–0·1	–0·1	0·0
LOCH GAIRLOCH							
–0020	–0020	–0010	–0010	0·0	+0·1	–0·3	–0·1

Ullapool is a Standard Port and detailed tidal predictions for each day of the year are given below.

SHELTER
Good in ⚓ E of pier; access at all tides. See Hr Mr for temp moorings. From Aug to Mar Ullapool is mainly a FV port and the pier is extremely congested. Loch Kanaird (N of ent to Loch Broom) has good ⚓ E of Isle Martin. Possible ⚓s 6ca S of Ullapool Pt, and beyond the narrows 3ca ESE of W cottage. The upper loch is squally in strong winds.

NAVIGATION
WPT L Broom ent 57°55'·80N 05°15'·00W, 309°/129° from/ to Ullapool Pt lt, 3.5M. N of Ullapool Pt extensive drying flats off the mouth of Ullapool R are marked by QR buoy. Beware fish pens and unlit buoys SE of narrows off W shore.

LIGHTS AND MARKS
Rhubha Cadail, N of L. Broom ent, Fl WRG 6s 11m 9/6M. Cailleach Hd, W of ent, Fl (2) 12s 60m 9M. Ullapool Pt Iso R 4s 8m 6M; grey mast, vis 258°-108°. Pier SE corner, Fl R 3s 6m 1M; SW corner 2FR (vert).

RADIO TELEPHONE
VHF Ch 14 16 12 (July-Nov: H24. Dec-June: HO).

TELEPHONE (01854)
Hr Mr 612091/612165; MRSC (01851) 702013; ⌗ (0141) 887 9369; Marinecall 0891 500464; Police 612017; Dr 612015.

FACILITIES
Pier AB £5 for 1 or more nights, D, FW, CH; **Ullapool YC** Gas; **Services:** ME, EI, Ⓔ, Sh, ACA. **Town** EC Tues (winter); P, Ⓟ, V, R, Bar, ⊠, Ⓑ, ⇌ (bus to Garve). Daily buses to Inverness (✈), ferries twice daily (summer) to Stornoway.

ADJACENT ANCHORAGES TO THE SOUTH-WEST

LOCH EWE, Ross & Cromarty, 57°52'·00N 05°40'·00W. AC 3146, 2509. Tides (Mellon Charles): See 10.8.8; HW –0415 on Dover; ML 2·9m; Duration 0610. Shelter in all winds. Easy ent with no dangers in loch. Rhubha Reidh lt, Fl (4) 15s 37m 24M, W tr, is 4·5M W of ent. Loch approx 7M long with Isle Ewe and 2 small islets about 2M from ent in centre; can be passed on either side. Beware unlit buoys E side Isle Ewe. Excellent ⚓ in Loch Thurnaig to S. Aultbea Pier, partly derelict, to NE. Beware fish farms. Boor Rks on W shore about 7ca from loch hd. Fairway buoy SWM L Fl 10s; No 1 lt buoy Fl (3) G 10s; NATO fuelling jetty and dolphins, all Fl G 4s. Facilities: Dr, P, ⊠, R, V, Bar. S of Poolewe Bay (3·5m), **Inverewe Gdns** FW, D, L on pier, P (at garage), ⊠, R, Bar, V, Gas; **Aultbea** V.

LOCH GAIRLOCH, Ross & Cromarty, 57°43'·00N 05°45'·00W. AC 2528, 2210. HW –0440 on Dover; ML no data; Duration 0600. See 10.8.8. A wide loch facing W. Ent clear of dangers. Quite heavy seas enter in bad weather. Good shelter in Badachro, to SW of Eilean Horrisdale on S side of loch or in Loch Shieldaig at SE end of the loch. Or ⚓ in approx 6m near Gairloch pier (NB: proposed marina at river mouth). Lts: Glas Eilean Fl WRG 6s 9m 6/4M, W080°-102°, R102°-296°, W296°- 333°, G333°-080°. Pier hd, QR 9m. VHF Ch 16 (occas). Gairloch Pier: AB fees charged. Facilities: P, D, FW, Hotel, Gas, V.

8

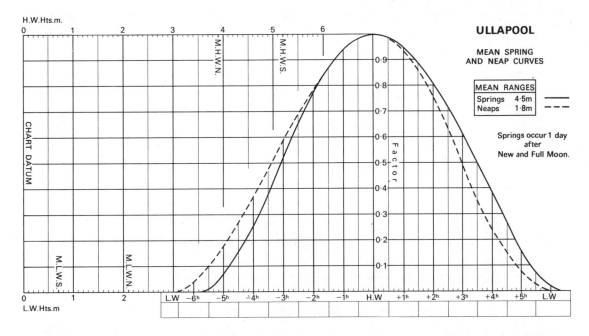

ULLAPOOL

MEAN SPRING AND NEAP CURVES

MEAN RANGES	
Springs	4·5m
Neaps	1·8m

Springs occur 1 day after New and Full Moon.

SCOTLAND – ULLAPOOL

LAT 57°54'N   LONG   5°10'W

TIMES AND HEIGHTS OF HIGH AND LOW WATERS

YEAR **1996**

TIME ZONE (UT)
For Summer Time add ONE hour in non-shaded areas

JANUARY

Day	Time	m	Day	Time	m
1 M	0410 / 1013 / 1620 / 2234	4.3 / 2.1 / 4.3 / 1.9	**16** TU	0254 / 0853 / 1516 / 2147	4.3 / 2.0 / 4.3 / 1.8
2 TU	0458 / 1108 / 1707 / 2322	4.4 / 1.9 / 4.4 / 1.8	**17** W	0359 / 1011 / 1624 / 2251	4.5 / 1.8 / 4.6 / 1.5
3 W	0535 / 1154 / 1747	4.6 / 1.7 / 4.6	**18** TH	0455 / 1114 / 1722 / 2344	4.9 / 1.4 / 4.9 / 1.2
4 TH	0002 / 0606 / 1234 / 1823	1.6 / 4.7 / 1.5 / 4.7	**19** F	0544 / 1208 / 1812	5.2 / 1.0 / 5.2
5 F O	0039 / 0638 / 1311 / 1858	1.5 / 4.9 / 1.4 / 4.8	**20** SA ●	0032 / 0629 / 1257 / 1858	0.9 / 5.5 / 0.7 / 5.4
6 SA	0113 / 0708 / 1345 / 1932	1.4 / 5.0 / 1.3 / 4.8	**21** SU	0118 / 0713 / 1344 / 1943	0.7 / 5.7 / 0.4 / 5.5
7 SU	0146 / 0737 / 1418 / 2004	1.3 / 5.0 / 1.2 / 4.8	**22** M	0203 / 0756 / 1429 / 2027	0.6 / 5.8 / 0.4 / 5.4
8 M	0220 / 0807 / 1451 / 2036	1.2 / 5.0 / 1.2 / 4.7	**23** TU	0246 / 0839 / 1514 / 2113	0.6 / 5.7 / 0.4 / 5.2
9 TU	0253 / 0839 / 1525 / 2111	1.2 / 4.9 / 1.2 / 4.6	**24** W	0330 / 0925 / 1558 / 2200	0.7 / 5.4 / 0.6 / 4.9
10 W	0327 / 0914 / 1559 / 2151	1.3 / 4.8 / 1.3 / 4.5	**25** TH	0414 / 1014 / 1642 / 2252	1.0 / 5.1 / 1.0 / 4.6
11 TH	0404 / 0953 / 1637 / 2236	1.4 / 4.7 / 1.4 / 4.3	**26** F	0500 / 1109 / 1729 / 2350	1.3 / 4.8 / 1.3 / 4.3
12 F	0444 / 1037 / 1719 / 2329	1.6 / 4.5 / 1.6 / 4.2	**27** SA	0549 / 1213 / 1819	1.7 / 4.4 / 1.7
13 SA	0530 / 1131 / 1809	1.8 / 4.3 / 1.8	**28** SU	0058 / 0647 / 1325 / 1920	4.1 / 2.1 / 4.1 / 2.1
14 SU	0032 / 0626 / 1240 / 1910	4.1 / 2.0 / 4.2 / 1.9	**29** M	0215 / 0804 / 1441 / 2039	3.9 / 2.3 / 4.0 / 2.2
15 M	0143 / 0734 / 1358 / 2026	4.1 / 2.1 / 4.2 / 1.9	**30** TU	0333 / 0940 / 1552 / 2202	4.0 / 2.3 / 4.0 / 2.2
			31 W	0434 / 1048 / 1648 / 2300	4.1 / 2.1 / 4.1 / 2.0

FEBRUARY

Day	Time	m	Day	Time	m
1 TH	0517 / 1137 / 1730 / 2344	4.3 / 1.8 / 4.3 / 1.8	**16** F	0441 / 1105 / 1708 / 2332	4.7 / 1.3 / 4.7 / 1.2
2 F	0551 / 1217 / 1806	4.5 / 1.6 / 4.5	**17** SA	0531 / 1158 / 1802	5.1 / 0.9 / 5.0
3 SA	0021 / 0621 / 1253 / 1840	1.5 / 4.7 / 1.3 / 4.7	**18** SU ●	0020 / 0616 / 1246 / 1845	0.8 / 5.4 / 0.6 / 5.3
4 SU O	0055 / 0651 / 1325 / 1911	1.3 / 4.9 / 1.1 / 4.8	**19** M	0105 / 0657 / 1330 / 1926	0.6 / 5.6 / 0.3 / 5.4
5 M	0128 / 0717 / 1357 / 1939	1.1 / 5.0 / 1.0 / 4.9	**20** TU	0148 / 0737 / 1412 / 2005	0.5 / 5.7 / 0.2 / 5.4
6 TU	0200 / 0745 / 1428 / 2009	1.0 / 5.1 / 0.9 / 4.9	**21** W	0229 / 0817 / 1453 / 2045	0.4 / 5.6 / 0.3 / 5.2
7 W	0233 / 0815 / 1500 / 2043	0.9 / 5.1 / 0.9 / 4.8	**22** TH	0309 / 0858 / 1532 / 2126	0.5 / 5.4 / 0.5 / 5.0
8 TH	0306 / 0848 / 1533 / 2119	0.9 / 5.0 / 0.9 / 4.7	**23** F	0349 / 0942 / 1612 / 2209	0.8 / 5.1 / 0.8 / 4.7
9 F	0341 / 0923 / 1609 / 2200	1.0 / 4.8 / 1.1 / 4.5	**24** SA	0430 / 1030 / 1652 / 2257	1.1 / 4.7 / 1.2 / 4.3
10 SA	0419 / 1003 / 1648 / 2248	1.2 / 4.6 / 1.3 / 4.3	**25** SU	0513 / 1127 / 1736 / 2359	1.5 / 4.3 / 1.7 / 4.0
11 SU	0502 / 1053 / 1734 / 2348	1.5 / 4.4 / 1.5 / 4.2	**26** M	0603 / 1238 / 1828	1.9 / 4.0 / 2.1
12 M	0553 / 1159 / 1832	1.7 / 4.2 / 1.8	**27** TU	0118 / 0709 / 1359 / 1941	3.8 / 2.3 / 3.8 / 2.4
13 TU	0102 / 0658 / 1325 / 1947	4.1 / 1.9 / 4.0 / 2.0	**28** W	0245 / 0855 / 1519 / 2121	3.7 / 2.4 / 3.8 / 2.3
14 W	0224 / 0821 / 1458 / 2123	4.1 / 2.0 / 4.1 / 1.9	**29** TH	0400 / 1022 / 1623 / 2234	3.9 / 2.2 / 3.9 / 2.1
15 TH	0339 / 0956 / 1615 / 2237	4.4 / 1.8 / 4.4 / 1.6			

MARCH

Day	Time	m	Day	Time	m
1 F	0450 / 1115 / 1708 / 2321	4.1 / 1.9 / 4.1 / 1.8	**16** SA	0426 / 1053 / 1706 / 2318	4.6 / 1.2 / 4.6 / 1.2
2 SA	0527 / 1154 / 1744 / 2358	4.3 / 1.6 / 4.4 / 1.5	**17** SU	0517 / 1145 / 1751	4.9 / 0.9 / 4.9
3 SU	0559 / 1228 / 1817	4.6 / 1.3 / 4.6	**18** M	0006 / 0600 / 1231 / 1830	0.8 / 5.2 / 0.5 / 5.1
4 M	0032 / 0626 / 1300 / 1845	1.2 / 4.8 / 1.0 / 4.8	**19** TU ●	0050 / 0640 / 1312 / 1907	0.6 / 5.4 / 0.3 / 5.3
5 TU O	0105 / 0652 / 1331 / 1913	1.0 / 5.0 / 0.8 / 4.9	**20** W	0131 / 0718 / 1352 / 1942	0.4 / 5.5 / 0.3 / 5.3
6 W	0137 / 0720 / 1402 / 1943	0.8 / 5.1 / 0.7 / 5.0	**21** TH	0210 / 0756 / 1429 / 2018	0.4 / 5.4 / 0.3 / 5.2
7 TH	0209 / 0750 / 1434 / 2016	0.7 / 5.1 / 0.6 / 5.0	**22** F	0248 / 0834 / 1506 / 2054	0.5 / 5.2 / 0.6 / 4.9
8 F	0243 / 0823 / 1508 / 2052	0.7 / 5.1 / 0.7 / 4.9	**23** SA	0326 / 0914 / 1542 / 2130	0.7 / 4.9 / 0.9 / 4.7
9 SA	0319 / 0900 / 1544 / 2132	0.8 / 4.9 / 0.8 / 4.7	**24** SU	0404 / 0957 / 1619 / 2209	1.0 / 4.6 / 1.2 / 4.3
10 SU	0358 / 0941 / 1624 / 2219	0.9 / 4.7 / 1.1 / 4.5	**25** M	0444 / 1047 / 1659 / 2258	1.4 / 4.2 / 1.6 / 4.0
11 M	0441 / 1032 / 1709 / 2318	1.2 / 4.4 / 1.4 / 4.2	**26** TU	0529 / 1155 / 1745	1.8 / 3.9 / 2.0
12 TU	0532 / 1140 / 1807	1.5 / 4.1 / 1.7	**27** W	0023 / 0627 / 1317 / 1849	3.8 / 2.1 / 3.6 / 2.3
13 W	0036 / 0636 / 1313 / 1924	4.1 / 1.8 / 3.9 / 2.0	**28** TH	0154 / 0801 / 1440 / 2029	3.7 / 2.3 / 3.6 / 2.4
14 TH	0203 / 0804 / 1451 / 2107	4.1 / 1.9 / 4.0 / 1.9	**29** F	0313 / 0938 / 1548 / 2152	3.7 / 2.2 / 3.8 / 2.2
15 F	0322 / 0945 / 1610 / 2223	4.3 / 1.7 / 4.3 / 1.6	**30** SA	0411 / 1038 / 1637 / 2246	3.9 / 1.9 / 4.0 / 1.9
			31 SU	0454 / 1120 / 1716 / 2326	4.2 / 1.6 / 4.3 / 1.6

APRIL

Day	Time	m	Day	Time	m
1 M	0528 / 1156 / 1748	4.5 / 1.3 / 4.5	**16** TU	0544 / 1211 / 1814	5.0 / 0.7 / 5.0
2 TU	0002 / 0556 / 1229 / 1817	1.3 / 4.7 / 1.0 / 4.8	**17** W ●	0032 / 0622 / 1252 / 1847	0.7 / 5.2 / 0.5 / 5.1
3 W	0037 / 0624 / 1301 / 1846	1.0 / 4.9 / 0.7 / 5.0	**18** TH	0113 / 0659 / 1330 / 1920	0.6 / 5.2 / 0.5 / 5.1
4 TH O	0111 / 0654 / 1334 / 1918	0.8 / 5.1 / 0.6 / 5.1	**19** F	0152 / 0736 / 1406 / 1954	0.6 / 5.2 / 0.6 / 5.0
5 F	0145 / 0728 / 1408 / 1953	0.6 / 5.1 / 0.5 / 5.1	**20** SA	0229 / 0813 / 1440 / 2027	0.6 / 5.0 / 0.7 / 4.9
6 SA	0222 / 0804 / 1444 / 2031	0.5 / 5.1 / 0.6 / 5.0	**21** SU	0306 / 0852 / 1515 / 2101	0.8 / 4.8 / 1.0 / 4.7
7 SU	0300 / 0844 / 1523 / 2113	0.6 / 4.9 / 0.7 / 4.8	**22** M	0342 / 0933 / 1551 / 2137	1.1 / 4.5 / 1.3 / 4.4
8 M	0342 / 0930 / 1605 / 2202	0.8 / 4.7 / 1.0 / 4.6	**23** TU	0421 / 1020 / 1629 / 2221	1.4 / 4.2 / 1.6 / 4.1
9 TU	0428 / 1026 / 1653 / 2304	1.0 / 4.4 / 1.3 / 4.3	**24** W	0504 / 1119 / 1712 / 2326	1.7 / 3.9 / 1.9 / 3.9
10 W	0521 / 1140 / 1753	1.3 / 4.1 / 1.7	**25** TH	0556 / 1232 / 1807	2.0 / 3.7 / 2.2
11 TH	0022 / 0628 / 1311 / 1912	4.2 / 1.6 / 3.9 / 1.9	**26** F	0057 / 0709 / 1351 / 1930	3.7 / 2.1 / 3.6 / 2.3
12 F	0146 / 0755 / 1445 / 2048	4.1 / 1.7 / 4.0 / 1.9	**27** SA	0217 / 0835 / 1502 / 2056	3.7 / 2.1 / 3.7 / 2.3
13 SA	0304 / 0927 / 1558 / 2204	4.2 / 1.5 / 4.2 / 1.6	**28** SU	0320 / 0943 / 1558 / 2158	3.8 / 1.9 / 3.9 / 2.0
14 SU	0408 / 1034 / 1652 / 2300	4.5 / 1.2 / 4.5 / 1.2	**29** M	0409 / 1034 / 1640 / 2246	4.1 / 1.6 / 4.2 / 1.7
15 M	0500 / 1126 / 1736 / 2348	4.8 / 0.9 / 4.8 / 0.9	**30** TU	0448 / 1116 / 1715 / 2327	4.3 / 1.3 / 4.5 / 1.4

Chart Datum: 2·75 metres below Ordnance Datum (Newlyn)

SCOTLAND – ULLAPOOL

LAT 57°54'N   LONG 5°10'W

TIMES AND HEIGHTS OF HIGH AND LOW WATERS   YEAR 1996

TIME ZONE (UT)
For Summer Time add ONE hour in non-shaded areas

Chart Datum: 2·75 metres below Ordnance Datum (Newlyn)

MAY

Day	Time	m	Day	Time	m
1 W	0522 / 1154 / 1747	4.6 / 1.1 / 4.8	**16** TH	0013 / 0605 / 1231 / 1829	1.0 / 4.8 / 0.9 / 4.9
2 TH	0005 / 0555 / 1231 / 1821	1.1 / 4.8 / 0.8 / 5.0	**17** F	0056 / 0642 / 1309 / 1901 ●	0.9 / 4.9 / 0.8 / 4.9
3 F O	0043 / 0632 / 1307 / 1857	0.8 / 5.0 / 0.6 / 5.1	**18** SA	0135 / 0719 / 1344 / 1934	0.8 / 4.8 / 0.9 / 4.9
4 SA	0122 / 0710 / 1345 / 1935	0.6 / 5.1 / 0.5 / 5.2	**19** SU	0212 / 0757 / 1418 / 2007	0.9 / 4.8 / 1.0 / 4.8
5 SU	0203 / 0752 / 1425 / 2016	0.5 / 5.1 / 0.6 / 5.1	**20** M	0248 / 0835 / 1452 / 2041	1.0 / 4.6 / 1.1 / 4.7
6 M	0246 / 0837 / 1507 / 2101	0.5 / 4.9 / 0.7 / 5.0	**21** TU	0325 / 0915 / 1528 / 2116	1.1 / 4.4 / 1.3 / 4.5
7 TU	0331 / 0928 / 1553 / 2154	0.7 / 4.7 / 1.0 / 4.8	**22** W	0402 / 0957 / 1605 / 2157	1.3 / 4.2 / 1.5 / 4.3
8 W	0420 / 1029 / 1644 / 2257	0.9 / 4.4 / 1.3 / 4.5	**23** TH	0443 / 1046 / 1646 / 2248	1.5 / 4.0 / 1.7 / 4.0
9 TH	0516 / 1140 / 1744	1.1 / 4.2 / 1.6	**24** F	0528 / 1144 / 1733 / 2352	1.7 / 3.8 / 2.0 / 3.9
10 F	0009 / 0621 / 1302 / 1857	4.3 / 1.4 / 4.0 / 1.8	**25** SA	0622 / 1251 / 1833	1.9 / 3.7 / 2.1
11 SA	0126 / 0737 / 1426 / 2020	4.2 / 1.5 / 4.0 / 1.8	**26** SU	0104 / 0728 / 1401 / 1947	3.8 / 2.0 / 3.7 / 2.2
12 SU	0240 / 0858 / 1537 / 2137	4.3 / 1.4 / 4.2 / 1.6	**27** M	0212 / 0838 / 1504 / 2059	3.8 / 1.9 / 3.9 / 2.1
13 M	0345 / 1007 / 1633 / 2237	4.4 / 1.3 / 4.4 / 1.4	**28** TU	0310 / 0940 / 1555 / 2158	4.0 / 1.7 / 4.1 / 1.8
14 TU	0440 / 1103 / 1718 / 2328	4.6 / 1.1 / 4.6 / 1.2	**29** W	0400 / 1032 / 1639 / 2247	4.2 / 1.5 / 4.4 / 1.5
15 W	0526 / 1149 / 1756	4.7 / 1.0 / 4.8	**30** TH	0446 / 1118 / 1719 / 2333	4.4 / 1.2 / 4.7 / 1.2
			31 F	0530 / 1201 / 1759	4.7 / 1.0 / 5.0

JUNE

Day	Time	m	Day	Time	m
1 SA O	0017 / 0613 / 1244 / 1839	0.9 / 4.9 / 0.8 / 5.2	**16** SU ●	0120 / 0704 / 1324 / 1918	1.1 / 4.6 / 1.1 / 4.8
2 SU	0102 / 0658 / 1326 / 1921	0.7 / 5.1 / 0.6 / 5.3	**17** M	0157 / 0741 / 1358 / 1950	1.0 / 4.6 / 1.1 / 4.8
3 M	0147 / 0744 / 1410 / 2004	0.5 / 5.1 / 0.6 / 5.3	**18** TU	0232 / 0817 / 1433 / 2022	1.0 / 4.6 / 1.1 / 4.7
4 TU	0234 / 0833 / 1455 / 2052	0.5 / 5.0 / 0.7 / 5.2	**19** W	0306 / 0854 / 1507 / 2055	1.1 / 4.5 / 1.2 / 4.6
5 W	0322 / 0925 / 1542 / 2144	0.5 / 4.9 / 0.8 / 5.0	**20** TH	0342 / 0931 / 1543 / 2131	1.2 / 4.3 / 1.3 / 4.4
6 TH	0412 / 1023 / 1633 / 2243	0.7 / 4.6 / 1.1 / 4.8	**21** F	0418 / 1012 / 1620 / 2213	1.3 / 4.2 / 1.5 / 4.3
7 F	0506 / 1127 / 1730 / 2349	0.9 / 4.4 / 1.4 / 4.5	**22** SA	0457 / 1058 / 1701 / 2302	1.4 / 4.0 / 1.7 / 4.1
8 SA	0605 / 1238 / 1834	1.1 / 4.2 / 1.6	**23** SU	0540 / 1152 / 1749 / 2359	1.6 / 3.9 / 1.9 / 4.0
9 SU	0059 / 0709 / 1355 / 1945	4.4 / 1.4 / 4.1 / 1.7	**24** M	0630 / 1255 / 1846	1.7 / 3.8 / 2.0
10 M	0211 / 0820 / 1507 / 2102	4.3 / 1.5 / 4.1 / 1.7	**25** TU	0103 / 0729 / 1401 / 1952	3.9 / 1.8 / 3.9 / 2.0
11 TU	0318 / 0933 / 1609 / 2211	4.3 / 1.5 / 4.2 / 1.6	**26** W	0211 / 0838 / 1506 / 2103	3.9 / 1.8 / 4.0 / 1.9
12 W	0418 / 1035 / 1659 / 2307	4.3 / 1.4 / 4.4 / 1.4	**27** TH	0315 / 0947 / 1603 / 2208	4.1 / 1.6 / 4.3 / 1.7
13 TH	0507 / 1126 / 1740 / 2356	4.4 / 1.3 / 4.5 / 1.3	**28** F	0415 / 1046 / 1653 / 2305	4.3 / 1.4 / 4.6 / 1.3
14 F	0550 / 1210 / 1814	4.5 / 1.3 / 4.6	**29** SA	0509 / 1137 / 1739 / 2357	4.6 / 1.1 / 4.9 / 1.0
15 SA	0039 / 0627 / 1249 / 1845	1.2 / 4.6 / 1.2 / 4.7	**30** SU	0559 / 1224 / 1824	4.8 / 0.9 / 5.2

JULY

Day	Time	m	Day	Time	m
1 M O	0046 / 0646 / 1311 / 1907	0.7 / 5.1 / 0.7 / 5.4	**16** TU	0138 / 0722 / 1339 / 1932	1.1 / 4.6 / 1.2 / 4.8
2 TU	0134 / 0734 / 1356 / 1951	0.5 / 5.2 / 0.6 / 5.4	**17** W	0211 / 0755 / 1412 / 2000	1.0 / 4.6 / 1.1 / 4.8
3 W	0222 / 0822 / 1442 / 2037	0.3 / 5.2 / 0.6 / 5.4	**18** TH	0243 / 0827 / 1446 / 2029	1.0 / 4.6 / 1.1 / 4.7
4 TH	0310 / 0912 / 1528 / 2127	0.3 / 5.0 / 0.7 / 5.2	**19** F	0316 / 0900 / 1519 / 2102	1.0 / 4.5 / 1.1 / 4.6
5 F	0358 / 1004 / 1617 / 2220	0.5 / 4.8 / 0.9 / 5.1	**20** SA	0350 / 0936 / 1554 / 2138	1.1 / 4.4 / 1.2 / 4.5
6 SA	0447 / 1102 / 1708 / 2321	0.7 / 4.6 / 1.2 / 4.7	**21** SU	0425 / 1018 / 1631 / 2219	1.3 / 4.2 / 1.4 / 4.3
7 SU	0539 / 1205 / 1803	1.0 / 4.3 / 1.5	**22** M	0503 / 1105 / 1713 / 2308	1.4 / 4.1 / 1.6 / 4.1
8 M	0027 / 0635 / 1315 / 1907	4.4 / 1.3 / 4.1 / 1.7	**23** TU	0547 / 1202 / 1803	1.6 / 4.0 / 1.8
9 TU	0138 / 0738 / 1430 / 2022	4.2 / 1.6 / 4.0 / 1.9	**24** W	0010 / 0640 / 1311 / 1904	4.0 / 1.7 / 3.9 / 2.0
10 W	0249 / 0851 / 1541 / 2144	4.1 / 1.8 / 4.0 / 1.8	**25** TH	0123 / 0746 / 1424 / 2017	3.9 / 1.8 / 4.0 / 2.0
11 TH	0355 / 1005 / 1639 / 2249	4.1 / 1.8 / 4.2 / 1.7	**26** F	0241 / 0906 / 1532 / 2137	4.0 / 1.8 / 4.2 / 1.8
12 F	0451 / 1104 / 1723 / 2340	4.2 / 1.7 / 4.3 / 1.5	**27** SA	0353 / 1021 / 1631 / 2246	4.2 / 1.6 / 4.5 / 1.4
13 SA	0535 / 1151 / 1758	4.3 / 1.6 / 4.5	**28** SU	0454 / 1119 / 1722 / 2342	4.5 / 1.2 / 4.9 / 1.0
14 SU	0024 / 0612 / 1231 / 1830	1.4 / 4.4 / 1.4 / 4.6	**29** M	0547 / 1209 / 1808	4.8 / 0.9 / 5.2
15 M ●	0103 / 0647 / 1306 / 1901	1.2 / 4.5 / 1.3 / 4.7	**30** TU O	0033 / 0634 / 1256 / 1852	0.6 / 5.1 / 0.6 / 5.5
			31 W	0121 / 0719 / 1341 / 1935	0.4 / 5.3 / 0.5 / 5.6

AUGUST

Day	Time	m	Day	Time	m
1 TH	0207 / 0804 / 1426 / 2018	0.2 / 5.3 / 0.4 / 5.6	**16** F	0215 / 0756 / 1421 / 2001	0.8 / 4.8 / 0.9 / 4.9
2 F	0252 / 0850 / 1510 / 2103	0.2 / 5.2 / 0.5 / 5.4	**17** SA	0246 / 0827 / 1453 / 2032	0.8 / 4.7 / 0.8 / 4.8
3 SA	0337 / 0937 / 1555 / 2152	0.3 / 5.0 / 0.7 / 5.1	**18** SU	0319 / 0902 / 1526 / 2106	0.9 / 4.6 / 1.0 / 4.7
4 SU	0422 / 1028 / 1641 / 2248	0.6 / 4.7 / 1.0 / 4.8	**19** M	0352 / 0941 / 1602 / 2143	1.0 / 4.5 / 1.2 / 4.5
5 M	0508 / 1126 / 1731 / 2352	1.0 / 4.4 / 1.4 / 4.4	**20** TU	0429 / 1026 / 1642 / 2229	1.2 / 4.3 / 1.4 / 4.3
6 TU	0558 / 1232 / 1828	1.4 / 4.1 / 1.8	**21** W	0512 / 1121 / 1730 / 2331	1.5 / 4.1 / 1.7 / 4.1
7 W	0103 / 0654 / 1348 / 1940	4.1 / 1.8 / 3.9 / 2.0	**22** TH	0603 / 1232 / 1830	1.7 / 4.0 / 1.9
8 TH	0218 / 0806 / 1508 / 2117	3.9 / 2.0 / 3.9 / 2.1	**23** F	0053 / 0710 / 1353 / 1946	3.9 / 1.9 / 4.0 / 2.0
9 F	0333 / 0934 / 1616 / 2232	3.9 / 2.1 / 4.0 / 1.9	**24** SA	0222 / 0838 / 1510 / 2120	3.9 / 1.9 / 4.2 / 1.8
10 SA	0433 / 1043 / 1705 / 2324	4.0 / 2.0 / 4.2 / 1.7	**25** SU	0341 / 1005 / 1614 / 2235	4.2 / 1.7 / 4.5 / 1.4
11 SU	0518 / 1131 / 1740	4.1 / 1.8 / 4.4	**26** M	0444 / 1105 / 1707 / 2330	4.5 / 1.3 / 4.9 / 1.0
12 M	0006 / 0553 / 1210 / 1811	1.5 / 4.3 / 1.5 / 4.6	**27** TU	0535 / 1154 / 1753	4.9 / 0.9 / 5.3
13 TU	0042 / 0626 / 1244 / 1840	1.2 / 4.5 / 1.3 / 4.8	**28** W O	0018 / 0619 / 1240 / 1834	0.6 / 5.2 / 0.6 / 5.6
14 W ●	0114 / 0658 / 1317 / 1908	1.1 / 4.6 / 1.1 / 4.9	**29** TH	0104 / 0701 / 1324 / 1915	0.3 / 5.4 / 0.4 / 5.7
15 TH	0145 / 0727 / 1349 / 1934	0.9 / 4.7 / 1.0 / 4.9	**30** F	0147 / 0743 / 1407 / 1956	0.2 / 5.4 / 0.3 / 5.7
			31 SA	0230 / 0824 / 1449 / 2038	0.2 / 5.3 / 0.4 / 5.5

8

SCOTLAND – ULLAPOOL

LAT 57°54′N   LONG 5°10′W

TIMES AND HEIGHTS OF HIGH AND LOW WATERS

YEAR **1996**

SEPTEMBER

Time	m		Time	m
1 0311	0.3	**16** 0249	0.8
0906	5.1	0833	4.9
SU 1531	0.6	M 1501	0.9
2123	5.2	2039	4.9
2 0352	0.7	**17** 0323	0.9
0951	4.8	0911	4.7
M 1613	1.0	TU 1537	1.1
2214	4.8	2117	4.7
3 0434	1.1	**18** 0401	1.1
1043	4.5	0955	4.5
TU 1658	1.4	W 1618	1.3
2315	4.4	2205	4.4
4 0519	1.5	**19** 0444	1.4
1147	4.1	1052	4.3
W 1750	1.8	TH 1706	1.6
		2311	4.1
5 0027	4.0	**20** 0536	1.8
0611	2.0	1207	4.1
TH 1305	3.9	F 1807	1.9
1859	2.2		
6 0146	3.8	**21** 0041	3.9
0721	2.3	0646	2.0
F 1430	3.8	SA 1333	4.1
2043	2.3	1929	2.0
7 0306	3.8	**22** 0215	4.0
0857	2.3	0822	2.1
SA 1546	3.9	SU 1452	4.3
2211	2.1	2111	1.8
8 0410	3.9	**23** 0335	4.2
1017	2.2	0950	1.8
SU 1638	4.1	M 1557	4.6
2302	1.8	2223	1.4
9 0455	4.1	**24** 0435	4.6
1106	1.9	1049	1.4
M 1715	4.4	TU 1650	5.0
2341	1.5	2316	1.0
10 0530	4.3	**25** 0522	4.9
1144	1.6	1137	1.0
TU 1746	4.6	W 1736	5.3
11 0014	1.3	**26** 0002	0.6
0602	4.5	0604	5.2
W 1218	1.4	TH 1223	0.7
1815	4.8	1817	5.6
12 0045	1.1	**27** 0045	0.4
0631	4.7	0643	5.4
TH 1250	1.1	F 1305	0.5
● 1841	5.0	○ 1856	5.7
13 0115	0.9	**28** 0126	0.3
0658	4.9	0720	5.4
F 1322	1.0	SA 1347	0.5
1906	5.1	1935	5.6
14 0145	0.8	**29** 0206	0.3
0726	5.0	0757	5.4
SA 1354	0.9	SU 1427	0.5
1934	5.1	2015	5.4
15 0216	0.7	**30** 0245	0.5
0758	5.0	0836	5.2
SU 1426	0.8	M 1507	0.8
2005	5.0	2057	5.1

OCTOBER

Time	m		Time	m
1 0323	0.8	**16** 0259	0.9
0916	4.9	0849	5.0
TU 1547	1.1	W 1519	1.0
2144	4.8	2103	4.8
2 0402	1.2	**17** 0340	1.2
1000	4.6	0936	4.8
W 1630	1.5	TH 1602	1.3
2240	4.4	2156	4.5
3 0443	1.7	**18** 0425	1.5
1058	4.2	1034	4.5
TH 1718	1.9	F 1652	1.5
2351	4.0	2308	4.2
4 0531	2.1	**19** 0519	1.8
1219	4.0	1151	4.3
F 1821	2.2	SA 1756	1.8
5 0109	3.8	**20** 0037	4.1
0635	2.4	0631	2.1
SA 1344	3.9	SU 1314	4.3
1956	2.4	1919	1.9
6 0228	3.8	**21** 0206	4.1
0809	2.5	0805	2.1
SU 1501	3.9	M 1431	4.4
2131	2.2	2054	1.8
7 0334	3.9	**22** 0323	4.3
0935	2.4	0929	1.8
M 1558	4.1	TU 1538	4.7
2228	2.0	2204	1.4
8 0423	4.1	**23** 0421	4.6
1030	2.1	1029	1.5
TU 1641	4.4	W 1632	5.0
2307	1.7	2257	1.1
9 0501	4.4	**24** 0508	4.9
1110	1.8	1119	1.2
W 1716	4.6	TH 1719	5.2
2340	1.4	2343	0.8
10 0534	4.6	**25** 0548	5.2
1146	1.5	1204	0.9
TH 1746	4.8	F 1800	5.4
11 0012	1.2	**26** 0025	0.7
0602	4.8	0625	5.3
F 1220	1.2	SA 1247	0.8
1812	5.0	○ 1838	5.5
12 0044	1.0	**27** 0105	0.6
0629	5.0	0700	5.4
SA 1253	1.0	SU 1328	0.7
● 1839	5.1	1917	5.5
13 0115	0.8	**28** 0143	0.7
0659	5.2	0734	5.3
SU 1327	0.9	M 1408	0.8
1910	5.2	1955	5.3
14 0148	0.8	**29** 0220	0.8
0733	5.2	0810	5.2
M 1402	0.9	TU 1447	1.0
1944	5.2	2036	5.1
15 0222	0.8	**30** 0256	1.1
0809	5.1	0847	5.0
TU 1439	0.9	W 1525	1.2
2021	5.0	2120	4.7
		31 0333	1.4
		0926	4.7
		TH 1606	1.5
		2210	4.4

NOVEMBER

Time	m		Time	m
1 0412	1.7	**16** 0412	1.4
1013	4.4	1022	4.8
F 1651	1.9	SA 1644	1.4
2313	4.1	2305	4.4
2 0456	2.1	**17** 0508	1.7
1124	4.2	1133	4.6
SA 1746	2.2	SU 1746	1.6
3 0026	3.9	**18** 0024	4.3
0551	2.4	0616	2.0
SU 1250	4.0	M 1249	4.5
1901	2.3	1901	1.8
4 0140	3.8	**19** 0146	4.2
0710	2.5	0737	2.1
M 1406	4.0	TU 1405	4.5
2025	2.3	2023	1.7
5 0247	3.9	**20** 0300	4.4
0836	2.5	0859	1.9
TU 1509	4.1	W 1513	4.7
2133	2.1	2137	1.5
6 0342	4.1	**21** 0401	4.6
0941	2.3	1005	1.7
W 1559	4.3	TH 1612	4.8
2222	1.9	2234	1.3
7 0426	4.4	**22** 0451	4.8
1030	2.0	1059	1.4
TH 1639	4.5	F 1702	5.0
2301	1.6	2322	1.2
8 0502	4.6	**23** 0533	5.0
1111	1.7	1147	1.2
F 1713	4.8	SA 1745	5.2
2338	1.3		
9 0533	4.9	**24** 0005	1.0
1149	1.4	0609	5.2
SA 1744	5.0	SU 1231	1.1
		1824	5.2
10 0013	1.1	**25** 0046	1.0
0603	5.1	0643	5.2
SU 1226	1.2	M 1313	1.0
1816	5.1	○ 1902	5.2
11 0048	0.9	**26** 0123	1.0
0637	5.3	0716	5.2
M 1303	1.0	TU 1352	1.0
● 1851	5.2	1940	5.1
12 0124	0.8	**27** 0159	1.1
0713	5.4	0751	5.2
TU 1341	0.9	W 1430	1.1
1930	5.2	2019	5.0
13 0201	0.8	**28** 0234	1.2
0752	5.3	0825	5.0
W 1422	0.9	TH 1508	1.3
2012	5.1	2100	4.8
14 0242	0.9	**29** 0310	1.4
0835	5.2	0902	4.8
TH 1505	1.0	F 1546	1.5
2059	4.9	2144	4.5
15 0325	1.1	**30** 0348	1.7
0924	5.0	0942	4.6
F 1552	1.1	SA 1627	1.7
2156	4.7	2233	4.3

DECEMBER

Time	m		Time	m
1 0428	1.9	**16** 0454	1.5
1030	4.4	1108	4.9
SU 1712	1.9	M 1730	1.3
2331	4.1	2358	4.5
2 0513	2.2	**17** 0554	1.8
1135	4.2	1218	4.7
M 1806	2.1	TU 1833	1.6
3 0038	4.0	**18** 0112	4.3
0609	2.4	0702	2.0
TU 1252	4.1	W 1332	4.6
1913	2.2	1944	1.7
4 0147	4.0	**19** 0228	4.3
0722	2.5	0820	2.0
W 1403	4.1	TH 1444	4.5
2025	2.2	2100	1.7
5 0249	4.1	**20** 0336	4.4
0838	2.4	0937	1.9
TH 1503	4.2	F 1550	4.6
2128	2.0	2207	1.6
6 0341	4.3	**21** 0433	4.6
0941	2.2	1040	1.7
F 1553	4.4	SA 1646	4.7
2220	1.8	2302	1.5
7 0424	4.5	**22** 0520	4.8
1033	1.9	1132	1.5
SA 1636	4.6	SU 1733	4.8
2304	1.6	2348	1.4
8 0503	4.8	**23** 0558	4.9
1118	1.6	1218	1.4
SU 1717	4.8	M 1813	4.9
2345	1.3		
9 0541	5.1	**24** 0029	1.3
1200	1.3	0630	5.0
M 1757	5.1	TU 1300	1.2
		○ 1849	4.9
10 0024	1.1	**25** 0107	1.3
0619	5.3	0702	5.1
TU 1243	1.1	W 1339	1.2
● 1838	5.2	1926	4.9
11 0105	0.9	**26** 0142	1.2
0659	5.5	0735	5.1
W 1325	0.9	TH 1415	1.2
1921	5.3	2002	4.9
12 0146	0.8	**27** 0217	1.3
0740	5.5	0808	5.1
TH 1409	0.8	F 1450	1.2
2006	5.2	2039	4.8
13 0229	0.9	**28** 0251	1.3
0824	5.5	0840	5.0
F 1455	0.8	SA 1526	1.3
2055	5.1	2115	4.6
14 0314	1.0	**29** 0327	1.4
0912	5.3	0914	4.8
SA 1543	0.9	SU 1602	1.4
2149	4.9	2153	4.5
15 0401	1.2	**30** 0403	1.6
1007	5.1	0952	4.6
SU 1634	1.1	M 1639	1.6
2250	4.7	2236	4.3
		31 0441	1.8
		1037	4.4
		TU 1720	1.8
		2328	4.1

Chart Datum: 2·75 metres below Ordnance Datum (Newlyn)

PORTREE   10-8-9

Skye 57°24'·75N 06°11'·00W

CHARTS

AC 2534, 2208; Imray C66; OS 23

TIDES

–0445 Dover; ML no data; Duration 0610; Zone 0 (UT)

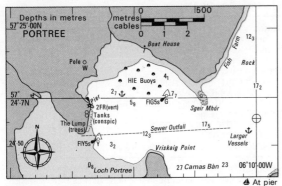

Standard Port ULLAPOOL (←—)

Times				Height (metres)			
High Water		Low Water		MHWS	MHWN	MLWN	MLWS
0000	0600	0300	0900	5·2	3·9	2·1	0·7
1200	1800	1500	2100				
Differences PORTREE (Skye)							
–0025	–0025	–0025	–0025	+0·1	–0·2	–0·2	0·0
SHIELDAIG (Loch Torridon)							
–0020	–0020	–0015	–0015	+0·4	+0·3	+0·1	0·0
LOCH A'BHRAIGE (Rona)							
–0020	0000	0000	0000	–0·1	–0·1	–0·1	–0·2
PLOCKTON (Loch Carron)							
+0005	–0025	–0005	–0010	+0·5	+0·5	+0·5	+0·2
LOCH SNIZORT (Uig Bay, Skye)							
–0045	–0020	–0005	–0025	+0·1	–0·4	–0·2	0·0
LOCH DUNVEGAN (Skye)							
–0105	–0030	–0020	–0040	0·0	–0·1	0·0	0·0
LOCH HARPORT (Skye)							
–0115	–0035	–0020	–0100	–0·1	–0·1	0·0	+0·1
SOAY (Camus nan Gall)							
–0055	–0025	–0025	–0045	–0·4	–0·2	No data	
KYLE OF LOCHALSH							
–0040	–0020	–0005	–0025	+0·1	0·0	+0·1	+0·1
DORNIE BRIDGE (Loch Alsh)							
–0040	–0010	–0005	–0020	+0·1	–0·1	0·0	0·0
GLENELG BAY (Kyle Rhea)							
–0105	–0035	–0035	–0055	–0·4	–0·4	–0·9	–0·1
LOCH HOURN							
–0125	–0050	–0040	–0110	–0·2	–0·1	–0·1	+0·1

SHELTER

Secure in all but strong SW winds, when holding ground not reliable. In the N of the bay there are 8 HIE Øs for <15 tons.

NAVIGATION

WPT 57°24'·60N 06°10'·00W, 095°/275° from/to pier, 0·72M Appr from S, avoid rks off An Tom Pt (off chartlet).

LIGHTS AND MARKS

The only lts are a SHM buoy Fl G 5s near centre of B, 2 FR (vert) 6m 4M (occas) on the pier and a SPM buoy Fl Y 5s.

RADIO TELEPHONE

VHF Ch 16 12 (occas).

TELEPHONE (01478)

Hr Mr ☎ 612926; Moorings 612341; MRSC (01631) 563720; ‡ (0141) 887 9369; Marinecall 0891 500464; Police 612888; Dr 612013; Ⓗ 612704.

FACILITIES

Pier D (cans), L, FW. **Town** EC Wed; P, V, Gas, Gaz, Ⓞ, R, Bar, ✉, Ⓑ, ⇌ (bus/ferry to Kyle of Lochalsh).

LOCH TORRIDON, Ross & Cromarty, 57°36'N 05°49'W. AC 2210. Tides as above. Three large lochs: ent to outer loch (Torridon) is 3M wide, with isolated Sgeir na Trian (2m) almost in mid-chan; ⚓s on SW side behind Eilean Mór and in L Beag. L Sheildaig is middle loch with good ⚓ between the Is and village. 1M to the N, a 2ca wide chan leads into Upper L Torridon; many fish cages and prone to squalls. Few facilities, except Shieldaig: FW, V, R, Bar, ✉, Garage.

ANCHORAGES AROUND OR NEAR SKYE

LOCH A'BHRAIGE, Rona, 57°34'·63N 05°57'·87W. AC 2534, 2479. HW –0438 on Dover; ML 2·8m; Duration 0605. See 10.8.9. A good ⚓ in NW of the island safe except in NNW winds. Beware rks on the NE side lying up to 1ca off shore. Hbr in NE corner of loch head. Ldg lts 137°, see 10.8.4. Few facilities: jetty, FW and a helipad, all owned by MOD (DRA). Call *Rona* on VHF Ch 16 before ent. **Acarseid Mhor** is ⚓ on W of Rona. App S of Eilean Garbh marked by W arrow. SD sketch of rks at ent is necessary. 5M SE of Portree at Churchton B, SW tip of Raasay, there are 4 HIE Øs; ☎ (01478) 612341.

LOCH DUNVEGAN, 4 HIE Øs off Stein, 57°30'·9N 06°34'·5W. 3 HIE Øs off Dunvegan, 57°26'·3N 06°35'·2W. Fuel, FW, R. ☎ (01478) 612341.

LOCH HARPORT, Isle of Skye, 57°20'·60N 06°25'·80W. AC 1795. HW –0447 (Sp), –0527 (Np) on Dover. See 10.8.9. On E side of Loch Bracadale, entered between Oronsay Is and Ardtreck Pt (W lt ho, Iso 4s 17m 9M). SW end of Oronsay has conspic rk pillar, called The Castle; keep ¼ M off-shore here and off E coast of Oronsay which is joined to Ullinish Pt by drying reef. ⚓ Oronsay Is, N side of drying reef (4m), or on E side, but beware rk (dries) 0·5ca off N shore of Oronsay. Fiskavaig Bay 1M S of Ardtreck (7m); Loch Beag on N side of loch, exposed to W winds; Port na Long E of Ardtreck, sheltered except from E winds (beware fish farm); Carbost on SW shore. Facilities: EC Wed (Carbost); V (local shop), Bar, R, P (garage), ✉, FW. (Port na Long) Bar, FW, V (shop).

SOAY HARBOUR, Skye, 57°09'·50N 06°13'·40W. AC 2208. Tides see 10.8.9. Narrow inlet on NW side of Soay; enter from Soay Sound above half flood to clear bar, dries 0·6m. Appr on 135° from 5ca out to avoid reefs close each side of ent. Cross bar slightly E of mid-chan, altering 20° stbd for best water; ent is 15m wide between boulder spits. ⚓ in 3m mid-pool or shoal draft boats can enter inner pool. Good shelter and holding. Camas nan Gall (poor holding) has public ☎; no other facilities.

CROWLIN ISLANDS, Ross & Cromarty, 57°21'·08N 05°50'·59W. AC 2498, 2209. HW –0435 on Dover, –0020 on Ullapool; HW +0·3m on Ullapool. See 10.8.9. ⚓ between Eilean Meadhonach and Eilean Mor, appr from N, keep E of Eilean Beg. Excellent shelter except in strong N winds. There is an inner ⚓ with 3½m but ent chan dries. Eilean Beg lt ho Fl 6s 32m 6M, W tr. There are no facilities.

PLOCKTON, LOCH CARRON, Ross & Cromarty, 57°20'·35N 05°38'·33W. AC 2528, 2209. HW –0435 on Dover; ML 3·5m; Duration 0600. See 10.8.9. Good ⚓ on S side of Outer Loch Carron, open only to N/NE'lies. Safest ent is ENE between Sgeir Bhuidhe and Sgeir Golach, marked by SHM buoy Fl G 3s (the only lt); thence 170° between Bogha Dubh Sgeir (1·5m, PHM bn) and Hawk Rk (0·7m) off Cat Is, (conspic disused lt ho). A shorter appr is E between High Stone (rk with bn, S of Sgeir Golach) and Cat Island. Beware Plockton Rks (2·7m) on E side of bay. ⚓ in centre of bay in approx 3·5m or moor close E of tiny slip. SW part of bay dries. Facilities: **Village** D, CH, Bar, FW, ✉, R, ⇌, Gas, V, airstrip.

LOCH ALSH, Ross & Cromarty, 57°16'·50N 05°43'·00W. AC 2540, 2541. HW –0450 on Dover; ML 3·0m; Duration 0555. See 10.8.9. Almost land-locked between the SE corner of Skye and mainland. Bridge to Skye at W end of Kyle Akin has 24·8m clearance. Safe ⚓s can be found for most winds (clockwise from Kyle of Lochalsh): off the hotel there in 11m; in Avernish Bay (2ca N of Racoon Rk) in 3m clear of power cables (open to SW); off NW side of Eilean Donnan Castle (conspic); in Ratagan Bay at head of L Duich in 7m; in Totaig (or Ob Aoinidh) Bay opposite Loch Long ent in 3·5m; on S shore in Ardintoul Bay (7ca S of Racoon Rk) in 5·5m; at head of Loch na Béiste in 7m close inshore and W of fish cages; inside the pier at Kyleakin hbr. Kyle of Lochalsh is a useful railhead. Old Ferry pier, two lts 2 FG (vert). Fish pier, unlit, where yachts can refuel. Admty pier, three lts Oc G 6s. Eileanan Dubha Fl (2) 10s 9m 8M. Hr Mr ☎ (01599) 534167. Facilities (Kyle of Lochalsh): Bar, D, FW, ✉, R, ⇌, V, CH, P, Bus to Glasgow or Inverness.

8

ANCHORAGES IN THE SOUND OF SLEAT AND IN THE SMALL ISLANDS

SOUND OF SLEAT: There are ⚓s at: **Glenelg Bay** (57°12'·58N 05°37'·88W) SW of pier out of the tide, but only moderate holding. Usual facilities in village. At **Sandaig Bay** (57°10'·00N 05°41'·43W), exposed to SW. Sandaig Is are to NW of the bay; beware rks off Sgeir nan Eun. Eilean Mór has lt Fl 6s. At **Isleornsay Hbr** (57°09'N 05°47'·7W) 2ca N of pier, 2FR (vert) and floodlit. Give drying N end of Ornsay Is a wide berth. Lts: SE tip of Ornsay, Oc 8s 18m 15M, W tr; N end, Fl R 6s 8m 4M. Facilities: FW, P, V, ✉, Hotel.

LOCH HOURN, Inverness, 57°08'N 05°42'W. AC 2541, 2208. Tides see 10.8.9. Ent is S of Sandaig Is and opposite Isle Ornsay, Skye. Loch extends 11M inland via 4 narrows to Loch Beag; it is scenically magnificent, but violent squalls occur in strong winds. Sgeir Ulibhe, drying 2·1m, bn, lies almost in mid-ent; best to pass S of it to clear Clansman Rk, 2·1m, to the N. ⚓s on N shore at Eilean Ràrsaidh and Camas Bàn, within first 4M. For pilotage further E, consult SDs. Facilities at Arnisdale (Camas Bàn): FW, V, R, Bar, ✉.

LOCH NEVIS, Inverness, 57°02'·20N 05°43'·34W. AC 2541, 2208. HW −0515 on Dover. See 10.8.10. ⚓ NE of Eilean na Glaschoille, good except in S winds; or 1M further E off Inverie, but holding poor. Beware rks Bogha cas Sruth (dries 1·8m), Bogha Don and Sgeirean Glasa both marked by bns. Upper parts of the loch are subject to very violent unpredictable squalls. Yachts can enter the inner loch with caution, and ⚓ N or SE of Eilean Maol.

ARMADALE BAY, Skye, 4M NW of Mallaig. AC 2208. 6 HIE 🛟s in 2 trots at 57°04'·0N 05°53'·6W (☎ (01478) 612341). Bay is sheltered from SE to N winds but subject to swell in winds from N to SE. From S, beware the Eilean Maol and Sgorach rocks. Ferry pier, Oc R 6s 6m 6M, with conspic W shed. Facilities: FW at ferry pier or on charter (☎ 01471 844216) moorings from long hose on old pier; D (cans), V, Gas, showers at Ardvasar ¾ mile; P (cans), Gaz at ¼ mile; R, Bar, ferry to Mallaig for ⇌.

CANNA, The Small Islands, 57°03'·30N 06°29'·40W. AC 2208, 1796. HW −0457 (Sp), −0550 (Np) on Dover; HW −0035 and −0·4m on Ullapool; Duration 0605. Good holding and shelter, except in strong E'lies, in hbr between Canna and Sanday Is. Appr along Sanday shore, keeping N of Sgeir a' Phuirt, dries 4·6m. Ldg marks as in SDs. ⚓ in 3 - 4m W of Canna pier, off which beware drying rky patch. ⚓ Lt is advised due to FVs. Conspic W lt bn, Fl 6s 32m 9M, vis 152°-061°, at E end of Sanday Is. Magnetic anomaly off NE Canna. Facilities: FW only. Note: National Trust for Scotland runs island; please do not ditch rubbish.

RHUM, The Small Islands, 57°00'·08N 06°15'·70W. AC 2207, 2208. HW −0500 on Dover; −0035 and −0·3m on Ullapool; ML 2·4m; Duration 0600. Nature Conservancy Council owns Is. The mountains (809m) are unmistakeable. Landing is only allowed at L Scresort on E side; no dogs. Beware drying rks 1ca off N point of ent and almost 3ca off S point. The head of the loch dries 2ca out; ⚓ off slip on S side or further in, to NE of jetty. Hbr is open to E winds/swell. Facilities: Hotel, ✉, FW, V, R, Bar, ferry to Mallaig.

EIGG HARBOUR, The Small Islands, 56°52'·64N 06°07'·60W. AC 2207. HW −0523 on Dover. See 10.8.10. Coming from N or E enter between Garbh Sgeir and Flod Sgeir (bn, ○ topmark), drying rks. An Sgùrr is a conspic 391m high peak/ridge brg 290°/1.3M from pier. Most of hbr dries, but good ⚓ 1ca NE of Galmisdale Pt pier, except in NE winds when yachts should go through the narrows and ⚓ in South Bay in 6-8m; tide runs hard in the narrows. Also ⚓ in 2·5m at Poll nam Partan, about 2ca N of Flod Sgeir. SE point of Eilean Chathastail Fl 6s 24m 8M, vis 181°-shore, W tr. VHF Ch 08 *Eigg Hbr*. Hr Mr ☎ via (01687) 482428. FW, repairs. **Cleadale village** (2M to N) Bar, ✉, R, V, Gas.

MUCK, The Small Islands, 56°49'·80N 06°13'·33W. AC 2207. Tides approx as Eigg, see 10.8.10. Port Mór at the SE end is the main hbr, with a deep pool inside offlying rks, but exposed to S'lies. Appr with tree plantation bearing exactly 329°; this leads between Dubh Sgeir and Bogha Ruadh rks. ⚓ towards the NW side of inlet; NE side has drying rks. On N side of Is, Bagh a' Ghallanaich is ⚓ protected from S; entrance needs SDs and careful identification of marks. Few facilities.

MALLAIG   10-8-10

Inverness 57°00'·48N 05°49'·40W

CHARTS
AC 2500, 2208; Imray C65, C66; OS 40
TIDES
−0515 Dover; ML 2·9; Duration 0605; Zone 0 (UT)

Standard Port OBAN (⟶)

Times				Height (metres)			
High Water		Low Water		MHWS	MHWN	MLWN	MLWS
0000	0600	0100	0700	4·0	2·9	1·8	0·7
1200	1800	1300	1900				
Differences MALLAIG							
+0017	+0017	+0017	+0017	+1·0	+0·7	+0·3	+0·1
INVERIE BAY (Loch Nevis)							
+0030	+0020	+0035	+0020	+1·0	+0·9	+0·2	0·0
BAY OF LAIG (Eigg)							
+0015	+0030	+0040	+0005	+0·7	+0·6	−0·2	−0·2
LOCH MOIDART							
+0015	+0015	+0040	+0020	+0·8	+0·6	−0·2	−0·2

SHELTER
Good in SW winds but open to the N. Access H24. ⚓ in SE part of hbr or berth on Fish Pier. No 🛟s. Hbr is often congested with FVs; also Skye ferry.
NAVIGATION
WPT 57°01'·08N 05°50'·00W, 333°/153° from/to Steamer Pier lt, 0·67M. Red Rks in ent (bn on centre rk) can be passed either side, the E side being easier.

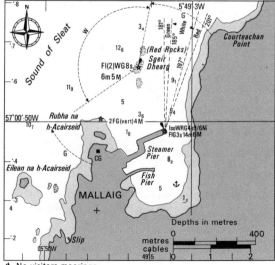

▲ No visitors moorings

LIGHTS AND MARKS
Lts as chartlet and 10.8.4. Sgeir Dhearg may be obsc by town lts. IPTS for ferries (Easter-Oct).
RADIO TELEPHONE
Call: *Mallaig Hbr Radio* VHF Ch 09 16 (office hrs).
TELEPHONE (01687)
Hr Mr 462154 (HO), 462249 (OT); MRSC (01631) 563720; ⌗ (0141) 887 9369; Marinecall 0891 500464; Police 462177.
FACILITIES
Jetty Slip, M, P (cans), D (tanker), L, FW, ME, El, Sh, C (10 ton mobile), CH, AB; **Services:** Ⓔ, ACA.
Town EC Wed; Dr 462202. V, R, Gas, Gaz, Bar, ✉, Ⓑ, ⇌.

ADJACENT ANCHORAGE

ARISAIG HARBOUR, (Loch nan Ceall), Inverness, 56°53'·78N 05°54'·50W. AC 2207. HW −0515 on Dover; +0030 and +0·9m on Oban; ML 2·9m; Duration 0605. Ldg line 256° into loch is S point of Eigg and N point of Muck. There are many unmarked rks, but no lts. S Chan is winding, but marked by perches. ⚓ above Cave Rk, approx 1M within the ent, is well sheltered. Access HW −3 to +2. Call *Arisaig Hbr* VHF Ch 16 32. **Arisaig Marine** ☎ (01687) 450224, Fax 450678, 20 x M, C (10 ton), CH, D at pier (HW), P (cans), El, ME, Sh. **Village** EC Thurs; FW at hotel, Bar, ✉, R, V, ⇌.

LOCH SUNART   10-8-11
Argyll 56°39'·50N 06°00'·00W

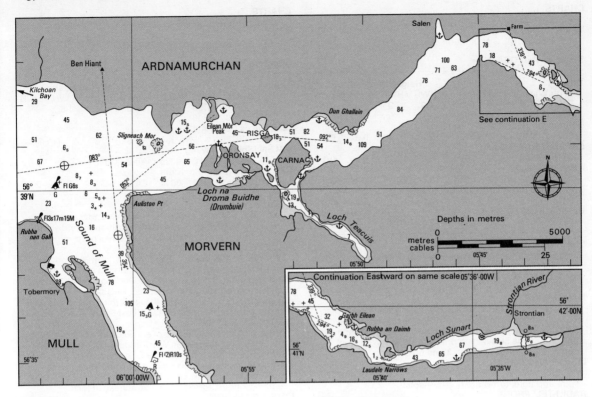

CHARTS
AC 2394, 2392, 2171; Imray C65; OS 45, 47, 49
TIDES
Salen –0500 Dover; ML 2·0; Zone 0 (UT)

Standard Port OBAN (→)

Times				Height (metres)			
High Water		Low Water		MHWS	MHWN	MLWN	MLWS
0100	0700	0100	0800	4·0	2·9	1·8	0·7
1300	1900	1300	2000				
Differences SALEN (L Sunart)							
–0015	+0015	+0010	+0005	+0·6	+0·5	–0·1	–0·1
LOCH EATHARNA (Coll)							
+0025	+0010	+0015	+0025	+0·4	+0·3	No data	
GOTT BAY (Tiree)							
0000	+0010	+0005	+0010	0·0	+0·1	0·0	0·0

SHELTER
8 HIE Øs at Kilchoan B (56°24'·5N 06°07'·3W); ☎ (01972) 510209. ⮑s in Loch na Droma Buidhe (S of Oronsay) sheltered in all winds; in Sailean Mór (N of Oronsay) convenient and easy ent; between Oronsay and Carna; in Loch Teacuis (very tricky ent); E of Carna; Salen Bay, with Øs; Garbh Eilean (NW of Rubha an Daimh), and E of sand spit by Strontian R.
NAVIGATION
West WPT, 56°39'·70N 06°03'·00W, 263°/083° from/to Creag nan Sgarbh (NW tip of Orinsay), 3·7M.
South WPT, 56°38'·00N 06°00'·65W, 1M S of Auliston Pt; there are extensive rky reefs W of this pt. Chart 2394 and detailed directions are needed to navigate the 17M long loch, particularly in its upper reaches. Beware Ross Rk, S of Risga; Broad Rk, E of Risga; Dun Ghallain Rk; shoals extending 3ca NNW from Eilean mo Shlinneag off S shore; drying rk 1ca W of Garbh Eilean and strong streams at sp in Laudale Narrows.
LIGHTS AND MARKS
Unlit. Transits as on the chart: from W WPT, Risga on with N pt of Oronsay at 083°; N pt of Carna on with top of Risga 092°. From S WPT, Ben Hiant bearing 354°, thence Eilean Mor Peak at 052°. Further up the loch, 339° and 294°, as on chartlet, are useful. Many other transits are shown on AC 2394.

RADIO TELEPHONE
None.
TELEPHONE (01967)
MRSC (01631) 563720; ⌗ (0141) 887 9369; Marinecall 0891 500463; Dr 431231.
FACILITIES
SALEN
Services: FW, CH, Gas, Gaz, M, Diver, D by hose, limited V, R, Bar, ME, El; **Acharacle** (2½M), P, V, ⊠, Ⓑ (Tues/Wed, mobile), ⇌ (bus to Loch Ailort/Ft William), → (Oban).
STRONTIAN
FW, P, V, hotel, ⊠, Gas, Gaz, Bar. Bus to Fort William.

ANCHORAGES IN COLL AND TIREE

ARINAGOUR, Loch Eatharna, Coll, 56°37'·00N 06°31'·20W. AC 2474, 2171. HW –0530 on Dover; ML 1·4m; Duration 0600; see 10.8.11. Good shelter except with SE swell or strong winds from ENE to SSW. Enter at SHM buoy, Fl G 6s, marking Bogha Mòr. Thence NW to Arinagour ferry pier, 2 FR(vert) 10m. Beware McQuarrie's Rk (dries 2·9m) 1ca E of pier hd and unmarked drying rks further N on E side of fairway. Ch and hotel are conspic ahead. Continue N towards old stone pier; ⮑ S of it or pick up a buoy. Six HIE Øs on W side of hbr, between the two piers. Also ⮑ E of Eilean Eatharna. Piermaster ☎ (01879) 220347; VHF Ch 31. Facilities: **HIE Trading Post** ☎ 220349, M, D, FW, Gas, V, CH, R. **Village** Ⓧ, FW, P, ⊠, ferry to Oban (⇌).

GOTT BAY, Tiree, 56°30'·75N 06°48'·00W. AC 2474. Tides as 10.8.11; HW –0540 on Dover. Adequate shelter in calm weather, but exposed in winds ENE to S. The bay, at NE end of island, can be identified by conspic latticed tr at Scarinish about 8ca SW of ent, with lt Fl 3s 11m 16M close by (obscd over hbr). Appr on NW track, keeping to SW side of bay which is obstructed on NE side by Soa Is and drying rks. The ferry pier at S side of ent has FR ldg lts 286½°. ⮑ about 1ca NW of pier head in 3m on sand; dinghy landing at pier. Facilities: P & D (cans), Gas, V, R, Bar, ⊠ at Scarinish (½M), ferry to Oban (⇌).

TOBERMORY   10-8-12
Mull 56°37'·60N 06°03'·15W

CHARTS
AC 2474, 2390, 2171; Imray C65; OS 47
TIDES
–0519 Dover; ML 2·4; Duration 0610; Zone 0 (UT)

Standard Port OBAN (→)

Times				Height (metres)			
High Water		Low Water		MHWS	MHWN	MLWN	MLWS
0100	0700	0100	0800	4·0	2·9	1·8	0·7
1300	1900	1300	2000				
Differences TOBERMORY (Mull)							
+0025	+0010	+0015	+0025	+0·4	+0·4	0·0	0·0
CARSAIG BAY (S Mull)							
–0015	–0005	–0030	+0020	+0·1	+0·2	0·0	–0·1
IONA (SW Mull)							
–0010	–0005	–0020	+0015	0·0	+0·1	–0·3	–0·2
BUNESSAN (Loch Lathaich, SW Mull)							
–0015	–0015	–0010	–0015	+0·3	+0·1	0·0	–0·1
ULVA SOUND (W Mull)							
–0010	–0015	0000	–0005	+0·4	+0·3	0·0	–0·1

SHELTER
Good, except for some swell in strong N/NE winds. ‡ off Old Pier clear of fairway, marked by Y buoys. To the SE are 8 Bu HIE ‡s. Other ‡s off Aros pier (beware fish farms); at SE end of The Doirlinn; or in bay on W side of Calve Is.
NAVIGATION
WPT 56°38'·00N 06°02'·00W, 058°/238° from/to ferry pier, 1·1M. N ent is wide and clear of dangers. From S beware Sgeir Calve on NE of Calve Is. S ent via The Doirlinn is only 80m wide at HW, and dries at LW; at HW±2 least depth is 2m. Enter between 2 bns on 300°.
LIGHTS AND MARKS
Rhubha nan Gall, Fl 3s 17m 15M, W tr is 1M N of ent. Ch spire and hotel turret are both conspic.
RADIO TELEPHONE
VHF Ch 16 12 (HO), M.
TELEPHONE (01688)
Hr Mr 302017; MRSC (01631) 563720; Local CG 302200; Marinecall 0891 500463; Police 302016; Dr 302013.
FACILITIES
Ferry Pier, temp AB for P, D, FW; **Old Pier** for FVs; **Western Isles YC ☎** 302420; **Services**: ME, CH, ACA, Gaz, Gas, Divers. **Town** EC Wed (winter); FW, P, Dr, V, R, Bar, ⊠, Ⓑ, ▯, ⊯ (ferry to Oban), ✈ (grass strip; helipad on golf course).

SOUND OF MULL. 8M SE of Tobermory at **Salen Bay** (Mull, 56°31'·45N 05°56'·75W) are 8 HIE ‡s. Beware drying rks 6ca E of the bay; ent on SE side. Land at jetty in SW corner. At **Craignure**, (Mull, 56°28'·37N 05°42'·25W) 9M SE, are 8 more HIE ‡s, N of ferry pier; ldg lts 241°, both FR 10/12m. Facilities: V, Bar, ⊠, Gas, ferry to Oban. Tides, see 10.8.13. There are 2 Historic Wrecks (see 10.0.3g) at the SE end of the Sound: *Dartmouth* at 56°30'·19N 05°41'·95W on W side of Eilean Rubha an Ridire; and *Speedwell* on Duart Point at 56°27'·45N 05°39'·32W.

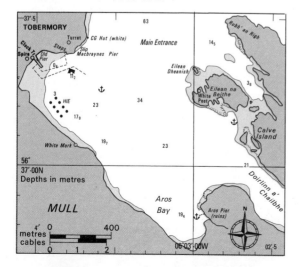

LOCH ALINE   10-8-13
Argyll 56°32'·10N 05°46'·40W

CHARTS
AC 2390; Imray C65; OS 49
TIDES
–0523 Dover; Duration 0610; Zone 0 (UT)

Standard Port OBAN (→)

Times				Height (metres)			
High Water		Low Water		MHWS	MHWN	MLWN	MLWS
0100	0700	0100	0800	4·0	2·9	1·8	0·7
1300	1900	1300	2000				
Differences LOCH ALINE							
+0012	+0012	No data		+0·5	+0·3	No data	
SALEN (Sound of Mull)							
+0045	+0015	+0020	+0030	+0·2	+0·2	–0·1	0·0
CRAIGNURE (Sound of Mull)							
+0030	+0005	+0010	+0015	0·0	+0·1	–0·1	–0·1

SHELTER
Very good. ‡s in SE end of loch and in N and E part of loch are restricted by fish farms. Temp berth on the old stone slip in the ent on W side, depth and ferries permitting.
NAVIGATION
WPT 56°31'·50N 05°46'·30W, 356°/176° from/to front ldg bn, 0·9M. Bns lead 356°, 100m W of Bogha Lurcain, drying rk off Bolorkle Pt on E side of ent. The buoyed ent is easy, but narrow with a bar (min depth 2·1m); stream runs 2½kn at sp. Beware coasters from the sand mine going to/from the jetty and ferries to/from Mull. Last 5ca of loch dries.
LIGHTS AND MARKS
Ardtornish Pt lt ho, 1M SSE of ent, Fl (2) WRG 10s 7m 8/5M. Lts and buoys as chartlet. War Memorial Cross (conspic, 9m high) stands on W side of ent. Ldg lts are FW 2/4m (H24). 1M up the loch on E side a Y bn with ● topmark marks a reef, and ½M further up similar bn marks a larger reef on W side. Clock tr is conspic at head of loch.
RADIO TELEPHONE
None.
TELEPHONE (01967)
MRSC (01631) 563720; ⌗ (0141) 887 9369; Marinecall 0891 500463; Ⓗ (01631) 563727; Dr 421252.
FACILITIES
Village Gas, V, R, Bar, P, ⊠, (Ⓑ, ⊯, ✈ at Oban), Ferry to Fishnish Bay (Mull).

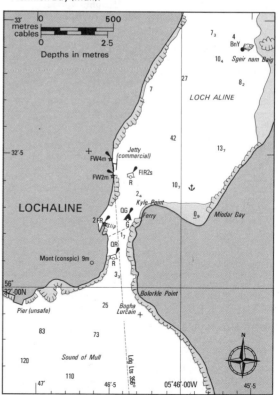

ANCHORAGES on WEST and SOUTH COASTS OF MULL
(Anti-clockwise from the North. SDs essential)

TRESHNISH ISLES, 56°30'N 06°24'W. AC 2652. The main Is (N to S) are: Cairn na Burgh, Fladda, Lunga, Bac Mòr and Bac Beag. Tides run hard and isles are exposed to swell, but merit a visit in calm weather. Appr with caution on ldg lines as in CCC SDs; temp ⚓ off Lunga's N tip in 4m.

STAFFA, 56°25'.97N 06°20'.27W. AC 2652. Spectacular isle with Fingal's Cave, but same caveats as above. Very temp ⚓ off SE tip where there is landing; beware unmarked rks.

GOMETRA, 56°28'.86N 06°16'W. AC 2652. Tides as 10.8.12. The narrow inlet between Gometra and Ulva Is offers sheltered ⚓, except in S'lies. Appr on 020° between Staffa and Little Colonsay, or N of the former. Beware rks drying 3·2m, to stbd and 5ca S of ent. Inside, E side is cleaner.

LOCH NA KEAL, 56°27'N 06°11'W (ent). AC 2652. Tides in 10.8.12. Appr S of Geasgill Is and N of drying rks off **Inch Kenneth**; E of this Is and in **Sound of Ulva** are sheltered ⚓s, except in S'lies. Beware MacQuarrie's Rk, dries 0·8m.

LOCH LATHAICH, Mull, 56°19'.30N 06°15'.40W. AC 2617. HW –0545 on Dover; ML 2·4. See 10.8.12. Excellent shelter with easy access; good base for cruising W Mull. Eilean na Liathanaich (a group of islets) lie off the ent, marked by a W bn at the E end, Fl WR 6s 12m 8/6M, R088°-108°, W108°-088°. Keep to W side of loch and ⚓ off Bendoran BY in SW, or SE of Eilean Ban off the pier in approx 5m. Facilities: **Bendoran BY** ☎ (01681) 700435 AB, M, P (cans), D, FW, CH, 🅖, Slip, Sh. (Bunessan) Shop, ✉, Bar, R, FW.

SOUND OF IONA, 56°19'.46N 06°23'.05W. AC 2617. Tides see 10.8.12. From N, enter in mid-chan; from S keep clear of Torran Rks. Cathedral brg 012° closes the Iona shore past 2 SHM buoys and SCM buoy. Beware a bank 0·1m in mid-sound, between cathedral and Fionnphort; also tel cables and ferries. ⚓ S of ferry close in to Iona, or in Bull Hole. Consult SDs. Crowded in season; limited facilities.

TINKER'S HOLE, Ross of Mull, 56°17'.50N 06°23'.00W. AC 2617. Beware Torran Rks, reefs extending 5M S and SW of Erraid. Usual app from S, avoiding Rankin's Rks, dry 0·8m, and Rk, dries 2·3m, between Eilean nam Muc and Erraid. Popular ⚓ in mid-pool twixt Eilean Dubh and Erraid.

CARSAIG BAY, Ross of Mull, 56°19'.20N 05°59'.00W. Tides see 10.8.12. AC 2386. Temp, fair weather ⚓s to N of Gamhnach Mhòr, reef 2m high, or close into NW corner of bay. Landing at stone quay on NE side. No facilities.

LOCH SPELVE, Mull, 56°23'N 05°41'W. AC 2387. Tides as Oban. Landlocked water, prone to squalls off surrounding hills. Ent narrows to ½ca due to shoal S side and drying rk N side. CCC SDs give local ldg lines. ⚓s in SW and NW arms, clear of fish farms. Pier at Croggan; no facilities.

ANCHORAGES ALONG LOCH LINNHE (AC 2378, 2379, 2380)

LYNN OF LORN, 56°33'N 05°25'.2W: At NE end are ⚓s off **Port Appin**, clear of ferry and cables (beware Appin Rks); and in **Airds Bay**, open to SW. At NW tip of Lismore, **Port Ramsey** offers good ⚓s between the 3 main islets.

LOCH CRERAN, 56°32'.15N 05°25'.15W. Ent at Airds Pt lt, Fl WRG 2s 2m 3/1M, W041°-058°. Caution: Chan turns 90° stbd and streams runs 4kn. Sgeir Callich, rky ridge juts out NE to SHM buoy, Fl G 3s; ⚓ W of it. Moorings (max LOA 7m) off Barcaldine; also off Creagan Inn, ☎ (01631) 573250, 3 ⚓s max LOA 9m. Bridge has 12m clearance.

LOCH LEVEN, 56°41'.62N 05°12'W. Ballachulish Bay has fair weather ⚓s at Kentallen B (deep), Onich and off St Brides on N shore. App bridge (17m clnce) on 114°; 4ca ENE of br are moorings and ⚓ at Poll an Dùnan, entered W of perch. Facilities at Ballachulish: Hotels, V, R, ✉, 🅑. Loch is navigable 7M to Kinlochleven.

CORRAN NARROWS, 56°43'.28N 05°14'.27W. AC 2372. Sp rate 6kn. Well buoyed; Corran Pt lt ho, Iso WRG 4s, and lt bn 5ca NE. ⚓ 5ca NW of Pt, off Camas Aiseig pier/slip.

FORT WILLIAM/CORPACH 10-8-14
Inverness 56°49'.00N 05°07'.00W (off Fort William)

CHARTS
AC 2372, 2380; Imray C65; OS 41
TIDES
–0535 Dover; ML 2·3; Duration 0610; Zone 0 (UT)

Standard Port OBAN (→)

Times				Height (metres)			
High Water		Low Water		MHWS	MHWN	MLWN	MLWS
0100	0700	0100	0800	4·0	2·9	1·8	0·7
1300	1900	1300	2000				
Differences CORPACH							
0000	+0020	+0040	0000	0·0	0·0	–0·2	–0·2
LOCH EIL (Head)							
+0025	+0045	+0105	+0025	No data		No data	
CORRAN NARROWS							
+0007	+0007	+0004	+0004	+0·4	+0·4	–0·1	0·0
LOCH LEVEN (Head)							
+0045	+0045	+0045	+0045	No data		No data	
LOCH LINNHE (Port Appin)							
–0005	–0005	–0030	0000	+0·2	+0·2	+0·1	+0·1
LOCH CRERAN (Barcaldine Pier)							
+0010	+0020	+0040	+0015	+0·1	+0·1	0·0	+0·1
LOCH CRERAN (Head)							
+0015	+0025	+0120	+0020	–0·3	–0·3	–0·4	–0·3

SHELTER
Exposed to winds SW thro' N to NE. ⚓s off Fort William pier; in Camus na Gall; SSW of Eilean A Bhealaidh; and off Corpach Basin, where there is also a waiting pontoon; or inside the canal. For Caledonian Canal see 10.8.15.
NAVIGATION
Corpach WPT 56°50'.30N 05°07'.00W, 135°/315° from/to lock ent, 0·30M. Beware McLean Rk, dries 0·3m, buoyed, 8ca N of Fort William. Lochy Flats dry 3ca off the E bank. In Annat Narrows at ent to Loch Eil streams reach 5kn.
LIGHTS AND MARKS
Iso WRG 4s lt is at N jetty of sea-lock ent, W310°-335°. A long pier/viaduct off Ft William is unlit.
RADIO TELEPHONE
Call: *Corpach Lock* VHF Ch 74 16 (during canal hours).
TELEPHONE (01397)
Hr Mr 772249 (Corpach); MRSC (01631) 563720; ⌗ (0141) 887 9369; Marinecall 0891 500463; Police 702361; Dr 703136.
FACILITIES
FORT WILLIAM. **Pier** ☎ 703881, AB; **Services:** Slip, L, CH, ACA. **Town** EC Wed; P, ME, El, Sh, YC, V, R, Bar, 🅗, ✉, 🅑, 🚂. CORPACH. **Corpach Basin** ☎ 772249, AB, L, FW; **Lochaber YC** ☎ 703576, M, FW, L, Slip; **Services:** ME, El, Sh, D (cans), M, CH, C, (18 ton), Slip, Divers. **Village** P, V, R, Bar, ✉, 🅑, 🚂.

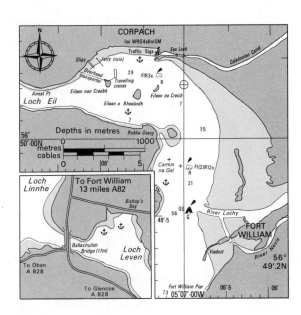

CALEDONIAN CANAL   10-8-15
Inverness

CHARTS
AC 1791; OS 41, 34, 26

TIDES
Tidal differences: Corpach –0455 on Dover; See 10.8.14.
Clachnaharry: +0116 on Dover; See 10.7.16.

SHELTER
Corpach is at the SW ent of the Caledonian Canal, which is available for vessels up to 45m LOA, 10m beam, 4m draft and max mast ht 27·4m. Access from HW–4 to HW+4 (sp); H24 (nps); the sea locks at both ends do not open LW±2 at springs. For best shelter transit the sea lock and lie above the double lock. Numerous pontoons along the canal; cost is included in the canal dues. For Inverness see 10.7.16.

NAVIGATION
The 60M canal consists of 38M through 3 lochs, (Lochs Lochy, Oich and Ness), connected by 22M through canals. Loch Oich is part of a hydro-electric scheme which may vary the water level. The passage normally takes two full days, possibly longer in the summer; absolute minimum is 14 hrs. Speed limit is 5kn in the canal sections. There are 10 swing bridges. Do not pass bridges at either end without the keeper's instructions.

LOCKS
There are 29 locks: 14 between Loch Linnhe (Corpach), through Lochs Lochy and Oich up to the summit (106′ above sea level); and 15 locks from the summit down through Loch Ness to Inverness. All locks are manned and operate early May to early Oct, 0800-1800LT daily. Contact canal office for reduced hrs in autumn, winter and spring; closed Christmas and New Year. Last lockings are 1 hr before close on main flights and ½ hr on other locks. Sea locks will open outside hrs for extra payment. Dues, payable at Corpach, at 1995 rates, inc VAT: £4.24 per metre for 1 day; £10.12 for 3 days, plus special offers. For regulations and a booklet *Skipper's Guide* apply to Canal Manager, Canal Office, Seaport Marina, Muirtown Wharf, Inverness IV3 5LS, ☎ (01463) 233140/Fax 710942.

LIGHTS & MARKS
See 10.8.14 and 10.7.16 for ent lts. Chan is marked by posts, cairns and unlit buoys, PHM on the NW side of the chan and SHM on the SE side.

RADIO TELEPHONE
Call all locks VHF Ch **74** during opening hours.

TELEPHONE
Corpach Sea Lock/Basin (01397) 772249; Canal Office, Inverness (01463) 233140; Clachnaharry Sea Lock (01463) 713896.

FACILITIES
For details see *Skipper's Guide* (using the maps).
– Corpach see 10.8.14.
– Banavie (Neptune's Staircase) AC, CH, V, ✉.
– Gairlochy AB, R.
– NE end of Loch Lochy V, M, AB, R.
– Oich Bridge D, AB, R.
– Invergarry V, L, FW, AB.
– Fort Augustus FW, P, L, ME, EI, AB, P, V, ✉, Dr, Bar.
– Dochgarroch FW, AC, P, V.
At Inverness (10.7.16):
– Caley Marina (25+25 visitors) ☎ (01463) 236539, (Muirtown top lock), FW, C (20 ton), ACA, CH, D, ME, EI, Sh, AC.
– Seaport Marina (20 + 20 visitors) ☎ (01463) 239475, D, EI, ME, Sh, FW, Gas, Gaz, ▣, C (40 ton), AC.

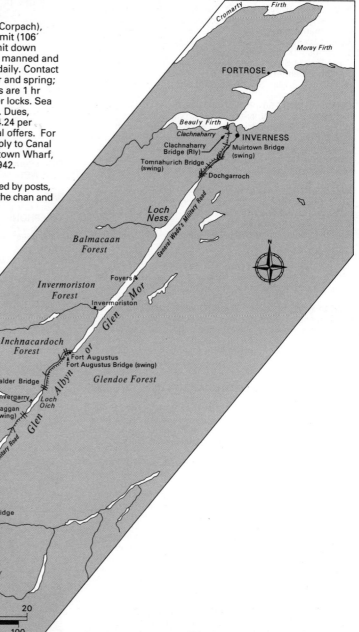

SCOTLAND – OBAN

LAT 56°25'N   LONG 5°29'W

TIMES AND HEIGHTS OF HIGH AND LOW WATERS

YEAR **1996**

TIME ZONE (UT)
For Summer Time add ONE hour in non-shaded areas

JANUARY

Day	Time / m	Time / m	Time / m	Time / m
1 M	0218 3.0	0850 1.7	1510 3.3	2103 1.7
2 TU	0311 3.2	0953 1.6	1552 3.4	2152 1.6
3 W	0354 3.4	1042 1.5	1628 3.5	2234 1.4
4 TH	0434 3.6	1122 1.4	1704 3.7	2313 1.3
5 F O	0513 3.8	1158 1.4	1740 3.8	2350 1.1
6 SA	0550 3.9	1231 1.4	1816 3.9	
7 SU	0027 1.1	0625 4.0	1305 1.4	1850 3.9
8 M	0104 1.1	0659 4.0	1338 1.4	1923 3.9
9 TU	0137 1.1	0731 3.9	1411 1.5	1953 3.8
10 W	0208 1.2	0801 3.8	1438 1.6	2023 3.6
11 TH	0238 1.3	0832 3.7	1502 1.7	2057 3.5
12 F	0314 1.4	0908 3.6	1538 1.8	2137 3.3
13 SA	0358 1.5	0952 3.5	1632 1.9	2228 3.2
14 SU	0455 1.6	1049 3.3	1746 1.9	2335 3.1
15 M	0604 1.7	1209 3.2	1906 1.8	
16 TU	0117 3.1	0721 1.6	1358 3.3	2021 1.6
17 W	0251 3.3	0837 1.4	1514 3.5	2127 1.4
18 TH	0350 3.6	0947 1.2	1610 3.7	2223 1.0
19 F	0438 3.9	1047 0.9	1657 3.9	2313 0.8
20 SA ●	0523 4.1	1140 0.7	1740 4.0	2359 0.5
21 SU	0606 4.3	1228 0.5	1822 4.1	
22 M	0045 0.4	0648 4.3	1314 0.5	1902 4.0
23 TU	0130 0.4	0729 4.3	1358 0.6	1942 3.9
24 W	0214 0.5	0810 4.1	1441 0.8	2020 3.7
25 TH	0257 0.7	0851 3.8	1524 1.0	2059 3.5
26 F	0342 1.0	0934 3.5	1609 1.3	2139 3.3
27 SA	0430 1.3	1022 3.3	1659 1.5	2226 3.0
28 SU	0524 1.6	1127 3.0	1756 1.7	2337 2.9
29 M	0630 1.6	1323 2.9	1901 1.8	
30 TU	0125 2.8	0810 1.9	1454 3.0	2016 1.8
31 W	0242 3.0	0942 1.8	1545 3.1	2126 1.7

FEBRUARY

Day	Time / m	Time / m	Time / m	Time / m
1 TH	0336 3.2	1034 1.6	1618 3.3	2217 1.5
2 F	0419 3.4	1113 1.5	1652 3.5	2257 1.3
3 SA	0458 3.6	1147 1.3	1727 3.7	2334 1.1
4 SU O	0536 3.8	1217 1.2	1802 3.9	
5 M	0009 1.0	0610 3.9	1247 1.2	1835 3.9
6 TU	0043 0.9	0642 4.0	1318 1.1	1905 3.9
7 W	0114 0.9	0711 4.0	1346 1.2	1931 3.8
8 TH	0142 0.9	0738 3.9	1408 1.2	1958 3.7
9 F	0211 1.0	0807 3.8	1431 1.3	2029 3.6
10 SA	0245 1.1	0841 3.7	1505 1.4	2107 3.5
11 SU	0328 1.2	0921 3.5	1552 1.6	2154 3.3
12 M	0422 1.4	1013 3.3	1659 1.7	2256 3.1
13 TU	0534 1.6	1129 3.1	1829 1.7	
14 W	0036 3.0	0659 1.6	1337 3.0	1954 1.6
15 TH	0238 3.2	0824 1.4	1515 3.2	2110 1.3
16 F	0343 3.5	0940 1.2	1611 3.5	2211 1.0
17 SA	0431 3.8	1040 0.9	1654 3.7	2302 0.7
18 SU ●	0514 4.1	1130 0.6	1732 3.9	2348 0.4
19 M	0554 4.3	1215 0.5	1809 3.9	
20 TU	0032 0.3	0633 4.3	1257 0.4	1845 4.0
21 W	0114 0.3	0710 4.3	1337 0.5	1921 4.0
22 TH	0155 0.4	0747 4.1	1415 0.7	1955 3.8
23 F	0234 0.6	0822 3.9	1453 0.9	2028 3.6
24 SA	0314 0.9	0858 3.6	1534 1.2	2101 3.4
25 SU	0355 1.2	0937 3.2	1619 1.4	2140 3.2
26 M	0443 1.6	1025 3.0	1712 1.7	2230 2.9
27 TU	0542 1.8	1150 2.7	1815 1.8	
28 W	0009 2.8	0706 2.0	1429 2.8	1928 1.8
29 TH	0213 2.9	0928 1.9	1528 2.9	2052 1.7

MARCH

Day	Time / m	Time / m	Time / m	Time / m
1 F	0318 3.0	1019 1.7	1602 3.2	2152 1.5
2 SA	0400 3.3	1055 1.5	1633 3.4	2235 1.2
3 SU	0438 3.5	1126 1.3	1707 3.6	2311 1.0
4 M	0515 3.7	1154 1.1	1741 3.8	2344 0.8
5 TU O	0549 3.9	1222 1.0	1813 3.9	
6 W	0016 0.7	0620 4.0	1250 0.9	1840 3.9
7 TH	0047 0.7	0647 4.0	1317 0.9	1905 3.9
8 F	0117 0.7	0714 3.9	1341 0.9	1933 3.8
9 SA	0149 0.7	0744 3.8	1409 1.0	2006 3.7
10 SU	0225 0.8	0819 3.7	1445 1.1	2045 3.5
11 M	0309 1.0	0900 3.4	1532 1.3	2132 3.3
12 TU	0405 1.3	0952 3.2	1638 1.5	2236 3.1
13 W	0521 1.5	1110 2.9	1807 1.6	
14 TH	0020 3.0	0648 1.5	1338 2.9	1934 1.5
15 F	0225 3.2	0816 1.4	1510 3.1	2054 1.3
16 SA	0328 3.5	0931 1.1	1603 3.3	2156 1.0
17 SU	0416 3.8	1027 0.8	1642 3.6	2246 0.7
18 M	0458 4.0	1113 0.6	1716 3.8	2331 0.4
19 TU ●	0536 4.2	1155 0.5	1750 4.0	
20 W	0014 0.3	0612 4.2	1235 0.4	1823 4.0
21 TH	0055 0.3	0647 4.2	1312 0.5	1857 4.0
22 F	0133 0.5	0721 4.0	1347 0.6	1929 3.9
23 SA	0211 0.7	0754 3.8	1423 0.9	2000 3.7
24 SU	0247 1.0	0827 3.5	1502 1.1	2032 3.5
25 M	0326 1.3	0903 3.3	1545 1.4	2109 3.3
26 TU	0411 1.6	0946 3.0	1636 1.6	2155 3.0
27 W	0508 1.9	1050 2.7	1736 1.8	2304 2.8
28 TH	0624 2.0	1345 2.7	1845 1.8	
29 F	0124 2.8	0856 1.9	1452 2.8	2002 1.7
30 SA	0247 3.0	0950 1.7	1532 3.0	2111 1.5
31 SU	0332 3.2	1024 1.5	1606 3.3	2159 1.3

APRIL

Day	Time / m	Time / m	Time / m	Time / m
1 M	0410 3.4	1053 1.2	1639 3.5	2237 1.0
2 TU	0446 3.7	1121 1.0	1713 3.7	2312 0.8
3 W	0521 3.8	1149 0.9	1745 3.8	2345 0.7
4 TH O	0553 3.9	1218 0.7	1812 3.9	
5 F	0019 0.5	0621 4.0	1247 0.7	1839 3.9
6 SA	0055 0.5	0652 3.9	1318 0.7	1911 3.9
7 SU	0133 0.6	0726 3.8	1354 0.8	1948 3.8
8 M	0215 0.7	0805 3.6	1435 0.9	2031 3.6
9 TU	0303 0.9	0850 3.4	1526 1.1	2122 3.4
10 W	0403 1.1	0945 3.1	1631 1.3	2228 3.1
11 TH	0517 1.3	1105 2.8	1751 1.4	
12 F	0013 3.0	0638 1.4	1327 2.8	1913 1.4
13 SA	0203 3.2	0803 1.3	1450 3.0	2032 1.2
14 SU	0306 3.4	0914 1.1	1543 3.2	2135 1.0
15 M	0354 3.7	1007 0.9	1621 3.5	2226 0.7
16 TU	0436 3.9	1051 0.7	1653 3.7	2311 0.6
17 W ●	0513 4.0	1131 0.6	1726 3.8	2353 0.5
18 TH	0549 4.1	1208 0.6	1800 3.9	
19 F	0033 0.6	0623 4.0	1245 0.6	1832 3.9
20 SA	0112 0.7	0656 3.9	1320 0.7	1904 3.9
21 SU	0148 0.9	0729 3.7	1356 0.9	1936 3.8
22 M	0224 1.1	0803 3.5	1434 1.1	2010 3.6
23 TU	0302 1.4	0840 3.3	1516 1.3	2048 3.4
24 W	0346 1.7	0922 3.1	1604 1.5	2131 3.2
25 TH	0440 1.9	1016 2.8	1659 1.7	2228 3.0
26 F	0548 2.0	1200 2.7	1800 1.8	2359 2.9
27 SA	0719 2.0	1400 2.8	1906 1.8	
28 SU	0147 2.9	0850 1.8	1450 3.0	2011 1.4
29 M	0248 3.1	0935 1.6	1530 3.2	2107 1.4
30 TU	0332 3.4	1010 1.3	1606 3.4	2153 1.1

Chart Datum: 2·10 metres below Ordnance Datum (Newlyn)

SCOTLAND – OBAN

LAT 56°25′N   LONG 5°29′W

TIMES AND HEIGHTS OF HIGH AND LOW WATERS

YEAR 1996

TIME ZONE (UT)
For Summer Time add ONE hour in non-shaded areas

Chart Datum: 2·10 metres below Ordnance Datum (Newlyn)

MAY

Day	Time	m	Time	m	Time	m	Time	m
1 W	0412	3.6	1042	1.1	1641	3.6	2234	0.9
2 TH	0449	3.8	1113	0.9	1714	3.8	2313	0.7
3 F O	0524	3.9	1146	0.7	1745	3.9	2354	0.5
4 SA	0558	3.9	1221	0.6	1819	3.9		
5 SU	0036	0.5	0634	3.9	1300	0.6	1856	3.9
6 M	0121	0.5	0713	3.8	1342	0.6	1937	3.8
7 TU	0208	0.6	0757	3.6	1429	0.7	2024	3.7
8 W	0301	0.8	0845	3.3	1521	0.9	2117	3.5
9 TH	0400	1.0	0943	3.1	1622	1.1	2222	3.3
10 F	0507	1.2	1058	2.9	1732	1.3	2355	3.1
11 SA	0622	1.3	1254	2.8	1848	1.3		
12 SU	0132	3.2	0739	1.3	1418	2.9	2004	1.2
13 M	0238	3.3	0848	1.2	1513	3.1	2110	1.1
14 TU	0329	3.5	0942	1.1	1553	3.3	2204	1.0
15 W	0412	3.6	1026	1.0	1627	3.5	2250	0.9
16 TH	0451	3.8	1105	0.9	1702	3.7	2333	0.8
17 F ●	0527	3.8	1142	0.8	1736	3.8		
18 SA	0013	0.9	0601	3.8	1219	0.8	1810	3.9
19 SU	0051	1.0	0635	3.8	1256	0.9	1844	3.9
20 M	0128	1.1	0710	3.7	1333	1.0	1918	3.9
21 TU	0205	1.3	0746	3.6	1411	1.1	1954	3.7
22 W	0243	1.5	0823	3.4	1451	1.3	2031	3.5
23 TH	0324	1.7	0904	3.2	1533	1.5	2111	3.3
24 F	0412	1.8	0950	3.0	1620	1.6	2157	3.2
25 SA	0509	1.9	1051	2.9	1713	1.7	2255	3.1
26 SU	0615	2.0	1225	2.8	1810	1.7		
27 M	0015	3.0	0726	1.9	1352	2.9	1910	1.7
28 TU	0143	3.1	0829	1.7	1445	3.1	2009	1.5
29 W	0245	3.3	0919	1.5	1528	3.3	2105	1.3
30 TH	0334	3.5	1001	1.2	1608	3.5	2157	1.0
31 F	0418	3.7	1040	1.0	1646	3.7	2246	0.8

JUNE

Day	Time	m	Time	m	Time	m	Time	m
1 SA O	0500	3.8	1120	0.7	1725	3.9	2334	0.6
2 SU	0541	3.9	1201	0.6	1805	4.0		
3 M	0022	0.5	0622	3.9	1245	0.5	1846	4.0
4 TU	0111	0.5	0706	3.8	1331	0.5	1931	4.0
5 W	0201	0.5	0751	3.7	1420	0.6	2019	3.8
6 TH	0254	0.7	0840	3.4	1511	0.7	2110	3.6
7 F	0349	0.9	0934	3.2	1607	0.9	2210	3.4
8 SA	0449	1.1	1039	3.0	1709	1.1	2325	3.2
9 SU	0555	1.3	1206	2.9	1816	1.3		
10 M	0053	3.2	0704	1.4	1331	2.9	1929	1.3
11 TU	0206	3.2	0813	1.4	1435	3.0	2041	1.3
12 W	0304	3.3	0912	1.3	1522	3.2	2142	1.3
13 TH	0351	3.4	1000	1.2	1607	3.4	2233	1.2
14 F	0432	3.5	1042	1.1	1639	3.5	2317	1.2
15 SA	0509	3.6	1120	1.0	1717	3.7	2357	1.1
16 SU ●	0545	3.7	1157	1.0	1753	3.8		
17 M	0034	1.2	0620	3.7	1235	1.0	1828	3.8
18 TU	0111	1.2	0656	3.7	1313	1.0	1903	3.8
19 W	0148	1.3	0732	3.6	1350	1.1	1939	3.8
20 TH	0224	1.4	0808	3.5	1426	1.2	2014	3.7
21 F	0302	1.6	0844	3.4	1502	1.4	2049	3.5
22 SA	0340	1.7	0921	3.2	1540	1.5	2126	3.4
23 SU	0422	1.8	1004	3.1	1624	1.6	2210	3.3
24 M	0515	1.9	1058	3.0	1717	1.7	2305	3.2
25 TU	0619	1.9	1212	2.9	1817	1.7		
26 W	0019	3.1	0725	1.9	1346	3.0	1921	1.6
27 TH	0151	3.2	0829	1.6	1451	3.2	2026	1.4
28 F	0301	3.4	0925	1.3	1542	3.4	2129	1.2
29 SA	0356	3.6	1015	1.0	1628	3.7	2227	0.9
30 SU	0444	3.7	1102	0.8	1712	3.9	2321	0.7

JULY

Day	Time	m	Time	m	Time	m	Time	m
1 M O	0530	3.9	1148	0.5	1756	4.1		
2 TU	0013	0.5	0614	3.9	1235	0.4	1840	4.1
3 W	0103	0.4	0658	3.9	1321	0.4	1924	4.1
4 TH	0152	0.4	0742	3.8	1408	0.4	2010	4.0
5 F	0241	0.6	0828	3.6	1456	0.6	2057	3.8
6 SA	0331	0.8	0915	3.4	1547	0.8	2148	3.5
7 SU	0423	1.0	1008	3.1	1641	1.0	2246	3.3
8 M	0520	1.3	1113	2.9	1741	1.3		
9 TU	0004	3.1	0621	1.4	1237	2.9	1848	1.5
10 W	0130	3.0	0730	1.5	1353	2.9	2008	1.6
11 TH	0242	3.0	0838	1.5	1454	3.0	2125	1.5
12 F	0337	3.1	0936	1.4	1541	3.2	2222	1.5
13 SA	0418	3.3	1022	1.3	1622	3.4	2307	1.4
14 SU	0455	3.5	1102	1.2	1701	3.6	2346	1.3
15 M ●	0531	3.6	1140	1.0	1738	3.7		
16 TU	0021	1.2	0607	3.7	1217	1.0	1814	3.8
17 W	0055	1.2	0642	3.8	1253	1.0	1849	3.9
18 TH	0129	1.2	0716	3.8	1328	1.0	1922	3.9
19 F	0203	1.3	0749	3.7	1400	1.1	1953	3.8
20 SA	0235	1.4	0819	3.6	1431	1.2	2023	3.7
21 SU	0303	1.5	0850	3.4	1503	1.3	2055	3.6
22 M	0330	1.6	0925	3.3	1542	1.4	2133	3.4
23 TU	0413	1.7	1010	3.1	1631	1.5	2220	3.3
24 W	0517	1.8	1109	3.0	1733	1.6	2324	3.1
25 TH	0635	1.8	1239	3.0	1846	1.6		
26 F	0102	3.1	0751	1.6	1426	3.1	2000	1.5
27 SA	0242	3.2	0900	1.4	1530	3.4	2113	1.3
28 SU	0347	3.4	1000	1.1	1620	3.7	2218	1.0
29 M	0437	3.7	1051	0.8	1705	4.0	2314	0.7
30 TU O	0523	3.8	1138	0.5	1748	4.2		
31 W	0004	0.5	0605	3.9	1224	0.3	1830	4.3

AUGUST

Day	Time	m	Time	m	Time	m	Time	m
1 TH	0052	0.4	0646	4.0	1309	0.2	1912	4.3
2 F	0137	0.4	0727	3.9	1353	0.3	1953	4.1
3 SA	0221	0.5	0807	3.7	1438	0.5	2035	3.9
4 SU	0306	0.7	0848	3.5	1523	0.7	2118	3.6
5 M	0352	1.0	0930	3.3	1611	1.0	2204	3.3
6 TU	0441	1.3	1019	3.0	1704	1.4	2304	3.0
7 W	0538	1.5	1131	2.8	1806	1.6		
8 TH	0045	2.8	0642	1.7	1313	2.8	1929	1.8
9 F	0225	2.9	0758	1.7	1432	2.9	2115	1.8
10 SA	0332	3.0	0912	1.6	1526	3.1	2215	1.6
11 SU	0408	3.2	1004	1.4	1607	3.3	2257	1.5
12 M	0440	3.4	1046	1.2	1644	3.6	2332	1.3
13 TU	0514	3.6	1123	1.0	1721	3.8		
14 W ●	0004	1.2	0549	3.8	1158	0.9	1756	3.9
15 TH	0034	1.1	0623	3.8	1232	0.9	1830	4.0
16 F	0105	1.1	0655	3.9	1304	0.9	1900	4.0
17 SA	0136	1.1	0723	3.8	1333	0.9	1928	3.9
18 SU	0204	1.2	0749	3.7	1400	1.0	1955	3.8
19 M	0226	1.3	0818	3.6	1431	1.1	2025	3.7
20 TU	0252	1.4	0852	3.4	1509	1.3	2100	3.5
21 W	0332	1.5	0935	3.3	1558	1.5	2145	3.3
22 TH	0432	1.7	1032	3.1	1703	1.6	2248	3.1
23 F	0559	1.7	1202	3.0	1825	1.7		
24 SA	0037	3.0	0726	1.7	1420	3.1	1948	1.6
25 SU	0243	3.1	0844	1.4	1523	3.4	2107	1.3
26 M	0347	3.4	0947	1.1	1612	3.8	2211	1.0
27 TU	0433	3.6	1039	0.7	1654	4.1	2304	0.7
28 W	0512	3.8	1126	0.5	1734	4.3	2350	0.5
29 TH	0550	4.0	1210	0.3	1813	4.4		
30 F	0034	0.3	0627	4.0	1253	0.2	1851	4.4
31 SA	0116	0.4	0704	4.0	1335	0.3	1929	4.2

SCOTLAND – OBAN

LAT 56°25′N   LONG 5°29′W

TIMES AND HEIGHTS OF HIGH AND LOW WATERS   YEAR 1996

TIME ZONE (UT)
For Summer Time add ONE hour in non-shaded areas

SEPTEMBER

Day	Time / m	Day	Time / m
1 SU	0156 0.5; 0741 3.9; 1416 0.5; 2006 4.0	16 M	0132 1.0; 0728 3.8; 1334 0.9; 1928 3.9
2 M	0236 0.7; 0816 3.7; 1458 0.8; 2043 3.7	17 TU	0156 1.1; 0750 3.7; 1407 1.0; 1959 3.7
3 TU	0318 1.0; 0852 3.4; 1541 1.1; 2123 3.3	18 W	0227 1.2; 0826 3.6; 1447 1.2; 2036 3.5
4 W	0404 1.3; 0933 3.2; 1630 1.5; 2210 3.0	19 TH	0308 1.4; 0910 3.4; 1538 1.4; 2122 3.3
5 TH	0457 1.6; 1027 2.9; 1728 1.8; 2330 2.8	20 F	0407 1.6; 1009 3.2; 1648 1.6; 2227 3.0
6 F	0600 1.7; 1221 2.8; 1850 2.0	21 SA	0536 1.7; 1146 3.0; 1815 1.7
7 SA	0206 2.8; 0715 1.8; 1416 2.9; 2105 1.9	22 SU	0031 2.9; 0705 1.6; 1408 3.2; 1941 1.6
8 SU	0314 2.9; 0840 1.7; 1513 3.1; 2200 1.7	23 M	0241 3.1; 0826 1.4; 1508 3.5; 2059 1.3
9 M	0350 3.1; 0940 1.5; 1549 3.3; 2238 1.5	24 TU	0338 3.3; 0930 1.1; 1556 3.8; 2159 1.0
10 TU	0419 3.4; 1023 1.2; 1624 3.6; 2310 1.3	25 W	0420 3.6; 1022 0.8; 1636 4.1; 2247 0.7
11 W	0451 3.6; 1059 1.1; 1659 3.8; 2339 1.2	26 TH	0456 3.8; 1108 0.5; 1714 4.3; 2330 0.5
12 TH ●	0525 3.8; 1133 0.9; 1733 3.9	27 F ○	0530 4.0; 1151 0.4; 1751 4.4
13 F	0007 1.0; 0558 3.9; 1205 0.8; 1805 4.0	28 SA	0011 0.5; 0604 4.1; 1233 0.4; 1827 4.4
14 SA	0036 1.0; 0629 3.9; 1236 0.8; 1834 4.0	29 SU	0050 0.5; 0639 4.1; 1314 0.5; 1902 4.2
15 SU	0106 0.9; 0654 3.9; 1305 0.8; 1900 4.0	30 M	0128 0.6; 0713 4.0; 1353 0.7; 1936 4.0

OCTOBER

Day	Time / m	Day	Time / m
1 TU	0206 0.8; 0747 3.8; 1432 1.0; 2011 3.7	16 W	0135 0.9; 0728 3.9; 1352 1.0; 1941 3.8
2 W	0246 1.1; 0821 3.6; 1513 1.3; 2048 3.4	17 TH	0212 1.1; 0808 3.7; 1436 1.2; 2022 3.6
3 TH	0330 1.3; 0859 3.4; 1600 1.7; 2130 3.1	18 F	0258 1.3; 0856 3.5; 1532 1.4; 2111 3.3
4 F	0421 1.6; 0947 3.1; 1657 1.9; 2231 2.8	19 SA	0358 1.4; 0957 3.3; 1643 1.6; 2220 3.0
5 SA	0521 1.8; 1106 2.9; 1814 2.1	20 SU	0517 1.6; 1134 3.2; 1805 1.6
6 SU	0130 2.8; 0631 1.9; 1346 2.9; 2037 2.0	21 M	0022 2.9; 0641 1.6; 1344 3.3; 1928 1.6
7 M	0238 2.9; 0752 1.8; 1447 3.1; 2134 1.8	22 TU	0222 3.0; 0802 1.4; 1445 3.6; 2042 1.3
8 TU	0319 3.1; 0902 1.6; 1523 3.3; 2209 1.6	23 W	0318 3.3; 0908 1.2; 1534 3.8; 2139 1.1
9 W	0351 3.4; 0949 1.4; 1556 3.6; 2239 1.4	24 TH	0400 3.6; 0930 0.9; 1615 4.1; 2226 0.9
10 TH	0424 3.6; 1027 1.2; 1652 3.8; 2307 1.2	25 F	0433 3.8; 1048 0.7; 1652 4.2; 2307 0.7
11 F	0457 3.8; 1101 1.0; 1705 4.0; 2335 1.0	26 SA ○	0506 4.0; 1131 0.6; 1728 4.3; 2346 0.7
12 SA ●	0530 3.9; 1133 0.9; 1737 4.1	27 SU	0541 4.1; 1213 0.6; 1803 4.2
13 SU	0004 0.9; 0559 4.0; 1206 0.8; 1806 4.1	28 M	0024 0.7; 0615 4.1; 1253 0.8; 1836 4.1
14 M	0034 0.9; 0626 4.0; 1239 0.8; 1834 4.1	29 TU	0101 0.9; 0649 4.1; 1332 1.0; 1910 4.0
15 TU	0103 0.9; 0654 3.9; 1313 0.9; 1905 4.0	30 W	0139 0.9; 0722 3.9; 1410 1.2; 1945 3.7
		31 TH	0218 1.1; 0757 3.8; 1449 1.5; 2022 3.5

NOVEMBER

Day	Time / m	Day	Time / m
1 F	0301 1.4; 0835 3.6; 1534 1.8; 2103 3.2	16 SA	0251 1.1; 0848 3.7; 1528 1.3; 2106 3.3
2 SA	0349 1.6; 0920 3.3; 1628 2.0; 2155 3.0	17 SU	0348 1.3; 0948 3.5; 1633 1.4; 2210 3.1
3 SU	0444 1.8; 1019 3.1; 1735 2.2; 2325 2.9	18 M	0457 1.5; 1111 3.3; 1745 1.5; 2342 2.9
4 M	0546 1.9; 1158 3.0; 1911 2.2	19 TU	0613 1.5; 1307 3.4; 1903 1.5
5 TU	0148 2.9; 0654 1.9; 1358 3.1; 2044 2.0	20 W	0143 3.0; 0730 1.4; 1416 3.5; 2014 1.4
6 W	0239 3.1; 0803 1.8; 1445 3.3; 2127 1.8	21 TH	0249 3.2; 0841 1.3; 1510 3.7; 2113 1.3
7 TH	0317 3.3; 0901 1.6; 1523 3.5; 2200 1.6	22 F	0333 3.4; 0939 1.1; 1553 3.9; 2201 1.1
8 F	0353 3.5; 0945 1.4; 1559 3.7; 2230 1.3	23 SA	0409 3.6; 1029 1.0; 1632 4.0; 2243 1.0
9 SA	0427 3.7; 1024 1.2; 1634 3.9; 2300 1.1	24 SU	0443 3.8; 1113 1.0; 1708 4.1; 2322 0.9
10 SU	0501 3.9; 1100 1.0; 1708 4.0; 2331 1.0	25 M ○	0519 4.0; 1155 1.0; 1743 4.1
11 M ●	0532 4.0; 1138 0.9; 1741 4.1	26 TU	0000 0.9; 0554 4.1; 1235 1.0; 1817 4.0
12 TU	0004 0.9; 0603 4.0; 1217 0.8; 1813 4.1	27 W	0038 0.9; 0629 4.1; 1314 1.2; 1851 3.9
13 W	0040 0.8; 0636 4.0; 1258 0.8; 1849 4.0	28 TH	0116 1.0; 0704 4.0; 1351 1.4; 1927 3.8
14 TH	0119 0.7; 0715 4.0; 1342 0.9; 1929 3.8	29 F	0155 1.2; 0740 3.9; 1430 1.6; 2004 3.6
15 F	0202 0.9; 0758 3.9; 1431 1.1; 2014 3.6	30 SA	0235 1.3; 0817 3.7; 1511 1.8; 2043 3.4

DECEMBER

Day	Time / m	Day	Time / m
1 SU	0318 1.5; 0857 3.6; 1557 2.0; 2127 3.2	16 M	0334 1.0; 0935 3.7; 1614 1.2; 2151 3.2
2 M	0405 1.7; 0943 3.4; 1652 2.1; 2222 3.1	17 TU	0434 1.2; 1041 3.5; 1717 1.4; 2300 3.1
3 TU	0458 1.9; 1041 3.2; 1757 2.2; 2346 3.0	18 W	0540 1.4; 1216 3.3; 1825 1.5
4 W	0555 1.9; 1204 3.2; 1911 2.1	19 TH	0037 3.0; 0653 1.5; 1341 3.4; 1936 1.6
5 TH	0133 3.0; 0656 1.9; 1339 3.2; 2018 2.0	20 F	0202 3.1; 0809 1.5; 1445 3.4; 2042 1.5
6 F	0233 3.2; 0757 1.8; 1439 3.4; 2108 1.8	21 SA	0301 3.2; 0918 1.4; 1536 3.5; 2136 1.4
7 SA	0317 3.4; 0853 1.6; 1524 3.6; 2149 1.5	22 SU	0345 3.4; 1013 1.3; 1618 3.7; 2222 1.3
8 SU	0356 3.6; 0944 1.4; 1605 3.8; 2226 1.3	23 M	0424 3.6; 1101 1.2; 1654 3.8; 2302 1.2
9 M	0434 3.8; 1030 1.1; 1644 3.9; 2303 1.0	24 TU ○	0502 3.8; 1143 1.2; 1730 3.9; 2341 1.1
10 TU ●	0510 3.9; 1115 0.9; 1722 4.0; 2342 0.8	25 W	0539 3.9; 1222 1.2; 1804 3.9
11 W	0547 4.1; 1200 0.8; 1800 4.1	26 TH	0019 1.0; 0614 4.0; 1300 1.3; 1838 3.9
12 TH	0023 0.7; 0626 4.1; 1247 0.7; 1840 4.0	27 F	0058 1.0; 0650 4.0; 1336 1.4; 1913 3.9
13 F	0106 0.7; 0707 4.1; 1334 0.8; 1922 3.9	28 SA	0135 1.1; 0725 4.0; 1411 1.5; 1948 3.8
14 SA	0152 0.7; 0751 4.0; 1424 0.9; 2007 3.7	29 SU	0212 1.2; 0800 3.9; 1447 1.6; 2024 3.6
15 SU	0241 0.8; 0840 3.9; 1516 1.0; 2056 3.5	30 M	0249 1.4; 0834 3.7; 1525 1.8; 2100 3.5
		31 TU	0327 1.6; 0910 3.6; 1605 1.9; 2139 3.3

8

Chart Datum: 2·10 metres below Ordnance Datum (Newlyn)

OBAN   10-8-16

Argyll 56°25′·00N 05°29′·00W

CHARTS
AC 1790, 2387, 2171; Imray C65; OS 49

TIDES
–0530 Dover; ML 2·4; Duration 0610; Zone 0 (UT)

Standard Port OBAN (←—)

Times				Height (metres)			
High Water		Low Water		MHWS	MHWN	MLWN	MLWS
0100	0700	0100	0800	4·0	2·9	1·8	0·7
1300	1900	1300	2000				
Differences DUNSTAFFNAGE BAY							
+0005	0000	0000	+0005	+0·1	+0·1	+0·1	+0·1
CONNEL							
+0020	+0005	+0010	+0015	–0·3	–0·2	–0·1	+0·1
BONAWE							
+0150	+0205	+0240	+0210	–2·0	–1·7	–1·3	–0·5

Oban is a Standard Port and tidal predictions for each day
of the year are given above.

SHELTER
Good except in strong SW/NW winds. See chartlet for ⚓s.
⚓s off town, but water is deep; or at Ardantrive (also 20
⚓s, some pontoon berths and Water Taxi 0800-2300). ⚓ or
M off Brandystone and in Kerrera Sound at: Horseshoe B,
Gallanachbeg (rk dries 0·3m) and Little Horseshoe B.
Dunstaffnage Bay, 3M NE: see next column. 37 ⚓s and
landing pontoon are approved in bay 8ca to E.

NAVIGATION
WPT 56°25′·80N 05°30′·00W, 306°/126° from/to Dunollie
lt, 0·71M. Beware Sgeir Rathaid, buoyed, in middle of the
bay; also CalMacBrayne's ferries run from Railway Quay.

LIGHTS AND MARKS
N Spit of Kerrera Fl R 3s 9m 5M, W col, R bands. Dunollie
Fl (2) WRG 6s 7m 5/4M; G351°-009°, W009°-047°, R047°-
120°, W120°-138°, G138°-143°. N Pier 2FG (vert). S Quay
2FG (vert). Northern Lights Wharf Oc G 6s.

RADIO TELEPHONE
Call *Oban Yachts* Ch 80. Call *North Pier* Ch 12 16 (0900-1700).
For Railway Quay, call *CalMac* Ch 16 06 12.

TELEPHONE (01631)
Pier 562892; Marinecall 0891 500 463; ⌗ (0141) 8879369;
MRSC 563720; Police 562213; Dr 563175.

FACILITIES
N Pier ☎ 562892, L, FW, C (15 ton mobile) via Piermaster;
Rly Quay, L, Slip, D, FW, CH;
Services: BY, Slip, ACA, Gas, ME, El, divers;
Oban Yachts (Ardantrive B) ☎ 565333, Fax 565888, AB
£10, M, D, FW, ME, Sh, C, CH, Slip, BH (16 ton), Gas.
Town EC Thurs; P, V, R, Bar, ✉, ⑧, ▣, ⇌, ✈.

ADJACENT ANCHORAGES/HAVEN

DUNSTAFFNAGE BAY, Argyll, 56°27′·05N 05°25′·90W. AC
2378, 2387. HW –0530 on Dover; differences, see 10.8.16.
Good shelter at pontoons on SE side of bay entered 'twixt
Rubha Garbh and Eilean Mór; little room to ⚓, but 7 Y ⚓s
available. No navigational hazards; W and SW sides of bay
dry. Private pier on NW side has 2 FG (vert) 4m 2M.
Dunstaffnage Yacht Haven ☎ (01631) 566555, Fax 565620,
AB, FW, Slip, BH (10 ton), SM, R, Bar; **Alba Yachts** ☎ 565630,
VHF Ch M call *Alba*, ME, El, Sh, CH, Gas. Facilities: P & D
(cans, ¾M), V (½M), Bus, ⇌ Oban (2M) & Connel (airstrip).
LOCH ETIVE, AC 2378 to Bonawe, thence 5076. Connel Br,
15m clrnce, and Falls of Lora can be physical and tidal
barriers. HT cables at Bonawe have 13m clrnce. See SDs.

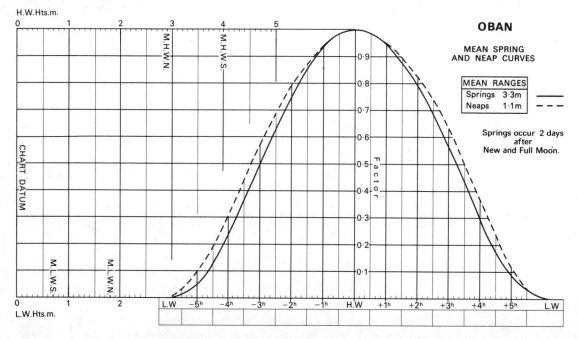

Dunstaffnage Yacht Haven

Depths in metres

LOCH FEOCHAN, Argyll, 56°21′·40N 05°29′·70W. AC 2387.
HW = HW Oban; flood runs 4 hrs, ebb for 8 hrs. Caution:
strong streams off Ardentallan Pt. Good shelter, 5M S of
Oban and 1·5M SE of Kerrera. Best appr at local slack LW
= LW Oban +0200. Narrow chan marked by 3 PHM buoys,
2 PHM perches onshore and 5 SHM buoys. ⚓ off pier, or
moor/berth at **Ardoran Marine** ☎ (01631) 566123, Fax
566611 AB, M, D, FW, ME, Gas, Sh, Slip, CH, Showers, V.
Royal Highland YC, Ardentallan Ho ☎ (01631) 563309.

OBAN

MEAN SPRING
AND NEAP CURVES

MEAN RANGES	
Springs	3·3m
Neaps	1·1m

Springs occur 2 days
after
New and Full Moon.

H.W.Hts.m.

CHART DATUM

M.H.W.N. M.H.W.S.

Factor

M.L.W.S. M.L.W.N.

L.W.Hts.m.

L.W. –5h –4h –3h –2h –1h H.W. +1h +2h +3h +4h +5h L.W.

OBAN *continued*

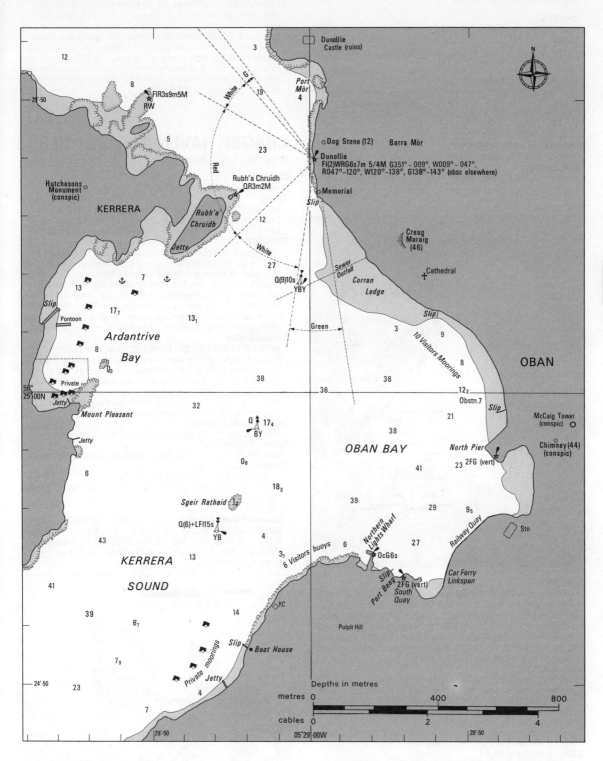

PUILLADOBHRAIN, Argyll, 56°19'·48N 05°35'·15W. AC 2386/2387. Tides as Oban. A popular ⚓ on the SE shore of the Firth of Lorne, approx 7M S of Oban, sheltered by the islets to the W of it. At N end of Ardencaple Bay identify Eilean Dùin (18m) and steer SE keeping 1½ca off to clear a rk awash at its NE tip. Continue for 4ca between Eilean nam Beathach, with Orange drum on N tip, and Dun Horses rks drying 2·7m. Two W cairns on E side of Eilean nam Freumha lead approx 215° into the inner ⚓ in about 4m. Landing at head of inlet. Nearest facilities: Bar, P at Clachan Br (½M); ☎, ✉ at Clachan Seil.

CUAN SOUND, Argyll, 56°15'·85N 05°37'·40W. AC 2326, 2386. Tides see 10.8.17 Seil Sound. Streams run up to 6kn at sp; N-going starts at Oban +0420, S-going at Oban −0200. The Sound is a useful doglegged short cut from Firth of Lorne to Lochs Melfort and Shuna, but demands care due to rks and tides. There are ⚓s at either end to await the tide. At the 90° dogleg, pass close N of Cleit Rk onto which the tide sets; it is marked by a Y △ perch. The chan is only ¾ca wide here due to rks off Seil. Overhead cables (35m) cross from Seil to Luing. There are ⚓s clear of the tide to the S of Cleit Rk. No lts/facilities. CCC SDs are recommended.

LOCH MELFORT   10-8-17

Argyll 56°14'·60N 05°34'·00W

CHARTS
AC *2326, 2169*; Imray C65; OS 55

TIDES
Loch Shuna –0615 Dover; ML Loch Melfort 1·7; Duration Seil Sound 0615; Zone 0 (UT)

Standard Port OBAN (←—)

Times				Height (metres)			
High Water		Low Water		MHWS	MHWN	MLWN	MLWS
0100	0700	0100	0800	4·0	2·9	1·8	0·7
1300	1900	1300	2000				
Differences LOCH MELFORT							
–0055	–0025	–0040	–0035	–1·2	–0·8	–0·5	–0·1
SEIL SOUND							
–0035	–0015	–0040	–0015	–1·3	–0·9	–0·7	–0·3

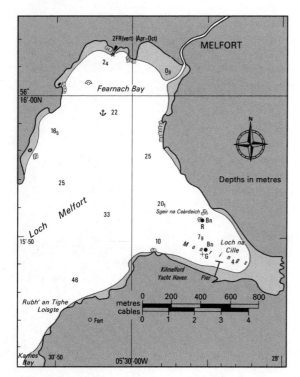

MELFORT

Depths in metres

Loch Melfort

SHELTER
Good at Kilmelford Yacht Haven in Loch na Cille; access H24 for 3m draft. Or at Melfort Pier (Fearnach Bay at N end of loch): pier/pontoons in 2m, but chan to inner hbr has only 1m; good ⚓ in N winds. ⚓s sheltered from S – W at: a bay with moorings ½M inside the ent on S shore, but beware rk drying 1·5m; in Kames Bay (1·5M further E) clear of moorings, rks and fish farm.

NAVIGATION
WPT 56°14'·00N 05°35'·00W, 210°/030° from/to summit Eilean Gamhna, 4ca. Pass either side of Eilean Gamhna. 8ca NE lies Campbell Rk (1·8m). A rk drying 1m lies 1½ca ESE of the FS on Eilean Coltair. The S side of L Melfort is mostly steep-to, except in Kames Bay. At Loch na Cille, beware drying reef ¾ca off NE shore (PHM perch), and rk near S shore (SHM perch); boats may obscure perches.

LIGHTS AND MARKS
2FR (vert) 6m 3M on Melfort pier; also depth gauge.

RADIO TELEPHONE
Kilmelford VHF Ch **80** M (HO). *Melfort Pier* Ch 12 16.

TELEPHONE (01852)
MRSC (01631) 563720; ✠ (0141) 887 9369; Police (01631) 562213; Marinecall 0891 500463; Ⓗ (01546) 602323.

FACILITIES
Kilmelford Yacht Haven ☎ 200248, £9.90, M, D, FW, BH (12 ton), Slip, ME, El, Sh, Gas; **Melfort Pier** ☎ 200333, Fax 200329, AB £10.50, M, D, P, AC, Gas, FW, ME, SM, Sh, Slip, R, Bar, ▣. **Village** (¾M) V, Bar, ✉.

ADJACENT ANCHORAGE

ARDINAMAR, Luing/Torsa, 56°14'·93N 05°36'·97W. AC *2326*. HW –0555 on Dover; ML 1·7m; see 10.8.17 SEIL SOUND. A small cove and popular ⚓ between Luing and Torsa, close W of ent to L. Melfort. Appr with conspic W paint mark inside cove on brg 290°. Narrow, shallow (approx 1m CD) ent has drying rks either side, those to N marked by 2 SHM perches. Keep about 15m S of perches and ⚓ in 2m in centre of cove; S part dries. Few facilities: V, ✉, ☎, at Cullipool 1½M WNW. Gas at Cuan Sound ferry 2M NNW.

CRAOBH HAVEN (L Shuna) 10-8-18

Argyll 56°12'·81N 05°33'·47W

CHARTS
AC *2326, 2169*; Imray C65; OS 55

TIDES
HW Loch Shuna –0615 Dover; ML Seil Sound 1·4; Duration Seil Sound 0615; Zone 0 (UT). For tidal figures see 10.8.17. Tidal streams in Loch Shuna are weak.

SHELTER
Very good. Craobh (pronounced Croove) Haven (access H24) is a marina on SE shore of Loch Shuna. It is formed by Eilean Buidhe on the NE side, by Eilean an Duin and Fraoch Eilean to the NW and W; each island is joined to the shore by a causeway. On the N side the ent is formed by bkwtrs. There are ⚓s in Asknish Bay 1M to the N, and in the bays E of Eilean Arsa and at Bàgh an Tigh-Stòir, S of Craobh Haven. Beware lobster pots in approaches.

NAVIGATION
WPT 56°13'·00N 05°34'·42W, 275°/095° from/to N tip of Eilean Buidhe, 0·7M. Beware un-marked reef (dr 1·5m) at Eich Donna NNE of Eilean Creagach and rks (dr 1·5m) 4ca N of ent. An unlit SHM buoy marks a rk (1m) ¾ca NNW of the N bkwtr. PHM buoys mark a shoal area between ent and pontoons. A pink perch on W corner of hbr marks a spit; elsewhere ample depth in the marina.

LIGHTS AND MARKS
None. A night approach would present problems.

RADIO TELEPHONE
VHF Ch M, 80 (summer 0830-2000LT; winter 0830-1800).

TELEPHONE (01852)
Hr Mr 500222; MRSC (01631) 563720; ✠ (0141) 887 9369; Marinecall 0891 500463; Police (01546) 602222; Ⓗ (01546) 602323.

FACILITIES
Craobh Haven Marina (200+50 visitors) ☎ 500222, Fax 500252, £12.34, AC, D, FW, SM, BY, CH, Slip, BH (15 ton), C (12 ton), Gas, Gaz, ME, El, Sh, R, SC, Ⓔ, ▣, Divers. **Village** V, Bar, Ⓑ (Wed), ✉ (Kilmelford), ⇌ (Oban by bus), ✈ (Glasgow).

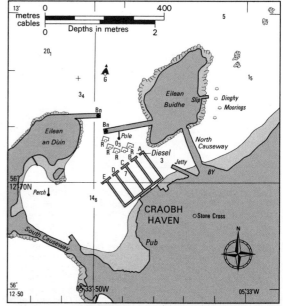

Depths in metres

Eilean Buidhe

Eilean an Dùin

CRAOBH HAVEN

Pub

South Causeway

LOCH CRAIGNISH   10-8-19

Argyll 56°08'·00N 05°35'·00W

CHARTS
AC *2326, 2169*; Imray C63, C65; OS 55

TIDES
+0600 Dover; ML (Loch Beag)1·2; Duration (Seil Sound) 0615; Zone 0 (UT)

Standard Port OBAN (←—)

Times				Height (metres)			
High Water		Low Water		MHWS	MHWN	MLWN	MLWS
0100	0700	0100	0800	4·0	2·9	1·8	0·7
1300	1900	1300	2000				
Differences LOCH BEAG (Sound of Jura)							
–0110	–0045	–0035	–0045	–1·6	–1·2	–0·8	–0·4

Note: HW Ardfern is approx HW Oban –0045; times/heights much affected by local winds and barometric pressure

SHELTER
Good at Ardfern, 56°11'·0N 05°31'·8W, access H24; ⚓s at:
– Eilean nan Gabhar; appr from E chan and ⚓ E of island.
– Eilean Righ; midway up the E side of the island.
– Bàgh na Cille, NNE of Craignish Pt.
– Eilean Dubh in the "lagoon" between the Is and mainland.
Beware squalls in E'lies, especially on E side of loch.

NAVIGATION
WPT 56°07'·60N 05°35'·30W (off chartlet) between Dorus Mór and Liath-sgier Mhòr. Beware: strong tidal streams (up to 8kn) in Dorus Mór; a reef extending 1ca SSW of the SE chain of islands; rk 1½ca SSW of Eilean Dubh; fish cages especially on E side of loch; a drying rk at N end of Ardfern ⚓ with a rk awash ¼ca E of it. (These 2 rks are ½ca S of the more S'ly of little islets close to mainland). The main fairway is free from hazards, except for Sgeir Dhubh, a rk 3½ca SSE of Ardfern, with a reef extending about ½ca all round. Ardfern is 1ca W of Eilean Inshaig.

LIGHTS AND MARKS
No lts.

RADIO TELEPHONE
Ardfern Yacht Centre VHF Ch 80 M (office hrs).

TELEPHONE (01852)
Hr Mr (Yacht Centre) 500247/500636; MRSC (01631) 563720; Marinecall 0891 500 463; ⌗ (0141) 887 9369; Dr (01546) 602921; Ⓗ (01546) 602449.

FACILITIES
Ardfern Yacht Centre (87+20 visitors); ☎ 500247/500636, Fax 500624, AB £10.57, M, FW, AC, D, BH (20 ton), Slip, ME, EI, Sh, ACA, C (12 ton), CH, Gas, Gaz.
Village R, V, Ⓑ (Wed), ✉ , ⇌ (Oban), ✈ (Glasgow).

SUBMARINE EXERCISE AREAS (SUBFACTS)   10-8-20

Those areas N of Mull where submarine activity is planned for the next 16 hrs are broadcast by Coast Radio Stns at the times and freqs shown below. The areas are referred to not by numbers, but by names as listed overleaf; see also 8.4.10. Stornoway CG will also supply Subfacts on request Ch 16. For Areas 26 – 81, S of Mull, see 10.9.22. Subfacts follow after the forecast. A Fisherman's Hotline ☎ (01374) 613097 can answer queries. Submarines on the surface and at periscope depth always listen on Ch 16. The former will comply strictly with IRPCS; the latter will not close to within 1500 yds of a FV without its express permission.

SUBFACTS ARE BROADCAST:
by the following **CRS** at 0303, 0703, 1103, 1503, 1903, 2303UT:
Lewis Ch 05. **Hebrides** Ch 26 and 1866kHz. **Skye** Ch 24; and by **Stornoway CG** on request Ch 16.

Continued

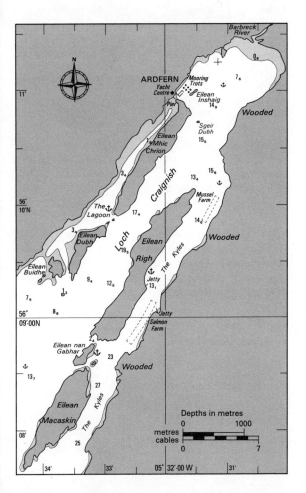

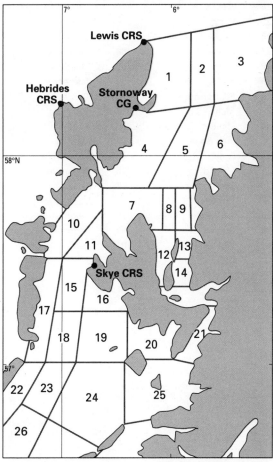

SUBFACTS continued

All references to Submarine Exercise Areas (off the West coast of Scotland and in the Irish Sea), by either BT Coast Radio Stations or the Coastguard, are to the geographic name of the area rather than to the area number (as shown, for lack of space, on the chartlets overleaf and at 10.9.22). The following are the area numbers and names:

1	Tiumpan	42	Long
2	Minch North	43	Cove
3	Stoer	44	Gareloch
4	Shiant	45	Rosneath
5	Minch South	46	Cumbrae
6	Ewe	47	Garroch
7	Trodday	48	Laggan
8	Rona West	49	Blackstone
9	Rona North	50	Place
10	Lochmaddy	51	Colonsay
11	Dunvegan	52	Boyle
12	Portree	53	Orsay
13	Rona South	54	Islay
14	Raasay	55	Otter
15	Neist	56	Gigha
16	Bracadale	57	Earadale
17	Ushenish	58	Lochranza
18	Hebrides North	59	Davaar
19	Canna	60	Brodick
20	Rhum	61	Irvine
21	Sleat	62	Lamlash
22	Barra	63	Ayr
23	Hebrides Central	64	Skerries
24	Hawes	65	Rathlin
25	Eigg	66	Kintyre
26	Hebrides South	67	Sanda
27	Ford	68	Stafnish
28	Tiree	69	Pladda
29	Staffa	70	Turnberry
30	Mackenzie	71	Torr
31	Mull	72	Mermaid
32	Linnhe	73	Ailsa
33	Jura Sound	74	Maiden
34	Fyne	75	Corsewall
35	Minard	76	Ballantrae
36	Tarbert	77	Magee
37	Skipness	78	Londonderry
38	West Kyle	79	Beaufort
39	Striven	80	Ardglass
40	East Kyle	81	Peel
41	Goil		

FERRIES ON THE WEST COAST OF SCOTLAND   10-8-21

The following is a brief summary of the many ferries plying between mainland and island harbours. It supplements the UK and Continental ferry services listed in 10.0.4, and may prove useful when cruise plans or crews change, often in remote places. It covers Area 8 (Stornoway to Oban) and Area 9 (Jura to the Clyde).
The major operator is Caledonian MacBrayne: Head Office, The Ferry Terminal, Gourock PA19 1QP; ☎ 01475-650000 for reservations, Fax 637607. Many routes are very short and may not be pre-booked; seasonal routes are *asterisked.

From	To	Time	Remarks
Area 8			
Ullapool	Stornoway	3½ hrs	See 10.0.4
Kyles Scalpay	Scalpay (Lewis)	10 mins	Not Sun
Uig (Skye)	Tarbert (Harris)	1¾ hrs	Not Sun
Uig	Lochmaddy (N Uist)	1¾ hrs	
Tarbert	Lochmaddy	1¾ hrs	Not Sun
Oban/Mallaig	Castlebay/Lochboisdale	5 hrs/1hr 50m	
Sconser (Skye)	Raasay	15 mins	Not Sun
Mallaig*	Kyle of Lochalsh	2 hrs	Fri only
Mallaig*	Armadale (Skye)	30 mins	
Mallaig	Eigg-Muck-Rhum-Canna	Varies	Not Sun
Oban	Tobermory-Coll-Tiree	Varies	Not Sun
Tobermory	Kilchoan	35 mins	
Fionnphort	Iona	5 mins	
Lochaline	Fishnish (Mull)	15 mins	
Oban	Craignure (Mull)	40 mins	
Oban	Lismore	50 mins	Not Sun
Areas 8/9			
Oban	Colonsay	2h10m	M/W/Fri
Area 9			
Kennacraig	Port Askaig/Colonsay	Varies	Wed
Kennacraig	Port Ellen	2h 10m	
Kennacraig	Port Askaig	2 hrs	
Tayinloan	Gigha	20 mins	
Ardrossan*	Douglas (IoM)	8 hrs	Sat/Sun
Ardrossan	Brodick	55 mins	
Rothesay*	Brodick (Arran)	1h50m	Mon/Thur
Claonaig	Lochranza (Arran)	30 mins	
Largs	Cumbrae Slip	15 mins	
Tarbert (L Fyne)	Portavadie*	20 mins	
Colintraive	Rhubodach (Bute)	5 mins	
Wemyss Bay	Rothesay (Bute)	30 mins	
Gourock	Kilcreggan	10 mins	Not Sun
Gourock	Helensburgh	30 mins	Not Sun
Gourock	Dunoon	20 mins	

Other Operators/services

Western Ferries (Argyll Ltd), ☎ 01496 840681:
Port Askaig	Feolin (Jura)	Short

Strathclyde Regional Council ☎ 01853 300252:
Seil	Luing	Short

D.A.MacAskill, ☎ 01867 540230:
North Uist	Berneray
North Uist	Leverburgh (S Harris)

D.J.Rodgers, ☎ 01878 720261:
South Uist	Eriskay

W. Rusk, ☎ 01878 720233:
South Uist	Barra

Volvo Penta service

Sales and service centres in area 9

STRATHCLYDE *J. N. MacDonald & Co Ltd*, 47-49 Byron Street, Glasgow
G11 6LP Tel 0141-334 6171 **RENFREWSHIRE** *J. N. MacDonald & Co Ltd*,
Units B & C, The Yacht Harbour, Inverkip, Greenock, PA16 0AS
Tel (01475) 522450

**VOLVO
PENTA**

Area 9

South-West Scotland
Crinan Canal to Mull of Galloway

9

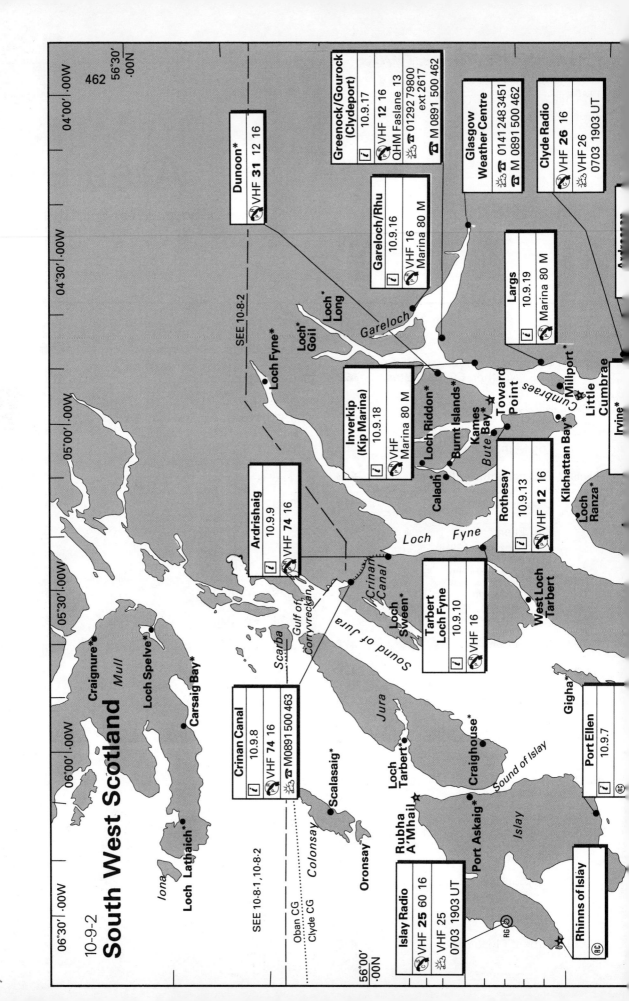

10-9-2
South West Scotland

462

Islay Radio
VHF **25** 60 16
☎ VHF 25
0703 1903 UT

Crinan Canal
10.9.8
VHF **74** 16
☎ M0891 500 463

Ardrishaig
10.9.9
VHF **74** 16

Tarbert
Loch Fyne
10.9.10
VHF 16

Port Ellen
10.9.7

Rothesay
10.9.13
VHF **12** 16

Inverkip
(Kip Marina)
10.9.18
VHF
Marina 80 M

Gareloch/Rhu
10.9.16
VHF 16
Marina 80 M

Greenock/Gourock
(Clydeport)
10.9.17
VHF **12** 16
QHM Faslane 13
☎ 01292 79800
ext 2617
M 0891 500 462

Dunoon*
VHF **31** 12 16

Glasgow
Weather Centre
☎ 0141 248 3451
M 0891 500 462

Clyde Radio
VHF **26** 16
☎ VHF 26
0703 1903 UT

Largs
10.9.19
Marina 80 M

SEE 10-8-2

SEE 10-8-1, 10-8-2

Oban CG
Clyde CG

Mull

Craignure*

Iona

Loch Lathaich*

Loch Spelve*

Carsaig Bay*

Scarba

Gulf of
Corryvreckan

Loch
Sween*

Crinan
Canal

Loch Fyne*

Loch
Goil*

Loch
Long*

Gareloch

Loch Fyne

Caladh

Loch Riddon*

Burnt Islands*

Kames

Bute Bay*

Toward
Point

Millport*

Cumbraes

Little
Cumbrae

Kilchattan Bay*

Irvine*

Loch
Ranza*

West Loch
Tarbert

Gigha*

Sound of Jura

Jura

Loch
Tarbert*

Craighouse*

Sound of Islay

Islay

Port Askaig*

Rubha
A'Mhail*

Scalasaig*

Colonsay

Oronsay

Rhinns of Islay

RG

56°30'N
.00N

56°00'N
.00N

06°30'W .00W
06°00'W .00W
05°30'W .00W
05°00'W .00W
04°30'W .00W
04°00'W .00W

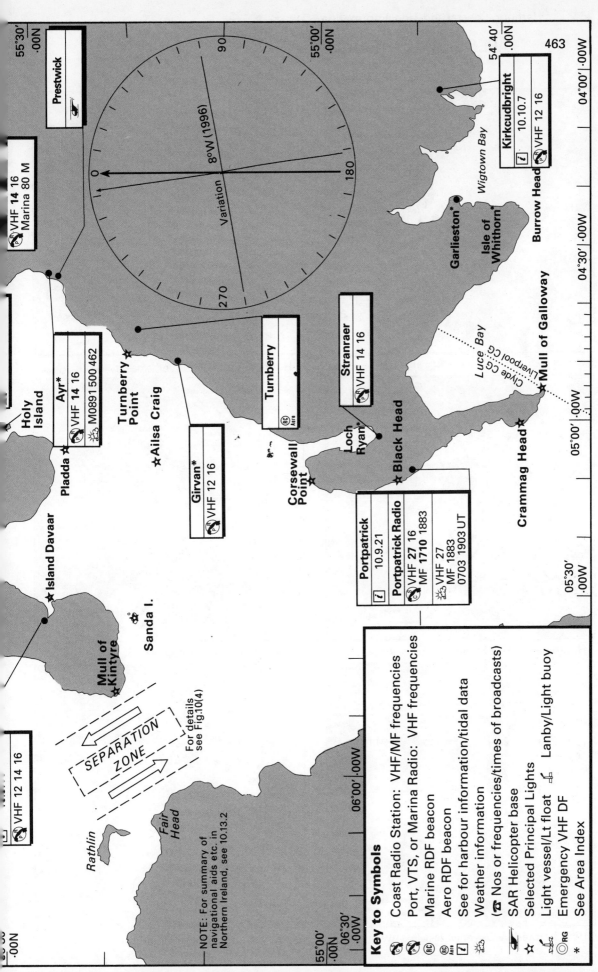

9

10-9-3   AREA 9 TIDAL STREAMS

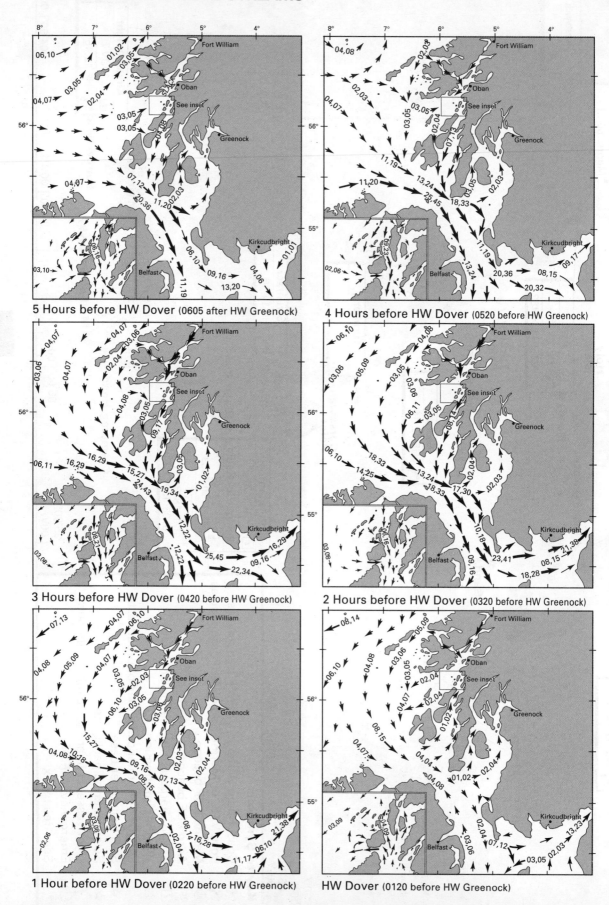

5 Hours before HW Dover (0605 after HW Greenock)

4 Hours before HW Dover (0520 before HW Greenock)

3 Hours before HW Dover (0420 before HW Greenock)

2 Hours before HW Dover (0320 before HW Greenock)

1 Hour before HW Dover (0220 before HW Greenock)

HW Dover (0120 before HW Greenock)

Northward   10.8.3   Irish Sea 10.10.3   North Ireland 10.13.3

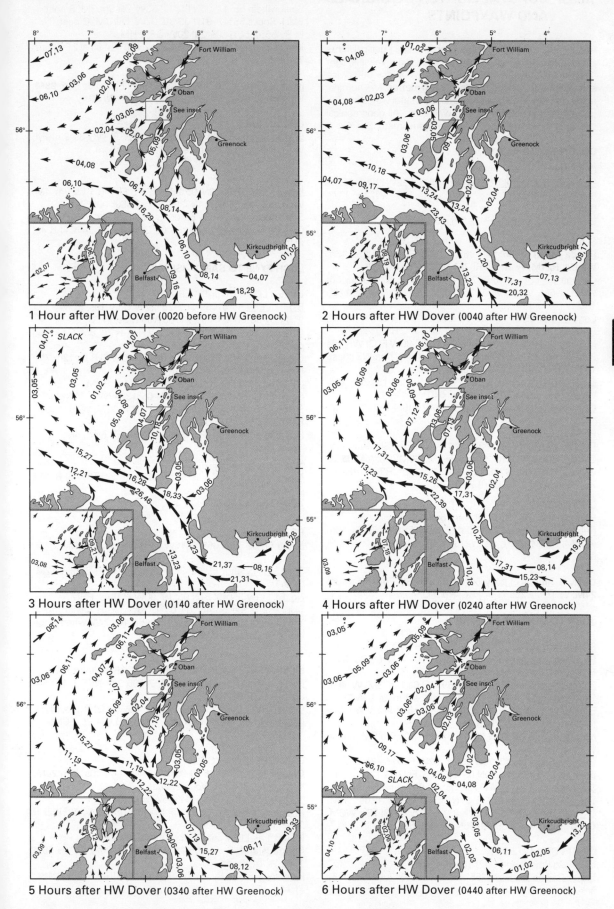

1 Hour after HW Dover (0020 before HW Greenock)

2 Hours after HW Dover (0040 after HW Greenock)

3 Hours after HW Dover (0140 after HW Greenock)

4 Hours after HW Dover (0240 after HW Greenock)

5 Hours after HW Dover (0340 after HW Greenock)

6 Hours after HW Dover (0440 after HW Greenock)

9

10.9.4 COASTAL LIGHTS, FOG SIGNALS AND WAYPOINTS

Abbreviations used below are given in 1.4.1. Principal lights are in **bold** print, places in CAPITALS, and light-vessels, light floats and Lanbys in *CAPITAL ITALICS*. Unless otherwise stated lights are white. m – elevation in metres; M – nominal range in miles. Fog signals are in *italics*. Useful waypoints are underlined – use those on land with care. All geographical positions should be assumed to be approximate. See 4.4.1.

COLONSAY TO ISLAY

COLONSAY
Scalasaig, Rubha Dubh 56°04'·02N 06°10'·83W Fl (2) WR 10s 6m W8M, R5M; W bldg; vis R shore-230°, W230°-337°, R337°-354°.
Pier Hd Ldg Lts 262°, FR 8/10m (occas).

SOUND OF ISLAY
Rhuda Mhail 55°56'·20N 06°07'·35W Fl (3) WR 15s 45m **W24M, R21M**; W Tr; vis R075°-180°, W180°-075°.
Carragh an t'Struith 55°52'·3N 06°05'·7W Fl WG 3s 8m W9M, G6M, W Tr; vis W354°-078°, G078°-170°, W170°-185°.
Carragh Mòr 55°50'·4N 06°06'·0W Fl (2) WR 6s 7m W8M, R6M; W Tr; vis R shore-175°, W175°-347°, R347°-shore.
McArthur's Hd S end 55°45'·85N 06°02'·80W Fl (2) WR 10s 39m W14M, R11M; W Tr; W in Sound of Islay from NE coast-159°, R159°-244°, W244°-E coast of Islay.
Eilean a Chùirn 55°40'·14N 06°01'·15W Fl (3) 18s 26m 8M; W Bn; obsc when brg more than 040°.
Otter Rock Lt By 55°33'·92N 06°07'·80W Q (6) + L Fl 15s; SCM.

PORT ELLEN
Port Ellen Lt By 55°37'·00N 06°12'·22W QG; SHM.
Carraig Fhada Fl WRG 3s 20m W8M, R6M, G6M; W ■ Tr; vis W shore-248°, G248°-311°, W311°-340°, R340°-shore.
Ro-Ro terminal 2 FG (vert) 7/6m 3M.

LOCH INDAAL
Bruichladdich Pier Hd 2 FR (vert) 6m 5M.
Rubh'an Dùin 55°44'·70N 06°22'·35W Fl (2) WR 7s 15m W13M, R12M; W Tr; vis W218°-249°, R249°-350°, W350°-036°.

Orsay Is, **Rhinns of Islay** 55°40'·38N 06°30'·70W Fl 5s 46m **24M**; W Tr; vis 256°-184°; RC; *Horn (3) 45s.*

JURA TO MULL OF KINTYRE

SOUND OF JURA/CRAIGHOUSE/LOCH SWEEN/GIGHA
Reisa an t-Struith, S end of Is 56°07'·78N 05°38'·84W Fl (2) 12s 12m 7M; W col.
Ruadh Sgeir 56°04'·32N 05°39'·69W Fl 6s 13m 8M; W ●Tr.
Skervuile 55°52'·47N 05°49'·80W Fl 15s 22m 9M; W Tr.
Eilean nan Gabhar 55°50'·05N 05°56'·15W Fl 5s 7m 8M; framework Tr; vis 225°-010°.
Na Cùiltean 55°48'·65N 05°54'·85W Fl 10s 9m 9M; col on W bldg.
Gamhna Gigha 55°43'·78N 05°41'·02W Fl (2) 6s 7m 5M.
Badh Rk Lt By 55°42'·30N 05°41'·18W Fl (2) G 12s; SHM.
Sgeir Nuadh Lt By 55°41'·78N 05°42'·00W Fl R 6s; PHM.
Sgeir Gigalum Lt By 55°39'·97N 05°42'·60W Fl G 6s; SHM.
Gigalum Rks Lt By 55°39'·20N 05°43'·62W Q (9) 15s; WCM.
Caolas Gigalum Bn 55°39'·16N 05°44'·50W; NCM.

WEST LOCH TARBERT
Dunskeig Bay, N end Q (2) 10s 11m 8M.
Eileen Tràighe (off S side) 55°45'·40N 05°35'·70W Fl (2) R 5s 5m 3M; R post; Ra refl.

Corran Pt 55°46'·12N 05°34'·28W QG 3m 3M; G post.
Sgeir Mhein 55°47'·06N 05°32'·33W QR 3m 3M; R post.
Black Rocks 55°47'·91N 05°30'·07W QG 3M; G post.
Lt By 55°48'·61N 05°29'·20W QR; PHM.
Kennacraig ferry terminal 55°48'·42N 05°28'·94W 2 FG (vert) 7m 3M; silver post.

Mull of Kintyre 55°18'·6N 05°48'·1W Fl (2) 20s 91m **29M**; W Tr on W bldg; vis 347°-178°; *Horn Mo(N) 90s.*

CRINAN CANAL
E of lock ent 56°05'·48N 05°33'·30W Fl WG 3s 8m 4M; W Tr, R band; vis W shore-146°, G146°-shore.

ARDRISHAIG
Bkwtr Hd 56°00'·76N 05°26'·53W L Fl WRG 6s 9m 4M; W Tr; vis G287°-339°, W339°-350°, R350°-035°.
Sgeir Sgalag No. 49 By 56°00'·36N 05°26'·23W; SHM.
Gulnare Rk No. 48 Lt By 56°00'·18N 05°26'·24W Fl R 4s; PHM.

LOCH FYNE TO SANDA ISLAND

UPPER LOCH FYNE/INVERARY
Big Rk Lt By 55°57'·89N 05°25'·27W Q (3) 10s; ECM.
'P' Lt By 56°00'·23N 05°21'·98W Fl R 3s; PHM.
Otter Spit 56°00'·63N 05°21'·03W Fl G 3s 7m 8M; G tank on pyramid.
Glas Eilean S end 56°01'·10N 05°21'·10W Fl R 5s 12m 7M; R col on pedestal.
'Q' Lt By 56°00'·97N 05°20'·60W Fl R 3s; PHM.
Sgeir an Eirionnaich 56°06'·49N 05°13'·47W Fl WR 3s 7m 8M; B Tr on B l Tr, W stripes; vis R044°-087°, W087°-192°, R192°-210°, W210°-044°.
Furnace Pier 56°09'·06N 05°10'·38W 2 FR (vert) 5M.

EAST LOCH TARBERT
Madadh Maol ent S side 55°52'·02N 05°24'·18W Fl R 2·5s 4m 3M; R col.
Eilean a'Choic SE side QG 3m 2M; G col.

PORTAVADIE
Bkwtr 55°52'·52N 05°19'·16W 2 FG (vert) 6/4m 4M.

Sgat Mór (S end) 55°50'·85N 05°18'·42W Fl 3s 9m 12M; W ● Tr.
No. 51 Lt By 55°45'·57N 05°19'·60W Fl R 4s; PHM.
Skipness range 55°46'·7N 05°19'·0W Iso R 8s 7m 10M; Y ◆ on bldg; vis 292·2°-312·2°. Oc (2) Y 10s **24M** when range in use (occas).

KILBRANNAN SOUND/CRANNAICH/CARRADALE BAY
Port Crannaich, bkwtr Hd 55°35'·7N 05°27'·8W Fl R 10s 5m 6M; vis 099°-279°.
Crubon Rk Lt By 55°34'·48N 05°27'·00W Fl (2) R 12s; PHM.
Otterard Lt By 55°27'·07N 05°31'·04W Q (3) 10s; ECM.

CAMPBELTOWN LOCH
Davaar N Pt 55°25'·69N 05°32'·37W Fl (2) 10s 37m **23M**; W Tr; vis 073°-330°; *Horn (2) 20s.*
"C" Lt By 55°25'·30N 05°34'·35W Fl (2) 6s; IDM.
Arranman's Barrels Lt By 55°19'·40N 05°32'·80W Fl (2) R 12s; PHM.
Macosh Rk Lt By 55°17'·95N 05°36'·90W Fl R 6s; PHM.
Sanda Island, S side 55°16'·50N 05°34'·90W Fl 10s 50m **15M**; W Tr; Racon (T).
Patersons Rk Lt By 55°16'·90N 05°32'·40W Fl (3) R 18s; PHM.

KYLES OF BUTE TO RIVER CLYDE

KYLES OF BUTE/CALADH
Ardlamont Pt No. 47 Lt By 55°49'·59N 05°11'·70W Fl R 4s; PHM.
Carry Pt No. 46 Lt By 55°51'·40N 05°12'·18W Fl R 4s; PHM.
Rubha Ban Lt By 55°54'·95N 05°12'·33W Fl R 4s; PHM.
Burnt Is Lt By (NE of Eilean Fraoich) 55°55'·79N 05°10'·43W Fl G 3s; SHM.
Burnt Islands No. 42 Lt By (S of Eilean Buidhe) 55°55'·77N 05°10'·32W Fl R 2s; PHM.
Creyke Rk No. 45 By 55°55'·68N 05°10'·82W; PHM.
Beere Rk No. 44 By 55°55'·56N 05°10'·57W; SHM.
Wood Farm Rk No. 43 By 55°55'·42N 05°10'·27W; SHM.
Rubha Bodach Lt By 55°55'·39N 05°09'·53W Fl G; SHM.
Ardmaleish Pt No. 41 Lt By 55°53'·03N 05°04'·63W Q; NCM.

ROTHESAY
Front Pier E end 55°50'·32N 05°03'·03W 2 FG (vert) 7m 5M.
Pier W end 2 FR (vert) 7m 5M.
Albert Pier near N end 2 FR (vert) 8m 5M.

FIRTH OF CLYDE
Ascog Patches No. 13 Lt Bn 55°49'·71N 05°00'·17W Fl (2) 10s 5m 5M; IDM.
Toward Pt 55°51'·73N 04°58'·73W Fl 10s 21m **22M**; W Tr.
No. 34 By 55°51'·44N 04°59'·04W; ECM.
Toward Bank No. 35 Lt By 55°51'·05N 04°59'·93W Fl G 3s; SHM.
Skelmorlie Lt By 55°51'·65N 04°56'·28W Iso 5s; SWM.

WEMYSS BAY/INVERKIP
Pier 55°52'·57N 04°53'·39W 2 FG (vert) 7/5m 5M.
No. 12 55°52'·96N 04°53'·70W Oc (2) Y 10s 5m 3M; SPM.
Inverkip oil jetty, S and N ends 2 FG (vert) 11m 2M.
'M' Lt By 55°53'·52N 04°54'·34W Fl G 5s; SHM.
Kip Lt By 55°54'·49N 04°52'·95W QG; SHM.
Cowal Lt By 55°56'·00N 04°54'·77W L Fl 10s; SWM.
Lunderston Bay No. 8 55°55'·5N 04°52'·9W Fl (4) Y 10s 5m 3M.

The Gantocks 55°56'·45N 04°55'·00W Fl R 6s 12m 6M;● Tr.

DUNOON
Pier, S end and N end 2 FR (vert) 5m 6M.
Cloch Pt 55°56'·55N 04°52'·67W Fl 3s 24m 8M; W ● Tr, B band, W dwellings.
McInroy's Pt Ro-Ro terminal 55°57'·09N 04°51'·20W 2 FG (vert) 5/3m 6M.
No. 5 55°56'·97N 04°51'·62W Oc (2) Y 10s 5m 3M; SPM.

HOLY LOCH
Hunter's Quay Ro-Ro terminal 55°58'·27N 04°54'·42W 2 FR (vert) 6/4m 6M.

LOCH LONG/LOCH GOIL
Loch Long Lt By 55°59'·17N 04°52'·33W Oc 6s; SWM.
Baron's Pt No. 3 55°59'·2N 04°51'·0W Oc (2) Y 10s 5m 3M.
Ravenrock Pt 56°02'·17N 04°54'·32W Fl 4s 12m 10M; W Tr on W col. Dir Lt 204°, Dir WRG 9m (same Tr); vis R201·5°-203°, Al WR203°-203·5° (W phase incr with brg), F W203·5°-204·5°, Al WG204·5°-205° (G phase incr with brg), FG205°-206·5°.
Port Dornaige 56°03·76N 04° 53'·60W Fl 6s 11m 11M; W col. vis 026°-206°.
Carraig nan Ron (Dog Rock) 56°06'·01N 04°51'·60W Fl 2s 7m 11M; W col.
Finnart Oil Terminal, Cnap Pt 56°07'·41N 04°49'·88W Ldg Lts 031°. Front Q 8m 10M; W col. Rear, 87m from front F 13m; R line on W Tr.
Ashton Lt By 55°58'·11N 04°50'·58W Iso 5s; SWM.

GOUROCK
Railway Pier Hd 55°57'·8N 04°49'·0W 2 FG (vert) 10/8m 3M; Gy Tr.
Kempock Pt No. 4 55°57'·72N 04°49'·27W Oc (2) Y 10s 6m 3M.
Whiteforeland Lt By 55°58'·11N 04°47'·20W L Fl 10s; SWM.
Rosneath Patch, S end 55°58'·52N 04°47'·37W Fl (2) 10s 5m 10M.

ROSNEATH/RHU NARROWS/GARELOCH
Ldg Lts 356°. **Front No. 7N** 56°00'·06N 04°45'·28W Dir Lt 356°. Dir WRG 3m **W16M**, R13M, G13M; vis Al G/W 353°-355°, FW 355°-357°, Al W/R 357°-000° .
Dir Lt 115° WRG 3m **W16M**, R13M, G13M; vis Al WG 111°-114°; F 114°-116°, Al W/R 116°-119°; FR 119°-121°. Passing Lt Oc G 6s 3m 3M; vis 360°; G △ on G pile structure. Rear, Ardencaple Castle Centre 56°00'·55N 04°45'·35W 2 FG (vert) 26m 12M; Tr on Castle NW corner; vis 335°-020°.
No. 8N Lt Bn. Dir Lt 080° 55°59'·09N 04°44'·13W Dir WRG 3m; vis F & Al **W16M**, R13M, G13M; vis FG 075°-077·5°, Al WG 077·5°-079·5°, FW 079·5°-080·5°, Alt WR 080·5°-082·5°, FR 082·5°-085°,°. Dir Lt 138° WRG 3m F & Al; **W16M**, R13M, G13M; vis FG 132°-134°, Al WG134°-137°, FW 137°-139°, Al WR 139°-142°. Fl Y 3s 3m 3M; vis 360°; Y ✖ on Y pile structure..
Gareloch No. 1 Lt Bn 55°59'·12N 04°43'·81W VQ (4) Y 5s 9m; Y ✖ on Y metal structure.
Row Lt By 55°59'·85N 04°45'·05W Fl G 5s; SHM.
Cairndhu Lt By 56°00'·36N 04°45'·93W Fl G 2·5s; SHM.
Castle Pt 56°00'·20N 04°46'·43W Fl (2) R 10s 8m 6M; R mast.
Lt By 56°00'·60N 04°46'·49W Fl G; SHM.
No. 3 N Lt Bn 56°00'·08N 04°46'·64W Dir Lt 149° WRG 9m **W16M**, R13M, G13M F & Al ; vis FG44°-145°, AlWG145°-148°, F148°-150°, Al WR150°-153°, FR153°-154°. Passing Lt Oc R 8s 9m 3M.
Rosneath DG Jetty 56°00'·40N 04°47'·43W 2 FR (vert) 5M; W col; vis 150°-330°.
Rhu SE Lt By 56°00'·65N 04°47'·09W Fl G 3s; SHM.
Rhu Pt 56°00'·96N 04°47'·12W Q (3) WRG 6s 9m W10M, R7M, G7M; vis G270°-000°, W000°-114°, R114°-188°, Al Dir Lt 318° Dir WRG **W16M**, R13M,G13M; vis Al WG 315°-317°, F317°-319°, Al WR319°-321°, FR321°-325°.
Limekiln No. 2N Lt Bn 56°00'·67N 04°47'·64W Dir Lt 295° WRG 5m **W16M**, R13M, G13M F & Al ; R □ on R Bn; vis AlWG291°-294°,F294°-296°, Al WR 296°-299°, FR299°-301°.
Rhu NE Lt By 56°01'·03N 04°47'·50W QG; SHM.
Rhu Narrows Lt Bn 56°00'·85N 04°47'·27W Fl 3s 6m 6M.
Mambeg Dir Lt 331° 56°03'·77N 04°50'·39W Dir Q (4) WRG 8s 8m 14M; W **I**; vis G328·5°-330°, W330°-332°, R332°-333°; shown H24.
Faslane Base, wharf, S elbow 56°03'·17N 04°49'·12W Fl G 5s 11m 5M.
Floating Barrier 56°03'·85N 04°49'·54W Fl Y 5s 3M.
Garelochhead, S Fuel Jetty 56°04'·23N 04°49'·62W 2 FG (vert) 10m 5M.
N Fuel Jetty, elbow 56°04'·35N 04°49'·66W Iso WRG 4s 10m; vis G351°-356°, W356°-006°, R006°-011°.

GREENOCK
Anchorage Lts in line 196°. Front 55°57'·6N 04°46'·5W FG 7m 12M; Y col. Rear, 32m from front, FG 9m 12M. Y col.
Lts in line 194·5°. Front 55°57'·4N 04°45'·8W FG 18m. Rear, 360m from front, FG 33m.
Clydeport Container Terminal NW corner QG 8m 8M.
Victoria Hbr ent W side 2 FG 5m (vert).
Garvel Embankment, W end 55°56'·81N 04°43'·48W Oc G 10s 9m 4M.
E end, Maurice Clark Pt 55°56'·61N 04°42'·78W QG 7m 2M; G Tr.

9

PORT GLASGOW

Bn off ent   55°56'·25N 04°41'·18W FG 7m 9M; B&W chequered Tr and cupola.

Steamboat Quay W end FG 12m 12M; B&W chequered col; vis 210°-290°. From here to Glasgow Lts on S bank are Fl G and Lts on N bank are Fl R.

CLYDE TO MULL OF GALLOWAY

LARGS

Marina S Bkwtr Hd 55°46'·35N 04°51'·67W Oc G 10s 4m 4M; G △ on l.

W Bkwtr Hd Oc R 10s 4m 4M; R ■ on col.

Approach Lt By 55°46'·40N 04°51'·78W L Fl 10s; SWM.

Largs Pier Hd N end 2 FG (vert) 7/5m 5M (H24).

FAIRLIE

Hunterston Jetty S end 55°45'·10N 04°52'·80W 2 FG (vert).

Pier N end 2 FG (vert) 7m 5M.

NATO Pier Hd 2 FG (vert) N and S ends.

MILLPORT, GREAT CUMBRAE

The Eileans W end 55°44'·89N 04°55'·52W QG 5m 2M; (shown 1/9-30/4).

Ldg Lts 333°. Pier Hd front 55°45'·04N 04°55'·78W FR 7m 5M. Rear, 137m from front, FR 9m 5M.

Mountstuart Lt By 55°48'·00N 04°57'·50W L Fl 10s; SWM.

Portachur Lt By 55°44'·35N 04°58'·44W Fl G 3s; SHM.

Runnaneun Pt (Rubha'n Eun) 55°43'·79N 05°00'·17W Fl R 6s 8m 12M; W Tr.

Little Cumbrae, Cumbrae Elbow 55°43'·27N 04°57'·95W Fl 3s 31m **23M**; W Tr; vis 334°-210°. Shown by day when))) operating.

ARDROSSAN

Approach Dir Lt 055°. 55°38'·66N 04°49'·14W Dir F WRG 15m W14M, R11M, G11M; vis FG 050°-051·2°, Alt WG 051·2°-053·8°,W phase increasing with Brg; FW 053·8°-056·2°; Alt WR 056·2°-058·8°. R phase increasing with Brg; FR 058·8°-060°. FR 13m 6M; vis 325°-145°.

N Bkwtr Hd Fl WR 2s 7m 5M; R gantry; vis R041°-126°, W126°-041°.

Lighthouse Pier Hd 55°38'·47N 04°49'·50W Iso WG 4s 11m 9M; W Tr; vis W035°-317°, G317°-035°.

Eagle Rk Lt By 55°38'·21N 04°49'·62W Fl G 5s; SHM.

IRVINE

Ent N side 55°36'·21N 04°42'·01W Fl R 3s 6m 5M; R col.

S side Fl G 3s 6m 5M; G col.

Ldg Lts 051°. Front 55°36'·41N 04°41'·50W FG 10m 5M. Rear, 101m from front, FR 15m 5M; G masts, vis 019°-120°.

TROON

Troon Lt By 55°33'·07N 04°41'·28W Fl G 4s; SHM.

West Pier Hd 55°33'·07N 04°40'·95W Oc WG 6s 11m 5M; W Tr; vis G036°-090°, W090°-036°.

E Pier Hd Fl R 10s 6m 3M.

Lady Is 55°31'·63N 04°43'·95W Fl (4) 30s 19m 8M; W Bn.

ARRAN/RANZA/LAMLASH/BRODICK

Brodick Bay, Pier Hd 2 FR (vert) 9m 4M.

Pillar Rk Pt (Holy Island), 55°31'·05N 05°03'·57W Fl (2) 20s 38m **25M**; W ■ Tr.

Holy Is SW end Fl G 3s 14m 10M; W Tr; vis 282°-147°.

Pladda 55°25'·50N 05°07'·07W Fl (3) 30s 40m **17M**; W Tr .

AYR

Bar Lt By 55°28'·12N 04°39'·38W Fl G 2s; SHM.

N Bkwtr Hd 55°28'·22N 04°38'·71W QR 9m 5M.

S Pier Hd Q 7m 7M; R Tr; vis 012°-161°. FG 5m 5M; same Tr; vis 012°-082°.

Ldg Lts 098°. Front 55°28'·16N 04°38'·31W FR 10m 5M; R Tr. Rear 130m from front Oc R 10s 18m 9M.

Turnberry Pt, near castle ruins 55°19'·55N 04°50'·60W Fl 15s 29m **24M**; W Tr.

Ailsa Craig 55°15'·12N 05°06'·42W Fl 4s 18m **17M**; W Tr; vis 145°-028°.

GIRVAN

N groyne Hd 55°14'·71N 04°51'·64W Iso 4s 3m 4M.

S pier Hd 2 FG (vert) 8m 4M; W Tr.

N Bkwtr Hd 55°14'·74N 04°51'·77W Fl (2) R 6s 7m 4M.

LOCH RYAN

Cairn Pt 54°58'·48N 05°01'·77W Fl(2) R 10s 14m 12M; W Tr.

Cairnryan 54°57'·77N 05°00'·92W Fl R 5s 5m 5M.

Stranraer No. 1 Bn 54°56'·69N 05°01'·30W Oc G 6s; SHM.

No. 3 Bn 54°55'·89N 05°01'·52W QG; SHM.

No. 5 54°55'·09N 05°01'·80W Fl G 3s; SHM.

STRANRAER

Ross Pier Hd 2 F Bu (vert).

E pier Hd 54°54'·62N 05°01'·52W 2 FR (vert) 9m.

W Pier Hd 2 FG (vert) 8m 4M; Gy col.

Corsewall Pt 55°00'·43N 05°09'·50W Fl (5) 30s 34m **22M**; W Tr; vis 027°-257°.

Killantringan Black Hd 54°51'·71N 05°08'·75W Fl (2) 15s 49m **25M**; W Tr.

PORTPATRICK

Ldg Lts 050·5°. Front 54°50'·50N 05°06'·95W FG (occas). Rear, 68m from front, FG 8m (occas).

Crammag Hd 54°39'·90N 04°57'·80W Fl 10s 35m **18M**; W Tr.

Mull of Galloway, SE end 54°38'·05N 04°51'·35W Fl 20s 99m **28M**; W Tr; vis 182°-105°.

10.9.5   PASSAGE INFORMATION

Although conditions in the South-West of Scotland are in general less rugged than from Mull northwards, some of the remarks at the start of 10.8.5 are equally applicable to this area. Refer to the Admiralty *West Coast of Scotland Pilot*; to *Yachtsman's Pilot to the W Coast of Scotland, Clyde to Colonsay*, Imray/Lawrence, and to the Clyde Cruising Club's SDs. Submarines exercise throughout these waters; see 10.8.20 and 10.9.22 for information on active areas (Subfacts).

Some of the more common Gaelic terms may help with navigation: *Acairseid*: anchorage. *Ailean*: meadow. *Aird, ard*: promontory. *Aisir, aisridh*: passage between rocks. *Beag*: little. *Beinn*: mountain. *Bo, boghar, bodha*: rock. *Cala*: harbour. *Camas*: channel, bay. *Caol*: strait. *Cladach*: shore, beach. *Creag*: cliff. *Cumhamn*: narrows. *Dubh, dhubh*: black. *Dun*: castle. *Eilean, eileanan*: island. *Garbh*: rough. *Geal, gheal*: white. *Glas, ghlas*: grey, green. *Inis*: island. *Kyle*: narrow strait. *Linn, Linne*: pool. *Mor, mhor:* large. *Mull*: promontory. *Rinn, roinn*: point. *Ruadh*: red, brown. *Rubha, rhu*: cape. *Sgeir*: rock. *Sruth*: current. *Strath*: river valley. *Tarbert*: isthmus. *Traigh*: beach. *Uig*: bay.

CORRYVRECKAN TO CRINAN (charts *2326, 2343*)

Between Scarba and Jura is the Gulf of Corryvreckan (chart 2343) which is best avoided, and should never be attempted by yachts except at slack water and in calm conditions. (In any event the Sound of Luing is always a safer and not much longer alternative). The Gulf has a least width of 6ca and is free of dangers, other than its very strong tides which, in conjunction with a very uneven bottom, cause extreme turbulence. This is particularly dangerous with strong W winds over a W-going (flood) tide which spews out several miles to seaward of the gulf, with overfalls extending 5M from the W of ent (The Great Race). Keep to the S side of the gulf to avoid the worst turbulence and the whirlpool known as The Hag, caused by depths of only 29m, as opposed to more than 100m in the fairway. The W-going stream in the gulf begins at HW Oban + 0410, and the E-going at HW Oban – 0210. Sp rate W-going is 8·5kn, and E-going about 6kn.

The range of tide at sp can vary nearly 2m between the E end of the gulf (1·5m) and the W end (3·4m), with HW ½ hr earlier at the E end. Slack water occurs at HW Oban +4 and –2½ and lasts almost 1 hr at nps, but only 15 mins at sps. On the W-going (flood) stream eddies form both sides of the gulf, but the one on the N (Scarba) shore is more important. Where this eddy meets the main stream of Camas nam Bairneach there is violent turbulence, with heavy overfalls extending W at the division of the eddy and the main stream. There are temp anchs with the wind in the right quarter in Bàgh Gleann a' Mhaoil in the SE corner of Scarba, and in Bàgh Gleann nam Muc at N end of Jura but the latter has rks in approaches E and SW of Eilean Beag.

SE of Corryvreckan is Loch Crinan, which leads to the Crinan Canal (10.9.8). Beware Black Rk, 2m high and 2ca N of the canal sea lock, and dangers extending 100m from the rk.

WEST OF JURA TO ISLAY (charts 2481, 2168)

The W coasts of Colonsay and Oronsay (chart *2169*) are fringed with dangers up to 2M offshore. The two islands are separated by a narrow chan which dries and has an overhead cable (10m). There are HIE ⚓s at Scalasaig; see 10.9.7.

The Sound of Islay presents no difficulty; hold to the Islay shore, where all dangers are close in. The N-going stream begins at HW Oban + 0440, and the S-going at HW Oban – 0140. The sp rates are 2·5kn at N entrance and 1·5kn at S entrance, but reaching 5kn in the narrows off Port Askaig.

There are anchs in the Sound, but mostly holding ground is poor. The best places are alongside at Port Askaig (10.9.7), or at anch off the distillery in Bunnahabhain B, 2·5M to N. There are overfalls off McArthur's Hd (Islay side of S entrance) during the S-going stream.

The N coast of Islay and Rhinns of Islay are very exposed. In the N there is anch SE of Nave Is at entrance to Loch Gruinart; beware Balach Rks which dry, just to N. To the SW off Orsay (lt), Frenchman's Rks and W Bank there is a race and overfalls which should be cleared by 3M. Here the NW-going stream begins at HW Oban + 0530, and the SE-going at HW Oban – 0040; sp rates are 6-8kn inshore, but decrease to 3kn 5M offshore. Loch Indaal gives some shelter; beware rks extending from Laggan Pt on E side of ent. Off the Mull of Oa there are further overfalls. Port Ellen, the main hbr on Islay, has HIE ⚓s; there are some dangers in approach, and it is exposed to S; see 10.9.7 and chart 2474.

SOUND OF JURA TO GIGHA (charts 2397, 2396, 2168)

From Crinan to Gigha the Sound of Jura is safe if a mid-chan course is held. Ruadh Sgeir (lt) are rky ledges in mid-fairway, about 3M W of Crinan. Loch Sween (chart 2397) can be approached N or SE of MacCormaig Islands, where there is an attractive anch on NE side of Eilean Mor, but exposed to NE. Coming from N beware Keills Rk and Danna Rk. Sgeirean a Mhain is a rk in fairway 1·5M NE of Castle Sween (conspic on SE shore). Anch at Tayvallich, near head of loch on W side. See 10.9.7.

W Loch Tarbert (chart 2477) is long and narrow, with good anchs and lts near ent, but unmarked shoals. On entry give a berth of at least 2½ca to Eilean Traighe off N shore, E of Ardpatrick Pt. Dun Skeig, an isolated hill, is conspic on S shore. Good anch near head of loch, 1M by road from E Loch Tarbert, see 10.9.10.

On W side of Sound, near S end of Jura, are The Small Is (chart 2396) across the mouth of Loch na Mile. Beware Goat Rk (dries 0·3m) 1½ca off southernmost Is, Eilean nan Gabhar, behind which is good anch. Also possible to go alongside Craighouse Pier (HIE ⚓) (10.9.7). Another anch is in Lowlandman's B, about 3M to N, but exposed to S winds; Ninefoot Rks with depth of 2·4m and ECM lt buoy lie off ent. Skervuile (lt) is a reef to the E, in middle of the Sound.

S of W Loch Tarbert, and about 2M off the Kintyre shore, is Gigha Is (chart 2475 and 10.9.7). Good anchs on E side in Druimyeon B and Ardminish B (HIE ⚓s), respectively N and S of Ardminish Pt. Outer and Inner Red Rks (least depth 2m) lie 2M SW of N end of Gigha Is. Dangers extend 1M W off S end of Gigha Is. Gigalum Is and Cara Is are off the S end. Gigha Sound needs very careful pilotage, since there are several dangerous rks, some buoyed/lit, others not. The N-going stream begins at HW Oban + 0430, and S-going at HW Oban – 0155, sp rates 1·3kn.

MULL OF KINTYRE (charts 2126, 2199, 2798)

From Crinan to Mull of Kintyre is about 50M. This long peninsula has great effect on tidal stream in North Chan. Off Mull of Kintyre (lt, fog sig) the N-going stream begins at HW Oban + 0400, and the S-going at HW Oban – 0225, sp rate 5kn. A strong race and overfalls exist S and SW of Mull of Kintyre, dangerous in strong S winds against S-going tide. Careful timing is needed, especially W-bound. The Traffic Separation Scheme in North Chan, see Fig. 10 (4), may restrict sea-room off the Mull.

Sanda Sound separates Sanda Is (lt) and its rks and islets, from Kintyre. On the mainland shore beware Macosh Rks (dry, PHM lt buoy) forming part of Barley Ridges, 2ca offshore; Arranman Barrels, drying and submerged, marked by PHM lt

9

buoy; and Blindman Rk (depth 2m) 1·3M N of Ru Stafnish, where 3 radio masts are 5ca inland. Sanda Is has Sheep Is 3ca to the N; Paterson's Rk (dries) is 1M E. There is anch in Sanda hbr on N side. In Sanda Sound the E-going stream begins at HW Greenock + 0340, and the W-going at HW Greenock − 0230, sp rates 5kn. Tide races extend W, N and NE from Sanda, and in strong S or SW winds the Sound is dangerous. In these conditions pass 2M S of Mull of Kintyre and Sanda and E of Paterson's Rk.

MULL OF KINTYRE TO UPPER LOCH FYNE
(charts *2126, 2383, 2381, 2382*).

Once E of Mull of Kintyre, tidal conditions and pilotage much improve. Campbeltown (10.9.11) is entered N of Island Davaar (lt, fog sig). 1·5M N of lt ho is Otterard Rk (depth 3·8m), with Long Rk (dries 1·1m) 5ca W of it; both are buoyed. E of Is Davaar tide runs 3kn at sp, and there are overfalls.

Kilbrannan Sound runs 21M from Is Davaar to Skipness Pt, where it joins Inchmarnock Water, Lower L. Fyne and Bute Sound. There are few dangers apart from overfalls on Erins Bank, 10M S of Skipness, on S-going stream. Good anch in Carradale B (10.9.11), off Torrisdale Castle. There are overfalls off Carradale Pt on S-going stream.

Lower L. Fyne (chart 2381) is mainly clear of dangers to East L. Tarbert (10.9.10). On E shore beware rks off Ardlamont Pt; 4M to NW is Skate Is which is best passed to W. 3M S of Ardrishaig (10.9.9) beware Big Rk (depth 2·1m). Further N, at entrance to Loch Gilp (mostly dries) note shoals (least depth 1·5m) round Gulnare Rk, PHM lt buoy; also Duncuan Is with dangers extending SW to Sgeir Sgalag (depth 0·6m), buoyed.

Where Upper L. Fyne turns NE (The Narrows) it is partly obstructed by Otter Spit (dries 0·9m), extending 8ca WNW from E shore and marked by lt bn. The stream runs up to 2kn here. A buoyed/lit rk, depth less than 2m, lies about 7ca SW of Otter Spit bn. In Upper L. Fyne (chart 2382) off Minard Pt, the chan between rks and islands in the fairway is buoyed/lit. For Inveraray, see 10.9.10.

ARRAN, BUTE AND FIRTH OF CLYDE (charts 1906, 1907)

Bute Sound leads into Firth of Clyde, and is clear in fairway. Arran's mountains tend to cause squalls or calms, but it has good anchs at Lamlash (10.9.12), Brodick and Loch Ranza. Sannox Rock (depth 1·5m) is 2½ca off Arran coast 8M N of Lamlash (10.9.12). 1ca off W side of Inchmarnock is Tra na-h-uil, a rk drying 1·5m. In Inchmarnock Sound, Shearwater Rk (depth 0·9m) lies in centre of S entrance.

Kyles of Bute are attractive chan N of Bute from Inchmarnock Water to Firth of Clyde, and straightforward apart from Burnt Islands. Here it is best to take the north channel, narrow but well buoyed, passing S of Eilean Buidhe, and N of Eilean Fraoich and Eilean Mor. Care is needed, since sp stream may reach 5kn. Caladh Hbr is beautiful anch 7ca NW of Burnt Is.

In contrast, the N lochs in Firth of Clyde are less attractive. Loch Goil is worth a visit but Loch Long is squally and has few anchs, while Gareloch (10.9.16) has little to attract cruising yachts other than Rhu marina. Navigation in Firth of Clyde is easy since tidal streams are weak, seldom exceeding 1kn and chans are well marked; but beware commercial and naval shipping and also unlit moorings, see 10.9.17. There are marinas on the mainland at Inverkip (10.9.18) and Largs (10.9.19). Rothesay hbr (10.9.13) on E Bute, and Kilchattan B (anch 6M to S) are both sheltered from SSE to WNW.

FIRTH OF CLYDE TO MULL OF GALLOWAY
(charts *2131, 2126*, 2199, 2198)

Further S the coast is less inviting, with mostly commercial hbrs such as Ardrossan until reaching Troon (10.9.20), NW of which there are various dangers: beware Troon Rk (depth 5·6m, but sea can break), Lappock Rk (dries 0·6m, marked by bn), and Mill Rk (dries 0·4m, buoyed). Lady Isle (lt), shoal to NE, is 2M WSW of Troon.

There is a severe race off Bennane Hd (8M SSE of Ailsa Craig, conspic) when tide is running strongly. Loch Ryan offers little for yachtsmen but there is anch S of Kirkcolm Pt, inside the drying spit which runs in SE direction 1·5M from the point. There is also useful anch in Lady Bay, sheltered except from NE. Between Corsewall Pt and Mull of Galloway the S-going stream begins HW Greenock + 0310, and the N-going at HW Greenock − 0250. Sp rate off Corsewall Pt is 2-3 kn, increasing to 5kn off and S of Black Hd. Portpatrick (10.9.21) is a useful passage hbr, but not in onshore winds. Races occur off Morroch B, Money Hd, Mull of Logan and SSE of Crammag Hd.

Mull of Galloway (lt) is S point of Scotland, a high (82m) headland and steep-to, but beware dangerous race extending nearly 3M to S. On E-going stream the race extends NNE into Luce B; on W-going stream it extends SW and W. Best to give the race a wide berth, or pass close inshore at slack water nps and calm weather.

See 10.10.5 for continuation eastward to Solway Firth and south into the Irish Sea. For notes on crossing the Irish Sea, see 10.13.5.

10.9.6   DISTANCE TABLE

Approximate distances in nautical miles are by the most direct route, whilst avoiding dangers and allowing for Traffic Separation Schemes. Places in *italics* are in adjoining areas; places in **bold** are in 10.0.5, Distances across the Irish Sea.

1. *Loch Craignish*	**1**																			
2. **Port Ellen (Islay)**	42	**2**																		
3. Crinan	5	39	**3**																	
4. Ardrishaig	14	48	9	**4**																
5. East Loch Tarbert	24	58	19	10	**5**															
6. **Campbeltown**	55	47	50	39	31	**6**														
7. Mull of Kintyre	56	27	51	54	45	20	**7**													
8. Lamlash	48	61	43	34	25	24	34	**8**												
9. Largs	48	94	43	34	24	39	47	17	**9**											
10. Rothesay	49	95	44	35	25	43	48	23	9	**10**										
11. Kip Marina	53	85	48	39	28	50	58	25	10	8	**11**									
12. Greenock	59	90	54	45	36	53	63	31	16	14	6	**12**								
13. Rhu (Helensburgh)	62	94	57	48	37	59	67	33	19	17	9	4	**13**							
14. **Troon**	54	71	49	40	33	33	44	16	20	25	29	34	38	**14**						
15. Girvan	67	58	62	53	43	29	31	20	33	40	46	49	51	21	**15**					
16. Stranraer	89	62	84	75	65	34	35	39	56	63	69	65	74	44	23	**16**				
17. **Portpatrick**	88	63	83	74	66	39	36	44	61	67	68	77	77	49	28	23	**17**			
18. **Mull of Galloway**	104	78	99	90	82	56	52	60	78	82	84	93	93	65	62	39	16	**18**		
19. *Kirkcudbright*	136	111	131	122	114	88	84	92	110	114	116	124	125	97	94	71	48	32	**19**	
20. *Douglas (IoM)*	146	120	141	132	124	106	94	102	141	130	126	141	135	107	104	84	60	42	45	**20**

HARBOURS AND ANCHORAGES IN COLONSAY, JURA, ISLAY AND THE SOUND OF JURA

SCALASAIG, Colonsay, 56°04'·15N 06°10'·80W. AC 2474, *2169*. HW +0542 on Dover; ML 2·2m. See 10·9·7. Conspic monument ½M SW of hbr. Beware group of rks N of pier hd marked by bn. 2 HIE **✪** berths on N side of pier, inner end approx 2·5m. Inner hbr to SW of pier is safe, but dries. Ldg lts 262°, both FR 8/10m on pier. Also ⚓ clear of cable in **Loch Staosnaig**; SW of Rubha Dubh lt, Fl (2) WR 10s 6m 8/5M; R shore-230°, W230°-337°, R337°-354°. Facilities: D, P, V (all at ✉), FW, Hotel ☎ (01951) 200316.

LOCH TARBERT, W. Jura, 55°57'·70N 06°00'·00W. AC 2481, *2169*. Tides as Rubha A'Mhàil (N tip of Islay). See 10·9·7. HW –0540 on Dover; ML 2·1m; Duration 0600. Excellent shelter inside the loch, but subject to squalls in strong winds; ⚓ outside in Glenbatrick Bay in approx 6m in S winds, or Bagh Gleann Righ Mor in approx 2m in N winds. To enter inner loch via Cumhann Beag, there are four pairs of ldg marks (W stones) at approx 120°, 150°, 077°, and 188°, the latter astern, to be used in sequence; pilot book required. There are no facilities.

PORT ASKAIG, Islay, 55°50'·88N 06°06'·20W. AC 2481, 2168. HW +0610 on Dover; ML 1·2m. See 10·9·7. Hbr on W side of Sound of Islay. ⚓ close inshore in 4m or secure to ferry pier. Beware strong tides/eddies. Facilities: FW (hose on pier), Gas, P, R, Hotel, V, ✉, ferries to Jura and Kintyre. Other ⚓s in the Sound are at: Bunnahabhain (2M N); Whitefarland Bay, Jura, opp Caol Ila distillery; NW of Am Fraoch Eilean (S tip of Jura); Aros Bay, N of Ardmore Pt.

CRAIGHOUSE, SE Jura, 55°50'·00N 05°56'·25W. AC 2396, 2481, 2168. HW +0600 on Dover; ML 0·5m; Duration 0640 np, 0530 sp. See 10·9·7. Good shelter, but squalls occur in W winds. Enter between lt bn on SW end of Eilean nan Gabhar, Fl 5s 7m 8M vis 225°-010°, and unlit bn close SW. There are 8 HIE **✪**s N of pier (☎ (01496) 810332), where yachts may berth alongside; or ⚓ in 5m in poor holding at the N end of Loch na Mile. Facilities: very limited, Bar, FW, ✉, R, V, Gas, P & D (cans). **Lowlandman's Bay** is 1M further N, with ECM buoy, Q (3) 10s, marking Nine Foot Rk (2·4m) off the ent. ⚓ to SW of conspic houses, off stone jetty.

LOCH SWEEN, Argyll, 55°55'·70N 05°41'·20W. AC 2397. HW +0550 on Dover; ML 1·5m; Duration 0610. See 10·9·8 Carsaig Bay. Off the ent to loch, **Eilean Mòr** (most SW'ly of MacCormaig Isles) has tiny anchorage on N side in 3m; local transit marks keep clear of two rks, 0·6m and 0·9m. Inside the loch, beware Sgeirean a'Mhain, a rk in mid-chan to S of Taynish ls, 3M from ent. Good shelter in Loch a Bhealaich (⚓ outside **Tayvallich** in approx 7m on boulders) or enter inner hbr to ⚓ W of central reef. There are no lts. Facilities: Gas, Bar, ✉, FW (⚓ by ✉), R, V. Close to NE are ⚓s at **Caol Scotnish** and **Fairy ls**, the former obstructed by rks 3ca from ent.

WEST LOCH TARBERT, Argyll, (Kintyre), 55°45'N 05°36'W. AC 2477. Tides as Gigha Sound, 10·9·7. Good shelter. Ent is S of Eilean Traighe, Fl (2) R 5s, and NW of Dun Skeig, Q (2) 10s, where there is also conspic conical hill (142m). Loch is lit for 5M by 3 bns, QG, QR and QG in sequence, up to Kennacraig ferry pier, 2FG (vert). PHM buoy, QR, is 2½ca NW of pier. Caution: many drying rks and fish farms outside the fairway and near head of loch. ⚓s are NE of Eilean Traighe (beware weed and ferry wash); near Rhu Pt, possible **✪**s; NE of Eilean dà Gallagain, and at loch hd by pier (ru). Tarbert is 1·5M walk/bus; facilities as 10·9·10.

GIGHA ISLAND, Argyll, 55°40'·60N 05°44'·00W. AC 2475, 2168. HW +0600 on Dover; ML 0·9m; Duration 0530. See 10·9·7. Main ⚓ is **Ardminish Bay**: 12 HIE **✪**s in the centre; call ☎ (01583) 545254. Reefs extend off both points, the S'ly reef marked by an unlit PHM By. Kiln Rk (dries 1·5m) is close NE of the old ferry jetty. **Druimyeon Bay** is more sheltered in E'lies, but care needed entering from S. Port Mór (S-W), Bàgh na Dòirlinne (SE-S), W Tarbert Bay (NE) are ⚓s sheltered from winds in ( ). Caolas Gigalum (⚓ 50m SE of pier) is good in all but NE-E winds. Beware many rks in Gigha Sound. Lts: Fl (2) 6s, on Gamhna Gigha (off NE tip); WCM By Fl (9) 15s marks Gigalum Rks, at S end of Gigha. **Ardminish**: Bar, FW, ✉, R, V, Gas, P & D (cans).

PORT ELLEN   10-9-7

Islay, 55°37'·30N 06°12'·20W

CHARTS
AC 2474, 2168

TIDES
HW +0620 np, +0130 sp on Dover; ML 0·6. Sea level is much affected by the weather, rising by 1m in S/E gales; at nps the tide is sometimes diurnal and range negligible.

Standard Port OBAN (←—)

Times				Height (metres)			
High Water		Low Water		MHWS	MHWN	MLWN	MLWS
0100	0700	0100	0800	4·0	2·89	1·8	0·7
1300	1900	1300	2000				

Differences PORT ELLEN (S Islay)

–0530	–0050	–0045	–0530	–3·1	–2·1	–1·3	–0·4

SCALASAIG (E Colonsay)

–0020	–0005	–0015	+0005	–0·1	–0·2	–0·2	–0·2

GLENGARRISDALE BAY (N Jura)

–0020	0000	0000	0000	–0·4	–0·2	0·0	–0·2

CRAIGHOUSE (SE Jura)

–0230	–0250	–0150	–0230	–3·0	–2·4	–1·3	–0·6

RUBHA A'MHÀIL (N Islay)

–0020	0000	+0005	–0015	–0·3	–0·1	–0·3	–0·1

ARDNAVE POINT (NW Islay)

–0035	+0010	0000	–0025	–0·4	–0·2	–0·3	–0·1

ORSAY ISLAND (SW Islay)

–0110	–0110	–0040	–0040	–1·4	–0·6	–0·5	–0·2

BRUICHLADDICH (Islay, Loch Indaal)

–0100	–0005	–0110	–0040	–1·7	–1·4	–0·4	+0·1

PORT ASKAIG (Sound of Islay)

–0110	–0030	–0020	–0020	–1·9	–1·4	–0·8	–0·3

GIGHA SOUND (Sound of Jura)

–0450	–0210	–0130	–0410	–2·5	–1·6	–1·0	–0·1

MACHRIHANISH

–0520	–0350	–0340	–0540	Mean range 0·5 metres.

SHELTER
Good shelter close S of pier and clear of ferries/FVs, but in S winds swell sets into the bay. 10 HIE **✪**s to W of Rubha Glas; adjacent rks are marked by 3 perches with reflective topmarks. Inner hbr dries. In W'lies ⚓ in Kilnaughton Bay, N of Carraig Fhada lt ho; or 4M ENE at Loch-an-t-Sàilein.

NAVIGATION
WPT 55°36'·70N 06°12'·00W, 146°/326° from/to Carraig Fhada lt ho, 0·63M. Beware Otter Rk 4M SE of hbr, and rks closer in on both sides of ent and in NE corner of bay.

LIGHTS AND MARKS
On W side 10 Radio masts (103m) and Carraig Fhada lt ho (conspic), Fl WRG 3s 20m 8/6M; W shore-248°, G248°-311°, W311°-340°, R340°-shore; keep in W sector until past the SHM buoy, QG. Ro Ro pier shows 2 FG (vert).

RADIO TELEPHONE
Nil.

TELEPHONE (01496)
Moorings 810332; ⌗ (0141) 887 9369.

FACILITIES
Village Bar, FW, ✉, R, V, Gas.

CRINAN CANAL   10-9-8

Argyll 56°05·50N 05°33'·31W

CHARTS

AC 2320, *2326*; Imray C65; OS 55

TIDES

−0608 Dover; ML 2·1; Duration 0605; Zone 0 (UT)
HW Crinan is at HW Oban −0045

Standard Port OBAN (←—)

Times				Height (metres)			
High Water		Low Water		MHWS	MHWN	MLWN	MLWS
0100	0700	0100	0800	4·0	2·89	1·8	0·7
1300	1900	1300	2000				

Differences CARSAIG BAY (4·5M SSW of Loch Crinan)

| −0105 | −0040 | −0050 | −0050 | −2·1 | −1·6 | −1·0 | −0·4 |

Note: In the Sound of Jura, S of Loch Crinan, the rise of tide occurs mainly during the 3½hrs after LW; the fall during the 3½hrs after HW. At other times the changes in level are usually small and irregular.

SHELTER

Complete shelter in canal basin; yachts are welcome, but often many FVs lie there. Good shelter in Crinan Hbr to E of Eilean da Mheim, but full of moorings. Except in strong W/N winds, ‡ E of the canal ent, clear of fairway. Berths may be reserved at Bellanoch Bay (see chartlet).

NAVIGATION

WPT 56°05'·70N 05°33'·57W, 326°/146° from/to Fl WG 3s lt, 0·27M. Beware the Black Rks and other rks in appr and near sector line 146° of dir Fl WG 3s lt. Off NW corner of chartlet, in the centre of Loch Crinan, a rectangular area, 6ca by 6ca, is devoted to shellfish beds (‡ prohib). SPM lt buoys mark each corner: Fl (4) Y 12s at the NE and NW corners, Fl Y 6s at the SW and SE corners; the latter being about 100m NE of Black Rk.

CANAL

Canal runs 9M to Ardrishaig and has 15 locks. It can be entered at all tides. All 7 bridges open. Max size: 26·5m LOA, 6m beam, 2·9m draught, mast ht 28·9m. Vessels NW-bound have right of way. Canal dues are payable at Ardrishaig or Crinan sea locks. Total transit/lock fee in 1995 was £6·88/metre, inc VAT, for 2 days. Passage time is 5 to 6 hrs. Sea locks open 0800-2100 daily in season, but only HW±3 in drought. Sea lock outer gates are left open after hours for yachts to shelter in the locks. Inland locks and bridges operate 0800-1800 daily; lock 14 and Crinan Bridge open 0800-2100 Fri-Sun. Last locking 30 mins before close. For reduced hrs in autumn, winter and spring, contact canal office. Canal shut Xmas/New Year.

LIGHTS AND MARKS

Crinan Hotel is conspic W bldg. A conspic chy, 3ca SW of hotel, leads 187° into Crinan Hbr. E of sea-lock: Dir Fl WG 3s 8m 4M, vis W shore-146°, G146°-shore. Ent: 2 FG (vert) and 2FR (vert).

RADIO TELEPHONE

VHF Ch **74** (throughout the canal) 16.

TELEPHONE (01546)

Sea lock 83(0)*285; Canal HQ 603210; MRCC (01475) 729988; ⌖ (01631) 563079; Marinecall 0891 500463; Police 602222; Dr 602921. *Extra 0 to be inserted at future date.

FACILITIES

Canal HQ ☎ 603210, M, L, FW; **Sea Basin** AB £14.53, D;
Services: BY, Slip, ME, El, Sh, Gas, ACA, C (5 ton), ⌖, CH, P (cans), V, R, Bar.
Village ✉, Ⓑ (Ardrishaig), ⇌ (Oban), ✈ (Glasgow or Macrihanish). There is a wintering park, plus BY and CH, at Cairnbaan for yachts <10m LOA.

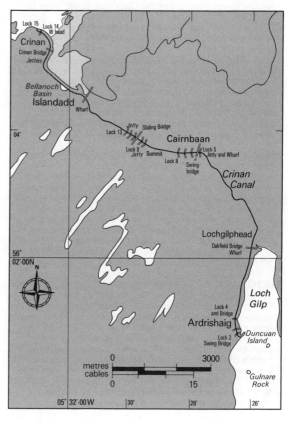

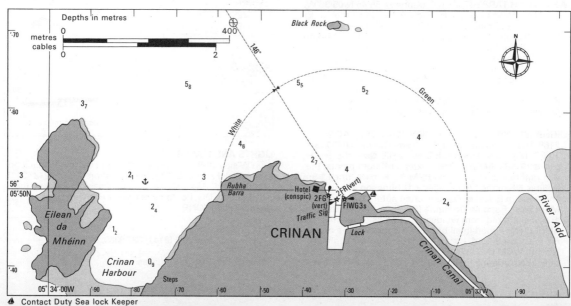

▲ Contact Duty Sea lock Keeper

ARDRISHAIG   10-9-9

Argyll 56°00'·78N 05°26'·55W

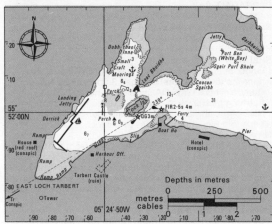

▲ Contact Duty Sea lock Keeper

CHARTS
AC 2381, *2131*; Imray C63; OS 55
TIDES
+0120 Dover; ML 1·9; Duration 0640; Zone 0 (UT)

Standard Port GREENOCK (→)

Times				Height (metres)			
High Water		Low Water		MHWS	MHWN	MLWN	MLWS
0000	0600	0000	0600	3·4	2·8	1·0	0·3
1200	1800	1200	1800				
Differences ARDRISHAIG							
+0006	+0006	–0015	+0020	0·0	0·0	+0·1	–0·1
INVERARAY							
+0011	+0011	+0034	+0034	–0·1	+0·1	–0·5	–0·2

SHELTER
Hbr is sheltered except from strong E winds. Sea lock into the Crinan Canal is normally left open; access at all tides. Complete shelter in the canal basin, or beyond lock No 2; see 10.9.8. Also ‡ 2ca N of hbr, off the W shore of L Gilp.
NAVIGATION
WPT No 48 PHM buoy, Fl R 4s, 56°00'·18N 05°26'·24W, 165°/345° from/to bkwtr lt, 0·61M. Dangerous drying rks to E of appr chan are marked by No 49 unlit SHM buoy.
LIGHTS AND MARKS
Conspic W Ho on with block of flats leads 315°between Nos 48 & 49 buoys. Bkwtr lt, L Fl WRG 6s, W339°-350°.
RADIO TELEPHONE
VHF Ch 74 16.
TELEPHONE (01546)
Hr Mr 603210; MRCC (01475) 729988; ‡ (0141) 887 9369; Marinecall 0891 500462; Police 603233; Dr 602921.
FACILITIES
Pier/Hbr ☎ 603210, AB, Slip, L, FW; **Sea Lock** ☎ 602458, AB £14.53; **Crinan Canal** AB, M, L, FW, R, Bar; **Services:** BY, ME, EI, Sh, CH, D (cans), Gas; C up to 20 ton available Lochgilphead (2M).
 Village EC Wed; P & D (cans), V, R, Bar, ⊠, ⑧, ≷ (bus to Oban), ✈ (Glasgow or Campbeltown).

TARBERT, LOCH FYNE   10-9-10

Argyll 55°52'·05N 05°24'·15W

CHARTS
AC 2381, *2131*; Imray C63; OS 62
TIDES
+0120 Dover; ML 1·9; Duration 0640; Zone 0 (UT)

Standard Port GREENOCK (→)

Times				Height (metres)			
High Water		Low Water		MHWS	MHWN	MLWN	MLWS
0000	0600	0000	0600	3·4	2·8	1·0	0·3
1200	1800	1200	1800				
Differences EAST LOCH TARBERT							
+0005	+0005	–0020	+0015	0·0	0·0	+0·1	–0·1

SHELTER
Very good in all weathers but gets crowded. Access H24. Visitors berth only on SE side of yacht pontoons in 5m. Note: also known as East Loch Tarbert.
NAVIGATION
WPT 55°52'·02N 05°22'·96W, 090°/270° from/to Fl R 2·5s lt, 0·70M. Ent is very narrow. Cock Isle divides the ent in half: Main hbr to the S, Buteman's Hole to the N, where ‡s are fouled by heavy moorings and lost chains.
LIGHTS AND MARKS
Outer ldg lts 252° to S ent: Fl R 2·5s on with Cock Is lt QG. Inner ldg line 239°: same QG, G column, on with conspic ✠ tr. Note: The W sector, 065°-078°, of Eilean na Beithe ☆, Fl WRG 3s 7m 5M (on E shore of Lower Loch Fyne), could be used to position for the initial appr to Tarbert.
RADIO TELEPHONE
VHF Ch 16 (0900-1700LT).
TELEPHONE (01880)
Hr Mr 820344, Fax 820719; MRCC (01475) 729988; ‡ (0141) 887 9369; Marinecall 0891 500462; Police 820200; Ⓗ (01546) 602323.
FACILITIES
Yacht Berthing Facility 100 visitors, AB £8.55, FW, AC; **Old Quay** D, FW; **Tarbert YC** Slip, L; **Services:** SM, ⊙, ACA, Sh, CH. **Town** EC Wed; P & D (cans), Gas, Gaz, L, V, R, Bar, ⊠, ⑧, ≷ (bus to Glasgow), ✈ (Glasgow/Campbeltown).

ANCHORAGES IN LOCH FYNE

INVERARAY, Argyll, 56°13'·95N 05°04'·00W. AC 2382, *2131*. HW +0126 on Dover. See 10.9.9. For Upper Loch Fyne see 10.9.5. Beyond Otter Spit, are ‡s on NW bank at Port Ann, Loch Gair and Minard Bay; and on SE bank at Otter Ferry, Strachur Bay (5 Ⓐs off Creggans Inn, ☎ (01369) 860279) and St Catherine's. Inveraray: beware An Oitir drying spit 2ca offshore, ½M S of pier. Some Ⓐs or ‡ SSW of pier in 4m or dry out NW of the pier. FW (on pier), ⊠, V, R, Bar, Gas, bus to Glasgow. In Lower L Fyne, 6M NNE of East Loch Tarbert there is a Ⓐ at Kilfinan Bay, ☎ (01700) 821201.

9

CAMPBELTOWN   10-9-11

Argyll 55°25'·90N 05°32'·50W (Seaward limit of hbr)

CHARTS
AC 1864, *2126*; Imray C63; OS 68

TIDES
+0125 Dover; ML 1·8; Duration 0630; Zone 0 (UT)

Standard Port GREENOCK (→)

Times				Height (metres)			
High Water		Low Water		MHWS	MHWN	MLWN	MLWS
0000	0600	0000	0600	3·4	2·8	1·0	0·3
1200	1800	1200	1800				
Differences CAMPBELTOWN							
−0025	−0005	−0015	+0005	−0.5	−0.3	+0.1	+0.2
CARRADALE BAY							
−0015	−0005	−0005	+0005	−0.3	−0.2	+0.1	+0.1
SOUTHEND, (Mull of Kintyre)							
−0030	−0010	+0005	+0035	−1.3	−1.2	−0.5	−0.2

SHELTER
Good, but gusts off the hills in strong SW'lies. Yacht pontoon (6+34 visitors) dredged 3·0m is close NW of Old Quay. Yachts >12m LOA should pre-notify ETA to Berthing Master by ☎ (below). Excellent ⚓ and moorings NNE of the hbr. S of Island Davaar there is a temp ⚓ in Kildalloig Bay, but no access to the loch.

NAVIGATION
WPT 55°26'·30N 05°31'·39W, 060°/240° from/to front ldg lt, 2·6M. The ent is easily identified by radio masts N and NE of Trench Pt (conspic W bldg) and conspic lt ho on N tip of Island Davaar off which streams are strong (4kn sp). Caution: The Dhorlin, a bank drying 2·5m which covers at HW, is close S of the ldg line.

LIGHTS AND MARKS
Davaar Fl (2) 10s 37m 23M. Otterard Rk (3·8m depth), 1·5M NNE of Island Davaar, is marked by ECM buoy Q (3) 10s. Ldg lts 240°, both FY 7/28m 6M; H24, sodium vapour lts.

RADIO TELEPHONE
VHF Ch 12 13 16 (Mon-Thurs 0845-1645; Fri 0845-1600LT).

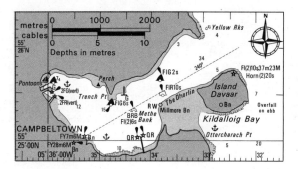

TELEPHONE (01586)
Hr Mr 552552; Berthing Master 554381, 554782 (night); MRCC (01475) 729988; ⌗ (0141) 887 9369; Marinecall 0891 500462; Police 552253; Dr 552105.

FACILITIES
Yacht pontoon £8, FW, AC; **Old Quay** ☎ 552552, D, FW, AB; **New Quay** Slip; **Campbeltown SC** Slip (dinghies); **Town** EC Wed; BY, ACA, C (25 ton); CH, P, D, El, Ⓔ, Gas, Gaz, V, R, Bar, ✉, Ⓑ, ⇌ (Air or bus to Glasgow), ✈.
Almost an Island – Always a Welcome.

ADJACENT ANCHORAGE IN KILBRANNAN SOUND

CARRADALE BAY, Argyll, 55°34'·40N 05°28'·60W. AC *2131*, HW+0115 on Dover. ML 1·8m. See 10.9.11. Good ⚓ in 7m off Torrisdale Castle in SW corner of bay. In N & E winds ⚓ in NE corner of Carradale Bay, W of Carradale Pt. 3ca E of this Pt, a PHM buoy Fl (2) R 12s marks Crubon Rk. With S & SE winds a swell sets into bay, when good shelter can be found 1M N in Carradale Hbr (Port Crannaich); if full of FVs, ⚓ 100m N of Hbr. Bkwtr lt, Fl R 10s 5m 6M. Facilities: D & P (cans), Gas, V, R, Bar, ✉.

LAMLASH   10-9-12

Isle of Arran, Bute 55°32'·00N 05°07'·00W

CHARTS
AC 1864, 2220, *2131*; Imray C63; OS 69

TIDES
+0115 Dover; ML no data; Duration 0635; Zone 0 (UT)

Standard Port GREENOCK (→)

Times				Height (metres)			
High Water		Low Water		MHWS	MHWN	MLWN	MLWS
0000	0600	0000	0600	3·4	2·8	1·0	0·3
1200	1800	1200	1800				
Differences LAMLASH							
−0016	−0036	−0024	−0004	−0.2	−0.2	No data	
BRODICK BAY							
0000	0000	+0005	+0005	−0.2	−0.2	0.0	0.0
LOCH RANZA							
−0015	−0005	−0010	−0005	−0.4	−0.3	−0.1	0.0

SHELTER
Very good in all weathers. ⚓ off Lamlash except in E'lies; off Kingscross, good except in strong N/NW winds; off the Farm at NW of Holy Island in E'lies; or Loch Ranza 14M to the N (opposite). (The large Warship buoys may be lifted).

NAVIGATION
WPT 55°32'·63N 05°03'·00W, 090°/270° from/to N Chan buoy (Fl R 6s), 1·0M. Beware submarines which exercise frequently in this area (see 10.9.20), and also wk of landing craft (charted) off farmhouse on Holy Is.

LIGHTS AND MARKS
Lts as on chartlet. There are two consecutive measured miles marked by poles north of Sannox, courses 322°/142° (about 12M N of Lamlash).

RADIO TELEPHONE
None.

TELEPHONE (01770)
MRCC (01475) 729988; ⌗ (0141) 887 9369; Marinecall 0891 500462; Police 302573; Ⓗ 600777.

FACILITIES
Lamlash Old Pier Slip, L, FW, CH, 5 x M = ☎ 302140.
Village EC Wed (Lamlash/Brodick); ME, P & D (cans), Bar, R, V, ✉, Ⓑ, ⇌ (bus to Brodick, ferry to Ardrossan), ✈ (Glasgow or Prestwick).

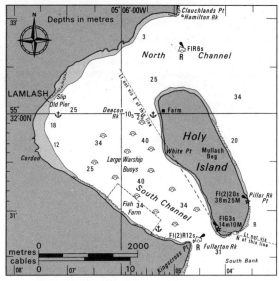

ADJACENT HARBOURS ON ARRAN

BRODICK, Arran, 55°35'·50N 05°08'·60W. AC 1864, 2220, *2131*. HW +0115 on Dover; ML 1·8m; Duration 0635. See 10.9.12. Shelter is good except in E winds. ‡ W of ferry pier in 3m; on NW side just below the Castle in 4·5m, or further N off Merkland Pt in 3-4m. Also 5 🛟s: contact ☎ (01770) 302140. There are no navigational dangers but the bay is in a submarine exercise area; see 10.9.22. Only lts are 2FR (vert) 9/7m 4M on pier hd and Admiralty buoy, Fl Y 2s, 5ca N of pier . Facilities: EC Wed; Ⓑ, Bar, P and D (cans), FW (at pier hd), ME, ⊠, R, V. Ferry to Rothesay and Ardrossan.

LOCH RANZA, Arran, 55°42'·60N 05°17'·90W. AC 2221, 2383, *2131*. HW +0120 on Dover; ML 1·7m; Duration 0635. See 10.9.12. Good shelter, but swell enters loch with N winds. The 850m mountain 4M to S causes fierce squalls in the loch with S winds. Beware Screda Reef extending SW off Newton Pt. 5 🛟s; call ☎ (01770) 302140. ‡ in 5m off castle (conspic); holding is suspect in soft mud. S shore dries. Facilities: Bar, FW at ferry slip, ⊠, R, V. Ferry to Claonaig.

HARBOURS AND ANCHORAGES AROUND BUTE
(Clockwise from Garroch Head, S end of island)

ST NINIAN'S BAY, Bute, 55°48'·15N 05°07'·80W. AC 2383, 2221. Inchmarnock Is gives some shelter from the W, but Sound is exposed to S'lies. At S end, beware Shearwater Rk, 0·9m, almost in mid-sound. ‡ in about 7m, 2ca E of St Ninian's Pt; beware drying spit to S of this Pt. Or ‡ off E side of Inchmarnock, close abeam Midpark Farm.

WEST KYLE, Bute, 55°54'N 05°12'·7W. AC1906. Tides, see 10.9.13 (Tighnabruaich). On W bank PHM buoys, each Fl R 4s, mark Ardlamont Pt, Carry Pt and Rubha Ban; N of which are two Fl Y buoys (fish farms). ‡ close off Kames or Tighnabruaich, where space allows; or in Black Farland Bay (N of Rubha Dubh). There are 24 HIE 🛟s (4 groups of 6) on W side, linked to Kames Hotel ☎ (01700) 811489; Kyles of Bute Hotel 811350; Royal Hotel 811239; and Tighnabruaich Hotel 811615. Facilities: FW, D (cans), BY, V.

CALADH HARBOUR, Argyll, 55°56'·00N, 05°11'·67W. AC 1906. HW (Tighnabruaich) +0015 on Dover; ML 2·1m. See 10.9.13. Perfectly sheltered natural hbr on W side of ent to Loch Riddon. There are two passages into Caladh Hbr: N or S of Eilean Dubh; keep to the middle of the S passage; between R and G bns when using the N, avoiding a drying rk marked by perch. ‡ in the middle of hbr; land at a stone slip on SW side. No facilities/stores; see West Kyle above.

LOCH RIDDON, Argyll, 55°57'N 05°11'·6W. AC 1906. Tides, see 10.9.13. Water is deep for 1·3M N of Caladh and shore is steep-to; upper 1·5M of loch dries. ‡ on W side close N of Ormidale pier; on E side at Salthouse; off Eilean Dearg (One Tree Is); and at NW corner of Fearnoch Bay.

BURNT ISLANDS, Bute, 55°55'·76N 05°10'·33W. AC 1906. Tides, see 10.9.13. The three islands (Eilean Mor, Fraoich and Buidhe) straddle the East Kyle. There are 2 channels: North, between Buidhe and the other 2 islets, is narrow, short and marked by 2 SHM buoys (the NW'ly one is Fl G 3s), and one PHM buoy, Fl R 2s. South chan lies between Bute and Fraoich/Mor; it is unlit, but marked by one PHM and two SHM buoys. A SHM buoy, Fl G 3s, is off Rubha a' Bhodaich, 4ca ESE. Direction of buoyage is to SE. Sp streams reach 5kn in N Chan and 3kn in S Chan. ‡ in Wreck Bay, Balnakailly Bay or in the lee of Buidhe and Mor in W'lies; also W of Colintraive Pt, clear of ferry and cables. There are 4 🛟s off the hotel, ☎ (01700) 84207.

KAMES BAY, Bute, 55°51'·7N 05°04'·75W. AC 1867, 1906. Tides as Rothesay. Deep water bay, but dries 2ca off head of loch and 1ca off NW shore. ‡ off Port Bannatyne (S shore) as space permits W of ruined jetty. Beware drying rks 1ca off Ardbeg Pt and 3 large unlit mooring buoys in mid-bay. No lts. Facilities: BY, FW, Gas, V, Bar, ⊠.

KILCHATTAN BAY, Bute, 55°45'N 05°01'·1W. AC 1907. Bay is deep, but dries 3ca off the W shore. Temp ‡s only in offshore winds: off the village on SW side, or on N side near Kerrytonlia Pt. 🛟s for hotel guests. Rubh' an Eun Lt, Fl R 6s, is 1·1M to SSE. Facilities: FW, V, ⊠, bus Rothesay.

ROTHESAY   10-9-13
Isle of Bute, Bute 55°50'·32N 05°03'·01W

CHARTS
AC 1867, 1906, 1907, *2131*; Imray C63; OS 63

TIDES
+0100 Dover; ML 1·9; Duration 0640; Zone 0 (UT)

Standard Port GREENOCK (→)

Times				Height (metres)			
High Water		Low Water		MHWS	MHWN	MLWN	MLWS
0000	0600	0000	0600	3·4	2·8	1·0	0·3
1200	1800	1200	1800				
Differences ROTHESAY BAY							
−0020	−0015	−0010	−0002	+0·2	+0·2	+0·2	+0·2
RUBHA A'BHODAICH (Burnt Is)							
−0020	−0010	−0007	−0007	−0·2	−0·1	+0·2	+0·2
TIGHNABRUAICH							
+0007	−0010	−0002	−0015	0·0	+0·2	+0·4	+0·5

SHELTER
Good on yacht pontoons in Outer Hbr (2m) and at W end inside the Front pier (2m). 40 🛟s WNW of pier or good ‡ in bay ¼M W, off Isle of Bute SC; except in strong N/NE'lies when Kyles of Bute or Kames Bay offer better shelter.

NAVIGATION
WPT 55°51'·00N 05°02'·69W, 014°/194° from/to Outer hbr ent, 0·69M. From E keep 1ca off Bogany Pt, and off Ardbeg Pt from N.

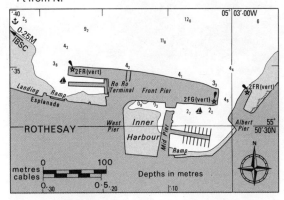

LIGHTS AND MARKS
Lts as chartlet, hard to see against shore lts. Conspic Ch spire leads 190° to outer hbr; at night beware large, unlit Admiralty buoy "MX" on this brg 5½ca from hbr.

RADIO TELEPHONE
VHF Ch 12 16 (1 May-30 Sept: 0600-2100; 1 Oct-30 Apl: 0600-1900 LT).

TELEPHONE (01700)
Hr Mr 503842; Moorings 504750; MRCC (01475) 729988; ⌗ (0141) 887 9369; Marinecall 0891 500462; Police 502121; Dr 503985; Ⓗ 503938.

FACILITIES
Outer Hbr AB, AC, FW, Slip, D*, L, FW, ME, EI, CH; **Inner Hbr** L, FW, AB, Note: due to be dredged in slow time; **Front Pier (W)** FW, AC, R; **Albert Pier** D*, L, FW, C (4 ton mobile). **Town** EC Wed; P, D, CH, V, R, Bar, ⊠, Ⓑ, ⇌ (ferry to Wemyss Bay), ✈ (Glasgow).
*By arrangement (min 200 galls).

FIRTH OF CLYDE AREA   10-9-14

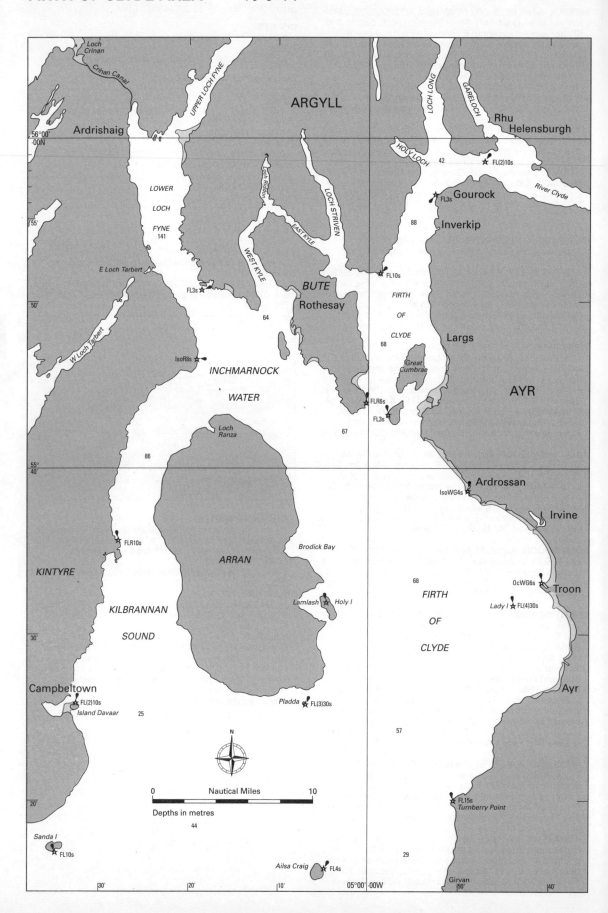

Loch Crinan
Crinan Canal
UPPER LOCH FYNE
ARGYLL
LOCH LONG
GARELOCH
Rhu
Helensburgh
56°00'
-00N
Ardrishaig
HOLY LOCH
42
FL(2)10s
River Clyde
LOWER
LOCH
FYNE
141
Loch Riddon
FL3s
Gourock
Inverkip
88
55'
E Loch Tarbert
WEST KYLE
EAST KYLE
LOCH STRIVEN
BUTE
Rothesay
FL10s
FIRTH
OF
CLYDE
50'
FL3s
64
68
Largs
W Loch Tarbert
IsoR8s
INCHMARNOCK
Great
Cumbrae
AYR
WATER
FLR6s
FL3s
Loch
Ranza
67
55°
40'
86
Ardrossan
IsoWG4s
Irvine
KINTYRE
FLR10s
ARRAN
Brodick Bay
68
FIRTH
OcWG6s
Troon
KILBRANNAN
Lamlash
Holy I
Lady I
FL(4)30s
OF
SOUND
30'
CLYDE
Campbeltown
FL(2)10s
Island Davaar
25
Pladda
FL(3)30s
57
Ayr
N
20'
FL15s
Turnberry Point
0   Nautical Miles   10
Depths in metres
44
Sanda I
FL10s
Ailsa Craig
FL4s
29
Girvan
30'   20'   10'   05°00'·00W   50'   40'

CLYDE AREA WAYPOINTS
10-9-15

Selected waypoints for use in the SW Scotland area are listed in alphabetical order below. Further waypoints for use in coastal waters are given in section 4 of each relevant area.

AE Lt Buoy	55°51'·68N 05°02'·32W
Ailsa Craig Lt	55°15'·12N 05°06'·42W
Ardgowan Outfall By	55°54'·92N 04°53'·04W
Ardlamont Pt No. 47 Lt By	55°49'·59N 05°11'·68W
Ardmaleish No.41 Lt By	55°53'·02N 05°04'·62W
Ardmore No. 4 Lt By	55°58'·75N 04°48'·30W
Ardmore No. 5 Lt By	55°58'·67N 04°47'·43W
Ardmore No. 8 Lt By	55°58'·95N 04°46'·67W
Ardmore No.10 Lt By	55°59'·03N 04°45'·62W
Ardyne Lt By	55°52'·10N 05°03'·12W
Arranman's Barrels Lt By	55°19'·40N 05°32'·80W
Ascog Patches Lt Bn (No. 13)	55°49'·71N 05°00'·17W
Ashton Lt By	55°58'·12N 04°50'·58W
Ayr Bar Lt By	55°28'·12N 04°39'·38W
Beere Rk By	55°55'·56N 05°10'·56W
Big Rock Lt By	55°57'·89N 05°25'·27W
Burnt Islands No. 43 Lt By	55°55'·43N 05°10'·27W
Burnt Islands No. 44 Lt By	55°55'·56N 05°10'·57W
Cairndhu Lt By	56°00'·36N 04°45'·93W
Carry Pt No. 46 Lt By	55°51'·42N 05°12'·17W
Cowal Lt By	55°56'·00N 04°54'·75W
Creyke Rk By	55°55'·67N 05°10'·80W
Crubon Rk Lt By	55°34'·48N 05°27'·00W
Dunoon Bank Lt By	55°56'·65N 04°54'·08W
Eagle Rk Lt By	55°38'·22N 04°49'·62W
Eilean Buidhe Lt By	55°55'·77N 05°10'·32W
Eilean Fraoich Lt By	55°55'·78N 05°10'·43W
Fairlie Patch Lt By	55°45'·37N 04°52'·27W
Fullerton Rk Lt By	55°30'·65N 05°04'·50W
Gantock Bn	55°56'·57N 04°55'·05W
Green Isle Lt By	55°59'·40N 04°45'·47W
Gulnare Rk No. 48 Lt By	56°00'·18N 05°26'·24W
Hotel Lt By	56°00'·67N 04°47'·45W
Hun 1 Lt By	55°48'·12N 04°54'·14W
Hun 3 Lt By	55°47'·61N 04°53'·44W
Hun 5 Lt By	55°45'·87N 04°52'·45W
Hun 7 Lt By	55°44'·97N 04°53'·87W
Hun 8 Lt By	55°44'·79N 04°53'·64W
Hun 9 Lt By	55°44'·67N 04°54'·37W
Hun 10 Lt By	55°44'·16N 04°54'·79W
Hun 11 Lt By	55°43'·46N 04°55'·10W
Hun 12 Lt By	55°43'·46N 04°55'·57W
Hun 13 Lt By	55°42'·53N 04°55'·10W
Hun 14 Lt By	55°42'·53N 04°55'·56W
Ironotter Outfall Lt By	55°58'·37N 04°48'·33W
Iron Rk Ledges Lt By	55°26'·83N 05°18'·80W
Kilcreggan No. 1 Lt By	55°58'·68N 04°50'·20W
Kilcreggan No. 3 Lt By	55°59'·20N 04°51'·38W
Kilcreggan No. 3 Lt Bn	55°59'·18N 04°51'·03W
Kip Lt By	55°54'·49N 04°52'·95W
Lady Isle Lt	55°31'·63N 04°43'·95W
Lamlash N Chan Lt By	55°32'·65N 05°04'·85W
Lamlash S Chan Lt By	55°30'·66N 05°04'·50W
Largs Lt By	55°46'·40N 04°51'·78W
Loch Long Lt By	55°59'·17N 04°52'·33W
Macosh Rk Lt By	55°17'·95N 05°36'·90W
Methe Bank Lt By	55°25'·30N 05°34'·36W
Millbeg Bank Lt By	55°25'·53N 05°33'·93W
Mountstuart Lt By	55°48'·00N 04°57'·50W
Otterard Lt By	55°27'·07N 05°31'·04W
Outer St Nicholas Lt By	55°28'·11N 04°39'·37W
Outfall Lt By	55°43'·58N 04°54'·70W
Patersons Rk Lt By	55°16'·90N 05°32'·40W
Pillar Rk Lt Ho	55°31'·05N 05°03'·57W
Perch Rk By	55°59'·45N 04°45'·58W
Pladda Lt Ho	55°25'·50N 05°07'·07W
Portachur Lt By	55°44'·35N 04°58'·44W
"Q" Loch Fyne Narrows Lt By	56°00'·97N 05°20'·60W
Rhu NE Lt By	56°01'·03N 04°47'·50W
Rhu SE Lt By	56°00'·65N 04°47'·09W
Rosneath Patch Lt Bn	55°58'·52N 04°47'·37W
Rosneath Patch No. 27 Lt By	55°58'·31N 04°47'·19W
Row Lt By	55°59'·85N 04°45'·05W
Rubha Ban Lt By	55°54'·96N 05°12'·33W
Skelmorlie Bank Lt By	55°51'·64N 04°55'·84W
Skelmorlie 'A' Lt By	55°46'·50N 04°57'·70W
Skelmorlie 'B' Lt By	55°47'·13N 04°57'·47W
Skelmorlie 'C' Lt By	55°48'·11N 04°55'·23W
Skelmorlie 'D' Lt By	55°47'·85N 04°56'·22W
Skelmorlie 'F' Lt By	55°48'·63N 04°54'·90W
Skelmorlie 'G' Lt By	55°49'·00N 04°54'·15W
Skelmorlie 'H' Lt By	55°49'·00N 04°54'·63W
Skelmorlie 'J' Lt By	55°51'·53N 04°54'·63W
Skelmorlie 'L' Lt By	55°52'·38N 04°54'·42W
Skelmorlie 'M' Lt By	55°53'·53N 04°54'·35W
Skelmorlie 'N' Lt By	55°53'·80N 04°55'·10W
Skelmorlie 'O' Lt By	55°54'·55N 04°54'·47W
Skipness Pt No. 51 Lt By	55°45'·57N 05°19'·60W
Strone Lt By	55°58'·77N 04°53'·77W
Tann Spit (No. 38) By	55°44'·42N 04°57'·06W
Toward Bank Lt By No.35	55°51'·04N 04°59'·93W
Troon Lt By	55°33'·07N 04°41'·28W
Warden Bank Lt By	55°55'·78N 04°54'·48W
Wemyss Bay No. 12 Lt Bn	55°52'·96N 04°53'·70W
West Crinan Lt By	55°38'·47N 04°49'·82W
Whiteforeland Lt By	55°58'·12N 04°47'·20W
Wood Farm Rk By	55°55'·43N 05°10'·25W
7N Lt Bn	56°00'·06N 04°45'·28W
8N Lt Bn	55°59'·09N 04°44'·13W

9

GARELOCH/RHU　　10-9-16

Dumbarton 56°00'·80N 04°47'·35W (E side of Rhu Narrows)

CHARTS
AC 2000, 1994, *2131*; Imray C63; OS 56, 63

TIDES
+0110 Dover; ML 1·9; Duration 0640; Zone 0 (UT). Tides at Helensburgh are the same as at Greenock

Standard Port GREENOCK (→)

Times				Height (metres)			
High Water		Low Water		MHWS	MHWN	MLWN	MLWS
0000	0600	0000	0600	3·4	2·8	1·0	0·3
1200	1800	1200	1800				
Differences ROSNEATH (Rhu pier)							
−0005	−0005	−0005	−0005	0·0	−0·1	0·0	0·0
FASLANE							
−0010	−0010	−0010	−0010	0·0	0·0	−0·1	−0·2
GARELOCHHEAD							
0000	0000	0000	0000	0·0	0·0	0·0	−0·1
COULPORT							
−0011	−0011	−0008	−0008	0·0	0·0	0·0	0·0
LOCHGOILHEAD							
+0015	−0005	−0005	−0005	−0·2	−0·3	−0·3	−0·3
ARROCHAR							
−0005	−0005	−0005	−0005	0·0	0·0	−0·1	−0·1

NAVIGATION
WPT 55°59'·30N 04°45'·19W, 176°/356° from/to bn No 7, 1·3M. Beaches between Cairndhu Pt and Helensburgh Pier (dries almost to the head) are strewn with large boulders above and below MLWS. Gareloch ent narrowed to about 225m by drying spit off Rhu Pt. Beware large unlit MoD mooring buoys and barges off W shore of Gareloch; if going to Garelochhead keep to W shore until well clear of Base area.

LIGHTS AND MARKS
Ldg/dir lts into Gareloch 356°, 318°, 295°, 329° and 331°. Gareloch Fuel Depot lt, Iso WRG 4s 10m 14M, G351°-356°, W356°-006°, R006°-011°, is clearly visible from S of the area. Lts and unlit floating boom make night sailing in the Base area inadvisable.

RADIO TELEPHONE
VHF Ch 16. Rhu Marina Ch **80** M (H24). See also 10.19.15.

TELEPHONE (01436)
Marina 820652; Queen's Hr Mr 74321; MRCC (01475) 729988 and 729014; ⊞ (0141) 887 9369; Marinecall 0891 500462; Police 72141; Ⓗ (0389) 54121; Dr 72277.

FACILITIES
Rhu Marina (150) ☎ 820238, AB £13.04, D, FW, AC, BH (4½ ton), Gas, Gaz; **Royal Northern & Clyde YC** ☎ 820322, L, R, Bar; **Helensburgh SC** ☎ 72778 Slip (dinghies) L, FW; **Services:** CH, ME, Sh, El, Slip, Ⓔ, L, M, BH (18 ton), SM, C hire; **Dumbarton Marina**, ☎ (01389) 762396, Fax 732605, M, FW, D, Slip, BH (10 ton), CH, Sh, ME, El. **Helensburgh** (1M) EC Wed; all services, ≥, ✈ (Glasgow).

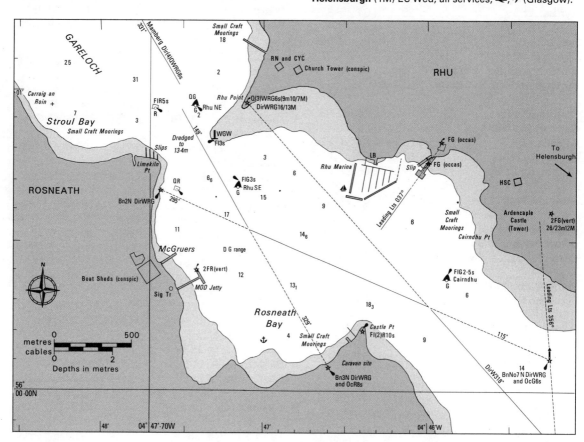

BYELAWS
Loch Long and Gareloch are classified as Dockyard Ports under the jurisdiction of the Queen's Harbour Master. Do not impede the passage of submarines/large warships.

SHELTER
Good in Gareloch. Rhu Marina has easy entrance between floating wavebreaks on its S and W sides; on SE side a drying stone bkwtr covers at half tide. Helensburgh Pier may be used, but rather exposed; keep clear of RCT craft and occas steamer. ⚓ E of marina or in Rosneath Bay. There are moorings N of the narrows at Stroul B; N of Rhu Pt; at Clynder and at the head of the loch. See also under Loch Long/Loch Goil.

Naval activity: Beware submarines from Faslane Base. See 10.9.22 for submarine activity (Subfacts) in the Clyde and offshore or call Faslane Ops ☎ (01346) 4321 Ext 6100.

Protected Areas: Vessels are never allowed within 150m of naval shore installations at Faslane and Coulport.

Restricted Areas (Faslane, Rhu Chan and Coulport): These are closed to all vessels during submarine movements (see below and *W Coast of Scotland Pilot*, App 2). MoD Police patrols enforce areas which are shown on charts. The S limit of Faslane Restricted area is marked by two Or posts with X topmarks on Shandon foreshore. The W limit is marked by Iso WRG 4s, vis W356°-006°, at Gareloch Oil fuel depot N jetty. The following signals are shown when restrictions are in force:

1. Entrance to Gareloch
   by day : Ⓡ Ⓖ Ⓖ (vert), supplemented by R flag with
   W diagonal bar.
   by night : Ⓡ Ⓖ Ⓖ (vert).
2. Faslane and Coulport
   by day : 3 Ⓖ (vert), supplemented by International
   Code pendant over pendant Nine.
   by night : 3 Ⓖ (vert) in conspic position.

HOLY LOCH, Argyll, 55°58'·5N 04°54'·0W is no longer a
restricted or protected area. There are some moorings on
the S side, and AB for about 4 boats on former USN jetty.
Possible development plans include a 400 berth marina.

LOCH LONG/LOCH GOIL, Argyll/Dumbartonshire, approx
56°00'N 04°52'·5W to 56°12'·00N 04°45'·00W. AC 3746.
Tides: See 10·9·16 for differences. ML 1·7m; Duration 0645.

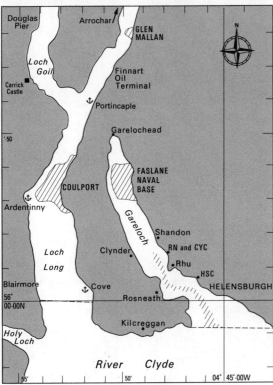

▨▨▨ Restricted Area-Max Speed 7Kn
– – – Southern Limit of Dockyard Port

Shelter: Loch Long is about 15M long. Temp ⚓s (S→N) at
Cove, Blairmore (not in S'lies), Ardentinny, Portincaple,
Coilessan (about 1M S of Ardgartan Pt), and near head of
loch (Arrochar) on either shore.
In Loch Goil ⚓ at Swines Hole and off Carrick Castle (S of
the pier, in N'lies a swell builds). Avoid ⚓ near Douglas
Pier. The head of the loch is crowded with private/dinghy
moorings, and is either too steep-to or too shallow.
Lights: Coulport Jetty, 2FG (vert) each end and two Fl G
12s on N jetty; Port Dornaige Fl 6s 8m 11M, vis 026°-206°;
Dog Rock (Carraig nan Ron) Fl 2s 11M; Finnart Oil
Terminal has FG lts and ldg lts 031° QW/FW on Cnap Pt.
Facilities: Loch Long (Cove), Cove SC, FW, Bar; V, FW
(pier); (Portincaple) shops, hotel, ✉, FW; (Ardentinny)
shop, V, R, hotel, M; (Blairmore) shops, ✉, Slip, FW;
(Arrochar) shops, hotel, FW, Gas, ✉.
Loch Goil (Carrick Castle) has ✉, shop, hotel;
(Lochgoilhead) has all stores, ✉, hotel, FW, Gas.

GREENOCK/GOUROCK   10-9-17
Renfrew 55°58'·00N 04°49'·00W (As WPT)

CHARTS
AC 1994, *2131*; Imray C63; OS 63
TIDES
+0122 Dover; ML 2·0; Duration 0640; Zone 0 (UT)

Standard Port GREENOCK (→)

Times				Height (metres)			
High Water		Low Water		MHWS	MHWN	MLWN	MLWS
0000	0600	0000	0600	3·4	2·8	1·0	0·3
1200	1800	1200	1800				
Differences PORT GLASGOW							
+0010	+0005	+0010	+0020	+0·2	+0·1	0·0	0·0
BOWLING							
+0020	+0010	+0030	+0055	+0·6	+0·5	+0·3	+0·1
RENFREW							
+0025	+0015	+0035	+0100	+0·9	+0·8	+0·5	+0·2
GLASGOW							
+0025	+0015	+0035	+0105	+1·3	+1·2	+0·6	+0·4

Greenock is a Standard Port and tidal predictions for each
day of the year are given below.

SHELTER
Gourock: good ⚓ in West Bay, but open to N/NE winds.
Greenock is a commercial port. Up-river, possible AB at
Dumbarton (McAlister's BY), Bowling Hbr and at Renfrew
Hbr, but the R Clyde is only suitable for laying-up/repairs.
NOTE: Possible marina in Gourock (Cardwell) Bay. Hbrs
are controlled by Clyde Port Authority.

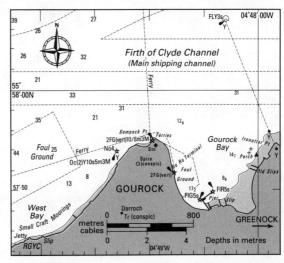

NAVIGATION
Gourock WPT 55°58'·00N 04°49'·00W, 000°/180° from/to
Kempock Pt lt, 0·22M. No navigational dangers, but much
shipping and ferries in the Clyde. Beware foul ground in
Gourock Bay. Cardwell Bay pier (lit) is disused.
LIGHTS AND MARKS
As chartlet. Note Ashton and Whiteforeland SWM buoys.
RADIO TELEPHONE
Call: *Clydeport Estuary Radio* VHF Ch 12 16 (H24). Info on
weather and traffic available on request.
TELEPHONE (Gourock/Greenock 01475; Glasgow 0141)
General Mgr Marine 725775; Estuary Control 726221;
MRCC 729988; ⌗ (0141) 8879369; Weather (0141) 246
8091; Police 724444; Marinecall 0891 500462; Dr 634617.
FACILITIES
GOUROCK: **Royal Gourock YC** ☎ 632983 M, L, FW, ME, V,
R, Bar; **Services:** SM.
Town EC Wed; P, D, V, R, Bar, ✉, Ⓑ, ⇌, ✈ (Glasgow).
GREENOCK: All facilities, but small craft not particularly
emcouraged. **Services:** AB, FW, AC, D, CH, Gas, ME, Sh,
El, Ⓔ, SM, C (45 ton).
GLASGOW (0141)
Clyde Yacht Clubs Ass'n is at Anchor Ho, Blackhall Lane,
Paisley ☎ 887 8296. Clyde Cruising Club is at Suite 408,
Pentagon Centre, 36 Washington St, Glasgow G3 8AZ
☎ 221 2774. **Services:** ACA, CH.

SCOTLAND – GREENOCK

LAT 55°57′N   LONG 4°46′W

TIMES AND HEIGHTS OF HIGH AND LOW WATERS

YEAR **1996**

TIME ZONE (UT)
For Summer Time add ONE hour in non-shaded areas

JANUARY

Day	Time	m	Time	m	Time	m	Time	m
1 M	0224	0.8	0903	3.1	1455	1.1	2148	3.1
2 TU	0320	0.8	1009	3.2	1550	0.9	2246	3.2
3 W	0410	0.7	1059	3.3	1636	0.8	2334	3.2
4 TH	0453	0.7	1141	3.4	1716	0.7		
5 F O	0017	3.2	0532	0.7	1220	3.5	1750	0.6
6 SA	0057	3.2	0607	0.6	1254	3.5	1822	0.6
7 SU	0131	3.2	0640	0.6	1325	3.6	1852	0.5
8 M	0203	3.1	0713	0.6	1356	3.6	1924	0.5
9 TU	0234	3.1	0748	0.6	1430	3.6	1959	0.5
10 W	0307	3.1	0826	0.6	1506	3.6	2037	0.5
11 TH	0344	3.1	0906	0.7	1544	3.5	2119	0.5
12 F	0423	3.1	0951	0.7	1624	3.4	2207	0.5
13 SA	0505	3.0	1041	0.8	1707	3.3	2301	0.6
14 SU	0552	2.9	1139	0.9	1757	3.2		
15 M	0001	0.7	0649	2.9	1244	1.0	1857	3.1
16 TU	0106	0.7	0805	2.9	1352	0.9	2016	3.0
17 W	0212	0.7	0931	3.0	1501	0.7	2141	3.1
18 TH	0317	0.6	1036	3.2	1602	0.5	2249	3.2
19 F	0415	0.5	1129	3.4	1654	0.3	2346	3.4
20 SA ●	0508	0.4	1217	3.6	1742	0.1		
21 SU	0039	3.5	0556	0.3	1303	3.8	1828	0.0
22 M	0130	3.5	0644	0.3	1348	3.9	1914	0.0
23 TU	0218	3.5	0731	0.3	1432	3.9	2000	0.0
24 W	0301	3.5	0817	0.4	1514	3.9	2048	0.1
25 TH	0342	3.5	0904	0.5	1555	3.8	2136	0.3
26 F	0423	3.4	0952	0.7	1638	3.7	2230	0.5
27 SA	0505	3.3	1045	0.9	1723	3.4	2333	0.8
28 SU	0550	3.2	1149	1.1	1812	3.2		
29 M	0046	0.9	0743	3.0	1310	1.2	1912	2.9
30 TU	0155	1.0	0743	2.9	1426	1.1	2112	2.8
31 W	0256	0.9	0927	3.0	1527	1.0	2228	2.9

FEBRUARY

Day	Time	m	Time	m	Time	m	Time	m
1 TH	0349	0.8	1034	3.1	1616	0.8	2318	3.0
2 F	0434	0.7	1121	3.3	1657	0.6		
3 SA	0001	3.1	0514	0.6	1201	3.4	1732	0.5
4 SU O	0041	3.1	0548	0.5	1236	3.4	1803	0.5
5 M	0116	3.1	0620	0.5	1305	3.4	1832	0.4
6 TU	0146	3.1	0650	0.5	1335	3.5	1902	0.4
7 W	0213	3.1	0723	0.4	1408	3.5	1934	0.3
8 TH	0243	3.1	0759	0.4	1444	3.5	2011	0.2
9 F	0315	3.1	0838	0.4	1521	3.5	2051	0.2
10 SA	0350	3.1	0920	0.4	1559	3.5	2136	0.3
11 SU	0427	3.1	1008	0.6	1639	3.3	2228	0.5
12 M	0508	3.0	1104	0.7	1724	3.2	2326	0.6
13 TU	0559	2.8	1209	0.8	1820	3.0		
14 W	0032	0.7	0711	2.8	1322	0.8	1935	2.9
15 TH	0145	0.8	0902	2.8	1441	0.7	2124	2.9
16 F	0300	0.7	1019	3.1	1548	0.4	2240	3.1
17 SA	0403	0.6	1113	3.4	1641	0.2	2337	3.2
18 SU ●	0456	0.4	1202	3.6	1728	0.0		
19 M	0029	3.3	0542	0.3	1249	3.7	1811	-0.1
20 TU	0116	3.4	0626	0.2	1333	3.8	1854	-0.1
21 W	0159	3.5	0709	0.2	1415	3.9	1937	0.0
22 TH	0238	3.5	0752	0.3	1455	3.9	2020	0.1
23 F	0314	3.5	0834	0.3	1533	3.8	2104	0.3
24 SA	0351	3.5	0917	0.5	1611	3.6	2150	0.5
25 SU	0429	3.4	1002	0.7	1651	3.4	2242	0.8
26 M	0510	3.2	1055	0.9	1735	3.1	2353	1.0
27 TU	0557	3.1	1212	1.1	1828	2.8		
28 W	0119	1.1	0652	2.9	1352	1.1	1937	2.6
29 TH	0227	1.1	0806	2.8	1457	1.0	2204	2.7

MARCH

Day	Time	m	Time	m	Time	m	Time	m
1 F	0323	0.9	1001	2.9	1548	0.8	2256	2.8
2 SA	0410	0.7	1054	3.1	1630	0.6	2338	3.0
3 SU	0449	0.6	1135	3.2	1706	0.6		
4 M	0016	3.0	0523	0.5	1210	3.3	1737	0.4
5 TU O	0051	3.0	0554	0.4	1239	3.3	1806	0.3
6 W	0121	3.0	0624	0.3	1310	3.4	1835	0.2
7 TH	0147	3.1	0656	0.2	1345	3.4	1908	0.1
8 F	0215	3.1	0732	0.2	1421	3.5	1945	0.1
9 SA	0247	3.2	0811	0.2	1459	3.5	2026	0.1
10 SU	0321	3.2	0854	0.2	1537	3.4	2112	0.2
11 M	0357	3.2	0943	0.3	1617	3.3	2202	0.4
12 TU	0437	3.0	1039	0.5	1642	3.1	2300	0.5
13 W	0527	2.9	1146	0.7	1758	2.9		
14 TH	0008	0.8	0637	2.7	1303	0.7	1916	2.8
15 F	0126	0.9	0840	2.8	1427	0.6	2117	2.8
16 SA	0248	0.8	1001	3.0	1533	0.3	2231	3.0
17 SU	0352	0.6	1056	3.3	1625	0.1	2325	3.2
18 M	0442	0.4	1145	3.5	1710	0.0		
19 TU ●	0013	3.3	0525	0.2	1231	3.6	1751	-0.1
20 W	0056	3.3	0606	0.2	1315	3.7	1832	-0.1
21 TH	0135	3.4	0646	0.1	1355	3.7	1912	0.0
22 F	0211	3.5	0725	0.2	1433	3.7	1952	0.0
23 SA	0245	3.5	0804	0.2	1510	3.6	2033	0.1
24 SU	0320	3.5	0844	0.4	1546	3.5	2115	0.5
25 M	0356	3.4	0926	0.5	1625	3.3	2200	0.8
26 TU	0436	3.3	1013	0.8	1708	3.0	2255	1.0
27 W	0520	3.1	1112	1.0	1758	2.8		
28 TH	0021	1.2	0613	2.9	1259	1.1	1901	2.6
29 F	0147	1.2	0718	2.8	1417	1.0	2102	2.6
30 SA	0248	1.0	0848	2.8	1511	0.8	2221	2.7
31 SU	0337	0.8	1011	2.9	1555	0.6	2305	2.9

APRIL

Day	Time	m	Time	m	Time	m	Time	m
1 M	0418	0.6	1056	3.1	1632	0.4	2344	3.2
2 TU	0453	0.4	1132	3.2	1705	0.3		
3 W	0018	3.0	0525	0.3	1206	3.2	1735	0.2
4 TH O	0049	3.1	0556	0.2	1246	3.3	1807	0.1
5 F	0118	3.1	0630	0.1	1320	3.4	1843	0.1
6 SA	0149	3.2	0708	0.0	1400	3.4	1923	0.0
7 SU	0222	3.3	0749	0.0	1440	3.4	2007	0.1
8 M	0258	3.3	0835	0.1	1520	3.4	2054	0.2
9 TU	0335	3.3	0926	0.2	1603	3.3	2146	0.4
10 W	0417	3.1	1024	0.4	1651	3.1	2244	0.6
11 TH	0510	3.0	1133	0.5	1752	2.9	2353	0.8
12 F	0624	2.8	1252	0.5	1920	2.7		
13 SA	0113	0.9	0819	2.8	1411	0.4	2106	2.8
14 SU	0232	0.8	0939	2.8	1513	0.3	2214	3.0
15 M	0335	0.6	1035	3.3	1605	0.1	2306	3.1
16 TU	0425	0.4	1124	3.4	1649	0.0	2351	3.2
17 W ●	0508	0.3	1210	3.5	1731	0.0		
18 TH	0032	3.3	0547	0.2	1253	3.5	1810	0.1
19 F	0109	3.4	0624	0.2	1334	3.5	1848	0.2
20 SA	0144	3.4	0701	0.2	1411	3.4	1927	0.3
21 SU	0218	3.5	0738	0.2	1448	3.4	2006	0.4
22 M	0253	3.5	0817	0.3	1524	3.3	2047	0.6
23 TU	0328	3.4	0858	0.5	1603	3.1	2130	0.7
24 W	0406	3.3	0942	0.6	1646	3.0	2219	0.9
25 TH	0449	3.1	1035	0.8	1736	2.8	2319	1.1
26 F	0539	2.9	1146	0.9	1834	2.6		
27 SA	0038	1.1	0639	2.8	1316	0.9	1942	2.6
28 SU	0154	1.1	0747	2.8	1421	0.8	2113	2.7
29 M	0252	0.9	0902	2.8	1510	0.6	2218	2.8
30 TU	0338	0.7	1003	3.0	1552	0.4	2303	2.9

Chart Datum: 1·62 metres below Ordnance Datum (Newlyn)

SCOTLAND – GREENOCK

LAT 55°57′N   LONG 4°46′W

TIMES AND HEIGHTS OF HIGH AND LOW WATERS

YEAR **1996**

TIME ZONE (UT)
For Summer Time add ONE hour in non-shaded areas

9

MAY

Day	Time	m	Day	Time	m
1 W	0418	0.5	**16** TH	0450	0.4
	1049	3.1		1148	3.3
	1629	0.3		1711	0.2
	2340	3.0			
2 TH	0454	0.3	**17** F ●	0007	3.2
	1131	3.2		0530	0.3
	1704	0.2		1233	3.3
				1750	0.2
3 F O	0015	3.1	**18** SA	0045	3.3
	0530	0.2		0607	0.3
	1214	3.3		1314	3.3
	1741	0.1		1829	0.3
4 SA	0051	3.2	**19** SU	0120	3.4
	0608	0.0		0642	0.3
	1257	3.3		1352	3.2
	1822	0.1		1907	0.4
5 SU	0127	3.3	**20** M	0155	3.4
	0649	0.0		0718	0.3
	1341	3.4		1428	3.2
	1905	0.1		1946	0.5
6 M	0204	3.4	**21** TU	0229	3.5
	0734	0.0		0755	0.3
	1425	3.4		1505	3.1
	1952	0.1		2025	0.6
7 TU	0242	3.4	**22** W	0304	3.4
	0822	0.0		0834	0.4
	1510	3.3		1543	3.0
	2042	0.3		2107	0.6
8 W	0323	3.4	**23** TH	0340	3.3
	0915	0.1		0917	0.5
	1557	3.2		1625	2.9
	2136	0.4		2152	0.7
9 TH	0408	3.3	**24** F	0420	3.2
	1015	0.2		1005	0.6
	1651	3.1		1713	2.8
	2235	0.6		2242	0.9
10 F	0503	3.1	**25** SA	0507	3.0
	1123	0.4		1102	0.7
	1756	2.9		1805	2.7
	2341	0.8		2340	1.0
11 SA	0617	3.0	**26** SU	0601	2.9
	1238	0.4		1207	0.8
	1915	2.8		1902	2.7
12 SU	0054	0.9	**27** M	0044	1.0
	0753	2.9		1315	0.7
	1348	0.3		2004	2.7
	2040	2.8			
13 M	0208	0.8	**28** TU	0150	0.9
	0912	3.1		0807	2.8
	1449	0.3		1415	0.6
	2148	3.0		2113	2.7
14 TU	0313	0.7	**29** W	0249	0.8
	1011	3.2		0913	2.9
	1542	0.2		1506	0.5
	2241	3.1		2215	2.9
15 W	0406	0.5	**30** TH	0340	0.6
	1102	3.3		1010	3.1
	1628	0.1		1552	0.3
	2326	3.2		2303	3.0
			31 F	0425	0.3
				1101	3.2
				1635	0.2
				2346	3.1

JUNE

Day	Time	m	Day	Time	m
1 SA O	0507	0.2	**16** SU ●	0024	3.3
	1149	3.3		0554	0.3
	1719	0.1		1258	3.1
				1814	0.4
2 SU	0028	3.3	**17** M	0101	3.3
	0550	0.0		0628	0.3
	1237	3.3		1336	3.0
	1804	0.1		1851	0.5
3 M	0109	3.4	**18** TU	0135	3.4
	0634	-0.1		0702	0.3
	1326	3.3		1412	3.0
	1851	0.1		1927	0.5
4 TU	0151	3.5	**19** W	0208	3.4
	0722	-0.1		0736	0.4
	1415	3.4		1447	3.0
	1941	0.2		2005	0.5
5 W	0233	3.6	**20** TH	0242	3.4
	0812	-0.1		0813	0.4
	1505	3.3		1524	3.0
	2033	0.3		2044	0.5
6 TH	0316	3.5	**21** F	0317	3.4
	0905	0.0		0852	0.4
	1556	3.2		1603	2.9
	2126	0.4		2125	0.6
7 F	0403	3.4	**22** SA	0355	3.3
	1003	0.1		0935	0.5
	1650	3.1		1645	2.9
	2222	0.5		2209	0.7
8 SA	0457	3.3	**23** SU	0436	3.2
	1106	0.2		1024	0.6
	1748	3.0		1731	2.8
	2323	0.7		2259	0.7
9 SU	0600	3.2	**24** M	0523	3.0
	1215	0.3		1120	0.6
	1850	3.0		1821	2.8
				2354	0.8
10 M	0029	0.8	**25** TU	0618	2.9
	0717	3.0		1220	0.6
	1322	0.4		1915	2.7
	1959	2.9			
11 TU	0140	0.8	**26** W	0054	0.8
	0839	3.0		0720	2.9
	1423	0.4		1322	0.6
	2112	2.9		2018	2.7
12 W	0248	0.7	**27** TH	0159	0.8
	0946	3.1		0829	2.9
	1519	0.3		1421	0.5
	2211	3.0		2129	2.8
13 TH	0346	0.6	**28** F	0302	0.6
	1041	3.1		0937	3.0
	1608	0.3		1518	0.4
	2301	3.1		2231	3.0
14 F	0435	0.4	**29** SA	0358	0.4
	1130	3.1		1036	3.1
	1654	0.3		1610	0.3
	2345	3.2		2322	3.1
15 SA	0516	0.4	**30** SU	0448	0.2
	1215	3.1		1130	3.2
	1735	0.4		1700	0.2

JULY

Day	Time	m	Day	Time	m
1 M O	0009	3.3	**16** TU	0044	3.3
	0535	0.0		0614	0.4
	1223	3.3		1322	3.0
	1749	0.2		1833	0.5
2 TU	0055	3.5	**17** W	0117	3.3
	0621	-0.1		0645	0.4
	1316	3.3		1357	3.0
	1838	0.2		1907	0.5
3 W	0140	3.6	**18** TH	0148	3.4
	0709	-0.2		0716	0.4
	1408	3.3		1429	3.0
	1928	0.2		1940	0.5
4 TH	0224	3.7	**19** F	0219	3.4
	0758	-0.1		0748	0.3
	1458	3.4		1501	3.0
	2018	0.2		2016	0.5
5 F	0308	3.7	**20** SA	0253	3.4
	0849	-0.1		0824	0.3
	1546	3.3		1535	3.0
	2109	0.3		2055	0.5
6 SA	0353	3.6	**21** SU	0329	3.3
	0942	0.0		0903	0.4
	1634	3.3		1613	3.0
	2201	0.4		2136	0.5
7 SU	0441	3.5	**22** M	0408	3.3
	1041	0.2		0947	0.4
	1723	3.2		1653	2.9
	2256	0.5		2222	0.6
8 M	0533	3.3	**23** TU	0449	3.2
	1146	0.4		1038	0.5
	1813	3.1		1738	2.8
	2358	0.8		2314	0.7
9 TU	0634	3.1	**24** W	0538	3.0
	1254	0.5		1137	0.6
	1909	3.0		1828	2.8
10 W	0108	0.9	**25** TH	0013	0.8
	0753	3.0		0636	2.9
	1358	0.6		1240	0.6
	2018	2.9		1930	2.7
11 TH	0222	0.9	**26** F	0118	0.8
	0921	2.9		0748	2.8
	1457	0.6		1345	0.6
	2138	2.9		2049	2.8
12 F	0327	0.7	**27** SA	0229	0.7
	1025	3.0		0910	2.9
	1550	0.5		1450	0.6
	2237	3.0		2205	2.9
13 SA	0419	0.6	**28** SU	0337	0.5
	1116	3.0		1020	3.1
	1637	0.5		1551	0.4
	2324	3.2		2303	3.2
14 SU	0503	0.5	**29** M	0432	0.2
	1202	3.0		1119	3.2
	1720	0.5		1645	0.3
				2353	3.4
15 M ●	0006	3.2	**30** TU O	0521	0.0
	0540	0.4		1213	3.3
	1244	3.0		1735	0.3
	1758	0.5			
			31 W	0041	3.5
				0607	-0.1
				1305	3.4
				1823	0.2

AUGUST

Day	Time	m	Day	Time	m
1 TH	0127	3.7	**16** F	0125	3.3
	0653	-0.2		0651	0.3
	1356	3.4		1405	3.0
	1910	0.2		1912	0.4
2 F	0211	3.8	**17** SA	0155	3.4
	0739	-0.2		0720	0.3
	1442	3.4		1433	3.0
	1957	0.2		1946	0.4
3 SA	0254	3.8	**18** SU	0228	3.4
	0826	0.0		0753	0.3
	1526	3.4		1504	3.1
	2045	0.3		2023	0.4
4 SU	0336	3.7	**19** M	0304	3.4
	0915	0.1		0831	0.3
	1607	3.4		1538	3.1
	2133	0.4		2103	0.4
5 M	0418	3.6	**20** TU	0341	3.4
	1008	0.3		0913	0.4
	1649	3.3		1615	3.1
	2223	0.6		2148	0.5
6 TU	0503	3.4	**21** W	0420	3.2
	1110	0.6		1002	0.5
	1733	3.2		1655	3.0
	2321	0.8		2240	0.6
7 W	0553	3.1	**22** TH	0503	3.1
	1223	0.8		1100	0.6
	1821	3.1		1743	2.9
				2340	0.8
8 TH	0034	1.0	**23** F	0558	2.9
	0653	2.9		1205	0.8
	1333	0.8		1846	2.8
	1917	2.9			
9 F	0157	1.0	**24** SA	0047	0.8
	0851	2.7		0712	2.8
	1435	0.8		1316	0.8
	2048	2.9		2016	2.8
10 SA	0305	0.9	**25** SU	0205	0.7
	1011	2.8		0851	2.8
	1530	0.8		1430	0.8
	2212	3.0		2145	3.0
11 SU	0359	0.7	**26** M	0320	0.5
	1103	3.0		1011	3.0
	1618	0.7		1536	0.6
	2303	3.1		2246	3.2
12 M	0443	0.5	**27** TU	0417	0.2
	1146	3.0		1111	3.2
	1701	0.6		1631	0.5
	2346	3.3		2337	3.5
13 TU	0521	0.4	**28** W O	0505	0.0
	1226	3.0		1202	3.3
	1738	0.5		1719	0.3
14 W ●	0024	3.3	**29** TH	0024	3.6
	0553	0.4		0549	-0.1
	1304	3.0		1251	3.4
	1810	0.5		1804	0.3
15 TH	0057	3.3	**30** F	0110	3.8
	0623	0.4		0632	-0.1
	1337	3.0		1337	3.5
	1841	0.5		1848	0.3
			31 SA	0154	3.8
				0715	-0.1
				1419	3.5
				1932	0.3

Chart Datum: 1·62 metres below Ordnance Datum (Newlyn)

SCOTLAND – GREENOCK

LAT 55°57'N   LONG 4°46'W

TIMES AND HEIGHTS OF HIGH AND LOW WATERS

YEAR 1996

TIME ZONE (UT)
For Summer Time add ONE hour in non-shaded areas

Chart Datum: 1·62 metres below Ordnance Datum (Newlyn)

SEPTEMBER

Day	Time	m	Time	m	Time	m	Time	m
1 SU	0235	3.8	0759	0.1	1458	3.5	2016	0.3
16 M	0203	3.5	0724	0.3	1433	3.3	1953	0.4
2 M	0314	3.8	0844	0.3	1535	3.5	2100	0.5
17 TU	0240	3.5	0803	0.3	1507	3.3	2034	0.4
3 TU	0353	3.6	0931	0.5	1613	3.5	2147	0.6
18 W	0317	3.4	0846	0.4	1542	3.2	2120	0.5
4 W	0433	3.4	1026	0.8	1655	3.3	2239	0.9
19 TH	0356	3.3	0934	0.6	1621	3.2	2213	0.6
5 TH	0518	3.1	1141	1.0	1741	3.2	2351	1.1
20 F	0438	3.2	1031	0.8	1707	3.0	2315	0.8
6 F	0611	2.9	1303	1.1	1834	3.0		
21 SA	0532	3.0	1139	0.9	1811	2.9		
7 SA	0127	1.1	0728	2.7	1408	1.1	1942	2.9
22 SU	0027	0.8	0649	2.8	1255	1.0	1950	2.9
8 SU	0237	1.0	0953	2.8	1505	1.0	2137	3.0
23 M	0150	0.8	0842	2.8	1415	1.0	2126	3.1
9 M	0332	0.8	1043	2.9	1553	0.8	2236	3.1
24 TU	0304	0.5	1003	3.1	1522	0.8	2228	3.3
10 TU	0416	0.7	1124	3.1	1635	0.6	2320	3.3
25 W	0359	0.3	1059	3.3	1616	0.6	2319	3.6
11 W	0454	0.5	1202	3.1	1712	0.6	2358	3.3
26 TH	0446	0.1	1147	3.4	1701	0.4		
12 TH ●	0527	0.4	1237	3.2	1743	0.5		
27 F O	0006	3.7	0528	0.0	1232	3.5	1743	0.3
13 F	0029	3.3	0555	0.4	1310	3.2	1812	0.5
28 SA	0051	3.8	0609	0.0	1313	3.6	1825	0.4
14 SA	0057	3.4	0622	0.3	1336	3.2	1842	0.4
29 SU	0133	3.8	0650	0.1	1352	3.6	1906	0.4
15 SU	0129	3.4	0651	0.3	1403	3.2	1916	0.4
30 M	0213	3.8	0732	0.3	1428	3.7	1947	0.4

OCTOBER

Day	Time	m	Time	m	Time	m	Time	m
1 TU	0251	3.7	0813	0.5	1504	3.7	2029	0.5
16 W	0219	3.5	0741	0.4	1441	3.5	2012	0.4
2 W	0328	3.6	0857	0.7	1541	3.6	2112	0.7
17 TH	0258	3.5	0826	0.5	1518	3.5	2100	0.5
3 TH	0407	3.4	0945	1.0	1621	3.5	2200	0.9
18 F	0339	3.4	0916	0.7	1558	3.4	2155	0.6
4 F	0450	3.2	1045	1.2	1706	3.3	2301	1.1
19 SA	0424	3.2	1013	0.9	1646	3.2	2259	0.8
5 SA	0542	2.9	1218	1.4	1758	3.2		
20 SU	0521	3.0	1121	1.1	1751	3.1		
6 SU	0042	1.2	0648	2.7	1332	1.3	1900	3.0
21 M	0013	0.8	0643	2.9	1240	1.2	1929	3.0
7 M	0159	1.2	0911	2.7	1431	1.2	2025	3.0
22 TU	0134	0.7	0830	2.9	1358	1.1	2103	3.2
8 TU	0255	1.0	1010	2.9	1522	1.0	2155	3.1
23 W	0243	0.6	0947	3.1	1504	0.9	2206	3.4
9 W	0342	0.8	1053	3.1	1604	0.8	2244	3.3
24 TH	0338	0.4	1041	3.3	1558	0.7	2258	3.6
10 TH	0421	0.6	1131	3.2	1641	0.7	2322	3.3
25 F	0425	0.2	1127	3.5	1643	0.6	2345	3.7
11 F	0454	0.5	1206	3.3	1713	0.6	2355	3.4
26 SA O	0508	0.2	1209	3.6	1725	0.5		
12 SA ●	0524	0.4	1237	3.3	1744	0.4		
27 SU	0030	3.7	0548	0.2	1249	3.6	1804	0.4
13 SU	0027	3.4	0552	0.4	1306	3.3	1815	0.4
28 M	0113	3.7	0628	0.3	1325	3.7	1843	0.4
14 M	0102	3.5	0624	0.3	1334	3.4	1849	0.4
29 TU	0152	3.7	0707	0.5	1401	3.7	1922	0.5
15 TU	0140	3.5	0700	0.3	1406	3.4	1928	0.4
30 W	0230	3.6	0748	0.6	1437	3.8	2002	0.6
31 TH	0307	3.5	0830	0.8	1514	3.7	2044	0.7

NOVEMBER

Day	Time	m	Time	m	Time	m	Time	m
1 F	0346	3.4	0914	1.0	1553	3.6	2129	0.9
16 SA	0330	3.4	0904	0.7	1546	3.6	2143	0.5
2 SA	0428	3.2	1005	1.2	1635	3.5	2222	1.1
17 SU	0419	3.3	1002	0.9	1635	3.4	2246	0.6
3 SU	0518	3.0	1111	1.4	1724	3.3	2332	1.2
18 M	0518	3.1	1107	1.1	1738	3.3	2357	0.7
4 M	0617	2.9	1235	1.4	1821	3.1		
19 TU	0633	3.0	1220	1.2	1903	3.2		
5 TU	0102	1.2	0730	2.8	1345	1.4	1926	3.1
20 W	0111	0.7	0802	3.0	1334	1.1	2033	3.3
6 W	0208	1.1	0910	2.9	1440	1.2	2042	3.1
21 TH	0217	0.6	0919	3.2	1441	1.0	2141	3.4
7 TH	0258	0.9	1010	3.1	1527	1.0	2150	3.2
22 F	0314	0.5	1016	3.3	1538	0.8	2236	3.5
8 F	0341	0.8	1053	3.2	1607	0.8	2238	3.3
23 SA	0404	0.4	1104	3.5	1626	0.7	2326	3.6
9 SA	0418	0.6	1131	3.3	1642	0.7	2318	3.4
24 SU	0448	0.4	1146	3.6	1709	0.6		
10 SU	0451	0.5	1204	3.4	1716	0.5	2357	3.4
25 M O	0011	3.6	0530	0.4	1226	3.6	1748	0.5
11 M ●	0525	0.5	1236	3.5	1751	0.4		
26 TU	0055	3.6	0610	0.5	1303	3.7	1826	0.5
12 TU	0038	3.5	0626	0.6	1310	3.5	1829	0.4
27 W	0135	3.5	0649	0.6	1339	3.8	1903	0.6
13 W	0120	3.5	0641	0.4	1346	3.6	1911	0.3
28 TH	0212	3.5	0728	0.7	1415	3.8	1941	0.6
14 TH	0202	3.4	0725	0.4	1423	3.7	1957	0.3
29 F	0249	3.4	0808	0.8	1451	3.8	2021	0.7
15 F	0245	3.5	0813	0.6	1503	3.6	2047	0.4
30 SA	0327	3.3	0850	0.9	1528	3.7	2103	0.8

DECEMBER

Day	Time	m	Time	m	Time	m	Time	m
1 SU	0408	3.2	0934	1.1	1608	3.6	2149	0.9
16 M	0414	3.4	0948	0.8	1627	3.6	2228	0.5
2 M	0453	3.1	1025	1.2	1651	3.4	2242	1.0
17 TU	0508	3.3	1048	0.9	1723	3.5	2334	0.6
3 TU	0545	3.0	1125	1.3	1741	3.3	2346	1.1
18 W	0609	3.2	1154	1.0	1829	3.3		
4 W	0642	2.9	1233	1.4	1838	3.1		
19 TH	0043	0.6	0717	3.1	1305	1.1	1952	3.2
5 TH	0056	1.1	0746	2.9	1340	1.3	1940	3.1
20 F	0150	0.7	0838	3.1	1416	1.0	2113	3.2
6 F	0200	1.0	0900	3.0	1438	1.1	2048	3.1
21 SA	0251	0.6	0946	3.2	1519	0.9	2216	3.3
7 SA	0252	0.9	1005	3.1	1528	0.9	2151	3.2
22 SU	0345	0.6	1040	3.3	1611	0.7	2310	3.4
8 SU	0338	0.7	1052	3.3	1611	0.7	2244	3.3
23 M	0433	0.6	1126	3.5	1657	0.6	2358	3.4
9 M	0419	0.6	1133	3.4	1652	0.6	2331	3.4
24 TU O	0516	0.6	1207	3.6	1737	0.6		
10 TU ●	0500	0.5	1212	3.5	1732	0.4		
25 W	0042	3.4	0556	0.6	1814	0.5		
11 W	0017	3.5	0542	0.4	1251	3.6	1813	0.3
26 TH	0123	3.3	0634	0.7	1322	3.7	1849	0.5
12 TH	0104	3.5	0626	0.4	1331	3.7	1858	0.2
27 F	0200	3.3	0711	0.7	1357	3.7	1924	0.6
13 F	0151	3.5	0713	0.4	1412	3.8	1945	0.2
28 SA	0234	3.3	0748	0.7	1431	3.7	2000	0.6
14 SA	0237	3.5	0802	0.5	1454	3.8	2036	0.3
29 SU	0309	3.2	0826	0.8	1506	3.7	2037	0.6
15 SU	0324	3.5	0854	0.6	1538	3.7	2129	0.3
30 M	0346	3.2	0905	0.8	1542	3.7	2118	0.7
31 TU	0425	3.1	0948	0.9	1621	3.5	2202	0.8

GREENOCK/GOUROCK *continued*

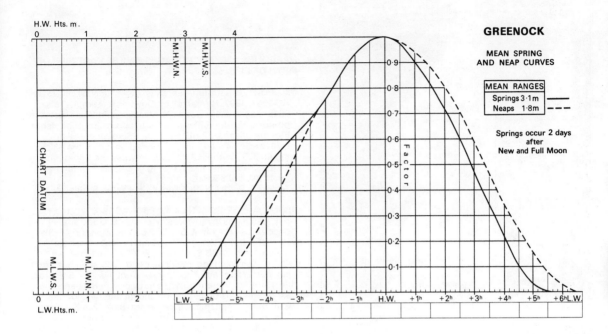

H.W. Hts. m.

GREENOCK

MEAN SPRING
AND NEAP CURVES

MEAN RANGES	
Springs 3·1m	
Neaps 1·8m	

Springs occur 2 days
after
New and Full Moon

INVERKIP (KIP MARINA)   10-9-18

Renfrew 55°54'·50N 04°53'·00W

CHARTS
AC 1907, *2131*; Imray C63; OS 63
TIDES
+0110 Dover; ML 1·8; Duration 0640; Zone 0 (UT)

Standard Port GREENOCK (←—)

Times				Height (metres)			
High Water		Low Water		MHWS	MHWN	MLWN	MLWS
0000	0600	0000	0600	3·4	2·8	1·0	0·3
1200	1800	1200	1800				
Differences WEMYSS BAY							
−0005	−0005	−0005	−0005	0·0	0·0	+0·1	+0·1

SHELTER
Excellent. Chan is navigable at all tides and dredged 1·5m; marina has 2·4m. Inverkip Bay exposed to SW/NW winds.
NAVIGATION
WPT 55°54'·48N 04°52'·95W, Kip SHM buoy, QG, at ent to buoyed chan; beware shifting bank to the N.
LIGHTS AND MARKS
Ent is ½M N of conspic chey (238m). SPM buoy marks sewer outfall off Ardgowan Pt. From Kip SHM buoy, 3 SHM and 3 PHM buoys mark 365m long appr chan.
RADIO TELEPHONE
VHF Ch **80** M (H24).
TELEPHONE (01475)
Hr Mr 521485; MRCC 729988; ✄ (0141) 887 9369; Marinecall 0891 500462; Police 521222; Dr 520248; Ⓗ 33777.
FACILITIES
Kip Marina (700+40 visitors), ☎ 521485, Fax 521298, £13.75 inc AC, D, FW, P (cans), Sh, BH (40 ton), SM, CH, V, R, Bar, Ⓞ, Gas, Gaz, YC; **Services:** ME, EI, Ⓔ.
Town EC Wed; ✉, Ⓑ (Gourock), ⇌, ✈ (Glasgow).

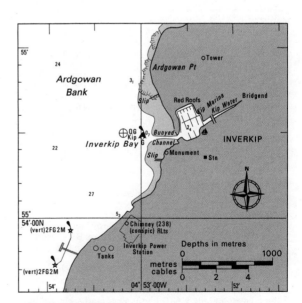

ADJACENT ANCHORAGE

DUNOON, Argyll, 55°56'·70N 04°55'·20W. AC 1994, 1907, *2131*. See 10.9.16 for tides. Temp ⚓ in either West or East Bays (S and N of Dunoon Pt). The former is open to the S; the latter more shoal. Six HIE ⚓s (free) in each bay; call ☎ (01369) 703785. The Gantocks, drying rks 3ca SE of Dunoon Pt, have W ○ bn tr, Fl R 6s 12m 6M. 2FR (vert) on ferry pier. Facilities: P & D (cans), V, R, Bar, ✉, Gas, ferry to Gourock. 3 ⚓s off Inellan, 3·7M S of Dunoon, ☎ (01369) 830445.

LARGS   10-9-19
Ayr 55°46'·40N 04°51'·77W

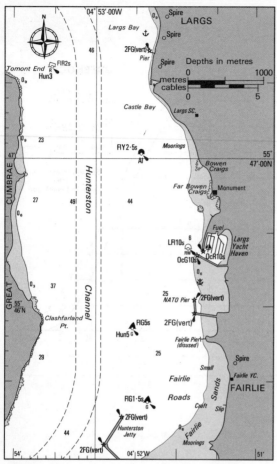

CHARTS
AC 1867, 1907, *2131*; Imray C63; OS 63
TIDES
+0105 Dover; ML 1·9; Duration 0640; Zone 0 (UT)

Standard Port GREENOCK (←)

Times				Heights (metres)			
High Water		Low Water		MHWS	MHWN	MLWN	MLWS
0000	0600	0000	0600	3·4	2·8	1·0	0·3
1200	1800	1200	1800				
Differences MILLPORT							
−0005	−0025	−0025	−0005	0·0	−0·1	0·0	+0·1
ARDROSSAN							
−0020	−0010	−0010	−0010	−0·2	−0·2	+0·1	+0·1
IRVINE							
−0020	−0020	−0030	−0010	−0·3	−0·3	−0·1	0·0

SHELTER
Excellent in Yacht Haven (1·4M S of Largs Pier) accessible at all tides (3·4m in ent; 2·0m inside). Largs B exposed to winds from S to N. Temp ‡ in 10m about ½ca N of pier.
NAVIGATION
WPT 55°46'·40N 04°51'·77W, SWM buoy off yacht haven. From S beware Hunterston and Southannan sands and outfalls from Hunterston Power Stn. The area between the S bkwtr and the NATO pier is restricted and ‡ prohib.
LIGHTS AND MARKS
"Pencil" monument (12m) is conspic 4ca N of ent. Yacht Haven SWM buoy RW, L Fl 10s; S bkwtr Oc G 10s; N bkwtr Oc R 10s 4m 4M. Largs Pier, 2 FG (vert) 7/5m 5M, when vessel expected.
RADIO TELEPHONE
Marina Ch 80 M (H24).
TELEPHONE (01475)
Yacht Haven 675333; MRCC 729988; ‡ (0141) 887 9369; Marinecall 0891 500462; Dr 673380; ⊞ 33777.

FACILITIES
Largs Yacht Haven (600, some visitors) ☎ 675333, Fax 672245, £12.94, FW, D, P, BH (45 ton), ⊚, CH, AC, SM, BY, C (17 ton), Gas, Gaz, Slip (Access H24), Bar, R;
Largs SC ☎ 520826; **Fairlie YC;**
Services: ME, Divers, El, Sh, Ⓔ.
Town EC Wed; LB, V, R, Bar, ⊠, Ⓑ, ⇌, ✈ (Glasgow).

HARBOURS AND ANCHORAGES ON THE EAST SIDE OF FIRTH OF CLYDE

MILLPORT, Great Cumbrae, Bute, 55°45'·00N 04°55'·75W. AC 1867, 1907. HW +0100 on Dover; ML 1·9m; Duration 0640. See 10.9.19. Good shelter, except in S'lies. Berth at pontoon N side of pier hd or ‡ in approx 3m S of pier or E of the Eileans. 12 HIE ⚓s 1½ca SSE of pier; call ☎ (01475) 530741. Ldg marks: pier hd on with ✠ twr 333°; or ldg lts 333°, both FR 7/9m 5M, between the Spoig and the Eileans, QG. Unmarked, drying rk is close E of ldg line. Hr Mr ☎ (01475) 530826.
Town EC Wed; CH, Bar, Gas, D, P, FW, ⊠, R, Slip, V.

IRVINE, Ayr, 55°36'·17N 04°42'·00W. AC 1866, 2220, *2126*. HW +0055 on Dover. Tides: see 10.9.19. Good shelter once across the bar (0·5m CD); access approx HW ±3½ for 1·4m draft. Do not attempt ent in heavy onshore weather. The 1-BB SPM buoy, Fl Y 3s, is 1·15M from hbr ent, close NW of ldg line. 5 blocks of flats and chys are conspic ENE of ent. Ldg lts 051°: front, FG 10m 5M; rear, FR 15m 5M. The ent groynes have bns, Fl R 3s and Fl G 3s; groynes inside the ent have unlit perches. W Pilot tr with mast is conspic 3ca inside ent. Berth 2ca beyond this on S side at visitors' quay (2·2m). ‡ prohib. VHF Ch 12 (0800-1600 Tues and Thurs; 0800-1300 Wed). Hr Mr ☎ (01294) 487254/278132. Facilities: **Quay** AB, FW, Slip, C (3 ton), Showers, SM. **Town** P & D (cans, 1·5km), Gas, V, R, ⇌, ✈ (Prestwick).

AYR, Ayr, 55°28'·22N 04°38'·71W. AC 1866, 2220, *2126*. HW +0050 on Dover; ML 1·8m. Duration 0630. See 10.9.20. Good shelter except in W winds when shelter can be found in the dock. Beware St Nicholas Rk to S of ent and large amounts of debris being washed down the R Ayr after heavy rains. Ent is not easy for larger yachts. Ldg lts 098°: front, by Pilot Stn, FR 10m 5M R tr, also tfc sigs; rear (130m from front), Oc R 10s 18m 10M. N bkwtr hd, QR 9m 5M. S pier hd, Q 7m 7M, vis 012°-161°, and FG 5m 5M, vis 012°-082°, over St Nicholas Rk. N Quay hd, 2 B ●s (vert) or 2FR (vert) = hbr closed. 1 B ● (1 Ⓡ or 1 Ⓖ) = proceed with care. Hr Mr ☎ (01292) 281687; VHF Ch 14 16; ‡ (0141) 887 9369; **Services:** Sh, ME, El, CH. **Town** EC Wed; Ⓑ, ⊠, Bar, Gas, D, FW, ⊠, R, ⇌, V.

GIRVAN, Ayr, 55°14'·77N 04°51'·80W. AC 1866, 2199. HW +0043 on Dover; ML 1·8m; Duration 0630. See 10.9.20. Good shelter for 16 yachts on 60m pontoon in 1·7m. Coasters and FVs berth on quay. No access LW±2 over bar 1·5m. Beware Girvan Patch, 2·4m, 4ca SW of ent, and Brest Rks, 3·5M N of hbr extending 6ca offshore. Ch spire (conspic) brg 104° leads between N bkwtr, Fl (2) R 6s 7m 4M, and S pier, 2 FG (vert) 8m 4M. Tfc sigs at S pier: 2 B discs (hor), at night 2 Ⓡ (hor) = hbr shut. VHF Ch 12 16 (HO). Hr Mr ☎ (01465) 713048; FW, Slip. **Town** EC Wed; Ⓑ, ⊠, R, ⇌, P & D (cans), V.

LOCH RYAN, Wigtown, 55°01'·00N 05°05'·00W. AC 1403, 2198. HW (Stranraer) +0055 on Dover; ML 1·6m; Duration 0640. See 10.9.20. Very good shelter except in strong NW winds. Ent between Milleur Pt and Finnarts Pt. ‡s in Lady Bay, 1·3M SSE of Milleur Pt, but exposed to heavy wash from fast catamaran ferries; in The Wig in 3m (avoid weed patches); or off Stranraer 3ca NW of W pier hd. Larger yachts berth on NE side of E pier, by arrangement with Hr Mr, VHF Ch 14 (H24) or ☎ (01776) 702460. Beware The Beef Barrel, rk 1m high 6ca SSE of Milleur Pt; the sand spit running 1·5M to SE from W shore opposite Cairn Pt lt ho Fl (2) R 10s 14m 12M. Lt at Cairnryan ferry terminal Fl R 5s 5m 5M. Lts at Stranraer: centre pier hd 2FBu (vert), E pier hd 2FR (vert), W pier hd 2 FG (vert) 8m 4M. Facilities (Stranraer): EC Wed; Ⓑ, Bar, D, FW, P, ⊠, R, ⇌, V.

TROON   10-9-20

Ayr 55°33'·10N 04°40'·90W

CHARTS
AC 1866, 2220, *2126*; Imray C63; OS 70

TIDES
+0050 Dover; ML 1·9; Duration 0630; Zone 0 (UT)

Standard Port GREENOCK (←)

Times				Height (metres)			
High Water		Low Water		MHWS	MHWN	MLWN	MLWS
0000	0600	0000	0600	3·4	2·8	1·0	0·3
1200	1800	1200	1800				
Differences TROON							
–0025	–0025	–0020	–0020	–0·2	–0·2	0·0	0·0
AYR							
–0025	–0025	–0030	–0015	–0·4	–0·3	+0·1	+0·1
GIRVAN							
–0025	–0040	–0035	–0010	–0·3	–0·3	–0·1	0·0
LOCH RYAN (Stranraer)							
–0020	–0020	–0017	–0017	–0·4	–0·4	–0·4	–0·2

SHELTER
Complete in marina (2·3m); 5kn speed limit. Strong SW/NW winds cause heavy seas in the apprs. Inside hbr, keep clear of Ailsa Shipyard.

NAVIGATION
WPT 55°33'·20N 04°42'·00W, 283°/103° from/to W pier lt, 0·61M. Appr in sector SW to NW. Beware Lady Isle, Fl (4) 30s, 2·2M SW; Troon Rk (5·6m) 1·1M W; Lappock Rk (G bn) 1·6M NNW; Mill Rk ½M NNE of hbr ent, PHM buoy.

LIGHTS AND MARKS
No ldg lts. Sheds (35m) at Ailsa Shipyard are conspic and floodlit at night. Ent sigs (not applicable to yachts): 2B ●s or 2F® lts (vert) = ent/exit prohib. W pier hd Oc WG 6s 11m 5M, G036°-090°, W090°-036°. 14m SE of this lt there is a floodlit dolphin, W with dayglow patches.

RADIO TELEPHONE
Marina VHF Ch 80 M (H24). Other station: Ardrossan Ch 16; 12 14 (H24).

TELEPHONE (01292)
Hr Mr 315553; MRCC (01475) 729988; ⌗ (0141) 887 9369; Marinecall 0891 500462; Police 313100; Dr 313593/312489; Ⓗ 610553.

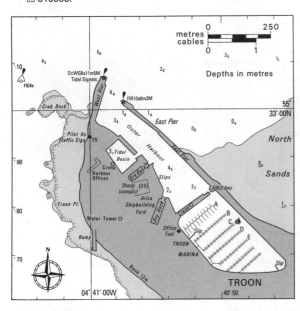

FACILITIES
Troon Yacht Haven (marina: 345+40 visitors) ☎ 315553, Fax 312836, £12.16, access all tides, D, FW, ME, El, Ⓔ, CH, AC, Sh (on-site repairs ☎ 316180), BH (12 ton), C (2 ton), Slip, V, R, Bar, ⌷, Gas, Gaz; **Hbr Pier** FW, Sh, AB, V; **Troon Cruising Club** ☎ 311190; **Ailsa Shipyard** has all normal 'big ship' repair facilities.
Town EC Wed; ✉, Ⓑ, ⇌, ✈ (Prestwick/Glasgow).

PORTPATRICK   10-9-21

Wigtown 50°50'·42N 05°07'·11W

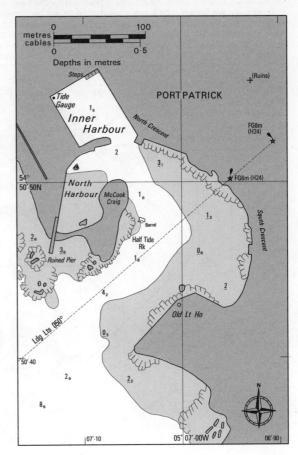

CHARTS
AC 2198, *2724*; Imray C62; OS 82

TIDES
+0032 Dover; ML 2·1; Duration 0615; Zone 0 (UT)

Standard Port LIVERPOOL (→)

Times				Heights (metres)			
High Water		Low Water		MHWS	MHWN	MLWN	MLWS
0000	0600	0200	0800	9·3	7·4	2·9	0·9
1200	1800	1400	2000				
Differences PORTPATRICK							
+0018	+0026	0000	–0035	–5·5	–4·4	–2·0	–0·6

SHELTER
Good in Inner hbr, but ent is difficult in strong SW/NW winds. Beware cross tides off ent, up to 3kn at springs.

NAVIGATION
WPT 54°50'·00N 05°08'·00W, 235°/055° from/to ent, 0·70M. Ent to outer hbr by short narrow chan with hazards either side, including rky shelf covered at HW. Barrel buoy marks end of Half Tide Rk.

LIGHTS AND MARKS
Killantringan lt ho, Fl (2) 15s 49m 25M, is 1.6M NW of ent. Ldg lts 050°, FG (H24) 6/8m: Front on sea wall; rear on bldg; 2 vert orange stripes by day. Conspic features include: TV mast 1M NE, almost on ldg line; large hotel on cliffs about 1½ca NNW of hbr ent; Dunskey Castle (ru) 4ca SE of hbr.

RADIO TELEPHONE
None. Portpatrick Coast Radio Stn VHF Ch 27 16.

TELEPHONE (01776)
Hr Mr 810355; MRSC (01475) 729988; ⌗ (0141) 887 9369; Marinecall 0891 500462; Police 810222; Ⓗ 702323.

FACILITIES
Hbr Slip (small craft), M, FW, L, AB £6. Note: Pontoons are planned in inner hbr, to be dredged approx 2·5m.
Village EC Thurs; P (cans), D (bulk tanker), Gas, V, R, Bar, ✉, Ⓑ (Stranraer), ⇌ (bus to Stranraer), ✈ (Carlisle).

9

SUBMARINE EXERCISE AREAS (SUBFACTS)

Those areas where submarine activity is planned for the next 16 hrs are broadcast by Coast Radio Stns at the times and on the channels shown below. The areas are referred to not by numbers, but by names as listed in 10.8.20 (Areas 1 – 26, N of Mull). Clyde, Oban and Belfast CG will supply Subfacts on request Ch 16. Clyde CG also broadcasts Subfacts on Ch 67 for the Clyde Areas (out to the SW boundary of Areas 67, 72 and 75), at the times below. Subfacts follow after the forecast. A Fisherman's Hotline ☎ (01374) 613097 can answer queries. Submarines on the surface and at periscope depth always listen on Ch 16. The former will comply strictly with IRPCS; the latter will not close to within 1500 yds of a FV without its express permission.

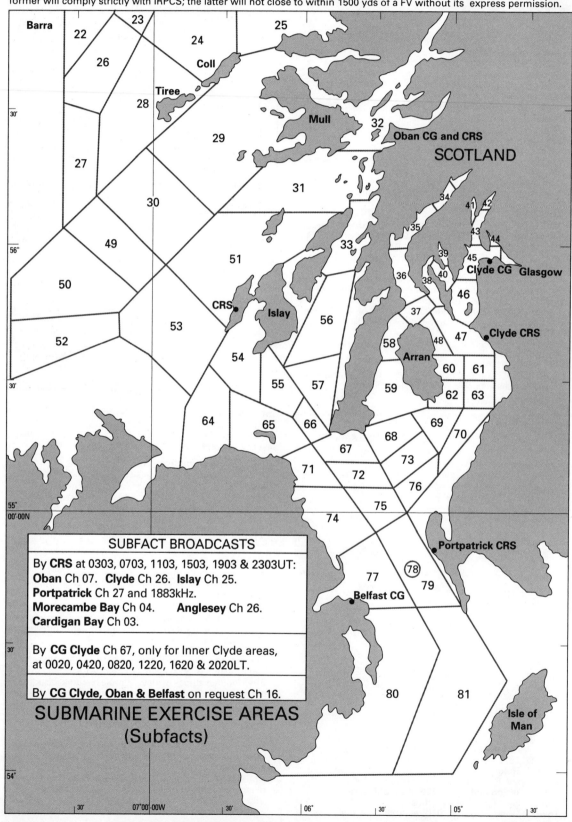

SUBFACT BROADCASTS

By **CRS** at 0303, 0703, 1103, 1503, 1903 & 2303UT:
Oban Ch 07.   **Clyde** Ch 26.   **Islay** Ch 25.
Portpatrick Ch 27 and 1883kHz.
Morecambe Bay Ch 04.   **Anglesey** Ch 26.
Cardigan Bay Ch 03.

By **CG Clyde** Ch 67, only for Inner Clyde areas,
at 0020, 0420, 0820, 1220, 1620 & 2020LT.

By **CG Clyde, Oban & Belfast** on request Ch 16.

SUBMARINE EXERCISE AREAS
(Subfacts)

Area 10

North-West England,
Isle of Man and North Wales
Mull of Galloway to Bardsey Island

10

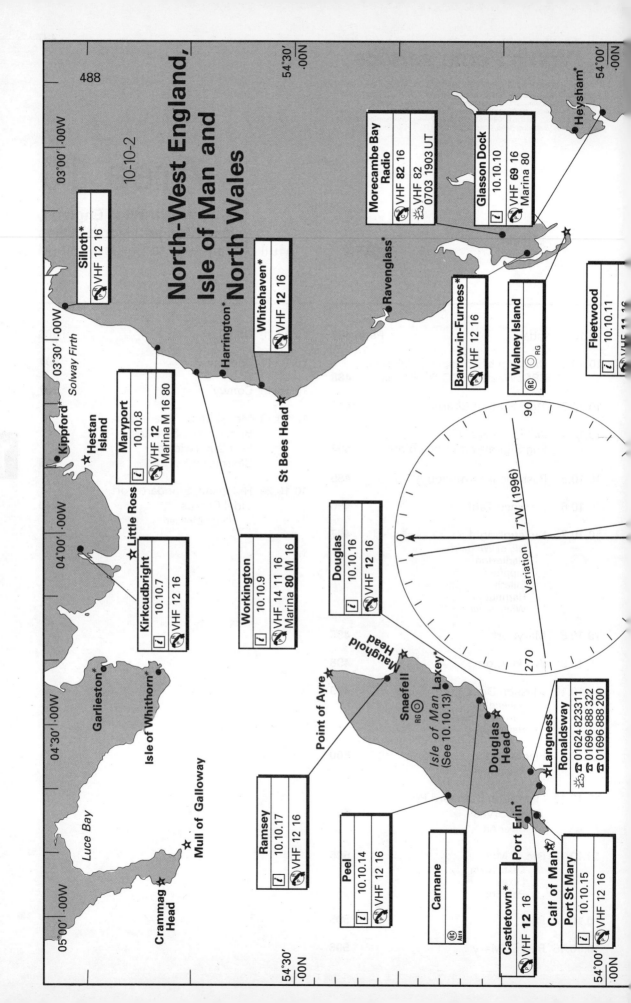

488

10-10-2

North-West England, Isle of Man and North Wales

Silloth*
🅿️🔧 VHF 12 16

Maryport
ℹ️ 10.10.8
🅿️🔧 VHF 12
Marina M 16 80

Whitehaven*
🅿️🔧 VHF 12 16

Morecambe Bay Radio
📡 VHF 82 16
🌦️ VHF 82
0703 1903 UT

Glasson Dock
ℹ️ 10.10.10
🅿️🔧 VHF 69 16
Marina 80

Barrow-in-Furness*
🅿️🔧 VHF 12 16

Walney Island
🆁🅲 ⊙ RG

Fleetwood
ℹ️ 10.10.11
🅿️🔧 VHF 11 16

Solway Firth

Kippford*

☆ Hestan Island

☆ Little Ross

Harrington*

St Bees Head ☆

Ravenglass*

Heysham*

Kirkcudbright
ℹ️ 10.10.7
🅿️🔧 VHF 12 16

Workington
ℹ️ 10.10.9
🅿️🔧 VHF 14 11 16
Marina 80 M 16

Douglas
ℹ️ 10.10.16
🅿️🔧 VHF 12 16

Garlieston*

☆ Isle of Whithorn*

Maughold Head ☆

Snaefell ⊙ RG

Point of Ayre

Isle of Man Laxey*
(See 10.10.13)

Douglas Head ☆

Ramsey
ℹ️ 10.10.17
🅿️🔧 VHF 12 16

Peel
ℹ️ 10.10.14
🅿️🔧 VHF 12 16

Carnane
🆁🅲 Aero

Castletown*
🅿️🔧 VHF 12 16

Port Erin*

Calf of Man ☆

Port St Mary
ℹ️ 10.10.15
🅿️🔧 VHF 12 16

Langness ☆

Ronaldsway
🌦️ ☎ 01624 823311
☎ 01696 888 322
☎ 01696 888 200

Mull of Galloway ☆

Luce Bay

Crammag Head ☆

Variation
7°W (1996)

0

90

270

54°30′
.00N

54°00′
.00N

54°30′
.00N

54°00′
.00N

03°00′ .00W

03°30′ .00W

04°00′ .00W

04°30′ .00W

05°00′ .00W

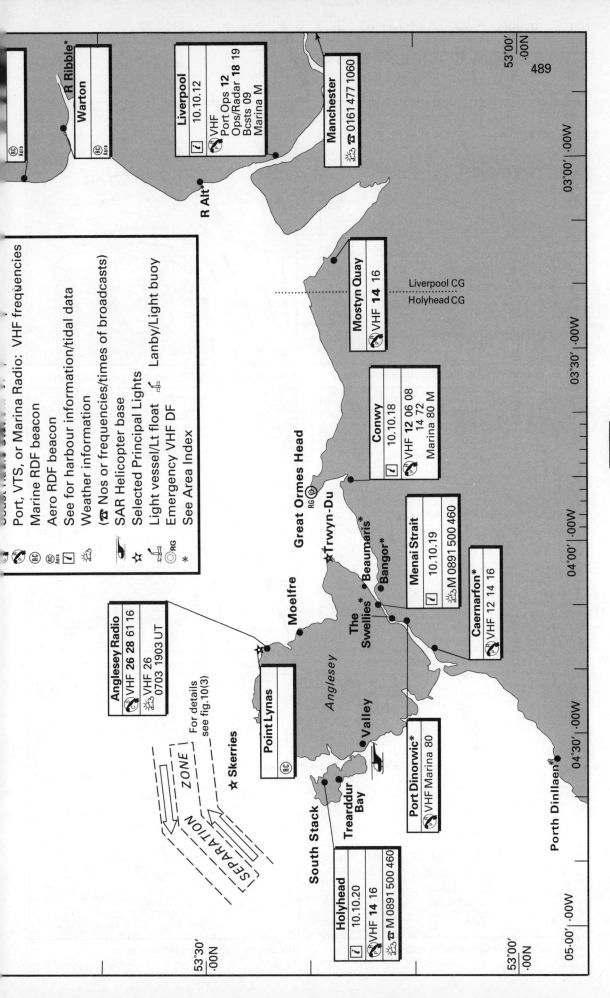

R Ribble

Warton

Liverpool 10.10.12

ℹ️ 🚢 VHF
Port Ops **12**
Ops/Radar **18** 19
Bcsts 09
Marina M

R Alt*

Manchester

☎ 0161 477 1060

Mostyn Quay

🚢 VHF **14** 16

Liverpool CG

Holyhead CG

Port, VTS, or Marina Radio: VHF frequencies

Marine RDF beacon

Aero RDF beacon

ℹ️ See for harbour information/tidal data

Weather information
(☎ Nos or frequencies/times of broadcasts)

SAR Helicopter base

☆ Selected Principal Lights

Light vessel/Lt float   Lanby/Light buoy

Emergency VHF DF

* See Area Index

10

Conwy 10.10.18

ℹ️ 🚢 VHF **12** 06 08
14 72
Marina 80 M

Great Ormes Head

RG⊚

☆Trwyn-Du

Moelfre

Beaumaris*

Bangor*

Menai Strait 10.10.19

ℹ️ 🚢 M 0891 500 460

Caernarfon*

🚢 VHF 12 14 16

Anglesey Radio

🚢 VHF 26 28 61 16

🚢 VHF 26
0703 1903 UT

The
Swellies*

Anglesey

For details
see fig.10(3)

Point Lynas

RC

☆ Skerries

ZONE

SEPARATION

Valley

Port Dinorwic*

🚢 VHF Marina 80

South Stack

Trearddur
Bay

Holyhead 10.10.20

ℹ️ 🚢 VHF **14** 16
🚢 M 0891 500 460

Porth Dinllaen*

53°30′
.00N

53°00′
.00N

05·00′·00W   04°30′·00W   04·00′·00W   03°30′·00W   03·00′·00W

53°00′
.00N

10-10-3 AREA 10 TIDAL STREAMS

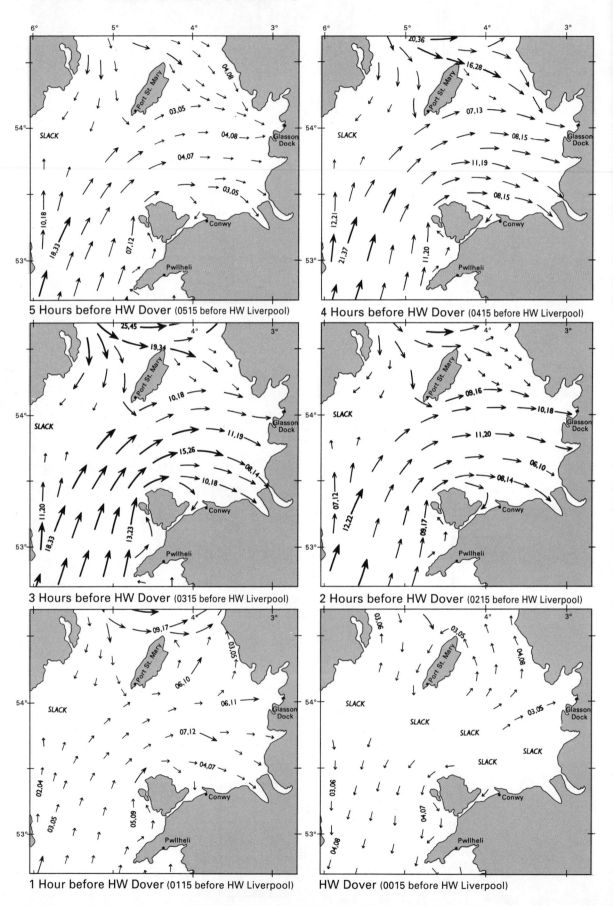

5 Hours before HW Dover (0515 before HW Liverpool)

4 Hours before HW Dover (0415 before HW Liverpool)

3 Hours before HW Dover (0315 before HW Liverpool)

2 Hours before HW Dover (0215 before HW Liverpool)

1 Hour before HW Dover (0115 before HW Liverpool)

HW Dover (0015 before HW Liverpool)

Northward 10.9.3   Southward 10.11.3   North Ireland 10.13.3   South Ireland 10.12.3

1 Hour after HW Dover (0045 after HW Liverpool)

2 Hours after HW Dover (0145 after HW Liverpool)

3 Hours after HW Dover (0245 after HW Liverpool)

4 Hours after HW Dover (0345 after HW Liverpool)

5 Hours after HW Dover (0445 after HW Liverpool)

6 Hours after HW Dover (0545 after HW Liverpool)

10.10.4 COASTAL LIGHTS, FOG SIGNALS AND WAYPOINTS

Abbreviations used below are given in 1.4.1. Principal lights are in **bold** print, places in CAPITALS, and light-vessels, light floats and Lanbys in *CAPITAL ITALICS*. Unless otherwise stated lights are white. m – elevation in metres; M – nominal range in miles. Fog signals are in *italics*. Useful waypoints are underlined – use those on land with care. All geographical positions should be assumed to be approximate. See 4.4.1.

SOLWAY FIRTH TO BARROW-IN-FURNESS

ISLE OF WHITHORN/GARLIESTON
Port William Ldg Lts 105°. Front Pier Hd 54°45'·65N 04°35'·10W Fl G 3s 7m 3M. Rear, 130m from front, FG 10m 2M.
Isle of Whithorn Hbr E Pier Hd 54°41'·8N 04°21'·7W QG 4m 5M; Gy col.
Ldg Lts 335°. Front 54°42'·01N 04°22'·00W Oc R 8s 7m 7M; Or ◆. Rear, 35m from front, Oc R 8s 9m 7M; Or ◆, synch.
Garlieston Pier Hd 54°47'·30N 04°21'·70W 2 FR (vert) 8m 3M.

Little Ross 54°45'·93N 04°05'·02W Fl 5s 50m 12M; W Tr; obsc in Wigtown B when brg more than 103°.

KIRKCUDBRIGHT BAY/KIPPFORD
No. 1 Lifeboat House 54°47'·68N 04°03'·66W Fl 3s 7m 3M.
Perch No.12 54°49'·13N 04°04'·76W Fl R 3s 3m.
Perch No.14 54°49'·25N 04°04'·76W Fl 3s 5m.
Perch No. 22 54°50'·08N 04°03'·93W Fl R 3s 2m.
Outfall 54°50'·18N 04°03'·76W Fl Y 5s 3m 2M; Y Tr.
Hestan I E end 54°49'·90N 03°48'·40W Fl (2) 10s 38m 7M; W house.

Barnkirk Pt 54°58'·00N 03°15'·90W Fl 2s 18m 2M.

SILLOTH
Two Feet Bank By 54°42'·40N 03°44'·40W; WCM.
Solway Lt By 54°46'·80N 03°30'·05W Fl G; SHM.
Corner Lt By 54°48'·90N 03°29'·45W Fl G; SHM.
Lees Scar Lt Bn 54°51'·80N 03°24'·75W QG 11m 8M; W structure on piles; vis 005°-317°.
E Cote 50°52'·78N 03°22'·78W FG 15m 12M; vis 046°-058°.
Groyne Hd 54°52'·14N 03°23'·84W 2 FG (vert) 4m 4M; Fl Bu tfc signals close by.

MARYPORT
S Pier Hd 54°43'·05N 03°30'·60W Fl 1·5s 10m 4M.

WORKINGTON/HARRINGTON
N Workington By 54°40'·10N 03°38'·10W; NCM.
S Workington Lt By 54°37'·00N 03°38'·50W Q (6) + L Fl 15s; SCM.
S Pier 54°39'·13N 03°34'·71W Fl 5s 11m 8M; R bldg; *Siren 20s.*
Ldg Lts 131·8°. Front 54°38'·92N 03°34'·12W FR 10m 3M. Rear, 134m from front, FR 12m 3M; both on W pyramidal Tr, Or bands.

WHITEHAVEN
W Pier Hd 54°33'·16N 03°35'·84W Fl G 5s 16m 13M; W● Tr.
N Pier Hd 54°33'·17N 03°35'·67W 2 FR (vert) 8m 9M; W● Tr.

Saint Bees Hd 54°30'·80N 03°38'·15W Fl (2) 20s 102m **21M**; W ● Tr; obsc shore-340°.

RAVENGLASS
Blockhouse 54°20'·15N 03°25'·27W FG; occasl.
Selker Lt By 54°16'·13N 03°29'·50W Fl (3) G 10s; SHM; *Bell.*

BARROW-IN-FURNESS
Lightning Knoll Lt By 53°59'·83N 03°14'·20W L Fl 10s; SWM; *Bell.*
Halfway Lt By 54°01'·40N 03°11'·87W Fl R 5s; PHM.
Outer Bar Lt By 54°02'·00N 03°11'·05W Fl (4) R 10s; PHM.
Bar Lt By 54°02'·61N 03°10'·15W Fl (2) R 5s; PHM.
Isle of Walney 54°02'·92N 03°10'·65W Fl 15s 21m **23M**; stone Tr; obsc 122°-127° within 3M of shore; RC.
Walney Chan Ldg Lts 040·7°. No. 1 Front 54°03'·33N 03°08'·93W Q 7m 10M; Pile, Or daymark. No. 2 Rear, 0·61M from front, Iso 2s 13m 10M; Pile, Or daymark.
Haws Pt Bn 54°02'·98N 03°10'·03W QR 8m 6M.
Rampside Sands Ldg Lts 005·1°. No. 3 Front 54°04'·40N 03°09'·70W Q 9m10M; W ● Tr. No. 4 Rear, 0·77M from front, Iso 2s 14m 6M; R col, W face.

BARROW TO RIVERS MERSEY AND DEE

MORECAMBE
Morecambe Lt By 53°52'·00N 03°24'·00W Q (9) 15s; WCM; *Whis.*
Lune Deep Lt By 53°55'·80N 03°11'·00W Q (6) + L Fl 15s; SCM; *Whis;* Racon.
Shell Wharf Lt By 53°55'·45N 03°08'·88W Fl G 2·5s; SHM
King Scar Lt By 53°56'·95N 03°04'·30W Fl G 2·5s; SHM.
Sewer outfall 54°04'·33N 02°53'·74W Fl G 2s 4m 2M; Tr.
Lts in line about 090°. Front 54°04'·40N 02°52'·52W FR 10m 2M; G mast. Rear, 140m from front, FR 14m 2M; G mast.

HEYSHAM
S Outfall 54°01'·73N 02°55'·73W Fl (2) G 10s 5m 2M.
N Outfall 54°01'·85N 02°55'·69W Fl G 5s 5m 2M; metal post.
S Bkwtr Hd 54°01'·90N 02°55'·64W 2 FG (vert) 9m 5M; W Tr; Ra refl; *Siren 30s.*
SW Quay Ldg Lts 102·2°. Front 54°01'·90N 02°55'·13W both F Bu 11/14m 2M; Or & B ◆ on masts.
S Pier Hd 54°01'·90N 02°55'·35W Oc G 7·5s 9m 6M.

RIVER LUNE/GLASSON DOCK
R Lune No.1 Lt By 53°58'·62N 02°59'·99W Q (9) 15s; WCM.
Ldg Lts 083·7°. Front, Plover Scar 53°58'·87N 02°52'·88W Fl 2s 6m 6M; W Tr, B lantern. Rear, 854m from front, Cockersand Abbey F 18m 8M; R Tr (chan liable to change).
Crook Perch, No. 7   53°59'·45N 02°52'·28W Fl G 5s 3M; G ▲ on mast.
Bazil Perch, No. 16 54°00'·19N 02°51'·58W Fl (3) R 10s 3M.
Glasson Quay 54°00'·02N 02°50·94W FG 1M.

FLEETWOOD
Fairway No. 1 Lt By 53°57'·65N 03°02'·15W Q; NCM; *Bell .*
Esplanade Ldg Lts 156°. Front 53°55'·70N 03°00'·47W Fl G 2s 14m. Rear, 320m from front, Fl G 4s 28m. Both stone Trs. Vis on Ldg line only. (H24) (chan liable to change).
Steep Breast Perch 53°55'·73N 03°00'·49W Iso G 2s 3m 2M.
Knott End slip Hd 53°55'·72N 03°00'·02W 2 FR (vert) 3m 2M.

BLACKPOOL
N Pier Hd 53°49'·16N 03°03'·83W 2 FG (vert) 3M.
Central Pier Hd 53°48'·65N 03°03'·55W 2 FG (vert) 4M.
Obstn By 53°48'·45N 03°04'·22W; SHM.
S Pier Hd 53°47'·72N 03°03'·60W 2 FG (vert) 4M.
Blackpool Tr 53°48'·95N 03°03'·26W Aero FR 158m.

RIVER RIBBLE
Gut Lt By 53°41'·75N 03°08'·90W L Fl 10s, SWM.
Perches show Fl R on N side, and Fl G on S side of chan.
S side, 14·3M Perch 53°42'·75N 03°04'·85W Fl G 5s 6m 3M.
Southport Pier Hd 52°39'·35N 03°01'·25W 2 FG (vert) 6m 5M; W post; vis 033°-213°.

El Oso Wreck Lt By 53°37'·55N 03°23'·45W Q; NCM.
Jordan's Spit Lt By 53°35'·75N 03°19'·20W Q (9) 15s; WCM.
FT Lt By 53°34'·55N 03°13'·12W Q; NCM.
Spoil Ground Lt By 53°34'·25N 03°17'·30W Fl Y 3s; SPM.

RIVER MERSEY/LIVERPOOL
BARLtF 53°32'·00N 03°20'·90W Fl 5s 10m 12M; R structure
on By; Racon (T); *Horn (2) 20s.*
Q 1 Lt F 53°31'·00N 03°16'·62W VQ; NCM.
Q 2 Lt F 53°31'·47N 03°14'·87W VQ R; PHM.
Q 3 Lt By 53°30'·95N 03°15'·00W Fl G 3s; SHM.
Burbo Trs Lt By 53°30'·41N 03°17'·52W Fl (3) G 9s; SHM.
FORMBY Lt F 53°31'·10N 03°13'·45W Iso 4s 11m 6M; R
hull, W stripes.
C 4 Lt F 53°31'·82N 03°08'·42W Fl R 3s; PHM.
CROSBY Lt F 53°30'·72N 03°06'·21W Oc 5s 11m 8M; R hull,
W stripes.
C 14 Lt F 53°29'·91N 03°05'·27W Fl R 3s; PHM.
BRAZIL Lt F 53°26'·83N 03°02'·18W QG; SHM.
Seacombe Ferry N and S corners 53°24'·6N 03°00'·8W 3 FG
5m 5M; near N corner FY 8m 6M; *Bell (3) 20s* .
Birkenhead, Woodside Landing Stage N end 53°23'·7N
03°00'·4W 3 FG 5m 4M and S end 2 FG (vert) with *Bell (4) 15s.*
Cammell Laird slip, SE corner 53°23'·96N 03°00'·22W
Fl (2) G 6s 5m 5M.
Pluckington Bk Lt By 53°22'·99N 02°59'·48W VQ (9) 10s; WCM.
Brombro Lt By 53°21'·81N 02°58'·59W Q (3) 10s; ECM.
Eastham Locks E Dn 53°19'·57N 02°56'·92W Fl (2) R 6s 5m 8M.
Garston NW Dn 53°20'·87N 02°54'·54W 2 FG (vert) 12m 9M;
Horn 11s.

RIVER DEE
HE1 Lt By 53°26'·31N 03°18'·00W Q (9) 15s; WCM.
HE2 Lt By 53°26'·20N 03°16'·80W Q (3) 10s; ECM.
HE3 Lt By 53°24'·75N 03°12'·90W; SHM.
Hilbre I 53°22'·97N 03°13'·70W Fl R 3s 14m 5M; W Tr.
HE 4 By 53°22'·30N 03°14'·20W; SHM.

MOSTYN/CONNAH'S QUAY
Mostyn Training wall Hd 53°19'·52N 03°15'·62W 2 FR (vert)
10m 3M; B mast.
Mostyn Ldg Lts 215·7°. Front 53°19'·18N 03°16'·15W FR
12m; W ♦ on B mast. Rear, 135m from front, FR 22m; W ♦
on B mast.
Flint Sands N Training wall Hd 53°15'·05N 03°06'·40W Fl R 3s
4m 6M; Tr.
Connah's Quay S Training wall Hd 53°13'·75N 03°04'·02W
Fl G 10s 3m 6M; Tr.

WELSH CHANNEL
Bank Lt By 53°20'·31N 03°15'·96W Fl R 5s; PHM.
Mostyn Lt By 53°21'·00N 03°16'·40W Fl (4) G 15s; SHM.
NE Mostyn Lt By 53°21'·48N 03°17'·73W Fl (3) G 10s; SHM.
Air By 53°21'·83N 03°19'·20W SHM.
Dee Lt By 53°21'·97N 03°18'·78W Q (6) + L Fl 15s; SCM.
E Hoyle Lt By 53°22'·03N 03°21'·03W Fl (4) R 15s; PHM.
Earwig Lt By 53°21'·37N 03°23'·50W Fl (2) G 5s; SHM.
S Hoyle Lt By 53°21'·40N 03°24'·78W Fl (3) R 10s; PHM.
Mid Hoyle By 53°22'·90N 03°19'·63W; PHM.
Hoyle Lt By 53°23'·14N 03°21'·30W QR; PHM.
NW Hoyle Lt By 53°26'·67N 03°50'·50W VQ; NCM.
N Hoyle Lt By 53°26'·67N 03°50'·50W VQ; NCM.

ISLE OF MAN

Point of Ayre 54°24'·95N 04°22'·03W Fl (4) 20s 32m **19M**;
W Tr, two R bands; Racon (M); *Horn (3) 60s.*
Low Lt 54°25'·05N 04°21'·80W Fl 3s 10m 8M; R Tr, lower
part W, on B Base; part obsc 335°-341°.

JURBY/PEEL
Cronk y Cliwe 54°22'·30N 04°31'·40W 2 Fl R 5s (vert); synch.
Orrisdale 54°19'·30N 04°34'·10W 2 Fl R 5s (vert); synch.
Peel Bkwtr Hd 54°13'·67N 04°41'·62W Oc 7s 11m 6M; W Tr;
Bell (4)12s (occas).
Peel Groyne Hd 54°13'·55N 04°41'·60W Iso R 2s 4m.

PORT ERIN
Ldg Lts 099·1°. Front 54°05'·23N 04°45'·49W FR 10m 5M; W
Tr, R band. Rear, 39m from front, FR 19m 5M; W col, R band.
Raglan Pier Hd 54°05'·11N 04°45'·79W Oc G 5s 8m 5M.

Thousla Rk 54°03'·71N 04°47'·97W Fl R 3s 9m 4M.
Calf of Man W Pt 54°03'·20N 04°49'·70W Fl 15s 93m **26M**;
W 8-sided Tr; vis 274°-190°; *Horn 45s.*
Chicken Rk 54°02'·30N 04°50'·20W Fl 5s 38m 13M; Tr; *Horn 60s.*

PORT ST MARY
The Carrick 54°04'·30N 04°42'·60W Q (2) 5s 6m 3M; IDM.
Alfred Pier Hd 54°04'·32N 04°43'·74W Oc R 10s 8m 6M;
W Tr, R band; *Bell (3) 12s* (occas).
Inner Pier Hd 54°04'·42N 04°44'·07W Oc R 3s 8m 5M.

CASTLETOWN/DERBY HAVEN
Lt By 54°03'·72N 04°38'·54W Fl R 3s; PHM; *Bell.*
New Pier Hd 54°04'·32N 04°38'·89W Oc R 15s 8m 5M.

Langness, Dreswick Pt 54°03'·28N 04°37'·45W Fl (2) 30s
21m 10M; W Tr.
Derby Haven, Bkwtr SW end 54°04'·57N 04°36'·98W
Iso G 2s 5m 5M; W Tr, G band.

DOUGLAS
Douglas Hd 54°08'·58N 04°27'·88W Fl 10s 32m **24M**; W Tr;
obsc brg more than 037°. FR Lts on radio masts 1 and 3M
West.
No. 1 Lt By 54°09'·03N 04°27'·61W Q (3) G 5s; SHM.
Princess Alexandra Pier Hd 54°08'·85N 04°27'·80W Fl R 5s
16m 8M; R mast; *Whis (2) 40s.*
Ldg Lts 229·3°, Front 54°08'·71N 04°28'·17W Oc 10s 9m
5M; W ▲ R border on mast. Rear, 62m from front, Oc 10s
12m 5M; W ▼ on R border; synch with front.
Victoria Pier Hd 54°08'·83N 04°28'·01W Oc G 8s 10m 3M; W
col; vis 225°-327°; Intnl Port Tfc Signals; *Bell (1) 2s.*

LAXEY
Pier Hd 54°13'·45N 04°23'·20W Oc R 3s 7m 5M; W Tr, R
band; obsc when brg less than 318°.
Bkwtr Hd 54°13'·50N 04°23'·30W Oc G 3s 7m; W Tr, G band.

Maughold Hd 54°17'·70N 04°18'·50W Fl (3) 30s 65m **21M.**
Bahama Lt By 54°20'·00N 04°08'·50W Q (6) + L Fl 15s; SCM;
Bell.

RAMSEY
Queens Pier Lt By 54°19'·28N 04°21'·79W Fl R 5s; PHM.
S Pier Hd 54°19'·42N 04°22'·42W QR 8m 10M; W Tr,
R band, B base; *Bell (2)10s* (occas).
N Pier Hd 54°19'·44N 04°22'·42W QG 9m 5M; W Tr, B base.

Whitestone Bk Lt By 54°24'·55N 04°20'·20W Q (9) 15s; WCM.
King William Bk Lt By 54°26'·00N 04°00'·00W Q (3) 10s; ECM.

WALES – NORTH COAST

Chester Flat Lt By 53°21'·65N 03°27'·40W Fl (2) R 5s; PHM.
Mid Patch Spit Lt By 53°21'·80N 03°31'·50W Fl R 5s; PHM.
N Rhyl Lt By 53°22'·75N 03°34'·50W Q; NCM.
W Constable Lt By 53°23'·13N 03°49'·17W Q (9) 15s; WCM.

RHYL/LLANDUDNO/CONWY
River Clwyd Bkwtr Hd 53°19'·50N 03°30'·30W QR 7m 2M.
Llanddulas, Llysfaen Jetty 53°17'·55N 03°39'·45W Fl G 10s.
Raynes Quarry Jetty Hd 53°17'·60N 03°40'·28W 2 FG (vert).
Llandudno Pier Hd 53°19'·90N 03°49'·40W 2 FG (vert) 8m 4M.
Great Ormes Hd Lt Ho 53°20'·55N 03°52'·10W (unlit).
Conwy Fairway By 53°17'·90N 03°55'·50W; SWM.
Conway R ent S side 53°17'·98N 03°50'·90W Fl WR 5s 5m
2M; vis W076°-088°, R088°-171°, W171°-319°, R319°-076°.

10

ANGLESEY

Pilot Station Pier 54°24'·90N 04°17'·20W 2 FR (vert).
Pt Lynas 53°24'·97N 04°17'·30W Oc 10s 39m **20M**; W castellated Tr; vis 109°-315°; (H24). Fog Det Lt F 25m 16M vis 211·8°-214·3°; RC; *Horn 45s.*

AMLWCH

Main Bkwtr 53°25'·01N 04°19'·80W Fl G 15s 11m 3M; W mast; vis 141°-271°.
Inner Bkwtr 53°24'·98N 04°19'·85W 2 FR (vert) 12m 5M; W mast; vis 164°-239°.
Inner Hbr 53°24'·94N 04°19'·90W F 9m 8M; W post; vis 233°-257°.

Wylfa power station 53°25'·06N 04°29'·17W 2 FG (vert) 13m 6M.
Furlong By 53°25'·40W 04°30'·40W; SHM.
Archdeacon Rk By 53°26'·70N 04°30'·80W; NCM.
Victoria Bank By 53°25'·60N 04°31'·30W; NCM.
Coal Rk By 53°25'·90N 04°32'·72W; SCM.
Ethel Rk By 53°26'·63N 04°33'·60W; NCM.
W Mouse Bn 53°25'·03N 04°33'·20W; SWM.
The Skerries 53°25'·25N 04°36'·45W Fl (2) 10s 36m **22M**; W ● Tr, R band; Racon (T). FR 26m **16M**; same Tr; vis 231°-254°; *Horn (2) 20s.*
Langdon Lt By 53°22'·74N 04°38'·58W Q (9) 15s; WCM.
Bolivar Rk By 53°21'·50N 04°35'·23W; SHM.
Wk Lt By 53°20'·43N 04°36'·40W Fl (2) R 10s; PHM.
Clipera Lt By 53°20'·08N 04°36'·15W Fl (4) R 15s; PHM; *Bell.*

HOLYHEAD

Bkwtr Hd 53°19'·83N 04°37'·08W Fl (3) 15s 21m 14M; W ■ Tr, B band; *Siren 20s.*
Old Hbr, Admiralty Pier Dn 53°18'·85N 04°37'·00W 2 FG (vert) 8m 5M; *Horn 15s (occas).*

S Stack 53°18'·39N 04°41'·91W Fl 10s 60m **23M**; (H24); W ● Tr; obsc to N by N Stack and part obsc in Penrhos bay. *Horn 30s.* Fog Det Lt vis 145°-325°.

Ynys Meibion 53°11'·40N 04°30'·20W Fl R 5s 37m 10M; (occas) 2 FR (vert) shown from flagstaffs 550m NW and 550m SE when firing taking place.
Llanddwyn I Lt 53°08'·00N 04°24'·70W Fl WR 2·5s 12m W7M, R4M; W Tr; vis R280°-013°, W015°-120°.

MENAI STRAIT TO BARDSEY ISLAND

Trwyn-Du 53°18'·76N 04°02'·38W Fl 5s 19m 12M castellated Tr, B bands; vis 101°-023°; *Bell (1) 30s,* sounded continuously. FR on radio mast 2M SW.
Ten Feet Bank By 53°19'·45N 04°02'·66W; PHM.
Dinmor By 53°19'·33N 04°03'·20W; SHM.

BEAUMARIS/BANGOR

(Direction of buoyage NE to SW)

Perch Rk Bn 53°18'·73N 04°02'·09W; PHM.
B2 Lt By 53°18'·32N 04°02'·00W Fl (2) R 5s; PHM.
B1 Lt By 53°18'·11N 04°02'·28W Fl (2) G 10s; SHM.

B3 Lt By 53°17'·68N 04°02'·68W QG; SHM.
B8 By 53°16'·48N 04°04'·40W; PHM.
B5 Lt By 53°17'·77N 04°04'·83W Fl G 5s; SHM.
B6 Lt By 53°17'·14N 04°03'·42W Fl R 3s; PHM.
Beaumaris Pier 53°15'·67N 04°05'·33W F WG 5m 6M; vis G212°-286°, W286°-014°, G014°-071°.
B10 Lt By 53°15'·59N 04°05'·15W Fl (2) R 10s; PHM.
B12 Lt By 53°15'·47N 04°05'·00W QR; PHM.
B7 Lt By 53°15'·00N 04°06'·05W Fl (2) G 5s; SHM.
Bangor By 53°14'·47N 04°07'·00W; PHM.
St George's Pier 53°13'·53N 04°09'·50W Fl G 10s.
E side of chan 53°13'·20N 04°09'·53W QR 4m; R mast; vis 064°-222°. (0·1M E of Menai Suspension Bridge).
Price's Pt 53°13'·10N 04°10'·44W Fl WR 2s 5m 3M; W Bn; vis R059°-239°, W239°-259°.
Britannia tubular bridge, S chan Ldg Lts 231° E side. Front 53°12'·90N 04°10'·97W FW. Rear, 45m from front, FW. Centre span of bridge Iso 5s 27m 3M, one either side. SE end of bridge, FR 21m 3M either side, NW end of bridge section FG 21m 3M either side.

PORT DINORWIC

Port Dinorwic Lt By 53°11'·22N 04°13'·64W Fl R; PHM.
Pier Hd 53°11'·18N 04°12'·56W F WR 5m 2M; vis R225°-357°, W357°-225°.
C9 By 53°10'·63N 04°13'·91W; SHM.
Channel By 53°10'·34N 04°15'·19W; SHM.
C14 By 53°10'·17N 04°15'·31W; PHM.
C11 By 53°09'·90N 04°15'·61W; SHM.
C13 By 53°09'·50N 04°15'·87W; SHM.

(Direction of buoyage SW to NE)

Change By 53°08'·80N 04°16'·67W; SCM.

CAERNARFON

Caernarfon S Pier Hd 53°08'·59N 04°16'·60W 2 FG (vert) 5m 2M.
C10 Lt By 53°07'·94N 04°18'·20W QR; PHM.
Abermenai Pt 53°07'·60N 04°19'·64W Fl WR 3·5s 6m 3M; W mast; vis R065°-245°, W245°-065°.
Mussel Bk Lt By 53°07'·23N 04°20'·85W Fl (2) R 5s; PHM.
C6 Lt By 53°07'·07N 04°22'·25W Fl R 5s; PHM.
C5 By 53°07'·04N 04°22'·60W; SHM.
C4 Lt By 53°07'·21N 04°23'·06W QR; PHM.
C3 Lt By 53°07'·33N 04°23'·80W QG; SHM.
C1 Lt By 53°07'·18N 04°24'·37W Fl G 5s; SHM.
C2 Lt By 53°07'·28N 04°24'·42W Fl R 10s; PHM.

Poole Lt By 53°00'·00N 04°34'·00W Fl Y 6s; SPM (Apr-Oct).

PORTH DINLLÄEN

CG Stn 52°56'·80N 04°33'·81W FR when firing taking place 10M N.
Careg y Chwislen 52°56'·96N 04°33'·44W; IDM (unlit).

Bardsey I 52°44'·97N 04°47'·93W Fl (5) 15s 39m **26M**; W ■ Tr, R bands; obsc by Bardsey I 198°-250° and in Tremadoc B when brg less than 260°; *Horn Mo (N) 45s.*

10.10.5   PASSAGE INFORMATION

For detailed directions covering these waters and harbours refer to the Admiralty Pilot *W Coast of England and Wales*; *A Cruising Guide to NW England & Wales* (Griffiths/Imray) and *Lundy and Irish Sea Pilot* (Taylor/Imray).

SCOTLAND – SW COAST

The Scares, two groups of rocks, lie at the mouth of Luce Bay which elsewhere is clear more than 3ca offshore; but the whole bay is occupied by a practice bombing range, marked by 12 DZ SPM lt buoys. Good anch at E Tarbert B to await the tide around the Mull of Galloway, or dry out alongside in shelter of Drummore. Off Burrow Hd there is a bad race in strong W winds with W-going tide. In Wigtown B the best anch is in Isle of Whithorn B, but exposed to S. It is also possible to dry out in Garlieston, see 10.10.7.

A tank firing range, between the E side of ent to Kirkcudbright Bay (10.10.7) and Abbey Hd, 4M to E, extends 14M offshore. If unable to avoid the area, cross it at N end close inshore. For information contact Range Control ☎ (01557) 323236 or call the Range safety boat "Gallovidian" on VHF Ch 16, 73. The range operates 0900-1600LT Mon-Fri, but weekend and night firing may also occur.

SOLWAY FIRTH (chart 1346)

Between Abbey Head and St Bees Head lies the Solway Firth, most of which is encumbered by shifting sandbanks. Off the entrances to the Firth, and in the approaches to Workington (10.10.9) beware shoals over which strong W winds raise a heavy sea. There are navigable, buoyed chans as far as Annan on the N shore, but buoys are laid primarily for the aid of Pilots. Local knowledge is required, particularly in the upper Firth, where streams run very strongly in the chans when the banks are dry, and less strongly over the banks when covered. In Powfoot chan for example the in-going stream begins at HW Liverpool – 0300, and the outgoing at HW Liverpool + 0100, sp rates up to 6kn. South along the Cumbrian coast past St Bees Hd to Walney Is there are no dangers more than 2M offshore, but no shelter either. For Silloth, Maryport, Workington, Harrington, Whitehaven and Ravenglass, see 10.10.7 to 10.10.10.

BARROW TO CONWY (AC 2010, 1981, *1978*)

Ent to Barrow-in-Furness (10.10.10 and chart 3164) is about 1M S of Hilpsford Pt at S end of Walney Island. Two chys of Roosecote power station are conspic, 3·25M N of Walney Lt Ho (Lt, RC). The stream sets across the chan, which is narrow and shallow but well marked. W winds cause rough sea in the ent. Moorings and anch off Piel Is, but space is limited and stream runs hard on ebb, see 10.10.10. Coming from S it is possible to cross the sands between Fleetwood (10.10.11) and Barrow with sufficient rise of tide.

Lune Deep, 2M NW of Rossall Pt, is ent to Morecambe B (chart 2010), and gives access to the ferry/commercial port of Heysham, Glasson Dock (10.10.10) and Fleetwood (10.10.11); it is well buoyed. Streams run 3·5kn at sp. Most of Bay is encumbered with drying sands, intersected by chans which are subject to change. S of Morecambe B, beware shoals extending 3M W of Rossall Pt. Further S, R. Ribble (10.10.11) gives access to the marina at Preston.

Queen's Chan and Crosby Chan (charts 1951 and *1978*) are entered E of the Bar Lanby. They are well buoyed, dredged and preserved by training banks, and give main access to R. Mersey and Liverpool (10.10.12). Keep clear of commercial shipping. From the N the old Formby chan is abandoned, but possible near HW. Towards HW and in moderate winds a yacht can cross the training bank (level of which varies between 2m and 3m above CD) E of Great Burbo Bank, if coming from the W. Rock Chan, parts of which dry and which is unmarked, may also be used but beware wrecks.

In good weather and at nps, the Dee Estuary (charts 1953, *1978*) is accessible for boats able to take the ground. But most of estuary dries and banks extend 6M seaward. Chans shift, and buoys are moved as required. Stream runs hard in chans when banks are dry. Main ent is Welsh Chan, but if coming from N, Hilbre Swash runs W of Hilbre Is (lit).

Sailing W from the Dee on the ebb, it is feasible to take the Inner Passage (buoyed) S of West Hoyle Spit, and this enjoys some protection from onshore winds at half tide or below. Rhyl is a tidal hbr, not accessible in strong onshore winds, but gives shelter for yachts able to take the ground. Abergele Road, Colwyn B and Llandudno B are possible anchs in settled weather and S winds. Conwy (10.10.18) offer good shelter in both marina and harbour.

Between Pt of Ayre and Great Ormes Hd the E-going stream begins at HW Liverpool + 0600, and the W-going at HW Liverpool – 0015, sp rates 3kn.

ISLE OF MAN (IOM) (charts 2094, 2696)

For general pilotage information, tidal streams and hbr details of IOM, see *IOM Sailing Directions*, *Tidal Streams and Anchorages*, published by the Manx Sailing and Cruising Club. For notes on crossing the Irish Sea, see 10.13.5.

There are four choices when rounding South of Isle of Man: i, In bad weather, or at night, keep S of Chicken Rk (Lt, fog sig). ii, In good conditions, take the chan between Chicken Rk and Calf of Man (Lt, fog sig). iii, Alternatively, with winds of Force 3 or less and a reliable engine capable of producing a speed of at least 5kn, by day only use Calf Sound between Calf of Man and IOM, passing W of Kitterland Island but E of Thousla Rock, which is marked by Lt Bn and is close to Calf of Man shore. iv, There is also a minor chan, called Little Sound, E of Kitterland Is.

The stream runs strongly through Calf Sound, starting N-going at HW Liverpool – 0145, and S-going at HW Liverpool + 0345, sp rates 3·5kn. W of Calf of Man the stream runs N and S, but changes direction off Chicken Rk and runs W and E between Calf of Man and Langness Pt 6M to E. Overfalls extend E from Chicken Rk on E-going stream, which begins at HW Liverpool + 0610, and N from the rk on W-going stream, which begins at HW Liverpool.

Off Langness Pt (Lt) the Skerranes (dry) extend 1ca SW, and tidal stream runs strongly, with eddies and a race. E side of Langness peninsula is foul ground, over which a dangerous sea can build in strong winds. Here the NE-going stream begins at HW Liverpool + 0545, and the SW-going at HW Liverpool – 0415, sp rates 2·25kn.

There is anch in Derby Haven, N of St Michael's Is, but exposed to E. From here to Douglas (10.10.16) and on to Maughold Hd (Lt), there are no dangers more than 4ca offshore. Near the coast the SW-going stream runs for 9 hours and the NE-going for 3 hours, since an eddy forms during the second half of the main NE-going stream. Off Maughold Hd the NE-going stream begins at HW Liverpool + 0500, and the SW-going at HW Liverpool – 0415.

SE, E and NW of Pt of Ayre are dangerous banks, on which seas break in bad weather. These are Whitestone Bk (least depth 2·0m), Bahama Bk (1·5m, buoy), Ballacash Bk (2·7m), King William Bks (3·3m, buoy), and Strunakill Bk (6·7m).

The W coast of IOM has few pilotage hazards. A spit with depth of 1·4m runs 2ca offshore from Rue Pt. Jurby Rk (depth 2·7m) lies 3ca off Jurby Hd. Craig Rk (depth 4 m) and shoals lie 2·5M NNE of Peel (10.10.14).

MENAI STRAIT (10.10.19 and chart *1464*)

The main features of this narrow chan include: Puffin Is, seaward of NE end; Beaumaris; Garth Pt at Bangor, where NE end of Strait begins; Menai Suspension Bridge (30·5m); The Swellies, a narrow 1M stretch with strong tide and dangers mid-stream; Britannia Rail Bridge (27·4m), with cables close W at elevation of 22m; Port Dinorwic and Caernarfon (10.10.19); Abermenai Pt and Fort Belan, where narrows mark SW end of Strait; and Caernarfon Bar.

10

The following brief notes only cover very basic pilotage. For detailed directions see *W Coasts of England and Wales Pilot*, or *Cruising Anglesey and N Wales* (NW Venturers Yacht Club). The Swellies should be taken near local HW slack, and an understanding of tidal streams is essential. The tide is about 1 hour later, and sp range about 2·7m more, at NE end of Strait than at SW end. Levels differ most at about HW +1 (when level at NE end is more than 1·8m above level at SW end); and at about HW – 0445 (when level at NE end is more than 1·8m below level at SW end). Normally the stream runs as follows (times referred to HW Holyhead). HW – 0040 to HW + 0420: SW between Garth Pt and Abermenai Pt. HW + 0420 to HW + 0545: outwards from about The Swellies, ie NE towards Garth Pt and SW towards Abermenai Pt. HW + 0545 to HW – 0040: NE between Abermenai Pt and Garth Pt. Sp rates are generally about 3kn, but more in narrows, ie 5kn off Abermenai Pt, 6kn under the bridges, and 8kn at The Swellies. The timings and rates of streams may be affected by strong winds in either direction.

From NE, enter chan W of Puffin Island, taking first of ebb to arrive Swellies at slack HW (HW Holyhead – 0100). Slack HW only lasts about 20 mins at sps, a little more at nps. Pass under centre of suspension bridge span, and steer to leave Platters (dry) on mainland shore to port and Swellies Lt Bn close to stbd. From Swellies Lt Bn to Britannia Bridge hold mainland shore, leaving Bn on Price Pt to port, and Gored Goch and Gribbin Rk to stbd. Leave Britannia Rk (centre pier of bridge) to stbd. Thence to SW hold to buoyed chan near mainland shore. (Note: A Historic Wreck (see 10.0.3g) is 4ca SW of Britannia Bridge at 53°12'·77N 04°11'·72W). Port Dinorwic is useful to await right tidal conditions for onward passage in either direction.

Note that direction of lateral buoyage changes at Caernarfon.

Caernarfon Bar is impassable even in moderately strong winds against ebb, but narrows at Abermenai Pt demand a fair tide, or slackish water, since tide runs strongly here. Going seaward on first of ebb, when there is water over the banks, it may not be practicable to return to the Strait if conditions on the bar are bad. Then it is best to anch near Mussel Bank By and await slack water, before returning to Caernarfon (say). Leaving Abermenai Pt on last of ebb means banks to seaward are exposed and there is little water in chan or over bar.

Going NE it is safe to arrive at Swellies with last of flood, leaving Caernarfon about HW Holyhead – 0230. Do not leave too late, or full force of ebb will be met before reaching Bangor.

ANGLESEY TO BARDSEY ISLAND (AC *1977*, 1970, 1971)

On N coast of Anglesey, a race extends 5ca off Pt Lynas (Lt, fog sig, RC) on E-going stream. Amlwch is a small hbr (partly dries) 1·5M W of Pt Lynas. A drying rk lies 100m offshore on W side of appr, which should not be attempted in strong onshore winds. From here to Carmel Hd beware E Mouse (and shoals to SE), Middle Mouse, Harry Furlong's Rks (dry), Victoria Bank (least depth 1·8m), Coal Rk (awash), and W Mouse (with dangers to W and SW). The outermost of these dangers is 2M offshore. There are overfalls and races at headlands and over many rks and shoals along this coast.

Between Carmel Hd and The Skerries (Lt, fog sig, Racon) the NE-going stream begins at HW Holyhead + 0550, and the SW-going at HW Holyhead – 0010, sp rates 5kn. 1M NW of Skerries the stream turns 1½ hours later, and runs less strongly. Note: A Historic Wreck (*Mary*; see 10.0.3g) is on The Skerries. Simplest passage, or at night or in bad weather, is to pass 1M off Skerries, in the TSS ITZ (see Fig. 10(3)). In good conditions by day and at slack water, Carmel Hd can be rounded close inshore; but beware short, steep, breaking seas here in even moderate winds against tide.

Holyhead (10.10.20) is a harbour of refuge, access H24 in all weathers, with new marina in New Harbour; beware fast ferries. Races also occur off N Stack and (more severe) off S Stack (Lt, fog sig), up to 1·5M offshore on NNE-going stream which begins at HW Holyhead – 0605, sp rate 5kn. Races do not extend so far on SSW-going stream which begins at HW Holyhead + 0020, sp rate 5kn.

The W coast of Anglesey is rugged with rks, some drying, up to 1·5M offshore. There are races off Penrhyn Mawr and Rhoscolyn Hd. Pilot's Cove, E of Llanddwyn Is, is good anch while waiting right conditions for Menai Strait.

On the Lleyn Peninsula Porth Dinllaen (10.10.20) is good anch, but exposed to N and NE. Braich y Pwll is the steep, rky point at end of Lleyn Peninsula (chart 1971). About 1M N of it and up to 1M offshore lie The Tripods, a bank on which there are overfalls and a bad sea with wind against tide.

Bardsey Sound, 1·5M wide, can be used by day in moderate winds. Stream reaches 6kn at sp, and passage should be made at slack water, – 0015 HW or + 0035 LW Holyhead. Avoid Carreg Ddu on N side and Maen Bugail Rk (dries 4·1m) on S side of Sound, where there are dangerous races. If passing outside Bardsey Is (Lt, fog sig) make a good offing to avoid overfalls which extend 1·5M W and 2·5M S of Island. Turbulence occurs over Bastram Shoal, Devil's Tail and Devil's Ridge, which lie SSE and E of Bardsey Is.

10.10.6   DISTANCE TABLE

Approximate distances in nautical miles are by the most direct route, whilst avoiding dangers and allowing for Traffic Separation Schemes. Places in *italics* are in adjoining areas; places in **bold** are in 10.0.6, Distances across the Irish Sea.

	1	2	3	4	5	6	7	8	9	10	11	12	13	14	15	16	17	18	19	20
1. *Portpatrick*	1																			
2. *Mull of Galloway*	16	2																		
3. **Kirkcudbright**	48	32	3																	
4. **Maryport**	65	49	26	4																
5. Workington	63	47	25	6	5															
6. Ravenglass	70	54	40	30	23	6														
7. **Point of Ayre**	38	22	28	37	31	34	7													
8. Peel	41	26	46	55	49	52	18	8												
9. **Port St Mary**	56	41	61	63	57	50	35	18	9											
10. Douglas	60	42	46	50	44	39	19	30	13	10										
11. Ramsey	44	28	34	41	35	34	6	24	27	15	11									
12. Glasson Dock	101	85	74	66	60	37	64	85	69	63	61	12								
13. **Fleetwood**	95	79	68	59	53	30	58	80	63	57	55	10	13							
14. **Liverpool**	118	102	97	89	83	60	80	86	76	70	77	52	46	14						
15. Conwy	111	95	95	92	86	58	72	72	57	59	68	62	56	46	15					
16. Beaumaris	109	93	94	95	89	72	71	73	58	58	70	66	60	49	12	16				
17. Caernarfon	117	103	104	105	99	82	81	73	68	68	80	76	70	59	22	10	17			
18. **Holyhead**	93	81	94	96	90	69	68	62	46	50	65	79	73	68	36	32	26	18		
19. Bardsey Island	127	113	129	129	123	114	107	94	80	88	98	107	101	90	53	41	31	43	19	
20. *Fishguard*	171	158	175	175	169	160	153	140	126	134	144	153	147	136	100	88	78	89	45	20

KIRKCUDBRIGHT   10-10-7

Kirkcudbrightshire 54°50'·30N 04°03'·40W

CHARTS
AC1344, 1346, 2094, *1826*; Imray C62; OS 84

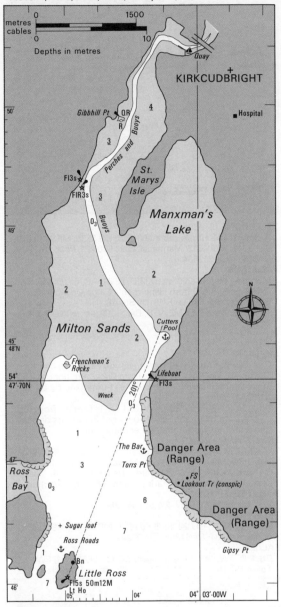

metres / cables
Depths in metres
Quay
KIRKCUDBRIGHT
Hospital
Gibbhill Pt QR R
Perches and Buoys
Fl3s
FlR3s
St. Marys Isle
Manxman's Lake
Buoys
Milton Sands
Cutters Pool
Frenchman's Rocks
Lifeboat Fl3s
Wreck
Danger Area (Range)
Ross Bay
The Bar
Torrs Pt
FS Lookout Tr (conspic)
Danger Area (Range)
Sugar loaf
Ross Roads
Gipsy Pt
Bn
Little Ross
Fl5s 50m12M
Lt Ho

TIDES
+0030 Dover; ML 4·1; Duration 0545; Zone 0 (UT).

Standard Port LIVERPOOL (→)

Times				Height (metres)			
High Water		Low Water		MHWS	MHWN	MLWN	MLWS
0000	0600	0200	0800	9·3	7·4	2·9	0·9
1200	1800	1400	2000				
Differences KIRKCUDBRIGHT BAY							
+0015	+0015	+0010	+0000	−1·8	−1·5	−0·5	−0·1
GARLIESTON							
+0025	+0035	+0030	+0005	−2·3	−1·7	−0·5	No data
ISLE OF WHITHORN							
+0020	+0025	+0025	+0005	−2·4	−2·0	−0·8	−0·2
HESTAN ISLET (Kippford)							
+0025	+0025	+0020	+0025	−1·0	−1·1	−0·5	0·0

SHELTER
Very good at floating pontoon/jetty, at pile moorings in 1-3m or drying out on town quays. Good ⚓s behind Ross Is and ½ca N of Torrs Pt, except in S'lies which cause heavy swell.

NAVIGATION
WPT 54°45'·50N 04°04'·00W, 185°/005° from/to Torrs Pt, 1·4M. The Bar is 1ca N of Torrs Pt; access HW±3. Spring tides run up to 3kn. A firing range crosses the ent; contact Range Safety Officer ☎ (01557) 323236 or VHF.

LIGHTS AND MARKS
Little Ross lt ho, W of ent, Fl 5s 50m 12M, (obscured in Wigtown bay when brg more than 103°). Upriver there are Fl G lts on the piles securing the mooring pontoons.

RADIO TELEPHONE
VHF Ch 12 16 (HW±2). *Range Control* Ch 16 73.

TELEPHONE (01557)
Hr Mr 331135; ⌗ (01671) 402718; MRCC 0151-931 3341; Marinecall 0891 500 461; Police 330600; Dr 330755.

FACILITIES
Pontoon/jetty AB £5, FW; **Town Quay** AB, P, D, FW, El, CH, ME. **Kirkcudbright YC** ☎ 330963; SC ☎ 330032, Slip, M, FW; **Town** EC Thurs; V, R, Bar, ✉, Ⓑ, ⇌ (Dumfries), ✈ (Glasgow).

OTHER HARBOURS ON THE SOUTH GALLOWAY COAST

ISLE OF WHITHORN, Wigtown, 54°41'·90N 04°21'·80W. AC 2094, *1826*. HW +0035 on Dover; ML 3·7m; Duration 0545. See 10.10.7. Shelter good but hbr dries, having approx 2·5m at HW±3. On W side of ent beware the Skerries, a ledge with pole/radar reflector. St Ninian's Tr (W☐ tr) is conspic at E side of ent. E pier hd has QG 4m 5M; ldg lts 335°, both Oc R 8s 7/9m 7M, synch, Or masts and ◇.
Hr Mr ☎ (01988) 500246; Facilities: AB on quay £3, Slip, P, D, FW, ME, Sh, CH, V, Bar, ✉, VHF Ch 80 (occas).

GARLIESTON, Kirkcudbrightshire, 54°47'·35N 04°21'·75W. AC 2094, *1826*. HW +0035 on Dover; ML no data; Duration 0545. See 10.10.7. Hbr affords complete shelter but dries. Access (2m) HW±3. Pier hd lt 2FR (vert) 5m 3M. Beware rky outcrops in W side of bay marked by a perch. Hr Mr ☎ (01988) 600274. Facilities: M £3, FW, AC on quay, Slip. **Town** V, ME, P, D.

KIPPFORD, Kirkcudbrightshire, 54°52'·35N 03°48'·85W. AC 1346, *1826*. HW +0040 on Dover; ML 4·2m (Hestan Is). See 10.10.7. Good shelter on drying moorings/pontoons off Kippford, 2·75M up drying Urr Estuary from Hestan Is lt ho Fl (2) 10s 38m 7M. Access HW±2 via marked, unlit chan. CCC or Solway SDs (from Solway YC) are strongly advised. Beware Craig Roan on E side of ent. Temp ⚓s NE or W of Hestan Is to await tide. VHF: Ch M call *Kippford Startline* (YC) HW±2 in season. Ch 16 *Kippford Slipway* (Pilotage). Facilities: **Solway YC** (01556) 62312, AB, AC, FW, M; **Services:** AB £6, M, Slip, D (cans), CH, BY, ME. **Town** P, SM, V, ✉, Bar, Slip.

OTHER HARBOURS EAST OF THE SOLWAY FIRTH

SILLOTH, Cumbria, 54°52'·15N 03°23'·78W. AC 2013, 1346, *1826*. HW −0050 on Dover; ML no data; Duration 0520. See 10·10·8. Appr via English or Middle Chans, approx 8M long, requires local knowledge. Beware constantly shifting chans and banks. Yachts are not encouraged. ⚓ SW of ent in about 4m off Lees Scar, QG 11m 8M; exposed to SW winds. Outer hbr dries; lock into New Dock, which is mainly commercial. East Cote Dir lt 052° FG 15m 12M; vis 046°-058°, intens 052°. Ldg lts, both F, 115°. Groyne 2 FG (vert). Tfc sigs on mast at New Dock: no entry unless Y signal arm raised by day or Q Bu lt by night. VHF Ch 16 12 (HW−2½ to HW+1½). Hr Mr ☎ (016973) 31358. Facilities: EC Tues; FW, Ⓑ, Bar, ✉, R, V.

HARRINGTON, Cumbria, 54°36'·76N 03°34'·21W. AC 2013, 1346, *1826*. HW +0025 on Dover; Duration 0540; Use Workington 10.10.9. Good shelter in small hbr only used by local FVs and yachts; dries 3ca offshore. Ent difficult in strong W winds. Berth on N wall of inner hbr (free). Call ☎ (01946) 823741 Ext 148 for moorings. Limited facilities. **SC**.

WHITEHAVEN, Cumbria, 54°33'·17N 03°35'·74W. AC 2013, 1346, *1826*. HW +0015 on Dover; ML 4·5m; Duration 0550. See 10·10·9. Very good shelter; ent safe in most wx. Hbr dries, access HW±2½; or lock into Queens Dock, HW±1, by consent of Hr Mr ☎ (01946) 692435. VHF Ch 12 16 (HW −2½ to +1½). Lts: SHM bn, Fl G 2·5s, is 4½ca S of ent, close inshore; W pier Fl G 5s 16m 13M; N pier 2 FR (vert) 8m 9M; Inner Hbr 2 FR (vert) 8m 2M, and 2 FG (vert) 8m 2M. Facilities: AB in S Hbr is usually free, FW, D & P (on Old Tongue), Slip, C (7½ ton). **Town** EC Wed; Bar, Ⓑ, CH, ✉, R, V.

10

MARYPORT   10-10-8

Cumbria 54°43'·03N 03°30'·38W

CHARTS
AC 2013, 1346, *1826*; Imray C62; OS 89
TIDES
+0038 Dover; ML no data; Duration 0550; Zone 0 (UT)

Standard Port LIVERPOOL (→)

Times				Height (metres)			
High Water		Low Water		MHWS	MHWN	MLWN	MLWS
0000	0600	0200	0800	9·3	7·4	2·9	0·9
1200	1800	1400	2000				
Differences MARYPORT							
+0017	+0032	+0020	+0005	−0·7	−0·8	−0·4	0·0
SILLOTH							
+0030	+0040	+0045	+0055	−0·1	−0·3	−0·6	−0·1
TORDUFF POINT							
+0105	+0140	+0520	+0410	−4·1	−4·9	Not below CD	

Note: At Torduff Point the LW time differences are for the start of the rise, which at sp is very sudden.

SHELTER
Good shelter in Marina (Senhouse Dock), access HW ±3 over sill 1·75m; or in Elizabeth Basin (commercial) which dries, access HW±1½, (not normally used by yachts).
NAVIGATION
WPT 54°43'·08N 03°32'·39W, 270°/090° from/to S pier lt, 1·0M. 1·8m over bar between piers at ent at half tide and in river chan. Mud banks cover HW −2. Chan not buoyed.
LIGHTS AND MARKS
S pier Fl 1·5s 10m 4M.
RADIO TELEPHONE
Port VHF Ch 12 (occas) 16. Marina (H24) Ch M 80 16.

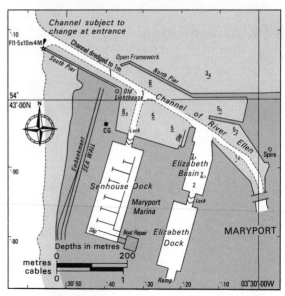

TELEPHONE (01900)
Hr Mr 817440; Hbr Authority 604351; CG 2238; MRSC (0151) 931 3341; ⌗ 604611; Marinecall 0891 500 461; Police 812601; Dr 815544; Ⓗ 812634.
FACILITIES
Maryport Marina (200) ☎ 813331, £8.81, AC, BY, CH, El, FW, Ⓖ, ME, Slip, (P & D from Fisherman's Co-op via marina); **Elizabeth Dock** Slip (at HW), M, Sh, AB.
Town EC Wed; P, D, ME, V, R, Bar, ✉, Ⓑ, ⇌, ✈ (Newcastle).

WORKINGTON   10-10-9

Cumbria 54°39'·02N 03°34'·30W

CHARTS
AC 2013, 1346, *1826*; Imray C62; OS 89
TIDES
+0025 Dover; ML 4·5; Duration 0545; Zone 0 (UT)

Standard Port LIVERPOOL (→)

Times				Height (metres)			
High Water		Low Water		MHWS	MHWN	MLWN	MLWS
0000	0600	0200	0800	9·3	7·4	2·9	0·9
1200	1800	1400	2000				
Differences WORKINGTON							
+0020	+0020	+0020	+0010	−1·2	−1·1	−0·3	0·0
WHITEHAVEN							
+0005	+0015	+0010	+0005	−1·3	−1·1	−0·5	+0·1
TARN POINT							
+0005	+0005	+0010	0000	−1·0	−1·0	−0·4	0·0

SHELTER
Good, but hbr dries. Berth where you can (free) or ⚓ in Turning Basin. Lock (HW±1½) into Dock 1·8m (for coasters). Inner tidal hbr is restricted by low (1·8m) fixed rly bridge.
NAVIGATION
WPT 54°39'·58N 03°35'·30W, 311°/131° from/to front ldg lt, 1·0M. No navigational dangers but in periods of heavy rain a strong freshet may be encountered.
LIGHTS AND MARKS
Unlit NCM buoy and SHM buoy, Fl G 5s, are 2·2M WNW and 1·3M NW of hbr ent respectively. Ldg lts 132°, both FR 10/12m 3M, on W pyramidal trs with Y bands. Two sets of F Bu lts in line mark NE and SW edges of chan.
RADIO TELEPHONE
VHF Ch 11 14 16 (HW−2½ to HW+2).
TELEPHONE (01900)
Hr Mr 602301; CG 2238; ⌗ 604611; MRSC 0151-931 3341; Police 812601; Dr 64866; Ⓗ 602244.
FACILITIES
Dock D, FW, ME, El; **Vanguard SC** ☎ 826886, M, FW.
Town EC Thurs; P, V, R, Bar, ✉, Ⓑ, ⇌, ✈ (Carlisle).

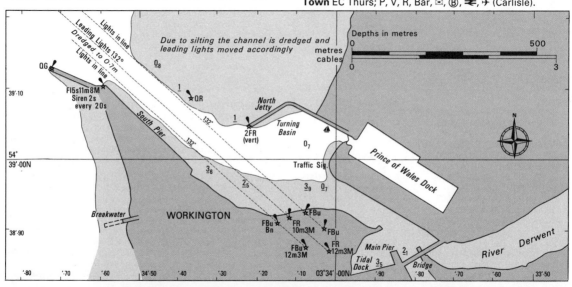

GLASSON DOCK   10-10-10

Lancashire 53°59'·97N 02°50'·85W

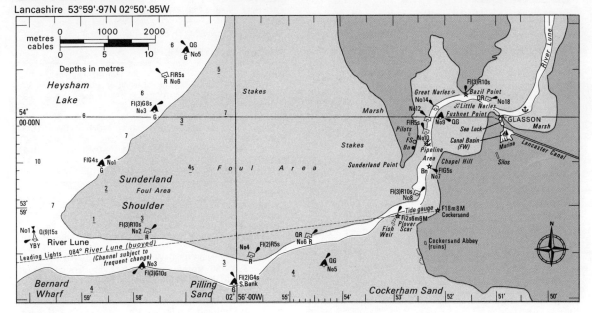

CHARTS
AC 1552, 2010, *1826*; Imray C62; OS 102, 97
TIDES
+0020 Dover; ML No data; Duration 0535; Zone 0 (UT)

Standard Port LIVERPOOL (→)

Times				Height (metres)			
High Water		Low Water		MHWS	MHWN	MLWN	MLWS
0000	0600	0200	0700	9·3	7·4	2·9	0·9
1200	1800	1400	1900				
Differences GLASSON DOCK							
+0020	+0030	+0220	+0240	−2·7	−3·0	No data	
LANCASTER							
+0110	+0030	No data		−5·0	−4·9	Dries out	
BARROW-IN-FURNESS (Ramsden Dock)							
+0015	+0015	+0015	+0015	0·0	−0·3	+0·1	+0·2
ULVERSTON							
+0020	+0040	No data		0·0	−0·1	No data	
ARNSIDE							
+0100	+0135	No data		+0·5	+0·2	No data	
MORECAMBE							
+0005	+0010	+0030	+0015	+0·2	0·0	0·0	+0·2
HEYSHAM							
+0005	+0005	+0015	0000	+0·1	0·0	0·0	+0·2

Note: At Glasson Dock LW time differences give the end of
a LW stand which lasts up to 2 hours at sp.

SHELTER
Very good in marina; also sheltered ⚓ in R Lune to await
sea lock, opens HW Liverpool −0045 to HW, into Glasson
Dock. Inner lock/swing bridge lead into BWB basin.
NAVIGATION
WPT 53°58'·40N 03°00'·00W (2ca S of R. Lune No 1 WCM
By), 264°/084° from/to front ldg lt 084°, 4·2M. Leave WPT
at HW−2 via buoyed/lit chan. Plover Scar lt bn has a tide
gauge showing depth over the lock sill at Glasson Dock. ⚓
is prohib between Sutherland Pt and No 10 PHM lt buoy.
Beyond this a training wall, marked by PHM lt buoys/bn,
extends to lock ent. R Lune is navigable to Lancaster.
LIGHTS AND MARKS
Ldg lts (hard to see from WPT): Plover Scar, Fl 2s, on with
Cockersand, FW, leads 084° up to Nos 2 /3 buoys; thence
follow buoyed chan which shifts.
Tfc Sigs by day (night) at E side of lock:
1 ● (Ⓡ)   = lock manned, but shut
R flag (Ⓡ over Ⓦ)   = lock open, clear to enter
R flag over ● (2 Ⓡ vert) = lock open, vessels leaving
RADIO TELEPHONE
VHF Ch 69 16 (HW−2 to HW+1). Marina Ch 80.
TELEPHONE (01524)
Hr Mr 751724; MRSC 0151-931 3341; ⌗ 851013; Marinecall
0891 500 461; Police 791239; Ⓗ 65944.

FACILITIES
Marina (240+20 visitors) ☎ 751491, Slip, D, FW, ME, El, Ⓔ,
Sh, C, (50 ton), BH (50 ton), AC, CH; **Glasson Basin**, M, AB;
Glasson SC ☎ 751089 Slip, M, C; **Lune CC** Access HW±2.
Town EC Lancaster Wed; P (cans), V, R, Bar, ✉, Ⓑ
(Lancaster), ⇌ (bus to Lancaster 4M), ✈ (Blackpool).

ADJACENT HARBOURS

RAVENGLASS, Cumbria, 54°20'·80N 03°24'·87W. AC 1346,
1826. HW +0020 on Dover; ML no data; Duration 0545.
See 10.10.9 (Tarn Point). Large drying hbr, formed by
estuaries of R Mite, Irt and Esk, has approx 2·5m in ent at
HW−2. There is a FG lt (occas) on blockhouse at S side of
ent. Local knowledge advised. From N beware Drigg Rk
and from S Selker Rks, marked by SHM buoy Fl (3) G 10s,
5M SSW of ent. A firing range is close S at Eskmeals (R
flags flown when in use), ☎ (01229) 717631 Ext 245.
Village: EC Wed; FW, Slip, Bar, V, ✉.

BARROW-IN-FURNESS, Cumbria, 54°05'·63N 03°13'·36W.
AC 3164, 2010, *1826*. HW +0030 on Dover; See 10·10·10.
ML 5·0m; Duration 0530. Good shelter. Hbr dries except
for appr chan and Walney Chan, dredged 3·5m, buoyed/
lit, which must be kept clear. Landings at Piel Is and Roa
Is. Lts: Walney Is, Fl 15s 21m 23M (obsc 122°-127° within
3M of shore), RC. From Lightning Knoll SWM buoy (L Fl
10s) ldg lts, front Q 7m 10M; rear (6ca from front), Iso 2s
13m 10M (both lattice structures) lead 041°/3·7M to Bar
buoy Fl (2) R 5s (abeam Walney Lt Ho). Inner Chan ldg
lts, front Q 9m 10M, rear Iso 2s 14m 6M, lead 006° past
Piel Is with conspic ruined castle; slip and moorings on E
side. Roa Island is 5ca N; jetty at S end and moorings on
E side; causeway connects to mainland. Commercial
docks are 3M NW. VHF *Ramsden Dock* Ch 16; 12 (H24).
Facilities: Piel Is, Bar; Roa, Hotel, V. **Town** EC Thurs; SM,
all needs.

HEYSHAM, Lancashire, 54°02'·00N 02°55'·88W. AC 1552,
2010, *1826*. HW +0015 on Dover; ML 5·1m; Duration 0545.
See 10·10·10. Good shelter, but yachts not normally
accepted without special reason. Beware ferries and 'rig'
supply ships. Ldg lts 102°, both F Bu 11/14m 2M, Y+B ◇
on masts. S jetty lt 2 FG (vert), Siren 30s. S pier hd ,Oc G
7·5s 9m 6M. N pier hd, 2FR (vert) 11m, obsc from
seaward. Ent sigs: R flag or Ⓡ = no entry; no sig = no
dep; 2 R flags or 2 Ⓡ = no ent or dep. VHF Ch 14 74 16
(H24). Hr Mr ☎ (01524) 52373. Facilities: EC Wed
(Morecambe also); Bar, FW, R, V at Morecambe (2M).

10

FLEETWOOD   10-10-11

Lancashire 53°55'·48N 03°00'·07W

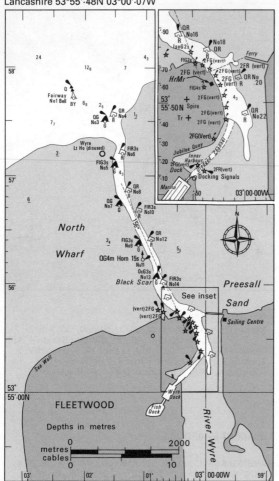

FLEETWOOD

Depths in metres

CHARTS
AC 1552, 2010, *1826*; Imray C62; OS 102

TIDES
+0015 Dover; ML 5.0; Duration 0530; Zone 0 (UT)

Standard Port LIVERPOOL (→)

Times				Height (metres)			
High Water		Low Water		MHWS	MHWN	MLWN	MLWS
0000	0600	0200	0700	9·3	7·4	2·9	0·9
1200	1800	1400	1900				
Differences FLEETWOOD							
0000	0000	+0005	0000	−0·1	−0·1	+0·1	+0·3
BLACKPOOL							
−0015	−0005	−0005	−0015	−0·4	−0·4	−0·1	+0·1
PRESTON							
+0010	+0010	+0335	+0310	−4·0	−4·1	−2·8	−0·8

SHELTER
Very good in Wyre Dock Marina, access HW±2 via chan dredged 3m and lock. Sheltered ⌕ off Knot End pier on E bank to await tide. Up river to Skippool (5M) needs local knowledge and shoal draft; access HW±1 (if ht of tide >8·0m).

NAVIGATION
WPT 53°57'·78N 03°02'·04W (abeam Fairway No 1 NCM lt buoy), 336°/156° from/to front ldg lt, 2·25M. For best water keep close to the 300m long training wall on SE side of chan to marina. Beware ferries/dredgers turning in hbr.

LIGHTS AND MARKS
Chan well buoyed and lit. Ldg lts, front Fl G 2s and rear Fl G 4s, 156° (only to be used between Nos 8 and 13 buoys). Lock sigs (only enter on instructions): 1 ● (1 Ⓡ) = Gates open for entry; 2 ● (2 Ⓡ) = open for deps.

RADIO TELEPHONE
Call *Fleetwood Hbr Control* Ch 11, when ferries under way. Call *Fleetwood Dock* Ch **12** 16, HW±2 for marina or Fish Dock.

TELEPHONE (01253)
Hr Mr 872323; MRSC 0151- 933 7075; ⌗ (01524) 851013; Marinecall 0891 500 461; Police 876611; Dr 873312.

FACILITIES
Marina (210) ☎ 872323, Fax 777549, D, FW, AC, Ⓞ, C (25 ton); **Services:** CH, SM, ACA, ME, EI, Sh, C (mobile 50 ton by arrangement), Ⓔ. **Blackpool & Fleetwood YC** (Skippool) ☎ 884205, AB, Slip, FW, Bar; **Town** EC Wed; P & D (cans), ME, EI, Sh, CH, V, R, Bar, ✉, Ⓑ, ⇌ (bus: Poulton-le-Fylde or Blackpool), ✈ (Blackpool).

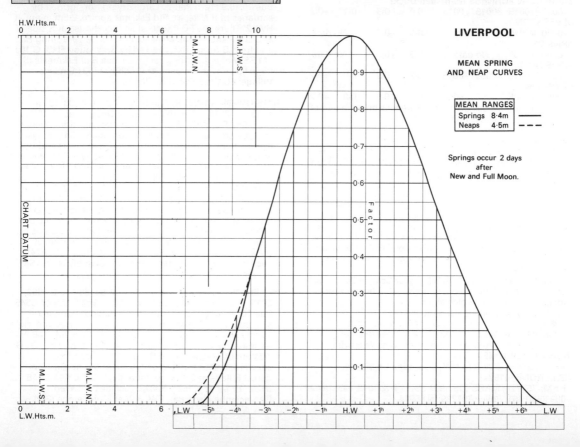

LIVERPOOL

MEAN SPRING AND NEAP CURVES

MEAN RANGES

| Springs | 8·4m | —— |
| Neaps | 4·5m | - - - |

Springs occur 2 days after New and Full Moon.

ADJACENT HARBOUR

RIVER RIBBLE, Lancashire, 53°43'·50N 03°00'·00W, AC 1981, *1826*. HW +0013 on Dover; ML no data; Duration St Anne's 0520. See 10.10.11 for Preston differences. Note: LW time differences give the end of a LW stand lasting about 3½ hrs. Good shelter 13M up river in Preston marina; lock in HW±1½, (no commercial traffic). Gut SWM buoy L Fl 10s is 2M W of chan ent, but lit chan has silted and is no longer dredged. Best water is now via S Gut (locally buoyed) to a breach in the training wall. For local knowledge/sketch contact **Ribble Cruising Club** ☎ (01253) 739983. Possible berths at Lytham or Freckleton on the N bank or 2M up R. Douglas. Facilities: **Douglas BY**, ☎ (01772) 812462, access HW±1, VHF Ch 16, AB, C (7 ton), CH, D, FW, Sh, Slip, ME. PRESTON: Hr Mr ☎ (01772) 726711; ⌖ (0151) 933 7075; **Preston Marina** (250) ☎ 733595, Fax 731881, VHF Ch **80** 14 16 call *Riversway*; CH, D, C (250 ton), R, V, AC, FW, ACA. SOUTHPORT: ACA.

LIVERPOOL   10-10-12

Merseyside 53°24'·20N 03°00'·20W (Abeam Liver Bldg)

CHARTS
AC 3490, 1951, *1978, 1826*; Imray C62; OS 108
TIDES
+0015 Dover; ML 5·2; Duration 0535; Zone 0 (UT)

Standard Port LIVERPOOL (ALFRED DOCK) (→)

Times				Height (metres)			
High Water		Low Water		MHWS	MHWN	MLWN	MLWS
0000	0600	0200	0700	9·3	7·4	2·9	0·9
1200	1800	1400	1900				
Differences SOUTHPORT							
−0020	−0010	No data		−0.3	−0.3	No data	
FORMBY							
−0015	−0010	−0020	−0020	−0.3	−0.1	0·0	+0·1
GLADSTONE DOCK							
−0003	−0003	−0003	−0003	−0.1	−0.1	0·0	−0.1
EASTHAM (River Mersey)							
+0010	+0010	+0009	+0009	+0.3	+0.1	−0.1	−0.3
WIDNES (River Mersey)							
+0040	+0045	+0400	+0345	−4.2	−4.4	−2.5	−0.3
HILBRE ISLAND (River Dee)							
−0015	−0012	−0010	−0015	−0.3	−0.2	+0.2	+0.4
MOSTYN QUAY (River Dee)							
−0020	−0015	−0020	−0020	−0.8	−0.7	No data	
CONNAH'S QUAY (River Dee)							
0000	+0015	+0355	+0340	−4.6	−4.4	Dries out	
CHESTER (River Dee)							
+0105	+0105	+0500	+0500	−5.3	−5.4	Dries out	
COLWYN BAY							
−0035	−0025	No data		−1.5	−1.3	No data	
LLANDUDNO							
−0035	−0025	−0025	−0035	−1.9	−1.5	−0.5	−0.2

NOTE: LW time differences at Connah's Quay give the end of a LW stand lasting about 3¾hrs at sp and 5hrs at nps. A bore occurs in the R Dee at Chester.

SHELTER
Good at marina in the Coburg and Brunswick docks. Ent is 1M S of Liver Bldg and abeam the Pluckington Bank WCM; access HW ±2 approx. Good shelter also in Canning and Albert Docks but access HW−2 to HW. ⚓ on the SW side of river but only in fair wx.
NAVIGATION
WPT Bar PHM Lt F 53°32'·00N 03°20'·90W, 280°/100° from/to Queen's Chan, 3M. From Bar Lt F to marina ent is 17M via Queen's and Crosby Chans. Wind against tide causes steep seas in outer reaches of Mersey. The whole area (R Mersey to R Alt and N to Morecambe B) is littered with sandbanks. The Mersey is safe inside buoyed chan, but elsewhere local knowledge and great caution needed.
For R Dee: WPT 53°26'·20N 03°16'·80W, Hilbre Swash HE2 PHM buoy, QR, (chan shifts).
LIGHTS AND MARKS
The ent to R Mersey is at the Bar PHM lt F, Fl 5s 12m 21M, Horn (2) 20s, Racon. Queen's Chan and Crosby Chan are marked by Boat lt bns to port, normal buoys to stbd.

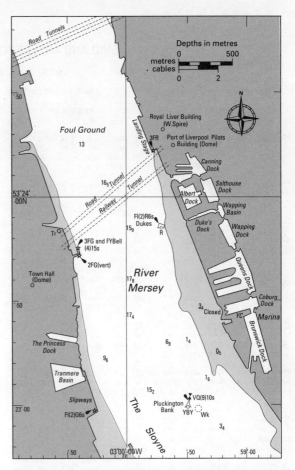

Formby and Crosby lt Floats are mid-chan SWMs. See also 10.10.4. Both chans have training banks which cover. Conspic black control bldg at lock ent has 3 R/G lts (vert).
RADIO TELEPHONE
Call: *Mersey Radio* VHF Ch **12** 16 (H24). Radar Ch 18. Marina Ch M. Tfc movements, nav warnings and wx reports broadcast on Ch 09 at HW−3 and −2. Local nav and gale warnings broadcast on receipt on Ch 12; also on Ch 09 every 4hrs from 0000LT, except HW −4 to HW −1. Eastham Locks Ch 07 (H24). Manchester Ship Canal Ch 14.
TELEPHONE (0151)
Hr Mr 200 4124; MRSC 931 3341; ⌖ 933 7075; Marinecall 0891 500 461; Police 709 6010; Ⓗ 709 0141.
FACILITIES
Marina (300 + 50) ☎ 708 5228, (0600-2130 Mar–Oct). Ent via Brunswick Dock lock, min depth 3·5m. £10.57, D, P (½M) AC, FW, BH (60 ton), Slip, CH, SM, Bar, ▣, R, V; **Albert Dock** ☎ 236 6090, VHF Ch M when ent manned, AB, FW, AC; **W Kirby SC** ☎ 625 5579, Slip, M (in Dee Est), L, FW, C (30ton), AB (at HW), Bar; **Blundellsands SC** ☎ 929 2101; Slip, L (at HW), FW, Bar; **Hoylake SC** ☎ 632 2616, Slip, M, FW, Bar; **Royal Mersey YC** ☎ 645 3204, Slip, M, P, D, L, FW, R, Bar. **Services:** CH, SM, ME, El, Sh, ACA, Ⓔ. **City** EC Wed; ✉, Ⓑ, ⇌, ✈. Note: Access to E Coast via Leeds & Liverpool Canal (BWB). Liverpool to Goole 161M, 103 locks. Max draft 0·9m, air draft 2·4m, beam 4·1m, LOA 18·3m.

ADJACENT ANCHORAGE

RIVER ALT, Merseyside, 53°31'·40N 03°03'·72W. AC 1951, *1978*. HW −0008 on Dover; see 10·10·12. Good shelter but only for LOA <8·5m x 1·2m draft on a HW of at least 8m. Mersey E training wall can be crossed HW±2. Ent to chan (shifts frequently) is E of C14 PHM lt float, thence marked by locally-laid Y Fairway buoy and perches on the training wall. Unsafe to ⚓ in R Alt; pick up a free mooring off the SC and contact club. Local knowledge advised. Facilities very limited. **Blundellsands SC** ☎ (0151) 929 2101 (occas).

ENGLAND – LIVERPOOL (ALFRED DOCK)

LAT 53°24′N   LONG 3°01′W

TIMES AND HEIGHTS OF HIGH AND LOW WATERS

YEAR **1996**

TIME ZONE (UT)
For Summer Time add ONE hour in non-shaded areas

Chart Datum: 4·93 metres below Ordnance Datum (Newlyn)

JANUARY

Day	Time	m	Time	m	Time	m	Time	m
1 M	0152	2.7	0753	7.8	1432	2.8	2018	8.0
16 TU	0054	2.8	0645	7.9	1321	2.8	1912	8.1
2 TU	0300	2.6	0850	8.1	1534	2.5	2112	8.3
17 W	0212	2.5	0756	8.3	1440	2.4	2023	8.5
3 W	0352	2.3	0937	8.5	1623	2.2	2159	8.5
18 TH	0321	1.9	0900	8.9	1549	1.8	2127	9.0
4 TH	0434	2.1	1019	8.8	1704	1.9	2239	8.7
19 F	0420	1.4	0955	9.5	1648	1.2	2222	9.5
5 F O	0511	1.9	1056	9.0	1741	1.8	2316	8.9
20 SA ●	0513	0.9	1047	9.9	1742	0.7	2314	9.8
6 SA	0544	1.8	1130	9.1	1817	1.7	2350	8.9
21 SU	0603	0.6	1136	10.2	1832	0.3		
7 SU	0615	1.7	1204	9.1	1849	1.6		
22 M	0002	10.0	0650	0.5	1224	10.3	1919	0.2
8 M	0023	8.9	0646	1.7	1239	9.1	1920	1.6
23 TU	0050	9.9	0735	0.5	1311	10.3	2004	0.3
9 TU	0058	8.8	0719	1.7	1313	9.0	1952	1.7
24 W	0136	9.8	0818	0.7	1356	10.0	2046	0.6
10 W	0132	8.8	0755	1.8	1348	8.9	2027	1.8
25 TH	0219	9.4	0900	1.1	1441	9.6	2127	1.1
11 TH	0208	8.7	0833	2.0	1426	8.8	2104	2.0
26 F	0303	8.9	0943	1.7	1525	9.0	2210	1.7
12 F	0247	8.5	0913	2.2	1507	8.6	2145	2.3
27 SA	0348	8.4	1029	2.2	1613	8.4	2257	2.4
13 SA	0331	8.2	0959	2.6	1555	8.3	2234	2.6
28 SU	0440	7.8	1124	2.8	1711	7.8	2353	2.9
14 SU	0426	7.9	1055	2.8	1653	8.1	2338	2.8
29 M	0549	7.4	1227	3.1	1827	7.4		
15 M	0532	7.8	1204	3.0	1801	7.9		
30 TU	0057	3.2	0712	7.3	1343	3.2	1946	7.5
31 W	0211	3.1	0822	7.7	1502	2.9	2048	7.8

FEBRUARY

Day	Time	m	Time	m	Time	m	Time	m
1 TH	0320	2.8	0915	8.1	1600	2.5	2138	8.2
16 F	0305	2.2	0845	8.6	1538	1.8	2117	8.8
2 F	0411	2.4	0959	8.6	1645	2.1	2221	8.6
17 SA	0408	1.5	0943	9.3	1624	1.1	2212	9.4
3 SA	0451	2.0	1038	8.9	1723	1.8	2258	8.8
18 SU ●	0502	0.9	1034	9.9	1730	0.5	2301	9.8
4 SU O	0526	1.8	1114	9.1	1758	1.6	2333	8.9
19 M	0550	0.5	1121	10.2	1818	0.1	2347	10.0
5 M	0559	1.6	1147	9.2	1830	1.4		
20 TU	0635	0.3	1206	10.4	1902	0.0		
6 TU	0006	9.0	0630	1.4	1220	9.2	1901	1.3
21 W	0030	10.0	0717	0.3	1250	10.3	1942	0.2
7 W	0039	9.0	0704	1.4	1253	9.2	1933	1.3
22 TH	0112	9.8	0757	0.5	1332	10.0	2021	0.6
8 TH	0111	9.0	0739	1.4	1327	9.2	2006	1.4
23 F	0151	9.5	0836	0.9	1412	9.6	2057	1.1
9 F	0145	9.0	0814	1.5	1403	9.1	2040	1.6
24 SA	0230	9.0	0914	1.5	1452	9.0	2134	1.7
10 SA	0221	8.8	0850	1.7	1441	8.9	2115	1.9
25 SU	0308	8.5	0955	2.1	1533	8.4	2214	2.4
11 SU	0302	8.6	0930	2.1	1526	8.6	2157	2.3
26 M	0351	7.9	1044	2.7	1621	7.7	2304	3.0
12 M	0351	8.2	1020	2.5	1621	8.2	2255	2.7
27 TU	0441	7.4	1145	3.2	1729	7.1		
13 TU	0455	7.8	1128	2.8	1730	7.8		
28 W	0009	3.4	0614	7.1	1257	3.1	1906	7.0
14 W	0015	2.9	0613	7.7	1251	2.8	1848	7.8
29 TH	0121	3.4	0746	7.3	1418	3.1	2020	7.4
15 TH	0145	2.7	0734	8.0	1422	2.5	2009	8.1

MARCH

Day	Time	m	Time	m	Time	m	Time	m
1 F	0238	3.1	0847	7.8	1529	2.7	2113	7.9
16 SA	0251	2.3	0831	8.5	1526	1.7	2105	8.6
2 SA	0341	2.6	0934	8.3	1618	2.1	2156	8.4
17 SU	0354	1.5	0928	9.2	1624	1.0	2158	9.2
3 SU	0426	2.1	1014	8.7	1657	1.7	2234	8.7
18 M	0446	0.9	1018	9.7	1713	0.5	2244	9.6
4 M	0503	1.7	1050	9.0	1732	1.4	2309	9.0
19 TU ●	0533	0.5	1103	10.0	1758	0.2	2327	9.8
5 TU O	0537	1.4	1124	9.2	1805	1.2	2342	9.1
20 W	0616	0.3	1146	10.1	1839	0.3		
6 W	0611	1.2	1156	9.3	1838	1.0		
21 TH	0007	9.8	0656	0.3	1227	10.0	1916	0.4
7 TH	0014	9.2	0645	1.1	1230	9.3	1911	1.0
22 F	0046	9.6	0734	0.5	1306	9.7	1952	0.7
8 F	0048	9.2	0720	1.0	1304	9.3	1944	1.1
23 SA	0122	9.3	0811	0.9	1343	9.3	2025	1.2
9 SA	0122	9.0	0755	1.1	1341	9.3	2017	1.3
24 SU	0158	9.0	0846	1.4	1420	8.8	2056	1.8
10 SU	0159	9.1	0831	1.3	1421	9.0	2051	1.6
25 M	0234	8.5	0923	2.0	1459	8.3	2128	2.4
11 M	0239	8.8	0910	1.7	1505	8.7	2132	2.1
26 TU	0314	8.0	1005	2.6	1543	7.7	2211	3.0
12 TU	0328	8.4	1000	2.2	1600	8.1	2228	2.6
27 W	0403	7.5	1102	3.1	1640	7.1	2317	3.4
13 W	0431	7.9	1107	2.6	1711	7.7	2349	2.9
28 TH	0511	7.1	1212	3.3	1807	6.8		
14 TH	0552	7.7	1233	2.7	1835	7.6		
29 F	0032	3.5	0652	7.1	1327	3.2	1938	7.1
15 F	0125	2.8	0718	7.9	1410	2.4	1959	8.0
30 SA	0146	3.3	0807	7.5	1440	2.8	2037	7.6
31 SU	0255	2.8	0859	8.0	1537	2.2	2123	8.2

APRIL

Day	Time	m	Time	m	Time	m	Time	m
1 M	0348	2.3	0942	8.5	1620	1.7	2203	8.6
16 TU	0426	1.1	0958	9.4	1651	0.7	2223	9.4
2 TU	0430	1.8	1019	8.8	1658	1.3	2238	8.9
17 W ●	0511	0.7	1042	9.6	1734	0.5	2304	9.5
3 W	0509	1.4	1054	9.1	1734	1.0	2313	9.1
18 TH	0553	0.6	1124	9.7	1812	0.5	2342	9.5
4 TH O	0546	1.1	1128	9.3	1811	0.9	2347	9.3
19 F	0632	0.6	1203	9.6	1848	0.7		
5 F	0624	0.9	1204	9.4	1847	0.8		
20 SA	0018	9.3	0709	0.8	1241	9.3	1921	1.1
6 SA	0023	9.4	0701	0.8	1243	9.4	1922	0.9
21 SU	0054	9.1	0746	1.1	1317	9.0	1952	1.4
7 SU	0101	9.3	0739	0.9	1323	9.3	1957	1.1
22 M	0129	8.9	0820	1.5	1353	8.7	2019	1.9
8 M	0141	9.2	0817	1.1	1406	9.0	2035	1.5
23 TU	0205	8.6	0853	1.9	1431	8.3	2047	2.3
9 TU	0225	8.9	0900	1.4	1454	8.6	2119	1.9
24 W	0245	8.2	0930	2.4	1513	7.8	2127	2.8
10 W	0316	8.5	0951	1.9	1550	8.1	2217	2.4
25 TH	0330	7.7	1020	2.8	1603	7.3	2226	3.2
11 TH	0420	8.0	1058	2.3	1701	7.7	2335	2.8
26 F	0426	7.3	1125	3.1	1709	7.0	2341	3.4
12 F	0539	7.8	1221	2.4	1825	7.6		
27 SA	0542	7.1	1234	3.1	1836	7.0		
13 SA	0106	2.7	0701	8.0	1353	2.2	1943	8.0
28 SU	0053	3.3	0706	7.3	1342	2.8	1947	7.8
14 SU	0231	2.2	0811	8.4	1507	1.6	2046	8.5
29 M	0200	2.9	0809	7.7	1444	2.3	2040	7.9
15 M	0334	1.6	0908	9.0	1604	1.1	2138	9.0
30 TU	0259	2.4	0858	8.4	1536	1.8	2123	8.4

ENGLAND – LIVERPOOL (ALFRED DOCK)

LAT 53°24′N   LONG 3°01′W

TIMES AND HEIGHTS OF HIGH AND LOW WATERS   YEAR **1996**

TIME ZONE (UT)
For Summer Time add ONE hour in non-shaded areas

MAY

Day	Time	m	Day	Time	m
1 W	0350	1.9	16 TH	0447	1.2
	0940	8.6		1021	9.2
	1621	1.4		1708	1.1
	2202	8.9		2241	9.1
2 TH	0436	1.4	17 F	0529	1.0
	1020	9.0		1103	9.2
	1703	1.1		1745	1.1
	2241	9.2		● 2318	9.1
3 F	0519	1.1	18 SA	0609	1.0
	1059	9.2		1142	9.1
	1743	0.8		1820	1.2
	O 2319	9.4		2354	9.1
4 SA	0602	0.8	19 SU	0647	1.1
	1140	9.4		1218	9.0
	1824	0.8		1853	1.4
5 SU	0000	9.5	20 M	0029	9.0
	0643	0.7		0722	1.3
	1224	9.4		1254	8.8
	1903	0.8		1921	1.6
6 M	0043	9.5	21 TU	0105	8.8
	0726	0.7		0756	1.6
	1309	9.3		1330	8.6
	1943	1.0		1948	1.9
7 TU	0128	9.4	22 W	0142	8.6
	0809	0.9		0828	1.9
	1356	9.1		1407	8.4
	2025	1.3		2019	2.2
8 W	0216	9.1	23 TH	0220	8.4
	0856	1.2		0902	2.2
	1447	8.8		1448	8.1
	2113	1.8		2059	2.5
9 TH	0310	8.7	24 F	0302	8.1
	0949	1.6		0945	2.5
	1544	8.3		1533	7.7
	2211	2.2		2149	2.9
10 F	0413	8.4	25 SA	0351	7.7
	1052	1.9		1040	2.8
	1651	8.0		1626	7.4
	2321	2.5		2252	3.1
11 SA	0524	8.1	26 SU	0450	7.5
	1206	2.1		1143	2.9
	1806	7.8		1731	7.3
12 SU	0041	2.5	27 M	0001	3.2
	0637	8.1		0557	7.4
	1326	2.0		1248	2.8
	1918	8.0		1842	7.4
13 M	0201	2.3	28 TU	0108	3.0
	0745	8.4		0705	7.6
	1439	1.8		1352	2.5
	2021	8.3		1946	7.8
14 TU	0307	1.9	29 W	0211	2.6
	0844	8.7		0805	8.0
	1538	1.4		1451	2.1
	2113	8.7		2039	8.3
15 W	0401	1.5	30 TH	0309	2.1
	0935	9.0		0858	8.5
	1626	1.2		1544	1.6
	2159	9.0		2126	8.8
			31 F	0403	1.6
				0946	8.9
				1633	1.2
				2210	9.2

JUNE

Day	Time	m	Day	Time	m
1 SA	0453	1.2	16 SU	0548	1.4
	1033	9.2		1123	8.8
	1719	1.0		1755	1.6
	O 2255	9.5		● 2334	8.9
2 SU	0541	0.9	17 M	0626	1.5
	1120	9.4		1204	8.8
	1804	0.8		1827	1.7
	2340	9.6			
3 M	0629	0.7	18 TU	0009	8.9
	1208	9.5		0701	1.5
	1848	0.8		1235	8.7
				1856	1.8
4 TU	0027	9.7	19 W	0045	8.8
	0716	0.6		0735	1.7
	1258	9.5		1310	8.6
	1932	0.9		1924	1.9
5 W	0117	9.6	20 TH	0121	8.7
	0804	0.7		0808	1.8
	1348	9.3		1346	8.5
	2018	1.1		1957	2.0
6 TH	0208	9.4	21 F	0158	8.6
	0853	0.9		0838	2.0
	1439	9.1		1424	8.3
	2107	1.5		2036	2.2
7 F	0302	9.1	22 SA	0237	8.4
	0945	1.2		0917	2.2
	1533	8.7		1504	8.1
	2201	1.8		2120	2.5
8 SA	0359	8.8	23 SU	0319	8.2
	1040	1.5		1002	2.4
	1632	8.3		1549	7.9
	2302	2.2		2211	2.8
9 SU	0501	8.5	24 M	0409	7.9
	1142	1.9		1056	2.6
	1738	8.0		1643	7.6
				2313	3.0
10 M	0009	2.4	25 TU	0507	7.8
	0608	8.2		1158	2.7
	1250	2.1		1746	7.6
	1846	7.9			
11 TU	0122	2.4	26 W	0019	2.9
	0715	8.2		0610	7.7
	1402	2.1		1305	2.6
	1951	8.1		1852	7.8
12 W	0235	2.2	27 TH	0127	2.7
	0817	8.3		0716	8.0
	1507	2.0		1411	2.3
	2048	8.3		1956	8.2
13 TH	0335	1.9	28 F	0233	2.3
	0912	8.5		0820	8.3
	1559	1.8		1512	1.9
	2137	8.6		2053	8.7
14 F	0424	1.7	29 SA	0335	1.8
	1001	8.7		0918	8.8
	1642	1.7		1608	1.5
	2220	8.8		2145	9.2
15 SA	0508	1.5	30 SU	0432	1.3
	1044	8.8		1012	9.2
	1720	1.6		1659	1.1
	2258	8.9		2235	9.6

JULY

Day	Time	m	Day	Time	m
1 M	0526	0.9	16 TU	0607	1.6
	1104	9.5		1142	8.7
	1748	0.9		1805	1.8
	O 2324	9.8		2352	9.0
2 TU	0618	0.6	17 W	0641	1.6
	1154	9.6		1217	8.7
	1836	0.7		1835	1.7
3 W	0014	9.9	18 TH	0026	8.9
	0708	0.4		0713	1.6
	1245	9.7		1251	8.7
	1923	0.7		1905	1.7
4 TH	0104	9.9	19 F	0100	8.9
	0757	0.4		0743	1.6
	1335	9.6		1324	8.7
	2010	0.9		1938	1.8
5 F	0155	9.8	20 SA	0134	8.8
	0844	0.5		0815	1.7
	1424	9.4		1359	8.6
	2056	1.1		2014	1.9
6 SA	0245	9.5	21 SU	0210	8.7
	0931	0.9		0850	1.9
	1513	9.0		1435	8.5
	2144	1.5		2053	2.1
7 SU	0336	9.1	22 M	0249	8.5
	1019	1.3		0929	2.1
	1605	8.6		1515	8.2
	2236	2.0		2136	2.4
8 M	0431	8.6	23 TU	0333	8.3
	1112	1.8		1014	2.4
	1703	8.1		1602	8.0
	2335	2.4		2228	2.7
9 TU	0533	8.2	24 W	0426	8.0
	1211	2.3		1110	2.7
	1809	7.8		1701	7.8
				2334	2.9
10 W	0042	2.6	25 TH	0529	7.8
	0642	7.9		1221	2.8
	1317	2.5		1810	7.8
	1919	7.7			
11 TH	0158	2.7	26 F	0049	2.9
	0750	7.9		0639	7.8
	1429	2.6		1336	2.6
	2022	8.0		1921	8.0
12 F	0308	2.4	27 SA	0205	2.5
	0850	8.1		0751	8.1
	1531	2.4		1447	2.2
	2116	8.3		2027	8.5
13 SA	0404	2.1	28 SU	0315	2.0
	0941	8.3		0858	8.6
	1619	2.2		1549	1.7
	2201	8.6		2126	9.1
14 SU	0449	1.9	29 M	0417	1.4
	1026	8.6		0957	9.1
	1658	2.0		1645	1.2
	2241	8.8		2219	9.7
15 M	0529	1.7	30 TU	0514	0.8
	1106	8.7		1050	9.5
	1733	1.8		1736	0.8
	● 2318	8.9		O 2309	10.0
			31 W	0606	0.4
				1140	9.8
				1824	0.6
				2358	10.2

AUGUST

Day	Time	m	Day	Time	m
1 TH	0655	0.2	16 F	0004	9.1
	1229	9.9		0648	1.4
	1911	0.5		1228	8.8
				1845	1.5
2 F	0046	10.2	17 SA	0036	9.0
	0742	0.2		0718	1.4
	1316	9.8		1259	8.8
	1954	0.6		1919	1.5
3 SA	0134	10.0	18 SU	0109	9.0
	0826	0.3		0750	1.5
	1402	9.6		1332	8.8
	2037	0.9		1953	1.6
4 SU	0221	9.7	19 M	0143	8.9
	0909	0.8		0824	1.6
	1446	9.2		1406	8.7
	2120	1.4		2029	1.8
5 M	0307	9.2	20 TU	0219	8.7
	0952	1.3		0859	1.9
	1532	8.7		1443	8.5
	2207	1.9		2107	2.1
6 TU	0356	8.6	21 W	0301	8.5
	1038	2.0		0937	2.3
	1622	8.1		1528	8.2
	2301	2.5		2152	2.5
7 W	0452	8.0	22 TH	0352	8.1
	1132	2.6		1027	2.7
	1724	7.6		1625	7.9
				2255	2.8
8 TH	0004	2.9	23 F	0457	7.8
	0604	7.5		1141	2.9
	1235	3.0		1737	7.7
	1843	7.4			
9 F	0120	3.0	24 SA	0018	2.9
	0723	7.5		0612	7.6
	1346	3.1		1309	2.9
	1956	7.6		1855	7.9
10 SA	0241	2.8	25 SU	0145	2.6
	0828	7.7		0732	7.9
	1501	2.8		1429	2.4
	2054	8.0		2009	8.4
11 SU	0344	2.4	26 M	0302	2.0
	0921	8.1		0845	8.5
	1556	2.5		1536	1.8
	2141	8.5		2111	9.1
12 M	0430	2.1	27 TU	0406	1.3
	1006	8.4		0944	9.1
	1638	2.2		1632	1.2
	2222	8.8		2205	9.7
13 TU	0509	1.8	28 W	0501	0.6
	1046	8.7		1035	9.6
	1713	1.9		1722	0.7
	2259	9.0		O 2253	10.1
14 W	0545	1.6	29 TH	0550	0.2
	1122	8.8		1123	9.9
	1747	1.7		1809	0.4
	● 2332	9.1		2340	10.3
15 TH	0618	1.5	30 F	0637	0.0
	1155	8.8		1208	9.9
	1815	1.6		1853	0.3
			31 SA	0025	10.3
				0720	0.1
				1252	9.8
				1934	0.5

Chart Datum: 4·93 metres below Ordnance Datum (Newlyn)

ENGLAND – LIVERPOOL (ALFRED DOCK)

LAT 53°24′N   LONG   3°01′W

TIMES AND HEIGHTS OF HIGH AND LOW WATERS

YEAR 1996

TIME ZONE (UT)
For Summer Time add ONE hour in non-shaded areas

SEPTEMBER

Day	Time / m	Time / m	Time / m	Time / m
1 SU	0110 10.0	0801 0.4	1334 9.5	2014 0.8
16 M	0042 9.1	0725 1.3	1304 9.0	1933 1.3
2 M	0152 9.6	0840 0.9	1415 9.1	2054 1.3
17 TU	0117 9.0	0759 1.5	1339 8.9	2008 1.5
3 TU	0234 9.1	0919 1.5	1455 8.6	2137 1.9
18 W	0155 8.9	0832 1.8	1417 8.7	2045 1.9
4 W	0318 8.4	1002 2.2	1539 8.1	2226 2.6
19 TH	0237 8.5	0910 2.2	1502 8.4	2129 2.3
5 TH	0407 7.8	1052 2.9	1632 7.5	2328 3.1
20 F	0329 8.1	0959 2.6	1600 8.0	2231 2.7
6 F	0517 7.2	1154 3.3	1755 7.2	
21 SA	0436 7.7	1113 3.0	1713 7.7	2357 2.9
7 SA	0041 3.3	0650 7.1	1305 3.4	1924 7.3
22 SU	0556 7.5	1247 3.0	1837 7.8	
8 SU	0205 3.1	0802 7.4	1422 3.2	2027 7.8
23 M	0131 2.6	0722 7.8	1413 2.5	1954 8.3
9 M	0315 2.6	0856 7.9	1527 2.7	2116 8.3
24 TU	0250 1.9	0833 8.4	1521 1.8	2056 9.0
10 TU	0403 2.2	0941 8.3	1612 2.3	2157 8.7
25 W	0352 1.2	0929 9.1	1616 1.2	2148 9.6
11 W	0442 1.8	1020 8.7	1648 1.9	2234 9.0
26 TH	0444 0.6	1017 9.6	1647 0.7	2235 10.0
12 TH ●	0516 1.5	1056 8.9	1721 1.6	2307 9.1
27 F O	0530 0.2	1102 9.8	1750 0.4	2319 10.2
13 F	0548 1.3	1128 9.0	1752 1.4	2338 9.1
28 SA	0614 0.1	1145 9.8	1832 0.4	
14 SA	0620 1.2	1200 9.0	1825 1.3	
29 SU	0002 10.1	0654 0.3	1226 9.7	1911 0.6
15 SU	0009 9.1	0652 1.2	1231 9.0	1858 1.3
30 M	0044 9.8	0733 0.6	1305 9.4	1950 0.9

OCTOBER

Day	Time / m	Time / m	Time / m	Time / m
1 TU	0123 9.4	0809 1.1	1343 9.1	2028 1.4
16 W	0056 9.2	0737 1.4	1317 9.1	1952 1.4
2 W	0202 8.9	0845 1.7	1420 8.6	2107 2.0
17 TH	0137 8.9	0813 1.7	1359 8.9	2032 1.7
3 TH	0242 8.3	0923 2.4	1501 8.1	2152 2.6
18 F	0223 8.6	0854 2.1	1447 8.6	2119 2.1
4 F	0327 7.7	1007 3.0	1548 7.6	2249 3.1
19 SA	0317 8.2	0946 2.6	1546 8.2	2221 2.5
5 SA	0425 7.2	1109 3.5	1654 7.2	
20 SU	0423 7.7	1058 2.9	1658 7.9	2342 2.7
6 SU	0000 3.3	0558 6.9	1221 3.6	1835 7.1
21 M	0544 7.6	1227 2.9	1820 7.9	
7 M	0116 3.2	0725 7.1	1335 3.4	1950 7.5
22 TU	0113 2.4	0707 7.9	1353 2.5	1934 8.4
8 TU	0229 2.8	0823 7.6	1444 3.0	2043 8.0
23 W	0231 1.9	0815 8.4	1501 1.9	2036 8.9
9 W	0324 2.3	0909 8.2	1535 2.5	2125 8.5
24 TH	0332 1.3	0910 9.0	1557 1.3	2129 9.4
10 TH	0406 1.8	0949 8.6	1616 2.0	2203 8.8
25 F	0423 0.8	0957 9.4	1645 0.9	2215 9.8
11 F	0442 1.5	1024 8.9	1651 1.6	2236 9.1
26 SA O	0508 0.5	1041 9.6	1740 0.7	2259 9.9
12 SA ●	0516 1.2	1057 9.1	1727 1.3	2309 9.2
27 SU	0549 0.5	1121 9.6	1810 0.7	2340 9.8
13 SU	0551 1.1	1130 9.2	1802 1.2	2342 9.2
28 M	0628 0.7	1200 9.5	1849 0.8	
14 M	0627 1.2	1203 9.2	1839 1.1	
29 TU	0019 9.5	0704 1.0	1237 9.3	1927 1.1
15 TU	0017 9.2	0702 1.2	1239 9.2	1915 1.2
30 W	0057 9.2	0739 1.4	1314 9.0	2004 1.5
31 TH	0135 8.8	0812 1.9	1351 8.7	2041 2.0

NOVEMBER

Day	Time / m	Time / m	Time / m	Time / m
1 F	0213 8.3	0844 2.4	1430 8.3	2119 2.5
16 SA	0215 8.8	0847 1.9	1440 8.9	2117 1.7
2 SA	0256 7.9	0921 2.9	1515 7.9	2208 2.9
17 SU	0309 8.4	0940 2.3	1537 8.6	2216 2.1
3 SU	0345 7.4	1015 3.3	1608 7.5	2311 3.2
18 M	0412 8.0	1045 2.6	1643 8.3	2326 2.3
4 M	0451 7.0	1126 3.6	1720 7.2	
19 TU	0526 7.8	1200 2.7	1757 8.2	
5 TU	0021 3.3	0622 7.0	1239 3.5	1848 7.3
20 W	0045 2.3	0642 7.9	1321 2.6	1909 8.3
6 W	0130 3.0	0735 7.4	1346 3.2	1954 7.7
21 TH	0203 2.0	0751 8.3	1435 2.2	2013 8.7
7 TH	0231 2.6	0827 7.9	1445 2.7	2043 8.2
22 F	0308 1.6	0848 8.7	1534 1.7	2108 9.1
8 F	0321 2.1	0911 8.4	1535 2.2	2124 8.6
23 SA	0400 1.3	0937 9.1	1624 1.3	2156 9.3
9 SA	0404 1.6	0949 8.8	1618 1.8	2202 9.0
24 SU	0445 1.1	1021 9.3	1709 1.1	2240 9.4
10 SU	0444 1.3	1025 9.1	1659 1.4	2239 9.2
25 M O	0526 1.0	1101 9.4	1750 1.1	2321 9.4
11 M ●	0524 1.1	1102 9.3	1740 1.2	2317 9.3
26 TU	0604 1.1	1139 9.3	1830 1.2	2359 9.2
12 SU	0603 1.0	1139 9.4	1821 1.1	2357 9.4
27 W	0640 1.1	1215 9.2	1908 1.3	
13 W	0642 1.1	1219 9.4	1902 1.1	
28 TH	0036 9.0	0713 1.6	1251 9.1	1944 1.6
14 TH	0040 9.3	0721 1.3	1303 9.4	1943 1.2
29 F	0112 8.8	0744 1.9	1328 8.9	2018 1.9
15 F	0126 9.1	0802 1.5	1349 9.2	2027 1.4
30 SA	0150 8.5	0814 2.3	1406 8.6	2051 2.3

DECEMBER

Day	Time / m	Time / m	Time / m	Time / m
1 SU	0229 8.2	0848 2.6	1447 8.3	2130 2.6
16 M	0259 8.9	0931 1.8	1524 9.1	2205 1.6
2 M	0313 7.8	0933 3.0	1533 7.9	2220 2.9
17 TU	0355 8.5	1027 2.2	1623 8.7	2304 1.9
3 TU	0405 7.5	1031 3.3	1627 7.6	2322 3.1
18 W	0459 8.1	1130 2.5	1728 8.4	
4 W	0508 7.2	1138 3.4	1732 7.5	
19 TH	0010 2.2	0610 8.0	1242 2.6	1838 8.2
5 TH	0028 3.1	0623 7.3	1246 3.3	1842 7.6
20 F	0125 2.3	0721 8.0	1401 2.5	1946 8.3
6 F	0133 2.8	0731 7.6	1351 3.0	1947 7.9
21 SA	0237 2.1	0824 8.3	1510 2.2	2047 8.6
7 SA	0233 2.6	0826 8.1	1451 2.5	2040 8.3
22 SU	0337 1.9	0917 8.7	1606 1.9	2139 8.8
8 SU	0326 2.0	0912 8.6	1545 2.0	2128 8.8
23 M	0425 1.7	1004 9.0	1653 1.6	2225 9.0
9 M	0414 1.5	0955 9.1	1634 1.6	2212 9.1
24 TU O	0507 1.5	1045 9.1	1735 1.5	2306 9.1
10 TU ●	0459 1.2	1037 9.4	1721 1.2	2257 9.4
25 W	0544 1.5	1123 9.2	1814 1.4	2344 9.1
11 W	0543 1.1	1120 9.6	1807 1.0	2342 9.5
26 TH	0620 1.6	1159 9.2	1851 1.5	
12 TH	0627 1.0	1205 9.7	1853 0.9	
27 F	0019 9.0	0653 1.7	1234 9.1	1926 1.6
13 F	0029 9.5	0711 1.1	1252 9.7	1938 0.9
28 SA	0054 8.9	0721 1.5	1309 9.0	1958 1.8
14 SA	0117 9.4	0755 1.2	1341 9.6	2025 1.0
29 SU	0129 8.7	0751 2.0	1345 8.9	2027 2.0
15 SU	0207 9.2	0842 1.5	1431 9.4	2113 1.3
30 M	0206 8.5	0824 2.2	1423 8.7	2100 2.2
31 TU	0245 8.3	0903 2.5	1502 8.4	2140 2.5

Chart Datum: 4·93 metres below Ordnance Datum (Newlyn)

ISLE OF MAN   10-10-13

CHARTS
AC 2696 (ports), 2094 (small scale). Irish Sea *1826, 1411*

The Isle of Man is one of the British Islands, set in the Irish Sea almost equidistant from England, Scotland and Ireland but it is not part of the UK. It has a large degree of self-government. The IOM comes under the same customs umbrella as the rest of the UK, but there are no formalities on landing from or returning to UK.

Harbours and anchorages. Manx hbrs are administered by the IOM Government and lights are maintained by the Commissioners of Northern Lighthouses in Scotland. Besides the four main hbrs given below, there are good ⚓s at Castletown in the SE, Laxey Bay in the E and Port Erin in the SW; see below. There are also good ⚓s in Derby Haven in the SE; this is a rather bleak area and the inner hbr dries. Most of the hbrs are on the E and S sides but a visit to the W coast with its characteristic cliffs is worth while. All IOM hbrs charge the same berthing fee, ie £5.30 regardless of LOA; or £21.20 weekly fee allows use of all hbrs.

Passage information. Including Calf Sound, see 10·10·5.

R/T. If contact with local Hr Mrs cannot be established on VHF, vessels should call *Douglas Hbr Control* Ch 12 16 for urgent messages or other info.

Coastguard. Call Liverpool MRSC Ch 16 67; there is no loss of VHF coverage as the Snaefell (IoM) aerial is linked to Liverpool by land line.

Weather. Forecasts can be obtained from Manx Radio, see Table 7 (5); or direct from the forecaster, Ronaldsway Met Office ☎ 0696 888 200, (0700-2030LT). Recorded shipping forecast (updated 3 times daily) ☎ 0696 888 322; recorded general forecast ☎ 0696 888 320.

Directions. The *Isle of Man SDs, Tidal streams and Anchorages* by the Manx Sailing and Cruising Club in Ramsey, ☎ 01624-813494, are recommended .

Distances. See 10.10.6 for distances between ports in Area 10 and 10.0.6 for distances across the Irish Sea, North Channel and St George's Channel.

MINOR HARBOURS IN THE ISLE OF MAN

PORT ERIN, Isle of Man, 54°05´·30N 04°46´·27W. AC 2696, 2094. HW −0020 on Dover; ML 2·9m; Duration 0555. See 10·10·14. The bay has good ⚓ in 3-8m, but exposed to all W winds. Ldg lts, both FR 10/19m 5M, lead 099° into the bay. Beware the ruined bkwtr extending N from the SW corner, marked by an unlit SHM buoy. A small hbr on the S side dries 0·8m. Raglan Pier (E arm of hbr) Oc G 5s 8m 5M. Two ⚓s W of Raglan Pier; call Hr Mr Port St. Mary (VHF Ch 12). Facilities: EC Thurs; Bar, D, P, FW, R, Slip, V.

LAXEY, Isle of Man, 54°13´·45N 04°23´·25W. AC 2094. HW +0025 on Dover, +0010 on Liverpool; HW ht −2·0m on Liverpool; ML 4·0m; Duration 0550. The bay gives good shelter in SW to N winds. The hbr dries 3·0m to rk and is only suitable for small yachts; access HW±3 for 1·5m draft. Beware rks on N side of the narrow ent. Keep close to pier after entering to avoid training wall to N. Pier hd lt Oc R 3s 7m 5M, obsc when brg <318°. Bkwtr hd lt Oc G 3s 7m. Facilities: FW, R, ✉, Ⓑ, Bar.

CASTLETOWN, Isle of Man, 54°03´·50N 04°38´·50W. AC 2696, 2094. HW +0025 on Dover; ML 3·4m; Duration 0555. See 10.10.14. Hbr dries (level sand). Access HW±2½. Berth in Outer Hbr or go via swing bridge (manually operated) into Inner Hbr below fixed bridge. ⚓ between Lheeah-rio Rks and pier in 3m; off Langness Pt; or in Derby Haven (dries). The bay gives good shelter except in SE to SW winds. Beware Lheeah-rio Rks in W of bay, marked by PHM Fl R 3s, Bell. Keep inside the race off Dreswick Pt, or give it a wide berth. Langness lt , on Dreswick Pt, Fl (2) 30s 23m 21M. S side of ent: New Pier Oc R 15s 8m 5M; then Irish Quay, Oc R 4s 5m 5M, vis 142°-322°. 150m NW is swing bridge marked by 2 FR (hor). N side of ent Oc G 4s 3m (W metal post on concrete column). VHF Ch 12 16 (when vessel due). Hr Mr ☎ 823549. Facilities: **Outer Hbr** Slip, L, C (20 ton) AB; **Irish Quay** AB, C, FW; **Inner Hbr** AB, C, FW; **Services:** P, D, Gas, ME. **Town** EC Thurs; Dr 823597.

PEEL   10-10-14

Isle of Man 54°13'·60N 04°41'·61W

CHARTS
AC 2696, 2094; Imray C62; Y70; OS 95

TIDES
+0005 Dover; ML 2·9; Duration 0545; Zone 0 (UT)

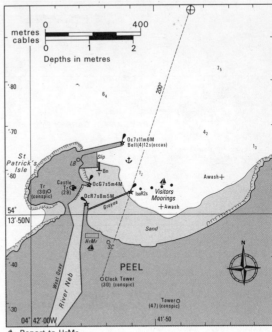

▲ Report to HrMr

Standard Port LIVERPOOL (←—)

Times				Height (metres)			
High Water		Low Water		MHWS	MHWN	MLWN	MLWS
0000	0600	0200	0700	9·3	7·4	2·9	0·9
1200	1800	1400	1900				
Differences PEEL							
−0015	+0010	0000	−0010	−4·0	−3·2	−1·4	−0·4
PORT ERIN							
−0005	+0015	−0010	−0050	−4·1	−3·2	−1·3	−0·5

SHELTER
Good, except in strong NW to NE winds when ent should not be attempted. 3 R ⚓s off S groyne in about 2m. Fin keelers may be able to berth on N bkwtr in 5m. Hbr dries; very crowded Jun-Oct. Inner hbr dries approx 2·8m to flat sand; access HW±3, possible AB on W quay.

NAVIGATION
WPT 54°13'·96N 04°41'·36W, 020°/200° from/to groyne lt, 0·42M. When approaching, a rky coastline indicates that you are S of Peel; a sandy coastline means you are to the N. When close in, beware groyne on S side of hbr ent, submerged at half tide.

LIGHTS AND MARKS
Power stn chy (80m, grey with B top; R lts) at S end of inner hbr is conspic from W and N; chy brg 203° leads to hbr ent. Groyne lt and Clock Tr (conspic) in transit 200° are almost on same line. Peel Castle and 2 twrs are conspic on St Patrick's Isle to NW of hbr. No ldg lts. N bkwtr Oc 7s 11m 6M. Groyne Iso R 2s 4m. S pier hd Oc R 7s 8m 5M; vis 156°-249°. Castle jetty Oc G 7s 5m 4M.

RADIO TELEPHONE
VHF Ch 12 16 (when vessel expected; at other times call *Douglas Hbr Control* Ch 12).

TELEPHONE (01624)
Hr Mr ☎/Fax 842338; MRSC·0151-931 3341; ⌗ 674321; Weather 0696 888322; Marinecall 0891 500 461; Police 842208; Dr 843636.

FACILITIES
Outer & Inner Hbrs, AB £5.30, M, Slip, FW, ME, El, Sh, C (30 ton mobile); **Peel Sailing and Cruising Club** ☎ 842390, P & D (cans), R, ✉, Bar; **Services:** ME, Gas, BY, CH, ACA. **Town** EC Thurs; CH, V, R, Bar, ✉, Ⓑ, ⇌ (bus to Douglas, ferry to Heysham), ✈ Ronaldsway.

10

PORT ST MARY   10-10-15

Isle of Man 54°04'·42N 04°43'·64W

CHARTS

AC 2696, 2094; Imray C62; Y70; OS 95

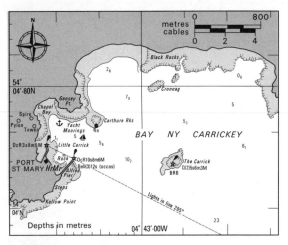

TIDES

+0020 Dover; ML 3·2; Duration 0605; Zone 0 (UT)

Standard Port LIVERPOOL (←—)

Times				Height (metres)			
High Water		Low Water		MHWS	MHWN	MLWN	MLWS
0000	0600	0200	0700	9·3	7·4	2·9	0·9
1200	1800	1400	1900				
Differences PORT ST MARY							
+0005	+0015	−0010	−0030	−3·4	−2·7	−1·2	−0·3
CALF SOUND							
+0005	+0005	−0015	−0025	−3·2	−2·6	−0·9	−0·3

SHELTER

Very good except in E or SE winds. Inner hbr dries 2·4m on sand. ‡ S of Gansey Pt, but poor holding. 8 R ♠s in same area.

NAVIGATION

WPT 54°04'·20N 04°43'·30W, 115°/295° from/to Alfred Pier lt, 0·30M. Rky outcrops to SE of pier to 2ca offshore. Beware lobster/crab pots, especially from Calf Is to Langness Pt.

LIGHTS AND MARKS

Alfred Pier, Oc R 10s 8m 6M. Inner pier, Oc R 3s 8m 5M; both lts on W trs + R band, in transit 295° lead clear S of The Carrick Rk, in centre of bay, which is marked by IDM bn, Q (2) 5s 6m 3M. A conspic TV mast, (133m, R lts) 5ca WNW of hbr, in transit 290° with Alfred Pier lt also leads clear of Carrick Rk.

RADIO TELEPHONE

Call *Port St Mary Hbr* VHF Ch 12 16 (when vessel due or through Douglas Hbr Control Ch 12).

TELEPHONE (01624)

Hr Mr 833206; MRSC 0151-931 3341; ⌗ 674321; Marinecall 0891 500 461; Police 822222; Dr 832281.

FACILITIES

Alfred Pier AB £5.30 (see 10.10.13), Slip, D (by road tanker), L, FW, C (20 ton mobile); **Inner Hbr** AB, Slip, D, L, FW; **Isle of Man YC** ☎ 832088, FW, Bar; **Services:** ME, CH, D, El, SM.
Town EC Thurs; CH, V, R, Bar, ✉, Ⓑ, ⇌ (bus to Douglas, ferry to Heysham); ✈ Ronaldsway.

DOUGLAS   10-10-16

Isle of Man 54°08'·86N 04°27'·89W

CHARTS

AC 2696, 2094; Imray C62; Y70; OS 95

TIDES

+0009 Dover; ML 3·8; Duration 0600; Zone 0 (UT)

Standard Port LIVERPOOL (←—)

Times				Height (metres)			
High Water		Low Water		MHWS	MHWN	MLWN	MLWS
0000	0600	0200	0700	9·3	7·4	2·9	0·9
1200	0800	1400	1900				
Differences DOUGLAS							
−0004	−0004	−0022	−0032	−2·4	−2·0	−0·5	−0·1

SHELTER

Good except in NE winds. Very heavy seas run in during NE gales. The Hbr Board provides a B can ♠, close NW of front ldg lt; yachts should moor stern-to the ♠, bower ‡ laid out radially. A small mooring pontoon at inner end of Battery Pier offers rafting for about 6 yachts; untenable in NE/E winds. Complete shelter, but very full in summer, at drying inner hbr W of swing bridge which opens 2300-0700 for shipping, and on request HW±3.

NAVIGATION

WPT 54°09'·00N 04°27'·60W (abeam No 1 SHM By, Q (3) G 5s), 049°/229° from/to front ldg lt, 0·47M. Appr from NE of No 1 buoy (to avoid overfalls E of Princess Alexandra Pier) and await port entry sig, or call on VHF Ch 12. There is no bar. Keep clear of large vessels and ferries. Beware swing bridge and also concrete step at end of dredged area (◊ mark on King Edward Pier).

LIGHTS AND MARKS

Douglas Head Fl 10s 32m 24M. Ldg lts 229°, both Oc 10s 9/12m 5M, synch; front W △; rear W ▽, both on R border. IPTS Nos 2, 3 & 5 shown from mast on Victoria Pier. Dolphin at N end of Alexandra Pier 2FR (vert). Corners of linkspan, S of K. Edward Pier, marked with 2 FG (vert).

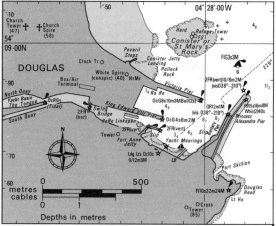

RADIO TELEPHONE

Douglas Hbr Control VHF Ch **12** 16 (H24); also broadcasts nav warnings for IoM coastal waters on Ch 12 at 0133, 0533, 0733, 0933, 1333, 1733 and 2133; met & tidal info on request.

TELEPHONE (01624)

Hr Mr 686628 (H24); MRSC 0151-931 3341; ⌗ 674321; Marinecall 0891 500 461; Police 631212; Ⓗ 663322.

FACILITIES

Outer Hbr AB £5.30 (see 10.10.13), M, FW at pontoon, P & D (cans) across the road from pontoon, ME, El, Sh, C (10, 5 ton), Slip; **Inner Hbr (N and S Quays)** AB, M, AC, FW, ME, C, El, Sh, CH, Slip; **Douglas Bay YC** (S side of inner hbr) ☎ 673965, Bar, Slip, L.
Services: P & D (cans), CH, ACA, El, Divers, Gas, Gaz, Kos.
Town EC Thurs; V, R, Bar, ✉, Ⓑ, ▣, Ferry to Heysham; also in summer to Belfast and Liverpool; ✈ Ronaldsway.

RAMSEY   10-10-17

Isle of Man 54°19'·43N 04°22'·42W

CHARTS
AC 2696, 2094; Imray C62; Y70; OS 95
TIDES
+0020 Dover; ML 4·2; Duration 0545; Zone 0 (UT)

Standard Port LIVERPOOL (◄——)

Times				Height (metres)			
High Water		Low Water		MHWS	MHWN	MLWN	MLWS
0000	0600	0200	0700	9·3	7·4	2·9	0·9
1200	1800	1400	1900				
Differences RAMSEY							
+0005	+0015	−0005	−0015	−1·7	−1·5	−0·6	+0·1

SHELTER
Very good except in strong NE/SE winds. Hbr dries 1·8m.
Access and ent only permitted HW −2½ to HW +2. Berth
on Town quay (S side) or as directed by Hr Mr on entry.
There are Y ⚓s SE of Queens Pier hd (summer only). Note:
Queens Pier is unsafe for landing.
NAVIGATION
WPT 54°19'·40N 04°21'·60W, 095°/275° from/to ent, 0·48M.
The foreshore dries out 1ca to seaward of the pier hds.
LIGHTS AND MARKS
No ldg lts/marks. Relative to hbr ent, Pt of Ayre, Fl (4)
20s 32m 19M, is 5·5M N; Maughold Hd, Fl (3) 30s 65m
21M, is 3M SE; Albert Tr (□ stone tr 14m, on hill 130m)
is conspic 7ca S; and Snaefell (617m) bears 220°/5M.
The Iso G 4s inside the hbr is not visible from seaward;
it is on a W post with violet band and marks the S tip of
Mooragh Bank. 2FR (hor) mark the centre of swing
bridge on each side.
RADIO TELEPHONE
VHF Ch 12 16 (0830-1700 LT and when commercial
vessels due; or via Douglas Hbr Control Ch 12).
TELEPHONE (01624)
Hr Mr 812245; MRSC 0151-931 3341; ⌗ 674321;
Marinecall 0891 500 461; Police 812234; Dr 813881;
Ⓗ 813254.
FACILITIES
Outer Hbr: E Quay ☎ 812245, AB (but mainly FVs), FW;
Town Quay (S side) AB £5.30 (see 10.10.13), FW, C*;
Inner Hbr, W Quay AB, FW, Slip (Grid); N Quay AB, FW;
Shipyard Quay Slip; Old Hbr AB, Slip, M;
Manx Sailing & Cruising Club ☎ 813494, Bar.
Services: P & D (cans) from garages; none located at
hbr. Gas, ME, El, Ⓔ, Sh.
Town EC Wed; V, R, Gas, Gaz, Kos, Bar, ⊠, ✉, Ⓑ, ⇌
(bus to Douglas, ferry to Heysham), ✈ Ronaldsway.
*Mobile cranes for hire from Douglas.

CONWY   10-10-18

Gwynedd 53°17'·70N 03°50'·30W

CHARTS
AC 1978, 1977, 1826; Imray C61; OS 115
TIDES
−0015 Dover; ML 4·3; Duration 0545; Zone 0 (UT)

Standard Port HOLYHEAD (——►)

Times				Height (metres)			
High Water		Low Water		MHWS	MHWN	MLWN	MLWS
0000	0600	0500	1100	5·6	4·4	2·0	0·7
1200	1800	1700	2300				
Differences CONWY							
+0020	+0020	No data	+0050	+2·1	+1·6	+0·3	No data

NOTE: HW Conwy is approx HW Liverpool −0040 sp and
−0020 nps.

SHELTER
Good in hbr and marina, except in strong NW winds.
Berth in marina (to stbd past the Narrows) or ask Hbr Mr
for ⚓ or berth at pontoon between marina and castle.
NAVIGATION
WPT Fairway SWM By, 53°17'·90N 03°55'·47W, 294°/114°
from/to No 2 PHM It By, 0·88M. Chan is marked by 4 PHM
buoys (Nos 2 & 8 are lit) and 3 unlit SHM buoys all with
radar reflectors. The Scabs, between No 6 & 8 Bys, have
least depth 0·1m and strong streams. Access HW±2; if
Conwy Sands (to N) are covered, there is enough water
in chan for 2m draft boat. Leave Perch It approx 30m to
stbd. Beware unlit moorings. Entry via "Inshore Passage"
(close SW of Gt Orme's Hd) is not advised without local
knowledge. Speed limit in estuary above Perch It is 10kn.
LIGHTS AND MARKS
Ent chan is mainly within W sector of Perch It, Fl WR 5s
5m 2M, vis W076°-088°, R088°-171°, W171°-319°, R319°-
076°. Unlit PHM & SHM Bys at the Narrows, then marina
bkwtr marked by Fl G It and ent by PHM and SHM piles.
RADIO TELEPHONE
Hr Mr Ch 12 06 08 14 71 80 16 (Summer 09-1700LT every
day; winter, same times Mon-Fri). Conwy Marina Ch 80
(H24). N Wales CA Ch 80 M. Conwy YC Ch M (water taxi).
TELEPHONE (01492)
Hr Mr 596253; MRSC (01407) 762051; ⌗ (01407) 762714;
Marinecall 0891 500 460; Police 2222; Dr 593385.
FACILITIES
Marina (420) ☎ 593000, Fax 572111, £12.69, AC, FW, D,
P, BH (30 ton), CH, Gas, R, Bar;
Harbour ☎ 596253, M, D, FW, Quay AB dries (12·3m
max LOA; short stay for loading), Pontoon AB £6.85;
Deganwy Dock (dries), AB, Slip, FW, C (mobile);
Conwy YC ☎ 583690, Slip, M, L, FW, R, Bar, water taxi;
N Wales Cruising Ass'n ☎ 593481, AB, M, FW, Bar.
Services: ME, Gas, Gaz, Sh, El, Ⓔ.
Town EC Wed; P & D (cans), V, R, Bar, ✉, Ⓑ, ⇌, ✈
(Liverpool).

10

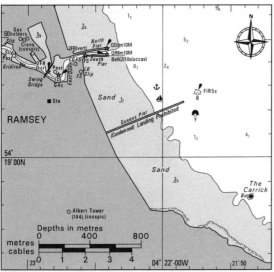

⚓ Report to HrMr

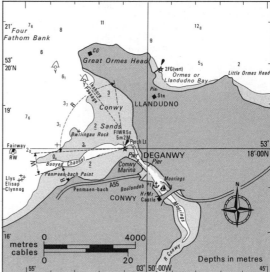

MENAI STRAIT   10-10-19
Gwynedd

CHARTS
AC *1464*, Imray C61; OS 114, 115. NOTE: The definitive Pilot book is *Cruising Anglesey and the North Wales Coast* by R.Morris, 4th edition 1993: North West Venturers YC

TIDES
Beaumaris –0025 Dover; ML Beaumaris 4·2; Duration 0540
Standard Port HOLYHEAD (⟶)

Times				Height (metres)			
High Water		Low Water		MHWS	MHWN	MLWN	MLWS
0000	0600	0500	1100	5·6	4·4	2·0	0·7
1200	1800	1700	2300				

Differences BEAUMARIS

+0025	+0010	+0055	+0035	+2·0	+1·6	+0·5	+0·1

MENAI BRIDGE

+0030	+0010	+0100	+0035	+1·7	+1·4	+0·3	0·0

PORT DINORWIC

–0015	–0025	+0030	0000	0·0	0·0	0·0	+0·1

CAERNARFON

–0030	–0030	+0015	–0005	–0·4	–0·4	–0·1	–0·1

FORT BELAN

–0040	–0015	–0025	–0005	–1·0	–0·9	–0·2	–0·1

LLANDDWYN ISLAND

–0115	–0055	–0030	–0020	–0·7	–0·5	–0·1	0·0

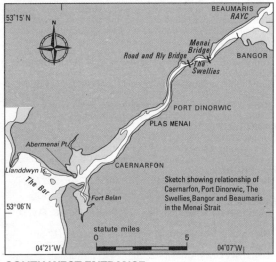

Sketch showing relationship of Caernarfon, Port Dinorwic, The Swellies, Bangor and Beaumaris in the Menai Strait

SOUTH WEST ENTRANCE
NAVIGATION
WPT 53°07'·60N 04°26'·00W, 270°/090° from/to Abermenai Pt lt, 3·8M. Wind against tide can build dangerous seas even in moderate breezes, especially if a swell is running in the Irish Sea. Caernarfon Bar shifts often and unpredictably.
LIGHTS AND MARKS
Llanddwyn Is lt, Fl WR 2·5s 12m 7/4M, R280°-015°, W015°-120°. Abermenai Pt lt, Fl WR 3·5s; R065°-245°, W245°-065°.
Direction of buoyage changes at Caernarfon.

PORT DINORWIC 53°11'·22N 04°13'·62W

TELEPHONE (01248)
Hr Mr 670441; MRSC (01407) 762051; Dr 670423.
FACILITIES
Port Dinorwic Yacht Hbr (fresh water marina, 230 berths) lock opens HW±2; ☎ 670559 D, P (cans), AC, CH, SM; Call *Dinorwic Marine* VHF Ch **80** M (HO). **Tidal basin** dries at sp. Pier hd F WR 5m 2M, vis R225°-357°, W357°-225°;
Services: SM, ME, El, Sh, Slip, C, CH. **Town** Ⓔ, ✉ (Bangor or Caernarfon), Ⓑ, ⇌ (Bangor), ✈ (Liverpool).
Note: Between Port Dinorwic and Caernarfon is **Plas Menai** ☎ 670964, the Sport Council for Wales Sailing and Sports Centre. *Menai Base* Ch **80** M. Day moorings only.

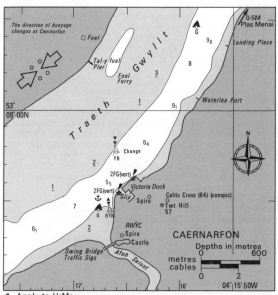

⚓ Apply to HrMr

CAERNARFON 53°08'·50N 04°16'·75W

SHELTER
Very good in river hbr, access HW±3 via swing bridge. Or in Victoria dock on NE wall, only near HW due silt. ⚓ off Foel Ferry, with local knowledge; or temp ⚓ inside Abermenai Pt in fair holding, sheltered from W'lies, but strong streams.
RADIO TELEPHONE
VHF Ch 12 14 16 (HJ).
TELEPHONE (01286)
Hr Mr 672118; MRSC (01407) 762051; ⌗ (01407) 762714; Police 673333; Dr 672236; Ⓗ 384384.
FACILITIES
Hbr AB, FW, Slip, C (2 ton), V, D (tanker), ME, El, Ⓔ, Sh, CH; **Caernarfon SC** ☎ 672861, L, Bar; **Royal Welsh YC** ☎ 672599, P, FW, Bar; **Town** P & D (cans), ✉, Ⓑ.

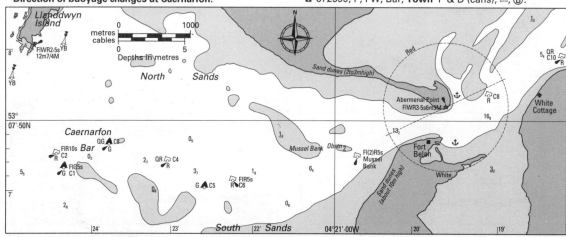

NORTH EAST ENTRANCE

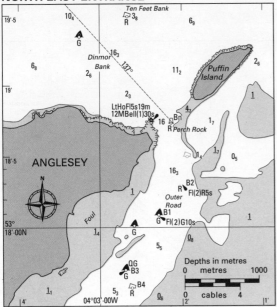

NAVIGATION

WPT 53°19'·47N 04°03'·20W, 317°/137° from/to Perch Rk PHM bn, 1·0M. From N end of Strait keep to buoyed chan near Anglesey shore. Night pilotage not recommended; many unlit buoys and moorings. See also 10·10·5.

LIGHTS AND MARKS

At NE end of Strait, Trwyn-Du lt, W tr/B bands, Fl 5s 19m 12M, vis 101°-023° (282°), Bell 30s. Conspic tr on Puffin Is. Chan is laterally buoyed, some lit. Beaumaris pier has FWG sectored lt (see 10.10.4). **Direction of buoyage changes at Caernarfon.**

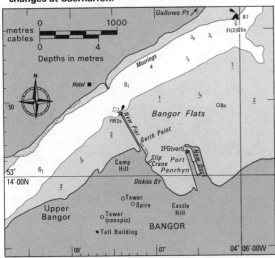

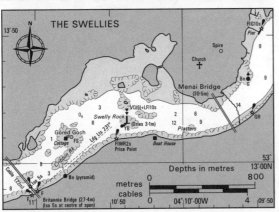

MENAI BRIDGE/BEAUMARIS 53°15'·65N 04°05'·30W

SHELTER

Reasonable off Beaumaris except from NE winds. ⚓ S of B10 PHM By or contact YCs for mooring. At Menai Bridge, call Hr Mr VHF Ch 69 16 for mooring or berth temp'y on St George's Pier (S of which a marina is planned for 1997).

TELEPHONE (01248)

Hr Mr Menai 712312; MRSC (01407) 762051; Marinecall 0891 500 460; ⌗ (01407) 762714; Police (01407) 762323; Dr 810501.

FACILITIES

St George's Pier (Fl G 10s) L at all tides; **Royal Anglesey YC** ☎ 810295, Slip, M, L, R, Bar, P; **North West Venturers YC** ☎ 810023, M, L, FW, water taxi at w/ends only; **Menai Bridge SC. Services:** Slip, P & D (cans), FW, ME, BH (20 ton), Sh, C (2 ton), CH, El, Ⓔ, Gas.
Both towns EC Wed; ✉, Ⓑ, ⇌ (bus to Bangor), ✈ (Liverpool).

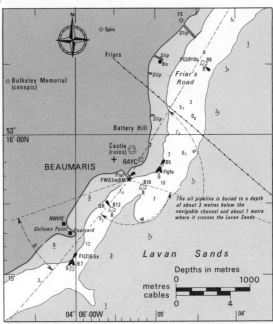

⚓ Apply to Royal Anglesey YC.

BANGOR 53°14'·45N 04°07'·50W

SHELTER

Good, except in E'lies, at Dickies BY or Port Penrhyn dock (both dry; access HW±2).

RADIO TELEPHONE

Dickies VHF Ch 09 M 16, all year.

TELEPHONE (01248)

Penrhyn Hr Mr 352525; MRSC (01407) 762051; ⌗ (01407) 762714; Dr 362055.

FACILITIES

Services: Slip, D, P (cans), FW, ME, El, Sh, C, CH, Ⓔ, SM, BH (30 ton), Gas, Gaz, ACA; **Port Penrhyn**, Slip, AB, D.
Town ✉, Ⓑ, ⇌, ✈ (Chester).

THE SWELLIES 53°13'·13N 04°10'·38W

NAVIGATION

For pilotage notes, see 10·10·5. The passage should only be attempted at slack HW, which is –0200 HW Liverpool. The shallow rky narrows between the bridges are dangerous for yachts at other times, when the stream can reach 8kn. At slack HW there is 3m over The Platters and the outcrop off Price Pt, which can be ignored. For shoal-draft boats passage is also possible at slack LW nps, but there are depths of 0·5m close E of Britannia Bridge. The bridges and power cables have a least clearance of 22m at MHWS. Night passage is not recommended.

LIGHTS AND MARKS

SE side of chan QR 4m, R mast, vis 064°-222°. Price Pt, Fl WR 2s 5m 3M, W Bn, vis R059°-239°, W239°-259°. Britannia Bridge, E side, ldg lts 231°, both FW. Bridge lts, both sides: Centre span Iso 5s 27m 3M; S end, FR 21m 3M; N end, FG 21m 3M.

HOLYHEAD   10-10-20
Gwynedd 53°19'·70N 04°37'·00W

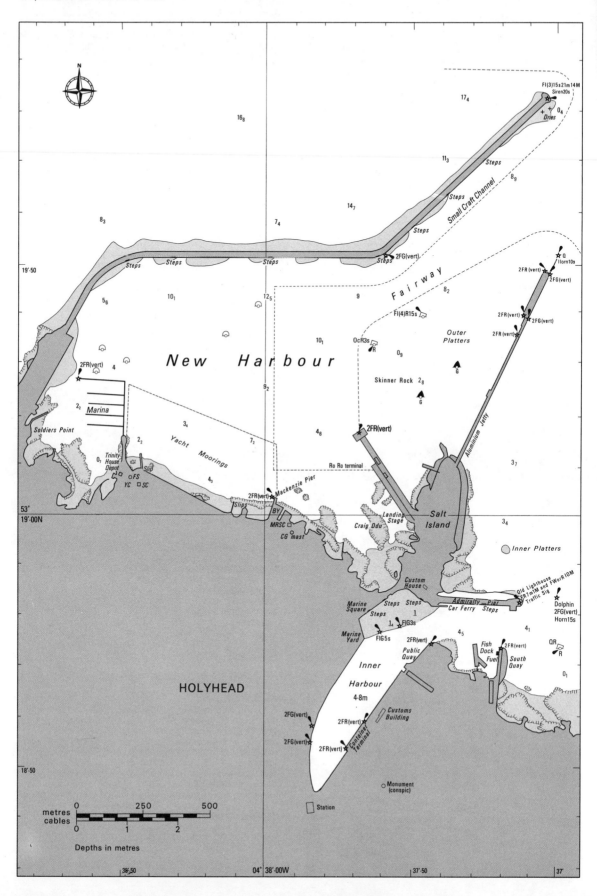

N

16₈

17₄

Fl(3)15s21m14M
Siren20s
0₄
Dries

11₃

8₉

Steps

Small Craft Channel

14₇

Steps

8₃

7₄

Steps

Steps   2FG(vert)

Fairway

Q
Horn10s
2FR(vert)   2FG(vert)

19'·50

5₆

10₁

12₅

9   8₂

Steps   Steps   Steps

Fl(4)R15s

2FR(vert)   2FG(vert)

2FR(vert)

New   Harbour

10₁   OcR3s
R   0₉   Outer
Platters
G

2FR(vert)

4

Skinner Rock   2₈
G

Marina

2₃

9₂

Aluminium Jetty

Soldiers Point

3₄   2FR(vert)

3₇

Trinity
House
Depot   2₂   Yacht
Moorings   7₂

0₇   Slip   4₆   Ro Ro terminal

FS
YC   SC   4₃

Slips

2FR(vert)   Mackenzie Pier

BY

MRSC

CG mast   Landing
Stage   Salt
Island   3₄

Craig Ddu

Inner Platters

Custom
House

Old Lighthouse
FR7mM and FWorR10M
Traffic Sig

Marine
Square   Steps   Steps
Admiralty   Pier
Car Ferry   Steps   Dolphin
2FG(vert)
Horn15s

53°
19'·00N   1

Steps

Marine
Yard   1₄   FlG3s
FlG5s   4₅   QR
R
2FR(vert)   4₁

HOLYHEAD   Public
Quay   Fish
Dock   2FR(vert)
Fuel   South
Quay   0₁

Inner

Harbour

4·8m   Customs
Building

2FG(vert)

2FR(vert)
2FG(vert)   Container
Terminal
2FR(vert)

18'·50   Monument
(conspic)

Station

metres
cables   0   250   500

0   1   2

Depths in metres

38'·50   04° 38'·00W   37'·50   37'

CHARTS
AC 2011, 1413, *1977*, 1970, *1826*; Imray C61; OS 114

TIDES
–0035 Dover; ML 3·2; Duration 0615; Zone 0 (UT)

Standard Port HOLYHEAD (→)

Times				Height (metres)			
High Water		Low Water		MHWS	MHWN	MLWN	MLWS
0000	0600	0500	1100	5·6	4·4	2·0	0·7
1200	1800	1700	2300				
Differences TRWYN DINMOR (W of Puffin Is)							
+0025	+0015	+0050	+0035	+1·9	+1·5	+0·5	+0·2
MOELFRE (NE Anglesey)							
+0025	+0020	+0050	+0035	+1·9	+1·4	+0·5	+0·2
AMLWCH (N Anglesey)							
+0020	+0010	+0035	+0025	+1·6	+1·3	+0·5	+0·2
CEMAES BAY (N Anglesey)							
+0020	+0025	+0040	+0035	+1·0	+0·7	+0·3	+0·1
TREARDDUR BAY (W Anglesey)							
–0045	–0025	–0015	–0015	–0·4	–0·4	0·0	+0·1
PORTH TRECASTELL (SW Anglesey)							
–0045	–0025	–0005	–0015	–0·6	–0·6	0·0	0·0
TREFOR (Lleyn peninsula)							
–0115	–0100	–0030	–0020	–0·8	–0·9	–0·2	–0··1
PORTH DINLLAEN (Lleyn peninsula)							
–0120	–0105	–0035	–0025	–1·0	–1·0	–0·2	–0·2
PORTH YSGADEN (Lleyn peninsula)							
–0125	–0110	–0040	–0035	–1·1	–1·0	–0·1	–0·1
BARDSEY ISLAND							
–0220	–0240	–0145	–0140	–1·2	–1·2	–0·5	–0·1

Holyhead is a Standard Port and tidal predictions for each day of the year are given below.

SHELTER
Very good in proposed new marina (3m) at SW corner of New Hbr, access H24; 160 berths are planned for spring 1996. Alternatives: ⚓ or moor off HSC (Ch M); or temp AB on bkwtr; or in Fish Dock (also D). Strong NE winds raise a slight sea.

NAVIGATION
WPT 53°20'·10N 04°37'·20W, 345°/165° from/to bkwtr lt ho, 0·28M. Beware very fast catamaran ferries in approaches. Yachts entering/leaving New Hbr should use the Small Craft Chan, parallel to and within 0·4ca of the bkwtr; but beware shoal, drying 0·5m, which extends 0·2ca SE of bkwtr head. Ferries enter within 2½ca of bkwtr hd for Inner Hbr or Ro-Ro terminal in New Hbr; outbound ferries pass within 2½ca WSW of Cliperau PHM buoy, Fl (4) R 15s. Keep clear of the Aluminium Jetty (Ore terminal), Outer Platters (buoyed) and 5 large unlit mooring buoys in New Hbr.

LIGHTS AND MARKS
Ldg marks 165°, bkwtr lt ho on with chy (127m) R lts. Tfc sigs on Admty pier: R Flag (Ⓡ) = Inner hbr closed. 2 R Flags (2 Ⓡ) = Old and Inner hbrs blocked.

RADIO TELEPHONE
Call *Holyhead* VHF Ch 14 16 (H24) before entering Old and Inner Hbrs. Marina and Holyhead SC: Ch M.

TELEPHONE (01407)
Port Control 766700; MRSC 762051; ⌗ 762714; Marinecall 0891 500 460; Police 762323; Dr via MRSC.

FACILITIES
Holyhead Marina (up to 300 berths) ☎ 764242, AC, FW, D, P, (more details, when available, will be in Supplements); **Holyhead SC** ☎ 762526, M, L, FW, Slip, launch, R (season only), Bar; **Inner Hbr** ☎ 762304, Slip, M, D, L, FW, C (many), CH, AB, ME, EI, Sh; **Fish Dock** ☎ 760139 AB on pontoons, FW, D by hose. **Services:** BY, ACA, CH, ME, EI, Sh, C (100 ton), BH, Slip, Ⓔ. **Town** EC Tues; P, V, R, Bar, 🗐, ✉, Ⓑ, ⇌, ✈ (Liverpool). Ferry/Fast Cat to Dun Laoghaire and Dublin. **Trearddur Bay** (3M south) M (small craft only), L; **BY** ☎ 860501, D, FW, Sh, CH. **Village** P, V, R, Bar.

MINOR HARBOUR ON THE LLEYN PENINSULA

PORTH DINLLAEN, Gwynedd, 52°56'·66N 04°33'·59W. AC 1512, 1971. HW –0240 on Dover; ML 2·5m; Duration 0535. See 10.10.19. Shelter good in S to W winds but strong NNW to NNE winds cause heavy seas in the bay. Beware Carreg-y-Chad (1·8m) 0·75M SW of the point, and Carreg-y-Chwislen (dries, with unlit IDM Bn) 2ca ENE of the point. From N, Carn Fadryn (369m) brg 182° leads into the bay. Best ⚓ 1ca S of LB ho in approx 2m, or ⚓ 1½ca E of ruined jetty. Hr Mr ☎ (01758) 720295; CG ☎ 720204. Facilities: EC Wed; Bar, V by landing stage. At Morfa Nefyn (1M), Bar, P, R, V.

10

At last about tea-time, when land began to loom vaguely to port, to starboard, and also ahead, we realized that we were near the head of Cardigan Bay, two points off course and some forty miles from Holyhead. Currents, the compass, the helmsman, even the navigator, may be responsible for these anomalies. It is not, however, for the navigator to accept responsibility for them or to show surprise, or he may sap what confidence the crew have in him. Attack is the best form of defence. A few remarks about the impossibility of navigating the ship if it is not steered straight will restore his own confidence and subdue and mystify the crew.

Mostly Mischief: H.W.Tilman

With acknowledgements to the Executors of the estate of H.W.Tilman and to Hollis & Carter (Publishers 1966).

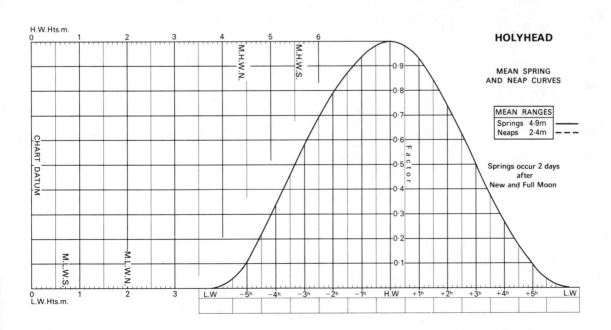

HOLYHEAD

MEAN SPRING AND NEAP CURVES

MEAN RANGES	
Springs	4·9m
Neaps	2·4m

Springs occur 2 days after New and Full Moon

WALES – HOLYHEAD

LAT 53°19′N   LONG 4°37′W

TIMES AND HEIGHTS OF HIGH AND LOW WATERS

YEAR 1996

TIME ZONE (UT)
For Summer Time add ONE hour in non-shaded areas

Chart Datum: 3·05 metres below Ordnance Datum (Newlyn)

JANUARY

Day	Time	m	Time	m	Time	m	Time	m
1 M	0047	1.7	0715	4.7	1320	1.8	1933	4.8
2 TU	0145	1.7	0810	4.9	1415	1.7	2026	4.9
3 W	0234	1.6	0854	5.1	1501	1.5	2110	5.0
4 TH	0315	1.4	0930	5.2	1541	1.3	2146	5.1
5 F O	0350	1.3	1003	5.3	1616	1.2	2219	5.1
6 SA	0422	1.2	1035	5.4	1649	1.1	2253	5.2
7 SU	0452	1.2	1108	5.5	1721	1.1	2327	5.1
8 M	0524	1.1	1142	5.5	1754	1.1		
9 TU	0003	5.2	0558	1.2	1217	5.4	1828	1.1
10 W	0040	5.1	0634	1.2	1253	5.3	1905	1.2
11 TH	0117	5.1	0712	1.3	1330	5.2	1945	1.3
12 F	0157	4.9	0753	1.5	1410	5.1	2029	1.4
13 SA	0242	4.8	0841	1.7	1457	4.9	2121	1.6
14 SU	0337	4.7	0939	1.9	1556	4.8	2226	1.7
15 M	0446	4.6	1052	2.0	1710	4.7	2339	1.7
16 TU	0602	4.7	1209	1.8	1830	4.8		
17 W	0048	1.6	0712	5.0	1318	1.5	1940	5.1
18 TH	0151	1.3	0812	5.3	1419	1.1	2039	5.4
19 F	0245	0.9	0903	5.7	1512	0.7	2131	5.6
20 SA ●	0335	0.6	0951	5.9	1602	0.4	2220	5.8
21 SU	0422	0.5	1037	6.1	1650	0.2	2307	5.8
22 M	0508	0.4	1123	6.2	1737	0.2	2353	5.8
23 TU	0554	0.4	1209	6.1	1824	0.3		
24 W	0039	5.6	0639	0.6	1255	5.9	1910	0.5
25 TH	0125	5.4	0726	0.8	1342	5.7	1958	0.8
26 F	0212	5.1	0814	1.2	1431	5.3	2047	1.2
27 SA	0303	4.8	0908	1.5	1525	5.0	2143	1.6
28 SU	0404	4.6	1013	1.9	1631	4.6	2250	1.9
29 M	0520	4.4	1131	2.0	1750	4.4		
30 TU	0007	2.0	0637	4.4	1249	2.0	1905	4.5
31 W	0117	2.0	0742	4.6	1353	1.8	2006	4.6

FEBRUARY

Day	Time	m	Time	m	Time	m	Time	m
1 TH	0212	1.8	0832	4.9	1442	1.6	2053	4.8
2 F	0255	1.6	0911	5.1	1523	1.3	2129	4.9
3 SA	0332	1.3	0944	5.2	1558	1.2	2201	5.0
4 SU O	0403	1.2	1016	5.3	1629	1.0	2232	5.1
5 M	0433	1.0	1047	5.4	1659	0.9	2305	5.2
6 TU	0503	0.9	1120	5.5	1730	0.8	2339	5.3
7 W	0535	0.9	1153	5.5	1803	0.8		
8 TH	0014	5.3	0609	0.9	1228	5.4	1837	0.8
9 F	0050	5.2	0646	1.0	1303	5.4	1915	0.9
10 SA	0127	5.1	0726	1.1	1341	5.2	1957	1.1
11 SU	0208	5.0	0810	1.3	1425	5.0	2045	1.4
12 M	0257	4.8	0904	1.6	1521	4.8	2146	1.7
13 TU	0402	4.6	1015	1.8	1636	4.6	2304	1.8
14 W	0525	4.6	1141	1.8	1807	4.6		
15 TH	0025	1.7	0648	4.8	1301	1.5	1927	4.8
16 F	0135	1.4	0755	5.1	1407	1.1	2030	5.2
17 SA	0233	1.0	0850	5.5	1502	0.7	2122	5.5
18 SU ●	0323	0.7	0938	5.9	1550	0.3	2208	5.7
19 M	0408	0.4	1023	6.1	1640	0.1	2251	5.8
20 TU	0451	0.3	1106	6.1	1718	0.1	2333	5.8
21 W	0534	0.3	1149	6.1	1800	0.2		
22 TH	0014	5.7	0615	0.4	1231	5.9	1842	0.5
23 F	0055	5.5	0658	0.7	1313	5.6	1924	0.8
24 SA	0135	5.2	0742	1.0	1356	5.3	2008	1.2
25 SU	0217	4.9	0829	1.4	1443	4.9	2056	1.6
26 M	0307	4.6	0927	1.8	1541	4.5	2157	2.0
27 TU	0416	4.3	1042	2.1	1703	4.2	2317	2.3
28 W	0549	4.3	1210	2.1	1832	4.2		
29 TH	0041	2.2	0706	4.4	1324	1.9	1940	4.4

MARCH

Day	Time	m	Time	m	Time	m	Time	m
1 F	0144	2.0	0802	4.7	1416	1.6	2028	4.6
2 SA	0230	1.7	0844	4.9	1457	1.3	2104	4.8
3 SU	0307	1.4	0918	5.1	1531	1.1	2136	5.0
4 M	0338	1.1	0950	5.3	1601	0.9	2207	5.2
5 TU O	0407	0.9	1021	5.4	1631	0.8	2239	5.3
6 W	0437	0.8	1053	5.5	1702	0.7	2312	5.4
7 TH	0510	0.7	1127	5.5	1735	0.6	2347	5.4
8 F	0545	0.6	1202	5.5	1811	0.6		
9 SA	0023	5.4	0623	0.7	1239	5.4	1849	0.8
10 SU	0101	5.3	0703	0.8	1319	5.3	1931	1.0
11 M	0142	5.1	0749	1.1	1404	5.0	2019	1.3
12 TU	0231	4.9	0843	1.4	1501	4.7	2121	1.6
13 W	0335	4.6	0954	1.6	1619	4.5	2241	1.8
14 TH	0500	4.5	1124	1.7	1755	4.5		
15 F	0008	1.8	0627	4.7	1248	1.4	1917	4.7
16 SA	0122	1.5	0738	5.1	1354	1.0	2018	5.1
17 SU	0220	1.1	0834	5.5	1448	0.6	2108	5.4
18 M	0309	0.7	0922	5.8	1534	0.4	2151	5.6
19 TU ●	0352	0.5	1005	5.9	1616	0.2	2232	5.7
20 W	0433	0.2	1047	6.0	1656	0.2	2310	5.7
21 TH	0512	0.3	1127	5.9	1735	0.3	2348	5.6
22 F	0552	0.4	1206	5.8	1813	0.6		
23 SA	0024	5.5	0631	0.7	1245	5.5	1851	0.9
24 SU	0101	5.3	0712	1.0	1324	5.2	1931	1.3
25 M	0140	5.0	0757	1.3	1407	4.8	2015	1.7
26 TU	0224	4.7	0848	1.7	1458	4.4	2109	2.1
27 W	0320	4.4	0955	2.0	1611	4.2	2222	2.3
28 TH	0445	4.2	1118	2.1	1746	4.1	2349	2.4
29 F	0615	4.3	1238	2.0	1900	4.3		
30 SA	0102	2.1	0719	4.5	1337	1.7	1952	4.5
31 SU	0153	1.8	0806	4.8	1420	1.4	2031	4.8

APRIL

Day	Time	m	Time	m	Time	m	Time	m
1 M	0232	1.5	0844	5.0	1455	1.1	2105	5.0
2 TU	0305	1.2	0918	5.2	1527	0.9	2137	5.2
3 W	0337	0.9	0951	5.4	1559	0.7	2210	5.4
4 TH O	0410	0.7	1025	5.5	1632	0.5	2245	5.5
5 F	0445	0.5	1101	5.6	1708	0.5	2321	5.6
6 SA	0523	0.5	1139	5.6	1746	0.5	2359	5.5
7 SU	0603	0.5	1219	5.5	1827	0.7		
8 M	0039	5.4	0647	0.7	1304	5.3	1912	0.9
9 TU	0125	5.3	0736	0.9	1353	5.0	2004	1.3
10 W	0217	5.0	0833	1.2	1454	4.7	2107	1.6
11 TH	0322	4.8	0946	1.4	1614	4.5	2228	1.8
12 F	0444	4.7	1112	1.5	1717	4.5	2352	1.7
13 SA	0608	4.8	1231	1.3	1903	4.7		
14 SU	0103	1.5	0717	5.1	1336	1.0	2002	5.0
15 M	0202	1.1	0814	5.4	1429	0.7	2050	5.3
16 TU	0251	0.8	0902	5.6	1515	0.5	2132	5.5
17 W ●	0334	0.6	0946	5.7	1556	0.5	2211	5.6
18 TH	0413	0.5	1026	5.7	1633	0.5	2247	5.6
19 F	0452	0.5	1105	5.7	1710	0.5	2323	5.5
20 SA	0530	0.6	1142	5.5	1746	0.8	2357	5.4
21 SU	0608	0.8	1219	5.3	1823	1.1		
22 M	0033	5.3	0647	1.0	1258	5.1	1900	1.3
23 TU	0111	5.1	0730	1.3	1338	4.8	1941	1.7
24 W	0152	4.8	0817	1.6	1425	4.5	2029	2.0
25 TH	0242	4.6	0913	1.9	1525	4.3	2132	2.3
26 F	0346	4.4	1023	2.0	1645	4.2	2249	2.4
27 SA	0509	4.3	1137	2.0	1805	4.2		
28 SU	0002	2.2	0622	4.4	1241	1.8	1904	4.5
29 M	0102	2.0	0718	4.6	1332	1.5	1950	4.7
30 TU	0148	1.6	0803	4.9	1414	1.2	2029	5.0

WALES – HOLYHEAD

LAT 53°19′N   LONG 4°37′W

TIMES AND HEIGHTS OF HIGH AND LOW WATERS   YEAR **1996**

TIME ZONE (UT)
For Summer Time add ONE hour in non-shaded areas

MAY

#	Day	Time	m	#	Day	Time	m
1	W	0228 / 0842 / 1451 / 2105	1.3 / 5.1 / 0.9 / 5.3	16	TH	0315 / 0926 / 1535 / 2151	0.9 / 5.4 / 0.8 / 5.4
2	TH	0305 / 0920 / 1528 / 2141	1.0 / 5.4 / 0.7 / 5.5	17	F	0356 / 1007 / 1612 / ●2227	0.8 / 5.4 / 0.8 / 5.4
3	F	0343 / 0958 / 1606 / ○2219	0.7 / 5.5 / 0.5 / 5.6	18	SA	0434 / 1045 / 1648 / 2301	0.8 / 5.4 / 0.9 / 5.4
4	SA	0422 / 1038 / 1645 / 2258	0.5 / 5.6 / 0.5 / 5.7	19	SU	0511 / 1122 / 1722 / 2335	0.9 / 5.3 / 1.0 / 5.4
5	SU	0504 / 1120 / 1727 / 2340	0.4 / 5.6 / 0.5 / 5.7	20	M	0548 / 1158 / 1758	1.0 / 5.2 / 1.2
6	M	0549 / 1205 / 1812	0.4 / 5.5 / 0.7	21	TU	0010 / 0626 / 1235 / 1835	5.3 / 1.1 / 5.1 / 1.4
7	TU	0025 / 0636 / 1255 / 1900	5.6 / 0.6 / 5.3 / 0.9	22	W	0048 / 0707 / 1315 / 1914	5.2 / 1.3 / 4.9 / 1.6
8	W	0114 / 0730 / 1349 / 1955	5.4 / 0.8 / 5.1 / 1.2	23	TH	0128 / 0749 / 1358 / 1957	5.0 / 1.5 / 4.7 / 1.8
9	TH	0210 / 0830 / 1451 / 2058	5.2 / 1.0 / 4.8 / 1.5	24	F	0212 / 0837 / 1448 / 2048	4.8 / 1.7 / 4.5 / 2.0
10	F	0314 / 0939 / 1605 / 2213	5.0 / 1.2 / 4.6 / 1.7	25	SA	0303 / 0934 / 1548 / 2152	4.6 / 1.8 / 4.3 / 2.2
11	SA	0428 / 1055 / 1727 / 2330	4.9 / 1.3 / 4.6 / 1.7	26	SU	0405 / 1038 / 1659 / 2301	4.5 / 1.9 / 4.3 / 2.2
12	SU	0544 / 1208 / 1840	4.9 / 1.2 / 4.7	27	M	0515 / 1142 / 1808	4.5 / 1.8 / 4.4
13	M	0039 / 0652 / 1312 / 1939	1.5 / 5.0 / 1.1 / 5.0	28	TU	0005 / 0621 / 1240 / 1904	2.0 / 4.6 / 1.6 / 4.7
14	TU	0139 / 0751 / 1407 / 2029	1.3 / 5.1 / 0.9 / 5.1	29	W	0101 / 0717 / 1331 / 1952	1.8 / 4.8 / 1.3 / 5.0
15	W	0230 / 0842 / 1454 / 2112	1.1 / 5.3 / 0.8 / 5.3	30	TH	0150 / 0806 / 1417 / 2035	1.4 / 5.1 / 1.0 / 5.2
				31	F	0235 / 0851 / 1500 / 2116	1.1 / 5.3 / 0.8 / 5.5

JUNE

#	Day	Time	m	#	Day	Time	m
1	SA	0319 / 0935 / 1543 / ○2157	0.8 / 5.5 / 0.6 / 5.7	16	SU	0419 / 1027 / 1629 / ●2243	1.1 / 5.2 / 1.1 / 5.3
2	SU	0404 / 1020 / 1627 / 2240	0.5 / 5.6 / 0.5 / 5.8	17	M	0455 / 1103 / 1703 / 2317	1.0 / 5.1 / 1.1 / 5.3
3	M	0450 / 1106 / 1712 / 2325	0.4 / 5.7 / 0.5 / 5.8	18	TU	0531 / 1138 / 1737 / 2351	1.1 / 5.1 / 1.2 / 5.3
4	TU	0538 / 1155 / 1800	0.4 / 5.6 / 0.6	19	W	0607 / 1214 / 1812	1.1 / 5.1 / 1.3
5	W	0014 / 0629 / 1247 / 1850	5.8 / 0.4 / 5.4 / 0.8	20	TH	0027 / 0644 / 1252 / 1848	5.3 / 1.2 / 5.0 / 1.4
6	TH	0105 / 0723 / 1341 / 1945	5.6 / 0.6 / 5.2 / 1.0	21	F	0105 / 0722 / 1332 / 1928	5.1 / 1.3 / 4.9 / 1.5
7	F	0200 / 0821 / 1440 / 2045	5.4 / 0.8 / 5.0 / 1.3	22	SA	0145 / 0804 / 1414 / 2011	5.0 / 1.4 / 4.7 / 1.7
8	SA	0300 / 0924 / 1546 / 2151	5.2 / 1.0 / 4.8 / 1.5	23	SU	0228 / 0850 / 1503 / 2101	4.9 / 1.6 / 4.6 / 1.9
9	SU	0405 / 1030 / 1658 / 2301	5.1 / 1.2 / 4.7 / 1.6	24	M	0317 / 0944 / 1600 / 2202	4.7 / 1.7 / 4.5 / 2.0
10	M	0515 / 1138 / 1810	5.0 / 1.3 / 4.7	25	TU	0416 / 1047 / 1707 / 2311	4.6 / 1.8 / 4.5 / 2.0
11	TU	0010 / 0623 / 1244 / 1913	1.6 / 4.9 / 1.3 / 4.8	26	W	0524 / 1151 / 1815	4.6 / 1.7 / 4.6
12	W	0113 / 0727 / 1342 / 2007	1.5 / 5.0 / 1.3 / 4.9	27	TH	0016 / 0631 / 1252 / 1915	1.8 / 4.7 / 1.5 / 4.9
13	TH	0209 / 0822 / 1433 / 2054	1.3 / 5.1 / 1.2 / 5.1	28	F	0116 / 0733 / 1347 / 2007	1.5 / 5.0 / 1.2 / 5.2
14	F	0257 / 0909 / 1516 / 2133	1.2 / 5.1 / 1.1 / 5.2	29	SA	0210 / 0828 / 1437 / 2055	1.2 / 5.2 / 0.9 / 5.5
15	SA	0340 / 0950 / 1555 / 2209	1.1 / 5.1 / 1.1 / 5.3	30	SU	0300 / 0918 / 1525 / ●2140	0.8 / 5.5 / 0.7 / 5.7

JULY

#	Day	Time	m	#	Day	Time	m
1	M	0349 / 1007 / 1612 / ○2226	0.5 / 5.6 / 0.5 / 5.9	16	TU	0439 / 1043 / 1644 / 2257	1.1 / 5.1 / 1.2 / 5.3
2	TU	0438 / 1055 / 1659 / 2313	0.3 / 5.7 / 0.5 / 6.0	17	W	0512 / 1116 / 1715 / 2330	1.1 / 5.1 / 1.1 / 5.4
3	W	0528 / 1144 / 1747	0.3 / 5.7 / 0.5	18	TH	0544 / 1151 / 1748	1.1 / 5.1 / 1.1
4	TH	0001 / 0618 / 1235 / 1836	5.9 / 0.3 / 5.6 / 0.6	19	F	0004 / 0617 / 1227 / 1822	5.3 / 1.0 / 5.1 / 1.2
5	F	0052 / 0710 / 1326 / 1928	5.8 / 0.4 / 5.4 / 0.8	20	SA	0040 / 0653 / 1304 / 1858	5.3 / 1.1 / 5.0 / 1.3
6	SA	0143 / 0803 / 1419 / 2022	5.7 / 0.6 / 5.2 / 1.1	21	SU	0116 / 0730 / 1342 / 1937	5.2 / 1.2 / 4.9 / 1.4
7	SU	0238 / 0858 / 1517 / 2121	5.4 / 0.9 / 4.9 / 1.3	22	M	0154 / 0811 / 1424 / 2021	5.1 / 1.3 / 4.8 / 1.6
8	M	0336 / 0959 / 1622 / 2227	5.1 / 1.2 / 4.7 / 1.6	23	TU	0237 / 0858 / 1513 / 2113	4.9 / 1.5 / 4.6 / 1.8
9	TU	0442 / 1104 / 1734 / 2339	4.9 / 1.4 / 4.6 / 1.7	24	W	0330 / 0956 / 1614 / 2221	4.7 / 1.7 / 4.5 / 1.9
10	W	0554 / 1213 / 1844	4.7 / 1.6 / 4.6	25	TH	0437 / 1107 / 1728 / 2337	4.6 / 1.8 / 4.6 / 1.8
11	TH	0047 / 0703 / 1317 / 1945	1.7 / 4.7 / 1.6 / 4.8	26	F	0554 / 1218 / 1842	4.6 / 1.7 / 4.8
12	F	0149 / 0804 / 1412 / 2036	1.6 / 4.8 / 1.5 / 4.9	27	SA	0048 / 0709 / 1323 / 1944	1.6 / 4.9 / 1.4 / 5.1
13	SA	0241 / 0854 / 1458 / 2117	1.4 / 4.9 / 1.4 / 5.1	28	SU	0150 / 0812 / 1419 / 2038	1.3 / 5.1 / 1.1 / 5.4
14	SU	0325 / 0935 / 1538 / 2152	1.3 / 5.0 / 1.3 / 5.2	29	M	0246 / 0906 / 1510 / 2126	0.9 / 5.4 / 0.7 / 5.8
15	M	0404 / 1010 / 1612 / ●2224	1.2 / 5.0 / 1.2 / 5.3	30	TU	0336 / 0955 / 1558 / ○2213	0.5 / 5.7 / 0.5 / 6.0
				31	W	0425 / 1043 / 1644 / 2258	0.2 / 5.8 / 0.4 / 6.1

AUGUST

#	Day	Time	m	#	Day	Time	m
1	TH	0513 / 1129 / 1731 / 2345	0.1 / 5.8 / 0.3 / 6.1	16	F	0517 / 1125 / 1721 / 2338	0.9 / 5.2 / 1.0 / 5.4
2	F	0600 / 1216 / 1817	0.2 / 5.7 / 0.5	17	SA	0548 / 1159 / 1754	0.9 / 5.2 / 1.0
3	SA	0032 / 0648 / 1303 / 1904	6.0 / 0.3 / 5.5 / 0.7	18	SU	0012 / 0621 / 1235 / 1829	5.4 / 0.9 / 5.2 / 1.1
4	SU	0120 / 0736 / 1350 / 1954	5.8 / 0.6 / 5.3 / 1.0	19	M	0047 / 0657 / 1311 / 1907	5.3 / 1.0 / 5.1 / 1.2
5	M	0209 / 0826 / 1441 / 2047	5.5 / 0.9 / 5.0 / 1.3	20	TU	0123 / 0736 / 1350 / 1949	5.2 / 1.2 / 5.0 / 1.4
6	TU	0303 / 0921 / 1539 / 2150	5.1 / 1.3 / 4.7 / 1.7	21	W	0204 / 0821 / 1435 / 2038	5.0 / 1.4 / 4.8 / 1.6
7	W	0406 / 1025 / 1652 / 2305	4.8 / 1.7 / 4.5 / 1.9	22	TH	0255 / 0917 / 1534 / 2143	4.8 / 1.7 / 4.6 / 1.9
8	TH	0522 / 1139 / 1812	4.5 / 1.9 / 4.5	23	F	0403 / 1030 / 1651 / 2307	4.6 / 1.9 / 4.5 / 1.9
9	F	0022 / 0640 / 1252 / 1921	1.9 / 4.5 / 1.9 / 4.6	24	SA	0529 / 1152 / 1816	4.6 / 1.8 / 4.7
10	SA	0129 / 0747 / 1351 / 2015	1.8 / 4.6 / 1.8 / 4.8	25	SU	0028 / 0654 / 1304 / 1926	1.7 / 4.8 / 1.6 / 5.1
11	SU	0223 / 0838 / 1439 / 2057	1.6 / 4.7 / 1.6 / 5.0	26	M	0136 / 0800 / 1405 / 2022	1.3 / 5.1 / 1.2 / 5.5
12	M	0307 / 0917 / 1518 / 2132	1.4 / 4.9 / 1.4 / 5.2	27	TU	0233 / 0854 / 1456 / 2111	0.8 / 5.4 / 0.8 / 5.8
13	TU	0344 / 0950 / 1552 / 2202	1.2 / 5.0 / 1.2 / 5.3	28	W	0323 / 0942 / 1543 / ○2157	0.5 / 5.7 / 0.5 / 6.1
14	W	0417 / 1020 / 1622 / ●2233	1.1 / 5.1 / 1.1 / 5.4	29	TH	0409 / 1026 / 1627 / 2241	0.2 / 5.8 / 0.3 / 6.2
15	TH	0447 / 1052 / 1651 / 2305	1.0 / 5.2 / 1.0 / 5.4	30	F	0454 / 1110 / 1711 / 2324	0.1 / 5.9 / 0.3 / 6.2
				31	SA	0538 / 1152 / 1754	0.2 / 5.8 / 0.4

10

Chart Datum: 3·05 metres below Ordnance Datum (Newlyn)

WALES – HOLYHEAD

LAT 53°19′N   LONG   4°37′W

TIMES AND HEIGHTS OF HIGH AND LOW WATERS

YEAR 1996

TIME ZONE (UT)
For Summer Time add ONE hour in non-shaded areas

Chart Datum: 3·05 metres below Ordnance Datum (Newlyn)

SEPTEMBER

Day	Time	m	Time	m	Time	m	Time	m
1 SU	0008	6.0	0621	0.4	1235	5.6	1838	0.6
16 M	0551	0.8	1206	5.4	1803	0.9		
2 M	0053	5.8	0705	0.7	1318	5.4	1923	1.0
17 TU	0019	5.4	0628	0.9	1243	5.3	1841	1.0
3 TU	0138	5.4	0751	1.1	1403	5.1	2013	1.4
18 W	0057	5.3	0708	1.1	1322	5.2	1925	1.3
4 W	0227	5.0	0840	1.6	1454	4.7	2111	1.8
19 TH	0140	5.1	0754	1.4	1408	5.0	2016	1.5
5 TH	0326	4.6	0941	2.0	1603	4.5	2226	2.1
20 F	0233	4.8	0850	1.7	1507	4.8	2122	1.8
6 F	0446	4.4	1059	2.2	1732	4.4	2352	2.1
21 SA	0344	4.6	1005	1.9	1627	4.6	2249	1.9
7 SA	0614	4.3	1220	2.2	1850	4.5		
22 SU	0516	4.5	1132	1.9	1755	4.8		
8 SU	0104	2.0	0723	4.5	1326	2.0	1947	4.8
23 M	0014	1.7	0643	4.8	1249	1.7	1907	5.1
9 M	0159	1.7	0814	4.7	1414	1.8	2030	5.0
24 TU	0123	1.3	0748	5.1	1350	1.3	2005	5.5
10 TU	0242	1.4	0852	4.9	1453	1.5	2105	5.2
25 W	0219	0.8	0840	5.5	1441	0.9	2054	5.9
11 W	0317	1.2	0923	5.1	1526	1.3	2135	5.3
26 TH	0307	0.5	0925	5.7	1526	0.6	2139	6.1
12 TH ●	0349	1.1	0953	5.2	1555	1.1	2206	5.4
27 F ○	0351	0.3	1007	5.9	1609	0.4	2221	6.2
13 F	0417	0.9	1024	5.3	1623	1.0	2237	5.5
28 SA	0432	0.3	1048	5.9	1650	0.4	2303	6.1
14 SA	0446	0.8	1056	5.4	1653	0.9	2310	5.5
29 SU	0513	0.4	1127	5.8	1731	0.5	2344	6.0
15 SU	0517	0.8	1130	5.4	1727	0.9	2343	5.5
30 M	0553	0.6	1206	5.7	1812	0.7		

OCTOBER

Day	Time	m	Time	m	Time	m	Time	m
1 TU	0025	5.7	0633	0.9	1246	5.4	1855	1.1
16 W	0604	0.9	1219	5.5	1823	1.0		
2 W	0108	5.4	0715	1.3	1327	5.2	1941	1.4
17 TH	0038	5.4	0647	1.1	1302	5.4	1909	1.2
3 TH	0153	5.0	0801	1.7	1414	4.9	2035	1.8
18 F	0126	5.1	0735	1.4	1352	5.2	2003	1.4
4 F	0246	4.6	0855	2.1	1512	4.6	2143	2.1
19 SA	0223	4.9	0833	1.7	1453	4.9	2111	1.7
5 SA	0400	4.3	1008	2.4	1638	4.4	2307	2.2
20 SU	0336	4.6	0948	1.9	1610	4.8	2235	1.7
6 SU	0533	4.3	1135	2.4	1804	4.5		
21 M	0505	4.6	1114	1.9	1733	4.9	2357	1.6
7 M	0026	2.1	0646	4.4	1248	2.3	1907	4.7
22 TU	0627	4.8	1230	1.7	1846	5.2		
8 TU	0124	1.9	0739	4.7	1340	2.0	1954	4.9
23 W	0105	1.3	0731	5.1	1332	1.4	1945	5.5
9 W	0208	1.6	0819	4.9	1421	1.7	2031	5.2
24 TH	0201	0.9	0822	5.4	1423	1.1	2035	5.8
10 TH	0244	1.3	0852	5.1	1441	1.4	2104	5.3
25 F	0249	0.7	0907	5.6	1509	0.8	2120	5.9
11 F	0316	1.1	0923	5.3	1525	1.2	2136	5.5
26 SA ○	0332	0.6	0948	5.8	1551	0.7	2203	6.0
12 SA ●	0346	0.9	0955	5.5	1555	1.0	2208	5.6
27 SU	0412	0.5	1027	5.8	1631	0.7	2243	5.9
13 SU	0416	0.8	1028	5.6	1627	0.9	2242	5.6
28 M	0450	0.7	1105	5.8	1710	0.7	2323	5.8
14 M	0449	0.8	1103	5.6	1703	0.8	2318	5.6
29 TU	0528	0.8	1142	5.7	1750	0.9		
15 TU	0525	0.8	1140	5.6	1741	0.8	2357	5.5
30 W	0002	5.6	0606	1.1	1220	5.5	1831	1.2
31 TH	0042	5.3	0645	1.4	1259	5.3	1915	1.4

NOVEMBER

Day	Time	m	Time	m	Time	m	Time	m
1 F	0124	5.0	0727	1.7	1341	5.0	2003	1.8
16 SA	0119	5.2	0723	1.3	1342	5.4	1957	1.2
2 SA	0212	4.7	0815	2.1	1432	4.8	2101	2.0
17 SU	0217	5.0	0822	1.6	1442	5.2	2102	1.4
3 SU	0312	4.5	0916	2.4	1537	4.6	2211	2.2
18 M	0326	4.8	0932	1.8	1552	5.0	2217	1.5
4 M	0432	4.3	1032	2.5	1700	4.5	2326	2.2
19 TU	0446	4.7	1050	1.8	1708	5.0	2333	1.5
5 TU	0551	4.4	1149	2.4	1813	4.6		
20 W	0603	4.8	1205	1.7	1819	5.2		
6 W	0032	2.0	0651	4.6	1252	2.2	1907	4.8
21 TH	0041	1.3	0708	5.0	1309	1.5	1921	5.4
7 TH	0123	1.8	0738	4.8	1339	1.9	1952	5.0
22 F	0139	1.1	0802	5.3	1404	1.3	2015	5.5
8 F	0204	1.5	0817	5.1	1418	1.6	2030	5.3
23 SA	0230	1.0	0849	5.5	1453	1.1	2103	5.6
9 SA	0240	1.2	0853	5.3	1453	1.3	2106	5.4
24 SU	0314	0.9	0931	5.6	1536	1.0	2146	5.7
10 SU	0314	1.0	0928	5.5	1528	1.1	2142	5.6
25 M ○	0354	0.9	1010	5.7	1616	0.9	2227	5.7
11 M ●	0349	0.8	1003	5.7	1605	0.9	2219	5.7
26 TU	0431	0.8	1047	5.7	1655	0.9	2305	5.6
12 TU	0426	0.8	1040	5.7	1644	0.8	2259	5.7
27 W	0507	1.1	1123	5.6	1733	1.0	2343	5.4
13 W	0505	0.8	1120	5.8	1725	0.8	2341	5.6
28 TH	0543	1.2	1158	5.5	1812	1.2		
14 TH	0547	0.9	1202	5.7	1811	0.8		
29 F	0020	5.3	0620	1.4	1236	5.4	1853	1.4
15 F	0027	5.5	0632	1.1	1250	5.6	1901	1.0
30 SA	0100	5.1	0659	1.6	1316	5.2	1935	1.6

DECEMBER

Day	Time	m	Time	m	Time	m	Time	m
1 SU	0143	4.9	0742	1.9	1359	5.0	2022	1.8
16 M	0206	5.2	0808	1.3	1427	5.4	2047	1.1
2 M	0231	4.7	0830	2.1	1449	4.8	2117	2.0
17 TU	0307	5.0	0910	1.5	1529	5.2	2152	1.3
3 TU	0329	4.5	0929	2.3	1549	4.6	2220	2.1
18 W	0416	4.8	1020	1.7	1637	5.1	2302	1.4
4 W	0440	4.4	1039	2.4	1700	4.6	2326	2.1
19 TH	0530	4.8	1133	1.7	1749	5.0		
5 TH	0551	4.5	1148	2.3	1809	4.7		
20 F	0011	1.4	0640	4.9	1244	1.7	1857	5.1
6 F	0027	1.9	0650	4.7	1248	2.1	1906	4.8
21 SA	0115	1.4	0741	5.0	1345	1.5	1958	5.2
7 SA	0119	1.7	0739	5.0	1338	1.8	1954	5.1
22 SU	0211	1.3	0833	5.2	1438	1.3	2049	5.3
8 SU	0204	1.4	0822	5.2	1422	1.4	2037	5.3
23 M	0258	1.2	0917	5.4	1524	1.2	2134	5.3
9 M	0246	1.1	0902	5.5	1504	1.1	2119	5.5
24 TU ○	0340	1.1	0956	5.5	1605	1.1	2214	5.3
10 TU ●	0326	0.9	0941	5.7	1546	0.9	2201	5.6
25 W	0417	1.1	1032	5.5	1643	1.1	2250	5.3
11 W	0407	0.7	1022	5.8	1629	0.7	2244	5.7
26 TH	0451	1.1	1106	5.6	1719	1.1	2325	5.3
12 TH	0450	0.7	1105	5.9	1715	0.6	2330	5.7
27 F	0525	1.2	1141	5.5	1755	1.1		
13 F	0534	0.7	1150	5.9	1803	0.6		
28 SA	0001	5.2	0559	1.2	1216	5.5	1830	1.2
14 SA	0019	5.6	0622	0.8	1239	5.8	1853	0.7
29 SU	0037	5.1	0634	1.4	1252	5.3	1908	1.3
15 SU	0111	5.4	0713	1.0	1331	5.6	1948	0.9
30 M	0115	5.0	0712	1.5	1330	5.2	1947	1.5
31 TU	0156	4.9	0752	1.7	1411	5.0	2030	1.7

Volvo Penta service

VOLVO PENTA

Area 11

South Wales and Bristol Channel
Bardsey Island to Lands End

11

10-11-2

South Wales
and Bristol Channel

Pwllheli
10.11.8
VHF 80 M

Porthmadog
10.11.9
VHF **14** 12 16
YC 80 M

Abersoch
10.11.7
VHF YC 80 M

Bardsey Island

St Tudwal's Island

Mochras*

Barmouth
10.11.10
VHF 12 16

Cardigan Bay Radio
VHF **03** 16
VHF 03
0703 1933 UT
RG

Aberdovey
10.11.11
VHF 12 16

Aberystwyth
10.11.12
VHF **14** 16

Aberaeron*
VHF 14 16

New Quay*
VHF 14 16

Aberporth
RC Aero

Sharpness
10.11.20
VHF **17** 09 16
Canal 74

Cardiff
10.11.19
VHF **14** 13 16
Marina 80
01222 397020
RC Aero

Newport*
VHF 09 11 16

Barry
10.11.18
VHF 11 10 16

Port Talbot
VHF 12 16

Neath*

Swansea
10.11.17
VHF 14
Marina 80
M 0891 500 459
RC Aero

Mumbles*

Swansea CG

Fishguard
10.11.13
VHF 14 16

Strumble Head

St David's Head

Solva*

St Brides Bay*

Skomer*

Skokholm Island

Cardigan*

Tenby
10.11.15
VHF 16

Carmarthen*

Saundersfoot*
VHF 11 16

Caldey I

Burry Inlet
10.11.16

St Gowan Lt.By

Holyhead CG
Milford Haven CG

Variation 7°W(1996)

270   90

0

180

South Bishop
RC

Milford Haven
10.11.14
VHF **12** 09 10
11 14 67
16
Marinas 80 M

Celtic Radio
VHF **24** 16
VHF 24
0733 1933 UT

St Ann's Head

53°00'·00N

05°00'·00W   04°30'·00W   03°00'·00W   02°30'·00W

52°30'·00N

52°00'·00N

52°30'N·00N

52°00'N

51°30'·00N

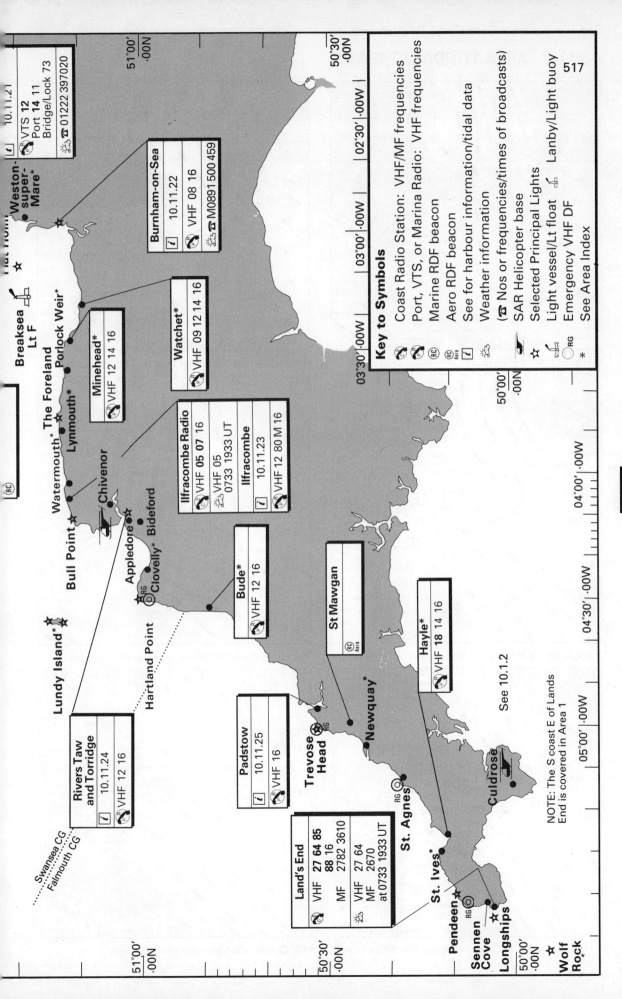

Weston-super-Mare*

⌐ 10.11.21
📻 VTS **12**
Port **14** 11
Bridge/Lock 73
☎ 01222 397020

Burnham-on-Sea

ⓘ 10.11.22
📻 VHF 08 16
☎ M0891 500 459

Watchet*
📻 VHF 09 12 14 16

Minehead*
📻 VHF 12 14 16

Porlock Weir*

Breaksea Lt F

The Foreland

Watermouth*

Lynmouth*

Chivenor

Bull Point

Ilfracombe Radio
📻 VHF 05 07 16
📻 VHF 05
☼ 0733 1933 UT

Ilfracombe
ⓘ 10.11.23
📻 VHF 12 80 M 16

Lundy Island*

Appledore • **Bideford**
Clovelly*

Rivers Taw and Torridge
ⓘ 10.11.24
📻 VHF 12 16

Swansea CG
Falmouth CG

Hartland Point

Bude*
📻 VHF 12 16

St Mawgan
Ⓡ Aero

Hayle*
📻 VHF 18 14 16

Padstow
ⓘ 10.11.25
📻 VHF 16

Newquay*

Trevose Head
Ⓡ RG

Culdrose

See 10.1.2

NOTE: The S coast E of Lands
End is covered in Area 1

Land's End
📻 VHF **27 64 85**
       88 16
   MF **2782** 3610
📻 VHF **27 64**
   MF 2670
☼ at 0733 1933 UT

St. Agnes RG

St. Ives*

Pendeen RG

Sennen Cove
Longships

Wolf Rock

11

51°00'
.00N

50°30'N

50°00'
.00N

51°00'
.00N

50°30'N

50°00'
.00N

03°30'.00W
03°00'.00W
02°30'.00W

04°00'.00W
04°30'.00W
05°00'.00W

10-11-3 AREA 11 TIDAL STREAMS

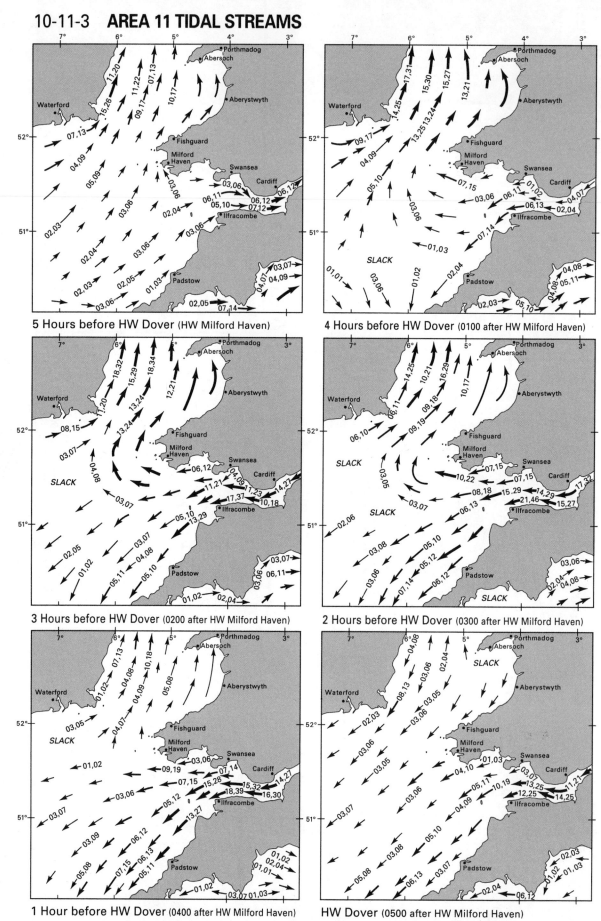

5 Hours before HW Dover (HW Milford Haven)

4 Hours before HW Dover (0100 after HW Milford Haven)

3 Hours before HW Dover (0200 after HW Milford Haven)

2 Hours before HW Dover (0300 after HW Milford Haven)

1 Hour before HW Dover (0400 after HW Milford Haven)

HW Dover (0500 after HW Milford Haven)

Southward 10.1.3   Northward   10.10.3   South Ireland 10.12.3

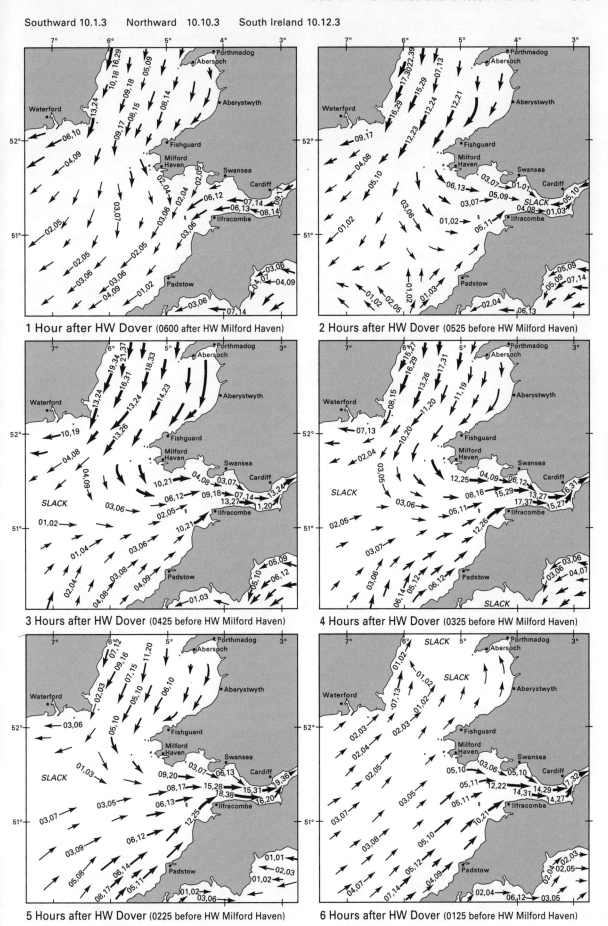

1 Hour after HW Dover (0600 after HW Milford Haven)

2 Hours after HW Dover (0525 before HW Milford Haven)

3 Hours after HW Dover (0425 before HW Milford Haven)

4 Hours after HW Dover (0325 before HW Milford Haven)

5 Hours after HW Dover (0225 before HW Milford Haven)

6 Hours after HW Dover (0125 before HW Milford Haven)

11

10.11.4 COASTAL LIGHTS, FOG SIGNALS AND WAYPOINTS

Abbreviations used below are given in 1.4.1. Principal lights are in **bold** print, places in CAPITALS, and light-vessels, light floats and Lanbys in *CAPITAL ITALICS*. Unless otherwise stated lights are white. m – elevation in metres; M – nominal range in miles. Fog signals are in *italics*. Useful waypoints are underlined – use those on land with care. All geographical positions should be assumed to be approximate. See 4.4.1.

CARDIGAN BAY (see also 10.10.4)

Bardsey I 52°44'.97N 04°47'.93W Fl (5) 15s 39m **26M**; W ■ Tr, R bands; obsc by Bardsey I 198°-250° and in Tremadoc B when brg less than 260°; *Horn Mo(N) 45s.*

St Tudwal's, 52°47'.88N 04°28'.20W Fl WR 20s 46m **W15, R13M**; W● Tr; vis W349°-169°, R169°-221°, W221°-243°, R243°-259°, W259°-293°, R293°-349°; obsc by East I 211°-231°.

PWLLHELI/PORTHMADOG/MOCHRAS LAGOON
Pwllheli App Lt By 52°53'.00N 04°23'.00W Iso 2s; SWM.
Training Arm Hd 52°53'.23N 04°23'.67W QG 3m 3M.
Sewer Outfall 52°53'.18N 04°23'.69W Fl R 2·5s.
Abererch By 52°53'.50N 04°23'.00W; SPM (Apr-Oct).
Butlins By 52°53'.00N 04°22'.00W; SPM (Apr-Oct).
West End By 52°52'.40N 04°25'.50W; SPM (Apr-Oct).
Porthmadog Fairway Lt By 52°52'.49N 04°10'.98W L Fl 10s; SWM.
Shell I NE Corner 52°49'.53N 04°07'.64W Fl WRG 4s; vis G079°-124°, W124°-134°, R134°-179°; (Mar- Nov).

BARMOUTH
Diffuser Lt By 52°43'.17N 04°05'.31W Fl Y 5s; SPM.
Barmouth Outer Lt By 52°42'.90N 04°04'.90W L Fl 10s; SWM.
N Bank Y Perch 52°42'.81N 04°03'.67W QR 4m 5M.
Ynys y Brawd SE end 52°42'.97N 04°03'.07W Fl R 5s 5M.

Sarn Badrig Causeway Lt By 52°41'.17N 04°25'.30W Q (9) 15s; WCM; *Bell.*
Sarn-y-Bwch. Bwch By 52°34'.80N 04°13'.50W; WCM.

ABERDOVEY
Aberdovey Outer By 52°31'.75N 04°06'.00W; SWM.
Cynfelyn Patches. Patches By 52°25'.80N 04°16'.30W; WCM.

ABERYSTWYTH/ABERAERON/NEW QUAY
Aberystwyth S Bkwtr Hd 52°24'.39N 04°05'.46W Fl (2) WG 10s 12m 10M; B col; vis G030°-053°, W053°-210°. (TE 1992).
Ldg Lts 138°. Front 52°24'.35N 04°05'.32W FR 4m 5M. Rear, 52m from front, FR 7m 6M.
Aberaeron S Pier 52°14'.60N 04°15'.87W Fl (3) G 10s 6M; vis 125°-200°. (TE 1994)
N Pier Fl (4) WRG 15s 6M; vis G050°-104°, W104°-178°, R178°-232°.
Carreg Ina By 52°13'.09N 04°20'.47W; NCM.
New Quay Pier Hd 52°12'.94N 04°21'.27W Fl WG 3s 12m W8M, G5M; G △; vis W135°-252°, G252°-295°.

CARDIGAN
CG Bldg 52°06'.98N 04°41'.14W 2 FR (vert).
Channel Bn 52°06'.44N 04°41'.32W Fl (2) 5s; IDM. (TE 1992).
Bridge, Iso Y 2s on upstream and downstream sides.

FISHGUARD
N Bkwtr Hd 52°00'.74N 04°58'.15W Fl G 4·5s 18m 13M; 8-sided Tr; *Bell (1) 8s .*
E Bkwtr Hd Fl R 3s 10m 5M.
Lts in line 282°. Front 52°00'.65N 04°59'.20W FG 77m 5M; W ◊ on W mast. Rear, 46m from front, FG 89m 5M; W ◊ on W mast.
Penanglas, 152m S of Pt, *Dia (2) 60s;* W obelisk.

Strumble Hd 52°01'.78N 05°04'.35W Fl (4) 15s 45m **26M**; W ● Tr; vis 038°-257°; (H24).

BISHOPS AND SMALLS

South Bishop 51°51'.15N 05°24'.65W Fl 5s 44m **24M**; W ● Tr; (H24); RC; *Horn (3) 45s.*
Brawdy. St Brides Bay. Research Area, seaward Lt Bys.
Lt By A1 51°49'.30N 05°20'.00W Fl (4) Y 20s; SPM.
Lt By B1 51°48'.30N 05°20'.00W Fl (4) Y 20s; SPM.

The Smalls 51°43'.25N 05°40'.15W Fl (3) 15s 36m **25M**; W ● Tr, R bands; Racon (T); *Horn (2) 60s.* Same Tr, FR 33m 13M; ; vis 253°-285° over Hats and Barrels Rk; both Lts shown H24.

Skokholm I, SW end 51°41'.60N 05°17'.17W Fl R 10s 54m **17M**; W 8-sided Tr; part obsc 226°-258°; (H24); *Horn 15s.*

WALES – SOUTH COAST – BRISTOL CHANNEL

MILFORD HAVEN
St Ann's Hd 51°40'.85N 05°10'.35W Fl WR 5s 48m **W18M, R17**/14M; W 8-sided Tr; vis W233°-247°, R247°-285°, R (intens) 285°-314°, R314°-332°, W332°-124°, W129°-131°; *Horn (2) 60s.*
W Blockhouse Pt Ldg Lts 022·5°. Front 51°41'.30N 05°09'.40W F 54m 13M; B stripe on W Tr; vis 004·5°-040·5°. By day 10M.
Watwick Pt Rear, 0·5M from front F 80m **15M**; vis 013·5°-031·5°. By day 10M.
W Blockhouse Pt 51°41'.26N 05°09'.40W Q WR 21m 9/7M; R lantern on W base.
Dale Fort 51°42'.13N 05°08'.93W Fl (2) WR 5s 20m W5M, R3M; vis R222°-276°, W276°-019°.
Great Castle Hd 51°42'.60N 05°07'.00W F WRG 27m W5M, R3M, G3M; W ■ Tr, B stripe; vis R243°-281°, G281°-299°, W299°-029°. Same Tr Ldg Lts 039·8° Oc 4s 27m **15M**; vis 031·2°-048·2°. **Rear**, 890m from front, **Little Castle Hd** 51°43'.02N 05°06'.52W Oc 8s 53m **15M**; vis 031·2°-048·2°.
St Anne's Hd Lt By 51°40'.23N 05°10'.43W Fl R 2·5s; PHM.
Mid Channel Rks Lt By 51°40'.16N 05°10'.07W Q (9) 15s; WCM.
Middle Chan Rks Lt Tr 51°40'.28N 05°09'.77W Fl (3) G 7s 18m 8M; B ●Tr, lantern.
Sheep Lt By 51°40'.03N 05°08'.23W QG; SHM.
Millbay Lt By 51°41'.02N 05°09'.38W Fl (2) R 5s; PHM.
W Chapel Lt By 51°40'.97N 05°08'.60W Fl G 10s; SHM.
E Chapel Lt By 51°40'.85N 05°08'.08W Fl R 5s; PHM.
Rat Lt By 51°40'.77N 05°07'.80W Fl G 5s; SHM.
Angle Lt By 51°41'.60N 05°08'.20W VQ; WCM.
Thorn Rock Lt By 51°41'.50N 05°07'.70W Q (9) 15s; WCM.
Dakotian Lt By 51°42'.13N 05°08'.22W Q (3) 10s; ECM.
Chapel Lt By 51°41'.63N 05°06'.80W Fl G 5s; SHM.
Stack Lt By 51°42'.00N 05°06'.46W Fl R 2·5s; PHM.
S Hook Lt By 51°40'.80N 05°06'.03W Q (6) +L Fl 15s; WCM.
Esso Lt By 51°41'.72N 05°05'.17W Q; NCM.
E Angle Lt By 51°41'.68N 05°04'.20W Fl (3) G 10s; SHM.

Turbot Bank Lt By 51°37'.40N 05°10'.00W VQ (9) 10s; WCM.

St Gowan Lt By 51°31'.90N 04°59'.70W Q (6) + L Fl 15s; Racon (T); *Whis;* SCM.
Caldey I 51°37'.86N 04°41'.00W Fl (3) WR 20s 65m W14M, R12M; W ● Tr; vis R173°-212°, W212°-088°, R088°- 102°.
Eel Pt By 51°38'.83N 04°42'.17W; SHM.
Giltar Spit By 51°39'.00N 04°42'.05W; PHM.
Spaniel By 51°38'.03N 04°39'.67W; ECM.
Woolhouse By 51°39'.32N 04°39'.62W; WCM.
North Highcliff By 51°39'.35N 04°40'.70W; NCM.

TENBY/SAUNDERSFOOT/CARMARTHEN BAY/BURRY INLET
Tenby Pier Hd 51°40'.37N 04°41'.81W FR 7m 7M.
Saundersfoot Pier Hd 51°42'.55N 04°41'.68W Fl R 5s 6m 7M.
DZ1 By 51°42'.02N 04°35'.55; SPM.

DZ2 Lt By 51°39'·75N 04°37'·45W Fl Y 2·5s; SPM.
DZ3 By 51°37'·35N 04°37'·70W; SPM.
DZ7 Lt By 51°38'·08N 04°30'·05W Fl Y 10s; SPM.
DZ4 Lt By 51°35'·42N 04°30'·00W Fl Y 5s; SPM.
DZ8 By 51°41'·50N 04°24'·30W; SPM.
DZ6 By 51°38'·00N 04°24'·17W; SPM.
DZ5 Lt By 51°36'·35N 04°24'·28W Fl Y 2·5s; SPM.
Burry Port Barrel Post 51°40'·47N 04°14'·92W QR 1M (occas).
Burry Port W Bkwtr 51°40'·60N 04°14'·97W FR 7M.
Whiteford Lt Tr 51°39'·12N 04°14'·99W Fl 5s 7m 7M; Tr; (occas).
West Helwick (W HWK) Lt By 51°31'·37N 04°23'·58W Q (9) 15s; Racon (T);Whis; WCM .
E Helwick Lt By 51°31'·77N 04°12'·60W VQ (3) 5s; Bell; ECM.

SWANSEA BAY/SWANSEA
Ledge Lt By 51°29'·90N 03°58'·70W VQ (6) + L Fl 10s; SCM.
Mixon By 51°33'·10N 03°58'·70W; Bell; PHM.
Outer Spoil Gnd Lt By 51°32'·08N 03°55'·67W Fl Y 2·5s; SPM.
Grounds Lt By 51°32'·90N 03°53'·40W VQ (3) 5s; ECM.

Mumbles 51°34'·00N 03°58'·20W Fl (4) 20s 35m **16M**; W Tr; Fog Det Lt Fl 5s 28m; vis 331·5°-336·5°; Horn(3) 60s.
Railway Pier Hd 51°34'·19N 03°58'·36W 2 FR (vert) 11m 9M.
SW Inner Green Grounds Lt By 51°34'·04N 03°56'·95W Q (6) + L Fl 15s; Bell; SCM.

Outer Fairway Lt By 51°35'·50N 03°56'·01W QG; Bell; SHM.
W Pier Hd 51°36'·47N 03°55'·67W Fl (2) R 10s 11m 9M; FR Lts on radio mast 014° 1·3M.
Swansea Inner Fairway Lt By 51°36'·20N 03°55'·60W Fl G 2·5s; Bell; SHM.
E Bkwtr Hd 51°36'·35N 03°55'·55W 2 FG (vert) 10m 6M; W Tr; Siren 30s.
Lts in line 020°. Jetty Hd Front 51°36'·51N 03°55'·43W Oc G 4s 5m 2M. Rear, 260m from front, FG 6M.

SWANSEA BAY/RIVER NEATH/PORT TALBOT
Neath App Chan Lt By 51°35'·70N 03°52'·75W Fl G 5s; SHM.
Neath SE Training Wall near S end 51°36'·30N 03°51'·89W 2 FG (vert) 6m 5M R mast.
Neath SE Training Wall Middle 51°36'·68N 03°51'·33W FG 6m 5M; R mast.
Neath SE Training Wall N End 51°37'·07N 03°50'·77W 3 FG (vert) 6m 5M; R mast.
Cabenda Lt By 51°33'·43N 03°52'·25W VQ (6) + L Fl 10s; SCM.
P Talbot S Outer Lt By 51°33'·66N 03°51'·20W Fl G 5s; SHM.
P Talbot N Outer Lt By 51°33'·76N 03°51'·30W Fl R 5s; PHM.
P Talbot N Inner Lt By 51°34'·19N 03°50'·17W Fl R 3s; PHM; Horn.
Ldg Lts 059·8° (occas). Front 51°34'·89N 03°48'·02W Oc R 3s 12m 6M; Y & Or ◆ on Tr. Rear, 400m from front, Oc R 6s 32m 6M; Y & Or ◆ on Tr.
N Bkwtr Hd 51°34'·73N 03°48'·93W Fl (4) R 10s 11m 3M.
S Bkwtr Hd 51°34'·43N 03°48'·95W Fl G 3s 11m 3M.

BRISTOL CHANNEL – EASTERN PART (NORTH SHORE)

Kenfig Lt By 51°29'·71N 03°46'·43W Q (3) 10s; ECM.
W Scarweather (W SCAR) Lt By 51°28'·28N 03°55'·50W Q (9) 15s; Racon (T); Bell; WCM.
S Scarweather (S SCAR) Lt By 51°27'·58N 03°51'·50W Q (6) + L Fl 15s; SCM.
Hugo By 51°28'·80N 03°48'·30W; PHM.
E Scarweather By 51°28'·12N 03°46'·23W; ECM.

PORTHCAWL
Fairy By 51°27'·83N 03°42'·00W; WCM.
Tusker Lt By 51°26'·82N 03°40'·67W Fl (2) R 5s; PHM.
Porthcawl Bkwtr Hd 51°28'·33N 03°41'·95W F WRG 10m W6M, R4M, G4M; W 6-sided Tr, B base; vis G302°-036°, W036°-082°, R082°-122°.

W Nash Lt By 51°25'·95N 03°45'·88W VQ(9) 10s; WCM.
Middle Nash By 51°24'·80N 03°39'·34W; WCM.
E Nash Lt By 51°24'·03N 03°34'·03W Q (3) 10s; ECM.

Nash 51°24'·00N 03°33'·05W Fl (2) WR 10s 56m **W21M, R20/17M**; W I Tr; vis R280°-290°, W290°-097°, R097°-100°, R (intens) 100°-104°, R104°-120°, W120°-128°; Siren (2) 45s, RC.

Saint Hilary 51° 27'·40N 03°24'·10W Aero QR 346m 11M; radio mast; 4 FR (vert) on same mast 6M.
Breaksea Pt intake 51°22'·50N 03°24'·45W Fl R 11m; Tr.

BREAKSEA Lt F 51°19'·85N 03°19'·00W Fl 15s 11m 12M; F riding Lt; Racon(T); Horn (2) 30s;
Wenvoe 51°27'·50N 03°16'·80W Aero Q 365m 12M; radio mast (H24).
Merkur Lt By 51°21'·85N 03°15'·87W Fl R 2·5s; PHM.
Welsh Water Barry W Lt By 51°22'·23N 03°16'·84W Fl R 5s; PHM.

BARRY
W Bkwtr Hd 51°23'·43N 03°15'·43W Fl 2·5s 12m 10M.
E Bkwtr Hd 51°23'·50N 03°15'·37W QG 7m 8M.
Lavernock Spit Lt By 51°22'·99N 03°10'·74W VQ (6) + L Fl 10s; SCM.
One Fathom N Lt By 51°20'·91N 03°12'·08W Q; NCM.
Mackenzie Lt By 51°21'·72N 03°08'·15W QR; PHM.
Holm Middle Lt By 51°21'·69N 03°06'·64W Fl G 2·5s; SHM.
Wolves Lt By 51°23'·10N 03°08'·80W VQ; NCM.

Flat Holm, SE Pt 51°22'·52N 03°07'·05W Fl (3) WR 10s 50m **W16M**, R13M; W ● Tr; vis R106°-140°, W140°-151°, R151°-203°, W203°-106°; (H24); Horn 30s.
Weston Lt By 51°22'·58N 03°05'·66W Fl (2) R 5s; PHM.
Monkstone Rock Lt 51°24'·87N 03°05'·92W Fl 5s 13m 12M; R col on ● Tr.

CARDIFF AND PENARTH ROADS
Lavernock Outfall Lt By 51°23'·92N 03°09'·41W QR; PHM.
Ranie Lt By 51°24'·22N 03°09'·30W Fl (2) R 5s; PHM.
S Cardiff Lt By 51°24'·15N 03°08'·48W Q (6) + L Fl 15s; SCM; Bell.
Mid Cardiff Lt By 51°25'·57N 03°08'·00W Fl (3) G 10s; SHM.
Cardiff Spit By 51°25'·53N 03°06'·42W; PHM.
N Cardiff Lt By 51°27'·77N 03°05'·28W QG; SHM.

PENARTH/CARDIFF
Penarth Promenade Pier near Hd 51°26'·06N 03°09'·82W 2 FR (vert) 8/6m 3M; Reed Mo(BA) 60s, sounded 10 min before a steamer expected.
Penarth Sailing Club pontoon 51°26'·80N 03°10'·50W Q.
Ldg Lts 349°. **Front** 51°27'·67N 03°09'·90W F 4m **17M**. **Rear,** 520m from front, F 24m **17M**.
Outer Wrach Lt By 51°26'·17N 03°09'·38W Q (9) 15s; WCM.
Inner Wrach Lt By 51°26'·71N 03°09'·57W Fl G 2·5s; SHM.
Queen Alexandra Dock ent S Jetty Hd 51°27'·06N 03°09'·50W 2 FG (vert); Tfc sigs; Dia 60s.
Tail Patch Lt By 51°23'·50N 03°03'·59W QG; SHM.
Hope Lt By 51°24'·82N 03°02'·60W Q (3) 10s; ECM.
NW Elbow Lt By 51°26'·48N 02°59'·61W VQ (9) 10s; WCM; Bell.
English and Welsh Grounds Lt By 51°26'·90N 03°00'·10W L Fl 10s 7M; Racon (O); SWM;Whis.

NEWPORT DEEP
Newport Deep Lt By 51°29'·33N 02°59'·03W Fl (3)G 10s; Bell; SHM.

RIVER USK/NEWPORT
East Usk 51°32'·38N 02°57'·93W Fl (2) WRG 10s 11m **W15M**, R11M, G11M; W ● Tr; vis W284°-290°, R290°-017°, W017°-037°, G037°-115°, W115°-120°. Also Oc WRG 10s 10m W11M, R9M, G9M; vis G018°-022°, W022°-024°, R024°-028°.

11

Alexandra Dock, S Lock W Pier Hd 51°32'·84N 02°59'·18W 2 FR (vert) 9m 6M; *Horn 60s*.

E Pier Hd 51°32'·93N 02°59'·03W 2 FG (vert) 9m 6M.

Julians Pill Ldg Lts about 057°. Common Front 51°33'·28N 02°57'·85W FG 5m 4M. Rear, 61m from front, FG 8m 4M. Ldg Lts 149°. Rear, 137m from common front FG 9m 4M.

Birdport Jetty 51°33'·64N 02°58'·01W 2 FG (vert) 6m.

Dallimores Wharf 51°33'·85N 02°58'·51W 2 FG (vert).

Transporter Bridge W side 2 FR (vert); 2 FY (vert) shown on transporter car.

E side 2 FG (vert). Centres of George Street and Newport Bridges marked by FY Lts.

BRISTOL CHANNEL – EASTERN PART (SOUTH SHORE)

BRISTOL DEEP

N Elbow Lt By 51°27'·12N 02°58'·10W QG; *Bell;* SHM.

S Mid Grounds Lt By 51°27'·66N 02°58'·34W VQ (6) + L Fl 10s; SCM.

E Mid-Grounds Lt By 51°27'·90N 02°55'·00W Fl R 5s; PHM.

Clevedon Lt By 51°27'·40N 02°54'·84W VQ; NCM.

Welsh Hook Lt By 51°28'·49N 02°51'·78W Q (6) + L Fl 15s; *Bell;* SCM.

Avon Lt By 51°27'·90N 02°51'·65W Fl G 2·5s; SHM.

Clevedon Pier 51°26'·61N 02°51'·82W 2 FG (vert) 7m 3M. (TE 1992).

Walton Bay, Old signal station 51°27'·86N 02°49'·71W Fl 2·5s 35m 2M.

Black Nore Pt 51°29'·05N 02°47'·95W Fl (2) 10s 11m **15M**; W ● Tr; obsc by Sand Pt when brg less than 049°; vis 044°-243°.

Newcome Lt By 51°29'·98N 02°46'·63W Fl (3) R 10s; PHM.

Firefly Lt By 51°29'·93N 02°45'·27W Fl (2) G 5s; SHM.

Outer Lt By 51°29'·97N 02°44'·71W IQ G 12s; SHM.

Middle Lt By 51°29'·90N 02°44'·13W Fl G 5s; SHM.

Inner Lt By 51°29'·83N 02°43'·78W Fl (3) G 15s; SHM.

Cockburn Lt By 51°30'·43N 02°44'·00W Fl R 2·5s; PHM.

Portishead Pt 51°29'·64N 02°46'·34W Q (3) 10s 9m **16M**; B Tr, W base; vis 060°-262°; *Horn 20s*.

PORTISHEAD

Pier Hd 51°29'·66N 02°45'·18W Iso G 2s 5m 3M; W col; *Horn 15s*, sounded when vessel expected.

Lock E side 51°29'·54N 02°45'·33W 2 FR (vert) 7m 1M; Gy col; (occas).

Lock W side 2 FG (vert) 7m 1M; Gy col; (occas).

Seabank. Lts in line 086·8°. Front 51°29'·99N 02°43'·66W IQ 13m 5M; vis 070·3°-103·3°, 076·8°-096·8°. Rear, 500m from front, IQ W 16m 5M; vis 070·3°-103·3°, 076·8°-096·8°. By day, both 1M.

Royal Portbury Dock Pier end 51°30'·13N 02°43'·64W L Fl G 15s 5m 6M; Gy pillar.

Pier corner 51°30'·10N 02°43'·77W Fl G 2s 7m 7M; Gy pillar; *Dia 30s*, sounded HW-4 to HW+3.

Knuckle Lts in line 099·6° 51°29'·92N 02°43'·60W Oc G 5s 6m 6M, rear, 165m from front, FG 13m 6M; vis 044°-134°.

AVONMOUTH

Royal Edward Dock N Pier Hd 51°30'·47N 02°43'·00W Fl 10s 15m 10M; ● Tr; vis 060°-228·5°.

King Road Ldg Lts 072·4°. N Pier Hd Front 51°30'·47N 02°43'·00W Oc R 5s 5m 9M; W obelisk, R bands; vis 062°-082°. Rear, 546m from front, QR 15m 10M; B&W striped ● on Tr, Or bands; vis 066°-078°.

Oil Jetty Hd 51°30'·62N 02°42'·85W 2 FG (vert) 6m 2M.

Gypsum effluent pipe 51°31'·31N 02°41'·62W Fl Y 3s 3m 2M; Y Bn.

Effluent pipe Lt By 51°31'·34N 02°42'·28W Fl G 5s; SHM.

RIVER AVON

S Pier Hd (see above)

Ldg Lts 127·2°. Front 51°30'·05N 02°42'·47W FR 7m 3M; W □, R stripes; vis 010°-160°. Rear 142m from front FR 17m 3M; W ○, vis 048°-138°.

Monoliths 51°30'·23N 02°42'·68W Fl R 5s 5m 3M; W □, B stripes on W col; vis 317°-137°.

Saint George Ldg Lts 173·3°, 51°29'·73N 02°42'·58W both Oc G 5s 6m 1M, on Or cols; vis 158°-305°; synch.

Nelson Pt 51°29'·82N 02°42'·43W Fl R 3s 9m 3M; W mast.

Broad Pill 51°29'·6N 02°41'·8W QY 11m 1M; W Tr.

Avonmouth Bridge, NE end 51°29'·36N 02°41'·45W L Fl R 10s 5m 3M, SW end L Fl G 10s 5m 3M, showing up and downstream. From here to City Docks, Oc G Lts are shown on S bank, and R or Y Lts on N bank.

CUMBERLAND BASIN

Ent N side 51°26'·95N 02°37'·36W 2 FR (vert) 6m 1M; S side W end 2 FG (vert) 7m 1M;

AVON BRIDGE

N side 51°26'·79N 02°37'·34W FR 6m 1M on Bridge pier. Centre of span Iso 5s 6m 1M. S side FG 6m 1M on Bridge pier.

SEVERN ESTUARY

THE SHOOTS

Lower Shoots Bn 51°33'·62N 02°42'·05W Q (9) 15s 6m 7M; WCM.

Upper Shoots Bn 51°34'·20N 02°41'·79W (unlit); WCM.

Charston Rk 51°35'·32N 02°41'·60W Fl 2·5s 5m 13/8M; W ● Tr, B stripe; vis (13M) 343°-043°, (8M) 043°-343°.

Redcliffe Ldg Lts 012·9° Front 51°36'·17N 02°41'·29W F Bu 16m; vis 358°-028°. Rear, 320m from front, F Bu 33m 10M.

Chapel Rk 51°36'·40N 02°39'·13W Fl WRG 2·6s 6m W8M, R5M, G5M; B Tr, W lantern; vis W213°-284°, R284°-049°, W049°-051·5°, G051·5°-160°.

RIVER WYE

Wye Bridge 51°37'·03N 02°39'·54W 2F Bu (hor); centre of span.

SEVERN BRIDGE

West Tr 3QR (hor) on upstream and downstream sides; *Horn (3) 45s*; obscured 040°-065°.

Centre of span 51°36'·57N 02°38'·32W Q Bu, each side.

E Tr 3 QG (hor) on upstream and downstream sides.

Aust 51°36'·13N 02°37'·91W 2 QG (vert) 11/5m 6M; power cable pylon.

Lyde Rk 51°36'·85N 02°38'·58W QR 5m 5M; B Tr, W lantern.

Sedbury 51°37'·75N 02°38'·93W 2 FR (vert) 10m 3M.

Slime Road Ldg Lts 210·4°. Front 51°37'·21N 02°39'·00W F Bu 9m 5M. Rear, 91 m from front, F Bu 16m 5M; B Tr.

Inward Rocks Ldg Lts 252·5°. Front 51°39'·23N 02°37'·37W F 6m 6M; B Tr. Rear, 183m from front, F 13m 2M.

Counts Lt By 51°39'·45N 02°35'·74W Q; NCM.

Sheperdine Ldg Lts 070·4°. Front 51°40'·03N 02°33'·22W F 7m 5M; B Tr, W lantern. Rear, 168m from front, F 13m 5M; B Tr, W lantern; *Bell (26) 60s*.

Ledges Lt By 51°39'·75N 02°34'·06W Fl (3) G 10s; SHM.

Narlwood Rks Ldg Lts 224·9°. Front 51°39'·54N 02°34'·68W Fl 2s 5m 8M; Y Bn, B lantern. Rear, 198m from front Fl 2s 9m 8M; Y Bn, B lantern.

Hills Flats Lt By 51°40'·66N 02°32'·59W Fl G 4s; SHM.

Hayward Rk Lt By 51°41'·24N 02°31'·00W Q; NCM.

Conigre Ldg Lts 077·5°. Front 51°41'·43N 02°29'·92W F Vi 21m 8M. Rear, 213m from front F Vi 29m 8M.

Fishing House Ldg Lts 217·7°. Front 51°40'·95N 02°30'·91W F 5m 2M: W hut and post. Rear F 11m 2M; W hut and mast.

BERKELEY

Power Station Centre 51°41'·62N 02°29'·97W 3x2 FG (vert); *Siren (2) 30s*.

Bull Rk 51°41'·78N 02°29'·80W Iso 2s 6m 8M.
Berkeley Pill Ldg Lts 187·8°. Front 51°41'·95N 02°29'·32W
FG 5m 2M. Rear, 152m from front, FG 11m 2M; both B Trs,
W lanterns.
Panthurst Pill 51°42'·56N 02°28'·93W F Bu 6m 1M; Y pillar.
Lydney Docks Pier Hd 51°42'·60N 02°30'·27W FW or R
(tidal); *Gong (tidal)*.

SHARPNESS DOCKS
S Pier Hd 51°42'·93N 02°29'·01W 2 FG (vert) 6m 3M; *Siren 20s*.
N Pier 2 FR (vert) 6m 3M.
Old ent S side, 51°43'·49N 02°28'·82W S*iren 5s* (tidal).

BRISTOL CHANNEL (SOUTH SHORE)
WESTON-SUPER-MARE
Pier Hd 51°20'·85N 02°59'·17W 2 FG (vert) 6m.
E Culver Lt By 51°17'·70N 03°14'·50W Q (3) 10s; ECM.
W Culver Lt By 51°16'·85N 03°19'·20W VQ (9) 10s; WCM.
Gore Lt By 51°13'·93N 03°09'·70W Iso 5s; *Bell*; SWM.

BURNHAM-ON-SEA/RIVER PARRETT
Ent 51°14'·86N 03°00'·26W Fl 7·5s 7m 12M; vis 074°-164°.
Dir Lt 076°. Dir F WRG 4m W12M, R10M, G10M; same Tr;
vis G071°-075°, W075°-077°, R077°-081°.
Seafront Lts in line 112°, moved for changing chan, Front
51°14'·38N 02°59'·86W FR 6m 3M W □, Or stripe on sea
wall. Rear FR 12m 3M; church Tr.
Brue Bn 51°13'·50N 03°00'·20W QR 4m 3M; W mast,
R bands. (TE 1992).
Stert Reach 51°11'·32N 03°01'·90W Fl 3s 4m 7M; vis 187°-
217°.

Hinkley Pt,intake 51°12'·90N 03°07'·96W 2 FG (vert) 7m 3M.
DZ No. 2 Lt By 51°12'·87N 03°14'·35W Fl Y 10s; SPM.

WATCHET
W Bkwtr Hd 51°11'·03N 03°19'·67W FG 9m 9M.
FR Lts on radio masts 1·6M SSW.
E Pier 51°10'·97N 03°19'·63W 2 FR (vert) 3M.

MINEHEAD/PORLOCK WEIR
Bkwtr Hd 51°12'·78N 03°28'·28W Fl (2) G 5s 4M; vis 127°-262°.
Sewer Outfall 51°12'·95N 03°28'·22W QG 6m 7M; SHM Bn.
Lynmouth Foreland 51°14'·70N 03°47'·15W Fl (4) 15s 67m
18M; W ● Tr; vis 083°-275°;(H24).

LYNMOUTH/WATERMOUTH
River training arm 51°13'·88N 03°49'·77W 2 FR (vert) 6m 5M.
Harbour arm 51°13'·89N 03°49'·78W 2 FG (vert) 6m 5M.
Sand Ridge By 51°14'·98N 03°49'·70W; SHM.
Copperas Rock By 51°13'·77N 04°00'·50W; SHM.
Watermouth 51°12'·90N 04°04'·50W Oc WRG 5s 1m; W △;
vis G149·5°-151·5°, W151·5°-154·5°, R154·5°-156·5°.

ILFRACOMBE
Lantern Hill 51°12'·64N 04°06'·70W FR 39m 6M.
Promenade Pier N end 51°12'·66N 04°06'·60W 2 FG (vert)
Siren 30s (occas).

Horseshoe Lt By 51°15'·00N 04°12'·85W Q; NCM.

Bull Point 51°11'·95N 04°12'·05W Fl (3) 10s 54m **25M**; W ●
Tr, obscd shore-056°. Same Tr; FR 48m 12M; vis 058°-096°.
Morte Stone By 51°11'·30N 04°14'·85W; SHM.
Baggy Leap By 51°08'·90N 04°16'·90W; SHM.

BIDEFORD, RIVERS TAW AND TORRIDGE
Bideford Fairway Lt By 51°05'·23N 04°16'·17W L Fl 10s; *Bell*;
SWM.
Bideford Bar By 51°04'·93N 04°14'·76W; NCM.
Instow Ldg Lts 118°. **Front** 51°03'·59N 04°10'·60W Oc 6s
22m **15M**; vis 104·5°-131·5°. **Rear**, 427m from front, Oc 10s
38m **15M**; vis 103°-133°; (H24).
Crow Pt 51°03'·93N 04°11'·32W Fl R 5s 8m 4M; W Tr; vis
225°-045°.
Clovelly Hbr Quay Hd 50°59'·85N 04°23'·75W Fl G 5s 5m 5M.

LUNDY
Near North Pt 51°12'·07N 04°40'·57W Fl 15s 48m **17M**;
W ● Tr; vis 009°-285°.
SE Pt 51°09'·70N 04°39'·30W Fl 5s 53m **15M**; W ● Tr;
vis 170°-073°; *Horn 25s*.

Hartland Pt 51°01'·27N 04°31'·50W Fl (6) 15s 37m **25M**;
(H24); W ● Tr; *Horn 60s*.

NORTH CORNWALL

BUDE
Compass Pt Tr 50°49'·70N 04°33'·35W.

PADSTOW
Stepper Pt 50°34'·11N 04°56'·63W L Fl 10s 12m 4M.
St Saviour's Pt 50°32'·72N 04°56'·00W L Fl G 10s 1M; G △.
N Quay Hd 50°32'·48N 04°56'·10W 2 FG (vert) 6m 2M.
Trevose Hd 50°32'·93N 05°02'·06W Fl R 5s 62m **25M**;
W ● Tr. *Horn (2) 30s*.

NEWQUAY
N Pier Hd 50°25'·04N 05°05'·12W 2 FG (vert) 5m 2M.
S Pier Hd 50°25'·02N 05°05'·13W 2 FR (vert) 4m 2M; ● Tr.

The Stones Lt By 50°15'·60N 05°25'·40W Q; NCM; *Bell*; *Whis*.
Godrevy I 50°14'·50N 05°23'·95W Fl WR 10s 37m W12M,
R9M; W 8-sided Tr; vis W022°-101°, R101°-145°, W145°-272°.

HAYLE
App Lt By 50°12'·25N 05°26'·18W Fl (2) R 5s; PHM.
Lts in line 180°. Front 50°11'·55N 05°26'·14W F 17m 4M.
Rear, 110m from front, F 23m 4M.

ST IVES
E Pier Hd 50°12'·77N 05°28'·53W 2 FG (vert) 8m 5M; W ● Tr.
W Pier Hd 50°12'·74N 05°28'·67W 2 FR (vert) 5m 3M Gy col.

Pendeen 50°09'·80N 05°40'·20W Fl (4) 15s 59m **18M**; W ●
Tr; vis 042°-240°; in B between Gurnard Hd and Pendeen it
shows to coast; *Horn 20s*. For Lts further SW see 10.1.4.

11

10.11.5 PASSAGE INFORMATION

For directions on this coast refer to the Admiralty *W Coasts of England and Wales Pilot. A Cruising Guide to NW England & Wales* (Imray/Griffiths) covers as far S as Tenby; *Lundy and Irish Sea Pilot* (Imray/Taylor) continues to Land's End.

It is useful to know some Welsh words with navigational significance. *Aber:* estuary. *Afon:* river. *Bach, bychan, fach:* little. *Borth:* cove. *Bryn:* hill. *Careg, craig:* rock. *Coch, goch:* red. *Dinas:* fort. *Ddu:* black. *Fawr, Mawr:* big. *Ffrydiau:* tiderip. *Llwyd:* grey. *Moel:* bare conical hill. *Mor:* sea. *Morfa:* sandy shore. *Mynydd:* mountain. *Penrhyn:* headland. *Porth:* cove. *Ynys, Ynysoedd:* island(s).

CARDIGAN BAY (charts 1971, 1972, 1973)

Hbrs are mostly on a lee shore, and/or have bars which make them dangerous to approach in bad weather. Abersoch (10.11.7) and Pwllheli (10.11.8) offer best shelter from prevailing W'lies. There may be overfalls off Trwyn Cilan, SW of St Tudwal's Is (lit). In N part of bay there are three major dangers to coasting yachts, as described briefly below: St Patrick's Causeway (Sarn Badrig) runs 12M SW from Mochras Pt. It is mostly large loose stones, and dries (up to 1·5m) for much of its length. In strong winds the sea breaks heavily at all states of tide. The outer end is marked by a WCM lt buoy. At the inner end there is a chan about 5ca offshore, which can be taken with care at half tide.

Sarn-y-Bwch runs 4M WSW from Pen Bwch Pt. It is composed of rky boulders, drying in places close inshore and with least depth 0·3m over 1M offshore. There is a WCM buoy off W end. NW of Aberystwyth (10.11.12), Sarn Cynfelyn and Cynfelyn Patches extend a total of 6·5M offshore, with depths of 1·5m in places. A WCM buoy is at the outer end. Almost halfway along the bank is Main Channel, 3ca wide, running roughly N/S, but not marked.

A military firing area occupies much of Cardigan B. Beware targets and buoys, some unlit. Range activity is broadcast on VHF Ch 16, 0800-1600LT Mon-Fri or ☎ (01239) 813219.

If on passage N/S through St George's Chan (i.e. not bound for Cardigan B or Milford Haven) the easiest route, and always by night, is W of the Bishops and the Smalls, but note the TSS, see Fig 10 (3). If bound to/from Milford Haven or Cardigan B, passage inside both the Smalls and Grassholm is possible.

RAMSEY SOUND AND THE BISHOPS (chart 1482)

The Bishops and the Clerks are islets and rks 2·5M W and NW of Ramsey Is, a bird sanctuary SSW of St David's Hd. N Bishop is the N'ly of the group, 3ca ENE of which is Bell Rk (depth 1·9m). S Bishop (Lt, fog sig, RC) is 3M to the SSW.

Between S Bishop and Ramsey Is the dangers include Daufraich with offliers to the E and heavy overfalls; Llech Isaf and Llech Uchaf drying rks are further ENE. Carreg Rhoson and offliers are between Daufraich and N Bishop. There are navigable routes between most of these islets and rocks, but only by day in good vis and with local knowledge. The N/S route close W of Ramsey Island is said to be easier than Ramsey Sound (see below).

2M W of The Bishops the S-going stream begins at HW Milford Haven + 0400, and the N-going at HW Milford Haven − 0225, sp rates 2kn. Between The Bishops and Ramsey Is the SW-going stream begins at HW Milford Haven + 0330, and the NE-going at HW Milford Haven − 0255, sp rates 5kn.

Ramsey Sound should be taken at slack water. The S-going stream begins at HW Milford Haven + 0300, and the N-going at HW Milford Haven − 0325, sp rates 6kn at The Bitches, where chan is narrowest (2ca), decreasing N and S. The Bitches are rks extending 2ca from E side of Ramsey Is. Other dangers are: Gwahan and Carreg-gafeiliog, at N end of Sound, to W and E; Horse Rk (dries 0·9m) almost in mid-chan about 5ca NNE of The Bitches, with associated overfalls; Shoe Rk (dries 3m) at SE end of chan; and rks extending 5ca SSE from S end of Ramsey Is.

THE SMALLS TO MILFORD HAVEN (chart 1478)

St Brides B (10.11.13) provides anch in settled weather or offshore winds, but is a trap in westerlies. Solva is a little hbr with shelter for boats able to take the ground, or anch behind Black Rk (dries 3·6m) in the middle of the entrance.

The Smalls Lt, where there is a Historic Wreck (see 10.0.3g) is 13M W of the Welsh mainland (Wooltack Pt). 2M and 4M E of The Smalls are the Hats and Barrels, rky patches on which the sea breaks. 7M E of The Smalls is Grassholm Island with a race either end and strong tidal eddies so that it is advisable to pass about 1M off. The chan between Barrels and Grassholm is 2·5M wide, and here the S-going stream begins at HW Milford Haven + 0440, and the N-going at HW Milford Haven − 0135, sp rates 5kn. 5M of clear water lie between Grassholm and Skomer Is/Skokholm Is to the E. But Wildgoose Race, which forms W of Skomer and Skokholm is very dangerous, so keep 2M W of these two Islands.

To E of Skomer is Midland Is, and between here and Wooltack Pt is Jack Sound which is only 2ca wide and should not be attempted without chart 1482, detailed pilotage directions, and only at slack water nps; it is a testing passage. Dangers which must be identified include: The Crab Stoncs, E from Midland Is; The Cable, a drying rk on E side of chan; Tusker Rk, steep-to on its W side, off Wooltack Pt; the Black Stones; and The Anvil and other rks off Anvil Pt. In Jack Sound the S-going stream begins at HW Milford Haven + 0200, and the N-going at HW Milford Haven − 0425, sp rates 6kn.

MILFORD HAVEN TO MUMBLES HD (charts 1179, 1076)

Milford Haven (10.11.14) is a long natural, all-weather hbr with marinas beyond the oil terminals. 3M S of the ent, beware Turbot Bank (WCM lt buoy). Crow Rk (dries 5·5m) is 5ca SSE of Linney Hd, and The Toes are dangerous submerged rks close W and SE of Crow Rk. There is a passage inshore of these dangers. There are overfalls on St Gowan Shoals which extend 4M SW of St Govan's Hd, and the sea breaks on the shallow patches in bad weather. For firing areas from Linney Hd to Carmarthen Bay, see 10.11.14.

Caldey Is (Lt) lies S of Tenby (10.11.15). Off its NW pt is St Margaret's Is connected by a rky reef. Caldey Sound, between St Margaret's Is and Giltar Pt (chart 1482), is buoyed, but beware Eel Spit near W end of Caldey Is where there can be a nasty sea with wind against tide, and Woolhouse Rks (dry 3·6m) 1ca NE of Caldey Is. Saundersfoot hbr (dries) is 2M N of Tenby, with anch well sheltered from N and W but subject to swell. Streams are weak here. Carmarthen Bay has no offshore dangers for yachts, other than the extensive drying sands at head of B and on its E side off Burry Inlet (10.11.16).

S of Worms Head, Helwick Sands (buoyed at each end) extend 7M W from Port Eynon Pt; least depth of 1·3m is near their W end. Stream sets NE/SW across the sands. There is a narrow chan inshore, close to Port Eynon Pt. Between here and Mumbles Hd the stream runs roughly along coast, sp rates 3kn off Pts, but there are eddies in Port Eynon B and Oxwich B (both yacht anchs), and overfalls SSE of Oxwich Pt.

MUMBLES HEAD TO CARDIFF (charts 1165, 1182)

Off Mumbles Hd (Lt, fog sig) beware Mixon Shoal (dries 0·3m), marked by PHM buoy. In good conditions pass N of shoal, 1ca off Mumbles Hd. Anch N of Mumbles Hd, good holding but exposed to swell. At W side of Swansea Bay, Green Grounds, rky shoals, lie in appr's to Swansea (10.11.17).

Scarweather Sands, much of which dry (up to 3·3m) and where sea breaks heavily, extend 7M W from Porthcawl (10.11.17) and are well buoyed (chart 1161). There is a chan between the sands and coast to E, but beware Hugo Bank (dries 2·6m) and Kenfig Patches (0·5m) with overfalls up to 7ca offshore between Sker Pt and Porthcawl.

Nash Sands extend 7·5M WNW from Nash Pt. Depths vary and are least at inshore end (dries 3m), but Nash Passage, 1ca wide, runs close inshore between E Nash ECM buoy and rky ledge off Nash Pt. On E-going stream there are heavy overfalls off Nash Pt and at W end of Nash Sands. Between Nash Pt and Breaksea Pt the E-going stream begins at HW Avonmouth + 0535, and the W-going at HW Avonmouth – 0035, sp rates 3kn. Off Breaksea Pt there may be overfalls.

From Rhoose Pt to Lavernock Pt the coast is fringed with foul ground. Lavernock Spit extends 1·75M S of Lavernock Pt, and E of the spit is main chan to Cardiff (10.11.19); the other side of the chan being Cardiff Grounds, a bank drying 5·4m which lies parallel with the shore and about 1·5M from it.

SEVERN ESTUARY (charts 1176, 1166)

Near the centre of Bristol Chan, either side of the buoyed fairway are the islands of Flat Holm (Lt, fog sig) and Steep Holm. 7M SW of Flat Holm lies Culver Sand (0·9m), 3M in length, with W & ECM bys. Monkstone Rk (Lt, dries) is 2M NW of the buoyed chan to Avonmouth and Bristol (10.11.21). Extensive drying banks cover the N shore of the estuary, beyond Newport and the Severn bridges (chart 1176).

The range of tide in the Bristol Chan is exceptionally large, 12·2m sp and 6·0m np, and tidal streams are very powerful, particularly above Avonmouth. Between Flat Holm and Steep Holm the E-going stream begins at HW Avonmouth – 0610, sp 3kn, and the W-going at HW Avonmouth + 0015, sp 4kn.

The ent to the R. Avon is just to the S of Avonmouth S Pier Hd. Bristol City Docks lie some 6M up river. Approach the ent via King Road and the Newcombe and Cockburn Lt Bys and thence via the Swash chan into the Avon. The ent dries at LW but the river is navigable at about half tide. Tidal streams are strong in the approaches to Avonmouth, up to 5kn at sp. The tide is also strong in the R. Avon which is best entered no earlier than HW Avonmouth – 0200.

From Avonmouth it is 16M to Sharpness which yachts should aim to reach at about HW Avonmouth. Tidal streams can reach 8kn at The Shoots, and 6kn at the Severn bridges at sp. At the Shoots the flood begins at HW Avonmouth –0430 and the ebb at HW Avonmouth + 0045. The Severn Bore can usually be seen if Avonmouth range is 13·5m or more.

AVONMOUTH TO HARTLAND POINT (AC 1152, 1165)

From Avonmouth to Sand Pt, the part-drying English Grounds extend 3M off the S shore. Extensive mud flats fill the bays S to Burnham-on-Sea (10.11.22). Westward, the S shore of Bristol Chan is cleaner than N shore. But there is less shelter since hbrs such as Watchet (marina planned), Minehead, Porlock Weir and Watermouth dry out, see 10.11.22. In bad weather dangerous overfalls occur NW and NE of Foreland Pt. 5M to W there is a race off Highveer Pt. Between Ilfracombe (10.11.23) and Bull Pt the E-going stream begins at HW Milford Haven + 0540, and the W-going at HW Milford Haven – 0025, sp rates 3kn. Overfalls occur up to 1·5M N of Bull Pt and over Horseshoe Rks, which lie 3M N. There is a dangerous race off Morte Pt, 1·5M to W of Bull Pt.

Shelter is available under lee of Lundy Is (10.11.23); but avoid bad races to NE (White Horses), the NW (Hen and Chickens), and to SE; also overfalls over NW Bank. W of Lundy streams are moderate, but strong around the Is and much stronger towards Bristol Chan proper.

Proceeding WSW from Rivers Taw/Torridge (10.11.24), keep 3M off to avoid the race N of Hartland Pt (Lt, fog sig). There is shelter off Clovelly in S/SW winds.

HARTLAND POINT TO LAND'S END (charts 1156, 1149)

The N coast of Cornwall and SW approaches to Bristol Chan are very exposed. Yachts need to be sturdy and well equipped, since if bad weather develops no shelter may be at hand. Bude (10.11.25) dries, and is not approachable in W winds; only accessible in calm weather or offshore winds. Boscastle is a tiny hbr (dries) 3M NE of Tintagel Hd. Only approach in good weather or offshore winds; anch off or dry out alongside.

Padstow is a refuge, but in strong NW winds the sea breaks on bar and prevents entry. Off Trevose Hd (Lt) beware Quies Rks which extend 1M to W. From here S the coast is relatively clear to Godrevy Is, apart from Bawden Rks 1M N of St Agnes Hd. Newquay B (10.11.25) is good anch in offshore winds, and the hbr (dries) is sheltered but uncomfortable in N winds. Off Godrevy Is (Lt) are The Stones, drying rky shoals extending 1·5M offshore and marked by NCM lt buoy.

In St Ives Bay (chart 1168), Hayle (10.11.25) is a commercial port (dries); seas break heavily on bar at times, especially with a ground swell. Stream is strong, so enter just before HW. The bottom is mostly sand. St Ives (10.11.25) gives shelter from winds E to SW, but is very exposed to N; there is sometimes a heavy breaking sea if there is ground swell.

From St Ives to Land's End coast is rugged and exposed. There are overfalls SW of Pendeen Pt (Lt, fog sig). Vyneck Rks lie awash about 3ca NW of C Cornwall. The Brisons are two high rky islets 5ca SW of C Cornwall, with rky ledges inshore and to the S. The Longships (Lt, fog sig) group of rks is about 1M W of Land's End. The inshore passage (001° on Brisons) is about 4ca wide with unmarked drying rks on the W side; only to be considered in calm weather.

For Isles of Scilly and South Cornwall, see 10.1.5.

10.11.6   DISTANCE TABLE

Approximate distances in nautical miles are by the most direct route, whilst avoiding dangers and allowing for Traffic Separation Schemes. Places in *italics* are in adjoining areas; places in **bold** are in 10.0.7, Distances across the Irish Sea.

1.	*Bardsey Island*	1																		
2.	Abersoch	14	2																	
3.	**Pwllheli**	18	5	3																
4.	Barmouth	27	18	18	4															
5.	Aberdovey	31	26	25	14	5														
6.	Aberystwyth	33	30	30	20	10	6													
7.	**Fishguard**	45	54	58	56	47	40	7												
8.	South Bishop	60	70	74	74	67	61	25	8											
9.	**Milford Haven**	83	93	97	97	90	84	48	23	9										
10.	Tenby	106	116	120	120	113	107	71	46	28	10									
11.	**Swansea**	129	139	143	143	136	130	94	69	55	36	11								
12.	Barry	151	161	165	165	158	152	116	91	77	57	37	12							
13.	Cardiff	160	170	174	174	167	161	125	100	86	66	46	9	13						
14.	Sharpness	191	201	205	205	198	192	156	131	117	106	75	39	33	14					
15.	**Avonmouth**	174	184	188	188	181	175	139	114	100	89	58	22	20	18	15				
16.	Burnham-on-Sea	168	178	182	182	175	169	133	108	94	70	48	18	53	50	33	16			
17.	**Ilfracombe**	127	137	141	141	134	128	92	67	53	35	25	35	44	74	57	45	17		
18.	Lundy Island	110	120	124	124	117	111	75	50	38	30	37	54	63	95	78	66	22	18	
19.	**Padstow**	141	151	155	155	148	142	106	81	70	70	76	88	97	127	110	98	55	39	19
20.	*Longships*	168	178	182	182	175	169	133	108	105	110	120	130	139	169	152	140	95	82	50	20

ABERSOCH   10-11-7

Gwynedd 52°49'·29N 04°29'·20W (Visitors' Buoy)

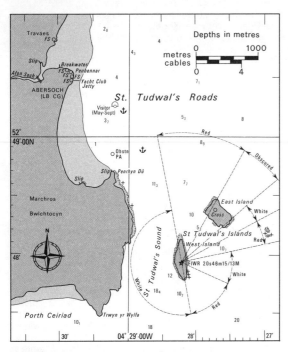

CHARTS

AC 1512, 1971, *1410*; Imray C61; OS 123

TIDES

−0315 Dover; ML 2·5; Duration 0520; Zone 0 (UT)

Standard Port MILFORD HAVEN (→)

Times				Height (metres)			
High Water		Low Water		MHWS	MHWN	MLWN	MLWS
0100	0800	0100	0700	7·0	5·2	2·5	0·7
1300	2000	1300	1900				
Differences ST TUDWAL'S ROADS							
+0155	+0145	+0240	+0310	−2·2	−1·9	−0·7	−0·2
ABERDARON							
+0210	+0200	+0240	+0310	−2·4	−1·9	−0·6	−0·2

SHELTER

There are few moorings for visitors. Apply to Hr Mr or SC. ⌕ in St Tudwal's Roads clear of moored yachts; sheltered from SSE through S to NE.

NAVIGATION

WPT 52°48'·50N 04°26'·06W, 113°/293° from/to YC jetty, 2·4M. There are no navigational dangers, but steer well clear of the drying rks to the E of East Island; a PHM buoy is 2ca E of these rks (just off chartlet). St Tudwal's islands themselves are fairly steep-to, except at N ends. St Tudwal's Sound is clear of dangers.

LIGHTS AND MARKS

The only lt is on St Tudwal's West Island (see chartlet).

RADIO TELEPHONE

S Caernarfon YC Ch **80** M.

TELEPHONE (01758)

Hr Mr 812684; MRSC (01407) 762051; ✠ (01407) 762714; Marinecall 0891 500 460; Police 2022; Dr 612535.

FACILITIES

S. Caernarvonshire YC ☎ 812338, Slip, M, L, FW, R, Bar (May-Sept), D; **Abersoch Power Boat Club** ☎ 812027. **Services:** BY, Slip, ME, El, Sh, ACA, CH, P, C (12 ton).
Town EC Wed; CH, V, R, Bar, ✉, Ⓑ, ≥ (Pwllheli), ✈ (Chester).

PWLLHELI   10-11-8

Gwynedd 52°53'·21N 04°23'·68W

CHARTS

AC 1512, 1971, *1410*; Imray C61; OS 123

TIDES

−0300 Dover; ML 2·6; Duration 0510; Zone 0 (UT)

Standard Port MILFORD HAVEN (→)

Times				Height (metres)			
High Water		Low Water		MHWS	MHWN	MLWN	MLWS
0100	0800	0100	0700	7·0	5·2	2·5	0·7
1300	2000	1300	1900				
Differences PWLLHELI							
+0210	+0150	+0245	+0320	−2·0	−1·8	−0·6	−0·2
CRICCIETH							
+0210	+0155	+0255	+0320	−2·0	−1·8	−0·7	−0·3

SHELTER

Good in hbr and marina. Pile berths on S side of chan, but visitors must report to marina. No ⌕ in hbr; 4kn speed limit. Drying moorings in inner hbr (SW and NW bights).

NAVIGATION

WPT 52°53'·00N 04°23'·00W, SWM lt buoy, Iso 2s, 119°/299° from/to QG lt at head of Training Arm, 0·47M. Ent is safe in most winds, but in strong E to SW winds sea breaks on offshore shoals. Bar and hbr chan are dredged to at least 1·0m; 3 tide gauges. Max tidal stream 2kn.

LIGHTS AND MARKS

No ldg lts/marks, but ent chan well marked (see chartlet). Gimblet Rk (30m) is conspic conical rk 3ca SW of ent.

RADIO TELEPHONE

VHF Ch 16 (occas). Ch **80** M H24.

TELEPHONE (01758)

Hr Mr 701219; MRSC (01407) 762051; CG 701589; ✠ (01407) 762714; Marinecall 0891 500 460; Police 701177; Dr 612535.

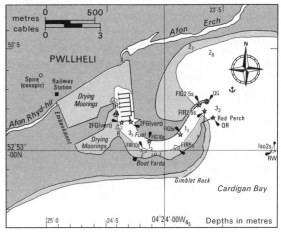

FACILITIES

Marina (400) ☎ 701219, Fax 701443, £9.67, FW, P, D, AC, BH (40 ton), C, Slip, ▣; **Marina Club** ☎ 612271, Slip, FW; **Hbr Authority** Slip, M, L, FW, AB; **S Caernarvonshire YC** ☎ 812338; **Pwllheli SC** ☎ 612219; **Services:** BY, Slip, L, FW, ME, Gas, Sh, CH, ACA, D, C (14 ton), El, Ⓔ, SM.
Town EC Thurs; V, R, Bar, ✉, Ⓑ, ≥, ✈ (Chester).

ADJACENT HARBOUR

MOCHRAS, Gwynedd, 52°49'·55N 04°07'·70W. AC 1512, 1971. HW −0245 on Dover. Small yacht hbr on SE side of Shell Is. Mochras lagoon dries. Bar, about 2ca seaward. Entry advised HW±2. Tide runs strongly in the narrows on the ebb; at sp beware severe eddies inside ent. Ent between Shell Is (lt Fl WRG 4s; G079°-124°, W124°-134°, R134°-179°; shown mid Mar-Nov) and sea wall. 3 grey posts, R topmarks, mark N side of chan. Shifting chan, marked by posts & buoys, runs NE to Pensarn, where permanent moorings limit space. To S, buoyed chan runs to Shell Is Yacht Hbr ☎ (0134123) 453 with facilities: M, FW, Slip, R, Bar, shwrs. Pensarn: drying AB, ≥.

PORTHMADOG   10·11·9

Gwynedd   52°55'·30N 04°07'·70W

CHARTS ·
AC 1512, 1971, *1410*; Imray C61; OS 124

TIDES
−0232 Dover; ML no data; Duration 0455; Zone 0 (UT)

Standard Port MILFORD HAVEN (→)

Times				Height (metres)			
High Water		Low Water		MHWS	MHWN	MLWN	MLWS
0100	0800	0100	0700	7·0	5·2	2·5	0·7
1300	2000	1300	1900				
Differences PORTHMADOG							
+0235	+0210	No data		−1·9	−1·8		No data

SHELTER
Inner hbr (N of Cei Ballast): Good all year round; visitors' drying AB adjacent Madoc YC or afloat rafted on moored yachts off YC. (Greaves Wharf is obstructed by dinghies and salmon nets). Outer hbr: Summer only and exposed to S winds. Speed limit 6kn in hbr upstream of No. 11 buoy.

NAVIGATION
WPT Fairway SWM buoy, 52°52'·87N 04°11'·02W, approx 2M SW of conspic white Ho at W side of ent (chan shifts and may divide). Bar changes frequently, but is close to No 3 and 4 buoys; dries approx 0·3m. Latest info from Hr Mr on request. Advise entering HW±1½. In SW'ly winds, waves are steep-sided and close, especially on the ebb.

LIGHTS AND MARKS
Fairway buoy RW, L Fl 10s. Chan marker buoys (16) have R/G reflective top marks and numbers in W reflective tape. Moel-y-Gest is conspic hill (259m) approx 1M WNW of hbr. Harlech Castle (ru) is about 3M SE of appr chan.

RADIO TELEPHONE
Hr Mr Ch 14 12 16 (0900-1715 and when vessel due). Madoc YC: Ch **80** M 16.

TELEPHONE (01766)
Hr Mr 512927, mobile (0374) 631844; MRSC (01407) 762051; Pilot 514939, Home 75684; Hbr Authority Dwyfor District Council (01758) 613131; ⌗ (01407) 762714; Marinecall 0891 500 460; Police 512226; Dr 512239.

FACILITIES
Hbr (265 berths) ☎ 512927, £4.35, D, FW, C, Slip; **Madoc YC** ☎ 512976, AB, M, FW, Bar; **Porthmadog and Transfynydd SC** ☎ 513546, AB, M, FW, Slip; **Services:** CH, ACA, Sh, D, P (45 gall drums), C (3½ ton), M, BY, El, Pilot.
Town EC Wed; ⌧, Ⓑ, ⇌, ✈ (Chester).

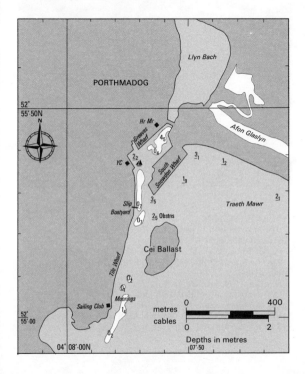

BARMOUTH   10·11·10

Gwynedd   52°42'·95N 04°03'·00W

CHARTS
AC 1484, 1971, *1410*; Imray C61; OS 124

TIDES
−0250 Dover; ML 2·6; Duration 0515; Zone 0 (UT)

Standard Port MILFORD HAVEN (→)

Times				Height (metres)			
High Water		Low Water		MHWS	MHWN	MLWN	MLWS
0100	0800	0100	0700	7·0	5·2	2·5	0·7
1300	2000	1300	1900				
Differences BARMOUTH							
+0215	+0205	+0310	+0320	−2·0	−1·7	−0·7	0·0

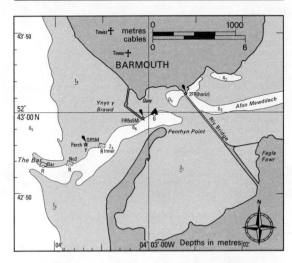

SHELTER
Good. Entry HW±2½ safe, but impossible with strong SW winds. Exposed ⚓ W of Barmouth Outer buoy in 6 to 10m. In hbr there are 3 ⚓s; secure as directed by Hr Mr, because of submarine cables and strong tidal streams. A quay, drying at half-tide, fronts the town. The estuary and river (Afon Mawddach) are tidal and can be navigated for about 7M above railway bridge (clearance approx 5·5m); but chan is not buoyed, and sandbanks move constantly - local knowledge essential.

NAVIGATION
WPT, Barmouth Outer SWM buoy, L Fl 10s, 52°42'·90N 04°04'·90W, 277°/097° from/to Y perch lt, QR, 0·75M. Appr from SW between St Patrick's Causeway (Sarn Badrig) and Sarn-y-Bwch (see 10·11·5). Barmouth can be identified by Cader Idris, a mountain 890m high, 5M ESE. Fegla Fawr, a rounded hill, lies on S side of hbr. The Bar, 0·75M W of Penrhyn Pt, with min depth 0·3m is subject to considerable change. Chan marked by 3 unlit PHM Bys, moved as necessary. Spring ebb runs 3 - 5kn. Note: A Historic Wreck (see 10.0.3g) is at 52°46'·73N 04°07'·53W, 4·5M NNW of Barmouth Outer SWM buoy.

LIGHTS AND MARKS
Y perch, QR 4m 5M, marks S end of stony ledge extending 3ca SW from Ynys y Brawd across N Bank. Ynys y Brawd groyne, SE end, marked by bn with lt, Fl R 5s 5M. NW end of rly bridge 2 FR (hor).

RADIO TELEPHONE
Call *Barmouth Hbr* VHF Ch **12** 16 (Apl-Sept 0900-2200LT; Oct-Mar 0900-1600LT); wind and sea state are available.

TELEPHONE (01341)
Hr Mr 280671; MRSC (01407) 762051; ⌗ (01407) 762714; Marinecall 0891 500460; Police 280222; Dr 280521.

FACILITIES
Quay £6.50, M (contact Hr Mr in advance if deep water ⚓ required), D, FW, El, AC, Slip; **Merioneth YC** ☎ 280000; **Services:** CH, ACA.
Town EC Wed; P, D, V, R, Bar, ⌧, Ⓑ, ⇌, ✈ (Chester), Ferry across to Penrhyn Pt.

11

ABERDOVEY   10-11-11

Gwynedd 52°32'·55N 04°02'·65W (Jetty)

CHARTS
AC 1484, 1972, *1410*; Imray C61; OS 135

TIDES
–0320 Dover; ML 2·6; Duration 0535; Zone 0 (UT)

Standard Port MILFORD HAVEN (→)

Times				Height (metres)			
High Water		Low Water		MHWS	MHWN	MLWN	MLWS
0100	0800	0100	0700	7·0	5·2	2·5	0·7
1300	2000	1300	1900				
Differences ABERDOVEY							
+0215	+0200	+0230	+0305	–2·0	–1·7	–0·5	0·0

SHELTER
Good except in strong W/SW winds. Berth on jetty; to the E there is heavy silting .

NAVIGATION
WPT Aberdovey Outer SWM buoy, 52°31'·75N 04°06'·22W, 250°/070° from/to jetty, 2·3M (chan shifts). Bar is hazardous below half-tide and constantly shifts. Visitors should ☎ the Pilot or call Hr Mr on VHF before entering. Submarine cables (prohib ⚓s) marked by bns with R ◊ top marks.

LIGHTS AND MARKS
No daymarks. 3 SHM buoys (Bar QG 5s, S Spit QG 10s and Inner, unlit) lead via dogleg chan to jetty.

RADIO TELEPHONE
Call *Aberdovey Hbr* VHF Ch 12 16.

TELEPHONE (01654)
Hr Mr 767626; MRSC (01646) 690909; Pilot 767247; ⌗ (01407) 762714 Ext 262; Marinecall 0891 500 460; Police 767222; Dr 710414; Ⓗ 710411.

FACILITIES
Jetty AB £6.50, M, FW; **Wharf** Slip, AB, L, FW, C;
Dovey YC ☎ (01827) 286514, Bar, Slip, L, FW;
Services: BY, ME, El, Sh, CH, ACA, Ⓔ.
Town EC Wed (winter only); P & D (cans), ME, El, CH, V, R, Bar, ✉, Ⓑ, ⇌, ✈ (Chester).

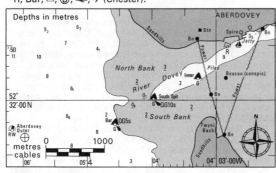

OTHER HARBOURS IN SOUTH CARDIGAN BAY

ABERAERON, Dyfed, 52°14'·60N 04°15'·87W. AC 1484, 1972, *1410*. HW –0325 on Dover; +0140 and –1·9m on Milford Haven; ML 2·7m; Duration 0540. A small, but popular drying hbr at the mouth of the R Aeron; access HW±1½. Short drying piers extend each side of river ent. In strong NW'lies there is little shelter. AB £2.50 on NW wall. Foul ground with depths of 1·5m extend 3ca offshore to SW of Aberaeron. Beware Carreg Gloyn (0·3m) 4ca WSW of hbr, and Sarn Cadwgan (1·8m) extending ½M offshore from Cadwgan Pt to NE. Lts: N pier Fl (4) WRG 15s 6M, G050°-104°, W104°-178°, R178°-232°. S pier Fl (3) G 10s 7m 6M, vis 050°-243°. VHF 12 80. Hr Mr ☎ (01545) 571645; **YC** ☎ 570077.

NEW QUAY, Dyfed, 52°12'·90N 04°21'·15W. AC 1484, 1972, *1410*. HW –0335 on Dover; Duration 0540; see 10.11.12. The bay is sheltered in offshore winds, but in NW'lies is untenable. On E side of bay Carreg Ina, rks drying 1·3m, are marked by NCM buoy. 2 Y bns indicate a sewer outfall extending 7ca NNW from Ina Pt. The hbr (dries 1·6m) is protected by a pier with lt, Fl WG 3s 12m 8/5M; W135°-252°, G252°-295°. Groyne extends 50m SSE of pierhd to a SHM bn; close ENE of which is a ECM bn, Q (3) 10s. There are ⚓s 1ca E of pier; £2.50. VHF Ch 12 16 80. Hr Mr ☎ (01545) 560368. CG ☎ 560212; Dr ☎ 560203; YC ☎ 560516; Facilities: D (from fishermen). **Town** FW, P (3M), ✉, R, Bar.

ABERYSTWYTH   10-11-12

Dyfed 52°24'·40N 04°05'·40W

CHARTS
AC 1484, 1972, *1410*; Imray C61; OS 135

TIDES
–0330 Dover; ML 2·7; Duration 0540; Zone 0 (UT)

Standard Port MILFORD HAVEN (→)

Times				Height (metres)			
High Water		Low Water		MHWS	MHWN	MLWN	MLWS
0100	0800	0100	0700	7·0	5·2	2·5	0·7
1300	2000	1300	1900				
Differences ABERYSTWYTH							
+0145	+0130	+0210	+0245	–2·0	–1·7	–0·7	0·0
NEW QUAY							
+0150	+0125	+0155	+0230	–2·1	–1·8	–0·6	–0·1
ABERPORTH							
+0135	+0120	+0150	+0220	–2·1	–1·8	–0·6	–0·1

SHELTER
Good in marina on E side of chan, dredged 1·6m. Access approx HW –4 to +5 for 1m draft in calm conditions.

NAVIGATION
WPT 52°24'·80N 04°06'·00W, 318°/138° from/to ent, 0·6M. Approach dangerous in strong on-shore winds. From N, beware Castle Rks and shoal NW of ent. The Bar, close off S pier hd, carries 0·7m MLWS. Beware cross-tides and boulders around S Pier hd. Turn 90° port in narrow ent.

LIGHTS AND MARKS
Hbr located by Wellington Monument on top of Pendinas, conspic hill 124m high, 0·5M SE of ent. N bkwtr head on with monument leads 140°, to S of Cas Rks. Ldg lts 138°, both FR on Ystwyth Bridge; white daymarks. N jetty QWR 9m 2M, R141°-175° covers Castle Rks. S jetty Fl (2) WG 10s 12m 10M. 4 FR (vert) on radio twr, 2·8M to S.

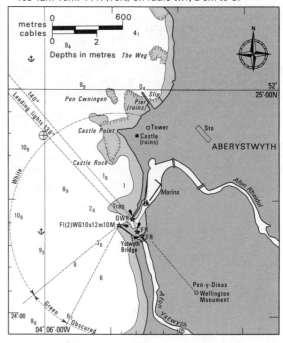

RADIO TELEPHONE
VHF (portable) Ch 16 14 (for hbr control only).

TELEPHONE (01970)
Hr Mr 611433; MRSC (01646) 690909; ⌗ (01646) 685807; Marinecall 0891 500460; Police 612791; Dr 4855.

FACILITIES
Marina, (104, inc 12+ visitors), FW, D, Slip, ▣, C (max 15 ton by arrangement); **Town Quay** AB £3.50;
YC ☎ 612907, Slip, M, L, FW, Bar;
Services: El, CH, D, Ⓔ, ME, Sh, M, Slip, C (25 ton), Gas.
Town P & D (cans), CH, V, R, Bar, ✉, Ⓑ, ⇌, ✈ (Swansea).

FISHGUARD   10-11-13

Dyfed   52°00'·10N 04°58'·33W (Lower Hbr)

CHARTS
AC 1484, 1973, *1410, 1178*; Imray C61/60; OS 157

TIDES
–0347 Dover; ML 2·6; Duration 0550; Zone 0 (UT)

Standard Port MILFORD HAVEN (→)

Times				Height (metres)			
High Water		Low Water		MHWS	MHWN	MLWN	MLWS
0100	0800	0100	0700	7·0	5·2	2·5	0·7
1300	2000	1300	1900				
Differences FISHGUARD							
+0115	+0100	+0110	+0135	–2·2	–1·8	–0·5	+0·1
PORT CARDIGAN							
+0140	+0120	+0220	+0130	–2·3	–1·8	–0·5	0·0
CARDIGAN (Town)							
+0220	+0150	No data		–2·2	–1·6	No data	
PORTHGAIN							
+0055	+0045	+0045	+0100	–2·5	–1·8	–0·6	0·0
RAMSEY SOUND							
+0030	+0030	+0030	+0030	–1·9	–1·3	–0·3	0·0
SOLVA							
+0015	+0010	+0035	+0015	–1·5	–1·0	–0·2	0·0
LITTLE HAVEN							
+0010	+0010	+0025	+0015	–1·1	–0·8	–0·2	0·0
MARTIN'S HAVEN							
+0010	+0010	+0015	+0015	–0·8	–0·5	+0·1	+0·1

SHELTER
Good, except in strong NW/NE winds. Access H24 to upper (commercial) hbr with only 2 Ⓥ berths; no ⚓, except SW of ferry terminal. Lower hbr at Abergwaun dries; access HW±1, limited AB. Good holding in most of the bay; ⚓ off Saddle Pt in 2m or as shown. Strong S'lies funnel down the hbr.

NAVIGATION
WPT 52°01'·00N 04°57'·50W, 057°/237° from/to N bkwtr lt, 0·48m. Beware large swell, especially in N winds. Keep clear of ferries manoeuvring.

LIGHTS AND MARKS
Strumble Hd Lt, Fl (4) 15s 45m 26M, is approx 4M WNW of hbr. N bkwtr Fl G 4·5s 18m 13M, Bell 8s. E bkwtr Fl R 3s 10m 5M. Ldg lts 282° (to ferry berths), both FG; W ◊ on masts.

RADIO TELEPHONE
Hr Mr Ch 14 16. Goodwick Marine Ch M (occas).

TELEPHONE (01348)
Commercial Hbr Supervisor 872881; Hr Mr (Lower hbr) 874616/873231; MRSC (01646) 690909; ⌗ (01646) 685807; Marinecall 0891 500 460; Police 873073; Dr 872802.

FACILITIES
Lower Hbr, M (free o'night) via Hr Mr; **Fishguard Bay YC** ☎ 872866, FW, Bar; **Services**: BY, D (cans), Sh, ME, ACA, Slip, CH, El, Gas. **Town** EC Wed; P & D (cans), V, R, Gas, Bar, ✉, ⬚, Ⓑ, ⇌, ✈ (Cardiff), Ferry–Rosslare.

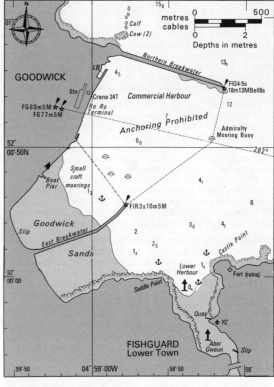

ADJACENT HARBOUR

CARDIGAN, Dyfed, 52°07'·00N 04°42'·00W. AC 1484, 1973. HW –0350 on Dover; ML 2·4m; Duration 0550; See above. Shelter is good, but ent dangerous in strong N/NW winds. Large scale chart (1484) and local advice essential. Bar has 0·3m or less; breakers form esp on sp ebb. ⚓ near Hotel (conspic) on E side of ent by 2 FR (vert). Chan is close to E side; IDM bn, Fl (2) 5s, should be left to stbd. From Pen-yr-Ergyd to Bryn-Du chan is unmarked and shifts constantly. ⚓ in pools off Pen-yr-Ergyd or near St Dogmaels. Possible ⚓s off Teifi Boating Club. Hr Mr ☎ as Aberaeron or New Quay. Facilities: **Moorings**: at Gwbert (drying) ☎ (01239) 612832, at Netpool (afloat) ☎ 612166; **Teifi BC** Hon Sec ☎ 612361 FW, Bar; **Services**: ME, Sh. **Town** EC Wed; Ⓑ, V, CH, P, D, FW, ME, Bar, R, ⇌.

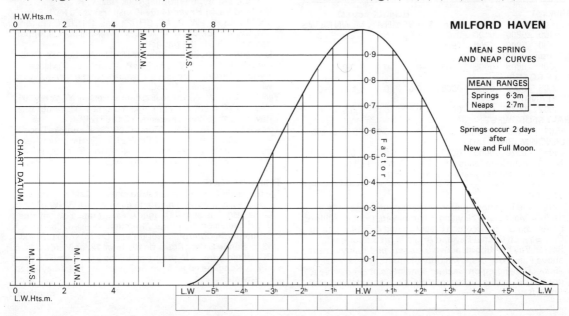

MILFORD HAVEN

MEAN SPRING AND NEAP CURVES

MEAN RANGES	
Springs	6·3m
Neaps	2·7m

Springs occur 2 days after New and Full Moon.

ADJACENT HARBOURS IN ST BRIDES BAY

SOLVA, Dyfed, 51°52′00N 05°11′·60W. AC *1478*. HW −0450 on Dover; ML 3·2m; Duration 0555. See 10.11.13. Good shelter for small boats that can take the ground; access HW±3. Avoid in strong S winds. Black Scar, Green Scar and The Mare are rks 5ca S. Ent via SSE side; best water near Black Rk in centre of ent. Beware stone spit at Trwyn Caws on W just inside ent. There are 9 R ♉s and some drying moorings available; or ⚓ behind the rk in approx 3m. Small craft can go up to the quay. Facilities limited; stores in village. FW on quay. Hr Mr (01437) 720153, M, CH. **Solva Boat Owners Assn ☎** 721489.

ST BRIDES BAY, Dyfed, 51°49′00N 05°10′·00W. AC *1478*. HW (Little Haven) −0450 on Dover; ML 3·2m; Duration 0555. See 10.11.13. Keep at least 100m off coastline 1/9-28/2 to avoid disturbing seals, and ditto nesting sea birds 1/3-31/7. Many good ⚓s, especially from Little Haven to Borough Head in S or E winds or between Solva and Dinas Fawr in N or E winds; but in W'lies boats should shelter in Solva (above), Skomer (below) or Pendinas Bach. For apprs from the N or S see 10·11·5. In the middle of the bay keep clear of Oceanographic Research Area (approx 51°51′·00N 05°09′·00W), marked by buoys. Facilities: (Little Haven) CH, V, R, Bar, FW (cans).

SKOMER, Dyfed, 51°44′·40N 05°16′·70W. AC 2878, *1478*. HW −0455 Dover. See 10.11.14. The island is a National Nature Reserve (fee payable to Warden on landing) and also a Marine Nature Reserve, extending to Marloes Peninsula. Keep at least 100m offshore 1/9-28/2 to avoid disturbing seals and ditto nesting sea birds 1/3-31/7. There is a 5kn speed limit within 100m of the island. ⚓ in N or S Haven. Enter N Haven close to W shore, and land on W side of bay on beach or at steps. In N Haven pick up ♉s provided or ⚓ to seaward of them. No access to the island from S Haven. For Jack Sound see 10·11·5. There are no lts, marks or facilities. For info, Marine Conservation Officer ☎ (01646) 636736.

MILFORD HAVEN   10-11-14

Dyfed 51°40′·10N 05°08′·10W

CHARTS
AC 3274, 3275, *2878, 1478, 1178, 1410*; Imray C60; OS 157

TIDES
−0454 Dover; ML 3·8; Duration 0605; Zone 0 (UT)

Standard Port MILFORD HAVEN (⟶)

Times				Height (metres)			
High Water		Low Water		MHWS	MHWN	MLWN	MLWS
0100	0800	0100	0700	7·0	5·2	2·5	0·7
1300	2000	1300	1900				
Differences SKOMER IS							
−0005	−0005	+0005	+0005	−0·4	−0·1	0·0	0·0
DALE ROADS							
−0005	−0005	−0008	−0008	0·0	0·0	0·0	−0·1
NEYLAND							
+0002	+0010	0000	0000	0·0	0·0	0·0	0·0
HAVERFORDWEST							
+0010	+0025	Dries		−4·8	−4·9	Dries out	
LLANGWM (Black Tar)							
+0010	+0020	0000	0000	+0·1	+0·1	0·0	−0·1

NOTE: Milford Haven is a Standard Port and all tidal predictions for the year are given below.

SHELTER
Very good in various places round the hbr, especially in Milford Marina and Neyland Yacht Haven. Contact Milford Haven Sig Stn to ascertain most suitable ⚓ or berth. ⚓s in Dale Bay; off Chapel Bay and Angle Pt on S shore; off Scotch Bay by Milford, above the town; and many others above Pembroke Dock. Majority of moorings are 'all-tide afloat'. Depending on weather conditions, it is possible to dry out safely at inshore areas of Dale, Sandy Haven and Angle Bay.

NAVIGATION
WPT 51°40′·18N, 05°10′·22W, 040°/220° from/to Great Castle Hd ldg lt, 3·18M. There is considerable tidal set across the ent to the Haven particularly at sp. In bad weather avoid passing over Mid Chan Rks and St Ann's Hd shoal, where a confused sea and swell will be found and give St Ann's Head a wide berth. Beware large tankers entering and leaving the haven and ferries moving at high speed in lower Haven. Caution: Only 15m clearance below cables between Thorn Is and Thorn Pt. NOTE: The Milford Haven Port Authority has a jetty, Sig Stn and offices near Hubberston Pt. Their launches have G hulls and W upperworks with the word 'Harbourmaster' in white letters and fly a Pilot flag (HOTEL) or a Bu flag while on patrol. Their instructions must be obeyed. No vessel may operate within 100 metres of any terminal or any tanker whether at ⚓ or under way.
River Cleddau is navigable up to Haverfordwest, at certain tides, for boats with moderate draughts. Clearance under Cleddau Bridge above Neyland is 37m; under power cable 1M upstream, 25m. Check low headroom under bridges and cables approaching Haverfordwest.

LIGHTS AND MARKS
St Ann's Hd Fl WR 5s 48m 18/14M, Horn (2) 60s. Middle Chan Rks Fl (3) G 7s 18m 8M; B tr, steel lantern. Ldg lts (for W chan) 040°: Front Oc 4s 27m 15M; rear Oc 8s 53m 15M; both vis 031°-048° (H24). Milford Dock ldg lts 348°, both FG, with W ● daymarks. Dock entry sigs on E side of lock: 2 FG (vert) = gates open, vessels may enter. Exit sigs are given via VHF Ch12. VHF is normally used for ent/exit by day and night.

RADIO TELEPHONE
Call: *Milford Haven Radio* (Port Sig Stn), VHF Ch **12** 11 14 16 (H24); 09 10 67. Local weather forecasts broadcast on Ch 12 and 14 at approx. 0300, 0900, 1500 and 2100 UT. Gale Warnings broadcast on receipt Ch 12 and 14. Shipping movements broadcast on Ch 12 0800–0830 & 2000–2030LT and on request.
Milford Haven Patrol Launches, Ch 11 12 (H24). Milford Docks Ch 09 12 14 16 (HW−2 to HW). Milford Marina Ch M, M2, 80, 12. Neyland Yacht Haven Ch **80** M. Lawrenny Yacht Stn Ch M.

TELEPHONE (01646)
Hr Mr 692342/3, Fax 690179; Lock 692275/1; Sig Stn 692343; Port Authority 693091; MRSC 690909; ⌗ 681310; Marinecall 0891 500 459; Police (Milford Haven) 692351; Police (Pembroke) 682121, (Neyland) 600221; Dr 600314.

FACILITIES
Marinas/ Berthing (from seaward):
Dale YC ☎ 636362 @ Neyland, C (23 ton), BY, ME, El, Sh, CH, D, V, FW, M, Ⓔ, P (Dale, cans), R (Dale), Slip (Dale), Gas, Gaz.
Milford Haven Port Authority Jetty ☎ 692342/3 (occas use by visitors with approval from Hr Mr), AB, FW.
Milford Marina (200) Access HW −2 to HW (free flow), also one entry and exit approx HW+2 to HW+2½; ☎ 692271/2, Fax 692274 or VHF Ch 12. FW, D, AC, CH, El, ME, Sh, SM, Ⓔ, C (various), Gas, Gaz, V, R, ▣.
Neyland Yacht Haven (410+40 visitors) ☎ 601601, Fax 600713, £8.80, FW, D, AC, CH, Ⓔ, Gas, Gaz, ▣, C (15 ton), SM, SC, ME, El, Sh, R, V; Access lower basin H24, upper basin HW±3½ (sill + gauge);
Lawrenny Yacht Station (100) ☎ 651637, AB, Bar, BY, C (30 ton), CH, D, Sh, ▣, FW, L, M, ME, P, R, Slip, V , ✉ in village.
Services: All marine services are available in the Haven; check with Hr Mr, marina or YC/SC.
Yacht Clubs: Dale YC ☎ 636362; Pembrokeshire YC ☎ 692799; Neyland YC ☎ 600267; Pembroke YC ☎ 684403; Pembroke Haven YC ☎ 651959; Lawrenny YC ☎ 651212.
Towns: Milford Haven, EC Thurs; ✉, Ⓑ, ⇌. Pembroke Dock, EC Wed; ✉, Ⓑ, ⇌, Ⓗ. Neyland, EC Wed; ✉, Ⓑ. Haverfordwest, EC Thurs; ✉, Ⓗ, ⇌, ✈ (Swansea or Cardiff); also a small airfield (Withybush) near Haverfordwest . Ferry: Pembroke Dock–Rosslare.

FIRING RANGES:
Castlemartin Range Danger Area extends 12M S from St Govans Hd, thence in an arc to a point 12M WNW of Linney Hd. The actual Danger Area operative on any one day depends on the ranges/ammunition used. Call Castlemartin Control Tower on VHF Ch 16, ☎ 661321 Ext 4336, Range Safety Boats on Ch 16 or 12, or Milford Haven CG. When firing is in progress R flags are flown (Fl R lts at night) along the coast from St Govans Hd to Linney Hd to Freshwater West.

Continued

MILFORD HAVEN *continued*

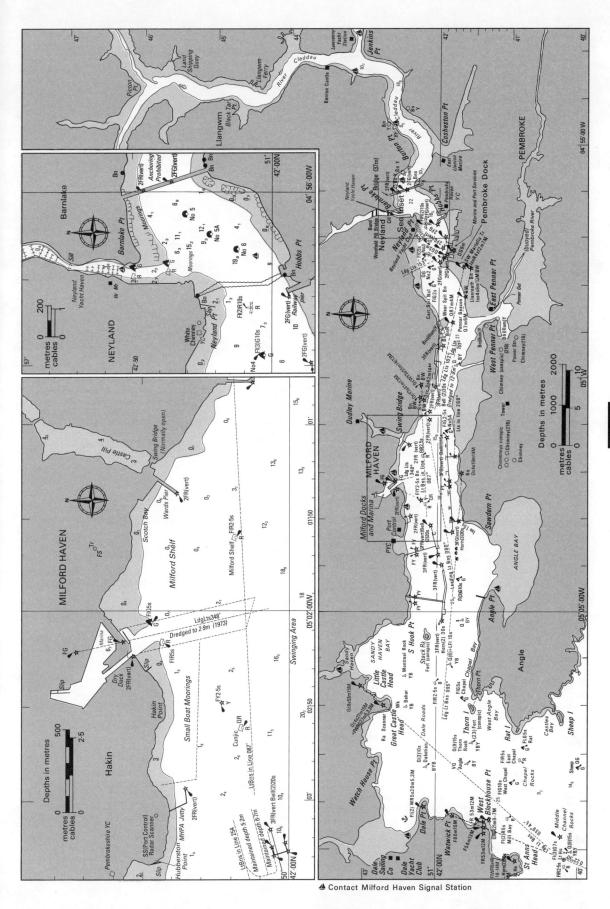

⚓ Contact Milford Haven Signal Station

MILFORD HAVEN *continued*

Times of firing are published locally and can be obtained from the Range Officer ☎ as above, or Ext 4364 (the Chief Clerk). During the firing period (Apr - Dec), firing takes place 0900 -1630; Jul-Nov, there is a break 1200-1300 when vessels may safely transit. Night firing takes place 1830 - 2359, normally on Tues and Thurs. (These times vary according to the hours of darkness). Firing also takes place for two weeks in Jan and Feb. Yachts are requested to keep clear of active ranges whenever possible.

Manorbier Range (further E at Old Castle Hd) partly overlaps Castlemartin Range. Info ☎ (01834) 871283 (HJ)/ 871282 (HN).

Pendine Range (between Tenby and Burry Inlet). Info ☎ (019945) 243 Ext 358. Broadcasts on VHF Ch 16, 73 at 0900 and 1400LT.

Pembrey Range is approx 5M NW of Burry Inlet. Info ☎ (01437) 764571 or (01554) 890420.

TENBY   10-11-15

Dyfed 51·40'·40N 04°41'·85W

CHARTS
AC 1482, 1076, *1179*; Imray C60; Stanfords 14; OS 158

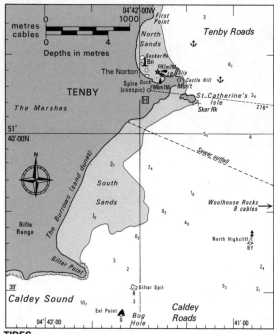

TIDES
–0510 Dover; ML 4·5; Duration 0610; Zone 0 (UT)

Standard Port MILFORD HAVEN (◄—)

Times				Height (metres)			
High Water		Low Water		MHWS	MHWN	MLWN	MLWS
0100	0800	0100	0700	7·0	5·2	2·5	0·7
1300	2000	1300	1900				
Differences TENBY							
–0015	–0010	–0015	–0020	+1·4	+1·1	+0·5	+0·2
STACKPOLE QUAY							
–0005	+0025	–0010	–0010	+0·9	+0·7	+0·2	+0·3

SHELTER
Hbr dries but shelter good; access HW±2½. Sheltered ⚓s, depending on wind direction, in Tenby Roads, Lydstep Haven (2·5M SW), and around Caldey Island as follows: Priory Bay (shallow, to the N), Jone's Bay (NE), Drinkim Bay (E) or Sandtop Bay (W). See Saundersfoot below.

NAVIGATION
WPT 51°40'·00N 04°38'·00W, 099°/279° from/to FS on Castle Hill, 2·2M. Beware Woolhouse Rks (SCM unlit) and Sker Rk (unbuoyed). On appr Tenby Roads, keep outside the line of mooring buoys. For Firing ranges, see 10.11.14.

LIGHTS AND MARKS
Church spire and N side of St Catherine's Is in line at 276°. FR 7m 7M on pier hd. Inside hbr, FW 6m 1M marks landing ↖. PHM Bn (unlit) marks outcrop from Gosker Rk on beach close N of hbr ent. Hbr is floodlit.

RADIO TELEPHONE
VHF Ch 16 (listening during HO).

TELEPHONE (01834)
Hr Mr 842717 (end May-end Sept); MRSC (01646) 690909; ☷ (01646) 681310; Marinecall 0891 500459; Police 842303; Dr 844161; Ⓗ 842040.

FACILITIES
Hbr ☎ 842717, Slip (up to 4·2m), L, AB, Sh, FW; **Tenby YC** ☎ 842762;
Town EC Wed; P & D (cans), ▣, CH, V, R, Bar, Gas, ✉, Ⓑ, ⇌, ✈ (Swansea; and a small airfield at Haverfordwest).

ADJACENT HARBOUR

SAUNDERSFOOT, Dyfed, 51°42'·58N 04°41'·68W. AC 1482, 1076, *1179*. HW –0510 on Dover; ML 4·4m; Duration 0605. See Tenby 10.11.15. A half-tide hbr with good shelter, but there may be a surge in prolonged E winds. On appr, beware buoys marking restricted area (power boats, etc) between Coppett Hall Pt and Perry's Pt. AB may be available (see Hr Mr), or moorings in the middle. Pier hd lt Fl R 5s 6m 7M on stone cupola. VHF: Hr Mr 11 16. Hr Mr ☎/Fax (01834) 812094/(Home 813782). Facilities: CH, FW (on SW wall), Slip, P & D (cans); **Services:** ME, BH. **Town** EC Wed; V, R, Bar, ✉, Ⓑ, ⇌ (Tenby/Saundersfoot).

WALES – MILFORD HAVEN

LAT 51°42′N LONG 5°01′W

TIMES AND HEIGHTS OF HIGH AND LOW WATERS

YEAR **1996**

TIME ZONE (UT)
For Summer Time add ONE hour in non-shaded areas

JANUARY

Day	Time	m		Day	Time	m
1 M	0239 / 0906 / 1508 / 2133	5.6 / 2.3 / 5.7 / 2.1		**16** TU	0127 / 0757 / 1404 / 2041	5.5 / 2.1 / 5.7 / 2.0
2 TU	0340 / 1006 / 1605 / 2227	5.8 / 2.1 / 5.9 / 1.9		**17** W	0247 / 0916 / 1520 / 2155	5.8 / 1.8 / 6.0 / 1.6
3 W	0430 / 1056 / 1653 / 2311	6.1 / 1.8 / 6.2 / 1.6		**18** TH	0356 / 1023 / 1625 / 2254	6.2 / 1.3 / 6.4 / 1.1
4 TH	0513 / 1137 / 1734 / 2349	6.4 / 1.5 / 6.4 / 1.4		**19** F	0453 / 1119 / 1719 / 2346	6.8 / 0.9 / 6.9 / 0.7
5 F ○	0552 / 1214 / 1812	6.6 / 1.3 / 6.5		**20** SA ●	0543 / 1210 / 1808	7.2 / 0.5 / 7.2
6 SA	0024 / 0626 / 1249 / 1846	1.2 / 6.7 / 1.2 / 6.6		**21** SU	0033 / 0630 / 1259 / 1855	0.4 / 7.5 / 0.2 / 7.4
7 SU	0058 / 0700 / 1322 / 1920	1.1 / 6.7 / 1.2 / 6.5		**22** M	0119 / 0716 / 1345 / 1941	0.3 / 7.6 / 0.2 / 7.4
8 M	0131 / 0733 / 1356 / 1952	1.1 / 6.6 / 1.2 / 6.4		**23** TU	0204 / 0802 / 1430 / 2026	0.3 / 7.6 / 0.4 / 7.2
9 TU	0205 / 0805 / 1430 / 2024	1.2 / 6.5 / 1.3 / 6.3		**24** W	0248 / 0848 / 1514 / 2110	0.5 / 7.4 / 0.7 / 7.0
10 W	0238 / 0839 / 1503 / 2058	1.3 / 6.4 / 1.4 / 6.2		**25** TH	0332 / 0933 / 1557 / 2154	0.8 / 7.1 / 0.9 / 6.6
11 TH	0312 / 0915 / 1537 / 2135	1.5 / 6.3 / 1.5 / 6.0		**26** F	0415 / 1018 / 1640 / 2239	1.2 / 6.6 / 1.4 / 6.2
12 F	0349 / 0954 / 1615 / 2216	1.6 / 6.1 / 1.7 / 5.8		**27** SA	0502 / 1106 / 1728 / 2328	1.7 / 6.2 / 1.9 / 5.8
13 SA	0432 / 1040 / 1700 / 2307	1.8 / 5.9 / 1.9 / 5.6		**28** SU	0556 / 1200 / 1824	2.2 / 5.7 / 2.3
14 SU	0526 / 1135 / 1800	2.1 / 5.7 / 2.1		**29** M	0029 / 0703 / 1309 / 1934	5.4 / 2.5 / 5.4 / 2.5
15 M	0010 / 0636 / 1245 / 1916	5.5 / 2.2 / 5.6 / 2.2		**30** TU	0149 / 0821 / 1429 / 2051	5.2 / 2.6 / 5.3 / 2.5
				31 W	0308 / 0936 / 1539 / 2159	5.4 / 2.4 / 5.5 / 2.2

FEBRUARY

Day	Time	m		Day	Time	m
1 TH	0407 / 1035 / 1632 / 2250	5.7 / 2.0 / 5.8 / 1.9		**16** F	0342 / 1011 / 1614 / 2243	6.0 / 1.4 / 6.2 / 1.2
2 F	0454 / 1119 / 1715 / 2330	6.1 / 1.7 / 6.1 / 1.5		**17** SA	0441 / 1109 / 1708 / 2334	6.6 / 0.8 / 6.8 / 0.7
3 SA	0533 / 1156 / 1752	6.4 / 1.4 / 6.4		**18** SU ●	0530 / 1156 / 1755	7.2 / 0.4 / 7.2
4 SU	0005 / 0607 / 1229 / 1826	1.2 / 6.6 / 1.1 / 6.5		**19** M	0019 / 0615 / 1243 / 1839	0.3 / 7.5 / 0.1 / 7.4
5 M	0039 / 0640 / 1302 / 1859	1.0 / 6.7 / 1.0 / 6.6		**20** TU	0103 / 0659 / 1326 / 1922	0.3 / 7.6 / 0.0 / 7.4
6 TU	0111 / 0712 / 1334 / 1930	0.9 / 6.7 / 0.9 / 6.6		**21** W	0145 / 0742 / 1408 / 2003	0.1 / 7.6 / 0.1 / 7.3
7 W	0144 / 0743 / 1407 / 2001	0.9 / 6.7 / 0.9 / 6.5		**22** TH	0225 / 0824 / 1447 / 2044	0.3 / 7.4 / 0.4 / 7.1
8 TH	0216 / 0815 / 1439 / 2034	0.9 / 6.7 / 1.0 / 6.5		**23** F	0304 / 0905 / 1526 / 2123	0.6 / 7.1 / 0.8 / 6.7
9 F	0249 / 0850 / 1510 / 2109	1.0 / 6.6 / 1.1 / 6.4		**24** SA	0343 / 0945 / 1603 / 2202	1.1 / 6.6 / 1.3 / 6.3
10 SA	0323 / 0927 / 1544 / 2148	1.2 / 6.4 / 1.3 / 6.2		**25** SU	0421 / 1026 / 1643 / 2243	1.6 / 6.1 / 1.8 / 5.8
11 SU	0402 / 1009 / 1625 / 2234	1.5 / 6.2 / 1.6 / 5.9		**26** M	0506 / 1112 / 1730 / 2333	2.1 / 5.6 / 2.3 / 5.4
12 M	0450 / 1101 / 1719 / 2332	1.8 / 5.9 / 1.9 / 5.6		**27** TU	0605 / 1214 / 1836	2.5 / 5.2 / 2.7
13 TU	0556 / 1207 / 1836	2.1 / 5.5 / 2.2		**28** W	0047 / 0729 / 1343 / 2002	5.1 / 2.7 / 5.0 / 2.8
14 W	0050 / 0725 / 1336 / 2013	5.4 / 2.2 / 5.4 / 2.1		**29** TH	0228 / 0908 / 1509 / 2124	5.1 / 2.6 / 5.1 / 2.5
15 TH	0224 / 0857 / 1505 / 2139	5.5 / 1.9 / 5.7 / 1.7				

MARCH

Day	Time	m		Day	Time	m
1 F	0340 / 1007 / 1607 / 2222	5.4 / 2.2 / 5.6 / 2.1		**16** SA	0328 / 0959 / 1602 / 2229	6.0 / 1.4 / 6.1 / 1.2
2 SA	0429 / 1053 / 1651 / 2305	5.8 / 1.8 / 6.0 / 1.6		**17** SU	0427 / 1055 / 1654 / 2319	6.6 / 0.8 / 6.7 / 0.7
3 SU	0508 / 1130 / 1727 / 2340	6.2 / 1.4 / 6.3 / 1.2		**18** M	0515 / 1142 / 1738	7.1 / 0.4 / 7.1
4 M	0542 / 1203 / 1801	6.5 / 1.1 / 6.6		**19** TU ●	0002 / 0558 / 1224 / 1820	0.3 / 7.4 / 0.2 / 7.3
5 TU ○	0013 / 0614 / 1235 / 1833	1.0 / 6.7 / 0.8 / 6.7		**20** W	0043 / 0639 / 1304 / 1900	0.2 / 7.5 / 0.1 / 7.3
6 W	0046 / 0645 / 1308 / 1904	0.8 / 6.9 / 0.7 / 6.8		**21** TH	0122 / 0719 / 1342 / 1938	0.2 / 7.4 / 0.2 / 7.2
7 TH	0119 / 0717 / 1341 / 1936	0.7 / 6.9 / 0.7 / 6.8		**22** F	0200 / 0758 / 1419 / 2016	0.4 / 7.2 / 0.5 / 7.0
8 F	0152 / 0751 / 1413 / 2009	0.7 / 6.9 / 0.8 / 6.8		**23** SA	0236 / 0836 / 1454 / 2052	0.9 / 6.9 / 0.9 / 6.7
9 SA	0226 / 0826 / 1446 / 2046	0.8 / 6.8 / 0.9 / 6.6		**24** SU	0311 / 0913 / 1528 / 2127	1.1 / 6.5 / 1.3 / 6.3
10 SU	0301 / 0905 / 1521 / 2126	1.0 / 6.6 / 1.1 / 6.4		**25** M	0346 / 0951 / 1603 / 2205	1.5 / 6.1 / 1.8 / 5.9
11 M	0341 / 0948 / 1603 / 2212	1.2 / 6.3 / 1.5 / 6.1		**26** TU	0425 / 1032 / 1644 / 2249	2.0 / 5.6 / 2.2 / 5.5
12 TU	0429 / 1039 / 1656 / 2309	1.6 / 5.9 / 1.9 / 5.7		**27** W	0516 / 1125 / 1741 / 2350	2.5 / 5.1 / 2.6 / 5.1
13 W	0535 / 1146 / 1814	2.0 / 5.5 / 2.2		**28** TH	0633 / 1246 / 1907	2.7 / 4.8 / 2.8
14 TH	0028 / 0708 / 1321 / 1958	5.4 / 2.2 / 5.3 / 2.2		**29** F	0126 / 0806 / 1425 / 2035	4.9 / 2.7 / 4.9 / 2.7
15 F	0208 / 0844 / 1454 / 2126	5.5 / 1.9 / 5.6 / 1.8		**30** SA	0257 / 0923 / 1531 / 2141	5.2 / 2.4 / 5.3 / 2.2
				31 SU	0352 / 1015 / 1617 / 2228	5.6 / 1.9 / 5.8 / 1.8

APRIL

Day	Time	m		Day	Time	m
1 M	0433 / 1054 / 1655 / 2307	6.1 / 1.5 / 6.2 / 1.3		**16** TU	0455 / 1121 / 1718 / 2342	6.9 / 0.6 / 6.9 / 0.6
2 TU	0509 / 1130 / 1729 / 2343	6.5 / 1.1 / 6.5 / 1.0		**17** W ●	0538 / 1202 / 1758	7.1 / 0.4 / 7.1
3 W	0543 / 1205 / 1803	6.7 / 0.8 / 6.8		**18** TH	0021 / 0618 / 1240 / 1837	0.5 / 7.2 / 0.4 / 7.1
4 TH ○	0018 / 0616 / 1240 / 1836	0.8 / 6.9 / 0.7 / 6.9		**19** F	0059 / 0657 / 1316 / 1914	0.5 / 7.1 / 0.5 / 7.0
5 F	0054 / 0651 / 1315 / 1911	0.6 / 7.0 / 0.6 / 7.0		**20** SA	0135 / 0734 / 1351 / 1949	0.6 / 7.0 / 0.7 / 6.9
6 SA	0130 / 0728 / 1351 / 1948	0.6 / 7.0 / 0.7 / 7.0		**21** SU	0210 / 0810 / 1425 / 2024	0.9 / 6.9 / 1.0 / 6.6
7 SU	0207 / 0808 / 1427 / 2028	0.7 / 6.9 / 0.8 / 6.9		**22** M	0244 / 0845 / 1458 / 2059	1.2 / 6.4 / 1.4 / 6.3
8 M	0247 / 0850 / 1507 / 2112	0.9 / 6.7 / 1.1 / 6.6		**23** TU	0318 / 0921 / 1532 / 2135	1.6 / 6.0 / 1.7 / 6.0
9 TU	0331 / 0936 / 1552 / 2201	1.1 / 6.4 / 1.4 / 6.3		**24** W	0355 / 1001 / 1610 / 2217	1.9 / 5.6 / 2.1 / 5.6
10 W	0422 / 1030 / 1649 / 2301	1.5 / 6.0 / 1.8 / 5.9		**25** TH	0441 / 1048 / 1701 / 2310	2.3 / 5.2 / 2.5 / 5.3
11 TH	0530 / 1139 / 1808	1.9 / 5.5 / 2.1		**26** F	0544 / 1153 / 1814	2.5 / 4.9 / 2.7
12 F	0019 / 0658 / 1311 / 1944	5.6 / 2.0 / 5.4 / 2.1		**27** SA	0023 / 0705 / 1318 / 1936	5.1 / 2.6 / 4.9 / 2.6
13 SA	0151 / 0827 / 1437 / 2106	5.6 / 1.8 / 5.6 / 1.8		**28** SU	0148 / 0822 / 1434 / 2046	5.1 / 2.4 / 5.2 / 2.3
14 SU	0308 / 0940 / 1542 / 2209	6.0 / 1.4 / 6.1 / 1.3		**29** M	0255 / 0922 / 1529 / 2141	5.5 / 2.0 / 5.6 / 1.9
15 M	0406 / 1035 / 1634 / 2259	6.5 / 1.0 / 6.5 / 0.9		**30** TU	0346 / 1011 / 1613 / 2227	5.9 / 1.6 / 6.1 / 1.5

Chart Datum: 3·71 metres below Ordnance Datum (Newlyn)

TIME ZONE (UT)
For Summer Time add ONE hour in non-shaded areas

WALES – MILFORD HAVEN

LAT 51°42′N LONG 5°01′W

TIMES AND HEIGHTS OF HIGH AND LOW WATERS

YEAR **1996**

MAY

Day	Time	m	Time	m	Day	Time	m	Time	m
1 W	0429 / 1054 / 1653 / 2309	6.3 / 1.2 / 6.5 / 1.1			16 TH	0515 / 1138 / 1736 / 2359	6.7 / 0.9 / 6.7 / 0.8		
2 TH	0509 / 1134 / 1731 / 2349	6.7 / 0.9 / 6.8 / 0.8			17 F ●	0557 / 1215 / 1814	6.8 / 0.8 / 6.8		
3 F O	0548 / 1213 / 1809	6.9 / 0.7 / 7.0			18 SA	0036 / 0635 / 1252 / 1851	0.8 / 6.8 / 0.8 / 6.8		
4 SA	0029 / 0628 / 1253 / 1849	0.6 / 7.1 / 0.6 / 7.1			19 SU	0112 / 0712 / 1326 / 1926	0.9 / 6.6 / 1.0 / 6.7		
5 SU	0111 / 0710 / 1333 / 1931	0.6 / 7.1 / 0.6 / 7.1			20 M	0147 / 0748 / 1400 / 2000	1.0 / 6.5 / 1.1 / 6.5		
6 M	0154 / 0754 / 1415 / 2016	0.6 / 7.0 / 0.8 / 7.0			21 TU	0221 / 0823 / 1433 / 2035	1.2 / 6.2 / 1.4 / 6.3		
7 TU	0239 / 0841 / 1500 / 2105	0.8 / 6.8 / 1.0 / 6.8			22 W	0255 / 0858 / 1508 / 2112	1.5 / 6.0 / 1.6 / 6.0		
8 W	0328 / 0931 / 1550 / 2157	1.0 / 6.5 / 1.3 / 6.5			23 TH	0333 / 0936 / 1546 / 2152	1.7 / 5.7 / 1.9 / 5.7		
9 TH	0422 / 1027 / 1649 / 2257	1.3 / 6.1 / 1.7 / 6.1			24 F	0415 / 1019 / 1631 / 2239	2.0 / 5.4 / 2.2 / 5.5		
10 F	0526 / 1133 / 1801	1.6 / 5.7 / 1.9			25 SA	0506 / 1111 / 1728 / 2337	2.2 / 5.2 / 2.4 / 5.3		
11 SA	0008 / 0642 / 1252 / 1922	5.9 / 1.8 / 5.6 / 2.0			26 SU	0610 / 1216 / 1838	2.3 / 5.1 / 2.4		
12 SU	0126 / 0801 / 1409 / 2037	5.8 / 1.8 / 5.7 / 1.8			27 M	0044 / 0720 / 1327 / 1947	5.3 / 2.3 / 5.2 / 2.3		
13 M	0238 / 0911 / 1514 / 2141	6.0 / 1.6 / 5.9 / 1.5			28 TU	0152 / 0826 / 1431 / 2050	5.4 / 2.0 / 5.5 / 2.0		
14 TU	0339 / 1009 / 1608 / 2234	6.3 / 1.3 / 6.3 / 1.2			29 W	0253 / 0925 / 1527 / 2146	5.8 / 1.7 / 5.9 / 1.6		
15 W	0430 / 1056 / 1654 / 2319	6.5 / 1.0 / 6.5 / 1.0			30 TH	0347 / 1017 / 1616 / 2236	6.1 / 1.3 / 6.3 / 1.2		
					31 F	0436 / 1104 / 1702 / 2323	6.5 / 1.0 / 6.7 / 0.9		

JUNE

Day	Time	m			Day	Time	m		
1 SA O	0523 / 1149 / 1747	6.8 / 0.7 / 7.0			16 SU ●	0016 / 0615 / 1230 / 1830	1.1 / 6.4 / 1.1 / 6.6		
2 SU	0009 / 0609 / 1234 / 1831	0.6 / 7.0 / 0.6 / 7.2			17 M	0052 / 0652 / 1305 / 1906	1.1 / 6.4 / 1.1 / 6.5		
3 M	0056 / 0656 / 1320 / 1918	0.5 / 7.1 / 0.6 / 7.2			18 TU	0127 / 0728 / 1338 / 1940	1.1 / 6.3 / 1.1 / 6.4		
4 TU	0144 / 0744 / 1406 / 2007	0.5 / 7.0 / 0.6 / 7.2			19 W	0200 / 0802 / 1412 / 2014	1.2 / 6.2 / 1.2 / 6.3		
5 W	0233 / 0834 / 1455 / 2057	0.6 / 6.9 / 0.8 / 7.0			20 TH	0235 / 0837 / 1447 / 2050	1.3 / 6.0 / 1.4 / 6.1		
6 TH	0323 / 0925 / 1546 / 2150	0.8 / 6.6 / 1.1 / 6.7			21 F	0311 / 0913 / 1523 / 2127	1.5 / 5.9 / 1.6 / 5.9		
7 F	0416 / 1019 / 1641 / 2246	1.0 / 6.3 / 1.4 / 6.4			22 SA	0349 / 0951 / 1602 / 2209	1.6 / 5.7 / 1.8 / 5.8		
8 SA	0513 / 1117 / 1743 / 2347	1.3 / 6.0 / 1.7 / 6.1			23 SU	0431 / 1034 / 1648 / 2256	1.8 / 5.5 / 2.0 / 5.6		
9 SU	0617 / 1222 / 1851	1.6 / 5.8 / 1.9			24 M	0520 / 1126 / 1745 / 2352	2.0 / 5.4 / 2.1 / 5.5		
10 M	0054 / 0725 / 1332 / 2001	5.9 / 1.8 / 5.7 / 1.9			25 TU	0621 / 1228 / 1851	2.1 / 5.3 / 2.1		
11 TU	0203 / 0833 / 1439 / 2107	5.9 / 1.8 / 5.7 / 1.8			26 W	0057 / 0729 / 1336 / 2000	5.5 / 2.0 / 5.4 / 2.0		
12 W	0307 / 0936 / 1538 / 2206	5.9 / 1.7 / 5.9 / 1.6			27 TH	0205 / 0839 / 1443 / 2107	5.6 / 1.8 / 5.7 / 1.7		
13 TH	0404 / 1029 / 1629 / 2255	6.1 / 1.5 / 6.2 / 1.4			28 F	0310 / 0943 / 1544 / 2208	5.9 / 1.5 / 6.1 / 1.3		
14 F	0453 / 1114 / 1713 / 2338	6.3 / 1.3 / 6.4 / 1.2			29 SA	0410 / 1040 / 1639 / 2303	6.3 / 1.1 / 6.5 / 1.0		
15 SA	0536 / 1153 / 1754	6.4 / 1.2 / 6.5			30 SU	0504 / 1131 / 1729 / 2354	6.7 / 0.8 / 6.9 / 0.6		

JULY

Day	Time	m			Day	Time	m		
1 M O	0554 / 1219 / 1818	7.0 / 0.5 / 7.2			16 TU	0033 / 0633 / 1245 / 1847	1.2 / 6.4 / 1.1 / 6.5		
2 TU	0043 / 0643 / 1308 / 1906	0.4 / 7.1 / 0.4 / 7.3			17 W	0107 / 0708 / 1318 / 1920	1.1 / 6.4 / 1.0 / 6.5		
3 W	0133 / 0732 / 1355 / 1955	0.3 / 7.1 / 0.4 / 7.3			18 TH	0140 / 0741 / 1351 / 1953	1.1 / 6.3 / 1.1 / 6.4		
4 TH	0222 / 0822 / 1444 / 2044	0.3 / 7.1 / 0.5 / 7.2			19 F	0213 / 0814 / 1424 / 2026	1.1 / 6.2 / 1.1 / 6.3		
5 F	0311 / 0911 / 1532 / 2134	0.5 / 6.9 / 0.8 / 7.0			20 SA	0247 / 0847 / 1458 / 2100	1.2 / 6.1 / 1.3 / 6.2		
6 SA	0400 / 1001 / 1621 / 2225	0.8 / 6.6 / 1.1 / 6.7			21 SU	0321 / 0921 / 1533 / 2137	1.3 / 5.9 / 1.4 / 6.0		
7 SU	0450 / 1052 / 1715 / 2319	1.1 / 6.2 / 1.5 / 6.3			22 M	0356 / 1000 / 1611 / 2219	1.5 / 5.8 / 1.6 / 5.9		
8 M	0545 / 1147 / 1814	1.5 / 5.9 / 1.8			23 TU	0437 / 1044 / 1658 / 2308	1.7 / 5.6 / 1.9 / 5.7		
9 TU	0018 / 0645 / 1251 / 1921	5.9 / 1.8 / 5.6 / 2.1			24 W	0529 / 1140 / 1800	1.9 / 5.5 / 2.0		
10 W	0124 / 0752 / 1400 / 2031	5.6 / 2.0 / 5.5 / 2.1			25 TH	0010 / 0637 / 1249 / 1917	5.5 / 2.1 / 5.4 / 2.1		
11 TH	0234 / 0900 / 1508 / 2138	5.6 / 2.1 / 5.6 / 2.0			26 F	0125 / 0759 / 1408 / 2037	5.5 / 2.0 / 5.5 / 1.9		
12 F	0338 / 1002 / 1606 / 2234	5.7 / 1.9 / 5.8 / 1.8			27 SA	0242 / 0917 / 1521 / 2149	5.7 / 1.7 / 5.9 / 1.5		
13 SA	0432 / 1052 / 1654 / 2319	5.9 / 1.7 / 6.1 / 1.5			28 SU	0352 / 1023 / 1623 / 2249	6.1 / 1.3 / 6.4 / 1.0		
14 SU	0517 / 1133 / 1735 / 2358	6.1 / 1.4 / 6.3 / 1.3			29 M	0450 / 1117 / 1716 / 2341	6.6 / 0.8 / 6.9 / 0.6		
15 M ●	0557 / 1210 / 1812	6.3 / 1.2 / 6.5			30 TU O	0542 / 1206 / 1805	6.9 / 0.4 / 7.3		
					31 W	0030 / 0629 / 1254 / 1851	0.2 / 7.2 / 0.2 / 7.5		

AUGUST

Day	Time	m			Day	Time	m		
1 TH	0118 / 0717 / 1340 / 1938	0.1 / 7.3 / 0.2 / 7.5			16 F	0116 / 0716 / 1328 / 1928	0.9 / 6.5 / 0.9 / 6.6		
2 F	0205 / 0803 / 1425 / 2025	0.1 / 7.2 / 0.3 / 7.4			17 SA	0148 / 0747 / 1400 / 1959	0.9 / 6.4 / 1.0 / 6.5		
3 SA	0250 / 0849 / 1510 / 2111	0.3 / 7.0 / 0.6 / 7.1			18 SU	0220 / 0818 / 1432 / 2032	1.0 / 6.4 / 1.1 / 6.4		
4 SU	0335 / 0935 / 1555 / 2157	0.6 / 6.7 / 0.9 / 6.8			19 M	0252 / 0852 / 1505 / 2107	1.2 / 6.3 / 1.2 / 6.3		
5 M	0420 / 1021 / 1641 / 2245	1.1 / 6.4 / 1.4 / 6.3			20 TU	0324 / 0928 / 1540 / 2146	1.3 / 6.1 / 1.5 / 6.1		
6 TU	0507 / 1109 / 1733 / 2338	1.6 / 5.9 / 1.9 / 5.8			21 W	0402 / 1011 / 1623 / 2233	1.6 / 5.9 / 1.7 / 5.8		
7 W	0602 / 1206 / 1837	2.0 / 5.5 / 2.3			22 TH	0450 / 1104 / 1722 / 2333	1.9 / 5.6 / 2.0 / 5.5		
8 TH	0042 / 0708 / 1319 / 1953	5.4 / 2.4 / 5.3 / 2.5			23 F	0559 / 1213 / 1845	2.2 / 5.4 / 2.2		
9 F	0200 / 0823 / 1439 / 2111	5.2 / 2.4 / 5.3 / 2.4			24 SA	0055 / 0732 / 1344 / 2019	5.3 / 2.2 / 5.4 / 2.1		
10 SA	0314 / 0935 / 1544 / 2215	5.4 / 2.3 / 5.6 / 2.1			25 SU	0227 / 0902 / 1508 / 2137	5.5 / 1.9 / 5.8 / 1.6		
11 SU	0412 / 1031 / 1635 / 2302	5.6 / 1.9 / 5.9 / 1.7			26 M	0342 / 1011 / 1612 / 2238	6.0 / 1.4 / 6.4 / 1.0		
12 M	0457 / 1113 / 1716 / 2339	6.0 / 1.6 / 6.3 / 1.4			27 TU	0440 / 1105 / 1704 / 2329	6.5 / 0.8 / 7.0 / 0.5		
13 TU	0536 / 1150 / 1753	6.3 / 1.3 / 6.5			28 W O	0529 / 1153 / 1750	7.0 / 0.3 / 7.4		
14 W	0012 / 0611 / 1223 / 1826	1.2 / 6.4 / 1.0 / 6.6			29 TH	0015 / 0614 / 1237 / 1834	0.2 / 7.3 / 0.2 / 7.6		
15 TH	0044 / 0645 / 1256 / 1857	1.0 / 6.5 / 0.9 / 6.7			30 F	0100 / 0657 / 1321 / 1918	0.0 / 7.4 / 0.1 / 7.7		
					31 SA	0143 / 0741 / 1403 / 2001	0.1 / 7.4 / 0.3 / 7.5		

Chart Datum: 3·71 metres below Ordnance Datum (Newlyn)

WALES – MILFORD HAVEN

LAT 51°42′N   LONG 5°01′W

TIMES AND HEIGHTS OF HIGH AND LOW WATERS

YEAR **1996**

TIME ZONE (UT)
For Summer Time add ONE hour in non-shaded areas

SEPTEMBER

Day	Time	m	Time	m	Time	m	Time	m
1 SU	0225	0.3	0824	7.2	1444	0.6	2044	7.2
2 M	0306	0.7	0905	6.8	1525	1.0	2127	6.8
3 TU	0346	1.2	0947	6.4	1606	1.5	2210	6.3
4 W	0428	1.7	1030	6.0	1651	1.9	2257	5.7
5 TH	0517	2.2	1121	5.5	1750	2.5	2358	5.3
6 F	0622	2.6	1232	5.2	1912	2.8		
7 SA	0124	5.0	0744	2.8	1407	5.1	2041	2.7
8 SU	0250	5.2	0905	2.6	1520	5.4	2151	2.3
9 M	0350	5.5	1006	2.2	1612	5.9	2239	1.9
10 TU	0435	5.9	1049	1.7	1653	6.3	2315	1.5
11 W	0512	6.3	1125	1.4	1728	6.6	2347	1.2
12 TH ●	0546	6.6	1158	1.1	1800	6.8		
13 F	0018	1.0	0618	6.7	1230	0.9	1831	6.9
14 SA	0050	0.9	0649	6.8	1303	0.9	1901	6.9
15 SU	0122	0.9	0719	6.7	1335	0.9	1933	6.8
16 M	0154	0.9	0751	6.7	1408	1.0	2006	6.7
17 TU	0226	1.1	0826	6.6	1441	1.2	2042	6.6
18 W	0259	1.3	0904	6.4	1518	1.4	2122	6.3
19 TH	0337	1.6	0947	6.1	1602	1.7	2209	5.9
20 F	0426	2.0	1040	5.8	1701	2.1	2311	5.5
21 SA	0537	2.3	1152	5.5	1829	2.3		
22 SU	0039	5.3	0719	2.4	1329	5.5	2008	2.2
23 M	0219	5.5	0851	2.0	1456	5.9	2126	1.7
24 TU	0332	6.0	0958	1.5	1559	6.5	2226	1.1
25 W	0427	6.6	1051	0.9	1649	7.1	2314	0.6
26 TH	0513	7.1	1136	0.5	1733	7.5	2358	0.3
27 F O	0556	7.4	1219	0.3	1816	7.6		
28 SA	0039	0.2	0637	7.5	1300	0.3	1857	7.6
29 SU	0119	0.3	0717	7.4	1340	0.4	1937	7.4
30 M	0158	0.5	0757	7.2	1419	0.7	2017	7.1

OCTOBER

Day	Time	m	Time	m	Time	m	Time	m
1 TU	0236	0.9	0836	6.9	1457	1.1	2057	6.7
2 W	0314	1.4	0915	6.5	1535	1.6	2136	6.2
3 TH	0352	1.8	0954	6.1	1615	2.1	2219	5.7
4 F	0434	2.3	1040	5.6	1706	2.5	2314	5.2
5 SA	0533	2.7	1142	5.2	1823	2.9		
6 SU	0036	4.9	0658	2.9	1319	5.1	1957	2.8
7 M	0214	5.0	0823	2.8	1445	5.4	2113	2.5
8 TU	0319	5.4	0928	2.4	1540	5.8	2204	2.1
9 W	0405	5.9	1016	2.0	1622	6.2	2242	1.6
10 TH	0443	6.3	1054	1.5	1658	6.5	2316	1.3
11 F O	0517	6.6	1129	1.2	1731	6.8	2349	1.0
12 SA ●	0549	6.8	1203	1.0	1803	7.0		
13 SU	0023	0.9	0621	7.0	1238	0.9	1835	7.0
14 M	0057	0.9	0653	7.0	1313	0.9	1909	7.0
15 TU	0131	0.9	0728	7.0	1348	1.0	1945	6.9
16 W	0205	1.1	0806	6.8	1426	1.1	2025	6.7
17 TH	0242	1.3	0847	6.6	1507	1.4	2108	6.4
18 F	0325	1.6	0934	6.3	1554	1.7	2158	6.0
19 SA	0417	2.0	1030	6.0	1706	2.5	2302	5.6
20 SU	0531	2.3	1142	5.7	1820	2.2		
21 M	0030	5.4	0707	2.4	1315	5.7	1952	2.1
22 TU	0204	5.6	0833	2.1	1436	6.0	2108	1.7
23 W	0314	6.0	0939	1.6	1539	6.5	2207	1.2
24 TH	0408	6.5	1032	1.1	1630	7.0	2256	0.8
25 F	0454	7.0	1118	0.8	1715	7.3	2339	0.6
26 SA O	0536	7.2	1200	0.6	1757	7.4		
27 SU ●	0018	0.5	0616	7.4	1240	0.6	1836	7.4
28 M	0056	0.6	0655	7.3	1319	0.7	1915	7.2
29 TU	0133	0.8	0733	7.1	1356	0.9	1954	7.0
30 W	0210	1.1	0810	6.9	1432	1.2	2031	6.6
31 TH	0245	1.5	0847	6.6	1509	1.6	2109	6.2

NOVEMBER

Day	Time	m	Time	m	Time	m	Time	m
1 F	0321	1.9	0925	6.2	1547	2.0	2149	5.8
2 SA	0401	2.3	1008	5.8	1633	2.4	2237	5.4
3 SU	0452	2.6	1101	5.4	1735	2.7	2342	5.1
4 M	0604	2.9	1214	5.2	1856	2.8		
5 TU	0111	5.0	0727	2.8	1341	5.3	2013	2.6
6 W	0229	5.3	0837	2.6	1449	5.6	2114	2.3
7 TH	0323	5.7	0932	2.2	1539	6.0	2201	1.9
8 F	0405	6.1	1017	1.8	1620	6.4	2242	1.5
9 SA	0443	6.5	1057	1.4	1658	6.7	2320	1.2
10 SU	0519	6.8	1136	1.1	1734	6.9	2357	1.0
11 M ●	0555	7.0	1215	1.0	1812	7.1		
12 TU	0035	0.9	0631	7.1	1254	0.9	1850	7.1
13 W	0113	0.9	0711	7.2	1335	0.9	1931	7.0
14 TH	0153	1.0	0753	7.1	1417	1.0	2015	6.9
15 F	0235	1.2	0838	6.9	1503	1.2	2102	6.6
16 SA	0322	1.5	0928	6.6	1554	1.5	2155	6.2
17 SU	0416	1.8	1025	6.3	1653	1.8	2256	5.9
18 M	0524	2.1	1132	6.0	1806	2.0		
19 TU	0013	5.7	0645	2.2	1251	5.9	1925	2.0
20 W	0135	5.7	0804	2.1	1407	6.1	2039	1.8
21 TH	0246	6.0	0912	1.8	1512	6.3	2142	1.5
22 F	0344	6.3	1009	1.5	1607	6.6	2234	1.2
23 SA	0433	6.7	1058	1.2	1655	6.9	2319	1.0
24 SU	0517	6.9	1142	1.0	1738	7.1	2358	0.9
25 M O	0557	7.1	1222	0.9	1819	7.1		
26 TU	0036	0.9	0636	7.1	1301	0.9	1857	7.0
27 W	0113	1.0	0713	7.0	1337	1.1	1934	6.8
28 TH	0148	1.2	0749	6.8	1413	1.3	2010	6.5
29 F	0223	1.4	0825	6.6	1448	1.5	2047	6.2
30 SA	0258	1.7	0902	6.3	1525	1.8	2124	5.9

DECEMBER

Day	Time	m	Time	m	Time	m	Time	m
1 SU	0336	2.0	0941	6.0	1606	2.1	2206	5.6
2 M	0420	2.3	1027	5.7	1654	2.4	2256	5.3
3 TU	0514	2.5	1121	5.5	1754	2.5	2359	5.2
4 W	0622	2.7	1228	5.4	1905	2.6		
5 TH	0113	5.2	0734	2.6	1338	5.4	2013	2.4
6 F	0222	5.4	0838	2.4	1441	5.7	2113	2.1
7 SA	0318	5.8	0935	2.0	1536	6.1	2205	1.7
8 SU	0406	6.2	1024	1.6	1624	6.4	2251	1.4
9 M	0450	6.6	1110	1.3	1709	6.8	2334	1.1
10 TU ●	0532	7.0	1154	1.0	1752	7.0		
11 W	0017	0.9	0613	7.2	1239	0.8	1835	7.1
12 TH	0100	0.8	0657	7.3	1324	0.7	1920	7.2
13 F	0144	0.8	0743	7.3	1410	0.8	2007	7.0
14 SA	0229	0.9	0831	7.2	1458	0.9	2056	6.8
15 SU	0318	1.1	0921	7.0	1548	1.1	2147	6.6
16 M	0409	1.4	1014	6.7	1641	1.4	2242	6.2
17 TU	0507	1.7	1113	6.4	1741	1.7	2345	5.9
18 W	0614	2.0	1218	6.1	1849	1.9		
19 TH	0056	5.7	0726	2.1	1330	6.0	2001	1.9
20 F	0210	5.8	0838	2.0	1440	6.0	2110	1.9
21 SA	0316	6.0	0943	1.8	1542	6.2	2210	1.6
22 SU	0411	6.3	1039	1.6	1636	6.4	2300	1.4
23 M	0459	6.5	1126	1.3	1721	6.6	2341	1.2
24 TU O	0541	6.8	1207	1.2	1803	6.7		
25 W	0019	1.1	0619	6.9	1245	1.1	1841	6.7
26 TH	0055	1.1	0656	6.9	1321	1.1	1917	6.7
27 F	0130	1.1	0732	6.8	1355	1.2	1952	6.5
28 SA	0204	1.2	0806	6.6	1429	1.3	2026	6.3
29 SU	0238	1.4	0840	6.4	1503	1.5	2101	6.1
30 M	0312	1.6	0916	6.2	1539	1.7	2137	5.9
31 TU	0349	1.8	0954	6.0	1618	1.9	2216	5.6

11

Chart Datum: 3·71 metres below Ordnance Datum (Newlyn)

BURRY INLET　　　　　10-11-16

Dyfed 51°40'·50N 04°14'·85W (Burry Port)

CHARTS
AC 1167, 1076, *1179*; Imray C59, C60; Stanfords 14; OS 159

TIDES
–0500 Dover; ML 4·7; Duration 0555; Zone 0 (UT)

Standard Port MILFORD HAVEN (←)

Times				Height (metres)			
High Water		Low Water		MHWS	MHWN	MLWN	MLWS
0100	0800	0100	0700	7·0	5·2	2·5	0·7
1300	2000	1300	1900				
Differences BURRY PORT							
+0003	+0003	+0007	+0007	+1·6	+1·4	+0·5	+0·4
LLANELLI							
–0003	–0003	+0150	+0020	+0·8	+0·6	No data	
FERRYSIDE							
0000	–0010	+0220	0000	–0·3	–0·7	–1·7	–0·6
CARMARTHEN							
+0010	0000	Dries out		–4·4	–4·8	Dries out	

SHELTER
Good in Burry Port hbr (dries); access HW±2. Inspect before entry as it is entirely filled with moorings, none for visitors. ‡ 1 to 2ca E of barrel post. Sp tides run hard. Note: If bad weather precludes access to Burry Inlet, see 10.11.15 for ‡ s around Caldey Island, especially in W'lies.

NAVIGATION
WPT DZ5 SPM buoy, Fl Y 2·5s, 51°36'·35N 04°24'·30W, 267°/087° from/to Burry Holms 3·3M; thence 4·5M to Burry Port. Carmarthen Bar, extending from the R Towy ent SE to Burry Holms, should not be attempted in W winds >F5 nor at night. Best entry is close NW of Burry Holms at HW–2; thence track 018° with Worms Hd on a stern transit (198°) between Burry Holms and Limekiln Pt. When Whiteford Lt Ho bears about 082°, alter approx 050° into deeper water for St. Mary's spire and the barrel post. Chan is not buoyed/lit and is liable to shift. Before appr, check Firing range activity (10.11.14).

LIGHTS AND MARKS
Whiteford lt ho Fl 5s 7m 7M occas. Barrel post, QR, is 1½ca S of conspic lt tr, FR, and FS on W bkwtr.

RADIO TELEPHONE
None.

TELEPHONE (01554)
Superintendent 758181; MRCC (01792) 366534; ⌗ (01446) 420241; Proof & Experimental Stn (019945) 243; Marinecall 0891 500459; Police 772222; Dr 832240.

FACILITIES
Outer Hbr W pier and Basin ☎ 833342, Slip, M, L, CH; **E Pier** Slip; **Burry Port YC** Bar;
Services: D, ME, El, Sh, C, Gas.
Town EC Tues; P, D, V, R, Bar, ⊠, Ⓑ, ⇌, ✈ (Cardiff).

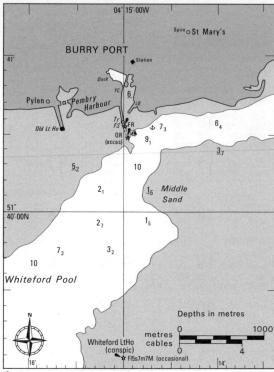

⏶ Report to Burry Port Yacht Services

ADJACENT HARBOUR

CARMARTHEN, Dyfed, 51°46'·25N 04°22'·45W. AC 1076, *1179*. HW –0455 on Dover. See 10.11.16. R Towy dries out, except for river water; access HW±2. Beware Carmarthen Bar off mouth of R Towy and Taf. Local knowledge or a pilot are essential. Chan into rivers changes frequently and is not buoyed. Six electric cables, min clearance 15m, cross between the mouth and the fixed rly bridge in Carmarthen. Visitors berths at R Towy YC at Ferryside (9M below Carmarthen), access HW±3 (liable to dry). Facilities:
R Towy BC ☎ (0126783) 755, Bar, FW, M.
Town Usual facilities, Ⓑ, Bar, Gas, ⊠, V, ⇌, ✈ (Swansea).

SWANSEA   10-11-17

West Glamorgan 51°36'·40N 03°55'·60W

CHARTS
AC 1161, 1165, *1179*; Imray C59; Stanfords 14; OS 159
TIDES
−0515 Dover; ML 5·2; Duration 0620; Zone 0 (UT)

Standard Port MILFORD HAVEN (←)

Times				Height (metres)			
High Water		Low Water		MHWS	MHWN	MLWN	MLWS
0100	0800	0100	0700	7·0	5·2	2·5	0·7
1300	2000	1300	1900				
Differences SWANSEA							
+0004	+0006	−0006	−0003	+2·6	+2·1	+0·7	+0·3
MUMBLES							
+0005	+0010	−0020	−0015	+2·3	+1·7	+0·6	+0·2
PORT TALBOT							
+0003	+0003	−0013	−0007	+2·7	+2·2	+1·0	+0·3
PORTHCAWL							
0000	0000	−0007	−0015	+2·9	+2·3	+0·8	+0·3

SHELTER
Very good in marina; enter via R Tawe Barrage lock, which operates on request HW±4½ (co-ordinated with the marina lock), 0700-2200BST; out of season, 0700-1900UT, but to 2200 at w/ends. At sp, yachts should not enter river until LW+2. Two large Or holding buoys below barrage in mid-stream; also landing pontoon (dries, foul ground) at W side of barrage lock. Pontoons to N of marina ent have no ❻ berths.
NAVIGATION
WPT SHM By, QG, Bell, 51°35'·50N 03°56'·06W, 200°/020° from/to E bkwtr lt, 0·92M. In Swansea Bay tidal streams flow anti-clockwise for 9½ hrs (Swansea HW −3½ to +6), with at times a race off Mumbles Hd. From HW−6 to −3 the stream reverses, setting N past Mumbles Hd towards Swansea. Keep seaward of Mixon Shoal. When N of SW Inner Green Grounds (SWIGG) SCM lt buoy, Q (6)+L Fl 15s, keep to W of dredged chan and clear of commercial ships. Yachts must motor in hbr and appr, max speed 4kn.
LIGHTS AND MARKS
Mumbles Hd, Fl (4) 20s 35m 16M, is 3M SSW of hbr ent. A conspic TV mast (R lts) NNE of hbr is almost aligned with the fairway. Ldg lts 020°: front Oc G 4s 5m 2M; rear FG 6M; these mark E side of chan dredged 3m. From E, keep well seaward of the inner fairway buoy (SHM, Fl G 2·5s).
Port Traffic sigs are conspic at W side of ent to King's Dock; there are 9 lts, Ⓡ or Ⓖ, arranged in a 3 x 3 frame. Yachts arriving must obey the middle lt in left column:
Ⓡ = Do not enter the river; hold SW of W Pier.
Ⓖ = yachts may enter the river, keeping to mid-chan, then to W of holding buoys.
Lock Master will advise on tfc movements Ch 18.
Lock sigs for barrage and marina locks alike are:
2 Ⓡ = Lock closed. Do not proceed
Ⓡ = Wait
Ⓖ = Enter with caution
Ⓡ
Ⓖ } = Free flow operating; proceed with caution
Barrage lock lit by 2FR/FG (vert) to seaward.
RADIO TELEPHONE
Call *Swansea Docks Radio* VHF Ch14 (H24). For barrage, call *Tawe Lock* Ch 18. For marina call *Swansea Marina* Ch 80.
TELEPHONE (01792)
Hr Mr 650855 Ext 260; Barrage 456014; MRCC 366534; Police 456999; ⚓ (01446) 420241; Marinecall 0891 500 459; Ⓗ 205666; Dr 653452; DVLA (for SSR) 783355.
FACILITIES
Swansea Marina (350+50 visitors) ☎ 470310, Fax 463948, £10.69, D (no P), AC, FW, C (1 ton), BH (18 ton), Gas, Gaz, CH, ME, EI, Ⓔ, Sh, Ⓖ, Bar, R;
Swansea Yacht & Sub Aqua Club ☎ 654863, M, L, (no visitors' berths), FW, C (5 ton static), R, Bar;
Services: ME, SM, ACA, CH, EI, Ⓔ, Sh.
City ME, EI, Sh, CH, V, R, Bar, ✉, Ⓑ, ⇌, ✈.

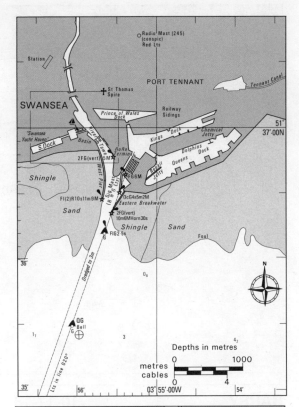

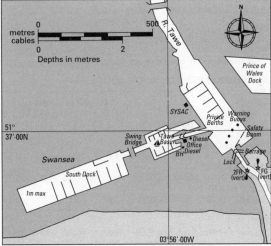

ADJACENT HARBOURS AND ANCHORAGES

MUMBLES, 51°34'·2N 03°58'·2W. Good ⚓ in W'lies 5ca N of Mumbles Hd lt ho. **Bristol Chan YC** ☎ (01792) 366000, Slip, M; **Mumbles YC** ☎ 369321, Slip, M, L, FW, C (hire).

R. NEATH, 51°37'·85N 03°49'·9W. **Monkstone Marina**, W bank just S of bridge, has about 1m. Ent over bar HW±2½ via 1·5M chan, marked/lit training wall. Facilities: AB, M, D, FW, Slip, BH (15 ton), R, Bar, Visitors welcome; **Monkstone C & SC**, ☎ (01792) 812229; VHF Ch M (occas).

PORTHCAWL, Mid Glamorgan, 51°28'·45N 03°41'·95W. AC 1169, 1165. HW −0505 on Dover; ML 5·3m. See 10·11·17. A tiny drying hbr (access HW±2) protected by bkwtr running SE from Porthcawl Pt. Beware rk ledge (dries) W of bkwtr. Porthcawl lt ho, W 6-sided tr with B base, F WRG 10m 6/4M, vis G302°-036°, W036°-082°, R082°-122°; in line 094° with St Hilary radio mast (QR & FR) leads through Shord chan. Tidal streams can reach 6kn at sp off end of bkwtr. ⚓ approx 3ca SSE of lt ho. Hr Mr ☎ (01656) 782756, 3 ❻s; Facilities: **Porthcawl Hbr B C** ☎ 782342. **Town** EC Wed; P & D (cans), CH, V, R, Bar, ✉, Ⓑ, ⇌ (Bridgend), ✈ (Cardiff).

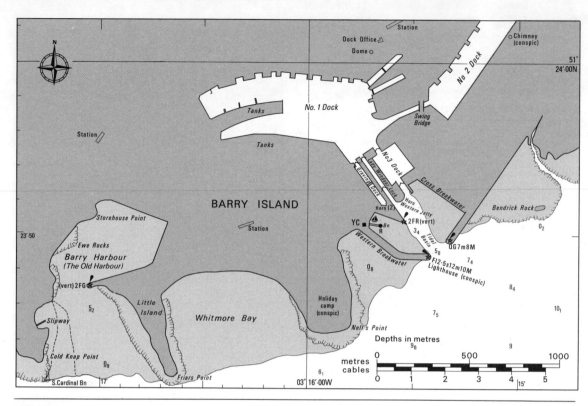

BARRY   10-11-18

South Glamorgan 51°23'·45N 03°15'·37W

CHARTS
AC 1182, 1152, *1179*; Imray C59; Stanfords 14; OS 171
TIDES
−0423 Dover; ML 6·1; Duration 0630; Zone 0 (UT)

Standard Port BRISTOL (AVONMOUTH) (→)

Times				Height (metres)			
High Water		Low Water		MHWS	MHWN	MLWN	MLWS
0600	1100	0300	0800	13·2	9·8	3·8	1·0
1800	2300	1500	2000				
Differences BARRY							
−0030	−0015	−0125	−0030	−1·8	−1·3	+0·2	0·0
FLAT HOLM							
−0015	−0015	−0045	−0045	−1·3	−1·1	−0·2	+0·2
STEEP HOLM							
−0020	−0020	−0050	−0050	−1·6	−1·2	−0·2	−0·2

SHELTER
Good, except in strong E/SE winds. In these winds
yachts are advised to enter the dock (HW±3) by prior
arrangement; yachts > 12m LOA should do so anyway.
Outer hbr: pick up a mooring (free) and see YC; access
HW±3. Old hbr to W of Barry Island dries and is not used.
NAVIGATION
WPT 51°23'·00N 03°15'·00W, 152°/332° from/to ent, 0·53M.
Beware heavy merchant traffic. Approaching from E keep
well out from the shore. Strong tidal stream across ent.
LIGHTS AND MARKS
W bkwtr Fl 2·5s 10M. E bkwtr QG 8M.
RADIO TELEPHONE
Call: *Barry Radio* VHF Ch **11** 10 16 (HW−4 to HW+3). Tidal
info available on request.
TELEPHONE (01446)
Hr Mr 700754; MRCC (01792) 366534; ⌗ 420241;
Marinecall 0891 500 459; Police 734451; Dr 739543.
FACILITIES
Barry YC (130) ☎ 735511, Slip, M, Bar, FW, access HW±3½;
Services: Slip, D, FW, Gas, ME, El, Sh, CH, SM.
Town EC Wed; P (cans, 1M away), D, CH, V, R, Bar, ✉, Ⓑ,
⇌, ✈ (Cardiff).

CARDIFF   10-11-19

South Glamorgan 51°27'·10N 03°09'·55W

CHARTS
AC 1182, 1176, *1179*; Imray C59; Stanfords 14; OS 171
TIDES
–0425 Dover; ML 6·4; Duration 0610; Zone 0 (UT)

Standard Port BRISTOL (AVONMOUTH) (→)

Times				Height (metres)			
High Water		Low Water		MHWS	MHWN	MLWN	MLWS
0600	1100	0300	0800	13·2	9·8	3·8	1·0
1800	2300	1500	2000				

Differences CARDIFF

–0015	–0015	–0100	–0030	–1·0	–0·6	+0·1	0·0

NEWPORT

–0020	–0010	0000	–0020	–1·1	–1·0	–0·6	–0·7

Note: At Newport the height of LW does not normally fall below MLWS. Tidal hts are based on a minimum river flow; max flow may raise ht of LW by as much as 0·3m.

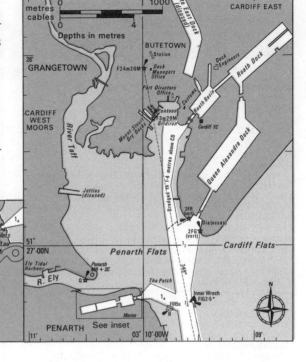

SHELTER
Very good in marina (open H24). Access approx HW±3¼, via lock with sill 3·5m above CD. Depth gauge on outer wall shows ht of water above sill. Waiting ⚓ in R Ely in W'lies; in E'lies cramped ⚓ off Alexandra Dock ent in 2m.
NAVIGATION
WPT 51°24'·00N 03°08'·73W (2½ca SW of S. Cardiff SCM lt buoy), 169°/349° from/to front ldg lt, 3·7M. Outer appr's from W or SW are via Breaksea lt F and N of One Fathom Bank. Keep S of Lavernock Spit (SCM lt By) and NW of Flat Holm and Wolves drying rk (NCM lt buoy). On the ldg line, Ranny Spit (dries) is 3½ca to the W, and Cardiff Grounds same distance to the E. From NE, drying ledges and shoals extend >1M offshore. From E, route via Monkstone lt ho and S of Cardiff Grounds. The Wrach Chan is buoyed/lit and dredged 1·2m; it passes 1½ca off Penarth Head. Give way to all commercial shipping, which can be heavy.
Note: Cardiff Barrage (from close SE of marina ent to 2FR (vert) at ent to Queen Alexandra Dock) is due to complete in 1998; for latest info consult marina, NMs or dredgers VHF Ch 72 (major dredging and piling work in progress).
LIGHTS AND MARKS
Ldg lts 349°, both FW 3/24m 20M. Marina lock sigs: ⓖ = enter lock. Ⓡ = Keep clear, lock in use. 2 Ⓡ = Keep clear; fast freeflow in progress, or no water.
RADIO TELEPHONE
VHF Ch **14** 13 16 (HW–4 to HW+3). Penarth marina Ch 80.
TELEPHONE (01222)
Hr Mr 471311; Marina 705021; MRCC (01792) 366534; ⌗ (01446) 420241; Weather Centre 397020; Marinecall 0891 500 459; Police 373934; Dr 415258.
FACILITIES
Penarth Marina (350 + some visitors; max draft 3m), ☎ 705021, Fax 712170, £11.88, FW, AC, P, D, El, ME, Sh, C, CH, BY, Gas, ▣, R;
Penarth YC ☎ 708196, Slip, FW, Bar; **Cardiff YC** ☎ 387697, Slip, M, FW, L (floating pontoon), Bar; **Penarth MB & SC** ☎ 226575, M, L, C, FW, Bar, Slip;
Services: D, SM, Sh, C (20 ton), CH, ACA, ME, El, Ⓔ, BY, Slip, BH (10 ton), Gas.
City EC Wed; P, D, ME, El, V, R, Bar, ✉, Ⓑ, ⇌, ✈.

ADJACENT HARBOUR

NEWPORT, Gwent, 51°32'·95N 02°59'·13W. AC 1176, 1152, *1179*. HW –0425 on Dover; ML 6·0m; Duration 0620. See 10·11·19. A commercial port controlled by ABP, but a safe shelter for yachts. Enter R Usk over bar (approx 0·5m) E of West Usk buoy, QR Bell) and follow buoyed and lit chan to S Lock ent; turn NE (ldg lts 057°) for yacht moorings on S side between power stn pier and YC. Beware overhead cables in Julian's Pill, clearance 3·8m. East Usk lt ho Fl (2) WRG 10s 11m 15/11M, W284°-290°, R290°-017°, W017°-037°, G037°-115°, W115°-120°. Ldg lts 057°, both FG. Alexandra Dock, S lock W pier head 2 FR (vert) 9/7m 6M. E pier head 2 FG (vert) 9/7m 6M. Port VHF Ch 09 11 16 (HW ±4). There is also a VTS, not compulsory for yachts; call *Newport Pier Head* VHF Ch 69, 71, 16, HW±4. Hr Mr (ABP) ☎ (01633) 244411. ⌗ ☎ 273709; Facilities: **Newport and Uskmouth SC** Bar, M; **Services:** CH, El, ME, Sh, Ⓔ. **Town** EC Thurs; all facilities.

11

SHARPNESS   10-11-20

Gloucestershire 51°43'·00N 02°29'·00W

Note: The new Severn Bridge, from 51°34'·9N 02°43'·8W to 51°34'·1N 02°39'·8W, is due to complete in summer 1996. For latest info call *Marine Base* Ch 15 prior to The Shoots.

CHARTS
AC 1166, Imray C59; Stanfords 14; OS 162

TIDES
−0315 Dover; Duration 0415; Zone 0 (UT). Note: Tidal regime is irregular and deviates from Avonmouth curve.

Standard Port BRISTOL (AVONMOUTH) (→)

Times				Height (metres)			
High Water		Low Water		MHWS	MHWN	MLWN	MLWS
0000	0600	0000	0700	13·2	9·8	3·8	1·0
1200	1800	1200	1900				
Differences SHARPNESS DOCK							
+0035	+0050	+0305	+0245	−3·9	−4·2	−3·3	−0·4
SUDBROOK							
+0010	+0010	+0025	+0015	+0·2	+0·1	−0·1	+0·1
NARLWOOD ROCKS							
+0025	+0025	+0120	+0100	−1·9	−2·0	−2·3	−0·8

SHELTER
Very good. The lock into Commercial Docks opens HW −2 to HW, but prompt arrival is not advised due to lack of water; the flood starts to make much later in the upper river. Pass 2 swing bridges for marina or Gloucester & Sharpness Canal.

NAVIGATION
WPT 51°42'·80N 02°29'·20W, 208°/028° from/to ent, 2ca. Leave King Road, Avonmouth (17M downriver) not before HW Sharpness −3, to be off hbr ent about HW −½. Stem strong flood S of F Bu lt; beware cross tide. Low-powered craft arriving any earlier may be unable to stem the tide.

LIGHTS AND MARKS
Berkeley Power Stn is conspic 1·5M S of lock. Lts as chartlet, but night passage not advised without local knowledge/pilot.

RADIO TELEPHONE
Call: *Sharpness Pierhead* VHF Ch 17 16 (HW −6 to +2) for lock. Gloucester & Sharpness Canal Ch 74 for bridges; no locks.

TELEPHONE (01453)
Pierhead 511968 (HW−6 to HW+2); Hr Mr 811644 (HO); ⌗ (01446) 420241; Marinecall 0891 500 459; MRCC (01792) 366534; Police 810477; Ⓗ 810777.

FACILITIES
Sharpness Marine (100+15) ☎ 811476, £4, D, AC, FW, Sh, CH, Gas; **Services:** ME, El, C. **Town** EC Sat; V, R, Bar, ✉, Ⓑ (Berkeley), ⇌ (Stonehouse), ✈ (Bristol). ACA, Gloucester.

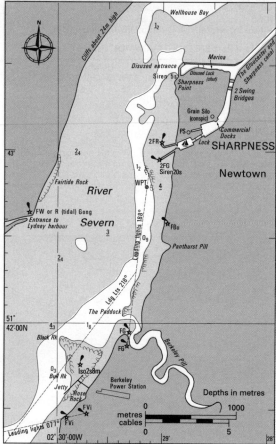

⚓ Report to Docks Hr Mr

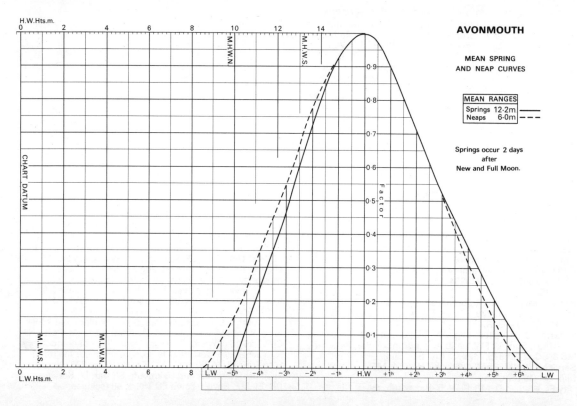

AVONMOUTH

MEAN SPRING AND NEAP CURVES

MEAN RANGES	
Springs 12·2m	———
Neaps 6·0m	– – –

Springs occur 2 days after New and Full Moon.

TIME ZONE (UT)
For Summer Time add ONE hour in non-shaded areas

ENGLAND – PORT OF BRISTOL (AVONMOUTH)

LAT 51°30'N   LONG 2°43'W

TIMES AND HEIGHTS OF HIGH AND LOW WATERS

YEAR **1996**

JANUARY

Day	Time	m	Day	Time	m
1 M	0320 / 0942 / 1554 / 2216	10.6 / 3.6 / 10.9 / 3.2	**16** TU	0207 / 0840 / 1451 / 2134	10.6 / 3.5 / 10.8 / 3.4
2 TU	0420 / 1055 / 1650 / 2319	11.0 / 3.0 / 11.4 / 2.6	**17** W	0335 / 1020 / 1614 / 2300	11.0 / 3.0 / 11.4 / 2.7
3 W	0513 / 1150 / 1740	11.7 / 2.4 / 11.9	**18** TH	0450 / 1133 / 1721	11.9 / 2.2 / 12.3
4 TH	0011 / 0600 / 1239 / 1825	1.9 / 12.2 / 1.8 / 12.3	**19** F	0006 / 0550 / 1236 / 1818	1.9 / 12.9 / 1.4 / 13.2
5 F O	0059 / 0642 / 1326 / 1906	1.5 / 12.6 / 1.6 / 12.5	**20** SA ●	0106 / 0643 / 1334 / 1910	1.2 / 13.7 / 0.9 / 13.8
6 SA	0144 / 0722 / 1410 / 1945	1.3 / 12.8 / 1.5 / 12.5	**21** SU	0201 / 0821 / 1428 / 2000	0.7 / 14.3 / 0.4 / 14.2
7 SU	0226 / 0759 / 1450 / 2021	1.4 / 12.7 / 1.7 / 12.4	**22** M	0252 / 0821 / 1517 / 2047	0.4 / 14.6 / 0.2 / 14.3
8 M	0304 / 0834 / 1524 / 2055	1.6 / 12.5 / 1.9 / 12.2	**23** TU	0337 / 0907 / 1600 / 2130	0.7 / 14.5 / 0.3 / 14.1
9 TU	0333 / 0906 / 1549 / 2125	1.9 / 12.3 / 2.2 / 12.0	**24** W	0416 / 0950 / 1636 / 2210	0.7 / 14.2 / 0.9 / 13.6
10 W	0353 / 0935 / 1606 / 2154	2.1 / 12.1 / 2.2 / 11.9	**25** TH	0447 / 1030 / 1705 / 2247	1.2 / 13.5 / 1.3 / 12.8
11 TH	0415 / 1005 / 1632 / 2227	2.1 / 12.0 / 2.2 / 11.8	**26** F	0512 / 1107 / 1732 / 2323	1.7 / 12.7 / 1.9 / 12.1
12 F	0447 / 1042 / 1707 / 2306	2.1 / 11.8 / 2.3 / 11.5	**27** SA	0541 / 1146 / 1805	2.3 / 11.7 / 2.5
13 SA	0526 / 1126 / 1748 / 2353	2.3 / 11.5 / 2.5 / 11.1	**28** SU	0003 / 0619 / 1236 / 1848	11.1 / 3.0 / 10.7 / 3.1
14 SU	0612 / 1220 / 1839	2.8 / 11.1 / 3.0	**29** M	0058 / 0710 / 1352 / 1946	10.3 / 3.6 / 10.1 / 3.7
15 M	0052 / 0711 / 1327 / 1944	10.7 / 3.2 / 10.7 / 3.4	**30** TU	0226 / 0819 / 1515 / 2100	10.0 / 4.0 / 10.1 / 3.8
			31 W	0344 / 0952 / 1620 / 2232	10.3 / 3.8 / 10.6 / 3.3

FEBRUARY

Day	Time	m	Day	Time	m
1 TH	0444 / 1118 / 1715 / 2339	11.0 / 3.0 / 11.2 / 2.5	**16** F	0433 / 1120 / 1709 / 2353	11.4 / 2.4 / 11.9 / 2.1
2 F	0536 / 1212 / 1802	11.7 / 2.2 / 11.9	**17** SA	0538 / 1223 / 1807	12.6 / 1.5 / 13.0
3 SA	0032 / 0620 / 1302 / 1844	1.8 / 12.3 / 1.7 / 12.3	**18** SU ●	0052 / 0631 / 1320 / 1857	1.2 / 13.6 / 0.7 / 13.8
4 SU O	0121 / 0701 / 1348 / 1924	1.5 / 12.7 / 1.4 / 12.5	**19** M	0147 / 0719 / 1413 / 1944	0.5 / 14.3 / 0.2 / 14.3
5 M	0207 / 0739 / 1432 / 2001	1.4 / 12.8 / 1.6 / 12.6	**20** TU	0236 / 0805 / 1501 / 2028	0.2 / 14.7 / 0.0 / 14.4
6 TU	0248 / 0815 / 1511 / 2036	1.5 / 12.7 / 1.7 / 12.5	**21** W	0321 / 0848 / 1542 / 2109	0.1 / 14.6 / 0.1 / 14.3
7 W	0323 / 0848 / 1541 / 2107	1.7 / 12.7 / 1.9 / 12.5	**22** TH	0358 / 0928 / 1616 / 2145	0.4 / 14.3 / 0.6 / 13.8
8 TH	0345 / 0918 / 1557 / 2136	1.6 / 12.6 / 2.0 / 12.4	**23** F	0427 / 1003 / 1640 / 2218	1.0 / 13.6 / 1.2 / 13.1
9 F	0402 / 0948 / 1615 / 2207	1.8 / 12.6 / 1.9 / 12.4	**24** SA	0446 / 1035 / 1659 / 2247	1.6 / 12.8 / 1.8 / 12.3
10 SA	0429 / 1023 / 1645 / 2244	1.7 / 12.4 / 1.9 / 12.1	**25** SU	0508 / 1107 / 1727 / 2320	2.1 / 11.8 / 2.3 / 11.4
11 SU	0503 / 1104 / 1721 / 2327	1.8 / 12.0 / 2.1 / 11.7	**26** M	0540 / 1145 / 1805	2.7 / 10.7 / 3.0
12 M	0544 / 1152 / 1805	2.3 / 11.4 / 2.6	**27** TU	0002 / 0624 / 1242 / 1859	10.4 / 3.4 / 9.8 / 3.7
13 TU	0020 / 0635 / 1254 / 1902	11.0 / 3.0 / 10.8 / 3.3	**28** W	0114 / 0732 / 1422 / 2014	9.6 / 4.0 / 9.4 / 4.0
14 W	0131 / 0748 / 1419 / 2042	10.5 / 3.6 / 10.4 / 3.8	**29** TH	0300 / 0854 / 1547 / 2138	9.7 / 4.1 / 9.9 / 3.7
15 TH	0308 / 1001 / 1555 / 2244	10.5 / 3.4 / 10.9 / 3.1			

MARCH

Day	Time	m	Day	Time	m
1 F	0411 / 1033 / 1646 / 2303	10.4 / 3.4 / 10.7 / 2.9	**16** SA	0419 / 1105 / 1655 / 2336	11.2 / 2.4 / 11.7 / 2.0
2 SA	0506 / 1143 / 1735	11.2 / 2.5 / 11.6	**17** SU	0522 / 1205 / 1751	12.4 / 1.3 / 12.8
3 SU	0003 / 0552 / 1235 / 1817	2.1 / 12.0 / 1.9 / 12.2	**18** M	0032 / 0614 / 1300 / 1839	1.1 / 13.4 / 0.5 / 13.7
4 M	0055 / 0634 / 1323 / 1858	1.6 / 12.5 / 1.5 / 12.6	**19** TU ●	0125 / 0700 / 1350 / 1923	0.4 / 14.1 / 0.1 / 14.1
5 TU O	0142 / 0714 / 1409 / 1936	1.4 / 12.8 / 1.4 / 12.8	**20** W	0213 / 0744 / 1436 / 2005	0.1 / 14.4 / 0.0 / 14.3
6 W	0226 / 0751 / 1450 / 2012	1.4 / 12.9 / 1.5 / 12.8	**21** TH	0257 / 0825 / 1517 / 2043	0.1 / 14.4 / 0.2 / 14.1
7 TH	0304 / 0826 / 1523 / 2044	1.5 / 12.9 / 1.7 / 12.8	**22** F	0334 / 0903 / 1550 / 2118	0.4 / 14.0 / 0.7 / 13.6
8 F	0331 / 0857 / 1543 / 2115	1.6 / 13.0 / 1.8 / 12.9	**23** SA	0402 / 0936 / 1612 / 2148	1.0 / 13.3 / 1.3 / 13.0
9 SA	0349 / 0930 / 1558 / 2148	1.5 / 12.9 / 1.7 / 12.8	**24** SU	0419 / 1005 / 1629 / 2215	1.6 / 12.6 / 1.8 / 12.2
10 SU	0413 / 1006 / 1625 / 2225	1.4 / 12.8 / 1.6 / 12.5	**25** M	0437 / 1034 / 1653 / 2244	1.9 / 11.7 / 2.2 / 11.4
11 M	0444 / 1046 / 1659 / 2307	1.5 / 12.3 / 1.9 / 11.9	**26** TU	0506 / 1107 / 1726 / 2320	2.4 / 10.8 / 2.8 / 10.5
12 TU	0523 / 1132 / 1741 / 2358	2.0 / 11.5 / 2.2 / 11.1	**27** W	0545 / 1152 / 1815	3.1 / 9.8 / 3.5
13 W	0611 / 1232 / 1835	2.8 / 10.7 / 3.3	**28** TH	0014 / 0647 / 1315 / 1931	9.7 / 3.8 / 9.2 / 4.1
14 TH	0108 / 0722 / 1400 / 2012	10.4 / 3.6 / 10.1 / 4.0	**29** F	0204 / 0812 / 1501 / 2055	9.3 / 4.1 / 9.4 / 3.9
15 F	0251 / 0949 / 1543 / 2231	10.3 / 3.4 / 10.3 / 3.2	**30** SA	0330 / 0935 / 1608 / 2215	9.9 / 3.6 / 10.3 / 3.2
			31 SU	0429 / 1059 / 1700 / 2325	10.8 / 2.8 / 11.2 / 2.4

APRIL

Day	Time	m	Day	Time	m
1 M	0519 / 1159 / 1745	11.6 / 2.1 / 12.0	**16** TU	0006 / 0550 / 1232 / 1814	1.1 / 13.1 / 0.6 / 13.3
2 TU	0020 / 0602 / 1250 / 1827	1.8 / 12.3 / 1.6 / 12.5	**17** W ●	0057 / 0636 / 1321 / 1858	0.5 / 13.6 / 0.3 / 13.7
3 W	0109 / 0644 / 1337 / 1906	1.4 / 12.7 / 1.4 / 12.9	**18** TH	0144 / 0719 / 1407 / 1939	0.3 / 13.9 / 0.2 / 13.8
4 TH O	0155 / 0723 / 1420 / 1944	1.3 / 13.0 / 1.4 / 13.1	**19** F	0228 / 0800 / 1448 / 2016	0.3 / 13.8 / 0.4 / 13.6
5 F	0236 / 0800 / 1456 / 2019	1.2 / 13.1 / 1.4 / 13.2	**20** SA	0307 / 0837 / 1522 / 2050	0.7 / 13.4 / 0.9 / 13.2
6 SA	0309 / 0837 / 1524 / 2055	1.2 / 13.2 / 1.4 / 13.2	**21** SU	0337 / 0910 / 1546 / 2121	1.2 / 12.9 / 1.4 / 12.7
7 SU	0335 / 0914 / 1546 / 2132	1.2 / 13.2 / 1.4 / 13.1	**22** M	0357 / 0940 / 1604 / 2149	1.6 / 12.3 / 1.8 / 12.1
8 M	0402 / 0952 / 1613 / 2211	1.2 / 13.0 / 1.5 / 12.7	**23** TU	0414 / 1009 / 1626 / 2217	1.9 / 11.6 / 2.1 / 11.4
9 TU	0434 / 1034 / 1647 / 2254	1.4 / 12.4 / 1.8 / 12.1	**24** W	0440 / 1040 / 1657 / 2249	2.3 / 10.9 / 2.5 / 10.7
10 W	0513 / 1122 / 1729 / 2346	1.9 / 11.6 / 2.4 / 11.2	**25** TH	0517 / 1118 / 1739 / 2333	2.8 / 10.1 / 3.1 / 10.0
11 TH	0603 / 1221 / 1824	2.7 / 10.7 / 3.3	**26** F	0608 / 1216 / 1843	3.4 / 9.5 / 3.8
12 F	0057 / 0721 / 1350 / 2033	10.5 / 3.4 / 10.2 / 3.8	**27** SA	0047 / 0726 / 1352 / 2009	9.5 / 3.8 / 9.3 / 3.9
13 SA	0239 / 0930 / 1524 / 2209	10.4 / 3.1 / 10.6 / 3.0	**28** SU	0233 / 0846 / 1515 / 2125	9.7 / 3.6 / 9.9 / 3.4
14 SU	0358 / 1041 / 1632 / 2311	11.2 / 2.2 / 11.6 / 2.0	**29** M	0341 / 1000 / 1616 / 2234	10.4 / 3.0 / 10.8 / 2.7
15 M	0459 / 1139 / 1727	12.2 / 1.3 / 12.5	**30** TU	0437 / 1109 / 1706 / 2335	11.2 / 2.4 / 11.6 / 2.0

11

Chart Datum: 6·50 metres below Ordnance Datum (Newlyn)

TIME ZONE (UT)
For Summer Time add ONE hour in non-shaded areas

ENGLAND – PORT OF BRISTOL (AVONMOUTH)

LAT 51°30′N   LONG 2°43′W

TIMES AND HEIGHTS OF HIGH AND LOW WATERS

YEAR 1996

Chart Datum: 6·50 metres below Ordnance Datum (Newlyn)

MAY

Day	Time	m		Day	Time	m
1 W	0525 / 1207 / 1752	12.0 / 1.8 / 12.4		16 TH	0026 / 0610 / 1250 / 1831	1.0 / 12.9 / 0.8 / 13.1
2 TH	0028 / 0610 / 1258 / 1834	1.6 / 12.6 / 1.5 / 12.9		17 F ●	0114 / 0654 / 1336 / 1912	0.8 / 13.1 / 0.7 / 13.2
3 F O	0118 / 0653 / 1345 / 1915	1.2 / 13.0 / 1.2 / 13.3		18 SA	0159 / 0735 / 1419 / 1951	0.8 / 13.1 / 0.8 / 13.1
4 SA	0204 / 0735 / 1427 / 1956	1.0 / 13.5 / 1.1 / 13.5		19 SU	0240 / 0813 / 1456 / 2026	1.0 / 12.8 / 1.1 / 12.8
5 SU	0245 / 0817 / 1505 / 2037	0.9 / 13.4 / 1.1 / 13.5		20 M	0315 / 0848 / 1525 / 2059	1.4 / 12.5 / 1.5 / 12.5
6 M	0323 / 0900 / 1538 / 2119	0.9 / 13.4 / 1.1 / 13.4		21 TU	0340 / 0920 / 1547 / 2129	1.7 / 12.0 / 1.8 / 12.0
7 TU	0358 / 0943 / 1611 / 2202	0.9 / 13.1 / 1.3 / 13.0		22 W	0359 / 0950 / 1609 / 2159	2.0 / 11.6 / 2.0 / 11.5
8 W	0435 / 1028 / 1647 / 2248	1.2 / 12.6 / 1.7 / 12.3		23 TH	0423 / 1021 / 1638 / 2229	2.2 / 11.1 / 2.3 / 11.0
9 TH	0516 / 1116 / 1730 / 2341	1.7 / 11.8 / 2.3 / 11.6		24 F	0457 / 1056 / 1715 / 2308	2.5 / 10.6 / 2.7 / 10.5
10 F	0608 / 1215 / 1827	2.4 / 11.1 / 3.0		25 SA	0540 / 1141 / 1804	2.9 / 10.1 / 3.2
11 SA	0050 / 0720 / 1334 / 2004	10.9 / 2.9 / 10.6 / 3.3		26 SU	0000 / 0639 / 1243 / 1913	10.1 / 3.3 / 9.8 / 3.5
12 SU	0217 / 0753 / 1456 / 2136	10.8 / 2.8 / 10.8 / 2.9		27 M	0113 / 0753 / 1401 / 2032	10.0 / 3.4 / 9.9 / 3.4
13 M	0329 / 1008 / 1601 / 2240	11.2 / 2.3 / 11.4 / 2.3		28 TU	0236 / 0908 / 1518 / 2144	10.3 / 3.1 / 10.5 / 2.9
14 TU	0430 / 1107 / 1658 / 2335	11.9 / 1.7 / 12.1 / 1.5		29 W	0345 / 1018 / 1621 / 2250	11.0 / 2.6 / 11.3 / 2.3
15 W	0523 / 1200 / 1747	12.5 / 1.1 / 12.7		30 TH	0444 / 1123 / 1715 / 2349	11.7 / 2.0 / 12.1 / 1.7
				31 F	0536 / 1220 / 1804	12.5 / 1.6 / 12.8

JUNE

Day	Time	m		Day	Time	m
1 SA O	0044 / 0625 / 1313 / 1850	1.3 / 13.0 / 1.2 / 13.4		16 SU ●	0132 / 0712 / 1352 / 1928	1.3 / 12.5 / 1.1 / 12.7
2 SU	0137 / 0714 / 1403 / 1937	1.0 / 13.4 / 1.0 / 13.7		17 M	0216 / 0751 / 1433 / 2006	1.3 / 12.4 / 1.2 / 12.6
3 M	0226 / 0801 / 1450 / 2023	0.8 / 13.6 / 0.9 / 13.8		18 TU	0255 / 0828 / 1509 / 2041	1.5 / 12.2 / 1.5 / 12.4
4 TU	0313 / 0849 / 1533 / 2109	0.7 / 13.6 / 0.9 / 13.7		19 W	0328 / 0902 / 1537 / 2113	1.8 / 12.0 / 1.8 / 12.1
5 W	0357 / 0936 / 1613 / 2156	0.7 / 13.4 / 1.1 / 13.4		20 TH	0353 / 0934 / 1559 / 2144	2.1 / 11.7 / 2.0 / 11.8
6 TH	0438 / 1022 / 1652 / 2243	0.9 / 13.0 / 1.4 / 12.9		21 F	0413 / 1005 / 1623 / 2213	2.2 / 11.4 / 2.1 / 11.5
7 F	0519 / 1109 / 1733 / 2333	1.3 / 12.4 / 1.9 / 12.2		22 SA	0440 / 1036 / 1655 / 2247	2.3 / 11.1 / 2.3 / 11.2
8 SA	0605 / 1202 / 1822	1.9 / 11.6 / 2.5		23 SU	0517 / 1114 / 1736 / 2330	2.4 / 10.8 / 2.6 / 10.9
9 SU	0033 / 0700 / 1307 / 1924	11.5 / 2.4 / 11.1 / 2.9		24 M	0602 / 1202 / 1827	2.7 / 10.5 / 3.0
10 M	0146 / 0809 / 1420 / 2048	11.1 / 2.7 / 10.8 / 3.1		25 TU	0026 / 0659 / 1303 / 1933	10.6 / 3.0 / 10.4 / 3.2
11 TU	0256 / 0925 / 1526 / 2202	11.1 / 2.7 / 11.0 / 2.8		26 W	0134 / 0811 / 1416 / 2054	10.5 / 3.1 / 10.5 / 3.1
12 W	0357 / 1030 / 1625 / 2302	11.4 / 2.3 / 11.4 / 2.3		27 TH	0251 / 0932 / 1533 / 2211	10.8 / 2.9 / 11.0 / 2.6
13 TH	0453 / 1127 / 1718 / 2356	11.8 / 1.9 / 11.9 / 1.8		28 F	0404 / 1047 / 1641 / 2319	11.4 / 2.4 / 11.8 / 2.0
14 F	0544 / 1219 / 1805	12.2 / 1.5 / 12.4		29 SA	0508 / 1151 / 1739	12.2 / 1.8 / 12.6
15 SA	0045 / 0629 / 1307 / 1848	1.4 / 12.4 / 1.2 / 12.7		30 SU	0020 / 0629 / 1251 / 1831	1.4 / 12.9 / 1.3 / 13.3

JULY

Day	Time	m		Day	Time	m
1 M O	0118 / 0657 / 1347 / 1921	1.0 / 13.4 / 1.0 / 13.8		16 TU	0154 / 0731 / 1413 / 1946	1.4 / 12.3 / 1.3 / 12.6
2 TU	0214 / 0748 / 1440 / 2011	0.7 / 13.7 / 0.7 / 14.1		17 W	0238 / 0809 / 1454 / 2023	1.5 / 12.3 / 1.4 / 12.5
3 W	0306 / 0838 / 1528 / 2059	0.5 / 13.9 / 0.6 / 14.1		18 TH	0316 / 0844 / 1528 / 2056	1.7 / 12.1 / 1.7 / 12.3
4 TH	0353 / 0926 / 1611 / 2146	0.4 / 13.8 / 0.7 / 13.9		19 F	0346 / 0917 / 1553 / 2126	2.0 / 11.9 / 2.0 / 12.1
5 F	0435 / 1011 / 1649 / 2231	0.6 / 13.5 / 1.0 / 13.4		20 SA	0406 / 0946 / 1610 / 2154	2.2 / 11.8 / 2.1 / 11.9
6 SA	0513 / 1055 / 1725 / 2316	1.0 / 12.9 / 1.5 / 12.7		21 SU	0423 / 1015 / 1636 / 2225	2.2 / 11.6 / 2.1 / 11.7
7 SU	0550 / 1140 / 1801	1.5 / 12.2 / 2.1		22 M	0453 / 1049 / 1710 / 2304	2.2 / 11.4 / 2.2 / 11.4
8 M	0006 / 0629 / 1231 / 1844	11.9 / 2.1 / 11.4 / 2.7		23 TU	0531 / 1132 / 1752 / 2352	2.3 / 11.1 / 2.5 / 11.1
9 TU	0107 / 0717 / 1336 / 1941	11.2 / 2.7 / 10.7 / 3.3		24 W	0617 / 1224 / 1845	2.7 / 10.7 / 3.0
10 W	0218 / 0819 / 1448 / 2103	10.7 / 3.1 / 10.5 / 3.5		25 TH	0053 / 0716 / 1331 / 1959	10.7 / 3.1 / 10.5 / 3.3
11 TH	0325 / 0942 / 1552 / 2227	10.7 / 3.1 / 10.8 / 3.2		26 F	0209 / 0843 / 1455 / 2139	10.6 / 3.3 / 10.7 / 3.1
12 F	0425 / 1050 / 1650 / 2327	11.0 / 2.7 / 11.3 / 2.5		27 SA	0334 / 1020 / 1615 / 2258	11.0 / 2.9 / 11.4 / 2.4
13 SA	0519 / 1149 / 1741	11.5 / 2.1 / 11.9		28 SU	0448 / 1133 / 1720	11.8 / 2.1 / 12.4
14 SU	0019 / 0607 / 1240 / 1826	2.0 / 11.9 / 1.6 / 12.3		29 M	0005 / 0549 / 1236 / 1816	1.6 / 12.7 / 1.5 / 13.3
15 M ●	0108 / 0650 / 1328 / 1907	1.6 / 12.2 / 1.4 / 12.6		30 TU O	0106 / 0644 / 1335 / 1908	1.0 / 13.4 / 0.9 / 14.0
				31 W	0203 / 0735 / 1430 / 1958	0.5 / 13.9 / 0.5 / 14.4

AUGUST

Day	Time	m		Day	Time	m
1 TH	0256 / 0824 / 1519 / 2045	0.2 / 14.1 / 0.3 / 14.5		16 F	0259 / 0822 / 1514 / 2035	1.5 / 12.4 / 1.6 / 12.5
2 F	0343 / 0910 / 1601 / 2130	0.1 / 14.1 / 0.4 / 14.3		17 SA	0334 / 0855 / 1542 / 2106	1.8 / 12.2 / 1.9 / 12.4
3 SA	0423 / 0953 / 1637 / 2212	0.4 / 13.8 / 0.8 / 13.8		18 SU	0355 / 0924 / 1557 / 2133	2.1 / 12.1 / 2.0 / 12.2
4 SU	0457 / 1033 / 1707 / 2252	0.9 / 13.2 / 1.4 / 13.0		19 M	0405 / 0952 / 1616 / 2204	2.2 / 12.0 / 2.1 / 12.1
5 M	0525 / 1111 / 1733 / 2332	1.5 / 12.4 / 2.0 / 12.0		20 TU	0429 / 1025 / 1646 / 2241	2.1 / 11.8 / 2.0 / 11.8
6 TU	0554 / 1151 / 1806	2.2 / 11.4 / 2.7		21 W	0502 / 1105 / 1723 / 2325	2.2 / 11.5 / 2.3 / 11.3
7 W	0018 / 0632 / 1243 / 1852	11.0 / 2.9 / 10.6 / 3.4		22 TH	0543 / 1154 / 1810	2.6 / 10.9 / 2.9
8 TH	0128 / 0725 / 1403 / 1955	10.2 / 3.5 / 10.0 / 3.9		23 F	0021 / 0635 / 1259 / 1914	10.7 / 3.2 / 10.4 / 3.5
9 F	0252 / 0836 / 1520 / 2132	10.0 / 3.7 / 10.2 / 3.9		24 SA	0139 / 0751 / 1427 / 2117	10.3 / 3.7 / 10.3 / 3.6
10 SA	0358 / 1012 / 1623 / 2301	10.3 / 3.4 / 10.7 / 3.1		25 SU	0316 / 1007 / 1558 / 2248	10.5 / 3.3 / 11.1 / 2.7
11 SU	0455 / 1122 / 1717 / 2356	11.0 / 2.6 / 11.5 / 2.3		26 M	0436 / 1122 / 1707 / 2355	11.7 / 2.4 / 12.2 / 1.7
12 M	0545 / 1215 / 1803	11.7 / 1.9 / 12.2		27 TU	0538 / 1224 / 1804	12.6 / 1.4 / 13.3
13 TU	0045 / 0628 / 1305 / 1845	1.7 / 12.2 / 1.4 / 12.6		28 W O	0054 / 0630 / 1321 / 1854	0.8 / 13.5 / 0.7 / 14.1
14 W ●	0133 / 0708 / 1352 / 1924	1.3 / 12.4 / 1.3 / 12.8		29 TH	0149 / 0719 / 1414 / 1941	0.3 / 14.1 / 0.3 / 14.6
15 TH	0218 / 0746 / 1436 / 2001	1.4 / 12.5 / 1.3 / 12.7		30 F	0239 / 0805 / 1502 / 2026	0.0 / 14.3 / 0.1 / 14.7
				31 SA	0324 / 0849 / 1543 / 2108	0.0 / 14.3 / 0.3 / 14.4

TIME ZONE (UT)
For Summer Time add ONE hour in non-shaded areas

ENGLAND – PORT OF BRISTOL (AVONMOUTH)

LAT 51°30′N   LONG 2°43′W

TIMES AND HEIGHTS OF HIGH AND LOW WATERS   YEAR **1996**

SEPTEMBER

Day	Time	m	Day	Time	m
1 SU	0403 / 0929 / 1618 / 2148	0.3 / 13.9 / 0.8 / 13.8	**16** M	0337 / 0859 / 1541 / 2111	2.0 / 12.4 / 1.9 / 12.5
2 M	0433 / 1005 / 1643 / 2223	1.0 / 13.2 / 1.5 / 12.9	**17** TU	0346 / 0929 / 1558 / 2144	2.1 / 12.3 / 1.9 / 12.4
3 TU	0454 / 1038 / 1702 / 2256	1.7 / 12.4 / 2.1 / 11.9	**18** W	0408 / 1004 / 1626 / 2222	2.1 / 12.1 / 1.9 / 12.1
4 W	0518 / 1111 / 1730 / 2332	2.3 / 11.4 / 2.8 / 10.8	**19** TH	0439 / 1044 / 1702 / 2305	2.1 / 11.7 / 2.2 / 11.4
5 TH	0552 / 1152 / 1810	3.0 / 10.4 / 3.5	**20** F	0518 / 1132 / 1746	2.5 / 11.0 / 2.8
6 F	0025 / 0641 / 1304 / 1911	9.8 / 3.7 / 9.7 / 4.1	**21** SA	0000 / 0607 / 1236 / 1847	10.6 / 3.3 / 10.3 / 3.6
7 SA	0214 / 0752 / 1448 / 2033	9.4 / 4.1 / 9.7 / 4.3	**22** SU	0118 / 0720 / 1411 / 2109	10.0 / 4.0 / 10.1 / 3.8
8 SU	0331 / 0919 / 1555 / 2233	9.8 / 3.9 / 10.3 / 3.6	**23** M	0306 / 0958 / 1546 / 2237	10.3 / 3.5 / 10.9 / 2.7
9 M	0429 / 1053 / 1649 / 2331	10.6 / 3.0 / 11.2 / 2.5	**24** TU	0424 / 1109 / 1653 / 2340	11.3 / 2.4 / 12.1 / 1.6
10 TU	0518 / 1149 / 1736	11.5 / 2.1 / 12.0	**25** W	0523 / 1207 / 1747	12.5 / 1.3 / 13.3
11 W	0020 / 0601 / 1239 / 1818	1.7 / 12.2 / 1.5 / 12.6	**26** TH	0035 / 0613 / 1301 / 1835	0.7 / 13.5 / 0.6 / 14.1
12 TH ●	0107 / 0641 / 1326 / 1858	1.3 / 12.6 / 1.2 / 12.9	**27** F O	0127 / 0659 / 1351 / 1920	0.1 / 14.1 / 0.2 / 14.5
13 F	0153 / 0719 / 1411 / 1935	1.3 / 12.7 / 1.3 / 12.9	**28** SA	0215 / 0742 / 1437 / 2003	-0.1 / 14.3 / 0.1 / 14.5
14 SA	0235 / 0756 / 1451 / 2010	1.4 / 12.7 / 1.5 / 12.8	**29** SU	0259 / 0824 / 1519 / 2044	0.1 / 14.1 / 0.4 / 14.2
15 SU	0312 / 0829 / 1523 / 2042	1.7 / 12.5 / 1.7 / 12.6	**30** M	0337 / 0902 / 1553 / 2121	0.5 / 13.7 / 0.9 / 13.6

OCTOBER

Day	Time	m	Day	Time	m
1 TU	0405 / 0936 / 1617 / 2154	1.2 / 13.1 / 1.6 / 12.7	**16** W	0332 / 0911 / 1547 / 2129	1.8 / 12.7 / 1.7 / 12.7
2 W	0424 / 1007 / 1633 / 2224	1.8 / 12.3 / 2.2 / 11.8	**17** TH	0355 / 0948 / 1616 / 2209	1.9 / 12.5 / 1.8 / 12.3
3 TH	0445 / 1037 / 1658 / 2256	2.4 / 11.4 / 2.7 / 10.8	**18** F	0426 / 1030 / 1652 / 2254	2.0 / 11.9 / 2.1 / 11.6
4 F	0516 / 1112 / 1735 / 2339	2.9 / 10.5 / 3.4 / 9.8	**19** SA	0505 / 1119 / 1736 / 2348	2.5 / 11.2 / 2.8 / 10.7
5 SA	0601 / 1209 / 1831	3.6 / 9.6 / 4.1	**20** SU	0555 / 1223 / 1840	3.3 / 10.5 / 3.5
6 SU	0104 / 0711 / 1406 / 1952	9.1 / 4.2 / 9.4 / 4.4	**21** M	0105 / 0711 / 1400 / 2053	10.1 / 3.9 / 10.3 / 3.6
7 M	0254 / 0834 / 1520 / 2121	9.4 / 4.1 / 10.0 / 3.9	**22** TU	0250 / 0938 / 1528 / 2214	10.3 / 3.5 / 11.0 / 2.7
8 TU	0355 / 1003 / 1616 / 2255	10.2 / 3.4 / 10.9 / 2.9	**23** W	0403 / 1046 / 1631 / 2315	11.3 / 2.4 / 12.0 / 1.7
9 W	0445 / 1114 / 1704 / 2348	11.2 / 2.5 / 11.7 / 2.1	**24** TH	0501 / 1142 / 1725	12.3 / 1.4 / 13.0
10 TH	0530 / 1206 / 1748	12.0 / 1.8 / 12.4	**25** F	0009 / 0550 / 1234 / 1813	0.9 / 13.2 / 0.7 / 13.7
11 F	0035 / 0611 / 1254 / 1828	1.5 / 12.5 / 1.4 / 12.8	**26** SA O	0059 / 0635 / 1323 / 1857	0.4 / 13.8 / 0.4 / 14.1
12 SA ●	0121 / 0650 / 1339 / 1907	1.3 / 12.8 / 1.3 / 12.9	**27** SU	0146 / 0718 / 1409 / 1940	0.2 / 14.0 / 0.4 / 14.1
13 SU	0204 / 0727 / 1421 / 1943	1.4 / 12.9 / 1.4 / 13.0	**28** M	0230 / 0758 / 1451 / 2020	0.3 / 13.8 / 0.6 / 13.8
14 M	0242 / 0802 / 1456 / 2018	1.5 / 12.9 / 1.5 / 12.9	**29** TU	0309 / 0836 / 1527 / 2057	0.8 / 13.5 / 1.1 / 13.2
15 TU	0312 / 0836 / 1523 / 2053	1.7 / 12.8 / 1.6 / 12.9	**30** W	0339 / 0910 / 1553 / 2129	1.3 / 12.9 / 1.7 / 12.5
			31 TH	0400 / 0941 / 1611 / 2159	1.9 / 12.3 / 2.2 / 11.8

NOVEMBER

Day	Time	m	Day	Time	m
1 F	0420 / 1011 / 1635 / 2230	2.3 / 11.5 / 2.6 / 11.0	**16** SA	0426 / 1023 / 1654 / 2249	1.9 / 12.4 / 1.9 / 12.0
2 SA	0449 / 1044 / 1708 / 2307	2.7 / 10.8 / 3.1 / 10.2	**17** SU	0506 / 1113 / 1740 / 2341	2.4 / 11.7 / 2.5 / 11.4
3 SU	0529 / 1127 / 1756	3.3 / 10.0 / 3.6	**18** M	0555 / 1214 / 1841	3.0 / 11.1 / 3.0
4 M	0003 / 0626 / 1248 / 1906	9.5 / 3.9 / 9.4 / 4.1	**19** TU	0050 / 0708 / 1339 / 2016	10.6 / 3.5 / 10.8 / 3.3
5 TU	0145 / 0747 / 1429 / 2026	9.2 / 4.1 / 9.6 / 4.0	**20** W	0221 / 0902 / 1500 / 2140	10.6 / 3.4 / 11.1 / 2.8
6 W	0307 / 0904 / 1533 / 2144	9.8 / 3.7 / 10.4 / 3.4	**21** TH	0333 / 1014 / 1603 / 2243	11.1 / 2.7 / 11.8 / 2.1
7 TH	0404 / 1017 / 1625 / 2257	10.6 / 3.0 / 11.2 / 2.7	**22** F	0433 / 1112 / 1659 / 2339	11.9 / 1.9 / 12.5 / 1.4
8 F	0453 / 1120 / 1712 / 2353	11.5 / 2.3 / 11.9 / 2.0	**23** SA	0525 / 1205 / 1749	12.6 / 1.3 / 13.1
9 SA	0537 / 1213 / 1756	12.2 / 1.8 / 12.5	**24** SU	0029 / 0611 / 1255 / 1834	1.0 / 13.2 / 0.9 / 13.4
10 SU	0042 / 0618 / 1302 / 1837	1.6 / 12.7 / 1.5 / 12.9	**25** M O	0118 / 0654 / 1342 / 1917	0.7 / 13.4 / 0.8 / 13.5
11 M ●	0128 / 0658 / 1347 / 1917	1.4 / 13.1 / 1.3 / 13.1	**26** TU	0202 / 0735 / 1425 / 1958	0.7 / 13.4 / 1.0 / 13.3
12 TU	0210 / 0737 / 1428 / 1957	1.4 / 13.2 / 1.3 / 13.2	**27** W	0243 / 0813 / 1504 / 2036	1.0 / 13.2 / 1.3 / 12.9
13 W	0248 / 0816 / 1506 / 2038	1.4 / 13.3 / 1.5 / 13.2	**28** TH	0317 / 0849 / 1537 / 2110	1.4 / 12.8 / 1.7 / 12.4
14 TH	0321 / 0857 / 1540 / 2119	1.5 / 13.2 / 1.4 / 13.0	**29** F	0343 / 0921 / 1558 / 2141	1.8 / 12.3 / 2.1 / 11.9
15 F	0352 / 0939 / 1615 / 2203	1.6 / 12.9 / 1.6 / 12.6	**30** SA	0404 / 0952 / 1620 / 2212	2.1 / 11.8 / 2.4 / 11.3

DECEMBER

Day	Time	m	Day	Time	m
1 SU	0431 / 1024 / 1649 / 2245	2.4 / 11.2 / 2.7 / 10.8	**16** M	0509 / 1105 / 1739 / 2330	1.9 / 12.6 / 1.9 / 12.0
2 M	0504 / 1059 / 1727 / 2325	2.8 / 10.6 / 3.1 / 10.2	**17** TU	0552 / 1159 / 1827	2.4 / 11.9 / 2.4
3 TU	0548 / 1146 / 1818	3.3 / 10.1 / 3.5	**18** W	0027 / 0645 / 1307 / 1928	11.3 / 3.0 / 11.3 / 2.9
4 W	0021 / 0649 / 1259 / 1927	9.8 / 3.8 / 9.8 / 3.8	**19** TH	0141 / 0802 / 1424 / 2051	10.9 / 3.4 / 11.1 / 3.1
5 TH	0143 / 0806 / 1426 / 2043	9.7 / 3.8 / 10.0 / 3.7	**20** F	0257 / 0933 / 1531 / 2206	10.9 / 3.3 / 11.3 / 2.8
6 F	0304 / 0920 / 1533 / 2156	10.1 / 3.5 / 10.6 / 3.2	**21** SA	0401 / 1040 / 1631 / 2307	11.3 / 2.8 / 11.7 / 2.3
7 SA	0406 / 1028 / 1630 / 2304	10.9 / 2.9 / 11.4 / 2.6	**22** SU	0457 / 1136 / 1725	11.8 / 2.2 / 12.2
8 SU	0459 / 1130 / 1721	11.8 / 2.2 / 12.1	**23** M	0000 / 0547 / 1228 / 1813	1.8 / 12.4 / 1.6 / 12.6
9 M	0001 / 0547 / 1225 / 1808	2.0 / 12.5 / 1.7 / 12.8	**24** TU O	0051 / 0633 / 1317 / 1858	1.3 / 12.9 / 1.3 / 12.9
10 TU ●	0054 / 0632 / 1316 / 1854	1.6 / 13.1 / 1.3 / 13.2	**25** W	0137 / 0715 / 1402 / 1940	1.1 / 13.1 / 1.2 / 12.9
11 W	0142 / 0716 / 1406 / 1940	1.3 / 13.5 / 1.1 / 13.5	**26** TH	0221 / 0755 / 1444 / 2018	1.1 / 13.1 / 1.4 / 12.8
12 TH	0229 / 0801 / 1453 / 2026	1.2 / 13.7 / 1.0 / 13.6	**27** F	0259 / 0831 / 1520 / 2053	1.3 / 12.9 / 1.7 / 12.5
13 F	0312 / 0846 / 1536 / 2112	1.1 / 13.7 / 1.0 / 13.5	**28** SA	0331 / 0905 / 1549 / 2125	1.6 / 12.6 / 2.0 / 12.2
14 SA	0352 / 0932 / 1617 / 2157	1.2 / 13.5 / 1.1 / 13.2	**29** SU	0355 / 0936 / 1610 / 2155	1.9 / 12.2 / 2.2 / 11.8
15 SU	0430 / 1017 / 1657 / 2242	1.5 / 13.2 / 1.4 / 12.7	**30** M	0416 / 1006 / 1631 / 2224	2.2 / 11.8 / 2.4 / 11.4
			31 TU	0443 / 1035 / 1701 / 2257	2.4 / 11.3 / 2.6 / 11.0

11

Chart Datum: 6·50 metres below Ordnance Datum (Newlyn)

BRISTOL (CITY DOCKS)   10-11-21
Avon 51°26'·92N 02°37'·36W

CHARTS
AC 1859, 1176, *1179*; Imray C59; Stanfords 14; OS 172
TIDES
−0401 on Dover; ML 7·0; Duration 0620; Zone 0 (UT)

Standard Port BRISTOL (AVONMOUTH) (←)

Times				Height (metres)			
High Water		Low Water		MHWS	MHWN	MLWN	MLWS
0200	0800	0300	0800	13·2	9·8	3·8	1·0
1400	2000	1500	2000				

Differences CUMBERLAND BASIN (Ent)

+0010	+0010	Dries out		−2·9	−3·0	Dries out

NOTE: The Port of Bristol (Avonmouth) is a Standard Port and tidal predictions for each day are given above.

SHELTER
Excellent in Harbour and marina. For R. Avon, Cumberland Basin & Bristol Hbr refer to *Bristol Harbour: Info for Boat Owners*, (from Hr Mr). Pill Creek has drying moorings.

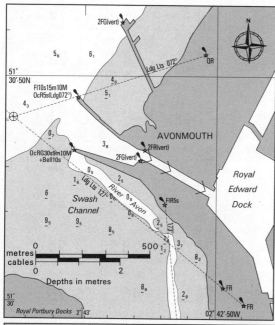

NAVIGATION
Avonmouth WPT 51°30'·42N 02°43'·25W, 307°/127° from/ to front ldg lt, 0·61M. The chan from Flatholm is buoyed. See R/T below for compliance with VTS and reporting. Avonmouth, Royal Portbury and Portishead Docks are prohib to yachts, except in emergency. Tidal stream across ent can run at >5kn. Best to reach ent lock into Cumberland Basin by HW (approx 7M upriver from WPT); waiting pontoon (dries). Ent lock opens at HW−2½, −1½ and −¼ hr for arrivals; departing craft lock out approx 15 mins after these times. Swing bridge opens in unison with lock, but not during road tfc rush hrs 0800-0900 and 1700-1800 Mon-Fri. Inner (Junction) lock is always open, except if ht of HW >9·5m ('stopgate' tide) when it closes.
LIGHTS AND MARKS
R Avon ent is abeam S pier lt Oc RG 30s, vis R294°-036°, G036°-194°. Ldg lts 127° both FR. St George ldg lts 173°, both Oc G 5s synch, Or daymarks. Above Pill Creek SHM lts are Oc G 5s, and PHM are mostly FY.
Ent sigs to Bristol Hbr are on E bank, 1½ and 2½ca beyond Clifton Suspension Bridge: Ⓖ = continue with caution; Ⓡ = stop and await orders.
Bridges: Prince St and Redcliffe bridges are manned 0600-2230 summer, 0900-1645 winter. Other bridges HW−3 to +1. Pre-notify Bridgemaster ☎ 9299338, or sound ·−·(R).
RADIO TELEPHONE
Yachts bound to/from Bristol should call *Avonmouth Radio* VHF Ch **12** 09 at English and Welsh Grounds SWM buoy and at Welsh Hook PHM buoy; comply with any VTS orders. On entering R Avon call again, low power, stating that you are bound for City Docks. (If no radio fitted, sig Avonmouth Sig Stn with Flag R or flash morse R (·−·). The sig stn will reply by light or loud hailer). Keep well clear of large vessels.
At Black Rks (0·8M to run) call *City Docks Radio* Ch **14** 11 (HW−3 to HW+1) for locking instructions.
For berths, call *Bristol Hbr* Ch 73 16 (HO), and/or Bristol Marina Ch **80** M. Prince St bridge, Netham lock Ch 73.
TELEPHONE (0117)
Hr Mr 9264797; Dock Master, Cumberland Basin 9273633; Prince St & Redcliffe Bridges 9299338; Netham Lock 9776590; ‡ (01752) 220661; MRCC (01792) 366534; Weather Centre 9279298; Marinecall 0891 500 459; Police 9277777; Ⓗ 9230000.
FACILITIES
Portishead CC (Pill Creek), M; **Bristol Hbr** ☎ 9264797, AB £5.40; gridiron outside Cumberland Basin;
Bristol Marina (150, inc visitors) ☎ 9265730, £6.90, D, FW, El, ME, Sh, AC, SM, Slip, C, BH (30 ton), access HW−3 to +1;
Baltic Wharf Leisure Centre ☎ 9297608, Slip, L, Bar;
Cabot Cruising Club ☎ 9268318, M, L, FW, AB, Bar;
Portavon Marina ☎ 9861626, Slip, M, FW, ME, Sh, CH, R;
Services: C (8 ton), FW, ME, El, Sh, CH, Ⓔ, ACA, P, D.
City EC Wed/Sat; all facilities, ✉, Ⓑ, ⇌, ✈.

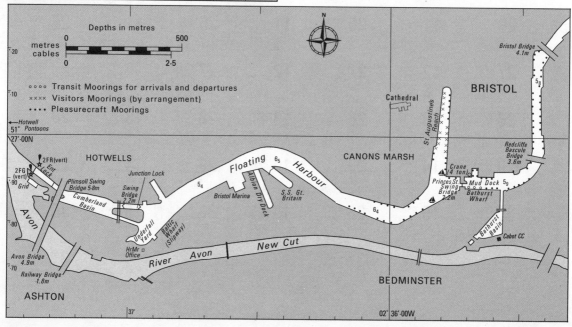

BURNHAM-ON-SEA   10-11-22

Somerset 51°14'·20N 03°00'·25W

CHARTS
AC 1152, *1179*; Imray C59; Stanfords 14; OS 182

TIDES
−0435 Dover; ML 5·4; Duration 0620; Zone 0 (UT)

Standard Port BRISTOL (AVONMOUTH) (←)

Times				Height (metres)			
High Water		Low Water		MHWS	MHWN	MLWN	MLWS
0200	0800	0300	0800	13·2	9·8	3·8	1·0
1400	2000	1500	2000				
Differences BURNHAM							
−0020	−0025	−0030	0000	−2·3	−1·9	−1·4	−1·1
WESTON-SUPER-MARE							
−0020	−0030	−0130	−0030	−1·2	−1·0	−0·8	−0·2
BRIDGWATER							
−0015	−0030	+0305	+0455	−8·6	−8·1		Dries out
WATCHET							
−0035	−0050	−0145	−0040	−1·9	−1·5	+0·1	+0·1
MINEHEAD							
−0037	−0052	−0155	−0045	−2·6	−1·9	−0·2	0·0
PORLOCK BAY							
−0045	−0055	−0205	−0050	−3·0	−2·2	−0·1	−0·1
LYNMOUTH							
−0055	−0115	No data		−3·6	−2·7	No data	

SHELTER
Ent is very choppy in strong winds, especially from SW to W and from N to NE. ‡ in 4m about 40m E of No 1 buoy or S of town jetty or for best shelter ⚓ in R. Brue (dries).

NAVIGATION
WPT 51°13'·35N 03°10'·00W, 256°/076° from/to Low lt, 6·2M. Enter HW −3 to HW; not advised at night. From 0·5M S of Gore SWM buoy pick up 076° transit of Low lt ho with High lt ho (disused). Approx 1·3M past No 1 buoy, steer on ldg line/lts 112°; thence alter 180° into the river chan. Beware unmarked fishing stakes outside appr chan.

LIGHTS AND MARKS
Low lt ho Dir 076° as chartlet and 10.11.4. Ldg lts/marks 112° (moved as chan shifts): front FR 6m 3M, Or stripe on □ W background on sea wall; rear FR 12m 3M, church tr.

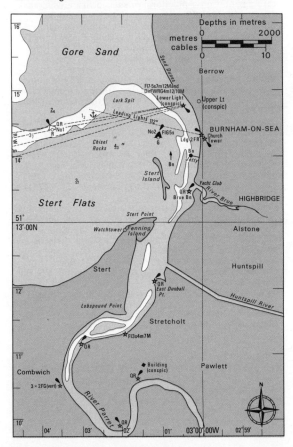

RADIO TELEPHONE
Hr Mr and Pilot VHF Ch 08 16 (when vessel expected).

TELEPHONE (01278)
Hr Mr and Pilot 782180; MRCC (01792) 366534; ⌗ (01752) 220661; Marinecall 0891 500 459; Police 782288; ⽥ 782262.

FACILITIES
Burnham-on-Sea SC ☎ 792911, M, few drying ⚓s in River Brue, L, Slip, Bar; **Jetty** Slip;
Services: ME, El, Sh, ACA (Bridgwater).
Town EC Wed; Gas, ✉, Ⓑ, ⇌ (Highbridge), ✈ (Bristol).
Note: No access to Bridgwater marina from sea/R Parrett.

OTHER HARBOURS ON S SHORE OF BRISTOL CHANNEL

WESTON-SUPER-MARE, Avon, 51°21'·00N 02°59'·20W. AC 1152, 1176, *1179*. HW −0435 on Dover; ML 6·1m; Duration 0655. See 10.11.22. Good shelter, except in S winds, in Knightstone Hbr (dries) at N end of bay; access HW±2. Causeway at ent marked by bn. Grand Pier hd 2 FG (vert) 6/5m. Alternative ‡ in good weather in R Axe (dries), entry HW±2. Facilities: **Weston Bay YC** ☎ 620772, FW, Bar, VHF Ch **80. Services**: AB, CH, El, D, BH (10 ton), FW, Slip, ME, Sh; **Town** EC Mon; Bar, Ⓑ, FW, P, ✉, R, ⇌, V.

WATCHET, Somerset, 51°11'·00N 03°19'·64W. AC 1160, 1152, *1179*. HW −0455 on Dover; ML 5·9m; Duration 0655. See 10.11.22. Culver Sand is approx 6M NNE. 2 radio masts (R lts) brg 210°/1·6M from ent a re conspic approach marks. Good shelter in semi-commercial hbr, dries 6·5m; access approx HW±2½. The ent has about 6m at MHWS. Rks/mud dry ½M to seaward. Beware tidal streams round W pier hd. Yachts berth on W pier; hd FG 9m 9M on Red (R) tr. E pier hd 2 FR (vert) 3M. VHF Ch 16 09 12 14 (from HW−2). On W bkwtr hd B ● (Fl G at night) and on E pier 2 FR (vert) = at least 2·4m on flood or 3m on ebb. Hr Mr ☎ (01984) 631264; ⌗ ☎ 631214; Facilities: **Watchet Boat Owners Assn**. **Town** EC Wed; FW, D, P, Slip, CH, V, R, Bar. Note: 288 berth marina planned to complete 1998.

MINEHEAD, Somerset, 51°12'·76N 03°28'·29W. AC 1160, 1165, *1179*. HW −0450 on Dover. ML 5·7m. See 10.11.22. Small hbr, dries 7·5m; access HW±2. Good shelter within pier curving E and then SE, over which seas may break in gales at MHWS; exposed to E'lies. Best appr from N or NW; beware The Gables, shingle bank (dries 3·7m) about 5ca ENE of pier. Keep E of a sewer outfall which passes ½ca E of pierhd and extends 1¾ca NNE of it; outfall is protected by rk covering, drying 2·8m and N end marked by SHM bn QG 6m 7M. There are 8 R ⚓s at hbr ent just seaward of 3 posts or dry out against pier. Hbr gets very crowded. Holiday camp is conspic 6ca SE. Pierhd lt Fl (2) G 5s 4M, vis 127°-262°. VHF Ch 16 12 14 (occas). Hr Mr ☎ (01643) 702566; Facilities: **Hbr** FW, Slip. **Town** EC Wed; D, P, El, Gas, ME, Sh, R, Bar, V, ✉, Ⓑ, ⇌ (Taunton).

PORLOCK WEIR, Somerset, 51°13'·14N 03°37'·57W. AC 1160, 1165, *1179*. HW −0500 on Dover; ML 5·6m. See 10.11.22. Access HW±1½. Ent chan (250°), about 15m wide marked by withies (3 PHM and 1 SHM), between shingle bank/ wood pilings to stbd and sunken wooden wall to port is difficult in any seas. A small pool (1m) just inside ent is for shoal draft boats; others dry out on pebble banks. Or turn 90° stbd, via gates (usually open), into inner drying dock with good shelter. No lts. Hr Mr ☎ (01643) 863277. **Porlock Weir SC** ☎ 862028. Facilities: FW and limited V.

LYNMOUTH, Devon, 51°14'·13N 03°49'·72W. AC 1160,1165. HW −0515 on Dover. See 10.11.22. Tiny hbr, dries approx 5m; access HW±1, but only in settled offshore weather. Appr from Sand Ridge SHM buoy, 1·6M W of Foreland Pt and 9ca N of hbr ent. The narrow appr chan between drying boulder ledges is marked by 7 unlit bns. Hbr ent is between piers, 2FR/FG lts, on W side of river course. Berth on E pier, which covers at MHWS. Resort facilities.

WATERMOUTH, Devon, 51°13'·00N 04°04'·60W. AC 1165, *1179*. HW −0525 on Dover; ML 4·9m; Duration 0625. Use 10.11.23. Good shelter in drying hbr, but heavy surge runs in strong NW winds. Access HW±3 at sp; only as far as inner bkwtr at np. Dir lt 153° Oc WRG 5s 1m, vis W151·5°-154·5°, W △ on structure, 1½ca inside ent on S shore. Bkwtr, covered at half tide, has Fl G 5s 2M. Eight Y ⚓s with B handles. Hr Mr ☎ (01271) 865422. Facilities: **Hbr** D (cans), FW (cans), CH, C (12 ton), Slip; **YC** ☎ 865048, Bar.

ILFRACOMBE   10-11-23

Devon 51°12'·62N 04°06'·58W

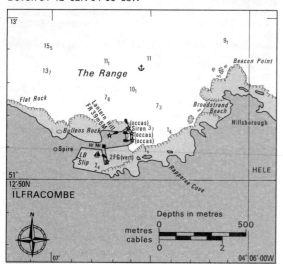

ILFRACOMBE

CHARTS

AC 1160, 1165, *1179* ; Imray C59; Stanfords 14; OS 180

TIDES

–0525 Dover; ML 5·0; Duration 0625; Zone 0 (UT)

Standard Port MILFORD HAVEN (←—)

Times				Height (metres)			
High Water		Low Water		MHWS	MHWN	MLWN	MLWS
0100	0700	0100	0700	7·0	5·2	2·5	0·7
1300	1900	1300	1900				
Differences ILFRACOMBE							
–0030	–0015	–0035	–0055	+2·2	+1·7	+0·5	0·0
LUNDY ISLAND							
–0030	–0030	–0020	–0040	+1·0	+0·7	+0·2	+0·1

SHELTER

Good except in NE/E winds. SW gales can cause surge in hbrs, which dry. 12 ⚓s in outer hbr; or ⚓ clear of pier and LB Slip. Possible AB on quays in inner hbr, access HW±3.

NAVIGATION

WPT 51°13'·20N 04°06'·60W, 000°/180° from/to pier hd, 0·55M. From E, beware Copperas Rks (4M to E), (SHM buoy) and tiderips on Buggy Pit, 7ca NE of ent. Beware lobster keep-pots obstructing hbr ent on SE side.

LIGHTS AND MARKS

No ldg marks/lts. Lantern Hill lt, FR 39m 6M, on conspic chapel. Promenade Pier has three 2FG (vert); shown 1/9-30/4. Siren 30s when vessel due. Inner bkwtr 2 FG (vert).

RADIO TELEPHONE

Call: *Ilfracombe Hbr* VHF Ch 12 16 (Apl-Oct 0800-2000 when manned; Nov-Mar occas). Ch **80** M (occas).

TELEPHONE (01271)

Hr Mr 862108; MRCC (01792) 366534; ⌖ (10752) 220661; Marinecall 0891 500 459; Police 863633; Dr 863119.

FACILITIES

Hbr M (see Hr Mr), D (cans), FW, CH, Slip, V, R, Bar; **Ilfracombe YC** ☎ 863969, M, FW, L, ▣, Bar, R, CH, C (35 ton, by arrangement). **Services:** ME, El, Sh. **Town** EC Thurs; ✉, Ⓑ, ⇌ (bus to Barnstaple), ✈ (Exeter).

LUNDY ISLAND, Devon, 51°09'·80N 04°39'·20W. AC 1164, *1179*. HW –0530 on Dover; ML 4·3m; Duration 0605. See above. Shelter good in lee of island's high ground (145m). In SSW to NW winds, ⚓ close inshore to N of SE Pt and Rat Is. In N'lies ⚓ in The Rattles, small bay on S side. In E winds Jenny's Cove is safe if there is no W'ly ground swell. Beware bad tide races, esp on E-going stream, off the N and SE tips of the Is; and to the SW on the W-going stream. A violent race forms over Stanley Bank 3M NE of the N tip. Waters off the Is are a Marine Nature Reserve. Lts: NW Pt, Fl 15s 48m 17M, vis 009°-285°, W ◯ tr. On SE Pt, lt Fl 5s 53m 15M, vis 170°-073°, W ◯ tr, horn 25s. Two Historic Wrecks (see 10.0.3g) are on the E side of island, one at 51°11'N 04°39'·4W, the other 4ca further E. Facilities: Landing by the ⚓ off SE end of Island; **Lundy Co Landmark Trust** ☎ (01271) 870870, CH, Gas, bar and hotel.

RIVERS TAW & TORRIDGE

Devon 51°04'·34N 04°12'·81W   10-11-24

CHARTS

AC 1160, 1164, 1179; Imray C58; Stanfords 14; OS 180

TIDES

–0516 (Bideford) Dover; ML 3·6; Duration 0600; Zone 0 (UT)

Standard Port MILFORD HAVEN (←—)

Times				Height (metres)			
High Water		Low Water		MHWS	MHWN	MLWN	MLWS
0100	0700	0100	0700	7·0	5·2	2·5	0·7
1300	1900	1300	1900				
Differences APPLEDORE							
–0020	–0025	+0015	–0045	+0·5	0·0	–0·9	–0·5
YELLAND MARSH (R Taw)							
–0010	–0015	+0100	–0015	+0·1	–0·4	–1·2	–0·6
FREMINGTON (R Taw)							
–0010	–0015	+0030	–0030	–1·1	–1·8	–2·2	–0·5
BARNSTAPLE (R Taw)							
0000	–0015	–0155	–0245	–2·9	–3·8	–2·2	–0·4
BIDEFORD (R Torridge)							
–0020	–0025	0000	0000	–1·1	–1·6	–2·5	–0·7
CLOVELLY							
–0030	–0030	–0020	–0040	+1·3	+1·1	+0·2	+0·2

SHELTER

Very well protected, but ent in strong on-shore winds is dangerous. Yachts can ⚓ or pick up buoy in Appledore Pool, N of Skern Pt where sp stream can reach 5kn. The quay at Bideford dries to soft mud; used by coasters.

NAVIGATION

WPT 51°05'·40N 04°16'·04W (abeam Fairway buoy, off chartlet), 298°/118° from/to Bar buoy, 0·9M. Bar and sands constantly shift and buoys are moved occasionally to comply. Advice on bar, where there are depths of 0·1 and 0·4m, from Pilot VHF Ch 12 or Swansea CG. Estuary dries; access is only feasible from HW–2 to HW. Once tide is ebbing, breakers quickly form between Bar buoy (unlit NCM) and Middle Ridge SHM buoy. 2M passage to Bideford is not difficult. If going 7M up to Barnstaple, take a pilot (from Appledore) or seek local knowledge.

LIGHTS AND MARKS

Entry at night is NOT advised. Apart from jetties etc, only the Bideford Fairway buoy L Fl 10s, Outer Pulley buoy QG, Crow Pt Fl R 5s, and the two ldg marks are lit. The latter are W trs, lit H24; front Oc 6s, rear Oc 10s. The ldg line 118° is only valid as far as Outer Pulley buoy after which the chan deviates to stbd toward Pulley unlit SHM buoy, Grey Sand Hill and Appledore. The Torridge is unlit, other than a QY on Bideford bridge showing the preferred chan.

RADIO TELEPHONE

Two Rivers Port/Pilots VHF Ch 12 16 (Listens from HW–2).

TELEPHONE (Instow/Barnstaple 01271; Bideford 01237)

Hr Mr Bideford 476711 Ext 317 or 477928; Barnstaple ring Amenities Officer 388327; Pilot (Appledore) (01237) 473806; MRCC (01792) 366534; ⌖ (01752) 220661; Marinecall 0891 500 459; Police (Bideford) 476896; Dr Appledore (01237) 474994, Bideford 471071/476363, Barnstaple 75221/473443.

FACILITIES

APPLEDORE: (01237) is a free port; no authority can charge for use of public facilities eg slips at town quay and AB.
 Services: CH, El, Ⓔ, BY, C (70 tons), Slip, ME, Sh.
BIDEFORD: AB (few/not encouraged; call Capt V. Harris ☎ 474569), V, R, Gas, Bar.
INSTOW: **N. Devon YC** FW ☎ 860367, Slip, R, Bar;
 Services: AB £5, D, ME, M, Ⓔ, C (4 ton). **Town** R, FW, Bar.
BARNSTAPLE: AB (see Hr Mr), V, Bar, Gas. Limited facilities for FW, D & P; small quantities in cans. Bulk D (min 500 ltrs/110 galls) by bowser, see Hr Mr.
 Towns: EC Barnstaple & Bideford = Wed; ✉ (all four), Ⓑ (Barnstaple, Bideford), ⇌ (Barnstaple,✈ (Exeter).

CLOVELLY, Devon, 51°00'·15N 04°23'·70W. AC 1164. Tides see above. HW –0524 on Dover. Tiny drying hbr 5M E of Hartland Pt has some AB £5 on pier, access only near HW; better to ⚓ off in 5m, sheltered from S/SW winds. Useful to await the tide around Hartland Pt or into Bideford. Lt Fl G 5s 5m 5M on hbr wall. Hr Mr via ☎ (01237) 431237 (Red Lion). Facilities: Slip, FW, ✉, limited V.

RIVERS TAW & TORRIDGE *continued*

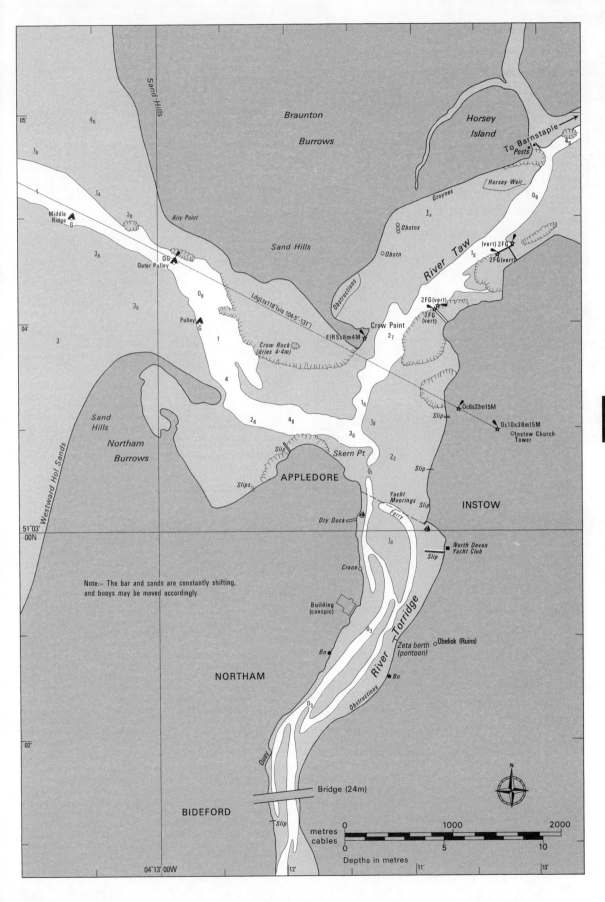

Note:– The bar and sands are constantly shifting,
and buoys may be moved accordingly.

11

metres
cables

Depths in metres

PADSTOW   10-11-25

Cornwall 50°32'·48N 04°56'·10W

CHARTS
AC 1168, 1156; Imray C58; Stanfords 13; OS 200

TIDES
−0550 Dover; ML 4·0; Duration 0600; Zone 0 (UT)

Standard Port MILFORD HAVEN (←)

Times				Height (metres)			
High Water		Low Water		MHWS	MHWN	MLWN	MLWS
0100	0700	0100	0700	7·0	5·2	2·5	0·7
1300	1900	1300	1900				
Differences PADSTOW							
−0055	−0050	−0040	−0050	+0·3	+0·4	+0·1	+0·1
WADEBRIDGE (R Camel)							
−0052	−0052	+0235	+0245	−3·8	−3·8	−2·5	−0·4
BUDE							
−0040	−0040	−0035	−0045	+0·7	+0·6		No data
BOSCASTLE							
−0045	−0010	−0110	−0100	+0·3	+0·4	+0·2	+0·2
NEWQUAY							
−0100	−0110	−0105	−0050	0·0	+0·1	0·0	−0·1
PERRANPORTH							
−0100	−0110	−0110	−0050	−0·1	0·0	0·0	+0·1
ST IVES							
−0050	−0115	−0105	−0040	−0·4	−0·3	−0·1	+0·1
CAPE CORNWALL							
−0130	−0145	−0120	−0120	−1·0	−0·9	−0·5	−0·1

Note: At Wadebridge LW time differences give the start of the rise, following a LW stand of about 5 hours.

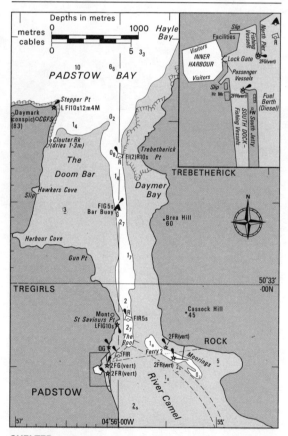

SHELTER
Good in inner hbr 3m+, access HW±2 via lock; or HW±4½ moor in the Pool or ⚓ just down-stream in 1·5m LWS. Drying moorings available for small vessels on passage.

NAVIGATION
WPT 50°35'·00N 04°58'·50W, 305°/125° from/to Stepper Pt, 1·5M. From S, beware Quies Rks, Gulland Rk, The Hen, Gurley Rk and Chimney Rks and a wreck 5ca W of Stepper Pt; all are hazardous (off the chartlet). From N, keep well clear of Newland Is and its offlying reef. Identify the first 2 buoys before entry. Heavy seas can break on Doom Bar

and in adjacent chan with strong onshore winds or heavy ground swell. Final appr S of St Saviours Pt runs close to W shore. Allow ample rise of tide (least depth in chan at MLWS, on the bar, is 0·5m). Shifting sandbanks in estuary require local knowledge, care and a rising tide; ditto the drying R.Camel to Wadebridge (4M). Consult Hr Mr (VHF).

LIGHTS AND MARKS
Conspic stone tr (83m daymark), 3ca W of Stepper Pt, L Fl 10s 12m 4M, marks the ent. Lock ent has 2 FG/FR (vert).

RADIO TELEPHONE
VHF Ch 12 16 (Mon-Fri 0830–1700 and HW±2).

TELEPHONE (01841; 01208 = Wadebridge)
Hr Mr 532239; MRCC (01326) 317575; ⌗ (01752) 220661; Marinecall 0891 500 458; Police (01566) 774211; Dr 532346.

FACILITIES
Hbr ☎ 532239, Fax 533346, Mobile (0374) 290771, AB £11.30, Slip, M, FW, El, C (6 ton), D, ME, ⌷, V, R, Bar, showers; **Rock SC** ☎ (01208) 862431, Slip; **Ferry 1** (to Rock, summer only) ☎ (01326) 317575 or VHF Ch 12 16; **Services:** BY, C, ME, CH, Slip, L, Sh. **Town** EC Wed; ⌷, P, ✉, Ⓑ, ⇌ (bus to Bodmin Road), ✈ (Newquay/Plymouth).

OTHER HARBOURS ON THE N COAST OF CORNWALL

BUDE, Cornwall, 50°49'·90N 04°33'·30W. AC 1156. HW −0540 on Dover. Duration 0605. See 10.11.25. Limited shelter in drying hbr, access for average yacht HW±2. Yachts can, by prior arrangement, lock into quiet canal berth (5·5m over CD required), but lock fees are high (£86 (HO); £125 outside HO; £167 Sun), and gates will only open if there is no swell. Conspic W radar dish aerials 3·3M N of hbr. Outer ldg marks 075°, front W spar with Y ◇ topmark, rear W flagstaff; hold this line until inner ldg marks in line at 131°, front W pile, rear W spar, both with Y △ topmarks. There are no lts. VHF Ch 16 12 (when vessel expected). Facilities: Hr Mr ☎ (01288) 353111; very limited facilities; **Town** EC Thurs; Ⓑ, Bar, ✉, R, V, Gas.

BOSCASTLE, Cornwall, 50°41'·45N 04°42·10W. AC 1156. HW −0543 on Dover; see 10.11.25. A tiny, picturesque hbr, almost a land-locked cleft in the cliffs. Access HW±2, but not in onshore winds when swell causes surge inside. An E'ly appr, S of Meachard Rk (37m high, 2ca NW of hbr), is best. 2 short bkwtrs at ent; moor bows-on to drying S quay.

NEWQUAY, Cornwall, 50°25'·03N 05°05'·12W. AC 1168, 1149. HW −0604 on Dover; ML 3·7m; see 10.11.25. Ent to drying hbr ('The Gap') between two walls, is 23m wide. Beware Old Dane Rk and Listrey Rk outside hbr towards Towan Hd. Swell causes a surge in the hbr. Enter HW±2 but not in strong onshore winds. Berth as directed by Hr Mr. Lts: N pier 2 FG (vert) 2M; S pier 2 FR (vert) 2M. VHF Ch16 14. Hr Mr ☎ (01637) 872809. Facilities: Gas, Gaz, CH. **Town** EC Wed (winter only); FW, Slip, D, V, R, Bar. Note: Shoal draft boats can dry out in Gannel Creek, close S of Newquay, but only in settled weather. Beware causeway bridge about half way up the creek.

HAYLE, Cornwall, 50°11'·74N 05°26'·10W (Chan ent). AC 1168, 1149. HW −0605 on Dover; ML 3·6m; Duration 0555. See 10.11.25. Shelter is very good in drying hbr, but in ground swell dangerous seas break on the bar, drying 2·7m; approx 4m at ent @ MHWS. Yachts may cross the bar in good weather HW±1, but hbr is not recommended for yachts. Charted aids do not necessarily indicate best water. Ldg lts 180°, both FW 17/23m 4M. A PHM lt buoy, Fl (2) R 5s, and a SHM lt buoy, Iso G 2s, are approx 0·75M N of the front ldg lt. Beware training bank W side of ent chan marked by 4 perches (FG lts). The hbr is divided by long pier (approx 300m, stretching almost to ldg lts), which should be left to W. E arm of hbr leads to Hayle, the W arm to Lelant Quay. VHF Ch 18 16 (0900-1700). Hr Mr ☎ (01736) 754043, AB £5. Facilities: EC Thurs; Ⓑ, Bar, FW, ⇌, R, V, P & D (cans).

ST IVES, Cornwall, 50°12'·76N 05°28'·60W. AC 1168, 1149. HW −0605 on Dover; ML 3·6m; Duration 0555. See 10.11.25. Shelter is good except in on-shore winds when heavy swell builds up. 7 ⚓s available, £5. Drying hbr with approx 4·5m at MHWS. Alternative ⚓ in 3m between the hbr and Porthminster Pt to S. From the NW beware Hoe Rk off St Ives Hd, and from SE The Carracks. Keep E of SHM buoy about 1½ ca ENE of E pier. Lts: E pier hd 2 FG (vert) 8m 5M. W pier hd 2 FR (vert) 5m 3M. VHF Ch 12 16. Hr Mr ☎ (01736) 795018. Facilities: **E Pier** FW. **Town** EC Thurs; Gas, Gaz, Ⓑ, ⌷, Bar, ✉, R, V, ⇌.

Volvo Penta service

Sales and service centres in area 12
Republic of Ireland *COUNTY DUBLIN* Western Marine Ltd, Bulloch Harbour, Dalkey, Dublin Tel 00 353 1 2800321 *COUNTY CORK* Kilmacsimon Boatyard Ltd, Kilmacsimon Quay, Bandon Tel 00 353 21 775134 *COUNTY CLARE* Derg Marine, Kilaloe Tel 00 353 61 376364

Area 12

South Ireland
Malahide, south to Liscanor Bay

VOLVO PENTA

12

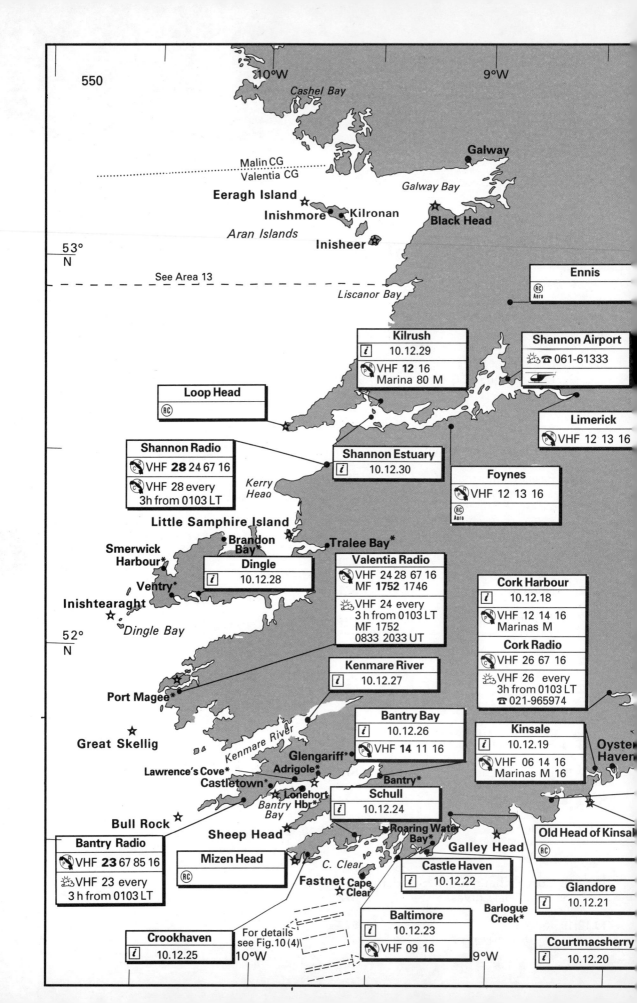

550

10°W   9°W

Cashel Bay

Malin CG
Valentia CG

Galway

Galway Bay

Eeragh Island ☆
Inishmore ● **Kilronan**
Aran Islands
Inisheer

☆ **Black Head**

53°
N

See Area 13

Liscanor Bay

Ennis
(RC) Aero

Kilrush	
ℹ	10.12.29
📻 VHF **12** 16 Marina 80 M	

Shannon Airport	
☼☎ 061-61333	
🚁	

Loop Head	
(RC)	

Limerick
📻 VHF 12 13 16

Shannon Radio	
📻 VHF **28** 24 67 16	
📻 VHF 28 every 3h from 0103 LT	

Kerry Head

Shannon Estuary	
ℹ	10.12.30

Foynes	
📻 VHF 12 13 16	
(RC) Aero	

Little Samphire Island

● **Brandon Bay***

Smerwick Harbour*

☆ **Tralee Bay***

Dingle	
ℹ	10.12.28

Valentia Radio	
📻 VHF 24 28 67 16 MF **1752** 1746	
☼ VHF 24 every 3 h from 0103 LT MF 1752 0833 2033 UT	

Ventry*

Inishtearaght ☆

Dingle Bay

52°
N

Cork Harbour	
ℹ	10.12.18
📻 VHF 12 14 16 Marinas M	
Cork Radio	
📻 VHF 26 67 16	
☼ VHF 26 every 3h from 0103 LT ☎ 021-965974	

Kenmare River	
ℹ	10.12.27

Port Magee* ☆

☆ **Great Skellig**

Kenmare River

Bantry Bay	
ℹ	10.12.26
📻 VHF **14** 11 16	

Kinsale	
ℹ	10.12.19
📻 VHF 06 14 16 Marinas M 16	

Oyster Haven

Glengariff* ●
Adrigole*
Lawrence's Cove*
Castletown*
Bull Rock ☆
● **Bantry***

Lonehort*
*Bantry Hbr***
Bantry Bay

Schull	
ℹ	10.12.24

Bantry Radio	
📻 VHF **23** 67 85 16	
☼ VHF 23 every 3 h from 0103 LT	

Sheep Head ☆

● **Roaring Water Bay***

☆ **Galley Head**

Old Head of Kinsale
(RC)

Mizen Head	
(RC)	

C. Clear

Fastnet ☆ **Cape Clear***

Castle Haven	
ℹ	10.12.22

Barlogue Creek*

Glandore	
ℹ	10.12.21

Baltimore	
ℹ	10.12.23
📻 VHF 09 16	

Crookhaven	
ℹ	10.12.25

For details see Fig.10 (4)
10°W

9°W

Courtmacsherry	
ℹ	10.12.20

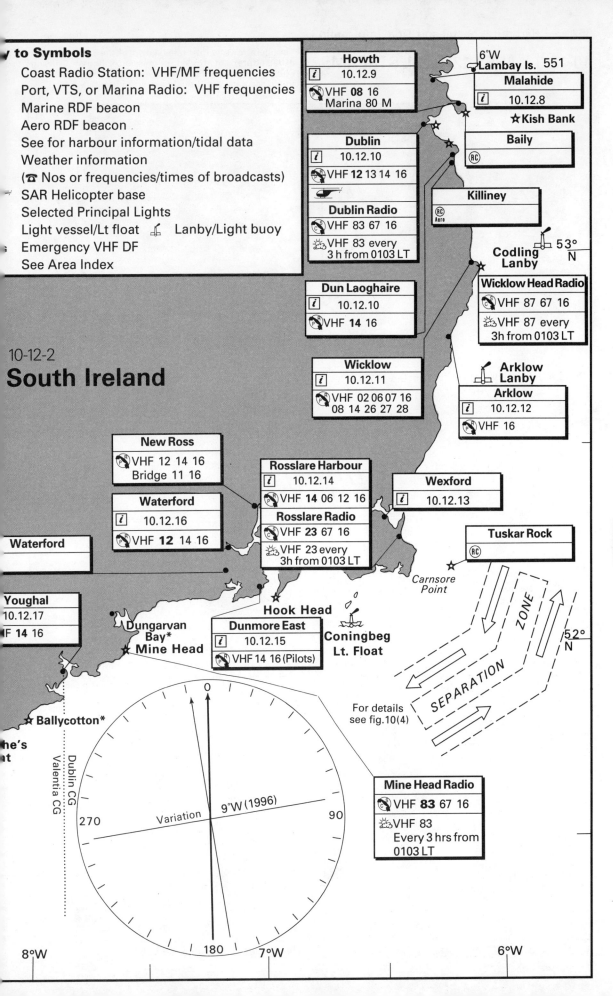

y to Symbols

Coast Radio Station: VHF/MF frequencies
Port, VTS, or Marina Radio: VHF frequencies
Marine RDF beacon
Aero RDF beacon
See for harbour information/tidal data
Weather information
(☎ Nos or frequencies/times of broadcasts)
SAR Helicopter base
Selected Principal Lights
Light vessel/Lt float   Lanby/Light buoy
Emergency VHF DF
See Area Index

10-12-2
South Ireland

Howth
ℹ	10.12.9
📞	VHF **08** 16
	Marina 80 M

6°W
Lambay Is. 551

Malahide
| ℹ | 10.12.8 |

☆ Kish Bank

Dublin
| ℹ | 10.12.10 |
| 📞 | VHF **12** 13 14 16 |

Baily
| 🅡🅒 |

Dublin Radio
| 📞 | VHF 83 67 16 |
| ☀ | VHF 83 every 3 h from 0103 LT |

Killiney
| 🅡🅒 Aero |

Dun Laoghaire
| ℹ | 10.12.10 |
| 📞 | VHF **14** 16 |

Codling Lanby   53° N

Wicklow Head Radio
| 📞 | VHF 87 67 16 |
| ☀ | VHF 87 every 3h from 0103 LT |

Wicklow
| ℹ | 10.12.11 |
| 📞 | VHF 02 06 07 16 08 14 26 27 28 |

Arklow Lanby

Arklow
| ℹ | 10.12.12 |
| 📞 | VHF 16 |

New Ross
| 📞 | VHF 12 14 16 |
| | Bridge 11 16 |

Rosslare Harbour
| ℹ | 10.12.14 |
| 📞 | VHF **14** 06 12 16 |

Wexford
| ℹ | 10.12.13 |

Waterford
| ℹ | 10.12.16 |
| 📞 | VHF **12** 14 16 |

Rosslare Radio
| 📞 | VHF **23** 67 16 |
| ☀ | VHF 23 every 3h from 0103 LT |

Waterford

Tuskar Rock
| 🅡🅒 |

Carnsore Point

Youghal
| 10.12.17 |
| F **14** 16 |

Dungarvan Bay*
☆ Mine Head

Dunmore East
| ℹ | 10.12.15 |
| 📞 | VHF 14 16 (Pilots) |

Hook Head

Coningbeg
Lt. Float

SEPARATION ZONE
52° N

For details
see fig.10(4)

☆ **Ballycotton***

he's
t

Dublin CG
Valentia CG

270

Variation   9°W (1996)

90

Mine Head Radio
| 📞 | VHF **83** 67 16 |
| ☀ | VHF 83 Every 3 hrs from 0103 LT |

180

8°W

7°W

6°W

12

10-12-3   AREA 12 TIDAL STREAMS

The tidal arrows (with no rates shown) off the S and W coasts of Ireland are printed by kind permission of the Irish Cruising Club, to whom the Editors are indebted. They have been found accurate, but should be used with caution.

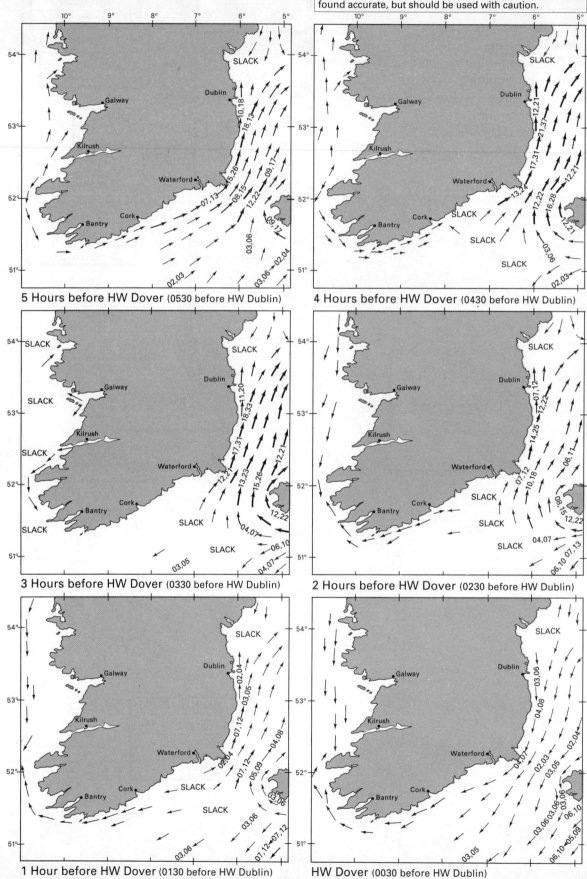

5 Hours before HW Dover (0530 before HW Dublin)

4 Hours before HW Dover (0430 before HW Dublin)

3 Hours before HW Dover (0330 before HW Dublin)

2 Hours before HW Dover (0230 before HW Dublin)

1 Hour before HW Dover (0130 before HW Dublin)

HW Dover (0030 before HW Dublin)

Northward 10.13.3   South Irish Sea 10.11.3

The tidal arrows (with no rates shown) off the S and W coasts of Ireland are printed by kind permission of the Irish Cruising Club, to whom the Editors are indebted. They have been found accurate, but should be used with caution.

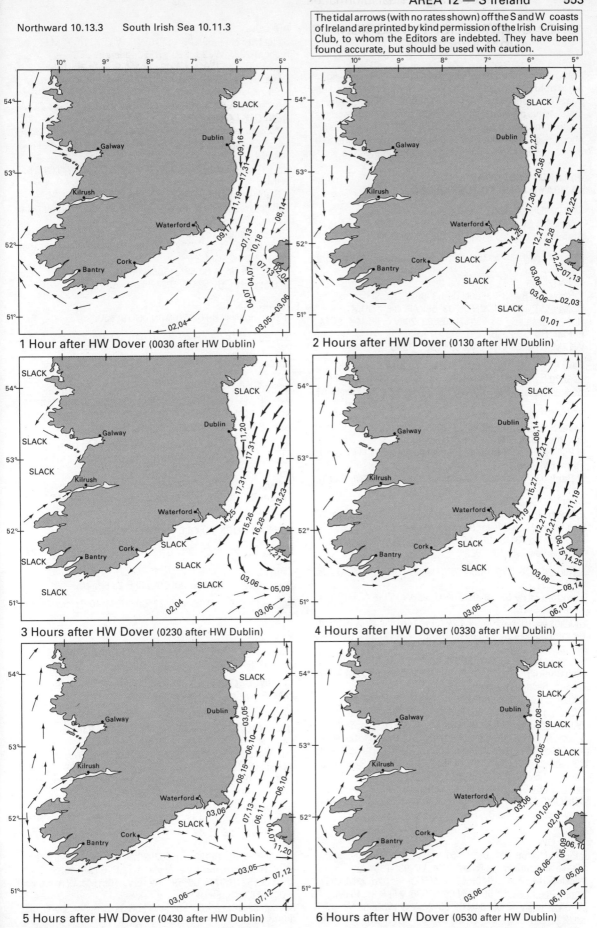

1 Hour after HW Dover (0030 after HW Dublin)

2 Hours after HW Dover (0130 after HW Dublin)

3 Hours after HW Dover (0230 after HW Dublin)

4 Hours after HW Dover (0330 after HW Dublin)

5 Hours after HW Dover (0430 after HW Dublin)

6 Hours after HW Dover (0530 after HW Dublin)

12

10.12.4 COASTAL LIGHTS, FOG SIGNALS AND WAYPOINTS

Abbreviations used below are given in 1.4.1. Principal lights are in **bold** print, places in CAPITALS, and light-vessels, light floats and Lanbys in *CAPITAL ITALICS*. Unless otherwise stated lights are white. m – elevation in metres; M – nominal range in miles. Fog signals are in *italics*. Useful waypoints are underlined – use those on land with care. All geographical positions should be assumed to be approximate. See 4.4.1.

IRELAND - EAST COAST
LAMBAY ISLAND TO TUSKAR ROCK

MALAHIDE/LAMBAY ISLAND
Taylor Rks By 53°30'·00N 06°01'·75W; SHM.
Burren Rks Bn 53°29'·34N 06°02'·40W; SHM.

Dublin Airport 53°25'·75N 06°14'·65W Aero Al Fl WG 4s 95m.

HOWTH
S Rowan Lt By 53°23'·80N 06°03'·89W QG; SHM.
Howth Lt By 53°23'·72N 06°03'·58W Fl G 5s; SHM.
Rowan Rks Lt By 53°23'·87N 06°03'·20W Q (3) 10s; ECM.
E Pier Hd 53°23'·64N 06°03'·97W Fl (2) WR 7·5s 13m W12M, R9M; W Tr; vis W256°-295°, R295°-256°.

Baily 53°21'·68N 06°03'·08W Fl 20s 41m **27M**; Tr; RC.
Rosbeg E Lt By 53°21'·00N 06°03'·39W Q (3) 10s; ECM.
Rosbeg S Lt By 53°20'·00N 06°04'·35W Q (6) + L Fl 15s; SCM.

PORT OF DUBLIN
Great S Wall Hd, **Poolbeg** 53°20'·52N 06°09'·02W Oc (2) R 20s 20m **15M**; R ● Tr; *Horn (2) 60s.*
N Bull Wall Hd, **N Bull** 53°20'·67N 06°08'·92W Fl (3) G 10s 15m **15M**; G ● Tr.
N Bank 53°20'·68N 06°10'·53W Oc G 8s 10m **16M**; G ■ Tr.

DUN LAOGHAIRE
E Bkwtr Hd 53°18'·13N 06°07'·56W Fl (2) 15s 16m **22M**; Tr, W lantern; *Horn 30s (or Bell (1) 6s).*
W Bkwtr Hd 53°18'·17N 06°07'·82W Fl (3) G 7·5s 11m 7M; Tr, W lantern; vis 188°-062°.

N Burford Lt By 53°20'·05N 06°01'·44W Q; *Horn Mo (N) 20s;* SWM.
S Burford Lt By 53°18'·05N 06°01'·21W VQ (6) + L Fl 10s; *Horn 20s;* SWM.
Muglins 53°16'·53N 06°04'·52W Fl 5s 14m 8M; W Tr, R band.
Bennett Bank Lt By 53°20'·15N 05°55'·05W Q (6) + L Fl 15s; *Whis;* SCM.
N Kish Lt By 53°18'·54N 06°56'·36W VQ; NCM.
Kish Bank 53°18'·68N 05°55'·38W Fl (2) 30s 29m **22M**; W Tr, R band; Racon (T); *Horn (2) 30s.*
E Kish Lt By 53°14'·33N 05°53'·50W Fl (2) R 10s; PHM.
E Codling Lt By 53°08'·52N 05°47'·05W Fl (4) R 10s; PHM.
W Codling Lt By 53°06'·95N 05°54'·45W Fl G 10s; SHM.
S Codling Lt By 53°04'·72N 05°49'·70W VQ (6) + L Fl 10s; SCM.
Moulditch Bk Lt By 53°08'·40N 06°01'·16W Fl R 10s; PHM.
Breaches Shoal Lt By 53°05'·65N 05°59'·75W Fl (2) R 6s; PHM.
India N Lt By 53°03'·15N 05°53'·40W Q; NCM.
India S Lt By 53°00'·34N 05°53'·25W Q (6) + L Fl 15s; SCM.
CODLING LANBY 53°03'·00N 05°40'·70W Fl 4s 12m **15M**; tubular structure on By; Racon (G); *Horn 20s.*

WICKLOW
E Pier Hd 52°58'·98N 06°02'·01W Fl WR 5s 11m 6M; W Tr, R base and cupola; vis R136°-293°, W293°-136°.
Wicklow Hd 52°57'·93N 05°59'·83W Fl (3) 15s 37m **23M**; W Tr.
Horseshoe Lt By 52°56'·60N 05°59'·30W Fl R 3s; PHM.
N Arklow Lt By 52°53'·84N 05°55'·20W Q; *Whis;* SCM.
No. 2 Arklow Lt By 52°50'·20N 05°54'·50W Fl R 6s; PHM.

ARKLOW
S Pier Hd 52°47'·59N 06°08'·16W Fl WR 6s 11m 13M; Tr; vis R shore-223°, W223°-350°; R350°-shore.
N Pier Hd 52°47'·61N 06°08'·23W L Fl G 7s 7m 10M.
Roadstone Jetty Hd 52°46'·68N 05°59'·30W Oc R 10s 9m 9M.
No. 1 Arklow Lt By 52°44'·30N 05°55'·96W Fl (3) R 10s; PHM.
S Arklow Lt By 52°40'·80N 05°59'·15W VQ (6) + L Fl 10s; SCM.
ARKLOW LANBY 52°39'·50N 05°58'·10W Fl (2) 12s 12m **15M**; tubular structure on By; Racon (O); *Horn Mo (A) 30s .*
No. 2 Glassgorman Lt By 52°44'·50N 06°05'·30W Fl (4) R 10s; PHM.
No. 1 Glassgorman Lt By 52°39'·06N 06°07'·40W Fl (2) R 6s; PHM.
N Blackwater Lt By 52°32'·20N 06°09'·50W Q; NCM.
E Blackwater Lt By 52°28'·00N 06°08'·00W Q (3) 10s; *Horn (3) 20s;* SCM.
SE Blackwater Lt By 52°25'·62N 06°09'·70W Fl R 10s; PHM.
S Blackwater Lt By 52°22'·74N 06°12'·80W Q (6) + L Fl 15s; *Whis (2) 30s;* SCM.
Rusk Chan No. 4 By 52°31'·05N 06°10'·75W; PHM.
W Blackwater By 52°25'·83N 06°13'·20W; SHM.

WEXFORD
N Training Wall Bn 52°20'·19N 06°13'·50W.

N Long Lt By 52°21'·42N 06°16'·90W Q; *Horn (3) 30s;* SCM.
West Long Lt By 52°18'·16N 06°17'·90W QG; SHM.
Lucifer Lt By 52°17'·00N 06°12'·61W VQ (3) 5s; ECM.

ROSSLARE
Pier Hd 52°15'·41N 06°20'·22W L Fl WRG 5s 15m W13M, R10M, G10M; R Tr; vis G098°-188°, W188°-208°, R208°-246°, G246°-283°, W283°-286°, R286°-320°.

W Holdens Lt By 52°15'·74N 06°18'·79W Fl (3) G 10s; SHM.
S Long Lt By 52°14'·81N 06°15'·58W VQ (6) + L Fl 10s; SCM; *Whis.*
Splaugh Lt By 52°14'·35N 06°16'·70W Fl R 6s; PHM.
Tuskar 52°12'·17N 06°12'·40W Q (2) 7·5s 33m **24M**; W Tr; RC; Racon (T); *Horn (4) 45s.*

TUSKAR ROCK TO OLD HEAD OF KINSALE

S Rock Lt By 52°10'·80N 06°12'·80W Q (6) + L Fl 15s; SCM.

CARNA
Pier Hd 52°11'·89N 06°20'·80W Fl R 3s 6m 4M.

Barrels Lt By 52°08'·33N 06°22'·00W Q (3) 10s; *Horn (2) 10s;* ECM.

KILMORE
Bkwtr Hd 52°10'·25N 06°35'·10W Q RG 6m 5M; vis R269°-354°, G354°-003°, R003°-077°.

CONINGBEG Lt F 52°02'·38N 06°39'·44W Fl (3) 30s 12m **24M**; R hull, and Tr, Racon (M); *Horn (3) 60s.*

WATERFORD
Hook Hd 52°07'·30N 06°55'·80W Fl 3s 46m **23M**; W Tr, two B bands; Racon (K).
Duncannon Dir Lt 002°. 52°13'·21N 06°56'·19W Oc WRG 4s 13m W11M, R8M, G8M; W Tr on fort; vis G358°-001·7°, W001·7°-002·2°, R002·2°-006°. Same Tr, Oc WR 4s 13m W9M, R7M; vis R119°-149°, W149°-172°.
Duncannon Bar Lt By 52°11'·27N 06°55'·90W Fl G 2s; SHM.
Duncannon Bar Lt By 52°11'·27N 06°56'·23W Fl R 2s; PHM.
Duncannon Spit Lt By 52°12'·67N 06°56'·00W Fl (2) G 5s; SHM.
Passage Pt 52°14'·23N 06°57'·70W Fl WR 5s 7m W6M, R5M; R pile structure; vis W shore-127°, R127°-302°.
Cheek Pt 52°16'·11N 06°59'·30W Q WR 6m 5M; W mast; vis W007°-289°, R289°-007°.
Sheagh 52°16'·29N 06°59'·38W Fl R 3s 29m 3M; Gy Tr; vis 090°-318°.

Kilmokea 52°16'·48N 06°58'·85W Fl 5s.

R. Barrow Railway Bridge 2 FR (Hor); tfc sigs.

Snowhill Pt Ldg Lts 255°. Front 52°16'·37N 07°00'·85W Fl WR 2·5s 5m 3M; vis W222°-020°, R020°-057°, W057°-107°. Rear, Flour Mill, 750m from front, Q 12m 5M.

Queen's Chan Ldg Lts 098°. Front 52°15'·30N 07°02'·32W QR 8m 5M; B Tr, W band; vis 030°-210°. Rear, 550m from front, Q 15m 5M; W mast.

Giles Quay 52°15'·47N 07°04'·15W Fl 3s 9m; vis 255°-086°.

Cove 52°15'·02N 07°05'·10W Fl WRG 6s 6m 2M; W Tr; vis R111°-161°, G161°-234°, W234°-111°.

Smelting Ho Pt 52°15'·13N 07°05'·20W Q 8m 3M; W mast.

Ballycar 52°15'·06N 07°05'·42W Fl RG 3s 5m; vis G127°-212°, R212°-284°.

DUNMORE EAST

Dunmore East, E Pier Hd 52°08'·91N 06°59'·32W Fl WR 8s 13m **W17M**, R13M; Gy Tr, vis W225°-310°, R310°-004°.

E Bkwtr extn 52°08'·96N 06°59'·32W Fl R 2s 6m 4M; vis 000°-310°.

DUNGARVAN

Ballinacourty Pt 52°04'·67N 07°33'·13W Fl (2) WRG 10s 16m W10M, R8M, G8M; W Tr; vis G245°-274°, W274°-302°, R302°-325°, W325°-117°.

Ballinacourty Ldg Lts 083°. Front 52°05'·01N 07°34'·23W Oc 5s 9m 2M; W col, B bands. Rear, 46m from front, Oc 5s 12m 2M; W col, B bands.

Esplanade Ldg Lts 297·5°. Front 52°05'·23N 07°36'·90W FR 8m 2M. Rear, 40m from front, FR 9m 2M.

Helvick Lt By 52°03'·59N 07°32'·20W Q (3) 10s; ECM.

Mine Hd 51°59'·50N 07°35'·20W Fl (4) 20s 87m **28M**; W Tr, B band; vis 228°-052°.

YOUGHAL

Bar Rocks By 51°54'·83N 07°50'·00W; SCM.

Blackball Ledge By 51°55'·32N 07°48'·48W; PHM.

W side of ent 51°56'·55N 07°50'·48W Fl WR 2·5s 24m **W17M**, R13M; W Tr; vis W183°-273°, R273°-295°, W295°-307°, R307°-351°, W351°-003°.

BALLYCOTTON

Ballycotton 51°49'·50N 07°59'·00W Fl WR 10s 59m **W21M**, **R17M**; B Tr, within W walls, B lantern; vis W238°-063°, R063°-238°; *Horn (4) 90s.*

Smiths Lt By 51°48'·56N 08°00'·66W Fl (3) R 10s; PHM.

Pollock Rk Lt By 51°46'·21N 08°07'·80W Fl R 6s; *Bell*; PHM.

CORK

Daunt Rk Lt By 51°43'·48N 08°17'·60W Fl (2) R 6s; PHM.

Cork Lt By 51°42'·89N 08°15'·55W L Fl 10s; *Whis;* Racon (T); SWM.

Fort Davis Ldg Lts 354·1°. Front 51°48'·79N 08°15'·77W Oc 5s 29m 10M; Or □. Rear. Dognose Landing Quay, 203m from front, Oc 5s 37m 10M; Or □, synch with front.

Roche's Pt 51°47'·51N 08°15'·24W Fl WR 3s 30m **W20M, R16M**; vis Rshore-292°, W292°-016°, R016°-033°, W(unintens) 033°-159°, R159°-shore.

Outer Hbr Lt By E2 51°47'·50N 08°15'·62W Fl R 2·5s; PHM.

Chicago Knoll Lt By E1 51°47'·66N 08°15'·50W Fl G 5s; SHM.

The Sound Lt By E4 51°47'·91N 08°15'·72W Q; NCM.

White Bay Ldg Lts 034·6°. Front 51°48'·51N 08°15'·18W Oc R 5s 11m 5M; W hut. Rear, 113m from front, Oc R 5s 21m 5M; W hut; synch with front.

Curraghbinney Ldg Lts 252°. Front 51°48'·63N 08°17'·56W F 10m 3M; W ◊ on col. Rear, 61m from front, F 15m 3M; W ◊ on col; vis 229·5°-274·5°.

Spit Bank Pile 51°50'·70N 08°16'·41W Iso WR 4s 10m W10M, R7M; W house on R piles; vis W087°-196°, W196°-221°, R221°-358°.

East Ferry Marina, E Passage 51°51'·90N 08°12'·75W 2 FR (Vert) at N and S ends.

KINSALE/OYSTER HAVEN

Bulman Lt By 51°40'·11N 08°29'·70W Q (6) + L Fl 15s; SCM.

Charle's Fort 51°41'·72N 08°29'·94W Fl WRG 5s 18m W8M, R5M, G6M; vis G348°-358°, W358°-004°, R004°-168°; H24.

IRELAND – SOUTH COAST
OLD HEAD OF KINSALE TO MIZEN HEAD

Old Hd of Kinsale, S point 51°36'·26N 08°31'·98W Fl (2) 10s 72m **25M**; B Tr, two W bands; RC; *Horn (3) 45s.*

COURTMACSHERRY

Black Tom By 51°36'·39N 08°37'·00W; SHM.

Wood Pt (Land Pt) 51°38'·3N 08°41'·0W Fl (2) WR 5s 15m 5M; vis W315°-332°, R332°-315°.

Galley Hd summit 51°31'·78N 08°57'·14W Fl (5) 20s 53m **23M**; W Tr; vis 256°-065°.

GLANDORE

Sunk Rk Lt By 51°33'·50N 09°06'·80W Q; NCM.

CASTLE HAVEN

Reen Pt 51°30'·95N 09°10'·46W Fl WRG 10s 9m W5M, R3M, G3M; W Tr; vis Gshore-338°, W338°-001°, R001°-shore.

Kowloon Bridge Lt By 51°27'·56N 09°13'·71W Q (6) + L Fl 15s; SCM.

BALTIMORE

Barrack Pt 51°28'·33N 09°23'·65W Fl (2) WR 6s 40m W6M, R3M; vis R168°-294°, W294°-038°.

Loo Rk Lt By 51°28'·42N 09°23'·42W Fl G 3s; SHM.

Fastnet, W end 51°23'·33N 09°36'·14W Fl 5s 49m **27M**; Gy Tr; Racon (G); *Horn (4) 60s.*

Copper Pt Long Island, E end 51°30'·22N 09°32'·02W Q (3) 10s 16m 8M; W ● Tr.

Amelia Rk Lt By 51°29'·95N 09°31'·42W Fl G 3s; SHM.

SCHULL

Ldg Lts 346° Front 51°31'·64N 09°32'·39W Oc 5s 5m 11M, W mast. Rear 91m from front, Oc 5s 8m 11M; W mast.

CROOKHAVEN

Rock Island Pt 51°28'·57N 09°42'·23W L Fl WR 8s 20m W13M, R11M; W Tr; vis W over Long Island B to 281°, R281°-340°; inside harbour R281°-348°, W348° towards N shore.

Mizen Hd 51°26'·97N 09°49'·18W Iso 4s 55m **15M**; vis 313°-133°; RC; Racon (T).

IRELAND – WEST COAST
MIZEN HEAD TO DINGLE BAY

Sheep's Hd 51°32'·57N 09°50'·89W Fl (3) WR 15s 83m **W18M**, **R15M**; W bldg; vis R007°-017°, W017°-212°.

BANTRY BAY/CASTLETOWN BEARHAVEN/WHIDDY ISLE/BANTRY/GLENGARIFF

Roancarrigmore 51°39'·17N 09°44'·79W Fl WR 3s 18m **W18M**, R14M; W ● Tr, B band; vis W312°-050°, R050°-122°, R(unintens) 122°-242°, R242°-312°. Reserve Lt W10M, R6M obsc 140°-220°.

Whiddy Island W clearing Lt 51°41'·01N 09°31'·81W Oc 2s 22m 3M; vis 073°-106°.

W ent, **Ardnakinna Pt** 51°37'·08N 09°55'·06W Fl (2) WR 10s 62m **W17M**, R14M; W ● Tr; vis R319°-348°, W348°-066°, R066°-shore.

FR on radio mast 3·45M 295°.

Castletown Dir Lt 024°. 51°31'·09N 09°54'·05W Dir Oc WRG 5s 4m W14M, R11M, G11M; W hut, R stripe; vis G020·5°-024°, W024°-024·5°, R024·5°-027·5°.

Perch Rk 51°38'·82N 09°54'·43W QG 4m 1M; G col.
Castletown Ldg Lts 010°. Front 51°39'·14N 09°54'·37W Oc 3s 4m 1M; W col, R stripe; vis 005°-015°. Rear, 80m from front, Oc 3s 7m 1M; W with R stripe; vis 005°-015°.

Bull Rock 51°35'·50N 10°18'·02W Fl 15s 83m **21M**; W Tr; vis 220°-186°.

KENMARE RIVER/DARRYNANE/BALLYCROVANE
Ballycrovane Hbr 51°42'·63N 09° 57'·53W Fl R 3s.
Darrynane Ldg Lts 034°. Front 51°45'·90N 10°09'·20W Oc 3s 10m 4M. Rear Oc 3s 16m 4M.

Skelligs Rk 51°46'·09N 10°32'·45W Fl (3) 10s 53m **27M**; W Tr; vis 262°-115°; part obsc within 6M 110°-115°.

VALENTIA/PORTMAGEE
Fort (Cromwell) Pt 51°56'·00N 10°19'·25W Fl WR 2s 16m **W17M**, **R15M**; W Tr; vis R102°-304°, W304°-351°; obsc from seaward by Doulus Hd when brg more than 180°.
FR Lts on radio masts on Geokaun hill 1·20M WSW.
Harbour Rk Lt 51°55'·79N 10°18'·91W Q (3) 10s 4m 5M; vis 080°-040°; ECM.
Ldg Lts 141°. Front 51°55'·49N 10°18'·39W Oc WRG 4s 25m W11M, R8M, G8M; W Tr, R stripe; vis G134°-140°, W140°-142°, R142°-148°. Rear, 122m from front, Oc 4s 43m 5M; vis 133°-233° synch with front.

DINGLE BAY TO LOOP HEAD

DINGLE BAY/VENTRY/DINGLE
Dingle, NE side of ent 52°07'·28N 10°15'·48W Fl G 3s 20m 6M.
Pier Hd 52°08'·21N 10°16'·49W.
Ldg Lts 182°. Front 52°07'·40N 10°16'·53W, rear 100m from front, both Oc 3s.

Inishtearaght, W end Blasket Islands 52°04'·51N 10°39'·66W Fl (2) 20s 84m **27M**; W Tr; vis 318°-221°; Racon (O).

BRANDON BAY
Brandon Pier Hd 52°16'·05N 10°09'·58W 2 FG (vert) 5m 4M.

TRALEE BAY
Little Samphire I 52°16'·23N 09°52'·88W Fl WRG 5s 27m **W16M**, R13M; G13M; Bu ● Tr; vis R262°-275°, R280°-090°, G090°-140°, W140°-152°, R152°-172°.
Gt Samphire I 52°16'·13N 09°51'·78W QR 15m 3M; vis 242°-097°.
Fenit Hbr Pier Hd 52°16'·22N 09°51'·51W 2 FR (vert) 12m 3M; vis 148°-058°.

RIVER SHANNON

Ballybunnion Lt By 52°32'·50N 09°46'·92W VQ; NCM; Racon.
Kilcredaune Hd 52°34'·79N 09°42'·58W Fl 6s 41m 13M; W Tr; obsc 224°-247° by hill within 1M .
Kilcredaune Lt By 52°34'·42N 09°41'·17W Fl (2+1) R 10s; PHM.
Tail of Beal Lt By 52°34'·37N 09°40'·71W Q (9) 15s; WCM.
Carrigaholt Lt By 52°34'·90N 09°40'·47W Fl (2) R 6s; PHM.
Beal Spit Lt By 52°34'·80N 09°39'·94W VQ (9) 10s; WCM.
Beal Bar Lt By 52°35'·16N 09°39'·19W Q; NCM.
Doonaha Lt By 52°35'·44N 09°38'·46W Fl (3) R 10s; PHM.
Letter Pt Lt By 52°35'·42N 09°35'·85W Fl R 7s; PHM.
Asdee Lt By 52°35'·07N 09°34'·51W Fl R 5s; PHM.
Rineanna Lt By 52°35'·51N 09°31'·20W QR; PHM.

Carrig Lt By 52°35'·59N 09°29'·72W Fl G 3s; SHM.
Scattery I Rineana Pt 52°36'·32N 09°31'·03W Fl (2) 7·5s 15m 10M; W Tr; vis 208°-092° (H24).

KILRUSH
Marina Ent Chan Ldg Lts 355°. Front 52°37'·93N 09°30'·26W Oc 3s. Rear, 75m from front, Oc 3s.
Tarbert I N Pt 52°35'·50N 09°21'·79W Iso WR 4s 18m W14M, R10M; W ● Tr; vis W069°-277°, R277°-287°, W287°-339°.
Tarbert (Ballyhoolahan Pt) Ldg Lts 128·2°. Front 52°34'·32N 09°18'·75W Iso 2s 13m 3M; △ on W Tr; vis 123·2°-133·2°. Rear, 400m from front, Iso 5s 18m 3M; G stripe on W Bn.
Garraunbaun Pt 51°35'·59N 09°13'·90W Fl (3) WR 10s 16m W8M, R5M; W ■ col, vis R shore-072°, W072°-242°, R242°-shore.
Rinealon Pt 52°37'·10N 09°09'·77W Fl 2·5s 4m 7M; B col, W bands; vis 234°-088°.

FOYNES
W Chan Ldg Lts 107·6° (may be moved for changes in chan). Front, Barneen Pt 52°36'·89N 09°06'·55W Iso WRG 4s 3m W4M, R3M, G3M; B △ with W stripe on W col with B bands; vis W273·2°-038·2°, R038·2°-094·2°, G094·2°-104·2°, W104·2°-108·2°, R108·2°-114·2°. Rear, E Jetty, 540m from front, Oc 4s 16m 10M; Or △ on post.
Colleen Pt No. 3 52°36'·89N 09°06'·81W QG 2m 2M; W col, B bands.
Hunts (Weir) Pt No. 4 52°37'·01N 09°06'·96W VQ (4) R 10s 2m 2M; W col, B bands.

Beeves Rk 52°39'·00N 09°01'·30W Fl WR 5s 12m W12M, R9M; vis W064·5°-091°, R091°-238°, W238°-265°, W(unintens) 265°-064·5°.
Shannon Airport 52°41'·71N 08°55'·66W Aero Al Fl WG 7·5s 40m.
Dernish I Pier Hd, 2 FR (vert) 4m 2M each end.
E Bkwtr Hd 52°40'·82N 08°54'·80W QR 3m 1M.
Conor Rock 52°40'·91N 08°54'·20W Fl R 4s 6m 6M; W Tr; vis 228°-093°.
N Channel Ldg Lts 093°. Front, Tradree Rk 52°40'·99N 08°49'·82W Fl R 2s 6m 5M; W Trs; vis 246°-110°. Rear 0·65M from front, Iso 6s 14m 5M; W Tr, R bands; vis 327°-190°.
Bird Rock 52°40'·93N 08°50'·22W QG 6m 5M; W Tr.
Grass I 52°40'·41N 08°48'·40W Fl G 2s 6m 4M; W col, B bands.
Laheen's Rk 52°40'·32N 08°48'·10W QR 4m 5M.
S side Spilling Rk 52°40'·0N 08°47'·1W Fl G 5s 5m 5M.
N side, Ldg Lts 061°. Front 52°40'·69N 08°45'·23W, Crawford Rk 490m from rear, Fl R 3s 6m 5M. Crawford No. 2, Common rear, 52°40'·83N 08°44'·84W Iso 6s 10m 5M.
Ldg Lts 302·1°. Flagstaff Rk, 670m from rear, Fl R 2s 7m 5M.
The Whelps 52°40'·67N 08°45'·05W Fl G 3s 5m 5M; W pile.
Ldg Lts 106·5°. Meelick Rk, front 52°40'·23N 08°42'·31W Iso 4s 6m 3M. Meelick No. 2, rear 275m from front Iso 6s 9m 5M; both W pile structures.
Ldg Lts 146°, Braemar Pt, front 52°39'·16N 08°41'·89W Iso 4s 5m 5M. Rear Braemar No. 2, 122m from front, Iso 6s 6m 4M; both W pile structures.
N side Clonmacken Pt 52°39'·50N 08°40'·64W Fl R 3s 7m 4M.
E side Spillane's Tr 52°39'·33N 08°39'·67W Fl 3s 11m 6M; turret on Tr.

LIMERICK DOCK
Lts in line 098·5°. Front 52°39'·48N 08°38'·76W. Rear 100m from front; both F; R ◊ on cols; occas.

Loop Head 52°33'·65N 09°55'·90W Fl (4) 20s 84m **23M**; RC.

10.12.5 PASSAGE INFORMATION

For all Irish waters the Sailing Directions published by the Irish Cruising Club are strongly recommended, and particularly on the W coast, where other information is scarce. They are published in two volumes: *E and N coasts of Ireland* which runs anti-clockwise from Carnsore Pt to Bloody Foreland, and *S and W coasts of Ireland* which goes clockwise. For notes on crossing the Irish Sea, see 10.13.5; and for Distances across it see 10.0.6.

MALAHIDE TO TUSKAR ROCK (charts 1468, 1787)

From the Dublin area (10.12.10) to Carnsore Pt the shallow offshore banks cause dangerous overfalls and dictate the route. This is not a good cruising area, but for passage making it is sheltered from the W winds. Tidal streams run mainly N and S, but the N-going flood sets across the banks on the inside, and the S-going ebb sets across them on the outside.

Malahide (10.12.8), 4M from both Lambay Is and Howth, can be entered in most weather via a chan dredged through drying sandbanks. Ireland's Eye, a rky Is which rises steeply to a height of 99m, lies about 7½ca N of Howth (10.12.9) with reefs running SE and SW from Thulla Rk at its SE end. Ben of Howth, on N side of Dublin B, is steep-to, with no dangers more than 1ca offshore.

Rosbeg Bank lies on the N side of Dublin B. Burford Bank, on which the sea breaks in E gales, and Kish Bank lie offshore in the approaches. The N-going stream begins at HW Dublin – 0600, and the S-going at HW Dublin, sp rates 3kn.

Leaving Dublin B, yachts normally use Dalkey Sound, but with a foul tide or light wind it is better to use Muglins Sound. Muglins (Lt) is steep-to except for a rk about 1ca WSW of the Lt. Beware Leac Buidhe (dries) 1ca E of Clare Rk. The inshore passage is best as far as Wicklow (10.12.11).

Thereafter yachts may take the offshore passage east of Arklow Bank and its Lanby to fetch Tuskar Rock or Greenore Pt. Alternatively the passage inshore of Arklow Bank, avoiding Glassgorman Banks, runs through the Rusk Channel, inside Blackwater and Lucifer Banks, to round Carnsore Pt NW of Tuskar Rock. Arklow (10.12.12) is safe in offshore winds; Wexford (10.12.13) has a difficult entrance. Rosslare (10.12.14) lacks yacht facilities, but provides good shelter to wait out a SW'ly blow.

TUSKAR ROCK TO OLD HEAD OF KINSALE (chart 2049)

Dangerous rks lie up to 2ca NW and 6½ca SSW of Tuskar Rk and there can be a dangerous race off Carnsore Pt. In bad weather or in poor vis, pass to seaward of Tuskar Rk (lt, RC), the Barrels ECM lt By and Coningbeg lt float, using the Inshore Traffic Zone of the Tuskar Rock TSS; see Fig. 10 (2).

If taking the inshore passage from Greenore Pt, stay inside The Bailies to pass 2ca off Carnsore Pt. Watch for lobster pots in this area. Steer WSW to pass N of Black Rk and the Bohurs, S of which are extensive overfalls. In settled weather the little hbr of Kilmore Quay (mostly dries) is available, but there are rks and shoals in the approaches.

Saltee Sound (chart 2740) is a safe passage, least width 3ca, between Great and Little Saltee, conspic islands to S and N. Sebber Bridge extends 7½ca N from the NE point of Great Saltee and Jackeen Rk is 1M NW of the S end of Little Saltee, so care is needed through the sound, where the stream runs 3·5 kn at sp. There are several rks S of the Saltees, but yachts may pass between Coningbeg Rk and the lt float. There are no obstructions on a direct course for a point 1M S of Hook Head, to avoid overfalls and Tower Race, which at times extend about 1M S of the Head.

Dunmore East (10.12.16 and chart 2046) is a useful passage port at the mouth of Waterford Hbr (10.12.15). To the W, beware salmon nets and Falskirt, a dangerous rk off Swines

Pt. There are few offlying rks from Tramore Bay to Ballinacourty Pt on the N side of Dungarvan Bay (10.12.17 and chart 2017). Helvick is a small sheltered hbr approached along the S shore of the bay, keeping S of Helvick Rk (ECM Lt By) and other dangers to the N.

Mine Hd (Lt) has two dangerous rks, The Rogue about 2½ca E and The Longship 1M SW. To the W, there is a submerged rk 100m SE of Ram Hd. Here the W-going stream starts at HW Cobh + 0230, and the E-going at HW Cobh –0215, sp rates 1·5 kn. For Youghal, see 10.12.17. Pass 1ca S of Capel Is. The sound is not recommended.

The N side of Ballycotton B is foul up to 5ca offshore. Ballycotton Hbr (10.12.18) is small and crowded, but usually there is sheltered anch outside. Sound Rk and Small Is lie between the mainland and Ballycotton Is (Lt, fog sig). From Ballycotton to Cork keep at least 5ca off for dangers including The Smiths (PHM Lt By) 1·5M WSW of Ballycotton Is. Pass between Hawk Rk, close off Power Hd, and Pollock Rk (PHM Lt By) 1.25M SE.

Near the easy entrance and excellent shelter of Cork Harbour (10.12.18 and chart 1777), Ringabella B offers temp anch in good weather. 7ca SE of Robert's Hd is Daunt Rk (3·5m) on which seas break in bad weather; marked by SHM lt buoy. Little Sovereign on with Reanies Hd 241° leads inshore of it. The Sovereigns are large rks off Oyster Haven, a good hbr but prone to swell in S'lies. The ent is clear except for Harbour Rk which must be passed on its W side, see 10.12.19. Bulman Rk (SCM Lt By) is 4ca S of Preghane Pt at the ent to Kinsale's fine harbour (10.12.19).

Old Head of Kinsale (Lt, fog sig, RC) is quite steep-to, but a race extends 1M to SW on W-going stream, and to SE on E-going stream. There is an inshore passage in light weather, but in strong winds keep 2M off.

OLD HEAD OF KINSALE TO MIZEN HEAD (chart 2424)

From Cork to Mizen Hd there are many natural hbrs. Only the best are mentioned here. Offshore the stream seldom exceeds 1·5kn, but it is stronger off headlands causing races and overfalls with wind against tide. Prolonged W winds increase the rate/duration of the E-going stream, and strong E winds have a similar effect on the W-going stream.

In the middle of Courtmacsherry B are several dangers, from E to W: Blueboy Rk, Barrel Rk (with Inner Barrels closer inshore), and Black Tom; Horse Rk is off Barry's Pt at the W side of the bay. These must be avoided going to or from Courtmacsherry, where the bar breaks in strong S/SE winds, but the river carries 2·5m; see 10.12.20. Beware Cotton Rk and Shoonta Rk close E of Seven Heads, off which rks extend 50m. Clonakilty B has little to offer. Keep at least 5ca off Galley Hd to clear Dhulic Rk, and further off in fresh winds. Offshore the W-going stream makes at HW Cobh + 0200, and the E-going at HW Cobh – 0420, sp rates 1·5 kn.

Across Glandore Bay there are good anchs off Glandore (10.12.21), or off Union Hall. Sailing W from Glandore, pass outside or inside High Is and Low Is, but if inside beware Belly Rk (awash) about 3ca S of Rabbit Is. On passage Toe Head has foul ground 100m S, and 7½ca S is a group of rks called the Stags. Castle Haven (10.12.22), a sheltered and attractive hbr, is entered between Reen Pt (Lt) and Battery Pt. Baltimore (10.12.23) is 10M further W.

Fastnet Rk (Lt, fog sig) is nearly 4M WSW of C Clear; one rk lies 2½ca NE of the Fastnet. Long Island Bay can be entered from C Clear or through Gascanane Sound, between Clear Is and Sherkin Is. Carrigmore Rks lie in the middle of this chan, with Gascanane Rk 1ca W of them. The chan between Carrigmore Rks and Badger Island is best. If bound for Crookhaven, beware Bullig Reef, N of Clear Is.

Schull (10.12.24) is N of Long Island, inside which passage can be made W'ward to Crookhaven (10.12.25). This is a well sheltered hbr, accessible at all states of tide, entered between

Rock Is Lt Ho and Alderman Rks, ENE of Streek Hd. Anch off the village.

Off Mizen Hd the W-going stream starts at HW Cobh + 0120, and the E-going at HW Cobh – 0500. The sp rate is 4 kn, which with wind against tide forms a dangerous race, sometimes reaching to Brow Hd or Three Castle Hd , with broken water right to the shore.

THE WEST COAST

This coast offers wonderful cruising, although exposed to the Atlantic and any swell offshore; but this diminishes mid-summer. In bad weather however the sea breaks dangerously on shoals with quite substantial depths. There is usually a refuge close by, but if caught out in deteriorating weather and poor vis, a stranger may need to make an offing until conditions improve, so a stout yacht and good crew are required. Even in mid-summer at least one gale may be meet in a two-week cruise. Fog is less frequent than in the Irish Sea. Listen regularly to the Radio Telefis Eireann forecasts; see Table 7(2).

Tidal streams are weak, except round headlands. There are few Lts, so inshore navigation is not wise after dark. Coastal navigation is feasible at night in good visibility. Keep a good watch for drift nets off the coast, and for lobster pots in inshore waters. Stores, fuel and water are not readily available.

MIZZEN HEAD TO DINGLE BAY (chart 2423)

At S end of Dunmanus B Three Castle Hd has rks 1ca W, and sea can break on S Bullig 4ca off Hd. Dunmanus B (chart 2552) has three hbrs: Dunmanus, Kitchen Cove and Dunbeacon. Carbery, Cold and Furze Is lie in middle of B, and it is best to keep N of them. Sheep's Hd (Lt) is at the S end of Bantry Bay (10.12.26; charts 1838, 1840) which has excellent hbrs, notably Glengariff and Castletown. There are few dangers offshore, except around Bear and Whiddy Islands. Off Blackball Hd at W entrance to Bantry B there can be a nasty race, particularly on W-going stream against the wind. Keep 3ca off Crow Is to clear dangers.

Dursey Island is steep-to except for rk 7½ca NE of Dursey Hd and Lea Rk (1.4m)1½ca SW . The Bull (Lt, fog sig) and two rks W of it lie 2·5M WNW of Dursey Hd. The Cow is midway between The Bull and Dursey Hd, with clear water each side. Calf and Heifer Rks are 7½ca SW of Dursey Hd, where there is often broken water. 2M W of The Bull the stream turns NW at HW Cobh + 0150, and SE at HW Cobh – 0420. Dursey Sound (chart 2495) is a good short cut, but the stream runs 4kn at sp; W-going starts at HW Cobh + 0135, and E-going at HW Cobh – 0450. Flag Rk lies almost awash in mid-chan at the narrows, which are crossed by cables 25m above MHWS. Hold very close to the Island shore. Beware wind changes in the sound, and broken water at N entrance.

Kenmare R. (chart 2495 and 10.12.27) has attractive hbrs and anchs, but its shores are rky, with no Lts. The best places are Sneem, Kilmakilloge and Ardgroom. Off Lamb's Head, Two Headed Island is steep-to; further W is Moylaun Is with a rk 300m SW of it. Little Hog (or Deenish) Island is rky 1·5M to W, followed by Great Hog (or Scariff) Is which has a rk close N, and a reef extending 2ca W.

Darrynane is an attractive, sheltered hbr NNW of Lamb Hd. The entrance has ldg lts and marks, but is narrow and dangerous in bad weather. Ballinskelligs Bay has an anch N of Horse Is, which has two rks close off E end. Centre of B is a prohib anch (cables reported).

Rough water is met between Bolus Hd and Bray Hd with fresh onshore winds or swell. The SW end of Puffin Island is steep-to, but the sound to the E is rky and not advised. Great Skellig (lit) is 6M, and Little Skellig 5M WSW of Puffin Is. Lemon Rk lies between Puffin Is and Little Skellig. Here the stream turns N at HW Cobh + 0500, and S at HW Cobh – 0110. There is a rk 3ca SW of Great Skellig. When very calm it is possible to go alongside at Blind Man's Cove on NE side of Great Skellig, where there are interesting ruins.

DINGLE BAY TO LISCANOR BAY (chart 2254)

Dingle Bay (charts 2789, 2790) is wide and deep, with few dangers around its shores. Dingle (10.12.28) has a small marina. The best anchs are at Portmagee and Ventry. At the NW ent to the bay, 2·5M SSW of Slea Hd, is Wild Bank (or Three Fathom Pinnacle), a shallow patch with overfalls. 3M SW of Wild Bank is Barrack Rk, which breaks in strong winds.

The Blasket Is are very exposed, with strong tides and overfalls, but worth a visit in settled weather (chart 2790). Gt Blasket and Inishvickillane each have anch and landing on their NE side. Inishtearaght is the most W Is (Lt), but further W lie Tearaght Rks, and 3M S are Little Foze and Gt Foze Rks. Blasket Sound is the most convenient N-S route, 1M wide, and easy in daylight and reasonable weather with fair wind or tide; extensive rks and shoals form its W side. The N-going stream starts at HW Galway + 0430, and the S-going at HW Galway – 0155, with sp rate 3 kn.

Between Blasket Sound and Sybil Pt there is a race in W or NW winds with N-going tide, and often a nasty sea. Sybil Pt has steep cliffs, and offlying rks extend 3½ca.

Smerwick hbr, entered between Duncapple Is and the E Sister is sheltered, except from NW or N winds. From here the scenery is spectacular to Brandon Bay on the W side of which there is an anch, but exposed to N winds and to swell.

There is no lt from Inishtearaght to Loop Hd, apart from Little Samphire Is in Tralee B, where Fenit hbr provides the only secure refuge until entering the Shannon Estuary. The coast from Loop Hd to Liscanor Bay has no safe anchs, and no lts. Take care not to be set inshore, although there are few offlying dangers except near Mutton Is and in Liscanor Bay.

THE SHANNON ESTUARY (charts 1819, 1547, 1548, 1549)

The estuary and lower reaches of the Shannon (10.12.30), are tidal for 50M, from its mouth between Loop Hd and Kerry Hd up to Limerick Dock, some 15M beyond the junction with R. Fergus. The tides and streams are those of a deep-water inlet, with roughly equal durations of rise and fall, and equal rates of flood and ebb streams. In the entrance the flood stream begins at HW Galway – 0555, and the ebb at HW Galway + 0015.

There are several anchs available for yachts on passage up or down the coast. Kilbaha Bay (chart 1819) is about 3M E of Loop Hd, and is convenient in good weather or in N winds, but exposed to SE and any swell. Carrigaholt B (chart 1547), entered about 1M N of Kilcredaun Pt, is well sheltered from W winds and has little tidal stream. In N winds there is anch SE of Querrin Pt (chart 1547), 4.5M further up river on N shore. At Kilrush (10.12.29) there is a marina and anchs E of Scattery Is and N of Hog Is. Note that there are overfalls 0·75M S of Scattery Is with W winds and ebb tide.

Off Kilcredaun Pt the ebb reaches 4kn at sp, and in strong winds between S and NW a bad race forms. This can be mostly avoided by keeping near the N shore, which is free from offlying dangers, thereby cheating the worst of the tide. When leaving the Shannon in strong W winds, aim to pass Kilcredaun Pt at slack water, and again keep near the N shore. Loop Hd (Lt, RC) marks the N side of Shannon est, and should be passed 3ca off. Here the stream runs SW from HW Galway + 0300, and NE from HW Galway – 0300.

Above the junction with R. Fergus (chart 1540) the tidal characteristics become more like those of most rivers, ie the flood stream is stronger than the ebb, but it runs for a shorter time. In the Shannon the stream is much affected by the wind. S and W winds increase the rate and duration of the flood stream, and reduce the ebb. Strong N or E winds have the opposite effect. Prolonged or heavy rain increases the rate and duration of the ebb. The Shannon is the longest river in Ireland, rising at Lough Allen 100M above Limerick, thence 50M to the sea.

10.12.6   DISTANCE TABLE

Approximate distances in nautical miles are by the most direct route, whilst avoiding dangers and allowing for Traffic Separation Schemes. Places in *italics* are in adjoining areas; places in **bold** are in 10.0.6, Distances across the Irish Sea.

	1	2	3	4	5	6	7	8	9	10	11	12	13	14	15	16	17	18	19	20
1. *Carlingford Lough*	1																			
2. Howth	39	2																		
3. Dun Laoghaire	48	8	3																	
4. Wicklow	63	25	21	4																
5. Arklow	75	37	36	15	5															
6. Tuskar Rock	113	73	70	52	37	6														
7. Rosslare	108	70	66	47	34	8	7													
8. Dunmore East	139	101	102	84	69	32	32	8												
9. Youghal	172	134	133	115	100	63	65	34	9											
10. Crosshaven	192	154	155	137	122	85	85	59	25	10										
11. Kinsale	202	164	168	150	135	98	95	69	35	17	11									
12. Baltimore	239	201	196	177	164	128	132	102	70	54	42	12								
13. Fastnet Rock	250	212	207	189	174	137	144	112	78	60	49	10	13							
14. Bantry	281	243	241	223	208	171	174	146	112	94	83	42	34	14						
15. Darrynane	283	245	240	221	208	172	176	146	114	98	86	44	39	38	15					
16. Valentia	295	257	252	242	227	184	188	165	131	113	102	56	48	55	16	16				
17. Dingle	308	270	265	246	233	197	201	171	139	123	111	69	61	63	29	13	17			
18. Kilrush	361	323	318	299	286	250	254	224	192	176	164	122	114	116	82	66	64	18		
19. *Galway*	366	362	357	339	324	287	291	262	228	210	199	159	150	155	119	103	101	76	19	
20. *Slyne Head*	317	351	346	328	313	276	283	251	217	199	188	153	139	144	113	97	95	75	49	20

SPECIAL NOTES FOR IRELAND
10.12.7

ORDNANCE SURVEY map numbers refer to the Irish OS maps, scale 1:12670 or ½ inch to 1 mile, which cover the whole island, including Ulster, in 25 sheets.

IRISH CUSTOMS: First port of call should preferably be at Customs posts in one of the following hbrs: Dublin, Dun Laoghaire, Waterford, New Ross, Cork, Ringaskiddy, Bantry, Foynes, Limerick, Galway, Sligo and Killybegs. Yachts may, in fact, make their first call anywhere and if no Customs officer arrives within a reasonable time, the skipper should inform the nearest Garda (Police) station of the yacht's arrival. Only non-EC members should fly flag Q or show Ⓡ over Ⓦ lts on arrival. Passports are not required by UK citizens.

IRISH MARINE EMERGENCY SERVICE (IMES): SAR ops anywhere in the Republic are controlled by the MRCC at Dublin ☎ (01) 6620922/0923. These ☎ No(s), as shown in each port, may be used routinely, but in emergency dial 999 and ask for *Marine Rescue.*
Dublin MRCC communicates/relays to vessels via the Coast Radio Stns at Dublin, Wicklow, Rosslare, Minehead, Cork, Bantry, Valentia, Shannon, Malin, Glenhead, Belmullet and Clifden (see 6.3.16 for VHF Chs).
(Note: Ultimately it is planned that the Coast Radio Stns at Valentia and Malin will be designated as MRSC).
The IMES can call out IMES helicopters, based at Dublin, Shannon and Finner (Donegal), the RNLI, Coast & Cliff Rescue Service, Irish Air Corps helicopters and search aircraft, Irish naval vessels, civil aircraft, the Irish lighthouse service and the Garda Siochana. The IMES liaises with UK and France and acts as a clearing house for all messages received during any rescue operation within 100M of the Irish coast.

COAST AND CLIFF RESCUE SERVICE: This is part of the IMES and comprises about 50 stations manned by volunteers, trained in first aid and equipped with inflatables, breeches buoys, cliff ladders etc. Their ☎ numbers (the Leader's residence) are given, where appropriate, under each port.

WEATHER: Weather bulletins (comprising gale warnings and a 24 hrs forecast for the Irish Sea and Irish waters up to 30M offshore) are broadcast by RTE Radio 1 at: 0633, 0755 (Mon-Sat), 0855 (Sun), 1253, 1823 (Sat/Sun), 1824 (Mon-Fri) and 2355, all LT; see Tables 7(1) & 7(2).

TELEPHONE: To call the Irish Republic from the UK, dial 00 (International Exchange), followed by 353 (Irish Republic), then the area code (given in UK ☎ directories or below) minus the initial 0, followed by the ☎ number. To call UK from the Irish Republic: dial 00, then 44 (UK), followed by the Area Code minus the initial 0, eg to call Southampton ☎ 123456, dial 00 44 703 123456.

SALMON DRIFT NETS are everywhere along the S and W coasts, off headlands and islands during the summer and especially May-Jul. They may be 1½ to 3M long and are hard to see. FVs may give warnings on VHF Ch 16, 06, 08.

LIQUIFIED PETROLEUM GAS: In the Republic of Ireland LPG is provided by Kosan, a sister company of Calor Gas Ltd, but the bottles have different connections, and the smallest bottle is taller than the normal Calor one fitted in most yachts. Yachts visiting the Irish Republic are advised to take an ample stock of Calor. Availability of Kosan gas is indicated by the symbol Kos.

INFORMATION: The Irish Cruising Club publishes two highly recommended books of Sailing Directions, one for the South and West coasts of Ireland, the other for the North and East coasts. For further information about the Republic of Ireland, write to Irish Yachting Association, 3 Park Road, Dun Laoghaire, Co Dublin ☎ (01) 2800239 or to Irish Tourist Board, 150 New Bond Street, London W1Y 0AQ ☎ (0171) 493 3201.
Note: Currency in the Republic of Ireland is the Punt (£IR) divided into 100p.

GAELIC: As in Scotland (see 10.8.5), it is helpful to understand some of the commoner words for navigational features (courtesy of the Irish Cruising Club):
Ail, alt: cliff, height. *Ath:* ford. *Barra:* sandbank. *Bel, beal:* river mouth, strait. *Beg:* little. *Bo:* (Cow), sunken rock. *Boy, bwee:* yellow. *Bullig:* shoal, rounded rock. *Caher:* fort. *Camus:* bay, river bend. *Carrick, carrig:* rock. *Cuan, coon:* harbour. *Derg,dearg:* red. *Drum:* hill, ridge. *Duff, dubh:* black. *Ennis:* island. *Fad, fadda:* long. *Fin:* white. *Freagh, free:* heather. *Glas, glass:* green. *Gorm:* blue. *Inish, innis, illaun:* island. *Inver:* river mouth. *Keal, keel:* narrow place, sound. *Kill:* church. *Kin, ken:* head, promontory. *Knock:* hill. *Lea:* grey. *Maan:* middle. *Maol, mwee:* bare. *More, mor:* big. *Rannagh, rin, rush:* point. *Roe, ruadh:* red. *Slieve:* mountain. *Stag, stac:* high rock. *Togher:* causeway.

NORTHERN IRELAND: Belfast CG (MRSC) is at Bangor, Co Down, ☎ (01247) 463933.
HM Customs should be contacted by ☎ at the following ports, if a local Customs Officer is not available:

Kilkeel	☎ (016937) 62158
Belfast	☎ (01232) 358250
Warrenpoint	)
Ardglass	)
Portavogie	) ☎ as Belfast
Larne	)
Londonderry	)
Coleraine	)

12

MALAHIDE   10-12-8

Dublin 53°27'·20N 06°08'·90W

CHARTS
AC 633, 1468; Imray C61, C62; Irish OS 13, 16
TIDES
+0030 Dover; ML 2·4; Duration 0615; Zone 0 (UT)

Standard Port DUBLIN (NORTH WALL) (→)

Times				Height (metres)			
High Water		Low Water		MHWS	MHWN	MLWN	MLWS
0000	0700	0000	0500	4·1	3·4	1·5	0·7
1200	1900	1200	1700				
Differences MALAHIDE							
–0019	–0013	+0014	+0006	+0·1	+0·1	0·0	0·0

SHELTER
Good in new marina, dredged approx 3·2m. Or safe ⚓ about 3ca E of conspic Grand Hotel. Caution: crowded moorings.

FACILITIES
Marina (150, increasing to 300 berths) ☎ 8450216, Fax 845 4255, £IR 11.88, FW, AC, D, P, Gas, BH (30 ton), BY, R, Bar, Ice, ▣;
Malahide YC ☎ 8450216, Slip, Scrubbing posts for <10m LOA; **Services:** Ⓔ, Sh, Kos.
Town ▣, ✉, Ⓑ, ⇌, ✈ (Dublin).

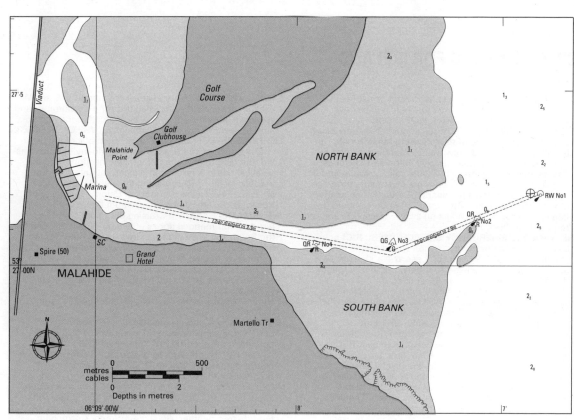

NAVIGATION
WPT 53°27'·20N 06°06'·80W, SWM lt buoy, 082°/262° from/to Grand Hotel, 1·2M. WPT is approx 2ca E of the Bar, dredged 2·9m; appr chan carries 3·3m across drying sandbanks. Do not attempt entry in thick weather or HN, nor in strong onshore winds. The flood reaches 3kn sp, and the ebb 3½kn. Speed limit 4kn in fairway and marina.
LIGHTS AND MARKS
Outer appr with ch spire on 266° just open N of Grand Hotel. The chan across the Bar to the marina is marked by 2 PHM lt buoys QR and 1 SHM lt buoy QG.
Note: Further details of buoys/lts and the alignment of the new dredged chan will appear in the Supplement(s).
RADIO TELEPHONE
Marina Ch **M** (H24) 80. MYC, call *Yacht Base* Ch M (occas).
TELEPHONE (01)
Marina 8450216/8451953/8377755; MRCC 6620922/3; ⌗ 8746571; Police 845 0216; Dr 845 1953; Ⓗ 837 7755.

HOWTH   10-12-9

Dublin 53°23'·60N 06°04'·00W

CHARTS
AC 1415, 1468; Imray C61, C62; Irish OS 16
TIDES
+0025 Dover; ML 2·4; Duration 0625; Zone 0 (UT)

Standard Port DUBLIN (NORTH WALL) (→)

Times				Height (metres)			
High Water		Low Water		MHWS	MHWN	MLWN	MLWS
0000	0700	0000	0500	4·1	3·4	1·5	0·7
1200	1900	1200	1700				
Differences HOWTH							
–0005	–0015	–0005	+0005	0·0	0·0	–0·3	0·0

SHELTER
Good, available at all tides and in almost any conditions.
Marina dredged to 3m. No ent to trawler dock for yachts.
Caution: many moorings in E part of outer hbr. Inside the
inner hbr keep strictly to chan to avoid drying shoals on
either side and a substantial wavebreak. 4kn speed limit.
NAVIGATION
WPT Howth SHM buoy, Fl G 5s, 53°23'·72N 06°03'·53W,
071°/251° from/to E pier lt, 0·27M. Beware Casana Rk 4ca
S of the Nose of Howth, where Puck's Rks extend about
50m off it. Ireland's Eye is 0·6M N of hbr, with the Rowan
Rks SE and SW from Thulla, marked by Rowan Rks ECM,
and S Rowan SHM lt buoys. The usual appr is S of
Ireland's Eye; to the W of which Howth Sound has 2·4m
min depth. Between the Nose and the hbr, watch out for
lobster pots. Beware rks off both pier hds. Give way to
FVs (constrained by draft) in the Sound and hbr entrance.

LIGHTS AND MARKS
E pier lt, Fl (2) WR 7·5s 13m 12/9M; W 256°–295°, R
elsewhere. W sector leads safely to NE pierhead which
should be rounded 50m off. Ent to Trawler Dock has QR
and Fl G 3s. The chan to marina is unlit, but marked by R
and G floating perches with W reflective tops; these are
reported to be difficult to discern at night.
RADIO TELEPHONE
Hr Mr VHF Ch 16 08 (Mon-Fri 0700–2300LT; Sat/Sun
occas). Marina Ch M 80 (H24).
TELEPHONE (01)
Hr Mr 832 2252; MRCC 6620922/3; ⌗ 8746571; Police 832
2806; Dr 832 3191; Ⓗ 837 7755.
FACILITIES
Howth YC Marina (300 inc Ⓥ) ☎ 839 2777, Fax 839 2430,
£10.50, D (H24), P (cans), FW, Slip, C (7 ton), AC, Ⓒ;
Howth YC ☎ 832 2141, Scrubbing posts <20m LOA, R (☎
839 2100), Bar, Ⓒ;
Services: Gas, Kos, ME, SM, CH, EI, Ⓔ.
Town EC Sat; P & D (cans), ✉, Ⓑ, Ⓒ, ⇌, ✈ (Dublin).

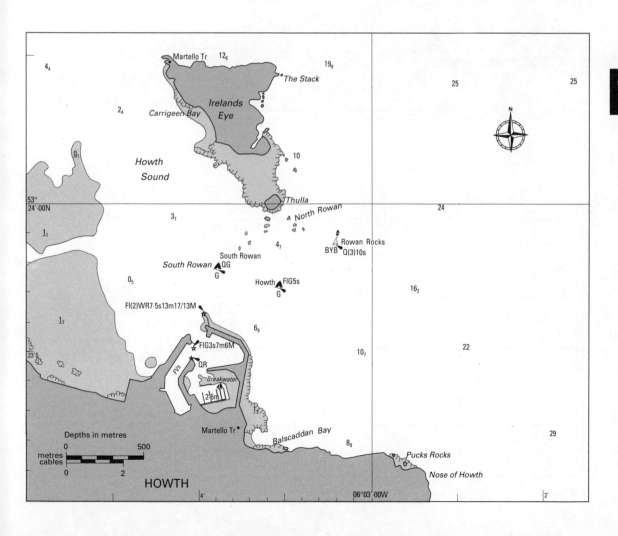

HOWTH

DUBLIN/DUN LAOGHAIRE

Dublin 53°20'·60N 06°08'·90W (Port ent)

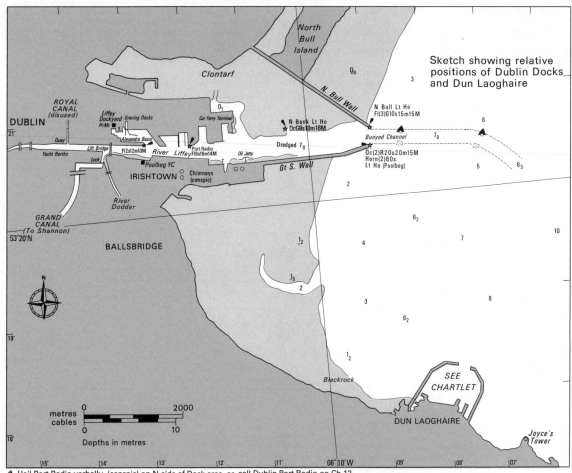

Sketch showing relative positions of Dublin Docks and Dun Laoghaire

⚓ Hail Port Radio verbally, (conspic) on N side of Dock area, or call Dublin Port Radio on Ch 12.

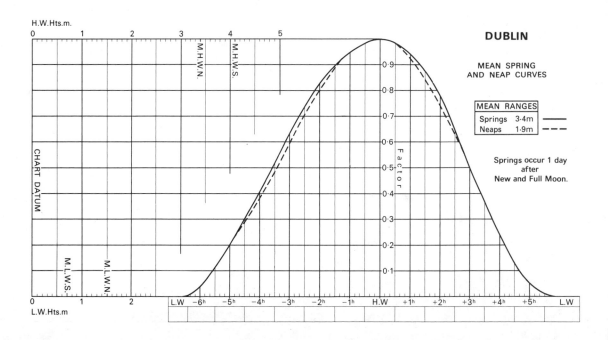

DUBLIN

MEAN SPRING AND NEAP CURVES

MEAN RANGES

Springs	3·4m	——
Neaps	1·9m	- - - -

Springs occur 1 day after New and Full Moon.

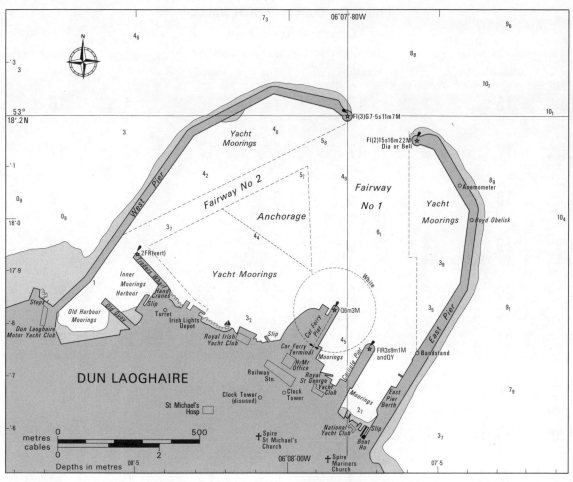

CHARTS
AC 1447, 1415, 1468; Imray C61, C62; Irish OS 16
TIDES
Dun Laoghaire +0042 Dover; ML 2·4; Duration 0640; Zone 0 (UT)

Standard Port DUBLIN (NORTH WALL) (→)

Times				Height (metres)			
High Water		Low Water		MHWS	MHWN	MLWN	MLWS
0000	0700	0000	0500	4·1	3·4	1·5	0·7
1200	1900	1200	1700				

Differences DUBLIN BAR and DUN LAOGHAIRE
–0006	–0001	–0002	–0003	0·0	0·0	0·0	+0·1

GREYSTONES (53°09'N 06°04'W)
–0008	–0008	–0008	–0008	–0·5	–0·4		No data

NOTE: Dublin is a Standard Port and daily predictions for the year are given below.

SHELTER
The following data refers to Dun Laoghaire which is one of the principal yachting centres for Dublin. The hbr is accessible H24, but is open to NE swell and ⚓ holding is poor. All YCs have pontoons, but only for fuelling/loading/ watering. Yachts (and FVs) may find berths SW of Traders Wharf. Do not ⚓ in areas marked 'moorings' nor in fairways.
In adverse conditions, unless YCs can provide sheltered moorings (the best option), yachts should go to Howth (10.12.9) or to Dublin Port. The latter is a commercial port and not very yacht orientated. Yachts must contact Dublin Port Radio Ch 12 for clearance to enter, keeping clear of the fairway and not impeding large vessels. The fairway starts at Rosbeg South SCM lt buoy, approx 2·7M NE of Dun Laoghaire. Expect to berth at the inner end of South Quay, near Poolbeg YC (see FACILITIES).

NAVIGATION
WPT 53°18'·40N 06°07'·00W, 060°/240° from/to ent, 0·47M. Keep clear of the many coasters and ferries, not least the HSS catamarans (41kn). Beware drying rks approx 10m off the end of the E Pier.
LIGHTS AND MARKS
There are no ldg lts/marks. Lt, Q, on Car Ferry Pier has a co-located QY = Ferries under way; small craft keep clear of No 1 Fairway. Other lts as chartlet.
RADIO TELEPHONE
Call *Hbr Office Dun Laoghaire* VHF Ch 14 16. YCs Ch M. At Dublin: call *Dublin Port Radio* Ch **12** 13 14 16 (H24). Lifting bridge (call *Eastlink*) Ch 12 13. Poolbeg YC Ch 12 16. Dublin Coast Radio Stn 16 67 83.
TELEPHONE (01)
Hr Mr 2801130, Dublin 8748772; MRCC 6620922/3; Coast/ Cliff Rescue Service 2803900; ⌗ 2803992; Weather 1550 123855 or 1850 24122; Police (Dublin) 6778141, (Dun Laoghaire) 2801285; Dr 2859244; Ⓗ 2806901.
FACILITIES
There are no overnight charges at either Dun Laoghaire or Dublin Port.
Yacht Clubs
National YC ☎ 2805725, Slip, M, L, C (7 ton), FW, D, R, Bar; **Royal St. George YC** ☎ 2801811, Slip, M, D, L, FW, C (5 ton), R, Bar; **Royal Irish YC** ☎ 2809452, Slip, M, D, L, FW, C (5 ton), R, Bar; **Dun Laoghaire Motor YC** ☎ 2801371, Slip, FW, AB, Bar; **Poolbeg YC** ☎ 6604681, M, Slip, AB, Bar, FW.
Services
FW, C (5 ton), AB, SM, CH, ACA, Sh, Ⓔ, El;, Gas.
City All needs, ⇌, ✈.

IRELAND – DUBLIN (NORTH WALL)

LAT 53°21′N   LONG 6°13′W

TIMES AND HEIGHTS OF HIGH AND LOW WATERS

YEAR 1996

TIME ZONE (UT)
For Summer Time add ONE hour in non-shaded areas

JANUARY

Day	Time	m	Time	m	Time	m	Time	m
1 M	0146	1.3	0833	3.7	1414	1.4	2050	3.6
2 TU	0247	1.3	0928	3.8	1511	1.3	2145	3.7
3 W	0336	1.2	1014	3.9	1559	1.2	2231	3.7
4 TH	0416	1.1	1052	3.9	1639	1.0	2308	3.7
5 F O	0452	1.1	1126	4.0	1715	1.0	2340	3.7
6 SA	0523	1.0	1157	4.0	1749	0.9		
7 SU	0011	3.8	0552	1.0	1228	4.0	1820	0.9
8 M	0043	3.8	0619	1.0	1259	4.0	1850	0.9
9 TU	0117	3.8	0648	1.0	1335	4.0	1921	0.9
10 W	0155	3.8	0724	1.0	1414	3.9	1958	0.9
11 TH	0237	3.7	0804	1.1	1457	3.9	2040	0.9
12 F	0322	3.7	0849	1.2	1542	3.8	2127	1.0
13 SA	0412	3.6	0940	1.3	1632	3.7	2221	1.1
14 SU	0508	3.5	1040	1.4	1729	3.6	2323	1.2
15 M	0612	3.5	1150	1.4	1835	3.6		
16 TU	0034	1.2	0720	3.6	1305	1.3	1948	3.6
17 W	0143	1.1	0825	3.7	1413	1.1	2055	3.8
18 TH	0245	0.9	0923	3.9	1512	0.9	2154	3.9
19 F	0338	0.7	1015	4.2	1605	0.6	2247	4.1
20 SA ●	0426	0.6	1103	4.3	1654	0.5	2335	4.2
21 SU	0511	0.4	1149	4.4	1740	0.2		
22 M	0022	4.2	0554	0.4	1235	4.5	1825	0.2
23 TU	0109	4.1	0639	0.5	1321	4.4	1912	0.3
24 W	0157	4.0	0726	0.6	1410	4.3	2001	0.4
25 TH	0247	3.9	0816	0.8	1501	4.1	2052	0.7
26 F	0340	3.7	0911	1.0	1555	3.9	2145	0.9
27 SA	0438	3.6	1008	1.2	1655	3.7	2241	1.2
28 SU	0541	3.5	1111	1.4	1802	3.5	2344	1.4
29 M	0647	3.4	1222	1.5	1910	3.4		
30 TU	0101	1.5	0751	3.5	1343	1.5	2016	3.4
31 W	0220	1.5	0852	3.6	1451	1.4	2118	3.5

FEBRUARY

Day	Time	m	Time	m	Time	m	Time	m
1 TH	0316	1.4	0945	3.7	1541	1.2	2208	3.5
2 F	0358	1.2	1027	3.8	1620	1.0	2247	3.6
3 SA	0433	1.1	1104	3.9	1654	0.9	2320	3.7
4 SU O	0503	1.0	1136	4.0	1725	0.8	2350	3.7
5 M	0530	0.9	1205	4.0	1753	0.8		
6 TU	0018	3.8	0554	0.8	1234	4.0	1819	0.7
7 W	0049	3.8	0622	0.8	1308	4.0	1850	0.7
8 TH	0125	3.8	0656	0.8	1346	4.0	1927	0.7
9 F	0205	3.8	0735	0.8	1428	3.9	2008	0.7
10 SA	0249	3.8	0819	0.9	1512	3.9	2054	0.8
11 SU	0336	3.7	0908	1.0	1601	3.7	2145	1.0
12 M	0430	3.6	1005	1.1	1657	3.6	2246	1.2
13 TU	0532	3.5	1115	1.3	1806	3.5		
14 W	0000	1.2	0646	3.5	1239	1.3	1927	3.5
15 TH	0120	1.2	0802	3.6	1357	1.1	2041	3.6
16 F	0231	1.0	0906	3.8	1503	0.8	2144	3.8
17 SA	0329	0.8	1002	4.1	1557	0.5	2238	4.0
18 SU ●	0417	0.6	1051	4.2	1644	0.3	2325	4.1
19 M	0500	0.4	1136	4.3	1727	0.2		
20 TU	0007	4.1	0540	0.3	1219	4.4	1809	0.1
21 W	0049	4.1	0621	0.3	1301	4.3	1851	0.3
22 TH	0129	4.0	0704	0.4	1345	4.2	1934	0.4
23 F	0212	3.9	0750	0.6	1431	4.0	2019	0.6
24 SA	0257	3.7	0840	0.8	1519	3.8	2107	0.7
25 SU	0348	3.6	0934	1.0	1614	3.6	2159	1.2
26 M	0448	3.4	1033	1.2	1719	3.4	2258	1.4
27 TU	0558	3.3	1139	1.4	1832	3.2		
28 W	0006	1.6	0708	3.3	1258	1.5	1941	3.2
29 TH	0139	1.6	0814	3.4	1420	1.3	2046	3.3

MARCH

Day	Time	m	Time	m	Time	m	Time	m
1 F	0250	1.5	0911	3.5	1514	1.2	2139	3.4
2 SA	0334	1.3	0959	3.7	1554	1.0	2221	3.5
3 SU	0408	1.1	1037	3.8	1626	0.8	2255	3.6
4 M	0437	0.9	1110	3.9	1655	0.7	2324	3.7
5 TU O	0502	0.8	1216	4.0	1722	0.6	2350	3.8
6 W	0527	0.7	1207	4.0	1749	0.5		
7 TH	0019	3.9	0555	0.6	1241	4.0	1821	0.5
8 F	0055	3.9	0630	0.5	1320	4.0	1858	0.5
9 SA	0136	3.9	0710	0.6	1402	4.0	1940	0.6
10 SU	0220	3.9	0755	0.6	1448	3.9	2028	0.7
11 M	0308	3.8	0846	0.8	1539	3.7	2121	0.9
12 TU	0401	3.6	0946	1.0	1638	3.6	2224	1.1
13 W	0505	3.5	1059	1.1	1750	3.4	2340	1.3
14 TH	0623	3.5	1224	1.1	1916	3.4		
15 F	0103	1.3	0743	3.6	1345	1.0	2032	3.6
16 SA	0217	1.1	0852	3.7	1452	0.7	2136	3.7
17 SU	0316	0.8	0950	4.0	1545	0.5	2229	3.9
18 M	0404	0.6	1040	4.1	1630	0.3	2313	4.0
19 TU ●	0446	0.4	1123	4.2	1712	0.2	2352	4.0
20 W	0525	0.3	1203	4.2	1751	0.2		
21 TH	0027	4.0	0604	0.3	1241	4.2	1829	0.3
22 F	0102	3.9	0644	0.4	1321	4.1	1908	0.5
23 SA	0140	3.8	0726	0.5	1404	3.9	1949	0.7
24 SU	0221	3.7	0813	0.7	1449	3.7	2033	0.9
25 M	0307	3.6	0904	0.9	1539	3.5	2122	1.2
26 TU	0359	3.4	1001	1.1	1639	3.3	2219	1.4
27 W	0508	3.3	1103	1.3	1752	3.1	2324	1.6
28 TH	0625	3.2	1212	1.4	1905	3.1		
29 F	0039	1.6	0734	3.3	1330	1.3	2010	3.2
30 SA	0203	1.5	0834	3.4	1433	1.2	2105	3.3
31 SU	0256	1.3	0924	3.5	1516	1.0	2149	3.5

APRIL

Day	Time	m	Time	m	Time	m	Time	m
1 M	0333	1.1	1005	3.7	1550	0.8	2224	3.6
2 TU	0404	0.9	1040	3.8	1620	0.6	2253	3.8
3 W	0431	0.7	1109	3.9	1649	0.5	2320	3.9
4 TH O	0459	0.6	1140	4.0	1720	0.4	2351	4.0
5 F	0531	0.4	1216	4.0	1755	0.4		
6 SA	0028	4.0	0608	0.4	1257	4.0	1834	0.4
7 SU	0110	4.0	0650	0.4	1342	4.0	1918	0.5
8 M	0157	4.0	0738	0.5	1431	3.9	2008	0.7
9 TU	0247	3.9	0834	0.7	1526	3.8	2105	0.9
10 W	0343	3.7	0939	0.8	1629	3.6	2211	1.1
11 TH	0448	3.6	1052	1.0	1744	3.5	2325	1.2
12 F	0606	3.6	1212	1.0	1906	3.5		
13 SA	0044	1.2	0725	3.6	1329	0.9	2019	3.6
14 SU	0157	1.1	0835	3.8	1433	0.7	2122	3.7
15 M	0256	0.9	0935	3.9	1526	0.5	2214	3.8
16 TU	0345	0.7	1027	4.0	1612	0.4	2259	3.9
17 W ●	0429	0.5	1110	4.1	1653	0.4	2336	3.9
18 TH	0509	0.5	1148	4.1	1732	0.4		
19 F	0007	3.9	0547	0.5	1224	4.0	1807	0.5
20 SA	0039	3.9	0626	0.5	1301	3.9	1844	0.6
21 SU	0114	3.8	0707	0.6	1341	3.8	1922	0.8
22 M	0153	3.7	0751	0.7	1424	3.7	2003	0.9
23 TU	0236	3.7	0840	0.8	1511	3.5	2050	1.1
24 W	0323	3.5	0932	1.0	1604	3.3	2143	1.3
25 TH	0420	3.4	1030	1.2	1709	3.2	2245	1.5
26 F	0533	3.3	1132	1.3	1821	3.1	2352	1.6
27 SA	0648	3.2	1236	1.3	1927	3.2		
28 SU	0100	1.5	0750	3.3	1338	1.2	2023	3.3
29 M	0201	1.4	0842	3.5	1428	1.0	2109	3.5
30 TU	0247	1.2	0926	3.6	1508	0.8	2147	3.6

Chart Datum: 0·20 metres above Ordnance Datum (Dublin)

IRELAND – DUBLIN (NORTH WALL)

LAT 53°21′N   LONG   6°13′W

TIMES AND HEIGHTS OF HIGH AND LOW WATERS

YEAR **1996**

TIME ZONE (UT)
For Summer Time add ONE hour in non-shaded areas

MAY

Day	Time	m	Day	Time	m
1 W	0323 / 1004 / 1543 / 2219	0.9 / 3.8 / 0.6 / 3.8	16 TH	0410 / 1055 / 1634 / 2318	0.8 / 3.9 / 0.6 / 3.9
2 TH	0357 / 1039 / 1617 / 2251	0.7 / 3.9 / 0.5 / 3.9	17 F ●	0453 / 1134 / 1713 / 2349	0.7 / 3.9 / 0.7 / 3.9
3 F O	0431 / 1115 / 1653 / 2326	0.5 / 4.0 / 0.4 / 4.1	18 SA	0532 / 1207 / 1748	0.6 / 3.9 / 0.7
4 SA	0509 / 1155 / 1732	0.4 / 4.1 / 0.4	19 SU	0018 / 0611 / 1242 / 1823	3.9 / 0.7 / 3.8 / 0.8
5 SU	0006 / 0550 / 1240 / 1814	4.1 / 0.4 / 4.1 / 0.4	20 M	0052 / 0650 / 1319 / 1858	3.9 / 0.7 / 3.7 / 0.9
6 M	0051 / 0636 / 1328 / 1902	4.1 / 0.4 / 4.0 / 0.5	21 TU	0130 / 0731 / 1400 / 1936	3.8 / 0.8 / 3.7 / 1.0
7 TU	0139 / 0729 / 1421 / 1954	4.1 / 0.5 / 3.9 / 0.7	22 W	0210 / 0816 / 1443 / 2018	3.8 / 0.9 / 3.5 / 1.1
8 W	0233 / 0828 / 1518 / 2054	4.0 / 0.6 / 3.8 / 0.9	23 TH	0254 / 0904 / 1530 / 2106	3.7 / 1.0 / 3.4 / 1.3
9 TH	0331 / 0933 / 1623 / 2158	3.9 / 0.7 / 3.7 / 1.1	24 F	0342 / 0955 / 1623 / 2201	3.5 / 1.1 / 3.3 / 1.4
10 F	0437 / 1043 / 1735 / 2308	3.8 / 0.8 / 3.6 / 1.2	25 SA	0438 / 1050 / 1724 / 2303	3.4 / 1.2 / 3.2 / 1.5
11 SA	0552 / 1155 / 1849	3.7 / 0.9 / 3.6	26 SU	0543 / 1148 / 1830	3.3 / 1.2 / 3.2
12 SU	0020 / 0706 / 1306 / 1958	1.2 / 3.7 / 0.9 / 3.6	27 M	0006 / 0651 / 1245 / 1930	1.5 / 3.3 / 1.2 / 3.3
13 M	0130 / 0814 / 1409 / 2100	1.2 / 3.8 / 0.8 / 3.7	28 TU	0105 / 0750 / 1338 / 2021	1.4 / 3.4 / 1.1 / 3.5
14 TU	0231 / 0915 / 1504 / 2154	1.0 / 3.9 / 0.7 / 3.8	29 W	0156 / 0841 / 1425 / 2105	1.3 / 3.6 / 0.9 / 3.6
15 W	0324 / 1009 / 1552 / 2240	0.9 / 3.9 / 0.7 / 3.8	30 TH	0242 / 0927 / 1508 / 2145	1.0 / 3.7 / 0.7 / 3.8
			31 F	0325 / 1010 / 1550 / 2225	0.8 / 3.9 / 0.6 / 4.0

JUNE

Day	Time	m	Day	Time	m
1 SA O	0407 / 1054 / 1631 / 2306	0.6 / 4.0 / 0.4 / 4.1	16 SU ●	0517 / 1150 / 1730	0.8 / 3.8 / 0.9
2 SU	0450 / 1139 / 1714 / 2349	0.4 / 4.1 / 0.4 / 4.2	17 M	0000 / 0555 / 1223 / 1803	3.9 / 0.8 / 3.7 / 0.9
3 M	0536 / 1226 / 1759	0.3 / 4.1 / 0.4	18 TU	0032 / 0614 / 1257 / 1835	3.9 / 0.8 / 3.7 / 1.0
4 TU	0035 / 0625 / 1316 / 1847	4.3 / 0.3 / 4.1 / 0.5	19 W	0107 / 0709 / 1334 / 1909	3.9 / 0.8 / 3.7 / 1.0
5 W	0126 / 0719 / 1410 / 1940	4.2 / 0.4 / 4.0 / 0.7	20 TH	0145 / 0748 / 1414 / 1945	3.8 / 0.9 / 3.6 / 1.1
6 TH	0220 / 0818 / 1508 / 2038	4.2 / 0.5 / 3.9 / 0.8	21 F	0225 / 0828 / 1456 / 2026	3.8 / 0.9 / 3.6 / 1.2
7 F	0318 / 0921 / 1610 / 2139	4.1 / 0.6 / 3.8 / 1.0	22 SA	0309 / 0912 / 1541 / 2112	3.7 / 1.0 / 3.5 / 1.3
8 SA	0422 / 1025 / 1716 / 2244	4.0 / 0.7 / 3.7 / 1.1	23 SU	0357 / 1001 / 1631 / 2204	3.6 / 1.1 / 3.4 / 1.4
9 SU	0532 / 1130 / 1824 / 2350	3.9 / 0.9 / 3.6 / 1.2	24 M	0449 / 1054 / 1728 / 2303	3.5 / 1.1 / 3.4 / 1.4
10 M	0642 / 1237 / 1931	3.8 / 0.9 / 3.6	25 TU	0549 / 1152 / 1829	3.4 / 1.2 / 3.4
11 TU	0058 / 0749 / 1341 / 2032	1.2 / 3.8 / 1.0 / 3.7	26 W	0007 / 0653 / 1251 / 1930	1.4 / 3.5 / 1.1 / 3.5
12 W	0204 / 0851 / 1440 / 2129	1.2 / 3.8 / 1.0 / 3.7	27 TH	0110 / 0757 / 1347 / 2026	1.3 / 3.6 / 1.0 / 3.6
13 TH	0302 / 0948 / 1531 / 2217	1.1 / 3.8 / 0.9 / 3.8	28 F	0206 / 0855 / 1439 / 2117	1.1 / 3.7 / 0.9 / 3.8
14 F	0352 / 1036 / 1615 / 2258	1.0 / 3.8 / 0.9 / 3.8	29 SA	0259 / 0947 / 1527 / 2204	0.9 / 3.9 / 0.7 / 4.0
15 SA	0437 / 1117 / 1654 / 2331	0.9 / 3.8 / 0.9 / 3.9	30 SU	0348 / 1037 / 1614 / 2250	0.7 / 4.0 / 0.5 / 4.2

JULY

Day	Time	m	Day	Time	m
1 M O	0437 / 1125 / 1659 / 2335	0.4 / 4.1 / 0.4 / 4.3	16 TU	0536 / 1202 / 1742	0.9 / 3.7 / 1.0
2 TU	0525 / 1213 / 1745	0.3 / 4.2 / 0.4	17 W	0011 / 0610 / 1234 / 1811	3.9 / 0.8 / 3.7 / 0.9
3 W	0021 / 0614 / 1303 / 1832	4.4 / 0.3 / 4.1 / 0.5	18 TH	0043 / 0642 / 1307 / 1839	3.9 / 0.8 / 3.7 / 0.9
4 TH	0111 / 0706 / 1355 / 1922	4.4 / 0.3 / 4.1 / 0.6	19 F	0117 / 0713 / 1343 / 1912	3.9 / 0.8 / 3.7 / 1.0
5 F	0203 / 0801 / 1449 / 2016	4.3 / 0.4 / 4.0 / 0.7	20 SA	0155 / 0748 / 1422 / 1950	3.9 / 0.9 / 3.7 / 1.0
6 SA	0259 / 0859 / 1546 / 2114	4.2 / 0.6 / 3.8 / 0.9	21 SU	0237 / 0827 / 1505 / 2032	3.8 / 0.9 / 3.6 / 1.1
7 SU	0358 / 0958 / 1648 / 2214	4.0 / 0.7 / 3.7 / 1.1	22 M	0322 / 0912 / 1551 / 2119	3.8 / 1.0 / 3.6 / 1.2
8 M	0504 / 1059 / 1752 / 2317	3.9 / 0.9 / 3.6 / 1.2	23 TU	0410 / 1003 / 1643 / 2213	3.7 / 1.1 / 3.5 / 1.3
9 TU	0613 / 1203 / 1857	3.8 / 1.1 / 3.6	24 W	0505 / 1101 / 1741 / 2317	3.5 / 1.2 / 3.4 / 1.4
10 W	0025 / 0720 / 1310 / 2000	1.3 / 3.7 / 1.2 / 3.6	25 TH	0610 / 1207 / 1848	3.5 / 1.2 / 3.5
11 TH	0136 / 0825 / 1415 / 2100	1.3 / 3.6 / 1.2 / 3.7	26 F	0029 / 0723 / 1314 / 1954	1.3 / 3.5 / 1.1 / 3.6
12 F	0242 / 0925 / 1511 / 2152	1.3 / 3.6 / 1.2 / 3.8	27 SA	0139 / 0831 / 1416 / 2054	1.2 / 3.6 / 1.0 / 3.8
13 SA	0336 / 1017 / 1557 / 2235	1.1 / 3.7 / 1.1 / 3.8	28 SU	0241 / 0930 / 1511 / 2147	0.9 / 3.8 / 0.8 / 4.0
14 SU	0421 / 1058 / 1636 / 2310	1.0 / 3.7 / 1.1 / 3.9	29 M	0336 / 1023 / 1600 / 2235	0.7 / 4.0 / 0.6 / 4.2
15 M ●	0501 / 1131 / 1710 / 2340	0.9 / 3.7 / 1.0 / 3.9	30 TU O	0426 / 1112 / 1646 / 2321	0.4 / 4.1 / 0.5 / 4.4
			31 W	0513 / 1159 / 1730	0.2 / 4.2 / 0.4

AUGUST

Day	Time	m	Day	Time	m
1 TH	0005 / 0559 / 1245 / 1814	4.5 / 0.2 / 4.2 / 0.4	16 F	0016 / 0609 / 1238 / 1810	4.0 / 0.8 / 3.8 / 0.8
2 F	0052 / 0647 / 1333 / 1901	4.4 / 0.2 / 4.1 / 0.5	17 SA	0049 / 0637 / 1312 / 1841	4.0 / 0.7 / 3.8 / 0.8
3 SA	0140 / 0737 / 1422 / 1951	4.4 / 0.3 / 4.0 / 0.6	18 SU	0125 / 0711 / 1350 / 1918	4.0 / 0.7 / 3.8 / 0.9
4 SU	0231 / 0830 / 1514 / 2044	4.2 / 0.5 / 3.8 / 0.8	19 M	0206 / 0750 / 1432 / 1959	3.9 / 0.8 / 3.8 / 0.9
5 M	0327 / 0925 / 1610 / 2141	4.0 / 0.8 / 3.7 / 1.0	20 TU	0250 / 0835 / 1518 / 2046	3.8 / 0.9 / 3.7 / 1.0
6 TU	0428 / 1022 / 1712 / 2242	3.8 / 1.0 / 3.6 / 1.2	21 W	0338 / 0925 / 1607 / 2139	3.7 / 1.0 / 3.6 / 1.2
7 W	0538 / 1123 / 1819 / 2349	3.6 / 1.3 / 3.5 / 1.4	22 TH	0433 / 1024 / 1705 / 2244	3.6 / 1.2 / 3.5 / 1.3
8 TH	0649 / 1232 / 1925	3.5 / 1.4 / 3.5	23 F	0539 / 1134 / 1814	3.5 / 1.3 / 3.5
9 F	0106 / 0757 / 1348 / 2028	1.4 / 3.5 / 1.4 / 3.6	24 SA	0002 / 0659 / 1250 / 1929	1.3 / 3.5 / 1.3 / 3.6
10 SA	0222 / 0902 / 1450 / 2124	1.4 / 3.5 / 1.4 / 3.7	25 SU	0122 / 0815 / 1359 / 2035	1.2 / 3.6 / 1.1 / 3.8
11 SU	0320 / 0955 / 1537 / 2210	1.2 / 3.6 / 1.2 / 3.8	26 M	0230 / 0918 / 1458 / 2131	0.9 / 3.8 / 0.9 / 4.0
12 M	0404 / 1036 / 1615 / 2247	1.1 / 3.6 / 1.1 / 3.9	27 TU	0327 / 1012 / 1548 / 2220	0.6 / 4.0 / 0.7 / 4.2
13 TU	0440 / 1110 / 1648 / 2319	1.0 / 3.7 / 1.0 / 4.0	28 W O	0416 / 1059 / 1633 / 2305	0.4 / 4.1 / 0.5 / 4.4
14 W ●	0513 / 1140 / 1718 / 2348	0.8 / 3.7 / 0.8 / 4.0	29 TH	0500 / 1143 / 1715 / 2348	0.2 / 4.2 / 0.4 / 4.5
15 TH	0543 / 1208 / 1744	0.8 / 3.8 / 0.9	30 F	0543 / 1225 / 1756	0.1 / 4.2 / 0.3
			31 SA	0031 / 0626 / 1308 / 1839	4.4 / 0.2 / 4.1 / 0.4

12

Chart Datum: 0·20 metres above Ordnance Datum (Dublin)

IRELAND – DUBLIN (NORTH WALL)

LAT 53°21′N   LONG 6°13′W

TIMES AND HEIGHTS OF HIGH AND LOW WATERS

YEAR **1996**

TIME ZONE (UT)
For Summer Time add ONE hour in non-shaded areas

SEPTEMBER

Day	Time	m	Time	m	Time	m	Time	m
1 SU	0115	4.3	0711	0.4	1352	4.0	1925	0.6
2 M	0202	4.2	0758	0.6	1439	3.9	2015	0.8
3 TU	0253	4.0	0849	0.9	1530	3.7	2110	1.0
4 W	0351	3.7	0943	1.1	1628	3.6	2209	1.2
5 TH	0459	3.5	1042	1.4	1736	3.4	2315	1.4
6 F	0614	3.3	1149	1.6	1846	3.4		
7 SA	0031	1.5	0726	3.3	1311	1.6	1952	3.5
8 SU	0157	1.4	0834	3.4	1424	1.5	2052	3.6
9 M	0256	1.2	0929	3.5	1513	1.3	2141	3.8
10 TU	0339	1.0	1011	3.6	1551	1.1	2220	3.9
11 W	0414	0.9	1045	3.7	1623	1.0	2254	4.0
12 TH ●	0444	0.8	1115	3.8	1651	0.9	2323	4.0
13 F	0512	0.7	1142	3.8	1716	0.8	2350	4.0
14 SA	0537	0.6	1209	3.9	1742	0.7		
15 SU	0020	4.0	0604	0.6	1242	3.9	1813	0.7
16 M	0057	4.0	0639	0.6	1321	3.9	1850	0.7
17 TU	0138	4.0	0719	0.7	1403	3.9	1933	0.8
18 W	0223	3.9	0804	0.8	1449	3.8	2021	0.9
19 TH	0313	3.8	0857	1.0	1540	3.7	2117	1.1
20 F	0410	3.6	0958	1.2	1638	3.6	2225	1.2
21 SA	0520	3.5	1112	1.3	1748	3.5	2347	1.3
22 SU	0645	3.5	1231	1.4	1907	3.6		
23 M	0109	1.1	0802	3.6	1344	1.2	2017	3.8
24 TU	0220	0.9	0907	3.8	1444	1.0	2116	4.0
25 W	0316	0.6	1001	4.0	1534	0.7	2206	4.2
26 TH	0403	0.4	1047	4.1	1618	0.5	2251	4.3
27 F O	0446	0.2	1128	4.2	1659	0.4	2332	4.4
28 SA	0526	0.2	1207	4.1	1739	0.4		
29 SU	0012	4.4	0605	0.3	1245	4.1	1820	0.4
30 M	0053	4.2	0646	0.5	1324	4.0	1903	0.6

OCTOBER

Day	Time	m	Time	m	Time	m	Time	m
1 TU	0137	4.1	0729	0.7	1407	3.9	1951	0.7
2 W	0225	3.9	0816	0.9	1454	3.8	2043	0.9
3 TH	0318	3.7	0908	1.2	1548	3.6	2140	1.2
4 F	0422	3.4	1005	1.4	1652	3.5	2242	1.3
5 SA	0536	3.3	1110	1.6	1805	3.4	2352	1.4
6 SU	0650	3.2	1223	1.7	1914	3.4		
7 M	0114	1.4	0757	3.3	1344	1.6	2015	3.6
8 TU	0221	1.3	0854	3.5	1440	1.4	2107	3.7
9 W	0306	1.1	0939	3.6	1520	1.2	2149	3.8
10 TH	0342	0.9	1016	3.8	1553	1.0	2225	3.9
11 F	0412	0.8	1047	3.9	1622	0.9	2256	4.0
12 SA ●	0439	0.7	1114	3.9	1725	0.8	2324	4.0
13 SU	0506	0.6	1142	4.0	1717	0.7	2355	4.1
14 M	0537	0.6	1215	4.1	1750	0.6		
15 TU	0033	4.1	0612	0.6	1254	4.1	1829	0.7
16 W	0116	4.0	0654	0.7	1338	4.0	1913	0.7
17 TH	0203	3.9	0741	0.9	1426	4.0	2005	0.9
18 F	0256	3.8	0836	1.1	1519	3.9	2105	1.0
19 SA	0357	3.7	0941	1.2	1619	3.8	2215	1.1
20 SU	0510	3.5	1054	1.4	1730	3.7	2334	1.2
21 M	0632	3.5	1212	1.4	1847	3.7		
22 TU	0054	1.1	0747	3.7	1324	1.3	1957	3.9
23 W	0202	0.9	0852	3.8	1425	1.1	2059	4.0
24 TH	0259	0.7	0946	4.0	1517	0.9	2152	4.2
25 F	0347	0.5	1033	4.1	1603	0.7	2238	4.2
26 SA O	0430	0.4	1114	4.1	1645	0.6	2319	4.3
27 SU	0509	0.4	1151	4.1	1725	0.5	2357	4.2
28 M	0547	0.5	1225	4.1	1805	0.6		
29 TU	0036	4.1	0624	0.6	1302	4.1	1846	0.6
30 W	0118	4.0	0703	0.8	1342	4.0	1931	0.8
31 TH	0202	3.8	0746	1.0	1426	3.9	2019	0.9

NOVEMBER

Day	Time	m	Time	m	Time	m	Time	m
1 F	0252	3.7	0835	1.2	1514	3.7	2112	1.1
2 SA	0348	3.5	0930	1.5	1611	3.6	2210	1.3
3 SU	0455	3.3	1032	1.6	1718	3.5	2312	1.4
4 M	0607	3.3	1139	1.7	1828	3.4		
5 TU	0020	1.4	0714	3.3	1249	1.7	1931	3.5
6 W	0127	1.3	0812	3.5	1352	1.6	2026	3.6
7 TH	0221	1.2	0900	3.6	1440	1.4	2113	3.7
8 F	0301	1.1	0941	3.8	1517	1.2	2152	3.8
9 SA	0335	0.8	1015	3.9	1550	1.0	2226	4.0
10 SU	0407	0.7	1045	4.0	1621	0.8	2259	4.0
11 M ●	0439	0.6	1116	4.1	1654	0.7	2334	4.1
12 TU	0513	0.6	1152	4.2	1732	0.5	2357	4.2
13 W	0015	4.1	0552	0.6	1233	4.2	1814	0.6
14 TH	0100	4.1	0635	0.7	1319	4.2	1901	0.6
15 F	0150	4.0	0724	0.8	1409	4.1	1955	0.7
16 SA	0245	3.9	0821	1.0	1504	4.0	2056	0.9
17 SU	0347	3.8	0925	1.2	1604	4.0	2203	1.0
18 M	0458	3.7	1035	1.3	1712	3.9	2316	1.0
19 TU	0613	3.7	1148	1.4	1824	3.9		
20 W	0030	1.0	0725	3.7	1259	1.3	1934	3.9
21 TH	0138	0.9	0830	3.8	1402	1.2	2039	4.0
22 F	0237	0.8	0926	4.0	1458	1.0	2136	4.0
23 SA	0329	0.7	1016	4.0	1547	0.9	2227	4.1
24 SU	0413	0.7	1100	4.1	1632	0.8	2310	4.1
25 M O	0454	0.7	1137	4.1	1713	0.7	2347	4.0
26 TU	0531	0.7	1209	4.1	1753	0.7		
27 W	0022	4.0	0606	0.8	1243	4.1	1832	0.7
28 TH	0100	3.9	0643	0.9	1320	4.0	1913	0.8
29 F	0141	3.8	0721	1.1	1401	3.9	1957	0.9
30 SA	0225	3.7	0804	1.2	1444	3.9	2044	1.0

DECEMBER

Day	Time	m	Time	m	Time	m	Time	m
1 SU	0314	3.5	0853	1.4	1531	3.7	2134	1.2
2 M	0408	3.4	0949	1.5	1625	3.6	2229	1.3
3 TU	0512	3.3	1051	1.7	1727	3.5	2328	1.4
4 W	0620	3.3	1154	1.7	1834	3.4		
5 TH	0028	1.4	0721	3.4	1256	1.7	1935	3.5
6 F	0125	1.3	0815	3.5	1350	1.5	2028	3.6
7 SA	0215	1.2	0900	3.7	1436	1.3	2114	3.7
8 SU	0258	1.0	0940	3.9	1517	1.1	2156	3.9
9 M	0337	0.8	1017	4.0	1556	0.9	2236	4.0
10 TU ●	0415	0.7	1054	4.2	1636	0.7	2318	4.1
11 W	0455	0.6	1134	4.3	1718	0.6		
12 TH	0001	4.2	0536	0.6	1217	4.3	1802	0.5
13 F	0048	4.2	0621	0.6	1304	4.3	1851	0.5
14 SA	0138	4.1	0710	0.7	1354	4.3	1944	0.6
15 SU	0233	4.0	0805	0.9	1448	4.2	2042	0.7
16 M	0333	3.9	0905	1.1	1547	4.1	2144	0.8
17 TU	0438	3.8	1010	1.2	1650	4.0	2250	0.9
18 W	0547	3.7	1118	1.3	1759	3.9	2359	1.0
19 TH	0657	3.7	1228	1.4	1909	3.8		
20 F	0109	1.1	0802	3.8	1337	1.3	2016	3.8
21 SA	0214	1.1	0903	3.9	1439	1.2	2119	3.9
22 SU	0311	1.0	0957	3.9	1533	1.1	2214	3.9
23 M	0358	1.0	1044	4.0	1620	1.0	2300	3.9
24 TU O	0440	0.9	1123	4.1	1702	0.9	2337	3.9
25 W	0517	0.9	1156	4.1	1741	0.8		
26 TH	0009	3.8	0551	0.9	1227	4.1	1818	0.8
27 F	0043	3.8	0624	1.0	1300	4.0	1855	0.8
28 SA	0119	3.8	0658	1.0	1336	4.0	1932	0.9
29 SU	0157	3.7	0733	1.1	1414	3.9	2011	0.9
30 M	0238	3.6	0811	1.2	1455	3.8	2052	1.0
31 TU	0322	3.6	0854	1.3	1539	3.7	2136	1.2

Chart Datum: 0·20 metres above Ordnance Datum (Dublin)

WICKLOW
10-12-11

Wicklow 52°58'·98N 06°02'·70W

CHARTS
AC 633, 1468; Imray C61; Irish OS 16
TIDES
–0010 Dover; ML 1·7; Duration 0640; Zone 0 (UT)

Standard Port DUBLIN (NORTH WALL) (←—)

Times				Height (metres)			
High Water		Low Water		MHWS	MHWN	MLWN	MLWS
0000	0700	0000	0500	4·1	3·4	1·5	0·7
1200	1900	1200	1700				
Differences WICKLOW							
–0019	–0019	–0024	–0026	–1·4	–1·1	–0·4	0·0

SHELTER
Very safe, and access H24. Outer hbr is open to NE winds which cause a swell. Moorings in NW of hbr belong to YC. Berths on E Pier (1·7m) are convenient and now well fendered; W pier is not recommended. Inner hbr (river) gives excellent shelter in 1·8m on New Quay (S), which is used by FVs. Packet Quay (N) is for ships (2·1m), but may be used if none due. ⌁ in hbr is restricted by ships' turning circle and foul ground. A rk, 5m NNW of Packet Quay point, should be avoided by at least 10m at LWS.
NAVIGATION
WPT 52°59'·20N 06°01'·80W, 040°/220° from/to ent, 0·27M. Appr presents no difficulty; keep in the R sector of the E pier lt to avoid Planet Rk and Pogeen Rk.
LIGHTS AND MARKS
No ldg marks/lts. The only lts are as on the chartlet.

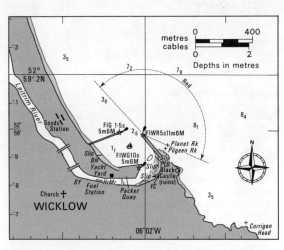

RADIO TELEPHONE
VHF Ch 16; 02 06 07 08 26 27 28. Wicklow SC Ch M 16.
TELEPHONE (0404)
Hr Mr 67455; MRCC (01) 6620922; Coast/Cliff Rescue Service 67310; # 67222; Police 67107; Dr 67381.
FACILITIES
East Pier L, AB; **New (S) Quay**, P & D (cans; bulk: see Hr Mr), L, FW, AB; **Wicklow SC** ☎ 67526, Slip (HW), M, L, FW, Bar; **Services:** M, ME, El, C, Sh, AB, Kos, Gaz.
Town EC Thurs; CH, V, R, Bar, ✉, Ⓑ, ⇌, ✈ (Dublin).

ARKLOW
10-12-12

Wicklow 52°47'·60N 06°08'·20W

CHARTS
AC 633, 1468; Imray C61; Irish OS 19

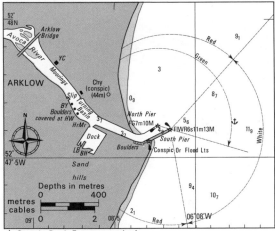

⚠ Stop in Dock Entrance and ask

TIDES
–0150 Dover; ML 1·0; Duration 0640; Zone 0 (UT)

Standard Port DUBLIN (NORTH WALL) (←—)

Times				Height (metres)			
High Water		Low Water		MHWS	MHWN	MLWN	MLWS
0000	0700	0000	0500	4·1	3·4	1·5	0·7
1200	1900	1200	1700				
Differences ARKLOW (Note small Range)							
–0315	–0201	–0140	–0134	–2·7	–2·2	–0·6	–0·1
COURTOWN							
–0328	–0242	–0158	–0138	–2·8	–2·4	–0·5	0·0

SHELTER
Good, access H24; but ent unsafe in strong NE to SE onshore winds, when seas break across the bar. Ent is difficult without power, due to blanking by piers. Once in Dock (3m), berth on SE wall in perfect shelter, but amidst FVs. One ⌁ in river off slipway and possible berth at YC quay, but Note: Due to obstructions it is dangerous to go up-river of Dock ent without local advice. Good ⌁ in bay; avoid whelk pots.
Arklow Rock Hbr, 1M S of Arklow, offers emergency ⌁ during SE winds off Roadstone Jetty (Oc R 10s 9m 9M). 2ca S of jetty a mole (QY) extends ENE for 3ca. Best ⌁ in 4m between jetty and mole, neither suitable for AB.
NAVIGATION
WPT 52°47'·60N 06°07'·50W, 090°/270° from/to ent, 0·40M. No navigational dangers, but beware ebb setting SE across hbr ent. The ent to the dock is 13·5m wide.
LIGHTS AND MARKS
No ldg lts/marks. 2 conspic factory chy's 2·5ca NW of piers. N pier L Fl G 7s 7m 10M, vis shore-287°, with Or flood lt at root of N pier; river banks are flood-lit. S pier Fl WR 6s 11m 13M; vis R shore–223°, W223°–350°, R350°–shore.
RADIO TELEPHONE
VHF Ch 16 (HJ).
TELEPHONE (0402)
Hr Mr 32426; MRCC (01) 6620922/3; Coast/Cliff Rescue Service 32430; RNLI 32001; # 32497; Police 2101; Dr 32421.
FACILITIES
Dock ☎ 32426, AB £9.75 for 1 week, FW, ME, El, C (1 ton), D (hose, as arranged), BH, Slip; **Arklow YC** (on NE bank, 2·6ca up-river of Dock) quay/jetty, M;
Services: BY, M, FW, ME, El, Sh, C (5 ton mobile), Kos.
Town EC Wed; CH, V, R, P & D (cans), Bar, ✉, Ⓑ, ⇌, ✈ (Dublin).

12

WEXFORD   10-12-13

Wexford 52°20'·10N 06°27'·00W

CHARTS

AC 1772, 1787; Imray C61; Irish OS 23

TIDES

–0450 Dover; ML 1·3; Duration 0630; Zone 0 (UT)

Standard Port COBH (→)

Times				Height (metres)			
High Water		Low Water		MHWS	MHWN	MLWN	MLWS
0500	1100	0500	1100	4·1	3·2	1·3	0·4
1700	2300	1700	2300				
Differences WEXFORD							
+0126	+0126	+0118	+0108	–2·1	–1·7	–0·3	+0·1

SHELTER

Safe sheltered ⚓ off town quays in 2·3m, but difficult ent; access approx HW±2. Do not attempt in strong E/S winds, when seas break on the bar. No commercial users, other than FVs. Some ⚓s are provided by WHBC. Note: A small marina is planned.

NAVIGATION

WPT 52°20'·55N 06°20'·15W, Bar buoy Iso Y, about 8ca ESE of The Raven Pt. Bar partly dries and shifts. Hbr Board has ceased to function, so in summer about 20 dayglow orange buoys are locally laid to mark the chan which has only 1m in places. The following directions are subject to change: After 3rd PHM buoy, N of ruins (awash at HW), head 325°. About ¼M off, keep along shore for approx 1M. After passing two W posts, head SW towards conspic chy, SE end of town. Turn stbd when 1ca off training wall. There are no pilots, but local advice is obtainable from Mr J. Sherwood ☎ 22875 (home 22713).

LIGHTS AND MARKS

Ldg marks and tracks on chartlet are approximate.

RADIO TELEPHONE

Wexford Hbr BC VHF Ch 16 occas.

TELEPHONE (053)

Hr Mr 33114; MRSC (01) 6620922/3; ⌗ 33116; Police 22333; Dr 31154; Ⓗ 42233.

FACILITIES

Wexford Quays Slip, P, D, L, FW, ME, El, AB, V, CH;
Wexford Hbr Boat Club ☎ 22039, Slip, C (5 ton), Bar;
Town ✉, Ⓑ, ≷, ✈ (Waterford).

AGENTS WANTED

If you are interested in becoming our agent for any of the following ports, please write to: The Editor, Edington House, Trent, Sherborne, Dorset DT9 4SR, England – and get your free copy of the almanac annually. You do not have to live in a port to be the agent, but at least a fairly regular visitor.

River Exe	Grandcamp-Maisy
Port Ellen (Islay)	Port-en-Bessin
Glandore/Union Hall	Courseulles
River Rance/Dinan	Boulogne
Lampaul	Dunkerque
Port Tudy	Terneuzen/Westerschelde
River Etel	Oudeschild
Le Palais (Belle Ile)	Lauwersoog
Le Pouliguen/Pornichet	Dornumer-Accumersiel
L'Herbaudière	Hooksiel
St Gilles-Croix-de-Vie	Langeoog
River Seudre	Bremerhaven
Royan	Helgoland
Anglet/Bayonne	Büsum
Hendaye	

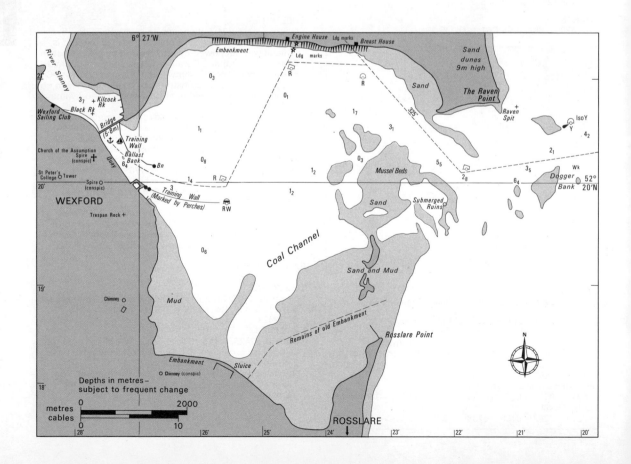

ROSSLARE HARBOUR   10-12-14

Dublin 52°15'·30N 06°20'·90W

CHARTS

AC 1772, 1787; Imray C61; Irish OS 23

TIDES

–0510 Dover; ML 1·1; Duration 0640; Zone 0 (UT)

Standard Port COBH (→)

Times				Height (metres)			
High Water		Low Water		MHWS	MHWN	MLWN	MLWS
0500	1100	0500	1100	4·1	3·2	1·3	0·4
1700	2300	1700	2300				
Differences ROSSLARE HARBOUR							
+0055	+0043	+0022	+0002	–2·2	–1·8	–0·5	–0·1
CARNSORE POINT							
+0029	+0019	–0002	+0008	–1·1	–1·0	No data	

SHELTER

Useful passage shelter from SW'lies, but few facilities for yachts. Rosslare is a busy port with 160 ferry/high-speed catamaran (41kn) movements per week. In WNW-NNE winds it is often uncomfortable and, if these winds freshen, dangerous; leave at once, via S Shear. Yachts may berth on E wall of marshalling area (⚓ on the chartlet, 3·7m), or ⚓ approx 0·5M W of hbr. Small craft hbr has 1m max at LW, bottom is reported foul; mainly used by local fishermen.

NAVIGATION

WPT 52°14'·70N 06°15·60W, (abeam S Long SCM buoy, VQ (6)+L Fl 10s), 105°/285° from/to bkwtr lt, 2·92M. Main appr from E, S and W is via S Shear, buoyed/lit chan to S of Holden's Bed, a shoal of varying depth; the tide sets across the chan. From S, beware rks off Greenore Pt, and overfalls here and over The Baillies. From the N, appr via N Shear. The Tuskar TSS is approx 8M ESE of the hbr.

LIGHTS AND MARKS

Tuskar Rk, Q (2) 7·5s 33m 28M, is 5·8M SE of hbr ent. Bkwtr lt, L Fl WRG 5s 15m 13/10M, shows G098°-188° over Rosslare B; W188°-208° through N Shear; R208°-246° over N part of Holdens Bed and Long Bank; G246°-283° over S part of Holdens Bed; W283 °–286° over S Shear, and R286°-320° over rks/shoals off Greenore Pt. Two sets of ldg lts lead 124° and 146° to ferry berths. At N corner of marshalling area, Oc WR 1·7s 7m 4M, is vis Rshore-152°, W152°-205° (unintens 200°-205°), R205°-shore. Water tr (R lt, 35m) is conspic 0·8M SSE of hbr ent. Note; powerful floodlights in the port make identification of navigational lights difficult.

RADIO TELEPHONE

Call: Rosslare Hbr VHF Ch 14 06 12 16 (H24).

TELEPHONE (053)

Hr Mr 33864/33162; MRCC (01) 6620922/3; LB Lookout Stn 33205; ⌗ 33116; Police 22333; Dr 31154; Ⓗ 42233.

FACILITIES

Pier ☎ 33114, No fee, M, P, D, L, FW, ME, C, Divers;
Services: Kos, BY, ME, Sh, El, Slip, C. (Marina planned)
Town EC Thurs; V, R, Bar, ✉, Ⓑ, ⇌, ✈ (Dublin). Ferries to Fishguard, Pembroke Dock, Cherbourg, Le Havre.

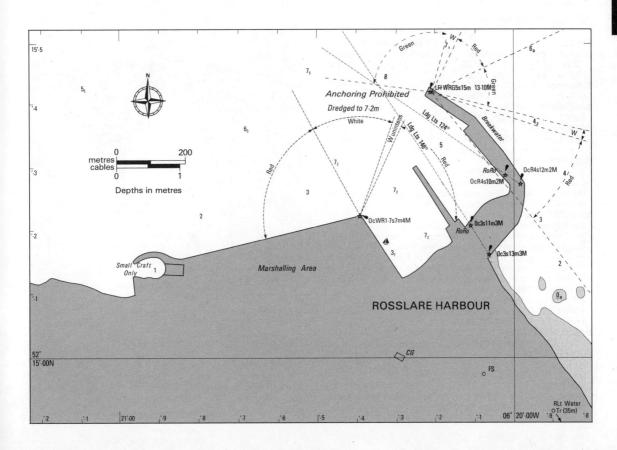

DUNMORE EAST   10-12-15

Waterford 52°08'·95N 06°59'·37W

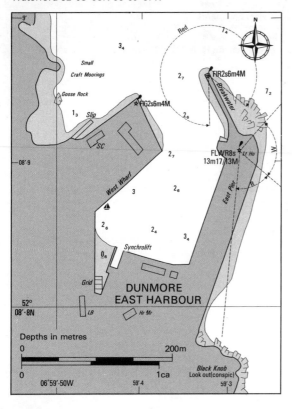

CHARTS
AC 2046, 2049; Imray C61, C57; Irish OS 23
TIDES
–0535 Dover; ML 2·4; Duration 0605; Zone 0 (UT)

Standard Port COBH (→)

Times				Height (metres)			
High Water		Low Water		MHWS	MHWN	MLWN	MLWS
0500	1100	0500	1100	4·1	3·2	1·3	0·4
1700	2300	1700	2300				
Differences DUNMORE EAST							
+0008	+0003	0000	0000	+0·1	+0·1	+0·2	0·0
BAGINBUN HEAD							
+0003	+0003	–0008	–0008	–0·2	–0·1	+0·2	+0·2
GREAT SALTEE							
+0019	+0009	–0004	+0006	–0·3	–0·4		No data

SHELTER
Very good, except in NE/SE winds. A useful passage port, but mainly a FV hbr, so limited AB for yachts on W wharf, clear of ice berth. Craft stay afloat in 2 - 3·4m at all times. No ⚓s, but ⚓ N of the hbr.
NAVIGATION
WPT (see also 10·12·16) 52°08'·00N, 06°58'·00W, 137°/ 317° from/to bkwtr lt, 1·2M. There are no navigational dangers, but clear Hook Hd and Tower Race by 1·5M min; then alter course for hbr in R sector of E pier lt ho. From W, beware Falskirt Rk; by night steer for Hook Hd until in R sector of E pier lt, then alter to N. Enter under power.
LIGHTS AND MARKS
E Pier lt ho Fl WR8s 13m 17/13M, W225°-310°, R310°- 004°. E bkwtr hd Fl R2s 6m 4M, vis 000°-310°. W wharf Fl G 2s 6m 4M, vis 165°–246°.
RADIO TELEPHONE
VHF Ch 14 16 (Pilot Station).
TELEPHONE (051)
Hr Mr 83166; Pilot 83119; ⌗ 75391; MRCC (01) 6620922/3; Coast Life Saving Service 83115; Dr 83194.
FACILITIES
Hbr ☎ 83166, BH (230 ton), D, FW (on E pier); **Waterford Hbr SC** ☎ 83389, R, Bar; **Services**: Kos, CH. **Village** D, P (cans), Slip, R, Bar, V, ⑧, ✉, ⇌ (Waterford), ✈ (Dublin).

WATERFORD   10-12-16

Waterford 52°15'·50N 07°06'·00W

CHARTS
AC 2046, 2049; Imray C57; Irish OS 23
TIDES
–0520 Dover; ML 2·4; Duration 0605; Zone 0 (UT)

Standard Port COBH (→)

Times				Height (metres)			
High Water		Low Water		MHWS	MHWN	MLWN	MLWS
0500	1100	0500	1100	4·1	3·2	1·3	0·4
1700	2300	1700	2300				
Differences WATERFORD							
+0057	+0057	+0046	+0046	+0·4	+0·3	–0·1	+0·1
CHEEK POINT							
+0022	+0020	+0020	+0020	+0·3	+0·2	+0·2	+0·1
KILMOKEA POINT							
+0026	+0022	+0020	+0020	+0·2	+0·1	+0·1	+0·1
NEW ROSS							
+0100	+0030	+0055	+0130	+0·3	+0·4	+0·3	+0·4

SHELTER
Very good, with many excellent ⚓s: off the quays just W of Cheek Pt (9M up the estuary); about 3M further W, on S side of R Suir in Kings Chan which should only be entered W of Little Is; in Waterford on a pontoon S bank, close downstream of clock tr; up the R Barrow near Marsh Pt (about 2M S of New Ross) and 0·5M S of New Ross fixed bridge.
Note: the rly swing bridge at the ent to R Barrow opens at its W end. Call bridge-keeper VHF Ch 16 or ☎ 88137.

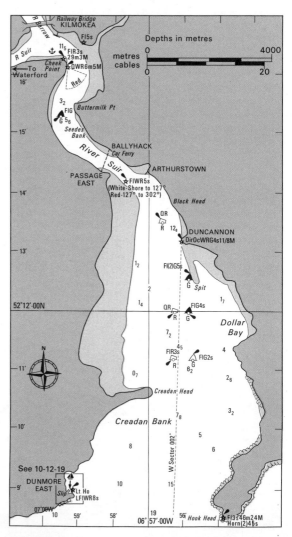

WATERFORD *Continued*

NAVIGATION
WPT 52°06'·50N 06°56'·50W, 182°/002° from/to Dir lt at Duncannon, 6·7M. From the W do not confuse Waterford ent with Tramore Bay; beware Falskirt Rk (2ca off Swine Hd). From the E, keep clear of Brecaun reef (2M NE of Hook Hd). Give Tower Race a wide berth; overfalls extend about 1·5M S of Hook Hd.

LIGHTS AND MARKS
The ent to R Suir lies between Dunmore East L Fl WR 8s 13m 16/12M; vis W225°–310°, R310°–004°; and Hook Hd, Fl 3s 46m 23M, W tr with 2 B bands. Duncannon Dir lt 002°, Oc WRG 4s 11/8M, G358°–001·7°, W001·7 °–002·2°, R002·2°–006°, leads up-river via well-buoyed lit chan. The R Barrow is also well lit/marked up to New Ross.

RADIO TELEPHONE
Waterford and New Ross VHF Ch 12 14 16.

TELEPHONE (051)
Hr Mr Waterford 74499/New Ross 21303; MRCC (01) 6620922/3; ⌗ 75391; Police 74888; Dr 83194; Ⓗ 75429.

FACILITIES
Services: BY (Ballyhack), ME, EI, Sh, C.
Town EC Thurs; AB, M, FW, P, D, Gaz, V, R, Bar, ⇌, ✈.

MINOR HARBOUR 15M ENE of YOUGHAL

DUNGARVAN BAY, Waterford, 52°05'·15N 07°36'·70W. AC 2017. HW –0540 on Dover; Duration 0600. See below. A large bay, drying to the W; Carrickapane Rk and Helvick Rk (ECM buoy Q (3) 10s) lie in the ent. The Gainers, an extensive unmarked rky patch (dries 0·8m), are 2 to 5ca NNW of Helvick pier head. ⌕ off Helvick hbr, in approx 4m, or go up to Dungarvan town hbr not later than HW+3½. Chan buoyed from Ballinacourty Pt, Lt Fl (2) WRG 10s 16m 12/9M, G245°–274°, W274°–302°, R302°–325°, W325°–117°. Ballinacourty ldg lts 083°/263°, both Oc 5s 9/12m 2M on W columns with B bands, 46m apart; Dungarvan ldg lts 298°, both FR 8/9m 2M. Beware salmon nets. Facilities: EC Thurs; AB, Bar, Ⓑ, D (cans), P (on quay), ⊠, R, V, Kos.

YOUGHAL   10-12-17

Cork 51°56'·54N 07°50'·20W

CHARTS
AC 2071, 2049; Imray C57; Irish OS 22

TIDES
–0556 Dover; ML 2·1; Duration 0555; Zone 0 (UT)

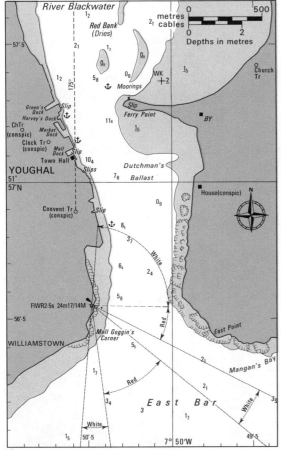

No special visitors berths

Standard Port COBH (→)

Times				Height (metres)			
High Water		Low Water		MHWS	MHWN	MLWN	MLWS
0500	1100	0500	1100	4·1	3·2	1·3	0·4
1700	2300	1700	2300				
Differences YOUGHAL							
0000	+0010	+0010	0000	–0·2	–0·1	–0·1	–0·1
DUNGARVAN HARBOUR							
+0004	+0012	+0007	–0001	0·0	+0·1	–0·2	0·0
BALLYCOTTON							
–0011	+0001	+0003	–0009	0·0	0·0	–0·1	0·0

SHELTER
Good, but strong S winds cause a swell inside the hbr. ⌕s as shown on chartlet. Caution strong tidal streams.

NAVIGATION
WPT, East Bar, 51°55'·62N 07°48'·00W, 122°/302° from/to Fl WR 2·5s lt, 1·8M. Beware Blackball Ledge (PHM buoy) and Bar Rks (SCM buoy), both outside hbr ent in R sector of lt ho. From W, appr via West Bar (1·7m) is shorter; E Bar has 2·0m. In winds E to SSW >F6 both Bars are likely to have dangerous seas. Beware salmon nets May-July.

LIGHTS AND MARKS
W of ent, Fl WR 2·5s 24m 17/14M, W tr (15m), has two W sectors ldg over the bars (see 10.12.4). Convent tr on with the town hall at 175° leads clear W of Red Bank up-river. Conspic water tr approx 0·65M WNW of clock tr.

RADIO TELEPHONE
VHF Ch 14 16 HW±3.

TELEPHONE (024)
Hr Mr 92820; MRCC (01) 6620922/3; Coast/Cliff Rescue Service 93252; ⌗ (021) 311024; Police 92200; Dr 92702.

FACILITIES
Services: ME, EI, Sh, CH, L, FW (see Hr Mr), Slip. **Town** P & D (cans), V, R, Bar, ⊠, Ⓑ, ⇌ (Cork/Waterford), ✈ (Cork).

MINOR HARBOUR 10M SOUTHWEST of YOUGHAL

BALLYCOTTON, Cork, 51°49'·70N 08°00'·19W. AC 2424. HW –0555 on Dover; ML no data; Duration 0550. See above. Small, N-facing hbr at W end of bay; suffers from scend in strong SE winds. 3m in ent and about 1·5m against piers. Many FVs alongside piers, on which yachts should berth, rather than ⌕ in hbr, which is foul with old ground tackle. Outside hbr, good ⌕ in offshore winds in 6m NE of bkwtr, protected by Ballycotton Is. Lt ho Fl WR 10s 59m 22/18M, B tr in W walls; W238°–063°, R063°–238°; Horn (4) 90s. Facilities: FW on pier. **Village** Bar, ⊠, R, V, LB, Kos.

12

CORK HARBOUR   10-12-18

Cork 51°47'·50N 08°15'·54W

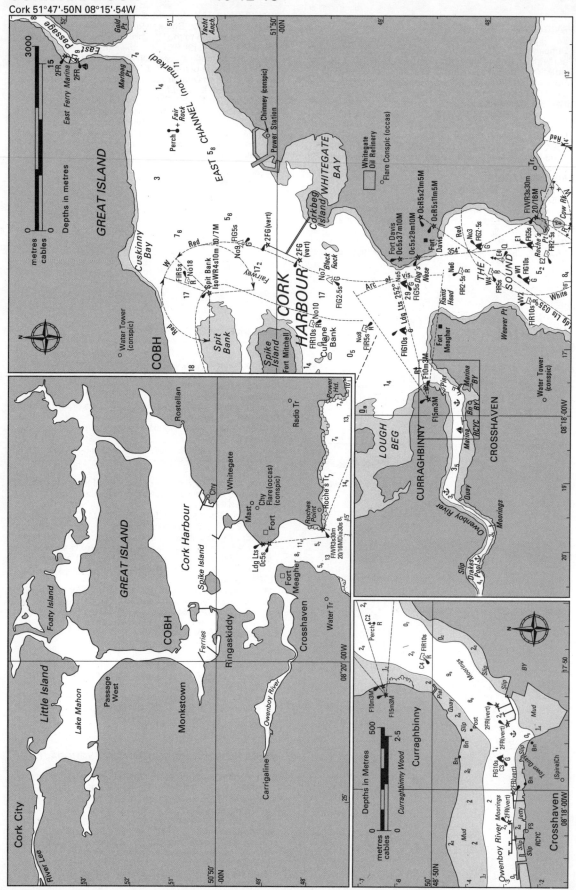

CHARTS
AC 1773, 1777, 1765; Imray C56, C57; Irish OS 25

TIDES
−0523 Dover; ML 2·3; Duration 0555; Zone 0 (UT)

Standard Port COBH (⟶)

Times				Height (metres)			
High Water		Low Water		MHWS	MHWN	MLWN	MLWS
0500	1100	0500	1100	4·1	3·2	1·3	0·4
1700	2300	1700	2300				
Differences RINGASKIDDY							
+0005	+0020	+0007	+0013	+0·1	+0·1	+0·1	+0·1
MARINO POINT							
0000	+0010	0000	+0010	+0·1	+0·1	0·0	0·0
CORK CITY							
+0005	+0010	+0020	+0010	+0·4	+0·4	+0·3	+0·2
ROBERTS COVE							
−0005	−0005	−0005	−0005	−0·1	0·0	0·0	+0·1

NOTE: Cobh is a Standard Port. Daily predictions are below.

SHELTER
Very good in all conditions, esp in Crosshaven and East Passage. There are 3 main marinas at Crosshaven (see Facilities), plus a small private marina and several ⚓s further up the Owenboy River, in particular at Drake's Pool. There is also a marina at E Ferry in E Passage at the E end of Great Island. Cobh and Cork City are ferry/commercial ports; before proceeding up river contact Port Operations for advice on possible yacht berths.

NAVIGATION
WPT 51°46'·00N, 08°15'·30W, 174°/354° from/to front ldg lt, 2·8M. There are no navigational dangers for yachts. It is one of the safest hbrs to enter in the world, being deep and well marked. Tidal streams run about 1½kn in ent at sp, but more between the forts. Ent to Owenboy River carries a minimum of 2m at LWS, and the chan is buoyed. Main chan up to Cork is buoyed.

LIGHTS AND MARKS
The hammerhead water tr S of Crosshaven is a very conspic mark, 24·5m high.
Ldg lts, two sets, both below Fort Davis on E shore:
(1) Oc 5s, 29/37m 10M lead 354° E of Hbr Rks.
(2) Oc R 5s, 11/21m 5M, lead 034° W of Hbr Rks.
Ldg lts, FW 10/15m 3M, with W ◇ day marks, lead 252° to Crosshaven, but hard to see.

RADIO TELEPHONE
Call: *Cork Hbr Radio* (Port Ops) VHF Ch 12 14 16 (H24); Crosshaven BY Ch M (Mon– Fri: 0830– 1700 LT). Royal Cork YC Marina Ch M (1000– 2359 LT). East Ferry Marina Ch M 80 (0800– 2200LT).

TELEPHONE (021)
Hr Mr 273125; Port Operations 811380; MRCC (01) 6620922/3; Coast/Cliff Rescue Service 831448; ⌗ 271322; Recorded Weather 964600; Police 831222; Dr 831716; Ⓗ + Emergency 546400.

FACILITIES
Royal Cork YC Marina (90 + 15 visitors) ☎ 831023, Fax 831586, £12, AC, FW, P (cans), Bar, R, Slip;
Crosshaven BY Marina (100 + 20 visitors) ☎ 831161, Fax 831603, £10, AC, BH (25 ton), C (1.5 tons), M, Ⓔ, CH, D, P, EI, FW, Gas, Gaz, ME, Sh, Slip (100 tons);
Salve Marine (28 + 12 visitors) ☎ 831145, Fax 831747, AB £10, M, FW, AC, BY, EI, ME, C, CH, D, P (cans), Slip;
East Ferry Marina (65 + 15 visitors) ☎ 811342, £10, D, AC, FW, Bar, R, Slip; access all tides, max draft 5·5m.
Services: EI, ME, Slip, SM, ACA, CH, BY, Ⓔ. **Crosshaven Village** Bar, Dr, L, ✉, R, V, Ⓥ, YC, Gas, Gaz.
Cork City All facilities. Ferries (to UK and France), ⇝, ✈.

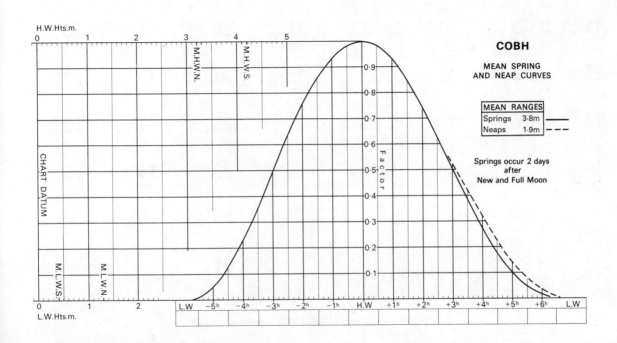

COBH

MEAN SPRING AND NEAP CURVES

MEAN RANGES	
Springs	3·8m
Neaps	1·9m

Springs occur 2 days after New and Full Moon

H.W.Hts.m.

CHART DATUM

M.H.W.N.   M.H.W.S.

M.L.W.S.   M.L.W.N.

Factor

L.W −5ʰ −4ʰ −3ʰ −2ʰ −1ʰ H.W +1ʰ +2ʰ +3ʰ +4ʰ +5ʰ +6ʰ L.W

L.W.Hts.m.

12

IRELAND – COBH

LAT 51°51'N   LONG   8°18'W

TIMES AND HEIGHTS OF HIGH AND LOW WATERS

YEAR **1996**

TIME ZONE (UT)
For Summer Time add ONE hour in non-shaded areas

JANUARY

Day	Time	m		Day	Time	m
1 M	0139 / 0822 / 1411 / 2049	3.4 / 1.1 / 3.5 / 1.1		16 TU	0031 / 0715 / 1308 / 1955	3.6 / 1.2 / 3.6 / 1.2
2 TU	0242 / 0922 / 1508 / 2145	3.5 / 1.1 / 3.6 / 1.0		17 W	0144 / 0827 / 1419 / 2104	3.7 / 1.1 / 3.7 / 1.0
3 W	0337 / 1014 / 1558 / 2233	3.7 / 1.0 / 3.8 / 0.9		18 TH	0255 / 0936 / 1527 / 2207	3.8 / 0.8 / 3.9 / 0.7
4 TH	0424 / 1058 / 1642 / 2312	3.9 / 0.9 / 3.9 / 0.8		19 F	0359 / 1037 / 1627 / 2302	4.1 / 0.6 / 4.1 / 0.4
5 F O	0506 / 1134 / 1721 / 2345	4.0 / 0.8 / 4.0 / 0.8		20 SA ●	0456 / 1130 / 1720 / 2352	4.3 / 0.3 / 4.2 / 0.2
6 SA	0543 / 1206 / 1756	4.1 / 0.8 / 4.0		21 SU	0547 / 1218 / 1808	4.4 / 0.2 / 4.3
7 SU	0014 / 0616 / 1236 / 1828	0.7 / 4.1 / 0.8 / 4.0		22 M	0039 / 0633 / 1304 / 1853	0.1 / 4.4 / 0.2 / 4.3
8 M	0044 / 0647 / 1307 / 1858	0.7 / 4.1 / 0.8 / 4.0		23 TU	0125 / 0718 / 1349 / 1937	0.1 / 4.4 / 0.2 / 4.2
9 TU	0116 / 0719 / 1342 / 1931	0.8 / 4.0 / 0.9 / 4.0		24 W	0209 / 0803 / 1433 / 2020	0.2 / 4.3 / 0.3 / 4.1
10 W	0152 / 0753 / 1419 / 2006	0.8 / 4.0 / 1.0 / 3.9		25 TH	0255 / 0847 / 1517 / 2103	0.4 / 4.1 / 0.5 / 3.9
11 TH	0231 / 0831 / 1458 / 2046	0.9 / 3.9 / 1.1 / 3.9		26 F	0340 / 0931 / 1602 / 2147	0.6 / 3.9 / 0.8 / 3.7
12 F	0314 / 0912 / 1541 / 2130	1.0 / 3.9 / 1.2 / 3.8		27 SA	0428 / 1018 / 1651 / 2235	0.8 / 3.7 / 1.0 / 3.5
13 SA	0402 / 0959 / 1630 / 2221	1.1 / 3.8 / 1.2 / 3.7		28 SU	0521 / 1110 / 1747 / 2333	1.0 / 3.5 / 1.2 / 3.3
14 SU	0457 / 1054 / 1730 / 2322	1.2 / 3.7 / 1.3 / 3.6		29 M	0623 / 1215 / 1853	1.2 / 3.3 / 1.3
15 M	0603 / 1158 / 1842	1.3 / 3.6 / 1.3		30 TU	0048 / 0732 / 1329 / 2004	3.2 / 1.3 / 3.3 / 1.3
				31 W	0206 / 0844 / 1437 / 2112	3.3 / 1.2 / 3.4 / 1.2

FEBRUARY

Day	Time	m		Day	Time	m
1 TH	0309 / 0947 / 1534 / 2209	3.5 / 1.1 / 3.6 / 1.0		16 F	0237 / 0919 / 1513 / 2151	3.7 / 0.9 / 3.7 / 0.7
2 F	0401 / 1036 / 1622 / 2253	3.7 / 0.9 / 3.8 / 0.8		17 SA	0346 / 1024 / 1615 / 2248	3.9 / 0.5 / 3.9 / 0.4
3 SA	0446 / 1116 / 1703 / 2328	3.9 / 0.8 / 3.9 / 0.7		18 SU ●	0443 / 1117 / 1707 / 2338	4.2 / 0.3 / 4.2 / 0.2
4 SU O	0524 / 1148 / 1739 / 2357	4.0 / 0.7 / 4.0 / 0.6		19 M	0531 / 1203 / 1753	4.3 / 0.1 / 4.3
5 M	0558 / 1217 / 1812	4.1 / 0.7 / 4.0		20 TU	0023 / 0615 / 1247 / 1835	0.0 / 4.4 / 0.1 / 4.3
6 TU	0025 / 0628 / 1248 / 1841	0.6 / 4.1 / 0.7 / 4.0		21 W	0106 / 0657 / 1328 / 1915	0.0 / 4.4 / 0.1 / 4.2
7 W	0056 / 0658 / 1320 / 1911	0.6 / 4.1 / 0.7 / 4.0		22 TH	0147 / 0738 / 1408 / 1954	0.1 / 4.3 / 0.2 / 4.1
8 TH	0130 / 0730 / 1355 / 1944	0.7 / 4.1 / 0.8 / 4.0		23 F	0228 / 0817 / 1448 / 2032	0.3 / 4.1 / 0.4 / 3.9
9 F	0207 / 0805 / 1432 / 2020	0.7 / 4.0 / 0.8 / 3.9		24 SA	0309 / 0857 / 1528 / 2111	0.5 / 3.9 / 0.7 / 3.8
10 SA	0248 / 0844 / 1511 / 2101	0.8 / 3.9 / 0.9 / 3.9		25 SU	0351 / 0937 / 1611 / 2153	0.7 / 3.6 / 0.9 / 3.5
11 SU	0332 / 0928 / 1556 / 2148	0.9 / 3.8 / 1.1 / 3.8		26 M	0438 / 1023 / 1700 / 2243	1.0 / 3.4 / 1.1 / 3.3
12 M	0423 / 1020 / 1651 / 2246	1.1 / 3.7 / 1.2 / 3.6		27 TU	0535 / 1120 / 1803 / 2352	1.2 / 3.2 / 1.3 / 3.1
13 TU	0526 / 1123 / 1802 / 2357	1.2 / 3.5 / 1.3 / 3.5		28 W	0643 / 1240 / 1917	1.3 / 3.1 / 1.4
14 W	0642 / 1238 / 1924	1.2 / 3.4 / 1.2		29 TH	0125 / 0759 / 1403 / 2032	3.1 / 1.3 / 3.2 / 1.3
15 TH	0117 / 0802 / 1358 / 2042	3.5 / 1.1 / 3.5 / 1.0				

MARCH

Day	Time	m		Day	Time	m
1 F	0239 / 0911 / 1507 / 2138	3.3 / 1.1 / 3.4 / 1.1		16 SA	0224 / 0903 / 1459 / 2135	3.6 / 0.8 / 3.6 / 0.7
2 SA	0335 / 1007 / 1557 / 2226	3.6 / 0.9 / 3.6 / 0.8		17 SU	0331 / 1008 / 1600 / 2233	3.8 / 0.5 / 3.9 / 0.4
3 SU	0420 / 1049 / 1639 / 2303	3.8 / 0.7 / 3.8 / 0.7		18 M	0426 / 1100 / 1650 / 2321	4.1 / 0.2 / 4.1 / 0.1
4 M	0459 / 1123 / 1716 / 2333	3.9 / 0.6 / 3.9 / 0.6		19 TU ●	0513 / 1145 / 1735	4.3 / 0.1 / 4.2
5 TU O	0533 / 1154 / 1749	4.0 / 0.5 / 4.0		20 W	0004 / 0555 / 1226 / 1814	0.0 / 4.3 / 0.0 / 4.2
6 W	0001 / 0604 / 1225 / 1819	0.5 / 4.1 / 0.5 / 4.0		21 TH	0045 / 0634 / 1305 / 1852	0.0 / 4.3 / 0.1 / 4.2
7 TH	0033 / 0633 / 1257 / 1849	0.5 / 4.1 / 0.5 / 4.0		22 F	0123 / 0712 / 1342 / 1928	0.1 / 4.2 / 0.2 / 4.1
8 F	0107 / 0705 / 1332 / 1922	0.5 / 4.1 / 0.6 / 4.0		23 SA	0201 / 0748 / 1419 / 2002	0.3 / 4.0 / 0.4 / 3.9
9 SA	0145 / 0741 / 1409 / 1958	0.5 / 4.0 / 0.6 / 4.0		24 SU	0239 / 0824 / 1457 / 2038	0.5 / 3.8 / 0.6 / 3.8
10 SU	0225 / 0820 / 1448 / 2038	0.6 / 3.9 / 0.7 / 3.9		25 M	0318 / 0901 / 1536 / 2118	0.7 / 3.6 / 0.9 / 3.6
11 M	0310 / 0904 / 1533 / 2126	0.7 / 3.8 / 0.9 / 3.8		26 TU	0402 / 0943 / 1621 / 2204	1.0 / 3.4 / 1.1 / 3.3
12 TU	0401 / 0956 / 1628 / 2223	0.9 / 3.6 / 1.0 / 3.6		27 W	0455 / 1034 / 1719 / 2303	1.2 / 3.2 / 1.3 / 3.1
13 W	0503 / 1100 / 1738 / 2334	1.1 / 3.4 / 1.2 / 3.4		28 TH	0600 / 1144 / 1832	1.3 / 3.0 / 1.3
14 TH	0619 / 1217 / 1901	1.1 / 3.3 / 1.1		29 F	0031 / 0712 / 1318 / 1946	3.1 / 1.3 / 3.0 / 1.3
15 F	0059 / 0742 / 1343 / 2024	3.4 / 1.1 / 3.4 / 1.0		30 SA	0159 / 0823 / 1430 / 2052	3.2 / 1.2 / 3.2 / 1.1
				31 SU	0258 / 0923 / 1523 / 2145	3.4 / 1.0 / 3.5 / 0.9

APRIL

Day	Time	m		Day	Time	m
1 M	0345 / 1010 / 1607 / 2226	3.6 / 0.7 / 3.7 / 0.7		16 TU	0405 / 1039 / 1630 / 2301	4.0 / 0.3 / 4.0 / 0.2
2 TU	0426 / 1049 / 1645 / 2301	3.8 / 0.6 / 3.9 / 0.5		17 W	0451 / 1124 / 1714 / 2344 ●	4.1 / 0.2 / 4.1 / 0.2
3 W	0501 / 1124 / 1720 / 2334	3.9 / 0.5 / 4.0 / 0.4		18 TH	0533 / 1204 / 1753	4.2 / 0.2 / 4.1
4 TH O	0534 / 1159 / 1753	4.0 / 0.4 / 4.0		19 F	0023 / 0611 / 1242 / 1829	0.2 / 4.1 / 0.2 / 4.1
5 F	0009 / 0607 / 1234 / 1826	0.4 / 4.0 / 0.4 / 4.1		20 SA	0100 / 0647 / 1317 / 1903	0.3 / 4.0 / 0.3 / 4.0
6 SA	0046 / 0643 / 1311 / 1902	0.4 / 4.1 / 0.4 / 4.1		21 SU	0135 / 0721 / 1353 / 1936	0.4 / 3.9 / 0.5 / 3.9
7 SU	0126 / 0721 / 1351 / 1941	0.4 / 4.0 / 0.5 / 4.0		22 M	0211 / 0755 / 1428 / 2011	0.6 / 3.8 / 0.7 / 3.8
8 M	0209 / 0804 / 1434 / 2025	0.5 / 3.9 / 0.6 / 3.9		23 TU	0248 / 0832 / 1505 / 2050	0.8 / 3.6 / 0.9 / 3.6
9 TU	0256 / 0851 / 1522 / 2114	0.6 / 3.8 / 0.7 / 3.8		24 W	0330 / 0912 / 1547 / 2133	1.0 / 3.5 / 1.0 / 3.4
10 W	0349 / 0944 / 1618 / 2212	0.8 / 3.6 / 0.9 / 3.6		25 TH	0419 / 0959 / 1640 / 2226	1.1 / 3.3 / 1.2 / 3.3
11 TH	0451 / 1048 / 1726 / 2323	0.9 / 3.4 / 1.0 / 3.4		26 F	0519 / 1058 / 1746 / 2333	1.3 / 3.1 / 1.3 / 3.2
12 F	0604 / 1204 / 1846	1.0 / 3.3 / 1.0		27 SA	0627 / 1214 / 1857	1.3 / 3.1 / 1.3
13 SA	0047 / 0726 / 1327 / 2006	3.4 / 0.9 / 3.4 / 0.9		28 SU	0056 / 0733 / 1334 / 2000	3.2 / 1.2 / 3.2 / 1.1
14 SU	0207 / 0844 / 1441 / 2116	3.6 / 0.7 / 3.6 / 0.6		29 M	0206 / 0832 / 1434 / 2055	3.3 / 1.0 / 3.4 / 0.9
15 M	0311 / 0947 / 1540 / 2213	3.8 / 0.5 / 3.8 / 0.4		30 TU	0258 / 0924 / 1523 / 2143	3.5 / 0.8 / 3.6 / 0.7

Chart Datum: 0·13 metres above Ordnance Datum (Dublin)

TIME ZONE (UT)
For Summer Time add ONE hour in non-shaded areas

IRELAND – COBH

LAT 51°51′N   LONG   8°18′W

TIMES AND HEIGHTS OF HIGH AND LOW WATERS

YEAR **1996**

MAY

Day	Time	m	Time	m	Time	m	Time	m
1 W	0343	3.7	1010	0.6	1606	3.8	2226	0.6
16 TH	0427	3.9	1101	0.4	1651	4.0	2323	0.4
2 TH	0424	3.9	1052	0.5	1647	3.9	2307	0.4
17 F ●	0510	4.0	1142	0.4	1731	4.0		
3 F O	0504	4.0	1133	0.4	1727	4.1	2347	0.3
18 SA	0001	0.4	0548	4.0	1219	0.4	1807	4.0
4 SA	0544	4.0	1214	0.3	1806	4.1		
19 SU	0037	0.5	0624	3.9	1254	0.5	1841	4.0
5 SU	0029	0.3	0625	4.1	1256	0.3	1847	4.1
20 M	0111	0.6	0657	3.9	1328	0.6	1914	3.9
6 M	0113	0.3	0708	4.0	1340	0.4	1931	4.1
21 TU	0145	0.7	0731	3.8	1401	0.7	1949	3.8
7 TU	0159	0.4	0754	3.9	1426	0.4	2018	4.0
22 W	0220	0.8	0807	3.7	1437	0.9	2026	3.7
8 W	0249	0.5	0844	3.8	1517	0.6	2109	3.8
23 TH	0300	1.0	0846	3.6	1517	1.0	2108	3.6
9 TH	0343	0.6	0939	3.6	1613	0.7	2207	3.7
24 F	0346	1.1	0930	3.5	1604	1.1	2155	3.5
10 F	0443	0.8	1040	3.5	1717	0.8	2314	3.5
25 SA	0439	1.2	1021	3.4	1701	1.2	2250	3.4
11 SA	0552	0.9	1149	3.4	1830	0.9		
26 SU	0540	1.2	1121	3.3	1805	1.2	2353	3.3
12 SU	0029	3.5	0707	0.8	1305	3.4	1945	0.8
27 M	0644	1.2	1229	3.3	1909	1.2		
13 M	0142	3.6	0819	0.7	1414	3.6	2052	0.6
28 TU	0100	3.4	0743	1.1	1335	3.4	2007	1.0
14 TU	0245	3.7	0921	0.6	1513	3.7	2149	0.5
29 W	0202	3.5	0840	0.9	1433	3.6	2101	0.8
15 W	0339	3.8	1014	0.5	1605	3.9	2239	0.4
30 TH	0257	3.7	0932	0.7	1525	3.8	2153	0.6
31 F	0347	3.8	1023	0.6	1615	3.9	2242	0.5

JUNE

Day	Time	m	Time	m	Time	m	Time	m
1 SA O	0436	4.0	1111	0.4	1703	4.1	2329	0.3
16 SU ●	0527	3.9	1158	0.6	1748	3.9		
2 SU	0524	4.1	1158	0.3	1749	4.2		
17 M	0015	0.6	0604	3.9	1232	0.6	1822	3.9
3 M	0016	0.2	0610	4.1	1244	0.2	1835	4.2
18 TU	0047	0.7	0638	3.9	1304	0.7	1855	3.9
4 TU	0103	0.2	0658	4.1	1331	0.2	1922	4.2
19 W	0119	0.7	0711	3.8	1336	0.7	1929	3.8
5 W	0151	0.3	0746	4.0	1419	0.3	2011	4.1
20 TH	0154	0.8	0745	3.8	1410	0.8	2004	3.8
6 TH	0241	0.3	0837	3.9	1510	0.4	2103	4.0
21 F	0232	0.9	0823	3.7	1448	0.9	2043	3.7
7 F	0334	0.5	0930	3.8	1604	0.5	2157	3.8
22 SA	0314	1.0	0903	3.6	1531	1.0	2125	3.7
8 SA	0431	0.6	1026	3.6	1703	0.7	2257	3.7
23 SU	0400	1.1	0949	3.6	1619	1.1	2213	3.6
9 SU	0533	0.8	1127	3.5	1808	0.8		
24 M	0452	1.2	1040	3.5	1714	1.1	2307	3.5
10 M	0002	3.6	0640	0.8	1234	3.5	1916	0.8
25 TU	0552	1.2	1138	3.5	1817	1.2		
11 TU	0110	3.5	0748	0.8	1341	3.5	2022	0.8
26 W	0008	3.5	0655	1.2	1243	3.5	1921	1.1
12 W	0213	3.6	0851	0.8	1443	3.6	2122	0.7
27 TH	0113	3.5	0758	1.0	1347	3.6	2023	0.9
13 TH	0310	3.7	0947	0.7	1538	3.7	2215	0.6
28 F	0216	3.6	0859	0.9	1449	3.7	2123	0.8
14 F	0401	3.8	1037	0.6	1627	3.8	2301	0.6
29 SA	0316	3.8	0957	0.7	1548	3.9	2220	0.5
15 SA	0447	3.8	1120	0.6	1710	3.9	2341	0.6
30 SU	0413	3.9	1051	0.5	1643	4.1	2314	0.4

JULY

Day	Time	m	Time	m	Time	m	Time	m
1 M O	0507	4.1	1142	0.3	1734	4.2		
16 TU	0545	3.9	1211	0.6	1804	3.9		
2 TU	0003	0.2	0557	4.1	1231	0.2	1822	4.3
17 W	0025	0.7	0619	3.9	1240	0.7	1836	3.9
3 W	0052	0.1	0646	4.2	1319	0.1	1911	4.3
18 TH	0055	0.7	0651	3.9	1310	0.7	1908	3.9
4 TH	0140	0.2	0734	4.1	1407	0.2	1959	4.2
19 F	0127	0.8	0723	3.8	1342	0.7	1940	3.9
5 F	0229	0.2	0823	4.0	1456	0.2	2048	4.1
20 SA	0203	0.8	0757	3.8	1419	0.8	2015	3.8
6 SA	0318	0.4	0912	3.9	1546	0.4	2138	3.9
21 SU	0242	0.9	0835	3.8	1458	0.9	2054	3.8
7 SU	0410	0.5	1002	3.7	1639	0.6	2230	3.7
22 M	0323	1.0	0916	3.7	1542	1.0	2137	3.7
8 M	0504	0.7	1056	3.6	1736	0.7	2328	3.6
23 TU	0409	1.1	1002	3.6	1631	1.1	2227	3.6
9 TU	0605	0.9	1157	3.4	1840	0.9		
24 W	0502	1.2	1056	3.6	1729	1.1	2325	3.5
10 W	0032	3.4	0710	1.0	1304	3.4	1946	0.9
25 TH	0608	1.2	1200	3.5	†838	1.2		
11 TH	0139	3.4	0817	1.0	1411	3.4	2051	0.9
26 F	0032	3.5	0720	1.1	1310	3.5	1950	1.1
12 F	0240	3.5	0919	0.9	1511	3.5	2150	0.9
27 SA	0143	3.6	0830	1.0	1421	3.7	2059	0.9
13 SA	0336	3.7	1014	0.8	1603	3.7	2240	0.8
28 SU	0252	3.7	0935	0.7	1527	3.9	2202	0.6
14 SU	0424	3.7	1058	0.7	1649	3.8	2321	0.7
29 M	0355	3.9	1034	0.5	1626	4.1	2258	0.4
15 M ●	0507	3.8	1138	0.7	1729	3.9	2355	0.7
30 TU O	0451	4.1	1126	0.2	1719	4.2	2349	0.2
31 W	0542	4.2	1215	0.1	1808	4.3		

AUGUST

Day	Time	m	Time	m	Time	m	Time	m
1 TH	0036	0.1	0630	4.2	1302	0.0	1854	4.3
16 F	0030	0.6	0628	3.9	1242	0.6	1843	4.0
2 F	0123	0.1	0716	4.2	1348	0.1	1939	4.3
17 SA	0101	0.7	0659	3.9	1314	0.7	1913	4.0
3 SA	0209	0.2	0801	4.1	1434	0.2	2024	4.1
18 SU	0135	0.7	0730	3.9	1349	0.7	1946	3.9
4 SU	0255	0.3	0847	4.0	1520	0.3	2110	3.9
19 M	0212	0.8	0805	3.8	1428	0.8	2023	3.9
5 M	0342	0.5	0932	3.8	1608	0.6	2156	3.7
20 TU	0251	0.9	0844	3.8	1510	0.9	2104	3.8
6 TU	0430	0.7	1020	3.6	1659	0.8	2247	3.5
21 W	0334	1.0	0928	3.7	1557	1.0	2152	3.7
7 W	0525	0.9	1115	3.4	1757	1.0	2348	3.3
22 TH	0425	1.1	1022	3.6	1654	1.1	2251	3.5
8 TH	0628	1.1	1224	3.2	1905	1.1		
23 F	0530	1.2	1127	3.5	1804	1.2		
9 F	0101	3.2	0739	1.2	1340	3.3	2017	1.1
24 SA	0001	3.4	0648	1.2	1243	3.5	1922	1.1
10 SA	0212	3.3	0850	1.1	1446	3.4	2124	1.0
25 SU	0119	3.5	0806	1.0	1402	3.6	2038	0.9
11 SU	0311	3.5	0951	0.9	1541	3.6	2217	0.9
26 M	0235	3.6	0916	0.8	1512	3.8	2146	0.6
12 M	0402	3.6	1039	0.8	1627	3.8	2259	0.8
27 TU	0340	3.9	1017	0.5	1611	4.1	2243	0.3
13 TU	0445	3.8	1117	0.7	1708	3.9	2333	0.7
28 W O	0436	4.1	1110	0.2	1703	4.3	2333	0.1
14 W ●	0524	3.9	1148	0.6	1743	3.9		
29 TH	0525	4.2	1157	0.0	1749	4.4		
15 TH	0001	0.6	0557	3.9	1215	0.6	1814	4.0
30 F	0018	0.0	0610	4.3	1242	0.0	1833	4.4
31 SA	0102	0.1	0654	4.3	1326	0.0	1915	4.3

Chart Datum: 0·13 metres above Ordnance Datum (Dublin)

12

TIME ZONE (UT)
For Summer Time add ONE hour in non-shaded areas

IRELAND – COBH

LAT 51°51'N   LONG 8°18'W

TIMES AND HEIGHTS OF HIGH AND LOW WATERS

YEAR **1996**

SEPTEMBER

Date	Day	Time	m	Time	m	Time	m	Time	m
1	SU	0145	0.2	0736	4.1	1408	0.2	1957	4.1
2	M	0227	0.3	0817	4.0	1451	0.4	2038	3.9
3	TU	0310	0.5	0859	3.8	1535	0.6	2120	3.7
4	W	0355	0.8	0943	3.6	1621	0.9	2206	3.5
5	TH	0446	1.0	1033	3.3	1716	1.1	2301	3.2
6	F	0547	1.2	1140	3.2	1822	1.3		
7	SA	0018	3.1	0700	1.3	1308	3.1	1938	1.3
8	SU	0141	3.2	0816	1.2	1420	3.3	2052	1.2
9	M	0245	3.4	0922	1.0	1516	3.5	2148	1.0
10	TU	0337	3.6	1011	0.8	1602	3.7	2231	0.8
11	W	0420	3.8	1050	0.7	1642	3.9	2305	0.7
12	TH	0458	3.9	1120	0.6	1717	4.0	● 2334	0.6
13	F	0532	4.0	1147	0.6	1748	4.0		
14	SA	0002	0.6	0602	4.0	1215	0.6	1816	4.0
15	SU	0034	0.6	0632	4.0	1247	0.6	1845	4.0
16	M	0108	0.6	0703	4.0	1323	0.6	1918	4.0
17	TU	0145	0.7	0738	3.9	1402	0.7	1955	4.0
18	W	0225	0.8	0817	3.9	1445	0.8	2037	3.9
19	TH	0309	0.9	0903	3.8	1533	1.0	2127	3.7
20	F	0401	1.1	0958	3.6	1631	1.1	2227	3.5
21	SA	0507	1.2	1105	3.5	1741	1.2	2339	3.4
22	SU	0627	1.3	1225	3.4	1903	1.2		
23	M	0102	3.4	0748	1.0	1348	3.6	2022	0.9
24	TU	0221	3.6	0900	0.8	1458	3.8	2130	0.6
25	W	0326	3.9	1000	0.5	1555	4.1	2226	0.4
26	TH	0419	4.1	1052	0.2	1645	4.3	2314	0.2
27	F	0507	4.3	1138	0.1	1730	4.4	O 2358	0.1
28	SA	0550	4.3	1221	0.1	1811	4.4		
29	SU	0039	0.1	0631	4.3	1302	0.1	1850	4.3
30	M	0119	0.3	0710	4.2	1342	0.3	1928	4.1

OCTOBER

Date	Day	Time	m	Time	m	Time	m	Time	m
1	TU	0159	0.4	0748	4.0	1422	0.5	2006	3.9
2	W	0240	0.6	0827	3.8	1503	0.8	2045	3.7
3	TH	0322	0.9	0908	3.6	1547	1.0	2127	3.5
4	F	0409	1.1	0955	3.4	1638	1.2	2217	3.3
5	SA	0507	1.3	1055	3.2	1741	1.4	2325	3.1
6	SU	0619	1.4	1222	3.1	1855	1.4		
7	M	0058	3.1	0734	1.3	1345	3.2	2007	1.3
8	TU	0211	3.3	0840	1.2	1443	3.5	2107	1.1
9	W	0304	3.5	0932	1.0	1530	3.7	2153	0.9
10	TH	0348	3.8	1013	0.8	1610	3.9	2230	0.7
11	F	0427	3.9	1047	0.7	1646	4.0	2304	0.5
12	SA	0502	4.0	1118	0.6	1718	4.1	● 2336	0.6
13	SU	0535	4.1	1149	0.5	1748	4.1		
14	M	0010	0.6	0607	4.1	1225	0.5	1821	4.1
15	TU	0046	0.6	0641	4.1	1303	0.6	1856	4.1
16	W	0125	0.6	0719	4.0	1344	0.7	1936	4.0
17	TH	0207	0.7	0801	4.0	1429	0.8	2021	3.9
18	F	0254	0.9	0849	3.8	1520	0.9	2112	3.7
19	SA	0349	1.0	0946	3.7	1618	1.1	2213	3.5
20	SU	0454	1.1	1053	3.5	1727	1.2	2325	3.4
21	M	0611	1.2	1212	3.5	1847	1.1		
22	TU	0046	3.4	0731	1.0	1333	3.6	2007	1.0
23	W	0204	3.6	0843	0.8	1440	3.9	2113	0.7
24	TH	0308	3.9	0943	0.5	1536	4.1	2208	0.5
25	F	0401	4.1	1034	0.3	1625	4.2	2255	0.3
26	SA	0448	4.2	1120	0.2	1710	4.3	O 2338	0.3
27	SU	0531	4.3	1202	0.3	1750	4.3		
28	M	0018	0.3	0610	4.2	1241	0.3	1827	4.2
29	TU	0056	0.4	0647	4.1	1319	0.5	1903	4.1
30	W	0133	0.6	0723	4.0	1356	0.7	1938	3.9
31	TH	0211	0.8	0759	3.9	1434	0.9	2014	3.8

NOVEMBER

Date	Day	Time	m	Time	m	Time	m	Time	m
1	F	0250	1.0	0839	3.7	1515	1.1	2054	3.6
2	SA	0334	1.1	0923	3.5	1602	1.3	2140	3.4
3	SU	0427	1.3	1015	3.3	1700	1.4	2237	3.2
4	M	0532	1.4	1122	3.2	1808	1.5	2352	3.2
5	TU	0643	1.4	1246	3.3	1917	1.4		
6	W	0115	3.3	0748	1.3	1355	3.4	2017	1.2
7	TH	0218	3.5	0843	1.1	1447	3.6	2108	1.0
8	F	0307	3.7	0930	0.9	1531	3.8	2152	0.7
9	SA	0350	3.9	1012	0.8	1610	4.0	2233	0.7
10	SU	0430	4.0	1051	0.7	1647	4.1	2312	0.6
11	M	0509	4.1	1129	0.6	1724	4.2	● 2350	0.5
12	TU	0547	4.3	1208	0.5	1750	4.3		
13	W	0030	0.5	0625	4.2	1250	0.5	1842	4.2
14	TH	0112	0.6	0707	4.2	1333	0.6	1925	4.1
15	F	0157	0.7	0753	4.1	1420	0.7	2012	4.0
16	SA	0247	0.8	0843	4.0	1512	0.8	2105	3.8
17	SU	0341	0.9	0939	3.8	1609	1.0	2204	3.6
18	M	0443	1.0	1043	3.7	1714	1.1	2310	3.5
19	TU	0554	1.1	1154	3.6	1829	1.1		
20	W	0025	3.5	0710	1.0	1309	3.7	1945	1.0
21	TH	0140	3.6	0821	0.9	1416	3.8	2051	0.8
22	F	0244	3.8	0922	0.7	1513	4.0	2147	0.7
23	SA	0340	4.0	1015	0.6	1604	4.1	2236	0.6
24	SU	0428	4.1	1102	0.5	1650	4.2	2319	0.5
25	M	0512	4.2	1144	0.5	1731	4.2	O 2359	0.5
26	TU	0552	4.2	1222	0.6	1808	4.1		
27	W	0035	0.6	0628	4.1	1258	0.7	1842	4.0
28	TH	0110	0.7	0703	4.1	1333	0.8	1915	4.0
29	F	0145	0.8	0738	3.9	1408	1.0	1950	3.8
30	SA	0220	0.8	0815	3.8	1445	1.1	2027	3.7

DECEMBER

Date	Day	Time	m	Time	m	Time	m	Time	m
1	SU	0300	1.1	0855	3.7	1528	1.3	2110	3.6
2	M	0346	1.3	0941	3.6	1618	1.4	2159	3.5
3	TU	0441	1.4	1034	3.5	1717	1.5	2257	3.4
4	W	0545	1.4	1135	3.4	1822	1.5		
5	TH	0004	3.4	0651	1.4	1244	3.4	1925	1.4
6	F	0115	3.5	0752	1.3	1348	3.6	2023	1.2
7	SA	0216	3.6	0847	1.1	1443	3.7	2115	1.0
8	SU	0309	3.8	0938	0.9	1532	3.9	2204	0.8
9	M	0358	4.0	1026	0.7	1619	4.1	2251	0.7
10	TU	0445	4.2	1112	0.6	1704	4.2	● 2335	0.5
11	W	0530	4.3	1156	0.5	1748	4.2		
12	TH	0019	0.4	0614	4.3	1241	0.5	1832	4.2
13	F	0103	0.4	0659	4.3	1326	0.5	1918	4.2
14	SA	0149	0.5	0747	4.2	1414	0.5	2005	4.1
15	SU	0238	0.6	0837	4.1	1504	0.7	2056	3.9
16	M	0331	0.7	0929	3.8	1557	0.8	2150	3.8
17	TU	0427	0.8	1026	3.8	1655	0.9	2249	3.6
18	W	0530	0.9	1128	3.7	1802	1.1	2354	3.6
19	TH	0641	1.0	1236	3.6	1914	1.1		
20	F	0106	3.6	0752	1.0	1345	3.7	2023	1.0
21	SA	0215	3.6	0858	0.9	1447	3.8	2124	0.9
22	SU	0316	3.8	0955	0.8	1542	3.9	2217	0.8
23	M	0409	3.9	1046	0.7	1630	4.0	2303	0.7
24	TU	0455	4.0	1129	0.7	1713	4.0	O 2342	0.7
25	W	0536	4.1	1206	0.7	1751	4.1		
26	TH	0017	0.7	0612	4.1	1240	0.7	1825	4.0
27	F	0050	0.7	0646	4.1	1312	0.8	1857	4.0
28	SA	0121	0.8	0719	4.0	1344	0.9	1930	3.9
29	SU	0154	0.9	0753	4.0	1418	1.0	2004	3.9
30	M	0229	1.0	0829	3.9	1456	1.1	2042	3.8
31	TU	0309	1.1	0909	3.8	1539	1.2	2125	3.7

Chart Datum: 0·13 metres above Ordnance Datum (Dublin)

KINSALE   10-12-19

Cork 51°40'·80N 08°30'·00W

CHARTS

AC 2053, 1765; Imray C56; Irish OS 25

TIDES

−0600 Dover; ML 2·2; Duration 0600; Zone 0 (UT)

Standard Port COBH (←——)

Times				Height (metres)			
High Water		Low Water		MHWS	MHWN	MLWN	MLWS
0500	1100	0500	1100	4·1	3·2	1·3	0·4
1700	2300	1700	2300				
Differences KINSALE							
−0019	−0005	−0009	−0023	−0·2	0·0	+0·1	+0·2

SHELTER

Excellent, except in very strong SE winds. Access H24 in all weathers/tides. Marinas at Kinsale YC and Castlepark. Small marina at Kinsale BY, opp Money Pt; Carrignarone Rk has been covered by infilling.

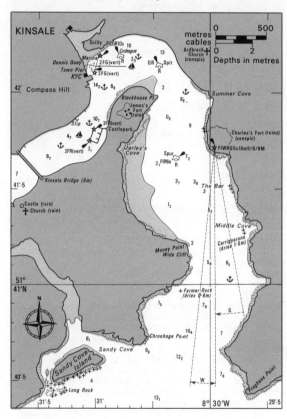

NAVIGATION

WPT 51°40'·00N 08°30'·00W, 181°/001° from/to Charles's Fort lt, 1·7M. Beware: Bulman Rk (0·9m; SCM lt buoy) 4ca S of Preghane Pt; and Farmer Rk (0·6m) ¾ca off W bank.

LIGHTS AND MARKS

Charles's Fort Dir 001°, Fl WRG 5s 18m 9/6M, vis G348°-358°, W358°-004°, R004°-168° (H24). Chan is marked by PHM lt buoys. Both marinas lit as on chartlet.

RADIO TELEPHONE

VHF Ch 06 14 16. Kinsale and Castlepark marinas M 16.

TELEPHONE (021)

Hr Mr 772503; MRCC (01) 6620922/3; Coast/Cliff Rescue Service 772133; ⌗ 968783; Police 772302; Dr 772253, 772717; Ⓗ 546400.

FACILITIES

Kinsale BY, ☎ 774774. AB (3m), M, P, D, FW, ME, Sh, El, C.
Kinsale YC Marina (170 + 50), ☎ 772196, Fax 774455, £11, 10m depth, M, FW, AC, D, P, M, Slip, C, R, Bar;
Castlepark Marina (70+20 visitors) ☎ 774959, Fax 774958, £11, 10m, FW, AC, M, Slip, Bar, El, Ⓖ; ferry (3 mins) to town.
Services: D, ME, El, Ⓔ, C (60 ton), CH, Gas, Gaz, SM.
Town EC Thurs; P, D, V, R, Bar, ✉, Ⓑ, ⇌, ✈ (bus to Cork).

MINOR HARBOUR 2M EAST OF KINSALE

OYSTER HAVEN, Cork, 51°41'·20N 08°26'·90W. AC 2053, 1765. HW −0600 on Dover; ML 2·2m; Duration 0600. See 10.12.19. Good shelter but subject to swell in S winds. Enter 0·5M N of Big Sovereign, a steep islet divided into two. Keep to S of Little Sovereign on E side of ent. There is foul ground off Ballymacus Pt on W side, and off Kinure Pt on E side. Pass W of Hbr Rk (0·9m) off Ferry Pt, the only danger within hbr. ⚓ NNW of Ferry Pt in 4–6m on soft mud/weed. NW arm shoals suddenly about 5ca NW of Ferry Pt. Also ⚓ up N arm of hbr in 3m off the W shore. Weed in higher reaches may foul ⚓. No lts, marks or radio telephone. Coast/Cliff Rescue Service ☎ (021) 770711. Facilities at Kinsale. See 10.12.19.

COURTMACSHERRY   10-12-20

Cork 51°38'·22N 08°40'·90W

CHARTS

AC 2081, 2092; Imray C56; Irish OS 25

TIDES

HW −0610 on Dover; Duration 0545; Zone 0 (UT)

Standard Port COBH (←——)

Times				Height (metres)			
High Water		Low Water		MHWS	MHWN	MLWN	MLWS
0500	1100	0500	1100	4·1	3·2	1·3	0·4
1700	2300	1700	2300				
Differences COURTMACSHERRY							
−0029	−0007	+0005	−0017	−0·4	−0·3	−0·2	−0·1

SHELTER

Good shelter in NW corner of bay, but seas break on the bar (2·3m) in strong S/SE winds, when ent must not be attempted. ⚓ NE of Ferry Pt in approx 2·5m or N of the quay. Weed may foul ⚓; best to moor up/down stream.

NAVIGATION

WPT, 51°37'·50N 08°40'·17W, 144°/324° from/to Wood Pt, 0·8M. Appr in the W sector of Wood Pt lt, between Black Tom and Horse Rk (dries 3·6m); the latter is 4½ca E of Barry Pt on the W shore. Black Tom (2·3m), with unlit SHM buoy 5ca SSE, is close NE of the appr. Beware other hazards further to NE: In centre of bay, Barrel Rk (dries 2·6m), has unlit SCM perch (no topmark). To NNW and E of it are Inner Barrels (0·5m) and Blueboy Rk. Courtmacsherry Hbr is entered between Wood Pt and a SHM buoy 2ca NE, Fl G 3s. Chan (2m) is marked by 4 unlit SHM spar buoys; keep about ½ – ¾ca off the S shore.

LIGHTS AND MARKS

Wood Pt Fl (2) WR 5s 15m 5M, W315°-332° (17°), R332°-315° (343°). Old Hd of Kinsale, Fl (2) 10s 72m 25M, RC.

RADIO TELEPHONE

None

TELEPHONE (023)

Hr Mr/RNLI 46311/46199; Dr 46185; Police 41145; Coast Rescue Service ☎ 40110.

FACILITIES

Quay Temp AB, FW, D, Slip, LB. **Village** P, V, ✉, Bar, R.

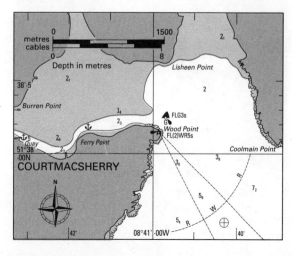

12

GLANDORE   10-12-21
Cork, 51°33'·70N 09°07'·20W

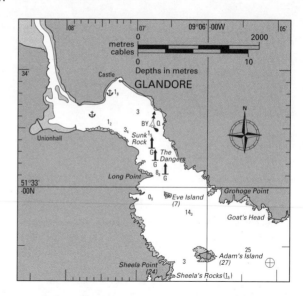

CHARTS
AC 2092; Imray C56; Irish OS 24
TIDES
Approx as for 10·12·22 Castletownshend. Zone 0 (UT)
SHELTER
Excellent. ‡ 1½ca SW of Glandore Pier in 2m or 1ca NE of
the pier (new) at Unionhall in 3m.
NAVIGATION
WPT 51°32'·35N 09°05'·10W, 309°/129° from/to Outer
Dangers 1·2M. Safer ent between Adam Is and Goat's Hd,
thence keep E of Eve Is and W of the chain of rks: Outer,
Middle and Inner Dangers and Sunk Rk. Before altering W
for Unionhall, stand on to clear mudbank 1ca off S shore.
LIGHTS AND MARKS
Galley Hd, Fl (5) 20s, is 5M E of the ent. The Outer Dangers
are marked by a SHM and PHM perch, Middle and Inner
Dangers by a SHM perch and Sunk Rk by NCM lt buoy, Q.
RADIO TELEPHONE
Nil.
TELEPHONE (028)
No Hr Mr; Police 48162; Dr 21488; Coast Rescue Service
☎ 33115.
FACILITIES
FW at both piers; **Glandore** CH, YC, ✉, R, V, Bar, Kos.
Unionhall D, P, ME, Gas, ✉, R, Bar, V.

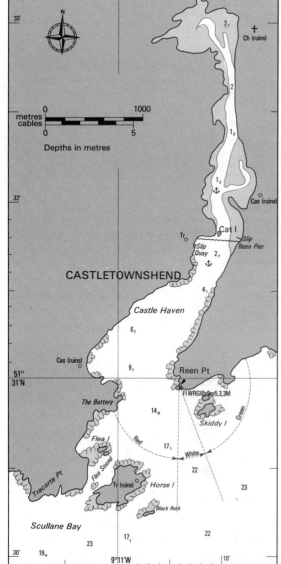

CASTLE HAVEN   10-12-22
Cork 51°30'·90N 09°10'·70W

CHARTS
AC 2129, 2092; Imray C56; Irish OS 24
TIDES
+0605 Dover; ML 2·2; Duration 0605; Zone 0 (UT)

Standard Port COBH (←—)

Times				Height (metres)			
High Water		Low Water		MHWS	MHWN	MLWN	MLWS
0500	1100	0500	1100	4·1	3·2	1·3	0·4
1700	2300	1700	2300				
Differences CASTLETOWNSHEND							
−0020	−0030	−0020	−0050	−0·4	−0·2	+0·1	+0·3
CLONAKILTY BAY							
−0033	−0011	−0019	−0041	−0·3	−0·2	No data	

SHELTER
Excellent ‡ protected from all weathers and available at
all tides, H24, although the outer part of hbr is subject to
swell in S winds. ‡ in midstream SE of Castletownshend
slip; N of Cat Island, or upstream as depth permits.
NAVIGATION
WPT 51°29'·00N, 09°10'·00W, 171°/351° from/to Reen Pt lt,
2M. Enter between Horse Is and Skiddy Is both of which
have foul ground all round. Black Rk lies off the SE side
of Horse Is and is steep-to along its S side. Inside Horse
Is, Flea Sound is a narrow boat chan, obstructed by rks.
Colonel Rk (0·5m) lies close to the E shore, 2ca N of Reen
Pt. A submarine cable runs E/W across the hbr from the
slip close N of Reen Pier to the slip at Castletownshend.
LIGHTS AND MARKS
Reen Pt lt, Fl WRG 10s 9m 5/3M; W tr; vis G shore– 338°,
W338°– 001°, R001°– shore. A ruined tr stands on E end
of Horse Is.
RADIO TELEPHONE
None.
TELEPHONE (028)
MRCC (01) 6620922/3; Coast/Cliff Rescue Service 21039;
⌗ Bantry (027) 50061; Police 36144; Dr 21488; Ⓗ 21677.
FACILITIES
Reen Pier L, FW; SC ☎ 36100. **Castletownshend Village**
Slip, Bar, R, V, FW, ✉, Ⓑ (Skibbereen), ⇌ , ✈ (Cork).

ANCHORAGE W OF TOE HEAD

BARLOGE CREEK, Cork, 51°29'·57N 09°17'·58W. AC 2129.
Tides approx as Castletownshend. A narrow creek, well-
sheltered except from S/SE winds. Appr with Gokane Pt
brg 120°. Enter W of Bullock Is, keeping to the W side to
clear rks S of the island. ‡ W of the Is in 3m. No facilities.

BALTIMORE   10-12-23

Cork 51°28'·30N 09°23'·40W

CHARTS
AC 3725, 2129; Imray C56; Irish OS 24

TIDES
−0605 Dover; ML 2·1; Duration 0610; Zone 0 (UT)

Standard Port COBH (←——)

Times				Height (metres)			
High Water		Low Water		MHWS	MHWN	MLWN	MLWS
0500	1100	0500	1100	4·1	3·2	1·3	0·4
1700	2300	1700	2300				
Differences BALTIMORE							
−0025	−0005	−0010	−0050	−0·6	−0·3	+0·1	+0·2

SHELTER
Excellent; access H24. Hbr, partly drying, is between N and S piers. A small marina (10 berths) is 50m NE of the N pier. Possible AB on N side of N pier for FW. ⚓ N or W of N pier, or in Church Strand Bay beyond LB slip in 2 to 3m. In strong W'ly winds ⚓ off ruined castle on Sherkin Is (off chartlet), 1ca N of ferry and submarine cable.

NAVIGATION
WPT 51°27'·80N 09°23'·42W, 180°/000° from/to Loo Rk SHM Fl G 3s, 0·62M. Beware Lousy Rks (SCM bn) and Wallis Rk (PHM buoy, QR) in the middle of the bay. Hbr can also be entered from the N via The Sound, but this is tricky and not recommended; ICC SDs essential. R Ilen is navigable on the flood for at least 4M above The Sound.

LIGHTS AND MARKS
Ent easily identified by conspic W tr (Lot's Wife) to stbd on Beacon Pt and Barrack Pt lt ho, Fl (2) WR 6s, to port.

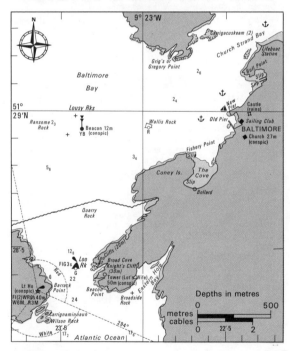

RADIO TELEPHONE
VHF Ch 09 16.

TELEPHONE (028)
Hr Mr 20132; MRCC (01) 6620922/3; Coast/Cliff Rescue Service 20125; ☰ (027) 50061; Police 20102; Dr 21488; Ⓗ 21677.

FACILITIES
Marina (20 inc visitors) ☎ 774959, Fax 774958, Slip, AB, FW; **Glenans Irish Sailing Club** ☎ 6611481. **Services:** P & D, CH, V, Gas, Gaz, Kos, Sh, ACA, ME;
Village EC None; P, Bar, ✉, ⇌ (bus to Cork), ✈ (Cork).

ADJACENT ANCHORAGES

HORSESHOE HARBOUR, 51°28'·20N 09°23'·86W. Small unlit hbr on Sherkin Is, 3ca WSW of ent to Baltimore. Keep to the W at narrow ent. ⚓ in about 5m in centre of cove.

CLEAR ISLAND, NORTH HARBOUR, 51°26'·60N 09°30'·20W. AC 2129. Tides approx as Schull, 10.12.23. A tiny, partly drying inlet on N coast of Clear Is, exposed to N'ly swell. There are rks either side of the outer appr 196°. Inside the narrow (30m), rky ent keep to the E. ⚓ fore & aft on E side in about 1·5m or berth at inner end of pier. Few facilities.

ROARING WATER BAY
Long Island Bay, entered between Cape Clear and Mizen Hd, extends NE into Roaring Water Bay (AC 2129). The Fastnet Rk, Fl 5s 49m 28M, Horn (4) 60s, is 4M to seaward. Safest appr, S of Schull, is via Carthy's Sound (51°30'N 09°30'W). From the SE appr via Gascanane Sound, but beware Toorane Rks, Anima Rk and outlying rks off many of the islands. Shelter in various winds at ⚓s clockwise from Horse Island: 3ca E and 7ca NE of E tip of Horse Is; in Ballydehob B 2m; Poulgorm B 2m; 5ca ENE of Mannin Is in 4m; 2ca SE of Carrigvalish Rks in 6m. Rincolisky Cas (ru) is conspic on S side of bay. The narrow chan E of Hare Is and N of Sherkin Is has two ⚓s; it also leads via The Sound into Baltimore hbr. Local advice is useful. There are temp fair weather ⚓s in the Carthy's Islands. Rossbrin Cove, 2·5M E of Schull, is a safe ⚓, but many local moorings; no access from E of Horse Is due to drying Horse Ridge. No facilities at most of the above ⚓s.

12

SCHULL　　　　　　　10-12-24

Cork 51°30'·80N 09°32'·00W

CHARTS
AC 2129, 2184; Imray C56; Irish OS 24
TIDES
+0610 Dover; ML 1·8; Duration 0610; Zone 0 (UT)

Standard Port COBH (←—)

Times				Height (metres)			
High Water		Low Water		MHWS	MHWN	MLWN	MLWS
0500	1100	0500	1100	4·1	3·2	1·3	0·4
1700	2300	1700	2300				
Differences SCHULL							
−0040	−0015	−0015	−0110	−0·9	−0·6	−0·2	0·0

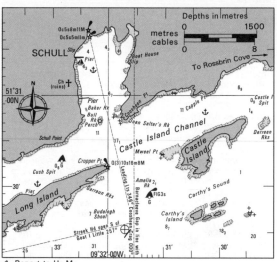

▲ Report to Hr Mr

SHELTER
Good, except in strong S/SE winds when best shelter is N of Long Island. Schull Hbr access H24. ‡ in 3m clear of fairway, 1ca SE of pier, usually lit by street lts all night.
NAVIGATION
WPT 51°29'·60N 09°31'·60W, 166°/346° from/to front ldg lt, 2·1M. In mid-chan between Schull Pt and Coosheen Pt, keep E of Bull Rk (dries 1·8m) marked by a R iron perch.
LIGHTS AND MARKS
Ldg Its, Oc 5s 5/8m 11M, lead 346° between Long Is Pt, Q (3) 10s 16m 8M, W ○ tr, and Amelia Rk SHM buoy Fl G 3s; thence E of Bull Rk and toward head of bay. By day 2 W radomes conspic on Mt Gabriel (2M N of Schull) lead 355° with Long Is Pt lt ho in transit.
RADIO TELEPHONE
None.
TELEPHONE (028)
Hr Mr 28136; MRCC (01) 6620922/3; Coast/Cliff Rescue Service 35117; ⌗ (027) 50061; Police 28111; Dr 28311; Ⓗ (027) 50133.

FACILITIES
Schull Pier Slip, M, D, L, FW, AC, AB; **Sailing Club** ☎ 28286; **Services**: Kos, BY, M, Sh, Slip, CH.
Village EC Tues; P, ME, El, Sh, V, R, Bar, ✉, Ⓑ, ⇌ (bus to Cork), ✈, car ferry (Cork).

CROOKHAVEN　　　　10-12-25

Cork 51°28'·50N 09°42'·00W

CHARTS
AC 2184; Imray C56; Irish OS 24
TIDES
+0550 Dover; ML 1·8; Duration 0610; Zone 0 (UT)

Standard Port COBH (←—)

Times				Height (metres)			
High Water		Low Water		MHWS	MHWN	MLWN	MLWS
0500	1100	0500	1100	4·1	3·2	1·3	0·4
1700	2300	1700	2300				
Differences CROOKHAVEN							
−0057	−0033	−0048	−0112	−0·8	−0·6	−0·4	−0·1
DUNMANUS HARBOUR							
−0107	−0031	−0044	−0120	−0·7	−0·6	−0·2	0·0
DUNBEACON HARBOUR							
−0057	−0025	−0032	−0104	−0·8	−0·7	−0·3	−0·1

SHELTER
Excellent. ‡s in middle of bay in 3m; off W tip of Rock Is; and E of Granny Is; latter two are far from the village. Beware weed.
NAVIGATION
WPT 51°28'·50N 09°40'·50W, 094°/274° from/to Rock Is lt ho, 1M. Ent between this lt and NCM bn on Black Horse Rks (3½ca ESE). From S, keep 1ca E of Alderman Rks and ½ca off Black Horse Rks bn. Passage between Streek Hd and Alderman Rks is not advised. Inside the bay the shores are steep to.
LIGHTS AND MARKS
Lt ho on Rock Is (conspic W tr) L Fl WR 8s 20m 13/11M; vis outside hbr: W over Long Is Bay–281°, R281°–340°; vis inside hbr: R 281°–348°, W348°–N shore.
RADIO TELEPHONE
None.
TELEPHONE (028)
MRCC (01) 6620922/3; Coast/Cliff Rescue Service Goleen 35318; ⌗ (027) 50061; Dr 35148.
FACILITIES
Services: Sh, ME. **Village** V, Kos, Ⓑ (Bantry), ✉, ⇌ and ✈ (Cork).

ADJACENT HARBOURS

GOLEEN (Kireal-coegea), Cork, 51°29'·65N 09°42'·21W. AC 2184. Tides as Crookhaven. A narrow inlet 6ca N of Spanish Pt; good shelter in fair weather, except from SE. 2 churches are easily seen, but ent not visible until close. Keep to S side of ent and ‡ fore-and-aft just below quay, where AB also possible. Facilities: P, V, Bar.

DUNMANUS BAY, Cork. AC 2552. Tides see 10.12.25. Appr between Three Castle Hd and Sheep's Hd, Fl (3) WR 15s 83m 18/15M; no other lts. Ent to **Dunmanus Hbr**, 51°32'·70N 09°39'·86W, is 1ca wide; breakers both sides. ‡ in 4m centre of B. **Kitchen Cove**, 51°35'·50N 09°38'·05W, is the best of the 3 hbrs; enter W of Owens Is and ‡ 1ca NNW of it or 2 ca further N in 3m. Exposed to S, but good holding. Quay at Ahakista village: V, R, Bar. **Dunbeacon Hbr**, 51°36'·35N 09°33'·60W, is shallow and rock-girt. ‡ E or SE of Mannion Is. At Durrus (1¼M): Fuel (cans), R, Bar.

BANTRY BAY

10-12-26

Cork 51°34'N 09°57'W

CHARTS
AC 1838, 1840, 2552; Imray C56; Irish OS 24

TIDES
+0600 Dover; ML 1·8; Duration 0610; Zone 0 (UT)

Standard Port COBH (←)

Times				Height (metres)			
High Water		Low Water		MHWS	MHWN	MLWN	MLWS
0500	1100	0500	1100	4·1	3·2	1·3	0·4
1700	2300	1700	2300				
Differences BANTRY							
–0045	–0025	–0040	–0105	–0·9	–0·8	–0·2	0·0
CASTLETOWN (Bearhaven)							
–0048	–0012	–0025	–0101	–0·9	–0·6	–0·1	0·0
BLACK BALL HARBOUR							
–0115	–0035	–0047	–0127	–0·7	–0·6	–0·1	+0·1

SHELTER/NAVIGATION
Bantry Bay extends 20M ENE from Sheep's Hd, Fl (3) WR 15s 83m 18/15M. Access is easy, but the B is exposed to W'lies. The shore is clean everywhere except off Bear Is and Whiddy Is. The many well sheltered ‡s on the N shore include: Castletown (major FV port) and Dunboy B; Lawrence's Cove and Lonehort Hbr on Bear Is; Adrigole Hbr (attractive ‡ 3M ENE of Bear Is). At the head of the B there are good ‡s off Whiddy Is and Bantry; Glengariff close to the N is a beautiful ‡. The S shore has few ‡s. See also chartlet 10.12.27.

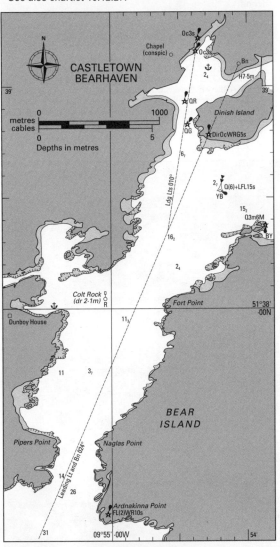

GLENGARIFF, 51°44'·20N 09°31'·90W. AC 1838. Tides as Bantry. Beautiful ‡ S of Bark Is in 7-10m; or to NE in 3m. Better for yachts than Bantry hbr. Ent between Big Pt and Gun Pt. No Its/marks. Keep 1ca E of rks off Garinish Island (Illnacullen) and Ship Is; beware marine farms. Rky chan W of Garinish, with HT cable 15m clearance, should not be attempted. Facilities: **Village** FW, Bar, D, P, ⊠, R, V, Kos.

BANTRY, 51°40'·85N 09°27'·85W. AC 1838. WPT 51 °42'·70N, 09°28'·45W, 335°/155° from/to SHM buoy, 0·7M. Beware Gerane Rks 1M W of Whiddy Is It, Oc 2s 22m 3M, vis 073°-106°. Main ent is the buoyed/lit N chan (10m) to E of Horse and Chapel Is; keep 2ca clear of all islands due to unlit mussel rafts. The S chan, fair weather only, has a bar 2m; Idg marks 091°, front RW post, FW It; rear W post, FR It. VHF Ch 14 11 16 (H24). Hr Mr (027) 505205;

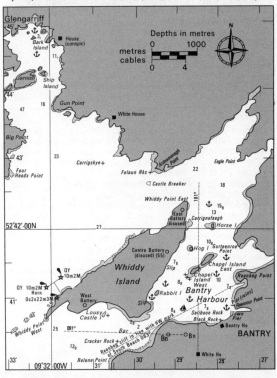

⚓ 50061; Police 50045; Dr 50405; Ⓗ 50133. MRCC (01) 6620922; Coast Rescue Service (028) 35115. Facilities: **Pier** L, FW; **Bantry Bay SC** ☎ 50081 Slip, L; **Town** EC Wed; P & D (cans), Kos, ME, CH, V, R, Bar, ⊠, Ⓑ, bus to Cork.

CASTLETOWN, 51°38'·80N 09°54'·45W. AC 1840. Good shelter at ‡ in 2·4m NW of Dinish Is, to E of 010° Idg I line; also at **Dunboy B**, W of Piper Sound (exposed to E). Lts: Ardnakinna Pt, Fl (2) WR 10s 62m 17/14M, at W ent. At E ent to Bearhaven: Roancarrigmore, Fl WR 3s 18m 18/14M. Appr W of Bear Is on 024° Dir It, Oc WRG 5s 4m 14/11M (W024°-024·5°); thence inner Idg Its 010°, both Oc 3s 4/7m 1M, vis 005°-015°, via ent chan which narrows to 50m abeam Perch Rk It bn. Beware Walter Scott Rk (2·7m), SCM buoy, Q (6) + L Fl 15s, and Carrigaglos (0·6m high) S of Dinish Is. VHF Ch 08 16. Hr Mr ☎ (027) 70220, Fax 70329. Facilities: FW & D on quay; BH on Dinish Is. **Town** EI, ME, Sh, P (cans), Bar, Ⓑ, ⊠, V, R, Kos.

LAWRENCE'S COVE, 51°38'·28N 09°49'·28W AC 1840. Good shelter on N side of Bear Is, open only to the N. ‡ in 4m to W of Turk Is or closer in, to NW of rky ridge off E shore. At Rerrin village: BY, Slip, V, R, Bar, ⊠; Glenans sailing school.

LONEHORT HARBOUR, 51°38'·12N 09°47'·80W. AC 1840. At E tip of Bear Is, good shelter but keep S at ent to clear unmarked rks; then turn ENE to ‡ in 2·7m at E end of cove.

ADRIGOLE, 51°40'·51N 09°43'·22W. AC 1840.1M SSW of ent beware Doucallia Rk, dries 1·2m. Beyond the 2ca wide ent, keep E of Orthons Is (rks on W side). ‡s to suit wind direction: off pier on E shore 4m; N or NW of Orthons Is. Good shelter, but squally in W/N gales. Drumlave (½M E): V.

12

KENMARE RIVER   10-12-27

Kerry 51°45'·00N 10°00'·00W

CHARTS
AC 2495; Imray C56; Irish OS 21/24
TIDES
+0515 Dover; Duration Dunkerron 0620; West Cove 0610.
Zone 0 (UT)

Standard Port COBH (←)

Times				Height (metres)			
High Water		Low Water		MHWS	MHWN	MLWN	MLWS
0500	1100	0500	1100	4·1	3·2	1·3	0·4
1700	2300	1700	2300				

Differences BALLYCROVANE HARBOUR (Coulagh Bay)

−0116	−0036	−0053	−0133	−0·6	−0·5	−0·1	0·0

DUNKERRON HARBOUR

−0117	−0027	−0050	−0140	−0·2	−0·3	+0·1	0·0

WEST COVE (51°46'N 10°03'W)

−0113	−0033	−0049	−0129	−0·6	−0·5	−0·1	0·0

BALLINSKELLIGS BAY

−0119	−0039	−0054	−0134	−0·5	−0·5	−0·1	0·0

VALENTIA HARBOUR (Knights Town)

−0118	−0038	−0056	−0136	−0·6	−0·4	−0·1	0·0

SHELTER
Garnish Bay: is only good in settled weather and W'ly winds. ⌇ either W or 1ca S of the Carrigduff concrete bn.
Ballycrovane: in NE of Coulagh B is a good ⌇, but open to W'ly swell which breaks on submerged rks in SE. N and E shores are foul. ⌇ ½ca NE of Bird Is.
Cleanderry: Ent NE of Illaunbweeheen (Yellow Is) is only 7m wide and rky. ⌇ ENE of inner hbr.
Ardgroom: excellent shelter, but intricate ent over rky bar. Appr with B bn brg 135°; then 2 W bns (front on Black Rk, rear ashore) lead 099° through bar. Alter 206° as two bns astern come in transit. When clear, steer WNW to ⌇ ½ca E of Reenavade pier; power needed. Beware fish farms.
Kilmakilloge: is a safe ⌇ in all winds. Beware mussel beds and rky shoals. On appr steer W of Spanish Is, but pass N of it. Ldg lts 041°, both Iso Y 8s, for Bunaw Hbr (access only near HW; AB for shoal draft). ⌇ 2ca E of Spanish Is; 2ca W of Carrigwee bn; S of Eskadawer Pt; or Colloru Hbr.
Ormond's Hbr: gives good shelter, but beware rk 2½ca ENE of Hog Is. ⌇ in S half of bay.

Kenmare: Good shelter. Access only near HW. 2 W piles in line astern mark max depth to the quay (AB) on N side of river, just below town.
Dunkerron Hbr: Ent between Cod Rks and The Boar to ⌇ 1ca NW of Fox Is in 3·2m; land at Templenoe pier. 4ca E of Reen Pt behind pier, AB (£6) at floating jetty in 1·5m.
Sneem: enter between Sherky Is and Rossdohan Is. Hotel conspic NE of hbr. ⌇ NE of Garinish Is; uncomfortable when considerable swell passes each side of Sherky Is.
Darrynane: 1½M NW of Lamb's Hd, is appr'd from the S between Deenish and Moylaun Islands, but not with high SW swell. Enter with care on the ldg marks/lts 034°, 2 W bns, both Oc 3s 10/16m 4M. Safe ⌇ (3m) NE of Lamb's Is. Other ⌇s include Lehid Hbr, R Blackwater, Coongar Hbr and W Cove.

NAVIGATION
WPT 51°41'·40N 10°10'·00W, 240°/060° from/to Sherky Is 11M. From SW, keep NW of The Bull and Dursey Is. From SE, Dursey Snd is possible in fair wx; to clear dangerous rks off Coulagh Bay, keep twr on Dursey Is well open of Cod's Hd 220°. From NW, there are three deep chans off Lamb's Hd: between Scarriff Is and Deenish Is which is clear; between Deenish and Moylaun Is which has rky shoals; and between Moylaun and Two Headed Is which is clear and 4½ca wide. Up-river from Sneem Hbr, keep N of Maiden Rk, dries 0·5m, and Church Rks; also Lackeen Rks. Beware salmon nets Jun–Sep. See also 10.12.5.

LIGHTS AND MARKS
Bull Rk lt, Fl 15s 83m 31M. On Dursey Is: Old Watch Twr (conspic) 250m. Eagle Hill (Cod's Hd) 216m. Ballycrovane Hbr lt, Fl R 3s, on S tip of Illaunnameanla (Bird Is).

RADIO TELEPHONE
None.

TELEPHONE (064)
MRCC (01) 6620922/3; Coast/Cliff Rescue Service (Waterville) (066) 74320; ⊞ Bantry (027) 50061; Ⓗ 41088.

FACILITIES
ARDGROOM (Pallas Hbr): D & P (cans), V, R, Bar, Kos, ⊠ at Ardgroom village (2M SSW of Reenavade pier), .
KILMAKILLOGE: **Bunaw Pier**, AB, V, Bar; 2M to D, Kos, ⊠.
KENMARE: AB. **Town** D & P (cans), Kos, Gaz, R, V, Bar, Ⓗ, ⊠, Ⓑ, ⇌ (bus to Killarney), ✈ (Cork or Killarney).
SNEEM: L at Hotel Parknasilla & Oysterbed Ho pier (FW).
Town (2M from hbr), P & D (cans), R, Bar, ⊠, Slip, V, Kos.

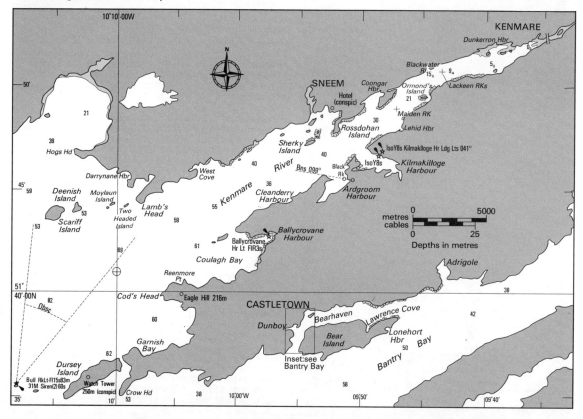

ANCHORAGES NEAR THE ENTRANCE TO DINGLE BAY

PORTMAGEE, Kerry, 51°53'·20N 10°22'·29W. AC 2125. HW +0550 on Dover; ML 2·0m; Duration 0610; See 10·12·27 under VALENTIA HBR. A safe ⚓ 2·5M E of Bray Hd in Portmagee Sound between the mainland and Valentia Is. The ent to the Sound often has bad seas, but dangers are visible. Care required E of Reencaheragh Pt (S side) due rks either side. Deepest water is N of mid-chan. ⚓ off the pier in 5m, opposite Skelling Heritage Centre (well worth a visit). AB on pier is not recommended due to strong tides. Facilities: ⚓, FW, V, R, Bar, Kos. 1ca E of pier, road bridge centre span opens, as pre-arranged with ☎ (066) 77174 or call *Valentia Radio* VHF Ch 24, 28; giving access to Valentia Hbr (Knight's Town) via intricate chan with 1·5m.

VALENTIA HARBOUR, Kerry, 51°56'·20N 10°19'·31W. AC 2125. Tides at 10.12.27. Main ent is at NE end of Valentia Is, between Fort Pt and Beginish Is. Easy access except in strong NW winds. Fort Pt It, Fl WR 2s 16m 17/15M, obsc'd from seaward when E of Doulus Head. Ldg Its 141°: Front Dir Oc WRG 4s 25m 11/8M, W sector 140°-142°; rear, Oc 4s 43m 5M, synch. Beware Hbr Rk, 2·6m, 3ca SE of Fort Pt and 100m W of ldg line; marked by ECM bn Q (3) 10s. Good shelter in ⚓s at: Glanleam B, 6ca S of Fort Pt in 4m; 1ca NW of LB slip in 2·5m (beware The Foot, spit drying 1·2m, marked by ECM buoy, Q (3) 5s); off the ferry pier at Knight's Town (E end of the island) in 4m; in bay on the S side of Beginish Is in 3m. Moorings via Hr Mr ☎ (066) 76124. Facilities (Knightstown): BY, Sh, ME, Gas, Fuel (cans), Kos, some V, R, Bar, ◻. Ferry/bus to Cahersiveen (2½M) for all normal shops; EC Thurs.

VENTRY Kerry, 52°06'·70N 10°20'·30W. AC 2790, 2789. HW +0540 on Dover; ML 2·1m; Duration 0605; See 10·12·28. Ent is 2M W of conspic Eask Tr. A pleasant hbr with easy ent 1M wide and good holding on hard sand; sheltered from SW to N winds, but open to swell from the SE, and in fresh W'lies prone to sharp squalls. Beware Reenvare Rks 1ca SE of Parkmore Pt; also a rky ridge 2·9m on which seas break, extends 2·5ca SSE of Ballymore Pt. ⚓ off Ventry Strand in approx 4m (⊕ brg W, the village NE) or in 3m S side of bay, 1ca N of pier. No Its. Facilities: L, P, Slip, V, Kos. Note: Castlemaine Hbr at the head of Dingle Bay should not be attempted.

ANCHORAGES BETWEEN THE BLASKETS AND KERRY HD

SMERWICK HARBOUR, Kerry, 52°13'·00N 10°24'·00W. AC 2789. Tides 10.12.28. Adequate shelter in this 1M wide bay, except from NW'ly when considerable swell runs in. Ent between East Sister (150m hill) and Dunacapple Is to the NE. ⚓s at: the W side close N or S of the Boat Hr in 3-10m; to the S, off Carrigveen Pt in 2·5m; or in N'lies at the bay in NE corner inside 10m line. Facilities: Ballynagall village on E side has pier (0·5m) and limited V, Bar, Bus.

BRANDON BAY, Kerry, 52°16'·10N 10°09'·92W. AC 2739. Tides as Fenit 10.12.28. A 4M wide bay, very exposed to the N, but in moderate SW-W winds there is safe ⚓ in 6m close E of drying Brandon Pier, 2FG (vert). Cloghane Inlet in SW of Bay is not advised. Facilities at Brandon: limited V, P (1M), ◻, R, Bar, bus.

TRALEE BAY, Kerry, 52°18'·00N 09°56'·00W. AC 2739. HW – 0612 on Dover; ML 2·6m; Duration 0605. See 10·12·28. Entering the bay from W, pass 3M N of Magharee Is. Lt on Little Samphire Is Fl WRG 5s 17m 16/13M, W140°-152° (ldg clear into bay), R152°-172°, obsc 172°-262°, R262°-275°, obsc 275°-280°, R280°-090°, G090°-140°.
Fenit Harbour is formed by a causeway from mainland to Samphire Is, thence a pier extending ENE. It is exposed to E/NE winds, but has good holding and is safe in most conditions. ⚓ off the pier hd in 4m or 1½ca further N in 2m. AB possible at W end of pier in 3m. ⚓s via Tralee SC VHF Ch 14 16 call *Neptune*. Samphire Is light QR 15m 3M vis 242°-097°. Fenit Pier hd 2 FR (vert) 12m 3M, vis 148°-058°. Hr Mr ☎ (066) 36046; ◻ ☎ 36115. Facilities: V, Bar, R, ◻, Slip, C, Fuel (cans), ME.

DINGLE   10-12-28

Kerry 52°07'·14N 10°15'·48W

CHARTS
AC 2790, 2789; Imray C55, 56; Irish OS 53
TIDES
+0540 Dover; ML 2·1m; Duration 0605; Zone 0 (UT)

Standard Port COBH (←→)

Times				Height (metres)			
High Water		Low Water		MHWS	MHWN	MLWN	MLWS
0500	1100	0500	1100	4·1	3·2	1·3	0·4
1700	2300	1700	2300				
Differences DINGLE							
–0111	–0041	–0049	–0119	–0·1	0·0	+0·3	+0·4
SMERWICK HARBOUR							
–0107	–0027	–0041	–0121	–0·3	–0·4	No data	
FENIT PIER (Tralee Bay)							
–0057	–0017	–0029	–0109	+0·5	+0·2	+0·3	+0·1

SHELTER
Excellent at marina (5m depth) in landlocked hbr. A busy fishing port. Also ⚓ 7ca S of pier, clear of dredged chan.
NAVIGATION
WPT 52°06'·20N 10° 15'·48W, 180°/360° from/to It Fl G 3s, 1·06M. Easy ent H24. Beware Crow Rk (dries 3·7m), 0·8M SW of Reenbeg Pt; also the rky ledge extending SW across ent at Black Pt.

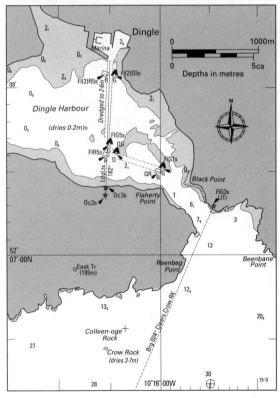

LIGHTS AND MARKS
Eask Twr (195m, with fingerpost pointing E) is conspic 0·85M WSW of ent. Lt tr, Fl G 3s 20m 6M, on NE side of ent. Ent chan, dredged 2·6m, is marked by 4 SHM It buoys and 3 PHM It buoys, as chartlet. Ldg Its, both Oc 3s, (◊ daymarks) lead from astern 182° to hbr bkwtrs.
RADIO TELEPHONE
Ch M, 14 (occas). Valentia Radio (Ch 24 28) has good VHF cover and will relay urgent messages to Dingle.
TELEPHONE (066)
Hr Mr 51629; MRCC (01) 6620922/3; ◻ 21480; Dr 51341; Ⓗ 51455; Police 51522. NB: 999 best for all emergencies.
FACILITIES
Marina (60 + 20 visitors) ☎/Fax 51629, £10, AC, FW, D, C (hire). **Town** EC Thurs; P (cans), Kos, ME, Ⓔ, SM, ◻, R, Bar, V, Ⓑ, ⇌ Tralee (by bus), ✈ (Kerry/Farranfore 30M).

KILRUSH 10-12-29

Clare 52°37'·90N 09°29'·70W

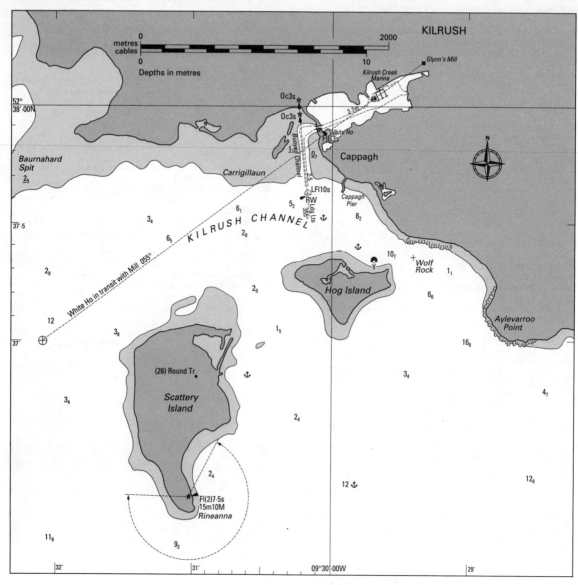

CHARTS
AC 1547, 1819; Imray C55; Irish OS 17
TIDES
−0555 Dover; ML 2·6; Duration 0610; Zone 0 (UT)

Standard Port GALWAY (→)

Times				Height (metres)			
High Water		Low Water		MHWS	MHWN	MLWN	MLWS
1000	0500	0000	0600	5·1	3·9	2·0	0·6
2200	1700	1200	1800				
Differences KILRUSH							
−0006	+0027	+0057	−0016	−0·1	−0·2	−0·3	−0·1

SHELTER
Excellent in Kilrush Creek Marina (2·7m), access via lock H24. Close to the E, Cappagh hbr partly dries, but is well sheltered except in SE winds; pier is constantly used by Shannon pilot boats and tugs. Day ⚓ in lee of Scattery Is.
NAVIGATION
WPT 52°37'·00N 09°32'·10W, 242°/062° from/to SWM buoy, 1·33M. See also 10·12·30. From seaward usual appr is N of Scattery Is (conspic Round Twr, 26m); beware Baurnahard Spit and Carrigillaun to the N. Coming down-river between Hog Is and mainland, beware Wolf Rk.

LIGHTS AND MARKS
Ldg marks 055° White Ho on with Glynn's Mill. SWM By L Fl 10s marks ent to buoyed chan (dredged 2·5m), with ldg lts 355°, both Oc 3s, to lock. Fl G 3s 2M, S side of lock.
RADIO TELEPHONE
VHF Ch 12 16. Marina Ch 80 M.
TELEPHONE (065)
Hr Mr 51327; Lock 52155; MRCC (01) 6620922/3; Coast/Cliff Rescue Service 51004; ⌗ (061) 415366; Weather (061) 62677; Police 51017; Dr (065) 51581.
FACILITIES
Marina (120+50) ☎ 52072, Fax 51692, £9.10, £2.50 for <6hrs, AC, FW, D, P (cans), Slip, BY, CH, Gas, Gaz, Kos, BH (45 ton), C (26 ton), ME, EI, ▣, V;
Cappagh, Slip, AB, L, FW, P, V.
Town EC Thurs; EI, CH, V, R, Bar, Dr, ✉, Ⓑ, ⇌ (bus to Limerick), ✈ (Shannon).

SHANNON ESTUARY   10-12-30

Clare (N); Kerry and Limerick (S) 52°35'·00N 09°40'·00W

CHARTS
AC 1819, 1547, 1548, 1549, 1540; L. Derg 5080 and L. Ree 5078. Imray C55.
Yachtsmen planning to visit the Shannon Estuary should study the ICC's *Sailing Directions for S and W Ireland* and/or the Admiralty *Irish Coast Pilot*.

TIDES

HW at	HW Galway	HW Dover
Kilbaha	−0015	+0605
Carrigaholt	−0015	+0605
Tarbert	+0035	−0530
Foynes	+0050	−0515
Limerick	+0130	−0435

At Limerick strong S-W winds increase the height and delay the times of HW; strong N-E winds do the opposite.

SHELTER
The Shannon Estuary is 50M long, from Loop Hd to Limerick. For boats on passage N or S the nearest ⚓ is Kilbaha B, 3M inside Loop Hd; it has ⚓s sheltered in winds from W to NE, but is exposed to swell and holding is poor. 6M further E, Carrigaholt B has ⚓s and good shelter from W'lies; ⚓ just N of the new quay, out of the tide.
From Kilconly and Kilcredaun Pts in the W to the R Fergus ent (about 25M) there are ⚓s or ⚓s, protected from all but E winds, at Tarbert Is, Glin, Labashadee, Killadysert and among the islands in the Fergus mouth. The best ⚓ in the estuary is at Foynes on the S bank, with also a pontoon off the YC. There are drying quays at Ballylongford Creek (Saleen), Knock and Clarecastle (S of Ennis, off chartlet). Yachts may go up to Limerick Dock, but this has all the drawbacks of a commercial port: frequent shifting of berth, dirt and someone constantly on watch.

NAVIGATION
WPT 52°32'·50N 09°46'·90W, Ballybunnion NCM By VQ, 244°/064° from/to Tail of Beal Bar buoy WCM, Q (9) 15s, 4·2M. For notes on ent and tidal streams see 10·12·5. The ebb can reach 4kn. The lower estuary is 9M wide between Kerry and Loop Heads narrowing to 2M off Kilcredaun Pt. Here the chan is well buoyed in midstream and then follows the Kerry shore, S of Scattery Is. From Tarbert Is to Foynes Is the river narrows to less than 1M in places, before widening where the R Fergus joins from the N, abeam Shannon airport.
Above this point the buoyed chan narrows and becomes shallower although there is a minimum of 2m at LWS. AC 1540 is essential for the final 15M stretch to Limerick.

RIVER SHANNON
Above Limerick navigation is inhibited by locks and bridges. The Shannon, which is the longest navigable river in the UK or Ireland, is controlled by the Limerick Hbr Commissioners up to Limerick; up-river it effectively becomes an inland waterway. Information on navigation and facilities can be obtained from the Office of Public Works (OPW), Shannon Navigation Branch, Athlone, Co Westmeath; or Inland Waterways Association of Ireland, Kingston Ho, Ballinteer, Dublin 4, ☎ 01-983392; also from Tourist Offices and inland marinas.

LIGHTS AND MARKS
Principal lts are listed in 10·12·4. There are QW (vert) aero hazard lts on tall chimneys at Money Pt power station 3M ESE of Kilrush. 2 chys at Tarbert Is are conspic (R lts).

RADIO TELEPHONE
Foynes Ch 12 13 16 (occas). Limerick Ch 12 13 16 (HO).

FACILITIES
Marine facilities have been provided at several communities on the Shannon Estuary. P & D (cans), FW, V, M are available at many villages. ⚓s are being laid at Labasheeda, Glin Pier (pontoon) and Foynes.
Facilities at the two major centres are:
Foynes Slip, L, AB, P & D (cans), FW, ✉, Ⓑ, Dr, V, R, Bar;
Foynes YC ☎ (069) 65261, Bar, R.
Limerick: Hbr Commissioners ☎ (061) 315377; ⌗ ☎ 415366.
City Slip, AB, L, FW, P & D (cans), Kos, Gas, Gaz, ME, El, Dr, Ⓗ, ✉, all usual city amenities, ⇌, ✈ (Shannon).

12

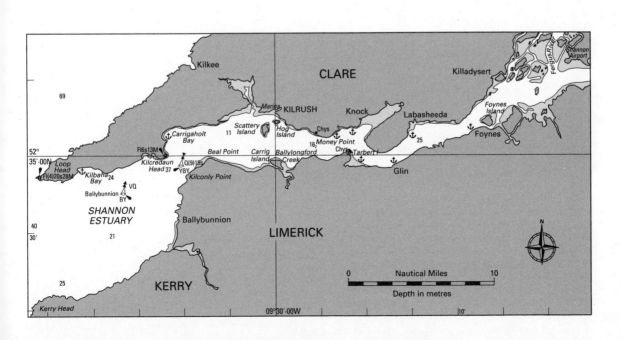

Volvo Penta service

Sales and service centres in area 13
Northern Ireland *Robert Craig & Sons Ltd,* 15-21 Great Georges Street,
Belfast BT15 1BW Tel (01232) 232971

Area 13

North Ireland
Lambay Island, north to Liscanor Bay

VOLVO PENTA

13

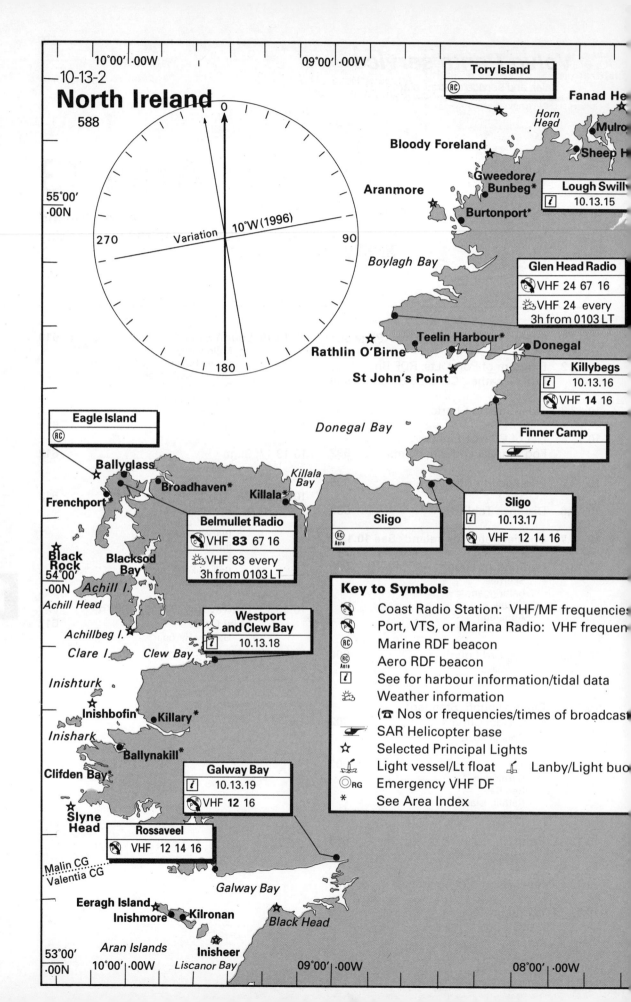

North Ireland

588

Tory Island
(RC)

Fanad He

Horn Head

Mulro

Bloody Foreland

Sheep H

Gweedore/ Bunbeg*

Lough Swill
(i) 10.13.15

Aranmore

Burtonport*

Boylagh Bay

Glen Head Radio
(C) VHF 24 67 16
(weather) VHF 24 every 3h from 0103 LT

Teelin Harbour*

Donegal

Rathlin O'Birne

St John's Point

Killybegs
(i) 10.13.16
(P) VHF **14** 16

Donegal Bay

Variation 10°W (1996)

270 — 90

0

90

180

55°00' ·00N

Finner Camp
(helicopter)

Eagle Island
(RC)

Killala Bay

Ballyglass

Broadhaven*

Killala*

Sligo
(RC Aero)

Sligo
(i) 10.13.17
(C) VHF 12 14 16

Frenchport*

Belmullet Radio
(C) VHF **83** 67 16
(weather) VHF 83 every 3h from 0103 LT

Black Rock

Blacksod Bay*

54°00' ·00N

Achill I.

Achill Head

Achillbeg I.

Westport and Clew Bay
(i) 10.13.18

Clare I.   *Clew Bay*

Inishturk

Key to Symbols

(C)   Coast Radio Station: VHF/MF frequencies
(P)   Port, VTS, or Marina Radio: VHF frequen
(RC)   Marine RDF beacon
(RC Aero)   Aero RDF beacon
(i)   See for harbour information/tidal data
(weather)   Weather information
    (☎ Nos or frequencies/times of broadcast
(helicopter)   SAR Helicopter base
☆   Selected Principal Lights
(light)   Light vessel/Lt float   (buoy) Lanby/Light buo
(RG)   Emergency VHF DF
*   See Area Index

Inishbofin   **Killary***

Inishark

Ballynakill*

Clifden Bay*

Galway Bay
(i) 10.13.19
(C) VHF **12** 16

Slyne Head

Rossaveel
(C) VHF 12 14 16

Malin CG
Valentia CG

Galway Bay

Eeragh Island
Inishmore   **Kilronan**

Black Head

Aran Islands   **Inisheer**

53°00' ·00N

10°00' ·00W   *Liscanor Bay*   09°00' ·00W   08°00' ·00W

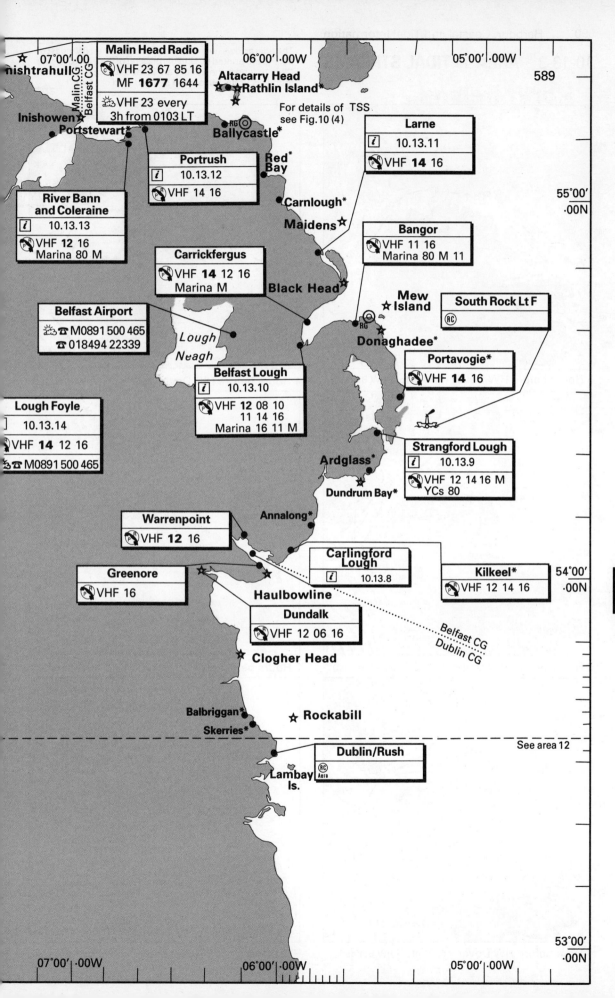

Malin Head Radio
☎ VHF 23 67 85 16
MF **1677** 1644
☼ VHF 23 every
3h from 0103 LT

589

Altacarry Head
Rathlin Island*

For details of TSS
see Fig.10 (4)

Inishowen
Portstewart*

Ballycastle*

Larne
ⓘ 10.13.11
☎ VHF **14** 16

Portrush
ⓘ 10.13.12
☎ VHF 14 16

Red*
Bay

**River Bann
and Coleraine**
ⓘ 10.13.13
☎ VHF **12** 16
Marina 80 M

Carnlough*

Maidens ☆

Bangor
☎ VHF 11 16
Marina 80 M 11

Carrickfergus
☎ VHF **14** 12 16
Marina M

Black Head*

**Mew
Island** ☆

South Rock Lt F
ⓡⓒ

Belfast Airport
☼☎ M0891 500 465
☎ 018494 22339

Lough
Neagh

Donaghadee*

Portavogie*
☎ VHF **14** 16

Belfast Lough
ⓘ 10.13.10
☎ VHF **12** 08 10
11 14 16
Marina 16 11 M

Lough Foyle
10.13.14
☎ VHF **14** 12 16
☼☎ M0891 500 465

Ardglass*

Strangford Lough
ⓘ 10.13.9
☎ VHF 12 14 16 M
YCs 80

Dundrum Bay*

Annalong*

Warrenpoint
☎ VHF **12** 16

**Carlingford
Lough**
ⓘ 10.13.8

Kilkeel*
☎ VHF 12 14 16

Greenore
☎ VHF 16

Haulbowline

Belfast CG
Dublin CG

Dundalk
☎ VHF 12 06 16

Clogher Head ☆

Balbriggan*

☆ **Rockabill**

Skerries*

See area 12

Dublin/Rush
ⓡⓒ Aero

**Lambay
Is.**

13

55°00'
·00N

54°00'
·00N

53°00'
·00N

07°00' ·00W   06°00' ·00W   05°00' ·00W

10-13-3   AREA 13 TIDAL STREAMS

The tidal arrows (with no rates shown) off the NW coast of Ireland are printed by kind permission of the Irish Cruising Club, to whom the Editors are indebted. They have been found accurate, but should be used with caution.

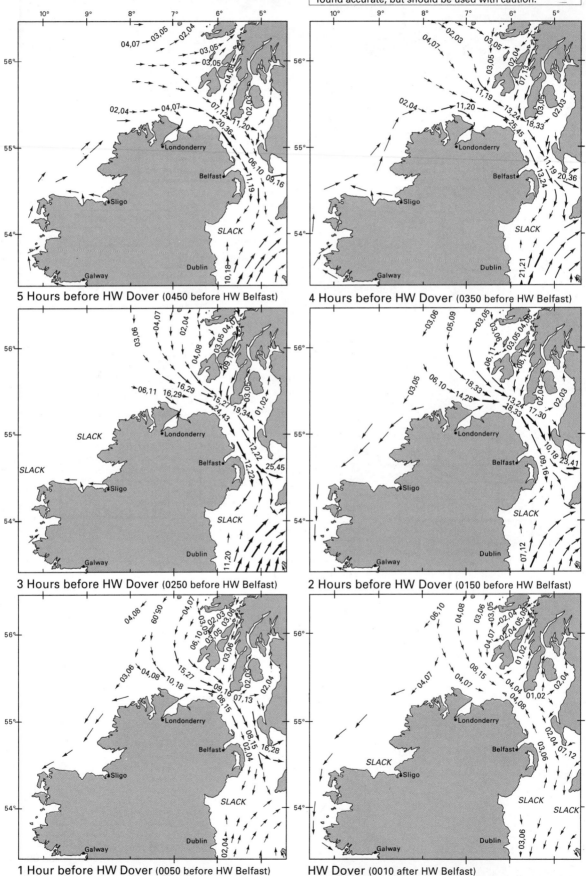

5 Hours before HW Dover (0450 before HW Belfast)

4 Hours before HW Dover (0350 before HW Belfast)

3 Hours before HW Dover (0250 before HW Belfast)

2 Hours before HW Dover (0150 before HW Belfast)

1 Hour before HW Dover (0050 before HW Belfast)

HW Dover (0010 after HW Belfast)

Southward 10.12.3   North Irish Sea 10.10.3
SW Scotland 10.9.3

The tidal arrows (with no rates shown) off the NW coast of Ireland are printed by kind permission of the Irish Cruising Club, to whom the Editors are indebted. They have been found accurate, but should be used with caution.

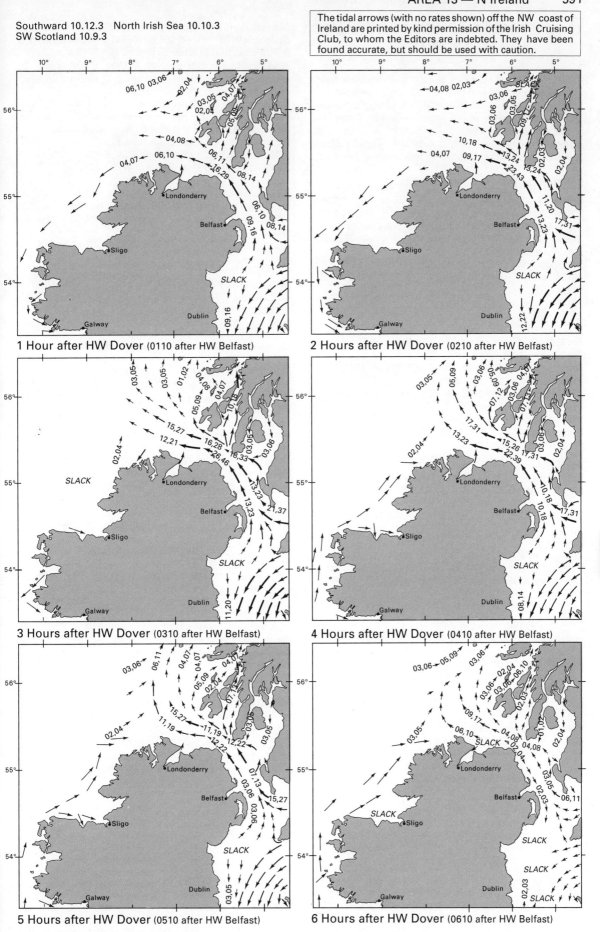

1 Hour after HW Dover (0110 after HW Belfast)

2 Hours after HW Dover (0210 after HW Belfast)

3 Hours after HW Dover (0310 after HW Belfast)

4 Hours after HW Dover (0410 after HW Belfast)

5 Hours after HW Dover (0510 after HW Belfast)

6 Hours after HW Dover (0610 after HW Belfast)

13

10.13.4 COASTAL LIGHTS, FOG SIGNALS AND WAYPOINTS

Abbreviations used below are given in 1.4.1. Principal lights are in **bold** print, places in CAPITALS, and light-vessels, light floats and Lanbys in *CAPITAL ITALICS*. Unless otherwise stated lights are white. m – elevation in metres; M – nominal range in miles. Fog signals are in *italics*. Useful waypoints are underlined – use those on land with care. All geographical positions should be assumed to be approximate. See 4.4.1.

LAMBAY ISLAND TO DONAGHADEE

Rockabill 53°35'·80N 06°00'·20W Fl WR 12s 45m **W22M, R18M**; W Tr, B band; vis W178°-329°, R329°-178°; *Horn (4) 60s*. Also shown by day when))) is operating.
Skerries Bay Pier Hd 53°35'·08N 06°06'·43W Oc R 6s 7m 7M; W col; vis 103°-154°.
Balbriggan 53°36'·75N 06°10'·75W Fl (3) WRG 20s 12m W13M, R10M, G10M; W Tr; vis G159°-193°, W193°-288°, R288°-305°.

DROGHEDA
Lts in line about 248°: **Front** 53°43'·14N 06°14'·80W Oc 12s 8m **15M**; Tr, W lantern; vis 203°-293°. **Rear**, 85m from front, Oc 12s 12m **17M**; Tr; vis 246°-252°.
North Light 53°43'·43N 06°15'·20W Fl R 4s 7m **15M**; Tr, W lantern; vis 282°-288°; tfc sigs.
Aleria Lt Bn 53°43'·34N 06°14'·27W QG 11m 3M; G Bn.
Lyons Lt Bn 53°43'·24N 06°41'·20W Fl (3) R 5s 2m. Above this Pt Lts on stbd hand when ent are G, and on port hand R.
Dunany Lt By 53°53'·55N 06°09'·40W Fl R 3s; PHM.

DUNDALK
N training wall Hd, **Pile Lt** 53°58'·54N 06°17'·68W Fl WR 15s 10m **W21M, R18M**; W Ho; vis W124°-151°, R151°-284°, W284°-313°, R313°-124°. Oc G 5s 8m; same Tr; vis 331°-334°; Fog Det Lt VQ 7m, vis when brg 358°; *Horn (3) 60s*.
No. 2 Bn 53°58'·33N 06°17'·73W Fl (2) R 5s 4m 3M; 2 in R□.
No. 8 Bn 53°59'·30N 06°18'·91W Fl R 3s; R pile. Above this Pt Lts on stbd hand when ent are QG, and on port hand QR.
Imogene Lt By 53°57'·04N 06°06'·95W Fl (2) R 10s; PHM.
Carlingford Lt By 53°58'·75N 06°01'·06W L Fl 10s; *Whis*; SWM.

CARLINGFORD LOUGH/NEWRY RIVER
Hellyhunter Lt By 54°00'·34N 06°01'·99W Q (6) + L Fl 15s; *Whis*; SCM.
Haulbowline 54°01'·18N 06°04'·68W Fl (3) 10s 32m **17M**; Gy Tr; reserve Lt 15M; Fog Det Lt VQ 26m; vis 330°.
Turning Lt FR 21m 9M; same Tr; vis 196°-208°; *Horn 30s*.
Ldg Lts 310·7° Front 54°01'·78N 06°05'·37W Oc 3s 7m 11M; R △ on Tr; vis 295°-325°. Rear, 457m from front, Oc 3s 12m 11M; R ▽ on Tr; vis 295°-325°; both H24.
Greenore Pt 54°02'·06N 06°07'·91W Fl R 7·5s 10m 5M.
Carlingford Quay Hd 54°02'·59N 06°11'·01W Fl 3s 5m 2M.
Newry River Ldg Lts 310·4°. Front 54°06'·37N 06°16'·46W. Rear, 274m from front. Both Iso 4s 5/15m 2M; stone cols.
Warren Pt Bkwtr Hd 54°05'·78N 06°15'·20W Fl G 3s 6m 3M.

KILKEEL
Pier Hd 54°03'·45N 05°59'·27W Fl WR 2s 8m 8M; vis R296°-313°, W313°-017°.
Meeney's Pier Hd Fl G 3s 6m 2M.

ANNALONG
E Bkwtr Hd 54°06'·50N 05°53'·65W Oc WRG 5s 8m 9M; Tr; vis G204°-249°, W249°-309°, R309°-024°.

DUNDRUM BAY
St John's Pt 54°13'·60N 05°39'·23W Q (2) 7·5s 37m **23M**; B ● Tr, Y bands; H24 when))) operating.
Auxiliary Lt Fl WR 3s 14m **W15M**, R11M; same Tr, vis W064°-078°, R078°-shore; Fog Det Lt VQ 14m vis 270°; *Horn (2) 60s*.
Dundrum Hbr FR on W side of chan outside Hbr and 3 FR on W side of chan inside Hbr when local vessels expected. FR on flagstaffs S and E of ent when firing takes place.
DZ East By 54°13'·50N 05°46'·16W; SPM.
DZ Middle By 54°13'·00N 05°48'·50W; SPM.
DZ West By 54°13'·34N 05°50'·00W; SPM.

ARDGLASS
Inner Pier Hd 54°15'·78N 05°36'·28W Iso WRG 4s 10m W8M, R7M, G5M; Tr; vis G shore-308°, W308°-314°, R314°-shore.
Outer Pier Hd 54°15'·62N 05°36'·07W Fl R 3s 10m 5M.

STRANGFORD LOUGH
Strangford Lt By 54°18'·60N 05°28'·59W L Fl 10s; *Whis*; SWM.
Bar Pladdy Lt By 54°19'·34N 05°30'·48W Q (6) + LFl 15s; SCM.
Angus Rk 54°19'·83N 05°31'·48W Fl R 5s 15m 6M shown H24.
Dogtail Pt Ldg Lts 341° Front 54°20'·78N 05°31'·78W Oc (4) 10s 2m 5M. Rear, Gowlands Rk, 0·8M from front, Oc (2) 10s 6m 5M.
Salt Rk 56°21'·41N 05°32'·60W Fl R 3s 8m 3M.
Swan I 54°22'·37N 05°33'·10W Fl (2) WR 6s 5m; W col; vis W115°-334°, R334°-115°.
Church Pt Bn 54°22'·59N 05°33'·35W Fl (4) R 10s.
Portaferry Pier Hd 54°22'·81N 05°32'·94W Oc WR 10s 9m W9M, R6M; Or mast; vis W335°-005°, R005°-017°, W017°-128°.
Killyleagh Town Rk Bn 54°23'·61N 05°38'·47W Q 4M; PHM.
Limestone Rk 54°25'·13N 05°36'·04W QR 3m 3M.
Butter Pladdy Lt By 54°22'·43N 05°25'·68W Q (3) 10s; ECM.

SOUTH ROCK Lt F 54°24'·47N 05°21'·92W Fl(3) R 30s 12m **20M**; R hull and Lt Tr, W Mast; RC; Racon (T); *Horn (3) 45s*.

PORTAVOGIE/BALLYWATER/DONAGHADEE
Plough Rk Lt By 54°27'·39N 05°25'·08W QR; PHM; *Bell*.
S Pier Hd 54°27'·44N 05°26'·08W, Iso WRG 5s 9m 9M; ■ Tr; vis G shore-258°, W258°-275°, R275°-348°.
Skulmartin Lt By 54°31'·83N 05°24'·83W L Fl 10s; *Whis*; SWM.
Ballywalter Bkwtr Hd 54°32'·67N 05°28'·75W Fl WRG 1·5s 5m 9M; vis G240°-267°, W267°-277°, R277°-314°. Unreliable.
Donaghadee, S Pier Hd 54°38'·70N 05°31'·80W Iso WR 4s 17m **W18M**, R14M; W Tr; vis W shore-326°, R326°-shore; *Siren 12s*.

DONAGHADEE TO RATHLIN ISLAND

Governor Rks Lt By 54°39'·36N 05°31'·93W Fl R 3s; PHM.
Deputy Reefs Lt By 54°39'·51N 05°31'·88W Fl G 2s; SHM.
Foreland Spit Lt By 54°39'·64N 05°32'·25W Fl R 6s; PHM.
Ninion Bushes By 54°41'·07N 05°30'·40W; PHM.

BELFAST LOUGH
Mew I NE end 54°41'·91N 05°30'·73W Fl (4) 30s 37m **24M**; B Tr, W band; Racon (O).
S Briggs Lt By 54°41'·19N 05°35'·66W Fl (2) R 10s; PHM.

BANGOR
N Pier Hd 54°40'·02N 05°40'·30W Iso R 12s 9m14M.
Dir Lt 105°. 54°39'·98N 05°40'·08W Dir Oc 10s WRG 12M; vis G093°-104·8°, W104·8°-105·2°, R105·2°-117°.
Marina ent 54°39'·90N 05°40'·20W Fl G 3s 5m 1M.

Belfast No. 1 Chan Lt By 54°41'·67N 05°46'·30W I QG; *Bell*; SHM.

Cloghan Jetty Lt By 54°44'·10N 05°41'·52W QG; SHM.

Kilroot power station intake 54°43'·20N 05°45'·82W Oc G 4s; 2 QR on chy 500m N.

CARRICKFERGUS

E Pier Hd 54°42'·63N 05°48'·30W Fl G 7·5s 5m 4M; G col.

Marina E Bkwtr Hd 54°42'·71N 05°48'·63W QG 8m 3M; G ● pillar.

W Bkwtr QR 7m 3M; R ● pillar.

Pier Hd 54°42'·58N 05°48'·71W F WRG 5m 3M; vis G308°-317·5°, W317·5°-322·5°, R322·5°-332°.

Black Hd 54°45'·99N 05°41'·27W Fl 3s 45m **27M**; W 8-sided Tr; RC.

N Hunter Rk Lt By 54°53'·04N 05°45'·06W Q; NCM.

S Hunter Rk Lt By 54°52'·69N 05°45'·22W Q (6) + L Fl 15s; *Horn(3) 30s*; SCM.

LARNE

Barr Pt 54°51'·50N 05°46'·73W; *Horn 30s*. Fog Det Lt VQ.

No. 1 Lt By 54°51'·62N 05°47'·53W Q (3) 10s; ECM.

No. 3 Lt By 54°51'·27N 05°47'·56W Fl (2) G 6s; SHM.

Chaine Tr 54°51'·27N 05°47'·82W Iso WR 5s 23m 11M; Gy Tr; vis W230°-240°, R240°-shore.

Larne No. 2 Lt Bn 54°51'·07N 05°47'·47W Fl R 3s.

Ent Ldg Lts 184°. No. 11 Front 54°49'·59N 05°47'·74W Oc 4s 6m 12M; W ◊ with R stripe on R pile structure; vis 179°-189°. No. 12 Rear, 610m from front, Oc 4s 14m 12M; W ◊ with R stripe on R ● Tr; synch with front, vis 179°-189°.

Maidens 54°55'·73N 05°43'·60W Fl (3) 20s 29m **24M**; W Tr, B band. Auxiliary Lt Fl R 5s 15m 8M; same Tr; vis 142°-182° over Russel and Highland Rks.

CARNLOUGH/RED BAY

Carnlough Hbr N Pier 54°59'·58N 05°59'·20W Fl G 3s 4m 5M; W col, B bands.

Red Bay Pier 55°03'·92N 06°03'·12W Fl 3s 10m 5M.

RATHLIN ISLAND TO INISHTRAHULL

RATHLIN ISLAND

Rue Pt 55°15'·53N 06°11'·40W Fl (2) 5s 16m 14M; W 8-sided Tr, B bands.

Drake Lt By 55°17'·00N 06°12'·41W Q (6) + L Fl 15s; SCM.

Altacarry Hd   Rathlin E 55°18'·06N 06°10'·23W Fl (4) 20s 74m **26M**; W Tr, B band; vis 110°-006° and 036°-058°; Racon (O).

Rathlin W 0·5M NE of Bull Pt 55°18'·05N 06°16'·75W Fl R 5s 62m **22M**; W Tr, lantern at base; vis 015°-225°; H24 when ⟫ operating; *Horn (4) 60s*.

Manor House Pier 55°17'·52N 06°11'·60W Fl (2) R 6s 5m 4M.

Ballycastle Pier Hd 55°12'·45N 06°14'·25W L Fl WR 9s 6m 5M; vis R110°-212°, W212°-000°.

PORTRUSH

N Pier Hd 55°12'·35N 06°39'·52W Fl R 3s 6m 3M; vis 220°-160°.

Portstewart Pt 55°11'·32N 06°43'·20W Oc R 10s 21m 5M; R ■ hut; vis 040°-220°.

RIVER BANN/COLERAINE

Ldg Lts 165°. Front 55°09'·95N 06°46'·17W Oc 5s 6m 2M; W Tr. Rear, 245m from front, Oc 5s 14m 2M; W ■ Tr. R. marked by Fl G on stbd hand, and Fl R on port.

W Pier 56°10'·32N 06°46'·40W Fl G 5s 2M; Gy mast; vis 350°-180°.

Lough Foyle Lt By 55°15'·29N 06°52'·51W L Fl 10s; *Whis*; SWM;

Tuns Lt By 55°14'·00N 06°53'·38W Fl R 3s; PHM.

Inishowen 55°13'·56N 06°55'·69W Fl (2) WRG 10s 28m **W18M**, R14M, G14M; W Tr, 2 B bands; vis G197°-211°, W211°-249°, R249°-000°; *Horn (2) 30s*. Fog Det Lt VQ 16m vis 270°.

LOUGH FOYLE

Greencastle Ldg Lts 022°. Front 55°12'·20N 06°58'·90W Fl 3s 11m 2M; Or ◊ on mast. Rear, 50m from front, Fl 3s 13m 2M; Or ◊ on mast. F WR 10m; vis R072°-082°, W082°-072°. F WR 5m; vis R037°-052°, W052°-037°.

Warren Pt Lt Bn Tr 55°12'·58N 06°57'·06W Fl 1·5s 9m 10M; W ● Tr, G abutment. G; vis 232°-061°.

Magilligan Pt 55°11'·74N 06°57'·97W QR 7m 4M; R structure. FR, 700m SE, when firing taking place.

McKinney's Bk 55°10'·92N 07°00'·50W Fl R 5s 6m 4M; R pile structure.

Moville 55°11'·00N 07°02'·06W Fl WR 2·5s 11m 4M; W house on G piles vis W240°-064°, R064°-240°.

Above this point the chal to R.Foyle is marked by Lts Fl G, when entering, on stbd hand, and Fl R on port hand. G Lts are shown from W structures on G or B piles; R Lts from W structures on R piles.

Kilderry 55°04'·09N 07°13'·95W Fl G 2s 6m 6M; W structure.

Muff 55°03'·63N 07°14'·21W Fl G 2s 5m 3M; G structure.

Coneyburrow 55°03'·32N 07°14'·42W Fl G 2·5s 5m 3M.

Faughan 55°03'·12N 07°14'·42W Fl R 4s 8m 3M.

Culmore Pt 55°02'·78N 07°15'·20W Q 6m 5M; G ● Tr.

Culmore Bay 55°02'·72N 07°15'·65W Fl G 5s 4m 2M.

Lisahally 55°02'·52N 07°05'·72W QR 2M; PHM Lt Bn; R refl; (TE 1991).

Ballynagard 55°02'·28N 07°16'·37W Fl 3s 6m 3M; W lantern on G ● house.

Otter Bank 55°01'·95N 07°16'·65W Fl R 4s 4m 3M; W structure on R ● Tr.

Brook Hall 55°01'·70N 07°17'·07W QG 4m 3M; W structure on G base.

Mountjoy 55°01'·25N 07°17'·49W QR 5m 3M; W lantern on R piles.

Inishtrahull 55°25'·85N 07°14'·60W Fl (3) 15s 59m **25M**; W Tr; Racon (T).

INISHTRAHULL TO BLOODY FORELAND

LOUGH SWILLY/BUNCRANA/RATHMULLAN

Fanad Hd 55°16'·57N 07°37'·86W Fl (5) WR 20s 39m **W18M**, R14M; W Tr; vis R100°-110°, W110°-313°, R313°-345°, W345°-100°. FR on radio mast 3·08M 200°.

Swilly More Lt By 55°15'·12N 07°35'·74W Fl G 3s; SHM.

Dunree 55°11'·88N 07°33'·20W Fl (2) WR 5s 46m W12M, R9M; vis R320°-328°, W328°-183°, R183°-196°.

Colpagh Lt By 55°10'·42N 07°31'·50W; Fl R 6s; PHM.

White Strand Rks Lt By 55°09'·06N 07°29'·90W Fl R 10s; PHM.

Buncrana Pier near Hd 55°07'·61N 07°29'·82W Iso WR 4s 8m W14M, R11M; vis R shore-052° over Inch spit, W052°-139°, R139°-shore over White Strand Rk.

Rathmullan Pier Hd 55°05'·70N 07°31'·66W Fl G 3s 5M; vis 206°-345°.

MULROY BAY

Limeburner Lt By 55°18'·54N 07°48'·36W Q Fl; NCM; *Whis*.

Ravedy I 55°15'·15N 07°46'·80W Fl 3s 9m 3M; Tr; vis 177°-357°.

Dundooan Rks 55°13'·14N 07°47'·91W QG 4m 1M; G Tr.

Crannoge Pt 55°12'·29N 07°48'·37W Fl G 5s 5m 2M; G Tr.

SHEEPHAVEN

Downies Bay Pier Hd 55°11'·36N 07°50'·42W Fl R 3s 5m 2M; vis 283° through N till obsc by Downies Pt.

Portnablahy Ldg Lts 125·3°. Front 55°10'·80N 07°55'·60W Oc 6s 7m 2M; B col, W bands. Rear, 81m from front, Oc 6s 12m 2M; B col, W bands.

Tory I NW Pt 55°16'·36N 08°14'·92W Fl (4) 30s 40m **27M**; B Tr, W band; vis 302°-277°; RC; H24.

13

Inishbofin Pier 55°10'·1N 08°10·5W Fl 8s 3m 3M; part obsc.
Ballyness Hbr. Ldg Lts 119·5°. Front 55°09'·0N 08°06'·9W
Iso 4s 25m 1M. Rear, 61m from front, Iso 4s 26m 1M.
Bloody Foreland 55°09'·51N 08°16'·98W Fl WG 7·5s 14m
W6M, G4M; vis W062°-232°, G232°-062°.

BLOODY FORELAND TO RATHLIN O'BIRNE

Glassagh. Ldg Lts 137·4°. Front 55°06'·85N 08°18'·90W Oc 8s
12m 3M. Rear, 46m from front, Oc 8s 17m 3M, synch with front.
Inishsirrer, NW end 55°07'·41N 08°20'·89W Fl 3·7s 20m 4M;
W ■ Tr vis 083°-263°.

BUNBEG/MULLAGHDOO/OWEY SOUND
Gola I Ldg Lts 171·2°. Front 55°05'·12N 08°21'·02W Oc 3s
9m 2M; W Bn, B band. Rear, 86m from front, Oc 3s 13m 2M;
B Bn, W band; synch with front.
Bo I E Pt 55°04'·78N 08°20'·08W Fl G 3s 3m; G Bn.
Inishinny No. 1 55°04'·48N 08°19'·78W QG 3m 1M; ■ col.

Inishcoole No. 4   55°03'·98N 08°18'·88W QR 4m 2M; R ■
col on base.
Yellow Rks No. 6 55°03'·67N 08°18'·90W QR 3m 1M; ■ col
with steps; Neon.
Cruit I. Owey Sound Ldg Lts 068·3°. Front 55°03'·07N
08°25'·79W Oc 10s. Rear, 107m from front, Oc 10s.
Rinnalea Pt 55°02'·60N 08°23'·67W Fl 7·5s 19m 9M; ■ Tr; vis
132°-167°.

Aranmore, Rinrawros Pt 55°00'·90N 08°33'·60W Fl (2) 20s
71m **29M**; W Tr; obsc by land about 234°-007° and about
013°. Auxiliary Lt Fl R 3s 61m 13M, same Tr; vis 203°-234°.

NORTH SOUND OF ARAN/RUTLAND NORTH CHANNEL
Ldg Lts 186°. Front 54°58'·94N 08°29'·22W Oc 8s 8m 3M; B
Bn, W band. Rear, 395m from front, Oc 8s 17m 3M; B Bn.
Ballagh Rks 54°59'·96N 08°28'·80W Fl 2·5s 13m 5M; W
structure, B band.
Black Rks 54°59'·43N 08°29'·59W Fl R 3s 3m 1M; R col.
Inishcoo Ldg Lts 119·3°. Front 54°59'·12N 08°27'·70W Iso 6s
6m 1M; W Bn, B band. Rear, 248m from front, Iso 6s 11m
1M; B Bn, Y band.
Carrickatine No. 2 Bn 54°59'·26N 08°28'·06W QR 6m 1M;
R Bn with steps; Neon.
Rutland I Ldg Lts 137·6°. Front 54°58'·97N 08°27'·63W Oc 6s
8m 1M; W Bn, B band. Rear, 330m from front, Oc 6s 14m
1M; B Bn, Y band.

BURTONPORT
Ldg Lts 068·1°. Front 54°58'·96N 08°26'·36W FG 17m 1M; Gy
Bn, W band. Rear, 355m from front, FG 23m 1M; Gy Bn,
Y band.

SOUTH SOUND OF ARAN/RUTLAND SOUTH CHANNEL
Illancrone I 54°56'·28N 08°28'·53W Fl 5s 7m 6M; W ■ Tr.
Wyon Pt 54°56'·50N 08°27'·50W Fl (2) WRG 10s 8m W6M,
R3M; W ■ Tr; vis G shore-021°, W021°-042°, R042°-121°,
W121°-150°, R 150°-shore.
Turk Rks 54°57'·30N 08°28'·15W Fl G 5s 6m 2M; G ■ Tr.
Aileen Reef 54°58'·18N 08°28'·78W QR 6m 1M. R ■ Bn.
Leac na bhFear 54°82'·1N 08°29'·2W Q (2) 5s 4m 2M.
Carrickbealatroha Fl 5s 3m 2M.
Carrickbealatroha, Upper 54°58'·64N 08°28'·58W Fl 5s 3m
2M; W ■ brickwork Tr.
Corren's Rk 54°58'·12N 08°26'·68W Fl R 3s 4m 2M; R ■ Tr.
Teige's Rk 54°58'·61N 08°26'·75W Fl 3s 4m 2M; W ● Tr, ■
base.
Dawros Hd 54°49'·60N 08°33'·60W L Fl 10s 39m 4M; W ■ col.
Dawros Bay 54°49'·3N 08°32'W Fl (2) 10s 5m 3M.
Rathlin O'Birne. W side 54°39'·80N 08°49'·90W Fl WR 15s

35m **W18M, R14M**; W Tr; vis R195°-307°, W307°-195°;
Racon (O).

RATHLIN O'BIRNE TO EAGLE ISLAND

DONEGAL BAY, TEELIN/KILLYBEGS
Teelin Hbr 54°37'·32N 08°37'·72W Fl R 10s; R structure.
St John's Pt 54°34'·15N 08°27'·60W Fl 6s 30m 14M; W Tr.
Bullockmore Lt By 54°33'·98N 08°30'·06W Qk Fl (9) 15s;
WCM.
Rotten I 54°36'·87N 08°26'·39W Fl WR 4s 20m **W15M**,
R11M; W Tr; vis W255°-008°, R008°-039°, W039°-208°.
Ldg Lts 338°. Pier, Front 54°38'·13N 08°26'·33W Oc R 8s
5m 2M. Rear, 65m from front, Oc R 8s 7m 2M. Both Y ◆, on
buildings.
Killybegs Outer Lt By 54°37'·91N 08°26'·10W V Q (6) + L Fl 10s;
SCM.
Black Rk Jetty 54°38'·3N 08°26'·5W Fl RG 5s; Gy col; vis
R254°-204°, G204°-254°.

SLIGO
Wheat Rk Lt By 54°18'·82N 08°39'·02W Q (6) + LFl 15s; SCM.
Black Rock 54°18'·45N 08°37'·03W Fl 5s 24m 13M; W Tr, B
band. Auxiliary Lt Fl R 3s 12m 5M; same Tr; vis 107°-130°
over Wheat and Seal rks.
Lower Rosses N of Pt (Cullaun Bwee) 54°19'·71N 08°34'·36W
Fl (2) WRG 10s 8m W10M, R8M, G8M; W hut on piles; vis G
over Bungar bank-066°, W066°-070°, R070° over Drumcliff
bar; shown H24.
Ldg Lts 125°. Front Metal Man 54°18'·23N 08°34'·51W Fl 4s
3m 7M. Rear Oyster I, 365m from front, Oc 4s 13m 10M.
Both shown H24.

KILLALA
Inishcrone Pier Root 54°13'·20N 09°05'·74W Fl WRG 1·5s
8m 2M; vis W098°-116°, G116°-136°, R136°-187°.
Ldg Lts 230°. Rinnaun Pt, Front No. 1 54°13'·53N 09°12'·21W
Oc 10s 7m 5M; ■ Tr. Rear, 150m from front, No. 2 Oc 10s 12m
5M; ■ Tr.
Dir Lt 215°, Inch I, 54°13'·29N 09°12'·25W Fl WRG 2s 6m
3M; ■ Tr; vis G205°-213°, W213°-217°, R217°-225°.
Ldg Lts 196°. Kilroe, Front 54°12'·62N 09°12'·28W Oc 4s 5m
2M; ■ Tr. Rear,120m from front, Oc 4s 10m 2M; ■ Tr.
Ldg Lts 236°. Pier, Front 54°13'·01N 09°12'·80W Iso 2s 5m
2M; W ◊ on Tr. Rear, 200m from front, Iso 2s 7m 2M; W ◊ on
pole.
Killala Bay. Bone Rk, NE end 54°15'·80N 09°11'·20W Q 7m;
NCM.

BROAD HAVEN BAY
Gubacashel Pt 54°16'·05N 09°53'·28W Iso WR 4s 27m W12M,
R9M; W Tr; vis W shore (S side of bay)-355°, R355°-shore.
Ballyglass 54°15'·28N 09°53'·38W Fl G 3s.

Eagle I, W end 54°17'·02N 10°05'·51W Fl (3) 10s 67m **23M**;
W Tr; RC. Shown H24.

EAGLE ISLAND TO SLYNE HEAD

Black Rk 54°04'·00N 10°19'·20W Fl WR 12s 86m **W22M,
R16M**; W Tr; vis W276°-212°, R212°-276°.

BLACKSOD BAY
Blacksod Lt By 54°05'·87N 10°02'·96W Q (3) 10s, ECM.
Blacksod Pier Root 54°05'·91N 10°03'·60W Fl (2) WR 7·5s
13m W12M, R9M; W Tr on dwelling; vis R189°-210°, W210°-
018°.
Achill I Ridge Pt. 54°01'·80N 09°58'·50W Fl 5s 21m 5M.
ACHILL SOUND
Achill Sound 53°56'·06N 09°55'·21W QR; R Bn.
Ldg Lts 330° Whitestone Pt, Front and rear both Oc 4s 5/6m;
W ◊, B stripe.

Saulia Pier 53°57'·03N 09°55'·53W Fl G 3s 12m.
Achillbeg E Lt Bn 53°52'·12N 09°56'·50W Fl R 2s 5m; R ■ Tr.
Carrigin-a-tShrutha 53°52'·29N 09°56'·70W Q (2) R 5s; R Bn.

Achill I Ldg Lts 310° Purteen 53°57'·79N 10°05'·92W (PA) Oc 8s 5m. Rear, 46m from front Oc 8s 6m.

CLEW BAY/WESTPORT
Achillbeg I S Pt 53°51'·50N 09°56'·80W Fl WR 5s 56m **W18M, R18M, R15M**; W ● Tr on ■ building; vis R262°-281°, W281°-342°, R342°-060°, W060°-092°, R(intens) 092°-099°, W099°-118°.
Clare I, E Pier 53°48'·00N 09°57'·00W Fl R 3s 5m 3M.
Cloghcormick By 53°50'·56N 09°43'·18W; WCM.
Dorinish Lt By 53°49'·47N 09°40'·45W Fl G 3s; SHM.
Inishgort S Pt 53°49'·60N 09°40'·20W L Fl 10s 11m 10M; W Tr. Shown H24.
Westport Appr 53°47'·97N 09°34'·30W Fl 3s; G box on conical Bn.
Roonagh Quay Ldg Lts 144°. Front 53°45'·80N 09°54'·20W. Rear, 54m from front, both Iso 10s 9/15m.

INISHBOFIN/CLIFDEN BAY
Inishlyon Lyon Hd 53°36'·70N 10°09'·50W Fl WR 7·5s 13m W7M, R4M; W post; vis W036°-058°, R058°-184°, W184°-325°, R325°-036°.
Gun Rk 53°36'·58N 10°13'·18W Fl (2) 6s 8m 4M; W col; vis 296°-253°.

Cleggan Pt 53°34'·50N 10°07'·70W Fl (3) WRG 15s 20m W6M, R3M, G3M; W col on W hut; vis W shore-091°, R091°-124°, G124°-221°.
Carrickrana Rks Bn 53°29'·20N 10°09'·50W; large W Bn.
Slyne Hd, N Tr, Illaunamid 53°23'·98N 10°14'·02W Fl (2) 15s 35m **24M**; B Tr.

SLYNE HEAD TO BLACK HEAD

Inishnee 53°22'·75N 09°54'·40W Fl (2) WRG 10s 9m W5M, R3M, G3M; W col on W ■ base; vis G314°-017°, W017°-030°, R030°-080°, W080°-194°.
Croaghnakeela Is 53°19'·40N 09°58'·11W Fl 3·7s 7m 5M; W col; vis 034°-045°, 218°-286°, 311°-325°.

GALWAY BAY/INISHMORE
Eeragh, Rock Is 53°08'·90N 09°51'·34W Fl 15s 35m **23M**; W Tr, two B bands; vis 297°-262°.

Straw Is 53°07'·05N 09°37'·80W Fl (2) 5s 11m **17M**; W Tr. Ldg Lts 192°. Front 53°06'·25N 09°39'·70W Oc 5s 6m 3M; W

col on W ■ base; vis 142°-197°. Rear 43m from front Oc 5s 8m 2M; W col on W ■ base; vis 142°-197°.
Killeany Lt By 53°07'·25N 09°38'·19W Fl G 3s; SHM.

Kilronan Pier Hd 53°07'·10N 09°39'·95W Fl WG 1·5s 5m 3M; W col; vis G240°-326°, W326°-000°.

KIGGAUL BAY
Kiggaul Bay 53°14'·01N 09°43'·00W Fl WR 3s 5m W5M, R3M; vis W329°-359°, R359°-059°, part obsc by W shore of bay.

CASHLA BAY/SPIDDLE
Ent W side 53°14'·23N 09°35'·14W Fl (3) WR 10s 8m W6M, R3M; W col on concrete structure; vis W216°-000°, R000°-069°.
Cannon Rk Lt By 53°14'·05N 09°34'·29W Fl G 5s; SHM.
Lion Pt Dir Lt 53°15'·83N 09°33'·93W Dir Iso WRG 4s 6m W8M, R6M, G6M; W ■ Tr on col; vis G357·5°-008·5°, W008·5°-011·5°, R011·5°-017·5°.
Rossaveel Pier Ldg Lts 116° Front 53°15'·98N 09°33'·36W Oc 3s 7m 3M; W mast. Rear, 90m from front, Oc 3s 8m 3M; W mast.
Spiddle Pier Hd 53°14'·42N 09°18'·50W Fl WRG 3·5s 11m W6M, R4M, G4M; Y col; vis G102°-282°, W282°-024°, R024°-066°.

GALWAY
Margaretta Shoal Lt By 53°13'·67N 09°05'·95W Fl G 3s; SHM; *Whis.*
Black Rock Lt By 53°13'·99N 09°06'·51W Fl R 3s; PHM.
Tawin Shoals Lt By 53°14'·27N 09°04'·24W Fl (3) G 10s; SHM.
Mutton Is Lt By 53°15'·06N 09°02'·89W Fl (2) R 6s; PHM.
Peter Rk By 53°15'·15N 09°01'·07W; SCM.
Leverets 53°15'·32N 09°01'·87W Q WRG 9m 10M; B ● Tr, W bands; vis G015°-058°, W058°-065°, R065°-103°, G103°-143·5°, W143·5°-146·5°, R146·5°-015°.
Rinmore 53°16'·11N 09°01'·93W Iso WRG 4s 7m 5M; W ■ Tr; vis G359°-008°, W008°-018°, R018°-027°.
Nimmo's Pier Hd 53°15'·99N 09°02'·77W Iso Y 6s 7m 6M. Approach chan Ldg Lts 325°. Front 53°16'·12N 09°02'·80W Fl R 1·5s 12m 7M; R ◆, Y diagonal stripes on mast; vis 315°-345°. Rear 310m from front Oc R 10s 19m 7M; R ◆, Y diagonal stripes on framework Tr; vis 315°-345°.

Black Hd 53°09'·25N 09°15'·78W Fl WR 5s 20m W11M, R8M, W ■ Tr; vis 045°-268°, R268°-276°.

Inisheer 53°02'·8N 09°31'·5W Iso WR 20s 34m **W20M, R16M**; Vis 225°-231°, W231°-245°, R245°-269°, W280°-218°; Racon (K).

13

10.13.5   PASSAGE INFORMATION

For all Irish waters the Sailing Directions published by the Irish Cruising Club are strongly recommended, and particularly on the N and W coasts, where other information is scarce. They are published in 2 volumes: *E and N coasts of Ireland* which runs anti-clockwise from Carnsore Pt to Bloody Foreland, and *S and W coasts of Ireland* which goes clockwise.

CROSSING THE IRISH SEA (charts 1123, 1121, 1411)

Passages across the Irish Sea can range from the fairly long haul from Land's End to Cork (140M), to the relatively short hop from Mull of Kintyre to Torr Pt (11M). But such distances are deceptive, because the average cruising yacht needs to depart from and arrive at a reasonably secure hbr; also in the North Chan strong tidal streams can cause heavy overfalls. So each passage needs to be treated on its merits. See 10.0.6 for distances across the Irish Sea.

Many yachts use the Land's End/Cork route on their way to (and from) the delightful cruising ground along the S coast of Ireland, see 10.12.5. Penzance Bay, or one of the Scilly Is anchs, make a convenient place from which to leave, with good lights to assist departure.

Although the Celtic Sea is exposed to the Atlantic, there are no dangers on passage and the tidal streams are weak. A landfall between Ballycotton and Old Hd of Kinsale (RC) (both have good Lts) presents no offlying dangers, and in poor vis decreasing soundings indicate approach to land. There is a likelihood, outward bound under sail, that the boat will be on the wind – a possible benefit on the return passage. If however the wind serves, and if it is intended to cruise along the southern coast, a landfall at the Fastnet with arrival at (say) Baltimore will place the yacht more to windward, for little extra distance.

From Land's End the other likely destination is Dun Laoghaire. A stop at (say) Milford Haven enables the skipper to select the best time for passing the Smalls or Bishops (see 10.11.5) and roughly divides the total passage into two equal parts. From S Bishop onwards there are the options of making the short crossing to Tuskar Rk and going N inside the banks (theoretically a good idea in strong W winds), or of keeping to seaward. But in bad weather the area off Tuskar is best avoided; apart from the Traffic Separation Scheme, the tide is strong at sp and the sea can be very rough.

The ferry route Holyhead/Dun Laoghaire is another typical crossing, and is relatively straightforward with easy landfalls either end. The tide runs hard round Anglesey at sp, so departure just before slack water minimises the set N or S. Beware also the TSS off The Skerries, see Fig. 10(3).

The Isle of Man (10.10.5) is a good centre for cruising in the Irish Sea, and its hbrs provide convenient staging points whether bound N/S or E/W.

CROSSING TO SCOTLAND (charts 2198, 2199, 2724)

Between Scotland and Northern Ireland there are several possible routes, but much depends on weather and tide. Time of departure must take full advantage of the stream, and avoid tide races and overfalls (see 10.9.5). Conditions can change quickly, so a flexible plan is needed.

From Belfast Lough ent, the passage distance to Mull of Kintyre is about 35M and, with a departure at HW Dover (also local HW) providing at least 6hrs of N-going tides, fair winds make it possible to get past the Mull or Sanda Is on one tide. But to be more confident of reaching Port Ellen or Gigha Is a departure from Carnlough or Red Bay at HW makes a shorter passage with better stream advantage. The inshore side of the TSS (Fig. 10(4)) coincides with the outer limit of the race S and SW off the Mull of Kintyre; this occurs between HW Dover + 0430 and + 0610 when a local S-going stream opposes the main N-going stream.

For information on submarine hazards see 10.9.22.

LAMBAY ISLAND TO FAIR HEAD (AC 44, 2093, 2198/9)

The coast is fairly steep-to except in larger Bs, particularly Dundalk. Streams offshore run up to 2·5kn as far as Rockabill, but are weaker further N until approaching Belfast Lough. Lambay Island is private, and steep-to except on W side, where there can be overfalls. Skerries Is (Colt, Shenick's and St Patrick's) are 1M E and SE of Red Is, to E of Skerries hbr. Shenick's Is is connected to shore at LW. Pass between Colt Is and St Patrick's Is, but the latter has offliers 3ca to S. Rockabill, two steep-to rks with Lt Ho, is 2·5M E of St Patrick's Is.

Going NE from Carlingford Lough (10.13.8), after rounding Hellyhunter By there are no offshore dangers until Strangford Lough (10.13.9). For Kilkeel and Ardglass, see 10.13.8. N of Strangford keep 5ca off Ballyquintin Pt. 3M to NE are Butter Pladdy Rks; keep to E of these. 2M further N is South Rk, with disused Lt Ho, part of group of rks to be avoided in poor vis or bad weather by closing South Rk Lt F. In good vis pass inshore of South Rk, between it and North Rks (chart 2156).

Three routes lead into Belfast Lough (10.13.10): E of Mew Is, but beware Ram Race (to the N on the ebb, and the S on the flood); Copeland Sound, between Mew Is and Copeland Is, is passable but not recommended; Donaghadee Sound is buoyed and a good short cut for yachts. Here the stream runs SSE from HW Belfast + 0530 and NW from HW Belfast – 0030, 4·5kn max. An eddy extends S to Ballyferris Pt, and about 1M offshore. For Donaghadee, see 10.13.10 and chart 3709.

N from Belfast Lough, Black Hd is clean. Pass E of Muck Is, which is steep-to. Hunter Rk (0·8m), 2·5M NE of Larne, is marked by N & S cardinals. 2M further N are the Maidens, two dangerous groups of rks extending 2·5M N/S; E Maiden is lit.

The very small hbr of Carnlough (10.13.11) provides shelter for small yachts, but should not be approached in strong onshore winds. Other anchs in offshore winds are at Red Bay (10.13.11) 5M further N, and in Cushendun B, 5M NNW of Garron Pt. All provide useful anch or passage to/from the Clyde or Western Is. Fair Hd is a bold 190m headland, steep-to all round, but with extensive overfalls in Rathlin Sound.

FAIR HEAD TO BLOODY FORELAND (chart 2723)

This is a good cruising area, under the lee of land in SW'lies, but very exposed to NW or N. Beware fishing boats and nets in many places and the North Channel TSS, see Fig. 10(4).

A fair tide is essential through Rathlin Sound where the stream runs 6kn at sp, and causes dangerous overfalls. The main stream runs NW from HW Galway – 0600 for 5hrs, and SE from HW Galway + 0100 for 4hrs. A W-going eddy runs from Fair Hd close inshore towards Carrickmannanon Rk from HW Galway + 0100, and an E-going eddy runs from HW Galway – 0500 to – 0100. The worst overfalls in the chan are from HW Galway – 0500 to – 0300, and it is best to enter W-bound at the end of this period, on the last of fair tide. Keep seaward of Carrickmannanon Rk and Sheep Is. There is a hbr in Church Bay, on the W side of Rathlin Is.

Proceeding to Portrush (10.13.12), use Skerries Sound in good weather. Enter Lough Foyle by either the North Chan W of The Tuns, or S chan passing 2ca N of Magilligan Pt and allowing for set towards The Tuns on the ebb (up to 3·5kn).

Tor Rks, Inishtrahull and Garvan Isles lie NE and E of Malin Hd. In bad weather it is best to pass at least 3M N of Tor Rks. Inishtrahull is lit and about 1M long; rks extend N about 3ca into Tor Sound. Inishtrahull Sound, between Inishtrahull and Garvan Isles, is exposed; tidal stream up to 4kn sp can raise a dangerous sea with no warning. Stream also sets hard through Garvan Isles, S of which Garvan Sound can be passed safely in daylight avoiding two sunken rks, one 1½ca NE of Rossnabarton, and the other 5ca NW. The main stream runs W for only 3hrs, from HW Galway – 0500 to – 0200. W of Malin Hd a W-going eddy starts at HW Galway + 0400, and an E-going one at HW Galway – 0300.

Note that direction of buoyage changes off Malin Head.

From Malin Head SW to Dunaff Head, at ent to Lough Swilly (10.13.15), keep 5ca offshore. Trawbreaga Lough (AC 2697) gives shelter, but is shallow, and sea can break on bar; only approach when no swell, and at half flood. Ent to L Swilly is clear except for Swilly Rks off the W shore, SSE of Fanad Hd.

W from Lough Swilly the coast is very foul. Beware Limeburner Rk (2m), 6·8M WNW of Fanad Hd. Mulroy Bay (10.13.15) has good anchs but needs accurate pilotage, as in *ICC SDs*.

Between Mulroy B and Sheephaven there is inshore passage S of Frenchman's Rk, and between Guill Rks and Carnabollion, safe in good weather; otherwise keep 1M offshore. Sheep Haven B (10.13.15) is easy to enter between Rinnafaghla Pt and Horn Hd, and has good anchs except in strong NW or N winds. Beware Wherryman Rks, dry 1·5m, 1ca off E shore.

Between Horn Hd and Bloody Foreland (chart 2752) are three low-lying islands: Inishbeg, Inishdooey and Inishbofin. The latter is almost part of the mainland; it has a temp anch on S side and a more sheltered anch on NE side in Toberglassan B. 6M offshore is Tory Is (Lt, fog sig, RC) with rks for 5ca off SW side. Temp anch in good weather in Camusmore B. In Tory Sound the stream runs W from HW Galway + 0230, and E from HW Galway – 0530, sp rates 2kn.

BLOODY FORELAND TO EAGLE ISLAND (chart 2725)

Off low-lying Bloody Foreland (Lt) there is often heavy swell. The coast and islands 15M SW to Aran Is give good cruising (chart 1883). An inshore passage avoids offlying dangers: Buniver and Brinlack shoals, which can break; Bullogconnell 1M NW of Gola Is; and Stag Rks 2M NNW of Owey Is. Anchs include Bunbeg and Gweedore hbr, and Cruit B which has easier access. Behind Aran Is are several good anchs. Use N ent, since S one is shallow (chart 2792). Rutland N Chan is main appr to Burtonport (10.13.15).

Boylagh B has shoals and rks N of Roaninish Is. Connell Rk (0·3m) is 1M N of Church Pool, a good anch, best approached from Dawros Hd 4·5M to W. On S side of Glen B a temp anch (but not in W or NW winds) is just E of Rinmeasa Pt. Rathlin O'Birne Is has steps E side; anch SE of them 100m offshore. Sound is 5ca wide; hold Is side to clear rks off Malin Beg Hd.

In Donegal B (chart 2702) beware uncharted rks W of Teelin, a good natural hbr but exposed to S/SW swell. Killybegs (10.13.16) has better shelter and is always accessible. Good shelter with fair access in Donegal Hbr (chart 2715). Good anch or ⚓ via YC at Mullaghmore in fair weather; sea state is calm with winds from SE through S to NW. Inishmurray is worth a visit in good weather, anch off S side. There are shoals close E and NE of the Is, and Bomore Rks 1·5M to N. Keep well clear of coast S to Sligo (10.13.17) in onshore winds, and watch for lobster pots.

Killala B has temp anch 1M S of Kilcummin Hd, on W side. Proceeding to Killala beware St Patrick's Rks. Ent has ldg lts and marks, but bar is dangerous in strong NE winds.

The coast W to Broadhaven is inhospitable. Only Belderg and Portacloy give a little shelter. Stag Rks are steep-to and high. Broadhaven (chart 2703) is good anch and refuge, but in N/NW gales sea can break in ent. In approaches beware Slugga Rk on E side with offlier, and Monastery Rk (0·3m) on S side.

EAGLE ISLAND TO SLYNE HEAD (chart 2420)

This coast has many inlets, some sheltered. Streams are weak offshore. There are few Lts. Keep 5ca off Erris Hd, and further in bad weather. Unless calm, keep seaward of Eagle Is (Lt, RC) where there is race to N. Frenchport (chart 2703) is good temp anch except in strong W winds. Inishkea Is (chart 2704) can be visited in good weather; anch N or S of Rusheen Is. On passage keep 5ca W of Inishkea to avoid bad seas if wind over tide. The sound off Mullet Peninsula is

clear, but for Pluddany Rk 6ca E of Inishkea N.
Blacksod B (chart 2704 and 10.13.18) has easy ent (possible at night) and good shelter. In the approaches Black Rk (Lt) has rks up to 1·25M SW. From N, in good weather, there is chan between Duvillaun Beg and Gaghta Is, but in W gales beware breakers 1M SE of Duvillaun More.

Rough water is likely off impressive Achill Hd. Achill Sound (chart 2667) is restricted by cables 11m high at swing bridge. Anchs each end of Sound, but the stream runs strongly.

Clare Is has Two Fathom Rk (3·4m) 5ca off NW coast, and Calliaghcrom Rk 5ca to the N; anch on NE side. In Clew Bay Newport and Westport (AC 2667, 2057 and 10.13.18) need detailed pilotage directions. S of Clare Is beware Meemore Shoal 1·5M W of Roonagh Hd. 2M further W is the isolated rk Mweelaun. The islands of Caher, Ballybeg, Inishturk (with anch on E side) and Inishdalla have few hidden dangers, but the coast to the E must be given a berth of 1·5M even in calm weather; in strong winds seas break much further offshore.

Killary B (chart 2706) and Little Killary both have good anchs in magnificent scenery. Consult sailing directions, and only approach in reasonable weather and good vis.

Ballynakill Hbr (chart 2706), easily entered either side of Freaghillaun South, has excellent shelter; Tully mountain is conspic to N. Beware Mullaghadrina and Ship Rk in N chan. Anch in Fahy, Derryinver or Barnaderg B. There is anch on S side of Inishbofin (Lt), but difficult access/exit in strong SW wind or swell (10.13.18). Rks and breakers exist E of Inishbofin and S of Inishshark; see chart 2707 for clearing lines. Lecky Rks lie 1M SSE of Davillaun. Carrickmahoy is a very dangerous rk (1·9m) between Inishbofin and Cleggan Pt.

Cleggan B is moderate anch, open to NW but easy access. High Is Sound is usual coasting route, not Friar Is Sound or Aughrus Passage. Clifden B (chart 2708) has offlying dangers with breakers; enter 3ca S of Carrickrana Bn and anch off Drinagh Pt, in Clifden Hbr or Ardbear B; see 10.13.18.

Slyne Hd (Lt) marks SW end of Rks and Is's stretching 2M WSW from coast. Here the stream turns N at HW Galway – 0320, and S at HW Galway + 0300. It runs 3kn at sp, and in bad weather causes a dangerous race. The sea may break on Barret Shoals, 3M NW of Slyne Hd.

SLYNE HEAD TO LISCANNOR BAY (chart 2173)

The Connemara coast (charts 2709, 2096) and Aran Islands (chart 3339) give excellent cruising in good vis. But there are many rks, and few navigational marks. Between Slyne Head and Roundstone B are many offlying dangers. If coasting, keep well seaward of Skerd Rks. A conspic Twr (24m) on Golan Head is a key feature. Going E the better hbrs are Roundstone B, Cashel B, Killeany B, Greatman B and Cashla B. Kilronan (Killeany B) on Inishmore is only reasonable hbr in Aran Islands, but is exposed in E winds. Disused Lt Ho on centre of island is conspic.

Normal approach to Galway B is through N Sound or S Sound. N Sound is 4M wide from Eagle Rk and other dangers off Lettermullan shore, to banks on S side which break in strong winds. S Sound is 3M wide, with no dangers except Finnis Rk (0·4m) 5ca SE of Inisheer. The other channels are Gregory Sound, 1M wide between Inishmore and Inishmaan, and Foul Sound between Inishmaan and Inisheer. The latter has one danger, Pipe Rk and the reef inshore of it, extending 3ca NW of Inisheer.

The N side of Galway Bay is exposed, with no shelter. Galway (10.13.19) is a commercial port, with possible marina plans. 3M SE, New Hbr (chart 1984) is a more pleasant anch with moorings off Galway Bay SC. Westward to Black Hd there are many bays and inlets, often poorly marked, but providing shelter and exploration. The coast SW to Liscannor Bay is devoid of shelter. O'Brien's Twr is conspic just N of the 199m high Cliffs of Moher.

13

10.13.6   DISTANCE TABLE

Approximate distances in nautical miles are by the most direct route, whilst avoiding dangers and allowing for Traffic Separation Schemes. Places in *italics* are in adjoining areas; places in **bold** are in 10.0.6, Distances across the Irish Sea.

1. *Dun Laoghaire*	**1**																			
2. **Carlingford Lough**	50	**2**																		
3. **Strangford Lough**	71	36	**3**																	
4. **Bangor**	96	61	34	**4**																
5. **Carrickfergus**	101	66	39	6	**5**															
6. **Larne**	108	73	45	16	16	**6**														
7. **Carnlough**	118	78	50	25	26	11	**7**													
8. Altacarry Head	135	102	74	45	45	31	21	**8**												
9. **Portrush**	150	115	87	58	60	48	35	19	**9**											
10. **Lough Foyle**	157	121	92	72	73	55	47	30	11	**10**										
11. L Swilly (Fahan)	200	166	138	109	104	96	81	65	48	42	**11**									
12. **Tory Island**	209	174	146	117	113	105	90	74	57	51	35	**12**								
13. Burtonport	218	182	153	130	130	116	108	90	74	68	49	18	**13**							
14. Killybegs	267	232	204	175	171	163	148	132	115	109	93	58	43	**14**						
15. Sligo	281	246	218	189	179	177	156	146	123	117	107	72	51	30	**15**					
16. Eagle Island	297	262	234	205	198	193	175	162	147	136	123	88	72	62	59	**16**				
17. Westport	337	323	295	266	249	240	226	207	193	187	168	137	120	108	100	57	**17**			
18. Slyne Head	352	317	289	260	257	248	234	217	201	195	178	143	128	117	114	55	44	**18**		
19. Galway	348	366	338	309	307	297	284	266	253	245	227	192	178	166	163	104	94	49	**19**	
20. *Kilrush*	318	361	364	335	332	323	309	291	276	270	251	220	203	191	183	142	119	75	76	**20**

10.13.7   Special Notes for Ireland: see 10.12.7

MINOR HARBOURS AND ANCHORAGES TO THE NORTH WEST OF LAMBAY ISLAND

SKERRIES, Dublin, 53°35'·1N 06°06'·66W. AC 633. Tides as Balbriggan, 10.13.8. E & SE of Red Island (a peninsula) lie Colt, Shenick's and St Patrick's Islands, the latter foul to S and SW. Inshore passage between Colt and St Patrick's Is uses transit/brg as on chart to clear dangers. Good shelter and holding in 3m at Skerries Bay, W of Red Is. Appr from E or NE outside PHM buoy, Fl R 10s, off Red Is. ‡ WNW of pier, Oc R 6s 7m 7M, vis 103°-154°; clear of moorings. Most facilities; Skerries SC ☎ 1-849 1233. Rockabill Lt, Fl WR 12s 45m 23/19M, is conspic 2·4M ExN of St Patrick's Is.

BALBRIGGAN, Dublin, 53°36'·8N 06°10'·7W. AC 1468, 44. Tides see 10.13.8. Good shelter in small hbr, dries about 0·9m, access approx HW ±2. Appr on SW, to open the outer hbr which is entered on SE; thence to inner hbr and AB on SE quay. Beware shoaling on both sides of outer hbr. Lt, Fl (3) WRG 20s 12m 13/10M, conspic W tr on E bkwtr head, vis G159°-193°, W193°-288°, R288°-305°. Facilities: FW, D, Gas, Slip, BH (9 ton), R, Bar, V. EC Thurs.

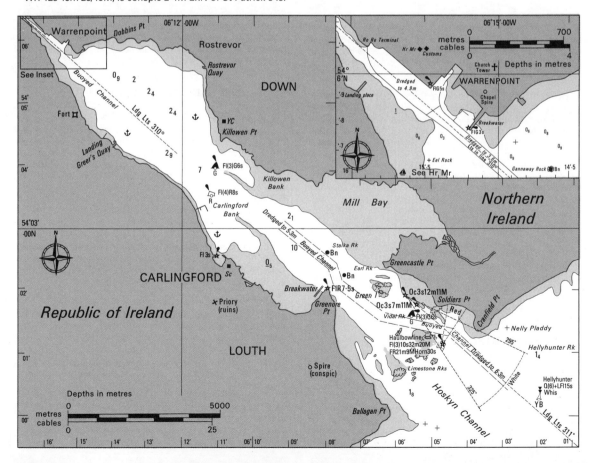

CARLINGFORD LOUGH   10-13-8

Louth/Down 54°01'·25N 06°04'·30W

CHARTS
AC 2800, 44; Imray C62; Irish OS 9

TIDES
Cranfield Pt +0025 and Warrenpoint +0035 Dover; ML 2·9;
Duration Cranfield Pt 0615, Warrenpoint 0540; Zone 0 (UT)

Standard Port DUBLIN (NORTH WALL) (←)

Times				Height (metres)			
High Water		Low Water		MHWS	MHWN	MLWN	MLWS
0000	0700	0000	0500	4·1	3·4	1·5	0·7
1200	1900	1200	1700				
Differences CRANFIELD POINT							
–0027	–0011	+0017	–0007	+0·7	+0·9	+0·3	+0·2
WARRENPOINT							
–0020	–0010	+0040	+0040	+1·0	+0·9	+0·1	+0·2
NEWRY (VICTORIA LOCK)							
–0010	–0010	+0040	Dries	+1·1	+1·0	+0·1	Dries
KILKEEL							
+0010	+0010	0000	0000	+1·8	+1·4	+0·8	+0·3
NEWCASTLE							
+0025	+0035	+0020	+0040	+1·6	+1·1	+0·4	+0·1
DUNDALK (SOLDIERS POINT)							
–0010	–0010	0000	+0045	+1·0	+0·8	+0·1	–0·1
DUNANY POINT							
–0028	–0018	–0008	–0006	+0·7	+0·9	No data	
RIVER BOYNE BAR							
–0025	–0015	+0110	0000	+0·4	+0·3	No data	
BALBRIGGAN							
–0021	–0015	+0010	+0002	+0·3	+0·2	No data	

SHELTER
Good. Options clockwise from ent include: ‡ at Greenore Pt, between SW end of quay and bkwtr, in 3m clear of commercial tfc. Carlingford Hbr (dries 2·2m), AB at piers. Carlingford Marina (pontoons: 1·4m; max depth 3·5m), protected on S side by sunken barges; appr from NE to clear the tail of Carlingford Bank (dries). Nos 18 and 23 buoys, on 012° astern, lead to marina. ‡ off Greer's Quay in 2m. Warrenpoint has pontoons on NW side of bkwtr (Fl G 3s); access dredged 1·1m. Caution: much shipping in narrow chan dredged 5·4m, outside which the head of the lough is shallow. ‡s off Rostrevor Quay, Killowen Pt (YC) and off derelict pier at Greencastle Pt (beware rks).

NAVIGATION
WPT 54°00'·23N 06°02'·20W, (abm Hellyhunter SCM buoy) 131°/311° from/to first chan buoys, 1·1M. The main chan is Carlingford Cut (6·3m), about 3ca SW of Cranfield Pt, and passing 2ca NE of Haulbowline lt ho. Drying rks/shoals obstruct most of the ent. Caution: NE bank is Ulster, SW bank the Republic of Ireland. Fly flag Q and courtesy ensign. Yachts may be stopped by Naval vessels. The lough becomes choppy in S winds and with on-shore winds the ent is impassable. Beware sudden squalls and waterspouts. Tides run up to 5kn off Greenore Pt and entry against the ebb is impracticable.

LIGHTS AND MARKS
Haulbowline Fl (3) 10s 32m 19M; granite tr; also turning lt FR 21m 9M, vis 196°-208°, horn 30s. Ldg lts 311°: both Oc 3s 7/12m 11M, vis 295°-325°; R △ front, ▽ rear, on framework trs. Greenore Pier Fl R 7·5s 10m 5M. Newry R: Ldg lts 310°, both Iso 4s 5/15m 2M, stone columns.

RADIO TELEPHONE
Monitor VHF Ch 16, 10. Greenore (call: *Ferry Greenore*) Ch 12 16 (HJ). Carlingford marina Ch M 16. Warrenpoint Ch 12 16 (H24). Other stns: Dundalk Ch 06 12 16 (HW±3).

TELEPHONE (Greenore/Carlingford 042; Warrenpoint 016937) Hr Mr Warrenpoint 73381; MRCC (01) 6620922/3 or (01247) 463933; ☷ (01232) 358250; Irish ☷ Dundalk (042) 34114; Marinecall 0891 500 465; Dr (042) 73110; Ⓗ Newry 65511, (042) 34701; Police (Carlingford) 73102, (Warrenpoint) 722222.

FACILITIES
Carlingford Marina (50 + 30 visitors), ☎/Fax 73492, £9.10, AC, D, FW, P, C, CH, Divers, Slip. **Village** V, R, Bar, ✉.
Hbr AB, Slip; **Carlingford YC** ☎ 38604, Slip, Bar, M, V, FW; **Dundalk SC** FW, Slip; **Services**: ME, EI, Sh, Kos, Gas. **Warrenpoint** EC Wed; FW, P, D, AB, ✉ (also at Rostrevor, Carlingford), Ⓑ (also Dundalk), ⇌ (Dundalk, Newry), ✈ (Dublin).

MINOR HARBOURS BETWEEN CARLINGFORD LOUGH AND ST. JOHN'S POINT

KILKEEL, Down, 54°03'·47N 05°59'·26W. AC 2800, 44. HW +0015 on Dover; ML 2·9m; Duration 0620. See 10·13·8. Inner basin is completely sheltered, but gets crowded by FVs. Depth off quays approx 1m. There are drying banks both sides of ent chan and SW gales cause a sandbank right across ent. This is dredged or slowly washed away in E winds. Secure in inner basin and see Hr Mr. S bkwtr lt Fl WR 2s 8m 8M, R296°-313°, W313°-017°, storm sigs. Meeney's pier (N bkwtr) Fl G 3s 6m 2M. VHF Ch 12 14 16 (Mon-Fri: 0900-2000). Hr Mr ☎ (016937) 62287; ☷ 62158; Facilities: FW on quay, BY (between fish market and dock), EI, ME, Sh, Slip. **Town** (¾M) EC Thurs; Bar, ✉, R, V, Gas, ▣.

ANNALONG HBR, Down, 54°06'·50N 05°53'·65W. AC 44. Tides as Kilkeel, see 10.13.8. Excellent shelter in small drying hbr, approx 2m from HW±3. Appr in W sector of S bkwtr lt, Oc WRG 5s 8m 9M, vis G204°-249°, W249°-309°, R309°-024°. Keep close N of the bkwtr to avoid rky shore to stbd. 40m beyond a spur on N side, turn hard port into the basin; berth as available. Facilities: V, Bar, ✉.

DUNDRUM BAY, Down. AC 44. Tides see 10.13.8. This 8M wide bay to the W of St John's Pt is shoal to 5ca offshore and unsafe in onshore winds. The small drying hbr at **Newcastle** (54°11'·8N 05°53'·0W) is for occas use in fair wx. **Dundrum Hbr** (54°14'·2N 05°49'·4W) provides ‡ in 2m for shoal draft; the bar carries about 0·3m. HW Dundrum is approx that of HW Liverpool; see also 10.13.8. ICC SDs are essential for the 1M long, buoyed appr chan. 3 unlit DZ buoys offshore are part of the Ballykinler firing range, 2M E of hbr; R flag/lts indicate range active.

AGENTS WANTED

If you are interested in becoming our agent for any of the following ports, please write to: The Editor, Edington House, Trent, Sherborne, Dorset DT9 4SR, England – and get your free copy of the almanac annually. You do not have to live in a port to be the agent, but at least a fairly regular visitor.

River Exe	Grandcamp-Maisy
Port Ellen (Islay)	Port-en-Bessin
Glandore/Union Hall	Courseulles
River Rance/Dinan	Boulogne
Lampaul	Dunkerque
Port Tudy	Terneuzen/Westerschelde
River Etel	Oudeschild
Le Palais (Belle Ile)	Lauwersoog
Le Pouliguen/Pornichet	Dornumer-Accumersiel
L'Herbaudière	Hooksiel
St Gilles-Croix-de-Vie	Langeoog
River Seudre	Bremerhaven
Royan	Helgoland
Anglet/Bayonne	Büsum
Hendaye	

13

MINOR HARBOURS BETWEEN ST. JOHN'S POINT AND BELFAST LOUGH

ARDGLASS, Down, 54°15'·63N 05°36'·00W. AC 633, 2093. HW +0025 on Dover; ML 3·0m; Duration 0620. See 10.13.9. A busy fishing port in rky bay; good shelter in S Hbr, with quays (2·1m) on inside of extended S bkwtr. In mid-hbr avoid Churn Rk, unlit SCM bn. Further up hbr on NW side old drying N Dock gives excellent shelter; yachts can berth on its E wall, but consult Hr Mr who will allocate berth or ⚓ clear of FVs. VHF Ch 16 14 12. Dir lt, 311° at N Dock, Iso WRG 4s 10m 8/7/5M, Gshore-308°, W308°-314°, R314°-shore. Outer bkwtr Fl R 3s 10m 5M. On NE side of ent, SHM bn Fl G 5s 10m 4M. Hr Mr ☎ (01396) 613844. Facilities: FW (on quay). **Town** P & D (cans), Bar, ✉, R, V, Gas. Note: A 55 berth marina is planned on W side of hbr.

PORTAVOGIE, Down, 54°27'·45N 05°26'·08W. AC 2156. HW +0016 on Dover; ML 2·6m; Duration 0620. See 10·13·9. Good shelter, but hbr so full of FVs as to risk damage; best only for overnight or emergency. Ent dangerous in strong onshore winds. Beware Plough Rks to SE marked by PHM lt buoy QR, Bell, and McCammon Rks to N of ent. Keep in W sector of outer bkwtr lt, Iso WRG 5s 9m 9M, G shore-258°, W258°-275°, R275°-348°. W bkwtr 2 FG (vert) 6m 4M. VHF Ch 12 14 16 (Mon-Fri: 0900-1700 LT). Hr Mr ☎ (012477) 71470. Facilities: Slip, FW (on central quay) Sh, ME, El. **Town** EC Thurs; CH, D & P (cans), ✉, R, Gas, V. No licenced premises.

STRANGFORD LOUGH   10-13-9

Down 54°19'·33N 04°30'·85W

CHARTS
AC 2159, 2156; Imray C62; Irish OS 5, 9
TIDES
Killard Pt 0000, Strangford Quay +0200 Dover; ML 2·0; Duration 0610; Zone 0 (UT)

Standard Port BELFAST (⟶)

Times				Height (metres)			
High Water		Low Water		MHWS	MHWN	MLWN	MLWS
0100	0700	0000	0600	3·5	3·0	1·1	0·4
1300	1900	1200	1800				
Differences STRANGFORD							
+0147	+0157	+0148	+0208	+0·1	+0·1	−0·2	0·0
KILLARD POINT							
+0011	+0021	+0005	+0025	+1·0	+0·8	+0·1	+0·1
QUOILE BARRIER							
+0150	+0200	+0150	+0300	+0·2	+0·2	−0·3	−0·1
KILLYLEAGH							
+0157	+0207	+0211	+0231	+0·3	+0·3	No data	
KILLOUGH HARBOUR							
0000	+0020	No data		+1·8	+1·6	No data	
ARDGLASS							
+0010	+0015	+0005	+0010	+1·7	+1·2	+0·6	+0·3
SOUTH ROCK							
+0023	+0023	+0025	+0025	+1·0	+0·8	+0·1	+0·1
PORTAVOGIE							
+0010	+0020	+0010	+0020	+1·2	+0·9	+0·3	+0·2

SHELTER
Excellent; largest inlet on E coast. Good ⚓ s in the Narrows at Cross Roads; in Strangford Creek (NW of Swan Is, which is marked by 3 lt bns to S, E and N); and in Audley Roads and Ballyhenry Bay. Berthing at piers in Strangford or Portaferry dependent on state of tide. Good ⚓ s up the lough in Quoile, Ringhaddy Sound and Whiterk. Some ⬤s.
NAVIGATION
WPT Strangford Fairway SWM buoy, L Fl 10s, Whis, 54°18'·62N 05°28'·62W, 126°/306° from/to Angus Rk lt tr, 2·05M. Visitors should use the E Chan. Beware overfalls in the SE apprs and at the bar, which can be dangerous when ebb from narrows is running against strong E to SSW winds. During flood the bar presents no special problem, but preferably enter on the young flood or when tide in the narrows is slack. Strong (up to 7kn at sp) tidal streams flow through the Narrows. Tidal flow in narrows, and hence the overfalls, relates to HW Strangford Quay (+0200 Dover) not to Killard Pt (0000). Beware St Patricks Rk, Bar Pladdy and Pladdy Lug and whirlpool at Routen Wheel. Beware car ferry plying from Strangford, S & E of Swan Is, to Portaferry. Swan Is, seen as grassy mound at HW, is edged with rks and a reef extends 32m E ending at W bn Fl (2) WR 6s. Up the lough, beware drying patches, known as pladdies and often un-marked.
LIGHTS AND MARKS
See Chartlet. Ent identified by Fairway buoy (SWM), W tr on Angus Rk, Pladdy Lug bn (W) and St Patrick's Rock perch. From NE, St Patrick's Rk perch on with Gun Island obelisk 224° clears Quintin Rk. For E Chan, Fairway By, Bar Pladdy SCM and Angus Rk tr give an approx transit on 324°. Thence Dogtail Pt, Oc (4) 10s, on with Gowland Rk bn, Oc (2) 10s, leads 341° up The Narrows.
RADIO TELEPHONE
Strangford FerryTerminal Ch 12 14 16 M (Mon-Fri 0900-1700 LT). In Strangford Lough most YCs and Seaquip Ch **80** M. Killyleagh Port VHF Ch 12 16 (occas).
TELEPHONE (01396)
Hr Mr 881637; MRSC (01247) 463933; ⌗ (01232) 358250; Marinecall 0891 500 465; Police 615011; Medical Clinic 313016; Casualty 613311.
FACILITIES
STRANGFORD M, L, FW, CH, AB, V, R, Bar, ✉, D (cans), El, Ⓔ, Sh, Gas.
PORTAFERRY M, L, Gas, Gaz, P & D (cans), V, R, Bar, ✉, Ⓑ.
KILLYLEAGH M, P & D (cans), L, C (mobile), CH, V, R, Ⓑ, Bar, ✉; **East Down YC** ☎ 828375; **Services:** Gas, Gaz, Kos.
SKETRICK ISLAND R, Bar, L.
KIRCUBBIN Gas, P & D (cans).

STRANGFORD LOUGH *continued*

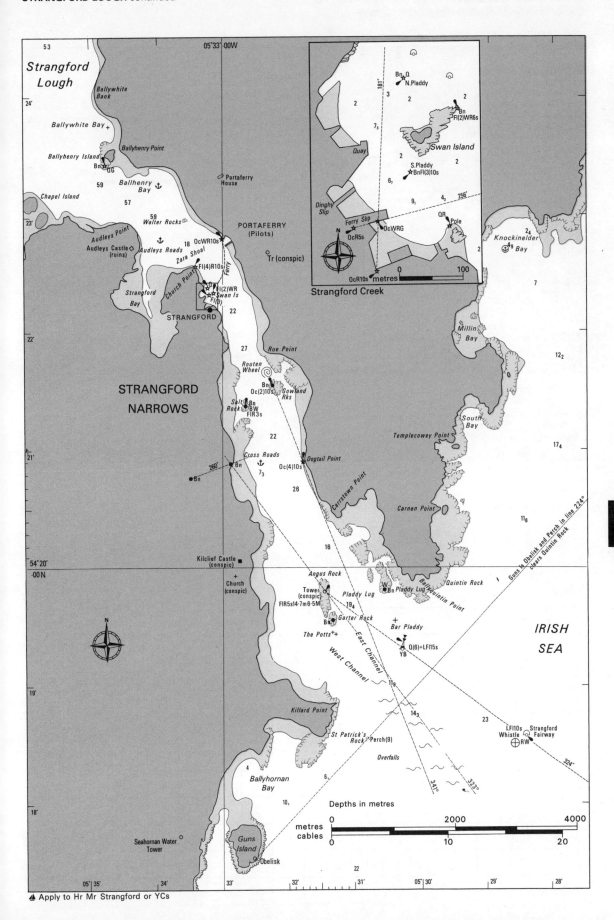

Strangford Lough

53

05°33'·00W

Ballywhite
Bank

24'

Ballywhite Bay

Ballyhenry Point

Ballyhenry Island   Ballyhenry Point

Bn QG

59   Ballhenry Bay

Chapel Island

57

23'

Walter Rocks   59

Audleys Point

Audleys Castle
(ruins)   Audleys Roads

Zara Shoal   18 OcWR10s

Fl(4)R10s

Church Point   Oc Fl(2)WR
Swan Is
Fl(3)

STRANGFORD BAY

STRANGFORD   22

22'

STRANGFORD
NARROWS

27   Rue Point

Routen
Wheel

Bn
Oc(2)10s   Gowland Rks

Salt Bn
Rock BW
Fl R 3s

22

21'   Cross Roads

Bn   Dogtail Point
Oc(4)10s

Bn   7₃

26

Carstown Point

16

54°20'
·00N

Kilclief Castle
(conspic)

Church
(conspic)

Angus Rock

Tower
(conspic)
Fl R 5s14·7m6·5M

Pladdy Lug

Bn   Garter Rock

The Potts

West Channel   East Channel

Killard Point

St Patrick's
Rock Perch(9)

Overfalls

Ballyhornan
Bay

4

10₁

Seahornan Water
Tower

Guns
Island

Obelisk

Portaferry
House

Portaferry
(Pilots)

Tr (conspic)

Ferry

Templecowey Point

South Bay

Carnan Point

Pladdy Lug
W Bn   Ballyquintin Point

Quintin Rock

Bar Pladdy
YB   Q(6)+LFl15s

11₉

14₃

23   LFl10s Strangford
Whistle   Fairway
RW

Knockinelder
Bay
4₉

7

Millin
Bay

12₂

17₄

11₈

IRISH SEA

Inset: Strangford Creek

Bn Q
N.Pladdy

2   3   2

7₃   Bn
Fl(2)WR6s

Quay   2

2   Swan Island

S.Pladdy
BnFl(3)10s   2

4₃   256°
6₇

Dinghy   9₁
Slip

Ferry Slip   OcWRG   QR   Pole
OcR5s

OcR10s   metres   0   100

Strangford Creek

Depths in metres

metres   0   2000   4000
cables   0   10   20

22

324°

341°   323°

19'

18'

05'   35'   34'   33'   32'   31'   05'   30'   29'   28'

13

Guns Is Obelisk and Perch in line 224°
clears Quintin Rock

260°

181°

⚓ Apply to Hr Mr Strangford or YCs

BELFAST LOUGH   10-13-10

County Down and County Antrim 54°42'N 05°45'W

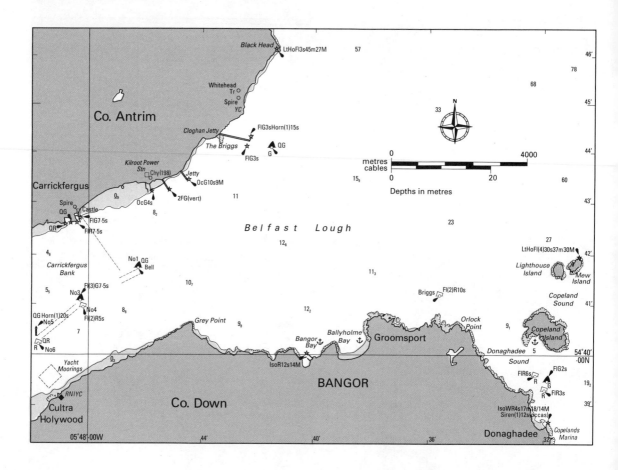

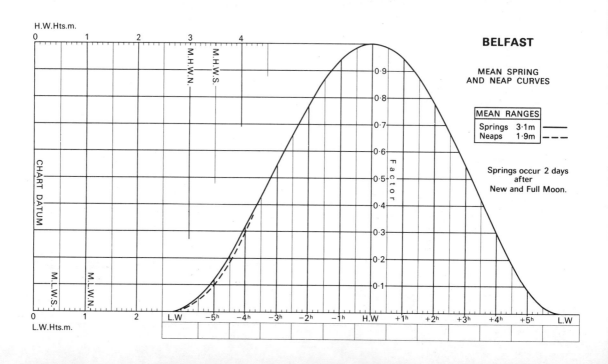

BELFAST

MEAN SPRING AND NEAP CURVES

MEAN RANGES	
Springs	3·1m
Neaps	1·9m

Springs occur 2 days
after
New and Full Moon.

BELFAST LOUGH *continued*

CHARTS
AC 1753, 2198; Imray C62, C64; Irish OS 5

TIDES
+0007 Dover; ML Belfast 2·0, Carrickfergus 1·8; Duration 0620; Zone 0 (UT)

Standard Port BELFAST (→)

Times				Height (metres)			
High Water		Low Water		MHWS	MHWN	MLWN	MLWS
0100	0700	0000	0600	3·5	3·0	1·1	0·4
1300	900	1200	1800				
Differences CARRICKFERGUS							
+0005	+0005	+0005	+0005	−0·3	−0·3	−0·2	−0·1
DONAGHADEE							
+0020	+0020	+0023	+0023	+0·5	+0·4	0·0	+0·1

NOTE: Belfast is a Standard Port and tidal predictions for every day of the year are given below.

SHELTER
Main sailing centres in Belfast Lough are at Bangor, Cultra and Carrickfergus. Belfast Harbour is a commercial port, not recommended for yachts except in emergency. See also 10.13.9 for Donaghadee at SE ent to the Lough.
Bangor: exposed to N winds; 4kn speed limit in well sheltered marina (depths 2·9m to 2·2m). 8kn speed limit between Luke's Pt and Wilson's Pt.
Cultra and **Ballyholme Bay:** good in offshore winds.
Carrickfergus: very good in marina, depths 1·9m to 2·4m. Good ⚓ SSE of Carrickfergus Pier, except in E winds.

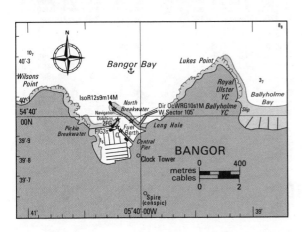

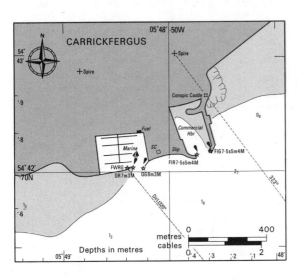

NAVIGATION
WPT Bangor 54°41'·00N 05°40'·00W, 010°/190° from/to bkwtr lt, 1·0M. Rounding Orlock Pt beware Briggs Rks extending ¾M offshore. The Lough is well marked. Beware between Carrickfergus and Kilroot Pt there is a sand bank drying up to 4ca from shore; and Carrickfergus Bank extends 1·5M SSW from the hbr.

LIGHTS AND MARKS
Bangor Dir Oc WRG 10s lt; W sector 105° leads through ent. Carrickfergus is easily recognised by conspic castle to E of commercial port. A Dir Lt 320°, F WRG 5m 3M, in lieu of the ldg bns, is 30m W of the ☆ QR 7m 3M on bkwtr; vis H24, G308°-317½°, W317½°-322½°, R322½°-332°. Carrick Hbr is manned only when commercial ship is expected. Chan up to Belfast is well marked by bys and bns. Once the pile bns are reached it is dangerous to leave the chan.

RADIO TELEPHONE
Bangor Hr Mr Ch 11 (H24); Marina Ch **80** M (H24). Copelands Marina, Royal Northern Ireland YC Ch **16**; 11 (H24) 80.
Carrickfergus Hbr Ch 12 14 16 (HW−3 to HW+1, when vessel expected); Marina Ch M.
Belfast Port Control (at Milewater Basin) Ch **12** 16 (H24); VTS provides info on request to vessels in port area. The greater part of Belfast Lough is under radar surveillance.

TELEPHONE (01232)
Hr Mr Bangor (01247) 453297; Hr Mr Belfast 553011/Fax 553017; MRSC (01247) 463933; ⌗ 358250; Weather (08494) 22339; Marinecall 0898 500 465; Police 58411, (019603) 62021, (01247) 464444; Dr 454444.

FACILITIES
GROOMSPORT (01247)
Hr Mr ☎ 464733, M, Slip, FW; **Cockle Island Boat Club**, Slip, M, FW, L, R; **Town:** see Bangor.
BANGOR (01247)
Bangor Marina (560 + 40 visitors) ☎ 453297, Fax 453450, £11.42 (£3 for 4 hrs), FW, AC, P, D, C, CH, BH (40 ton), ME, EI, Ⓔ, Sh, Gas, Gaz, Slip, SM, V, Ⓖ;
R Ulster YC ☎ 270568, R, Bar; **Ballyholme YC** ☎ 271467, M, L; **Todd Chart Agency** ☎ 466640, Fax 471070 ACA, CH.
Services: BY, Diving, Gas, ME, EI, Sh.
Town EC Thurs; V, R, Bar, ✉, Ⓑ, ⇌, ✈ (Belfast).
HOLYWOOD (01232)
Royal N of Ireland YC, Cultra ☎ 428041, Slip, M, P(½M), D, L, FW, AB, R, Bar. **Services:** ME, EI, Sh;
Town P, CH, V, R, Bar, ✉, Ⓑ, ⇌, ✈.
BELFAST (01232)
Hbr ☎ 554422, AB, P, D, FW, ME, EI, Sh, CH, C (up to 200 ton); **Services:** SM, Gas.
City EC Wed; All facilities, ⇌, ✈.
CARRICKFERGUS (01960)
Carrickfergus Marina (270+30 visitors) ☎ 366666, £13.50, AC, BH (30 ton), CH, D, EI, FW, Sh; **Carrick SC** ☎ 351402, M, L, FW, C, AB; **Services:** Gas, Rigging, ME, EI, Sh, Ⓔ.
Town EC Wed; V, R, Ⓑ, ✉, ⇌, ✈ (Belfast).

13

MINOR HARBOUR AT SE ENTRANCE TO BELFAST LOUGH

DONAGHADEE, Down, 54°38'·71N 05°31'·85W. AC 3709, 1753. HW +0025 on Dover; ML no data; Duration 0615. Hbr is small and very full; scend often sets in. Best berth alongside SE quay. Depth in hbr approx 3m. Beware ledge with less than 2m extends 1·5ca ENE from S pier hd. Or go to the small, well sheltered marina 3ca S of hbr, access HW±4. Excellent shelter and facilities but tricky ent (pilots available). S pier lt, Iso WR 4s 17m 18/14M, W shore–326°, R326°–shore. No lts at marina. Hr Mr ☎ (0247) 882377. Facilities: **Copelands Marina** ☎ 882184; all facilities, C (20 ton).
Town Bar, D, P, Gas, ✉, R, V, Ⓑ, ⇌ (Bangor), ✈ (Belfast).

NORTHERN IRELAND – BELFAST

LAT 54°36′N   LONG 5°55′W

TIMES AND HEIGHTS OF HIGH AND LOW WATERS

YEAR 1996

TIME ZONE (UT)
For Summer Time add ONE hour in non-shaded areas

JANUARY

Day	Time	m	Time	m	Time	m	Time	m
1 M	0129	0.9	0756	3.1	1352	1.1	2021	3.2
16 TU	0007	1.0	0639	3.0	1311	1.2	1910	3.2
2 TU	0228	0.9	0850	3.2	1451	1.0	2115	3.2
17 W	0129	1.0	0752	3.1	1422	1.0	2018	3.3
3 W	0318	0.9	0938	3.3	1541	1.0	2202	3.2
18 TH	0236	0.9	0857	3.3	1519	0.8	2119	3.4
4 TH	0359	0.9	1021	3.4	1621	0.9	2243	3.2
19 F	0330	0.7	0951	3.5	1609	0.6	2214	3.5
5 F ○	0436	0.9	1100	3.5	1655	0.9	2321	3.2
20 SA ●	0418	0.6	1042	3.7	1657	0.4	2305	3.6
6 SA	0509	0.9	1136	3.5	1727	0.8	2354	3.2
21 SU	0505	0.6	1130	3.8	1743	0.3	2355	3.6
7 SU	0541	0.9	1209	3.5	1759	0.8		
22 M	0551	0.5	1218	3.8	1828	0.3		
8 M	0024	3.2	0614	0.9	1241	3.6	1831	0.7
23 TU	0045	3.5	0637	0.6	1307	3.8	1913	0.3
9 TU	0052	3.2	0648	0.8	1312	3.6	1906	0.7
24 W	0134	3.5	0723	0.6	1355	3.8	2000	0.4
10 W	0122	3.2	0725	0.8	1345	3.6	1944	0.7
25 TH	0223	3.4	0811	0.6	1443	3.7	2049	0.5
11 TH	0157	3.2	0804	0.8	1422	3.6	2025	0.7
26 F	0313	3.3	0902	0.7	1533	3.5	2144	0.6
12 F	0239	3.2	0848	0.9	1505	3.5	2111	0.7
27 SA	0404	3.2	0958	0.9	1625	3.4	2243	0.8
13 SA	0328	3.1	0937	1.0	1555	3.4	2202	0.8
28 SU	0459	3.1	1102	1.0	1722	3.2	2347	1.0
14 SU	0424	3.1	1032	1.1	1653	3.3	2259	0.9
29 M	0605	3.0	1210	1.1	1837	3.0		
15 M	0528	3.0	1138	1.2	1800	3.2		
30 TU	0052	1.1	0721	3.0	1318	1.1	1955	3.0
31 W	0156	1.1	0823	3.1	1423	1.1	2055	3.0

FEBRUARY

Day	Time	m	Time	m	Time	m	Time	m
1 TH	0251	1.0	0915	3.2	1518	1.0	2143	3.1
16 F	0225	1.0	0841	3.3	1507	0.8	2109	3.3
2 F	0335	0.9	1000	3.3	1600	0.9	2225	3.1
17 SA	0320	0.8	0938	3.5	1559	0.5	2203	3.4
3 SA	0412	0.9	1040	3.4	1634	0.8	2303	3.1
18 SU ●	0409	0.6	1028	3.7	1647	0.4	2253	3.5
4 SU ○	0447	0.8	1116	3.5	1707	0.7	2336	3.1
19 M	0455	0.5	1115	3.8	1732	0.3	2340	3.5
5 M	0522	0.8	1148	3.5	1740	0.7		
20 TU	0539	0.5	1202	3.8	1815	0.2		
6 TU	0002	3.2	0555	0.7	1216	3.5	1812	0.6
21 W	0026	3.5	0621	0.5	1249	3.8	1856	0.3
7 W	0023	3.2	0629	0.7	1243	3.6	1845	0.6
22 TH	0112	3.5	0703	0.5	1334	3.8	1937	0.4
8 TH	0051	3.2	0702	0.7	1317	3.6	1919	0.5
23 F	0157	3.3	0746	0.5	1420	3.7	2020	0.5
9 F	0127	3.3	0738	0.7	1355	3.6	1957	0.6
24 SA	0242	3.3	0831	0.6	1506	3.5	2106	0.7
10 SA	0208	3.3	0819	0.8	1439	3.5	2040	0.6
25 SU	0327	3.2	0920	0.8	1553	3.3	2159	0.9
11 SU	0254	3.2	0905	0.9	1528	3.4	2129	0.8
26 M	0415	3.1	1018	0.9	1644	3.1	2303	1.1
12 M	0346	3.1	0958	1.0	1625	3.3	2226	0.9
27 TU	0509	3.0	1129	1.1	1745	2.9		
13 TU	0448	3.0	1103	1.1	1733	3.2	2333	1.1
28 W	0011	1.2	0620	2.9	1241	1.1	1921	2.8
14 W	0603	3.0	1247	1.2	1847	3.1		
29 TH	0118	1.2	0747	3.0	1348	1.1	2030	2.8
15 TH	0109	1.1	0727	3.1	1407	1.0	2003	3.2

MARCH

Day	Time	m	Time	m	Time	m	Time	m
1 F	0217	1.1	0846	3.1	1446	1.0	2120	2.9
16 SA	0211	1.0	0824	3.2	1452	0.6	2057	3.3
2 SA	0306	0.9	0933	3.2	1531	0.8	2202	3.1
17 SU	0308	0.8	0921	3.5	1544	0.4	2150	3.4
3 SU	0346	0.8	1013	3.3	1608	0.7	2238	3.1
18 M	0357	0.7	1010	3.6	1632	0.3	2237	3.5
4 M	0424	0.7	1049	3.4	1643	0.6	2310	3.2
19 TU ●	0442	0.5	1057	3.7	1716	0.3	2322	3.5
5 TU ○	0500	0.7	1118	3.5	1717	0.6	2333	3.2
20 W	0525	0.5	1142	3.8	1758	0.3		
6 W	0535	0.6	1143	3.5	1750	0.5	2353	3.3
21 TH	0006	3.5	0605	0.5	1227	3.7	1837	0.4
7 TH	0608	0.6	1213	3.6	1821	0.5		
22 F	0049	3.5	0644	0.5	1311	3.6	1914	0.5
8 F	0023	3.3	0640	0.6	1250	3.6	1854	0.5
23 SA	0130	3.5	0722	0.5	1354	3.5	1951	0.6
9 SA	0101	3.3	0715	0.6	1331	3.6	1932	0.5
24 SU	0211	3.4	0802	0.6	1438	3.4	2032	0.7
10 SU	0143	3.3	0755	0.6	1417	3.5	2015	0.6
25 M	0253	3.3	0846	0.7	1522	3.2	2117	0.9
11 M	0229	3.3	0841	0.7	1509	3.4	2104	0.8
26 TU	0338	3.2	0937	0.9	1610	3.0	2213	1.1
12 TU	0321	3.2	0935	0.9	1609	3.2	2202	1.0
27 W	0428	3.1	1044	1.0	1704	2.8	2324	1.2
13 W	0423	3.1	1045	1.0	1717	3.1	2312	1.1
28 TH	0525	3.0	1200	1.1	1810	2.7		
14 TH	0539	3.0	1234	1.0	1832	3.0		
29 F	0034	1.3	0635	2.9	1308	1.1	1950	2.7
15 F	0055	1.2	0708	3.0	1351	0.9	1951	3.1
30 SA	0137	1.2	0759	3.0	1406	0.9	2046	2.9
31 SU	0231	1.0	0854	3.1	1455	0.8	2129	3.0

APRIL

Day	Time	m	Time	m	Time	m	Time	m
1 M	0316	0.9	0935	3.3	1536	0.6	2204	3.1
16 TU	0339	0.7	0951	3.6	1611	0.3	2218	3.5
2 TU	0357	0.7	1010	3.4	1614	0.5	2235	3.2
17 W ●	0425	0.6	1037	3.6	1655	0.4	2301	3.5
3 W	0435	0.6	1040	3.5	1650	0.5	2259	3.3
18 TH	0508	0.5	1121	3.6	1737	0.4	2344	3.5
4 TH ○	0511	0.6	1110	3.5	1723	0.4	2326	3.4
19 F	0549	0.5	1204	3.6	1816	0.5		
5 F	0546	0.6	1146	3.5	1756	0.4		
20 SA	0024	3.5	0625	0.6	1247	3.5	1850	0.6
6 SA	0000	3.4	0620	0.5	1227	3.6	1832	0.5
21 SU	0104	3.5	0659	0.6	1328	3.4	1924	0.7
7 SU	0041	3.4	0656	0.5	1312	3.5	1912	0.5
22 M	0143	3.5	0735	0.6	1409	3.3	1959	0.8
8 M	0125	3.4	0738	0.6	1402	3.5	1957	0.6
23 TU	0223	3.4	0815	0.7	1452	3.1	2040	0.9
9 TU	0213	3.4	0827	0.6	1457	3.3	2049	0.8
24 W	0306	3.3	0900	0.8	1539	3.0	2128	1.1
10 W	0307	3.3	0926	0.8	1559	3.2	2149	1.0
25 TH	0353	3.2	0955	0.9	1630	2.9	2226	1.2
11 TH	0410	3.2	1043	0.9	1707	3.1	2302	1.1
26 F	0446	3.1	1106	1.0	1726	2.8	2341	1.2
12 F	0525	3.1	1217	0.8	1821	3.0		
27 SA	0544	3.0	1221	1.0	1829	2.8		
13 SA	0034	1.1	0650	3.1	1330	0.7	1937	3.1
28 SU	0051	1.2	0648	3.0	1323	0.9	1940	2.9
14 SU	0149	1.0	0803	3.3	1431	0.6	2040	3.3
29 M	0150	1.1	0752	3.1	1415	0.8	2037	3.0
15 M	0248	0.8	0901	3.4	1524	0.4	2131	3.4
30 TU	0241	0.9	0844	3.2	1500	0.6	2118	3.2

Chart Datum: 2·01 metres below Ordnance Datum (Belfast)

NORTHERN IRELAND – BELFAST

LAT 54°36′N   LONG 5°55′W

TIMES AND HEIGHTS OF HIGH AND LOW WATERS

YEAR **1996**

TIME ZONE (UT)
For Summer Time add ONE hour in non-shaded areas

MAY

Day	Time	m	Day	Time	m
1 W	0326	0.8	16 TH	0405	0.7
	0926	3.4		1017	3.5
	1541	0.5		1632	0.5
	2154	3.3		2240	3.5
2 TH	0407	0.7	17 F ●	0449	0.6
	1004	3.5		1101	3.5
	1619	0.4		1714	0.6
	2228	3.4		2321	3.5
3 F O	0446	0.6	18 SA	0530	0.6
	1042	3.5		1143	3.4
	1655	0.4		1752	0.7
	2304	3.5			
4 SA	0524	0.5	19 SU	0001	3.5
	1124	3.6		0606	0.7
	1733	0.4		1223	3.3
	2343	3.5		1825	0.8
5 SU	0603	0.5	20 M	0039	3.5
	1209	3.5		0637	0.7
	1814	0.5		1302	3.3
				1856	0.8
6 M	0026	3.5	21 TU	0117	3.5
	0644	0.5		0709	0.7
	1259	3.5		1342	3.2
	1858	0.5		1930	0.9
7 TU	0113	3.5	22 W	0156	3.5
	0730	0.5		0746	0.7
	1352	3.4		1423	3.1
	1947	0.6		2008	0.9
8 W	0204	3.5	23 TH	0237	3.4
	0822	0.5		0828	0.8
	1450	3.3		1508	3.0
	2041	0.8		2052	1.0
9 TH	0259	3.4	24 F	0321	3.3
	0923	0.6		0916	0.8
	1552	3.2		1557	3.0
	2142	0.9		2142	1.1
10 F	0402	3.3	25 SA	0409	3.2
	1038	0.7		1010	0.9
	1656	3.1		1648	2.9
	2252	1.0		2239	1.1
11 SA	0512	3.2	26 SU	0502	3.2
	1154	0.7		1114	0.9
	1805	3.1		1744	2.9
				2346	1.2
12 SU	0008	1.0	27 M	0601	3.1
	0628	3.2		1225	0.9
	1303	0.6		1842	2.9
	1916	3.1			
13 M	0120	1.0	28 TU	0100	1.1
	0739	3.3		0700	3.1
	1405	0.6		1329	0.8
	2017	3.2		1940	3.1
14 TU	0222	0.9	29 W	0201	1.0
	0839	3.4		0758	3.2
	1459	0.5		1421	0.7
	2109	3.3		2033	3.2
15 W	0316	0.8	30 TH	0252	0.9
	0930	3.5		0849	3.4
	1547	0.5		1507	0.6
	2156	3.4		2119	3.3
			31 F	0339	0.7
				0936	3.5
				1549	0.5
				2202	3.4

JUNE

Day	Time	m	Day	Time	m
1 SA O	0422	0.6	16 SU ●	0511	0.7
	1021	3.5		1124	3.3
	1727	0.8		1727	0.8
	2245	3.5		2339	3.5
2 SU	0505	0.5	17 M	0546	0.7
	1107	3.6		1201	3.2
	1714	0.5		1759	0.9
	2329	3.6			
3 M	0549	0.4	18 TU	0016	3.5
	1156	3.6		0615	0.7
	1759	0.5		1238	3.2
				1829	0.9
4 TU	0016	3.6	19 W	0053	3.5
	0633	0.4		0645	0.7
	1248	3.5		1315	3.1
	1846	0.6		1903	0.9
5 W	0106	3.6	20 TH	0130	3.5
	0721	0.4		0720	0.7
	1343	3.4		1353	3.1
	1936	0.6		1940	0.9
6 TH	0157	3.6	21 F	0207	3.5
	0813	0.5		0759	0.7
	1439	3.4		1434	3.1
	2030	0.7		2022	0.9
7 F	0252	3.5	22 SA	0245	3.5
	0913	0.5		0842	0.7
	1538	3.3		1518	3.1
	2129	0.8		2107	0.9
8 SA	0351	3.5	23 SU	0327	3.4
	1019	0.5		0929	0.7
	1639	3.2		1606	3.0
	2232	0.9		2157	1.0
9 SU	0454	3.4	24 M	0416	3.3
	1127	0.6		1022	0.8
	1743	3.2		1658	3.0
	2340	1.0		2252	1.1
10 M	0602	3.3	25 TU	0512	3.2
	1233	0.6		1122	0.9
	1849	3.2		1754	3.0
				2358	1.2
11 TU	0048	1.0	26 W	0615	3.2
	0713	3.3		1231	0.9
	1336	0.6		1854	3.1
	1950	3.2			
12 W	0153	0.9	27 TH	0117	1.1
	0816	3.3		0718	3.2
	1424	0.6		1341	0.8
	2045	3.3		1954	3.2
13 TH	0252	0.9	28 F	0221	1.0
	0910	3.4		0818	3.3
	1523	0.6		1437	0.7
	2133	3.4		2049	3.3
14 F	0344	0.8	29 SA	0315	0.8
	0959	3.4		0913	3.4
	1608	0.7		1526	0.6
	2218	3.4		2140	3.5
15 SA	0430	0.7	30 SU	0404	0.6
	1043	3.3		1004	3.5
	1650	0.7		1613	0.6
	2300	3.5		2228	3.6

JULY

Day	Time	m	Day	Time	m
1 M	0450	0.5	16 TU	0525	0.8
	1054	3.6		1142	3.2
	1658	0.5		1734	0.9
	2316	3.7		2354	3.5
2 TU	0536	0.4	17 W	0553	0.8
	1145	3.6		1216	3.2
	1745	0.5		1805	0.9
3 W	0005	3.7	18 TH	0028	3.5
	0621	0.3		0623	0.7
	1236	3.5		1248	3.2
	1832	0.5		1838	0.8
4 TH	0055	3.7	19 F	0101	3.6
	0708	0.3		0655	0.7
	1329	3.5		1319	3.2
	1921	0.6		1914	0.8
5 F	0145	3.7	20 SA	0133	3.6
	0758	0.3		0731	0.6
	1422	3.4		1351	3.2
	2012	0.6		1952	0.8
6 SA	0238	3.7	21 SU	0207	3.5
	0852	0.3		0809	0.6
	1517	3.3		1430	3.2
	2107	0.7		2033	0.9
7 SU	0332	3.6	22 M	0247	3.5
	0953	0.5		0852	0.7
	1614	3.3		1515	3.2
	2206	0.8		2119	0.9
8 M	0429	3.4	23 TU	0333	3.4
	1057	0.6		0940	0.8
	1713	3.2		1607	3.1
	2310	0.9		2210	1.1
9 TU	0532	3.3	24 W	0428	3.3
	1202	0.7		1034	0.9
	1817	3.1		1705	3.1
				2309	1.2
10 W	0017	1.0	25 TH	0532	3.2
	0643	3.2		1139	1.0
	1307	0.8		1809	3.1
	1921	3.2			
11 TH	0124	0.9	26 F	0032	1.2
	0753	3.2		0643	3.2
	1407	0.8		1302	1.0
	2020	3.2		1918	3.2
12 F	0228	1.0	27 SA	0157	1.1
	0851	3.2		0753	3.2
	1500	0.8		1415	0.9
	2111	3.3		2024	3.3
13 SA	0325	0.9	28 SU	0257	0.9
	0942	3.2		0856	3.3
	1547	0.8		1510	0.8
	2157	3.4		2121	3.5
14 SU	0413	0.8	29 M	0349	0.6
	1026	3.2		0951	3.5
	1627	0.8		1558	0.7
	2239	3.5		2212	3.6
15 M ●	0453	0.8	30 TU O	0437	0.4
	1106	3.2		1041	3.6
	1702	0.9		1644	0.6
	2318	3.5		2301	3.7
			31 W	0523	0.3
				1131	3.6
				1729	0.5
				2349	3.8

AUGUST

Day	Time	m	Day	Time	m
1 TH	0607	0.2	16 F	0000	3.5
	1220	3.6		0559	0.7
	1815	0.5		1218	3.2
				1814	0.8
2 F	0038	3.8	17 SA	0026	3.6
	0651	0.2		0630	0.6
	1309	3.5		1241	3.2
	1901	0.6		1848	0.8
3 SA	0127	3.8	18 SU	0057	3.6
	0737	0.3		0702	0.6
	1359	3.5		1313	3.3
	1949	0.6		1922	0.8
4 SU	0217	3.7	19 M	0133	3.6
	0826	0.4		0737	0.6
	1450	3.4		1351	3.3
	2039	0.7		2000	0.7
5 M	0308	3.6	20 TU	0215	3.5
	0920	0.6		0817	0.7
	1542	3.3		1435	3.3
	2133	0.8		2043	0.9
6 TU	0401	3.4	21 W	0301	3.4
	1021	0.7		0903	0.8
	1636	3.2		1525	3.2
	2235	0.9		2133	1.0
7 W	0458	3.2	22 TH	0355	3.3
	1127	0.9		0956	0.9
	1736	3.1		1623	3.1
	2343	1.0		2232	1.1
8 TH	0608	3.1	23 F	0500	3.2
	1233	1.0		1059	1.1
	1846	3.1		1730	3.1
				2353	1.2
9 F	0053	1.1	24 SA	0615	3.1
	0728	3.0		1223	1.2
	1339	1.0		1847	3.1
	1952	3.1			
10 SA	0203	1.1	25 SU	0136	1.1
	0833	3.0		0732	3.1
	1437	1.0		1357	1.1
	2048	3.2		2002	3.3
11 SU	0306	1.0	26 M	0241	0.9
	0924	3.1		0841	3.3
	1525	1.0		1456	0.9
	2135	3.4		2103	3.5
12 M	0355	0.9	27 TU	0335	0.6
	1008	3.2		0937	3.4
	1604	0.9		1545	0.8
	2218	3.4		2155	3.7
13 TU	0431	0.8	28 W O	0423	0.4
	1047	3.2		1027	3.6
	1637	0.9		1630	0.6
	2256	3.5		2243	3.8
14 W ●	0500	0.7	29 TH	0508	0.3
	1122	3.2		1114	3.6
	1709	0.8		1713	0.6
	2330	3.5		2331	3.8
15 TH	0529	0.7	30 F	0551	0.3
	1153	3.2		1200	3.6
	1742	0.8		1756	0.5
			31 SA	0018	3.8
				0632	0.3
				1247	3.6
				1839	0.6

13

Chart Datum: 2·01 metres below Ordnance Datum (Belfast)

NORTHERN IRELAND – BELFAST

LAT 54°36'N   LONG 5°55'W

TIMES AND HEIGHTS OF HIGH AND LOW WATERS   YEAR **1996**

TIME ZONE (UT)
For Summer Time add ONE hour in non-shaded areas

SEPTEMBER

Day	Time	m	Day	Time	m
1 SU	0106 / 0714 / 1334 / 1923	3.8 / 0.4 / 3.5 / 0.6	**16** M	0025 / 0632 / 1242 / 1854	3.6 / 0.6 / 3.4 / 0.7
2 M	0153 / 0758 / 1421 / 2009	3.7 / 0.5 / 3.5 / 0.7	**17** TU	0105 / 0707 / 1322 / 1931	3.6 / 0.6 / 3.4 / 0.8
3 TU	0241 / 0845 / 1508 / 2059	3.6 / 0.7 / 3.4 / 0.8	**18** W	0149 / 0747 / 1406 / 2015	3.5 / 0.7 / 3.4 / 0.8
4 W	0331 / 0940 / 1557 / 2156	3.4 / 0.9 / 3.3 / 0.9	**19** TH	0237 / 0834 / 1455 / 2105	3.4 / 0.8 / 3.3 / 1.0
5 TH	0423 / 1044 / 1651 / 2304	3.2 / 1.1 / 3.1 / 1.1	**20** F	0333 / 0928 / 1553 / 2206	3.3 / 1.0 / 3.2 / 1.1
6 F	0525 / 1154 / 1755	3.0 / 1.2 / 3.1	**21** SA	0440 / 1032 / 1701 / 2330	3.1 / 1.2 / 3.1 / 1.2
7 SA	0017 / 0656 / 1302 / 1916	1.1 / 2.8 / 1.2 / 3.1	**22** SU	0556 / 1157 / 1822	3.1 / 1.3 / 3.1
8 SU	0129 / 0809 / 1405 / 2019	1.1 / 2.9 / 1.2 / 3.2	**23** M	0115 / 0715 / 1338 / 1942	1.1 / 3.1 / 1.2 / 3.3
9 M	0235 / 0902 / 1456 / 2109	1.0 / 3.0 / 1.1 / 3.3	**24** TU	0222 / 0827 / 1439 / 2045	0.8 / 3.3 / 1.0 / 3.5
10 TU	0324 / 0945 / 1535 / 2152	0.9 / 3.1 / 1.0 / 3.4	**25** W	0317 / 0922 / 1529 / 2137	0.6 / 3.4 / 0.8 / 3.6
11 W	0359 / 1023 / 1610 / 2229	0.8 / 3.2 / 0.9 / 3.5	**26** TH	0405 / 1010 / 1614 / 2225	0.4 / 3.6 / 0.7 / 3.8
12 TH	0430 / 1057 / 1644 / ● 2300	0.7 / 3.2 / 0.8 / 3.5	**27** F	0450 / 1055 / 1657 / O 2311	0.4 / 3.6 / 0.6 / 3.8
13 F	0502 / 1126 / 1718 / 2324	0.7 / 3.3 / 0.8 / 3.5	**28** SA	0532 / 1140 / 1738 / 2357	0.4 / 3.6 / 0.6 / 3.8
14 SA	0534 / 1144 / 1750 / 2351	0.6 / 3.3 / 0.8 / 3.6	**29** SU	0612 / 1224 / 1818	0.4 / 3.6 / 0.6
15 SU	0603 / 1207 / 1822	0.6 / 3.3 / 0.7	**30** M	0043 / 0651 / 1308 / 1859	3.7 / 0.5 / 3.6 / 0.6

OCTOBER

Day	Time	m	Day	Time	m
1 TU	0129 / 0730 / 1351 / 1941	3.6 / 0.6 / 3.5 / 0.7	**16** W	0043 / 0642 / 1300 / 1910	3.6 / 0.7 / 3.5 / 0.7
2 W	0214 / 0812 / 1435 / 2027	3.5 / 0.8 / 3.4 / 0.8	**17** TH	0129 / 0725 / 1345 / 1956	3.5 / 0.7 / 3.4 / 0.8
3 TH	0300 / 0859 / 1520 / 2118	3.3 / 1.0 / 3.3 / 0.9	**18** F	0221 / 0814 / 1436 / 2049	3.4 / 0.9 / 3.4 / 0.9
4 F	0350 / 0957 / 1610 / 2221	3.1 / 1.2 / 3.2 / 1.1	**19** SA	0320 / 0911 / 1533 / 2153	3.3 / 1.1 / 3.3 / 1.0
5 SA	0445 / 1107 / 1705 / 2334	2.9 / 1.3 / 3.1 / 1.2	**20** SU	0427 / 1017 / 1641 / 2317	3.1 / 1.2 / 3.2 / 1.0
6 SU	0554 / 1217 / 1813	2.8 / 1.3 / 3.0	**21** M	0540 / 1140 / 1801	3.1 / 1.3 / 3.2
7 M	0043 / 0733 / 1321 / 1935	1.2 / 2.8 / 1.3 / 3.1	**22** TU	0046 / 0658 / 1311 / 1921	0.9 / 3.1 / 1.2 / 3.3
8 TU	0146 / 0831 / 1416 / 2033	1.1 / 2.9 / 1.2 / 3.2	**23** W	0156 / 0808 / 1416 / 2026	0.8 / 3.3 / 1.0 / 3.4
9 W	0238 / 0915 / 1501 / 2118	0.9 / 3.1 / 1.0 / 3.3	**24** TH	0253 / 0903 / 1509 / 2119	0.6 / 3.4 / 0.9 / 3.6
10 TH	0320 / 0953 / 1540 / 2154	0.8 / 3.2 / 0.9 / 3.4	**25** F	0342 / 0951 / 1556 / 2207	0.5 / 3.6 / 0.7 / 3.7
11 F	0357 / 1026 / 1617 / 2224	0.7 / 3.3 / 0.8 / 3.5	**26** SA	0428 / 1036 / 1639 / O 2253	0.5 / 3.6 / 0.7 / 3.7
12 SA	0431 / 1053 / 1652 / ● 2250	0.6 / 3.4 / 0.7 / 3.5	**27** SU	0510 / 1120 / 1721 / 2338	0.5 / 3.7 / 0.6 / 3.7
13 SU	0504 / 1113 / 1725 / 2322	0.6 / 3.4 / 0.7 / 3.6	**28** M	0551 / 1202 / 1800	0.6 / 3.6 / 0.6
14 M	0534 / 1142 / 1758	0.6 / 3.4 / 0.6	**29** TU	0022 / 0628 / 1244 / 1837	3.6 / 0.7 / 3.6 / 0.7
15 TU	0000 / 0605 / 1218 / 1831	3.6 / 0.6 / 3.5 / 0.7	**30** W	0106 / 0704 / 1324 / 1915	3.5 / 0.8 / 3.6 / 0.7
			31 TH	0148 / 0741 / 1405 / 1956	3.4 / 0.9 / 3.5 / 0.8

NOVEMBER

Day	Time	m	Day	Time	m
1 F	0232 / 0822 / 1448 / 2042	3.2 / 1.0 / 3.4 / 0.9	**16** SA	0210 / 0804 / 1424 / 2041	3.4 / 0.9 / 3.5 / 0.7
2 SA	0318 / 0910 / 1535 / 2134	3.1 / 1.2 / 3.3 / 1.0	**17** SU	0310 / 0902 / 1522 / 2145	3.3 / 1.0 / 3.4 / 0.8
3 SU	0409 / 1009 / 1626 / 2238	2.9 / 1.3 / 3.2 / 1.1	**18** M	0414 / 1007 / 1627 / 2300	3.2 / 1.1 / 3.3 / 0.8
4 M	0505 / 1122 / 1723 / 2350	2.8 / 1.4 / 3.1 / 1.1	**19** TU	0523 / 1121 / 1740	3.1 / 1.2 / 3.3
5 TU	0610 / 1231 / 1826	2.8 / 1.3 / 3.1	**20** W	0016 / 0636 / 1240 / 1857	0.8 / 3.1 / 1.2 / 3.3
6 W	0055 / 0734 / 1331 / 1932	1.1 / 2.9 / 1.3 / 3.1	**21** TH	0125 / 0745 / 1348 / 2005	0.8 / 3.2 / 1.1 / 3.4
7 TH	0151 / 0831 / 1422 / 2028	1.0 / 3.0 / 1.1 / 3.2	**22** F	0225 / 0842 / 1445 / 2101	0.7 / 3.4 / 0.9 / 3.5
8 F	0239 / 0913 / 1506 / 2112	0.8 / 3.2 / 1.0 / 3.3	**23** SA	0318 / 0932 / 1536 / 2151	0.6 / 3.5 / 0.8 / 3.6
9 SA	0320 / 0949 / 1547 / 2148	0.7 / 3.3 / 0.8 / 3.4	**24** SU	0405 / 1018 / 1622 / 2238	0.6 / 3.6 / 0.8 / 3.6
10 SU	0358 / 1020 / 1625 / 2223	0.7 / 3.4 / 0.8 / 3.5	**25** M	0449 / 1102 / 1705 / Q 2322	0.7 / 3.6 / 0.7 / 3.5
11 M	0434 / 1049 / 1702 / ● 2300	0.6 / 3.5 / 0.7 / 3.6	**26** TU	0530 / 1143 / 1744	0.8 / 3.6 / 0.7
12 TU	0509 / 1123 / 1739 / 2341	0.6 / 3.5 / 0.7 / 3.6	**27** W	0004 / 0606 / 1223 / 1819	3.4 / 0.8 / 3.6 / 0.7
13 W	0546 / 1202 / 1818	0.6 / 3.6 / 0.6	**28** TH	0045 / 0639 / 1302 / 1853	3.4 / 0.9 / 3.6 / 0.8
14 TH	0027 / 0627 / 1246 / 1900	3.5 / 0.7 / 3.6 / 0.6	**29** F	0124 / 0713 / 1341 / 1929	3.3 / 1.0 / 3.6 / 0.8
15 F	0117 / 0713 / 1333 / 1947	3.5 / 0.8 / 3.5 / 0.7	**30** SA	0205 / 0750 / 1421 / 2010	3.2 / 1.0 / 3.5 / 0.8

DECEMBER

Day	Time	m	Day	Time	m
1 SU	0248 / 0833 / 1504 / 2055	3.1 / 1.1 / 3.4 / 0.9	**16** M	0258 / 0850 / 1512 / 2131	3.3 / 0.9 / 3.5 / 0.6
2 M	0335 / 0921 / 1551 / 2146	3.0 / 1.2 / 3.3 / 1.0	**17** TU	0357 / 0950 / 1612 / 2238	3.2 / 1.0 / 3.4 / 0.7
3 TU	0426 / 1016 / 1642 / 2244	2.9 / 1.3 / 3.2 / 1.0	**18** W	0501 / 1057 / 1718 / 2347	3.2 / 1.0 / 3.3 / 0.8
4 W	0521 / 1121 / 1737 / 2350	2.9 / 1.3 / 3.1 / 1.1	**19** TH	0610 / 1209 / 1832	3.1 / 1.1 / 3.3
5 TH	0620 / 1235 / 1836	2.9 / 1.3 / 3.1	**20** F	0055 / 0720 / 1319 / 1943	0.8 / 3.2 / 1.1 / 3.3
6 F	0058 / 0724 / 1338 / 1936	1.0 / 3.0 / 1.2 / 3.2	**21** SA	0159 / 0821 / 1421 / 2044	0.8 / 3.3 / 1.0 / 3.3
7 SA	0156 / 0823 / 1431 / 2030	0.9 / 3.1 / 1.1 / 3.3	**22** SU	0256 / 0914 / 1517 / 2137	0.8 / 3.4 / 0.9 / 3.4
8 SU	0245 / 0911 / 1518 / 2117	0.8 / 3.3 / 0.9 / 3.4	**23** M	0346 / 1002 / 1607 / 2225	0.8 / 3.5 / 0.8 / 3.4
9 M	0329 / 0952 / 1602 / 2201	0.7 / 3.4 / 0.8 / 3.5	**24** TU	0431 / 1046 / 1651 / O 2309	0.8 / 3.6 / 0.8 / 3.4
10 TU	0410 / 1031 / 1643 / ● 2244	0.6 / 3.5 / 0.7 / 3.5	**25** W	0511 / 1127 / 1730 / 2349	0.8 / 3.6 / 0.7 / 3.3
11 W	0451 / 1110 / 1725 / 2329	0.6 / 3.6 / 0.6 / 3.5	**26** TH	0547 / 1206 / 1803	0.9 / 3.6 / 0.8
12 TH	0533 / 1152 / 1807	0.6 / 3.6 / 0.5	**27** F	0026 / 0617 / 1243 / 1833	3.2 / 0.9 / 3.6 / 0.8
13 F	0017 / 0617 / 1238 / 1851	3.5 / 0.7 / 3.7 / 0.5	**28** SA	0102 / 0648 / 1319 / 1906	3.2 / 0.9 / 3.6 / 0.8
14 SA	0108 / 0704 / 1325 / 1939	3.5 / 0.7 / 3.6 / 0.5	**29** SU	0138 / 0723 / 1356 / 1942	3.2 / 0.9 / 3.6 / 0.8
15 SU	0201 / 0755 / 1417 / 2032	3.4 / 0.8 / 3.6 / 0.5	**30** M	0216 / 0802 / 1434 / 2023	3.1 / 0.9 / 3.5 / 0.8
			31 TU	0257 / 0845 / 1513 / 2108	3.1 / 1.0 / 3.4 / 0.8

Chart Datum: 2·01 metres below Ordnance Datum (Belfast)

LARNE   10-13-11

Antrim 54°51'·20N 05°47'·50W

CHARTS
AC 1237, 2198; Imray C62, C64; Irish OS 5

TIDES
0000 Dover; ML 1·6; Duration 0620; Zone 0 (UT)

Standard Port BELFAST (←)

Times				Height (metres)			
High Water		Low Water		MHWS	MHWN	MLWN	MLWS
0100	0700	0000	0600	3·5	3·0	1·1	0·4
1300	1900	1200	1800				
Differences LARNE							
+0005	0000	+0010	−0005	−0·7	−0·5	−0·3	0·0
RED BAY							
+0022	−0010	+0007	−0017	−1·9	−1·5	−0·8	−0·2
CUSHENDUN BAY							
+0010	−0030	0000	−0025	−1·7	−1·5	−0·6	−0·2

SHELTER
Secure shelter in Larne Lough or ⌁ overnight outside hbr in Brown's Bay (E of Barr Pt) in 2–4m. Hbr can be entered H24 in any conditions. Larne is a busy ferry and commercial port; W side is commercial until Curran Pt where there are two YCs with congested moorings. ⌁ S of Ballylumford Power Stn. Yachts should not berth on any commercial quays including Castle Quay without Hr Mr's express permission. Boat Hbr (0·6m) 2ca S of Ferris Pt only for shoal draft craft.

Note: Work continues (started 1993) to extend the harbour southward and will eventually result in E Antrim BC moving to Curran Point, with fewer moorings.

NAVIGATION
WPT 54°51'·70N 05°47'·47W, 004°/184° from/to front ldg lt, 2·1M. Beware Hunter Rk 2M NE of hbr ent. Inside the narrow ent, the recommended chan is close to the E shore. Tide in the ent runs at up to 3½kn. Note: Magnetic abnomalies exist near Hunter Rk and between it and the mainland.

LIGHTS AND MARKS
Ldg lts 184°, Oc 4s 6/14m 12M, synch and vis 179°-189°; W ◊ with R stripes. Chaine Tr and fairway lts as chartlet. Note: Many shore lts on W side of ent may be mistaken for nav lts.

RADIO TELEPHONE
VHF Ch 14 16 *Larne Harbour*. Traffic, weather and tidal info available on Ch 14.

TELEPHONE (01574)
Hr Mr 279221; MRSC (01247) 463933; Pilot 273785; ⌗ (01232) 358250; Marinecall 0891 500 465; Police 272266; Dr 275331.

FACILITIES
Pier ☎ 279221, M, L, FW, C (32 ton); **E Antrim Boat Club ☎** 277204, Visitors should pre-contact Sec'y for advice on moorings; Slip, L, V, FW, Bar; **Services:** D, Gas, Sh, El. **Town** EC Tues; P & D (delivered, tidal), CH, V, R, Bar, ✉, Ⓑ, ⇌, Ferry to Stranraer and Cairnryan, ✈ (Belfast City and Belfast/Aldergrove).

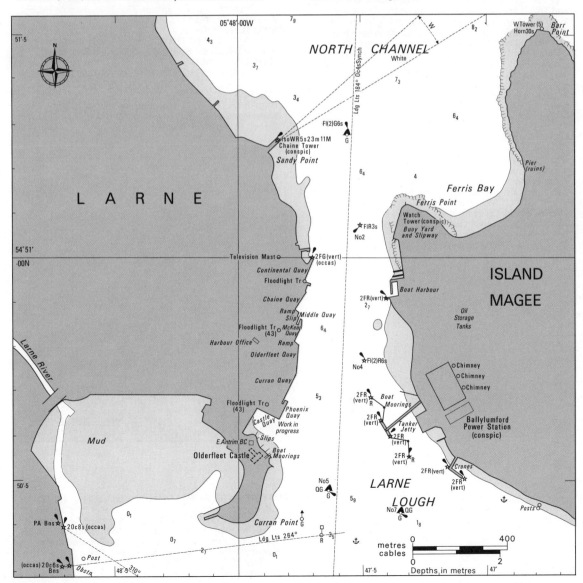

MINOR HARBOURS AND ANCHORAGES BETWEEN LARNE AND PORTRUSH

CARNLOUGH HARBOUR, Antrim, 54°59'·87N 05°59'·20W. AC 2198. HW +0006 on Dover, +0005 on Belfast; HW −1·6m on Belfast; ML no data; Duration 0625. Good shelter except in SE gales; do not ent in onshore winds >F6. Ldg marks 310°, R ▲s on B/W posts. Small hbr used by yachts and small FVs; visitors welcome. Ent and hbr dredged 2m every May. Beware fish farms in the bay marked by lt buoys (unreliable); also beware rks which cover at HW on either side of ent. N pier lt, Fl G 3s 4m 5M; S pier Fl R 3s 6m 5M. Hr Mr ☎ (01574) 272677. Facilities: **Quay** AB £2.50, AC (see Hr Mr), FW, Slip. **Town** P & D (cans), Gas, Gaz, ⊠, R, V, Bar.

RED BAY, Antrim, 55°03'·91N 06°03'·13W. AC 2199. HW +0006 on Dover; ML 1·1m; Duration 0625. See 10·13·11. Good holding, but open to E winds. Beware rks, 2 ruined piers W of Garron Pt and fish farms, marked by lt Bys, on S side of bay, approx ½M from shore. Glenariff pier has lt Fl 3s 10m 5M. In S and E winds ‡ 2ca off W stone arch near hd of bay in approx 3·5m; in N or W winds ‡ S of small pier in 2 – 5m, ½M NE of Waterfoot village. Facilities: **Cushendall** (1M N of pier) Bar, D & P (cans), ⊠, R, V, Gas; **Services:** CH, El, Slip. **Waterfoot** Bar, R, ⊠.

RATHLIN ISLAND, Antrim, 55°17'·52N 06°11'·60W. AC 2798. HW sp −0445, nps −0200 on Dover. Small hbr in NE corner of Church Bay, sheltered from winds NW through E to SSE. Beware sp streams up to 6kn in Rathlin Sound and TSS N of the ls. A wreck, marked by SCM buoy, is 1m SW of hbr. When clear, appr on 083° to cross The Bow (bar, approx 0·5m); keep very close to Manor Ho pier (N) and turn hard port into hbr ent dredged 2·5m. Outside hbr, ‡ close W of Sheephouse pier in about 5m. Lts: Rue Point (S tip), Fl (2) 5s 16m 14M, W 8-sided tr, B bands. Altacarry Head (Rathlin East) Fl (4) 20s 74m 26M, vis 110°−006°, 036°−058°, W tr, B band, Racon. Rathlin West, Fl R 5s 62m 22M, vis 015°−215°, W tr, lantern at base; Fog detector lt VQ; Horn (4) 60s. Manor Ho pier has Fl (2) R 6s 5m 4M. Church Bay R, Bar, ⊠.

BALLYCASTLE, Antrim, 55°12'·50N 06°14'·30W. AC 2798. Tides as for Rathlin Is (above); ML 0·8m. A fair weather ‡ on S side of Rathlin Sound. (New hbr planned). It is clear of strong tidal streams, but subject to swell. ‡ off the pier in 5m, sheltered from winds ENE to W; or berth on hd of pier (2·7m). Beware ferries at new pier with L Fl WR 9s 6m 5M, R110°−212°, W212°−000°, W col, B bands. Facilities: AB, FW, L, Slip. CG ☎ (012657) 62226; Ⓗ 62666. **Services:** P & D (cans), Gas. **Town** EC Wed; R, Bar, V, ⊠, Ⓑ. Note: A Historic Wreck (*Girona*; see 10.0.3g) is at Lacada Point, 55°14'·85N 06°30'·05W, 6M ENE of Portrush.

PORTRUSH 10-13-12

Antrim 55°12'·34N 06°39'·49W

CHARTS
AC 49, 2499, 2798; Imray C64; Irish OS 2
TIDES
−0410 Dover; ML 1·1; Duration 0610; Zone 0 (UT)

Standard Port BELFAST (←)

Times				Height (metres)			
High Water		Low Water		MHWS	MHWN	MLWN	MLWS
0100	0700	0000	0600	3·5	3·0	1·1	0·4
1300	1900	1200	1800				
Differences PORTRUSH							
−0433		−0433		−1·6	−1·6	−0·3	0·0

SHELTER
Good in hbr, except in strong NW/N winds. Berth on N quay or on pontoon at E end of N quay and see Hr Mr. A mooring may be available, but very congested in season. ‡ on E side of Ramore Hd in Skerries Roads 1ca S of Large Skerrie gives good shelter in most conditions, but open to NW sea/swell.
NAVIGATION
WPT 55°13'·00N 06°41'·00W, 308°/128° from/to N pier lt, 1·1M. Ent with on-shore winds >F 4 is difficult. Beware submerged bkwtr projecting 20m SW from N pier.
LIGHTS AND MARKS
Ldg lts 028° (occas, for LB use) both FR 6/8m 1M; R △ on metal bn and metal mast. N pier Fl R 3s 6m 3M; vis 220°-160°. S pier Fl G 3s 6m 3M; vis 220°-100°. Ramore Hd, FW lt (occas) on unmanned CG look-out.
RADIO TELEPHONE
VHF Ch 12 16 (0900-1700 LT, Mon-Fri; extended evening hrs June-Sept; Sat-Sun: 0900–1700, June-Sept only).
TELEPHONE (01265)
Hr Mr 822307; MRSC (01247) 463933; ⌗ 44803; Marinecall 0891 500 465; Police 822721; Dr 823767; Ⓗ 44177.
FACILITIES
Hbr AB £8, D, FW, M, Slip; **Portrush YC** ☎ 823932, Bar; **Services:** Gas, El, Ⓔ; **Town** EC Wed; V, R, Bar, ⊡, D & P (cans), ⊠, Ⓑ, ⇌, ✈ (Belfast).

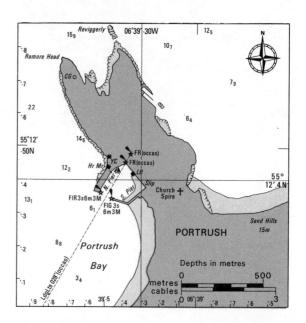

PORTSTEWART, Antrim, 55°11'·21N 06°43'·21W. AC 49. Tides as for Portrush. A tiny hbr 1·1ca S of Portstewart Pt lt, Oc R 10s 21m 5M, vis 040°−220°, obscd in final appr. A temp, fair weather berth (£8) at S end of inner basin in 0·8 – 1·7m; the very narrow ent is open to SW wind and swell. Beware salmon nets and rks close to S bkwtr. Facilities: EC Thurs; FW, Gas, D (tanker), Slip, Bar, V, R, convenient shops.

RIVER BANN   10-13-13

Londonderry/Antrim 55°10'·32N 06°46'·35W

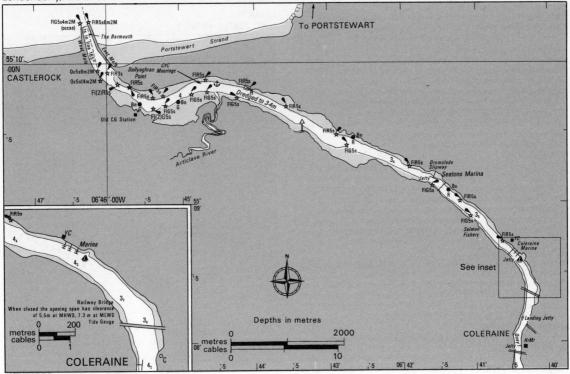

CHARTS
AC 2499, 2798, 2723; Imray C64; Irish OS 2
TIDES
–0345 Dover (Coleraine); ML 1·1; Duration 0540; Zone 0 (UT)

Standard Port BELFAST (◄—)

Times				Height (metres)			
High Water		Low Water		MHWS	MHWN	MLWN	MLWS
0100	0700	0000	0600	3·5	3·0	1·1	0·4
1300	1900	1200	1800				
Differences COLERAINE							
–0403		–0403		–1·3	–1·2	–0·2	0·0

SHELTER
Good, once inside the river ent (The Barmouth) between 2 training walls, extending 2ca N from the beaches. Do not try to enter in strong on-shore winds or when swell breaks on the pierheads. If in doubt call *Coleraine Hbr Radio* or ring Hr Mr. ⚓ upstream of old CG stn, or berth at Seaton's or Coleraine marinas, 3½M & 4½M from ent, on NE bank.
NAVIGATION
WPT 55°11'·00N, 06°46'·65W, 345°/165° from/to ent, 0·72M. Appr from E of N to bring ldg lts into line at bkwtr ends. The sand bar is constantly moving but ent is dredged to approx 3·5m. Beware salmon nets across the width of the river at 2M or 4M above ent, May to July. Also beware commercial traffic.
LIGHTS AND MARKS
Ldg lts 165°, front Oc 5s 6m 2M on W metal tower; rear Oc 5s 14m 2M. Portstewart Pt, Oc R 10s, is 2M ENE.
RADIO TELEPHONE
Coleraine Hbr Radio Ch 12 (Mon-Fri: HO and when vessel due). Coleraine Marina Ch M.
TELEPHONE (01265)
Hr Mr 42012; ✆ 44803; MRSC (01247) 463933; Marinecall 0891 500 465; Rly Bridge 42403; Police 44122; Ⓗ 44177; Dr 44831.
FACILITIES
Seatons Marina ☎ 832086, £5.40, CH, Slip.
Coleraine Hbr ☎ 42012, BH (35 ton); **Coleraine (Borough Council) Marina** (45+15 visitors), ☎ 44768, £9, Slip, D, FW, R, BH (15 ton), AC; **Coleraine YC** ☎ 44503, Bar, M;
Services: Gas, Kos, El, Ⓔ.
Town EC Thurs; P & D (cans), V, R, ✉, Ⓑ, ⇌, ✈ (Belfast).

LOUGH FOYLE   10-13-14

Londonderry (to SE)/Donegal (to NW) 55°14'N 06°54W

CHARTS
AC 2499, 2798, 2723; Imray C64; Irish OS 2
TIDES
Culmore Point –0025 Londonderry
Moville) –0055 Londonderry
Moville) –0300 Dover
Moville) –0400 Belfast
Warren Point –0400 Dover
Londonderry –0300 Dover
ML 1·6; Duration 0615; Zone 0 (UT)

Standard Port GALWAY (—►)

Times				Height (metres)			
High Water		Low Water		MHWS	MHWN	MLWN	MLWS
0200	0900	0200	0800	5·1	3·9	2·0	0·6
1400	2100	1400	2000				
Differences LONDONDERRY							
+0254	+0319	+0322	+0321	–2·4	–1·8	–0·8	–0·1
INISHTRAHULL							
+0100	+0100	+0115	+0200	–1·8	–1·4	–0·4	–0·2
PORTMORE							
+0120	+0120	+0135	+0135	–1·3	–1·1	–0·4	–0·1
TRAWBREAGA BAY							
+0115	+0059	+0109	+0125	–1·1	–0·8	No data	

SHELTER
The SE side of the Lough is low lying and shallow. The NW rises steeply and has a number of village hbrs between the ent and Londonderry (often referred to as Derry).
Greencastle: a busy fishing hbr, open to swell in winds SW to E. Not recommended for yachts unless in emergency.

13

LOUG FOYLE *continued*

Moville: the pier, with 1·5m at the end, is near the village (shops closed all day Wed), but is considerably damaged. ‡ outside hbr is exposed; inside for shoal draft only.
Carrickarory: pier/quay is condemned as unsafe. ‡ in bay is sheltered in winds from SW to NNW.
Culmore Bay: Complete shelter; ‡ 1½ca W of Culmore Pt in pleasant cove, 4M from Londonderry.
Londonderry: Rarely used by yachts, although commercial operations have been transferred to new facilities at Lisahally (55°02'·6N 07°15'·6W). ‡ close below Craigavon Bridge clearance 1·7m, or berth on non-commercial quay (down from Guildhall). Foyle Bridge at Rosses Pt about 2M downriver has 32m clearance.

NAVIGATION
WPT Tuns PHM buoy, Fl R 3s, 55°14'·01N 06°53'·38W, 055°/235° from/to Warren Pt lt, 2·5M. The Tuns bank lies 3M NE of Magilligan Pt. The main or N Chan, ¾M wide, runs NW of The Tuns; a lesser chan, min depth 4m, runs 3ca off shore around NE side of Magilligan Pt. Beware commercial traffic. In June and July the chan is at times obstructed by salmon nets at night. N Chan tides reach 3½kn, and up in the river the ebb runs up to 6kn.

LIGHTS AND MARKS
Inishowen Fl (2) WRG 10s 28m 18/14M; W tr, two B bands; vis G197°–211°, W211°–249°, R249°–000°; Horn (2) 30s. Warren Pt Fl 1·5s 9m 10M; W tr, G abutment; vis 232°–061°. Magilligan Pt QR 7m 4M; R structure. The main chan up to Londonderry is very well lit. Foyle Bridge centre FW each side; VQG on W pier; VQR on E pier.

RADIO TELEPHONE
VHF Ch **14** 12 16 (H24). Traffic and nav info Ch 14.

TELEPHONE (01504)
Hr Mr (Londonderry) 263680; MRSC (01247) 883184; ‡ 261937 or (01232) 358250; Marinecall 0891 500 465; Police 261893; Dr 264868; Ⓗ 45171.

FACILITIES (Londonderry)
Harbour Office ☎ 263680, M, FW, C (10 ton mobile), AB; **8 & 9 Sheds** M, FW, C (2 x 1½ ton elec), AB; **7 Shed** M, FW, AB; **14/15 Berth** M, FW, AB; **Dolphins** M, FW, El, AB; **NR Quay** P, D, ME, El; **Prehen Boat Club** ☎ 43405.
City EC Thurs; P, D, ME, El, CH, V, R, Bar, ⊠, Ⓑ, ⇌, ✈.

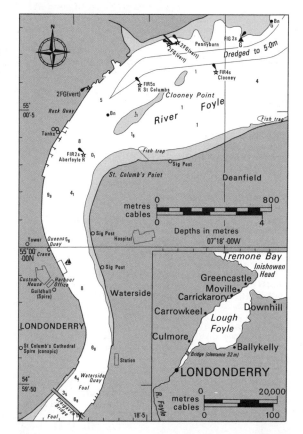

LOUG SWILLY   10-13-15
Donegal 55°17'N 07°34'W

CHARTS
AC 2697; Irish OS 1

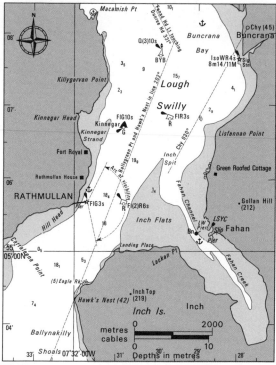

TIDES
–0500 Dover; ML 2·3; Duration 0605; Zone 0 (UT)

Standard Port GALWAY (⟶)

Times				Height (metres)			
High Water		Low Water		MHWS	MHWN	MLWN	MLWS
0200	0900	0200	0800	5·1	3·9	2·0	0·6
1400	2100	1400	2000				
Differences FANAD HEAD							
+0115	+0040	+0125	+0120	–1·1	–0·9	–0·5	–0·1
RATHMULLAN							
+0125	+0050	+0126	+0118	–0·8	–0·7	–0·1	–0·1
MULROY BAY (BAR)							
+0108	+0052	+0102	+0118	–1·2	–1·0	No data	
SHEEP HAVEN (DOWNIES BAY)							
+0057	+0043	+0053	+0107	–1·1	–0·9	No data	

SHELTER
Ent easy, but beware downdrafts on E side. ‡s N of Inch Is may suffer from swell. ‡ in Port Salon B (off chartlet to NW), except in E winds; off Macamish Pt sheltered from SE to N winds; Rathmullan Road N of pier, where there is AB on N/S yacht pontoon 3·6m MLWS; Fahan Creek, ent at HW–1.

NAVIGATION
WPT 55°17'·50N 07°34'·50W, 352°/172° from/to Dunree Hd lt, 5·7M. Main chan is well lit/buoyed. Beware Swilly More Rks, Kinnegar Spit, Colpagh Rks off E shore, Kinnegar Strand, Inch Flats and fish farms. Fahan Creek is buoyed by LSYC.

LIGHTS AND MARKS
Fanad Hd lt, Fl (5) WR 20s 39m 18/14M, touching Dunree Hd lt, Fl (2) WR 5s 46m 12/9M, leads 151° into the Lough. Thence Ballygreen Pt and Hawk's Nest in line at 202°.

RADIO TELEPHONE
None.

TELEPHONE (074)
Hr Mr 58177; MRCC (01) 6620922/3; ‡ 21935; Police 58113; Dr 58135; Pier Hotel, Rathmullan pontoon 58178.

FACILITIES
RATHMULLAN **Pier** AB (£10), AC, C (5 ton), FW, L, M, Slip; **Services:** CH, M, ⊡, R, Bar. **Town** EC Wed; D & P (cans), Kos, Bar, R, V, ⊠, Ⓑ, ⇌, ✈ (bus to Londonderry).
RAMELTON AB, L. **Town** Bar, P & D (cans), FW, Kos, R, V, ⊠.
FAHAN Slip, FW, L, R; **L Swilly YC** ☎ 60189, M, Bar; **Services:** (1M SE), Kos, V, P & D (cans). Marina planned.

OTHER HARBOURS AND ANCHORAGES IN DONEGAL

MULROY BAY, Donegal, 55°15′·30N 07°46′·30W. AC 2699; HW (bar) −0455 on Dover. See 10.13.15. Beware Limeburner Rk, (marked by NCM buoy, Q, whis) 3M N of ent and the bar which is dangerous in swell or onshore winds. Ent at half flood (not HN); chan lies between Bar Rks and Sessiagh Rks, thence through First, Second and Third Narrows (with strong tides) to Broad Water. HW at the head of the lough is 2¼ hrs later than at the bar. ‡s: Close SW of Ravedy Is (Fl 3s 9m 3M); Fanny's Bay (2m), excellent; Rosnakill Bay (3·5m) in SE side; Cranford Bay; Milford Port (3 to 4m). Beware power cable 6m, over Moross chan, barring North Water to masted boats. Facilities: **Milford Port** AB, FW, V; **Fanny's Bay** ✉, Shop at Downings village (1M), hotel at Rosepenna (¾M).

SHEEP HAVEN, Donegal, 55°11′·00N 07°51′·00W. AC 2699. HW −0515 on Dover. See 10·13·15. Bay is 4M wide with many ‡ s, easily accessible in daylight, but exposed to N winds. Beware rks for 3ca off Rinnafaghla Pt; also Wherryman Rks, which dry, 1ca off E shore 2¼M S of Rinnafaghla Pt. ‡ in Downies (or Downings) Bay to SW of pier; in Pollcormick Inlet close W in 3m; in Ards Bay for excellent shelter, but beware the bar in strong winds. Lts: Portnablahy ldg lts 125°, both Oc 6s 7/12m 2M, B col, W bands; Downies pier hd, Fl R 3s 5m 2M, R post. Facilities: (Downies) EC Wed; V, FW, P (cans 300m), R, Bar; (Portnablahy Bay) V, P (cans), R, Bar.

GWEEDORE HBR/BUNBEG, Donegal, 55°03′·75N 08°18′·87W. AC 1883. Tides see 10.13.16. Gweedore hbr, the estuary of the R Gweedore, has sheltered ‡s or temp AB at Bunbeg Quay, usually full of FVs. Apprs via Gola N or S Sounds are not simple especially in poor visibility. N Sound is easier with ldg Its 171°, both Oc 3s 9/13m 2M, B/W bns, on the SE tip of Gola Is. (There are also ‡s on the S and E sides of Gola Is). E of Bo is the bar 0·4m has a Fl G 3s and the chan, lying E of Inishinny Is and W of Inishcoole, is marked by a QG and 3 QR. A QG marks ent to Bunbeg. Night ent not advised. Facilities: FW, D at quay; V, ✉, Ⓑ, Bar at village ½M.

BURTONPORT, Donegal, 54°58′·93N 08°26′·60W. AC 2792, 1879. HW −0525 on Dover; ML 2·0m; Duration 0605. See 10·13·16. Normal ent via N Chan. Hbr very full, no space to ‡; berth on local boat at pier or go to Rutland Hbr or Aran Is. Ent safe in all weathers except NW gales. Ldg marks/lts: N Chan ldg lts on Inishcoo 119°, both Iso 6s 6/11m 1M; front W bn, B band; rear B bn, Y band. Rutland Is ldg lts 138°, both Oc 6s 8/14m 1M; front W bn, B band; rear B bn, Y band. Burtonport ldg lts 068°, both FG 17/23m 1M; front Gy bn, W band; rear Gy bn, Y band. Facilities: D (just inside pier), FW (root of pier), P (½M inland). **Village** Bar, ✉, R, V, Kos.

TEELIN HARBOUR, Donegal, 54°37′·50N 08°37′·87W. AC 2792. Tides as for Killybegs (below). A possible passage ‡, being mid-way between Rathlin O'Birne and Killybegs. But the hbr is open to S'ly swell and prone to squalls in NW winds. Ent, 1ca wide, is close E of Teelin Pt lt, Fl R 10s, which is hard to see by day. ‡ on W side in 3m to N of pier, or on E side near derelict pier. Many moorings and, in the NE, mussel rafts. Facilities: possible FW, D, V at Carrick, 3M inland.

KILLYBEGS   10-13-16

Donegal 54°36′·90N 08°26′·80W

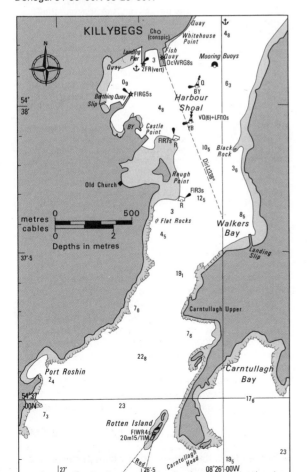

CHARTS
AC 2792, 2702; Irish OS 3
TIDES
−0520 Dover; ML 2·2; Duration 0620; Zone 0 (UT)

Standard Port GALWAY (→)

Times				Height (metres)			
High Water		Low Water		MHWS	MHWN	MLWN	MLWS
0600	1100	0000	0700	5·1	3·9	2·0	0·6
1800	2300	1200	1900				
Differences KILLYBEGS							
+0040	+0050	+0055	+0035	−1·0	−0·9	−0·5	0·0
GWEEDORE HARBOUR							
+0048	+0100	+0055	+0107	−1·3	−1·0	−0·5	−0·1
BURTONPORT							
+0042	+0055	+0115	+0055	−1·2	−1·0	−0·6	−0·1
DONEGAL HARBOUR (SALTHILL QUAY)							
+0038	+0050	+0052	+0104	−1·2	−0·9		No data

SHELTER
Secure natural hbr, but some swell in SSW winds. A busy major FV port, H24 access. ‡ about 2½ca NE of the Pier, off blue shed (Gallagher Bros) in 3m, clear of FV wash. Or **Bruckless Hbr**, about 2M E at the head of McSwyne's Bay, is a pleasant ‡ in 1·8m, sheltered from all except SW winds. Ent on 038° between rks; ICC SDs are essential.
NAVIGATION
WPT 54°36′·00N 08°27′·00W, 202°/022° from/to Rotten Is lt, 0·94M. From W, beware Manister Rk (covers at HW; dries at LW) off Fintragh B. Keep mid chan until off Rough Pt, then follow the Dir lt or Y ◊ ldg marks 338° into hbr.
LIGHTS AND MARKS
Rotten Is lt, Fl WR 4s 20m 15/11M, W tr, vis W255°−008°, R008°−039°, W039°−208°. Dir Lt 338°, Oc WRG 8s, and Al WG/WR 8s; Oc W 8s sector 336°-340° (see 10.13.4). Harbour Shoal is marked by a SCM and NCM lt buoy.
RADIO TELEPHONE
Hr Mr VHF Ch 16 14; essential to request a berth.
TELEPHONE (073)
Hr Mr 31032; MRCC (01) 6620922/3; Bundoran Inshore Rescue ☎ (072) 41713; ♯ 31070; Police 31002; Dr 31148 (Surgery).
FACILITIES
Landing Pier ☎ 31032, AB (free), M, D & P (cans), FW, ME, EI, CH, Slip, V, R, Bar; **Berthing Quay** AB, M, Slip, D; **Services:** Sh, C (12 ton), ME, EI, Sh, Kos, Ⓔ.
Town EC Wed; ✉, Ⓑ, ⇌ (bus to Sligo), ✈ (Strandhill).

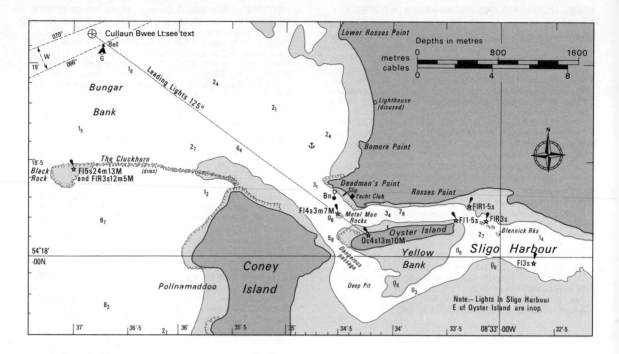

SLIGO   10-13-17

Sligo 54°18'·30N 08°34'·70W

CHARTS
AC 2852, 2767; Imray C54; Irish OS 7
TIDES
−0511 Dover; ML 2·3; Duration 0620; Zone 0 (UT)

Standard Port GALWAY (→)

Times				Height (metres)			
High Water		Low Water		MHWS	MHWN	MLWN	MLWS
0600	1100	0000	0700	5·1	3·9	2·0	0·6
1800	2300	1200	1900				
Differences SLIGO HARBOUR (Oyster Is)							
+0043	+0055	+0042	+0054	−1·0	−0·9	−0·5	−0·1
MULLAGHMORE							
+0036	+0048	+0047	+0059	−1·4	−1·0	−0·4	−0·2
BALLYSADARE BAY (Culleenamore)							
+0059	+0111	+0111	+0123	−1·2	−0·9	No data	
KILLALA BAY (Inishcrone)							
+0035	+0055	+0030	+0050	−1·3	−1·2	−0·7	−0·2

SHELTER
The lower hbr is fairly exposed; ⚓ along N side of Oyster Is, or proceed 4M (not at night) up to the shelter of Sligo town; 2nd berth below bridge for yachts.
NAVIGATION
WPT 54°19'·15N 08°36'·77W, 305°/125° from/to front ldg lt, 1·6M. The passage between Oyster Is and Coney Island is marked 'Dangerous'. Pass N of Oyster Is leaving Blennick Rks to port. Passage up to Sligo town between training walls. Some perches are in bad repair. Pilots at Raghly Pt and Rosses Pt. Chan up to quays dredged 1·6m.
LIGHTS AND MARKS
Cullaun Bwee Dir lt (off chartlet), Fl (2) WRG 10s 8m10/8M (H24), W sector 066°-070°: Ldg lts (H24) lead 125° into ent: front, Fl 4s 3m 7M, Metal Man Rks (statue of a man on a twr); rear, Oyster Is lt ho, Oc 4s 13m 10M. Lts up-channel are inop.
RADIO TELEPHONE
Pilots VHF Ch 12 16.
TELEPHONE (071)
Hbr Office 61197; MRCC (01) 6620922/3; ⌗ 61064; Police 42031; Dr 42886; Ⓗ 71111.
FACILITIES
Deepwater Pier AB, P & D (in cans), L, FW, ME, El, Sh, CH, C (15 ton); **Sligo YC** ☎ 77168, M, FW, Bar, Slip.
Services: Slip, D, ME, El, Sh, SM, Gas;
Town V, R, Bar, ✉, Ⓑ, ⇌ Irish Rail ☎ 69888, Bus ☎ 60066, ✈ (Strandhill) ☎ 68280.

MINOR HARBOUR/ANCHORAGE TO THE WEST

KILLALA BAY, Sligo/Mayo, 54°13'·02N 09°12'·80W. AC 2715. Tides, see 10.13.17. The bay, which is exposed to the N and NE, is entered between Lenadoon Pt and Kilcummin Hd, 6M to the W. Carrickpatrick ECM buoy, Q (3) 10s, in mid-bay marks St Patrick's Rks to the W. Thence, if bound for Killala hbr, make good Killala SHM buoy, Fl G 6s, 7½ca to the SSW. The Round Tr and cathedral spire at Killala are conspic. Four sets of ldg bns/lts lead via a narrow chan between sand dunes and over the bar (0·3m) as follows:
1. 230°, Rinnaun Pt lts Oc 10s 7/12m 5M, ☐ concrete trs.
2. 215°, Inch ls, ☐ concrete trs; the rear has Dir lt Fl WRG 2s, G205°-213°, W213°-217°, R217°-225°.
3. 196°, Kilroe lts Oc 4s 5/10m 2M, W ☐ trs, which lead to ⚓ in Bartragh Pool, 6ca NE of Killala hbr; thence
4. 236°, Pier lts Iso 2s 5/7m 2M, W ◇ daymarks, lead via narrow, dredged chan to pier where AB is possible in about 1·5m. Facilities: FW, P & D (cans), V in town ½M, EC Thurs. Other hbrs in the bay: R Moy leading to Ballina should not be attempted without pilot/local knowledge. Inishcrone in the SE has a pier and lt, Fl WRG 1·5s 8m 2M; see 10.13.4.

The West Coast of Ireland

The splendour of the mountains, their varying colours, whether in the rising or setting sunlight, by noonday or under the moon, the glory of the sea in fine weather at sundown, when it often resembles a lake of molten gold, the mighty cliffs, attaining in Donegal and Mayo to a height of nearly 2000 ft, and the secure harbours scattered with few exceptions at easy intervals, will well repay the efforts required to reach these waters.

Given a small seaworthy vessel, a careful skipper of experience, provided with charts and small auxiliary power, can navigate the coast with ease and confidence.

H.J.Hanson OBE, MA.

Reprinted from their Handbook by kind permission of the Cruising Association.

WESTPORT (CLEW BAY)   10-13-18

Mayo 53°47'·85N 09°35'·40W

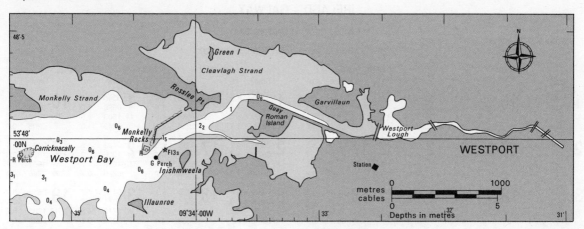

CHARTS
AC 2057, 2667; Imray C54; Irish OS 10 and 11
TIDES
−0545 Dover; ML 2·5; Duration 0610; Zone 0 (UT)

Standard Port GALWAY (→)

Times				Height (metres)			
High Water		Low Water		MHWS	MHWN	MLWN	MLWS
0600	1100	0000	0700	5·1	3·9	2·0	0·6
1800	2300	1200	1900				
Differences INISHRAHER							
+0030	+0012	+0058	+0026	−0·6	−0·5	−0·3	−0·1
BROADHAVEN							
+0040	+0050	+0040	+0050	−1·4	−1·1	−0·4	−0·1
BLACKSOD QUAY							
+0025	+0035	+0040	+0040	−1·2	−1·0	−0·6	−0·2
BLACKSOD BAY (BULL'S MOUTH)							
+0101	+0057	+0109	+0105	−1·5	−1·0	−0·6	−0·1
CLARE ISLAND							
+0019	+0013	+0029	+0023	−1·0	−0·7	−0·4	−0·1
KILLARY HARBOUR							
+0021	+0015	+0035	+0029	−1·0	−0·8	−0·4	−0·1
INISHBOFIN HARBOUR							
+0013	+0009	+0021	+0017	−1·0	−0·8	−0·4	−0·1
CLIFDEN BAY							
+0005	+0005	+0016	+0016	−0·7	−0·5	No data	
SLYNE HEAD							
+0002	+0002	+0010	+0010	−0·7	−0·5	No data	

SHELTER
Secure ⚓s amongst the islands at all tides, as follows: E of Inishlyre in about 2m; E of Collan More via narrow ent off Rosmoney Pt; and 2ca NE of Dorinish More, good holding in lee of Dorinish Bar (dries). Or go up to Westport Quay HW±1½, to dry out on S side. Newport Hbr (dries) can be reached above mid-flood with careful pilotage (AC 2667); dry out against N quay or ⚓ at E end of Rabbit Is.
NAVIGATION
WPT 53°49'·20N 09°42'·10W, 251°/071° from/to Inishgort lt ho, 1·2M. Contact Tom Gibbons (Inishlyre Is) ☎ (098) 26381 for pilotage advice. Beware of Monkellys Rks (PHM buoy) and the Spit (G perch).
LIGHTS AND MARKS
Westport Bay entered via Inishgort lt, L Fl 10s 11m 10M (H24), and a series of ldg lines, but not recommended at night. Final appr line 080° towards lt bn, Fl 3s. Passage from Westport Bay to Westport Quay, 1½M approx, is marked by bns.
RADIO TELEPHONE
None.
TELEPHONE (098)
MRCC (01) 6620922/3; ⌗ (094) 21131; Police 25555; ⊞ (094) 21733.
FACILITIES
Quays M, L, AB, Slip, V, R, Bar; **Mayo SC** ☎ 26160 L, Slip, Bar, at Rosmoney (safe for leaving boat); **Glénans Irish SC** ☎ 26046 on Collan More Is; **Services:** Kos, El, Ⓔ; **Town** EC Wed; P & D (cans), ✉, Ⓑ, ⇌, ✈ (Galway/Knock).

OTHER ANCHORAGES FROM EAGLE IS TO SLYNE HEAD

BROAD HAVEN, Mayo, 54°16'·00N 09°53'·20W. AC 2703. See 10.13.18 for tides; ML 1·9m. A safe refuge in all but N'lies. Easy appr across Broad Haven Bay to the ent between Brandy Pt and Gubacashel Pt, Iso WR 4s27m 12/9M, W tr. 7ca S of this lt is Ballyglas Fl G 3s on W side. ⚓ close N or S of Ballyglas which has pier (2m); or in E winds ⚓ 3ca S of Inver Pt out of the tide. Further S, the inlet narrows off Barrett Pt then turns W to Belmullet. Facilities: V, ✉.

PORTNAFRANKAGH Mayo, 54°14'·95N 10°06'·00W. AC 2703. Tides approx as Broad Haven. A safe passage ⚓, close to the coastal route, but swell enters in all winds. Appr toward Port Pt, thence keep to the N side for better water; middle and S side break in onshore winds. ⚓ in 4–5m on S side, close inshore. L and slip at new pier. Unlit, but Eagle Is lt, Fl (3) 10s 67m 26M H24, W tr, is 2M N. No facilities; Belmullet 4M, V.

BLACKSOD BAY, Mayo, 54°05'·00N 10°02'·00W. AC 2704. HW − 0525 on Dover; ML 2·2m; Duration 0610. See 10·13.18. Safe ⚓ with no hidden dangers, access day or night. Good ⚓s NW of Blacksod Quay (3m); at Elly B (1·8m); Elly Hbr; Saleen B; N of Claggan Pt. Beware drying rk 3·5ca SSE of Ardmore Pt. Lts: Blacksod Pt, Fl (2) WR 7·5s 13m 9M, R189°-210°, W210°-018°. ECM buoy Q (3) 10s.Blacksod pier hd, 2 FR (vert) 6m 3M. No facilities, but supplies, inc P & D (cans), at Belmullet 2·5M N.

KILLARY HARBOUR, Mayo/Galway, 53°37'·83N 09°54'·00W. AC 2706. Tides 10.13.18. A spectacular 7M long inlet, narrow and deep. Appr in good vis to identify ldg marks. Doonee Is and Inishbarna bns lead 099° to ent. (Lat/Long above is 4ca W of Doonee Is on the ldg line). Caution fish farms, some with Fl Y lts. ⚓s off Dernasliggaun, Bundorragha and Leenaun at head of inlet. (Village: V, Bar, hotel). Enter Little Killary Bay 4ca S of Doonee. Rks at ent do not cover. Good ⚓ in 3m at hd of bay.

BALLYNAKILL, Galway, 53°34'·95N 10°03'·00W. AC 2706. Tides as Inishbofin/Killary. Easy appr between Cleggan Pt, Fl (3) WRG 15s and Rinvyle Pt. Usual ent N of Freaghillaun South Is, E of which is good passage ⚓ in 7m. Further E, Carrigeen and Ardagh Rks lie in mid-chan. Keep N for ⚓ in Derryinver B. S chan leads to ⚓s off Ross Pt; S of Roeillaun; or, inside bar dries 0·2m, in complete shelter at Fahy B. No facilities.

INISHBOFIN, Mayo, 53°36'·60N 10°13'·20W. AC 2707, 1820.HW −0555 on Dover; ML 1·9m. See 10·13.18. Very safe hbr once inside narrow ent. 2 conspic W trs lead 032°. ⚓ between new pier and Port Is. Old pier to the E dries. Gun Rock, Fl (2) 6s 8m 4M, vis 296°-253°. Facilities: FW, R, Bar, V, Hotel ☎ (095) 45803.

CLIFDEN BAY, Galway, 53°29'·40N 10°05'·90W. AC 2708, 1820. HW −0600 on Dover; Duration 0610. Tides see 10·13.18. The high W bn on Carrickrana Rks, 2·8M WSW of Fishing Pt, must be identified before entering. Ldg marks 080°: W bn at Fishing Pt on with Clifden Castle. Beware bar at ent by Fishing Pt and another SE of creek going up to Clifden; also Doolick Rks, Coghan Rks and rks off Errislannon Pt. ⚓ between Larner Rks and Drinagh Pt; dry out against Clifden Quay (beware ruined training wall); or ⚓ in Ardbear Bay SE of Yellow Slate Rks in 3·4m. Keep clear of fish farms. Facilities: **Town** EC Thurs; Bar, Ⓑ, CH, D, P, ✉, R, V, Kos, FW, V, R, Dr, ⊞. Bus to Galway.

13

IRELAND – GALWAY

LAT 53°16′N   LONG   9°03′W

TIMES AND HEIGHTS OF HIGH AND LOW WATERS

YEAR **1996**

TIME ZONE (UT)
For Summer Time add ONE hour in non-shaded areas

JANUARY

Day	Time / m	Time / m	Time / m	Time / m
1 M	0148 4.2	0745 1.8	1409 4.1	2011 1.7
16 TU	0035 4.2	0642 1.8	1257 4.1	1925 1.6
2 TU	0244 4.3	0838 1.6	1503 4.3	2057 1.6
17 W	0146 4.4	0759 1.5	1416 4.3	2031 1.3
3 W	0330 4.5	0923 1.4	1549 4.4	2137 1.4
18 TH	0249 4.7	0857 1.1	1519 4.6	2123 1.0
4 TH	0411 4.6	1005 1.3	1630 4.5	2214 1.3
19 F	0343 5.0	0948 0.7	1613 4.9	2210 0.7
5 F ○	0449 4.7	1043 1.1	1709 4.6	2251 1.2
20 SA ●	0434 5.3	1035 0.4	1703 5.2	2256 0.4
6 SA	0526 4.8	1120 1.0	1747 4.7	2327 1.1
21 SU	0523 5.5	1120 0.1	1751 5.3	2341 0.3
7 SU	0603 4.8	1156 0.9	1825 4.7	
22 M	0611 5.5	1204 0.0	1837 5.3	
8 M	0002 1.1	0639 4.8	1230 0.9	1901 4.7
23 TU	0025 0.3	0656 5.5	1248 0.1	1921 5.2
9 TU	0038 1.1	0714 4.8	1303 0.9	1938 4.6
24 W	0109 0.5	0741 5.3	1330 0.3	2007 4.9
10 W	0113 1.2	0749 4.7	1337 1.0	2015 4.5
25 TH	0153 0.7	0827 5.0	1413 0.7	2055 4.6
11 TH	0150 1.4	0823 4.6	1413 1.2	2054 4.4
26 F	0240 1.1	0916 4.6	1459 1.1	2148 4.3
12 F	0231 1.5	0900 4.4	1455 1.4	2140 4.2
27 SA	0334 1.5	1011 4.3	1553 1.5	2249 4.0
13 SA	0318 1.7	0946 4.3	1543 1.6	2232 4.1
28 SU	0442 1.8	1112 4.0	1700 1.8	2356 3.8
14 SU	0414 1.9	1042 4.2	1641 1.7	2330 4.1
29 M	0558 1.9	1221 3.8	1822 2.0	
15 M	0520 1.9	1144 4.1	1753 1.8	
30 TU	0112 3.8	0710 1.9	1339 3.8	1938 1.9
31 W	0223 3.9	0815 1.8	1445 3.9	2036 1.7

FEBRUARY

Day	Time / m	Time / m	Time / m	Time / m
1 TH	0315 4.1	0905 1.5	1534 4.1	2119 1.5
16 F	0236 4.5	0846 1.1	1510 4.5	2112 1.0
2 F	0357 4.3	0947 1.3	1615 4.3	2157 1.3
17 SA	0332 4.8	0936 0.7	1602 4.8	2158 0.6
3 SA	0435 4.5	1025 1.0	1653 4.5	2234 1.0
18 SU ●	0422 5.2	1022 0.3	1650 5.1	2242 0.4
4 SU ○	0511 4.7	1101 0.8	1730 4.6	2310 0.9
19 M	0509 5.4	1105 0.1	1735 5.2	2325 0.2
5 M	0547 4.8	1136 0.7	1806 4.7	2344 0.8
20 TU	0555 5.5	1147 0.0	1818 5.3	
6 TU	0621 4.8	1208 0.6	1841 4.8	
21 W	0007 0.1	0638 5.4	1227 0.0	1900 5.2
7 W	0018 0.8	0654 4.8	1240 0.6	1914 4.7
22 TH	0049 0.3	0721 5.3	1307 0.2	1941 5.0
8 TH	0051 0.8	0726 4.8	1312 0.7	1947 4.6
23 F	0129 0.5	0802 5.0	1346 0.6	2023 4.7
9 F	0126 0.9	0757 4.7	1347 0.9	2020 4.5
24 SA	0212 0.9	0845 4.6	1426 1.0	2107 4.3
10 SA	0205 1.1	0829 4.5	1426 1.1	2100 4.3
25 SU	0259 1.3	0932 4.2	1512 1.5	2158 4.0
11 SU	0249 1.3	0911 4.4	1512 1.3	2152 4.2
26 M	0358 1.7	1026 3.9	1612 1.9	2301 3.7
12 M	0341 1.6	1010 4.1	1607 1.6	2255 4.0
27 TU	0515 1.9	1135 3.6	1737 2.1	
13 TU	0444 1.7	1119 4.0	1715 1.8	
28 W	0027 3.6	0632 2.0	1304 3.5	1859 2.1
14 W	0004 4.0	0606 1.8	1236 4.0	1901 1.7
29 TH	0157 3.7	0742 1.8	1424 3.7	2006 1.8
15 TH	0124 4.2	0742 1.5	1404 4.2	2019 1.4

MARCH

Day	Time / m	Time / m	Time / m	Time / m
1 F	0255 3.9	0839 1.6	1515 4.0	2054 1.5
16 SA	0223 4.4	0832 1.1	1459 4.5	2058 1.0
2 SA	0337 4.2	0922 1.3	1555 4.2	2134 1.2
17 SU	0318 4.8	0921 0.7	1548 4.8	2142 0.7
3 SU	0415 4.4	0959 1.0	1632 4.5	2211 0.9
18 M	0406 5.1	1004 0.4	1632 5.1	2225 0.4
4 M	0450 4.6	1035 0.7	1707 4.7	2247 0.7
19 TU ●	0452 5.3	1046 0.2	1715 5.2	2306 0.2
5 TU ○	0525 4.7	1110 0.5	1742 4.8	2322 0.6
20 W	0535 5.4	1126 0.1	1757 5.3	2347 0.2
6 W	0559 4.8	1143 0.5	1815 4.9	2355 0.5
21 TH	0618 5.3	1204 0.2	1837 5.2	
7 TH	0631 4.9	1214 0.4	1847 4.9	
22 F	0027 0.3	0658 5.2	1242 0.4	1915 5.0
8 F	0028 0.5	0702 4.9	1246 0.5	1919 4.8
23 SA	0106 0.5	0738 4.9	1318 0.7	1953 4.7
9 SA	0103 0.6	0734 4.8	1321 0.7	1951 4.7
24 SU	0146 0.8	0818 4.6	1356 1.1	2033 4.4
10 SU	0142 0.8	0807 4.6	1401 0.9	2029 4.5
25 M	0229 1.2	0900 4.2	1437 1.5	2117 4.1
11 M	0226 1.1	0850 4.4	1446 1.3	2121 4.2
26 TU	0322 1.6	0949 3.9	1529 1.9	2210 3.8
12 TU	0317 1.4	0950 4.1	1541 1.6	2229 4.1
27 W	0437 1.9	1049 3.6	1655 2.1	2319 3.6
13 W	0421 1.6	1104 3.9	1654 1.8	2344 4.0
28 TH	0555 2.0	1214 3.5	1821 2.1	
14 TH	0546 1.7	1226 3.9	1853 1.8	
29 F	0113 3.6	0701 1.9	1349 3.6	1928 2.0
15 F	0109 4.1	0728 1.5	1355 4.1	2006 1.5
30 SA	0222 3.8	0800 1.6	1446 3.9	2021 1.7
31 SU	0308 4.0	0848 1.3	1527 4.2	2104 1.3

APRIL

Day	Time / m	Time / m	Time / m	Time / m
1 M	0346 4.3	0928 1.0	1603 4.5	2143 1.0
16 TU	0346 5.0	0943 0.6	1612 5.0	2205 0.6
2 TU	0422 4.5	1006 0.8	1638 4.7	2220 0.7
17 W ●	0431 5.1	1024 0.5	1653 5.1	2246 0.4
3 W	0456 4.7	1041 0.6	1712 4.9	2256 0.5
18 TH	0514 5.2	1103 0.4	1733 5.2	2326 0.4
4 TH	0530 4.8	1115 0.4	1745 5.0	2330 0.4
19 F	0555 5.1	1140 0.5	1812 5.1	
5 F	0604 4.9	1147 0.4	1818 5.0	
20 SA	0006 0.5	0635 5.0	1217 0.7	1849 5.0
6 SA	0005 0.4	0638 5.0	1222 0.5	1853 5.0
21 SU	0045 0.7	0714 4.8	1252 0.9	1927 4.7
7 SU	0043 0.5	0715 4.9	1300 0.6	1929 4.9
22 M	0123 0.9	0753 4.6	1328 1.2	2006 4.5
8 M	0124 0.6	0754 4.7	1341 0.9	2011 4.7
23 TU	0204 1.2	0835 4.3	1408 1.5	2048 4.2
9 TU	0209 0.9	0841 4.5	1428 1.2	2105 4.4
24 W	0252 1.5	0921 4.0	1454 1.9	2136 4.0
10 W	0302 1.2	0942 4.2	1525 1.6	2214 4.2
25 TH	0357 1.8	1014 3.8	1605 2.1	2233 3.8
11 TH	0406 1.5	1055 4.0	1643 1.8	2331 4.1
26 F	0514 1.9	1116 3.6	1738 2.2	2340 3.7
12 F	0535 1.6	1216 4.0	1836 1.8	
27 SA	0619 1.9	1242 3.7	1845 2.1	
13 SA	0052 4.2	0707 1.4	1339 4.2	1945 1.5
28 SU	0122 3.7	0716 1.7	1358 3.9	1941 1.8
14 SU	0203 4.5	0810 1.1	1440 4.5	2038 1.1
29 M	0223 3.9	0808 1.5	1447 4.1	2029 1.5
15 M	0259 4.8	0900 0.8	1529 4.8	2123 0.8
30 TU	0307 4.1	0853 1.2	1526 4.4	2112 1.2

Chart Datum: 0·20 metres below Ordnance Datum (Dublin)

IRELAND – GALWAY

LAT 53°16′N   LONG   9°03′W

TIMES AND HEIGHTS OF HIGH AND LOW WATERS

YEAR **1996**

TIME ZONE (UT)
For Summer Time add ONE hour in non-shaded areas

MAY

Day	Time	m	Day	Time	m
1 W	0345 / 0933 / 1602 / 2151	4.4 / 0.9 / 4.7 / 0.9	**16** TH	0409 / 1002 / 1631 / 2226	4.9 / 0.8 / 5.0 / 0.7
2 TH	0421 / 1011 / 1637 / 2228	4.6 / 0.7 / 4.9 / 0.6	**17** F ●	0452 / 1040 / 1710 / 2307	4.9 / 0.8 / 5.0 / 0.7
3 F ○	0458 / 1046 / 1713 / 2305	4.8 / 0.5 / 5.1 / 0.4	**18** SA	0534 / 1117 / 1748 / 2346	4.9 / 0.8 / 4.9 / 0.7
4 SA	0537 / 1123 / 1751 / 2344	5.0 / 0.5 / 5.2 / 0.3	**19** SU	0614 / 1153 / 1826	4.8 / 1.0 / 4.9
5 SU	0618 / 1201 / 1832	5.0 / 0.5 / 5.2	**20** M	0025 / 0653 / 1229 / 1904	0.9 / 4.7 / 1.1 / 4.7
6 M	0025 / 0659 / 1243 / 1914	0.4 / 5.0 / 0.6 / 5.1	**21** TU	0103 / 0732 / 1305 / 1943	1.0 / 4.5 / 1.3 / 4.6
7 TU	0110 / 0744 / 1327 / 2000	0.5 / 4.8 / 0.8 / 4.9	**22** W	0142 / 0813 / 1344 / 2024	1.2 / 4.4 / 1.5 / 4.4
8 W	0157 / 0834 / 1416 / 2055	0.7 / 4.6 / 1.2 / 4.6	**23** TH	0225 / 0856 / 1427 / 2109	1.4 / 4.2 / 1.7 / 4.2
9 TH	0251 / 0933 / 1514 / 2202	1.0 / 4.3 / 1.5 / 4.4	**24** F	0315 / 0943 / 1517 / 2158	1.6 / 4.0 / 2.0 / 4.0
10 F	0354 / 1043 / 1631 / 2315	1.3 / 4.2 / 1.8 / 4.3	**25** SA	0417 / 1035 / 1630 / 2251	1.8 / 3.9 / 2.1 / 3.9
11 SA	0515 / 1157 / 1809	1.4 / 4.1 / 1.7	**26** SU	0526 / 1131 / 1753 / 2348	1.8 / 3.8 / 2.1 / 3.8
12 SU	0029 / 0639 / 1313 / 1919	4.3 / 1.4 / 4.3 / 1.5	**27** M	0628 / 1235 / 1856	1.8 / 3.9 / 1.9
13 M	0137 / 0744 / 1416 / 2015	4.5 / 1.2 / 4.5 / 1.3	**28** TU	0056 / 0724 / 1344 / 1950	3.9 / 1.6 / 4.1 / 1.7
14 TU	0235 / 0836 / 1506 / 2101	4.6 / 1.1 / 4.7 / 1.0	**29** W	0208 / 0815 / 1438 / 2038	4.0 / 1.4 / 4.3 / 1.3
15 W	0324 / 0921 / 1550 / 2144	4.8 / 0.9 / 4.9 / 0.8	**30** TH	0300 / 0900 / 1521 / 2121	4.3 / 1.1 / 4.6 / 1.0
			31 F	0345 / 0941 / 1602 / 2202	4.6 / 0.9 / 4.9 / 0.7

JUNE

Day	Time	m	Day	Time	m
1 SA ○	0429 / 1021 / 1645 / 2244	4.8 / 0.7 / 5.1 / 0.5	**16** SU ●	0514 / 1057 / 1728 / 2328	4.6 / 1.1 / 4.8 / 0.9
2 SU	0514 / 1102 / 1729 / 2327	5.0 / 0.5 / 5.3 / 0.3	**17** M	0555 / 1133 / 1806	4.6 / 1.1 / 4.8
3 M	0600 / 1145 / 1814	5.1 / 0.5 / 5.3	**18** TU	0006 / 0634 / 1209 / 1844	0.9 / 4.6 / 1.1 / 4.7
4 TU	0012 / 0646 / 1230 / 1900	0.2 / 5.1 / 0.5 / 5.2	**19** W	0043 / 0712 / 1245 / 1922	0.9 / 4.5 / 1.2 / 4.6
5 W	0058 / 0733 / 1316 / 1949	0.3 / 5.0 / 0.7 / 5.1	**20** TH	0120 / 0751 / 1322 / 2001	1.0 / 4.4 / 1.3 / 4.5
6 TH	0146 / 0823 / 1405 / 2043	0.5 / 4.8 / 1.0 / 4.8	**21** F	0158 / 0831 / 1400 / 2041	1.2 / 4.3 / 1.5 / 4.3
7 F	0238 / 0919 / 1500 / 2145	0.8 / 4.5 / 1.3 / 4.6	**22** SA	0237 / 0913 / 1442 / 2124	1.3 / 4.2 / 1.7 / 4.2
8 SA	0336 / 1022 / 1608 / 2253	1.1 / 4.3 / 1.6 / 4.4	**23** SU	0322 / 0957 / 1531 / 2212	1.5 / 4.1 / 1.8 / 4.0
9 SU	0445 / 1130 / 1733	1.3 / 4.2 / 1.7	**24** M	0413 / 1046 / 1632 / 2304	1.7 / 4.0 / 1.9 / 4.0
10 M	0001 / 0602 / 1240 / 1848	4.3 / 1.4 / 4.2 / 1.6	**25** TU	0513 / 1138 / 1748	1.7 / 4.0 / 1.9
11 TU	0108 / 0712 / 1347 / 1950	4.3 / 1.4 / 4.3 / 1.4	**26** W	0000 / 0625 / 1238 / 1903	3.9 / 1.7 / 4.1 / 1.8
12 W	0209 / 0809 / 1442 / 2040	4.4 / 1.4 / 4.5 / 1.3	**27** TH	0105 / 0732 / 1344 / 2003	4.0 / 1.6 / 4.2 / 1.5
13 TH	0302 / 0857 / 1529 / 2125	4.5 / 1.3 / 4.6 / 1.1	**28** F	0216 / 0828 / 1444 / 2054	4.2 / 1.3 / 4.5 / 1.1
14 F	0349 / 0940 / 1611 / 2207	4.6 / 1.2 / 4.7 / 1.0	**29** SA	0315 / 0916 / 1535 / 2141	4.4 / 1.0 / 4.8 / 0.7
15 SA	0433 / 1019 / 1650 / 2248	4.6 / 1.1 / 4.8 / 0.9	**30** SU	0406 / 1002 / 1623 / 2227	4.7 / 0.7 / 5.1 / 0.4

JULY

Day	Time	m	Day	Time	m
1 M ○	0456 / 1047 / 1711 / 2313	4.9 / 0.5 / 5.3 / 0.2	**16** TU	0537 / 1114 / 1749 / 2345	4.5 / 1.0 / 4.7 / 0.8
2 TU	0545 / 1132 / 1800 / 2359	5.1 / 0.4 / 5.4 / 0.1	**17** W	0615 / 1149 / 1826	4.6 / 1.0 / 4.7
3 W	0633 / 1217 / 1848	5.2 / 0.4 / 5.3	**18** TH	0020 / 0652 / 1224 / 1901	0.8 / 4.6 / 1.0 / 4.7
4 TH	0044 / 0719 / 1303 / 1935	0.1 / 5.1 / 0.5 / 5.2	**19** F	0055 / 0729 / 1259 / 1937	0.8 / 4.6 / 1.1 / 4.6
5 F	0131 / 0806 / 1349 / 2026	0.2 / 4.9 / 0.7 / 5.0	**20** SA	0129 / 0805 / 1334 / 2012	0.9 / 4.5 / 1.2 / 4.4
6 SA	0219 / 0857 / 1439 / 2122	0.5 / 4.7 / 1.0 / 4.7	**21** SU	0204 / 0841 / 1411 / 2049	1.1 / 4.4 / 1.3 / 4.3
7 SU	0311 / 0954 / 1538 / 2224	0.9 / 4.4 / 1.4 / 4.4	**22** M	0242 / 0920 / 1454 / 2133	1.3 / 4.2 / 1.5 / 4.1
8 M	0410 / 1057 / 1650 / 2329	1.2 / 4.2 / 1.6 / 4.2	**23** TU	0326 / 1005 / 1545 / 2225	1.5 / 4.1 / 1.7 / 4.0
9 TU	0520 / 1203 / 1811	1.5 / 4.1 / 1.7	**24** W	0418 / 1057 / 1646 / 2324	1.6 / 4.0 / 1.8 / 3.9
10 W	0035 / 0633 / 1314 / 1922	4.1 / 1.6 / 4.1 / 1.6	**25** TH	0521 / 1156 / 1805	1.7 / 4.0 / 1.8
11 TH	0142 / 0740 / 1419 / 2021	4.1 / 1.6 / 4.2 / 1.5	**26** F	0029 / 0646 / 1304 / 1933	3.9 / 1.7 / 4.2 / 1.6
12 F	0241 / 0834 / 1511 / 2108	4.1 / 1.5 / 4.4 / 1.3	**27** SA	0145 / 0802 / 1416 / 2034	4.1 / 1.5 / 4.4 / 1.2
13 SA	0332 / 0918 / 1555 / 2149	4.3 / 1.4 / 4.5 / 1.1	**28** SU	0254 / 0858 / 1516 / 2125	4.3 / 1.1 / 4.7 / 0.8
14 SU	0416 / 0959 / 1634 / 2229	4.4 / 1.3 / 4.6 / 1.0	**29** M	0350 / 0946 / 1607 / 2212	4.7 / 0.8 / 5.1 / 0.4
15 M ●	0457 / 1037 / 1712 / 2308	4.5 / 1.1 / 4.6 / 0.8	**30** TU	0441 / 1032 / 1656 / 2258	4.9 / 0.5 / 5.3 / 0.1
			31 W ○	0529 / 1117 / 1745 / 2343	5.1 / 0.3 / 5.4 / -0.1

AUGUST

Day	Time	m	Day	Time	m
1 TH	0616 / 1201 / 1832	5.2 / 0.2 / 5.4	**16** F	0629 / 1201 / 1838	4.7 / 0.8 / 4.8
2 F	0027 / 0701 / 1245 / 1917	-0.1 / 5.2 / 0.3 / 5.3	**17** SA	0026 / 0703 / 1234 / 1910	0.7 / 4.7 / 0.8 / 4.7
3 SA	0111 / 0745 / 1329 / 2004	0.1 / 5.0 / 0.5 / 5.1	**18** SU	0059 / 0736 / 1307 / 1941	0.8 / 4.6 / 0.9 / 4.6
4 SU	0155 / 0831 / 1414 / 2054	0.4 / 4.8 / 0.8 / 4.7	**19** M	0132 / 0808 / 1343 / 2012	0.9 / 4.5 / 1.1 / 4.4
5 M	0241 / 0921 / 1505 / 2150	0.8 / 4.4 / 1.2 / 4.3	**20** TU	0209 / 0842 / 1423 / 2052	1.1 / 4.4 / 1.3 / 4.3
6 TU	0334 / 1017 / 1608 / 2253	1.3 / 4.1 / 1.6 / 4.0	**21** W	0251 / 0925 / 1511 / 2149	1.4 / 4.2 / 1.5 / 4.1
7 W	0439 / 1122 / 1729 / 2256	1.6 / 3.9 / 1.8 / 3.9	**22** TH	0342 / 1020 / 1610 / 2256	1.6 / 4.1 / 1.8 / 3.9
8 TH	0001 / 0554 / 1239 / 1850	3.8 / 1.8 / 3.8 / 1.8	**23** F	0445 / 1124 / 1725	1.8 / 4.0 / 1.8
9 F	0115 / 0707 / 1356 / 2000	3.8 / 1.9 / 3.9 / 1.6	**24** SA	0006 / 0613 / 1236 / 1912	3.9 / 1.8 / 4.1 / 1.6
10 SA	0223 / 0808 / 1454 / 2050	3.9 / 1.7 / 4.1 / 1.4	**25** SU	0127 / 0746 / 1357 / 2020	4.0 / 1.6 / 4.4 / 1.2
11 SU	0315 / 0856 / 1539 / 2130	4.1 / 1.5 / 4.3 / 1.2	**26** M	0241 / 0843 / 1502 / 2111	4.4 / 1.2 / 4.7 / 0.8
12 M	0359 / 0937 / 1618 / 2207	4.3 / 1.3 / 4.5 / 1.0	**27** TU	0336 / 0931 / 1553 / 2156	4.7 / 0.8 / 5.1 / 0.4
13 TU	0438 / 1015 / 1654 / 2244	4.4 / 1.1 / 4.6 / 0.8	**28** W ○	0425 / 1016 / 1641 / 2240	5.0 / 0.5 / 5.4 / 0.1
14 W ●	0516 / 1052 / 1730 / 2319	4.6 / 0.9 / 4.7 / 0.7	**29** TH	0511 / 1059 / 1727 / 2323	5.2 / 0.2 / 5.5 / -0.1
15 TH	0553 / 1127 / 1805 / 2354	4.7 / 0.8 / 4.8 / 0.6	**30** F	0556 / 1142 / 1812	5.3 / 0.1 / 5.5
			31 SA	0005 / 0639 / 1224 / 1856	0.0 / 5.3 / 0.2 / 5.4

13

Chart Datum: 0·20 metres below Ordnance Datum (Dublin)

IRELAND – GALWAY

LAT 53°16′N   LONG 9°03′W

TIMES AND HEIGHTS OF HIGH AND LOW WATERS   YEAR **1996**

TIME ZONE (UT)
For Summer Time add ONE hour in non-shaded areas

SEPTEMBER

Day	Time	m	Time	m	Day	Time	m	Time	m
1 SU	0047 / 0721 / 1305 / 1939	0.1 / 5.1 / 0.4 / 5.1			**16** M	0028 / 0705 / 1240 / 1912	0.7 / 4.8 / 0.8 / 4.8		
2 M	0128 / 0802 / 1348 / 2024	0.5 / 4.9 / 0.8 / 4.7			**17** TU	0102 / 0737 / 1317 / 1944	0.9 / 4.7 / 0.9 / 4.6		
3 TU	0211 / 0846 / 1433 / 2114	0.9 / 4.5 / 1.2 / 4.3			**18** W	0140 / 0810 / 1358 / 2024	1.1 / 4.6 / 1.2 / 4.4		
4 W	0258 / 0934 / 1529 / 2213	1.4 / 4.2 / 1.6 / 4.0			**19** TH	0224 / 0853 / 1446 / 2123	1.4 / 4.4 / 1.4 / 4.2		
5 TH	0359 / 1034 / 1649 / 2325	1.8 / 3.9 / 1.9 / 3.7			**20** F	0316 / 0952 / 1544 / 2236	1.7 / 4.2 / 1.7 / 4.0		
6 F	0519 / 1156 / 1815	2.0 / 3.7 / 1.9			**21** SA	0421 / 1101 / 1700 / 2352	1.9 / 4.1 / 1.8 / 4.0		
7 SA	0046 / 0635 / 1329 / 1930	3.7 / 2.1 / 3.8 / 1.8			**22** SU	0605 / 1218 / 1857	2.0 / 4.2 / 1.7		
8 SU	0202 / 0738 / 1433 / 2026	3.8 / 1.9 / 4.0 / 1.6			**23** M	0116 / 0732 / 1343 / 2004	4.1 / 1.7 / 4.4 / 1.3		
9 M	0255 / 0830 / 1518 / 2105	4.0 / 1.7 / 4.2 / 1.3			**24** TU	0227 / 0827 / 1447 / 2054	4.5 / 1.3 / 4.8 / 0.9		
10 TU	0337 / 0912 / 1557 / 2141	4.3 / 1.4 / 4.5 / 1.0			**25** W	0320 / 0914 / 1537 / 2138	4.8 / 0.8 / 5.2 / 0.5		
11 W	0415 / 0950 / 1632 / 2216	4.5 / 1.1 / 4.6 / 0.8			**26** TH	0406 / 0957 / 1623 / 2220	5.1 / 0.6 / 5.4 / 0.2		
12 TH ●	0451 / 1027 / 1706 / 2251	4.7 / 0.9 / 4.8 / 0.6			**27** F ○	0450 / 1040 / 1707 / 2301	5.3 / 0.3 / 5.5 / 0.2		
13 F	0527 / 1102 / 1739 / 2325	4.8 / 0.8 / 4.9 / 0.6			**28** SA	0533 / 1121 / 1751 / 2341	5.4 / 0.3 / 5.5 / 0.2		
14 SA	0601 / 1135 / 1811 / 2357	4.9 / 0.7 / 4.9 / 0.6			**29** SU	0615 / 1202 / 1833	5.3 / 0.3 / 5.4		
15 SU	0634 / 1207 / 1842	4.9 / 0.7 / 4.8			**30** M	0021 / 0655 / 1242 / 1914	0.4 / 5.2 / 0.5 / 5.1		

OCTOBER

Day	Time	m	Time	m	Day	Time	m	Time	m
1 TU	0101 / 0734 / 1322 / 1956	0.7 / 4.9 / 0.9 / 4.8			**16** W	0037 / 0711 / 1257 / 1927	0.9 / 4.9 / 0.8 / 4.8		
2 W	0141 / 0814 / 1405 / 2042	1.1 / 4.6 / 1.2 / 4.4			**17** TH	0118 / 0749 / 1340 / 2012	1.1 / 4.8 / 1.0 / 4.6		
3 TH	0225 / 0858 / 1455 / 2135	1.5 / 4.3 / 1.7 / 4.0			**18** F	0203 / 0835 / 1428 / 2111	1.4 / 4.6 / 1.3 / 4.3		
4 F	0321 / 0949 / 1608 / 2243	1.9 / 4.0 / 2.0 / 3.8			**19** SA	0257 / 0935 / 1527 / 2223	1.7 / 4.4 / 1.6 / 4.1		
5 SA	0444 / 1055 / 1735	2.2 / 3.8 / 2.1			**20** SU	0406 / 1046 / 1643 / 2340	2.0 / 4.3 / 1.8 / 4.1		
6 SU	0007 / 0601 / 1245 / 1847	3.7 / 2.2 / 3.7 / 2.0			**21** M	0555 / 1203 / 1834	2.0 / 4.3 / 1.7		
7 M	0129 / 0704 / 1400 / 1946	3.8 / 2.1 / 3.9 / 1.7			**22** TU	0100 / 0711 / 1323 / 1943	4.3 / 1.7 / 4.5 / 1.4		
8 TU	0226 / 0758 / 1449 / 2031	4.1 / 1.8 / 4.2 / 1.5			**23** W	0208 / 0807 / 1427 / 2034	4.6 / 1.4 / 4.9 / 1.0		
9 W	0308 / 0843 / 1528 / 2110	4.3 / 1.5 / 4.4 / 1.2			**24** TH	0300 / 0854 / 1518 / 2118	4.9 / 0.7 / 5.2 / 0.7		
10 TH	0346 / 0922 / 1604 / 2146	4.6 / 1.2 / 4.6 / 0.9			**25** F	0345 / 0938 / 1603 / 2159	5.2 / 0.8 / 5.4 / 0.6		
11 F	0421 / 1000 / 1637 / 2222	4.8 / 1.0 / 4.8 / 0.8			**26** SA ○	0428 / 1020 / 1647 / 2239	5.3 / 0.6 / 5.4 / 0.5		
12 SA ●	0455 / 1035 / 1709 / 2255	4.9 / 0.8 / 4.9 / 0.7			**27** SU	0509 / 1101 / 1709 / 2318	5.4 / 0.5 / 4.9 / 0.6		
13 SU	0529 / 1109 / 1741 / 2327	5.0 / 0.7 / 5.0 / 0.7			**28** M	0550 / 1141 / 1811 / 2357	5.3 / 0.6 / 5.3 / 0.8		
14 M	0602 / 1142 / 1815	5.0 / 0.7 / 5.0			**29** TU	0630 / 1221 / 1852	5.2 / 0.8 / 5.1		
15 TU	0000 / 0636 / 1218 / 1849	0.7 / 5.0 / 0.7 / 4.9			**30** W	0035 / 0709 / 1301 / 1933	1.0 / 5.0 / 1.0 / 4.8		
					31 TH	0114 / 0749 / 1341 / 2016	1.3 / 4.7 / 1.3 / 4.5		

NOVEMBER

Day	Time	m	Time	m	Day	Time	m	Time	m
1 F	0157 / 0830 / 1427 / 2105	1.7 / 4.5 / 1.6 / 4.2			**16** SA	0150 / 0824 / 1417 / 2101	1.3 / 4.8 / 1.1 / 4.5		
2 SA	0246 / 0917 / 1525 / 2202	2.0 / 4.2 / 1.9 / 3.9			**17** SU	0245 / 0922 / 1513 / 2209	1.6 / 4.6 / 1.4 / 4.3		
3 SU	0356 / 1011 / 1646 / 2312	2.3 / 4.0 / 2.1 / 3.8			**18** M	0352 / 1031 / 1624 / 2322	1.9 / 4.5 / 1.6 / 4.3		
4 M	0519 / 1115 / 1759	2.3 / 3.8 / 2.1			**19** TU	0526 / 1144 / 1759	1.9 / 4.4 / 1.6		
5 TU	0030 / 0624 / 1255 / 1859	3.9 / 2.2 / 3.9 / 1.9			**20** W	0036 / 0644 / 1258 / 1916	4.4 / 1.8 / 4.5 / 1.5		
6 W	0139 / 0719 / 1404 / 1951	4.0 / 2.0 / 4.0 / 1.7			**21** TH	0144 / 0744 / 1403 / 2011	4.6 / 1.5 / 4.7 / 1.2		
7 TH	0229 / 0809 / 1450 / 2035	4.3 / 1.8 / 4.3 / 1.4			**22** F	0238 / 0834 / 1457 / 2057	4.9 / 1.3 / 5.0 / 1.1		
8 F	0310 / 0852 / 1528 / 2115	4.5 / 1.5 / 4.5 / 1.2			**23** SA	0325 / 0920 / 1544 / 2139	5.1 / 1.0 / 5.1 / 0.9		
9 SA	0346 / 0931 / 1603 / 2152	4.7 / 1.2 / 4.7 / 1.0			**24** SU	0408 / 1002 / 1627 / 2219	5.2 / 0.9 / 5.2 / 0.9		
10 SU	0420 / 1008 / 1637 / 2227	4.9 / 0.9 / 4.9 / 0.8			**25** M ○	0449 / 1044 / 1710 / 2258	5.2 / 0.8 / 5.1 / 0.9		
11 M ●	0456 / 1044 / 1713 / 2302	5.1 / 0.8 / 5.0 / 1.0			**26** TU	0529 / 1124 / 1751 / 2336	5.2 / 0.8 / 5.1 / 1.0		
12 TU	0533 / 1121 / 1752 / 2339	5.2 / 0.6 / 5.1 / 0.8			**27** W	0609 / 1204 / 1832	5.1 / 0.9 / 4.9		
13 W	0612 / 1200 / 1833	5.2 / 0.6 / 5.1			**28** TH	0013 / 0648 / 1243 / 1913	1.2 / 5.0 / 1.1 / 4.8		
14 TH	0019 / 0652 / 1242 / 1916	0.9 / 5.2 / 0.7 / 5.0			**29** F	0052 / 0727 / 1321 / 1954	1.4 / 4.8 / 1.2 / 4.6		
15 F	0103 / 0735 / 1327 / 2004	1.0 / 5.0 / 0.8 / 4.8			**30** SA	0133 / 0808 / 1402 / 2039	1.6 / 4.6 / 1.5 / 4.3		

DECEMBER

Day	Time	m	Time	m	Day	Time	m	Time	m
1 SU	0216 / 0850 / 1448 / 2128	1.8 / 4.4 / 1.7 / 4.1			**16** M	0232 / 0908 / 1458 / 2149	1.3 / 4.8 / 1.1 / 4.5		
2 M	0308 / 0936 / 1543 / 2223	2.1 / 4.2 / 1.9 / 4.0			**17** TU	0332 / 1011 / 1559 / 2257	1.6 / 4.6 / 1.4 / 4.4		
3 TU	0415 / 1026 / 1654 / 2321	2.2 / 4.0 / 2.0 / 3.9			**18** W	0448 / 1119 / 1715	1.8 / 4.5 / 1.6		
4 W	0530 / 1120 / 1804	2.3 / 3.9 / 2.0			**19** TH	0006 / 0609 / 1228 / 1840	4.3 / 1.8 / 4.4 / 1.6		
5 TH	0025 / 0633 / 1222 / 1904	4.0 / 2.2 / 3.9 / 1.9			**20** F	0115 / 0717 / 1336 / 1947	4.4 / 1.7 / 4.5 / 1.5		
6 F	0130 / 0729 / 1343 / 1957	4.1 / 2.0 / 4.1 / 1.7			**21** SA	0216 / 0814 / 1436 / 2038	4.6 / 1.5 / 4.6 / 1.4		
7 SA	0223 / 0819 / 1441 / 2043	4.4 / 1.7 / 4.3 / 1.4			**22** SU	0307 / 0903 / 1527 / 2122	4.7 / 1.3 / 4.7 / 1.3		
8 SU	0307 / 0903 / 1526 / 2124	4.6 / 1.4 / 4.5 / 1.2			**23** M	0352 / 0947 / 1612 / 2203	4.9 / 1.1 / 4.8 / 1.2		
9 M	0347 / 0944 / 1607 / 2203	4.9 / 1.1 / 4.8 / 0.9			**24** TU O	0433 / 1029 / 1654 / 2241	4.9 / 1.0 / 4.8 / 1.1		
10 TU ●	0427 / 1024 / 1650 / 2242	5.1 / 0.8 / 5.0 / 0.8			**25** W	0514 / 1110 / 1735 / 2319	5.0 / 1.0 / 4.8 / 1.0		
11 W	0510 / 1105 / 1734 / 2324	5.3 / 0.6 / 5.1 / 0.7			**26** TH	0553 / 1149 / 1815 / 2356	5.0 / 0.9 / 4.8 / 1.1		
12 TH	0554 / 1148 / 1820	5.4 / 0.4 / 5.2			**27** F	0632 / 1225 / 1855	4.9 / 1.0 / 4.7		
13 F	0007 / 0639 / 1232 / 1905	0.7 / 5.4 / 0.4 / 5.1			**28** SA	0033 / 0709 / 1301 / 1934	1.2 / 4.8 / 1.0 / 4.6		
14 SA	0053 / 0727 / 1317 / 1953	0.8 / 5.3 / 0.5 / 5.0			**29** SU	0111 / 0747 / 1338 / 2014	1.3 / 4.7 / 1.2 / 4.5		
15 SU	0140 / 0813 / 1405 / 2047	1.0 / 5.1 / 0.8 / 4.7			**30** M	0150 / 0825 / 1416 / 2056	1.5 / 4.5 / 1.3 / 4.3		
					31 TU	0230 / 0904 / 1456 / 2141	1.7 / 4.4 / 1.5 / 4.2		

Chart Datum: 0·20 metres below Ordnance Datum (Dublin)

GALWAY BAY   10-13-19

Galway 53°12'N 09°08'W

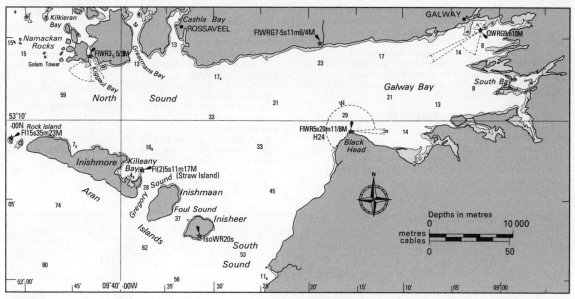

CHARTS
AC 1903, 1984, 3339, 2173; Imray C55; Irish OS 14
TIDES
−0555 Dover; ML 2·9; Duration 0620; Zone 0 (UT)

Standard Port GALWAY (←—)

Times				Height (metres)			
High Water		Low Water		MHWS	MHWN	MLWN	MLWS
0600	1100	0000	0700	5·1	3·9	2·0	0·6
1800	2300	1200	1900				
Differences KILKIERAN COVE							
+0005	+0005	+0016	+0016	−0·3	−0·2	−0·1	0·0
ROUNDSTONE BAY							
+0003	+0003	+0008	+0008	−0·7	−0·5	−0·3	−0·1
KILLEANY BAY (Aran Islands)							
−0008	−0008	+0003	+0003	−0·4	−0·3	−0·2	−0·1
LISCANNOR							
−0003	−0007	+0006	+0002	−0·4	−0·3		No data

NOTE: Galway is a Standard Port and tidal predictions for each day of the year are given above.

SHELTER
Galway B is sheltered from large swells by Aran Is, but seas get up in the 20M from Aran Is to Galway. Beware salmon drift nets in the apps to many bays. The better ⚓s clock-wise from Slyne Head and around Galway B are:
Bunowen B: Easy ent NE of Split Rk. ⚓ below conspic Doon Hill in 3-4m. Good shelter in W to NE winds; unsafe in S'ly.
Roundstone B: (Off chartlet). Safe shelter/access, except in SE'ly. ⚓ in 2m off N quay; other ⚓s E'ward in Cashel B.
Kilkieran B: A long (14M), sheltered bay with many ⚓s to suit wind conditions. Easy ent alongside Golam Tr (conspic).
Kiggaul B: Easy ent, H24; ⚓ close W/NW of lt Fl WR 3s 5/3M. Depth 3 to 4m; exposed to S/SE winds.
Greatman B: Beware English Rk (dries 1·2m), Keeraun Shoal (breaks in heavy weather), Arkeena Rk, Trabaan Rk, Rin Rks and Chapel Rks. ⚓ off Natawny Quay or go alongside at Maumeen Quay.
Cashla B: Easiest hbr on this coast; ent in all weather. ⚓ off Sruthan pier. Rossaveel, opposite, is busy fish and ferry hbr.
Note: There is no safe hbr from Cashla to Galway (20M).
Bays between Galway and Black Hd have rks and shallows, but give excellent shelter. Kinvarra B, Aughinish B, South B and Ballyvaghan B are the main ones. Enter Kinvarra B with caution on the flood; beware rks. Berth in small drying hbr. Ballvaghan B, entered either side of Illaunloo Rk, leads to two piers (both dry) or ⚓ close NE in pool (3m). Best access HW±2
Aran Islands: The only reasonable shelter is on Inishmore at Killeany Bay, but very crowded with FVs and exposed to E/NE winds. ⚓ S of Kilronan pier, or off Trawmore Strand; or in good weather at Portmurvy.

NAVIGATION
Enter the Bay by one of four Sounds:
(1)   N Sound between Inishmore and Golam Tr (conspic), 4½M wide, is easiest but beware Brocklinmore Bank in heavy weather.
(2)   Gregory Sound between Inishmore and Inishmaan, is free of dangers, but give Straw Is a berth of 2 to 3ca.
(3)   Foul Sound between Inishmaan and Inisheer; only danger is Pipe Rk (dries) at end of reef extending 3ca NW of Inisheer.
(4)   S Sound between Inisheer and mainland. Only danger Finnis Rk (dries 0·4m) 4½ca SE of E point of Inisheer (marked by ECM buoy Q (3) 10s). From S, beware Kilstiffin Rks off Liscanor B.

LIGHTS AND MARKS
Roundstone B: Croaghnakeela Is Fl 3·7s 7m 5M. Inishnee lt Fl (2) WRG 10s 9m 5/3M has W sector 017°-030°.
Kiggaul B: Fl WR 3s 5m 5/3M, W329°-359°, R359°-059°.
Cashla B: Killeen Pt Fl (3) WR 10s 6/3M; Lion Pt Dir (010°) Iso WRG 4s 8/6M, W008·5°-011·5°. Rossaveel ldg lts 116°, Oc 3s; pier hd 2FW (hor).
Black Hd lt Fl WR 5s 20m 11/8M H24, vis W045°-268°, R268°-276° covers Illanloo Rk.
Aran Islands:
Inishmore: Eeragh Island (Rk Is) Fl 15s 35m 23M, W tr, B bands. Killeany B: Straw Is, Fl (2) 5s 11m 17M. Kilronan pier Fl WG 1·5s. Ldg lts 192° both Oc 5s for Killeany hbr.
Inisheer: Iso WR 20s 34m 20/16M, Racon, vis W225°-245° (partially obscd 225°-231° beyond 7M), R245°-269° covers Finnis Rk, W269°-115°; obscd 115°-225°.

FACILITIES
BUNOWEN B: No facilities.
ROUNDSTONE B: V, FW, Bar, ✉, Bus to Galway.
KILKIERAN B: Bar, ☎, P, V, Bus to Galway.
KIGGAUL B: Bar (no ☎), shop at Lettermullen (1M).
GREATMAN B: Maumeen V, P (1M), Bar.
CASHLA B: **Carraroe** (1M SW) V, Hotel, ☎; **Rossaveel** Hr Mr ☎ 091-72109, FW, D, ME; **Costelloe** (1½M E), Hotel, ✉, Gge.
KILRONAN: (Killeany B, Inishmore) V, D, FW, ✉, Ferry to Galway, ✈ to Galway from airstrip on beach.

13

GALWAY HARBOUR 53°16'·07N 09°02'·74W

SHELTER
Very good protection in Galway hbr, being sheltered from SW by Mutton Is. Dock gates open HW−2 to HW, when min depth is 6m. Enter Galway dock and secure in SW corner of basin. It is dangerous to lie in the 'Layby' (a dredged cut NE of New pier) when wind is SE or S; if strong from these points, seas sweep round the pierhead.
Note: Marina in Canal basin is under discussion.
New Harbour (2·5M ESE, and home of Galway Bay SC) is nearest safe ⌕ to Galway.

NAVIGATION
Galway WPT 53°14'·80N 09°03'·40W, 241°/061° from/to Leverets lt, 1·1M.

LIGHTS AND MARKS
Leverets Q WRG 9m 10M; B tr, W bands; G015°-058°, W058°-065°, R065°-103°, G103°-143°, W143°-146°, R146°-015°.
Rinmore Iso WRG 4s 7m 5M; W□ tr ; G359°-008°, W008°-018°, R018°-027°.

Appr chan ldg lts 325°: front Fl R 1·5s, rear Oc R 10s; both R ◇ with Y diagonal stripes on masts, vis 315°-345°.
Note: Below the front ldg lt an experimental Dir lt (FW 325°) has the following characteristics and sectors: FG 322¼°-323¾°, Al GW 3s 323¾°-324¾°, FW 324¾°-325¼°, Al RW 3s 325¼°-326¼°, FR 326¼°-331¼°, Fl R 3s 331¼°-332¼°.

RADIO TELEPHONE
Call *Hr Mr Galway* VHF Ch 12 16 (HW−2½ to HW+1).

TELEPHONE (091)
Hr Mr 61874; MRCC (01) 6620922/3; Coast/Cliff Rescue Service (099) 61107/9/31; Police 63161; Dr 62453.

FACILITIES
Dock AB £IR5 (see Hr Mr), FW, EI, ME, C (35 ton), CH, V, R, Bar; **Galway YC** Slip, M, L, FW, C, CH, Bar; **Galway Bay SC** ☎ 94527, M, CH, Bar; **Services:** CH, ACA.
Town EC Mon; Slip, P, D, L, FW, ME, EI, C, V, R, Bar, ✉, Ⓑ, ⇌, ✈ Inverin (10M to the W of Galway City).

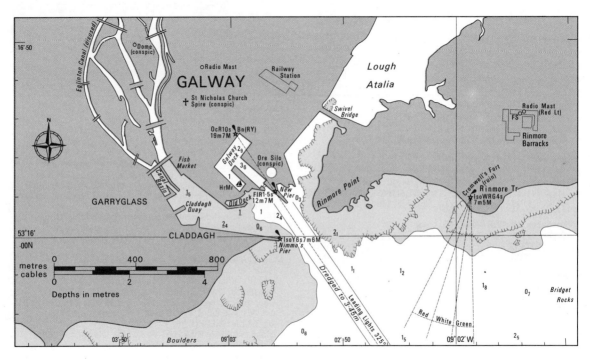

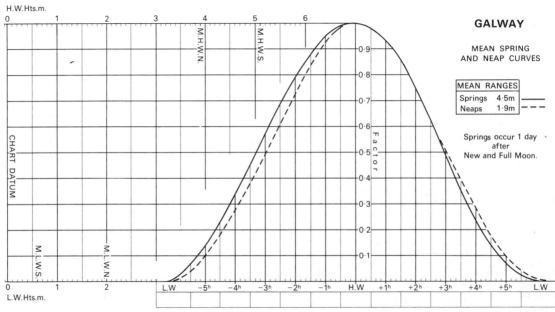

GALWAY

MEAN SPRING AND NEAP CURVES

MEAN RANGES	
Springs	4·5m
Neaps	1·9m

Springs occur 1 day after New and Full Moon.

Volvo Penta service

Sales and service centres in area 14
Channel Islands GUERNSEY *Chicks Marine Ltd,* Collings Road, St. Peter Port
GY1 1FL Tel (01481) 723716/724536 **JERSEY** *D. K. Collins Marine Ltd,* South
Pier, St. Helier, JE2 3NB Tel (01534) 32415

**VOLVO
PENTA**

Area 14

Channel Islands
Alderney to Jersey

14

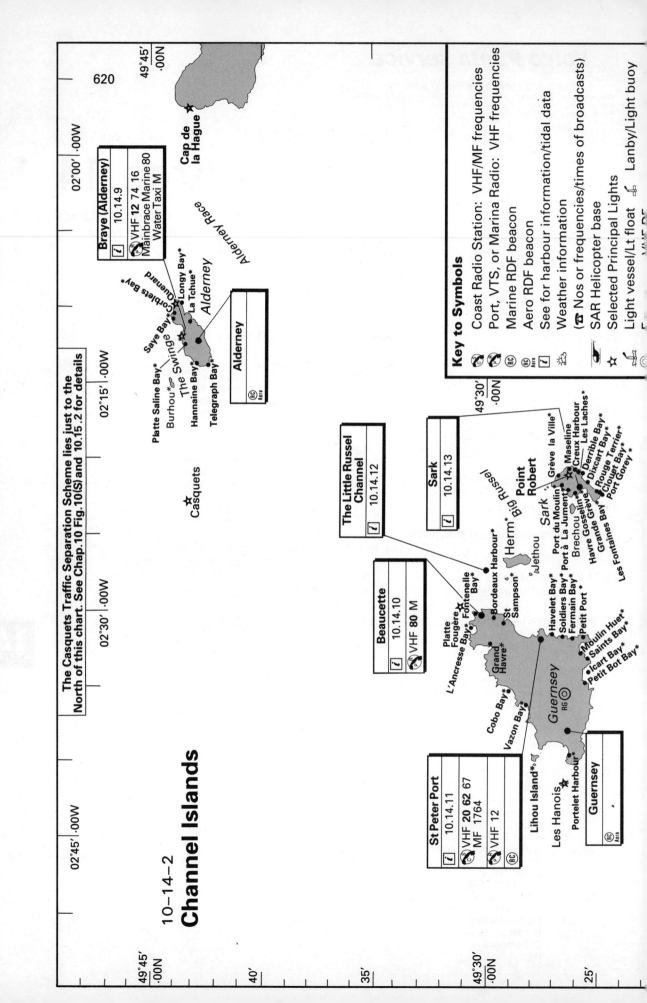

10-14-2
Channel Islands

620

The Casquets Traffic Separation Scheme lies just to the
North of this chart. See Chap.10 Fig.10(S) and 10.15.2 for details

Braye (Alderney)

i	10.14.9
	VHF **12** 74 16
	Mainbrace Marine 80
	Water Taxi M

Cap de
la Hague

Alderney Race

Save Bay*
The Swinge
Burhou*
Platte Saline Bay*
Hannaine Bay*
Telegraph Bay*

Corblets Bay*
Longy Bay*
La Tchue*
Alderney
Quenard

Alderney

Casquets

The Little Russel Channel

i	10.14.12

Sark

i	10.14.13

Maseline
Creux Harbour
Les Laches*
Derrible Bay*
Dixcart Bay*
Rouge Terrier*
Clouet Bay*
Port Gorey*

Grève la Ville*
Point
Robert
Port du Moulin*
Port à La Jument*
Brechou
Havre Gosselin*
Grande Grève*
Les Fontaines Bay*
Sark

Big Russel
Herm*
Jethou

Beaucette

i	10.14.10
	VHF 80 M

Bordeaux Harbour*
St
Sampson*

Platte
Fougère*
L'Ancresse Bay*
Grand
Havre*
Cobo Bay*
Vazon Bay*

Fontenelle
Bay*

Havelet Bay*
Soldiers Bay*
Fermain Bay*
Petit Port

Moulin Huet*
Saints Bay*
Icart Bay*
Petit Bot Bay*

Guernsey
RG

Lihou Island*

Les Hanois
Portelet Harbour*

St Peter Port

i	10.14.11
	VHF 20 62 67
	MF 1764
	VHF 12
	RC Aero

Guernsey

RC
Aero

Key to Symbols

Coast Radio Station: VHF/MF frequencies

Port, VTS, or Marina Radio: VHF frequencies

RC — Marine RDF beacon

RC Aero — Aero RDF beacon

i — See for harbour information/tidal data

Weather information
(☎ Nos or frequencies/times of broadcasts)

SAR Helicopter base

☆ Selected Principal Lights

Light vessel/Lt float   Lanby/Light buoy

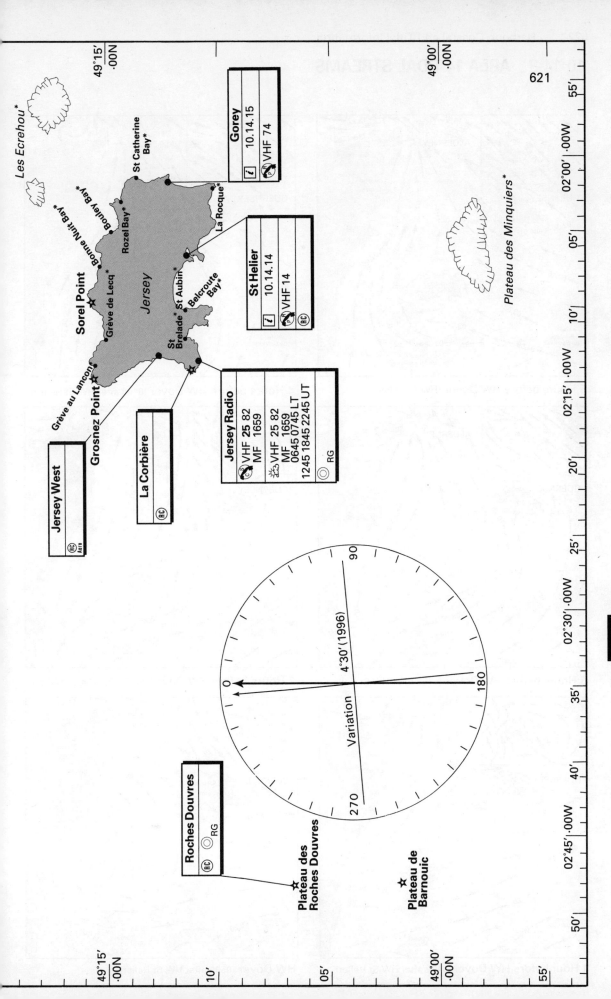

621

14

Les Ecrehou*

49°15'
·00N

Sorel Point

Grosnez Point

Jersey West

La Corbière

⒭ RC

Jersey Radio

📠 VHF 25 82
MF 1659

🌦 VHF 25 82
MF 1659
0645 0745 LT
1245 1845 2245 UT

◎ RG

Grève au Lanconf

Grève de Lecq*

Bonne Nuit Bay*

Bouley Bay*

Rozel Bay*

St Catherine
Bay*

Jersey

St Brelade*

St Aubin*

Belcroute
Bay*

La Rocque*

St Helier

10.14.14

ⓘ | 📠 | ⒭ RC

VHF 14

Gorey

10.14.15

ⓘ | 📠

VHF 74

Plateau des Minquiers*

Variation

4°30'(1996)

0

90

180

270

Roches Douvres

⒭ RC | ◎ RG

Plateau des
Roches Douvres

Plateau de
Barnouic

49°00'
·00N

49°15'
·00N

10'

05'

49°00'N
·00N

55'

55'   02°00'·00W   05'   10'   02°15'·00W   20'   25'   02°30'·00W   35'   40'   02°45'·00W   50'

10-14-3 **AREA 14 TIDAL STREAMS**

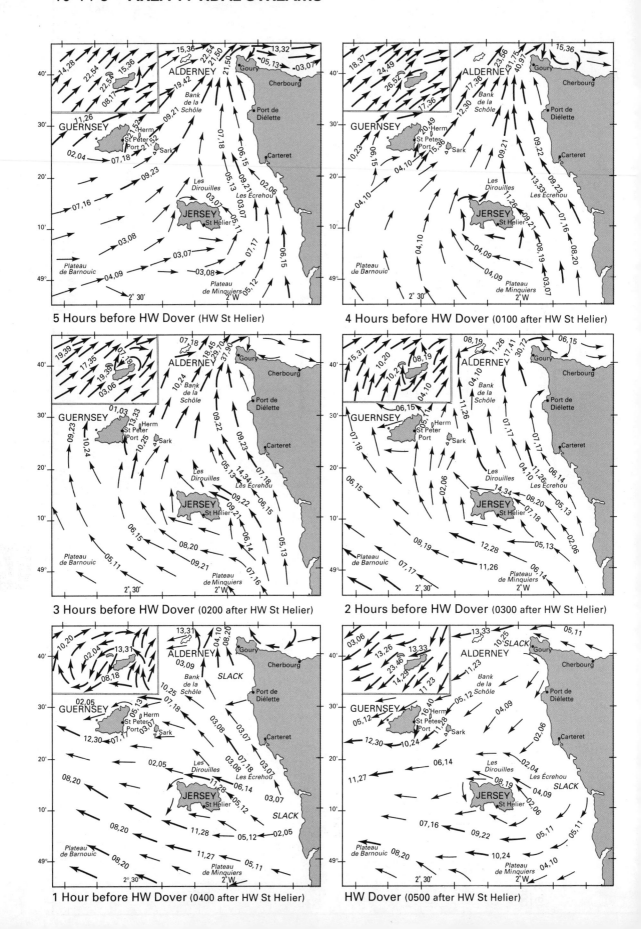

5 Hours before HW Dover (HW St Helier)

4 Hours before HW Dover (0100 after HW St Helier)

3 Hours before HW Dover (0200 after HW St Helier)

2 Hours before HW Dover (0300 after HW St Helier)

1 Hour before HW Dover (0400 after HW St Helier)

HW Dover (0500 after HW St Helier)

Westward 10.16.3   Southward 10.15.3   Northward 10.2.3   Eastward 10.19.3

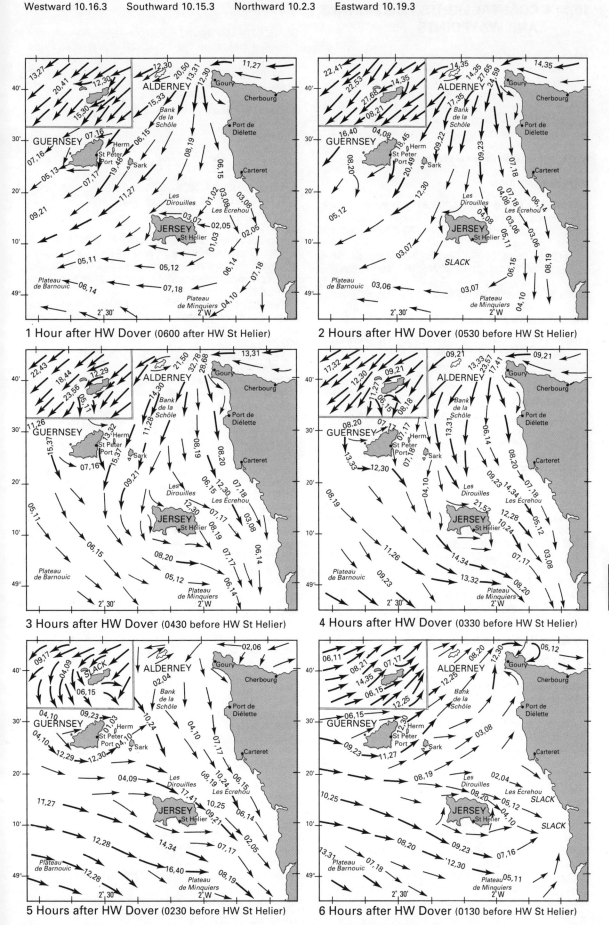

1 Hour after HW Dover (0600 after HW St Helier)

2 Hours after HW Dover (0530 before HW St Helier)

3 Hours after HW Dover (0430 before HW St Helier)

4 Hours after HW Dover (0330 before HW St Helier)

5 Hours after HW Dover (0230 before HW St Helier)

6 Hours after HW Dover (0130 before HW St Helier)

14

10.14.4 COASTAL LIGHTS, FOG SIGNALS AND WAYPOINTS

Abbreviations used below are given in 1.4.1. Principal lights are in **bold** print, places in CAPITALS, and light-vessels , light floats and Lanbys in *CAPITAL ITALICS*. Unless otherwise stated lights are white. m – elevation in metres; M – nominal range in miles. Fog signals are in *italics*. Useful waypoints are underlined – use those on land with care. All geographical positions should be assumed to be approximate. See 4.4.1.

NOTE: For English Channel Waypoints see 10.1.7

MID CHANNEL AIDS

CHANNEL Lt F 49°54'·42N 02°53'·67W Fl 15s 12m **25M**; R hull with Lt Tr amidships; Racon (O); *Horn (1) 20s.*
E CHANNEL Lt By 49°58'·67N 02°28'·87W Fl Y 5s; Racon (T); *Whis.*
EC 1 Lt By 50°05'·90N 01°48'·35W Fl Y 2·5s; Racon (T); *Whis.*
EC 2 Lt By 50°12'·10N 01°12'·40W Fl (4) Y 15s; Racon (T) ; *Whis.*
EC 3 Lt By 50°18'·30N 00°36'·10W Fl Y 5s; Racon (T); *Whis.*

THE CASQUETS AND ALDERNEY

Casquets 49°43'·38N 02°22'·55W Fl (5) 30s 37m **24M**; W Tr, the highest and NW of three; Racon (T); *Horn (2) 60s*; H24.

ALDERNEY

Alderney (Quenard Pt.) 49°43'·81N 02°09'·77W Fl (4) 15s 37m **28M**; W ● Tr, B band; vis 085°-027°; *Siren (4) 60s*.
Château à L'Etoc Pt 49°44'·00N 02°10'·55W Iso WR 4s 20m W10M, R7M; W col; vis R071·1°-111·1°, W111·1°-151·1°; in line 111·1° with main Lt.
Ldg Bns 142°. Front 49°43'·96N 02°10'·89W; W Bn, O topmark. Rear, 720m from front, BW Bn, △ topmark.

BRAYE

Ldg Lts 215°. **Front**, elbow of old pier, 49°43'·46N 02°11'·83W Q 8m **17M**; vis 210°-220°. **Rear** 335m from front Q 17m **18M**; vis 210°-220°. Both metal posts on W cols.
Bkwtr Hd 49°43'·87N 02°11'·59W L Fl 10s 13m 5M.
No. 1 Lt By 49°43'·78N 02°11'·63W QG; SHM.
Lt By 49°43'·63N 02°11'·90W Q (2) G 5S; SHM.
No. 2 Lt By 49°43'·66N 02°11'·67W QR; PHM.
Lt By 49°43'·60N 02°11'·85W Q (2) R 5S; PHM.
Braye Jetty Hd 49°43'·59N 02°11'·92W 2 FR (vert) 14m 5M.

APPROACHES TO GUERNSEY

LITTLE RUSSEL CHANNEL

Platte Fougère 49°30'·88N 02°29'·05W Fl WR 10s 15m **16M**; W 8-sided Tr, B band; vis W155°-085°, R085°-155°; Racon (P); *Horn 45s.*
Tautenay Lt Bn 49°30'·17N 02°26'·74W Q (3) WR 6s 7m W7M, R6M; B and W Bn; vis W050°-215°, R215°-050°.
Roustel Lt Bn Tr 49°29'·28N 02°28'·71W Q 10m 7M; Lantern on B & W chequered Tr.
Platte Lt Bn 49°29'·15N 02°29'·50W Fl WR 3s 6m W7M, R5M; G Tr; vis R024°-219°, W219°-024°.
Brehon Lt Bn 49°28'·34N 02°29'·20W Iso 4s 19m 9M; Bn on ● Tr.

BIG RUSSEL

Noire Pute 49°28'·27N 02°24'·93W Fl (2) WR 15s 8m 6M; vis W220°-040°, R040°-220°. Dest (T) 1987.
Fourquies Lt By 49°27'·40N 02°26'·40W Q; NCM.
Lower Heads Lt By 49°25'·91N 02°28'·48W Q (6) + L Fl 15s; SCM; *Bell* .

GUERNSEY

BEAUCETTE MARINA/BORDEAUX HARBOUR
Petite Canupe Lt Bn 49°30'·25N 02°29'·05W Q (6) + L Fl 15s; SCM.
Beaucette Ldg Lts 276°. Front 49°30'·25N 02°30'·13W FR; W board with R stripe. Rear, 185m from front, FR; R board with W stripe.
Bordeaux Hbr Bkwtr Hd 49°29'·38N 02°30'·30W; post.

ST SAMPSON
Ldg Lts 286°. Front Crocq Pier Hd 49°28'·97N 02°30'·66W FR 11m 5M; vis 250°-340°; Tfc sigs. Rear, 390m from front, FG 13m; clock Tr.
N Pier Hd 49°28'·98N 02°30'·62W FG 3m 5M; vis 230°-340°.
2 FR (vert) on chimneys (conspic) 300m NNW.

ST PETER PORT
Ldg Lts 220°. **Front**, Castle Bkwtr Hd 49°27'·36N 02°31'·34W Al WR 10s 14m **16M**; dark ● Tr, W on NE side; vis 187°-007°; RC (synch with ⠔); *Horn 15s.* Rear Belvedere Oc 10s 61m 14M; W ■ with Y stripe on W Tr; vis 179°-269°; both intens 217°-223°.
Reffée Lt By 49°27'·80N 02°31'·18W VQ (6) + L Fl 10s; SCM.
Queen Elizabeth II Marina 49°27'·79N 02°31'·78W. Dir Lt 270°. Dir Oc WRG 3s 5m 6M; vis G258°-268°, W268°-272°, R272°-282°.
Queen Elizabeth II Marina app Lt By 49°27'·78N 02°31'·66W QR; PHM.
White Rock Pier Hd 49°27'·43N 02°31'·60W Oc G 5s 11m 14M; ● stone Tr; intens 174°-354°; tfc sigs.
Victoria Marina Ldg Lts 265°. Front, S Pier Hd, 49°27'·38N 02°31'·95W Oc R 5s 10m 14M; W framework Tr. Rear, 160m from front, Iso R 2s 22m 3M; vis 260°-270°.
Albert Dock Fish Quay Hd 49°27'·30N 02°31'·39W FR.

HAVELET BAY
Oyster Rk Bn 49°27'·15N 02°31'·38W; Y Bn 'O'.
Oyster Rk Lt By 49°27'·10N 02°31'·39W QG; SHM.
Moulinet Lt By 49°27'·03N 02°31'·46W QR; PHM.
Moulinet Bn 49°27'·01N 02°31'·49W; Y Bn 'M'.

SOLDIERS BAY
Anfré Bn 49°26'·52N 02°31'·40W; Y Bn "A".

St Martin's Pt 49°25'·37N 02°31'·61W Fl (3) WR 10s 15m 14M; flat-roofed, W bldg; vis R185°-191°, W191°-011°, R011°-081°. Horn *(3) 30s.*

Les Hanois 49°26'·16N 02°42'·02W Q (2) 5s 33m **23M**; Gy ●Tr, B lantern, helicopter platform; vis 294°-237°; *Horn (2) 60s.* 4 FR on masts 1·27M ESE.

PORTELET HARBOUR
Portelet Hbr Bkwtr Bn 49°26'·22N 02°39'·74W.

COBO BAY/GRAND HAVRE
Grosse Rk Bn 49°29'·07N 02°36'·11W 11m; B Bn.
Rousse Pt Bkwtr Bn 49°29'·98N 02°32'·97W; B Bn.

HERM

Alligande Lt Bn 49°27'·91N 02°28'·69W Fl (3) G 5s; Or A on B mast; Ra refl.
Épec Lt Bn 49°28'·04N 02°27'·81W Fl G 3s; Black E on G mast.
Vermerette Lt Bn 49°28'·18N 02°27'·67W Fl (2) Y 5s; Or V on Bn.
Percée Pass, Gate Rk 49°27'·94N 02°27'·44W Q (9) 15s; WCM.

SARK

Courbée du Nez 49°27'·15N 02°22'·08W Fl (4) WR 15s 14m 8M; vis W057°-230°, R230°-057°.

GRÈVE LA VILLE/MASELINE

Pt Robert 49°26'·20N 02°20'·70W Fl 15s 65m **20M**; W 8-sided Tr; vis 138°-353°; *Horn (2) 30s.*

Blanchard Lt By 49°25'·43N 02°17'·33W Q (3) 10s; ECM; *Bell.*

JERSEY

Desormes Lt By 49°19'·00N 02°17'·90W Q (9) 15s; WCM.
Grosnez Pt 49°15'·55N 02°14'·75W Fl (2) WR 15s 50m **W19M**, **R17M**; W hut; vis W081°-188°, R188°-241°.

La Corbière 49°10'·85N 02°14'·90W Iso WR 10s 36m **W18M**, **R16M**; ● stone Tr; vis W shore-294°, R294°-328°, W328°-148°, R148°-shore; RC; *Horn Mo (C) 60s.*

WESTERN PASSAGE/ST BRELADE

Ldg Lts 082°. Front La Gréve d'Azette 49°10'·21N 02°05'·00W Oc 5s 23m 14M; vis 034°-129°. Rear, Mont Ubé 1M from front, Oc R 5s 46m 12M; vis 250°-095°; Racon (T).
Noirmont Pt 49°09'·97N 02°09'·94W Fl (4) 12s 18m 13M; B Tr, W band.
Passage Rk Lt By 49°09'·59N 02°12'·18W VQ Fl; NCM.
Les Fours Lt By 49°09'·65N 02°10'·08W Q Fl; NCM.
Ruaudière Rk Lt By 49°09'·80N 02°08'·51W Fl G 3s; SHM; *Bell.*
Diamond Rk Lt By 49°10'·18N 02°08'·56W Fl (2) R 6s; PHM.

SAINT AUBIN

North Pier Hd 49°11'·28N 02°09'·94W Iso R 4s 12m 10M; and Dir Lt 254° Dir F WRG 5m, vis G248°-253°, W253°-255°, R255°-260°.
Fort Pier Hd 49°11'·18N 02°09'·52W Fl R 4s 8m 1M.

ST HELIER

Red and Green Passage (Small Roads) Ldg Lts 022·7°. Front, Elizabeth East Berth Dn 49°10'·69N 02°06'·86W Oc G 5s 10m 11M; R stripe on framework Tr. Rear, Albert Pier elbow, 230m from front, Oc R 5s 18m 12M; R stripe on framework Tr; synch with front.
E Rock Lt By 49°10'·02N 02°07'·20W QG; SHM.
Platte Rock Lt Bn 49°10'·22N 02°07'·27W Fl R 1·5s 6m 5M; R metal col.
Ldg Lts 078°. Front 49°10'·68N 02°06'·58W FG. Rear, 80m from front, FG; both on W cols.
Victoria Pier Hd 49°10'·63N 02°06'·80W; *Bell*; tfc sigs.

EASTERN PASSAGE/VIOLET CHANNEL/LA ROCQUE

Hinguette Lt By 49°09'·39N 02°07'·22W Fl (4) R 15s; PHM.
Demie de Pas Lt Bn Tr 49°09'·07N 02°06'·05W Mo (D) WR 12s 11m W14M, R10M; B Tr, Y top; vis R130°-303°, W303°-130°; Racon (T); *Horn (3) 60s.*
Canger Rock Lt By 49°07'·41N 02°00'·30W Q (9) 15s; WCM.
Frouquier Aubert Lt By 49°06'·14N 01°58'·78W Q (6) + L Fl 15s; SCM.
Violet Lt By 49°07'·87N 01°57'·05W L Fl 10s; SWM.

GOREY

Ldg Lts 298°. Front, Pier Hd 49°11'·86N 02°01'·25W Oc RG 5s 8m 12M; W framework Tr; vis R304°-352°, G352°-304°. Rear, 490m from front, Oc R 5s 24m 8M.
Inner Road Lt By 49°11'·55N 02°00'·25W QG; SHM.

ST CATHERINE BAY/ROZEL BAY

Verclut Bkwtr Hd 49°13'·39N 02°00'·57W Fl 1·5s 18m 13M; framework Tr.
Rozel Bay Dir Lt 245° 49°14'·27N 02°02'·68W Dir F WRG 11m 5M; vis G240°-244°, W244°-246°, R246°-250°.

BONNE NUIT BAY TO GRÈVE AU LANCON

Bonne Nuit Bay Ldg Lts 223°. Front Pier Hd 49°15'·17N 02°07'·08W FG 7m 6M. Rear, 170m from front, FG 34m 6M.
Sorel Pt 49°15'·64N 02°09'·45W L Fl WR 7·5s 50m **15M**; B & W chequered ● Tr; vis W095°-112°, R112°-173°, W173°-230°, R230°-269°, W269°-273°.

OFFLYING ISLANDS

LES ÉCREHOU

Écrevière Lt By 49°15'·32N 01°52'·07W Q (6) + L Fl 15s; SCM.
Mâitre I Bn 49°17'·14N 01°55'·52W.

PLATEAU DES MINQUIERS

NW Minquiers Lt By 48°59'·70N 02°20'·50W Q; NCM; *Bell.*
SW Minquiers Lt By 48°54'·40N 02°19'·30W Q (9) 15s; WCM; *Whis.*
S Minquiers Lt By 48°53'·15N 02°10'·00W Q (6) + L Fl 15s; SCM.
SE Minquiers Lt By 48°53'·50N 02°00'·00W Q (3) 10s; ECM; *Bell.*
NE Minquiers Lt By 49°00'·90N 01°55'·20W VQ (3) 5s; ECM; *Bell.*
N Minquiers Lt By 49°01'·70N 02°00'·50W Q; NCM.
Demi de Vascelin By 49°00'·08N 02°05'·10W; SHM; (unlit).

14

10.14.5   PASSAGE INFORMATION

Current Pilots for this popular area include: *Shell Channel Pilot* (Imray/Cunliffe); *Normandy and CI Pilot* (Adlard Coles/ Brackenbury); *Brittany and CI Cruising Guide* (Adlard Coles/ Jefferson); *N Brittany and CI Cruising* (YM/Cumberlidge).

CHANNEL ISLANDS – GENERAL (chart 2669)

In an otherwise delightful cruising area, the main problems around the Channel Islands include fog and thick weather, the very big tidal range, strong tidal streams, overfalls and steep seas which get up very quickly. The shoreline is generally rugged with sandy bays and many offlying rks. It is important to use large scale charts, and recognised leading marks (of which there are plenty) when entering or leaving many of the hbrs and anchs. Several passages are marked by bns/perches which have an alphabetical letter in lieu of topmark.

From the N, note the Casquets TSS and ITZ – see Fig. 10 (3). Soundings of Hurd Deep can help navigation. The powerful lights at the Casquets, Alderney (Quenard Pt), Cap de la Hague, Cap Levi and Barfleur greatly assist a night or dawn landfall. buoy day Alderney is relatively high and conspic. Sark is often seen before Guernsey which slopes down from S to N. Jersey is low-lying in the SE. The islands are fringed by many rky dangers. In bad vis it is prudent to stay in hbr.

It is important to appreciate that over a 12 hour period tidal streams broadly rotate anti-clockwise around the Islands, particularly in open water and in wider chans (see 10.14.3). The E-going (flood) stream is of less duration than the W-going, but is stronger. The islands lie across the main direction of the streams, so eddies are common along the shores. The range of tide is most in Jersey, and least in Alderney. Streams run very hard through the chans and around headlands; they need to be worked carefully and neaps are best, particularly for a first visit. Strong W'lies cause a heavy sea, usually worst from local HW – 3 to + 3.

Apart from the main hbrs described in 10.14.9 – 10.14.15, there are many attractive minor hbrs and anchs, see Index. In the very nature of islands a lee can usually be found somewhere. Boats which can take the ground have an advantage for exploring the quieter hbrs. Be careful to avoid lobster pots and oyster beds.

THE CASQUETS AND ORTAC ROCK (chart 60)

Casquets lt ho (fog sig) is on the largest island of this group of rks 5·5M W of Braye, Alderney (10.14.9). Off-lying dangers extend 4ca W and WSW (The Ledge and Noire Roque) and 4ca E (Pte Colotte). The tide runs very hard round and between these various obstructions. A shallow bank, on which are situated Fourquie and l'Equet rks (dry), lies from 5ca to 1M E of Casquets, and should not be approached. Ortac rk (24m) is 3·5M E of Casquets. Ortac chan runs N/S 0·5M W of Ortac; here the stream begins to run NE at HW St Helier – 0230, and SW at HW St Helier + 0355, with sp rates 7kn. Ortac chan should not be used in bad weather, when there are very heavy overfalls in this area. Overfalls may also be met over Eight-fathom Ledge (8½ca W of Casquets), and over the Banks SW, SSW and SSE of the Casquets.

ALDERNEY AND THE SWINGE (chart 60)

See 10.14.9 for Braye Harbour (chart 2845) and approaches, together with pleasant bays and anchs around the island, offering shelter from different wind/sea directions.

The Swinge lies between Burhou with its bordering rks, and the NW coast of Alderney. It can be a dangerous chan, and should only be used in reasonable vis and fair weather. On N side of the Swinge the main dangers are Boues des Kaines, almost awash at LW about 7½ca ESE of Ortac, and North Rk 2½ca SE of Burhou. On S side of the Swinge beware Barsier Rk (dries) 3½ca NNW of Fort Clonque, and Corbet Rk, marked by a bn with a 'C' topmark, with outliers 5ca N of Fort Clonque.

The SW-going stream begins at HW St Helier + 0340, and the NE stream at HW St Helier – 0245, sp rates 7-8kn. On the NE-going stream, beware the very strong northerly set in vicinity of Ortac. The tide runs very hard, and in strong or gale force winds from S or W there are very heavy overfalls on the SW-going stream between Ortac and Les Etacs (off W end of Alderney). In strong E winds, on the NE-going stream, overfalls occur between Burhou and Braye breakwater. These overfalls can mostly be avoided by choosing the best time and route (see below), but due to the uneven bottom and strong tides broken water may be met even in calm conditions.

The best time to pass SW through the Swinge is at about HW St Helier +0400, when the SW-going stream starts; hold to the SE side of the chan. But after HW St Helier +0500, to clear the worst of the overfalls keep close to Burhou and Ortac, avoiding North Rk and Boues des Kaines.

Heading NE at about HW St Helier –0200, Great Nannel in transit with E end of Burhou clears Pierre au Vraic to the E, but passes close W of Les Etacs. On this transit, when Roque Tourgis fort is abeam, alter slightly to stbd to pass 1ca NW of Corbet Rk; keep near SE side of chan.

Pierre au Vraic (dries 1·2m) is an isolated, unmarked Rk 1·8M S of Ortac and 1·8M WSW of Les Étacs, almost in the fairway to/from the Swinge. On a fair tide from Guernsey it will be well covered, but it is a serious hazard if leaving the Swinge on a SW-going Spring tide close to LW (HWD to HWD +4). See AC 60 for clearing bearings.

THE ALDERNEY RACE (chart 3653)

The Alderney Race, so called due to very strong tidal streams, runs NE/SW between Alderney and Cap de la Hague. The fairway, approx 4M wide, is bounded by Race Rk and Alderney S Banks to the NW, and to the SE by rky banks 4M WSW of Cap de la Hague, Milieu and Banc de la Schôle (least depth 2·7m). These dangers which cause breaking seas and heavy overfalls should be carefully avoided. In bad weather and strong wind-against-tide conditions the seas break in all parts of the Race and passage is not recommended. Conditions are exacerbated at sp tides.

In mid-chan the NE-going stream starts at HW St Helier – 0210 (HWD + 0530) and the SW stream at HW St Helier +0430 (HWD), sp rates both 5·5kn. Times at which streams turn do not vary much for various places, but the rates do; for example, 1M W of C de la Hague the sp rates are 7-8kn.

To obtain optimum conditions, timing is of the essence. As a rule of thumb the Race should be entered on the first of the fair tide so as to avoid the peak tidal streams with attendant overfalls/breaking seas.

Thus, bound SW, arrive off C de la Hague at about HW St Helier +0430 (HW Dover) when the stream will be slack, whilst just starting to run SW off Alderney. A yacht leaving Cherbourg at HW Dover –0300 will achieve the above timing by utilising the inshore W-going tidal eddy.

Conversely, NE bound, leave St Peter Port at approx local HW –0425 (HW Dover+3) with a foul tide so as to pass Banc de la Schôle as the first of the fair tide starts to make. A later departure should achieve a faster passage, but with potentially less favourable conditions in the Race. On the NE stream the worst overfalls are on the French side.

APPROACHES TO GUERNSEY (charts 808, 3654)

From the N, The Little Russel Chan (chartlet at 10.14.12) between Guernsey and Herm gives the most convenient access to Beaucette Marina (10.14.10) and St Peter Port (10.14.11 and chart 3140). With lts on Platte Fougère, Tautenay, Roustel, Platte and Bréhon, plus the ldg lts (220°) for St Peter Port, the Little Russel can be navigated day or night in reasonable vis, even at LW. But it needs care, due to rks which fringe the chan and appr, and the strong tide which also sets across the ent. In mid chan, S of Platte and NW of Bréhon, the NE-going stream begins at HW St Peter Port – 0245, and the SW stream at HW St Peter Port +0330, sp rates both 5·25kn which can cause a very steep sea with wind against tide.

The Big Russel is wider and easier; in bad weather or poor vis it may be a better approach to St Peter Port, via Lower Heads SCM lt buoy. From the NW, Doyle Passage, which is aligned 146°/326° off Beaucette, should only be used with local knowledge by day. In onshore winds keep well clear of Guernsey's W coast, where in bad weather the sea breaks on dangers up to 4M offshore. From S or W, the natural route is around St Martin's Pt.

The minor hbrs and anchs (10.14.11) include Bordeaux, St Sampson, Havelet B, Soldiers B and Fermain B on the E coast. On the S coast Moulin Huet B and Icart B are good anchs in N and E winds. Portelet hbr and Lihou Is on the W coast and Grande Havre, L'Ancresse and Fontenelle B on the N coast also provide shelter.

HERM AND JETHOU (charts 807, 808).

Herm (10.14.11) and Jethou can be approached from the Little Russel via any of 7 passages all of which require reasonable vis and care with tidal streams. The appr from the Big Russel is more open and leads easily to pleasant anchs at Belvoir Bay and Shell Bay.

SARK (10.14.12 and chart 808)

La Maseline and Creux on the E coast are the only proper hbrs, the former much used by ferries. Elsewhere around the island, whatever the wind direction, a sheltered anch can usually be found in a lee: on the NW coast, Port à La Jument and Port du Moulin in Banquette Bay offer some shelter from S and E winds. Fontaines Bay and La Grève de la Ville offer different degrees of protection on the NE coast. Derrible B, Dixcart B and Rouge Terrier are good anchs on the SE coast. Port Gorey, Les Fontaines B, La Grande Grève and Havre Gosselin are all on the W coast; the last named is crowded in season due to easy access from Guernsey.

JERSEY (charts 3655, 1136, 1137, 1138)

To N and NE of Jersey, Les Pierres de Lecq, Les Dirouilles and Les Ecrehou are groups of drying rks, 2-4M offshore. On the N coast several bays (10.14.14) offer anchs sheltered in offshore winds. Coming from N, a convenient landfall is Desormes WCM buoy, 4M NNW of Grosnez Pt (conspic lookout tr). In St Ouen B on the W coast, which has drying rks almost 1M offshore, there are no good anchorages except NW of La Rocco tr which is sheltered in offshore winds.

To clear offlying dangers by 1M, keep the top of La Corbière lt ho (conspic) level with or below the clifftops behind (FR lt). The NW and W Passages (buoyed) lead E past Noirmont Pt toward St Helier (10.14.13). On the S coast, St Brelade B and St Aubin B (10.14.14) provide some shelter from W'lies.

SE of Jersey the Violet Bank extends 2M off La Rocque Pt with rky plateaux 1M further to seaward. The Violet Channel (chart 1138), although buoyed is best avoided in bad weather, wind-over-tide or poor vis. From St Helier make good Canger WCM buoy, thence track 078° for 2·2M to Violet SWM lt buoy. Turn N to pick up the charted ldg lines toward Gorey (10.14.14) or St Catherine Bay, both popular drying hbrs. The safe width of Violet Chan is only 5ca in places. Beware Decca problems due to being in baseline extension area. Anquette Chan leads NE from Violet buoy between the Petite and Grande Anquette bns, towards France.

Les Minquiers (10.14.14), 10-18M S of St Helier, should only be entered with extreme caution and in ideal weather.

14

10.14.6   DISTANCE TABLE

Approximate distances in nautical miles are by the most direct route, whilst avoiding dangers and allowing for Traffic Separation Schemes. Places in *italics* are in adjoining areas; places in **bold** are in 10.0.5, Cross-Channel Distances.

	1	2	3	4	5	6	7	8	9	10	11	12	13	14	15	16	17	18	19	20
1. *Cherbourg*	**1**																			
2. *Cap de la Hague*	14	**2**																		
3. *Carteret*	37	23	**3**																	
4. *Granville*	75	61	38	**4**																
5. ***St Malo***	87	73	38	23	**5**															
6. Casquets	31	17	32	63	70	**6**														
7. **Braye (Alderney)**	23	9	26	66	73	8	**7**													
8. Beaucette	39	25	34	59	58	15	19	**8**												
9. **St Peter Port**	42	28	31	55	54	18	23	4	**9**											
10. Les Hanois	49	35	37	58	56	23	29	14	10	**10**										
11. Creux (Sark)	37	23	23	50	52	18	22	11	10	16	**11**									
12. **St Helier**	59	45	28	30	38	43	46	33	29	32	24	**12**								
13. *Gorey (Jersey)*	47	33	16	29	38	36	35	32	29	35	20	13	**13**							
14. *Dahouet*	88	74	62	44	28	70	72	62	58	57	53	41	47	**14**						
15. ***St Quay-Portrieux***	88	74	64	54	35	71	73	55	56	48	51	46	52	12	**15**					
16. *Paimpol*	91	77	65	56	42	67	70	54	50	45	50	45	53	24	24	**16**				
17. *Lézardrieux*	88	74	68	54	49	65	68	52	48	42	38	47	55	33	21	14	**17**			
18. *Tréguier*	94	80	72	72	60	66	72	56	52	42	58	53	63	58	46	29	22	**18**		
19. *Roscoff*	117	103	95	96	84	87	94	77	73	63	79	80	93	71	59	58	54	41	**19**	
20. *L'Aberwrac'h*	145	131	126	128	116	115	122	107	103	93	109	110	123	103	91	88	84	72	32	**20**

SPECIAL NOTES FOR THE CHANNEL ISLANDS   10-14-8

The Channel Islands (Jersey, Guernsey, Alderney, Sark and other smaller islands) lie, not in the Channel, but in the Bay of St. Malo. Alderney is part of the Bailiwick of Guernsey and the States of Alderney have seats in the States of Guernsey. Brecqhou belongs to Sark which, in turn with Herm and Jethou, is part of Guernsey.

History Although the eastern ends of Jersey (15 miles) and Alderney (8.5 miles) are close to France, the Channel Islands were originally part of Normandy and therefore French. They could not be thought of as British until, at the earliest, the 13th century, after King John had lost mainland Normandy. The French call them Les Iles Anglo-Normandes (Jersey, Guernsey, Aurigny et Sercq).

Customs The Islands are British but are not part of the UK nor of the EC. They are self governing and have their own laws and customs regulations. British yachts entering Channel Island ports will be required to complete the local Customs declaration form and may have to produce the vessel's registration documents; they will also be subject to customs formalities on return to UK. Yachts going to France need the normal documents (passports etc) and British yachts returning to the Channel Islands from France, must, like all French yachts, wear the Q flag. (It is advisable to do so when arriving from UK, but not mandatory, except in Alderney). All Channel Islands have reciprocal medical arrangements with UK.

Ports of Entry are Braye, Beaucette, St Sampson, St Peter Port, St Helier and Gorey.

SAR operations are directed by the Hr Mrs of St Peter Port (for the N area) and St Helier (for the S area), via St Peter Port and Jersey Radio respectively. Major incidents are co-ordinated with CROSSMA Joburg and Falmouth MRCC. Unlike the UK there are no CGs, but there are LBs at Braye, St Peter Port, St Helier and St Catherines (Jersey).

Casquets TSS/ITZ is under radar surveillance by Jobourg Traffic (10.15.9). Portland CG provides radio cover only. See also diagrams in Fig 10 (5) and 10.15.2.

Telephones All CI telephones are part of the UK BT system.

Radio Telephone VHF Link calls to the UK made by British yachtsmen through St Peter Port or Jersey Radio will incur handling charges by British Telecom at the rate for foreign calls (see 6.3.5).

Courtesy Flags Further to 6·4·6, many yachts fly a courtesy flag in Channel Island ports as a mark of politeness but it is not de rigueur. The local flags are:
Jersey W flag with R diagonal cross, with the Jersey Royal Arms (three lions passant with gold crown above) in the canton.
Guernsey R ensign with Duke William's cross in the fly. Vessels owned by Guernsey residents may wear this ensign.
Sark The English (St George's) flag with the Normandy arms in the canton.
Alderney The English (St George's) flag and in the centre a G disc charged with a gold lion.
Herm The English (St George's) flag, and in the canton the Arms of Herm (three cowled monks on a gold diagonal stripe between blue triangles containing a silver dolphin).

Cars can be hired in Jersey, Guernsey and Alderney. All cars are forbidden in Sark.

Animals The rules regarding animals are as strict as they are in UK. Landing of animals from boats is permitted only from UK, Ireland, Isle of Man or other Channel Isles, but not if the boat has visited France. Unless expressly permitted by a Revenue Officer, no vessel may lie alongside a pontoon or quay with an animal on board.

Currency is interchangeable with UK currency except in coin. Using CI notes on return to UK is not always popular! Postage stamps, issued by Jersey, Guernsey and Alderney must be used in the appropriate island. There is only one class of post; it is cheaper than UK.

BRAYE   10-14-9

Alderney (Channel Islands) 49°43'·83N 02°11'·42W

CHARTS
AC *2845, 60, 3653, 2669*; SHOM 6934, 7158; ECM 1014; Imray C33A; Stanfords 7, 16

TIDES
−0400 Dover; ML 3·5; Duration 0545; Zone 0 (UT)

Standard Port ST HELIER (⟶)

Times				Height (metres)			
High Water		Low Water		MHWS	MHWN	MLWN	MLWS
0300	0900	0200	0900	11·0	8·1	4·0	1·4
1500	2100	1400	2100				
Differences BRAYE							
+0050	+0040	+0025	+0105	−4·8	−3·4	−1·5	−0·5

SHELTER
Good in Braye Hbr except in strong N/NE winds. There are 80 Y ⚓s parallel to the Admiralty bkwtr and near Fort Albert. ⚓ in hbr is good, but keep clear of the jetty and fairway because of steamer traffic. Hbr speed limit 4kn. Access to inner hbr HW±2 for D, FW. No landing on Admiralty bkwtr; at NE end beware submerged bkwtr extension.

NAVIGATION
WPT 49°44'·32N 02°10'·90W, 035°/215° from/to front ldg lt 215°, 1·05M. The main hazards are strong tidal streams and the many rocks encircling Alderney. The safest appr is from the NE. Take the Swinge and the Race at/near slack water to avoid the dangerous overfalls in certain wind and tide conditions (see 10.14.5). In the Swinge calmest area is often near Corbet Rk, bn 'C'. At mid-flood (NE-going) a strong eddy flows SW past the hbr ent. On the S side of the island during the ebb, a strong NE-going eddy runs close inshore of Coque Lihou. Give Brinchetais Ledge (E end) a wide berth to avoid heavy overfalls. An Historic Wreck is 5ca N of Quenard Pt lt ho (see 10.0.3g).

LIGHTS AND MARKS
From NW, N side of Ft Albert and end of Admiralty bkwtr 115° clear the Nannels. Iso WR 4s at Chateau à l'Etoc Pt, E of the hbr, vis R071°-111°, W111°-151°, in line 111° with Quenard Pt lt ho, Fl (4) 15s, clears sunken ruins of bkwtr. Ldg lts, both Q vis 210°-220°, lead 215° into hbr; front 8m 17M; rear 17m 18M. The Admty bkwtr hd has a lt, L Fl 10s 13m 5M. By day, St Anne's church spire on with W bn at Douglas Quay leads 210° to fairway which is marked by a QR and QG buoy and an inner pair of Q (2) R 5s and Q (2) G 5s buoys. End of steamer quay has 2 FR (vert) lts.

RADIO TELEPHONE
Call: *Alderney Radio* VHF Ch 12 16 74 (0800-1700, 7 days/wk, May to Sept; 0800-1700, Mon-Fri, Oct to Apr: all LT). Outside these hrs call St Peter Port. Mainbrayce Marine Ch 80 M (Apr-mid Sept: 0800-2000LT). Water taxi call *Mainbrayce* Ch M, 0800-2359. For Casquets TSS see Cherbourg (10.15.9).

TELEPHONE (01481)
Hr Mr and ▓ 822620; Marinecall 0898 500 457; Police 822731; Dr 822077; Ⓗ 822822; Visitor Info 822994 (H24).

FACILITIES
Hbr M (£8 for <12m LOA, £10 for >12m); **Jetty** , FW, C, Ⓓ; **Sapper Slip**, FW; **Alderney SC** ☎ 822758, Bar; **Services:** Slip, FW, ME, El, Ⓔ, Gas, SM, Sh, CH, ACA, D (Mainbrayce, inner hbr HW±2), P (cans).
Town EC Wed; V, R, Bar, ✉, Ⓑ, ✈ to Guernsey, Jersey, Dinard, Southampton and Cherbourg.
Ferry: via Guernsey – Weymouth.

ANCHORAGES AROUND ALDERNEY

There are several ⚓s, all picturesque but only safe in off-shore winds. None provide any facilities; clockwise from BRAYE:
SAYE BAY, Small sandy bay adjacent to Braye.
CORBLET BAY, A clear bay in NE corner of the island.
LONGY BAY, Wide sandy bay with good holding in sand. ⚓ between Essex Castle and Raz Is to await fair tide in the Race.
LA TCHUE, Good holding in small bay surrounded by cliffs.
TELEGRAPH BAY, Pleasant sandy bay on SW tip of the island.
HANNAINE BAY, A good place to wait for the flood tide.
PLATTE SALINE BAY, Good shelter from E winds.
BURHOU, ⚓ in bay in SW of the islands, below half tide.

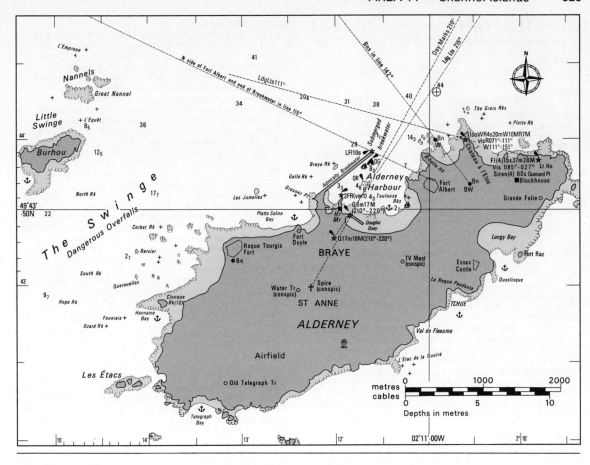

BEAUCETTE   10-14-10

Guernsey (Channel Islands) 49°30'.25N 02°30'·12W

CHARTS
AC *808, 807, 3654*; SHOM 6903, 6904, 7159; ECM 1014; Imray C33A; Stanfords 16

TIDES
−0450 Dover; ML 5·0; Duration 0550; Zone 0 (UT)

To find depth of water over the sill:
1. Note predicted time and ht of HW St Peter Port.
2. Enter table below on the line for ht of HW.
3. Extract depth (m) of water for time before/after HW.

Ht (m) of HW St Peter Port	Depth of Water over the Sill in metres (dries 2.37 m)						
	HW	±1hr	±2hrs	±2½hrs	±3hrs	±3½hrs	±4hrs
6·20	3·85	3·67	3·30	3·03	2·75	2·47	2·20
·60	4·25	4·00	3·50	3·13	"	2·37	2·00
7·00	4·65	4·34	3·70	3·23	"	2·27	1·80
·40	5·05	4·67	3·90	3·33	"	2·17	1·60
·80	5·45	5·00	4·10	3·43	"	2·07	1·40
8·20	5·85	5·34	4·30	3·53	"	1·97	1·20
·60	6·25	5·67	4·50	3·63	"	1·87	1·00
9·00	6·65	6·00	4·70	3·73	"	1·77	0·80
·40	7·05	6·34	4·90	3·83	"	1·67	0·60
·80	7·45	6·67	5·20	3·93	"	1·57	0·40

SHELTER
Excellent, but access as above table; entry not advised in strong onshore winds or heavy swell. There are 2 Y waiting buoys outside and tidal depth gauges outside/inside the ent.

NAVIGATION
WPT 49°30'·15N 02°28'·50W, 097°/277° from/to ent, 1·1M. Appr from Little Russel to mid-way between Platte Fougère lt tr (W with B band, 25m) and Roustel lt tr (BW checked). Pick up the ldg marks/lts, but beware cross tide and the Petite Canupe Rks (SCM lt bn) to the N, and rks and drying areas to the S. Chan has 5 pairs of unlit buoys. The ent is 18m wide.

LIGHTS AND MARKS
Petite Canupe SCM bn, Q (6) + L Fl 15s. Ldg lts 277°: Front FR, R arrow on W background to stbd of ent; rear FR, W arrow on R background, on roof of bldg, with windsock.

RADIO TELEPHONE
VHF Ch 80 M 16.

TELEPHONE (01481)
Hr Mr 45000; ⌗ 45000; Marinecall 0898 500 457; Police 25111; Dr 25211 (St John Ambulance).

FACILITIES
Beaucette Marina (200+50 visitors), ☎ 45000, Fax 47071, £13.69, D, FW, AC, Gas, Gaz, V, ▣, BH (16 ton), Slip, Bar, R; **Services** ME, El, Marine management. **Town** EC Thurs; ⊠, Ⓑ (St Sampson), ✈ (Guernsey). Ferry: St Peter Port – Weymouth.

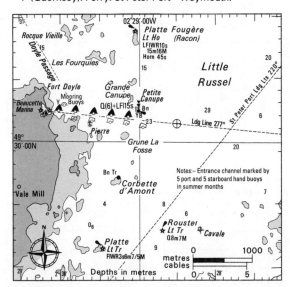

ST PETER PORT   10-14-11

Guernsey (Channel Islands) 49°27'·41N 02°31'·45W

CHARTS
AC *3140, 808, 807, 3654*; SHOM 6903, 6904, 7159;
ECM 1014; Imray C33A; Stanfords 16

TIDES
–0439 Dover; ML 5·2; Duration 0550; Zone 0 (UT)
NOTE: Predicted times and heights of HW and LW for
each day of the year are shown below.

SHELTER
Good, especially in Victoria Marina which has a sill 4·4m
above CD. Storm gates are fitted, with a fixed vert pillar
in mid-entrance. Access approx HW±2½ according to
draft; ent/exit controlled by R/G tfc lts. Appr via buoyed
chan along S side of hbr. No ⚓. Marina boat will meet
and direct yachts to waiting pontoon or Y ⚓s to E of
marina ent. Local moorings are in centre of hbr, with a
secondary fairway N of them. Albert and Queen Elizabeth
II marinas are for local boats only.
Havelet Bay: Enter between Oyster Rk and Moulinet Rk,
marked by SHM By QG and PHM By QR, with unlit SHM
and PHM buoy approx 100m further inshore. Crowded ⚓
in summer; no ⚓s. Landing slip close W of Castle Cornet.
Note: Other hbrs and ⚓s around Guernsey, Herm and
Sark are listed after the St Peter Port tidal predictions.

NAVIGATION
WPT 49°27'·88N 02°30'·70W, 040°/220° from/to front ldg lt,
0·68M. Offlying dangers, big tidal range and strong tidal
streams demand careful navigation. Easiest appr from N
is via Big Russel between Herm and Sark, passing S of
Lower Hds SCM lt buoy. The Little Russel is slightly more
direct, but needs care; see 10·14·5 and 10.14.12 chartlet.
From W and S of Guernsey, give Les Hanois a wide
berth. Beware ferries and shipping. Hbr speed limits: 6kn
from outer pier heads to line N/S from New Pier; 4kn W
of that line.

LIGHTS AND MARKS
Appr ldg lts 220°: Front, Castle bkwtr hd Al WR 10s 14m
16M (vis 187°-007°) Horn 15s; rear, Belvedere Oc 10s 61m
14M, intens 217°-223°. By day, White patch at Castle
Cornet in line 223° with Belvedere Ho (conspic).
Inner ldg lts 265°: Front, Oc R 5s 10m 14M; rear (160m
from front) Iso R 2s 22m 3M, vis 260°-270° (10°). Front lt
is at ent to Victoria Marina; rear is on W side of marina.
This line leads through moorings in The Pool; normal
appr to Victoria marina is via buoyed/lit S chan.
Traffic Signals on White Rock pierhead:
Ⓡ (vis from seaward)   = No ent
Ⓡ (vis from landward)   = No exit (also shown from SW
corner of New Pier).
These sigs do not apply to boats, <15m LOA, under
power and keeping clear of the fairways.

RADIO TELEPHONE
Call: *Victoria Marina* VHF Ch 20; Ch 80 may also be in use
Jul/Aug as overload channel. Water taxi Ch 10 (0800-
2359LT). For St Peter Port as a whole call *Port Control* Ch
12 (H24). If difficulty experienced in contacting *Port
Control* on VHF, messages may be sent via St Peter Port
Radio on VHF or MF; see 6·3·15. St Sampson Ch 12 (H24).

TELEPHONE (01481)
Hr Mr 720229, Fax 714177; Marina 725987; CG Sig Stn
720085; ⌗ 726911; Weather 37766/64033; Recorded
forecast for CI (06966) 0022; Marinecall 0898 500 457;
Police 725111; Dr 725211 (St Johns Ambulance).

FACILITIES
Victoria Marina (400, all visitors) ☎ 725987, £12, FW, AC,
Slip, ▣, R, Max LOA/draft = 12·8m/1·8m, Max stay 14 days;
N Pier ☎ 720085, C (32, 20 & 7 ton), AB; **Castle Pier** P, D,
approx HW±3, (also fuel pontoon at QE II marina).
Royal Chan Is YC ☎ 723154 Bar; **Guernsey YC** ☎ 722838;
Services: CH, Gas, Gaz, ACA, ME, EI, SM, BY, Ⓔ.
Town EC Thurs; P, D, V, CH, R, ▣, Bar, ✉, Ⓑ. Ferry to
Weymouth, Cherbourg, St. Malo; Hydrofoil/catamaran to
Sark, Weymouth, Jersey, St Malo; ✈ (Guernsey Airport).

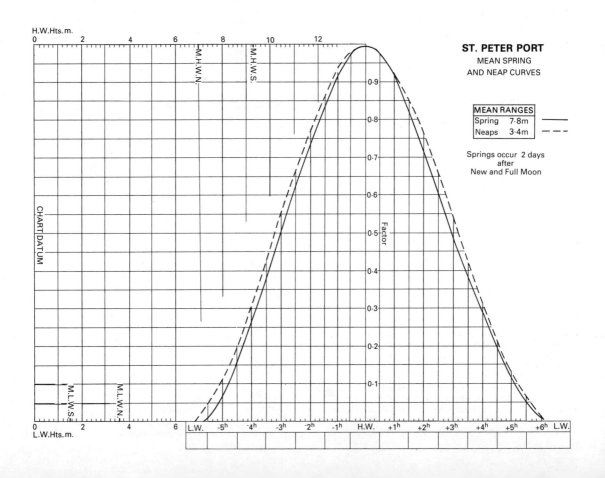

ST. PETER PORT
MEAN SPRING
AND NEAP CURVES

MEAN RANGES	
Spring	7·8m
Neaps	3·4m

Springs occur 2 days
after
New and Full Moon

ST. PETER PORT *continued*

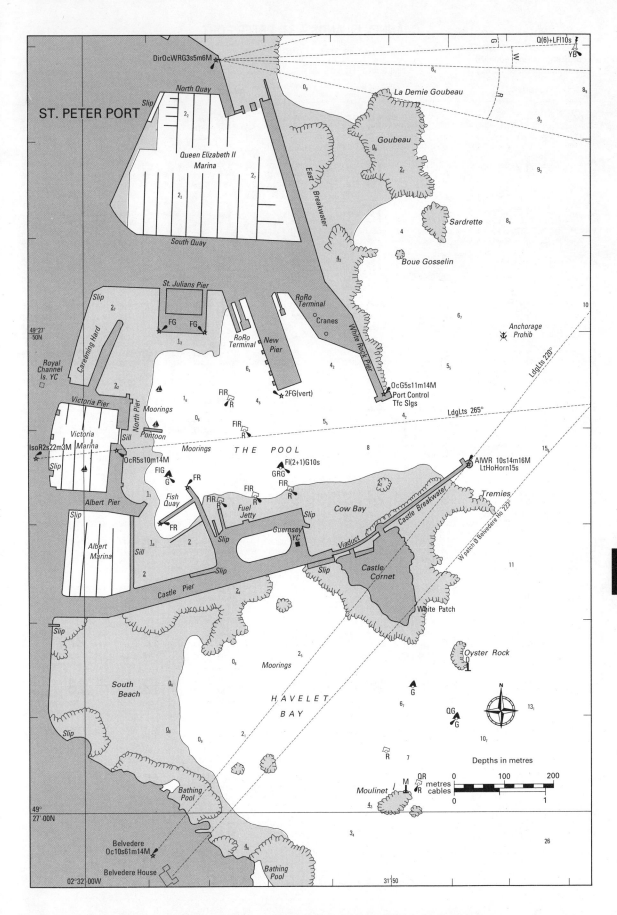

Q(6)+LFl10s

G

W

6₄

8₉

YB

DirOcWRG3s5m6M

La Demie Goubeau

0₉

ST. PETER PORT

North Quay

Slip

2₂

Queen Elizabeth II Marina

2₇

South Quay

2₂

2₇

Goubeau

0₈

2₇

9₂

9₂

Sardrette

8₉

4

Boue Gosselin

4₃

East Breakwater

St. Julians Pier

Slip

Careening Hard

2₇

FG   FG

1₃

RoRo Terminal

RoRo Terminal   New Pier

6₄

Cranes

RoRo Terminal

White Rock Pier

6₇

5₅

10

Anchorage Prohib

LdgLts 220°

Royal Channel Is. YC

2₂

Victoria Pier

North Pier

Moorings

Sill

Pontoon

FIR R

1₆

4₈

2FG(vert)

4₂

5₅

OcG5s11m14M Port Control Tfc Slgs

LdgLts 265°

49°27′ 50N

IsoR2s22m3M

Victoria Marina

OcR5s10m14M

Slip

FIG G

FR

FIR R

Moorings

0₆

FIR R

THE POOL

8

5₅

4₂

AIWR 10s14m16M LtHoHorn15s

15₈

Albert Pier

Slip

Albert Marina

Sill

1₁

Fish Quay

FR

1₆

2

FIR R

Slip

2

Fuel Jetty

Fl(2+1)G10s

GRG

FIR   FIR R

Cow Bay

Castle Breakwater

Tremies

11

Castle Pier

2₄

Slip

Guernsey YC

Viaduct

Slip

Castle Cornet

W patch Ø Belvedere Ho 223°

Slip

White Patch

Oyster Rock

South Beach

0₆

Moorings

2₅

0₈

0₈

2₁

0₉

HAVELET BAY

6₇

G

QG G

13₁

10₇

Depths in metres

R   7

Moulinet

4₃

M   QR
R

metres
cables

100   200
0

1

Bathing Pool

3₄

26

49° 27′·00N

Belvedere Oc10s61m14M

Belvedere House

Bathing Pool

02°32′·00W

31′50

14

CHANNEL ISLANDS – ST. PETER PORT

LAT 49°27'N   LONG   2°31'W

TIMES AND HEIGHTS OF HIGH AND LOW WATERS

YEAR 1996

TIME ZONE (UT)
For Summer Time add ONE hour in non-shaded areas

JANUARY

Day	Time	m		Day	Time	m
1 M	0300 / 0934 / 1531 / 2156	7.2 / 3.3 / 7.2 / 3.1		16 TU	0140 / 0817 / 1420 / 2054	7.3 / 3.2 / 7.4 / 3.0
2 TU	0358 / 1030 / 1625 / 2247	7.5 / 2.9 / 7.5 / 2.8		17 W	0301 / 0937 / 1536 / 2209	7.6 / 2.7 / 7.7 / 2.5
3 W	0445 / 1117 / 1711 / 2331	7.9 / 2.6 / 7.8 / 2.5		18 TH	0411 / 1043 / 1643 / 2311	8.1 / 2.1 / 8.2 / 1.9
4 TH	0528 / 1158 / 1753	8.2 / 2.3 / 8.1		19 F	0512 / 1142 / 1742	8.8 / 1.4 / 8.8
5 F O	0010 / 0606 / 1237 / 1832	2.2 / 8.5 / 2.0 / 8.4		20 SA ●	0008 / 0606 / 1238 / 1836	1.3 / 9.3 / 0.9 / 9.3
6 SA	0047 / 0644 / 1312 / 1909	2.0 / 8.7 / 1.8 / 8.5		21 SU	0101 / 0657 / 1329 / 1925	0.9 / 9.8 / 0.4 / 9.6
7 SU	0121 / 0720 / 1345 / 1944	1.8 / 8.8 / 1.8 / 8.6		22 M	0150 / 0745 / 1416 / 2011	0.5 / 10.0 / 0.2 / 9.7
8 M	0154 / 0753 / 1417 / 2016	1.8 / 8.8 / 1.8 / 8.5		23 TU	0235 / 0829 / 1500 / 2053	0.5 / 10.0 / 0.3 / 9.6
9 TU	0226 / 0824 / 1448 / 2046	1.9 / 8.7 / 1.9 / 8.4		24 W	0317 / 0911 / 1541 / 2133	0.7 / 9.7 / 0.7 / 9.3
10 W	0257 / 0855 / 1519 / 2116	2.1 / 8.5 / 2.1 / 8.2		25 TH	0357 / 0951 / 1620 / 2211	1.2 / 9.2 / 1.3 / 8.7
11 TH	0329 / 0927 / 1550 / 2149	2.4 / 8.3 / 2.4 / 7.9		26 F	0436 / 1031 / 1659 / 2250	1.8 / 8.5 / 2.0 / 8.0
12 F	0403 / 1005 / 1626 / 2229	2.7 / 8.0 / 2.7 / 7.7		27 SA	0517 / 1113 / 1741 / 2335	2.6 / 7.7 / 2.8 / 7.4
13 SA	0444 / 1049 / 1711 / 2318	2.9 / 7.7 / 2.9 / 7.4		28 SU	0607 / 1207 / 1834	3.2 / 7.1 / 3.4
14 SU	0537 / 1146 / 1808	3.2 / 7.4 / 3.2		29 M	0036 / 0713 / 1321 / 1941	6.8 / 3.6 / 6.6 / 3.7
15 M	0021 / 0646 / 1258 / 1923	7.2 / 3.3 / 7.3 / 3.2		30 TU	0200 / 0840 / 1452 / 2107	6.7 / 3.8 / 6.6 / 3.7
				31 W	0324 / 1001 / 1601 / 2218	6.9 / 3.5 / 6.9 / 3.3

FEBRUARY

Day	Time	m		Day	Time	m
1 TH	0422 / 1055 / 1652 / 2308	7.3 / 3.0 / 7.4 / 2.9		16 F	0357 / 1030 / 1633 / 2259	7.9 / 2.2 / 8.1 / 2.1
2 F	0508 / 1139 / 1734 / 2350	7.8 / 2.5 / 7.8 / 2.4		17 SA	0500 / 1131 / 1731 / 2356	8.6 / 1.5 / 8.7 / 1.4
3 SA	0549 / 1218 / 1814	8.3 / 2.1 / 8.2		18 SU ●	0554 / 1224 / 1823	9.3 / 0.8 / 9.3
4 SU O	0028 / 0627 / 1254 / 1851	2.0 / 8.6 / 1.8 / 8.5		19 M	0047 / 0643 / 1314 / 1909	0.8 / 9.8 / 0.4 / 9.7
5 M	0103 / 0703 / 1328 / 1927	1.7 / 8.9 / 1.5 / 8.7		20 TU	0134 / 0728 / 1358 / 1952	0.4 / 10.1 / 0.1 / 9.9
6 TU	0137 / 0737 / 1400 / 1958	1.5 / 9.0 / 1.4 / 8.8		21 W	0217 / 0810 / 1439 / 2031	0.3 / 10.1 / 0.2 / 9.8
7 W	0209 / 0807 / 1430 / 2027	1.5 / 9.0 / 1.5 / 8.7		22 TH	0256 / 0849 / 1517 / 2107	0.5 / 9.8 / 0.6 / 9.5
8 TH	0240 / 0837 / 1500 / 2056	1.6 / 8.9 / 1.6 / 8.6		23 F	0332 / 0924 / 1551 / 2140	0.9 / 9.3 / 1.2 / 8.9
9 F	0311 / 0908 / 1530 / 2127	1.8 / 8.7 / 1.8 / 8.4		24 SA	0405 / 0958 / 1623 / 2213	1.6 / 8.6 / 1.9 / 8.2
10 SA	0343 / 0943 / 1603 / 2203	2.1 / 8.4 / 2.2 / 8.1		25 SU	0438 / 1033 / 1657 / 2249	2.4 / 7.8 / 2.7 / 7.5
11 SU	0420 / 1023 / 1643 / 2248	2.4 / 8.0 / 2.6 / 7.7		26 M	0515 / 1116 / 1739 / 2335	3.1 / 7.1 / 3.4 / 6.9
12 M	0507 / 1115 / 1735 / 2346	2.8 / 7.6 / 3.0 / 7.3		27 TU	0612 / 1218 / 1843	3.7 / 6.5 / 3.9
13 TU	0611 / 1224 / 1846	3.2 / 7.2 / 3.3		28 W	0051 / 0735 / 1353 / 2005	6.5 / 4.0 / 6.3 / 4.0
14 W	0105 / 0742 / 1353 / 2024	7.2 / 3.7 / 7.1 / 3.2		29 TH	0235 / 0913 / 1531 / 2135	6.5 / 3.8 / 6.6 / 3.7
15 TH	0238 / 0918 / 1521 / 2153	7.4 / 2.9 / 7.5 / 2.7				

MARCH

Day	Time	m		Day	Time	m
1 F	0352 / 1026 / 1626 / 2239	7.0 / 3.3 / 7.1 / 3.2		16 SA	0344 / 1018 / 1621 / 2246	7.9 / 2.2 / 8.0 / 2.1
2 SA	0442 / 1112 / 1710 / 2323	7.5 / 2.7 / 7.7 / 2.6		17 SU	0445 / 1115 / 1716 / 2340	8.6 / 1.5 / 8.7 / 1.4
3 SU	0524 / 1152 / 1750	8.1 / 2.2 / 8.2		18 M	0537 / 1206 / 1804	9.2 / 0.9 / 9.2
4 M	0002 / 0603 / 1229 / 1827	2.0 / 8.5 / 1.7 / 8.6		19 TU ●	0028 / 0623 / 1252 / 1848	0.9 / 9.7 / 0.5 / 9.6
5 TU O	0040 / 0640 / 1303 / 1902	1.6 / 8.9 / 1.4 / 8.9		20 W	0113 / 0707 / 1335 / 1928	0.5 / 9.9 / 0.3 / 9.8
6 W	0115 / 0714 / 1337 / 1935	1.3 / 9.1 / 1.1 / 9.1		21 TH	0154 / 0747 / 1414 / 2006	0.4 / 9.9 / 0.4 / 9.7
7 TH	0148 / 0746 / 1409 / 2005	1.1 / 9.2 / 1.1 / 9.1		22 F	0232 / 0824 / 1449 / 2039	0.6 / 9.7 / 0.7 / 9.4
8 F	0221 / 0818 / 1440 / 2035	1.1 / 9.2 / 1.2 / 9.0		23 SA	0305 / 0857 / 1521 / 2110	1.0 / 9.2 / 1.3 / 9.0
9 SA	0253 / 0850 / 1511 / 2108	1.3 / 9.0 / 1.4 / 8.8		24 SU	0335 / 0928 / 1550 / 2140	1.6 / 8.6 / 2.0 / 8.4
10 SU	0326 / 0925 / 1544 / 2144	1.6 / 8.7 / 1.8 / 8.4		25 M	0403 / 1000 / 1618 / 2212	2.3 / 7.9 / 2.7 / 7.7
11 M	0403 / 1005 / 1623 / 2227	2.0 / 8.2 / 2.3 / 7.9		26 TU	0433 / 1037 / 1652 / 2250	3.0 / 7.2 / 3.4 / 7.1
12 TU	0449 / 1055 / 1714 / 2324	2.6 / 7.6 / 2.9 / 7.5		27 W	0518 / 1129 / 1748 / 2349	3.6 / 6.6 / 3.9 / 6.6
13 W	0552 / 1205 / 1825	3.0 / 7.2 / 3.3		28 TH	0644 / 1256 / 1917	4.0 / 6.3 / 4.1
14 TH	0044 / 0725 / 1338 / 2009	7.1 / 3.2 / 7.0 / 3.3		29 F	0131 / 0813 / 1438 / 2040	6.4 / 3.9 / 6.4 / 3.9
15 F	0223 / 0905 / 1512 / 2141	7.3 / 2.9 / 7.4 / 2.9		30 SA	0303 / 0933 / 1547 / 2152	6.8 / 3.5 / 6.9 / 3.4
				31 SU	0403 / 1030 / 1635 / 2244	7.3 / 2.9 / 7.5 / 2.8

APRIL

Day	Time	m		Day	Time	m
1 M	0449 / 1114 / 1717 / 2328	7.9 / 2.3 / 8.1 / 2.2		16 TU	0515 / 1142 / 1740	9.0 / 1.2 / 9.1
2 TU	0530 / 1154 / 1756	8.4 / 1.8 / 8.6		17 W ●	0005 / 0600 / 1227 / 1822	1.2 / 9.3 / 0.9 / 9.4
3 W	0008 / 0609 / 1233 / 1832	1.7 / 8.8 / 1.3 / 8.9		18 TH	0049 / 0643 / 1309 / 1902	0.9 / 9.5 / 0.8 / 9.5
4 TH O	0048 / 0646 / 1310 / 1907	1.3 / 9.2 / 1.0 / 9.2		19 F	0129 / 0722 / 1347 / 1938	0.8 / 9.5 / 0.8 / 9.5
5 F	0125 / 0722 / 1345 / 1942	1.0 / 9.3 / 0.9 / 9.3		20 SA	0206 / 0758 / 1421 / 2011	1.0 / 9.3 / 1.1 / 9.3
6 SA	0201 / 0758 / 1420 / 2016	0.9 / 9.4 / 1.0 / 9.3		21 SU	0239 / 0831 / 1452 / 2042	1.3 / 9.0 / 1.6 / 8.9
7 SU	0237 / 0834 / 1454 / 2052	1.0 / 9.2 / 1.2 / 9.1		22 M	0308 / 0902 / 1520 / 2113	1.7 / 8.5 / 2.1 / 8.4
8 M	0313 / 0912 / 1531 / 2131	1.3 / 8.8 / 1.6 / 8.7		23 TU	0335 / 0935 / 1548 / 2144	2.3 / 7.9 / 2.7 / 7.9
9 TU	0353 / 0955 / 1612 / 2216	1.8 / 8.3 / 2.2 / 8.2		24 W	0405 / 1010 / 1620 / 2220	2.9 / 7.4 / 3.2 / 7.4
10 W	0441 / 1047 / 1705 / 2314	2.3 / 7.7 / 2.8 / 7.6		25 TH	0444 / 1055 / 1706 / 2309	3.4 / 6.9 / 3.7 / 6.9
11 TH	0545 / 1157 / 1816	2.8 / 7.2 / 3.2		26 F	0551 / 1203 / 1823	3.8 / 6.5 / 4.0
12 F	0032 / 0714 / 1328 / 1957	7.3 / 3.0 / 7.1 / 3.3		27 SA	0024 / 0720 / 1333 / 1949	6.6 / 3.8 / 6.5 / 3.9
13 SA	0207 / 0849 / 1457 / 2125	7.4 / 2.8 / 7.4 / 2.8		28 SU	0158 / 0834 / 1450 / 2059	6.7 / 3.5 / 6.9 / 3.5
14 SU	0325 / 0959 / 1601 / 2227	7.9 / 2.2 / 8.0 / 2.2		29 M	0308 / 0937 / 1548 / 2158	7.2 / 3.0 / 7.4 / 3.0
15 M	0424 / 1054 / 1654 / 2318	8.5 / 1.6 / 8.6 / 1.6		30 TU	0403 / 1029 / 1635 / 2248	7.7 / 2.5 / 7.9 / 2.4

Chart Datum: 5·06 metres below Ordnance Datum (Local)

CHANNEL ISLANDS – ST. PETER PORT

LAT 49°27'N LONG 2°31'W

TIMES AND HEIGHTS OF HIGH AND LOW WATERS

YEAR **1996**

TIME ZONE (UT)
For Summer Time add ONE hour in non-shaded areas

MAY

Day		Time	m	Time	m	Time	m	Time	m
1	W	0450	8.2	1115	2.0	1718	8.4	2334	1.8
2	TH	0534	8.7	1159	1.5	1800	8.9		
3	F O	0018	1.3	0617	9.0	1242	1.1	1839	9.2
4	SA	0101	1.0	0658	9.3	1323	0.9	1919	9.4
5	SU	0142	0.8	0740	9.4	1403	0.9	1959	9.5
6	M	0223	0.8	0822	9.3	1443	1.1	2040	9.3
7	TU	0305	1.1	0905	8.9	1524	1.5	2123	8.9
8	W	0349	1.5	0951	8.5	1609	2.0	2211	8.5
9	TH	0439	2.0	1044	7.9	1702	2.5	2307	7.9
10	F	0541	2.5	1148	7.5	1809	3.0		
11	SA	0018	7.6	0658	2.8	1309	7.3	1936	3.1
12	SU	0143	7.5	0823	2.7	1430	7.5	2059	2.9
13	M	0258	7.8	0932	2.3	1534	7.9	2201	2.4
14	TU	0358	8.2	1027	2.0	1627	8.3	2253	2.0
15	W	0449	8.5	1116	1.6	1714	8.7	2340	1.6
16	TH	0536	8.8	1200	1.4	1756	9.0		
17	F ●	0023	1.4	0618	9.0	1242	1.3	1835	9.1
18	SA	0104	1.3	0658	9.0	1320	1.4	1912	9.1
19	SU	0141	1.4	0735	8.9	1355	1.5	1947	9.0
20	M	0214	1.6	0809	8.7	1427	1.8	2019	8.8
21	TU	0244	1.9	0842	8.4	1457	2.1	2051	8.5
22	W	0314	2.2	0915	8.0	1527	2.6	2123	8.1
23	TH	0345	2.6	0950	7.6	1600	3.0	2158	7.7
24	F	0421	3.1	1030	7.2	1639	3.4	2240	7.3
25	SA	0509	3.4	1120	6.9	1732	3.7	2335	7.0
26	SU	0618	3.6	1226	6.8	1847	3.8		
27	M	0046	6.9	0736	3.5	1341	6.9	2005	3.6
28	TU	0204	7.1	0843	3.2	1450	7.3	2110	3.1
29	W	0310	7.5	0943	2.7	1548	7.7	2208	2.6
30	TH	0407	8.0	1037	2.2	1639	8.2	2300	2.0
31	F	0500	8.4	1127	1.7	1727	8.7	2350	1.5

JUNE

Day		Time	m	Time	m	Time	m	Time	m
1	SA O	0550	8.8	1216	1.3	1814	9.1		
2	SU	0039	1.1	0638	9.1	1303	1.0	1900	9.4
3	M	0127	0.8	0725	9.3	1349	0.9	1946	9.6
4	TU	0213	0.7	0812	9.3	1434	0.9	2031	9.5
5	W	0259	0.8	0859	9.2	1519	1.2	2117	9.3
6	TH	0346	1.1	0946	8.8	1605	1.6	2204	8.9
7	F	0435	1.6	1036	8.3	1655	2.1	2256	8.3
8	SA	0529	2.1	1132	7.9	1754	2.6	2357	7.9
9	SU	0632	2.5	1238	7.5	1904	3.0		
10	M	0108	7.6	0745	2.7	1353	7.4	2023	3.0
11	TU	0224	7.5	0857	2.7	1501	7.6	2131	2.8
12	W	0329	7.7	0958	2.5	1558	7.9	2227	2.5
13	TH	0424	7.9	1049	2.2	1647	8.2	2316	2.2
14	F	0513	8.2	1135	2.0	1732	8.5		
15	SA	0000	1.9	0556	8.4	1218	1.9	1812	8.7
16	SU ●	0041	1.8	0637	8.5	1257	1.8	1850	8.8
17	M	0119	1.7	0715	8.6	1333	1.8	1926	8.8
18	TU	0153	1.7	0751	8.5	1406	1.9	2001	8.7
19	W	0225	1.9	0825	8.4	1438	2.1	2033	8.5
20	TH	0256	2.1	0858	8.2	1509	2.3	2105	8.3
21	F	0327	2.4	0931	7.9	1541	2.7	2137	8.0
22	SA	0400	2.7	1004	7.6	1616	3.0	2214	7.7
23	SU	0437	3.0	1045	7.3	1657	3.3	2259	7.4
24	M	0524	3.2	1135	7.2	1750	3.5	2355	7.2
25	TU	0626	3.3	1237	7.1	1858	3.5		
26	W	0103	7.2	0742	3.3	1349	7.2	2019	3.2
27	TH	0218	7.4	0857	3.0	1500	7.6	2129	2.8
28	F	0328	7.7	1002	2.5	1603	8.0	2231	2.2
29	SA	0430	8.2	1100	2.0	1700	8.6	2327	1.7
30	SU	0527	8.6	1155	1.5	1754	9.0		

JULY

Day		Time	m	Time	m	Time	m	Time	m
1	M O	0022	1.2	0621	9.0	1248	1.1	1844	9.5
2	TU	0114	0.7	0713	9.3	1338	0.8	1934	9.7
3	W	0204	0.5	0802	9.5	1426	0.7	2021	9.8
4	TH	0251	0.5	0849	9.5	1511	0.8	2106	9.7
5	F	0336	0.7	0934	9.2	1555	1.2	2151	9.3
6	SA	0421	1.1	1019	8.8	1641	1.7	2237	8.7
7	SU	0508	1.8	1106	8.2	1729	2.3	2327	8.1
8	M	0600	2.4	1200	7.7	1826	2.9		
9	TU	0028	7.5	0700	2.9	1307	7.3	1936	3.2
10	W	0142	7.2	0812	3.1	1422	7.2	2055	3.3
11	TH	0259	7.2	0925	3.1	1529	7.4	2202	3.0
12	F	0401	7.4	1024	2.9	1624	7.7	2255	2.7
13	SA	0453	7.7	1113	2.6	1711	8.1	2341	2.4
14	SU	0538	8.0	1156	2.3	1753	8.4		
15	M ●	0022	2.1	0618	8.3	1236	2.0	1832	8.6
16	TU	0100	1.9	0657	8.5	1313	1.9	1909	8.8
17	W	0135	1.8	0734	8.6	1347	1.8	1944	8.8
18	TH	0207	1.8	0808	8.6	1419	1.9	2016	8.7
19	F	0237	1.9	0839	8.4	1450	2.0	2045	8.6
20	SA	0307	2.1	0907	8.3	1520	2.3	2115	8.4
21	SU	0337	2.3	0938	8.0	1552	2.6	2148	8.1
22	M	0409	2.6	1013	7.8	1627	2.9	2227	7.8
23	TU	0448	2.9	1056	7.5	1711	3.1	2315	7.5
24	W	0539	3.2	1151	7.3	1810	3.3		
25	TH	0019	7.3	0646	3.3	1301	7.2	1928	3.3
26	F	0137	7.3	0814	3.2	1422	7.4	2057	3.0
27	SA	0258	7.5	0934	2.8	1536	7.9	2208	2.5
28	SU	0409	8.0	1040	2.2	1641	8.4	2311	1.8
29	M	0512	8.5	1139	1.7	1738	9.0		
30	TU O	0008	1.2	0608	9.1	1234	1.1	1831	9.6
31	W	0101	0.7	0700	9.5	1325	0.7	1920	10.0

AUGUST

Day		Time	m	Time	m	Time	m	Time	m
1	TH	0151	0.3	0748	9.8	1412	0.5	2006	10.1
2	F	0236	0.2	0832	9.8	1456	0.5	2050	10.0
3	SA	0319	0.5	0914	9.6	1538	0.9	2131	9.6
4	SU	0400	1.0	0955	9.1	1618	1.4	2212	8.9
5	M	0441	1.7	1035	8.4	1700	2.2	2254	8.2
6	TU	0524	2.4	1120	7.7	1747	2.9	2344	7.4
7	W	0615	3.1	1216	7.2	1847	3.5		
8	TH	0052	6.9	0721	3.6	1335	6.9	2007	3.7
9	F	0225	6.7	0846	3.7	1501	7.0	2136	3.6
10	SA	0341	7.0	1000	3.4	1603	7.3	2237	3.1
11	SU	0435	7.4	1053	2.9	1651	7.8	2323	2.7
12	M	0519	7.8	1136	2.5	1733	8.2		
13	TU	0003	2.3	0558	8.2	1216	2.1	1812	8.6
14	W ●	0040	1.9	0636	8.6	1252	1.8	1849	8.9
15	TH	0114	1.7	0712	8.8	1325	1.7	1923	9.0
16	F	0145	1.6	0745	8.8	1357	1.6	1954	9.0
17	SA	0215	1.6	0815	8.8	1428	1.7	2023	8.9
18	SU	0244	1.8	0842	8.6	1458	1.9	2052	8.7
19	M	0313	2.0	0911	8.4	1528	2.2	2123	8.5
20	TU	0343	2.3	0944	8.1	1601	2.5	2200	8.1
21	W	0419	2.7	1025	7.8	1642	2.9	2245	7.7
22	TH	0506	3.1	1118	7.4	1738	3.3	2347	7.3
23	F	0612	3.4	1229	7.2	1856	3.4		
24	SA	0110	7.2	0744	3.4	1357	7.3	2036	3.2
25	SU	0240	7.4	0918	3.0	1520	7.8	2154	2.6
26	M	0357	7.9	1027	2.4	1627	8.5	2258	1.9
27	TU	0459	8.6	1126	1.7	1724	9.1	2354	1.2
28	W O	0554	9.2	1219	1.1	1816	9.7		
29	TH	0045	0.6	0642	9.7	1308	0.6	1903	10.1
30	F	0132	0.3	0728	10.0	1354	0.4	1947	10.3
31	SA	0216	0.2	0810	10.0	1436	0.4	2029	10.1

14

Chart Datum: 5·06 metres below Ordnance Datum (Local)

CHANNEL ISLANDS – ST. PETER PORT

LAT 49°27′N   LONG 2°31′W

TIMES AND HEIGHTS OF HIGH AND LOW WATERS   YEAR **1996**

TIME ZONE (UT)
For Summer Time add ONE hour in non-shaded areas

SEPTEMBER

Day	Time	m	Time	m	Time	m	Time	m
1 SU	0256	0.5	0850	9.7	1515	0.8	2107	9.7
16 M	0220	1.5	0817	8.9	1436	1.6	2030	9.0
2 M	0334	1.0	0926	9.2	1552	1.4	2143	9.0
17 TU	0250	1.8	0847	8.7	1507	1.9	2103	8.7
3 TU	0410	1.8	1002	8.5	1628	2.2	2220	8.2
18 W	0321	2.1	0922	8.4	1541	2.3	2139	8.3
4 W	0447	2.6	1040	7.8	1708	3.0	2302	7.4
19 TH	0357	2.6	1002	8.0	1622	2.8	2225	7.8
5 TH	0532	3.4	1129	7.1	1802	3.7		
20 F	0444	3.1	1056	7.5	1718	3.2	2328	7.3
6 F	0003	6.7	0635	3.9	1243	6.7	1919	4.1
21 SA	0551	3.5	1209	7.2	1841	3.5		
7 SA	0140	6.4	0759	4.1	1425	6.7	2103	3.9
22 SU	0055	7.1	0731	3.6	1343	7.3	2024	3.2
8 SU	0318	6.7	0932	3.8	1538	7.1	2213	3.4
23 M	0232	7.4	0908	3.1	1509	7.8	2143	2.6
9 M	0412	7.3	1029	3.2	1627	7.6	2259	2.9
24 TU	0347	8.0	1015	2.4	1613	8.5	2244	1.9
10 TU	0455	7.8	1112	2.7	1708	8.2	2337	2.4
25 W	0445	8.7	1110	1.7	1707	9.0	2336	1.2
11 W	0533	8.3	1149	2.2	1747	8.6		
26 TH	0535	9.3	1200	1.1	1756	9.7		
12 TH	0013	1.9	0609	8.7	1225	1.8	● 1823	8.9
27 F	0024	0.7	0621	9.7	1248	0.7	O 1842	10.0
13 F	0046	1.6	0645	8.9	1259	1.6	1857	9.1
28 SA	0110	0.5	0704	10.0	1332	0.5	1925	10.1
14 SA	0118	1.5	0718	9.1	1332	1.4	1929	9.2
29 SU	0152	0.5	0745	9.9	1413	0.6	2005	9.9
15 SU	0150	1.4	0748	9.0	1404	1.5	2000	9.2
30 M	0230	0.8	0822	9.7	1450	1.0	2041	9.5

OCTOBER

Day	Time	m	Time	m	Time	m	Time	m
1 TU	0306	1.3	0857	9.2	1525	1.6	2115	8.9
16 W	0231	1.6	0829	9.0	1451	1.6	2048	8.8
2 W	0339	2.0	0930	8.6	1558	2.3	2149	8.2
17 TH	0306	2.0	0906	8.7	1529	2.0	2128	8.4
3 TH	0411	2.8	1005	7.9	1632	3.0	2227	7.4
18 F	0345	2.4	0950	8.2	1613	2.5	2216	7.9
4 F	0449	3.5	1047	7.2	1719	3.7	2320	6.8
19 SA	0434	3.0	1045	7.7	1711	3.0	2320	7.4
5 SA	0549	4.1	1151	6.7	1835	4.1		
20 SU	0542	3.4	1158	7.4	1833	3.3		
6 SU	0045	6.4	0713	4.3	1329	6.6	2003	4.1
21 M	0045	7.2	0721	3.5	1329	7.4	2010	3.1
7 M	0236	6.6	0843	4.1	1457	6.9	2131	3.7
22 TU	0219	7.5	0853	3.1	1452	7.9	2126	2.5
8 TU	0338	7.1	0951	3.5	1551	7.4	2222	3.1
23 W	0330	8.1	0958	2.4	1554	8.5	2225	1.9
9 W	0421	7.7	1037	2.9	1635	8.0	2302	2.5
24 TH	0425	8.7	1051	1.8	1647	9.0	2315	1.4
10 TH	0500	8.2	1116	2.4	1714	8.5	2338	2.1
25 F	0513	9.2	1140	1.3	1735	9.4		
11 F	0538	8.6	1153	1.9	1752	8.8		
26 SA	0002	1.0	0557	9.6	1226	1.0	O 1820	9.7
12 SA	0014	1.7	0614	9.0	1230	1.6	● 1828	9.1
27 SU	0046	0.9	0640	9.7	1309	0.9	1902	9.7
13 SU	0049	1.4	0648	9.2	1306	1.4	1903	9.3
28 M	0127	0.9	0719	9.7	1349	1.0	1941	9.5
14 M	0124	1.3	0721	9.2	1342	1.3	1937	9.3
29 TU	0204	1.4	0756	9.5	1426	1.3	2017	9.2
15 TU	0157	1.4	0754	9.2	1416	1.4	2012	9.1
30 W	0239	1.6	0830	9.1	1500	1.7	2050	8.7
31 TH	0310	2.2	0903	8.6	1532	2.3	2124	8.1

NOVEMBER

Day	Time	m	Time	m	Time	m	Time	m
1 F	0341	2.8	0936	8.0	1603	2.9	2200	7.5
16 SA	0341	2.1	0944	8.5	1612	2.1	2213	8.1
2 SA	0415	3.4	1014	7.4	1643	3.5	2245	7.0
17 SU	0431	2.6	1038	8.1	1708	2.6	2313	7.7
3 SU	0502	3.9	1105	6.9	1746	4.0	2352	6.6
18 M	0535	3.1	1145	7.7	1819	2.9		
4 M	0621	4.3	1224	6.7	1907	4.1		
19 TU	0027	7.4	0700	3.3	1306	7.6	1943	2.9
5 TU	0122	6.6	0743	4.2	1352	6.8	2022	3.8
20 W	0153	7.5	0828	3.0	1426	7.8	2100	2.6
6 W	0241	6.9	0854	3.8	1459	7.2	2126	3.4
21 TH	0305	7.9	0935	2.6	1530	8.2	2201	2.2
7 TH	0336	7.4	0950	3.2	1550	7.7	2216	2.8
22 F	0401	8.4	1029	2.1	1625	8.6	2252	1.8
8 F	0421	8.0	1036	2.6	1635	8.1	2259	2.3
23 SA	0450	8.8	1118	1.7	1714	8.9	2339	1.5
9 SA	0502	8.4	1118	2.1	1717	8.6	2340	1.9
24 SU	0535	9.1	1204	1.4	1759	9.1		
10 SU	0541	8.8	1200	1.7	1758	8.9		
25 M	0022	1.4	0617	9.3	1247	1.3	O 1841	9.1
11 M	0020	1.5	0619	9.1	1241	1.4	● 1838	9.2
26 TU	0104	1.4	0656	9.3	1328	1.3	1920	9.1
12 TU	0100	1.3	0657	9.3	1322	1.2	1918	9.3
27 W	0141	1.5	0733	9.2	1405	1.5	1957	8.9
13 W	0139	1.3	0736	9.4	1402	1.2	1958	9.2
28 TH	0216	1.8	0808	9.0	1439	1.8	2031	8.6
14 TH	0218	1.4	0816	9.2	1442	1.3	2039	9.0
29 F	0247	2.2	0841	8.6	1510	2.2	2105	8.2
15 F	0258	1.7	0858	9.0	1525	1.7	2123	8.6
30 SA	0318	2.6	0915	8.2	1541	2.7	2139	7.8

DECEMBER

Day	Time	m	Time	m	Time	m	Time	m
1 SU	0350	3.1	0950	7.7	1616	3.1	2217	7.3
16 M	0426	2.0	1029	8.6	1659	2.0	2258	8.1
2 M	0428	3.5	1030	7.3	1659	3.5	2303	7.0
17 TU	0522	2.5	1126	8.1	1757	2.4	2359	7.7
3 TU	0519	3.9	1123	7.0	1800	3.8		
18 W	0629	2.9	1234	7.7	1906	2.8		
4 W	0006	6.8	0634	4.0	1234	6.8	1916	3.8
19 TH	0114	7.5	0750	3.1	1351	7.6	2024	2.8
5 TH	0125	6.8	0752	3.9	1351	7.0	2025	3.6
20 F	0231	7.5	0905	2.9	1502	7.7	2133	2.7
6 F	0236	7.1	0857	3.5	1456	7.3	2125	3.1
21 SA	0335	7.8	1006	2.6	1602	7.9	2229	2.4
7 SA	0333	7.6	0953	3.0	1551	7.7	2218	2.6
22 SU	0428	8.2	1059	2.2	1655	8.2	2318	2.1
8 SU	0422	8.1	1044	2.4	1642	8.2	2307	2.1
23 M	0516	8.5	1146	1.9	1741	8.4		
9 M	0509	8.5	1132	1.9	1730	8.6	2354	1.7
24 TU	0003	1.9	0558	8.8	1230	1.7	O 1824	8.6
10 TU	0553	9.0	1219	1.4	● 1817	8.9		
25 W	0045	1.8	0638	8.9	1310	1.6	1904	8.7
11 W	0040	1.4	0638	9.3	1306	1.1	1903	9.2
26 TH	0122	1.7	0716	9.0	1348	1.6	1941	8.7
12 TH	0125	1.1	0722	9.5	1351	0.9	1948	9.3
27 F	0157	1.8	0751	8.9	1421	1.8	2015	8.6
13 F	0209	1.1	0807	9.5	1437	0.9	2033	9.2
28 SA	0229	2.0	0824	8.7	1452	2.0	2047	8.4
14 SA	0253	1.2	0852	9.4	1522	1.1	2119	9.0
29 SU	0259	2.2	0856	8.5	1521	2.3	2119	8.1
15 SU	0338	1.6	0939	9.0	1608	1.5	2206	8.6
30 M	0329	2.6	0927	8.1	1551	2.6	2150	7.8
31 TU	0400	2.9	1001	7.8	1623	3.0	2224	7.4

Chart Datum: 5·06 metres below Ordnance Datum (Local)

ANCHORAGES AROUND GUERNSEY, HERM AND SARK

GUERNSEY

⚓s, clockwise from St. Peter Port:

SOLDIERS BAY, Quiet ⚓, sandy bottom, no facilities.

FERMAIN BAY, Popular with tourists. Good shelter from SW/NW. Café.

PETIT PORT BAY ⎫
MOULIN HUET BAY ⎬ All tourist attractions with usual amenities.
SAINTS BAY ⎬ S coast bays with sandy bottoms.
PETIT BOT BAY ⎭ (Last is part of Icart Bay).

PORTELET HARBOUR, ⚓ on sandy bottom. Beware of fish farm. Stone Quay (dries) but not advisable to dry out alongside. Hotel, café/toilets. Bus to St. Peter Port.

LIHOU ISLAND, Privately owned, but visitors are welcome. ⚓ off NE corner.

VAZON BAY, Large sandy beach with long surf line. Beware surfers and bathers. Facilities: Hotel/Timeshare complex, bus to St. Peter Port.

COBO BAY, Sandy beach with many local moorings. Facilities: Hotel, bar, D, L, P, ✉, R, V. Bus to St. Peter Port.

GRANDE HAVRE, Very popular, many local moorings. ⚓ to W of Hommet de Greve. Stone slip; very busy in summer; lying alongside not recommended. Facilities: Hotel/Bar. Bus to St. Peter Port.

L'ANCRESSE BAY, Sandy bay, good shelter from S/SW.

FONTENELLE BAY, Good shelter but many rks.

BORDEAUX HARBOUR, Small drying hbr full of local moorings. Facilities: Café. Bus to St. Peter Port.

ST SAMPSON HARBOUR, Hbr dries. Official port of entry. Good shelter but the disadvantages of a commercial port. Ldg lts 286°: Front, FR 3m 5M, on S pier hd, vis 230°-340°; rear, FG 13m, 390m from front, on clocktower. Lt on Crocq pier hd, FR 11m 5M, vis 250°-340°, and tfc sigs. N pier hd FG 3m 5M, vis 230°-340°. VHF Ch 12 (H24). Facilities: See Hr Mr for AB, C, FW. No yacht facilities.
Services: Slip, ME, EI, Sh, C. Bus to St Peter Port.

HERM ISLAND

Herm hbr has ldg lts, both FW (occas) and W drums at 078°. Hbr used by local ferries above half tide. Very congested in summer. Facilities: Hr Mr ☎ 822377; Hotel/bar. Alternatively use Rosiére steps to the S; or ⚓ in the bight to W of Rosiére steps. Speed limit is 6kn. Other ⚓s are on the E coast in Belvoir and Shell bays.

Note: JETHOU, CREVICHON and GRANDE FAUCONNIERE islands are private and landing is forbidden.

SARK (See overleaf)

All moorings are private; use in emergency only. ⚓s (clock-wise from Creux) are unlit but safe in settled weather and off-shore winds:

LES LACHES, (outside Creux hbr) ⚓ E of white patch on pier. Note: Goulet passage is for N-bound traffic only.

DERRIBLE BAY. Good shelter and good holding on sand.

DIXCART BAY. Sandy and sheltered; good holding. 2 hotels.

ROUGE TERRIER, (in Little Sark). Sandy with cliff path to hotel.

CLOUET BAY, (good departure point for l'Etac). LW ⚓; swell unpleasant at HW.

PORT GOREY. Remains of quay exists but ⚓ in bay.

LES FONTAINES BAY. SW-facing small bay.

LA GRANDE GREVE. Big sandy bay with small drying rk in centre. Exposed to SW winds. Pub at cliff top.

HAVRE GOSSELIN. A safe small ⚓, exposed to SW winds. Crowded in summer. Landing, plus many steps.

PORT À LA JUMENT. Shingle bay with good holding.

PORT DU MOULIN. Shingle bay.

LES FONTAINES BAY. Exposed to NE winds.

GREVE DE LA VILLE. Sand and shingle close into stone steps with access to village at cliff top.

LITTLE RUSSEL CHANNEL   10-14-12

See 10.14.5

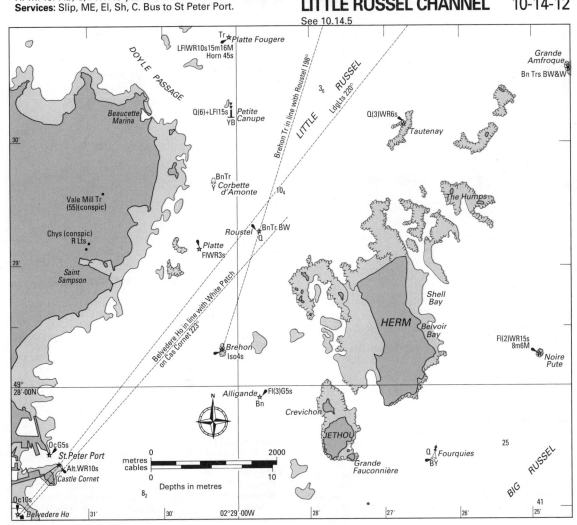

SARK   10-14-13

Sark (Channel Islands) 49°25'·87N 02°20'·35W (Creux)

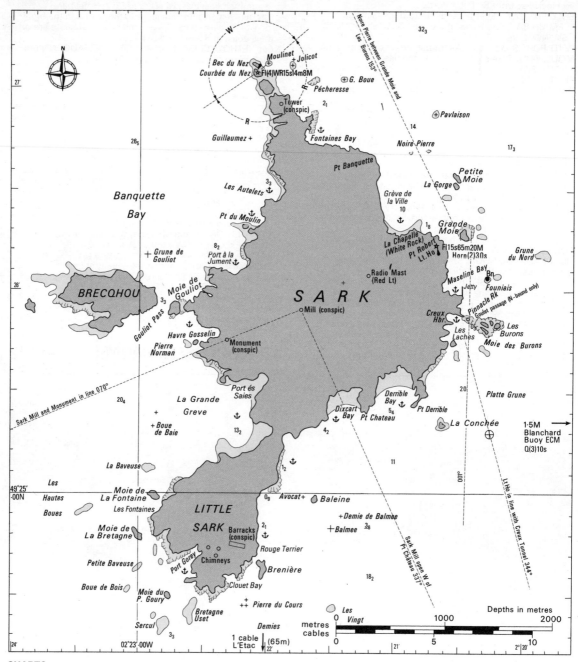

CHARTS
AC *808*; SHOM 6904; ECM 1014; Imray C33A; Stanfords 16
TIDES
−0450 Dover; ML 4·9; Duration 0550; Zone 0 (UT)

Standard Port ST HELIER (→)

Times				Height (metres)			
High Water		Low Water		MHWS	MHWN	MLWN	MLWS
0300	0900	0200	0900	11·0	8·1	4·0	1·4
1500	2100	1400	2100				
Differences SARK (MASELINE PIER)							
+0005	+0015	+0005	+0010	−2·1	−1·5	−0·6	−0·3

SHELTER
Many ⚓s (see overleaf) sheltered in various winds, but may be disturbed, except in settled wx. Only hbrs are Creux (dries) and Maseline. No AB at quay when ships due, or if boat is unattended. Do not stay in Creux (except to land people) unless authorised by Hr Mr or Tourist Office.

NAVIGATION
Creux WPT 49°25'·30N 02°20'·30W, 164°/344° from/to ent, 0·57M. Beware large tidal range, strong streams and many lobster pots. Sark is fringed by rks, but the centres of the bays are mainly clear of dangers.
LIGHTS AND MARKS
From S, Pinnacle Rk on with E side of Grand Moie at 001°; or W patch on Creux pier hd in line 350° with Pt Robert lt ho, Fl 15s 65m 20M; W 8-sided tr; vis 138°-353°; horn (2) 30s.
RADIO TELEPHONE
VHF Ch 74 occas; call *Tango Oscar* (Tourist Office).
TELEPHONE (01481)
Hr Mr 832323; ⌗ (Guernsey) 726911; Marinecall 0898 500457; Police (Guernsey) 725111; Dr 832045.
FACILITIES
Creux ☎ 832025, Slip, M, L, FW, C (1 ton), AB;
Maseline ☎ 832070, M, C (3 ton); **Services:** Gas, Gaz, Kos.
Village P & D (cans), V, R, Bar, ✉, Ⓑ. Ferry to Guernsey. Condor catamaran to Jersey and St Malo.

CHANNEL ISLANDS – ST. HELIER

LAT 49°11′N   LONG 2°07′W

TIMES AND HEIGHTS OF HIGH AND LOW WATERS   YEAR **1996**

TIME ZONE (UT)
For Summer Time add ONE hour in non-shaded areas

JANUARY

Day	Time	m	Time	m	Time	m	Time	m
1 M	0245	8.6	0928	3.9	1520	8.7	2153	3.7
16 TU	0136	8.6	0823	3.6	1414	8.7	2101	3.4
2 TU	0347	9.0	1030	3.6	1617	9.1	2249	3.3
17 W	0301	9.0	0944	3.1	1536	9.1	2217	2.9
3 W	0438	9.4	1121	3.2	1706	9.5	2336	2.9
18 TH	0414	9.6	1054	2.5	1646	9.8	2323	2.2
4 TH	0522	9.9	1205	2.7	1748	9.9		
19 F	0515	10.4	1156	1.7	1744	10.6		
5 F O	0018	2.6	0601	10.3	1245	2.4	1826	10.2
20 SA ●	0022	1.5	0608	11.2	1253	1.0	1835	11.2
6 SA	0057	2.3	0638	10.5	1322	2.2	1903	10.3
21 SU	0115	1.0	0656	11.7	1344	0.5	1921	11.7
7 SU	0134	2.2	0713	10.6	1358	2.1	1937	10.3
22 M	0204	0.7	0741	12.0	1430	0.8	2005	11.8
8 M	0209	2.2	0747	10.5	1432	2.1	2009	10.2
23 TU	0249	0.6	0824	12.0	1513	0.5	2046	11.6
9 TU	0242	2.3	0818	10.3	1503	2.2	2040	10.0
24 W	0330	0.9	0905	11.6	1553	0.9	2125	11.2
10 W	0312	2.5	0848	10.1	1532	2.4	2110	9.7
25 TH	0409	1.5	0944	11.0	1630	1.6	2204	10.5
11 TH	0342	2.7	0919	9.8	1603	2.7	2142	9.5
26 F	0446	2.3	1024	10.2	1707	2.4	2243	9.7
12 F	0416	3.0	0956	9.5	1639	2.9	2222	9.2
27 SA	0524	3.1	1107	9.3	1748	3.2	2327	8.9
13 SA	0457	3.2	1041	9.2	1723	3.2	2312	8.9
28 SU	0610	3.8	1200	8.6	1839	3.9		
14 SU	0550	3.5	1138	8.9	1820	3.5		
29 M	0027	8.3	0711	4.3	1313	8.1	1946	4.3
15 M	0015	8.6	0659	3.7	1251	8.6	1934	3.6
30 TU	0151	8.1	0830	4.4	1440	8.0	2105	4.2
31 W	0312	8.3	0952	4.1	1551	8.4	2215	3.8

FEBRUARY

Day	Time	m	Time	m	Time	m	Time	m
1 TH	0413	8.8	1053	3.6	1644	9.0	2309	3.3
16 F	0401	9.2	1039	2.5	1636	9.4	2310	2.1
2 F	0501	9.4	1141	3.0	1728	9.5	2354	2.7
17 SA	0505	10.1	1144	1.7	1734	10.3		
3 SA	0542	10.0	1223	2.5	1807	10.0		
18 SU ●	0010	1.5	0557	11.0	1240	0.9	1823	11.1
4 SU O	0036	2.3	0619	10.4	1303	2.0	1843	10.3
19 M	0103	0.8	0644	11.7	1330	0.3	1907	11.7
5 M	0116	2.0	0655	10.6	1341	1.8	1918	10.5
20 TU	0150	0.4	0727	12.1	1415	0.1	1948	11.9
6 TU	0154	1.8	0730	10.7	1416	1.7	1951	10.6
21 W	0233	0.3	0807	12.1	1456	0.2	2026	11.8
7 W	0228	1.8	0801	10.7	1448	1.7	2021	10.4
22 TH	0311	0.5	0844	11.8	1530	0.6	2101	11.3
8 TH	0258	1.9	0831	10.5	1516	1.8	2051	10.2
23 F	0345	1.1	0919	11.1	1602	1.3	2134	10.7
9 F	0327	2.0	0901	10.3	1545	2.1	2122	10.0
24 SA	0416	1.9	0953	10.3	1632	2.2	2206	9.9
10 SA	0358	2.3	0935	10.0	1617	2.4	2157	9.7
25 SU	0445	2.8	1027	9.4	1704	3.1	2242	9.0
11 SU	0434	2.7	1016	9.6	1655	2.9	2241	9.2
26 M	0520	3.6	1110	8.5	1745	3.8	2329	8.3
12 M	0519	3.1	1107	9.1	1746	3.2	2339	8.8
27 TU	0613	4.3	1214	7.8	1849	4.4		
13 TU	0622	3.5	1216	8.6	1858	3.6		
28 W	0046	7.7	0734	4.6	1351	7.6	2015	4.5
14 W	0059	8.4	0751	3.6	1347	8.2	2032	3.6
29 TH	0228	7.8	0905	4.4	1520	7.9	2135	4.1
15 TH	0238	8.6	0922	3.3	1521	8.7	2159	3.1

MARCH

Day	Time	m	Time	m	Time	m	Time	m
1 F	0343	8.3	1020	3.8	1618	8.5	2238	3.5
16 SA	0346	9.1	1023	2.4	1622	9.3	2253	2.2
2 SA	0434	9.0	1112	3.1	1702	9.2	2327	2.8
17 SU	0449	10.0	1126	1.6	1717	10.2	2352	1.4
3 SU	0517	9.7	1157	2.4	1742	9.8		
18 M	0540	10.8	1221	0.9	1805	10.9		
4 M	0011	2.2	0555	10.2	1239	1.9	1818	10.3
19 TU ●	0044	0.8	0625	11.4	1310	0.3	1847	11.5
5 TU O	0053	1.8	0632	10.6	1318	1.5	1854	10.6
20 W	0131	0.3	0707	11.8	1353	0.1	1926	11.7
6 W	0132	1.5	0707	10.9	1354	1.3	1927	10.8
21 TH	0212	0.2	0745	11.8	1431	0.2	2002	11.6
7 TH	0207	1.3	0740	10.9	1426	1.3	1959	10.8
22 F	0249	0.5	0821	11.5	1505	0.7	2035	11.2
8 F	0239	1.3	0811	10.9	1456	1.4	2029	10.7
23 SA	0320	1.0	0854	10.9	1534	1.3	2105	10.6
9 SA	0310	1.5	0842	10.7	1526	1.6	2101	10.4
24 SU	0348	1.8	0925	10.1	1601	2.1	2135	9.9
10 SU	0341	1.8	0917	10.3	1558	2.0	2136	10.0
25 M	0413	2.6	0956	9.3	1627	2.9	2205	9.1
11 M	0416	2.2	0957	9.8	1635	2.5	2220	9.4
26 TU	0442	3.3	1031	8.5	1702	3.7	2244	8.3
12 TU	0500	2.7	1048	9.1	1725	3.0	2317	8.8
27 W	0525	4.0	1125	7.7	1756	4.3	2348	7.7
13 W	0603	3.2	1159	8.4	1839	3.5		
28 TH	0642	4.5	1257	7.2	1924	4.6		
14 TH	0041	8.3	0733	3.5	1334	8.2	2016	3.6
29 F	0130	7.5	0814	4.4	1435	7.6	2049	4.3
15 F	0222	8.4	0906	3.1	1510	8.5	2143	3.0
30 SA	0258	7.9	0933	3.9	1541	8.2	2157	3.7
31 SU	0357	8.6	1032	3.2	1629	8.9	2251	3.0

APRIL

Day	Time	m	Time	m	Time	m	Time	m
1 M	0443	9.3	1121	2.5	1710	9.6	2339	2.3
16 TU	0517	10.4	1156	1.2	1741	10.7		
2 TU	0525	9.9	1205	1.9	1749	10.2		
17 W ●	0021	1.1	0602	11.0	1245	0.8	1822	11.1
3 W	0023	1.8	0604	10.5	1247	1.5	1825	10.6
18 TH	0108	0.7	0644	11.2	1328	0.6	1901	11.3
4 TH O	0104	1.3	0640	10.9	1325	1.2	1900	11.0
19 F	0149	0.7	0723	11.3	1407	0.7	1937	11.3
5 F	0142	1.1	0716	11.1	1401	1.0	1934	11.1
20 SA	0225	0.8	0759	11.0	1440	1.1	2010	11.0
6 SA	0218	1.0	0750	11.1	1434	1.1	2008	11.0
21 SU	0257	1.3	0831	10.6	1508	1.6	2040	10.5
7 SU	0253	1.1	0826	10.9	1508	1.3	2044	10.7
22 M	0323	1.8	0902	9.9	1534	2.2	2109	9.8
8 M	0328	1.4	0904	10.5	1544	1.8	2123	10.3
23 TU	0348	2.5	0932	9.2	1600	2.9	2139	9.2
9 TU	0406	1.9	0947	9.8	1625	2.3	2209	9.6
24 W	0416	3.1	1005	8.5	1632	3.5	2214	8.5
10 W	0454	2.5	1042	9.1	1718	3.0	2310	8.9
25 TH	0454	3.7	1049	7.9	1718	4.0	2304	8.0
11 TH	0600	3.0	1154	8.5	1835	3.4		
26 F	0553	4.1	1201	7.5	1830	4.4		
12 F	0032	8.5	0725	3.2	1324	8.3	2004	3.4
27 SA	0025	7.7	0718	4.2	1333	7.6	1956	4.3
13 SA	0203	8.6	0849	2.9	1451	8.7	2124	2.9
28 SU	0155	7.8	0836	3.9	1448	8.0	2107	3.8
14 SU	0323	9.1	1001	2.3	1600	9.3	2231	2.2
29 M	0305	8.3	0941	3.3	1545	8.6	2206	3.2
15 M	0425	9.8	1102	1.7	1654	10.0	2329	1.6
30 TU	0400	9.0	1037	2.7	1632	9.3	2259	2.5

14

Chart Datum: 5·88 metres below Ordnance Datum (Local)

CHANNEL ISLANDS – ST. HELIER

LAT 49°11'N   LONG   2°07'W

TIMES AND HEIGHTS OF HIGH AND LOW WATERS

YEAR **1996**

TIME ZONE (UT)
For Summer Time add ONE hour in non-shaded areas

Chart Datum: 5·88 metres below Ordnance Datum (Local)

MAY

Day	Time	m	Day	Time	m
1 W	0448 / 1126 / 1715 / 2348	9.6 / 2.1 / 10.0 / 1.9	**16** TH	0538 / 1218 / 1757	10.3 / 1.5 / 10.5
2 TH	0532 / 1212 / 1756	10.3 / 1.6 / 10.6	**17** F ●	0043 / 0621 / 1303 / 1837	1.5 / 10.6 / 1.4 / 10.8
3 F O	0034 / 0613 / 1256 / 1834	1.4 / 10.8 / 1.2 / 11.0	**18** SA	0126 / 0701 / 1342 / 1914	1.3 / 10.6 / 1.4 / 10.8
4 SA	0117 / 0653 / 1337 / 1913	1.0 / 11.1 / 1.0 / 11.3	**19** SU	0202 / 0738 / 1416 / 1948	1.4 / 10.5 / 1.6 / 10.7
5 SU	0159 / 0733 / 1417 / 1952	0.9 / 11.2 / 1.0 / 11.3	**20** M	0234 / 0812 / 1445 / 2019	1.6 / 10.2 / 1.9 / 10.3
6 M	0239 / 0814 / 1456 / 2033	0.9 / 11.0 / 1.2 / 11.0	**21** TU	0303 / 0843 / 1513 / 2049	2.0 / 9.8 / 2.3 / 9.9
7 TU	0320 / 0857 / 1537 / 2117	1.2 / 10.6 / 1.6 / 10.5	**22** W	0330 / 0914 / 1540 / 2120	2.4 / 9.3 / 2.8 / 9.4
8 W	0404 / 0945 / 1624 / 2207	1.5 / 10.0 / 2.2 / 9.9	**23** TH	0358 / 0946 / 1611 / 2153	2.6 / 8.8 / 3.2 / 8.9
9 TH	0456 / 1041 / 1720 / 2307	2.2 / 9.4 / 2.8 / 9.3	**24** F	0432 / 1025 / 1651 / 2235	3.3 / 8.4 / 3.6 / 8.4
10 F	0559 / 1148 / 1830	2.6 / 8.9 / 3.1	**25** SA	0518 / 1115 / 1745 / 2332	3.6 / 8.0 / 3.9 / 8.1
11 SA	0019 / 0712 / 1305 / 1947	8.9 / 2.8 / 8.7 / 3.2	**26** SU	0621 / 1223 / 1858	3.8 / 7.9 / 4.0
12 SU	0138 / 0826 / 1423 / 2100	8.8 / 2.8 / 8.8 / 2.9	**27** M	0044 / 0735 / 1339 / 2012	8.0 / 3.8 / 8.0 / 3.8
13 M	0253 / 0933 / 1530 / 2205	9.1 / 2.5 / 9.2 / 2.5	**28** TU	0159 / 0845 / 1448 / 2118	8.3 / 3.5 / 8.5 / 3.4
14 TU	0356 / 1034 / 1625 / 2303	9.5 / 2.1 / 9.7 / 2.1	**29** W	0307 / 0949 / 1548 / 2218	8.7 / 3.0 / 9.1 / 2.8
15 W	0450 / 1128 / 1714 / 2355	9.9 / 1.8 / 10.2 / 1.7	**30** TH	0407 / 1047 / 1640 / 2314	9.3 / 2.4 / 9.8 / 2.2
			31 F	0500 / 1140 / 1728	10.0 / 1.9 / 10.4

JUNE

Day	Time	m	Day	Time	m
1 SA O	0006 / 0549 / 1231 / 1813	1.6 / 10.5 / 1.4 / 11.0	**16** SU ●	0101 / 0640 / 1317 / 1852	2.0 / 10.1 / 2.0 / 10.4
2 SU	0056 / 0636 / 1318 / 1857	1.1 / 11.0 / 1.1 / 11.3	**17** M	0139 / 0718 / 1352 / 1928	1.9 / 10.2 / 2.0 / 10.5
3 M	0144 / 0721 / 1404 / 1941	0.8 / 11.2 / 1.0 / 11.5	**18** TU	0213 / 0753 / 1425 / 2001	1.9 / 10.1 / 2.1 / 10.3
4 TU	0230 / 0807 / 1449 / 2026	0.8 / 11.2 / 1.1 / 11.3	**19** W	0245 / 0826 / 1456 / 2033	2.1 / 9.9 / 2.3 / 10.0
5 W	0316 / 0853 / 1535 / 2112	0.9 / 10.9 / 1.4 / 11.0	**20** TH	0315 / 0858 / 1525 / 2104	2.3 / 9.6 / 2.5 / 9.7
6 TH	0403 / 0942 / 1623 / 2202	1.3 / 10.5 / 1.9 / 10.5	**21** F	0344 / 0929 / 1555 / 2135	2.6 / 9.2 / 2.8 / 9.3
7 F	0453 / 1034 / 1715 / 2256	1.8 / 9.9 / 2.4 / 9.9	**22** SA	0414 / 1002 / 1629 / 2210	2.9 / 8.9 / 3.2 / 9.0
8 SA	0548 / 1131 / 1815 / 2357	2.3 / 9.4 / 2.8 / 9.4	**23** SU	0451 / 1041 / 1711 / 2255	3.1 / 8.6 / 3.4 / 8.7
9 SU	0650 / 1235 / 1920	2.7 / 9.0 / 3.1	**24** M	0537 / 1131 / 1806 / 2351	3.4 / 8.4 / 3.7 / 8.5
10 M	0104 / 0755 / 1346 / 2028	9.0 / 2.9 / 8.9 / 3.2	**25** TU	0636 / 1234 / 1915	3.5 / 8.3 / 3.7
11 TU	0216 / 0900 / 1454 / 2133	8.9 / 2.9 / 9.0 / 3.1	**26** W	0100 / 0748 / 1348 / 2030	8.4 / 3.5 / 8.4 / 3.5
12 W	0323 / 1002 / 1554 / 2234	9.0 / 2.8 / 9.2 / 2.8	**27** TH	0215 / 0903 / 1503 / 2140	8.6 / 3.3 / 8.8 / 3.1
13 TH	0423 / 1100 / 1647 / 2329	9.3 / 2.6 / 9.6 / 2.5	**28** F	0328 / 1012 / 1608 / 2245	9.0 / 2.8 / 9.5 / 2.5
14 F	0514 / 1151 / 1733	9.6 / 2.4 / 10.0	**29** SA	0433 / 1114 / 1706 / 2344	9.6 / 2.2 / 10.2 / 1.8
15 SA	0018 / 0559 / 1237 / 1814	2.2 / 9.9 / 2.1 / 10.3	**30** SU	0531 / 1211 / 1758	10.3 / 1.6 / 10.8

JULY

Day	Time	m	Day	Time	m
1 M O	0039 / 0623 / 1305 / 1846	1.2 / 10.8 / 1.2 / 11.4	**16** TU	0115 / 0657 / 1329 / 1907	2.1 / 10.1 / 2.1 / 10.5
2 TU	0132 / 0713 / 1355 / 1933	0.9 / 11.3 / 0.9 / 11.7	**17** W	0151 / 0732 / 1405 / 1942	2.0 / 10.2 / 2.0 / 10.5
3 W	0221 / 0800 / 1442 / 2019	0.6 / 11.4 / 0.8 / 11.7	**18** TH	0226 / 0806 / 1438 / 2014	1.9 / 10.1 / 2.0 / 10.3
4 TH	0309 / 0845 / 1528 / 2104	0.6 / 11.3 / 1.0 / 11.5	**19** F	0258 / 0838 / 1509 / 2045	2.0 / 9.9 / 2.2 / 10.1
5 F	0354 / 0931 / 1613 / 2149	0.9 / 11.0 / 1.4 / 11.0	**20** SA	0326 / 0907 / 1537 / 2114	2.2 / 9.7 / 2.4 / 9.8
6 SA	0439 / 1017 / 1659 / 2236	1.4 / 10.5 / 2.0 / 10.3	**21** SU	0354 / 0937 / 1607 / 2145	2.5 / 9.4 / 2.7 / 9.5
7 SU	0526 / 1105 / 1747 / 2327	2.0 / 9.8 / 2.6 / 9.6	**22** M	0425 / 1010 / 1643 / 2224	2.7 / 9.1 / 3.0 / 9.2
8 M	0616 / 1158 / 1842	2.7 / 9.2 / 3.2	**23** TU	0503 / 1052 / 1727 / 2312	3.0 / 8.8 / 3.3 / 8.9
9 TU	0025 / 0713 / 1302 / 1945	9.0 / 3.2 / 8.7 / 3.6	**24** W	0553 / 1147 / 1826	3.3 / 8.6 / 3.6
10 W	0134 / 0819 / 1413 / 2056	8.6 / 3.5 / 8.6 / 3.7	**25** TH	0015 / 0658 / 1300 / 1945	8.6 / 3.5 / 8.4 / 3.6
11 TH	0248 / 0927 / 1522 / 2204	8.5 / 3.6 / 8.7 / 3.5	**26** F	0134 / 0822 / 1426 / 2109	8.5 / 3.5 / 8.6 / 3.3
12 F	0355 / 1030 / 1621 / 2303	8.7 / 3.3 / 9.1 / 3.2	**27** SA	0259 / 0944 / 1544 / 2222	8.7 / 3.1 / 9.1 / 2.7
13 SA	0451 / 1124 / 1710 / 2352	9.1 / 3.0 / 9.5 / 2.8	**28** SU	0415 / 1054 / 1650 / 2327	9.3 / 2.5 / 9.9 / 2.0
14 SU	0538 / 1210 / 1753	9.5 / 2.6 / 10.0	**29** M	0519 / 1156 / 1746	10.0 / 1.8 / 10.7
15 M ●	0036 / 0619 / 1251 / 1831	2.4 / 9.9 / 2.3 / 10.3	**30** TU O	0025 / 0613 / 1252 / 1835	1.3 / 10.8 / 1.1 / 11.4
			31 W O	0119 / 0701 / 1343 / 1922	0.7 / 11.4 / 0.6 / 11.9

AUGUST

Day	Time	m	Day	Time	m
1 TH	0209 / 0747 / 1430 / 2005	0.3 / 11.7 / 0.4 / 12.0	**16** F	0202 / 0741 / 1416 / 1951	1.7 / 10.4 / 1.7 / 10.6
2 F	0254 / 0830 / 1513 / 2047	0.3 / 11.7 / 0.6 / 11.8	**17** SA	0235 / 0813 / 1447 / 2021	1.7 / 10.3 / 1.8 / 10.4
3 SA	0336 / 0911 / 1554 / 2128	0.5 / 11.4 / 1.0 / 11.3	**18** SU	0303 / 0841 / 1516 / 2049	1.9 / 10.1 / 2.0 / 10.2
4 SU	0416 / 0951 / 1633 / 2209	1.1 / 10.8 / 1.7 / 10.6	**19** M	0330 / 0909 / 1544 / 2119	2.1 / 9.8 / 2.3 / 9.9
5 M	0454 / 1032 / 1711 / 2252	1.9 / 10.0 / 2.5 / 9.7	**20** TU	0359 / 0940 / 1616 / 2155	2.4 / 9.5 / 2.6 / 9.5
6 TU	0534 / 1116 / 1755 / 2342	2.8 / 9.2 / 3.3 / 8.9	**21** W	0434 / 1019 / 1656 / 2240	2.8 / 9.1 / 3.0 / 9.0
7 W	0623 / 1212 / 1852	3.6 / 8.5 / 4.0	**22** TH	0519 / 1111 / 1751 / 2343	3.2 / 8.7 / 3.4 / 8.5
8 TH	0048 / 0727 / 1328 / 2009	8.2 / 4.1 / 8.1 / 4.3	**23** F	0622 / 1225 / 1911	3.6 / 8.3 / 3.7
9 F	0212 / 0847 / 1449 / 2134	8.0 / 4.2 / 8.2 / 4.1	**24** SA	0107 / 0752 / 1402 / 2045	8.2 / 3.7 / 8.4 / 3.5
10 SA	0329 / 1000 / 1555 / 2238	8.3 / 3.9 / 8.7 / 3.6	**25** SU	0242 / 0924 / 1528 / 2205	8.4 / 3.3 / 8.9 / 2.8
11 SU	0428 / 1056 / 1647 / 2326	8.8 / 3.3 / 9.2 / 3.0	**26** M	0402 / 1038 / 1635 / 2312	9.1 / 2.6 / 9.8 / 2.0
12 M	0514 / 1143 / 1729	9.3 / 2.8 / 9.8	**27** TU	0505 / 1140 / 1731	10.0 / 1.8 / 10.7
13 TU	0009 / 0554 / 1225 / 1808	2.5 / 9.8 / 2.3 / 10.3	**28** W O	0009 / 0557 / 1236 / 1819	1.2 / 10.8 / 1.0 / 11.5
14 W ●	0049 / 0632 / 1304 / 1844	2.1 / 10.2 / 2.0 / 10.6	**29** TH	0102 / 0644 / 1326 / 1904	0.5 / 11.4 / 0.5 / 12.0
15 TH	0127 / 0707 / 1341 / 1919	1.8 / 10.4 / 1.8 / 10.7	**30** F	0149 / 0727 / 1411 / 1946	0.2 / 11.8 / 0.3 / 12.2
			31 SA	0232 / 0808 / 1452 / 2025	0.1 / 11.8 / 0.4 / 11.9

CHANNEL ISLANDS – ST. HELIER

LAT 49°11'N LONG 2°07'W

TIMES AND HEIGHTS OF HIGH AND LOW WATERS YEAR **1996**

TIME ZONE (UT)
For Summer Time add ONE hour in non-shaded areas

Chart Datum: 5·88 metres below Ordnance Datum (Local)

SEPTEMBER

Day	Time	m	Day	Time	m
1 SU	0311	0.5	**16** M	0236	1.7
	0846	11.5		0812	10.5
	1529	0.9		1451	1.7
	2103	11.4		2023	10.5
2 M	0346	1.1	**17** TU	0304	1.9
	0921	10.9		0841	10.2
	1602	1.6		1521	2.0
	2139	10.6		2055	10.2
3 TU	0419	2.0	**18** W	0334	2.2
	0956	10.1		0913	9.8
	1634	2.5		1554	2.4
	2216	9.6		2131	9.7
4 W	0451	2.9	**19** TH	0409	2.7
	1034	9.2		0952	9.3
	1708	3.4		1634	2.9
	2259	8.7		2217	9.1
5 TH	0531	3.8	**20** F	0454	3.2
	1123	8.4		1046	8.8
	1758	4.1		1729	3.4
				2322	8.5
6 F	0001	8.0	**21** SA	0559	3.7
	0633	4.4		1206	8.3
	1239	7.9		1852	3.7
	1916	4.6			
7 SA	0133	7.6	**22** SU	0054	8.1
	0801	4.6		0735	3.8
	1414	7.9		1346	8.4
	2056	4.4		2029	3.4
8 SU	0302	7.9	**23** M	0230	8.4
	0927	4.2		0908	3.4
	1527	8.4		1511	9.0
	2209	3.8		2149	2.7
9 M	0401	8.5	**24** TU	0347	9.2
	1027	3.6		1021	2.6
	1619	9.0		1617	9.8
	2258	3.2		2253	1.9
10 TU	0446	9.2	**25** W	0447	10.0
	1113	2.9		1121	1.7
	1701	9.7		1711	10.7
	2339	2.5		2349	1.2
11 W	0526	9.8	**26** TH	0537	10.8
	1155	2.4		1215	1.0
	1740	10.2		1759	11.4
12 TH	0019	2.1	**27** F	0039	0.6
	0602	10.2		0621	11.4
	1236	1.9		1304	0.6
	● 1816	10.6		○ 1842	11.8
13 F	0058	1.7	**28** SA	0125	0.3
	0638	10.5		0703	11.7
	1314	1.7		1348	0.4
	1851	10.8		1923	12.0
14 SA	0134	1.6	**29** SU	0207	0.3
	0712	10.7		0742	11.8
	1350	1.5		1427	0.5
	1924	10.9		2001	11.8
15 SU	0206	1.5	**30** M	0244	0.7
	0743	10.6		0818	11.4
	1422	1.6		1502	1.0
	1954	10.8		2036	11.2

OCTOBER

Day	Time	m	Day	Time	m
1 TU	0316	1.4	**16** W	0242	1.8
	0851	10.8		0818	10.6
	1533	1.7		1503	1.8
	2110	10.5		2036	10.4
2 W	0345	2.2	**17** TH	0315	2.1
	0923	10.1		0854	10.2
	1600	2.5		1539	2.2
	2143	9.6		2116	9.9
3 TH	0413	3.0	**18** F	0353	2.6
	0956	9.2		0937	9.6
	1629	3.4		1622	2.7
	2221	8.7		2206	9.2
4 F	0447	3.8	**19** SA	0441	3.2
	1038	8.4		1035	9.0
	1712	4.1		1720	3.2
	2316	7.9		2315	8.6
5 SA	0540	4.5	**20** SU	0550	3.7
	1147	7.8		1156	8.6
	1824	4.6		1842	3.5
6 SU	0046	7.5	**21** M	0043	8.4
	0708	4.8		0724	3.8
	1327	7.7		1329	8.6
	2001	4.6		2012	3.3
7 M	0223	7.7	**22** TU	0213	8.6
	0840	4.5		0850	3.3
	1447	8.1		1449	9.1
	2125	4.1		2128	2.7
8 TU	0326	8.3	**23** W	0325	9.3
	0947	3.9		1000	2.6
	1543	8.8		1553	9.8
	2220	3.4		2230	2.0
9 W	0412	9.0	**24** TH	0423	10.0
	1037	3.2		1059	1.9
	1627	9.5		1647	10.5
	2304	2.7		2325	1.4
10 TH	0452	9.7	**25** F	0512	10.7
	1122	2.5		1152	1.4
	1707	10.1		1735	11.1
	2345	2.2			
11 F	0530	10.2	**26** SA	0014	1.0
	1203	2.1		0556	11.2
	1745	10.5		1240	1.0
				○ 1819	11.4
12 SA	0024	1.8	**27** SU	0100	0.8
	0606	10.6		0638	11.5
	1243	1.7		1324	0.8
	● 1821	10.9		1900	11.5
13 SU	0102	1.5	**28** M	0141	0.9
	0640	10.9		0716	11.5
	1321	1.5		1404	0.9
	1855	11.0		1938	11.4
14 M	0137	1.5	**29** TU	0218	1.2
	0713	10.9		0752	11.2
	1356	1.4		1438	1.3
	1928	11.0		2013	10.9
15 TU	0209	1.5	**30** W	0249	1.7
	0745	10.9		0825	10.7
	1429	1.5		1507	1.9
	2001	10.8		2045	10.3
			31 TH	0317	2.4
				0855	10.1
				1534	2.6
				2117	9.6

NOVEMBER

Day	Time	m	Day	Time	m
1 F	0344	3.1	**16** SA	0349	2.5
	0927	9.4		0934	10.1
	1603	3.3		1620	2.4
	2152	8.8		2204	9.6
2 SA	0416	3.7	**17** SU	0440	3.0
	1003	8.7		1032	9.5
	1640	3.9		1718	2.9
	2237	8.1		2308	9.1
3 SU	0500	4.3	**18** M	0547	3.4
	1056	8.1		1143	9.1
	1736	4.4		1830	3.2
	2347	7.7			
4 M	0612	4.7	**19** TU	0023	8.8
	1220	7.8		0706	3.6
	1859	4.6		1303	9.0
				1947	3.2
5 TU	0120	7.7	**20** W	0144	8.9
	0739	4.7		0825	3.3
	1348	7.9		1418	9.2
	2021	4.3		2100	2.9
6 W	0235	8.1	**21** TH	0255	9.3
	0853	4.2		0933	2.9
	1454	8.4		1525	9.6
	2127	3.7		2203	2.5
7 TH	0329	8.7	**22** F	0355	9.8
	0952	3.6		1034	2.4
	1545	9.1		1622	10.1
	2220	3.1		2259	2.1
8 F	0414	9.4	**23** SA	0446	10.3
	1042	2.9		1128	2.0
	1630	9.7		1712	10.5
	2307	2.5		2350	1.8
9 SA	0455	10.0	**24** SU	0533	10.7
	1128	2.4		1218	1.7
	1712	10.3		1758	10.8
	2350	2.1			
10 SU	0534	10.6	**25** M	0037	1.6
	1211	1.9		0615	11.0
	1751	10.7		1303	1.5
				○ 1839	11.0
11 M	0031	1.7	**26** TU	0119	1.5
	0611	10.9		0654	11.1
	1253	1.5		1343	1.5
	● 1829	11.1		1918	10.9
12 TU	0111	1.5	**27** W	0155	1.7
	0648	11.2		0730	11.0
	1333	1.4		1417	1.7
	1907	11.2		1953	10.7
13 W	0149	1.5	**28** TH	0227	2.0
	0725	11.2		0804	10.7
	1412	1.4		1448	2.1
	1946	11.1		2027	10.2
14 TH	0227	1.6	**29** F	0257	2.4
	0804	11.0		0835	10.2
	1452	1.6		1516	2.5
	2027	10.7		2058	9.7
15 F	0306	2.0	**30** SA	0325	2.9
	0846	10.6		0906	9.7
	1533	1.9		1545	3.0
	2112	10.2		2131	9.2

DECEMBER

Day	Time	m	Day	Time	m
1 SU	0355	3.4	**16** M	0439	2.5
	0939	9.1		1023	10.2
	1618	3.5		1710	2.3
	2207	8.6		2253	9.7
2 M	0432	3.9	**17** TU	0535	3.0
	1019	8.6		1122	9.6
	1700	3.9		1809	2.8
	2254	8.2		2354	9.3
3 TU	0523	4.3	**18** W	0640	3.3
	1113	8.2		1229	9.3
	1758	4.2		1914	3.1
	2359	8.0			
4 W	0634	4.5	**19** TH	0105	9.0
	1226	8.1		0750	3.5
	1912	4.2		1341	9.1
				2024	3.2
5 TH	0117	8.0	**20** F	0218	9.0
	0751	4.3		0901	3.4
	1344	8.2		1452	9.2
	2025	4.0		2132	3.1
6 F	0229	8.4	**21** SA	0324	9.3
	0859	3.9		1007	3.1
	1451	8.7		1556	9.4
	2130	3.5		2233	2.9
7 SA	0327	9.0	**22** SU	0422	9.7
	0959	3.4		1106	2.7
	1547	9.2		1651	9.8
	2226	3.0		2328	2.5
8 SU	0418	9.7	**23** M	0512	10.1
	1053	2.7		1158	2.4
	1638	9.9		1739	10.1
	2317	2.4			
9 M	0504	10.3	**24** TU	0016	2.3
	1143	2.2		0556	10.5
	1725	10.5		1244	2.1
				○ 1822	10.4
10 TU	0005	1.9	**25** W	0058	2.1
	0547	10.9		0636	10.7
	1231	1.7		1324	1.9
	● 1809	10.9		1901	10.5
11 W	0051	1.6	**26** TH	0136	2.0
	0630	11.3		0713	10.8
	1317	1.3		1400	1.9
	1854	11.2		1937	10.5
12 TH	0135	1.4	**27** F	0210	2.1
	0713	11.5		0747	10.7
	1402	1.2		1432	2.0
	1938	11.3		2010	10.3
13 F	0219	1.4	**28** SA	0241	2.3
	0757	11.4		0819	10.4
	1446	1.2		1502	2.3
	2022	11.1		2042	10.0
14 SA	0303	1.6	**29** SU	0311	2.6
	0842	11.2		0850	10.0
	1531	1.5		1531	2.6
	2109	10.8		2112	9.6
15 SU	0349	2.0	**30** M	0340	2.9
	0930	10.7		0920	9.6
	1619	1.9		1600	2.9
	2158	10.3		2142	9.2
			31 TU	0411	3.3
				0951	9.2
				1632	3.3
				2216	8.8

14

ST HELIER 10-14-14

Jersey (Channel Islands) 49°10'·63N 02°06'·90W

CHARTS
AC *3278, 1137, 3655*; SHOM 6938, 7160, 7161; ECM 534,
1014; Imray C33B; Stanfords 16

TIDES
−0455 Dover; ML 6·1; Duration 0545; Zone 0 (UT)
NOTE: St Helier is a Standard Port and the tidal
predictions for each day of the year are shown above.

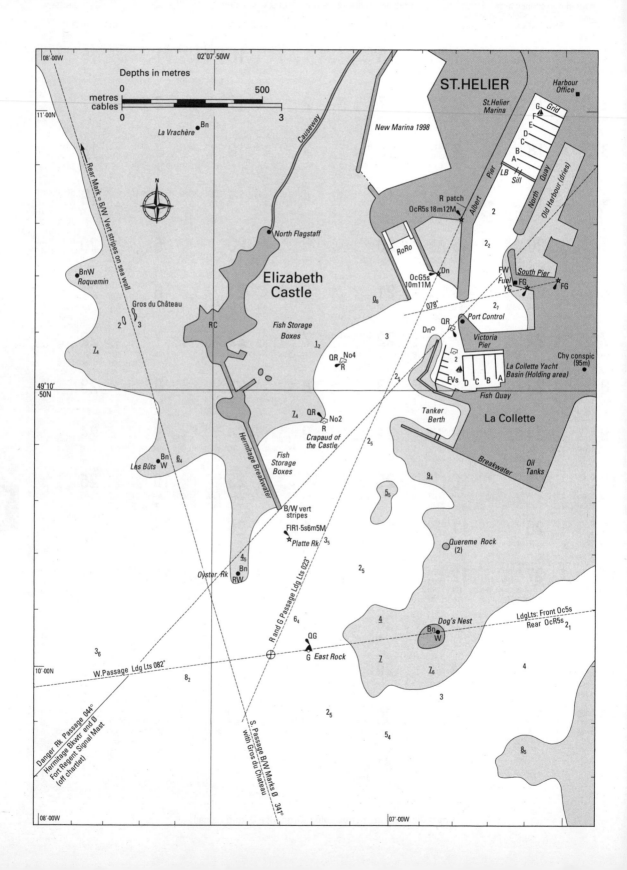

SHELTER

Excellent in **marina**, access HW±3 over sill (CD+3·6m); hinged gate rises 1·4m above sill to retain 5m. Depths in marina vary from 2·8m at ent to 2·1m at N end. **Ⓥ** berths at pontoons E, F & G; (yachts >12m LOA or >2·1m draft, use N side of pontoon A; check with staff). New marina, NW of ferry terminal, is planned to open 1998.

Good shelter in **La Collette waiting basin**, depth 1·8m; access H24. Caution: Ent narrow at LWS; keep close to W side; PHM buoys mark shoal on E side. Waiting berths on pontoon D and W side of C. FVs berth on W side of basin. No ⚓ in St Helier Rds due to shipping & fish storage boxes. Note: For other hbrs and ⚓s around Jersey, see 10.14.15.

NAVIGATION

WPT 49°10′·01N 02°07′·30W, 203°/023° from/to front ldg lt, 0·74M. This WPT is common to all eight appr chans:

(1)   W Passage (082°); beware race off Noirmont Pt, HW to HW +4.

(1A) NW Passage (095°, much used by yachts) passes 6ca S of La Corbière lt ho to join W Passage abm Noirmont Pt.

(2)   Danger Rk Passage (044°) unlit; and

(3)   Red and Green Passage (023°); both lead past rky, drying shoals (the latter over Fairway Rk 1·2m) and need precision and good vis.

(4)   Middle Passage (339°) unlit, for St Aubin Bay.

(5)   S Passage (341°) is clear but unlit. Alternatively, Demie de Pas on 350° with power stn Chy is easier to see D/N.

(6)   E Passage, 290° from Canger Rk WCM By, Q (9) 15s, passes S of Demie de Pas, B tr/Y top, Mo (D) WR 12s (at night stay in W sector); thence 314°.

(7)   Violet Passage around SE tip of Jersey, see 10.14.15.

Caution: very large tidal range, and many offlying reefs. Entering hbr, note Oyster Rk (W bn; R 'O' topmark) to W of Red and Green (R & G) Passage; and to the E, Dog's Nest Rk (W bn with globe topmark). Speed limit 10kn N of Platte Rk, and 5kn N of La Collette. Land reclamation WIP to the S and E of La Collette power stn.

LIGHTS AND MARKS

Power stn chy (95m, floodlit) and W concave roofs of Fort Regent are conspic, close E of R & G ldg line.

W Passage ldg lts: Front Oc R 5s 23m 14M; rear Oc R 5s 46m 12M and Dog's Nest bn (unlit) lead 082°, N of Les Fours NCM Q and Ruaudière SHM Fl G 3s buoys, to a

position close to E Rock SHM buoy QG, where course is altered to pick up the **Red & Green Passage** ldg lts 023°: Front Oc G 5s; rear Oc R 5s, synch; (now easier to see against town lts). Nos 2 and 4 PHM buoys (both QR) mark Small Roads chan beyond Platte Rk (Fl R 1·5s). Outer pier hds and dolphin are painted white and floodlit. Inner ldg lts 078°, both FG on W columns; not for yachts.

Entry Signals (at Port Control stn and marina)

Ⓖ lt (Oc , F or Fl)   = Enter, no exit
Ⓡ lt (Oc , F or Fl)   = Leave, no entry
Ⓡ and Ⓖ lts together   = No exit/entry

Q Ⓨ lts on Port Control Stn indicate that power-driven craft < 25m LOA may enter/dep against the displayed sigs (keeping to stbd at ent and well clear of ferries). Note: Entry sigs are repeated at marina ent, where a large digital tide gauge shows depth over sill.

RADIO TELEPHONE

Monitor *St Helier Port Control* VHF Ch 14 (H24) for ferry movements. No marina VHF, but call *Port Control* if necessary. If unable to pass messages to *Port Control*, these can be relayed via *Jersey Radio* CRS, Ch **82** 25 16 (H24) or ☎ 41121. Jersey Radio broadcasts wx forecasts on Ch 25, 82 at 0645 & 0745LT; and at 1245, 1845, 2245UT.

TELEPHONE (01534)

Hr Mr 885588, Fax 885599; Marina 885508; ⌗ 30232; Jersey Weather Centre *(06966) 7777; Recorded forecast *(06966) 0011 for Jersey and 0022 for CI; Marinecall 0898 500 457; Police 612612; Dr 835742 and 853178; Ⓗ 59000. *(06966) is a dialling code within the CI for info services.

FACILITIES

St Helier Marina (180+200 visitors), ☎ 885508, £11.00, FW, AC, CH, ME, El, Sh, Grid, Gas, Gaz, ◌, V, Kos;
La Collette Yacht Basin (130) ☎ 885529; (holding area when marina is inaccessible and a few visitors berths for up to 24 hrs), FW, AC, BH (18 ton), slip;
Hbrs Dept ☎ 885588, FW, C (various, max 32 ton), Slip, Grids, BH (18 ton), AC, **St Helier YC** ☎ 832229, R, Bar;
S Pier (below YC) P & D (Access approx HW±3), FW.
Royal Channel Islands YC, at St Aubin: see overleaf.
Services: SM, CH, Sh, ME, El, Ⓔ, Gas. **Town** EC Thurs; P, D, CH, V, R, Bar, ✉, Ⓑ, ✈. Ro Ro Ferry: Guernsey, St Malo, Weymouth. Fast ferries (Mar-Nov): St Malo, Granville, Weymouth, Sark, Guernsey.

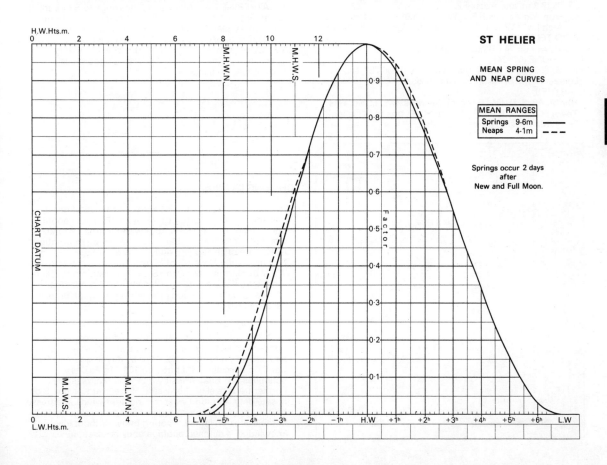

ST HELIER

MEAN SPRING AND NEAP CURVES

MEAN RANGES	
Springs	9·6m
Neaps	4·1m

Springs occur 2 days after New and Full Moon.

14

GOREY   10-14-15

Jersey (Channel Islands) 49°11'·84N 02°01'·28W

CHARTS
AC 1138, *3655*; SHOM 6939, 7157, 7160; ECM 534, 1014;
Imray C33A; Stanfords 16

TIDES
–0454 Dover; ML 6·0; Duration 0545; Zone 0 (UT)

Standard Port ST HELIER (⟵)

Times				Height (metres)			
High Water		Low Water		MHWS	MHWN	MLWN	MLWS
0300	0900	0200	0900	11·0	8·1	4·0	1·4
1500	2100	1400	2100				
Differences ST. CATHERINE BAY							
0000	+0010	+0010	+0010	0·0	–0·1	0·0	+0·1
BOULEY BAY							
+0002	+0002	+0004	+0004	–0·3	–0·3	–0·1	–0·1
LES ECREHOU							
+0005	+0009	+0011	+0009	+0·1	+0·5	–0·1	0·0
LES MINQUIERS							
–0014	–0018	–0001	–0008	+0·5	+0·6	+0·1	–0·1

SHELTER
Good in the hbr (dries completely), except in S/SE winds.
Access HW±3. There are 12 drying ⚓s 150m W of pier hd.
⚓ about 1½ca E of pier hd or in deeper water in the Roads;
also in St Catherine B to the N, except in S/SE winds.

NAVIGATION
WPT 49°10'·50N 01°57'·33W, 118°/298° from/to front ldg lt,
2·9M. Note the very large tidal range. On appr, keep well
outside all local bns until the ldg marks are identified, but
beware Banc du Chateau (0·4m) 1M offshore to N of 298°
ldg line and Azicot Rk (dries 2·2m) just S of ldg line, 2ca
from ent.
From/to St Helier the Violet Chan skirts Violet Bank, but
requires good vis and can be very rough in strong E'lies.

LIGHTS AND MARKS
(1) Ldg Its 298°: front, Gorey pier lt, Oc RG 5s 8m 12M, W
    framework tr, vis R304°-352°, G352°-304°; rear, 490m
    from front, Oc R 5s 24m 8M, W ☐ with Or border.
(2) Front ldg lt on with church spire 304° leads over Road
    Rk (3·3m), and Azicot Rk.
(3) Front ldg lt on with Fort William 250° leads close to Les
    Arch bn (B/W with A topmark) and Pacquet Rk (0·3m).

RADIO TELEPHONE
Gorey Hbr Ch 74 (HW±3 summer only).

TELEPHONE (01534)
Hr Mr 853616; ⌗ 30232; Marinecall 0898 500 457; Dr
contact Hr Mr, or Hr Mr St Helier 885588.

FACILITIES
Hbr M, AB, P, D, FW, C (7 ton); **Services:** ME, EI, Sh, Gas.
Town EC Thurs; P, CH, V, R, Bar, ✉, Ⓑ, bus to St Helier.
Ferry (Mar-Nov) to Portbail, Carteret.

OTHER HARBOURS AND ANCHORAGES AROUND JERSEY

Of the many ⚓s around the island, the following are the
main ones, clockwise from St. Helier.
ST. AUBIN, Quiet ⚓ with off-shore winds in bay (mostly
    dries) or yachts can dry out alongside N quay; access HW
    ±1. From seaward Middle Passage leads 339°, Mon
    Plaisir Ho in transit with tr at St Aubin Fort. Final appr is
    N of St. Aubin Fort, via fairway in W sector of N pier head
    dir lt 254°, F WRG 5m, G248°-253°, W253°-255°,
    R255°-260°; and, same structure, Iso R 4s 12m 10M. St
    Aubin Fort pier head Fl R 4s 8m 1M. Facilities: AB, FW on
    N quay, Slip, C (1 and 5 ton), Grid; **Royal Channel Islands
    YC**, ☎ 41023, Bar, R, M, Slip; **Services:** Sh, D, CH, BY,
    Gas, EI, ME, SM, Sh.
    Town Bar, D, FW, Ⓞ, P, R, V, buses to St. Helier.
BELCROUTE BAY, N of Noirmont Pt. Excellent shelter from
    W to SW winds, but dries 3·5m and many moorings; or ⚓
    further off in 2·4m, landing by dinghy.
PORTELET BAY, W of Noirmont Pt. Good ⚓ in N'lies, either
    side of Janvrin Tr.
ST. BRELADE BAY, Small stone pier in NW corner, local
    moorings in Bouilly Port. Good shelter from N and W,
    but open to SW'ly swell. A very popular sandy tourist
    beach with various hotels. A quiet ⚓ is in Beau Port.
GREVE AU LANCON (PLEMONT), A wide sandy bay E of
    Grosnez Pt, Fl (2) WR 15s, which covers at HW. Suitable
    for day visits on calm days. Exposed to swell. Beware
    discontinued submarine cables.
GREVE de LECQ, Ldg line 202°: ○ W tr in line with white ho
    with grey roof. Ruins extend E from present pier. Pub,
    and bus to St. Helier. Exposed to swell.
BONNE NUIT BAY, Ldg lts 223°, both FG 7/34m 6M.
    Conspic TV mast (232m) is ½M W of the bay. Avoid
    Cheval Rk (dries 10·1m) close SE of ldg line. Hbr dries to
    sand and shingle. Many local boat moorings. Hotel.
BOULEY BAY, Good ⚓. ML 5·8m. Rky bottom close to pier.
    Local boat moorings. Hotel.
ROZEL BAY, Dir lt 245° F WRG, 11m 5M, G240°-244°,
    W244°-246°, R246°-250°; W sector leads between pier
    heads and bn. Hbr dries to sand and shingle. Local boat
    moorings. Shops and pubs, bus to St. Helier.
ST. CATHERINE BAY, Many local moorings to S of Verclut
    bkwtr, Fl 1·5s 18m 13M. ML 6·0m. Beware St Catherine
    Bank, rocky plateau 3·3m in centre of bay. Landing on
    slip at root of bkwtr. Dinghy SC, RNLI ILB Station, café.
LA ROCQUE, Small pier, local boat moorings, sandy
    beach. Not suitable for visitors without good local
    knowledge. No facilities.

OFFLYING ISLANDS

LES ECREHOU, 49°17'·45N 01°55'·50W. 5M NE of Rozel,
    has about a dozen cottages. ML 6·2m. Arrive at about ½
    tide ebbing; see 10.14.15. Appr with Bigorne Rk on 022°;
    when SE of Ile Maitre alter to 330° for FS on Marmotière
    Is. Beware of strong and eddying tidal streams 4 - 8kn.
    Pick up a buoy close SE of Marmotière or ⚓ in a pool 4ca
    WSW of Marmotière (with FS and houses); other islands
    are Maitre Ile (one house), Blanche and 5 other small
    islands. Local knowledge or a detailed pilotage book is
    essential. No lts.

PLATEAU des MINQUIERS, 48°58'·10N 02°03'·63W. About
    12M S of Jersey (AC 3656) and ringed by 6 cardinal lt
    buoys. See 10.14.15 for tides. ML 6·4m. Beware of strong
    and eddying tidal streams. Appr by day in good vis from
    Demi de Vascelin SHM buoy on 161°, Jetée des
    Fontaines RW bn in transit with FS on Maîtresse Ile.
    Further transits skirt the W side of the islet to ⚓ due S of
    it; safe only in settled weather and light winds. Maitresse
    Ile has about a dozen cottages. Land at the slipway NW
    of the States of Jersey mooring buoy. Without local
    knowledge, a detailed pilotage book is essential.

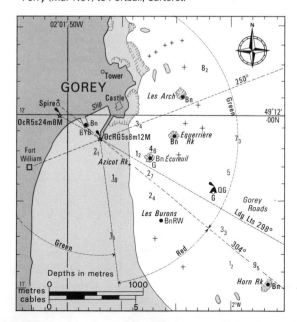

Volvo Penta service

Sales and service centres in area 15
France *Volvo Penta France SA*, 1 Rue de la Nouvelle, B. P. 49, 78133 Les
Mureaux Tel 33-1-30912799, Fax 33-1-34746415 Telex 695221 F.

**VOLVO
PENTA**

Area 15

Central North France
Pointe de Barfleur to
St. Quay-Portrieux

15

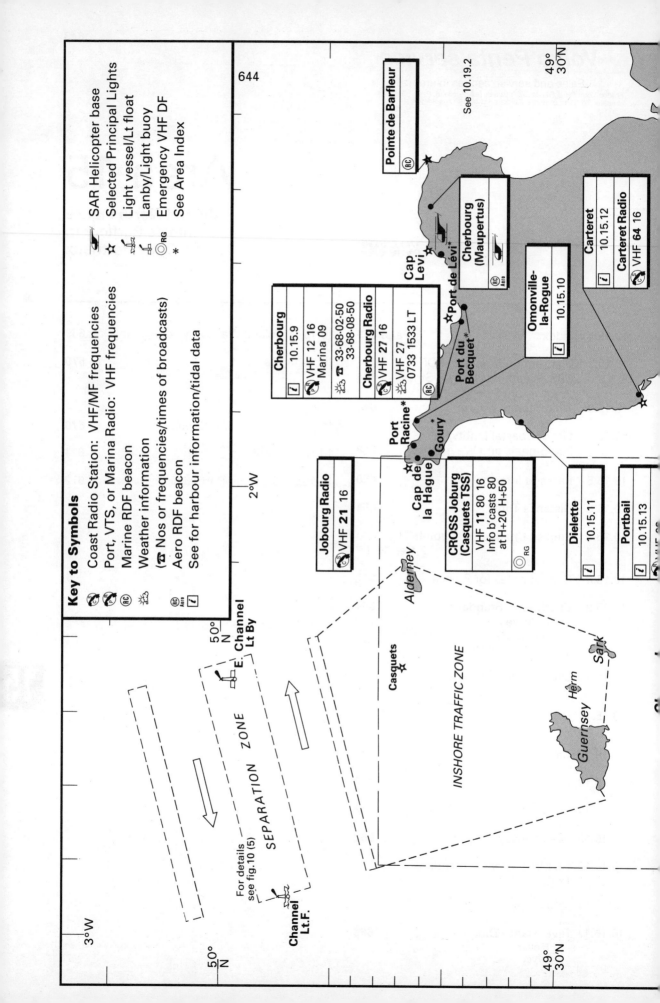

Key to Symbols

🕭	Coast Radio Station: VHF/MF frequencies
🕭	Port, VTS, or Marina Radio: VHF frequencies
⊙RC	Marine RDF beacon
🎣	Weather information
(☎ Nos or frequencies/times of broadcasts)	
⊙RC Aero	Aero RDF beacon
i	See for harbour information/tidal data

🚁	SAR Helicopter base
☆	Selected Principal Lights
🚢	Light vessel/Lt float
🛟	Lanby/Light buoy
⊙RG	Emergency VHF DF
*	See Area Index

644

Pointe de Barfleur ⊙RC

See 10.19.2

Cherbourg
10.15.9
| i |
| 🕭 VHF 12 16 Marina 09 |
| 🎣 ☎ 33·68·02·50 / 33·68·08·50 |
Cherbourg Radio
| 🕭 VHF 27 16 |
| 🎣 VHF 27 0733 1533 LT | ⊙RC

Cherbourg (Maupertus) ⊙RC Aero 🚁

Omonville-la-Rogue
10.15.10
| i |

Carteret
10.15.12
| i |
Carteret Radio
🕭 VHF 64 16

Cap Levi ☆

Port de Lévi *

Port du Becquet *

Port Racine *

Goury *

Cap de la Hague ☆

Jobourg Radio
🕭 VHF 21 16

CROSS Joburg (Casquets TSS)
VHF 11 80 16
Info b'casts 80 at H+20 H+50
⊙RG

Dielette
10.15.11
| i |

Portbail
10.15.13
| i |

Alderney

Casquets ☆

INSHORE TRAFFIC ZONE

Guernsey   Herm

Sark

SEPARATION ZONE

For details see fig.10 (5)

Channel Lt.F. 🎣

E. Channel Lt By 🛟

3°W   2°W

50° N

49° 30'N

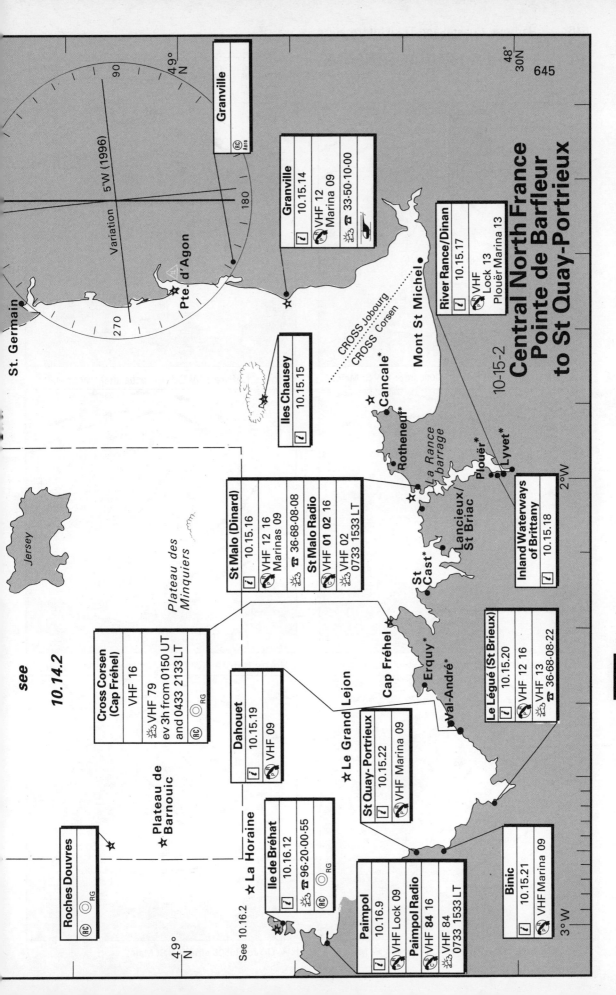

Roches Douvres
RC ◎ RG

see
10.14.2

St. Germain

☆ Plateau de Barnouic

49°
N

★ La Horaine

See 10.16.2

Jersey

Plateau des Minquiers

Cross Corsen (Cap Fréhel)
VHF 16
🔊 VHF 79 ev 3h from 0150 UT and 0433 2133 LT
RC ◎ RG

Dahouet
| *i* | 10.15.19 |
🛥 VHF 09

★ Le Grand Lejon

St Quay-Portrieux
| *i* | 10.15.22 |
🛥 VHF Marina 09

Ile de Bréhat
| *i* | 10.16.12 |
🔊 ☎ 96·20·00·55
RC ◎ RG

Paimpol
| *i* | 10.16.9 |
🛥 VHF Lock 09
Paimpol Radio
🛥 VHF 84 16
🔊 VHF 84 0733 1533 LT

Binic
| *i* | 10.15.21 |
🛥 VHF Marina 09

Le Légué (St Brieux)
| *i* | 10.15.20 |
🛥 VHF 12 16
🔊 VHF 13 ☎ 36·68·08·22

Cap Fréhel ★

● Erquy*

● Val-André*

St Cast*

Lancieux/ St Briac

Plouër*

☆ Lyvet*

Inland Waterways of Brittany
| *i* | 10.15.18 |

2°W

La Rance barrage

☆ Rotheneuf*

☆ Cancale*

● Mont St Michel

CROSS Jobourg,
CROSS Corsen

St Malo (Dinard)
| *i* | 10.15.16 |
🛥 VHF 12 16 Marinas 09
🔊 ☎ 36·68·08·08
St Malo Radio
🛥 VHF 01 02 16
🔊 VHF 02 0733 1533 LT

Iles Chausey
| *i* | 10.15.15 |

Pte. d'Agon

Variation 5°W (1996)

90
180
270

49° N

Granville
RC Aero

Granville
| *i* | 10.15.14 |
🛥 VHF 12 Marina 09
🔊 ☎ 33·50·10·00

River Rance/Dinan
| *i* | 10.15.17 |
🛥 VHF Lock 13 Plouër Marina 13

48°
30N

645

10-15-2

Central North France
Pointe de Barfleur
to St Quay-Portrieux

15

3°W
2°W

10-15-3   AREA 15 TIDAL STREAMS

Due to very strong tidal stream rates, eddies may occur. Where possible some indication of these has been shown, but in many areas there is either insufficient information or the eddies are unstable.

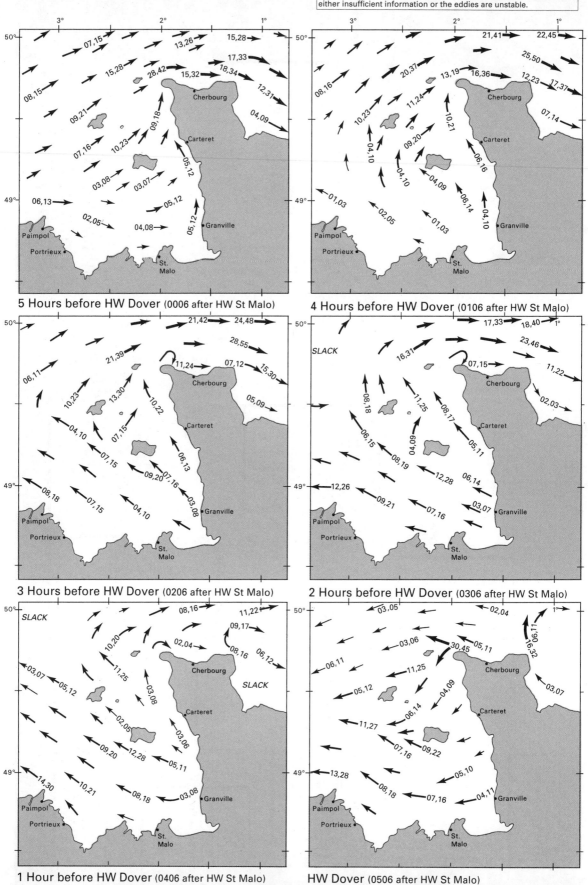

5 Hours before HW Dover (0006 after HW St Malo)

4 Hours before HW Dover (0106 after HW St Malo)

3 Hours before HW Dover (0206 after HW St Malo)

2 Hours before HW Dover (0306 after HW St Malo)

1 Hour before HW Dover (0406 after HW St Malo)

HW Dover (0506 after HW St Malo)

Westward 10.16.3   Channel Islands 10.14.3   Eastward 10.19.3   Northward 10.2.3

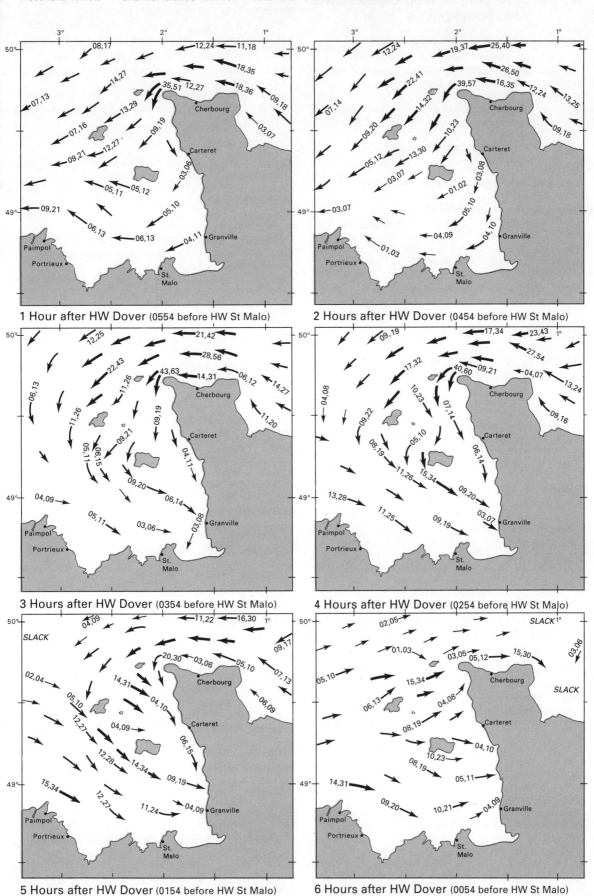

1 Hour after HW Dover (0554 before HW St Malo)

2 Hours after HW Dover (0454 before HW St Malo)

3 Hours after HW Dover (0354 before HW St Malo)

4 Hours after HW Dover (0254 before HW St Malo)

5 Hours after HW Dover (0154 before HW St Malo)

6 Hours after HW Dover (0054 before HW St Malo)

10.15.4 COASTAL LIGHTS, FOG SIGNALS AND WAYPOINTS

Abbreviations used below are given in 1.4.1. Principal lights are in **bold** print, places in CAPITALS, and light-vessels, light floats and Lanbys in *CAPITAL ITALICS*. Unless otherwise stated lights are white. m – elevation in metres; M – nominal range in miles. Fog signals are in *italics*. Useful waypoints are underlined – use those on land with care. All geographical positions should be assumed to be approximate. See 4.4.1.

NOTE: For English Channel Waypoints see 10.1.7.

POINTE DE BARFLEUR TO CAP DE LA HAGUE

Pte de Barfleur-Gatteville 49°41'·83N 01°15'·87W Fl (2) 10s 72m **29M**; Gy Tr, B top; obsc when brg less than 088°; RC; *Horn (2) 60s.*
Les Équets Lt By 49°43'·68N 01°18'·28W Q 8m 3M; NCM.
Basse du Rénier Lt By 49°44'·90N 01°22'·10W VQ 8m 4M; NCM; *Whis.*
La Pierre Noire Lt By 49°43'·57N 01°28'·98W Q (9) 15s 8m 4M; WCM.
Anse de Vicq Ldg Lts 158°. Front 49°42'·26N 01°23'·88W FR 8m 7M; ▲ on W pylon, R top. Rear, 403m from front, FR 14m 7M; ▲ on W pylon, R top.

PORT DE LÉVI/LE BECQUET

Cap Lévi 49°41'·80N 01°28'·40W Fl R 5s 36m **22M**; Gy ■ Tr, W top.
Port de Lévi 49°41'·30N 01°28'·27W F WRG 7m W10M, R7M, G7M; vis G050°-109°, R109°-140°, W140°-184°.
Le Becquet Ldg Lts 186·5°. Front 49°39'·30N 01°32'·80W Dir Oc (2+1) 12s 8m 10M; W 8-sided Tr; intens 183°-190°. Rear, 49m from front, Dir Oc (2+1) R 12s 13m 7M; W 8-sided Tr, R top; synch with front, intens 183°-190°.

CHERBOURG PASSE DE L'EST TO MARINA

Fort des Flamands 49°39'·16N 01°35'·53W Dir Q WRG 13m W12M, R10M, G10M; vis G173·5°-176°, W176°-183°, R183°-193°.
Fort de l'Est 49°40'·33N 01°35'·93W Iso WG 4s 19m W12M, G9M; W pylon, G top; vis W008°-229°, G229°-008°.
La Truite Lt By 49°40'·39N 01°35'·39W Fl (4) R 15s; PHM.
Forte d'Île Pelée Oc (2) WR 6s 19m W10M, R7M; W & R pedestal on fort; vis W055°-120°, R120°-055°.
Digue du Homet 49°39'·53N 01°36'·88W FG 10m 8M; W pylon, G top on blockhouse; *Horn (2+1) 60s.*
Gare Maritime NW corner QR 6m 6M; W col, R lantern.
Marina Môle Hd 49°38'·93N 01°37'·07W Oc (2) G 6s 7m 6M; G pylon.

CHERBOURG PASSE DE L'OUEST

CH1 Lt By 49°43'·30N 01°42'·10W L Fl 10s 8m 4M ; SWM; *Whis*, Ra refl.
Passe de l'Ouest Ldg Lts 140·3° and 142·2°. **Front**, two Lts at root of Digue du Homet Dir Q (2 hor) 5m **17M**; W ▲ on parapet; 63m apart; intens 137·3°-143·3° and 139·2°-145·2°. Rear, Gare Maritime 0·99M from front Dir Q 35m **19M**; Gy pylon with W ▲ on building; intens 140°-142·5°.
Fort de l'Ouest 49°40'·50N 01°38'·87W Fl (3) WR 15s 19m **W24M**, **R20M**; Gy Tr, R top, on fort; vis W122°-355°, R355°-122°; RC; *Horn (3) 60s.*
Digue de Querqueville Hd, 49°40'·36N 01°39'·72W Fl (4) WG 15s 8m W6M, G4M; W col, G top; vis W120°-290°, G290°-120°.
Le Tenarde Lt By 49°48'·78N 01°37'·67W VQ; NCM.
Ldg Lts 124·3°. Front Digue du Homet E Hd (see above). Rear, 0·75M from front, Terre-plein de Mielles Iso G 4s 16m 7M; W col, B bands; intens 114·3°-134·3°.

OMONVILLE-LA-ROGUE/PORT RACINE

Omonville-la-Rogue 49°42'·33N 01°50'·10W Iso WRG 4s 13m W10M, R7M, G7M; W pylon; vis G180°-252°, W252°-262°, R262°-287°.

Port Racine Bkwtr Hd (unlit) 49°42'·78N 01°53'·70W.
Basse Bréfort Lt By 49°43'·70N 01°51'·05W VQ 8m 6M; NCM; *Whis.*
La Plate Lt Bn Tr 49°44'·03N 01°55'·64W Fl (2+1) WR 12s 11m W9M, R6M; Y 8-sided Tr, with B top; vis W115°-272°, R272°-115°; NCM.

CAP DE LA HAGUE TO ST MALO

Cap de la Hague (Gros du Raz) 49°43'·37N 01° 57'·19W Fl 5s 48m **23M**; Gy Tr, W top; *Horn 30s.*
La Foraine By 49°42'·95N 01°58'·75W; WCM; *Whis*; (occasionally submerged).

GOURY/DIÉLETTE

Goury Ldg Lts 065·2°. Front 49°42'·95N 01°56'·55W QR 11m 8M; R □ on W □ on pier. Rear, 116m from front, Q 11m 8M; W pylon on hut.
Diélette Ldg Lts 125·5°. Front, Jetée Ouest 49°33'·23N 01°51'·73W Fl (2) WRG 6s 12m W7M, R4M, G4M; W Tr, G top; vi G shore-072°, W072°-138°, R138°-206°, G206°-shore. Rear, 460m from front, Dir Oc (2) 6s 23m 7M; intens 121°-130°.
Flamanville Lt By 49°32'·62N 01°53'·93W Q (9) 15s; WCM.

CARTERET/PORTBAIL

Cap de Carteret 49°22'·46N 01°48'·35W Fl (2+1) 15s 81m **26M**; Gy Tr, G top; *Horn (3) 60s.*
Trois-Grunes Lt By 49°21'·88N 01°55'·12W Q (9) 15s; WCM.
Carteret Jetée Ouest Hd 49°22'·20N 01°47'·40W Oc R 4s 6m 7M; W col, R top.
Carteret Training wall Hd 49°22'·35N 01°47'·20W Fl G 2·5s 1M; W mast, G top.
Portbail Ldg Lts 042°. Front La Caillourie 49°19'·79N 01°42'·40W Q 14m 10M; W pylon, R top. Rear, 870m from front, Oc 4s 20m 10M; belfry.
Portbail Training wall Hd Q (2) R 5s 5m 1M; W mast, R top.

REGNÉVILLE

La Catheue Lt By 48°57'·95N 01°42'·00W Q (6) + L Fl 15s; SCM.
Pte d'Agon 49°00'·25N 01°34'·60W Oc (2) WR 6s 12m W10M, R7M; W Tr, R top, W dwelling; vis R063°-110°, W110°-063°.
Dir Lt 028° 49°00'·77N 01°33'·28W Dir Oc WRG 4s 9m W13M, R9M, G9M; House; vis G024°-027°, W027°-029°, R029°-033°.

PASSAGE DE LA DÉROUTE

Écrévière Lt By 49°15'·32N 01°52'·07W Q (6) + L Fl 15s; SCM; *Bell.*
Bas Jourdan Lt By 49°06'·90N 01°44'·07W Q (3) 10s; ECM; *Whis.*
Le Sénéquet 49°05'·54N 01°39'·65W Fl (3) WR 12s 18m W13M, R10M; W Tr; vis R083·5°-116·5°, W116·5°-083·5°.
Basse le Marié Lt By 49°01'·89N 01°48'·76W Q (9) 15s; WCM.
Les Ardentes Lt By 48°57'·84N 01°51'·53W Q (3) 10s; ECM.
NE Minquiers Lt By 49°00'·90N 01°55'·20W VQ (3) 5s; ECM; *Bell.*
SE Minquiers Lt By 48°53'·50N 02°00'·00W Q (3) 10s; ECM; *Bell.*
S Minquiers Lt By 48°53'·15N 02°10'·00W Q (6) + L Fl 15s; SCM.

ÎLES CHAUSEY

La Petite Entrée Bn 48°54'·60N 01°49'·48W; WCM.
Le Pignon 48°53'·52N 01°43'·40 W Oc (2) WR 6s 10m W11M, R8M; B Tr, Y band; vis R005°-150°, W150°-005°.
Basse du Founet By 48°53'·34N 01°42'·22W; ECM.
Grande Île (Pte de la Tour) 48° 52'·25N 01°49'·27W Fl 5s 39m **23M**; Gy ■ Tr; *Horn 30s.*

Channel Lt By 48°52'·18N 01°49'·00W Fl G 2s; SHM.
La Crabière Est Lt Bn Tr 48°52'·52N 01°49'·30W Oc WRG 4s 5m W9M, R6M, G6M; B Tr, Y top; vis W079°-291°, G291°-329°, W329°-335°, R335°-079°.

Anvers Wk Lt By 48°53'·90N 01°40'·84W Q (3) 10s; ECM.
Le Videcoq Lt By 48°49'·70N 01°42'·02W VQ (9) 10s; WCM.

GRANVILLE
Tourelle Fourchie 48°50'·21N 01°36'·92W; PHM; *Horn (4) 60s*.
Pointe du Roc 48°50'·11N 01°36'·70W Fl (4) 15s 49m **23M**; Gy Tr, R top.
Le Loup Lt Bn 48°49'·63N 01°36'·17W Fl (2) 6s 8m 11M; IDM.
Hérel Marina Hd 48°49'·96N 01°35'·82W Fl R 4s 12m 8M; W ● Tr, R top; *Horn (2) 40s*.
Commercial Port Jetée Ouest Hd 48°49'·92N 01°36'·16W Iso R 4s 12m 6M; R pylon.

CANCALE/ROTHENEUF
La Pierre-de-Herpin 48°43'·83N 01°48'·83W Oc (2) 6s 20m **17M**; W Tr, B top and base; *Siren Mo (N) 60s*.
Cancale Jetty Hd 48°40'·16N 01°51'·04W Oc (3) G 12s 12m 7M; W pylon, G top, G hut; obsc when brg less than 223°.
Rothneuf Entrance Bn 48°41'·42N 01°57'·61W; SHM; (unlit).

ST MALO TO ST QUAY PORTRIEUX

APPROACHES TO ST MALO
La Plate Lt Bn Tr 48°40'·85N 02°01'·83W Fl WRG 4s 11m, W11M, R8M, G8M; vis W140°-203°, R203°-210°, W210°-225°, G225°-140°.
Brunel Lt By 48°40'·88N 02°05'·26W Q (9) 15s; WCM; *Bell*.

CHENAL DE LA PETITE PORTE/RADE DE ST MALO
Ldg Lts 130°. Front **Le Grand Jardin** 48°40'·27N 02°04'·90W Fl (2) R 10s 24m **15M**; Gy Tr, R top; RC. Rear **La Balue**, 4·08M from front, Dir FG 69m **24M**; Gy ■ Tr; intens 128·2°-129·7°.
Bassée NE Lt By 48°42'·51N 02°09'·34W Q; NCM; *Bell*.
Fairway Lt By 48°41'·42N 02°07'·21W L Fl 10s; SWM; *Whis*.
Les Courtis Lt Bn 48°40'·52N 02°05'·72W Fl (3) G 12s 14m 8M.

CHENAL DE LA GRANDE PORTE
Ldg Lts 089·1°. **Front Le Grand Jardin** Fl (2) R 10s 24m **15M** Rear **Rochebonne** 4·2M from front 48°40'·32N 01°58'·61W Dir FR 40m **24M**; Gy ■ Tr, R top; intens 088·2°-089·7°.
Le Sou Lt By 48°40'·17N 02°05'·16W VQ (3) 5s; ECM; *Bell*.
No. 1 Lt By 48°40'·24N 02°05'·97W Fl G 4s; SHM; *Whis*.
No. 2 Lt By 48°40'·27N 02°07'·48W Fl (3) R 12s; PHM; *Whis*.
Banchenou Lt By 48°40'·52N 02°11'·42W Fl (5) G 20s; SHM.
Ldg Lts 128·7°. Front **Les Bas-Sablons** 48°38'·22N 02°01'·23W Dir FG 20m **18M**; W ■ Tr, B top; intens 127·5°-130·5°. Common rear **La Balue**, 0·9M from front Dir FG 69m **24M**; Gy ■ Tr; intens 128·2°-129·7°.
Basse du Buron No.12 Lt By 48°39'·46N 02°03'·44W L Fl R 10s; PHM.
Le Buron Lt Bn 48°39'·38N 02°03'·60W Fl (2) 6s 15m 8M; G Tr.
Plateau Rance Nord 48°38'·71N 02°02'·27W VQ; NCM.
Plateau Rance Sud 48°38'·52N 02°02'·23W Q (6) + L Fl 15s; SCM.

ST MALO
Écluse du Naye Ldg Lts 070·7° Front 48°38'·64N 02°01'·46W FR 7m 3M. Rear FR 23m 8M vis 030°-120°.
La Grenouille Lt By 48°38'·44N 01°01'·92W Fl (4) 15s; SHM.
Môle des Noires Hd 48°38'·58N 02°01'·85W Fl R 5s 11m 13M; W Tr, R top; obsc 155°-159°, 171°-178°, and when brg more than 192°; *Horn(2) 20s*.
Bas-Sablons Marina Môle Hd 48°38'·48N 02°01'·63W Fl G 4s 7m 5M; Gy mast.

LA RANCE
La Jument Lt Bn Tr 48°37'·50N 02°01'·68W Fl (5) G 20s 6m 3M; G Tr, SHM.
Tidal barrage NW wall Fl G 4s 6m 5M, G pylon, vis 191°-291°.
NE dolphin Fl (2) R 6s 6m 5M; vis 040°-200°.

ST BRIAC/ST CAST
Embouchure du Fremur. Dir Lt 125° 48°37'·1N 02°08'·2W Dir Iso WRG 4s 10m W13M, R11M, G11M; W mast on hut, vis G121·5°-124·5°, W124·5°-125·5°, R125·5°-129·5°.
St Cast Môle Hd 48°38'·47N 02°14'·50W Iso WG 4s 11m W11M, G8M; G and W structure; vis W204°-217°, G217°-233°, W233°-245°, G245°-204°.
Cap Fréhel 48°41'·10N 02°19'·07W Fl (2) 10s 85m **29M**; Brown ■ Tr, G lantern; *Horn (2) 60s*; RC.

CHENAL D'ERQUY/ERQUY/VAL-ANDRÉ
Les Justières Lt By 48°40'·66N 02°26'·43W Q (6) + L Fl 15s; SCM.
Basses du Courant Lt By 48°39'·29N 02°29'·08W VQ (6) + L Fl 10s; SCM.
Erquy S Môle Hd 48°38'·13N 02°28'·60W Oc (2+1) WRG 12s 11m W11M, R8M, G8M; W Tr, R top; vis R055°-081°, W081°-094°, G094°-111°, W111°-120°, R120°-134°.
Erquy Inner Jetty Hd 48°38'·16N 02°28'·31W Fl R 2·5s 10m 3M; R and W Tr.
Val-Andre Jetty Hd 48°35'·89N 02°33'·24W.

PORT DE DAHOUET
La Dahouet By 48°35'·28N 02°35'·28W; NCM.
La Petite-Muette 48°34'·91N 02°34'·21W Fl WRG 4s 10m W9M, R6M, G6M; ▲ on G & W Tr; vis G055°-114°, W114°-146°, R146°-196°. Fl (2) G 6s; vis 156°-286° 240m SE.

BAIE DE SAINT BRIEUC
Grande Lejon 48°44'·95N 02°39'·90W Fl (5) WR 20s 17m **W18M**, R14M; R Tr, W bands; vis R015°-058°, W058°-283°, R283°-350°, W350°-015°.
Le Rohein Lt Bn Tr 48°38'·88N 02°37'·68W VQ (9) WRG 10s 13m W10M, R7M, G7M; WCM; vis R072°-105°, W105°-180°, G180°-193°, W193°-237°, G237°-282°, W282°-301°. G301°-330°, W330°-072°.

LE LÉGUÉ (St BRIEUC)
Le Légué Lt By 48°34'·38N 02°41'·07N Mo (A) 10s; SWM; *Whis*.
Pointe à l'Aigle Jetty 48°32'·15N 02°43'·05W VQG 13m 8M; W Tr, G top; vis 160°-070°.
Custom House Jetty 48°31'·96N 02°43'·34W Iso G 4s 6m 8M, W cols, G top.

BINIC
Binic, Môle de Penthièvre Hd 48°36'·13N 02°48'·84W Oc (3) 12s 12m 11M; W Tr, G gallery; unintens 020°-110°.

SAINT-QUAY-PORTRIEUX
Caffa Lt By 48°37'·89N 02°43'·00W Q (3) 10s; ECM.
La Roselière Lt By 48°37'·51N 02°46'·31W VQ (9) 10s; WCM.
Elbow 48°39'·05N 02°49'·01W Dir Iso WRG 4s **W15M**, R11M, G11M; vis 159°-179°, G179°-316°, W316°-320·5°, R320·5°-159°; Reserve Lt ranges 12/9M.
Île Harbour Roches de Saint-Quay 48°40'·05N 02°48'·42W Oc (2) WRG 6s 16m W10M, R8M, G8M; W Tr and dwelling, R top; vis R011°-133°, G133°-270°, R270°-306°, G306°-358°, W358°-011°.
NE Môle Hd 48°38'·90N 02°48'·84W Fl (3) G 12s 2M; G Tr.
Herflux Dir Lt 130° 48°39'·13N 02°47'·87W Dir Fl (2) WRG 6s W8M, R6M, G6M; vis G115°-125°, W125°-135°, R135°-145°; SCM.

15

10.15.5 PASSAGE INFORMATION

Current Pilots for this area include: *Shell Channel Pilot* (Imray/Cunliffe); *Normandy and CI Pilot* (Adlard Coles/Brackenbury) as far W as St Malo; *Brittany and CI Cruising Guide* (Adlard Coles/Jefferson); *N Brittany and CI Cruising* (YM/Cumberlidge); *N Brittany Pilot* (Imray/RCC) W'ward from St Malo; Admiralty *Channel Pilot*. Charts *2669* and *1106 cover* the whole area. For French Glossary see 1.4.2.

Along the French coastline between Pte de Barfleur and Cap Lévi rky shoals extend up to 2·5M seaward. From C. Lévi around C. de la Hague and S to C. de Flamanville the coast is cleaner with few dangers extending more than 1M offshore. Southward to Mont St Michel and W to St Malo the coast changes to extensive offshore shoals, sand dunes studded with rks and a series of drying hbrs. Continuing W, the coast from St Malo to St Quay-Portrieux is characterised by deep bays (often drying), a few rugged headlands and many offlying rks.

The sea areas around this coast, including the Channel Islands, are dominated by powerful tidal streams with an anti-clockwise rotational pattern and a very large tidal range. Across the top of the Cotentin Peninsula and between C. de la Hague and Alderney the main English Channel tidal streams are rectilinear E/W. Neap tides are best, particularly for a first visit, and tidal streams need to be worked carefully. Boats which can take the ground have an advantage for exploring the shallower hbrs. Be careful to avoid lobster pots, and oyster and mussel beds in some rivers and bays.

POINTE DE BARFLEUR TO CAP DE LA HAGUE (AC *1106*)

The N coast of the Cotentin Peninsula runs E/W for 26M, mostly bordered by rks which extend 2·5M offshore from Pte de Barfleur to C. Lévi, and 1M offshore between Pte de Jardeheu and C. de la Hague. Tidal streams reach 5kn at sp, and raise a steep sea with wind against tide.

Pte de Barfleur has dangers up to 2M offshore, and a race, in which the sea breaks heavily, extends 3-4M NE and E from the lt ho. In bad weather, particularly with winds from NW or SE against the tide, it is necessary to keep at least 6M to seaward to avoid the worst effects; in calmer conditions the Pte can be rounded close inshore. The inner passage between Pte de Barfleur and C. Lévi, keeping S of three cardinal buoys, is not recommended without local knowledge except in good weather and visibility when the transits shown on chart *1106* can be used. Tidal streams run strongly with considerable local variations.

Off C. Lévi a race develops with wind against tide, and extends nearly 2M to N. Port Lévi and Port de Becquet are two small drying hbrs E of Cherbourg. Off Cherbourg (10.15.9) the stream is E-going from about HW – 0430 and W-going from HW + 0230.

Close inshore between Cherbourg and C. de la Hague a back eddy runs W. As an alternative to Omonville (10.15.10) there is anch in Anse de St Martin, about 2M E of C. de la Hague, exposed to N, but useful to await the tide for the Alderney Race.

THE ALDERNEY RACE (chart *3653*)

The Alderney Race, so called due to very strong tidal streams, runs SW/NE between C. de la Hague and Alderney. The fairway, approx 4M wide, is bounded by Race Rk and Alderney S Banks to the NW, and to the SE by rky banks 4M WSW of C. de la Hague, Milieu and Banc de la Schôle (least depth

2·7m). These dangers which cause breaking seas and heavy overfalls should be carefully avoided. In bad weather and strong wind-against-tide conditions the seas break in all parts of the Race and passage is not recommended. Conditions are exacerbated at sp tides.

In mid-chan the the SW-going stream starts at HW St Helier + 0430 (HW Dover) and the NE-going stream at HW St Helier –0210 (HW Dover + 0530), sp rates both 5·5kn. The times at which the stream turns do not vary much for various places, but the rates do; for example, 1M W of C. de la Hague the sp rates reach 7 to 8kn.

To obtain optimum conditions, timing is of the essence. As a rule of thumb the Race should be entered on the first of the fair tide so as to avoid the peak tidal stream with attendant overfalls/seas.

Thus, bound SW, arrrive off C. de la Hague at around HW St Helier + 0430 (HW Dover) when the stream will be slack, whilst just starting to run SW off Alderney. A yacht leaving Cherbourg at HW Dover – 0300 will achieve the above timing by utilising the inshore W-going tidal eddy.

Conversely, NE bound, leave St Peter Port, say, at approx local HW St Helier – 0430 (HWD+3) with a foul tide so as to pass Banc de la Schôle as the first of the fair tide starts to make. A later departure should achieve a faster passage, but with potentially less favourable conditions in the Race. On the NE stream the worst overfalls are on the French side.

CAP DE LA HAGUE TO ST MALO
(charts *3659*, 3656, *3655*, *3653*)

The Jobourg radar surveillance station (CROSS) and atomic energy station Chy (R lts) are conspic about 3-4M SE of Gros du Raz (lt, fog sig), off C de la Hague. 5M S of C de la Hague beware Les Huquets de Jobourg, an extensive bank of drying and submerged rks, and Les Huquets de Vauville (dry) close SE of them.

The W coast of the Cotentin Peninsula is exposed, and is mostly rky and inhospitable; along much of this coast S of Carteret there is little depth of water, so that a nasty sea can build. The drying hbrs/non-tidal marinas* at Goury, Dielette* (10.15.11), Carteret* (10.15.12) and Portbail (10.15.13) are more readily accessible if cruising from S to N on the tide, since all hbrs are restricted by drying approaches.

The two main chans from/to the Alderney Race are Déroute de Terre and, further offshore, Passage de la Déroute. Neither chan are well marked in places, and are not advised at night. The former leads between Plateau des Trois Grunes and Carteret, between Basses de Portbail and Bancs Félés, between Le Sénéquet lt tr and Basse Jourdan, and E of Îles Chausey toward Pte du Roc, off Granville (10.15.14). The S end of this chan, E of Îles Chausey, is very shallow; for detailed directions see *Channel Pilot*.

The Passage de la Déroute passes W of Plateau des Trois Grunes, between Basses de Taillepied and Les Écrehou, between Chaussée de Boeufs and Plateau de l'Arconie, E and SE of Les Minquiers and Les Ardentes, and W of Îles Chausey (10.15.15).

To the S of Granville is the drying expanse of B du Mont St Michel. Proceeding W, the drying hbr of Cancale (10.15.16) with many oyster beds and a fair weather anch SE of Île des Rimains, lies 4M S of Pte du Grouin, off which the many dangers are marked by La Pierre-de-Herpin (lt, fog sig). The large drying inlet of Rothéneuf, with anch off in good weather, is 4M E of St Malo (10.15.16 and chart 2700).

ST MALO TO L'OST PIC (charts *3674, 3659*)

In the apprs to St Malo (chart 2700) are many islets, rks and shoals, between which are several chans that can be used in good vis. Tidal streams reach 4kn at sp, and can set across chans. From E and N, with sufficient rise of tide and good vis, Chenal de la Bigne, Chenal des Petits Pointus or Chenal de la Grande Conchée can be used, but they all pass over or near to drying patches. From the W and NW, Chenal de la Grande Porte and Chenal de la Petite Porte are the easiest routes and are well marked/lit. Chenal du Décollé is a shallow, demanding inshore route from the W, and no shorter than Chenal de la Grande Porte.

By passing through the lock at W end of the R. Rance barrage (10.15.17) it is possible to cruise up river to Dinan, via the lock at Châtelier (SHOM chart 4233). At Dinan is ent to Canal d'Ille et Rance to Biscay (10.15.18).

6M NW of St Malo beware Le Vieux-Banc (dries). Here the E-going stream begins at HW St Helier – 0555, and the W-going at HW St Helier – 0015, sp rates 2·5kn. There are W-going eddies very close inshore on the E-going stream. Between St Malo and C. Fréhel is St Cast hbr (10.15.20), and there are anchs S of Île Agot in the apprs to the drying hbr of St Briac, in B de l'Arguenon and B de la Fresnaye. From C. Fréhel to C. d'Erquy there are no worthwhile hbrs.

About 3ca off Cap d'Erquy, and inshore of the various rky patches close to seaward Chenal d'Erquy runs WSW/ENE into the E side of the B de St Brieuc. Erquy is a pleasant, drying hbr, but often crowded with fishing boats. The Plateau du Rohein (lt), at W end of a long ridge, is 6M W of C. d'Erquy. There are several rky shoals within the B itself, some extending nearly 2M offshore.

To seaward of B de St Brieuc is Grand Léjon (lt), a rky shoal 9M NE of St Quay-Portrieux. Rks extend 2½ca W and 8ca NNE of the lt ho. Petit Léjon (dries) lies 3·5M SSE of lt ho. From the N/NW, keep W of these dangers via a chan 3-4M wide which gives access to the shallow, partly drying S end of the B and the hbrs of Val André, Dahouet (10.15.19), Le Légué/St Brieux (10.15.20), and Binic (10.15.21). On the W side of B de St Brieuc, Roches de St Quay and offlying patches extend 4M E from St Quay-Portrieux (10.15.22) which can only be approached from NW or SE.

To the N and NE of L'Ost-Pic extensive offshore shoals guard the approaches to Paimpol (10.16.9), Ile de Bréhat and the Trieux river. Further N, the Plateau de Barnouic and Plateau des Roches Douvres (lt, fog sig, RC) should be avoided. Here the E-going stream begins at about HW St Malo – 0400 and the W-going at about HW St Malo +0100 with Sp rates exceeding 4kn.

10.15.6   DISTANCE TABLE

Approximate distances in nautical miles are by the most direct route, whilst avoiding dangers and allowing for Traffic Separation Schemes. Places in *italics* are in adjoining areas; places in **bold** are in 10.0.5, Cross-Channel Distances.

	1	2	3	4	5	6	7	8	9	10	11	12	13	14	15	16	17	18	19	20
1. *Calais*	1																			
2. *Barfleur*	148	2																		
3. **Cherbourg**	160	20	3																	
4. Omonville	163	27	10	4																
5. Cap de la Hague	167	32	18	6	5															
6. *Braye (Alderney)*	172	41	25	15	9	6														
7. **St Peter Port**	193	60	44	34	28	23	7													
8. *Creux (Sark)*	190	55	37	29	23	22	10	8												
9. **St Helier**	213	77	64	51	45	46	29	24	9											
10. Carteret	192	55	45	29	23	28	31	23	26	10										
11. Portbail	196	59	49	33	27	32	35	27	25	5	11									
12. Iles Chausey	222	87	69	61	55	58	48	43	25	33	30	12								
13. Granville	227	93	75	67	61	66	55	50	30	38	35	9	13							
14. Dinan	250	117	102	91	85	85	66	64	50	62	59	29	35	14						
15. **St Malo**	238	105	90	79	73	73	54	52	38	50	47	17	23	12	15					
16. Dahouet	240	106	88	80	74	72	54	52	41	60	59	37	45	41	29	16				
17. Le Légué/St Brieux	244	110	86	86	78	76	57	56	46	69	69	41	49	45	33	8	17			
18. Binic	244	115	95	84	78	75	56	55	46	70	70	43	51	46	33	10	8	18		
19. **St Quay-Portrieux**	244	106	88	80	74	73	56	51	46	64	64	47	54	47	35	11	7	4	19	
20. *Lézardrieux*	238	106	88	80	74	68	48	38	47	68	71	53	54	61	49	33	32	30	21	20

15

10.15.7 English Channel Waypoints: See 10.1.7

SPECIAL NOTES FOR FRANCE
(Areas 15 to 19)   10-15-8

There are some minor differences in the hbr information for French ports. Instead of 'County' the 'Département' is given. The Time Zone for France is –0100 (i.e. 1300 Standard Time in France is 1200UT), DST not having been taken into account (see 9·1·2.)
For details of documentation apply to the French Tourist Office, 178 Piccadilly, London, W1V 0AL, ☎ 0171-629 2869, Fax 0171-493 6594.

AFFAIRES MARITIMES
In every French port there is a representative of the central government, L'Administration Maritime, known as Affaires Maritimes. This organisation watches over all maritime activities (commercial, fishing, pleasure, etc) and helps them develop harmoniously. All information on navigation and any other maritime problems can be supplied by the local representative whose ☎ is given under each port. The Head office address is: Ministère Chargé de la Mer, Bureau de la Navigation de Plaisance, 3 Place Fontenoy, 75007 Paris, ☎ (1) 44·49·80·00.

CHARTS
Two types of French chart are shown: SHOM as issued by the *Service Hydrographique et Oceanographique de la Marine*, the French Navy's Hydrographic Service; ECM *Éditions Cartographiques Maritimes* are charts for sea and river navigation. Notes: Under 'Facilities', SHOM means a chart agent. Any new edition of a SHOM chart receives a new, different chart number. SHOM charts refer elevations of lights, bridges etc to Mean Level (ML), not to MHWS as on Admiralty charts.

TIDAL COEFFICIENTS
See 10.16.24 for Coefficients based on Brest, together with explanatory notes and French tidal terms.

METEO (Weather)
The BQR (*Bulletin Quotidien des Renseignements*) is a very informative daily bulletin displayed in Hr Mr Offices and YC's. Some weather terms are in the Glossary 1.4.2.
For each French port, under **TELEPHONE**, Météo is the ☎ of a local Met Office. Auto is the ☎ for recorded Inshore and Coastal forecasts. It will be ☎ 36.68.08.nn (nn being the Département No, as shown). To select either the Inshore (*rivage*) or Coastal (*côte;* out to 20M offshore) bulletin, say "STOP" as your choice is spoken.
Inshore bulletins are 5 day forecasts, also containing local info on tides, signals, sea temperature, surf conditions, etc. Coastal bulletins (for 5 areas from the Belgian to Spanish borders) contain strong wind/gale warnings, general synopsis, 24hrs forecast and outlook.
For recorded Offshore forecasts for North Sea, Channel and Atlantic sea areas, as in Fig 7(5), dial ☎ 36.68.08.08. To select your sea area say "STOP" as your area is named. Offshore bulletins contain strong wind/gale warnings, the general synopsis and forecast, and the 5 day outlook.

SAFETY AT SEA
CROSS (Centres Régionaux Opérationnel de Surveillance et de Sauvetage) equate to CG MRCCs; a Sous-CROSS is an MRSC. CROSS primarily controls SAR operations and monitors VHF Ch 16 and 2182 kHz H24. Geographic cover and dedicated VHF Ch's are as follows:
1. Belgian border to Antifer: *CROSS Gris Nez*, VHF Ch 15, 67 and 73; ☎ 21.87.21.87.
2. Antifer to Mont St Michel: *CROSS Jobourg*, (H24) VHF Ch 15, 67 and 73; ☎ 33.52.72.13.
3. Mont St Michel to Pointe du Raz: *CROSS Corsen*, VHF Ch 15, 67 and 73; ☎ 98.89.31.31.
4. Pointe du Raz to Spanish border: *CROSSA Etel*, VHF Ch 11; ☎ 97.55.35.35.
4A. 46°20'N to Spanish border: *Sous-CROSS Soulac*, Ch 11, 0700-2200LT; ☎ 56.09.82.00. Soulac, near Pte de Grave, is a subsidiary of Etel.
CROSS also provides marine and fishery surveillance and broadcasts urgent nav and weather info: Etel and Soulac broadcast on Ch 13, 79 and 80 on receipt, then every 2 hrs. CROSS stations, except Gris Nez, are shown on Fig 6 (4). Note: CROSS does not accept public correspondence (eg link calls) which is the task of Coast Radio Stations.

CROSS can be contacted by radiotelephone, by ☎, through Coast Radio stations, via the Semaphore system as shown below, or via the National Gendarmerie or Affaires Maritimes.
Call Naval 'Semaphore' (ie Signal) stations on Ch 16 (working Ch 10) or by ☎ as follows:

* Dunkerque	28·66·86·18	Ouessant Creach	98·48·80·49
Boulogne	21·31·32·10	St-Mathieu	98·89·01·59
Ault	22·60·47·33	Portzic (Vigie) (Ch 8)	98·22·90·01
Dieppe	35·84·23·82	Toulinguet	98·27·90·02
Fecamp	35·28·00·91	Cap-de-la-Chevre	98·27·09·55
* La Heve	35·46·07·81	* Pointe-du-Raz	98·70·66·57
Le Havre (Ch 12)	35·21·74·39	* Penmarch	98·58·61·00
Villerville	31·88·11·13	Beg Meil	98·94·98·92
* Port-en-Bessin	31·21·81·51	Port-Louis	97·82·52·10
St-Vaast	33·54·44·50	Etel	97·55·35·59
* Barfleur	33·54·04·37	Beg Melen (Groix)	97·86·80·13
Levy	33·54·31·17	Taillefer (Belle-Ile)	97·31·83·18
Le Homet	33·92·60·08	Talut (Belle-Ile)	97·31·85·07
La Hague	33·52·71·07	St-Julien	97·50·09·35
Carteret	33·53·85·08	Piriac-sur-Mer	40·23·59·87
Le Roc	33·50·05·85	* Chemoulin	40·91·99·00
Le Grouin	99·89·60·12	St-Sauveur (Yeu)	51·58·31·01
St-Cast	96·41·85·30	Les Baleines (Ré)	46·29·42·06
* St Quay-Portrieux	96·70·42·18	Chassiron(Oléron)	46·47·85·43
Brehat	96·20·00·12	* La Coubre	46·22·41·73
* Ploumanach	96·91·46·51	Pointe-de-Grave	56·09·60·03
Batz	98·61·76·06	Cap Ferret	56·60·60·03
* Brignogan	98·83·50·84	* Socoa	59·47·18·54
Ouessant Stiff	98·48·81·50		

* H24. Remainder sunrise to sunset.

Although the lifeboat service SNSM (Société Nationale de Sauvetage en Mer) comes under CROSS, it is best to contact local lifeboat stns direct, ☎ as listed under SNSM. Notes: There are strict penalties for infringing the IRPCS. Speed under power is limited in France to 5kn, when within 300m of the shore.

MEDICAL
Doctors and/or hospital ☎ are given for each port. Also, the Services d'Aide Médicale Urgente (SAMU), which liaises closely with CROSS, can be contacted as follows:

NORD (Lille)	20·54·22·22
PAS-DE-CALAIS (Arras)	21·71·51·51
SOMME (Amiens)	22·44·33·33
SEINE-MARITIME (Le Havre)	35·47·15·15
CALVADOS (Caen)	31·44·88·88
CÔTES D'ARMOR (Saint Brieuc)	96·94·28·95
FINISTERE (Brest)	98·46·11·33
MORBIHAN (Vannes)	97·54·22·11
LOIRE-ATLANTIQUE (Nantes)	40·08·37·77
VENDEE (La Roche-sur-Yon)	51·44·62·15
CHARENTE-MARITIME (La Rochelle)	46·27·32·15
GIRONDE (Bordeaux)	56·96·70·70
LANDES (Mont-de-Marsan)	58·75·44·44
PYRÉNÉES-ATLANTIQUE (Bayonne)	59·63·33·33

PUBLIC HOLIDAYS
New Year's Day, Easter Sunday and Monday, Labour Day (1 May), Ascension Day, Armistice Day 1945 (8 May), Whit Sunday and Monday, National (Bastille) Day (14 July), Feast of the Assumption (15 Aug), All Saints' Day (1 Nov), Remembrance Day (11 Nov), Christmas Day.

TELEPHONES
To telephone France from UK, dial 00 33 (for Paris, dial 00 33 1) followed by the 8 digit number (the first 2 digits of which act as an Area Code). The ringing tone consists of long, equal on/off tones (slower than UK engaged tone). Rapid pips indicates your call is being connected. Engaged tone is similar to that in UK. An unobtainable number is indicated by a recorded announcement.
To telephone UK from France dial 19 44 followed by the Area Code (omitting the first 0) and the number.
Emergencies: Dial 18 for Fire, 17 Police, 15 Ambulance; or 112 as used in all EC countries.
Phonecards for public 'phones may be bought at the PTT or at many cafés and tabacs. Cheap rates are 2130-0800 Mon-Sat; all day Sun.

FRENCH GLOSSARY: see 1.4.2.

FACILITIES.
At some marinas fuel can only be obtained/paid for by using a French credit card (of the smart variety) in a slot machine. If not in possession of such a card, it may be possible to persuade a Frenchman to use his card on your behalf and to reimburse him in cash.

The cost shown for a visitor's overnight berth is unavoidably the previous year's figure (as in similar publications). It is based on high season rates and is calculated on LOA, although beam may be taken into account at some ports. Low season rates and concessions can much reduce costs. The fee usually includes electricity, but rarely showers which average around FF10-12.

SIGNALS
Standard sets of Traffic, Storm Warning and Tidal signals apply in all French ports unless otherwise stated.

Traffic Signals

Day		Night	
Full Code	Simplified Code	Full Code	Simplified Code
●▲●	or **R** Flag	⑧⑩⑧	or ⑧ NO ENTRY
▼▲●	**R** Flag or over **G** Flag	⑤⑩⑧	or ⑧⑤ NO ENT/DEP
▼▲▼	or **G** Flag	⑩⑩⑤	or ⑤ NO DEP
●●●	**R** **R** Balls **R**	⑧⑧⑧	EMERGENCY NO ENTRY
INTERNATIONAL CODE SIGNAL		⑤⑤⑤	PORT OPEN

A Black Flag indicates a shipping casualty in the area. Flag 'P' sometimes indicates that lock or dock gates are open.

Storm Signals (International System)

Day	Night	
▲	⑧⑧	N.W. gale
▲▶▲	⑧⑩	N.E. gale
▼	⑩⑩	S.W. gale
▼▼	⑩⑧	S.E. gale
●	⑩⑤	Strong wind (force 6-7)
✚	⑧⑤⑧	Hurricane (force 12) any direction
■ ■	} colour of flags is variable	Wind veering
■ ■		Wind backing

In France, ⑩ Lts, Q or IQ, by day only, indicate forecast wind >F6, as follows: Q = within 3 hrs; IQ = within 6 hrs.

Tidal Signals
There are two sets of signals, one showing the state of the tide and the other showing the height of tide.

a.   State of the tide is shown by:

	Day		Night
High Water . . .	⊠	W Flag B Cross	⑩ ⑩
Tide falling . . .	▼		⑩ ⑩
Low Water . . .	▷	Bu Flag	⑤ ⑤
Tide rising . . .	▲		⑤ ⑩

b.   The height of tide signals show the height above CD by adding together the values of the various shapes. Day: ▼ = 0·2m; ■ = 1·0m; ● = 5·0m. Night: ⑤ = 0·2m; ⑧ = 1·0m; ⑩ = 5·0m. The three different shapes are shown horizontally, with ▼s to the left of ■s and ●s to the right, viewed from seaward. Lights are disposed similarly.
The following examples will help to explain:

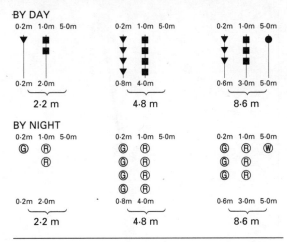

BY DAY

0·2m 1·0m 5·0m	0·2m 1·0m 5·0m	0·2m 1·0m 5·0m
0·2m 2·0m	0·8m 4·0m	0·6m 3·0m 5·0m
2·2 m	**4·8 m**	**8·6 m**

BY NIGHT

0·2m 1·0m 5·0m	0·2m 1·0m 5·0m	0·2m 1·0m 5·0m
0·2m 2·0m	0·8m 4·0m	0·6m 3·0m 5·0m
2·2 m	**4·8 m**	**8·6 m**

TOLLS AND QUALIFICATIONS ON INLAND WATERWAYS
Tolls are due on waterways managed by Voies Navigable de France (VNF), ie those E of a line Rouen to Arles; also the Canal Latéral à la Garonne, Canal du Midi and R. Loire. In 1995 licences were available for either one year, 30 days (not necessarily consecutive) or 15 consecutive days. The rates, were based on 5 categories of boat area, ie LOA x Beam (m) = m², as follows in French francs:

	<12m²	12-25m²	25-40m²	40-60m²	>60m²
1 Year	450	650	1300	2100	2600
30 days	250	450	800	1250	1550
15 days	100	200	300	400	500

Licence stickers, which must be visibly displayed stbd side forward, are obtainable from VNF offices at larger centres on the canals or from: Librairie VNF, 18 Quai d'Austerlitz, 75013 Paris; ☎ 44.24.57.94. Further info from: French Tourist Office, London; ☎ 0171 629 2869, Fax 0171 493 6594.

Helmsmen of craft <15m LOA and not capable of >20 kph (11kn) must have a Helmsman's Overseas Certificate of Competence or International Certificate of Competence, plus a copy of the French CEVNI rules. For larger, faster craft the requirements are under review.

Foreign vessels >25m LOA must get permission to navigate or ⚓ in French inland waters and must keep watch on Ch 16 or other nominated frequency.

15

CHERBOURG 10-15-9
Manche 49°39'·00N 01°37'·03W (Marina ent)

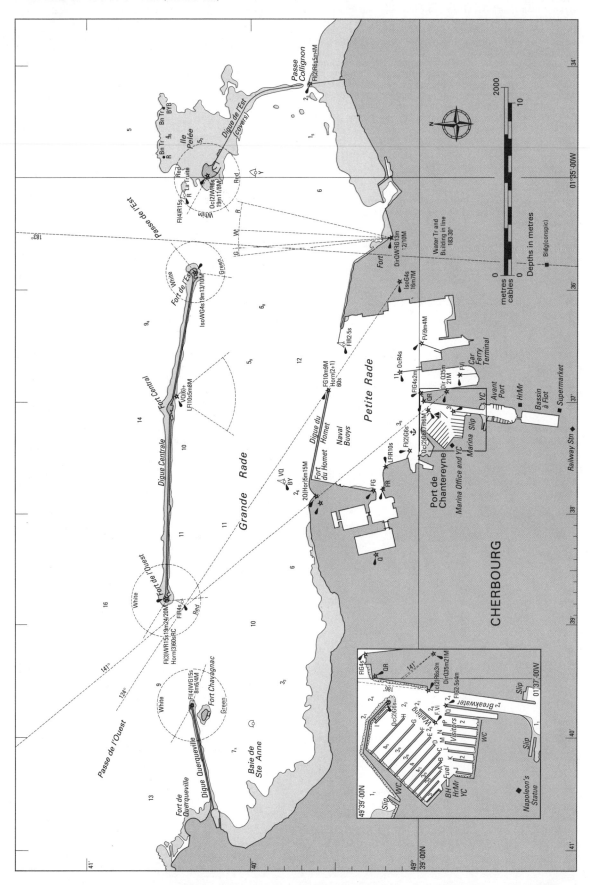

CHERBOURG *continued*

CHARTS
AC 2602, *1106, 2669*; SHOM 7086, 7092, 6737; ECM 528, 1014; Imray C32, C33A; Stanfords 7, 16
TIDES
−0308 Dover; ML 3·8; Duration 0535; Zone −0100

Cherbourg is a Standard Port and tidal predictions for every day of the year are given below.

SHELTER
Excellent; hbr accessible in all tides and weather. Visitors berth on pontoons M, N, P & Q, on S side of Chantereyne Marina. There is also a small craft ⚓ N of marina bkwtr. Lock into Bassin à Flot (HW±1) is normally for commercial vessels only.
NAVIGATION
WPT **Passe de l'Ouest** 49°41'·10N 01°39'·80W, 321°/141° from/to W ent, 0·85M. Note: CH1 SWM spar buoy, L Fl 10s, bears 323° from Fort de l'Ouest 3·5M.
WPT **Passe de l'Est** 49°41'·00N 01°35'·70W, 000°/180° from/to E ent, 0·65M. For coastal features from Cap de la Hague to Pte de Barfleur see 10·15·5.
There are 3 ents:
(1) Passe de l'Ouest (W ent) is the easiest. Rks extend about 80m from each bkwtr. From W, the white sector of Fort de l'Ouest lt (bearing more than 122° by day) keeps clear of offlying dangers E of Cap de la Hague.
(2) Passe de l'Est (E ent) carries 6m. Keep to W side of chan (but at least 80m off Fort de l'Est) to avoid dangers W of Ile Pelée marked by PHM buoy, Fl (4) R 15s, and by 2 unlit bn trs on N side which must be given a wide berth.
(3) Passe Collignon is a shallow (2m) chan, 93m wide, through Digue de l'Est (covers), near the shore. Not recommended except in good conditions and near HW.
LIGHTS AND MARKS
There are three powerful lts near Cherbourg:
(1) To the E, Cap Levi, Fl R 5s 36m 22M; and further E,
(2) Pte de Barfleur, Fl (2) 10s 72m 29M;
(3) To the W, Cap de la Hague, Fl 5s 48m 23M; further W, the lts of Alderney (Quenard Pt, Fl (4) 15s 37m 28M) and Casquets, Fl (5) 30s 37m 24M, can often be seen. See 10.14.4, 10.15.4 and 10.19.4 for details.
Fort de l'Ouest lt, at W end of Digue Centrale, Fl (3) WR 15s 19m 24/20M, vis W122°-355°, R355°-122°, RC, Reed (3) 60s. Close SSW is PHM buoy Fl R 4s.
Passe de l'Ouest ldg lts 140·5°: Gare Maritime lt, Dir Q 35m 21M, in line with centre of 2Q (hor) 5m 15M at base of Digue du Homet. Grande Rade ldg lts 124°: Front FG 10m 9M, W pylon, G top, on blockhouse; rear, 0·75M from front, Iso G 4s 16m 12M, W column, B bands, W top, intens 114°-134°.
Passe de l'Est is covered by W sector (176°-183°) of Dir lt, Q WRG 13m 12/10M, at Fort des Flamands.
Inside Petite Rade steer 200° for marina ent, QR and Oc (2) G 6s. Shore lights may be confusing and mask nav lts.
RADIO TELEPHONE
Marina: call *Chantereyne* Ch 09 (0800-2300LT).
Jobourg Traffic Ch **11** 16 (H24) provides radar surveillance of the Casquets TSS/ITZ and the waters from Mont St Michel to Antifer. (For diagrams of the Casquets TSS/ITZ see Fig 10 (5) and 10.15.2). It also broadcasts traffic, nav and weather info in English and French on Ch 80 at H+20 and H+50; and at H+05 and H+35, when visibility < 2M. Radar assistance is available on request, Ch 11 or 80, to vessels in the sector from due W to due N, out to 35M, from Jobourg Centre at 49°41'N 01°54'·5W.
TELEPHONE
Hr Mr (Port) 33·44·00·13; Hr Mr (Marina) 33·87·65·70; Aff Mar 33·23·36·12; CROSS 33·52·72·13; ⌗ 33·44·16·00; Météo 33·53·53·44; Auto 36.68.08.50; Police 33·44·20·22; Ⓗ 33·52·61·45; Dr 33·53·05·68; Brit Consul 33·44·20·13.
FACILITIES
Port de Plaisance ☎ 33.87.65.70, Fax 33.53.21.12, access H24, (1200+300 visitors), FF100, Slip, AC, FW, ME, El, Sh, BH (27 ton), CH, P & D (0800-1200; 1400-1900);
YC de Cherbourg ☎ 33·53·02·83, FW, R, Bar;
Services: ME, El, Ⓔ, Sh, CH, M, SM, SHOM.
City P, D, Gaz, V, R, Bar, ⊠, Ⓑ, ⇌, ✈ (☎ 33.22.91.32).
Ferry: Portsmouth, Southampton, Poole; Weymouth (summer only).

MINOR HARBOURS TO THE EAST OF CHERBOURG

PORT DU BECQUET, Manche, 49°39'·30N 01°32'·80W. AC *1106*; SHOM 7092. Tides as 10.15.9. Shelter is good except in winds from N to E when a strong scend occurs. Secure to S of jetty (which lies E/W). Ldg lts 186·5°: Front Dir Oc (2+1) 12s 8m 10M, W 8-sided tr, intens 183·5°-190·5°; rear, 48m from front, Dir Oc (2+1) R 12s 13m 7M, synch, also in W 8-sided tr. Facilities: very few; all facilities at Cherbourg 2·5M.

PORT DE LÉVI, Manche, 49°41'·30 N 01°28'·30W. AC *1106*; SHOM 7092, 5609; HW −0310 on Dover (UT); +0024 on Cherbourg. HW ht +0·2m on Cherbourg. Shelter good except in winds SW to N. Secure on NE side below white wall. Lt is F WRG 7m 11/8M, G050°-109°, R109°-140°, W140°-184°. Keep in G sector. By day keep the white wall and lt between the white marks on each pier hd. Beware lobster pots. Facilities: None. Fermanville (1·5M) has V, R, Bar.

Plus ça change ...

There are few things in this world that produce a greater sense of satisfaction than to sail your own boat across the sea and into a foreign port. She may be only ten tons, but you have most of the rights – as well as the responsibilities – inherent in captaining the largest ship afloat, including (bureaucracy be praised!) the right to take tobacco and liquor 'out of bond', in other words free of Customs Duty. To visit Monsieur Henri Ryst's ship-chandling office and see hard liquor, like Scotch and gin, listed at less than a quarter of the price ashore, cognac at a third, cigarettes at a fifth – it is enough to raise the morale of even the tiredest Scotsman; and then to have Monsieur Ryst apologise for not delivering until five p.m. – because he has to victual the Queen Mary! And finally the moment when all those beautiful bottles are collected in the dinghy and taken back to the ship to be stored lovingly away against the day they will be drunk, the crew all lending a willing hand amongst a litter of paper and straw.
It is for this that one puts in to Cherbourg ...... Why else, when close-by are such attractive little ports as Omonville-la-Rogue?

Harvest of Journeys: Hammond Innes/William Collins Sons & Co Ltd, 1960.

15

AGENTS WANTED

If you are interested in becoming our agent for any of the following ports, please write to: The Editor, Edington House, Trent, Sherborne, Dorset DT9 4SR, England – and get your free copy of the almanac annually. You do not have to live in a port to be the agent, but at least a fairly regular visitor.

River Exe	Grandcamp-Maisy
Port Ellen (Islay)	Port-en-Bessin
Glandore/Union Hall	Courseulles
River Rance/Dinan	Boulogne
Lampaul	Dunkerque
Port Tudy	Terneuzen/Westerschelde
River Etel	Oudeschild
Le Palais (Belle Ile)	Lauwersoog
Le Pouliguen/Pornichet	Dornumer-Accumersiel
L'Herbaudière	Hooksiel
St Gilles-Croix-de-Vie	Langeoog
River Seudre	Bremerhaven
Royan	Helgoland
Anglet/Bayonne	Büsum
Hendaye	

TIME ZONE –0100
(French Standard Time)
Subtract 1 hour for UT
For French Summer Time add
ONE hour in non-shaded areas

FRANCE – CHERBOURG

LAT 49°39′N   LONG   1°38′W

TIMES AND HEIGHTS OF HIGH AND LOW WATERS   YEAR 1996

JANUARY

Day	Time	m	Day	Time	m
1 M	0519 / 1218 / 1750	5.2 / 2.4 / 5.2	16 TU	0409 / 1102 / 1641 / 2339	5.2 / 2.3 / 5.2 / 2.2
2 TU	0044 / 0620 / 1315 / 1848	2.3 / 5.4 / 2.2 / 5.4	17 W	0525 / 1218 / 1758	5.4 / 2.0 / 5.5
3 W	0136 / 0709 / 1403 / 1936	2.2 / 5.6 / 2.0 / 5.6	18 TH	0050 / 0631 / 1324 / 1902	1.9 / 5.8 / 1.6 / 5.9
4 TH	0220 / 0752 / 1445 / 2017	2.0 / 5.8 / 1.7 / 5.8	19 F	0152 / 0728 / 1422 / 2000	1.5 / 6.2 / 1.2 / 6.2
5 F O	0258 / 0830 / 1522 / 2054	1.8 / 6.0 / 1.6 / 5.9	20 SA ●	0248 / 0822 / 1516 / 2054	1.2 / 6.5 / 0.8 / 6.5
6 SA	0334 / 0904 / 1556 / 2127	1.7 / 6.1 / 1.5 / 5.9	21 SU	0339 / 0914 / 1606 / 2144	0.9 / 6.8 / 0.6 / 6.6
7 SU	0408 / 0936 / 1629 / 2159	1.6 / 6.1 / 1.4 / 6.0	22 M	0428 / 1002 / 1653 / 2231	0.8 / 6.9 / 0.5 / 6.6
8 M	0441 / 1007 / 1701 / 2231	1.6 / 6.1 / 1.4 / 5.9	23 TU	0515 / 1048 / 1738 / 2315	0.8 / 6.8 / 0.6 / 6.5
9 TU	0513 / 1039 / 1733 / 2304	1.6 / 6.1 / 1.5 / 5.9	24 W	0558 / 1131 / 1820 / 2355	1.0 / 6.6 / 0.9 / 6.2
10 W	0546 / 1113 / 1805 / 2338	1.7 / 6.0 / 1.6 / 5.7	25 TH	0641 / 1212 / 1901	1.3 / 6.3 / 1.3
11 TH	0619 / 1147 / 1839	1.8 / 5.8 / 1.7	26 F	0034 / 0723 / 1252 / 1942	5.9 / 1.7 / 5.9 / 1.7
12 F	0015 / 0657 / 1224 / 1918	5.6 / 2.0 / 5.6 / 1.9	27 SA	0114 / 0808 / 1336 / 2027	5.5 / 2.1 / 5.4 / 2.2
13 SA	0055 / 0741 / 1307 / 2005	5.4 / 2.2 / 5.4 / 2.1	28 SU	0202 / 0901 / 1433 / 2124	5.2 / 2.5 / 5.0 / 2.6
14 SU	0145 / 0836 / 1404 / 2105	5.2 / 2.4 / 5.2 / 2.3	29 M	0308 / 1012 / 1549 / 2240	4.9 / 2.7 / 4.8 / 2.8
15 M	0250 / 0944 / 1517 / 2220	5.1 / 2.5 / 5.1 / 2.3	30 TU	0431 / 1134 / 1714	4.9 / 2.7 / 4.8
			31 W	0002 / 0548 / 1245 / 1824	2.7 / 5.0 / 2.5 / 5.0

FEBRUARY

Day	Time	m	Day	Time	m
1 TH	0112 / 0646 / 1340 / 1915	2.4 / 5.3 / 2.1 / 5.3	16 F	0033 / 0616 / 1309 / 1853	2.0 / 5.6 / 1.7 / 5.7
2 F	0202 / 0731 / 1425 / 1957	2.1 / 5.6 / 1.8 / 5.6	17 SA	0140 / 0717 / 1410 / 1951	1.6 / 6.1 / 1.2 / 6.1
3 SA	0241 / 0811 / 1503 / 2035	1.9 / 5.8 / 1.6 / 5.8	18 SU ●	0237 / 0812 / 1504 / 2043	1.2 / 6.5 / 0.8 / 6.4
4 SU O	0317 / 0846 / 1552 / 2109	1.7 / 6.0 / 1.4 / 6.0	19 M	0328 / 0902 / 1552 / 2130	0.9 / 6.7 / 0.5 / 6.6
5 M	0350 / 0919 / 1610 / 2141	1.5 / 6.2 / 1.3 / 6.0	20 TU	0414 / 0948 / 1636 / 2213	0.7 / 6.9 / 0.5 / 6.7
6 TU	0422 / 0951 / 1642 / 2213	1.4 / 6.2 / 1.2 / 6.1	21 W	0457 / 1031 / 1717 / 2252	0.7 / 6.8 / 0.6 / 6.6
7 W	0454 / 1023 / 1714 / 2245	1.3 / 6.2 / 1.2 / 6.1	22 TH	0536 / 1109 / 1755 / 2328	0.8 / 6.6 / 0.8 / 6.3
8 TH	0527 / 1055 / 1745 / 2318	1.3 / 6.2 / 1.2 / 6.0	23 F	0614 / 1145 / 1830	1.1 / 6.3 / 1.2
9 F	0559 / 1128 / 1817 / 2351	1.4 / 6.1 / 1.4 / 5.8	24 SA	0001 / 0650 / 1220 / 1905	6.0 / 1.5 / 5.9 / 1.7
10 SA	0634 / 1202 / 1853	1.6 / 5.8 / 1.6	25 SU	0034 / 0727 / 1256 / 1942	5.6 / 1.9 / 5.4 / 2.2
11 SU	0026 / 0715 / 1239 / 1936	5.6 / 1.8 / 5.6 / 1.9	26 M	0112 / 0811 / 1343 / 2029	5.2 / 2.4 / 5.0 / 2.6
12 M	0108 / 0803 / 1329 / 2030	5.4 / 2.1 / 5.3 / 2.1	27 TU	0207 / 0911 / 1455 / 2140	4.9 / 2.7 / 4.6 / 2.9
13 TU	0207 / 0907 / 1440 / 2143	5.2 / 2.3 / 5.0 / 2.4	28 W	0336 / 1040 / 1634 / 2317	4.6 / 2.8 / 4.6 / 2.9
14 W	0330 / 1029 / 1617 / 2312	5.1 / 2.4 / 5.0 / 2.4	29 TH	0509 / 1207 / 1755	4.7 / 2.6 / 4.8
15 TH	0502 / 1156 / 1744	5.2 / 2.1 / 5.3			

MARCH

Day	Time	m	Day	Time	m
1 F	0044 / 0616 / 1310 / 1850	2.6 / 5.0 / 2.3 / 5.1	16 SA	0021 / 0604 / 1256 / 1843	2.1 / 5.5 / 1.7 / 5.7
2 SA	0136 / 0705 / 1358 / 1932	2.3 / 5.4 / 1.9 / 5.5	17 SU	0128 / 0705 / 1356 / 1938	1.6 / 6.0 / 1.2 / 6.1
3 SU	0217 / 0746 / 1437 / 2010	1.9 / 5.7 / 1.6 / 5.8	18 M	0223 / 0758 / 1448 / 2027	1.2 / 6.4 / 0.9 / 6.4
4 M	0252 / 0823 / 1512 / 2046	1.6 / 6.0 / 1.3 / 6.0	19 TU ●	0312 / 0846 / 1533 / 2110	0.9 / 6.6 / 0.7 / 6.5
5 TU O	0326 / 0858 / 1545 / 2119	1.4 / 6.2 / 1.1 / 6.1	20 W	0355 / 0929 / 1615 / 2150	0.8 / 6.7 / 0.6 / 6.6
6 W	0359 / 0931 / 1618 / 2152	1.2 / 6.3 / 1.0 / 6.2	21 TH	0435 / 1008 / 1652 / 2226	0.7 / 6.7 / 0.7 / 6.5
7 TH	0433 / 1004 / 1651 / 2224	1.1 / 6.4 / 1.0 / 6.3	22 F	0512 / 1044 / 1727 / 2258	0.9 / 6.5 / 0.9 / 6.3
8 F	0506 / 1037 / 1724 / 2258	1.0 / 6.3 / 1.0 / 6.2	23 SA	0546 / 1118 / 1800 / 2329	1.1 / 6.2 / 1.3 / 6.0
9 SA	0540 / 1111 / 1757 / 2331	1.1 / 6.2 / 1.2 / 6.1	24 SU	0619 / 1151 / 1832	1.4 / 5.9 / 1.7
10 SU	0615 / 1145 / 1834	1.3 / 6.0 / 1.4	25 M	0000 / 0654 / 1224 / 1907	5.7 / 1.8 / 5.4 / 2.1
11 M	0006 / 0655 / 1224 / 1916	5.8 / 1.5 / 5.7 / 1.8	26 TU	0034 / 0733 / 1304 / 1950	5.3 / 2.2 / 5.0 / 2.5
12 TU	0048 / 0743 / 1313 / 2010	5.5 / 1.9 / 5.3 / 2.2	27 W	0119 / 0825 / 1405 / 2051	4.9 / 2.6 / 4.7 / 2.9
13 W	0144 / 0846 / 1425 / 2124	5.2 / 2.2 / 5.0 / 2.4	28 TH	0235 / 0941 / 1544 / 2223	4.6 / 2.8 / 4.5 / 3.0
14 TH	0309 / 1009 / 1607 / 2256	5.0 / 2.3 / 5.0 / 2.4	29 F	0417 / 1115 / 1714 / 2352	4.6 / 2.7 / 4.7 / 2.8
15 F	0447 / 1141 / 1736	5.2 / 2.1 / 5.2	30 SA	0534 / 1227 / 1813	4.8 / 2.4 / 5.0
			31 SU	0053 / 0628 / 1319 / 1858	2.4 / 5.2 / 2.0 / 5.4

APRIL

Day	Time	m	Day	Time	m
1 M	0140 / 0712 / 1401 / 1938	2.0 / 5.6 / 1.7 / 5.7	16 TU	0205 / 0738 / 1427 / 2005	1.4 / 6.2 / 1.1 / 6.2
2 TU	0219 / 0752 / 1439 / 2016	1.7 / 5.9 / 1.4 / 6.0	17 W ●	0252 / 0825 / 1510 / 2047	1.1 / 6.4 / 0.9 / 6.4
3 W	0256 / 0830 / 1515 / 2052	1.4 / 6.1 / 1.1 / 6.2	18 TH	0334 / 0907 / 1550 / 2124	1.0 / 6.5 / 0.9 / 6.4
4 TH O	0333 / 0906 / 1551 / 2127	1.1 / 6.3 / 1.0 / 6.3	19 F	0412 / 0945 / 1626 / 2158	0.9 / 6.4 / 1.0 / 6.3
5 F	0409 / 0942 / 1627 / 2202	0.9 / 6.4 / 0.9 / 6.4	20 SA	0447 / 1020 / 1700 / 2231	1.0 / 6.3 / 1.2 / 6.2
6 SA	0445 / 1019 / 1703 / 2238	0.9 / 6.4 / 0.9 / 6.4	21 SU	0521 / 1053 / 1732 / 2302	1.2 / 6.1 / 1.4 / 6.0
7 SU	0522 / 1056 / 1740 / 2314	0.9 / 6.3 / 1.1 / 6.2	22 M	0554 / 1126 / 1805 / 2334	1.4 / 5.8 / 1.7 / 5.7
8 M	0601 / 1135 / 1820 / 2353	1.1 / 6.1 / 1.4 / 6.0	23 TU	0628 / 1200 / 1840	1.7 / 5.5 / 2.1
9 TU	0644 / 1218 / 1905	1.4 / 5.8 / 1.7	24 W	0007 / 0705 / 1238 / 1921	5.4 / 2.1 / 5.1 / 2.4
10 W	0038 / 0734 / 1310 / 2002	5.7 / 1.7 / 5.4 / 2.1	25 TH	0049 / 0751 / 1328 / 2014	5.1 / 2.4 / 4.8 / 2.7
11 TH	0137 / 0838 / 1423 / 2117	5.3 / 2.0 / 5.1 / 2.4	26 F	0147 / 0852 / 1445 / 2128	4.8 / 2.6 / 4.6 / 2.9
12 F	0259 / 0959 / 1600 / 2246	5.1 / 2.1 / 5.0 / 2.4	27 SA	0311 / 1012 / 1615 / 2252	4.6 / 2.6 / 4.7 / 2.8
13 SA	0432 / 1126 / 1722	5.2 / 2.0 / 5.3	28 SU	0434 / 1128 / 1723	4.8 / 2.5 / 4.9
14 SU	0006 / 0546 / 1238 / 1825	2.1 / 5.5 / 1.7 / 5.7	29 M	0000 / 0537 / 1228 / 1815	2.5 / 5.0 / 2.2 / 5.3
15 M	0111 / 0646 / 1338 / 1918	1.7 / 5.9 / 1.3 / 6.0	30 TU	0053 / 0629 / 1317 / 1859	2.1 / 5.4 / 1.8 / 5.6

Chart Datum: 3·70 metres below Lallemand System (Mean Sea Level, Marseilles)

TIME ZONE –0100
(French Standard Time)
Subtract 1 hour for UT

For French Summer Time add
ONE hour in non-shaded areas

FRANCE – CHERBOURG

LAT 49°39′N   LONG 1°38′W

TIMES AND HEIGHTS OF HIGH AND LOW WATERS   YEAR 1996

MAY

Time	m	Time	m
1 0139 / 0715 / W 1401 / 1941	1.8 / 5.7 / 1.5 / 5.9	**16** 0229 / 0802 / TH 1446 / 2022	1.4 / 6.0 / 1.3 / 6.1
2 0222 / 0758 / TH 1442 / 2021	1.4 / 6.0 / 1.2 / 6.2	**17** 0311 / 0844 / F 1525 / ● 2100	1.3 / 6.1 / 1.3 / 6.2
3 0304 / 0840 / F 1523 / O 2100	1.1 / 6.2 / 1.0 / 6.4	**18** 0350 / 0923 / SA 1602 / 2135	1.2 / 6.1 / 1.3 / 6.2
4 0345 / 0920 / SA 1604 / 2140	0.9 / 6.4 / 0.9 / 6.5	**19** 0425 / 0958 / SU 1636 / 2208	1.2 / 6.0 / 1.4 / 6.1
5 0426 / 1002 / SU 1645 / 2220	0.8 / 6.4 / 0.9 / 6.5	**20** 0500 / 1032 / M 1710 / 2241	1.3 / 5.9 / 1.6 / 6.0
6 0508 / 1044 / M 1727 / 2302	0.8 / 6.3 / 1.1 / 6.4	**21** 0533 / 1106 / TU 1744 / 2313	1.4 / 5.7 / 1.8 / 5.8
7 0551 / 1128 / TU 1811 / 2346	0.9 / 6.1 / 1.3 / 6.1	**22** 0607 / 1140 / W 1819 / 2348	1.6 / 5.5 / 2.0 / 5.5
8 0638 / 1215 / W 1901	1.2 / 5.9 / 1.7	**23** 0643 / 1217 / TH 1857	1.9 / 5.3 / 2.3
9 0035 / 0731 / TH 1310 / 2000	5.8 / 1.5 / 5.5 / 2.0	**24** 0026 / 0723 / F 1300 / 1943	5.3 / 2.1 / 5.0 / 2.5
10 0133 / 0833 / F 1419 / 2111	5.5 / 1.8 / 5.3 / 2.2	**25** 0113 / 0812 / SA 1357 / 2041	5.0 / 2.3 / 4.8 / 2.7
11 0247 / 0947 / SA 1542 / 2230	5.3 / 1.9 / 5.2 / 2.3	**26** 0214 / 0914 / SU 1507 / 2151	4.8 / 2.5 / 4.8 / 2.7
12 0409 / 1104 / SU 1657 / 2344	5.3 / 1.9 / 5.3 / 2.1	**27** 0326 / 1025 / M 1620 / 2301	4.8 / 2.4 / 4.9 / 2.5
13 0520 / 1212 / M 1800	5.4 / 1.7 / 5.6	**28** 0436 / 1131 / TU 1722	4.9 / 2.2 / 5.2
14 0047 / 0621 / TU 1312 / 1853	1.8 / 5.7 / 1.5 / 5.8	**29** 0004 / 0539 / W 1230 / 1816	2.2 / 5.2 / 1.9 / 5.5
15 0142 / 0715 / W 1402 / 1940	1.6 / 5.9 / 1.4 / 6.0	**30** 0058 / 0634 / TH 1322 / 1904	1.9 / 5.5 / 1.6 / 5.8
		31 0148 / 0725 / F 1411 / 1950	1.5 / 5.8 / 1.3 / 6.1

JUNE

Time	m	Time	m
1 0237 / 0814 / SA 1458 / O 2035	1.2 / 6.1 / 1.1 / 6.3	**16** 0330 / 0904 / SU 1541 / ● 2115	1.4 / 5.9 / 1.6 / 6.0
2 0324 / 0901 / SU 1544 / 2120	1.0 / 6.3 / 1.0 / 6.5	**17** 0407 / 0940 / M 1617 / 2149	1.4 / 5.9 / 1.6 / 6.0
3 0410 / 0948 / M 1630 / 2206	0.8 / 6.4 / 0.9 / 6.5	**18** 0442 / 1014 / TU 1652 / 2222	1.4 / 5.8 / 1.6 / 6.0
4 0457 / 1034 / TU 1717 / 2252	0.7 / 6.4 / 1.0 / 6.5	**19** 0515 / 1048 / W 1725 / 2255	1.4 / 5.8 / 1.7 / 5.9
5 0544 / 1122 / W 1805 / 2340	0.8 / 6.3 / 1.2 / 6.3	**20** 0548 / 1121 / TH 1759 / 2329	1.5 / 5.6 / 1.9 / 5.7
6 0633 / 1211 / TH 1856	1.0 / 6.0 / 1.5	**21** 0622 / 1156 / F 1834	1.7 / 5.5 / 2.0
7 0030 / 0725 / F 1303 / 1952	6.1 / 1.2 / 5.7 / 1.8	**22** 0004 / 0657 / SA 1234 / 1914	5.5 / 1.9 / 5.3 / 2.2
8 0124 / 0821 / SA 1402 / 2055	5.8 / 1.5 / 5.5 / 2.0	**23** 0044 / 0737 / SU 1318 / 2000	5.3 / 2.0 / 5.1 / 2.4
9 0227 / 0924 / SU 1508 / 2204	5.5 / 1.8 / 5.3 / 2.2	**24** 0131 / 0826 / M 1411 / 2058	5.1 / 2.2 / 5.0 / 2.5
10 0336 / 1032 / M 1620 / 2313	5.3 / 2.0 / 5.3 / 2.2	**25** 0228 / 0927 / TU 1515 / 2205	5.0 / 2.3 / 5.0 / 2.5
11 0446 / 1139 / TU 1726	5.3 / 2.0 / 5.4	**26** 0336 / 1036 / W 1625 / 2315	4.9 / 2.3 / 5.1 / 2.3
12 0018 / 0551 / W 1241 / 1824	2.0 / 5.4 / 1.9 / 5.6	**27** 0448 / 1145 / TH 1731	5.1 / 2.1 / 5.3
13 0116 / 0649 / TH 1336 / 1915	1.9 / 5.6 / 1.8 / 5.7	**28** 0019 / 0555 / F 1247 / 1829	2.0 / 5.3 / 1.8 / 5.7
14 0206 / 0739 / F 1422 / 1959	1.7 / 5.7 / 1.7 / 5.9	**29** 0118 / 0656 / SA 1343 / 1923	1.7 / 5.7 / 1.5 / 6.0
15 0250 / 0825 / SA 1503 / 2039	1.5 / 5.8 / 1.6 / 6.0	**30** 0213 / 0752 / SU 1437 / 2014	1.3 / 6.0 / 1.2 / 6.3

JULY

Time	m	Time	m
1 0306 / 0845 / M 1528 / O 2105	1.0 / 6.2 / 1.0 / 6.5	**16** 0349 / 0923 / TU 1600 / 2132	1.4 / 5.8 / 1.6 / 6.0
2 0356 / 0936 / TU 1618 / 2154	0.7 / 6.4 / 0.9 / 6.6	**17** 0423 / 0956 / W 1633 / 2204	1.3 / 5.9 / 1.6 / 6.0
3 0446 / 1025 / W 1707 / 2243	0.6 / 6.5 / 0.9 / 6.7	**18** 0456 / 1028 / TH 1706 / 2235	1.4 / 5.8 / 1.6 / 6.0
4 0534 / 1113 / TH 1755 / 2331	0.6 / 6.4 / 1.0 / 6.5	**19** 0527 / 1059 / F 1737 / 2307	1.4 / 5.8 / 1.7 / 5.9
5 0622 / 1200 / F 1844	0.7 / 6.2 / 1.2	**20** 0558 / 1132 / SA 1810 / 2340	1.5 / 5.7 / 1.8 / 5.8
6 0018 / 0710 / SA 1247 / 1934	6.3 / 1.0 / 6.0 / 1.5	**21** 0630 / 1206 / SU 1845	1.6 / 5.6 / 1.9
7 0106 / 0759 / SU 1335 / 2028	6.0 / 1.4 / 5.6 / 1.9	**22** 0016 / 0705 / M 1243 / 1925	5.6 / 1.8 / 5.4 / 2.1
8 0158 / 0852 / M 1430 / 2129	5.6 / 1.8 / 5.4 / 2.2	**23** 0054 / 0747 / TU 1327 / 2014	5.3 / 2.0 / 5.2 / 2.3
9 0258 / 0953 / TU 1535 / 2236	5.3 / 2.1 / 5.2 / 2.3	**24** 0143 / 0840 / W 1422 / 2116	5.1 / 2.2 / 5.1 / 2.4
10 0407 / 1101 / W 1647 / 2346	5.1 / 2.3 / 5.1 / 2.3	**25** 0246 / 0948 / TH 1533 / 2231	5.0 / 2.4 / 5.0 / 2.4
11 0520 / 1209 / TH 1755	5.1 / 2.3 / 5.3	**26** 0405 / 1106 / F 1652 / 2347	5.0 / 2.3 / 5.2 / 2.2
12 0049 / 0626 / F 1313 / 1852	2.1 / 5.2 / 2.1 / 5.5	**27** 0527 / 1219 / SA 1803	5.2 / 2.0 / 5.5
13 0144 / 0721 / SA 1404 / 1939	1.9 / 5.4 / 2.0 / 5.7	**28** 0055 / 0636 / SU 1323 / 1903	1.8 / 5.6 / 1.7 / 5.9
14 0231 / 0807 / SU 1446 / 2021	1.7 / 5.6 / 1.8 / 5.9	**29** 0155 / 0736 / M 1421 / 1959	1.3 / 5.9 / 1.3 / 6.3
15 0312 / 0847 / M 1524 / ● 2058	1.6 / 5.7 / 1.7 / 6.3	**30** 0251 / 0832 / TU 1514 / O 2051	1.0 / 6.3 / 1.0 / 6.6
		31 0343 / 0924 / W 1605 / 2142	0.6 / 6.5 / 0.8 / 6.8

AUGUST

Time	m	Time	m
1 0432 / 1012 / TH 1653 / 2230	0.5 / 6.6 / 0.7 / 6.8	**16** 0432 / 1005 / F 1642 / 2212	1.3 / 6.0 / 1.4 / 6.2
2 0519 / 1058 / F 1739 / 2315	0.5 / 6.6 / 0.8 / 6.7	**17** 0502 / 1035 / SA 1713 / 2243	1.3 / 6.0 / 1.4 / 6.1
3 0603 / 1140 / SA 1823 / 2359	0.6 / 6.4 / 1.1 / 6.4	**18** 0532 / 1106 / SU 1744 / 2315	1.3 / 5.9 / 1.5 / 6.0
4 0646 / 1221 / SU 1908	1.0 / 6.1 / 1.4	**19** 0603 / 1138 / M 1817 / 2348	1.4 / 5.8 / 1.7 / 5.8
5 0040 / 0729 / M 1301 / 1954	6.1 / 1.4 / 5.7 / 1.8	**20** 0636 / 1212 / TU 1854	1.6 / 5.6 / 1.9
6 0124 / 0814 / TU 1346 / 2047	5.6 / 1.9 / 5.4 / 2.2	**21** 0023 / 0715 / W 1250 / 1939	5.5 / 1.9 / 5.4 / 2.1
7 0216 / 0909 / W 1446 / 2154	5.2 / 2.3 / 5.1 / 2.5	**22** 0107 / 0804 / TH 1340 / 2038	5.3 / 2.2 / 5.2 / 2.4
8 0327 / 1019 / TH 1605 / 2311	4.9 / 2.6 / 4.9 / 2.6	**23** 0210 / 0911 / F 1453 / 2157	5.0 / 2.4 / 5.0 / 2.5
9 0450 / 1137 / F 1726	4.8 / 2.6 / 5.0	**24** 0338 / 1037 / SA 1625 / 2324	4.9 / 2.5 / 5.1 / 2.3
10 0023 / 0606 / SA 1250 / 1830	2.4 / 5.0 / 2.4 / 5.3	**25** 0511 / 1200 / SU 1745	5.1 / 2.2 / 5.5
11 0122 / 0703 / SU 1343 / 1919	2.1 / 5.3 / 2.2 / 5.5	**26** 0038 / 0624 / M 1308 / 1849	1.8 / 5.5 / 1.8 / 5.9
12 0210 / 0748 / M 1428 / 2000	1.9 / 5.5 / 1.9 / 5.8	**27** 0140 / 0724 / TU 1407 / 1945	1.4 / 6.0 / 1.3 / 6.4
13 0251 / 0826 / TU 1504 / 2037	1.6 / 5.7 / 1.7 / 6.0	**28** 0236 / 0817 / W 1500 / O 2037	0.9 / 6.4 / 1.0 / 6.7
14 0327 / 0901 / W 1539 / ● 2111	1.4 / 5.9 / 1.6 / 6.1	**29** 0326 / 0907 / TH 1548 / 2125	0.6 / 6.6 / 0.8 / 6.9
15 0400 / 0934 / TH 1611 / 2142	1.3 / 6.0 / 1.5 / 6.1	**30** 0413 / 0953 / F 1634 / 2211	0.5 / 6.7 / 0.7 / 6.9
		31 0457 / 1035 / SA 1716 / 2253	0.5 / 6.7 / 0.8 / 6.8

15

Chart Datum: 3·70 metres below Lallemand System (Mean Sea Level, Marseilles)

TIME ZONE –0100
(French Standard Time)
Subtract 1 hour for UT

For French Summer Time add ONE hour in non-shaded areas

FRANCE – CHERBOURG

LAT 49°39′N   LONG   1°38′W

TIMES AND HEIGHTS OF HIGH AND LOW WATERS   YEAR 1996

SEPTEMBER

Day	Time / m	Day	Time / m
1 SU	0538 0.7 / 1114 6.5 / 1757 1.0 / 2332 6.5	**16** M	0506 1.2 / 1039 6.2 / 1720 1.3 / 2251 6.2
2 M	0616 1.1 / 1149 6.2 / 1836 1.4	**17** TU	0538 1.4 / 1112 6.0 / 1753 1.5 / 2325 6.0
3 TU	0010 6.1 / 0654 1.6 / 1224 5.8 / 1916 1.9	**18** W	0612 1.6 / 1145 5.8 / 1831 1.7
4 W	0048 5.6 / 0733 2.1 / 1303 5.4 / 2002 2.3	**19** TH	0001 5.7 / 0651 1.9 / 1224 5.6 / 1915 2.0
5 TH	0135 5.1 / 0821 2.5 / 1356 5.0 / 2104 2.7	**20** F	0047 5.4 / 0740 2.2 / 1315 5.3 / 2014 2.3
6 F	0243 4.8 / 0931 2.9 / 1518 4.8 / 2230 2.8	**21** SA	0152 5.1 / 0848 2.5 / 1430 5.1 / 2134 2.4
7 SA	0418 4.7 / 1102 2.9 / 1652 4.8 / 2352 2.6	**22** SU	0327 4.9 / 1019 2.6 / 1608 5.1 / 2307 2.3
8 SU	0542 4.8 / 1224 2.7 / 1802 5.1	**23** M	0502 5.2 / 1147 2.3 / 1731 5.5
9 M	0054 2.3 / 0638 5.2 / 1317 2.3 / 1852 5.4	**24** TU	0024 1.8 / 0612 5.6 / 1255 1.8 / 1834 6.0
10 TU	0143 2.0 / 0721 5.5 / 1403 2.0 / 1933 5.7	**25** W	0125 1.4 / 0709 6.1 / 1352 1.4 / 1929 6.4
11 W	0223 1.7 / 0759 5.8 / 1438 1.7 / 2010 6.0	**26** TH	0218 1.0 / 0800 6.4 / 1443 1.0 / 2019 6.7
12 TH	0259 1.5 / 0834 6.0 / 1512 1.5 / ●2044 6.2	**27** F	0306 0.7 / 0846 6.6 / 1529 0.8 / O2105 6.9
13 F	0332 1.3 / 0907 6.1 / 1544 1.4 / 2116 6.3	**28** SA	0351 0.6 / 0929 6.7 / 1612 0.8 / 2148 6.8
14 SA	0403 1.2 / 0938 6.2 / 1616 1.3 / 2147 6.3	**29** SU	0432 0.7 / 1008 6.7 / 1652 0.9 / 2227 6.7
15 SU	0435 1.2 / 1008 6.2 / 1648 1.3 / 2219 6.3	**30** M	0510 0.9 / 1043 6.5 / 1729 1.1 / 2304 6.4

OCTOBER

Day	Time / m	Day	Time / m
1 TU	0545 1.3 / 1117 6.2 / 1805 1.5 / 2339 6.0	**16** W	0517 1.3 / 1050 6.2 / 1736 1.3 / 2309 6.1
2 W	0620 1.7 / 1150 5.9 / 1842 1.9	**17** TH	0554 1.6 / 1128 6.0 / 1816 1.6 / 2350 5.8
3 TH	0015 5.6 / 0657 2.2 / 1226 5.5 / 1922 2.3	**18** F	0637 1.9 / 1210 5.8 / 1903 1.9
4 F	0057 5.1 / 0740 2.6 / 1311 5.1 / 2015 2.7	**19** SA	0040 5.5 / 0729 2.2 / 1304 5.4 / 2002 2.2
5 SA	0159 4.8 / 0841 3.0 / 1424 4.8 / 2135 2.9	**20** SU	0146 5.2 / 0838 2.5 / 1418 5.2 / 2121 2.3
6 SU	0334 4.6 / 1015 3.1 / 1604 4.7 / 2308 2.8	**21** M	0318 5.1 / 1006 2.6 / 1552 5.2 / 2250 2.2
7 M	0503 4.8 / 1144 2.9 / 1721 4.9	**22** TU	0447 5.3 / 1131 2.3 / 1712 5.5
8 TU	0016 2.5 / 0602 5.1 / 1245 2.5 / 1815 5.3	**23** W	0005 1.9 / 0554 5.7 / 1238 1.9 / 1815 5.9
9 W	0106 2.1 / 0646 5.4 / 1328 2.1 / 1858 5.6	**24** TH	0105 1.5 / 0649 6.1 / 1334 1.5 / 1909 6.3
10 TH	0148 1.8 / 0724 5.8 / 1405 1.8 / 1937 5.9	**25** F	0158 1.2 / 0737 6.4 / 1423 1.2 / 1958 6.5
11 F	0225 1.5 / 0801 6.0 / 1440 1.6 / 2013 6.2	**26** SA	0244 1.0 / 0801 6.5 / 1508 1.0 / O2042 6.7
12 SA	0300 1.3 / 0835 6.2 / 1514 1.3 / ●2048 6.3	**27** SU	0327 0.9 / 0903 6.6 / 1603 1.0 / 2123 6.6
13 SU	0334 1.2 / 0909 6.3 / 1549 1.2 / 2121 6.4	**28** M	0406 1.0 / 0940 6.5 / 1627 1.1 / 2201 6.5
14 M	0408 1.1 / 0941 6.4 / 1624 1.1 / 2156 6.4	**29** TU	0443 1.2 / 1014 6.4 / 1703 1.2 / 2237 6.3
15 TU	0442 1.2 / 1015 6.3 / 1659 1.2 / 2231 6.3	**30** W	0518 1.5 / 1047 6.2 / 1738 1.5 / 2312 6.0
		31 TH	0552 1.8 / 1121 5.9 / 1813 1.8 / 2347 5.6

NOVEMBER

Day	Time / m	Day	Time / m
1 F	0627 2.2 / 1155 5.6 / 1851 2.2	**16** SA	0630 1.8 / 1203 6.0 / 1857 1.6
2 SA	0027 5.3 / 0708 2.6 / 1237 5.2 / 1936 2.5	**17** SU	0037 5.7 / 0724 2.1 / 1258 5.7 / 1956 1.9
3 SU	0118 4.9 / 0759 2.9 / 1333 4.9 / 2037 2.8	**18** M	0140 5.4 / 0830 2.3 / 1406 5.4 / 2107 2.1
4 M	0233 4.7 / 0913 3.1 / 1456 4.7 / 2200 2.8	**19** TU	0300 5.3 / 0948 2.4 / 1528 5.4 / 2226 2.1
5 TU	0402 4.7 / 1040 3.0 / 1619 4.8 / 2319 2.7	**20** W	0420 5.4 / 1108 2.3 / 1645 5.5 / 2340 1.9
6 W	0510 5.0 / 1149 2.7 / 1723 5.1	**21** TH	0527 5.6 / 1215 2.0 / 1750 5.8
7 TH	0018 2.4 / 0601 5.3 / 1242 2.3 / 1814 5.4	**22** F	0042 1.7 / 0624 5.9 / 1313 1.7 / 1846 6.0
8 F	0105 2.0 / 0644 5.7 / 1325 2.0 / 1858 5.8	**23** SA	0135 1.5 / 0714 6.1 / 1403 1.5 / 1936 6.2
9 SA	0147 1.7 / 0724 6.0 / 1405 1.7 / 1939 6.0	**24** SU	0222 1.4 / 0759 6.3 / 1448 1.4 / 2021 6.3
10 SU	0226 1.5 / 0802 6.2 / 1445 1.4 / 2019 6.2	**25** M	0305 1.3 / 0839 6.4 / 1529 1.2 / O2102 6.3
11 M	0304 1.3 / 0839 6.4 / 1524 1.2 / ●2057 6.4	**26** TU	0344 1.3 / 0916 6.4 / 1607 1.3 / 2139 6.3
12 TU	0343 1.2 / 0916 6.5 / 1603 1.1 / 2136 6.4	**27** W	0421 1.4 / 0951 6.3 / 1643 1.3 / 2215 6.1
13 W	0422 1.2 / 0954 6.5 / 1643 1.1 / 2216 6.4	**28** TH	0456 1.6 / 1025 6.2 / 1717 1.5 / 2250 5.9
14 TH	0502 1.3 / 1034 6.4 / 1724 1.2 / 2259 6.2	**29** F	0530 1.8 / 1058 6.0 / 1752 1.7 / 2325 5.7
15 F	0544 1.5 / 1117 6.2 / 1808 1.4 / 2345 6.0	**30** SA	0605 2.1 / 1132 5.7 / 1827 2.0

DECEMBER

Day	Time / m	Day	Time / m
1 SU	0001 5.4 / 0642 2.3 / 1209 5.4 / 1905 2.2	**16** M	0030 5.9 / 0717 1.8 / 1249 6.0 / 1945 1.6
2 M	0043 5.2 / 0725 2.6 / 1253 5.2 / 1951 2.5	**17** TU	0125 5.7 / 0815 2.1 / 1348 5.7 / 2045 1.7
3 TU	0136 4.9 / 0818 2.8 / 1350 4.9 / 2050 2.7	**18** W	0230 5.4 / 0922 2.3 / 1456 5.4 / 2154 2.1
4 W	0244 4.8 / 0925 2.9 / 1502 4.8 / 2202 2.7	**19** TH	0343 5.3 / 1036 2.3 / 1610 5.4 / 2307 2.1
5 TH	0359 4.9 / 1040 2.8 / 1616 4.9 / 2314 2.5	**20** F	0453 5.4 / 1148 2.2 / 1720 5.5
6 F	0504 5.1 / 1147 2.5 / 1720 5.2	**21** SA	0014 2.0 / 0556 5.6 / 1250 2.0 / 1823 5.6
7 SA	0015 2.3 / 0558 5.4 / 1242 2.2 / 1816 5.5	**22** SU	0115 1.9 / 0651 5.8 / 1344 1.8 / 1917 5.8
8 SU	0106 1.9 / 0646 5.8 / 1331 1.8 / 1905 5.8	**23** M	0204 1.7 / 0739 6.0 / 1431 1.6 / 2004 6.0
9 M	0153 1.6 / 0730 6.1 / 1417 1.5 / 1951 6.1	**24** TU	0247 1.6 / 0821 6.1 / 1513 1.5 / 2046 6.0
10 TU	0238 1.4 / 0813 6.3 / 1502 1.2 / ●2036 6.3	**25** W	0327 1.6 / 0859 6.2 / 1550 1.4 / 2123 6.1
11 W	0322. 1.2 / 0856 6.5 / 1546 1.0 / 2121 6.4	**26** TH	0404 1.6 / 0934 6.2 / 1626 1.4 / 2158 6.0
12 TH	0407 1.1 / 0939 6.6 / 1631 0.9 / 2206 6.4	**27** F	0439 1.6 / 1007 6.2 / 1700 1.4 / 2232 6.0
13 F	0451 1.1 / 1024 6.6 / 1716 0.9 / 2252 6.4	**28** SA	0512 1.7 / 1040 6.1 / 1733 1.5 / 2304 5.8
14 SA	0537 1.3 / 1109 6.5 / 1802 1.0 / 2339 6.2	**29** SU	0545 1.8 / 1112 5.9 / 1805 1.7 / 2337 5.6
15 SU	0625 1.5 / 1157 6.3 / 1852 1.3	**30** M	0619 2.0 / 1145 5.7 / 1838 1.9
		31 TU	0012 5.4 / 0654 2.2 / 1220 5.5 / 1915 2.1

Chart Datum: 3·70 metres below Lallemand System (Mean Sea Level, Marseilles)

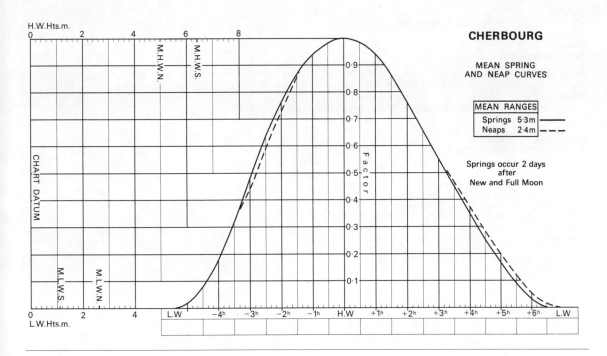

CHERBOURG

MEAN SPRING
AND NEAP CURVES

MEAN RANGES	
Springs	5·3m
Neaps	2·4m

Springs occur 2 days
after
New and Full Moon

OMONVILLE-LA-ROGUE 10-15-10

Manche 49°42'·34N 01°49'·78W

CHARTS
AC *1106, 2669*; SHOM 5636, 6737, 7158; ECM 528, 1014; Imray C33A; Stanfords 7, 16

TIDES
–0330 Dover; ML 3·6; Duration 0545; Zone –0100

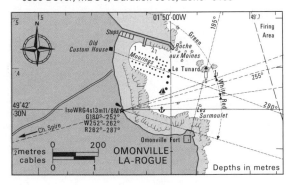

Standard Port CHERBOURG (←)

Times				Height (metres)			
High Water		Low Water		MHWS	MHWN	MLWN	MLWS
0300	1000	0400	1000	6·4	5·0	2·5	1·1
1500	2200	1600	2200				
Differences OMONVILLE							
–0025	–0030	–0022	–0022	–0·3	–0·2	–0·2	–0·1
GOURY							
–0100	–0040	–0105	–0120	+1·7	+1·6	+1·0	+0·3

SHELTER
Good, except in strong winds from N to SE. Pick up a vacant mooring or ⚓ S of bkwtr, but beware rks at outer end.

NAVIGATION
WPT 49°42'·50N 01°48'·60W, 075°/255° from/to Omonville lt, 1·0M. Ent is 100m wide, between rks extending N from Omonville Fort, and running ESE from bkwtr marked by

Le Tunard, G bn tr. From W or N, keep clear of Basse Bréfort (depth 1m, marked by NCM buoy, VQ) 0·6M N of Pte de Jardeheu. Appr on 195° transit (below), passing 100m E of Le Tunard and into W sector of lt before turning stbd 290° for old Custom Ho and moorings. From E, appr on 255° transit in W sector of lt, until S of Le Tunard.
To ENE of port is a military firing area; when active, a R flag is flown from the bkwtr head.

LIGHTS AND MARKS
Omonville lt, Iso WRG 4s 13m 11/8M, on W framework tr with R top, vis G180°-252°, W252°-262°, R262°-287°. Lt in transit 255° with ⊞ steeple, 650m beyond, leads S of Le Tunard. From N, Le Tunard leads 195° in transit with fort. Street lts adequately illuminate the hbr area.

RADIO TELEPHONE
None. For Casquets TSS see Cherbourg (10·15·9).

TELEPHONE
Aff Mar Cherbourg 33·53·21·76; ♯ Cherbourg 33·53·05·60; CROSS 33·52·72·13; 33·52·71·33; Meteo 33·22·91·77; Auto 36.68.08.50; Police 33·52·72·02; Dr 33·53·08·69; Brit Consul 33·44·20·13.

FACILITIES
Jetty M, L, FW, AB, V, R, Bar. **Village** V, Gaz, R, Bar, nearest fuel (cans) at Beaumont-Hague 5km, ⊠, Ⓑ, ⇌ (bus to Cherbourg), ✈. Ferry: See Cherbourg.

ADJACENT HARBOUR

PORT RACINE, Manche, 49°42'·78N 01°53'·70W. AC *1106, 3653;* SHOM 5636. Tides as 10.15.10. Port Racine (reputedly the smallest hbr in France) is in the SW corner of Anse de St.Martin. This bay, 2M E of Cap de la Hague, has ⚓s sheltered from all but onshore winds. From N, appr with conspic chy (279m) at atomic stn brg 175°; or from NE via Basse Bréfort NCM buoy, VQ, with St Germain des Vaux spire brg 240°. Both lines clear La Parmentière rks awash in centre of bay and Les Herbeuses and Le Grun Rks to W and E respectively. ⚓ or moor off the hbr which is obstructed by lines; only accessible by dinghy. R is only facility.

15

DIÉLETTE   10-15-11

Manche, 49°33′·30′N 01°51′·80′W

CHARTS
AC *3653*; SHOM 7133, 7158; ECM 528, 1014; Imray C33A;
Stanfords 16

TIDES
HW −0430 on Dover (UT); ML 5·2m.

Standard Port ST-MALO (→)

Times				Height (metres)			
High Water		Low Water		MHWS	MHWN	MLWN	MLWS
0100	0800	0300	0800	12·2	9·2	4·3	1·6
1300	2000	1500	2000				
Differences FLAMANVILLE							
+0050	+0050	+0025	+0045	−2·7	−1·8	−1·1	−0·5

SHELTER
Good. A marina is due to open in 1996. On completion,
the port will comprise 3 hbrs: the outer hbr (drying 5m)
for FVs/transient craft, enclosed by the original W bkwtr
from which a new spur extends N'wards; a new N bkwtr
extends W'ward to form the ent. Inside, the non-tidal
marina is entered via a lock; the new, first basin is for
visitors and the original, inner basin is for locals. *See the
Almanac Supplements for further details, as available.*

NAVIGATION
WPT 49°33′·46N 01°52′·21W, 305°/125° from/to front ldg
lt, 0·38M. Appr is exposed to W'ly winds/swell. A prohib
area from Diélette to C de Flamanville extends 5ca offshore.

LIGHTS AND MARKS
Two chys (72m) are conspic at power stn 1·2M to SW,
where 6ca offshore a WCM buoy, Q (9) 15s, bears 245°/
1·2M from hbr ent. Ldg lts 125·5°: Front on end of Jetée
Ouest, Fl (2) WRG 6s 12m, 7/4M on W tr with G top, G
shore -072°, W072°-138°, R138°-206°, G206°-shore; rear
(460m from front), Dir Oc (2) 6s 23m 7M, intens 121°-
130°, on house with W gable. Enter 50m NE of front lt.

RADIO TELEPHONE
Not known.

TELEPHONE
Users Assoc'n 33.04.15.25; YC ☎ 33·53·03·85; Meteo
33·42·20·40; CROSS 33.52.72.13; SNSM 33.53.83.69.

FACILITIES
Marina (350) AC, FW, Fuel, Slip, C (4 ton); **Village**, V, Bar,
R, ☎. Also facilities at Flamanville (1·3M).

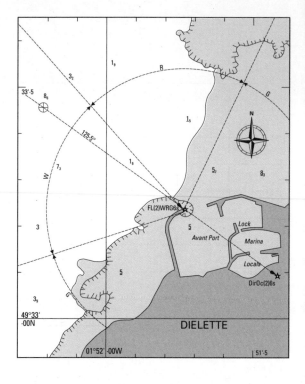

MINOR HARBOUR CLOSE SOUTH OF CAP DE LA HAGUE

GOURY, Manche, 49°43′·00N 01°56·70′W. AC *1106, 3653*;
SHOM 5636, 7158. HW −0410 on Dover (UT); ML 5·1m.
See 10.15.10. For visitors, a fair wx hbr only; dries to flat
sand/mud. Cap de la Hague lt, Fl 5s, is 0·5M NW of hbr
ent; La Foraine WCM unlit buoy is 1·3M to the W. Ldg lts:
Front QR 4m 7M, on bkwtr hd; rear (110m from front), Q
10m 12M, intens 057°-075°, lead 065° between Charlin
to stbd and Les Grois to port. By day, W patch with R ■ at
end of bkwtr on with RH edge of R roofed house, 063°.
There are 2 LB slips; inside these, berth or ⚓ on the NE
side of the bkwtr. Facilities: R, Bar at Auderville (0·5M).

CARTERET   10-15-12

Manche 49°22′·20N 01°47′·38W

CHARTS
AC *3655, 2669*; SHOM 7133, 7157, 7158; ECM 1014; Imray
C33A; Stanfords 16

TIDES
−0440 Dover; ML 5·9; Duration 0545; Zone −0100

Standard Port ST-MALO (→)

Times				Height (metres)			
High Water		Low Water		MHWS	MHWN	MLWN	MLWS
0100	0800	0300	0800	12·2	9·2	4·3	1·6
1300	2000	1500	2000				
Differences CARTERET							
+0035	+0025	+0020	+0035	−1·6	−1·1	−0·6	−0·3

SHELTER
Good in non-tidal marina (sill is 4m above CD; lifting gate
retains 2·3m within); access HW−2½ to +3 for 1·5m draft.
Visitors berth on far side of the most E'ly pontoon. If too
late on the tide for the marina, possible waiting berths on
W Jetty (clear of ferry) where a 1·5m draft boat can stay
afloat for 6 hrs np, 9hrs sp. The tiny Port des Américains
and drying basin, close W of marina, have up to 5m at HW.

NAVIGATION
WPT 49°21′·18N 01°47′·50W (off chartlet), 189°/009° from/
to W Jetty lt, 1M. From N/NW, keep well off shore on appr
to avoid rks 1M N of Cap de Carteret extending about 1M
from coast. From W, about 4M off shore, beware Trois
Grune Rks (dry 1·6m) marked by WCM buoy, Q (9) 15s.

Appr dries ½M offshore and is exposed to fresh W/SW
winds which can make ent rough. There are no safe ⚓s off
shore. Best appr at HW−2 to avoid max tidal stream, 4½kn
sp. Bar, at right angles to W Jetty, dries 4m; the chan dries
progressively to firm sand, and is reported to dry 4.5m
just W of the marina. Best water tends toward quays and
outside of bend. On E side beware old training wall which
partly covers. No ⚓ in river.

LIGHTS AND MARKS
Cap de Carteret, Fl (2+1) 15s 81m 26M, grey tr, G top, Horn
(3) 60s, and conspic Sig Stn are 8ca WxN of the ent.
W Jetty, Oc R 4s 6m 8M, W col, R top; E bkwtr, Fl G 2·5s.
These lts in transit lead about 009° to ent. The chan, to the
marina, approx 7ca up-river, is marked by bns, some lit.

RADIO TELEPHONE
VHF Ch 16 64. Marina Ch 09.

TELEPHONE
Hr Mr 33·44·00·13; CROSS 33·52·72·13; ⌗ 33·04·90·08;
Meteo 33·22·91·77; Auto 36.68.08.50; Police 33·53·80·17;
Ⓗ (Valognes) 33·40·14·39; Brit Consul 33·44·20·13.

FACILITIES
Port de Plaisance "Port des Iles" ☎ 33·04·70·84, (260 + 60
visitors), FF84-105, AC, FW, CH, Fuel; **West Jetty** AB free
for 6 hrs, then at 50% of marina rate, Slip, FW, R, Bar;
Cercle Nautique de Barneville-Carteret ☎ 33·53·88·29,
Slip, M, Bar;
Town ME, P & D (cans), V, Gaz, R, Bar, ✉, Ⓑ (Barneville),
➾ (Valognes), ✈ (Cherbourg). Ferry: Cherbourg, Jersey.

CARTERET *continued*

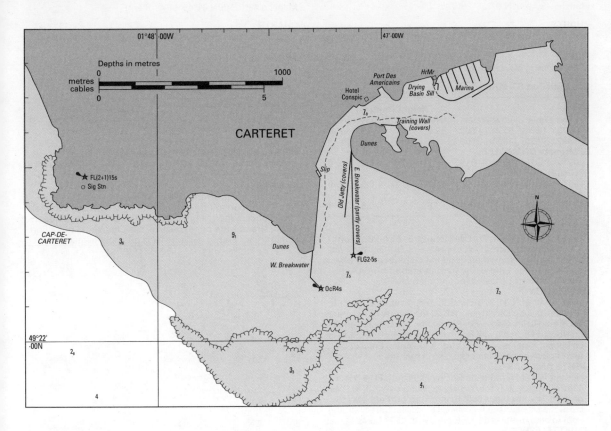

PORTBAIL   10-15-13

Manche 49°19'·46N 01°42'·85W

CHARTS

AC *3655, 2669*; SHOM 7133, 7157; ECM 1014; Imray C33A; Stanfords 16

TIDES

HW −0440 on Dover (UT); ML 6·3m; Duration 0545.

Standard Port ST-MALO (→)

Times				Height (metres)			
High Water		Low Water		MHWS	MHWN	MLWN	MLWS
0100	0800	0300	0800	12·2	9·2	4·3	1·6
1300	2000	1500	2000				
Differences PORTBAIL							
+0035	+0030	+0030	+0035	−0·8	−0·5	−0·3	−0·2
ST GERMAIN-SUR-AY							
+0030	+0030	+0040	+0040	−0·7	−0·4	−0·1	0·0
LE SÉNÉQUET							
+0020	+0026	+0028	+0028	−0·3	−0·2	0·0	0·0

SHELTER

Good. Hbr dries 7·0m, but access HW±½ at np, HW±2½ at sp for 1m draft. Drying basin to E of jetty: visitors berth on pontoon parallel with NW side of basin or moor on first line of buoys parallel to jetty. Portbail is 4M SE of Carteret.

NAVIGATION

WPT 49°18'·30N 01°44'·49W (off chartlet, abeam "PB" SWM buoy), 222°/042° from/to chan buoys, 1·4M. Beware very strong tide over bar. Ldg line crosses sand banks (drying about 8ca offshore) to a pair of unlit PHM/SHM buoys. Thence via chan dredged 5·2m; on port side a training wall (covers at HW) is marked by R spar bns, the first Q (2) R 5s.

LIGHTS AND MARKS

A blue Water Tr (43m) is conspic 6ca NNW of ent. Ldg lts 042°: Front (La Caillourie) QW 14m 10M, W pylon, R top; rear, 870m from front, Oc 4s 20m 10M (church spire). Training wall hd, Q (2) R 5s 5m 2M.

RADIO TELEPHONE

VHF Ch 09.

TELEPHONE

Hr Mr ☎ 33·04·83·48 (15 Jun-31Aug)

FACILITIES

Quay FF50, FW, D, P, AC, C (5 ton); **Cercle Nautique de Portbail-Denneville** ☎ 33·04·86·15, Bar, R; **YC de Portbail** ☎ 33·04·83·48, AB, C, Slip; **Services**: Sh, ME, El.
Town (½M by causeway) Bar, ⒷB, ✉, R, V, ⇌ (Valognes).

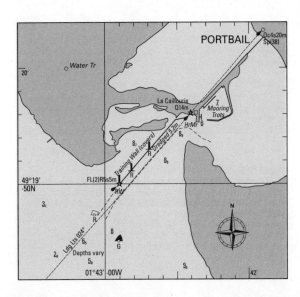

GRANVILLE   10-15-14

Manche 48°49'·97N 01°35'·88W

CHARTS
AC 3672, 3656, *3659*; SHOM 7341, 7156; ECM 534, 535;
Imray C33B; Stanfords 16
TIDES
−0510 Dover; ML 7·1; Duration 0525; Zone −0100

Standard Port ST-MALO (→)

Times				Height (metres)			
High Water		Low Water		MHWS	MHWN	MLWN	MLWS
0100	0800	0300	0800	12·2	9·2	4·3	1·6
1300	2000	1500	2000				
Differences GRANVILLE							
+0010	+0025	+0015	+0015	+0·7	+0·6	+0·2	0·0
REGNÉVILLE-SUR-MER							
+0018	+0018	+0028	+0028	−0··2	−0·1	0·0	0·0
CANCALE							
−0002	−0002	+0012	+0006	+0·8	+0·7	+0·3	+0·1

SHELTER
Good in the marina, Port de Hérel, 1·5–2·5m. Caution:
vis at ent is restricted. Access HW −2½ to +3½, over sill;
depth over sill shown on lit digital display atop S bkwtr:
eg 76=7·6m; 00 = no entry; hard to read in bright sun.
The Avant Port (dries) is for commercial/ FVs.
NAVIGATION
WPT 48°49'·40N 01°37'·00W, 235°/055° from/to S bkwtr lt
(Fl R 4s), 0·95M. Le Videcoq WCM, VQ (9) 10s Whis, marks
rks drying 0·8m, 3¼ M W of Pte du Roc. Beware rks off Pte
du Roc, La Fourchie and Banc de Tombelaine, 1M SSW of
Le Loup lt. Appr is rough in strong W winds. Ent/exit
under power; speed limit 4kn, 2kn in marina.
LIGHTS AND MARKS
Hbr ent is 0·6M E of Pte du Roc (conspic hd), Fl (4) 15s
49m 23M, grey tr, R top. No ldg lts, but S bkwtr lt, Fl R 4s,
on with TV mast leads 055° to ent. Turn port at bkwtr to
cross the sill between R/G piles, Oc R/G 4s. Sill of bathing
pool to stbd is marked by 5 R piles with lts Fl Bu 4s.
RADIO TELEPHONE
Port VHF Ch 12 16 (HW±1½). Marina Ch 09, H24 in season.
TELEPHONE
Hr Mr (Hérel) 33·50·20·06; Hr Mr (Port) 33·50·17·75; Aff
Mar 33·50·00·59; CROSS 33·52·72·13; SNSM 33·61·26·51;
⌗ 33·50·19·90; Meteo 33·22·91·77; Auto 36.68.08.50;
Police 33·50·01·00; Dr 33·50·00·07; Hosp 33·90·74·75;
Brit Consul 33·44·20·13.

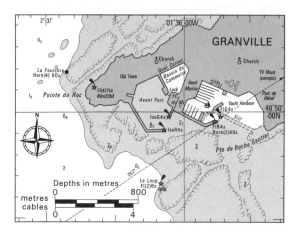

FACILITIES
Hérel Marina (850+150 visitors) ☎ 33·50·20·06, Slip, P, D,
FW, ME, AC, BH (12 ton), C (10 ton), CH, Gaz, R, ⌧, V, Bar,
SM, El, Sh; **YC de Granville** ☎ 33·50·04·25, L, M, BH, D, P,
CH, ⌧, Slip FW, AB, Bar;
Services: CH, M, ME, El, Ⓔ, Sh, SHOM, SM.
Town P, D, ME, V, Gaz, R, Bar, ⌧, Ⓑ, ⇌, ✈ (Dinard).
Ferry: UK via Jersey or Cherbourg.

ILES CHAUSEY   10-15-15

Manche 48°52'·20N 01°49'·00W (S ent)

CHARTS
AC 3656, *3659*; SHOM 7134, 7156, 7155; ECM 534, 535;
Imray C33B; Stanfords 16
TIDES
−0500 Dover; ML 7·4; Duration 0530; Zone −0100

Standard Port ST-MALO (→)

Times				Height (metres)			
High Water		Low Water		MHWS	MHWN	MLWN	MLWS
0100	0800	0300	0800	12·2	9·2	4·3	1·6
1300	2000	1500	2000				
Differences ILES CHAUSEY (Grande Ile)							
+0010	+0010	+0020	+0015	+0·8	+0·7	+0·5	+0·3

SHELTER
Good except in strong NW or SE winds. W ⚓s available
free for mooring fore-and-aft. Hbr very crowded summer
weekends. When ⚓ing, note the big tidal range, although
tidal streams are not excessive. Iles Chausey is not a Port
of Entry for France. Grande Ile is privately owned.

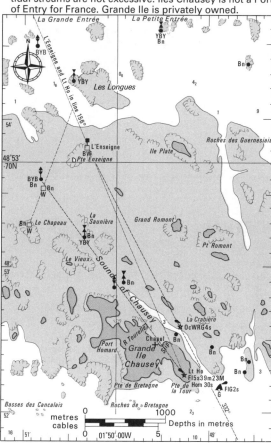

NAVIGATION
WPT 48°51'·50N 01°48'·48W, 152°/332° from/to La Crabière
lt, 1·2M. The easier route into the Sound is from the S,
but beware rks E and S of Pte de la Tour (conspic). The
route from N requires sufficient ht of tide; SHOM 7134 or
detailed SDs for transits, and local knowledge is advised.
Dangerous wk reported N of La Petite Entrée (off chartlet).
LIGHTS AND MARKS
Pte de la Tour, Fl 5s 39m 23M, Horn 30s. La Crabière, Oc
WRG 4s 5m 9/6M, B tr, Y top; sectors see 10.15.4. From N,
L'Enseigne bn tr (19m) on with Pte de la Tour lt ho leads
156°. From S, La Crabière on with L'Enseigne leads 332°.
RADIO TELEPHONE
None.
TELEPHONE
Police 33·52·72·02; CROSS 33·52·72·13; Auto 36.68.08.50.
FACILITIES
R. Tourelle L. **Village** FW, Gaz, V (limited), R, Bar. See
also Granville. Ferry to UK via Granville and Jersey.

TIME ZONE –0100
(French Standard Time)
Subtract 1 hour for UT

For French Summer Time add
ONE hour in non-shaded areas

FRANCE – ST. MALO

LAT 48°38′N   LONG 2°02′W

TIMES AND HEIGHTS OF HIGH AND LOW WATERS

YEAR **1996**

JANUARY

Day	Time	m	Day	Time	m
1 M	0322 / 1013 / 1557 / 2240	9.3 / 4.3 / 9.5 / 4.1	**16** TU	0205 / 0852 / 1442 / 2134	9.4 / 4.1 / 9.6 / 3.9
2 TU	0426 / 1117 / 1655 / 2339	9.8 / 3.9 / 10.0 / 3.6	**17** W	0329 / 1017 / 1602 / 2257	9.9 / 3.5 / 10.2 / 3.3
3 W	0517 / 1210 / 1742	10.4 / 3.4 / 10.4	**18** TH	0440 / 1133 / 1711	10.7 / 2.8 / 11.0
4 TH	0029 / 0600 / 1256 / 1824	3.2 / 10.8 / 3.0 / 10.8	**19** F	0007 / 0542 / 1240 / 1812	2.5 / 11.6 / 2.0 / 11.8
5 F	0111 / 0638 / 1336 / 1902	2.9 / 11.2 / 2.7 / 11.1	**20** SA	0110 / 0638 / 1341 / 1907	1.8 / 12.3 / 1.3 / 12.4
6 SA	0149 / 0714 / 1412 / 1937	2.6 / 11.4 / 2.5 / 11.2	**21** SU	0207 / 0729 / 1436 / 1957	1.3 / 12.9 / 0.9 / 12.7
7 SU	0224 / 0747 / 1446 / 2010	2.5 / 11.6 / 2.4 / 11.2	**22** M	0258 / 0817 / 1526 / 2043	1.0 / 13.1 / 0.7 / 12.8
8 M	0257 / 0818 / 1518 / 2041	2.4 / 11.6 / 2.4 / 11.2	**23** TU	0344 / 0901 / 1610 / 2125	1.0 / 13.1 / 0.9 / 12.6
9 TU	0329 / 0850 / 1549 / 2113	2.5 / 11.5 / 2.5 / 11.1	**24** W	0425 / 0943 / 1649 / 2205	1.3 / 12.6 / 1.4 / 12.1
10 W	0400 / 0922 / 1620 / 2145	2.6 / 11.3 / 2.7 / 10.9	**25** TH	0502 / 1022 / 1724 / 2241	2.0 / 11.9 / 2.2 / 11.3
11 TH	0432 / 0955 / 1651 / 2219	2.9 / 10.9 / 3.0 / 10.5	**26** F	0537 / 1059 / 1757 / 2317	2.8 / 11.0 / 3.1 / 10.5
12 F	0506 / 1030 / 1725 / 2255	3.2 / 10.5 / 3.4 / 10.0	**27** SA	0610 / 1129 / 1832 / 2358	3.7 / 10.1 / 3.9 / 9.7
13 SA	0544 / 1109 / 1805 / 2339	3.7 / 10.0 / 3.8 / 9.6	**28** SU	0652 / 1228 / 1918	4.4 / 9.3 / 4.5
14 SU	0631 / 1201 / 1858	4.0 / 9.6 / 4.1	**29** M	0054 / 0755 / 1342 / 2027	9.1 / 4.9 / 8.8 / 4.9
15 M	0041 / 0733 / 1314 / 2007	9.3 / 4.2 / 9.4 / 4.2	**30** TU	0221 / 0920 / 1518 / 2153	8.8 / 4.9 / 8.9 / 4.7
			31 W	0353 / 1042 / 1631 / 2308	9.2 / 4.4 / 9.4 / 4.2

FEBRUARY

Day	Time	m	Day	Time	m
1 TH	0454 / 1145 / 1723	9.8 / 3.8 / 10.0	**16** F	0427 / 1120 / 1704 / 2355	10.4 / 2.9 / 10.7 / 2.7
2 F	0006 / 0541 / 1236 / 1806	3.6 / 10.5 / 3.2 / 10.6	**17** SA	0533 / 1230 / 1804	11.4 / 2.0 / 11.6
3 SA	0054 / 0621 / 1320 / 1845	3.1 / 11.0 / 2.8 / 11.0	**18** SU	0100 / 0629 / 1332 / 1856	1.9 / 12.2 / 1.3 / 12.4
4 SU	0134 / 0658 / 1358 / 1921	2.7 / 11.4 / 2.5 / 11.3	**19** M	0157 / 0718 / 1425 / 1943	1.2 / 12.9 / 0.8 / 12.8
5 M	0210 / 0732 / 1432 / 1955	2.4 / 11.6 / 2.3 / 11.5	**20** TU	0246 / 0803 / 1511 / 2025	0.8 / 13.2 / 0.6 / 13.0
6 TU	0242 / 0804 / 1503 / 2026	2.2 / 11.8 / 2.1 / 11.6	**21** W	0328 / 0844 / 1550 / 2104	0.8 / 13.1 / 0.7 / 12.8
7 W	0314 / 0834 / 1534 / 2056	2.1 / 11.9 / 2.0 / 11.6	**22** TH	0405 / 0922 / 1624 / 2138	1.1 / 12.8 / 1.3 / 12.3
8 TH	0345 / 0905 / 1604 / 2127	2.1 / 11.8 / 2.1 / 11.5	**23** F	0438 / 0956 / 1654 / 2210	1.7 / 12.1 / 2.0 / 11.6
9 F	0416 / 0936 / 1633 / 2158	2.2 / 11.5 / 2.4 / 11.2	**24** SA	0506 / 1027 / 1720 / 2240	2.5 / 11.2 / 2.9 / 10.8
10 SA	0447 / 1008 / 1704 / 2230	2.5 / 11.1 / 2.8 / 10.7	**25** SU	0531 / 1059 / 1746 / 2311	3.4 / 10.3 / 3.7 / 10.0
11 SU	0521 / 1044 / 1739 / 2308	3.0 / 10.5 / 3.3 / 10.2	**26** M	0601 / 1136 / 1823 / 2354	4.2 / 9.4 / 4.5 / 9.2
12 M	0602 / 1129 / 1825	3.5 / 9.9 / 3.8	**27** TU	0653 / 1236 / 1926	4.8 / 8.7 / 5.0
13 TU	0001 / 0657 / 1237 / 1931	9.6 / 4.0 / 9.4 / 4.2	**28** W	0113 / 0820 / 1430 / 2102	8.6 / 5.1 / 8.4 / 5.1
14 W	0124 / 0817 / 1415 / 2104	9.3 / 4.1 / 9.3 / 4.2	**29** TH	0311 / 1002 / 1603 / 2234	8.7 / 4.8 / 9.0 / 4.6
15 TH	0304 / 0956 / 1549 / 2239	9.6 / 3.8 / 9.9 / 3.6			

MARCH

Day	Time	m	Day	Time	m
1 F	0426 / 1116 / 1659 / 2339	9.4 / 4.1 / 9.7 / 3.9	**16** SA	0416 / 1111 / 1653 / 2344	10.3 / 2.9 / 10.6 / 2.7
2 SA	0516 / 1211 / 1743	10.1 / 3.4 / 10.4	**17** SU	0520 / 1219 / 1750	11.2 / 2.0 / 11.5
3 SU	0029 / 0558 / 1256 / 1823	3.2 / 10.8 / 2.8 / 11.0	**18** M	0047 / 0614 / 1316 / 1839	1.9 / 12.1 / 1.3 / 12.2
4 M	0110 / 0636 / 1335 / 1859	2.7 / 11.3 / 2.4 / 11.4	**19** TU	0140 / 0701 / 1406 / 1922	1.3 / 12.6 / 1.0 / 12.6
5 TU	0147 / 0711 / 1410 / 1933	2.3 / 11.7 / 2.1 / 11.7	**20** W	0226 / 0743 / 1447 / 2002	0.9 / 12.9 / 0.8 / 12.8
6 W	0222 / 0744 / 1443 / 2005	2.0 / 11.9 / 1.8 / 11.9	**21** TH	0305 / 0822 / 1523 / 2037	0.9 / 12.9 / 0.9 / 12.6
7 TH	0255 / 0815 / 1515 / 2036	1.7 / 12.1 / 1.6 / 12.0	**22** F	0339 / 0856 / 1554 / 2109	1.1 / 12.5 / 1.3 / 12.3
8 F	0328 / 0847 / 1545 / 2106	1.6 / 12.1 / 1.7 / 11.9	**23** SA	0409 / 0928 / 1621 / 2138	1.6 / 12.0 / 2.0 / 11.7
9 SA	0359 / 0919 / 1615 / 2138	1.7 / 11.9 / 1.9 / 11.7	**24** SU	0435 / 0957 / 1645 / 2206	2.3 / 11.2 / 2.7 / 10.9
10 SU	0431 / 0952 / 1646 / 2211	2.0 / 11.4 / 2.4 / 11.2	**25** M	0459 / 1026 / 1710 / 2235	3.1 / 10.4 / 3.5 / 10.2
11 M	0504 / 1028 / 1721 / 2250	2.5 / 10.8 / 3.0 / 10.5	**26** TU	0526 / 1059 / 1743 / 2313	3.9 / 9.5 / 4.2 / 9.4
12 TU	0544 / 1114 / 1807 / 2342	3.1 / 10.1 / 3.6 / 9.8	**27** W	0610 / 1150 / 1839	4.5 / 8.8 / 4.9
13 W	0639 / 1223 / 1912	3.7 / 9.4 / 4.1	**28** TH	0019 / 0724 / 1331 / 2008	8.7 / 5.0 / 8.3 / 5.2
14 TH	0106 / 0801 / 1404 / 2049	9.3 / 4.1 / 9.2 / 4.2	**29** F	0213 / 0909 / 1519 / 2147	8.5 / 4.8 / 8.7 / 4.8
15 F	0250 / 0945 / 1541 / 2227	9.5 / 3.7 / 9.7 / 3.6	**30** SA	0343 / 1033 / 1624 / 2257	9.0 / 4.3 / 9.4 / 4.1
			31 SU	0440 / 1132 / 1711 / 2350	9.8 / 3.6 / 10.1 / 3.4

APRIL

Day	Time	m	Day	Time	m
1 M	0525 / 1219 / 1752	10.5 / 3.0 / 10.8	**16** TU	0025 / 0552 / 1253 / 1815	2.1 / 11.7 / 1.6 / 11.8
2 TU	0034 / 0606 / 1301 / 1830	2.8 / 11.1 / 2.5 / 11.3	**17** W	0116 / 0638 / 1339 / 1857	1.6 / 12.1 / 1.3 / 12.2
3 W	0115 / 0643 / 1340 / 1905	2.3 / 11.6 / 2.0 / 11.7	**18** TH	0200 / 0719 / 1418 / 1934	1.4 / 12.3 / 1.3 / 12.3
4 TH	0154 / 0719 / 1417 / 1939	1.8 / 11.9 / 1.6 / 12.1	**19** F	0237 / 0756 / 1452 / 2008	1.3 / 12.3 / 1.3 / 12.2
5 F	0232 / 0753 / 1452 / 2012	1.4 / 12.2 / 1.4 / 12.3	**20** SA	0310 / 0830 / 1523 / 2039	1.4 / 12.1 / 1.6 / 12.0
6 SA	0308 / 0827 / 1526 / 2046	1.3 / 12.3 / 1.4 / 12.2	**21** SU	0341 / 0901 / 1551 / 2109	1.7 / 11.7 / 2.0 / 11.6
7 SU	0343 / 0903 / 1559 / 2121	1.3 / 12.1 / 1.6 / 12.0	**22** M	0408 / 0931 / 1617 / 2138	2.3 / 11.1 / 2.6 / 11.0
8 M	0417 / 0940 / 1633 / 2158	1.6 / 11.7 / 2.1 / 11.5	**23** TU	0434 / 1001 / 1644 / 2209	2.9 / 10.4 / 3.3 / 10.4
9 TU	0454 / 1021 / 1711 / 2241	2.1 / 11.0 / 2.7 / 10.8	**24** W	0503 / 1036 / 1717 / 2247	3.5 / 9.7 / 3.9 / 9.7
10 W	0537 / 1112 / 1759 / 2338	2.8 / 10.2 / 3.4 / 10.0	**25** TH	0541 / 1122 / 1805 / 2342	4.1 / 9.1 / 4.5 / 9.0
11 TH	0635 / 1222 / 1906	3.4 / 9.5 / 4.0	**26** F	0640 / 1238 / 1916	4.6 / 8.6 / 4.9
12 F	0059 / 0757 / 1355 / 2040	9.5 / 3.8 / 9.3 / 4.0	**27** SA	0109 / 0805 / 1417 / 2044	8.6 / 4.8 / 8.6 / 4.8
13 SA	0235 / 0934 / 1524 / 2212	9.6 / 3.5 / 9.8 / 3.5	**28** SU	0241 / 0931 / 1532 / 2200	8.8 / 4.5 / 9.1 / 4.3
14 SU	0357 / 1054 / 1633 / 2325	10.2 / 2.8 / 10.5 / 2.7	**29** M	0349 / 1038 / 1627 / 2258	9.4 / 3.9 / 9.8 / 3.7
15 M	0500 / 1159 / 1728	11.0 / 2.1 / 11.3	**30** TU	0442 / 1131 / 1712 / 2348	10.0 / 3.3 / 10.5 / 3.0

15

Chart Datum: 6·60 metres below Lallemand System (Mean Sea Level, Marseilles)

TIME ZONE –0100
(French Standard Time)
Subtract 1 hour for UT
For French Summer Time add ONE hour in non-shaded areas

FRANCE – ST. MALO

LAT 48°38′N   LONG 2°02′W

TIMES AND HEIGHTS OF HIGH AND LOW WATERS   YEAR **1996**

MAY

Day	Time m	Time m	Time m	Time m	Day	Time m	Time m	Time m	Time m
1 W	0527 10.7	1219 2.6	1753 11.1		16 TH	0048 2.2	0612 11.4	1308 2.0	1830 11.6
2 TH	0036 2.4	0609 11.3	1304 2.1	1832 11.7	17 F ●	0131 2.0	0654 11.6	1347 1.9	1907 11.8
3 F O	0122 1.8	0650 11.8	1348 1.6	1911 12.1	18 SA	0209 1.9	0732 11.6	1422 1.8	1942 11.8
4 SA	0206 1.4	0730 12.1	1429 1.5	1949 12.4	19 SU	0243 1.8	0806 11.6	1454 1.9	2014 11.7
5 SU	0249 1.1	0810 12.3	1508 1.3	2027 12.4	20 M	0315 1.9	0839 11.4	1525 2.1	2045 11.5
6 M	0329 1.1	0851 12.2	1546 1.5	2108 12.2	21 TU	0346 2.2	0911 11.0	1556 2.5	2116 11.1
7 TU	0409 1.4	0934 11.8	1625 1.9	2151 11.8	22 W	0416 2.7	0943 10.6	1625 3.0	2150 10.6
8 W	0451 1.8	1020 11.2	1708 2.5	2238 11.1	23 TH	0446 3.2	1019 10.0	1658 3.6	2227 10.1
9 TH	0538 2.5	1113 10.5	1758 3.1	2336 10.4	24 F	0521 3.7	1100 9.5	1738 4.1	2312 9.5
10 F	0637 3.1	1218 9.9	1903 3.6		25 SA	0606 4.1	1156 9.0	1832 4.5	
11 SA	0048 9.9	0750 3.4	1335 9.6	2025 3.8	26 SU	0013 9.0	0707 4.4	1310 8.8	1940 4.6
12 SU	0210 9.8	0911 3.4	1455 9.8	2147 3.5	27 M	0130 8.9	0820 4.4	1428 9.0	2053 4.4
13 M	0328 10.1	1026 3.0	1604 10.3	2257 3.0	28 TU	0245 9.1	0933 4.1	1532 9.4	2200 3.9
14 TU	0432 10.6	1129 2.6	1700 10.8	2357 2.5	29 W	0348 9.7	1037 3.6	1626 10.1	2300 3.3
15 W	0526 11.1	1223 2.2	1748 11.3		30 TH	0443 10.3	1134 2.9	1714 10.8	2357 2.6
					31 F	0533 11.0	1228 2.3	1759 11.5	

JUNE

Day	Time m	Time m	Time m	Time m	Day	Time m	Time m	Time m	Time m
1 SA O	0051 1.9	0622 11.6	1320 1.7	1844 12.1	16 SU ●	0143 2.3	0711 11.1	1357 2.3	1920 11.5
2 SU	0143 1.4	0709 12.0	1408 1.4	1929 12.4	17 M	0220 2.2	0747 11.2	1432 2.2	1954 11.5
3 M	0233 1.1	0756 12.3	1454 1.2	2014 12.6	18 TU	0255 2.1	0821 11.2	1506 2.3	2027 11.5
4 TU	0320 1.0	0843 12.3	1538 1.3	2059 12.5	19 W	0328 2.2	0854 11.0	1538 2.4	2059 11.3
5 W	0405 1.1	0930 12.1	1622 1.6	2146 12.1	20 TH	0359 2.5	0927 10.8	1609 2.7	2131 11.0
6 TH	0451 1.5	1018 11.6	1707 2.1	2234 11.6	21 F	0430 2.8	1001 10.5	1640 3.1	2206 10.6
7 F	0539 2.0	1108 11.0	1755 2.7	2327 10.9	22 SA	0501 3.2	1037 10.0	1715 3.5	2244 10.1
8 SA	0631 2.6	1203 10.4	1852 3.3		23 SU	0538 3.6	1119 9.6	1756 3.9	2328 9.6
9 SU	0027 10.3	0731 3.2	1305 9.9	1958 3.7	24 M	0622 4.0	1211 9.2	1847 4.2	
10 M	0136 9.9	0837 3.4	1416 9.7	2111 3.8	25 TU	0024 9.2	0719 4.2	1316 9.0	1950 4.3
11 TU	0251 9.8	0947 3.5	1527 9.9	2221 3.5	26 W	0136 9.1	0828 4.2	1429 9.2	2103 4.1
12 W	0400 10.0	1052 3.2	1628 10.3	2324 3.2	27 TH	0251 9.4	0943 3.8	1536 9.8	2215 3.6
13 TH	0458 10.4	1148 3.0	1720 10.7		28 F	0359 10.0	1053 3.2	1636 10.5	2322 2.8
14 F	0017 2.8	0547 10.7	1237 2.7	1804 11.0	29 SA	0501 10.7	1157 2.5	1731 11.3	
15 SA	0103 2.6	0631 11.0	1319 2.5	1844 11.3	30 SU	0024 2.1	0559 11.4	1256 1.9	1824 12.0

JULY

Day	Time m	Time m	Time m	Time m	Day	Time m	Time m	Time m	Time m
1 M	0124 1.5	0653 12.0	1352 1.4	1915 12.5	16 TU	0202 2.4	0730 11.1	1415 2.4	1937 11.5
2 TU	0220 1.1	0745 12.4	1444 1.2	2004 12.8	17 W	0238 2.2	0804 11.2	1449 2.3	2010 11.6
3 W	0312 0.8	0835 12.6	1532 1.1	2051 12.9	18 TH	0311 2.2	0837 11.2	1521 2.3	2041 11.5
4 TH	0401 0.8	0922 12.5	1617 1.3	2138 12.6	19 F	0342 2.3	0908 11.1	1551 2.4	2112 11.4
5 F	0446 1.1	1008 12.1	1701 1.7	2223 12.1	20 SA	0411 2.5	0939 10.9	1621 2.6	2143 11.0
6 SA	0530 1.7	1052 11.5	1743 2.4	2309 11.3	21 SU	0440 2.8	1011 10.6	1652 3.0	2216 10.6
7 SU	0614 2.4	1138 10.8	1829 3.1	2358 10.5	22 M	0511 3.2	1045 10.1	1726 3.4	2251 10.1
8 M	0700 3.0	1228 10.1	1921 3.8		23 TU	0547 3.6	1124 9.7	1808 3.8	2335 9.6
9 TU	0055 9.8	0755 3.8	1329 9.6	2025 4.2	24 W	0633 4.0	1215 9.3	1901 4.2	
10 W	0206 9.4	0900 4.1	1443 9.4	2140 4.2	25 TH	0037 9.2	0735 4.2	1329 9.2	2012 4.2
11 TH	0325 9.4	1011 4.0	1556 9.6	2250 3.9	26 F	0201 9.2	0856 4.1	1452 9.5	2137 3.8
12 F	0432 9.7	1115 3.6	1655 10.1	2349 3.4	27 SA	0326 9.7	1020 3.6	1607 10.2	2256 3.1
13 SA	0526 10.2	1210 3.2	1743 10.6		28 SU	0440 10.5	1133 2.8	1712 11.1	
14 SU	0039 3.0	0611 10.6	1257 2.8	1825 11.1	29 M	0006 2.3	0544 11.3	1238 2.0	1810 12.0
15 M ●	0123 2.6	0652 10.9	1338 2.6	1902 11.4	30 TU O	0110 1.5	0642 12.0	1339 1.4	1903 12.6
					31 W	0209 0.9	0734 12.6	1433 1.0	1953 13.1

AUGUST

Day	Time m	Time m	Time m	Time m	Day	Time m	Time m	Time m	Time m
1 TH	0302 0.6	0823 12.9	1522 0.8	2040 13.2	16 F	0251 2.1	0815 11.5	1501 2.1	2020 11.8
2 F	0350 0.5	0908 12.9	1606 0.9	2123 13.0	17 SA	0320 2.1	0845 11.5	1531 2.1	2050 11.7
3 SA	0432 0.9	0949 12.5	1646 1.4	2204 12.4	18 SU	0349 2.1	0914 11.3	1600 2.2	2119 11.5
4 SU	0511 1.5	1029 11.8	1722 2.2	2244 11.5	19 M	0417 2.4	0944 11.1	1630 2.5	2149 11.0
5 M	0546 2.4	1106 11.0	1758 3.1	2324 10.6	20 TU	0446 2.8	1014 10.6	1701 3.0	2221 10.5
6 TU	0622 3.3	1147 10.1	1837 3.9		21 W	0519 3.3	1048 10.1	1738 3.5	2300 9.9
7 W	0010 9.6	0706 4.1	1238 9.4	1933 4.6	22 TH	0600 3.8	1133 9.5	1826 4.0	2357 9.3
8 TH	0115 9.0	0808 4.6	1353 8.9	2053 4.8	23 F	0657 4.2	1244 9.2	1935 4.3	
9 F	0249 8.8	0929 4.6	1524 9.1	2217 4.4	24 SA	0127 9.1	0822 4.3	1422 9.3	2110 4.0
10 SA	0410 9.2	1045 4.2	1633 9.7	2324 3.8	25 SU	0310 9.5	0958 3.8	1550 10.0	2240 3.3
11 SU	0507 9.8	1146 3.6	1723 10.4		26 M	0429 10.3	1117 2.9	1659 11.0	2353 2.3
12 M	0017 3.2	0552 10.5	1236 3.0	1805 10.9	27 TU	0533 11.3	1225 2.1	1758 12.0	
13 TU	0103 2.7	0632 10.9	1319 2.6	1843 11.4	28 W O	0058 1.4	0628 12.2	1325 1.3	1850 12.8
14 W ●	0143 2.4	0709 11.2	1356 2.4	1918 11.6	29 TH	0155 0.8	0718 12.8	1419 0.8	1937 13.2
15 TH	0219 2.2	0744 11.4	1429 2.2	1950 11.8	30 F	0246 0.5	0803 13.0	1506 0.7	2021 13.3
					31 SA	0330 0.5	0845 13.0	1546 0.8	2102 13.1

Chart Datum: 6·60 metres below Lallemand System (Mean Sea Level, Marseilles)

TIME ZONE –0100
(French Standard Time)
Subtract 1 hour for UT
For French Summer Time add ONE hour in non-shaded areas

FRANCE – ST. MALO

LAT 48°38′N   LONG 2°02′W

TIMES AND HEIGHTS OF HIGH AND LOW WATERS

YEAR **1996**

SEPTEMBER

	Time	m		Time	m
1 SU	0408 0923 1623 2139	0.9 12.6 1.4 12.4	**16** M	0325 0848 1538 2056	1.9 11.7 1.9 11.7
2 M	0442 0958 1654 2213	1.6 11.9 2.2 11.5	**17** TU	0354 0917 1609 2127	2.1 11.5 2.2 11.3
3 TU	0512 1031 1723 2247	2.6 11.0 3.1 10.5	**18** W	0424 0948 1641 2200	2.5 11.0 2.7 10.7
4 W	0540 1104 1753 2324	3.5 10.1 4.0 9.5	**19** TH	0457 1023 1718 2240	3.1 10.4 3.2 10.0
5 TH	0616 1147 1838	4.3 9.3 4.7	**20** F	0537 1110 1805 2339	3.7 9.8 3.8 9.4
6 F	0019 0714 1258 1959	8.7 4.9 8.7 5.1	**21** SA	0636 1223 1916	4.2 9.2 4.2
7 SA	0206 0845 1447 2141	8.4 5.1 8.7 4.9	**22** SU	0115 0804 1407 2057	9.0 4.4 9.3 4.1
8 SU	0346 1014 1606 2256	8.8 4.6 9.3 4.1	**23** M	0301 0945 1537 2230	9.4 3.9 10.0 3.2
9 M	0443 1118 1657 2351	9.6 3.8 10.1 3.4	**24** TU	0419 1105 1645 2342	10.3 3.0 11.0 2.2
10 TU	0527 1209 1739	10.4 3.2 10.8	**25** W	0519 1211 1742	11.4 2.1 12.0
11 W	0037 0606 1252 1818	2.8 10.9 2.7 11.3	**26** TH	0042 0610 1308 1832	1.4 12.2 1.4 12.7
12 TH ●	0117 0643 1330 1853	2.4 11.4 2.4 11.7	**27** F O	0136 0657 1359 1917	0.9 12.7 1.0 13.0
13 F	0152 0717 1404 1926	2.2 11.6 2.1 11.9	**28** SA	0223 0739 1443 1958	0.7 12.9 0.9 13.1
14 SA	0225 0749 1436 1956	2.0 11.7 1.9 12.0	**29** SU	0303 0818 1521 2036	0.8 12.8 1.0 12.8
15 SU	0255 0818 1508 2026	1.9 11.8 1.8 11.9	**30** M	0338 0853 1555 2111	1.2 12.5 1.5 12.2

OCTOBER

	Time	m		Time	m
1 TU	0409 0926 1624 2142	1.8 11.9 2.2 11.4	**16** W	0335 0856 1553 2111	1.9 11.8 2.0 11.6
2 W	0436 0956 1651 2213	2.7 11.1 3.1 10.5	**17** TH	0407 0932 1628 2150	2.3 11.4 2.4 11.0
3 TH	0502 1027 1718 2246	3.5 10.2 3.9 9.6	**18** F	0443 1012 1709 2235	2.9 10.8 3.0 10.2
4 F	0534 1104 1757 2332	4.3 9.4 4.6 8.8	**19** SA	0528 1104 1800 2338	3.5 10.1 3.6 9.5
5 SA	0626 1205 1905	5.0 8.7 5.1	**20** SU	0628 1218 1912	4.1 9.5 4.0
6 SU	0107 0754 1354 2050	8.3 5.3 8.5 5.1	**21** M	0110 0756 1353 2048	9.2 4.3 9.5 3.9
7 M	0304 0932 1524 2216	8.6 4.9 9.0 4.4	**22** TU	0246 0932 1519 2215	9.5 3.8 10.1 3.2
8 TU	0409 1041 1621 2315	9.3 4.2 9.8 3.7	**23** W	0400 1049 1626 2324	10.3 3.0 10.9 2.3
9 W	0455 1133 1706	10.1 3.5 10.5	**24** TH	0458 1152 1721	11.2 2.2 11.7
10 TH	0002 0535 1217 1746	3.0 10.8 2.9 11.1	**25** F O	0021 0548 1247 1810	1.7 11.9 1.7 12.2
11 F	0043 0612 1256 1823	2.6 11.3 2.5 11.5	**26** SA O	0112 0633 1335 1854	1.3 12.3 1.4 12.5
12 SA ●	0120 0647 1333 1858	2.2 11.7 2.1 11.8	**27** SU	0155 0713 1417 1933	1.2 12.5 1.4 12.5
13 SU	0155 0720 1409 1931	1.9 11.9 1.9 12.0	**28** M	0233 0750 1453 2010	1.3 12.4 1.5 11.9
14 M	0229 0751 1444 2003	1.7 12.0 1.7 12.0	**29** TU	0306 0824 1526 2043	1.6 12.2 1.8 11.9
15 TU	0302 0823 1519 2036	1.7 12.0 1.7 11.9	**30** W	0337 0855 1556 2115	2.0 11.8 2.3 11.3
			31 TH	0406 0926 1625 2146	2.7 11.2 3.0 10.6

NOVEMBER

	Time	m		Time	m
1 F	0433 0958 1653 2219	3.4 10.5 3.7 9.8	**16** SA	0439 1009 1709 2237	2.6 11.2 2.6 10.6
2 SA	0505 1034 1728 2301	4.1 9.7 4.3 9.1	**17** SU	0527 1102 1802 2338	3.2 10.6 3.2 10.0
3 SU	0549 1125 1821	4.7 9.1 4.8	**18** M	0627 1210 1908	3.7 10.0 3.6
4 M	0009 0658 1247 1943	8.5 5.1 8.7 5.0	**19** TU	0053 0744 1331 2029	9.6 4.0 9.8 3.6
5 TU ●	0155 0829 1421 2115	8.5 5.1 8.8 4.7	**20** W	0217 0909 1451 2149	9.7 3.8 10.1 3.3
6 W	0318 0946 1531 2223	9.0 4.6 9.4 4.1	**21** TH	0332 1024 1600 2258	10.2 3.3 10.6 2.8
7 TH	0413 1044 1624 2315	9.7 3.9 10.0 3.5	**22** F	0432 1128 1657 2356	10.8 2.7 11.1 2.3
8 F	0457 1133 1708	10.4 3.3 10.7	**23** SA	0523 1222 1746	11.3 2.3 11.5
9 SA	0001 0537 1217 1749	2.9 11.0 2.8 11.2	**24** SU	0045 0608 1310 1831	2.1 11.7 2.1 11.7
10 SU	0043 0614 1300 1828	2.4 11.5 2.3 11.6	**25** M O	0128 0649 1351 1911	1.9 11.9 2.0 11.8
11 M ●	0123 0650 1342 1905	2.0 11.9 1.9 11.9	**26** TU	0205 0726 1427 1947	1.9 12.0 2.0 11.7
12 TU	0203 0726 1423 1943	1.8 12.2 1.7 12.1	**27** W	0239 0800 1502 2021	2.0 11.9 2.1 11.5
13 W	0242 0803 1504 2022	1.7 12.3 1.6 12.1	**28** TH	0312 0832 1534 2054	2.2 11.7 2.3 11.2
14 TH	0320 0842 1543 2103	1.8 12.1 1.8 11.8	**29** F	0343 0904 1605 2127	2.6 11.3 2.8 10.8
15 F	0358 0920 1624 2147	2.1 11.8 2.1 11.3	**30** SA	0414 0937 1635 2200	3.1 10.8 3.3 10.2

DECEMBER

	Time	m		Time	m
1 SU	0445 1012 1707 2238	3.7 10.2 3.8 9.6	**16** M	0527 1057 1759 2327	2.7 11.2 2.6 10.7
2 M	0522 1053 1747 2326	4.2 9.7 4.3 9.1	**17** TU	0619 1154 1854	3.2 10.6 3.2
3 TU	0611 1149 1843	4.7 9.1 4.7	**18** W	0027 0722 1300 1959	10.1 3.7 10.1 3.6
4 W	0037 0717 1305 1955	8.7 4.9 8.9 4.8	**19** TH	0138 0835 1415 2112	9.8 3.9 9.9 3.7
5 TH	0205 0833 1425 2112	8.8 4.8 9.0 4.6	**20** F	0254 0952 1529 2224	9.8 3.8 10.0 3.5
6 F	0317 0944 1531 2218	9.2 4.4 9.5 4.1	**21** SA	0403 1100 1632 2327	10.1 3.4 10.4 3.2
7 SA	0411 1043 1625 2314	9.8 3.8 10.1 3.4	**22** SU	0500 1158 1726	10.6 3.0 10.7
8 SU	0458 1137 1713	10.5 3.2 10.7	**23** M	0019 0547 1247 1812	2.9 11.0 2.7 11.0
9 M	0005 0541 1228 1759	2.8 11.2 2.5 11.3	**24** TU O	0104 0629 1330 1853	2.6 11.4 2.5 11.3
10 TU ●	0054 0623 1318 1844	2.3 11.8 2.0 11.8	**25** W	0143 0707 1408 1931	2.4 11.6 2.3 11.4
11 W	0142 0706 1407 1929	1.9 12.2 1.6 12.1	**26** TH	0220 0742 1443 2006	2.3 11.7 2.3 11.4
12 TH	0228 0749 1454 2014	1.6 12.5 1.4 12.3	**27** F	0254 0815 1517 2039	2.3 11.7 2.3 11.3
13 F	0312 0833 1539 2059	1.6 12.5 1.4 12.2	**28** SA	0327 0847 1549 2111	2.5 11.5 2.5 11.1
14 SA	0356 0919 1624 2146	1.6 12.3 1.6 11.8	**29** SU	0358 0919 1618 2143	2.7 11.2 2.9 10.7
15 SU	0440 1006 1710 2235	2.1 11.8 2.1 11.3	**30** M	0428 0952 1647 2216	3.1 10.8 3.3 10.3
			31 TU	0459 1026 1719 2252	3.6 10.3 3.7 9.8

Chart Datum: 6·60 metres below Lallemand System (Mean Sea Level, Marseilles)

15

ST MALO/DINARD   10-15-16

Ille et Vilaine 48°38'·35N 02°01'·80W

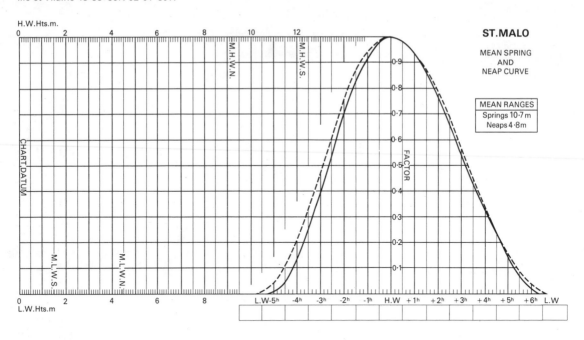

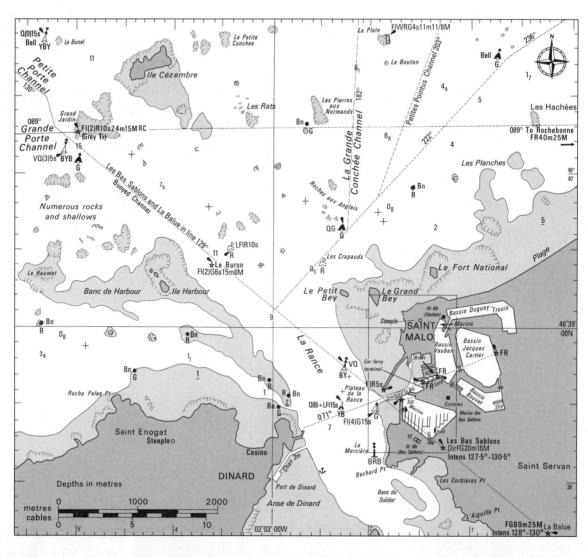

ST MALO/DINARD *continued*

CHARTS
AC 2700, *3659, 2669*; SHOM 7130, 7155, 7156, 6966; ECM 535; Imray C33B; Stanfords 16

TIDES
–0506 Dover; ML 6·8; Duration 0535; Zone –0100
Saint-Malo is a Standard Port and the tidal predictions for each day of the year are given above.

SHELTER
Two options: (1) Lock into the basins near the walled city; Excellent shelter in Bassin Vauban, min depth 6m. Outside lock are 3 waiting buoys N of appr chan; keep clear of ferry berths. Lock opens HW –2½ to HW+1½. No ⚓ in basins; 3kn speed limit. Bassin Duguay-Trouin, via bridge, is better for long stay.
(2) Good shelter nearer St Servan in Les Bas Sablons marina, entered over sill 2m above CD; but Ⓥ berths on N end of pontoon 'A' are exposed to NW winds. Caution: marina ent is only 40m wide, to S of ferry pier extending W from N corner of Bas-Sablons basin and beyond marina bkwtr, Fl G 4s 7m 5M. Two W waiting buoys outside. The depth of water over sill is shown on a digital gauge atop the bkwtr, visible only from seaward; from inside, a conventional gauge at base of bkwtr shows depths <3m. At **Dinard** there is a yacht ⚓ and moorings, reached by beaconed chan, all dredged 2m.

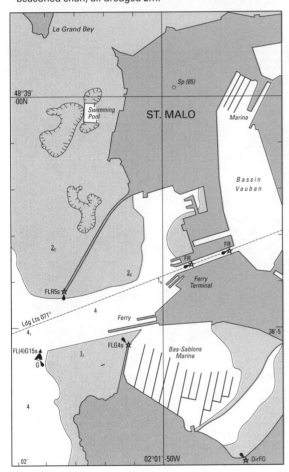

NAVIGATION
WPT Fairway SWM buoy, L Fl 10s Whis, 48°41´·42N 02°07´·20W, 307°/127° from/to Grand Jardin lt, 1·9M. Care is needed due to many dangerous rks around the appr chans, plus strong tidal streams. The 3 principal chans are:
1. Petite Porte (130°/129°); best from N or NW and at night.
2. Grande Porte (089°/129°); from the W.
These 2 chans meet at Le Grand Jardin lt and continue 129°.
3. La Grande Conchée (182°); most direct from N.
The first two are well lit. In fresh W'lies it can be quite rough abeam Le Grand Jardin.

LIGHTS AND MARKS
Chenal de la Petite Porte: Ldg lts 130°, front, Le Grand Jardin, Fl (2) R 10s 24m 15M, grey tr; rear, La Balue, FG 69m 25M.
Chenal de la Grande Porte: Ldg lts 089°, front, Le Grand Jardin; rear, Rochebonne, FR 40m 24M, (off chartlet) 4·2M from front; leads into Chenal de la Petite Porte.
Inner ldg lts 129° from Le Grand Jardin lt ho: Front, Les Bas Sablons, FG 20m 16M; rear, La Balue (as above).
La Plate lt, Fl WRG 4s 11m 9/6M, W140°-203°, R203°-210°, W210°-225°, G225°-140°.
Ldg lts, 2 FR, 071° into lock.

St Malo Lock sigs:

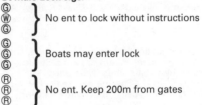

Ⓨ alongside the top lt shows that both gates are open but instructions are the same.
2 Ⓡ over Ⓖ = all movements prohib, except departure of large ships.

RADIO TELEPHONE
Call: *St Malo Port* or *Grand Jardin* VHF Ch **12** 16 (H24).
Port Vauban and Les Bas Sablons marinas Ch 09.

TELEPHONE
ST MALO: Hr Mr 99·81·62·86; Hr Mr (Sablons) 99·81·71·34; Hr Mr (Vauban) 99·56·51·91; Aff Mar 99·56·87·00; CROSS 98·89·31·31; SNSM 98·89·31·31; ⌗ 99·81·65·90; Meteo 99·46·10·46; Auto 36.68.08.35; Police 99·81·52·30; Ⓗ 99·56·56·19; Brit Consul 99·46·26·64.
DINARD: Hr Mr 99·46·65·55; ⌗ 99·46·12·42; Meteo 99·46·10·46; Auto 36.68.08.35; Ⓗ 99·46·18·68.

FACILITIES
ST MALO: **Bassin Vauban** (250 + 100 visitors) ☎ 99·56·51·91, FF86.50, FW, AC, C (1 ton); **Société Nautique de la Baie de St. Malo** ☎ 99·40·84·42, Bar (visitors welcome).
ST SERVAN: **Marina Les Bas-Sablons** (1216 + 64 visitors on Pontoon A, berths 43-75 and 32-64) ☎ 99·81·71·34, Fax 99.81.91.81, FF91.90, Slip, C, AC, FW, CH, BH (10 ton), Gaz, R, YC, Bar, P & D at Pontoon l; Note: Fuel may only be paid for by French credit card.
Services: El, Ⓔ, ME, CH, Sh, C, BY, SM, SHOM.
Town Slip, P, Gaz, D, ME, El, Sh, C, V, R, Bar, ✉, Ⓑ, ⇌, ✈ (Dinard). Ferry: Portsmouth, Poole or Jersey.
DINARD: **Port de Dinard** ☎ 99·46·65·55, Slip, ⚓, M FF83, P, D, L, FW, temp AB; **YC de Dinard** ☎ 99·46·14·32, Bar;
Services: ME, El, Ⓔ, Sh, M, SM.
Town P, D, ME, El, CH, V, Gaz, R, Bar, ✉, Ⓑ, ⇌, ✈.

OTHER HARBOURS EAST OF ST MALO

CANCALE, Ille-et-Vilaine, 48°40´·10N 01°51´·10W. AC *3659*; SHOM 7131, 7155. HW –0510 on Dover (UT); ML 7·2m; Duration 0535. See 10.15.14. A drying hbr just inside Bay of Mont St Michel, 1M SW of Pte de la Chaine. Area dries to about 1M off-shore; ⚓ off Pte de la Chaine in deep water. Drying berths usually available in La Houle, the hbr in Cancale. Exposed to winds SW to SE. Jetty hd lt Oc (3) G 12s 12m 8M, obsc when brg < 223°. Facilities: **Quay** D, P, C (1·5 ton), FW; **Club Nautique de Cancale** ☎ 99·89·90·22.
Services: El, M, ME, Sh;
Town (famous for oysters), Ⓑ, Bar, D, P, ✉, R, V.

ROTHENEUF, Ille-et-Vilaine, 48°41´·42N 01°57´·56W. AC 2700, *3659*; SHOM 7131, 7155. HW –0510 on Dover (UT); Tides as for St. Malo; ML 7·0m; Duration 0540. Complete shelter in hbr which dries completely. ⚓ outside in 4m just N of spar bn marking ent. Rks on both sides of ent which is less than 170m wide. Safest to enter when rks uncovered. Ldg line at 163°, W side of Pte Benard and old converted windmill. There are no lts. Facilities: FW, Slip.
Village Bar, D, P, R, V.

15

RIVER RANCE/DINAN   10-15-17

Ille-et-Vilaine 48°37'·10N 02°01'·62W (Barrage)

CHARTS
AC 2700, *3659*; SHOM 4233, 7130; Imray C33B; Stanfords 16

TIDES
Standard Port ST MALO (◄——) Zone –0100

Water levels up-river from the Rance hydro-electric tidal barrage are artificially maintained by sluice gates. From 0700 – 2100LT, 4m above CD is guaranteed, whilst from 0800 – 2000LT, during a specified 4 hour period, 8·5m above CD will be maintained.

Outside these hours levels may, exceptionally, drop by as much as 1·4m in 10 minutes. A French language pamphlet, issued by Électricité de France is available from Hr Mrs at St. Malo and Bas Sablons; it is essential for a detailed understanding of the barrage and water level schedule (also published daily in *Ouest-France*). A visit to the barrage display (on site) may be instructive.

SHELTER
Good shelter up-river dependent on wind direction. The principal ⚓s/moorings on the E bank are at St. Suliac and Mordreuc, and on the W bank at La Richardais, La Jouvente, Le Minihic and La Pommeraie. See below for marinas at Plouër, Lyvet (E bank, above the Chatelier lock) and Dinan.

NAVIGATION
From St. Malo/Dinard, appr the lock at the W end of the barrage between a prohib area to port, marked by PHM buoys and wire cables, and Pointe de La Jument to stbd. Waiting dolphins either side of the lock.

Lock opening by day on the hour, every hour provided the level is at least 4m above CD; from 2030 – 0430 opening is on request. Yachts should arrive at H –20 mins, ideally HW –3. The lifting road-bridge across the lock opens between H and H +15. Boats leaving the lock have priority. Up-river of the lock a further prohib area to port is marked as above.

The 3M chan to St. Suliac has min depth of 2m; the next 6M to the Chatelier lock partially dries. The suspension bridge at Port St. Hubert has 23m clearance, with a road bridge alongside it; whilst a railway viaduct 1M above Mordreuc has 19m clearance.

The Chatelier lock and swing bridge operate 0800-2000, provided there is at least 8·5m rise of tide. The final 3M to Dinan is canalised with min depth of approx 1·2m (check with lock-keeper). Dinan gives access to the Ille et Rance Canal and River Vilaine to Biscay (see 10.15.15).

LIGHTS AND MARKS
Approaching the barrage from seaward:

Pte de la Jument bn tr, Fl (5) G20s 6m 4M; PHM Prohib Area buoy opposite, Fl R 4s.

NW side of lock, Fl G 4s, with G △ on W background.

First dolphin, Fl R (2) 6s, with R □ on W background.

Approaching from Dinan:

PHM, Oc R 4s, at S end of Prohib Area.

Last dolphin, Oc R (2) 6s, with R □ on W background.

SE side of lock, Iso G4s, G △ on W background.

Lock entry sigs:

1 ▼ or Ⓡ = Passage permitted sea to river.

1 ● or Ⓖ = Passage permitted river to sea.

▼ & ● together or Ⓡ & Ⓖ = No entry to lock.

Additional sigs on the barrage to the E of the lock show the direction of flow through the turbines.

The chan up-river is partly buoyed and marked by stakes.

RADIO TELEPHONE
Barrage lock: VHF Ch 13.

TELEPHONE
Water levels/navigation 99·46·14·46; Barrage/lock info 99·46·21·87; Hr Mr (Richardais) 99·46·24·20; Hr Mr (Plouër) 96·86·83·15; Chatelier lock 96·39·55·66; Hr Mr (Lyvet) 96·83·35·57; Hr Mr (Dinan) 96·39·04·67; Meteo 99·46·10·46; Auto 36.68.08.35; Aff Mar 96·39·56·44; Police 99·81·52·30; Brit Consul 99·46·26·64.

FACILITIES
St. Suliac Slip, M, Bar, R, V, Divers (Convoimer); Mordreuc Slip, L, M, Bar, R, P, V; La Richardais CH, El, ME, Sh. Villages: Bar, D, P, ✉, R, V, Ⓑ; La Jouvente AB, Bar, R; Le Minihic M, L, Slip, ME, El, Sh; La Pommeraie M, L, SC, R.

MARINAS ON THE RIVER RANCE

PLOUËR, Côtes d'Armor, 49°32'·00N 01°58'·00W. Marina is on the W bank of the R Rance, 6M above the barrage and 0·5M above the two St Hubert bridges. Access approx HW±3, when tide is 8m above CD, giving at least 1·5m water above rising gate. Approach on about 285°, ent in line with Plouër church spire. Unlit PHM and SHM perches are 30m from ent at S end of bkwtr. Ent is marked by FR and FG lts which are lit, by day or night, whenever access is available. Depth gauge (hard to read) has W flood-light. Facilities: Marina (240+ visitors on pontoon B) ☎ 96·86·83·15. VHF Ch 09. AB FF 57, Slip, AC, FW, BY, R, Bar, limited V.

LYVET, Hr Mr ☎ 96·83·35·57; Marina (175 berths) AC, FW, R, Bar, limited V. Immediately upstream of Chatelier lock, on the E bank.

DINAN, Hr Mr ☎ 96·39·56·44; Marina AC, FW, P, D, C for masts, R, Bar. Berths line the W bank of the river, with finger pontoons close to the Port. Low bridge beyond Port has 2·5m headroom, giving access to the Ille et Rance canal. Town (75m above water level) V, R, ✉, Ⓑ, ⇌, ✈ (Dinard).

Ille et Rance canal (see opposite): On the Breton canals the tolls charged elsewhere in France (see 10.15.8) are not envisaged. A certificate of competence is not required, unless LOA >15m or speed >20kph/11kn.

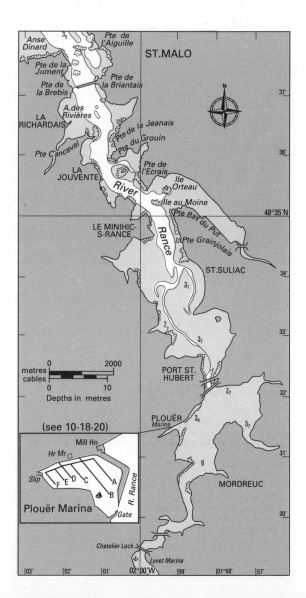

INLAND WATERWAYS OF BRITTANY

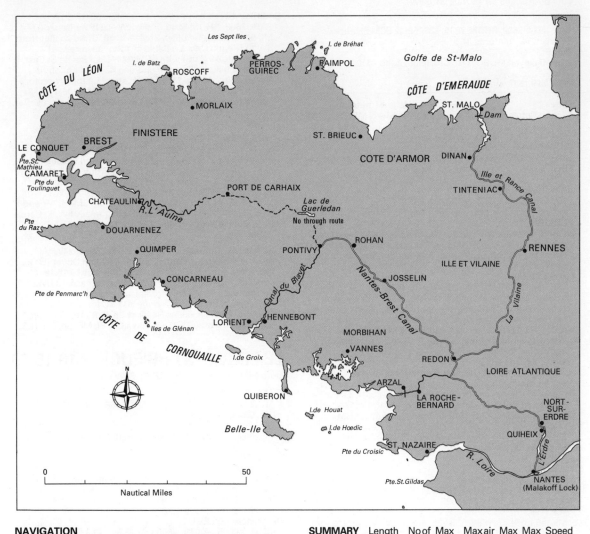

NAVIGATION

Canals and rivers across and within Brittany enable boats of limited water and air drafts to go from the Channel to the Bay of Biscay avoiding the passage around Finistere. Dinan to Arzal takes about 5 days. Distances, number of locks, boat size and speed limits are summarised opposite.

LOCKS

From Apr to Sept locks are worked 7 days a week 0800-1930LT, closing for lunch 1230-1330 approx. All locks are attended, but a fair measure of self-help is the order of the day. In Jul/Aug, in order to conserve water, locks may open on the hour only (and at H+30 if traffic demands).

ACCESS

For prior estimate of max draught possible, write:
  Equipement, Ille et Vilaine, 1 Avenue de Mail,
  35000 Rennes. (☎ 99.59.20.60; Fax 99.54.03.99).
Or obtain recorded information update on ☎ 99.59.11.12.
For latest info on the Ille et Rance Canal/R Vilaine, contact:
Rennes ☎ 99.59.20.60 or Redon ☎ 99.71.03.78.
For the Lorient-Nantes Canal, contact:
Nantes ☎ 40.71.02.00; Hennebont ☎ 97.85.15.15;
Lorient ☎ 97.21.21.54; Pontivy ☎ 97.25.55.21.
Closures *(Chômages)* for maintenance are scheduled in late autumn and in winter each Wednesday (approx first week in November to last week in March).

INFORMATION

For maps and guide books write (with SAE) to:
  Comité des Canaux Bretons,
  Service de Documentation du Comité,
  12 rue de Jemmapes, 44000 Nantes (☎ 40.47.42.94).
Inland Waterways of France: D Edwards-May (Imray) and the ECM Carte-Guide No 12 are recommended.
TOLLS may be due on the R Loire only; see 10.15.8 for rates.

SUMMARY	Length km	No of locks	Max draft m	Max air draft m	Max LOA m	Max beam m	Speed limit kn
St MALO-ARZAL (Ille et Rance Canal and La Vilaine)							
R Rance-Dinan	29·0	1	1·3	19	25	–	5·4
Ille et Rance Canal							
Dinan-Rennes	79·0	48	1·2	2·5	25	4·5	4·3
Rennes-Redon	89·0	13	1·2	3·2/2·6*	25	4·5	4·3
Redon-Arzal	42·0	1	1·3	–			
*Depending on water level							
LORIENT - NANTES (See 10.17.14)							
Canal du Blavet							
Lorient-Pontivy	70	28	1·4	2·6	25	4·6	4·3
Nantes-Brest Canal							
	184·3	106	–	3	25	4·6	4·3
Pontivy-Rohan			0·8 (possible closure)				
Rohan-Josselin			1·0				
Josselin-Redon			1·4				
Redon-Quiheix			1·1				
L'Erdre River	27·6	1	1·4	3·8	400	6·2	13·5
R Loire, above Nantes (10.17.26), may be navigable to Angers.							
R L'AULNE (See 10.16.28)							
Brest-Chateaulin	42	1	3·0	N/A	25	–	–
Chateaulin-Carhaix							
	72	33	1·1	2·5	25	4·6	4·3

DAHOUET   10-15-19

Côte d'Armor 48°34'·85N 02°34'·30W

CHARTS
AC *3674*, 2669; SHOM 7310, 833, 6966; ECM 536; Imray C33B, C34; Stanfords 16

TIDES
–0520 Dover; ML 6·3; Duration 0550; Zone –0100

Standard Port ST-MALO (←—)

Times				Height (metres)			
High Water		Low Water		MHWS	MHWN	MLWN	MLWS
0100	0800	0300	0800	12·2	9·2	4·3	1·6
1300	2000	1500	2000				
Differences DAHOUET							
–0006	–0006	–0020	–0015	–0.9	–0.6	–0.3	–0.3
ERQUY							
–0005	0000	–0018	–0012	–0.6	–0.4	–0.1	–0.1
SAINT CAST							
–0002	–0002	–0005	–0005	–0.2	–0.1	–0.1	–0.1

SHELTER
Good, but ent (dries <u>4</u>m) unsafe in fresh NW winds; a bar may form after strong NW'lies. Outer hbr (FVs) dries <u>5</u>·5m; access HW±2. Marina, min depth 2·5m, accessible over sill 5·5m above CD.

NAVIGATION
WPT 48°35'·28N 02°35'·28W, unlit NCM By, 297°/117° from/to La Petite Muette SHM lt tr, 0·8M; appr in W sector (see 10.15.20 chartlet) until close in. Hbr ent is a narrow break in the cliffs. Pick up 148° transit of 2 W bns, leaving these to port and Petite Muette to stbd. The W ent, S of Petite Muette is dangerous. There are rks W and SW of the ent.

LIGHTS AND MARKS
The wide beach at Val André and the W chapel at hbr ent are both conspic; see also 10.15.20 for other conspic marks in the bay. Appr is marked by G/W lt tr, La Petite Muette, Fl WRG 4s 10m 9/6M, G055°–114°, W114°–146°, R146°–196°. Stone pagoda is seen NE of ent. SHM bn, Fl (2) G 6s, vis 156°–286°, marks the narrow ent abeam the 2 W ldg bns. Sill ent has PHM and SHM perches.

RADIO TELEPHONE
VHF Ch 09 16.

TELEPHONE
Hr Mr 96·72·82·85; Meteo 36·65·02·22; ⌗ 96·74·75·32; Aff Mar 96·72·31·42; CROSS 98·89·31·31; Auto 36.68.08.22; Ⓗ 96·45·23·28; Brit Consul 99·46·26·64; Police 96·72·22·18.

FACILITIES
Marina (318+20) ☎ 96·72·82·85, FF87, FW, AC, BH (10 ton), Slip, C (14 ton); **Quay** P, D, C (4 ton); **YC du Val-André** ☎ 96·72·95·28;
Services: CH, El, ME, Sh. **Town**, V, R, Bar, ⇌ (Lamballe), ✈ (St. Brieuc). Ferry: St. Malo-Portsmouth.

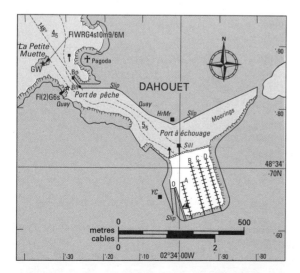

OTHER HARBOURS BETWEEN ST MALO AND DAHOUET

SAINT CAST, Côte d'Armor, 48°38'·45N 02°14'·51W. AC *3659*, 2669; SHOM 5646, 7155. HW –0515 on Dover (UT); ML 6·8m; Duration 0550. See 10·15·19. Good shelter from SW to N winds; ⚓s available in 1·8m. Beware Les Bourdinots (dry 2m) with ECM ¾M NE of Pte de St Cast, and La Feuillade (IDM bn) and Bec Rond (R bn) off hbr. Mole hd, Iso WG 4s 11m 11/8M; appr in either W sector (see 10.15.4). Hr Mr ☎ 96·41·88·34; SNSM ☎ 96·41·88·34; Facilities: **YC** ☎ 96·41·91·77. **Town** CH, El, ME, Sh, Ⓑ, Bar, D, P, ✉, R, V.

ERQUY, Côte d'Armor, 48°38'·10N 02°28'·60W. AC 3672, *3674*, 2669; SHOM 7310, 833. HW –0515 on Dover (UT); ML 6·5m; Duration 0550. See 10·15·19. Sheltered from E, but exposed to SW/W winds. Hbr dries and is usually full of FVs. Beware Plateau des Portes d'Erquy (dry) about 2M to W. From S, beware rks off Pte de la Houssaye. Mole hd lt Oc (3+1) WRG 12s 11m 11/8M; appr in either W sector (see 10.15.4). Inner jetty hd Fl R 2·5s 10m 3M. Hr Mr and ⌗ ☎ 96·72·19·32; Facilities: **Quay** C (3·5 ton), D, FW, P; **Cercle de la Voile d'Erquy** ☎ 96·72·32·40; **Town** CH, El, ME, Sh, R, V, Bar.

VAL-ANDRÉ, Côte d'Armor, 48°35'·88N 02°33'·24W. AC *3674*, 2669; SHOM 7310, 833. HW –0520 on Dover (UT); ML 6·1m; Duration 0550. Tides as Dahouet 10.15.19. A small drying hbr exposed to S/SW winds; access HW±3. From the E beware Le Verdelet, and Platier des Trois Têtes from the W. Berth on the quay, ask YC for mooring off Le Piegu or ⚓ off. Facilities: Hr Mr ☎ 96·72·83·20, FW, Slip; **YC du Val-André** ☎ 96·72·21·68; **Town** CH, El, ME, Sh, Bar, R, V.

LE LÉGUÉ (ST BRIEUC)   10-15-20

Côte d'Armor 48°31'·95N 02°43'·30W

CHARTS
AC *3674*, 2669; SHOM 833, 7128, 6966; ECM 536; Imray C34, C33B; Stanfords 16

TIDES
–0520 Dover; ML 6·5; Duration 0550; Zone –0100

Standard Port ST-MALO (←—)

Times				Height (metres)			
High Water		Low Water		MHWS	MHWN	MLWN	MLWS
0100	0800	0300	0800	12·2	9·2	4·3	1·6
1300	2000	1500	2000				
Differences LE LÉGUÉ							
+0005	+0005	–0013	–0003	–0.7	–0.3	–0.2	–0.2

SHELTER
Very good in Le Légué (the port for St Brieuc), especially in the wet basin. Yachts use Bassin No 2 (min 3m) near viaduct. Lock opens HW –2 to HW+1 sp; HW ±1 nps. The lock sill is 5·0m above CD. Yachts can wait against Le Quai Gilette (N bank), but soft mud slopes very steeply to chan.

NAVIGATION
WPT 48°34'·39N 02°41'·09W, Le Légué SWM buoy, Fl Mo (A) 10s, Whis, 030°/210° from/to Pte de l'Aigle lt, 2·6M. Appr via buoyed chan (with some gaps); not advised in strong N/NE winds. The area dries E/SE of conspic Pte du Roselier; see 10·18·5. Keep close to Pte à l'Aigle to avoid Les Galettes Rks.

LIGHTS AND MARKS
Conspic marks: Rohein tr, from N, and Le Verdelet ls from E (beware Plateau des Jaunes). No ldg lines; 2 lts on the NW bank of the river de Gouet ent: Pte de l'Aigle, QG 13m 8M, vis 160°–070°, W tr G top. Jetée de la Douane (W columns with G top), Iso G 4s 6m 8M.

RADIO TELEPHONE
Call: *Légué Port* VHF Ch 12 16 (approx HW–2 to +1½).

TELEPHONE
Hr Mr 96·33·35·41; Aff Mar 96·61·22·61; CROSS 98·89·31·31; Meteo 99·46·10·46 and VHF Ch 13; Auto 36·68·08·22; SNSM 96·88·35·47; ⌗ 96·33·33·03; Police 96·94·52·25; Dr St Brieuc 96·61·49·07; Brit Consul 99·46·26·64.

FACILITIES
Quai (100+20 visitors), AB FF56, C (30 ton), P & D (cans on quai or tanker); **Services:** Sh, ME, El, CH, SM, Ⓔ, El, CH.
Town (St Brieuc) P & D (cans), FW, Gaz, V, R, Bar, ✉, Ⓑ, ⇌, ✈. Ferry: St Malo.

LE LÉGUÉ/ST BRIEUC *continued*

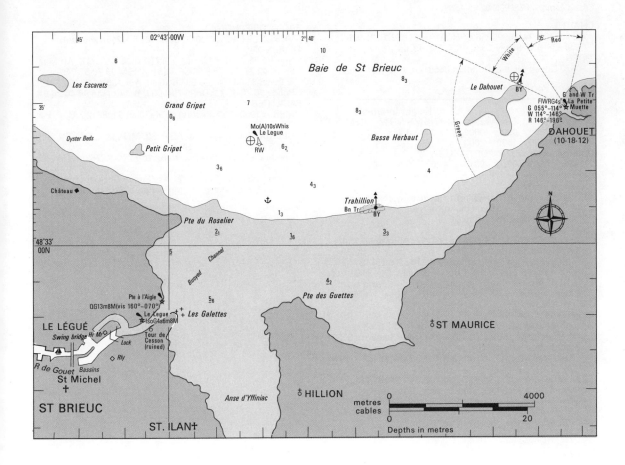

BINIC   10-15-21

Côte d'Armor 48°36′·12N 02°48′·90W

CHARTS
AC *3674*, 2669; SHOM 833, 7128, 6966; ECM 536; Imray C33B; Stanfords 16

TIDES
−0525 Dover; ML 6·3; Duration 0550; Zone −0100

Standard Port ST-MALO (←)

Times				Height (metres)			
High Water		Low Water		MHWS	MHWN	MLWN	MLWS
0100	0800	0300	0800	12·2	9·2	4·3	1·6
1300	2000	1500	2000				
Differences BINIC							
−0003	−0003	−0025	−0010	−0·8	−0·6	−0·3	−0·3

SHELTER
Good, especially in Bassin à Flot/marina (1·5-3m). Easy access HW±3 by day/night to Avant Port (dries), except in E winds. Lock opens, in working hrs, approx HW−1 to HW near sp, if tide reaches 9·5m; no opening near nps, when gate may be closed for 4 or 5 days.

NAVIGATION
WPT 48°37′·00N 02°42′·00W, 078°/258° from/to ent, 4·7M. Best appr from E, from Baie de St Brieuc (see 10·18·5) keeping E of Caffa ECM, from which ent is 246°; or from N through Rade de Portrieux. Ent between moles dries 4·2m.

LIGHTS AND MARKS
Ldg line 275°, N mole hd lt tr, Oc (3) 12s 12m 12M, W tr, G gallery, on with church spire.
Gate and sliding bridge sigs on mast N of gate:

By day: St Andrew's Cross, B on W flag	= Gate open
By night: Ⓦ and Ⓡ (hor)	= No entry
Ⓦ and Ⓖ (hor)	= No exit
Ⓡ and Ⓖ (hor)	= No exit/entry

RADIO TELEPHONE
VHF Ch 09.

TELEPHONE
Hr Mr 96·73·61·86; Aff Mar 96·70·42·27; SNSM 96·73·74·41; CROSS 98·89·31·31; ⊞ 96·74·75·32; Meteo 99·46·10·46; Auto 36·68·08·22; Police 96·73·60·32; Dr 96·42·61·05; Ⓗ 96·94·31·71; Brit Consul 99·46·26·64.

FACILITIES
Basin (540+60), FF73, FW, AC, C (20 ton), Slip;
Club Nautique de Binic ☎ 96·73·31·67;
Services: CH, ME, El, Ⓔ, Sh, SM, SHOM.
Town P, V, Gaz, ▣, R, Bar, ✉, Ⓑ, ⇌ (bus to St Brieuc), ✈ (St Brieuc). Ferry: St Malo.

15

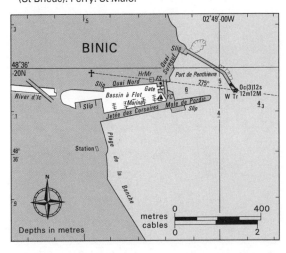

SAINT QUAY-PORTRIEUX 10-15-22
Côte d'Armor 48°38'·90N 02°48'·88W

CHARTS
AC 3672, *3674*, 2669, *2668*; SHOM 7128, 832, 833, 6966; ECM 536, 537; Imray C33B, C34; Stanfords 16, 17

TIDES
−0520 Dover; ML 6·3; Duration 0550; Zone −0100

Standard Port ST-MALO (←)

Times				Height (metres)			
High Water		Low Water		MHWS	MHWN	MLWN	MLWS
0100	0800	0300	0800	12·2	9·2	4·3	1·6
1300	2000	1500	2000				
Differences ST QUAY-PORTRIEUX							
−0005	0000	−0020	−0010	−1·0	−0·6	−0·3	−0·2

SHELTER
Excellent in the marina (3·5m). Yachts may also dry out in the Old Hbr. ⚓ in the Rade de Portrieux is good but affected by winds from N to SE.

NAVIGATION
WPT 48°41'·00N 02°49'·60W, 349°/169° from/to NE mole elbow, 2·0M. Portrieux lies inside the Roches de St Quay, the chan between being about ½M wide. To NE lie the rky Ile Harbour and to the E Rochers Déan. Due N beware the Moulières de Portrieux, unlit ECM bn tr. From E and SE appr via Caffa ECM Q (3) 10s and La Roselière WCM VQ (9) 10s (both off chartlet).

LIGHTS AND MARKS
At night, from the N, White sectors of 4 Dir lts lead safely to the marina in sequence 169°, 130°, 185° (astern), 318° (see chartlet and below):
(1) NE mole elbow, Dir Iso WRG 4s 15/11M, **W159°-179°**, G179°-316°, W316°-320.5°, R320.5°-159°.
(2) Herflux Dir lt, Fl (2) WRG 6s 8/6M, vis G115°-125°, **W125°-135°**, R135°-145°; on Rochers Déan.
(3) Ile Harbour Dir lt, Oc (2) WRG 6s 16m 11/8M, vis R011°-133°, G133°-270°, R270°-306°, G306°-358°, **W358°-011°**.
(4) NE mole elbow, as (1) above, **W316°-320·5°**.

RADIO TELEPHONE
VHF Ch 09 (0830-1230; 1330-1830LT. H24 in season).
TELEPHONE
Marina 96·70·49·51; Hr Mr (Old Hbr) 96·70·95·31; Aff Mar 96·70·42·27; CROSS 98·89·31·31; SNSM 96·70·52·04; ⌗ 96·33·33·03; Meteo 99·46·10·46; Auto 36.68.08.22; Police 96·70·61·24; Dr 96·70·41·31; Brit Consul 99·46·26·64.
FACILITIES
Marina (900+100 visitors) ☎ 96·70·49·51, FF120, D, P, FW, BH, AC, C (5 ton);
Old Hbr (500+8 visitors) AB FF60, M, P, D, L, FW, Sh, Slip, C (1·5 ton), ME, El, Ⓔ, Sh, CH, R, Bar;
Cercle de la Voile de Portrieux ☎ 96·70·41·76, M, FW, C (1 ton), Bar;
Town V, Gaz, R, Bar, ✉, Ⓑ, ⇌ (bus to St Brieuc), ✈ (St Brieuc/Armor). Ferry: St Malo–Poole, Portsmouth.

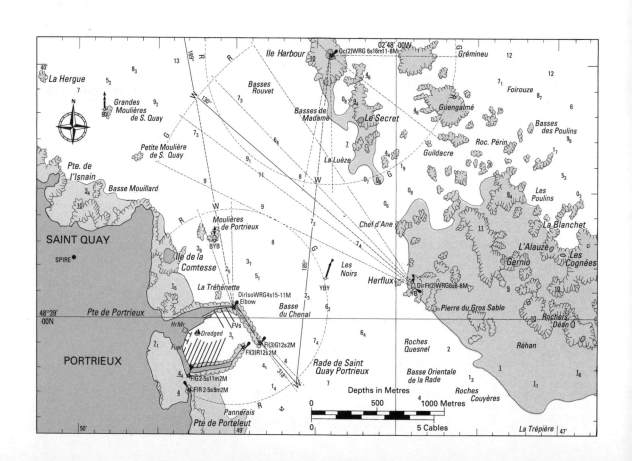

Volvo Penta service

Sales and service centres in area 16
Names and addresses of Volvo Penta dealers in
this area are available from:
France Volvo Penta France SA, 1 Rue de la Nouvelle, B. P. 49, 78133 Les
Mureaux Tel 33-1-30912799, Fax 33-1-34746415 Telex 695221 F.

Area 16

North Brittany
Paimpol to Raz de Sein

**VOLVO
PENTA**

16

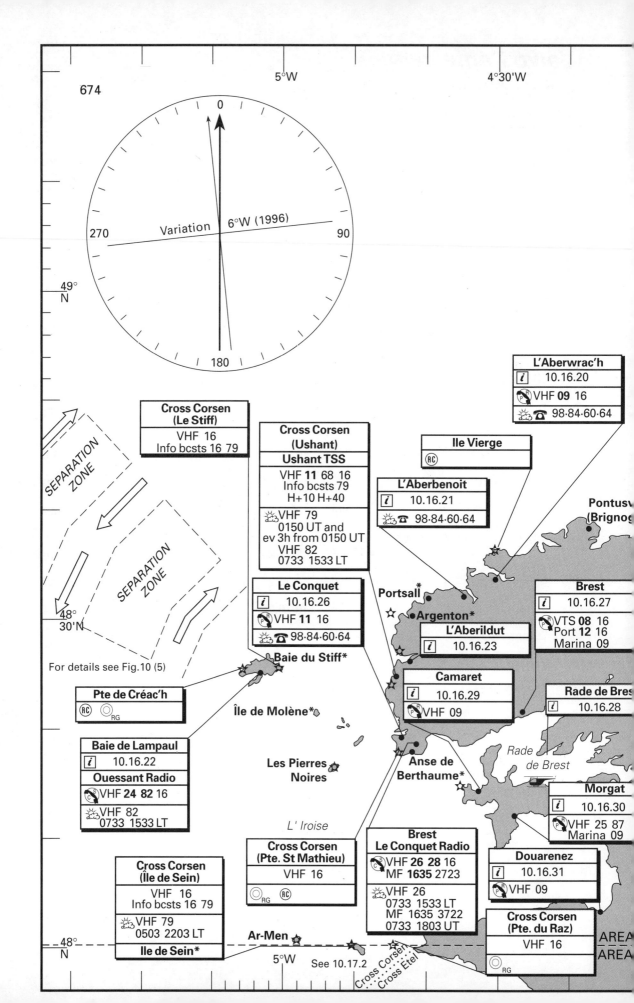

674

Variation 6°W (1996)

0
90
180
270

49°N

48°30'N

48°N

5°W

4°30'W

Cross Corsen (Le Stiff)
VHF 16
Info bcsts 16 79

Cross Corsen (Ushant)
Ushant TSS
VHF **11** 68 16
Info bcsts 79
H+10 H+40
VHF 79
0150 UT and
ev 3h from 0150 UT
VHF 82
0733 1533 LT

SEPARATION ZONE

SEPARATION ZONE

For details see Fig.10 (5)

Pte de Créac'h
(RC) (RG)

Baie de Lampaul
i 10.16.22
Ouessant Radio
VHF **24 82** 16
VHF 82
0733 1533 LT

Cross Corsen (Île de Sein)
VHF 16
Info bcsts 16 79
VHF 79
0503 2203 LT
Île de Sein*

Baie du Stiff*

Île de Molène*

Les Pierres Noires

L' Iroise

Cross Corsen (Pte. St Mathieu)
VHF 16
(RG) (RC)

Ar-Men

See 10.17.2

Cross Corsen Cross Etel

L'Aberwrac'h
i 10.16.20
VHF **09** 16
☎ 98·84·60·64

Ile Vierge
(RC)

L'Aberbenoit
i 10.16.21
☎ 98·84·60·64

Le Conquet
i 10.16.26
VHF **11** 16
☎ 98·84·60·64

Portsall*

Argenton*

L'Aberildut
i 10.16.23

Camaret
i 10.16.29
VHF 09

Anse de Berthaume*

**Brest
Le Conquet Radio**
VHF **26 28** 16
MF **1635** 2723
VHF 26
0733 1533 LT
MF 1635 3722
0733 1803 UT

Pontusv (Brignog

Brest
i 10.16.27
VTS **08** 16
Port **12** 16
Marina 09

Rade de Bres
i 10.16.28

Rade de Brest

Morgat
i 10.16.30
VHF 25 87
Marina 09

Douarenez
i 10.16.31
VHF 09

Cross Corsen (Pte. du Raz)
VHF 16
(RG)

AREA

AREA

10-16-2
North Brittany

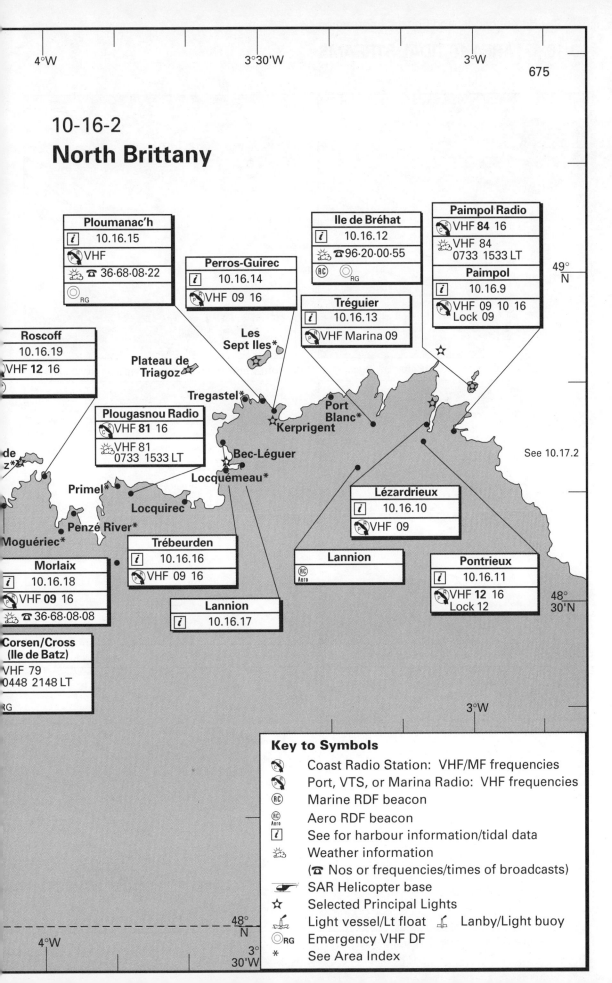

Ploumanac'h
i	10.16.15
VHF	
☎ 36·68·08·22	
RG	

Perros-Guirec
i	10.16.14
VHF 09 16	

Ile de Bréhat
i	10.16.12
☎ 96·20·00·55	
RC	RG

Paimpol Radio
VHF **84** 16	
VHF 84 0733 1533 LT	

Paimpol
i	10.16.9
VHF 09 10 16 Lock 09	

Tréguier
i	10.16.13
VHF Marina 09	

Roscoff
10.16.19
VHF **12** 16

49°N

Les Sept Iles*

Plateau de Triagoz

Tregastel*

Port Blanc*

Kerprigent

Plougasnou Radio
VHF **81** 16	
VHF 81 0733 1533 LT	

Bec-Léguer

Primel*

Locquirec

Locquémeau*

Penzé River*

Moguériec*

Lézardrieux
i	10.16.10
VHF 09	

See 10.17.2

Morlaix
i	10.16.18
VHF **09** 16	
☎ 36·68·08·08	

Trébeurden
i	10.16.16
VHF 09 16	

Lannion
RC Aero	

Pontrieux
i	10.16.11
VHF **12** 16 Lock 12	

48°30'N

Lannion
i	10.16.17

Corsen/Cross (Ile de Batz)
VHF 79
0448 2148 LT

RG

3°W

16

Key to Symbols
🅒	Coast Radio Station: VHF/MF frequencies
🅟	Port, VTS, or Marina Radio: VHF frequencies
RC	Marine RDF beacon
RC Aero	Aero RDF beacon
i	See for harbour information/tidal data
☁	Weather information (☎ Nos or frequencies/times of broadcasts)
🚁	SAR Helicopter base
☆	Selected Principal Lights
⚓	Light vessel/Lt float ⚓ Lanby/Light buoy
RG	Emergency VHF DF
*	See Area Index

10-16-3   AREA 16 TIDAL STREAMS

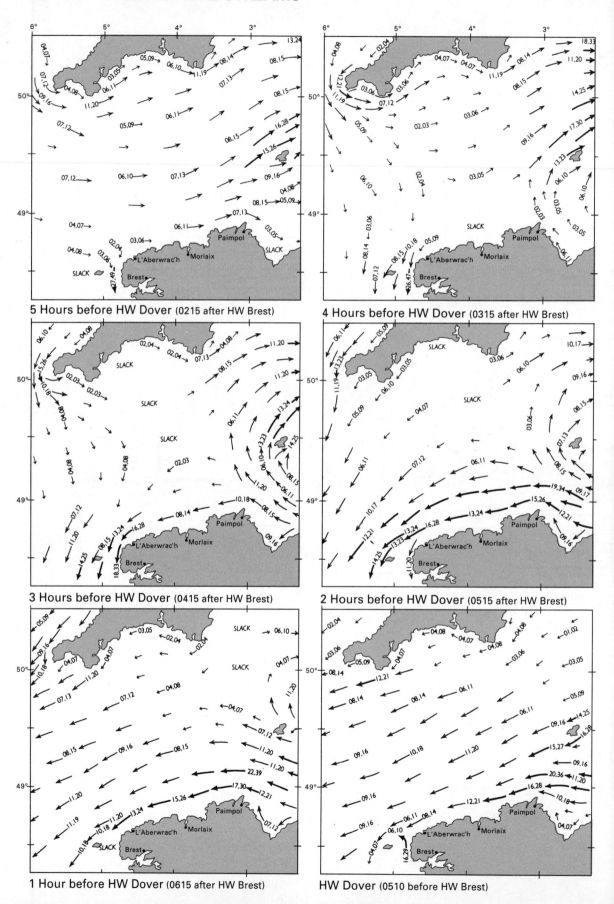

5 Hours before HW Dover (0215 after HW Brest)

4 Hours before HW Dover (0315 after HW Brest)

3 Hours before HW Dover (0415 after HW Brest)

2 Hours before HW Dover (0515 after HW Brest)

1 Hour before HW Dover (0615 after HW Brest)

HW Dover (0510 before HW Brest)

Southward 10.17.3   Eastward 10.15.3   Northward 10.1.3

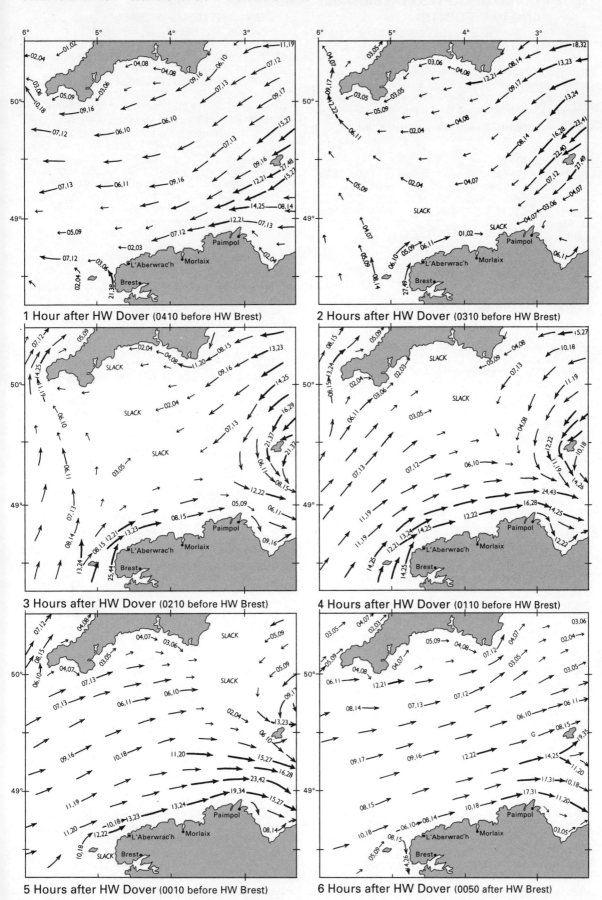

1 Hour after HW Dover (0410 before HW Brest)

2 Hours after HW Dover (0310 before HW Brest)

3 Hours after HW Dover (0210 before HW Brest)

4 Hours after HW Dover (0110 before HW Brest)

5 Hours after HW Dover (0010 before HW Brest)

6 Hours after HW Dover (0050 after HW Brest)

16

10.16.4 COASTAL LIGHTS,FOG SIGNALS AND WAYPOINTS

Abbreviations used below are given in 1.4.1. Principal lights are in **bold** print, places in CAPITALS, and light-vessels, light floats and Lanbys in *CAPITAL ITALICS*. Unless otherwise stated lights are white. m – elevation in metres; M – nominal range in miles. Fog signals are in *italics*. Useful waypoints are underlined – use those on land with care. All geographical positions should be assumed to be approximate. See 4.4.1.

NOTE: For English Channel Waypoints see 10.1.7.

OFFSHORE AIDS

Roches Douvres 49°06'·35N 02°48'·65W Fl 5s 60m **28M**; pink Tr on dwelling with G roof; RC; RG; *Siren 60s*.
Barnouic Lt Tr 49°01'·70N 02°48'·33W VQ (3) 5s 15m 7M; ECM.
Roche Gautier Lt By 49°00'·49N 02°52'·92W VQ (9) 10s; WCM; *Whis*.
Nord Horaine By 48°54'·48N 02°55'·08W; NCM.
La Horaine 48°53'·57N 02°55'·15W Fl (3) 12s 13m 11M; Gy 8-sided Tr on B hut.
Men-Marc'h By 48°52'·23N 02°51'·71W; ECM.

PAIMPOL TO ÎLE DE BRÉHAT

PAIMPOL
Les Calemarguiers By 48°47'·04N 02°54'·77W; ECM.
L'Ost Pic Lt Tr 48°46'·82N 02°56'·33W Oc WR 4s 20m W11M, R8M; 2 W Trs, R tops; vis W105°–116°, R116°–221°, W221°–253°, R253°–291°, W291°–329°; obsc by islets near Bréhat when brg less than 162°.
Les Charpentiers Bn 48°47'·95N 02°55'·92W; ECM.
La Gueule By 48°47'·48N 02°57'·25W; PHM.
La Jument Bn 48°47'·41N 02°57'·88W; PHM.

Pte de Porz-Don 48°47'·53N 03°01'·47W Oc (2) WR 6s 13m **W15M**, R11M; W house; vis W269°–272°, R272°–279°.
Ldg Lts 262·2°. Kernoa, front 48°47'·26N 03°02'·37W FR 5m 7M; W & R hut. Rear, 370m from front, Dir FR 12m 14M; W pylon, R top; intens 260·2°–264·2°.

CHENAL DU DENOU/CHENAL DE BRÉHAT
Roc'h Denou Bn 48°47'·90N 02°57'·96W; W Bn.
Roc'h Denou Vihan Bn 48°48'·50N 02°57'·87W; SHM.
La Petite Moisie Bn 48°48'·65N 02°57'·60W; PHM.
Cain Ar Monse By 48°50'·22N 02°56'·73W; NCM.
Roche Guarine By 48°51'·69N 02°57'·54W; ECM.

CHENAL DU FERLAS
Le Ar Serive By 48°50'·04N 02°58'·68W; SCM.
Cadenenou By 48°49'·87N 02°58'·97W; NCM.
Les Piliers Bn 48°49'·83N 02°59'·91W; NCM.
Réceveur Bihan Bn 48°49'·76N 03°01'·87W; SCM.
Roche Quinonec, Dir Lt 257·3°, 48°49'·43N 03°03'·58W Dir Q WRG 12m W10M, R8M, G8M; Gy Tr; vis G254°–257°, W257°–257·7°, R257·7°–260·7°.
Rompa Bn 48°49'·64N 02°02'·67W; IDM.
Kermouster, Embouchure du Trieux, Dir Lt 271°, 48°49'·62N 03°05'·11W Dir Fl WRG 2s 16m W10M, R8M, G8M; W col; vis G267°–270°, W270°–272°, R272°–274°.

ÎLE DE BRÉHAT
Rosédo 48°51'·51N 03°00'·21W Fl 5s 29m **20M**; W Tr; RC.
Le Paon 48°51'·98N 02°59'·08W F WRG 22m W11M, R8M, G8M; Y Tr; vis W033°–078°, G078°–181°, W181°–196°, R196°–307°, W307°–316°, R316°–348°.
Men-Joliguet 48°50'·18N 03°00'·12W Iso WRG 4s 6m W13M, R10M, G10M; WCM Bn Tr; vis R255°–279°, W279°–283°, G283°–175°.

LÉZARDRIEUX TO TRÉGUIER

LE TRIEUX RIVER, LÉZARDRIEUX/PONTRIEUX
Les Echaudés 48°53'·42N 02°57'·26W; PHM.
Les Sirlots By 48°53'·00N 02°59'·48W; SHM; *Whis*.
Vieille du Tréou Bn Tr 48°52'·05N 03°01'·00W; SHM.
Gosrod Bn 48°51'·48N 03°01'·14W; PHM.
Men Krenn Lt Bn Tr 48°51'·27N 03°03'·84W Q (9) 15s 7m 7M; WCM.
Ldg Lts 224·7°. Front **La Croix** 48°50'·28N 03°03'·16W Oc 4s 15m **19M**; two Gy ● Trs joined, W on NE side, R tops; intens 215°–235°. Rear **Bodic**, 2·1M from front Dir Q 55m **22M**; W house with G gable; intens 221°–229°.
Coatmer Ldg Lts 218·7°. Front 48°48'·32N 03°05'·67W F RG 16m R9M, G9M; W gable; vis R200°–250°, G250°–053°. Rear, 660m from front, FR 50m 9M; W gable; vis 197°–242°.
Les Perdrix Lt Tr 48°47'·80N 03°05'·71W Fl (2) WG 6s 5m W6M, G3M; G Tr; vis G165°–197°, W197°–202·5°, G202·5°–040°.
3 F Bu Lts mark Marina pontoons, 750m SSW.

LE TRIEUX RIVER TO TRÉGUIER RIVER
An Ogejou Bihan Bn 48°53'·44N 03°01'·83W; ECM.
La Moisie Bn 48°53'·89N 03°02'·15W; ECM.
Les Héaux de Bréhat 48°54'·57N 03°05'·10W Oc (3) WRG 12s 48m **W15M**, R11M, G11M; Gy ● Tr; vis R227°–247°, W247°–270°, G270°–302°, W302°–227°.
Basse des Héaux Bn 48°54'·13N 03°05'·20W; SHM.
Pont de la Gaîne Bn 48°53'·20N 03°07'·26W; PHM.

TRÉGUIER RIVER
La Jument des Héaux Lt By 48°55'·41N 03°07'·95W VQ; NCM; *Bell*.
Grande Passe Ldg Lts 137°. Front, Port de la Chaîne 48°51'·61N 03°07'·80W Oc 4s 12m 11M; W house. Rear **St Antoine** 0·75M from front Dir Oc R 4s 34m **15M**; R&W house; synch with front; intens 134°–140°.
Basse Crublent Lt By 48°54'·35N 03°11'·07W Fl (2) R 6s; PHM; *Whis*.
Le Corbeau By 48°53'·42N 03°10'·20W; PHM.
Pierre à l'Anglais By 48°53'·30N 03°10'·38W; SHM.
Petit Pen ar Guézec By 48°52'·58N 03°09'·34W; SHM.
La Corne Lt Tr 48°51'·40N 03°10'·53W Fl (3) WRG 12s 14m W11M, R8M, G8M; W Tr, R base; vis W052°–059°, R059°–173°, G173°–213°, W213°–220°, R220°–052°.

TRÉGUIER TO TRÉBEURDEN

PORT-BLANC
Le Voleur Lt Tr 48°50'·27N 03°18'·44W Fl WRG 4s 17m W14M, R11M, G11M; W Tr; vis G140°–148°, W148°–152°, R152°–160°.

PERROS-GUIREC
Basse Guazer By 48°51'·65N 03°20'·89W; PHM.
Passe de l'Est Ldg Lts 224·5°. Front **Le Colombier** 48°47'·93N 03°26'·58W Dir Oc (4) 12s 28m **15M**; W house; intens 214·5°–234·5°. Rear, **Kerprigent** 1·5M from front Dir Q 79m **21M**; W Tr; intens 221°–228°.
Pierre à Jean Rouzic By 48°49'·61N 03°24'·11W; SHM.
Pierre du Chenal Bn 48°49'·35N 03°24'·59W; IDM.
Passe de l'Ouest. **Kerjean** Dir Lt 143·6°. 48°47'·85N 03°23'·31W Dir Oc (2+1) WRG 12s 78m **W15M**, R12M, G12M; W Tr, B top; vis G133·7°–143·2°, W143·2°–144·8°, R144·8°–154·3°.
Roc'h Hu de Perros Bn 48°48'·88N 03°24'·87W; PHM.
Jetée Est (Linkin) Hd 48°48'·26N 03°26'·23W Fl (2) G 6s 4m 9M; W pile, G top.
Roche Bernard Bn 48°49'·50N 03°25'·38W; SHM.
La Fronde By 48°49'·93N 03°25'·90W; SHM.
Bilzic Bn 48°50'·27N 03°25'·65W; PHM.
La Horaine Bn 48°49'·95N 03°27'·18W; NCM.
Les Couillons de Tomé By 48°50'·95N 03°25'·60W; WCM.

PLOUMANAC'H
Men-Ruz 48°50'·32N 03°28'·90W Oc WR 4s 26m W12M, R9M; pink ■ Tr; vis W226°-242°, R242°-226°; obsc by Pte de Trégastel when brg less than 080°, and part obsc by Sept-Îles 156°-207°, and by Île Tomé 264°-278°.

LES SEPT-ÎLES
Île-aux-Moines 48°52'·78N 03°29'·33W Fl (3) 15s 59m **24M**; Gy Tr and dwelling; obsc by Îlot Rouzic and E end of Île Bono 237°-241°, and in Baie de Lannion when brg less than 039°.
Les Dervinis By 48°52'·41N 03°27'·23W; SCM.

TRÉGASTEL
Île Dhu Bn 48°50'·43N 03°31'·13W; PHM.
Le Taureau Bn 48°50'·47N 03°31'·51W; SHM.

Les Triagoz 48°52'·35N 03°38'·73W Oc (2) WR 6s 31m W14M, R11M; Gy ■ Tr, R lantern; vis W010°-339°, R339°-010°; obsc in places 258°-268° by Les Sept-Îles.
Bar all Gall Lt By 48°49'·80N 03°36'·00W VQ (9) 10s; WCMTr.
Le Crapaud Lt By 48°46'·65N 03°40'·40W Q (9) 15s; WCM.

TRÉBEURDEN
Ar Gouredec Lt By 48°46'·49N 03°36'·40W VQ (6) + L Fl 10s; SCM.
Lt By 48°46'·54N 03°35'·89W Fl (2) R 6s; PHM.
Pt de Lan Kerellec 48°46'·80N 03°34'·98W Iso WRG 4s; W8M, R5M, G5M; vis G058°-064°, W064°-069°, R069°-130°.

TRÉBEURDEN TO ROSCOFF

LÉGUER RIVER, LANNION
Kinierbel By 48°44'·20N 03°34'·95W; SHM; *Bell*.
Beg-Léguer 48°44'·40N 03°32'·83W Oc (4) WRG 12s 60m W12M, R9M, G9M; W face of W house, R lantern; vis G007°-084°, W084°-098°, R098°-129°.

LOCQUÉMEAU
Ldg Lts 121°. Front 48°43'·48N 03°34'·40W FR 21m 6M; W pylon, R top; vis 068°-228°. Rear, 484m from front Oc (2+1) R 12s 39m 7M; W gabled house; vis 016°-232°.
Locquémeau By 48°43'·94N 03°35'·73W; SHM; *Whis*.

PRIMEL
Ldg Lts 152°. Front 48°42'·52N 03°49'·10W FR 35m 6M; W ■, R stripe on pylon; vis 134°-168°. Rear, 172m from front, FR 56m 6M; W ■, R stripe.
Marina Jetty Hd 48°42'·82N 03°49'·53W Fl G 4s 6m 7M.

Méloine By 48°45'·65N 03°50'·55W; WCM; *Whis*.

BAIE DE MORLAIX
Chenal du Tréguier Ldg Lts 190·5°. Front, Île Noire 48°40'·41N 03°52'·44W Oc (2) WRG 6s 15m W11M, R8M, G8M; W ■ Tr, R top; vis G051°-135°, R135°-211°, W211°-051°; obsc in places. Common Rear, **La Lande** 48°38'·26N 03°53'·04W Fl 5s 85m **23M**; W ■ Tr, B top; obsc by Pte Annelouesten when brg more than 204°.
La Pierre Noire Bn 48°41'·71N 03°53'·97W; SHM.
La Chambre Bn 48°40'·80N 03°52'·41W; SHM.
Grande Chenal Ldg Lts 176·4°. Front **Île Louet** 48°40'·47N 03°53'·24W Oc (3) WG 12s 17m **W15M**; G10M; W ■ Tr, B top; vis W305°-244°, G244°-305°, vis 139°-223° from offshore, except when obsc by Is. Common Rear, **La Lande** above.
Pot de Fer By 48°44'·29N 03°53'·93W; ECM.
Vieille Bn 48°42'·66N 03°54'·03W; SHM.
Stolvezen By 48°42'·71N 03°53'·32W; PHM.
La Noire Bn 48°42'·61N 03°52'·11W; SHM.
Ricard Bn 48°41'·60N 03°53'·40W; SHM.
Barre de-Flot No. 1 By 48°40'·24N 05°52'·86W; SHM.

Marine farm prohib area Lt By 48°43'·00N 03°54'·10W VQ (6) + L Fl 10s; SCM.

BLOSCON/ROSCOFF
Le Menk Lt Bn Tr 48°43'·35N 03°56'·60W Q (9) WR 15s 6m W5M, R3M; vis W160°-188°; WCM.
Bloscon Jetty Hd 48°43'·27N 03°57'·59W Fl WG 4s 9m W10M, G7M; W Tr, G top, vis W206°-216°, G216°-206°; RC. In fog Fl 2s.
Ar Pourven Lt By 48°43'·10N 03°57'·61W Q; NCM.
Astan Lt By 48°44'·95N 03°57'·55W VQ (3) 5s 9m 6M; ECM; *Whis*; Ra refl.
Basse de Bloscon Lt By 48°43'·77N 03°57'·48W VQ; NCM.
Ar-Chaden Lt Bn 48°43'·99N 03°58'·15W Q (6) + L Fl WR 15s 14m W8M, R6M; vis R262°-289·5°, W289·5°-293°, R293°-326°, W326°-110°; SCM.
Men-Guen-Bras Lt Bn 48°43'·81N 03°57'·95W Q WRG 14m W9M, R6M, G6M; vis W068°-073°, R073°-197°, W197°-257°, G257°-068°; NCM.
Roscoff Ldg Lts 209°. Front, N Môle 48°43'·62N 03°58'·57W Oc (2+1) G 12s 7m 7M; W col, G top; vis 078°-318°. **Rear**, 430m from front, Oc (2+1) 12s 24m **15M**; Gy ■ Tr, W on NE side; vis 062°-242°.
Jetty Hd 48°43'·98N 03°58'·87W F Vi; W & Purple **l**.

ÎLE DE BATZ TO ÎLE VIERGE

ÎLE DE BATZ
Lt Ho 48°44'·78N 04°01'·55W Fl (4) 25s 69m **23M**; Gy Tr; auxiliary Lt FR 65m 7M; same Tr; vis 024°-059°.

CANAL DE L'ÎLE DE BATZ
Perroch Bn 48°44'·17N 03°59'·62W; NCM.
Île aux Moutons Ldg stage 48°44'·31N 04°00'·34W VQ (6) + L Fl 10s 3m 7M; SCM.
L'Oignon Bn 48°44'·10N 04°01'·27W; NCM.
Basse Plate Bn 48°44'·32N 04°02'·44W; NCM.

MOGUÉRIEC
Ldg Lts 162°. Front, Jetty Hd 48°41'·40N 04°04'·40W Iso WG 4s 9m W11M, G6M; W Tr, G top; vis W158°-166°, G166°-158°. Rear, 440m from front FG 22m 7M; W Col, G top; vis 142°-182°.

PONTUSVAL
Pointe de Pontusval By 48°41'·51N 04°19'·12W; ECM.
Ar Peich By 48°40'·95N 04°19'·08W; SHM.
An Neudenn Bn 48°40'·72N 04°19'·01W; PHM.
Pte de Beg-Pol 48°40'·73N 04°20'·70W Oc (3) WR 12s 16m W10M, R7M; W ■ Tr, B top, W dwelling; vis W shore-056°, R056°-096°, W096°-shore. QY and FR Lts on towers 2·4M S.

Aman-ar-Ross Lt By 48°41'·94N 04°26'·96W Q 9m 7M; NCM; *Whis*.
Barr. Ar-Skoaz By 48°38'·29N 04°29'·99W; PHM.
Lizen Ven Ouest Lt By 48°40'·55N 04°33'·68W VQ (9) 10s 8m 5M; WCM; *Whis*.
Île-Vierge 48°38'·38N 04°33'·97W Fl 5s 77m **27M**; Gy Tr; vis 337°-325°; RC; *Horn 60s*.

ÎLE VIERGE TO LE FOUR

L'ABERWRAC'H
Libenter Lt By 48°37'·57N 04°38'·35W Q (9) 15s 8m 6M; Ra refl; WCM; *Whis*.
Ldg Lts 100·1° Front Île Wrac'h 48°36'·95N 04°34'·47W QR 20m 7M; W ■ Tr, Or top, dwelling. Rear, Lanvaon 1·63M from front, Dir Q 55m 12M; W ■ Tr, Or ▲ on top; intens 090°-110°.
Trepied By 48°37'·35N 04°37'·47W; PHM.
Grand Pot de Beurre Bn 48°37'·27N 04°36'·39W; PHM.
Petit Pot de Beurre Bn 48°37'·18N 04°36'·13W; ECM.

16

Basse de la Croix Lt By 48°36'·98N 04°35'·90W Fl (3) G 12s; SHM.

Breac'h Ver Lt Tr 48°36'·70N 04°35'·30W Fl G 2·5s 6m 3M; ▲ on Tr, SHM.

Dir Lt 128°, N Bkwtr 48°35'·95N 04°33'·72W Dir Oc (2) WRG 6s 5m W13M, R11M, G11M; vis G125·7°-127·2°, W127·2°-128·7°, R128·7°-130·2°.

L'ABER BENOÎT

Petite Fourche By 48°37'·05N 04°38'·67W; WCM.
Ruzven Est By 48°36'·37N 04°38'·53W; SHM.
Poul Orvil By 48°35'·58N 04°38'·20W; WCM.
La Jument Bn 48°35'·19N 04°37'·30W; PHM.
Le Chien Bn 48°34'·73N 04°36'·80W; IDM.

Le Relec By 48°36'·05N 04°40'·76W; ECM.
Corn-Carhai 48°35'·25N 04°43'·86W Fl (3) 12s 19m 9M; W 8-sided Tr, B top.
Basse Paupian By 48°35'·38N 04°46'·20W; WCM.
Grande Basse de Portsall Lt By 48°36'·78N 04°46'·05W VQ (9) 10s 9m 4M; Ra refl; WCM; Whis.

PORTSALL/ARGENTON

Bosven Arval Bn 48°33'·88N 04°44'·18W; W Bn.
Men ar Pic Bn 48°33'·72N 04°43'·93W; G Bn.
Portsall 48°33'·89N 04°42'·18W Oc (4) WRG 12s 9m W13M, R10M, G10M; W col, R top; vis G058°-084°, W084°- 088°, R088°-058°.
Île Dolvez Front Ldg Mark (086°) 48°31'·32N 04°46'·13W; W Bn.

Le Four 48°31'·45N 04°48'·23W Fl (5) 15s 28m **18M**; Gy ● Tr; *Horn (3+2) 60s.*

Le Taureau Bn 48°31'·51N 04°47'·26W; WCM.

CHENAL DU FOUR

L'ABER-ILDUT

L'Aber-Ildut 48°28'·32N 04°45'·47W Dir Oc (2) WR 6s 12m **W25M, R20M**; W bldgs; vis W081°-085°, R085°-087°.

Ldg Lts 158·5°. Front **Kermorvan** 48°21'·80N 04°47'·31W Fl 5s 20m **22M**. Rear, **Pte de St Mathieu** Fl 15s 56m **29M**. Dir F 54m **28M**; same Tr; intens 157·5°-159·5° (see above).
Les Plâtresses 48°26'·35N 04°50'·85W Fl RG 4s 17m 6M; W Tr; vis R343°-153°, G153°-333°.
La Valbelle Lt By 48°26'·55N 04°49'·90W Fl (2) R 6s 8m 5M; PHM; *Whis.*
SE Plâtresses By 48°26'·03N 04°50'·43W; SHM.
Le Tendoc By 48°25'·73N 04°49'·36W; PHM.
Saint Paul Lt By 48°24'·93N 04°49'·08W Oc (2) R 9s; PHM.
Taboga By 48°23'·88N 04°47'·99W; IDM.

Pte de Corsen 48°24'·95N 04°47'·52W Dir Q WRG 33m W12M, R8M, G8M; W hut; vis R008°-012°, W012°-015°, G015°-021°.
Kermorvan 48°21'·80N 04°47'·31W Fl 5s 20m **22M**; W☐ Tr; obsc by Pte de St Mathieu when brg less than 341°.
Rouget Lt By 48°22'·10N 04°48'·79W Iso G 4s; SHM; *Whis.*
La Grande Vinotière Lt Tr 48°22'·00N 04°48'·32W `L Fl R 10s 15m 5M; R 8-sided Tr.

LE CONQUET

Môle Sainte Barbe 48°21'·64N 04°46'·94W Oc G 4s 5m 6M.

Bas. des Renards By 48°21'·05N 04°47'·50W; IDM.
Lochrist 48°20'·63N 04°45'·73W Dir Oc (3) 12s 49m **22M**; W 8-sided Tr, R top; intens 135°-140°.
Tournant et Lochrist Lt By 48°20'·70N 04°48'·03W Iso R 4s; PHM.
Ar C'hristian Braz Bn 48°20'·75N 04°50'·10W; ECM.

Ldg Lts 007°. Front, **Kermorvan** 48°21'·80N 04°47'·31W Fl 5s 20m **22M**. Rear, **Trézien** 48°25'·48N 04°46'·65W Dir Oc (2) 6s 84m **20M**; Gy Tr, W on S side; intens 003°-011°.
Pte de St Mathieu 48°19'·85N 04°46'·17W Fl 15s 56m **29M**; W Tr, R top. Dir F 54m **28M**; same Tr; intens 157·5°-159·5°; RC. 54m 291° from St Mathieu Q WRG 26m, W14M, R11M, G11M; W Tr; vis G085°-107°, W107°-116°, R116°-134°.
La Fourmi By 48°19'·31N 04°47'·88W; SHM.
Les Vieux-Moines 48°19'·40N 04°46'·55W Fl R 4s 16m 5M; R 8-sided Tr; vis 280°-133°; PHM.

CHENAL DE LA HELLE

Ldg Lt 137·9°. Front, **Kermorvan** 48°21'·80N 04°47'·31W Fl 5s 20m **22M**. Rear, **Lochrist** 48°20·63N 04°45'·73W Dir Oc (3) 12s 49m **22M** (see above).
Luronne By 48°26'·67N 04°53'·70W; WCM; *Bell.*
Ldg Lts 293·5°. Front, Le Faix Lt Tr 48°25'·78N 04°53'·82W VQ; 16m 8M; NCM. Rear, **Le Stiff** 48°28'·60N 05°03'·10W Fl (2) R 20s 85m **24M** (see below).
Ldg Lt 142·5° for Chenal de La Helle. Front **Kermorvan** 48°21'·80N 04°47'·31W Fl 5s 20m **22M** (see above). Rear, two W Bns 48°20'·17N 04°45'·44W.
Pourceaux Lt By 48°24'·07N 04°51'·22W Q; NCM.
S. Pierre By 48°23'·15N 04°49'·00W; SHM.

OUESSANT AND ÎLE DE MOLÈNE

Men-Korn Lt Bn Tr 48°27'·95N 05°01'·22W VQ (3) WR 5s 21m W8M, R8M; vis W145°-040°, R040°-145°; ECM.
Le Stiff 48°28'·60N 05°03'·10W Fl (2) R 20s 85m **24M**; two adjoining W Trs.
GorleVihan Bn 48°28'·40N 05°02'·50W; IDM.
Port du Stiff. Môle Est Hd 48°28'·18N 05°03'·16W Dir Q WRG 11m W10M, R7M, G7M; W Tr, G top; vis G251°-254°, W254°-264°, R264°-267°.

OUESSANT SW LANBY 48°31'·68N 05°49'·10W Fl 4s 12m **20M**; RC; Racon (M).
NE Lt By 48°45'·90N 05°11'·60W L Fl 10s 9m 8M; *Whis*; Racon.
Créac'h 48°27'·62N 05°07'·72W Fl (2) 10s 70m **34M**; W Tr, B bands; obsc 247°-255°; Racon (C), RC; RG; *Horn (2) 120s.*
Nividic Lt Tr 48°26'·80N 05°08'·95W VQ (9) 10s 28m 9M; W 8-sided Tr, R bands; obsc by Ouessant 225°-290°. Helicopter platform.
La Jument 48°25'·40N 05°07'·95W Fl (3) R 15s 36m **22M**; Gy 8-sided Tr, R Top; vis 241°-199°; *Horn (3) 60s.*
Men ar Froud Bn 48°26'·70N 05°03'·57W; SCM.

Kéréon (Men-Tensel) 48°26'·30N 05°01'·45W Oc (2+1) WR 24s 38m **W17M**, R7M; Gy Tr; vis W019°-248°, R248°-019°; *Horn (2+1) 120s.*
Pierres-Vertes Lt By 48°22'·26N 05°04'·68W VQ (9) 10s 9m 5M; WCM; *Whis*; Ra refl.

ÎLE DE MOLÈNE

Les Trois-Pierres 48°24'·75N 04°56'·75W Iso WRG 4s 15m W9M, R6M, G6M; W col; vis G070°-147°, W147°-185°, R185°-191°, G191°-197°, W197°-213°, R213°-070°.
Molène Old Môle Hd Dir Lt 191°, 48°23'·91N 04°57'·18W Dir Fl (3) WRG 12s 6m W9M, R7M, G7M; vis G183°-190°, W190°-192°, R192°-203°. Chenal des Laz Dir Lt 261°, Dir Fl (2) WRG 6s 9m W9M, R7M, G7M; same structure; vis G252·5°-259·5°, W259·5°-262·5°, R262·5°-269·5°.

L'IROISE/BREST AND APPROACHES

Pierres Noires By 48°18'·54N 04°58'·18W; SCM; *Bell.*
Les Pierres Noires 48°18'·73N 04°54'·80W Fl R 5s 27m **19M**; W Tr, R top; *Horn (2) 60s.*
Basse Royale Lt By 48°17'·52N 04°49'·52W Q (6) + L Fl 15s; SCM.

Vandrée Lt By 48°15'·30N 04°48'·17W VQ (9) 10s; *Whis*; WCM.

La Parquette 48°15'·96N 04°44'·25W Fl RG 4s 17m R6M, G5M; W 8-sided Tr, B diagonal stripes; vis R244°-285°, G285°-244°.

GOULET DE BREST
Roc du Charles Martel Lt By 48°18'·90N 04°42'·10W Fl (4) R; PHM; *Whis*.

Swansea Vale Lt By 48°18'·27N 04°38'·75W Fl (2) 6s; *Whis*; IDM.

CAMARET
Môle Nord Hd 48°16'·92N 04°35'·20W Iso WG 4s 7m W12M, G8M; W pylon, G top; vis W135°-182°, G182°-027°.

Môle Sud Hd 48°16'·69N 04°35'·25W Fl (2) R 6s 9m 5M; R pylon.

Pointe du Toulinguet 48°16'·88N 04°37'·64W Oc (3) WR 12s 49m **W15M**, R11M; W ■ Tr on bldg; vis W shore-028°, R028°-090°, W090°-shore.

Pte du Petit-Minou 48°20'·26N 04°36'·80W Fl (2) WR 6s 32m **W19M, R15M**; Gy Tr, R top; vis Rshore-252°, W252°-260°, R260°-307°, W(unintens) 307°-015°, W015°-065·5°, W070·5°-shore. Same structure, Ldg Lts 068°. **Front** Dir Q 30m **23M**, intens 067·3°-068·8°. **Rear, Pte du Portzic,** Dir Q 54m **22M**, intens 065°-071°

Fillettes Lt By 48°19'·81N 04°35'·58W VQ (9); WCM; *Whis*.

Kerviniou Lt By 48°19'·81N 04°35'·20W Fl (2) R 6s; PHM.

Roche Mengam 48°20'·40N 04°34'·48W Fl (3) WR 12s 11m W11M, R8M, R Tr, B bands, vis R034°-054°, W054°-034°.

Pte du Portzic 48°21'·55N 04°31'·96W Oc (2) WR 12s 56m **W19M, R15M**; Gy Tr; vis R219°-259°, W259°-338°, R338°-000°, W000°-065·5°, W070·5°-219°. Same structure Dir Q (6) + L Fl 15s 54m **24M**, intens 045°-050°.

BREST
Pénoupèle Lt By 48°28'·51N 04°30'·43W Fl (3) R 12s; PHM.

Port Militaire, Jetée Sud Hd 48°22'·17N 04°29'·37W QR 10m 5M; W Tr, R top; vis 094°-048°.

Jetée Est Hd 48°22'·22N 04°29'·12W QG 10m 5M; W Tr, G top; vis 299°-163°.

Ldg Lts 344°. Front 48°22'·85N 04°29'·53W Q WRG; W10M, R5M, G5M; vis G 334°-342°, W342°-346°, R346°-024°. Rear, 334° 118m from front, Dir Q 10M.

La Penfeld Ldg Lts 314° Front 48°22'·93N 04°29'·85W Dir Iso R 5s 9m 10M. Rear, 17m from front, Dir Iso R 5s 16m 12M; both intens 309°-319°.

Port de Commerce Jetée du Sud W Hd 48°22'·66N 04°29'·02W Fl G 4s 10m 6M; vis 022°-257°.

Port de Commerce Jeteé du Sud E Hd 48°22'·76N 04°28'·39W Oc (2) R 6s 8m 5M; W pylon, R top; vis 018°-301°.

R2 Lt By 48°22'·07N 04°28'·66W Fl (2) R 6s; PHM.

R1 Lt By 48°21'·80N 04°28'·22W Fl G 4s; SHM.

R4 Lt By 48°22'·28N 04°27'·91W Fl R 10s; PHM.

Lt Bn 48°22'·70N 04°26'·50W Oc (3) R 12s; R □ on pile.

Moulin Blanc Lt By 48°22'·85N 04°25'·90W Fl (3) R 12s; PHM.

LE MOULIN BLANC
MB 1 Lt By 48°23'·29N 04°25'·66W Fl G 2s; SHM.

L'IROISE/BAIE DE DOUARNENEZ
Basse Du Lis Lt By 48°13'·05N 04°44'·46W Q (6) + L Fl 15s 9m 8M; SCM HFP; *Whis*.

Le Chevreau By 48°13'·35N 04°36'·85W; WCM.

Le Bouc Lt By 48°11'·58N 04°37'·29W Q (9) 15s; WCM; *Whis*.

Basse Vieille Lt By 48°08'·30N 04°35'·68W Fl (2) 6s 8m 8M; IDM HFP; *Whis*; Ra refl.

MORGAT
Pointe de Morgat 48°13'·24N 04°29'·72W Oc (4) WRG 12s 77m **W15M**, R11M, G10M; W ■ Tr, R top, W dwelling; vis W shore-281°, G281°-301°, W301°-021°, R021°-043°; obsc by Pte du Rostudel when brg more than 027°.

Mole Hd 48°13'·57N 04°29'·92W Oc (2) WR 6s 8m W9M, R6M; W&R framework Tr; vis Wshore-257°, R257°-shore.

Marina ent through wavebreak pontoons marked by Fl G 4s to stbd and Fl R 4s to port.

DOUARNENEZ
Épi de Biron Hd 48°06'·15N 04°20'·38W QG 7m 6M; W col, G top.

Île Tristan 48°06'·20N 04°20'·17W Oc (3) WR 12s 35m W13M, R10M; Gy Tr, W band, B top; vis W shore-138°, R138°-153°, W153°-shore; obsc by Pte de Leidé when brg less than 111°.

Bassin Nord, N Mole E Hd 48°06'·02N 04°19'·20W Iso G 4s 9m 4M; W & G pylon.

S Mole N Hd Oc (2) R 6s 6m 6M; W&R pylon.

Elbow, Môle de Rosmeur Hd 48°05'·86N 04°19'·15W Oc G 4s 6m 6M; W pylon, G top; vis 170°-097°.

Pointe du Millier 48°05'·99N 04°27'·85W Oc (2) WRG 6s 34m **W16M**, R12M, G11M; W house; vis G080°-087°, W087°-113°, R113°-120°, W120°-129°, G129°-148°, W148°-251°, R251°-258°; part obsc 255·5°-081·5°.

Basse Jaune By 48°05'·25N 04°42'·35W; IDM.

Tévennec 48°04'·34N 04°47'·65W VQ WR 28m W10M, R7M; W Tr; viz W090°-345°, R345°-090°. Dir Iso 4s 24m 12M; same Tr intens 324°-332°.

16

10.16.5 PASSAGE INFORMATION

NORTH BRITTANY (charts 2643 *2644 2668*)

Refer to *North Brittany Pilot* (Imray/RCC); Admiralty *Channel Pilot* (NP 27); *North Brittany and CI Cruising* (YM/Cumberlidge); *Brittany and CI Cruising Guide* (Adlard Coles/Jefferson), and *Shell Channel Pilot* (Imray/Cunliffe). For French Glossary see 1.4.2, and 10.17.5 for Breton words with navigational value.

Good landfall marks must be carefully identified before closing this rock-strewn coast. Closer inshore the tidal streams and currents vary, and overfalls are best avoided. In rough weather, low visibility (fog and summer haze are frequent) or if uncertain of position, it may be prudent to lie off and wait for conditions to improve; there are few safe havens. A high degree of planning is needed to achieve safe pilotage. In the W of the area the size of Atlantic swells can much reduce the range at which objects, especially floating marks, are seen.

PAIMPOL TO PLOUMANAC'H (AC 3670)

In the offing, between 11M and 18M NNE of Île de Bréhat, are Plateau de Barnouic (lit) and Plateau des Roches Douvres (lt, fog sig, RC), both with drying and submerged rks, to be given a wide berth particularly in poor vis.

Approaching from the SE, keep to seaward of the three ECM buoys off L'Ost-Pic or enter B de Paimpol (10.16.9) from a point about 1M E of the most N'ly ECM (Les Charpentiers). The Ferlas chan (AC 3673) runs S of Île de Bréhat (10.16.12), and is useful if entering/leaving R. Trieux from/to the E. It is well marked and not difficult, but best taken at half tide due to unmarked rks in chan almost awash at or near LW.

For the many yachts approaching from Guernsey, Les Héaux-de-Bréhat lt ho is a conspic landfall day/night for either Tréguier or Lézardrieux. Closer in or from the E, La Horaine (lt bn) is the best landfall for the latter. It marks the Plateaux de la horaine and des Échaudés and other rks to the SE. In poor visibility it should be closed with caution and left at least 7ca to the SE, as the flood stream sets strongly onto it. The Grand Chenal is the main, lit chan into R. de trieux for Lézardrieux (10.16.10) and up-river to Pontrieux (10.16.11). From NW the unlit Chenal de La Moisie leads SSE to join the Grand Chenal at Ile de Bréhat (10.16.12).

Between Lézardrieux and Tréguier (10.16.13) the Passage de la Gaine is a useful inshore route, avoiding a detour round Les Heaux. It is unlit and needs good vis, but if taken at above half tide, presents no problem in fair weather. The Grande Passe into R. de Tréguier is well lit, but ldg marks are less easy to see by day. The NE Passage should be used with caution.

Between Basse Crublent lt buoy and Port Blanc unmarked rks extend 2M offshore. Port Blanc (AC 3672) can be difficult to identify by day. Perros-Guirec (10.16.14) is approached either side of Ile Tomé from NE or NW via well lit/marked chans (AC 3672). Ploumanac'h (10.16.15) can only be entered by day.

LES SEPT ÎLES TO BAIE DE MORLAIX (AC 3669)

Les Sept Îles (10.16.16 and AC 3670) consist of five main islands and several islets, through which the tide runs strongly. Île aux Moines is lit, and all the islands are bird sanctuaries. Further W, Plateau des Triagoz has offlying dangers WSW and NE of the lt, where the sea breaks heavily. Here the stream turns ENE at HW Brest – 0325, and WSW at HW Brest +0245, sp rates both 3·8kn.

Trégastel Ste Anne (10.16.16) is a small anchorage W of Ploumanac'h. To the SW the coast as far as Trébeurden (10.16.16) is not easily approached due to many offlying rks. The radome NE of Trébeurden is conspic. Further S in the B de Lannion is Locquémeau and anchs near the mouth of the drying R. Léguier up to Lannion (10.16.17). Primel (10.16.18), at the E ent to Baie de Morlaix, provides a good deep anch. To the N is the drying Plateau de la Méloine.

The B de Morlaix (10.16.18 and AC 2745) is bestrewn with drying rks and shoals, all marked. Careful pilotage and adequate visibility are needed to negotiate any of the chans which are narrow in parts. The Grand Chenal passes close E of Île Ricard with Île Louet and La Lande (both lit) in transit 176°; abeam Calhic bn tr alter to port to transit between Château du Taureau (conspic) and Île Louet. Continue SSE for the river up to Morlaix. The anchorage NE of Carantec is reached from Chenal Ouest de Ricard.

ÎLE DE BATZ TO LE FOUR (charts 3668, 3669)

N of Île de Batz the E-going stream begins at HW Brest – 0435, and the W-going stream at HW Brest +0105, sp rates 3·8kn. Approaching Roscoff (10.16.19) from NE, leave Basse Astan ECM lt buoy to stbd steering with Men Guen Bras NCM lt bn in transit 213° with Chapelle St Barbe to round Ar Chaden for Roscoff hbr (dries); or transit W via Canal de L'Île de Batz.

In daylight and above half tide Canal de L'Île de Batz is a useful short cut between the island and the mainland. From near Ar Chaden steer 275° for the Vi bn at end of the conspic Roscoff ferry pier. Pass 30m N of this bn, and at this point alter to 300° for Run Oan SCM. Thence steer 283°, leaving Perroch NCM bn 100m to port. When clear of this rky, drying shoal alter to 270°, leaving Por Kernock hbr bkwtrs well to stbd and aiming midway between L'Oignon NCM and La Croix SCM. When these are abeam steer 281° for Basse Plate NCM bn; thence West into open waters.

Proceeding W from Île de Batz toward Le Four there are many off-lying dangers, in places 3M offshore. Swell may break on shoals even further to seaward. The tide runs strongly, and in poor vis or bad weather it is a coast to avoid. But in good conditions this is an admirable cruising ground with delightful hbrs such as Moguériec and Pontusval (10.16.18), L'Aberwrac'h (10.16.20), L'Aberbenoit (10.16.21), Portsall and Argenton (10.16.25). N of L'Aberwrac'h is Île Vierge lt ho, reputedly the tallest in the world, and a conspic landmark. Off Le Libenter, at N side of L'Aberwrac'h ent, the E-going stream starts at HW Brest – 0500, sp rate 3·8kn, and the W-going stream at HW Brest + 0110.

W of L'Aberwrac'h is an inshore chan leading past Portsall to Le Four (lt bn). This is a sheltered short-cut, but must only be used by day and in good visibility. AC 1432 or SHOM 5772 and full directions, as in *North Brittany Pilot*, are needed.

OUESSANT (USHANT) (chart 2694)

Île Ouessant lies 10M off NW Brittany. It is a rky island, with dangers extending 5ca to NE, 7½ca to SE, 1·5M to SW and 1M to NW; here Chaussée de Keller is a dangerous chain of drying and submerged rks running 1M W of Île de Keller and into the ITZ. Apart from Lampaul (10.16.22) the only other anch is B du Stiff which gives some shelter in moderate winds between S and NW. Tidal streams are strong close to the island, and in chans between it and mainland. Off Pte de Créac'h (lt, fog sig, RC) the stream turns NNE at HW Brest – 0550, and SSW at HW Brest + 0045, sp rate 5·5kn.

The route outside Ouessant TSS has little to commend it. Unless bound to/from Spain/Portugal it adds much to the distance and is exposed to sea and swell. Yachts should round Ouessant via the ITZ. Besides being an important landfall Ouessant is something of a barrier between N and W coasts of France, but in fair weather and reasonable visibility the pilotage in the chans between it and the mainland is not very demanding. They are well buoyed and marked (see 10.16.26), but the tide runs hard in places, causing overfalls when against wind >F5. In thick weather this is an unhealthy area, and it is prudent to stay in harbour until the vis improves.

The three main chans between the island and mainland are: The Chenal du Four, inshore and most direct and popular; Chenal de la Helle, an alternative to N part of Chenal du Four (partly used for access to Île Moléne), is not so direct but better in bad weather. Passage du Fromveur, close SE of Ouessant, is easiest but longer and can become extremely rough; tidal streams may exceed 8kn.

CHENAL DU FOUR (10.16.24 and AC 3345, 2694)

It is imperative to work the tides to best advantage through this passage: 1M W of Le Four the S-going stream begins at HW Brest + 0130; the N-going stream at HW Brest – 0545, sp rates 3·6kn. Further S, off Pte de Corsen, the stream is weaker, max 2·3kn at sp. The tide runs strongest at S end of Chenal du Four, off Le Conquet. Here the S-going stream starts at HW Brest + 0015, max 5kn; the N-going stream begins at HW Brest – 0550, 5·2kn max at sp. Wind-over-tide effects may be considerable.

Yachts are less rigidly tied to transits/dir lts than large ships and the following pilotage sequence can be used day or night, buoy-hopping as necessary if transits are obscured:
From 1·2M W of Le Four, track 180° (04°50'W: clear of Les Liniou reef to port) for 5M to Valbelle PHM lt buoy. Here pick up the transit 158·5°of Pte de Kermorvan on with Pte St Mathieu. Maintain this transit until Pte de Corsen lt bears 012° astern; then alter 192° to pass between La Grande Vinotière lt bn and Roche du Rouget lt buoy. Stand on until Le Faix lt bn is on with Grand Courleau bn 325° astern; alter 145° to maintain this track for 2·3M when open water will be reached with Vieux-Moines lt bn 4ca abeam to port.

Double check all lt/marks; do not confuse St Mathieu with Lochrist. L'Aberildut (10.16.23), 3·5M SSE of Le Four, and Le Conquet (10.16.26), 3ca SE of Pte de Kermorvan are the only ports off the Chenal du Four; but in offshore winds anch can be found in Anse de Porsmoguer and Anse des Blancs-Sablons, both between Corsen and Kermorvan.

Homeward-bound, or along the N coast of France, enter the S end of Chenal du Four at LW Brest; a fair tide can then be carried through the chan and NE past Île Vierge. The reverse sequence of pilotage is followed.

CHENAL DE LA HELLE (10.16.24 and AC 3345, 2694)

At N end of Chenal de la Helle the ENE stream starts at HW Brest – 0520 (sp rate 2·8kn), and the SW stream at HW Brest – 0045 (sp rate 3·8kn). The Ch de la Helle converges at a 20° angle with the Ch du Four. From the N, steer SW from Le Four towards Ile de Molène lt to pick up the 138° transit of Pte de Kermorvan and Lochrist close to Luronne unlit WCM buoy. Maintain this transit until Le Faix lt bn and Le Stiff lt ho are in transit 293° astern; steer 113° for 8ca until Pte de Kermorvan is on with 2 W bns (Pignons de Kéravel) at 142°. This transit avoids Basse St Pierre (4·7m) and intercepts the Ch du Four 7ca N of Grande Vinotière.

APPROACHES TO BREST (charts 798, 3427, 3428)

The outer approaches lie between Chaussée des Pierres Noires and Pte St Mathieu to the N and Pte du Toulinguet to the S. From the W steer on the 068° transit of Petit Minhou and Portzic on the N shore. From the S steer NNE toward Petit Minhou to pick up the transit, but beware rks 7M W and SW of Pte du Toulinguet. Yachts <25m LOA are exempt from VTM, but should monitor VHF Ch 08 or 16.

Abeam Petit Minhou lt ho the Goulet (Narrows) de Brest narrows to 1M; there are well-marked drying rks almost in mid-stream. A course of 075° through the Passe Nord leaves Roc Mengam lt bn 2ca to stbd. Tidal streams attain 4·5kn in the Goulet. In Passe Sud there is a useful back-eddy close inshore which runs ENE during the ebb. Once beyond Pte du Portzic a buoyed chan leads ENE past the Naval and commercial hbrs to the Moulin Blanc marina (10.16.27). The Rade de Brest (10.16.28) opens to the S and E.

L'IROISE/BAIE DE DOUARNENEZ (charts 3427, 798)

L'Iroise is the area between Chaussée des Pierres Noires and Chaussée de Sein; the B de Douarnenez lies further E. On the NE side of L'Iroise (chart 3427) a chain of rks extends 7M W from Pte du Toulinguet. There are several chans through these rks, of which the simplest for Brest (10.16.27) and Camaret (10.15.29) is the 3ca wide Chenal du Toulinguet which runs NNW between La Louve bn tr (1ca W of Pte du Toulinguet) on E side and Le Pohen rk on the W side.

Here the N-going stream begins at HW Brest – 0550, and the S-going at HW Brest + 0015, sp rates 2·75kn. 2·5M NW of C. de la Chèvre is Le Chévreau (dries), with La Chèvre 5ca to NE of it (1·25M WSW of Pte de Dinan). 7M W of Pte de Dinan lies Basse du Lis, rky shoals with depth of 2·4m.

The B de Douarnenez is entered between C. de la Chèvre and Raz de Sein. Off C. de la Chèvre various dangers, on which the sea breaks, extend SW for 2·25M to Basse Vieille (dries), lt buoy. Morgat (10.16.30) lies 4M NNE of C. de la Chèvre. Beware group of drying rks, including La Pierre-Profonde and Le Taureau close SSW of Les Verrès (rk 9m high), which lies nearly 2·5M ESE of Morgat.

Approaching Douarnenez (10.16.31) beware Basse Veur and Basse Neuve. The S shore of the B is clear of dangers more than 2ca offshore, except for Duellou Rk (4m high) 5ca offshore, and other rks 1M eastward. Further W beware Basse Jaune, an isolated rk (dries) about 1M N of Pte du Van.

10.16.6   DISTANCE TABLE

Approximate distances in nautical miles are by the most direct route, whilst avoiding dangers and allowing for Traffic Separation Schemes. Places in *italics* are in adjoining areas; places in **bold** are in 10.0.5, Cross-Channel Distances.

1. *St Quay-Portrieux*	1																			
2. Paimpol	24	2																		
3. Bréhat (Port Clos)	15	8	3																	
4. **Lézardrieux**	21	14	6	4																
5. **Tréguier**	46	29	22	22	5															
6. Perros-Guirec	37	35	28	28	21	6														
7. Ploumanac'h	40	33	27	29	25	6	7													
8. Trébeurden	48	44	38	40	32	17	11	8												
9. **Lannion**	52	48	42	44	33	21	15	6	9											
10. Morlaix	67	64	58	60	46	36	30	23	24	10										
11. **Roscoff**	59	58	52	54	41	28	22	17	19	12	11									
12. **L'Aberwrac'h**	91	88	82	84	72	60	54	49	51	48	32	12								
13. L'Aberbenoit	92	89	83	85	76	61	55	50	52	45	33	7	13							
14. Lampaul	114	110	104	106	98	83	77	72	74	67	55	29	28	14						
15. **Le Conquet**	114	110	104	106	98	83	77	72	71	68	55	29	23	17	15					
16. Brest (marina)	125	119	114	114	107	92	86	83	87	79	67	42	41	31	18	16				
17. Camaret	124	120	114	116	108	93	87	82	81	78	65	39	33	27	13	10	17			
18. Morgat	134	130	124	126	118	103	97	92	91	88	75	49	43	37	20	24	16	18		
19. Douarnenez	139	135	129	131	123	108	102	97	96	93	80	54	48	42	25	29	21	11	19	
20. *Audierne*	144	139	133	135	128	113	108	102	101	98	86	55	53	40	30	34	28	27	30	20

10.16.7   English Channel Waypoints: See 10.1.7   **10.16.8**   Special Notes for France: See 10.15.8

PAIMPOL   10-16-9

Côte d'Armor 48°47'·06N 03°02'·47W

CHARTS
AC 3673, 3670, *2668*; SHOM 7127, 831, 832; ECM 537;
Imray C34; Stanfords 17

TIDES
Dover –0525; ML 6·1; Duration 0600; Zone –0100

Standard Port ST MALO (←)

Times				Height (metres)			
High Water		Low Water		MHWS	MHWN	MLWN	MLWS
0100	0800	0300	0800	12·2	9·2	4·3	1·6
1300	2000	1500	2000				
Differences PAIMPOL							
–0005	–0010	–0035	–0025	–1·4	–0·8	–0·5	–0·2

SHELTER
Good shelter from all winds in hbr, but few ⚓s as most of
the Anse de Paimpol dries, including the appr chan to hbr.
Lock opens HW ±2 when height of HW <10m; HW ±2½
when HW >10m. Visitors' berths at pontoon A, Basin No
2, min depth 3·8m. Larger yachts berth in Basin No 1.

NAVIGATION
WPT 48°47'·88N 02°54'·50W, 080°/260° from/to summit of
Pte Brividic 4·7M. Chenal de la Jument is the normal appr
from the E. After La Jument PHM bn tr, either ⚓ to await
the tide; or alter 262° for unlit bns/buoys marking final
1M of chan. The drying rks (El Paimpol, El Bras and Ar
Fav) are close N of the ldg line. An alternative appr from
Ile de Bréhat at HW+2 lies E of Les Piliers NCM bn tr,
thence S past Pte de la Trinité. Or appr from further E via
Chenal du Denou 193°. Bearing in mind the large tidal
range, there is enough water in the bay from half-flood
for most craft.

LIGHTS AND MARKS
4M E is L'Ost-Pic lt, Oc WR 4s 20m 11/8M, conspic □ W tr.
Pte de Porz-Don, Oc (2) WR 6s 13m 15/11M, vis W269°-
272°, R272°-279°, is 7ca ENE of hbr ent. W sector leads
270° to the inner ldg lts 262°. A conspic tr (52m) is 3ca W
of Porz -Don.
Outer ldg marks 260° for Chenal de la Jument: Paimpol ✠
spire on with the summit (27m) of Pte Brividic.
Inner ldg lts 262°: front, Jetée de Kernoa, FR 5m 7M; rear,
Dir FR 12m 14M, intens 260°-264°.

RADIO TELEPHONE
VHF Ch 09 (0800-1200LT and lock opening hrs).

TELEPHONE
Hr Mr 96.20.47.65; Port Mgr 96·20·80·77; ⌗ 96·20·81·87;
Aff Mar 96·20·84·30; CROSS 98·89·31·31; Auto 36·68.08.22;
Police 96·20·80·17; Ⓗ 96·20·86·02; Dr 96·20·80·04; Brit
Consul 99·46·26·64.

FACILITIES
Basin No 2 (marina 280+20 visitors), FF95, FW, AC, D
(quay), P (cans), ME, El; **Basin No 1** C (6 and 4 ton);
Quai de Kernoa P, ME; **Quai neuf** Slip, M, FW, AB;
Services: Sh, CH, SHOM, Ⓔ.
Town P, CH, V, R, Bar, Gaz, ⊘, ⊠, Ⓑ, ⇌, ✈ Dinard, Brest,
Rennes. Ferry: Roscoff, St Malo.

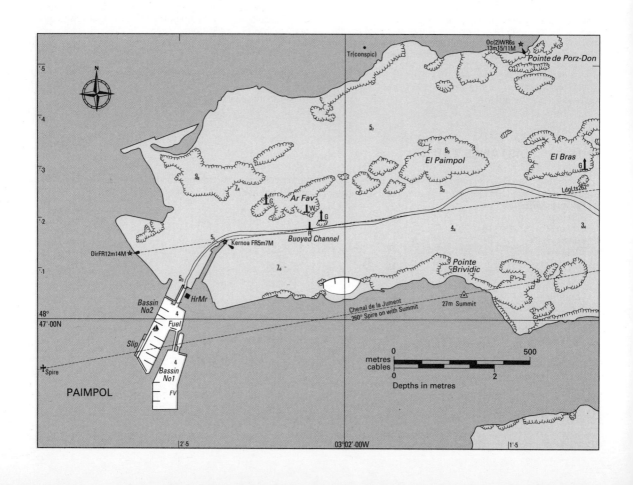

LÉZARDRIEUX   10-16-10
Côte d'Armor 48°47'·41N 03°05'·83W

CHARTS
AC 3673, 3670, *2668*; SHOM 7126, 7127, 831, 832, 967;
ECM 537; Imray C34; Stanfords 17

TIDES
−0510 Dover; ML 5·9; Duration 0610; Zone −0100

Standard Port ST MALO (←—)

Times				Height (metres)			
High Water		Low Water		MHWS	MHWN	MLWN	MLWS
0100	0800	0300	0800	12·2	9·2	4·3	1·6
1300	2000	1500	2000				
Differences LÉZARDRIEUX							
−0010	−0010	−0047	−0037	−1·7	−1·2	−0·6	−0·3
LES HEAUX DE BRÉHAT							
−0018	−0017	−0050	−0050	−2·4	−1·6	−0·7	−0·3
ILE DE BRÉHAT							
−0008	−0013	−0040	−0037	−1·8	−1·2	−0·5	−0·3

SHELTER
Very good in all weathers. The Trieux River and marina
pontoons are accessible H24. A marina extension (247
berths), very close SW of the pontoons, has some ♥
berths; access over sill 4·9m above CD (2·4m inside). As
sill covers on the flood, door automatically drops to give
1·35m clearance. A depth gauge shows water over sill.
IPTS in use. Multi-hulls and boats >12·5m LOA should
moor on ♂s in the stream, rather than berth on pontoons.
Yachts can go about 12km up river (bridge clearance
17m) to lock in at Pontrieux (10·16·11).

NAVIGATION
WPT 48°55'·00N 02°56'·20W, 045°/225° from/to front ldg lt
225° (La Croix), 6·7M. Roches Douvres and Barnouic are
dangers in the outer apps; closer in, are the Plateau de la
Horaine and rky shoals to the W. Off river ent beware
strong cross streams. The 3 well-marked ent chans are:
Ferlas Chan from the E, running S of Ile de Bréhat;
Grand Chenal, main chan from NE, best for strangers;
and Moisie, unlit from the NW, which also connects with
Passe de la Gaine from/to Tréguier (10.16.13).

LIGHTS AND MARKS
Offshore lts: Roches Douvres, Fl 5s 60m 28M, pink tr.
Barnouic ECM bn tr, VQ (3) 5s 15m 9M.
Les Héaux de Bréhat, Oc (3) WRG 12s 48m 17/12M, gy tr.
Pte du Paon and Rosédo, on Bréhat, see 10.16.4 and .12.
The ldg marks/lts for the ent chans are:
(1) Ferlas chan:
  W sector of Men Joliguet lt bn tr 271° (see 10.16.25).
  W sector of Roche Quinonec Dir Q WRG 257°.
  W sector of Kermouster Dir Fl WRG 2s leads 271° to
  join Coatmer ldg line.
(2) Grand Chenal ldg lts 225°: Front, La Croix Oc 4s 15m
  19M; two grey trs joined, W on NE side with R tops,
  intens 215°-235°; rear, Bodic (2·1M from front) Q 55m
  22M (intens 221°-229°).
(3) Moisie chan: Amer du Rosédo W obelisk on 159° with
  St Michael's chapel (both conspic on Ile de Bréhat).
Within the Trieux river:
(4) Coatmer ldg lts 219°: front F RG 16m 9/9M, vis R200°-
  250°, G250°-053°; rear, 660m from front, FR 50m 9M.
(5) W sector 200° of Les Perdrix G tr, Fl (2) WG 6s.
Beware, at night, the unlit Roc'h Donan 2½ca S of Perdrix.
The only lts beyond Perdrix are F Bu lts at the outboard
ends of the 3 'old' marina pontoons, and a Fl R 4s and Fl
G 4s buoy 50 - 100m E of the ent to new marina; also
unlit perches: PHM/SHM at ent; 1 ECM 50m NE of ent,
and 5 Y SPM marking the limits of the marina.

RADIO TELEPHONE
VHF Ch 09 (0800-2000 Jul/Aug. 0800-1200 and 1400-1800
rest of year).

TELEPHONE
Hr Mr 96·20·14·22; Aff Mar at Paimpol 96·20·84·30; CROSS
98·89·31·31; ⌗ at Paimpol 96·20·81·87; Auto 36·68.08.22;
Police 96·20·10·17; Dr 96·20·10·30; Brit Consul 99·46·26·64.

FACILITIES
Marina (477; visitors as directed by Hr Mr), ☎ 96·20·14·22,
FF86, Slip, P, D, FW, ME, El, CH, AC, Bar, Gaz, R, SM, Sh,
▣, C (6 ton);
YC de Trieux ☎ 96·20·10·39. **Services:** Divers, Ⓔ;
Town EC Sun; P, D, V, Gaz, R, Bar, ✉, Ⓑ, ⇌ (occas bus to
Paimpol), ✈ Lannion. Ferry: Roscoff.

---

*A Breton fishing-smack was working nets close to the
rocks. We sailed up to her and hailed:*
*Où sommes nous? The dripping men on board answered in
a chorus that came to us like the barking of sea lions. At
length we made out: Les Roches Douvres.*
*Now there was a flurry of charts and Sailing Directions.
Where was the nearest anchorage? (With us in such
circumstances the nearest is always the best). A place called
Lézardrieux situated some distance up the tidal Rivière de
Pontrieux, of whose dangers the Sailing Directions write in a
tone even more tartly warning than usual. Lézardrieux it
would have to be.*
*Fate is a strange bird. The night before I had ordered my
charts, Mr Adlard Coles had climbed down our ladder to have
a look at us. He happened to mention the anchorage at
Lézardrieux. So I had ordered a full-scale chart of the Pontrieux
River. On the chart the river looked small, but in the darkness
(and we were entering at approximately high water) it proved
to be vast.*
*A sea writhed and in places boiled on the bar, but we
buffeted through it. I had been so obsessed with navigation
and so keen to get somewhere as quickly as possible that it
had not occurred to me to reduce sail. Sailing at that speed
with breakers audible and sometimes visible on either hand
was too much for me, and I got down the mainsail. The engine
started at the first touch of the button.*
*We passed beacons, buoys, a cluster of wind-flattened
islands, and then entered the land between the hills. Leading
lights guided us up the main channel. A bend, more leading
lights, and the swell had changed to a ripple. The patent log
showed ninety-five miles for the day's run. We dropped
anchor in eight fathoms at the top of the last reach before the
village.*

A White boat from England (George Millar/Heinemann 1951)

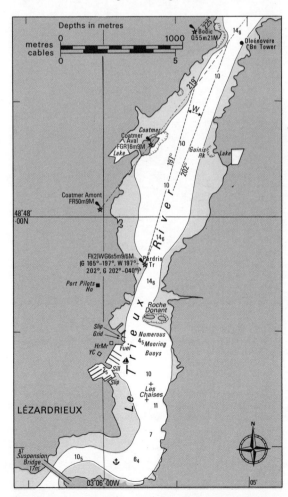

PONTRIEUX   10-16-11

Côte d'Armor 48°42'·80N 03°08'·90W

CHARTS

ECM 537; AC 3673 and SHOM 7126 downstream of
Lézardrieux

TIDES

HW at Pontrieux Lock is at HW ST MALO. See also 10·16·10.

SHELTER

Complete shelter in 2-4m depth alongside Quay (SE
bank), approx 1km above lock.

NAVIGATION

See 10·16·10 for approach up to Lézardrieux. Not before
HW –3, proceed via suspension bridge (17m clearance)
6M up-river, keeping to high, rky bank on bends. Lock
opens HW –2 (–1 at weekends) to HW+1. Waiting buoy (½
tide) close E and slip with FW and AC on the bend. Below
Château de la Roche Jagu there is also a waiting buoy
available HW±3.

LIGHTS AND MARKS

River is unlit (beware sand dredgers at night); few marks.

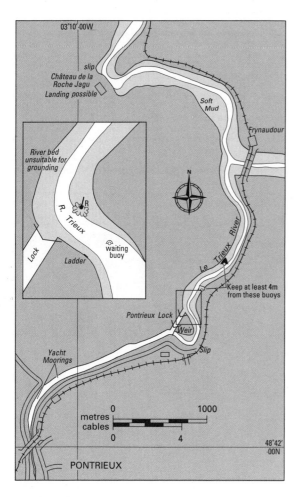

Lock VHF Ch 12, HW –2 to +1. ☎ link to Pontrieux Port.

TELEPHONE

Hr Mr 96·95·64·66; Lock 96·95·60·70; SNSM 92·20·00·45;
Auto 36·68.08.22. There is a ☎ at the Château Roche Jagu.

FACILITIES

Quay (100) AB FF58, FW, C (6 ton), AC, R, Bar.
Town Bar, FW, R, Slip, V, Gaz, P, D, Ⓑ, ✉, Ⓞ, ⇌ Paimpol/
Guingamp, ✈ Brest, Rennes & Dinard.

ILE DE BRÉHAT   10-16-12

Côte d'Armor 48°51'·00N 03°00'·00W

CHARTS

AC 3673, 3670, *2668*; SHOM 7127, 831, 832; ECM 537;
Imray C34; Stanfords 17

TIDES

–0525 Dover; ML 5·8; Duration 0605; Zone –0100
Differences see 10.16.10

SHELTER

Port Clos: drying main hbr; good shelter, but busy with
vedettes. No AB; ⚓ clear of fairway. (Due to cables across
the Ferlas Chan, ⚓ is prohib to the SW of Port Clos).
Port de la Corderie: hbr dries; get well out of strong tides.
Good shelter, except in W winds.
La Chambre in SE: ⚓ in upper reaches just S of the 'No ⚓'
area, close to the town of Le Bourg. Slipway can be
floodlit by pressing button on lamp post at top of slip.
Guerzido in the Chenal de Ferlas, is good holding
ground, partly out of the strong tides. There are ⚓s or ⚓ E
of Men Allan and close to the buoys of the boat barrier.

NAVIGATION

WPT Ferlas chan 48°49'·45N 02°55'·00W, 098°/278° from/to
La Croix lt, 5·5M. See also 10·16·10. On appr, beware La
Horaine, Men Marc'h and C'hign Bras closer in.

LIGHTS AND MARKS

For the three principal lts on Ile de Bréhat, see 10.16.4.

RADIO TELEPHONE

Sémaphore de Bréhat VHF Ch 16 10, Day only.

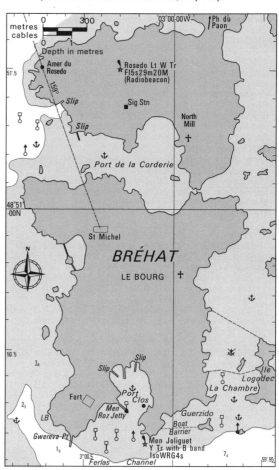

TELEPHONE

Hr Mr none; CROSS 98·89·31·31; SNSM 96·20·00·14;
Auto 36·68.08.22; ⌗ 96·20·81·87; Police 96·20·80·17;
Dr 96·20·00·99; Brit Consul 99·46·26·64.

FACILITIES

Hbrs M, FW, P from fuel barge at Port Clos, Slip, full
access at HW; **CN de Bréhat**, FW, Bar; **Services:** ME.
Village V, Gaz, Bar, ✉, Ⓑ (Paimpol), ⇌ (ferry to Pte de
l'Arcouest, bus to Paimpol), ✈ (Dinard, Brest, Rennes to
London). Ferry: Roscoff. No cars on Is.

TRÉGUIER   10-16-13

Côte d'Armor 48°47'·50N 03°12'·80W

CHARTS
AC 3672, 3670, *2668*; SHOM 7126, 967; ECM 537; Imray C34; Stanfords 17

TIDES
−0540 Dover; ML 5·7; Duration 0600; Zone −0100
Standard Port ST MALO (◀—)

Times				Height (metres)			
High Water		Low Water		MHWS	MHWN	MLWN	MLWS
0100	0800	0300	0800	12·2	9·2	4·3	1·6
1300	2000	1500	2000				
Differences TRÉGUIER							
−0005	−0010	−0055	−0040	−2·3	−1·5	−0·7	−0·3
PORT-BÉNI							
−0017	−0022	−0100	−0045	−2·4	−1·5	−0·6	−0·2

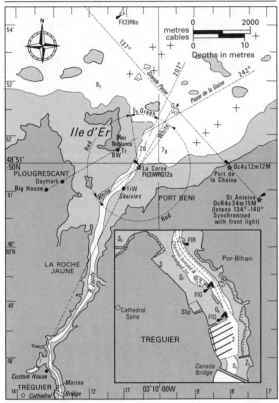

SHELTER
Good in marina; beware tide when berthing. Possible ⚓s, keeping clear of the chan: 7ca SW of La Corne lt tr, but exposed to N'lies; N and S of La Roche Jaune village; in pool 1ca NE of No 10 buoy (1M N of marina).

NAVIGATION
WPT 48°55'·25N 03°13'·00W, 317°/137° from/to front ldg lt, 5M (Grande Passe). There are three ent chans:
(1) Grande Passe: well marked/lit, but marks are hard to see by day. Caution: strong tidal streams across the chan.
(2) Passe de la Gaine: well marked, navigable with care by day in good vis. Unlit short cut to/from Lézardrieux.
(3) Passe du Nord-Est: unlit, dangerous with winds from W and NW as sea breaks across the chan.
Within the R. Jaudy it is important to heed chan buoys/bns. Speed limit is 6kn above La Roche Jaune.

LIGHTS AND MARKS
Important marks: La Corne WR lt tr, Fl (3) WRG 12s 11/8M; 6ca to the N is Men Noblance WB bn tr on SE corner of Ile d'Er; and 4ca SW is Skeiviec W bn tr. Spire of Tréguier cathedral is 4·6M SSW of La Corne.
Ldg lts/marks for the appr chans:
(1) For Grande Passe 137°: front, Port de la Chaine, Oc 4s 12m 12M, white ho; rear, St Antoine Dir Oc R 4s 34m 15M, RW ho. At Pen Guézec unlit SHM buoy steer 216° in the W sector of La Corne lt.

(2) For Passe de la Gaine 242°: Men Noblance bn tr, W with horiz B band, on with rear mark (W wall with B vert stripe) below the skyline and just right of conspic Plougrescant ✠. Hold this transit exactly to stay in narrow, marked chan; but marks hard to see from afar.
(3) Passe du Nord-Est, for direct appr to La Corne having cleared W of La Jument NCM By and adjacent rky shoals: Tréguier cathedral spire and Skeiviec at 207°.

RADIO TELEPHONE
Marina Ch 09 (In season: Mon-Sat 0800-1200, 1330-2100; Sun 0800-1000, 1600-1800. Out of season: Sun/Mon closed; Tue-Sat 0800-1200, 1330-1700).

TELEPHONE
Hr Mr 96·92·42·37; Aff Mar 96·92·30·38; CROSS 96·54·11·11; ⌗ 96·92·31·44; Auto 36·68.08.22; Police 96·92·32·17; Dr 96·92·32·14; Ⓗ 96·92·30·72; Brit Consul 99·46·26·64.

FACILITIES
Marina (200+130 visitors), ☎ 96·92·42·37, FF80, Slip, FW, ME, C (8 ton), D (on most N'ly pontoon HW±1), CH, El, Sh, AC, Bar, R, Gaz, Ⓒ;
Club Nautique du Tregor ☎ 96·92·42·37, excellent facilities, open all year.**Services:** M, CH;
Town EC Mon; Market Wed, P, FW, CH, V, Gaz, R, Bar, ✉, Ⓑ, V (small supermarket just E of cathedral delivers to boats), ⇌ (bus to Paimpol and Perros-Guirec), ✈ (St Brieuc, Lannion). Ferry: Roscoff.

ADJACENT HARBOUR

PORT BLANC, Côte d'Armor, 48°50'·60N 03°18'·80W, AC 3672, 3670; SHOM 974, 967. HW −0545 on Dover (UT); HW−0040 and ht −2·0m on St Malo; ML 5·3m; Duration 0600. Good natural hbr (known as Port Bago), but open to winds between NW and NNE. Appr on 150° toward Le Voleur Dir lt, Fl WRG 4s 17m 14/11M, G140°-148°, W148°-152°, R152°-160°. Note: the former rear ldg mark is reported ruined/obsc'd. The most conspic daymark is a 16m high W obelisk on Ile du Chateau Neuf, to stbd of appr chan; a less obvious W tr is to port on Ile St Gildas. There are 30 W ⚓s in the pool or yachts can ⚓ off or dry out alongside quays, 1·3m. Facilities: AB FF30, FW, AC, C (16 ton), Slip; **Services:** CH, El, ME, Sh. **Town** Bar, R, V.

16

PERROS-GUIREC   10-16-14

Côte d'Armor 48° 48'·23N 03° 26'·12W

CHARTS
AC 3672, 3670, *2668*; SHOM 974, 967; ECM 537, 538; Imray C34; Stanfords 17

TIDES
−0550 Dover; ML 5·4; Duration 0605; Zone −0100

Standard Port ST MALO (←—)

Times				Height (metres)			
High Water		Low Water		MHWS	MHWN	MLWN	MLWS
0100	0800	0300	0800	12·2	9·2	4·3	1·6
1300	2000	1500	2000				
Differences PERROS-GUIREC							
−0030	−0040	−0115	−0055	−2·9	−1·8	−0·9	−0·3

SHELTER
Very good in marina (2·5m). Enter via 6m wide gate, which is opened when rise of tide reaches 7m (there is no lock). Sill under gate is 3·5m above CD, giving 3·5m water inside gateway on first opening. Gate opens approx HW±1½ if Coeff >70; HW±1 for Coeff 60-70; HW−1 to +½ for Coeff 50-60; HW−½ to HW for Coeff 40-50. Caution: at Coeff <40 gate may never open for up to 4 days. Retaining wall is marked by R & W poles. ‡ prohib in basin. Drying moorings 1ca E of Jetée du Linkin. Good ‡ and about 20 W ⚓s in approx 3m off Pte du Chateau, except in NE'lies.

NAVIGATION
WPT 48°52'·40N 03°20'·00W, 045°/225° from/to front ldg lt (Le Colombier), 6·4M. Beware Ile Tomé in the ent to Anse de Perros. Rks extend 7ca (1300m) off the W side and 6ca (1110m) E of the N side.

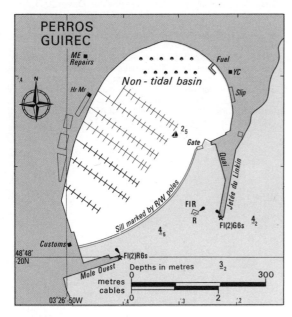

LIGHTS AND MARKS
From NE: Ldg lts 225°: front Le Colombier Dir Oc (4) 12s 28m 18M, intens 220°-230°; rear Kerprigent (1·5M from front) Q 79m 22M, intens 221°-228°.
Passe de l'Ouest: Kerjean Dir lt 144° Oc (2+1) WRG 12s 78m 15/13M, vis G134°-143°, W143°-144°, R144°-154°.
Gate sigs (flags/lts): Ⓖ over Ⓡ = closed;
Ⓖ = open, priority to enter; Ⓡ = open, priority to leave.

RADIO TELEPHONE
VHF Ch 09 16.

TELEPHONE
Hr Mr 96·23·37·82, Fax 96.23.37.19; Aff Mar 96·23·13·78; ☷ 96·23·18·12; CROSS 98·89·31·31; SNSM 96·20·00·45; Auto 36.68.08.22; Police 96·23·20·17; Dr 96·23·20·01; Brit Consul 99·46·26·64.

FACILITIES
Marina (600+50 visitors) ☎ 96·23·19·03, FF95, P, D, FW, ME, AC, El, Sh, C (7 ton), CH, V, R, SM, Gas, Gaz, Kos, ▣; **Services:** Ⓔ, SHOM; **Town** CH, V, Gaz, R, Bar, ✉, Ⓑ, ⇌ (Lannion), ✈ (Morlaix/Lannion). Ferry: Roscoff.

PLOUMANAC'H   10-16-15

Côte d'Armor 48° 50'·35N 03° 29'·14W

CHARTS
AC 3669, 3670, *2668*; SHOM 967; ECM 537, 538; Imray C34; Stanfords 17

TIDES
−0550 Dover; ML 5·5; Duration 0605; Zone −0100

Standard Port ST MALO (←—)

Times				Height (metres)			
High Water		Low Water		MHWS	MHWN	MLWN	MLWS
0100	0800	0300	0800	12·2	9·2	4·3	1·6
1300	2000	1500	2000				
Differences PLOUMANAC'H							
−0023	−0033	−0112	−0053	−2·9	−1·8	−0·7	−0·2

SHELTER
Good; ⚓s are first line of dumbell buoys. Ent is difficult in strong NW winds. A sill, 2·25m above CD retains at least 1·5m within. Depth gauges are on the 4th and the last PHM stakes. If the concrete base of the 3rd SHM stake is covered, depth over sill is >1·5m. Inside the sill, for best water keep to port and appr moorings from N. FV moorings to stbd of ent. SE and SW sides of hbr are very shallow.

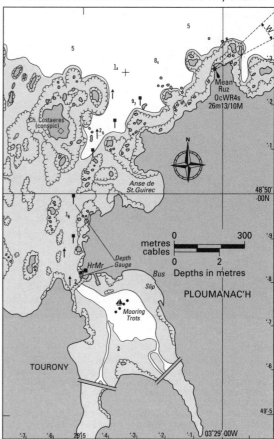

NAVIGATION
WPT 48°51'·50N 03°29'·00W, 008°/188°, 1·25M from/to ent between Mean Ruz lt ho and Chateau Costaeres (conspic). From NW, beware unmarked rk (dries about 1·4m), 100m NNE of No 1 SHM stake. Chan marked by unlit stakes.

LIGHTS AND MARKS
Mean Ruz lt ho, Oc WR 4s, to E with adjacent sig stn, conspic.

RADIO TELEPHONE
VHF Ch 09.

TELEPHONE
Hr Mr 96·91·44·31 or 96·23·37·82; SNSM 96·20·00·45; Auto 36·68.08.22; Dr 96·91·42·00; ME 96·23·31·40.

FACILITIES
Port de Plaisance (230 + 50 visitors) M FF100; **Quai Bellevue** FW, AC, L, Slip, P & D cans; Bus to Lannion and Perros; **YC Société Nautique de Perros Guirec.** Ferry: See Roscoff.

TRÉBEURDEN 10-16-16

Côte d'Armor 48°46′·35N 03°35′·06W

CHARTS
AC 3669; SHOM 7124, 7151; ECM 537, 538; Imray C34; Stanfords 17

TIDES
–0605 Dover; ML 5·5; Duration 0605; Zone –0100

Standard Port BREST (→)

Times				Height (metres)			
High Water		Low Water		MHWS	MHWN	MLWN	MLWS
0000	0600	0000	0600	6·9	5·4	2·6	1·0
1200	1800	1200	1800				
Differences TRÉBEURDEN							
+0100	+0110	+0120	+0100	+2·3	+1·9	+0·9	+0·4

SHELTER
Very good in marina (3·5m). Access HW±4¼ over moving sill (2m) at stbd side of ent; rest of sill is fixed 3·5m. Tide gauge floodlit at ent. Visitors berth on pontoon F (second from ent); due to strong underwater inrush, boats are advised not to manoeuvre within 10 minutes of the sill dropping. Deep-water waiting buoys outside. ‡ off NW tip of Ile Miliau, but exposed to W'lies.

NAVIGATION
WPT 48°45′·13N 03°40′·68W, 246°/066° from/to Lan Kerellec Dir lt, 4·1M. From W, appr is clear. From E and N, round Bar all Gall and Le Crapaud WCM buoys; continue S for 1·5M, then alter 066° toward Ile Miliau (conspic); thence as below to enter the marked chan to marina ent.

LIGHTS AND MARKS
Le Crapaud WCM buoy, Q (9) 15s. Lan Kerellec Dir lt, Iso WRG 4s 8/5M, G058°-064°, W064°-069°, R069°-130°, leads 066° past Ile Miliau. By day, appr on 075° with conspic villa open just left of Fornigo Rk. From Ar Gouredec SCM buoy, VQ (6) + L Fl 10s, church spire (conspic) brg 098° leads to ent. Chan buoyed as chartlet. IPTS, Sigs 2 & 4, on bkwtr. R/G tfc sigs at ent.

RADIO TELEPHONE
Call *Port Trébeurden* VHF Ch 09 16.

TELEPHONE
Hr Mr ☎ 96·23·64·00; Aff Mar 96.37.06.52; CROSS 98.89.31.31; SNSM 96·23·53·82; ☷ 96·92·31·44; Police 96.23.51.96 (Jul/Aug); Ⓗ (Lannion) 96.05.71.11.

FACILITIES
Marina (400 + 160 visitors), ☎ as Hr Mr, Fax 96.47.40.87, FF105, FW, AC, P, D, BY, C (20 ton);
YC de Trébeurden ☎ 96·37·00·40 (open July-Aug);
Services: BY, ME, EI, Sh, CH.
Town V, R, Bar, ✉, Ⓑ, ✈ (Lannion). Ferry: Roscoff/St.Malo.

ADJACENT HARBOUR AND ANCHORAGES

TRÉGASTEL, Côte d'Armor, 48°50′·10N 03°31′·20W, AC 3669, 3670; SHOM 967. HW –0550 on Dover (UT); +0005 and –1·8m on Brest HW; ML 5·1m; Duration 0605. Use 10·16·15 differences. Good ‡ in 2m but very exposed to winds from W to N. Ent, 2ca W of La Pierre Pendue (conspic), is marked by PHM bn on Ile Dhu and SHM buoy off Le Taureau, rk drying 4·5m (bn destroyed). Turreted house, conspic, brg approx 165° leads between Ile Dhu and Le Taureau. Thence keep between 2 more PHM and 1 SHM bns, turn E to the ‡ or W mooring buoys S of Ile Ronde. Facilities: Slip; **Club Nautique de Tregastel** ☎ 96·23·45·05; **Town** CH, Bar, Ⓑ, ✉, R, V.

LES SEPT ILES, Côte d'Armor, 48° 52′·80N 03°29′·10W, AC 3669, 3670; SHOM 967. HW-0550 on Dover (UT); +0005 on Brest. HW ht –1·8m on Brest. ML 5·2m. Use 10.16.15 differences. All 7 islands form a bird sanctuary. Main ‡ between Île aux Moines and Ile Bono. Landing on latter is prohib. ‡ due E of jetty; below the Old Fort, or close to S side of Ile Bono. Île aux Moines lt ho, grey tr, Fl (3) 15s 59m 24M, obsc 237°-241° and in Baie de Lannion when brg < 039°. No facilities.

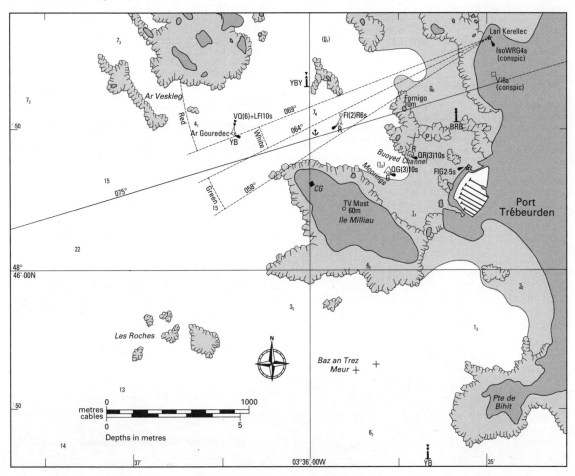

16

AGENTS WANTED

If you are interested in becoming our agent for any of the following ports, please write to: The Editor, Edington House, Trent, Sherborne, Dorset DT9 4SR, England – and get your free copy of the almanac annually. You do not have to live in a port to be the agent, but at least a fairly regular visitor.

River Exe	Grandcamp-Maisy
Port Ellen (Islay)	Port-en-Bessin
Glandore/Union Hall	Courseulles
River Rance/Dinan	Boulogne
Lampaul	Dunkerque
Port Tudy	Terneuzen/Westerschelde
River Etel	Oudeschild
Le Palais (Belle Ile)	Lauwersoog
Le Pouliguen/Pornichet	Dornumer-Accumersiel
L'Herbaudière	Hooksiel
St Gilles-Croix-de-Vie	Langeoog
River Seudre	Bremerhaven
Royan	Helgoland
Anglet/Bayonne	Büsum
Hendaye	

LANNION (Léguer River)

Côte d'Armor 48°44'.00N 03°33'.50W   **10-16-17**

CHARTS
AC 3669, *2668*; SHOM 7124, 7151; ECM 537, 538; Imray C34; Stanfords 17

TIDES
–0605 Dover; ML 5·4; Duration: no data; Zone –0100

Standard Port BREST (→)

Times				Height (metres)			
High Water		Low Water		MHWS	MHWN	MLWN	MLWS
0000	0600	0000	0600	6·9	5·4	2·6	1·0
1200	1800	1200	1800				
Differences LOCQUIREC							
+0058	+0108	+0120	+0100	+2·2	+1·8	+0·8	+0·3

SHELTER
Good, except in strong W/NW winds. ⚓ in estuary or in non-drying pools off Le Yaudet and Le Beguen. It may be possible to dry out on the N bank just below Lannion town.

NAVIGATION
WPT 48°44'.40N 03°36'.60W, 284°/104° from/to Pte de Dourven 1·9M (also on Locquemeau ldg lts 122°). Beware drying sandbank extending approx 2ca N/NE from Pte de Dourven. Enter chan close to two G bn trs. No access at very LW, esp with strong NW winds when seas break on the bar.

LIGHTS AND MARKS
Large W radome conspic 3·5M NNE of ent. Pte Beg-Léguer lt ho Oc (4) WRG 12s 60m 13/10M; vis W084°-098°, R098°-129°, G007°-084°. Chan up river is narrow but marked by trs/bns.

RADIO TELEPHONE
None.

TELEPHONE
Hr Mr 96·37·06·52; Aff Mar 96·37·06·52; CROSS 98·89·31·31; SNSM 96·23·52·07; ⌗ 96·37·45·32; Auto 36.68.08.22; Police 96·37·03·78; Dr 96·37·42·52; Brit Consul 99·46·26·64.

FACILITIES
Quai de Loguivy Slip, L, FW, C (1 ton mobile), AB; **Services**: M, ME, El, Sh, SHOM, Ⓔ, CH. **Town** M, CH, V, Gaz, R, Bar, ⊠, Ⓑ, ⇌, ✈ (Morlaix, Lannion). Ferry: Roscoff.

ADJACENT HARBOUR

LOCQUEMEAU, Côte d'Armor, 48°43'.60N 03°34'.70W, AC 3669, 2668; SHOM 7124. HW –0600 on Dover (UT); +0110 on Brest; HW ht +1·5m on Brest; ML 5·3m. A small drying hbr by ent to Lannion River (10·16·17). There are two quays: the outer is accessible at LW, but open to W 'lies. Yachts can dry out at inner quay, on S side. Ldg lts 122° to outer quay: front FR 21m 6M, vis 068°-228°, W pylon + R top; rear, 484m from front, Oc (2+1) R 12s 39m 7M, W gable and R gallery. **Services**: ME, El, Sh; **Town** Bar.

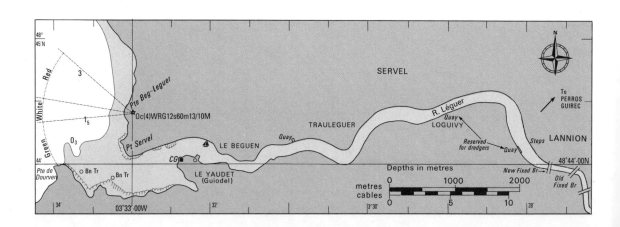

MORLAIX   10-16-18

Finistere 48°35'·50N 03°50'·50W

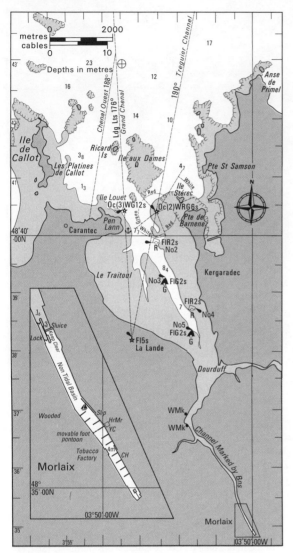

CHARTS

AC 2745, 3669; SHOM 7095, 7151; ECM 538; Imray C34, C35; Stanfords 17

TIDES

–0610 Dover; ML 5·3; Duration 0610; Zone –0100

Standard Port BREST (→)

Times				Height (metres)			
High Water		Low Water		MHWS	MHWN	MLWN	MLWS
0000	0600	0000	0600	6·9	5·4	2·6	1·0
1200	1800	1200	1800				
Differences MORLAIX (CHÂTEAU DU TAUREAU)							
+0055	+0105	+0115	+0055	+2·0	+1·7	+0·8	+0·3
ANSE DE PRIMEL							
+0100	+0110	+0120	+0100	+2·1	+1·7	+0·8	+0·3

SHELTER

Good in the bay (waiting buoys off Pen Lann) and at Dourduff (dries). Yachts can go 5M up to Morlaix town and lock in to the Bassin à Flot to berth in complete shelter at the marina. Lock opens at HW –1½, HW and HW+1, day only. Visitor's pontoon on E bank, just N of slip and YC. Note: a movable pontoon (passerelle) across the marina, opposite the YC, serves as a footbridge from E to W banks; it will normally be open during lock hours.

NAVIGATION

WPT Grand Chenal 48°43'·00N 03°53'·50W, 356°/176° from/to Ile Louet lt, 2·5M. Morlaix B is divided by the Ile de Callot, to the W of which lies the Penzé R and to the E the Morlaix R. The three ent channels all have rky dangers:
(1) Chenal Ouest 188°, W of Ricard Is. Deepest chan, but unlit.
(2) Grand Chenal 176°, E of Ricard Is, shallower but lit.
(3) Chenal de Tréguier, 190°, best at night, but almost dries.
Strong N'lies can raise a steep sea even in the estuary.

LIGHTS AND MARKS

Grand Chenal ldg lts 176°: front Ile Louet, Oc (3) WG 12s; rear La Lande, Fl 5s.
Chenal de Tréguier ldg lts 190°: Ile Noire, Oc (2) WRG 6s; rear La Lande, Fl 5s.
River up to Morlaix, 3M above Dourduff, is buoyed but unlit.

RADIO TELEPHONE

Port and marina VHF Ch 09 16.

TELEPHONE

Hr Mr 98·62·13·14; Lock 98·88·54·92; Aff Mar 98·62·10·47; CROSS 98·89·31·31; SNSM 98·88·00·76; ⌗ 98·88·06·31; Auto 36.68.08.29; Police 98·88·58·13; Ⓗ 98·62·61·60; Brit Consul 99·46·26·64.

FACILITIES

Marina (180+30 visitors) ☎ 98·62·13·14, access as lock times, FF70, AC, FW, C (8 ton), P & D; **YC de Morlaix** ☎ 98·62·08·51, Slip, M, P, D, L, FW, ME, El, Sh, CH, AB; **Services:** SM, Ⓔ, SHOM.
Town P, D, V, Gaz, R, Bar, ✉, Ⓑ, ▣, ⇌, ✈. Ferry: Roscoff.

OTHER HARBOURS AND ANCHORAGES N OF MORLAIX

PRIMEL, Finistere, 48°42'·80N 03°49'·30W, AC 2745, 3669; SHOM 7095, 7151. HW –0610 on Dover (UT); ML 5·3m; Duration 0600. See 10.16.18. Good deep ⚓ well protected, but seas break across ent in strong winds. Beware rks off Pte de Primel to E of ent, and Le Zamegues to W. Ldg lts 152°: both FR 35/56m 6M, vis 134°-168°; front W pylon, rear wall with W ☐ and R vert stripe. Jetty hd lt Fl G 4s 6m 7M. ⚓ in chan in 2-9m or 30 ⚓s, marked Passagers. VHF Ch 09 16 (season). Hr Mr ☎ 98.62.28.40. Facilities: C (12 ton), FW, Slip, CH, El, ME, Sh, Ⓔ, R, Bar.

PENZÉ RIVER, Finistere, Ent 48°42'·00N 03°56'·40W, AC 2745; SHOM 7095. HW –0610 on Dover (UT), +0105 on Brest; HW ht +1·2m Brest; ML 5·0m; Duration 0605. Appr at mid-flood from NNW between Cordonnier and Guerhéon bn trs or, for deeper water, from ENE between Les Bizeyer and Le Paradis bn tr; thence pass W of Ile Callot. The Passe aux Moutons, between Carantec and Ile Callot, is a short cut from Morlaix estuary to the Penzé with adequate rise. Yachts can dry out inside Pempoul bkwtr on the W shore. The ⚓ off Carentec is exposed, especially to NW; landing stage dries about 4·6m. Further S the chan narrows and is scantily marked only by oyster withies and local moorings. SW of Pte de Lingos shelter is better; or moor off St Yves where the old ferry slips provide landing places. S of the bridge (11m) the R is buoyed and navigable on the tide for 3M to complete shelter at Penzé. Facilities at Carantec: El, ME, Sh, M, CH, P, D, Ⓔ. **Town** Ⓑ, Bar, ✉, R, V. **Penzé** AB (drying), limited V, R, Bar.

OTHER HARBOURS WEST OF ROSCOFF

MOGUÉRIEC, Finistere, 48°40'·40N 04°04'·40W, AC 3669, 2668; SHOM 7151. Tides approx as for Ile de Batz (10.16.19). A small drying fishing hbr, 3M SSW of W ent to Canal de Batz, open to NW swell. Ldg lts 162°: front, W tr on jetty, Iso WG 4s 9m, W sector 158°-166°; rear FG 22m. Beware Méan Névez rk, dries 3·3m, to stbd of appr. ⚓ 2ca NNE of jetty or close SW of Ile de Siec or dry out against the jetty. Facilities: V, R, Bar, P.

PONTUSVAL, Finistere, 48°40'·65N 04°19'·08W, AC 3668, 2644; SHOM 7150. HW +0605 on Dover (UT); +0055 on Brest (Zone –0100); HW ht +0·7m on Brest; ML 4·7m; Duration 0600. Ent between An Neudenn bn tr to E and 3 white-topped rks to W. Hbr, port of Brignogan-Plage, is open to N winds and is often full of FVs. Ldg line into hbr: bn on shore on with ch spire at 178°. Entry at night prohib. Facilities: Bar, FW, R, V.

16

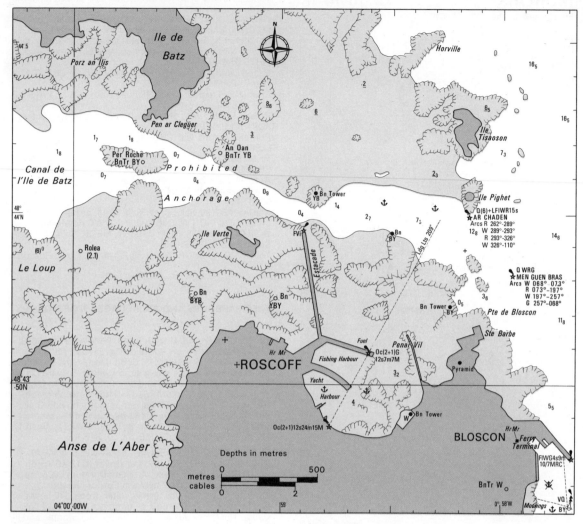

ROSCOFF   10-16-19

Finistere 48°43'·60N 03°58'·50W

CHARTS
AC 2745, 3669; SHOM 7095, 7151; ECM 538; Imray C35;
Stanfords 17

TIDES
−0605 Dover; ML 5·2; Duration 0600; Zone −0100

Standard Port BREST (→)

Times				Height (metres)			
High Water		Low Water		MHWS	MHWN	MLWN	MLWS
0000	0600	0000	0600	6·9	5·4	2·6	1·0
1200	1800	1200	1800				
Differences ROSCOFF							
+0055	+0105	+0115	+0055	+1·9	+1·6	+0·8	+0·3
ILE DE BATZ							
+0045	+0100	+0105	+0055	+2·0	+1·6	+0·9	+0·4

SHELTER
Good in Roscoff (dries 4·9m) except in strong winds from N
and E. Berth on inner side of jetty in Yacht hbr (Vieux Port) or
secure to ⚓ in SW corner. Access HW±2. There are W ⚓s
close W of Ar Chaden in 4-5m.
Entry to Bloscon ferry hbr only with Hr Mr's permission, but
yachts can moor or ⚓ to the S, well clear of ferries. Beware
foul ground close inshore and WIP.

NAVIGATION
WPT 48°46'·00N 03°55'·80W, 033°/213° from/to Men Guen
Bras lt, 2·6M. The ent to Roscoff needs care due to many
large rks in the area; best to enter near HW. See 10.16.5 for
pilotage notes on the Canal de l'Ile de Batz. The chans are
well marked and must be kept to. Appr to Bloscon is easier.

LIGHTS AND MARKS
Ile de Batz lt ho (conspic) Fl (4) 25s 69m 23M. Off Roscoff
at E end of Canal de l'Ile de Batz are Ar Chaden Q (6)+L Fl
WR 15s, SCM bn tr, and Men-Guen-Bras Q WRG, NCM.
Ldg lts/marks 209° for the hbr: both Oc (2+1) G 12s, front 7m
7M, W col, G top, with B/W vert stripes on end of mole;
rear conspic W lt ho 24m 15M. Bloscon jetty hd Fl WG 4s;
appr in W sector 206°-216°; in fog, Fl W 2s.

RADIO TELEPHONE
Roscoff Ch 09. *Bloscon* Ch 12 16; 0830-1200, 1330-1800LT.

TELEPHONE
Hr Mr (Port de Plaisance) 98·69·76·37; Hr Mr (Roscoff)
98·61·27·84; Aff Mar 98·69·70·15; CROSS 98·89·31·31;
SNSM 98·61·27·84; ⊞ (Roscoff) 98·69·19·67; ⊞ (Bloscon)
98·61·27·86; Auto 36.68.08.29; Police 98·69·00·48;
Ⓗ 98·88·40·22; Dr 98·69·71·18; Brit Consul 99·46·26·64.

FACILITIES
Vieux Port (220+30 visitors) ☎ 98·69·76·37, AB (with fender
board), FW, AC, M; **Quai Neuf** Reserved for FVs, C (5 ton);
Club Nautique de Roscoff ☎ 98·69·72·79, Bar; **Bloscon** M.
Services: BY, ME, El, Sh, CH. **Town** P, D, ME, El, Sh, CH, Gaz,
V, R, Bar, ✉, Ⓑ, ⇌, ✈ (Morlaix). Ferry: Plymouth.

HARBOUR/ANCHORAGE CLOSE NORTH

ILE DE BATZ, Finistere, 48°44'·50N 04°00'·50W, AC 2745, 3669;
SHOM 7095; HW +0610 Dover (UT); ML 5·2m. See 10·16·19.
Porz-Kernoc'h gives good shelter but dries. E slip is reserved
for ferries. ⚓ in E or W parts of the chan depending on wind,
but holding ground poor. ⚓ prohib in area W of Roscoff
landing slip. Ile de Batz lt ho Fl (4) 25s. Facilities: a few shops.

L'ABERWRAC'H   10-16-20

Finistere 48°36'·75N 04°35'·30W

CHARTS
AC 1432, 2644; SHOM 7094, 7150; ECM 539; Imray C35; Stanfords 17

TIDES
+0547 Dover; ML 4·5; Duration 0600; Zone –0100

Standard Port BREST (→)

Times				Height (metres)			
High Water		Low Water		MHWS	MHWN	MLWN	MLWS
0000	0600	0000	0600	6·9	5·4	2·6	1·0
1200	1800	1200	1800				
Differences L'ABERWRAC'H, ILE CÉZON							
+0030	+0030	+0038	+0037	+0·8	+0·7	+0·2	0·0

SHELTER
Good except in strong NW'lies. At La Palue either moor on 30 numbered W 🅐s; or berth bows on to a single pontoon (stern line to buoy); max LOA = 11m. Vessels at this pontoon may collide at slack water or if wind and tide conflict. Free water taxi in summer every H, 0800-2200. Excellent shelter in all winds at Paluden, 1·5M up-river (off chartlet), on dumbell 🅐s; plus landing jetty, but ⚓ prohib.

NAVIGATION
WPT Grand Chenal 48°37'·40N 04°38'·40W, 280°/100° from/to front ldg lt 2·6M. Beware Le Libenter shoal marked by WCM, Q (9) 15s (Whis), brg 254° from Ile Vierge lt 3·0M. Also beware Basse Trousquennou to S. Two chans lead to the inner 128° appr line:
(1) Grand Chenal 100° (from W and best for strangers) runs S of Libenter, Grand and Petit Pot de Beurre.
(2) Chenal de la Malouine (a narrow short cut from N, only by day and in good weather) 176° transit of Petit Pot de Beurre with Petite Ile de la Croix W bn; great precision is required.

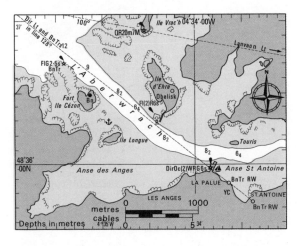

LIGHTS AND MARKS
Ile-Vierge lt ho Fl 5s 77m 27M, Gy tr, Horn 60s, RC, vis 337°–325° (348°). For the Grand Chenal the 100° ldg lts/ marks are: front QR, Ile Vrac' h, W ☐ tr orange top; and, 1·63M to the rear, Dir Q, Lanvaon, W ☐ tr orange △ on top. Then Dir Oc (2) WRG 6s, W127·2°-128·7°, leads 128 ° almost to the pontoon at La Palue. Unlit up river.

RADIO TELEPHONE
VHF Ch 09 16 (0700-2100 LT).

TELEPHONE
Hr Mr 98·04·91·62; Aff Mar 98·04·90·13; CROSS/SNSM 98·89·31·31; ⊞ 98·04·90·27; Meteo 98·84·60·64; Auto 36.68.08.29; Police 98·04·00·18; Ⓗ 98·46·11·33; Dr 98·04·91·87; SAMU 15; Brit Consul 99·46·26·64.

FACILITIES
Pontoon (30, some visitors) ☎ 98·04·91·62, FF84, M, D, FW, ME, El, CH, BH (12 ton); **YC des Abers** ☎ 98·04·92·60, Bar, 🅾; **Services:** Sh, Ⓔ, Slip, C (3 ton mobile).
Town P, V, Gaz, R, 🅾, P, Bar, ✉, Ⓑ (Landeda, every a.m. except Mon), ⇌, ✈, (bus to Brest). Ferry: Roscoff.

L'ABERBENOIT   10-16-21

Finistere 48°34'·65N 04°36'·80W

CHARTS
AC 1432, 2644; SHOM 7094, 7150; ECM 539, 540; Imray C35; Stanfords 17

TIDES
+0535 Dover; ML 4·7; Duration 0555; Zone –0100

Standard Port BREST (→)

Times				Height (metres)			
High Water		Low Water		MHWS	MHWN	MLWN	MLWS
0000	0600	0000	0600	6·9	5·4	2·6	1·0
1200	1800	1200	1800				
Differences L'ABERBENOIT							
+0022	+0025	+0035	+0020	+1·0	+0·9	+0·4	+0·2
PORTSALL							
+0015	+0020	+0025	+0015	+0·6	+0·5	+0·1	0·0

SHELTER
Excellent, but do not enter at night, in poor vis nor in strong WNW winds; best near LW when dangers can be seen. Six 🅐s and ⚓ as shown or further up-river. R navigable on the tide to Tréglonou bridge 3M upstream. Beware oyster beds.

NAVIGATION
WPT 48°37'·05N 04°38'·67W, Petite Fourche WCM, 337°/ 157° from/to Ile Guénioc, 1M. From WPT track 168° for 1M until abeam Ile Guénioc; thence 134° past Basse du Chenal and Karreg ar Poul Doun PHM bns to Men Renead SHM buoy. Alter stbd 160° to pass close to La Jument rk (PHM bn and R paint patch); thence 140°, passing 2 SHM buoys and leaving Le Chien IDM bn to port, leads to the fairway.

LIGHTS AND MARKS
Unlit. Chan bns and buoys must be carefully identified.

RADIO TELEPHONE
None.

TELEPHONE
Hr Mr none; CROSS/SNSM 98·89·31·31; ⊞ 98·04·90·27; Meteo 98·84·60·64; Auto 36.68.08.29; Police 98·48·10·10; Dr 98·89·75·67; Brit Consul 99·46·26·64.

FACILITIES
Le Passage Slip, M (free), L, FW; **Services:** Sh, ME, El.
Tréglonou Slip; **Town** Gaz, ✉, Ⓑ (Ploudalmezeau), ⇌, ✈ (bus to Brest). Ferry: Roscoff.

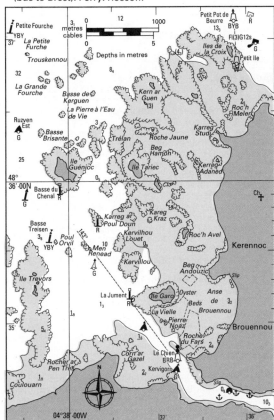

LAMPAUL (ILE D'OUESSANT)

Finistere 48°26'·70N 05°07'·40W   10-16-22

CHARTS
AC 2694; SHOM 7123, 7149; ECM 540; Imray C36; Stan 17
TIDES
+0522 Dover; ML 3·9; Duration 0555; Zone –0100

Standard Port BREST (→)

Times				Height (metres)			
High Water		Low Water		MHWS	MHWN	MLWN	MLWS
0000	0600	0000	0600	6·9	5·4	2·6	1·0
1200	1800	1200	1800				
Differences BAIE DE LAMPAUL							
+0005	+0005	–0005	+0003	0·0	–0·1	–0·1	0·0
ILE DE MOLENE							
+0012	+0012	+0017	+0017	+0·4	+0·3	+0·2	+0·1

SHELTER
Bay is open to SW winds and swell; only usable in settled weather, prone to poor vis, esp in July. There are approx 24 ⚓s to S of the small drying hbr to E of pier, ent 15m wide, which normally has no room for visitors.

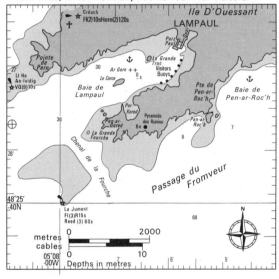

NAVIGATION
WPT 48°26'·30N 05°09'·00W, 250°/070° from/to Le Corce Rk, 1·4M. Bring Le Stiff lt ho 055° open N of Le Corce, which may be passed on either side. PHM/SHM bn trs mark Men-ar-Blank and Men-ar-Groas Rks further inshore. Beware ferries using the T-shaped quay; they also use the Ch de la Fourche, but this is not advised for yachts. The ITZ extends 5M NW of Ushant to the NE-bound lane of the TSS (see Fig 10 (5) and 10.16.2).
LIGHTS AND MARKS
La Jument Fl (3) R 15s 36m **22**M; grey 8-sided tr, R top; obsc 199°-241°; Horn (3) 60s. An-Ividig (Nividic) VQ (9) 10s 28m 9M; W 8-sided tr, R bands; obsc 225°-290°; helicopter platform. Creac'h Fl (2) 10s 70m **34**M; W tr, B bands; obsc 247°-255°; Horn (2) 120s; RC; Racon. Le Stiff Fl (2) R 20s 85m **24**M; close to conspic radar tr 72m.
RADIO TELEPHONE
None. For Ouessant TSS/ITZ see under Brest 10.16.27.
TELEPHONE
Hr Mr 98·89 20 05; Aff Mar 94·48·80·27; CROSS 98·89·31·31; Meteo 98·84·60·64; Auto 36·68·08·29; SNSM 98·89·70·04; Police 98·68·10·39; Dr 98·89·92·70; Brit Consul 99·46·26·64.
FACILITIES
Few facilities: L, AB, FW, P & D (cans), Slip. **Town** Gaz, ✉, Ⓑ, ferry to Le Conquet and Brest ⇌, ✈. UK Ferry: Roscoff.

ADJACENT HARBOUR

BAIE DU STIFF, 48°28'·13N 05°03'·18W, is sheltered in S to NW winds. Appr is clear apart from Gorle Vihan with IDM bn. Dir lt 259°, Q WRG 11m 10/7M, vis W254°-264°, is on the mole. S of the lt ho, Porz Liboudou is for ferries, but 9 R ⚓s are available in 5m. Holding is poor; little room to ⚓.

L'ABERILDUT

Finistere 48°28'·30N 04°45'·72W   10-16-23

CHARTS
AC 3345, 2694, *2644*; SHOM 7122, 7149; ECM 540; Imray C36; Stanfords 17
TIDES
+0520 on Dover (UT); ML 4·2m; Zone –0100

Standard Port BREST (→)

Times				Height (metres)			
High Water		Low Water		MHWS	MHWN	MLWN	MLWS
0000	0600	0000	0600	6·9	5·4	2·6	1·0
1200	1800	1200	1800				
Differences L'ABERILDUT							
+0010	+0010	+0023	+0010	+0·4	+0·3	0·0	0·0

SHELTER
Good inside, but appr is open to W winds; access at all tides and at night with care. Hbr partly dries, but a narrow chan at the ent has 2m, with pools to 6m inside. Beyond the FV quay (NW side) a pontoon provides landing and fuel. Some ⚓s; little room to ⚓, but ⚓ s outside as chartlet. A useful passage hbr to await the tide in the Ch du Four.
NAVIGATION
WPT 48°28'·12N 04°48'·13W, 263°/083° from/to Dir lt, 1·6M. From N beware Les Liniou Rks 1·5M NNW of the WPT and Plateau des Fourches 1·2M SSW. Appr is fairly easy in good vis, but beware strong cross tides. At the ent leave both Men Tassin PHM bn and La Roche du Crapaud, a large rounded rk, close to port to clear drying spit on S side of the narrow ent. For Chenal du Four see opposite and 10·16·5.

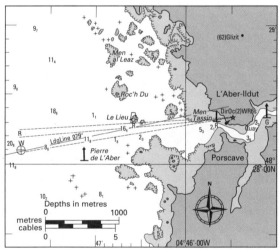

LIGHTS AND MARKS
Le Four tr, Fl (5) 15s 28m 18M, gy tr, siren (3+2) 60s, is 3·35M N of the WPT. Pointe de Corsen lt, Dir Q WRG 33m 12/8M, is 3·2M S of the WPT.
A stern transit 258° of Kéréon lt, gy tr, Oc (2+1) WR 24s 38m **17**M, with La Jument lt, Fl (3) R 15s 36m **22**M, gy tr + R top, (both off Ouessant) leads to the W sector of a powerful Dir lt 083°, Oc (2) WR 6s 12m **25/20**M, W bldgs, vis W081°-085°, R085°-087°, at hbr ent.
Ldg marks (difficult to see from afar): front, Lanildut spire on with Brélès spire leads 079° into fairway. Drying rks are marked by Pierre de l'Aber SHM bn and Le Lieu PHM bn tr 5m; the latter is easier to see.
RADIO TELEPHONE
None.
TELEPHONE
Hr Mr 98.04.41.31 (Jun-Sep); Aff Mar 98.48.66.54; Auto 36.68.08.29; ⌗ 98.44.35.20; CROSS/SNSM 98.89.31.31; Police 98.48.10.10; Dr 98.04.33.08.
FACILITIES
Hbr, M (300, inc 12 ⚓s; FF50); FW, D, slips, AC at FV quay; **Services:** BY, Sh, ME, El, CH, M.
Village V, R, Bar, ✉. All needs at Brest 25km. Ferry: Roscoff.

CHENAL DU FOUR and CHENAL DE LA HELLE

See 10.16.5 for notes on these passages

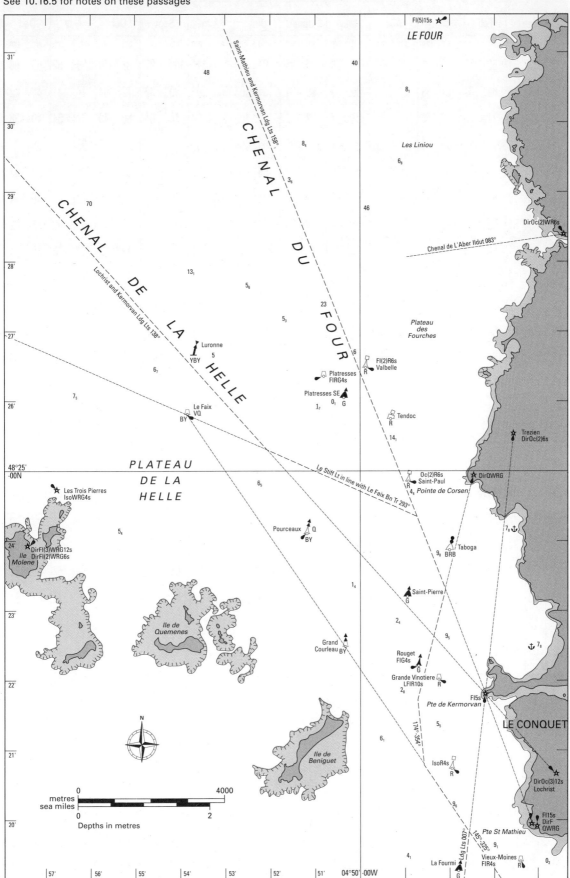

BREST TIDAL COEFFICIENTS 1996

Date	Jan am	Jan pm	Feb am	Feb pm	Mar am	Mar pm	Apr am	Apr pm	May am	May pm	June am	June pm	July am	July pm	Aug am	Aug pm	Sept am	Sept pm	Oct am	Oct pm	Nov am	Nov pm	Dec am	Dec pm
1	49	51	52	57	46	51	66	71	73	79	90	95	97	101	111	111	103	97	87	79	59	52	55	50
2	55	58	62	67	57	63	77	82	85	89	98	101	104	105	109	106	90	82	72	64	47	41	46	42
3	62	65	71	75	69	74	87	91	93	97	102	102	106	105	102	96	74	65	56	49	37	34	40	38
4	69	71	78	81	79	83	94	97	99	101	101	99	103	100	90	82	57	49	42	37	33		38	
5	74	76	84	85	86	90	99	99	101	100	96	93	96	91	75	67	43	37	33	32	35	38	39	42
6	78	79	87	88	92	94	99	98	98	95	88	83	86	79	60	53	35			33	42	47	46	51
7	80	81	88	87	95	95	95	92	91	87	78	73	73	67	47	43	35	37	37	41	52	58	56	62
8	81	80	86	84	94	93	88	83	81	76	68	64	62	57		41	41	46	47	53	64	70	68	74
9	79	78	82	79	90	87	77	71	70	65	61	59	53		41	44	51	57	59	64	75	80	79	85
10	76	73	75	71	83	78	65	59	61	58		58	51	51	47	52	62	68	70	75	85	89	89	93
11	70	67	66	61	73	67	55	52	58		59	60	51	53	56	61	72	76	79	84	92	94	96	99
12	64	60	57	53	61	55		52	58	61	62	65	56	60	65	69	80	83	87	90	96	97	100	100
13	57	53	50	49	51	49	55	60	64	68	68	71	63	66	73	76	86	88	92	94	96	95	99	97
14	51	49		50		49	66	72	72	76	73	75	69	72	79	81	90	90	95	94	93	90	95	91
15	49		54	60	53	59	79	85	80	83	77	79	74	76	83	84	91	90	93	91	86	81	87	82
16	50	54	67	75	66	74	90	94	86	87	79	80	78	79	85	85	88	86	88	85	76	71	77	72
17	59	65	83	91	82	89	97	100	89	89	80	79	79	80	85	84	83	80	80	75	66	62	67	63
18	72	79	98	104	96	101	101	101	89	88	78	77	79	79	82	80	75	70	69	64	58	57	60	58
19	86	93	108	112	105	108	99	97	86	84	75	73	77	76	77	73	65	60	58	54	57			58
20	99	104	113	113	110	110	94	90	81	78	71	68	74	71	69	65	54	50	51	50	59	62	59	61
21	108	110	112	109	108	105	86	81	74	70	65	62	68	65	61	56	47	47		52	66	70	63	67
22	112	111	104	99	101	96	75	70	66	62	59	56	62	58	52	49		49	57	62	75	79	70	73
23	109	106	92	85	91	84	63	58	58	53	52	50	55	52	47	47	55	61	69	76	83	86	76	79
24	101	96	77	69	77	70	52	46	49	46	47	46	49	48		50	69	77	83	89	89	91	81	82
25	89	82	61	53	62	55	41	37	43	41	46	47	48		54	61	86	93	94	98	92	92	83	84
26	74	67	46	39	48	41	35	34	40	41		49	49	53	69	77	99	104	101	102	91	90	84	83
27	59	52	34	32	36	32		36		43	53	57	58	64	85	93	108	110	103	102	87	85	82	80
28	46	41		33	31		39	44	47	51	63	69	71	78	100	105	111	110	100	97	81	78	78	75
29		39	36	40	32	36	49	55	57	62	75	81	85	92	110	113	108	104	93	89	73	69	72	69
30	38	40			41	47	61	67	68	74	87	92	98	103	114	113	99	93	83	78	64	60	65	61
31	43	48			53	59			80	86			107	110	111	108			71	65			57	53

TIDAL COEFFICIENTS   10-16-25

These indicate at a glance the magnitude of the tide on any particular day by assigning a non-dimensional coefficient to the twice-daily range of tide. The coefficient is based on a scale of 45 for mean neap (morte eau) and 95 for mean spring (vive eau) ranges. The coefficient is 70 for an average tide. A very small np tide may have a coefficient of only 20, whilst a very big sp tide might be as high as 120. The ratio of the coefficients of different tides equals the ratio of their ranges; the range, for example, of the largest sp tide (120) is six times that of the smallest np tide (20).

The table opposite is for Brest, but holds good elsewhere along the Channel and Atlantic coasts of France.

French tide tables, similar to Admiralty tide tables as in this Almanac, show for Secondary ports their time and height differences against the appropriate standard port for vive eau (springs) and for morte eau (neaps). The tidal coefficient for the day may be used to decide which correction(s) to apply. In general it is satisfactory to use the vive eau corrections for coefficients over 70 and the morte eau corrections for the others. Where it is necessary to obtain more accurate corrections (in estuaries for example) this can be done by interpolating or extrapolating.

Coefficients may also be used to determine rates of tidal streams on a given day, using a graph similar in principle to that shown in Table 9 (2). On the vertical axis plot tidal coefficients from 20 at the bottom to 120 at the top. The horizontal axis shows tidal stream rates from zero to (say) five knots. From the tidal stream atlas or chart, plot the np and sp rates against coefficient 45 and 95 respectively; join these two points. Entering with the tidal coefficient for the day in question, go horizontally to the sloping line, then vertically to read the required rate on the horizontal axis.

French translations of common tidal terms are as follows:

HW	Pleine mer (PM)
LW	Basse mer (BM)
Springs	Vive eau (VE)
Neaps	Morte eau (ME)
CD	Zero des cartes
MHWS	Pleine mer moyenne de VE
MHWN	Pleine mer moyenne de ME
MLWN	Basse mer moyenne de ME
MLWS	Basse mer moyenne de VE

ADJACENT HARBOURS

PORTSALL, Finistere, 48°33'·85N 04°42'·95W. AC 1432, 3688; SHOM 7094, 7150. HW +0535 on Dover (UT); ML 4·4m; Duration 0600. See 10.16.21. Small drying hbr at head of bay. Access HW±3. Good shelter except in strong N winds. Ldg marks: Le Yurc'h rk (7m) on with Ploudalmézeau spire leads 109°; thence 085° on W & RW marks. By night use W sector 084°-088° of lt Oc (4) WRG 12s 9m 13/10M, W col/R top. Appr marked by 5 bn trs. Beware many rks for about 2M off-shore. ⚓ to W of ent, or go alongside quay in hbr. Facilities: Aff Mar ☎ 98·48·66·54; SNSM ☎ 98·48·77·44; Dr ☎ 98·48·10·46; **Quay** C (0·5 ton), D, FW, P, Slip; **Club Nautique** ☎ 98·48·63·10; **Coop de Pêcheurs** ☎ 98·48·63·26, CH. **Town** Bar, ⊠, R, V.

ARGENTON, Finistere, 48°31'·32N 04°46'·25W. AC 3347, 2694; SHOM 7122. HW +0535 on Dover (UT); ML 4·6m; Duration 0600; use PORTSALL diffs 10.16.21. Small drying hbr; good shelter except in W winds when a swell comes up the bay into the hbr. Access HW±3. Appr 086° on 2 W bns & RW wall. Le Four lt Fl (5) 15s is 1·4M to W. Beware strong E-W tides. ⚓ in deep water off hbr ent. 10 ⚓s. Facilities: FW, P on quay; **SC** ☎ 98·89·54·04. **Town** Bar, R, V.

ILE DE MOLENE, Finistere, 48°24'·13N 04°57'·26W. AC 2694; SHOM 7123, 7122, 7149. HW +0520 on Dover (UT); ML 4·6m; see 10.16.22. Hbr, part-drying, is easier at nps, good wx/vis. Beware strong tidal streams. Best appr is via Ch de la Helle, twixt Le Faix bn tr, VQ 16m, and Luronne WCM buoy. Track W to pick up ldg marks 215°: front, Trois Pierres bn, Iso WRG 4s, 15m; rear, RW N.Mill bn tr. Nearing front mark, alter stbd to align spire 199° between ECM bn tr and WCM buoy. ⚓ S of N bkwtr hd in about 1·5m. Dir lt 191°, Fl (3) WRG 12s, W190°-192°, is on old S pier; same lt, but Fl (2) WRG 6s, also covers Chenal des Las (W259·5°-262·5°). Facilities: V, CH, R, Bar, ⊠.

LE CONQUET   10-16-26

Finistere 48°21'·60N 04°47'·15W

CHARTS
AC 3345, 2694; SHOM 7122, 7149; ECM 540; Imray C36; Stanfords 17

TIDES
+0535 Dover; ML 3·9; Duration 0600; Zone –0100

Standard Port BREST (⟶)

Times				Height (metres)			
High Water		Low Water		MHWS	MHWN	MLWN	MLWS
0000	0600	0000	0600	6·9	5·4	2·6	1·0
1200	1800	1200	1800				
Differences LE CONQUET							
–0005	0000	+0007	+0007	–0·1	–0·1	–0·1	0·0

SHELTER
Good except in strong W winds. A busy fishing port with few yacht facilities. AB only briefly at quay for loading. ⚓ prohib in Avant Port. Yachts can ⚓ further up hbr but it dries and may be foul.

NAVIGATION
WPT 48°21'·50N 04°48'·50W, 263°/083° from/to Mole Ste Barbe lt, 1M. From the NW, beware the Grande Vinotière rks. Also note strong cross streams in the Chenal du Four.

LIGHTS AND MARKS
Ldg line 095° lt on Mole Ste Barbe, Oc G 4s in line with spire of Le Conquet church. La Louve R bn tr and end of Mole St Christophe in line at 079°.

RADIO TELEPHONE
Le Conquet Port (Hr Mr) VHF 11 16. Call: *St Mathieu* VHF Ch 16 for Chenal du Four and Chenal de la Helle (see 10.16.9).

TELEPHONE
Hr Mr 98·89·08·07; Aff Mar 98·89·00·05; Meteo 98·84·60·64; Auto 36.68.08.29; CROSS 98·89·31·31; SNSM 98·89·02·07; Police 98·89·00·13; Dr 98·89·01·86; Brit Consul 99·46·26·64.

FACILITIES
Hbr Slip, M, L, D; **Services:** ME, El, P (cans), CH.
Town P, D, FW, ME, El, V, Gaz, R, Bar, ⊠, Ⓑ, ⇌ (bus to Brest), ✈ (Brest). Ferry: Roscoff.

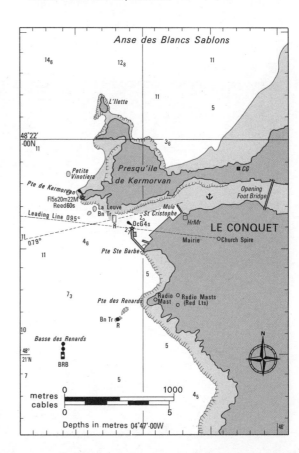

16

BREST   10-16-27

Finistere 48°21'·30N 04°25·70W (Moulin Blanc)

CHARTS
AC 3428, 3427, 798; SHOM 6542, 6426, 6427, 6678, 7149;
ECM 542; Imray C36; Stanfords 17

TIDES
+0520 Dover; ML 4·0; Duration 0605; Zone –0100
NOTE: Brest is a Standard Port. Tidal predictions for every
day are given below; tidal coefficients are above.

SHELTER
Excellent in Brest, and at many ⚓s in the Rade de Brest
(50 sq miles). Access at any tide H24. Yachts should use
Moulin Blanc marina, not the Port du Commerce. Brest is
a busy commercial, naval and fishing port. The Port
Militaire and a zone round Ile Longue are prohib areas.

NAVIGATION
WPT 48°18'·30N 04°44'·00W, 248°/068° from/to front ldg lt
(Pte du Petit Minou), 5·3M. Tidal streams run hard in the
Goulet de Brest. In mid-chan beware rks, well marked;
pass either side. As WPT to Marina, use Moulin Blanc
PHM buoy, Fl (3) R 12s, 48°22'·85N 04°25'·90W, 207°/027°
from/to MB1 and MB2 chan buoys, 0·55M.

LIGHTS AND MARKS
Apprs marked by lts at Pte St Mathieu, Pte du Petit Minou
and Pte du Portzic. Oceanopolis bldg, W roof, is conspic.
Marina, 2M E of the Port de Commerce, has buoyed chan;
MB4 lt and the ECM lt By can be obsc'd by berthed craft.

RADIO TELEPHONE
Call: *Brest Port* (at Pte du Portzic) VHF Ch 08 16 (controls
apprs to Brest). All vessels entering keep watch on Ch 16.
Marina Ch 09 16 (H24).
Ouessant Traffic provides radar surveillance/assistance
in the TSS/ITZ on Ch 11 16 68; it also broadcasts nav and
tfc reports, in English/French, on Ch 79 at H+10 and +40;
plus vis reports, when vis < 2M. *Saint Mathieu* Ch 16 is
part of Ouessant VTS, for vessels sailing in Ch de la Helle
and Ch du Four. In poor vis or in emergency it may give
radar assistance to small craft which should monitor Ch
16 throughout their transit.

TELEPHONE
Hr Mr Brest 98·44·13·44; Moulin Blanc 98·02·20·02;
Aff Mar 98·80·62·25; CROSS 98·89·31·31; ⌗ 98·44·35·20;
Meteo 98·84·60·64; Auto 36.68.08.29; Police 98·22·83·90;
Dr 98·44·38·70; Ⓗ 98·22·33·33; Brit Consul 99·46·26·64.

FACILITIES (MOULIN BLANC)
Marina (1225+100 visitors), ☎ 98·02·20·02, Fax 98.41.67.91,
FF89, P & D H24, FW, AC, Slip, ME, El, Ⓔ, SHOM, Sh, SM,
CH, BH (14 & 35 ton), C (3 & 12 ton), Gaz, R, ⊡, V, Bar;
Sté des Régates de Brest ☎ 98·02·53·36, R.
BREST **Services**: CH, SM, ME, El, Sh, Ⓔ, SHOM.
City all facilities, Gaz, ✉, Ⓑ, ⇌, ✈. Ferry: Roscoff.

ADJACENT ANCHORAGE TO THE WEST

ANSE DE BERTHAUME, 48°20'·50N 04°41'·75W. AC 3427.
A useful passage ⚓ if awaiting the tide E into Goulet de
Brest; N into Ch du Four, or S toward Raz de Sein. Good
shelter in W'lies. ⚓ in 5m off slip N of Fort de Berthaume
(conspic); 1ca NE, beware Le Chat rk, dries 6·8m. No lts.

RADE DE BREST   10-16-28

Finistere

TIDES
In most of the bays in the Rade de Brest tidal streams are
weak, but in the main rivers they can exceed 2kn at sp.

SHELTER AND NAVIGATION
The Rade de Brest offers a sheltered cruising ground,
useful in bad weather, with many attractive ⚓s.
To the NE, ½M beyond Pont Albert -Louppe (28m) is a
good ⚓ at Le Passage. It is possible to explore R L'Elorn
for about 6M to the drying port of Landerneau; keep well
inboard of chan buoys.
On the S side of Rade de Brest are various naval sites
with prohib ⚓ around Ile Longue. There are however ⚓s
at Le Fret, on SE side of Ile Longue, and at Roscanvel on
E side of the Quelern Peninsula.
To the SE, L'Aulne is a lovely river with steep wooded
banks. Near the mouth of its estuary, on the N shore, is a
good ⚓ in Anse de l'Auberlach. Further E, 3 small drying
rivers run into the Aulne from the north: R Daoulas, R de
l'Hôpital and R du Faou and provide shelter for boats
which can dry out.
Up the Aulne there are ⚓s near Landévennec, below
Térénez bridge (27m), and also 1½M above that bridge.
At Guily-Glaz, 14M above Landévennec, a lock (open HW
Brest –2 to +1½) opens into the canalised river to Port
Launay (AB on quay, FW, R) and 3M to Chateaulin, AB on
pontoons; most facilities.

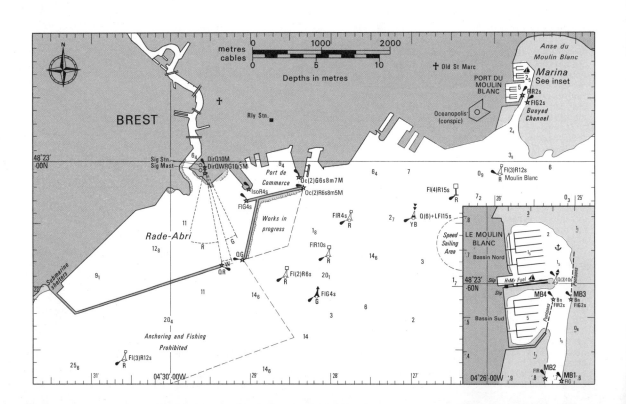

RADE DE BREST *continued*

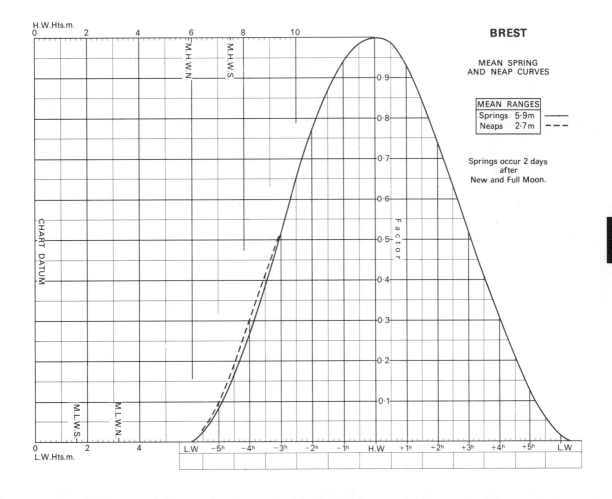

BREST

MEAN SPRING
AND NEAP CURVES

MEAN RANGES	
Springs	5·9m
Neaps	2·7m

Springs occur 2 days
after
New and Full Moon.

16

TIME ZONE –0100
(French Standard Time)
Subtract 1 hour for UT

For French Summer Time add
ONE hour in non-shaded areas

FRANCE – BREST

LAT 48°23′N   LONG   4°30′W

TIMES AND HEIGHTS OF HIGH AND LOW WATERS

YEAR **1996**

JANUARY

Day	Time	m	Day	Time	m
1 M	0133 / 0757 / 1402 / 2023	5.5 / 2.4 / 5.6 / 2.3	**16** TU	0019 / 0639 / 1252 / 1920	5.5 / 2.4 / 5.6 / 2.3
2 TU	0233 / 0855 / 1457 / 2115	5.7 / 2.2 / 5.8 / 2.1	**17** W	0133 / 0753 / 1410 / 2029	5.8 / 2.1 / 5.9 / 1.9
3 W	0321 / 0943 / 1542 / 2159	6.0 / 2.0 / 6.0 / 1.9	**18** TH	0239 / 0859 / 1511 / 2129	6.3 / 1.6 / 6.4 / 1.4
4 TH	0401 / 1025 / 1621 / 2238	6.2 / 1.8 / 6.2 / 1.8	**19** F	0337 / 0958 / 1606 / 2224	6.8 / 1.1 / 6.8 / 1.0
5 F O	0437 / 1101 / 1657 / 2313	6.4 / 1.6 / 6.3 / 1.7	**20** SA ●	0430 / 1051 / 1657 / 2315	7.2 / 0.7 / 7.1 / 0.7
6 SA	0511 / 1136 / 1730 / 2347	6.5 / 1.5 / 6.4 / 1.6	**21** SU	0520 / 1142 / 1745	7.5 / 0.4 / 7.3
7 SU	0544 / 1209 / 1803	6.6 / 1.5 / 6.4	**22** M	0004 / 0607 / 1230 / 1831	0.6 / 7.6 / 0.4 / 7.3
8 M	0020 / 0617 / 1242 / 1836	1.6 / 6.6 / 1.5 / 6.4	**23** TU	0051 / 0653 / 1316 / 1913	0.6 / 7.5 / 0.5 / 7.1
9 TU	0052 / 0649 / 1314 / 1909	1.6 / 6.5 / 1.6 / 6.3	**24** W	0136 / 0737 / 1401 / 1957	0.8 / 7.2 / 0.8 / 6.8
10 W	0126 / 0722 / 1348 / 1943	1.7 / 6.4 / 1.7 / 6.1	**25** TH	0221 / 0820 / 1445 / 2040	1.2 / 6.8 / 1.3 / 6.3
11 TH	0201 / 0757 / 1424 / 2021	1.8 / 6.2 / 1.9 / 6.0	**26** F	0307 / 0904 / 1530 / 2125	1.6 / 6.3 / 1.8 / 5.9
12 F	0240 / 0836 / 1505 / 2104	2.0 / 6.0 / 2.1 / 5.8	**27** SA	0355 / 0952 / 1620 / 2218	2.1 / 5.8 / 2.2 / 5.5
13 SA	0325 / 0923 / 1554 / 2158	2.2 / 5.8 / 2.3 / 5.6	**28** SU	0451 / 1050 / 1718 / 2323	2.5 / 5.4 / 2.6 / 5.2
14 SU	0419 / 1021 / 1653 / 2304	2.4 / 5.6 / 2.4 / 5.5	**29** M	0557 / 1829	2.7 / 2.8
15 M	0524 / 1132 / 1804	2.5 / 5.5 / 2.4	**30** TU	0047 / 0716 / 1325 / 1947	5.2 / 2.8 / 5.2 / 2.7
			31 W	0203 / 0827 / 1432 / 2050	5.4 / 2.5 / 5.4 / 2.5

FEBRUARY

Day	Time	m	Day	Time	m
1 TH	0258 / 0921 / 1522 / 2137	5.7 / 2.2 / 5.7 / 2.2	**16** F	0223 / 0845 / 1458 / 2116	6.1 / 1.7 / 6.2 / 1.6
2 F	0341 / 1004 / 1602 / 2217	6.0 / 1.9 / 6.0 / 1.9	**17** SA	0324 / 0945 / 1554 / 2211	6.6 / 1.2 / 6.7 / 1.1
3 SA	0418 / 1041 / 1638 / 2253	6.2 / 1.7 / 6.2 / 1.6	**18** SU ●	0417 / 1039 / 1644 / 2302	7.1 / 0.7 / 7.1 / 0.7
4 SU O	0452 / 1115 / 1711 / 2326	6.5 / 1.5 / 6.4 / 1.5	**19** M	0506 / 1127 / 1729 / 2348	7.4 / 0.4 / 7.3 / 0.5
5 M	0525 / 1148 / 1743 / 2359	6.6 / 1.3 / 6.5 / 1.3	**20** TU	0550 / 1212 / 1812	7.6 / 0.3 / 7.3
6 TU	0557 / 1221 / 1815	6.7 / 1.3 / 6.6	**21** W	0032 / 0632 / 1254 / 1851	0.5 / 7.5 / 0.5 / 7.2
7 W	0032 / 0629 / 1252 / 1847	1.3 / 6.8 / 1.3 / 6.6	**22** TH	0114 / 0712 / 1335 / 1929	0.7 / 7.3 / 0.8 / 6.9
8 TH	0104 / 0701 / 1325 / 1920	1.3 / 6.7 / 1.3 / 6.5	**23** F	0154 / 0750 / 1414 / 2006	1.0 / 6.9 / 1.2 / 6.5
9 F	0138 / 0734 / 1359 / 1955	1.4 / 6.6 / 1.5 / 6.3	**24** SA	0235 / 0828 / 1454 / 2044	1.5 / 6.4 / 1.7 / 6.0
10 SA	0216 / 0811 / 1438 / 2035	1.6 / 6.3 / 1.7 / 6.1	**25** SU	0317 / 0909 / 1537 / 2128	2.0 / 5.8 / 2.2 / 5.6
11 SU	0258 / 0854 / 1523 / 2123	1.9 / 6.0 / 2.0 / 5.8	**26** M	0406 / 0959 / 1628 / 2227	2.4 / 5.4 / 2.7 / 5.2
12 M	0348 / 0947 / 1619 / 2225	2.1 / 5.7 / 2.3 / 5.6	**27** TU	0506 / 1108 / 1735 / 2350	2.8 / 5.0 / 2.9 / 5.0
13 TU	0450 / 1056 / 1729 / 2343	2.4 / 5.5 / 2.5 / 5.5	**28** W	0625 / 1239 / 1900	2.9 / 4.9 / 3.0
14 W	0608 / 1223 / 1852	2.4 / 5.5 / 2.4	**29** TH	0122 / 0749 / 1401 / 2017	5.1 / 2.8 / 5.2 / 2.7
15 TH	0109 / 0731 / 1352 / 2010	5.7 / 2.2 / 5.7 / 2.1			

MARCH

Day	Time	m	Day	Time	m
1 F	0228 / 0851 / 1455 / 2109	5.4 / 2.4 / 5.5 / 2.3	**16** SA	0210 / 0832 / 1445 / 2103	6.1 / 1.7 / 6.2 / 1.6
2 SA	0314 / 0936 / 1536 / 2150	6.1 / 2.1 / 5.9 / 2.0	**17** SU	0310 / 0931 / 1539 / 2157	6.6 / 1.2 / 6.6 / 1.1
3 SU	0352 / 1014 / 1612 / 2227	6.1 / 1.7 / 6.2 / 1.6	**18** M	0402 / 1022 / 1627 / 2245	7.0 / 0.8 / 7.0 / 0.8
4 M	0427 / 1049 / 1646 / 2301	6.4 / 1.4 / 6.4 / 1.4	**19** TU ●	0448 / 1108 / 1709 / 2330	7.3 / 0.6 / 7.2 / 0.6
5 TU O	0501 / 1123 / 1719 / 2335	6.7 / 1.2 / 6.7 / 1.2	**20** W	0530 / 1150 / 1749	7.4 / 0.5 / 7.2
6 W	0533 / 1156 / 1752	6.9 / 1.1 / 6.8	**21** TH	0011 / 0609 / 1230 / 1825	0.6 / 7.4 / 0.6 / 7.1
7 TH	0009 / 0606 / 1229 / 1824	1.0 / 6.9 / 1.0 / 6.9	**22** F	0050 / 0645 / 1307 / 1901	0.7 / 7.1 / 0.9 / 6.9
8 F	0042 / 0639 / 1302 / 1858	1.0 / 6.9 / 1.1 / 6.8	**23** SA	0127 / 0721 / 1343 / 1935	1.0 / 6.8 / 1.3 / 6.5
9 SA	0118 / 0713 / 1338 / 1934	1.1 / 6.8 / 1.2 / 6.6	**24** SU	0205 / 0756 / 1420 / 2010	1.5 / 6.3 / 1.7 / 6.1
10 SU	0156 / 0751 / 1417 / 2014	1.3 / 6.5 / 1.5 / 6.3	**25** M	0244 / 0834 / 1500 / 2050	1.9 / 5.9 / 2.2 / 5.7
11 M	0239 / 0834 / 1502 / 2101	1.6 / 6.2 / 1.9 / 6.0	**26** TU	0328 / 0919 / 1546 / 2141	2.4 / 5.4 / 2.6 / 5.3
12 TU	0329 / 0927 / 1558 / 2203	1.9 / 5.8 / 2.2 / 5.7	**27** W	0422 / 1021 / 1646 / 2254	2.7 / 5.0 / 2.9 / 5.0
13 W	0431 / 1038 / 1709 / 2324	2.3 / 5.5 / 2.5 / 5.5	**28** TH	0531 / 1145 / 1805	2.9 / 4.9 / 3.0
14 TH	0550 / 1209 / 1835	2.4 / 5.4 / 2.5	**29** F	0025 / 0657 / 1314 / 1928	5.0 / 2.9 / 5.0 / 2.8
15 F	0053 / 0717 / 1338 / 1957	5.6 / 2.2 / 5.7 / 2.1	**30** SA	0141 / 0808 / 1416 / 2028	5.3 / 2.6 / 5.4 / 2.5
			31 SU	0234 / 0858 / 1501 / 2114	5.6 / 2.2 / 5.8 / 2.1

APRIL

Day	Time	m	Day	Time	m
1 M	0317 / 0939 / 1540 / 2154	6.0 / 1.8 / 6.2 / 1.7	**16** TU	0341 / 1002 / 1605 / 2226	6.8 / 1.0 / 7.0 / 1.0
2 TU	0355 / 1017 / 1616 / 2231	6.4 / 1.4 / 6.5 / 1.3	**17** W ●	0426 / 1046 / 1647 / 2308	7.0 / 0.9 / 7.0 / 0.8
3 W	0432 / 1053 / 1651 / 2308	6.7 / 1.2 / 6.8 / 1.1	**18** TH	0507 / 1127 / 1725 / 2348	7.1 / 0.8 / 7.0 / 0.8
4 TH O	0507 / 1129 / 1726 / 2344	6.9 / 1.0 / 7.0 / 0.9	**19** F	0544 / 1204 / 1800	7.0 / 0.9 / 6.9
5 F	0542 / 1204 / 1801	7.0 / 0.9 / 7.0	**20** SA	0026 / 0620 / 1240 / 1834	1.0 / 6.9 / 1.1 / 6.8
6 SA	0021 / 0618 / 1240 / 1837	0.9 / 7.0 / 0.9 / 7.0	**21** SU	0102 / 0654 / 1315 / 1908	1.2 / 6.6 / 1.4 / 6.5
7 SU	0059 / 0656 / 1319 / 1916	0.9 / 6.9 / 1.1 / 6.8	**22** M	0138 / 0729 / 1351 / 1943	1.5 / 6.3 / 1.8 / 6.2
8 M	0140 / 0737 / 1401 / 2000	1.1 / 6.6 / 1.4 / 6.5	**23** TU	0216 / 0806 / 1429 / 2022	1.9 / 5.9 / 2.1 / 5.8
9 TU	0226 / 0824 / 1450 / 2051	1.4 / 6.3 / 1.8 / 6.2	**24** W	0256 / 0849 / 1512 / 2107	2.2 / 5.5 / 2.5 / 5.5
10 W	0319 / 0920 / 1547 / 2154	1.8 / 5.8 / 2.2 / 5.8	**25** TH	0344 / 0942 / 1605 / 2207	2.6 / 5.2 / 2.8 / 5.2
11 TH	0423 / 1032 / 1659 / 2314	2.1 / 5.5 / 2.4 / 5.6	**26** F	0443 / 1053 / 1711 / 2322	2.8 / 5.0 / 2.9 / 5.1
12 F	0541 / 1202 / 1822	2.2 / 5.5 / 2.4	**27** SA	0556 / 1213 / 1827	2.8 / 5.0 / 2.9
13 SA	0038 / 0702 / 1322 / 1941	5.7 / 2.1 / 5.7 / 2.1	**28** SU	0043 / 0710 / 1322 / 1935	5.2 / 2.6 / 5.3 / 2.6
14 SU	0152 / 0814 / 1427 / 2045	6.1 / 1.7 / 6.1 / 1.7	**29** M	0143 / 0809 / 1416 / 2029	5.5 / 2.3 / 5.7 / 2.2
15 M	0251 / 0912 / 1519 / 2139	6.5 / 1.3 / 6.5 / 1.3	**30** TU	0234 / 0857 / 1501 / 2115	5.9 / 1.9 / 6.1 / 1.8

Chart Datum: 4·45 metres below Lallemand System (Mean Sea Level, Marseilles)

TIME ZONE –0100
(French Standard Time)
Subtract 1 hour for UT
For French Summer Time add
ONE hour in non-shaded areas

FRANCE – BREST

LAT 48°23′N   LONG 4°30′W

TIMES AND HEIGHTS OF HIGH AND LOW WATERS   YEAR **1996**

MAY

Day	Time m	Time m	Time m	Time m
1 W	0319 6.2	0940 1.5	1542 6.4	2158 1.4
16 TH	0403 6.6	1023 1.3	1624 6.6	2247 1.2
2 TH	0401 6.6	1021 1.2	1621 6.7	2239 1.1
17 F ●	0444 6.7	1103 1.2	1702 6.7	2326 1.2
3 F ○	0439 6.8	1100 1.0	1700 7.0	2319 0.9
18 SA	0522 6.7	1141 1.3	1737 6.7	
4 SA	0519 7.0	1140 0.9	1739 7.1	
19 SU	0003 1.2	0557 6.6	1216 1.4	1812 6.6
5 SU	0001 0.8	0559 7.0	1221 0.9	1820 7.1
20 M	0039 1.4	0632 6.4	1251 1.5	1846 6.4
6 M	0044 0.8	0642 6.9	1305 1.0	1904 7.0
21 TU	0115 1.6	0707 6.2	1327 1.8	1921 6.2
7 TU	0129 1.0	0728 6.7	1351 1.3	1952 6.4
22 W	0151 1.8	0744 5.9	1403 2.0	1958 6.0
8 W	0219 1.2	0819 6.3	1443 1.6	2046 6.4
23 TH	0229 2.1	0823 5.6	1443 2.3	2039 5.7
9 TH	0314 1.6	0917 6.0	1541 2.0	2149 6.0
24 F	0311 2.3	0909 5.4	1529 2.5	2128 5.4
10 F	0416 1.9	1025 5.7	1650 2.2	2301 5.8
25 SA	0401 2.5	1005 5.2	1624 2.7	2228 5.3
11 SA	0527 2.2	1142 5.6	1804 2.2	
26 SU	0501 2.6	1113 5.1	1728 2.7	2338 5.2
12 SU	0016 5.8	0641 2.0	1257 5.7	1918 2.1
27 M	0608 2.6	1223 5.3	1837 2.6	
13 M	0126 6.0	0749 1.8	1402 6.0	2022 1.8
28 TU	0046 5.4	0714 2.4	1325 5.5	1939 2.3
14 TU	0227 6.2	0848 1.6	1456 6.3	2116 1.5
29 W	0149 5.7	0811 2.1	1418 5.9	2034 1.9
15 W	0318 6.5	0939 1.4	1542 6.5	2204 1.3
30 TH	0242 6.0	0902 1.7	1506 6.3	2124 1.6
31 F	0329 6.4	0949 1.4	1552 6.6	2211 1.2

JUNE

Day	Time m	Time m	Time m	Time m
1 SA ○	0414 6.7	1034 1.1	1636 6.9	2257 0.9
16 SU ●	0502 6.3	1120 1.5	1718 6.5	2344 1.4
2 SU	0459 6.9	1120 0.9	1721 7.1	2344 0.7
17 M	0538 6.3	1155 1.5	1753 6.5	
3 M	0545 7.0	1206 0.8	1807 7.2	
18 TU	0019 1.5	0613 6.3	1230 1.6	1827 6.4
4 TU	0031 0.7	0632 7.0	1253 0.9	1855 7.1
19 W	0053 1.5	0647 6.2	1304 1.7	1901 6.1
5 W	0120 0.8	0721 6.8	1343 1.1	1946 6.9
20 TH	0128 1.7	0722 6.0	1339 1.8	1935 6.1
6 TH	0211 1.0	0813 6.5	1435 1.4	2039 6.6
21 F	0203 1.8	0758 5.8	1415 2.0	2012 5.9
7 F	0305 1.3	0908 6.2	1531 1.7	2137 6.3
22 SA	0240 2.0	0837 5.6	1455 2.2	2053 5.7
8 SA	0402 1.6	1007 5.9	1632 2.0	2239 6.0
23 SU	0322 2.2	0923 5.5	1542 2.4	2141 5.5
9 SU	0505 1.9	1114 5.7	1738 2.1	2346 5.8
24 M	0412 2.4	1018 5.3	1637 2.6	2240 5.4
10 M	0611 2.0	1224 5.6	1847 2.1	
25 TU	0511 2.5	1123 5.3	1740 2.5	2348 5.4
11 TU	0054 5.8	0717 2.0	1331 5.8	1953 2.0
26 W	0618 2.4	1231 5.5	1848 2.4	
12 W	0158 5.9	0820 1.9	1429 5.9	2052 1.8
27 TH	0057 5.5	0724 2.2	1335 5.7	1953 2.1
13 TH	0253 6.0	0914 1.8	1519 6.1	2142 1.7
28 F	0201 5.8	0825 1.9	1433 6.1	2052 1.7
14 F	0342 6.2	1001 1.7	1603 6.3	2227 1.5
29 SA	0300 6.2	0923 1.7	1526 6.5	2147 1.3
15 SA	0424 6.3	1042 1.6	1642 6.4	2307 1.5
30 SU	0354 6.5	1012 1.2	1617 6.9	2239 0.9

JULY

Day	Time m	Time m	Time m	Time m
1 M ○	0445 6.8	1103 0.9	1707 7.1	2330 0.6
16 TU	0519 6.3	1135 1.6	1734 6.5	2359 1.5
2 TU	0534 7.0	1152 0.7	1756 7.3	
17 W	0553 6.3	1209 1.5	1806 6.5	
3 W	0019 0.5	0622 7.1	1241 0.7	1845 7.3
18 TH	0032 1.5	0625 6.3	1242 1.6	1839 6.5
4 TH	0109 0.5	0710 7.0	1331 0.8	1934 7.2
19 F	0104 1.5	0658 6.2	1314 1.6	1911 6.4
5 F	0158 0.7	0758 6.7	1420 1.1	2023 6.9
20 SA	0136 1.6	0731 6.1	1348 1.7	1944 6.2
6 SA	0248 1.0	0848 6.4	1512 1.4	2114 6.5
21 SU	0210 1.8	0806 6.0	1425 1.9	2020 6.0
7 SU	0339 1.4	0940 6.0	1606 1.8	2209 6.1
22 M	0248 2.0	0846 5.8	1506 2.1	2103 5.8
8 M	0434 1.8	1036 5.7	1706 2.1	2310 5.7
23 TU	0332 2.2	0934 5.6	1555 2.3	2154 5.6
9 TU	0535 2.2	1144 5.5	1812 2.3	
24 W	0425 2.4	1033 5.4	1654 2.5	2259 5.4
10 W	0017 5.5	0641 2.3	1256 5.5	1922 2.3
25 TH	0530 2.4	1143 5.4	1804 2.4	
11 TH	0127 5.5	0750 2.3	1403 5.6	2027 2.2
26 F	0015 5.4	0644 2.4	1258 5.6	1919 2.2
12 F	0231 5.6	0850 2.1	1459 5.8	2122 2.0
27 SA	0131 5.7	0755 2.1	1407 6.0	2028 1.8
13 SA	0323 5.8	0940 2.0	1545 6.1	2208 1.8
28 SU	0242 6.1	0859 1.7	1508 6.4	2129 1.3
14 SU	0406 6.0	1023 1.8	1624 6.2	2248 1.6
29 M	0338 6.5	0955 1.2	1603 6.9	2224 0.9
15 M ●	0444 6.2	1101 1.7	1700 6.4	2325 1.5
30 TU ○	0430 6.9	1048 0.9	1654 7.2	2316 0.5
31 W	0520 7.1	1138 0.6	1743 7.5	

AUGUST

Day	Time m	Time m	Time m	Time m
1 TH	0005 0.4	0607 7.2	1227 0.5	1830 7.5
16 F	0007 1.3	0601 6.5	1217 1.4	1814 6.6
2 F	0052 0.4	0652 7.1	1314 0.6	1915 7.3
17 SA	0038 1.3	0632 6.5	1249 1.4	1845 6.6
3 SA	0139 0.6	0736 6.9	1400 0.9	2000 7.0
18 SU	0109 1.4	0704 6.4	1322 1.5	1917 6.5
4 SU	0224 1.0	0821 6.6	1442 1.3	2045 6.6
19 M	0142 1.6	0737 6.3	1357 1.7	1952 6.3
5 M	0310 1.4	0907 6.1	1536 1.8	2134 6.1
20 TU	0218 1.8	0814 6.0	1437 1.9	2031 6.0
6 TU	0400 1.9	0959 5.8	1630 2.2	2229 5.6
21 W	0300 2.0	0859 5.8	1523 2.2	2120 5.7
7 W	0456 2.4	1059 5.4	1734 2.5	2337 5.3
22 TH	0351 2.3	0955 5.5	1621 2.4	2224 5.4
8 TH	0602 2.6	1218 5.2	1848 2.6	
23 F	0455 2.5	1108 5.4	1733 2.5	2345 5.3
9 F	0056 5.2	0718 2.6	1337 5.4	2003 2.5
24 SA	0614 2.5	1232 5.5	1855 2.3	
10 SA	0209 5.4	0827 2.4	1438 5.6	2102 2.2
25 SU	0113 5.6	0734 2.2	1349 5.9	2011 1.9
11 SU	0304 5.6	0920 2.2	1525 5.9	2148 1.9
26 M	0224 6.0	0843 1.8	1453 6.4	2114 1.4
12 M	0347 5.9	1002 1.9	1604 6.2	2227 1.7
27 TU	0324 6.5	0941 1.3	1548 7.0	2209 0.9
13 TU	0424 6.1	1039 1.7	1639 6.4	2302 1.5
28 W ○	0415 7.0	1033 0.8	1639 7.4	2300 0.5
14 W ●	0458 6.3	1113 1.5	1711 6.5	2335 1.4
29 TH	0503 7.2	1122 0.6	1725 7.6	2347 0.3
15 TH	0530 6.4	1145 1.4	1743 6.6	
30 F	0548 7.3	1208 0.5	1810 7.6	
31 SA	0031 0.4	0630 7.3	1252 0.6	1852 7.4

16

Chart Datum: 4·45 metres below Lallemand System (Mean Sea Level, Marseilles)

TIME ZONE –0100
(French Standard Time)
Subtract 1 hour for UT

For French Summer Time add
ONE hour in non-shaded areas

FRANCE – BREST

LAT 48°23′N   LONG   4°30′W

TIMES AND HEIGHTS OF HIGH AND LOW WATERS   YEAR **1996**

SEPTEMBER

Day	Time	m	Day	Time	m
1 SU	0114 / 0709 / 1335 / 1932	0.6 / 7.0 / 0.9 / 7.0	16 M	0043 / 0638 / 1257 / 1852	1.3 / 6.7 / 1.3 / 6.7
2 M	0156 / 0750 / 1418 / 2013	1.0 / 6.6 / 1.3 / 6.5	17 TU	0117 / 0712 / 1333 / 1928	1.4 / 6.5 / 1.5 / 6.5
3 TU	0238 / 0831 / 1503 / 2056	1.6 / 6.2 / 1.8 / 6.0	18 W	0154 / 0749 / 1414 / 2008	1.7 / 6.3 / 1.8 / 6.1
4 W	0323 / 0917 / 1553 / 2148	2.1 / 5.7 / 2.3 / 5.5	19 TH	0236 / 0834 / 1502 / 2058	2.0 / 6.0 / 2.1 / 5.8
5 TH	0415 / 1016 / 1653 / 2255	2.5 / 5.3 / 2.7 / 5.1	20 F	0328 / 0931 / 1600 / 2204	2.3 / 5.7 / 2.4 / 5.5
6 F	0520 / 1135 / 1810	2.9 / 5.1 / 2.9	21 SA	0433 / 1047 / 1715 / 2330	2.6 / 5.5 / 2.5 / 5.3
7 SA	0021 / 0642 / 1304 / 1933	5.0 / 2.9 / 5.2 / 2.7	22 SU	0556 / 1217 / 1841	2.6 / 5.6 / 2.3
8 SU	0143 / 0758 / 1412 / 2036	5.2 / 2.7 / 5.5 / 2.4	23 M	0103 / 0721 / 1336 / 1958	5.6 / 2.3 / 6.0 / 1.9
9 M	0240 / 0853 / 1459 / 2122	5.5 / 2.4 / 5.8 / 2.1	24 TU	0212 / 0830 / 1439 / 2100	6.1 / 1.8 / 6.5 / 1.4
10 TU	0322 / 0935 / 1538 / 2200	5.9 / 2.0 / 6.1 / 1.8	25 W	0309 / 0927 / 1533 / 2153	6.6 / 1.3 / 7.0 / 0.9
11 W	0358 / 1012 / 1612 / 2235	6.2 / 1.7 / 6.4 / 1.5	26 TH	0359 / 1017 / 1621 / 2241	7.0 / 0.9 / 7.3 / 0.6
12 TH	0431 / 1046 / 1645 / ● 2308	6.4 / 1.5 / 6.6 / 1.3	27 F	0444 / 1104 / 1705 / O 2326	7.2 / 0.6 / 7.5 / 0.5
13 F	0503 / 1119 / 1718 / 2340	6.6 / 1.4 / 6.7 / 1.2	28 SA	0526 / 1148 / 1747	7.3 / 0.6 / 7.5
14 SA	0535 / 1152 / 1748	6.7 / 1.3 / 6.8	29 SU	0008 / 0606 / 1229 / 1827	0.6 / 7.2 / 0.7 / 7.3
15 SU	0012 / 0606 / 1224 / 1820	1.2 / 6.7 / 1.3 / 6.8	30 M	0048 / 0643 / 1310 / 1904	0.8 / 7.0 / 1.0 / 6.9

OCTOBER

Day	Time	m	Day	Time	m
1 TU	0127 / 0720 / 1350 / 1942	1.2 / 6.7 / 1.4 / 6.5	16 W	0056 / 0652 / 1316 / 1911	1.3 / 6.8 / 1.4 / 6.6
2 W	0207 / 0758 / 1432 / 2022	1.7 / 6.3 / 1.9 / 6.0	17 TH	0136 / 0733 / 1400 / 1955	1.6 / 6.5 / 1.6 / 6.3
3 TH	0248 / 0840 / 1518 / 2109	2.2 / 5.8 / 2.4 / 5.5	18 F	0221 / 0821 / 1449 / 2048	1.9 / 6.2 / 1.9 / 5.9
4 F	0336 / 0933 / 1613 / 2212	2.6 / 5.4 / 2.8 / 5.1	19 SA	0315 / 0920 / 1540 / 2156	2.2 / 5.9 / 2.2 / 5.6
5 SA	0436 / 1046 / 1724 / 2336	3.0 / 5.1 / 3.0 / 4.9	20 SU	0422 / 1037 / 1704 / 2321	2.5 / 5.6 / 2.4 / 5.4
6 SU	0554 / 1216 / 1849	3.1 / 5.1 / 2.9	21 M	0544 / 1202 / 1827	2.5 / 5.7 / 2.3
7 M	0103 / 0716 / 1331 / 1958	5.1 / 2.9 / 5.3 / 2.6	22 TU	0046 / 0705 / 1319 / 1941	5.7 / 2.3 / 6.1 / 1.9
8 TU	0204 / 0816 / 1423 / 2047	5.4 / 2.6 / 5.7 / 2.3	23 W	0155 / 0813 / 1421 / 2042	6.1 / 1.8 / 6.5 / 1.5
9 W	0248 / 0901 / 1504 / 2127	5.8 / 2.2 / 6.0 / 1.9	24 TH	0251 / 0909 / 1514 / 2134	6.5 / 1.4 / 6.9 / 1.1
10 TH	0326 / 0940 / 1541 / 2203	6.2 / 1.8 / 6.4 / 1.6	25 F	0339 / 0959 / 1601 / 2221	6.9 / 1.1 / 7.1 / 1.0
11 F	0401 / 1016 / 1616 / 2238	6.5 / 1.5 / 6.6 / 1.4	26 SA	0423 / 1044 / 1644 / O 2304	7.1 / 0.9 / 7.3 / 0.8
12 SA	0435 / 1051 / 1650 / ● 2312	6.7 / 1.3 / 6.8 / 1.2	27 SU	0504 / 1125 / 1725 / 2345	7.2 / 0.9 / 7.2 / 0.9
13 SU	0508 / 1126 / 1723 / 2346	6.9 / 1.2 / 6.9 / 1.2	28 M	0542 / 1207 / 1803	7.1 / 0.9 / 7.0
14 M	0541 / 1201 / 1757	6.9 / 1.2 / 6.9	29 TU	0023 / 0618 / 1246 / 1839	1.1 / 6.9 / 1.2 / 6.8
15 TU	0020 / 0615 / 1237 / 1833	1.2 / 6.9 / 1.2 / 6.8	30 W	0101 / 0654 / 1324 / 1916	1.4 / 6.7 / 1.5 / 6.4
			31 TH	0138 / 0731 / 1404 / 1954	1.8 / 6.3 / 1.9 / 6.0

NOVEMBER

Day	Time	m	Day	Time	m
1 F	0217 / 0810 / 1446 / 2037	2.2 / 5.9 / 2.3 / 5.6	16 SA	0213 / 0815 / 1443 / 2044	1.7 / 6.5 / 1.7 / 6.1
2 SA	0301 / 0856 / 1534 / 2131	2.6 / 5.5 / 2.7 / 5.2	17 SU	0308 / 0914 / 1542 / 2148	2.0 / 6.1 / 2.0 / 5.8
3 SU	0353 / 0955 / 1634 / 2242	2.9 / 5.2 / 2.9 / 5.0	18 M	0412 / 1024 / 1651 / 2304	2.3 / 5.9 / 2.1 / 5.6
4 M	0459 / 1111 / 1747	3.0 / 5.1 / 3.0	19 TU	0526 / 1140 / 1805	2.4 / 5.9 / 2.1
5 TU	0003 / 0615 / 1230 / 1902	5.0 / 3.0 / 5.2 / 2.8	20 W	0022 / 0642 / 1254 / 1916	5.7 / 2.2 / 6.0 / 2.0
6 W	0112 / 0724 / 1333 / 2000	5.3 / 2.7 / 5.5 / 2.5	21 TH	0131 / 0750 / 1358 / 2019	6.0 / 2.0 / 6.3 / 1.7
7 TH	0205 / 0817 / 1422 / 2046	5.6 / 2.4 / 5.8 / 2.1	22 F	0229 / 0849 / 1452 / 2113	6.3 / 1.6 / 6.6 / 1.4
8 F	0248 / 0902 / 1505 / 2127	6.0 / 2.0 / 6.2 / 1.8	23 SA	0319 / 0940 / 1541 / 2201	6.6 / 1.4 / 6.7 / 1.3
9 SA	0327 / 0943 / 1545 / 2206	6.4 / 1.7 / 6.5 / 1.5	24 SU	0403 / 1026 / 1625 / 2244	6.8 / 1.2 / 6.9 / 1.2
10 SU	0405 / 1022 / 1623 / 2244	6.7 / 1.4 / 6.7 / 1.3	25 M	0444 / 1108 / 1705 / O 2324	6.9 / 1.1 / 6.9 / 1.2
11 M	0442 / 1101 / 1700 / ● 2321	6.9 / 1.2 / 6.9 / 1.1	26 TU	0522 / 1148 / 1743	6.9 / 1.2 / 6.8
12 TU	0519 / 1140 / 1738	7.0 / 1.1 / 7.0	27 W	0002 / 0558 / 1225 / 1819	1.3 / 6.8 / 1.3 / 6.6
13 W	0000 / 0558 / 1221 / 1818	1.1 / 7.1 / 1.1 / 6.9	28 TH	0038 / 0634 / 1302 / 1855	1.5 / 6.6 / 1.5 / 6.4
14 TH	0041 / 0639 / 1304 / 1902	1.2 / 7.0 / 1.2 / 6.7	29 F	0115 / 0709 / 1339 / 1931	1.7 / 6.4 / 1.8 / 6.1
15 F	0125 / 0724 / 1351 / 1949	1.4 / 6.8 / 1.4 / 6.4	30 SA	0151 / 0746 / 1417 / 2010	2.0 / 6.1 / 2.1 / 5.8

DECEMBER

Day	Time	m	Day	Time	m
1 SU	0230 / 0825 / 1458 / 2054	2.3 / 5.8 / 2.4 / 5.5	16 M	0258 / 0903 / 1529 / 2133	1.6 / 6.5 / 1.6 / 6.1
2 M	0314 / 0911 / 1546 / 2147	2.6 / 5.5 / 2.7 / 5.2	17 TU	0357 / 1003 / 1630 / 2237	1.9 / 6.2 / 1.9 / 5.8
3 TU	0406 / 1008 / 1643 / 2254	2.8 / 5.3 / 2.8 / 5.1	18 W	0502 / 1110 / 1736 / 2348	2.2 / 5.9 / 2.1 / 5.7
4 W	0509 / 1118 / 1752	2.9 / 5.2 / 2.8	19 TH	0612 / 1221 / 1845	2.3 / 5.9 / 2.1
5 TH	0006 / 0619 / 1231 / 1900	5.2 / 2.8 / 5.3 / 2.6	20 F	0100 / 0722 / 1330 / 1953	5.8 / 2.2 / 5.9 / 2.0
6 F	0111 / 0724 / 1335 / 1958	5.4 / 2.6 / 5.6 / 2.3	21 SA	0205 / 0827 / 1431 / 2052	6.0 / 2.0 / 6.1 / 1.9
7 SA	0205 / 0820 / 1427 / 2048	5.8 / 2.2 / 5.9 / 2.0	22 SU	0259 / 0922 / 1523 / 2143	6.2 / 1.7 / 6.3 / 1.7
8 SU	0252 / 0909 / 1514 / 2134	6.1 / 1.9 / 6.3 / 1.6	23 M	0347 / 1010 / 1609 / 2227	6.4 / 1.6 / 6.4 / 1.5
9 M	0336 / 0954 / 1558 / 2217	6.5 / 1.5 / 6.6 / 1.3	24 TU	0428 / 1052 / 1649 / O 2307	6.6 / 1.4 / 6.5 / 1.5
10 TU	0419 / 1039 / 1640 / ● 2300	6.8 / 1.2 / 6.8 / 1.1	25 W	0506 / 1131 / 1727 / 2344	6.7 / 1.4 / 6.5 / 1.5
11 W	0501 / 1123 / 1724 / 2344	7.1 / 1.0 / 7.0 / 1.0	26 TH	0542 / 1207 / 1802	6.7 / 1.4 / 6.5
12 TH	0545 / 1208 / 1808	7.2 / 0.8 / 7.0	27 F	0019 / 0616 / 1242 / 1836	1.5 / 6.6 / 1.5 / 6.4
13 F	0029 / 0630 / 1255 / 1855	1.0 / 7.2 / 0.9 / 6.9	28 SA	0053 / 0649 / 1317 / 1910	1.6 / 6.5 / 1.6 / 6.2
14 SA	0116 / 0718 / 1343 / 1943	1.1 / 7.1 / 1.0 / 6.7	29 SU	0127 / 0723 / 1351 / 1944	1.8 / 6.3 / 1.8 / 6.0
15 SU	0205 / 0808 / 1434 / 2035	1.3 / 6.8 / 1.3 / 6.4	30 M	0202 / 0757 / 1426 / 2020	2.0 / 6.1 / 2.1 / 5.8
			31 TU	0239 / 0834 / 1505 / 2101	2.2 / 5.9 / 2.3 / 5.5

Chart Datum: 4·45 metres below Lallemand System (Mean Sea Level, Marseilles)

CAMARET   10-16-29

Finistere 48°16'·80N 04°35'·19W

CHARTS
AC 3427, 798; SHOM 6678, 7148, 7149; Imray C36; ECM 540, 542; Stanfords 17

TIDES
+0500 Dover; ML 3·8; Duration 0610; Zone –0100

Standard Port BREST (←—)

Times				Height (metres)			
High Water		Low Water		MHWS	MHWN	MLWN	MLWS
0000	0600	0000	0600	6·9	5·4	2·6	1·0
1200	1800	1200	1800				
Differences CAMARET							
–0010	–0010	–0013	–0013	–0·3	–0·3	–0·1	0·0

SHELTER
Good, except in strong E winds. Plaisance La Pointe (5m) is mainly for visitors, but Styvel has some visitors berths for smaller craft (0·9m) and is nearer town. SW side of hbr dries; FVs berth on SSE side.

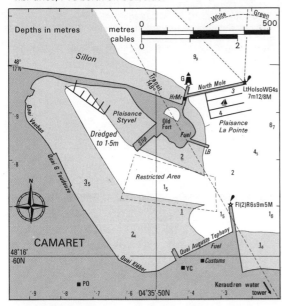

NAVIGATION
WPT 48°18'·00N 04°36'·00W, 335°/155° from/to N mole lt, 1·2M. Beware rks W of Pte du Grand Gouin. ⚓ in hbr prohib.

LIGHTS AND MARKS
Lt ho at E end of N mole, Iso WG 4s, W135°-182°, G182°-027°; appr in W sector. The G SHM bn tr at the W end of the N mole is very conspic; also Tour Vauban and chapel close SW. Ldg line at 148°: front mark = top of the old fort; rear = Keraudren water tr on hill behind.

RADIO TELEPHONE
VHF Ch 09. For Ouessant Traffic see Fig 10 (1).

TELEPHONE
Hr Mr 98·27·95·99; Aff Mar 98·27·93·28; SNSM 98·27·94·76; CROSS 98·89·31·31; ⌷ 98·27·93·02; Auto 36.68.08.29; Police 98·27·00·22;Dr 98·57·91·35; Brit Consul 40·63·16·02.

FACILITIES
Plaisance La Pointe (100+80 visitors) ☎ 98·27·95·99, FF88, FW, AC, C (8 ton), D, Access H24; **Plaisance 'Styvel'** (200+30 visitors), FW, AC, Access H24;
Services: M, ME, El, Ⓔ, Sh, CH, P, C (5 ton), SM, SHOM.
Town P, V, Gaz, R, Bar, ✉, Ⓑ, ⇌ (Brest), ✈ (Brest or Quimper). Ferry: Roscoff.

MORGAT   10-16-30

Finistere 48°13'·62N 04°29'·69W

CHARTS
AC 798; SHOM 6676, 6099; Imray C36; ECM 541, 542; Stanfords 17

TIDES
+0500 Dover; ML 3·8; Duration No data; Zone –0100

Standard Port BREST (←—)

Times				Height (metres)			
High Water		Low Water		MHWS	MHWN	MLWN	MLWS
0000	0600	0000	0600	6·9	5·4	2·6	1·0
1200	1800	1200	1800				
Differences MORGAT							
–0008	–0008	–0020	–0010	–0·4	–0·4	–0·2	0·0

SHELTER
The port is exposed to winds from the W and N, but the marina is protected by floating concrete wavebreaks. There are pleasant day ⚓s between Morgat and Cap de la Chèvre in the bays of St Hernot, St Norgard & St Nicolas; sheltered from the W. Also 2·5M to E in lee of Is de l'Aber.

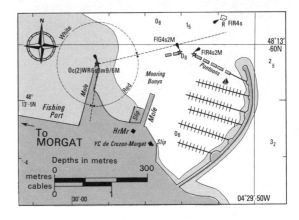

NAVIGATION
WPT 48°12'·00N 04°28'·00W, 147°/327° from/to E bkwtr hd, 1·9M. There are rks close under the cliffs S of Pte de Morgat, and Les Verres 2M ESE of ent. Ent chan, dredged 1·4m, is marked by PHM buoy Fl R 4s and Fl R/G 4s lts at end of wavebreaks.

LIGHTS AND MARKS
Pte de Morgat lt, Oc (4) WRG 12s 77m 15/10M, is 4ca S of hbr; G sector covers Les Verres. Appr in W sector, 007°-257°, of inner Mole lt, Oc (2) WR 6s 8m 9/6M.

RADIO TELEPHONE
VHF Ch 25 87. Marina 09 16.

TELEPHONE
Hr Mr 98·27·01·97; Aff Mar 98·27·09·95; CROSS 98·89·31·31; Auto 36.68.08.29; SNSM 98·27·00 41; ⌷ 98·27·93·02; Police 98·27·00·22; Ⓗ 98·27·05·33; Brit Consul 40·63·16·02.

FACILITIES
Marina (450+50 visitors), ☎ 98·27·01·97, Fax 98. 27.19.76, FF74, AC, FW, C (8 ton), Slip, CH, D, P, ME, Access H24;
YC du Crozon-Morgat ☎ 98·27·01·98;
Services: M, C (6 ton), El, Sh, Ⓔ.
Town (Crozon), V, Gaz, R, Bar, ✉, Ⓑ, ⇌, ✈ (Brest or Quimper). Ferry: Roscoff.

16

DOUARNENEZ   10-16-31

Finistere 48°06'·17N 04°20'·32W

CHARTS

AC 798; SHOM 6677, 6099; Imray C36; ECM 542; Stanfords 17

TIDES

+0500 Dover; ML 3·7; Duration 0615; Zone −0100

Standard Port BREST (←)

Times				Height (metres)			
High Water		Low Water		MHWS	MHWN	MLWN	MLWS
0000	0600	0000	0600	6·9	5·4	2·6	1·0
1200	1800	1200	1800				
Differences DOUARNENEZ							
−0010	−0015	−0018	−0008	−0·5	−0·5	−0·3	−0·1

SHELTER

Very good; access H24, all weathers and tides to visitors' berths in the marina (1·5m) at Tréboul, or in the river outside (subject to wash from passing traffic). About 2ca S of the marina the river has been dammed to form a non-tidal basin (3·2m), Port Rhu, as a museum for classic craft; limited access via a lock opening HW±1½ sp, HW±½ nps. The Fishing hbr is prohib to yachts and Port du Rosmeur is full of moorings.

NAVIGATION

WPT 48°07'·00N 04°20'·30W, 353°/173° from/to Ile Tristan lt, 0·81M. There are 3 rks, from 3 to 9ca NW of Ile Tristan lt (in R sector), Basse Veur, Petite Basse Neuve and Basse Neuve, least depth 1·8m.

LIGHTS AND MARKS

Approx 5M to W is Pte du Milier lt, Oc (2) WRG 6s 34m 16/11M, G080°-087°, W087°-113°, R113°-120°, W120°-129°, G129°-148°, W148°-251°, R 251°-258°.
Ile Tristan Oc (3) WR 12s 33m 13/10M, vis R138°-153°, W elsewhere; R sector covers Basse Veur and Basse Neuve, least depth 1·8m.
On the high road bridge at S end of Port Rhu, Dir lt 157°, Fl (5) WRG 20s 16m 5/4M, covers the Grande Passe and river; vis G154°-156°, W156°-158°, R158°-160°.
Port Rhu lock ent is marked by a Fl R 5s and a Fl G 5s.

RADIO TELEPHONE

Marina VHF Ch 09 (0700-1200 and 1330-2100LT in season; out of season 0830-1200, 1330-1730LT). Port Ch 12 16.

TELEPHONE

Hr Mr (Plaisance) 98·74·02·56; Aff Mar 98·92·00·91; CROSS 98·89·31·31; SNSM 98·89·63·16; ⌗ 98·92·01·45; Meteo 98·84·60·64; Auto 36.68.08.29; Police 98·92·01·22; Ⓗ 98·92·25·00; Brit Consul 40·63·16·02.

FACILITIES

Marina (380+30 visitors) ☎ 98·74·02·56, Fax 98.74.05.08, FF82, Slip, FW, AC, P, D, C (6 ton), ME, El, Sh, Ⓒ;
Sté des Regates de Douarnenez ☎ 98·92·02·03;
Services: M, CH, BH (12 ton), SM, Ⓔ.
Town Slip, P, D, Gaz, V, R, Bar, ✉, Ⓑ, ⇌ and ✈ (Quimper 22km). Ferry: Roscoff.

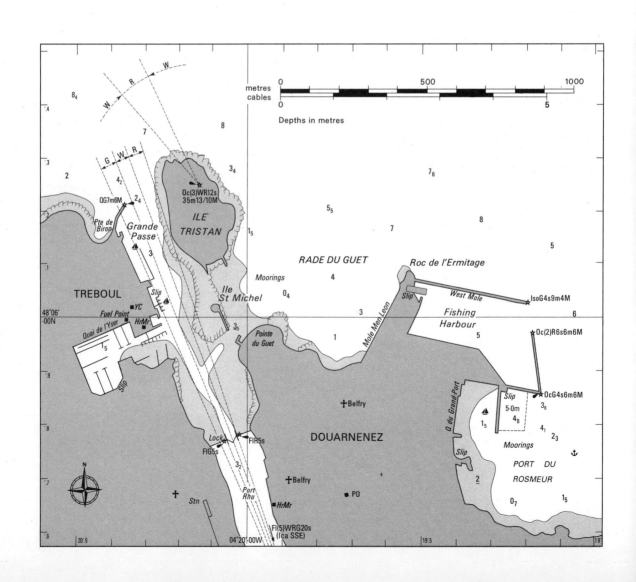

Volvo Penta service

Sales and service centres in area 17
Names and addresses of Volvo Penta dealers in
this area are available from:
France *Volvo Penta France SA,* 1 Rue de la Nouvelle, B. P. 49, 78133 Les
Mureaux Tel 33-1-30912799, Fax 33-1-34746415 Telex 695221 F.

Area 17

South Brittany
Raz de Sein to River Loire

**VOLVO
PENTA**

17

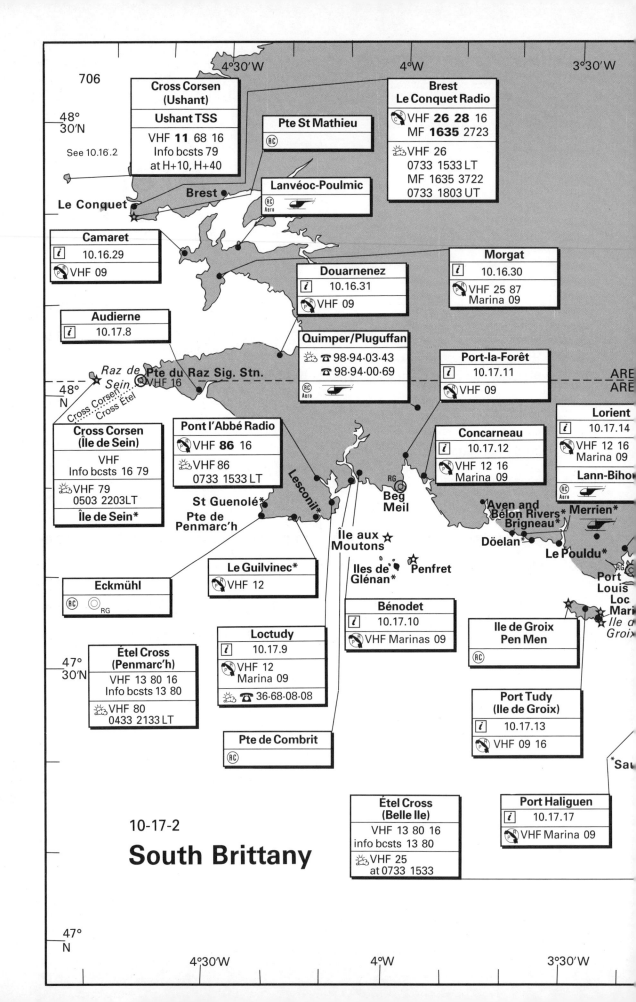

706

48°
30'N

See 10.16.2

Cross Corsen
(Ushant)

Ushant TSS

VHF **11** 68 16
Info bcsts 79
at H+10, H+40

Pte St Mathieu
RC

Brest
Le Conquet Radio

VHF **26 28** 16
MF **1635** 2723

VHF 26
0733 1533 LT
MF 1635 3722
0733 1803 UT

Le Conquet
Brest

Lanvéoc-Poulmic
RC
Aero

Camaret

i   10.16.29

VHF 09

Morgat

i   10.16.30

VHF 25 87
Marina 09

Douarnenez

i   10.16.31

VHF 09

Audierne

i   10.17.8

Raz de Pte du Raz Sig. Stn.
48° *Sein* VHF 16
N

Cross Corsen
Cross Etel

Quimper/Pluguffan

☎ 98·94·03·43
☎ 98·94·00·69

RC
Aero

Port-la-Forêt

i   10.17.11

VHF 09

ARE
ARE

Cross Corsen
(Île de Sein)

VHF
Info bcsts 16 79

VHF 79
0503 2203LT

Île de Sein*

Pont l'Abbé Radio

VHF **86** 16

VHF 86
0733 1533 LT

Concarneau

i   10.17.12

VHF 12 16
Marina 09

Lorient

i   10.17.14

VHF 12 16
Marina 09

Lann-Biho
RC
Aero

Lesconil*

RG
Beg
Meil

*Aven and
Bélon Rivers* Merrien*
Brigneau*

St Guenolé*
Pte de
Penmarc'h

Döelan*

Le Pouldu*

Eckmühl
RC ◎
RG

Le Guilvinec*

VHF 12

Île aux ☆
Moutons

Iles de ☆ Penfret
Glénan*

RG
Port
Louis
Loc
Mari
*Île a
Groi*

Bénodet

i   10.17.10

VHF Marinas 09

Ile de Groix
Pen Men

RC

47°
30'N

Étel Cross
(Penmarc'h)

VHF 13 80 16
Info bcsts 13 80

VHF 80
0433 2133 LT

Loctudy

i   10.17.9

VHF 12
Marina 09

☎ 36·68·08·08

Port Tudy
(Ile de Groix)

i   10.17.13

VHF 09 16

Pte de Combrit
RC

10-17-2

South Brittany

Étel Cross
(Belle Ile)

VHF 13 80 16
info bcsts 13 80

VHF 25
at 0733 1533

Port Haliguen

i   10.17.17

VHF Marina 09

*Sau

47°
N

4°30'W   4°W   3°30'W

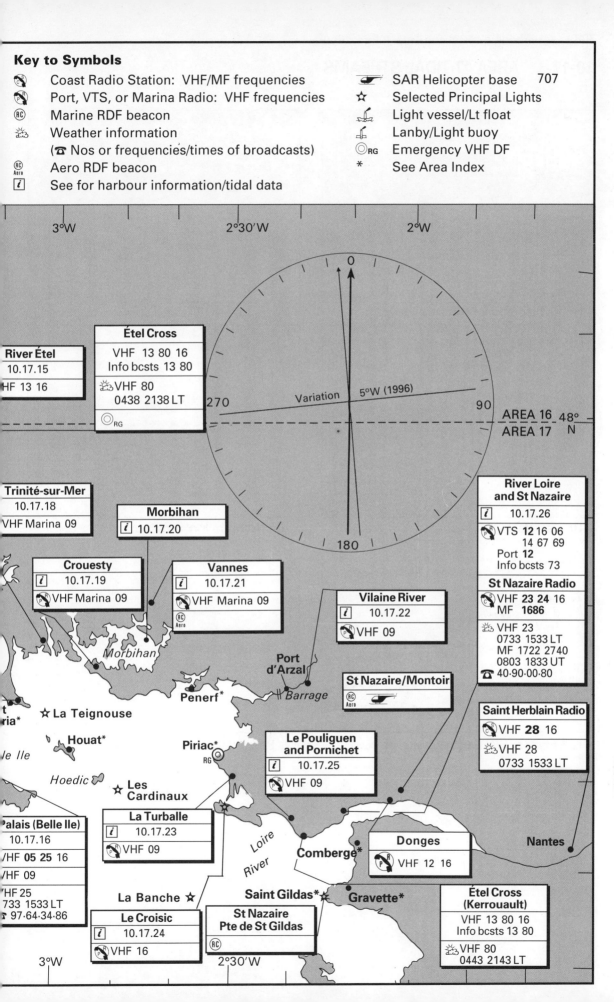

Key to Symbols

C	Coast Radio Station: VHF/MF frequencies	SAR Helicopter base	707
P/R	Port, VTS, or Marina Radio: VHF frequencies	☆ Selected Principal Lights	
RC	Marine RDF beacon	Light vessel/Lt float	
Weather information	(☎ Nos or frequencies/times of broadcasts)	Lanby/Light buoy	
RC Aero	Aero RDF beacon	©RG Emergency VHF DF	
i	See for harbour information/tidal data	* See Area Index	

River Étel
10.17.15
HF 13 16

Étel Cross
VHF 13 80 16
Info bcsts 13 80

VHF 80
0438 2138 LT
©RG

Variation 5°W (1996)

AREA 16
AREA 17
48° N

Trinité-sur-Mer
10.17.18
VHF Marina 09

Morbihan
i 10.17.20

Crouesty
i 10.17.19
VHF Marina 09

Vannes
i 10.17.21
VHF Marina 09
RC Aero

Morbihan

Vilaine River
i 10.17.22
VHF 09

River Loire and St Nazaire
i 10.17.26
VTS 12 16 06
14 67 69
Port 12
Info bcsts 73

St Nazaire Radio
VHF 23 24 16
MF 1686

VHF 23
0733 1533 LT
MF 1722 2740
0803 1833 UT
☎ 40·90·00·80

Port d'Arzal
Barrage

St Nazaire/Montoir
RC Aero

☆ La Teignouse

Penerf*

Saint Herblain Radio
VHF 28 16

VHF 28
0733 1533 LT

Houat*

Piriac*
RG

le Ile

Hoedic

☆ Les Cardinaux

Le Pouliguen and Pornichet
i 10.17.25
VHF 09

Nantes

alais (Belle Ile)
10.17.16
VHF 05 25 16
VHF 09
HF 25
733 1533 LT
☎ 97·64·34·86

La Turballe
i 10.17.23
VHF 09

Loire River

Comberge*

Donges
VHF 12 16

La Banche ☆

Saint Gildas*

Gravette*

Étel Cross (Kerrouault)
VHF 13 80 16
Info bcsts 13 80

VHF 80
0443 2143 LT

Le Croisic
i 10.17.24
VHF 16

St Nazaire Pte de St Gildas
RC

17

10·17·3   AREA 17 TIDAL STREAMS

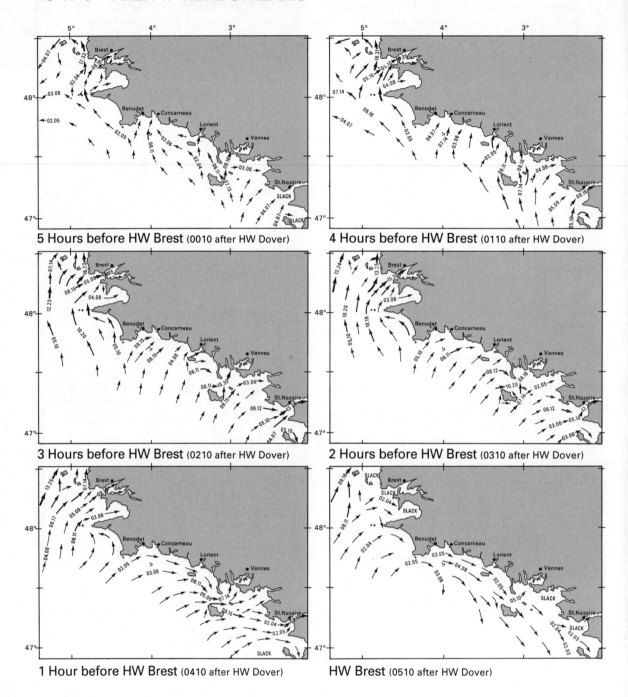

5 Hours before HW Brest (0010 after HW Dover)

4 Hours before HW Brest (0110 after HW Dover)

3 Hours before HW Brest (0210 after HW Dover)

2 Hours before HW Brest (0310 after HW Dover)

1 Hour before HW Brest (0410 after HW Dover)

HW Brest (0510 after HW Dover)

Northward 10.16.3   Southward 10.18.3

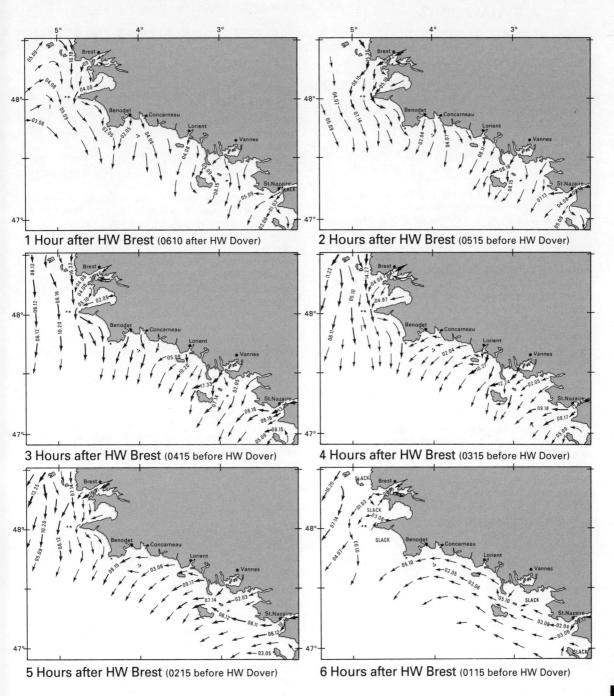

1 Hour after HW Brest (0610 after HW Dover)

2 Hours after HW Brest (0515 before HW Dover)

3 Hours after HW Brest (0415 before HW Dover)

4 Hours after HW Brest (0315 before HW Dover)

5 Hours after HW Brest (0215 before HW Dover)

6 Hours after HW Brest (0115 before HW Dover)

17

10.17.4 COASTAL LIGHTS, FOG SIGNALS AND WAYPOINTS

Abbreviations used below are given in 1.4.1. Principal lights are in **bold** print, places in CAPITALS, and light-vessels, light floats and Lanbys in *CAPITAL ITALICS*. Unless otherwise stated lights are white. m – elevation in metres; M – nominal range in miles. Fog signals are in *italics*. Useful waypoints are underlined – use those on land with care. All geographical positions should be assumed to be approximate. See 4.4.1.

RAZ DE SEIN TO LESCONIL

CHAUSSÉE DE SEIN/ÎLE DE SEIN
Chaussée de Sein Lt By 48°03'·80N 05°07'·70W VQ (9) 10s 9m 8M; WCM HFP;Racon (O); *Whis.*
Ar-Men 48°03'·06N 04°59'·80W Fl (3) 20s 29m **24M**; W Tr, B top. *Horn (3) 60s.*
Île de Sein 48°02'·70N 04°51'·95W Fl (4) 25s 49m **29M**; W Tr, B top; RC.
Ar Guéveur 48°02'·00N 04°51'·32W 20m; W Tr; *Dia 60s.*
Men-Brial, 0·8M 115° from main Lt, Oc (2) WRG 6s 16m W12M, R9M, G7M; G&W Tr; vis G149°-186°, W186°-192°, R192°-221°, W221°-227°, G227°-254°.
Cornoc-An-Ar-Braden Lt By 48°03'·30N 04°50'·80W Iso G 4s; SHM; *Whis.*

RAZ DE SEIN
Tévennec 48°04'·34N 04°47'·65W VQ WR 28m W10M R7M; W ■ Tr and dwelling; vis W090°-345°, R345°-090°; Dir Lt Iso 4s 24m 12M; same Tr; intens 324°-332°.
La Vieille 48°02'·49N 04°45'·31W Oc (2+1) WRG 12s 33m **W17M**, R14M, G13M; Gy ■Tr; vis W290°-298°, R298°-325°, W325°-355°, G355°-017°, W017°-035°, G035°-105°, W105°-123°, R123°-158°, W158°-205°; R Lt on radio mast 3·4M ENE; *Horn (2+1) 60s.*
La Plate 48°02'·36N 04°45'·50W VQ (9) 10s 19m 8M; WCM.
Le Chat 48°01'·44N 04°48'·80W Fl (2) WRG 6s 27m W9M, R6M, G6M; SCM; vis G096°-215°, W215°-230°, R230°-271°, G271°-286°, R286°-096°; Ra refl.

AUDIERNE
Pointe de Lervily 48°00'·11N 04°33'·84W Fl (2+1) WR 12s 20m W14M, R11M; W Tr, R top; vis W211°-269°, R269°-294°, W294°-087°, R087°-121°.
Gamelle W Lt By 47°59'·53N 04°32'·76W VQ (9) 10s; WCM; *Whis.*
Kergadec Dir Lt 006°. 48°01'·01N 04°32'·80W Dir Q WRG 43m W12M, R9M, G9M; vis G000°-005·3°, W005·3°-006·7° R006·7°-017°.
Jetée de Sainte-Évette 48°00'·38N 04°32'·98W Oc (2) R 6s 2m 7M; R lantern; vis 090°-270°.
Passe de l'Est Ldg Lts 331°. Front Jetée de Raoulic 48°00'·60N 04°32'·37W Oc (2+1) WG 12s 11m W14M, G9M; W ●Tr; vis W shore-034°, G034°-shore, but may show W037°-055°. Rear, Kergadec, 0·5M from front, Dir FR 44m 9M ; W 8-sided Tr, R top; intens 321°-341°.

PORS POULHAN
W side of ent 47°59'·15N 04°27'·80W QR 14m 9M; W ■ Tr, R lantern.

SAINT GUÉNOLÉ
Chenal de Groumilli Ldg Lts 123°. Front 47°48'·20N 04°22'·60W FG 9m 9M; Or ● on W Tr, B bands. Rear, 300m from front, FG 13m 9M ; Or ● on W Tr, B bands.
Basse Gaouac'h Lt By 47°48'·66N 04°24'·13W Fl (3) G 12s; SHM; *Whis.*
Scoedec 47°48'·46N 04°23'·10W Fl G 2·5s 6m 3M; G Tr.

Ldg Lts 055·4°. Front 47°48'·75N 04°22'·65W VQ 5m 2M; G &W col. Rear, 320m from front, F Vi 12m 1M; G&W col; vis 040°-070°.
Ldg Lts 026·5°. Front 47°49'·05N 04°22'·60W QR 8m 4M; R mast. Rear, 51m from front, QR 12m 4M; mast, R&W bands; synch with front.

POINTE DE PENMARC'H
Eckmühl 47°47'·95N 04°22'·35W Fl 5s 60m **24M**; Gy 8-sided Tr; RC; *Horn 60s.*
Menhir 47°47'·80N 04°23'·90W Fl (2) WG 6s 19m W8M, G5M; W Tr, B band; vis W135°-315°, W315°-135°.

LE GUILVINEC
Cap Caval Lt By 47°46'·52N 04°22'·60W Q (9) 15s; WCM; *Whis.*
Locarec 47°47'·33N 04°20'·30W Iso WRG 4s 11m W9M, R6M, G6M; W tank on rk; vis G063°-068°, R068°-271°, W271°-285°, R285°-298°, G298°-340°, R340°-063°.
Kérity. Men Hir 47°47'·3N 04°20'·6W Fl R 2·5s 6m 2M; R ■ on Bn.
Detached Bkwtr Hd 47°47'·6N 04°20'·9W Fl (2) G 6s 5m 1M.
Névez Lt By 47°46'·08N 04°19'·68W VQ; NCM.
Spinec Lt By 47°45'·24N 04°18'·80W Q (6) + L Fl 15s; SCM; *Whis.*
Le Guilvinec Ldg Lts 053°. Môle de Léchiagat, spur, front 47°47'·49N 04°17'·00W Q 7m 8M; W pylon; vis 233°-066°. Rocher Le Faoute's, Middle, 210m from front Q WG 12m W14M, G11M; R ● on W pylon; vis W006°-293°, G293°-006°; synch with front. Rear, 0·58M from front, Dir Q 26m 8M; R ● on W pylon; vis 051·5°-054·5°; synch with front.
Capelan Lt By 47°47'·21N 04°17'·47W Fl (2) G 6s; SHM.
Môle de Léchiagat Hd 47°47'·51N 04°17'·09W Fl G 4s 5m 7M; W hut, G top.
Lost Moan 47°47'·07N 04°16'·69W Fl (3) WRG 12s 8m W9M, R6M, G6M; ■ on W Tr, R top; vis R327°-014°, G014°-065°, R065°-140°, W140°-160°, R160°-268°, W268°-273°, G273°-317°, W317°-327°.
Ar Guisty Bn 47°45'·69N 04°15'·50W; SCM.

LESCONIL
Reissant Bn 47°46'·45N 04°13'·43W; SCM.
Men-ar-Groas 47°47'·86N 04°12'·60W Fl (3) WRG 12s 14m W13M, R9M, G9M; W Tr, G top; vis G268°-313°, W313°-333°, R333°-050°.
E Bkwtr Hd 47°47'·77N 04°12'·56W QG 5m 9M; G Tr.
Karek Greis Lt By 47°46'·10N 04°11'·30W Q (3) 10s; ECM; *Whis.*

LOCTUDY TO CONCARNEAU

LOCTUDY
Rostolou By 47°46'·70N 04°07'·20W; ECM.
Roc'h Hélou By 47°47'·17N 04°08'·00W; WCM.
Bas Boulanger Lt By 47°47'·40N 04°09'·05W VQ (6) + L Fl 10s; SCM.
Bilien Lt By 47°49'·17N 04°08'·02W VQ (3) 5s; ECM; *Whis.*
Chenal de Bénodet By 47°48'·60N 04°06'·96W; ECM.
Basse Malvic By 47°48'·52N 04°06'·53W; WCM.
Pointe de Langoz S side 47°49'·94N 04°09'·48W Fl (4) WRG 12s 12m **W15M**, R11M, G11M; W Tr, R top; vis W115°-257°, G257°-284°, W284°-295°, R295°-318°, W318°-328°, R328°-025°.
Men Audierne Bn 47°50'·37N 04°08'·98W; SHM.
Karek-Saoz 47°50'·08N 04°09'·30W QR 3m 1M; R Tr.
Les Perdrix 47°50'·31N 04°09'·88W Fl WRG 4s 15m W11M, R8M, G8M; ▲ on B&W Tr; vis G090°-285°, W285°-295°, R295°-090°.
Le Blas 47°50'·34N 04°10'·15W Fl (3) G 12s 5m 1M; G ▲ on truncated col

BENODET
Ldg Lts 345·5°. Front **Pte du Coq** 47°52'·38N 04°06'·61W, Dir Oc (2+1) G 12s 11m **17M**; W ● Tr, G stripe; intens 345°-347°. Common rear Pyramide, 336m from front, Oc (2+1) 12s 48m 11M; W Tr, G top; vis 338°-016°, synch with front.
Ldg Lts 000·5°. Front, Pte de Combrit 47°51'·92N 04°06'·70W, Oc (3+1) WR 12s 19m W12M , R9M; W ■ Tr, Gy corners; vis W325°-017°, R017°-325°; RC. Common rear Pyramide, 0·63M from front.
Les Verrés Bn 47°51'·61N 04°06'·06W; SHM.
Le Four Bn 47°51'·85N 04°06'·32W; SHM.
Pte du Toulgoet Fl R 2s 2m 2M; R mast.

Le Taro Bn 47°50'·57N 04°04'·86W; WCM.
Men Déhou Bn 47°48'·18N 04°04'·63W; ECM.
Les Poulains Bn 47°47'·75N 04°03'·40W; NCM.
La Voleuse Lt By 47°48'·81N 04°02'·40W Q (6) + L Fl 15s; SCM; _Whis_.
La Vache Bn 47°49'·60N 04°02'·53W; SHM.
Men Vras Bn 47°49'·72N 04°01'·50W; ECM.

BEG-MEIL
Linuen Bn 47°50'·71N 03°57'·70W; SCM.
Chaussée de Beg'Meil Lt By 47°50'·82N 03°57'·23W Q (3) 10s; ECM.
Laouen Pod Bn 47°51'·29N 03°57'·91W; ECM.
Quay Hd 47°51'·72N 03°58'·85W Fl R 2s 6m 2M; R&W col.

PORT-LA-FORÊT
Le Scoré Bn 47°52'·81N 03°57'·48W; SCM.
Les Ormeaux Bn 47°53'·33N 03°58'·25W; PHM.
Channel Lt By 47°53'·46N 03°58'·05W Fl (2) G 6s; SHM.
Ldg Lts 334°. Cap Coz Mole Hd Front 47°53'·55N 03°58'·20W Fl (2) R 6s 5m 6M. Rear, Kerleven Bkwtr Fl G 4s 8m 6M.

CONCARNEAU
Ldg Lts 028·5°. Front La Croix 47°52'·22N 03°55'·00W Oc (3) 12s 14m 13M; R&W Tr; vis 006·5°-093°. **Rear Beuzec**, 1·34M from front, Dir Q 87m **23M**; Spire; intens 026·5°-030·5°.
Le Cochon 47°51'·53N 03°55'·47W Fl (3) WRG 12s 5m W9M, R6M, G6M; G Tr; vis G048°-205°, R205°-352°, W352°-048°; SHM.
Basse du Chenal Lt Bn 47°51'·58N 03°55'·60W QR 6m 5M; PHM.
Men Fall Lt By 47°51'·82N 03°55'·20W Fl G 4s; SHM.
Kersos Bn 47°51'·87N 03°54'·85W; SHM.
Lanriec 47°52'·07N 03°54'·56W QG 13m 8M; G Lt window on W gable; vis 063°-078°.
La Medée 47°52'·12N 03°54'·71W Fl R 2·5s 6m 4M; R Tr: PHM.
Marina Hd 47°52'·20N 03°54'·72W Fl (3) R 12s; R □ on post.

BAIE DE POULDOHAN
Petit Taro Bn 47°51'·17N 03°55'·21W; WCM.
Pouldohan 47°51'·03N 03°53'·61W Fl G 4s 7m 8M; W ■ Tr, G top; vis 053°-065°.
Roché Tudy Bn 47°50'·58N 03°54'·41W; SHM.

ÎLES DE GLENAN

ÎLES DE GLÉNAN/ÎLE AUX MOUTONS
Basse Pérennès Lt By 47°41'·15N 04°06'·05W Q (9) 15s 8m 8M; WCM; _Whis_; Ra refl.
Jument de Glénan Lt By 47°38'·80N 04°01'·32W Q (6) + L Fl 15s 10m 8M; SCM; _Whis_; Ra Refl.
Penfret 47°43'·32N 03°57'·10W Fl R 5s 36m **21M**; W ■ Tr, R top; auxiliary Lt Dir Q 34m 12M; same Tr; vis 295°-315°.
Île Cigogne 47°43'·10N 03°59'·59W Q (2) RG 5s 2M; W Tr B top; vis G106°-108°, R108°-262°, G262°-268°, obsc 268°-106°; shown 1May to 1Oct.
Les Bluniers Bn 47°43'·42N 04°03'·73W; WCM.

Broc'h Bn 47°43'·22N 04°01'·31W; NCM.
La Pie Lt Bn 47°43'·81N 03°59'·65W; Fl (2) 6s 9m 3M. IDM.
Île de Bananec Bn 47°43'·32N 03°59'·11W; ECM.
Rouge de Glénan Lt By 47°45'·50N 04°03'·90W VQ (9) 10s 8m 8M ; WCM; _Whis_; Ra refl.
Île-aux-Moutons 47°46'·55N 04°01'·62W Oc (2) WRG 6s 18m **W15M**, R11M, G11M; W ■ Tr and dwelling; vis W035°-050°, G050°-063°, W063°-081°, R081°-141°, W141°-292°, R292°-035°; **auxiliary Lt** Dir Oc (2) 6s 17m **24M**; same Tr; synch with main Lt, intens 278·5°-283·5°.
Grand Pourceaux Lt By 47°46'·05N 04°00'·75W Q; NCM.
Rochers Leuriou Bn 47°45'·20N 03°59'·90W; ECM.
Jaune de Glénan Lt By 47°42'·60N 03°49'·75W Q (3) 10s; ECM; _Whis_.
Cor-Loch By 47°42'·28N 03°52'·22W; IDM.
Basse an Ero By 47°40'·47N 03°55'·38W; SCM.
Laoennou By 47°39'·70N 03°54'·60W; IDM.

CONCARNEAU TO ÎLE DE GROIX

TRÉVIGNON TO PORT MANECH
Les Soldats Lt Bn 47°47'·91N 03°53'·32W VQ (9) 10s; WCM.
Môle Hd 47°47'·72N 03°51'·20W Fl G 4s 5m 8M; W col, G top.
Trévignon Bkwtr root 47°47'·65N 03°51'·22W Oc (3+1) WRG 12s 11m W14M, R11M, G11M; W ■ Tr, G top; vis W004°-051°, G051°-085°, W085°-092°, R092°-127°, R322°-351°.
Men Du Bn 47°46'·44N 03°50'·40W; IDM.
Corn Vas By 47°45'·92N 03°50'·18W; WCM.
Men ar Tréas By 47°45'·84N 03°49'·58W; SCM.
Île Verte Bn 47°46'·35N 03°47'·95W.
Île de Raguénès By 47°46'·95N 03°47'·65W; SCM.

PORT MANECH/AVEN AND BÉLON RIVERS
Pointe de Beg-ar-Vechen 47°48'·03N 03°44'·30W Oc (4) WRG 12s 38m W10M, R7M, G7M; W & R Tr; vis W(unintens) 050°-140°, W140°-296°, G296°-303°, W303°-311°, R311°-328° over Les Verrès, W328°-050°; obsc by Pte de Beg-Morg when brg less than 299°.
Les Verrès Bn 47°46'·70N 03°42'·60W; IDM.

BRIGNEAU/MERRIEN/DOËLAN
Brigneau Mole Hd 47°46'·95N 03°40'·10W Oc (2) WRG 6s 7m W12M, R9M, G9M; W col, R top; vis G280°-329°, W329°-339°, R339°-034°.
Brigneau By 47°46'·15N 03°39'·99W; SWM; _Whis_.
Merrien Dir Lt 47°47'·05N 03°38'·82W QR 26m 7M; W ■ Tr, R top; vis 004°-009°.
Port de la Merrien By 47°46'·52N 03°39'·09W; SCM.
Doëlan Ldg Lts 013·8°. Front 47°46'·35N 03°36'·42W Oc (3) WG 12s 20m W13M, G10M; W Tr, G band and top; vis W shore-305°, G305°-314°, W314°-shore. Rear 326m from front, QR 27m 9M; W Tr, R band and top.

LE POULDU TO LOMENER/RIVIÈRE DE QUIMPERLÉ
Le Pouldu Ent Bn 47°45'·76N 03°32'·11W; PHM.
Grand Cochon By 47°43'·09N 03°30'·73W; SCM.
Kerroc'h 47°42'·00N 03°27'·53W Oc (2) WRG 6s 22m W11M, R8M, G8M; W Tr, R top; vis R096·5°-112°·5, G112·5°-132°, R132°-302°, W302°-096·5°.
Anse de Stole Dir Lt 357·2°. 47°42'·33N 03°25'·57W Dir Q WRG 18m W10M, R8M, G8M; W Tr, R top; vis G349·2°-355·2°, W355·2°-359·2°, R359·2°-005·2°.

ÎLE DE GROIX/PORT TUDY/LOCMARIA
Pen Men 47°38'·87N 03°30'·48W Fl (4) 25s 59m **29M**; W ■ Tr, B top; vis 309°-275°; RC.
Pointe des Chats 47°37'·30N 03°25'·25W Fl R 5s16m **19M**; W ■ Tr and dwelling.
Port Tudy Môle N Hd 47°38'·78N 03°26'·62W Iso G 4s 12m 6M; W Tr, G top.

17

Pointe de la Croix 47°38'·10N 03°25'·20W Oc WR 4s 16m W12M, R9M; W pedestal, R lantern; vis W169°-336°, R336°-345°, W345°-353°.
Edouard de Cougy By 47°37'·97N 03°23'·80W; ECM.
Les Chars Lt By 47°35'·74N 03°23'·50W Q (6) + L Fl 15s; SCM; *Whis*.

LORIENT

PASSE OUEST
Ldg Lts 057°. Front, Les Soeurs 47°42'·22N 03°21'·70W Dir Q 6m 13M, R Tr, W bands; vis intens 042·5°-058·5°, (4M) 058·5°-042·5°. Rear, **Port Louis** 740m from front, Dir Q **18M**; W daymark, R bands on bldg. Lts intens 042·5°-058·5°, (4M) 058·5°-042·5°.
'L' Banc des Truics Lt By 47°40'·82N 03°24'·40W Q (9) 15s; WCM.
A2 Locqueltas Lt By 47°41'·00N 03°24'·90W Fl R 2·5s; PHM.
A5 Lt By 47°41'·56N 03°23'·02W Fl (2) G 6s; SHM.
A7 Lt By 47°41'·77N 03°22'·58W Fl G 2·5s; SHM.
Les Trois Pierres 47°41'·58N 03°22'·40W Q RG 11m R6M, G6M; B Tr, R bands; vis G060°-196°, R196°-002°.
Île aux Souris 47°42'·22N 03°21'·43W Dir Q WG 6m W3M, G2W; G Tr; vis W041·5°-043·5°, G043·5°-041·5°.

PASSE DU SUD
Ldg Lts 008·5°. **Front**, Fish Market 47°43'·82N 03°21'·67W Dir QR 16m **15M**; R ■ on Gy Tr; intens 006°-011°. **Rear**, Kergroise-La Perrière 515m from front Dir QR 28m **16M**; R ■, W stripe on Gy Tr; synch with front; intens 006°-011°.
Bastresse Sud Lt By 47°40'·83N 03°22'·01W QG; SHM; *Bell*.
Les Errants Lt By 47°41'·16N 03°22'·29W Fl (2) R 6s; PHM.

ENTRANCE CHANNEL
Île Saint Michel Passe de la Citadelle Ldg Lts 016°. **Front** 47°43'·53N 03°21'·54W Dir Oc (3) G 12s 8m **16M**; W Tr, G top. **Rear**, 306m from front, Dir Oc (3) G 12s 14m **16M**; W Tr, G top; synch with front; both intens 014·5°-017·5°.
La Potée de Beurre Bn 47°42'·30N 03°21'·90W; SHM.
Chan W side, La Petite Jument 47°42'·63N 03°21'·98W Oc R 4s 5m 6M; R Tr; vis 182°-024°.
Chan E side, Tourelle de la Citadelle 47°42'·66N 03°21'·86W Oc G 4s 6m 6M; G Tr; vis 009°-193°.
Chan W side Le Cochon Fl R 4s 5m 5M; R Tr, G band.

KERNEVEL
Banc du Turc Lt By 47°43'·39N 03°21'·77W Fl (3) G 12s; SHM.
Port de Kernevel Marina ent Lt By 47°43'·47N 03°22'·01W Fl Y 2·5s; SPM with can topmark.
Ldg Lts 217°. 47°43'·08N 03°22'·23W Front Dir QR 10m 14M; R ■ on R&W Tr; intens 215°-219°. Rear, 290m from front, Dir QR 18m 14M; W ■Tr, R top; synch with front; intens 215°-219°.

PORT-LOUIS
Jetty 47°42'·76N 03°21'·29W Iso G 4s 7m 6M; W Tr, G top.

KÉROMAN/FISHING HARBOUR/RADE DE PENMANÉ
Submarine base Ldg Lts 350°. **Front** 47°43'·66N 03°21'·93W Dir Oc (2) R 6s 25m **17M**. **Rear**, 91m from front, Dir Oc (2) R 6s 31m **17M**; R&W topmark on Gy pylon, R top; Lts synch and intens 348°-353°.
E side of ent 47°43'·68N 03°21'·79W Fl RG 4s 7m 6M; W Tr, G top; vis G000°-235°, R235°-360°.
Pengarne 47°43'·94N 03°21'·13W Fl G 2·5s 3m 4M; G Tr.
Pointe de l'Espérance Dir Lt 037°. 47°44'·57N 03°20'·58W Dir Q WRG 8m W10M, R8M, G8M; W Tr, G top; vis G034·2°-036·7°, W036·7°-037·2°, R037·2°-047·2°.
Ro-Ro Terminal 47°44'·48N 03°20'·88W Oc (2) R 6s 7m 6M.
Lorient Marina ent Lt By No. 8 47°44'·61N 03°20'·90W Fl R 2·5s; PHM.

LORIENT TO BELLE ÎLE

RIVIÈRE D'ÉTEL
Roheu Bn 47°38'·57N 03°14'·68W; SCM.
W side ent 47°38'·75N 03°12'·82W Oc (2) WRG 6s 13m W9M, R6M, G6M; R Tr; vis W022°-064°, R064°-123°, W123°-330°, G330°-022°; 2 FR on radio Mast 2·3M NW; FR and F on radio masts 2·4M NW.
Les Pierres Noires Bn 47°35'·55N 03°13'·25W; IDM.

PORT MARIA
Le Pouilloux By 47°27'·97N 03°08'·93W; SCM.
Ldg Lts 006·5°. Front 47°28'·65N 03°07'·15W Dir QG 5m 13M; W Tr, B band. Rear, 230m from front, Dir QG 13m 13M; W Tr, B band; both intens 005°-008°.
Main light 47°28'·85N 03°07'·42W Q WRG 28m **W14M**, R10M, G10M; W Tr; vis W246°-252°, W291°-297°, G297°-340°, W340°-017°, R017°-051°, W051°-081°, G081°-098°, W098°-143°.
Baz an Tréac'h By 47°27'·98N 03°07'·10W; IDM.
S Bkwtr Hd 47°28'·60N 03°07'·23W Oc (2) R 6s 9m 7M; W Tr, R top.

PLATEAU DES BIRVIDEAUX
Tower 47°29'·20N 03°17'·45W Fl (2) 6s 24m 9M; B Tr, R bands; IDM.

BELLE ÎLE/SAUZON/LE PALAIS
Pte des Poulains 47°23'·37N 03°15'·08W Fl 5s 34m **24M**; W ■ Tr and dwelling; vis 023°-291°.
Les Poulains By 47°23'·42N 03°16'·65W; WCM.
Goulphar 47°18'·67N 03°13'·67W Fl (2) 10s 87m **24M**; Gy Tr.
La Truie Bn 47°17'·10N 03°11'·62W; IDM.
N Poulains By 47°23'·70N 03°14'·86W; NCM.
Bas. Gareau Bn 47°22'·85N 03°12'·97W; SHM.
Sauzon Jetée NW Hd 47°22'·58N 03°13'·00W Fl G 4s 8m 8M.
Jetée SE Hd Fl R 4s 8m 8M; W Tr, R top.
Le Palais Jetée Nord 47°20'·90N 03°09'·00W Fl (2+1) G 12s 11m 7M; W Tr; obsc 298°-170°.
La Truie du Bugul Bn 47°19'·60N 03°06'·50W; NCM.
Pointe de Kerdonis 47°18'·65N 03°03'·50W Fl (3) R 15s 35m **15M** ; W ■ Tr and dwelling; obsc by Pointes d'Arzic and de Taillefer 025°-129°.
Les Galères By 47°18'·80N 03°02'·75W; ECM.

BAIE DE QUIBERON AND MORBIHAN

CHAUSSÉE AND PASSAGE DE LA TEIGNOUSE
Le Four Bn 47°27'·80N 03°06'·48W; SCM.
Bas. Cariou By 47°27'·00N 03°06'·33W; WCM; *Bell*.
Bas. du Chenal By 47°26'·70N 03°05'·70W; SCM.
Goué Vaz N By 47°26'·27N 03°05'·35W; NCM.
Goué Vaz S Lt By 47°25'·84N 03°04'·80W Q (6) + L Fl 15s; SCM; *Whis*.
Basse du Milieu Lt By 47°26'·00N 03°04'·10W Fl (2) G 6s 9m 5M; SHM HFP.
Goué Vaz E Lt By 47°26'·30N 03°04'·20W Fl (3) R 12s; PHM.
La Teignouse 47°27'·50N 03°02'·67W Fl WR 4s 19m **15**/11M; W ●Tr, R top vis W033°-039°, R039°-033°.
NE Teignouse Lt By 47°26'·62N 03°01'·80W Fl (3) G 12s; SHM.
Basse Nouvelle Lt By 47°27'·02N 03°01'·85W Fl R 2·5s; PHM.
Quiberon S Lt By 47°30'·10N 03°02'·30W Q (6) + L Fl 15s; SCM.

PORT HALIGUEN
Outer S Bkwtr Hd 47°29'·36N 03°05'·90W Oc (2) WR 6s 10m W12M, R9M; W Tr, R top; vis W233°-240·5°, R240·5°-299°, W299°-306°, R306°-233°.

Quiberon N By 47°29'·68N 03°02'·52W; NCM.
Explosive Wk By 47°31'·25N 03°05'·36W; IDM.
Men er Roue Bn 47°32'·33N 03°06'·00W; IDM.

RIVIÈRE DE CRAC'H/LA TRINITÉ-SUR-MER
Ldg Lts 347°. Front 47°34'·14N 03°00'·29W Q WRG 11m
W10M, R7M, G7M; W Tr, G top; vis G321°-345°, W345°-
013·5°, R013·5°-080°. **Rear**, 560m from front, Dir Q 21m **15M**;
W ● Tr, G top; synch with front, intens 337°-357°.
Le Rat By 47°32'·89N 03°01'·69W; IDM.
Souris By 47°32'·03N 03°01'·14W; IDM.
Petit Trého Lt By 47°33'·55N 03°00'·67W Fl (4) R 15s; PHM.
La Trinité-sur-Mer Dir Lt 347°. 47°35'·09N 03°00'·90W Dir Oc
WRG 4s 9m W13M, R11M, G11M; W Tr; vis G345°-346°,
W346°-348°, R348°-349°.
S Pier Hd 47°35'·15N 03°01'·42W Oc (2) WR 6s 6m W10M,
R7M; W Tr, R top; vis R090°-293·5°, W293·5°-300·5°,
R300·5°-329°.

Buissons de Méaban By 47°31'·71N 02°58'·42W; SCM.
Méaban By 47°30'·83N 02°56'·14W; SCM.

MORBIHAN
Le Grand Mouton 47°33'·77N 02°54'·78W QG 4m 3M;
G tripod.
Le Grégan 47°33'·96N 02°54'·96W Q (6) + L Fl 15s 3m 8M;
SCM.
Auray No. 13 Bn 47°39'·53N 02°58'·57W; SHM.
Creizic S. By 47°34'·68N 02°52'·75W; SCM.
Creizic N. By 47°35'·00N 02°52'·12W; NCM.
Les Rechauds Bns 47°36'·25N 02°51'·20W; 2 x SHM.
Truie d'Arradon Bn 47°36'·63N 02°50'·18W; PHM.
Roguédas 47°37'·18N 02°47'·19W Fl G 2·5s 4m 4M; G Tr.

PLATEAU DU GRAND MONT
Basse de S Gildas By 47°29'·83N 02°52'·30W; WCM.
Roc de l' Epieu By 47°29'·55N 02°52'·86W; IDM.
Chimère By 47°28'·90N 02°53'·90W; SCM.
Basse du Grand Mont By 47°29'·05N 02°51'·08W; SCM.

CHAUSSÉE DU BÉNIGUET
Les Esclassiers W Bn 47°25'·72N 03°03'·00W; WCM.
Le Grand Coin Bn 47°24'·50N 03°00'·20W; ECM.

ÎLE DE HOUAT
Le Rouleau Bn 47°23'·74N 03°00'·20W; WCM.
Bonnenn Vraz Bn 47°24'·30N 02°59'·80W; WCM.
Port de Saint-Gildas Môle Nord 47°23'·63N 02°57'·26W
Fl (2) WG 6s 8m W9M, G6M; W Tr, G top; vis W168°-198°,
G198°-210°, W210°-240°, G240°-168°.
Men Grouiz Bn 47°22'·82N 02°54'·97W; ECM.
Er Rouzez Bn 47°22'·02N 02°54'·42W; ECM.

Pot de Feu By 47°21'·75N 02°59'·70W; IDM.

ÎLE DE HÖEDIC
Er Palaire Bn 47°20'·23N 02°54'·95W; WCM.
Les Sœurs Bn 47°21'·20N 02°54'·70W; WCM.
La Chèvre Bn 47°21'·16N 02°52'·50W; IDM.
Port de l'Argol Bkwtr Hd 47°20'·75N 02°52'·46W Fl WG 4s
10m W9M, G6M; W Tr, G top; vis W143°-163°, G163°-183°,
W183°-203°, G203°-143°.
Le Chariot By 47°18'·94N 02°52'·90W; SCM.
Les Grands Cardinaux 47°19'·35N 02°50'·08W Fl (4) 15s 28m
13M; R and W Tr.
Cohfournik Bn 47°19'·48N 02°49'·72W; ECM.
Er Guéranic Bn 47°20'·58N 02°50'·43W; ECM.

CROUESTY TO LE CROISIC
PORT NAVALO/CROUESTY EN ARZON
Pte de Port-Navalo 47°32'·93N 02°55'·02W Oc (3) WRG 12s
32m **W15M**, R11M , G11M ; W Tr and dwelling; vis W155°-
220°, G317°-359°, W359°-015°, R015°-105°.
Ldg Lts 058°. **Front** 47°32'·60N 02°53'·85W Dir Q 10m **19M**;
R panel with W vert stripe; intens 056·5°-059·5°. **Rear**, 315m
from front, Dir Q 27m **19M**; Gy Tr; intens 056·5°-059·5°.
N Jetty Hd Oc (2) R 6s 9m 7M; R and W ■ Tr, R top.
S Jetty Hd 47°32'·51N 02°54'·02W Fl G 4s 9m 7M; G&W
■ Tr.

PLATEAU DE S JACQUES/SAINT-JACQUES-EN-SARZEAU
Bas Rohaliguen S Jacques By 47°28'·25N 02°47'·45W; SCM.
Saint-Jacques-en-Sarzeau Lt Tr 47°29'·22N 02°47'·45W
Oc (2) R 6s 5m 6M; W 8-sided Tr, R top.

PLATEAU DE LA RECHERCHE
Recherche Lt By 47°25'·65N 02°50'·27W Q (9) 15s; WCM.
Locmariaquer By 47°25'·88N 02°47'·30W; IDM.

PÉNERF
Le Pignon 47°30'·10N 02°38'·85W Fl (3) WR 12s 6m W9M,
R6M ; R ■ on Tr; vis R028·5°-167°, W167°-175°, R175°-
349·5°, W349·5°-028·5°.

VILAINE RIVER
Basse de Kervoyal 47°30'·43N 02°32'·55W Dir Q WR W8M,
R6M; vis W269°-271°, R271°-269°; SCM on B Tr.
Basse Bertrand 47°31'·10N 02°30'·63W Iso WG 4s 6m
W9M, G6M; G Tr; vis W040°-054°, G054°-227°, W227°-234°,
G234°-040°.
Penlan 47°31'·05N 02°30'·06W Oc (2) WRG 6s 26m **W15M**,
R11M, G11M; W Tr, R bands; vis R292·5°-025°, G025°-052°,
W052°-060°, R060°-138°, G138°-180°.
Pointe du Scal, 47°29'·72N 02°26'·78W QG 12s 8m 6M;
W ■ Tr, G top.

ÎLE DUMET
Fort 47°24'·80N 02°37'·10W Fl (2+1) WRG 15s 14m W8M,
R6M, G6M; W col, G top on fort; vis G090°-272°, W272°-
285°, R285°-325°, W325°-090°.
E Île Dumet Lt By 47°25'·20N 02°35'·00W Q (3) 10s; ECM.

MESQUER
Jetty Hd 47°25'·32N 02°27'·95W Oc (3+1) WRG 12s 7m
W12M, R8M, G7M; W col and bldg; vis W067°-072°, R072°-
102°, W102°-118°, R118°-293°, W293°-325°, G325°-067°.

PIRIAC-SUR-MER
Inner Mole Hd 47°23'·00N 02°32'·65W Oc (2) WRG 6s 8m
W10M, R7M, G6M; W col; vis R066°-185°, W185°-201°,
G201°-224°; Siren 120s.
Les Bayonelles Lt By 47°22'·58N 02°34'·90W Q (9) 15s;
WCM; *Whis.*
Oil Pipeline 47°22'·15N 02°32'·70W Oc (2+1) WRG 12s 14m
W12M, R9M, G9M; W ■, R stripe on R Tr; vis G300°-036°,
W036°-068°, R068°-120°.

LA TURBALLE/LE CROISIC
La Turballe Ldg Lts 006·5° both Dir F Vi 11/19m 3M, both
intens 004°-009°.
Jetée de Garlahy 47°20'·77N 02°30'·83W Fl (4) WR 12s 13m
W10M, R7M; W pylon, R top; vis R060°-315°, W315°-060°.
Basse Hergo 47°18'·68N 02°31'·62W Fl G 2·5s 5m 3M; SHM.
Jetée de Tréhic Hd 47°18'·55N 02°31'·34W Iso WG 4s 12m
W13M, G10M; Gy Tr, G top; vis G042°-093°, W093°-137°,
G137°-345°; F Bu Fog Det Lt.
Le Grand Mabon 47°18'·11N 02°30'·94W Fl R 2·5s 6m 5M,
R pedestal.

17

LE CROISIC TO PTE DE ST GILDAS

PLATEAU DU FOUR/BANC DE GUÉRANDE
Bonen du Four Lt By 47°18'·60N 02°39'·20W Q; NCM; *Whis*.
Le Four 47°17'·94N 02°37'·96W Fl 5s 23m **19M** ; W Tr, B stripes, G top.
W Basse Capella Lt By 47°15'·67N 02°44'·66W Q (9) 15s; WCM; *Whis*.
Goué-Vas-du-Four Lt By 47°14'·96N 02°38'·13W Q (6) + L Fl 15s; SCM.
S Banc Guérande Lt By 47°08'·87N 02°42'·74W VQ (6) + L Fl 10s; SCM; *Whis*.

PLATEAU DE LA BANCHE
W Banche Lt By 47°11'·65N 02°32'·34W VQ (9) 10s; WCM; *Whis*.
NW Banche Lt By 47°12'·90N 02°30'·95W Q 8m 8M; NCM HFP; *Bell*.
La Banche 47°10'·70N 02°28'·00W Fl (2+1) WR 15s 22m **W17M**, R12M; B Tr, W bands; vis R266°-280°, W280°-266°.
SE Banche By 47°10'·47N 02°26'·02W; ECM.

BAIE du POULIGUEN (Baie de la Baule) APPROACHES
Penchateau Lt By 47°15'·36N 02°24'·30W Fl R 2·5s; PHM.
Les Guérandaises Lt By 47°15'·06N 02°24'·23W Fl G 4s; SHM.
Les Evens By 47°14'·47N 02°22'·46W; PHM.
Les Troves By 47°14'·25N 02°22'·30W; SHM.
NNW Pierre Percée 47°13'·67N 02°20'·54W; NCM.
La Vieille Bn 47°14'·09N 02°19'·43W; SCM.
Sud de la Vieille By 47°13'·81N 02°19'·41W; IDM.
Le Caillou By 47°13'·71N 02°19'·11W; NCM.
Le Petit Charpentier Bn 47°13'·40N 02°18'·87W; SCM.

LE POULIGUEN.
Les Petits Impairs 47°16'·08N 02°24'·53W Fl (2) G 6s 6m 6M; G ▲, on Tr; vis outside B. 298°-034°.
S Jetty 47°16'·48N 02°25'·30W QR 13m 9M; W col; vis 171°-081°.

PORT DE PORNICHET
La Baule S Bkwtr Hd 47°15'·55N 02°21'·07W Iso WG 4s 11m W11M, G8M; W Tr, G top; vis G084°-081°, W081°-084°.
South Ent Fl G 2s 3m 2M.
North Ent Fl R 2s 3m 2M.

Le Grand Charpentier 47°12'·90N 02°19'·05W Q WREG 22m W14M, R10M, G10M, Gy Tr, G lantern; vis G020°-049°, W049°-111°, R111°-310°, W310°-020°; Helicopter platform; Sig Stn 1·5M NE.

LOIRE APPROACHES
Loire Approach Lt By SN1 47°00'·15N 02°39'·75W L Fl 10s 8m 8M; SWM HFP; *Whis*; Racon (Z).
Loire Approach Lt By SN2 47°02'·15N 02°33'·45W Iso 4s 8m 5M; SWM HFP; Ra refl.
Thérésia Lt By 47°04'·92N 02°27'·20W Fl R 2·5s; PHM.
Les Chevaux Lt By 47°03'·58N 02°26'·29W Fl G 2·5s; SHM.
La Couronnée Lt By 47°07'·67N 02°20'·00W QG 8m 6M; SHM HFP; Racon.
Lancastria Lt By 47°08'·92N 02°20'·39W VQR 8m 2M; PHM HFP; Ra Refl.

PLATEAU DE LA LAMBARDE
SE Lambarde Lt By 47°10'·10N 02°20·72W Q (6) + L Fl 15s; SCM, *Bell*.
NW Lambard By 47°10'·88N 02°22'·78W; WCM.

PASSE DES CHARPENTIERS
Portcé Ldg Lts 025·5°. **Front** 47°14'·62N 02°15'·36W Dir Q 6m **22M** ; W col; intens 024·7°-026·2°. **Rear**, 0·75M from front, Q 36m **27M**; W Tr; intens 024·7°-026·2° (H24).
No. 1 Lt By 47°10'·02N 02°18'·35W VQ G; SHM.
No. 7 Lt By 47°13'·37N 02°16'·02W VQ G; SHM.
Pointe d'Aiguillon 47°14'·60N 02°15'·70W Oc (4) WR 12s 27m **W15M**, R11M; W Tr; vis W233°-293°, W297°-300°, R300°-327°, W327°-023°, W027°-089°.

VILLE-ES-MARTIN
Jetty Hd 47°15'·40N 02°13'·58W Fl (2) 6s 10m 12M; W Tr, R top.
Les Morées 47°15'·05N 02°12'·95W Oc (2) WR 6s 12m W9M, R6M; G Tr; vis W058°-224°, R300°-058°.

SAINT-NAZAIRE
W Jetty Oc (4) R 12s 11m 10M; W Tr, R top.
East Jetty 47°16'·05N 02°12'·06W Oc (4) G 12s 11m 11M; W Tr, G top.
Old Môle Hd 47°16'·33N 02°11'·74W Oc (2+1) 12s 18m 12M; W Tr, R top; vis 153·5°-063·5°; weather signals.
Basse Nazaire S Lt By 47°16'·27N 02°11'·57W Q (6) + L Fl 15s; SCM.

POINTE DE MINDIN
W Môle 47°16'·27N 02°10'·04W Fl G 2·5s 5m 2M.

LE POINTEAU/PORT DE COMBERGE/PORT DE LA GRAVETTE
Le Pointeau Digue S Hd 47°14'·08N 02°10'·89W Fl WG 4s 4m W10M, G6M; G&W ● hut; vis G050°-074°, W074°-149°, G149°-345°, W345°-050°.
Port de Comberge S Jetty 47°10'·60N 02°09'·95W Oc WG 4s 7m W9M , G5M; W Tr, G top; vis W123°-140°, G140°-123°.
Port de la Gravette Jetty Hd 47°09'·80N 02°12'·60W Fl (3) WG 12s 7m W8M, G5M; W structure, G top; vis G224°-124°, W124°-224°.

SAINT GILDAS (Anse de Boucau)
Pte de Saint Gildas 47°08'·10N 02°14'·67W Q WRG 23m W11M , R6M , G6M ; framework Tr on W house; vis R264°-308°, G308°-078°, W078°-088°, R088°-174°, W174°-180°, G180°-264°; RC.

RIVER LOIRE TO NANTES

Bridge (Chan centre) 47°17·16N 02°10'·16W Iso 4s 55m. (TD 1989.)

DONGES
SW dolphin 47°18'·12N 02°04'·90W Fl G 4s 12m 7M; Gy col.
NE dolphin (close ENE) Iso G 4s 12m 6M; G col.
Jetty Hd 47°18'·35N 02°04'·11W Fl (2) R 6s 9m 9M.

PAIMBŒUF
Môle Hd 47°17'·50N 02°01'·88W Oc (3) WG 12s 9m **W16M**, G11M; W ● Tr, G top; vis G shore-123°, W123°-shore.
Île du Petit Carnet 47°17'·29N 02°00'·29W Fl G 2·5s 8m 6M; W framework Tr, G top.
From Paimbœuf to Nantes Lts on S side are G, and N Red.

PORT DE TRENTE MOULT/NANTES
Trente Moult Bn off 47°11'·83N 01°34'·63W; SPM.
Quai du Président Wilson Hd 47°12'·02N 01°34'·37W Fl R 2·5s.

10.17.5   PASSAGE INFORMATION

SOUTH BRITTANY (charts 2643, 2646)

The *North Biscay Pilot* (Imray/RCC) or the Admiralty *Bay of Biscay Pilot* are recommended. The *French Pilot* (Vol 3) (Nautical/Robson), although out of print, contains many unique almost timeless sketches and transits. French charts (SHOM) are often larger scale than Admiralty charts, and hence more suitable for inshore waters. For French Glossary, see 1.4.2. The following Breton words have navigational significance: *Aber*: estuary. *Aven*: river, stream. *Bann*: hill. *Bian*: small. *Bras*: great. *Du*: black. *Enez, Inis*: island. *Garo*: rough, hard. *Glas*: green. *Goban*: shoal. *Gwenn*: white. *Karreg*: rock. *Ker*: house. *Men, mein*: rock, stone. *Morlenn*: creek. *Penn*: strait. *Porz*: harbour. *Raz*: tide race. *Ruz*: red. *Trez*: sand.

Mist and haze are quite common in the summer, fog less so. Winds are predominantly from SW to NW, often light and variable in summer, but in early and late season N or NE winds are common. Summer gales are infrequent, and are usually related to passing fronts. In summer the sea is often calm or slight, but swell, usually from W or NW, can severely affect exposed anchorages. When crossing B of Biscay, allow for a likely set to the E, particularly after strong W winds.

A particular feature of this coast during the summer is the sea and land breeze cycle, known locally as the *vent solaire*. After a quiet forenoon, a W'ly sea breeze sets in about midday, blowing onshore. It slowly veers to the NW, almost parallel to the coast, reaching F4 by late afternoon; it then veers further to the N, expiring at dusk. Around midnight a land breeze may pipe up from the NE and freshen sufficiently to kick up rough seas – with consequent disruption to moorings and anchs open to the NE. By morning the wind has abated.

Tidal streams are weak offshore, but can be strong in estuaries, channels and around headlands, especially nearer the English Chan. The tidal stream chartlets at 10.17.4 are based on NP 265 (Admiralty Tidal Stream Atlas for France, W Coast) which uses data from actual observations out to 15-25M offshore. The equivalent French Atlas gives more data, but based on computer predictions.

Inland waterways (10.15.18) can be entered from Lorient (10.17.14), Vilaine R (10.17.22) and the R. Loire (10.17.26).

RAZ DE SEIN TO BENODET (chart 2351)

Chaussée de Sein (chart 798) is a chain of islands, rks and shoals extending 15M W from the Pte du Raz. A WCM lt buoy marks the seaward end. For directions on Île de Sein (10.17.8) and Raz de Sein see *North Biscay Pilot* (RCC/Imray).

Raz de Sein (chart 798) is the chan between Le Chat bn tr (at E end of Chaussée de Sein) and the dangers extending 8ca off Pte du Raz, the extremity of which is marked by La Vieille lt ho and La Plate lt tr. The Plateau de Tévennec is 2M N of Raz de Sein; it consists of islets, rks and shoals which extend 5ca in all directions from the lt ho thereon. Other dangers on the N side of the Raz are rks and shoals extending nearly 1M W and WSW from Pte du Van, and Basse Jaune (dries) 1M to N. On the S side the main dangers, all 1·5M off La Vieille, are: to the SW, Kornog Bras, a rk with depth of 3m; to the S, Masklou Greiz, rky shoals on which sea can break heavily; and to the SE, Roche Moulleg.

In the middle of Raz de Sein the NE-going (flood) stream begins at HW Brest + 0550, sp rate 6·5kn; the SW-going (ebb) stream begins at HW Brest – 0030, sp rate 5·5kn. There are eddies near La Vieille on both streams. In good weather, near np, and with wind and tide together, the Raz presents no difficulty, but in moderately strong winds it should be taken at slack water, which lasts for about ½ hour at end of flood · stream. In strong winds the chan must not be used with wind against tide, when there are overfalls with a steep breaking sea.

The B des Trépassés (1·5M ENE of La Vieille) is possible anch to await the S-going tide. Port Bestrée or Anse du Loc'h (1M and 4M E of Pte du Raz) may be suitable anchs if N-bound.

Audierne (10.17.8) lies between Raz de Sein and Pte de Penmarc'h (lt, fog sig, RC) off which dangers extend 3M to SE, and 1M to S, W and NW, and breaking seas occur in strong winds. The fishing hbrs of St Guénolé, Le Guilvinec (10.17.8) and Lesconil provide excellent shelter, but have difficult ents. Loctudy (10.17.9) is well sheltered from W/SW.

BENODET TO LORIENT (chart 2352)

Îles de Glénan (chart 3640, SHOM 6648, 10.17.12), lie to seaward of Loctudy and Concarneau. With offlying dangers they stretch 5M from W to E and 4M from N to S. The islands are interesting to explore, but anchs are rather exposed. Between Îles de Glénan and Bénodet lie Les Pourceaux, reefs which dry, and Île aux Moutons which has dangers extending SW and NW.

Along the coast the larger ports are Bénodet (10.17.10), Port-la-Forêt (10.17.11) and Concarneau (10.17.12). Anse de Bénodet has rky shoals on both sides but is clear in the middle. The coast from Pte de Mousterlin to Beg Meil is fringed by rks, many of which dry, extending 1M offshore. Chaussée de Beg Meil extends 8½ca SE, where Linuen rk (dries) is marked by bn. From Concarneau to Pte de Trévignon rks extend nearly 1·5M offshore in places.

Between Pte de Trévignon and Lorient are rky cliffs and several interesting lesser hbrs and anchs, delightful in fair weather; but most dry and are dangerous to approach in strong onshore winds. These include the Aven and Belon rivers, Brigneau, Merrien (mostly dries), Doëlan (but most of hbr dries) and Le Pouldu (Rivière de Quimperlé). All are described in 10.17.12 and the *North Biscay Pilot*.

Hazards SE and E of Pte de Trévignon include: Men Du, a rk 0·3m high, marked by IDM bn, about 1·25M SE of the same pt. Corn Vas, depth 1·8m, and Men ar Tréas, a rk which dries, are close S, both buoyed. Île Verte lies 6ca S of Ile de Raguénès, with foul ground another 2ca to S. The approaches to Aven and Bélon Rivers are clear, except for Le Cochon and Les Verrés (IDM bn) to the SE. Between Le Pouldu and Lorient, Grand Cochon (SCM buoy) and Petit Cochon lie about 1M offshore.

LORIENT TO QUIBERON (charts 2352, 2353)

The great seaport of Lorient (10.17.14) has sheltered apprs and 4 marinas. Île de Groix lies 4M SW. Its main offlying dangers are to the E and SE: shoals off Pte de la Croix; Les Chats which extend 1M SE from Pte des Chats; and shoals extending 7½ca S of Loc Maria. Port Tudy (10.17.13), on N coast, is the main hbr, and is easy of access and well sheltered except from NE.

7M SE of Lorient, River Étel (10.15.19) is an attractive hbr with a difficult ent which must only be approached in good weather and on the last of the flood. Further S do not appr the isthmus of the Quiberon peninsula closely due to rky shoals. 6M W of Quiberon lies Plateau des Birvideaux (lt), a rky bank (depth 4·6m) on which the sea breaks in bad weather.

Belle Île has no dangers more than 2½ca offshore, apart from buoyed rks which extend 7½ca W of Pte des Poulains, and La Truie rk marked by IDM bn tr 5ca off the S coast. The S coast is much indented and exposed to swell from W. In good settled weather (only) and in absence of swell there is an attractive anch in Port du Vieux Château (Ster Wenn), 1M S of Pte des Poulains; see *North Biscay Pilot*. On the NE coast lie Le Palais (10.17.16) and Sauzon, which partly dries but has good anch off and is sheltered from S and W. Off Le Palais the ESE-going (flood) stream begins at HW Brest – 0610, and the WNW- going at HW Brest + 0125, sp rates 1·5kn.

17

BAIE DE QUIBERON (chart 2353)

B de Quiberon is an important and attractive yachting area, with centres at Port Haliguen (10.17.17), La Trinité (10.17.18), Crouesty (10.17.19) and the Morbihan (10.17.20). The S side of the bay is enclosed by a long chain of islands, islets, rks and shoals from Presqu'île de Quiberon to Les Grands Cardinaux 13M SE. This chain includes the attractive islands of Houat (10.17.19) and Hoëdic, well worth visiting, preferably mid-week. The Bay is open to the E and SE.

From W or S, enter the B via Passage de la Teignouse in W sector (033°-039°) of La Teignouse lt ho; thence 068° between Basse Nouvelle lt buoy and NE Teignouse lt buoy. In this chan the NE-going (flood) stream begins at HW Brest – 0610, and the SW-going at HW Brest – 0005, sp rates 3·75 kn; in strong winds it is best to pass at slack water. Good alternative chans are Passage du Béniguet, NW of Houat, and Passage des Soeurs, NW of Hoëdic.

The Golfe du Morbihan, on the N side of B de Quiberon, is an inland sea containing innumerable islands and anchs. Port Navalo anch is on the E side of the ent with Port du Crouesty close SE. Inside, River Auray flows in from the NW and the city of Vannes (10.17.21) is on the N side. Sp stream rates in the vicinity of Grand Mouton achieve 8kn and elsewhere in the ent can exceed 4kn. Flood commences HW Brest – 0400 and turns at HW Brest + 0200.

CROUESTY TO LE CROISIC (chart 2353)

Eastwards from the Morbihan, dangers extend 1M seaward of Pte de St Jacques, and 3M offshore lies Plateau de la Recherche with depths of 1·8m. SE of Penerf (10.17.22), which provides good anch, Plateau des Mats is an extensive rky bank, drying in places, up to 1·75M offshore.

Approaching the R. Vilaine (10.17.22) beware La Grande Accroche, a large shoal with least depth 1m, astride the ent. The main lit chan keeps NW of La Grande Accroche, to the bar on N side thereof. Here the flood begins at HW Brest – 0515, and the ebb at HW Brest + 0035, sp rates 2·5kn. In SW winds against tide the sea breaks heavily; when the Passe de la Varlingue, 5ca W of Pte du Halguen, is better, but beware La Varlingue (dries). At Arzal/Camoël yachts can lock into the non-tidal river for canal to Dinan/St Malo (see 10.15.18).

S of Pte du Halguen other dangers, close inshore, are the rky shoals, depth 0·6m, of Basse de Loscolo and Basse du Bile. Off Pte du Castelli, the Plateau de Piriac extends about 1·75M NW with depths of 2·3m and drying rks closer inshore. The small hbr of Piriac (10.17.23) lies on the N side of Pointe du Castelli and Les Bayonelles (dry) extend 5ca W. A chan runs between Plateau de Piriac and Île Dumet (lt), which is fringed by drying rks and shoals particularly on N and E sides.

In the Rade du Croisic are the hbrs of La Turballe (10.17.23) and Le Croisic (10.17.24). Off Pte du Croisic dangers extend 1M to N and W. Plateau du Four, a dangerous drying bank of rks, lies about 4M W and WSW of Pte du Croisic, marked by buoys and lt ho near N end. Between Pte du Croisic and Pte de Penchâteau, Basse Lovre is a rky shoal with depths of 1m, 5ca offshore.

LE CROISIC TO R. LOIRE (chart 2353, 3216)

From Chenal du Nord, B du Pouliguen (10.17.25) is entered between Pte de Penchâteau and Pte du Bec, 3M to E. In SE corner of bay is the yacht hbr of Pornichet. The B is partly sheltered from S by rks and shoals extending SE from Pte de Penchâteau to Le Grand Charpentier, but a heavy sea develops in strong S-SW winds. The W chan through these rks runs between Penchâteau and Les Guérandaises lateral buoys; other chans lie further E.

The River Loire estuary (chart 3216), which carries much commercial tfc, is entered via either the Chenal du Nord or the Chenal du Sud. The former runs ESE between the mainland and two shoals, Plateau de la Banche and Plateau de la Lambarde; these lie about 4M S of B du Pouliguen. Chenal du Sud, the main DW chan, leads NE between Plateau de la Lambarde and Pte de St Gildas. Here the in-going stream begins at HW Brest – 0500, and the out-going at HW Brest + 0050, sp rates about 2·75kn.

In the near apprs to St Nazaire (10.17.26 and charts 2985, 2989) beware Le Vert, Les Jardinets and La Truie (all dry) which lie close E of the chan. The river is navigable as far as Nantes. On the E side of the estuary, between the Loire bridge and Pte de St Gildas, are the small drying hbrs of Comberge, La Gravette and St Gildas (10.17.26).

10.17.6   DISTANCE TABLE

Approximate distances in nautical miles are by the most direct route, whilst avoiding dangers and allowing for Traffic Separation Schemes. Places in *italics* are in adjoining areas; places in **bold** are in 10.0.5, Cross-Channel Distances.

1.	*Le Conquet*	1																		
2.	*Camaret*	13	2																	
3.	*Morgat*	22	16	3																
4.	*Douarnenez*	29	21	11	4															
5.	Audierne	30	28	27	30	5														
6.	Loctudy	55	55	53	55	30	6													
7.	Bénodet	58	58	57	60	33	4	7												
8.	Port-la-Forêt	65	64	63	66	36	12	12	8											
9.	Concarneau	63	62	61	64	37	12	11	4	9										
10.	Lorient	84	86	85	88	61	38	36	33	32	10									
11.	Le Palais (Belle Ile)	95	99	98	101	74	54	52	48	47	26	11								
12.	Port Haliguen	100	105	104	107	80	59	57	55	53	32	11	12							
13.	La Trinité	108	110	109	112	85	64	62	60	58	37	16	8	13						
14.	Crouesty	108	110	109	112	85	64	62	60	58	37	16	9	8	14					
15.	*Vannes*	120	121	120	123	96	75	73	71	69	48	27	20	19	12	15				
16.	Arzal/Camoël	131	130	129	132	105	84	82	80	78	57	36	31	31	28	37	16			
17.	Le Croisic	124	125	124	127	100	79	77	75	73	48	27	26	26	22	33	18	17		
18.	La Baule/Pornichet	134	131	130	133	106	85	82	80	78	55	34	35	36	30	40	30	13	18	
19.	St Nazaire	145	138	137	140	113	95	91	90	87	66	41	42	45	40	50	39	24	12	19
20.	*Pornic*	146	149	148	151	124	105	101	100	97	72	45	47	49	43	55	42	24	18	16	20

10.17.7   Special notes for France: See 10.15.8

AUDIERNE   10-17-8
Finistere 48°00'·61N 04°32'·33W

CHARTS
AC 3640, 2351; SHOM 7147, 7148; Imray C36, C37; ECM 541

TIDES
+0440 Dover; ML 3·1; Duration 0605; Zone 0100

Standard Port BREST (←)

Times				Height (metres)			
High Water		Low Water		MHWS	MHWN	MLWN	MLWS
0000	0600	0000	0600	6·9	5·4	2·6	1·0
1200	1800	1200	1800				
Differences AUDIERNE							
−0035	−0030	−0035	−0030	−1·7	−1·3	−0·6	−0·2
ILE DE SEIN							
−0005	−0005	−0010	−0005	−0·7	−0·6	−0·2	−0·1
LE GUILVINEC							
−0010	−0025	−0025	−0015	−1·8	−1·4	−0·6	−0·1
LESCONIL							
−0008	−0028	−0028	−0018	−1·9	−1·4	−0·6	−0·1

SHELTER
Good in marina, 3 pontoons 2ca SW of the bridge. Access HW±3 in all but strong SE-SW winds when seas break at the ent. Chan is dredged about 1m; beware drying banks close to stbd. Quays reserved for FVs.
At Ste Evette a long bkwtr, Oc (2) R 6s, gives good shelter, except in SE-SW winds which cause swell. W 🛟s to the N are marked 'Payant-Visiteurs'. Keep clear of slip area as vedettes enter with much verve.

NAVIGATION
WPT 47°59'·54N 04°32'·91W, 186°/006° from/to Kergadec lt, 1·5M. Appr between La Gamelle, drying rks in the middle of the bay, and Le Sillon de Galets rks to the W. Or from the SE, leave La Gamelle to port. Appr is difficult in strong SE-SW winds. Inside the ent, dredged chan initially favours the W bank with ldg marks, vert R/W chevrons, in line 359°. After 2ca chan turns NE, with astern transit 225° on 2nd set of R/W chevrons. Hold 045° for 0·5M till abeam fish market on stbd side, then alter 90° port to marina, keeping close to quays and pontoons; banks dry to stbd.

LIGHTS AND MARKS
By day from the WPT, Kergadec, W 8-sided lt tr, R top, on with Old lt ho (difficult to see) leads 006°. At night stay in the W sector (005°-007°) of Kergadec, Dir Q WRG 43m 12/9M. From the SE, ldg marks/lts at 331°: Front Fl (3) WG 12s 11m 14/9M, W ○ tr on hbr bkwtr; rear FR 44m 9M (Kergadec).

RADIO TELEPHONE
None. Adjacent sig stn at Pte du Raz Ch 16.

TELEPHONE
Hr Mr 98·70·07·91; Aff Mar 98·70·03·33; CROSS 97·55·35·35; SNSM 98·70·03·31; ⊞ 98·70·70·97; Meteo 98·94·03·43; Auto 36.68.08.29; Police 98·70·06·38; Ⓗ 98·70·00·18; Brit Consul 40·63·16·02.

FACILITIES
Port de Plaisance (100+20 visitors) ☎ 98·70·08·47, AC, FW, CH, ME, El, Ⓔ, Sh, Bar, R, V; **Poulgoazec** C (15 ton), P & D (cans), Slip.**Town** V, Gaz, R, Bar, ✉, Ⓑ, bus to Quimper ⇌, ✈. Ferry: Roscoff.
Ste Evette, Hr Mr ☎ 98·70·00·28, access H24, M, Ⓒ.

ADJACENT HARBOURS AND ANCHORAGES

ILE DE SEIN, Finistere, 48°02'·40N 04°50'·80W. AC 798, 2351; SHOM 5252, 7148. Tides, see above; ML 3·8m. Ile de Sein is the only inhabited Is in the Chausée de Sein, a chain of islands, rks and shoals extending 15M W from the Pte du Raz. The outer end has a WCM lt buoy and 5M E is Ar-Men lt tr, Fl (3) 20s 29m, horn (3) 60s. The E end is separated from the mainland by the Raz de Sein; see 10.17.5 for passage details. Ile de Sein is worth visiting in fair weather, good vis and preferably near nps. Best appr is from the N, 187° via Chenal d'Ezaudi, with Men-Brial lt ho, Oc (2) WRG 6s, on with third house (W with B stripe) from left (close S of lt ho). Chan between drying rks is entered at Cornoc-An-Ar-Braden SHM By, Iso G 4s and tide sets across the chan, which is marked by bn trs. There are also chans from NE and E. ⚓ off or inside the mole, but open to N and E. Hbr partly dries. See *North Biscay Pilot* (RCC/Imray) for directions. Facilities: limited V, R, CH, Sh.

ST GUÉNOLÉ, Finistere, 47°48'·70N 04°22'·90W. AC 2351; SHOM 6645, 7147; ECM 541. Strictly a fishing port; yachts not welcomed. Access difficult in fresh W'lies, impossible in heavy weather. 3 sets of ldg marks/lts. Lts as in 10.17.4. Pilot book and SHOM 6645 essential. Hr Mr ☎ 98.58.60.43.

LE GUILVINEC, Finistere, 47°47'·52N 04°17'·10W. AC 3640, 2351; SHOM 6646, 7146. HW + 0447 on Dover (UT); ML 3·0m. See 10.17.8. Good shelter and useful passage port; hbr (3m) accessible H24 for <2·5m draft, but scant room for yachts due to FVs. At NE end of hbr (amongst hosts of lesser buoys), secure fore and aft to 2 large W 🛟s; max stay 24hrs. No ent/exit 1600-1830. Good ⚓ off ent in lee of reef but keep clear of fairway. Beware Lost Moan Rks SE of ent marked by RW bn tr, Fl (3) WRG 12s 8m 9/6M. Ent is easy if vis adequate to see ldg lts/marks. Three ldg lts, all synch, in line 053°: front, Mole de Lechiagat Q 7m 8m, W pylon, vis 233°-066°; middle, Rocher Le Faoutés, 210m from front, QWG 12m 14/11M, R □ on W pylon, vis W006°-293°, G293°-006°; rear, 0·58M from front, Dir Q 26m 8M, R □ on W pylon with R stripe, vis 051·5°-054·5°. VHF Ch 12. Facilities: Hr Mr ☎ 98·58·05·67; Aff Mar ☎ 98·58·13·13; ⊞, C, FW, D, P, El, ME, Sh, CH, Ⓔ.

LESCONIL, Finistere, 47°47'·76N 04°12'·57W. AC 3640, 2351; SHOM 6646, 7146; ECM 543. Tides, see opposite; ML 3m. Fishing port 3M SW of Loctudy; yachts tolerated at their own risk. Do not enter/leave 1630-1830LT due to FV inrush. Appr from Karek Greis ECM buoy, Q (3) 10s, on ldg line 325°, belfry just open W of Men ar Groas lt ho, Fl (3) WRG 12s 14m 13/9M; at night in W sector 313°-333°. Bkwtr lts are QG and Oc R 4s. Possible drying mooring inside S bkwtr; no 🛟s, no AB on quays. Hr Mr ☎ 98.82.22.97. Facilities of fishing port.

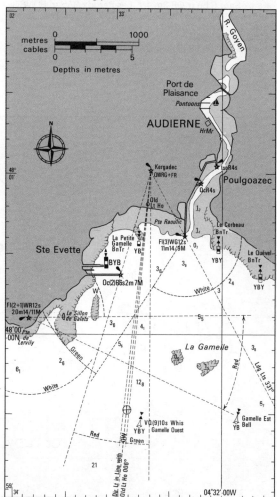

17

LOCTUDY   10-17-9

Finistere 47°50´.30N 04°10´.50W

CHARTS
AC 3641, 2351/2; SHOM 6649, 6679, 7146; ECM 543;
Imray C37, 38

TIDES
+0505 Dover (UT); ML 3·0; Duration 0615; Zone –0100

Standard Port BREST (←—)

Times				Height (metres)			
High Water		Low Water		MHWS	MHWN	MLWN	MLWS
0000	0600	0000	0600	6·9	5·4	2·6	1·0
1200	1800	1200	1800				
Differences LOCTUDY							
–0013	–0033	–0035	–0025	–1·9	–1·5	–0·7	–0·2

SHELTER
Excellent in marina and hbr, except in strong ESE winds. The
many 🛥s and moorings in the river leave little space to ⚓.
Keep clear of FVs, esp 17-1900LT daily when yachts are
discouraged from entering/leaving hbr.

NAVIGATION
WPT 47°50´.12N 04°08´.86W, 105°/285° from/to Les Perdrix
lt, 0·73M. From S and W, leave Bas Bilien ECM, VQ (3), to
port, thence to WPT. From E/NE, give Men Audierne SHM bn
a wide berth. Bar has least depth 0·9m, deeper to the N. Sp
ebb runs at 3½kn; enter under power only. Appr 285° (to clear
unmarked Karek Croisic rk) in W sector of Les Perdrix lt; when
300m short, alter port onto 274° as marina and Chateau
Laubrière (conspic) come in transit. Beware rky ledges
close S of Les Perdrix and SHM bn, Fl (3) G 12s.
Pont l'Abbé (3M up-river) dries about 2m, but is accessible
to shoal draft boats on the flood; chan marked by perches.

LIGHTS AND MARKS
Pte de Langoz Fl (4) WRG 12s 12m 15/11M (see 10.15.4).
Karek-Saoz R bn tr QR 3m 1M. Les Perdrix B/W tr, Fl WRG
4s 15m 11/8M, G090°-285°, W285°-295°, R295°-090°. Le
Blas Fl (3) G 12s 5m 1M.

RADIO TELEPHONE
Marina VHF Ch 09 (Office hrs); Port Ch 12.

TELEPHONE
Hr Mr 98·87·51·36; Aff Mar 98·87·41·79; CROSS 97·55·35·35;
SNSM 98·87·40·15; ⌗ 98·58·28·80; Auto 36·68·08·29;
Police 17; Fire 18; Dr 98·87·41·80; Ⓗ (6km) 98·82·40·40.

FACILITIES
Marina (450+80 visitors) ☎ 98·87·51·36, FW, AC, Slip, D &
P, C (9 tons), CH, Sh, ME, El. **Town** Bar, V, R, Dr, ▨, Ⓑ.

BÉNODET   10-17-10

Finistere 47°51´.80N 04°06´.40W

CHARTS
AC 3641, 2352; SHOM 6679, 6649, 7313, 7146; ECM 543;
Imray C37

TIDES
+0450 Dover; ML 3·1; Duration 0610; Zone –0100

Standard Port BREST (←—)

Times				Height (metres)			
High Water		Low Water		MHWS	MHWN	MLWN	MLWS
0000	0600	0000	0600	6·9	5·4	2·6	1·0
1200	1800	1200	1800				
Differences BÉNODET							
0000	–0020	–0023	–0013	–1·7	–1·3	–0·5	–0·1
CORNIGUEL							
+0015	+0010	–0015	–0010	–2·0	–1·6	–1·0	–0·7

SHELTER
Marinas at Ste Marine (W bank), access H24 at any tide and at
Anse de Penfoul (E bank). Caution: In both marinas, arr/dep at
slack water to avoid strong stream, esp ebb, through the
pontoons. Some 🛥s available. ⚓ in Anse du Trez in offshore
winds. Speed limit 3kn in hbr.

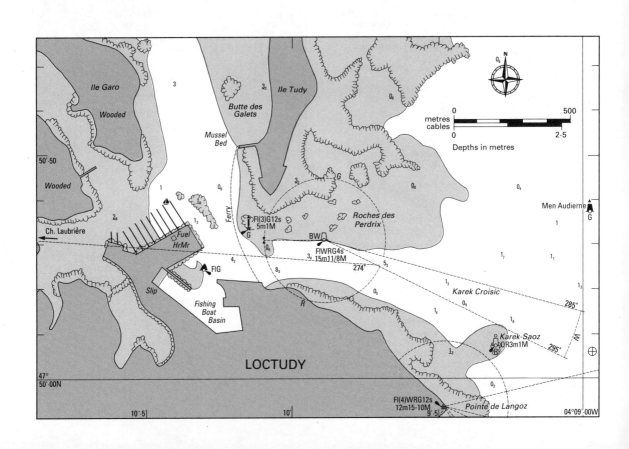

BENODET *continued*

R Odet is navigable near HW to Quimper, but masted vessels should stop at Corniguel due to a 5·8m clearance bridge at Poulguinan (0·5M below the city); pleasant ⚓s at Anse de Combrit, Anse de Kerautret, Porz Meilou, Anse de Toulven and SW of Lanroz. SHOM 6679 recommended.

NAVIGATION

WPT 47°51'·00N 04°06'·10W, 166°/346° from/to front ldg lt 346°, 1·43M. The centre of the B is clear for small craft. Beware Roches de Mousterlin at the SE end of the bay and various rks off Loctudy to the SW. There is a tanker chan past the Ile aux Moutons, 6M SSE of hbr.

LIGHTS AND MARKS

Ldg lts/daymarks 346°: Front, Oc (2+1) G 12s 11m 17M, intens 345°-347°, W ○ tr, G vert stripe, G top (hard to see until close); rear Oc (2+1) 12s 48m 11M, conspic W tr, G top, synch. Ile-aux-Moutons (6M SSE), Oc (2) WRG 6s 18m 15/11M + Dir Oc (2) 6s 17m 24M, intens 278°-283°.

RADIO TELEPHONE

Both marinas VHF Ch 09 (0800-2000LT in season).

TELEPHONE

Hr Mr 98·56·38·72; Aff Mar 98·57·03·82; CROSS 97·55·35·35; SNSM 98·57·02·00; ⌗ 98·55·04·19; Meteo 98·94·03·43; Police 17; Fire 18; Dr 98·57·22·21; Brit Consul 40·63·16·02.

FACILITIES

BENODET **Anse de Penfoul Marina** (250+40 visitors AB; 260 extra pontoon berths are 1ca S of marina; also 175 buoys +15 for visitors) ☎ 98·57·05·78, Fax 98.57.00.21, AC, FW, Ⓞ, R, CH, ME, V, P, D, M, El, Ⓔ, Sh, C, SM, Divers. **Quay** C (10 ton). **Town** All facilities, Gaz, ✉, Ⓑ, bus to Quimper ⇌, ✈.
SAINTE MARINE **Marina** (350+40 visitors) ☎ 98·56·38·72, Fax 98.51.95.17, FF72, AC, CH, FW. **Village** V, R, Bar, Ⓞ, Ⓔ.

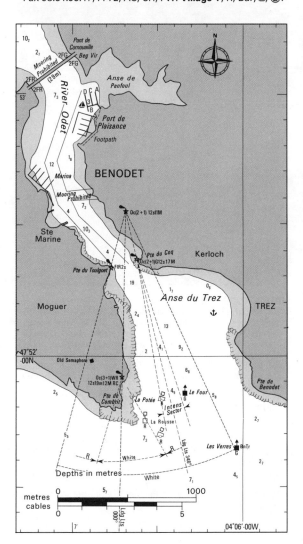

PORT-LA-FORÊT   10-17-11

Finistere 47°53'·55N 03°58'·17W

CHARTS

AC 3641, 2352; SHOM 6650, 7146; ECM 543, 544; Imray C38

TIDES

+0450 Dover; ML 2·9; Duration 0615; Zone –0100
Use Differences CONCARNEAU 10.17.12

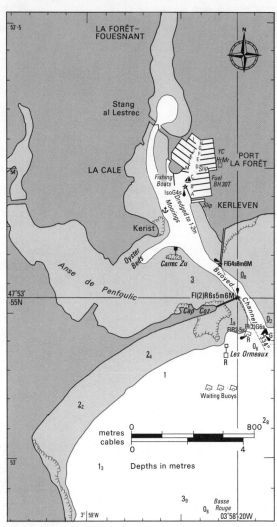

SHELTER

Very good in marina in all weathers. There is an ⚓ inside Cap Coz and moorings to port of the inner chan.

NAVIGATION

WPT 47°52'·77N 03°57'·62W, 154°/334° from/to Cap-Coz lt, 0·88M. Beware Basse Rouge 6·5ca S of Cap Coz, Le Scoré (unlit SCM bn) and buoyed oyster farms in apprs. At sp a shoal patch 0·9m just S of the ent denies access LW±1½; there are 3 W waiting buoys close WSW of the ent.

LIGHTS AND MARKS

Cap Coz, Fl (2) R 6s 5m 6M, and Kerleven bkwtr lt, Fl G 4s 8m 6M, lead 334° through chan marked with buoys and bns; only the first pair of chan buoys are lit, Fl R 2·5s and Fl (2) G 6s.

RADIO TELEPHONE

VHF Ch 09.

TELEPHONE

Hr Mr 98·56·98·45; Aff Mar 98·56·01·98; Rescue CROSS-Etel 97·55·35·35; Auto 36.68.08.29; SNSM 98·56·98·25; ⌗ (Concarneau) 98·97·01·73; Police 98·56·00·11; Ⓗ (Concarneau) 98·50·30·30; Brit Consul 40·63·16·02.

FACILITIES

Marina (900+100 visitors) ☎ 98·56·98·45, Fax 98.56.81.31, FF108, AC, D, P, FW, ME, El, Sh, CH, Gaz, R, Ⓞ, SM, V, Bar, BH (16 ton), C (30 ton), Slip (multi hull).
Town Gaz, ✉, Ⓑ, ⇌, ✈ Quimper. Ferry: Roscoff.

17

CONCARNEAU   10-17-12

Finistere 47°52'·10N 03°54'·68W

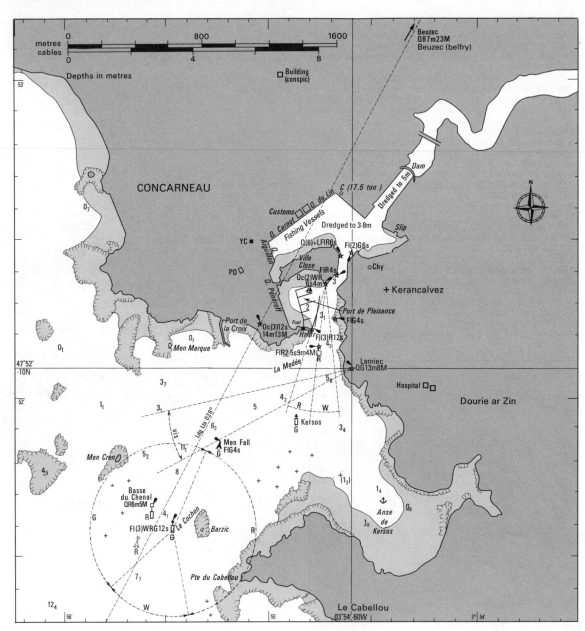

CHARTS
AC 3641, 2352; SHOM 6650, 7146; ECM 543/4; Imray C38

TIDES
+0455 Dover; ML 3·0; Duration 0615; Zone −0100

Standard Port BREST (←—)

Times				Height (metres)			
High Water		Low Water		MHWS	MHWN	MLWN	MLWS
0000	0600	0000	0600	6·9	5·4	2·6	1·0
1200	1800	1200	1800				
Differences CONCARNEAU							
−0010	−0030	−0030	−0020	−1·9	−1·5	−0·7	−0·2
ILE DE PENFRET (Iles de Glénan)							
−0005	−0030	−0028	−0018	−1·9	−1·5	−0·7	−0·2

SHELTER
Good, except in strong S winds. The marina (2m) has an anti-wash barrier. The Arrière Port quays are solely for FVs, but a yacht pontoon (locals) is on the NE corner of La Ville Close.

NAVIGATION
WPT 47°50'·00N 03°56'·80W, 208°/028° from/to front ldg lt 028°, 2·52M. Beware rks around Men Cren and Le Cochon.

LIGHTS AND MARKS
Ldg lts 028°: front Oc (3) 12s 14m 13M, RW tr which is hard to see against bldgs behind; rear, 1·35M from front, Q 87m 23M, spire on skyline. Steer between Le Cochon G bn tr (Fl WRG 12s) and Basse du Chenal R bn tr, QR, both of which are easier to see than the ldg marks. Past Men Fall SHM buoy Fl G 4s, steer 070° for Lanriec lt, QG 13m 8M, vis 063°-078°, G window on W gable, LANRIEC below.

RADIO TELEPHONE
Marina Ch 09 (0700-2100LT in season). FV hbr Ch **12** 16 (H24).

TELEPHONE
Marina Office 98·97·57·96; Hr Mr (FV hbr) 98·97·33·80; Aff Mar 98·97·53·45; CROSS 97·55·35·35; 97·64·32·42; Meteo 98·94·03·43; Auto 36.68.08.29; ⌗ 98·97·01·73; Police 17; Fire 18; Ⓗ 98·50·30·30; Brit Consul 40·63·16·02.

FACILITIES
Marina (267+40 visitors), P, D, FW, M, AC, Slip, C (17 ton), Sh, ME, El, CH, SHOM, ACA, SM.
Town Ⓔ, Gaz, V, R, Bar, ✉, Ⓑ, bus to Quimper ⇌ and ✈.
Ferry: Roscoff.

OTHER HARBOURS AND ANCHORAGES BETWEEN CONCARNEAU AND LORIENT

ILES DE GLÉNAN, 47°43'·04N 03°59'·51W (twr on Île Cigogne). A good Pilot and large-scale chart are essential: AC 3640; SHOM 6648 (larger scale than AC 3640), 7146, 7313; ECM 243. Tides see 10.17.12. A low-lying archipelago, 10M SSW of Concarneau, with Ile aux Moutons and Les Pourceaux, both rky plateaux, to the N. Cardinal buoys mark Basse Jaune, a partly drying shoal to the E, and the SE, S and SW limits of the Islands. Visit in settled weather as ⸆s are rather exposed. There is enough water HW±3 for most boats, but below half-tide careful pilotage is needed. **Conspic marks** are Penfret, highest island with Fl R 5s 36m 21M & Dir Q; and the tower (W with B top) on Ile Cigogne, where the Centre Nautique is based, Q (2) RG 5s 5m 2M. **Approaches**: Easiest is from the N, via WPT 47°44'·0N 03°57'·5W, to W side of Penfret, with bn on Ile Guéotec brg 192°. ⸆ there or proceed W to ⸸s and ⸆ in La Chambre, S of Ile de St Nicolas; at W end a wind turbine (5 FR) is conspic. Also from N, Cigogne tr in transit 181° with chy on Ile du Loc'h leads close E of La Pie IDM bn, Fl (2) 6s 9m 3M, to ⸆ NW of Ile de Bananec; or SE into the pool. From the W, Chenal des Bluiniers 095° dries 0·8m between Ile Drénec and St Nicolas. S apprs and night navigation are not advised. Other ⸆s: E side of Penfret; close E of Cigogne; and N of Ile du Loc'h. No facilities.

AVEN and BELON RIVERS, Finistere, 47°48'·05N 03°44'·20W, AC 2352; SHOM 7138, 7031; ECM 544. HW +0450 on Dover (UT), −0030 on Brest; HW ht −1·9m on Brest; ML 2·8m; Duration 0610. Both rivers are shallow in their upper reaches and have bars, shown on SHOM 7138 as dredged 0·6m. Seas rarely break on the Aven bar, but the Belon bar is impassable in bad weather. Beware Les Cochons de Rousbicout (drying 0·3m) to SW of ent and Les Verres to SE. Port Manech has ⸸s and a good ⸆ in 2·5m outside the bar which dries 0·9m. Very good shelter at Rosbras up the **Aven**; Pont-Aven, 3·6M up-river, only accessible for shoal craft. Moorings in 2·5m; or AB at the quay dries 2·5m. For the **Belon**, appr near HW from close to Pte de Kerhermen and hug the E shore to cross the bar (dries 0·3m); SHOM 7138/ pilot book is advisable. 1M up-river are 3 ⸸s or ⸆ in deep water; dumbell ⸸s further up. The only lt is at Port Manech Oc (4) WRG 12s 38m 10/7M, see 10.15.4 for sectors. Night entry not advised. Facilities: Aff Mar ☎ 98·06·00·73; **YC de l'Aven** at Port Manech. **Town** ME, Slip, C, FW, P & D, R, Bar.

BRIGNEAU, Finistere, 47°47'·82N 03°40'·00W. AC 2352; SHOM 7138, 7031; ECM 544. −0020 on Brest; ML 2·8m. Small drying, fair weather hbr. Strong onshore winds render the ent dangerous and the hbr untenable due to swell. Unlit RW buoy is 8ca S of hbr ent. By day bkwtr lt and rear W panel (hard to see) lead 331° to ent, close E of ruined factory. Dir lt on bkwtr, Oc (2) WRG 6s 7m 12/9M, W tr/R top, W329°- 339°. Some ⸸s or AB on W quay, dries. Facilities: FW, AC, V.

MERRIEN, Finistere, 47°46'·51N 03°38'·98W. AC 2352; SHOM 7138, 7031; ECM 544. HW −0020 on Brest; ML 2·8m. Drying inlet with rky ledges either side of apprs. Ldg marks 005°: front W □ lt ho; rear, house gable. Dir lt QR 26m 7M, vis 004°-009°. ⸆ outside ent or moor to ⸸ or AB on quay SE side. Avoid oyster beds beyond quay. Facilities: FW, AC, R.

DOËLAN, Finistere, 47°46'·20N 03°36'·45W. AC 2352; SHOM 7138, 7031; ECM 544. HW +0450 on Dover (UT), −0035 on Brest ; HW ht −2·2m on Brest; ML 3·1m; Duration 0607. Fair weather only, open to onshore winds. Drying AB at quays; or afloat on W buoys just N and S of bkwtr. Conspic factory chy E od front ldg lt. Daymark, W bn/B stripe, (about 1km NNE of rear ldg lt) on with ldg lts 014°: front Oc (3) WG 12s 20m 13/10M, W tr/G band & top, W shore -305°, G305°- 314°, W314°-shore; rear QR 27m 9M, W tr/R band & top. Facilities: Aff Mar ☎ 98·96·62·38; **Services:** CH, El, Ⓔ, ME, Sh. **Town** D, P, FW, Dr, ✉, R, V, Bar.

LE POULDU (La Laïta or Quimperlé River), Finistere, 47°45'·70N 03°32'·20W. AC 2352; SHOM 7138, 7031; ECM 544. HW − 0020 on Brest; ML 2·8m. Strictly a fair weather hbr, but once inside a small marina on the E bank provides adequate shelter for small yachts; or ⸆ in deeper pools upstream. At HW appr the estuary ent close E of a W ○ tr on low cliffs. The ent favours the W side, but chan shifts often and local advice is needed. In onshore winds the bar is dangerous on the ebb. Tides reach 6kn at sp. No lights. Facilities: FW, V, R, Bar.

PORT TUDY   10-17-13
Morbihan (Ile de Groix) 47°38'·74N 03°26'·63W

CHARTS
AC 2352, 2646; SHOM 7139, 7031, 7032; ECM 544; Imray C38
TIDES
+0505 Dover; ML 3·1; Duration 0610; Zone −0100

Standard Port BREST (←—)

Times				Height (metres)			
High Water		Low Water		MHWS	MHWN	MLWN	MLWS
0000	0600	0000	0600	6·9	5·4	2·6	1·0
1200	1800	1200	1800				
Differences PORT TUDY (Ile de Groix)							
0000	−0025	−0025	−0015	−1·8	−1·4	−0·6	−0·1

SHELTER
Very good in marina (Bassin à Flot), if any room; depths 1·7 to 3·2m. Access, via lock gate 7m wide, (0630–2200) HW −1½ to +2, or less at small coefficients. Outer hbr is open to swell in strong N/NE winds, access H24. Moor fore and aft to buoys; max draft 3m. No ⸆ in hbr, often very crowded. Caution: ferries navigating with panache.

NAVIGATION
WPT 47°39'·14N 03°26'·28W, (100m E of Speerbrecker unlit ECM buoy), 039°/219° from/to N mole hd lt, 0·5M. Remain in R sector of E mole hd lt. Beware 3 large unlit mooring buoys 0·6M NW of ent and rks SE of appr.

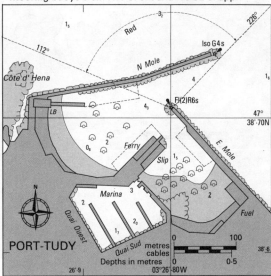

LIGHTS AND MARKS
Pen-Men lt ho (at NW end of island), Fl (4) 25s 59m 29M, W □ tr, B top. Pte de la Croix lt (at E end of island), Oc WR 4s 16m 12/9M. Ldg line at 220°, church spire in line with W end of N mole. By night, mole hd lts in transit 219° clears offlying rks to the NE. N mole hd, Iso G 4s 12m 6M. E mole hd, Fl (2) R 6s 11m 6M, vis 112°-226°.
RADIO TELEPHONE
VHF Ch 09 16 during lock opening times.
TELEPHONE
Hr Mr 97·86·54·62; Aff Mar 97·37·16·22; CROSS 97·55·35·35; SNSM 97·86·82·87; ⌗ 97·86·80·93; Auto 36·68·08·56; Police 97·86·81·17; Ⓗ (Lorient) 97·83·04·02.
FACILITIES
Marina (150), FF100, FF20 on buoy, FW, AC, **Quay** P & D (cans, 0800–1200 & 1400–1900, ☎ 97·86·80·96), ME, El, Sh, C (3 ton), CH. **Town** V, R, ▣, ✉, Bar. Ferry to Lorient.

OTHER HARBOUR ON ILE DE GROIX

LOCMARIA, Morbihan, 47°37'·85N 03°26'·28W. AC 2352, SHOM 7139; −0020 Brest; ML 2·8m. Appr is open to the S, but tiny drying hbr gives shelter in offshore winds. Steer N for G bn tr initially; then ldg line 350°, W bn on with conspic Ho. Close in, 2 PHM bns and a SCM and NCM bn mark the unlit chan. Limited space inside to dry out; or ⸆ outside the hbr W of the ldg line. Few facilities in village, V, R.

17

LORIENT

10-17-14

Morbihan 47°42'·64N 03°21'·92W

CHARTS

AC 304, 2352; SHOM 6470, 7139, 7031, 7032; ECM 544, 545; Imray C38

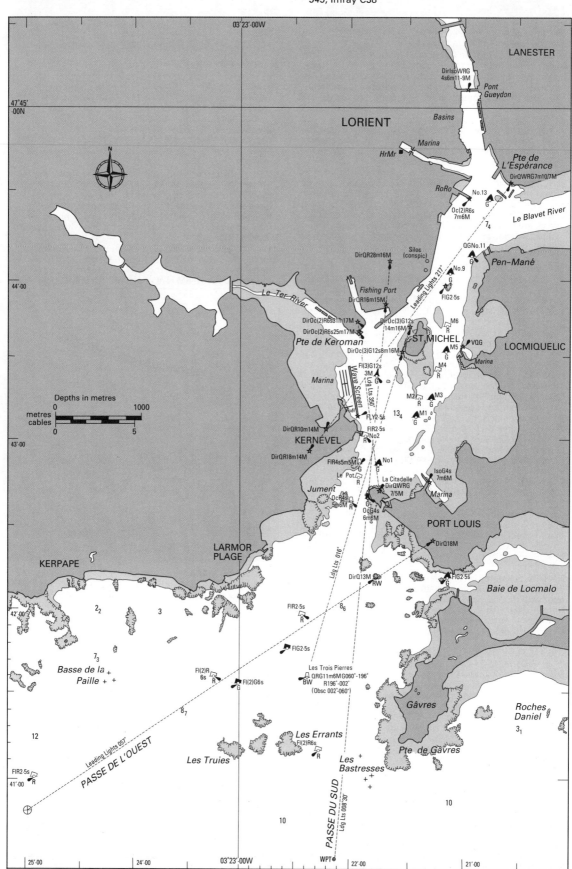

TIDES
+0455 Dover; ML 3·1; Duration 0620; Zone –0100

Standard Port BREST (←—)

Times				Height (metres)			
High Water		Low Water		MHWS	MHWN	MLWN	MLWS
0000	0600	0000	0600	6·9	5·4	2·6	1·0
1200	1800	1200	1800				
Differences LORIENT							
+0003	–0022	–0020	–0010	–1·8	–1·4	–0·6	–0·2
PORT LOUIS							
+0004	–0021	–0022	–0012	–1·8	–1·4	–0·6	–0·1
PORT D'ETEL							
+0020	–0010	+0030	+0010	–2·0	–1·3	–0·4	+0·5

SHELTER
Very good. Ile de Groix shelters the ent from SW'lies. Hbr access all tides/weather. 4 marinas at: **Kernével**, W of main chan (enter between 2 Y buoys at N end of wavebreak, thence ⑦ berths at S end); **Port Louis** (E of La Citadelle); **Locmiquélic** (E of Ile Ste Michel); and **Port du Lorient** in the city: berth in Avant Port or lock into the Bassin à Flot, HW±1 sp, ±15 mins nps; access HJ. No ⚓ in chans and hbr, but moorings ENE of La Citadelle and ⚓ for shoal draft in B de Locmalo. R. Blavet has excellent shelter; moorings below first of two bridges, both 22m clearance. River carries 2m to Hennebont (see 10.15.15) where there are ⚓s and pontoon.

NAVIGATION
WPT Passe du Sud 47°40'·50N 03°22'·40W, 188°/008° from/to front ldg lt, 3·35M. WPT Passe de l'Ouest, 47°40'·80N 03°24'·92W, 237°/057° from/to front ldg lt, 3·0M. There are few navigational dangers if ldg lines are kept to, but yachts must keep clear of shipping in the main chan. Abeam La Citadelle a secondary yacht chan parallels the main chan to W of La Jument R bn tr, Oc R 4s and Le Cochon RGR bn tr, Fl R 4s.

LIGHTS AND MARKS
Conspic daymarks are Water Tr 8ca W of Kernevel, La Citadelle to stbd of ent, submarine pens at Pte de Keroman and 2 silos N of Ile St Michel.
Ldg and Dir lts as seen from seaward in sequence:
(1) Passe du Sud: ldg lts 008·5°, both Dir QR, intens 006°-011°, synch; Front, 16m 15M; R □, G bands on Gy tr, . Rear, Kergroise, 515m from front, 28m 16M; R □, W stripe on Gy framework tr.
(2) Passe de l'Ouest: ldg lts 057°, both Dir Q; Front, Les Soeurs, 11m 13M; R tr, W bands. Rear, Port Louis 740m from front, 22m 18M; W daymark, R bands on bldg.
(3) Les Trois Pierres: QRG 11m 6M; conspic B tr, W bands, G 060°-196°, R196°-002°.
(4) Ile Saint-Michel: ldg lts 016·5°, both Dir Oc (3) G 12s 8/14m 16M, intens 015°-018°; W trs, G tops.
(5) Pte de Keroman: ldg lts 350°, both Dir Oc (2) R 6s 17M, synch, intens 349°-351°. Front, 25m; R ho, W bands; Rear, 31m; RW topmark on Gy pylon, R top.
(6) Kernével: ldg lts 217°, both Dir QR 14M, intens 215°-219°; Front, 10m. Rear, 18m; W □ tr, R top.
(7) Pte de l'Esperance: Dir lt 037°: Dir Q WRG 8m 10/7M; G034·2°-036·7°, W036·7°-037·2°, R037·2°-047·2°.
(8) Pont Gueydon: Dir lt 352°: Iso WRG 4s 6m 11/9M; G350°-351·5°, W351·5°-352·5°, R352·5°-355·5°.

RADIO TELEPHONE
Vigie Port Louis VHF Ch 11 16 (H24). Marinas Ch 09 (HO).

TELEPHONE
Hr Mr Port de Plaisance 97·21·10·14; Aff Mar 97·37·16·22; CROSS 97·55·35·35; SNSM 97·64·32·42; ⌗ 97·37·29·57; Meteo 97·64·34·86; Auto 36.68.08.56; Police 97·64·27·17; Ⓗ 97·37·51·33; Brit Consul 40·63·16·02.

FACILITIES
Kernével Marina (410+60 ⑦) ☎ 97·65·48·25; access H24, depth 3m; FW, AC, P & D (pontoon at S of marina), Ⓘ, Slip, BH (25 ton), C (100 ton), YC ☎ 97·47·47·25.
Port-Louis Marina (160+20 ⑦), ☎ 97.82.18.18, dredged 2m, FW, AC, C (150 ton).
Locmiquélic (S. Catherine) **Marina**, (217+10) ☎ 97.33.59.51, depth 1·5-3m, FW, AC, C (40 ton), Ⓘ.
Lorient Marina (320+50 ⑦) ☎ 97·21·10·14; Avant Port 2·5-3m depth, 2·3m in Bassin à Flot; P, D, FW, AC, Ⓘ, Slip, BH (25 ton), C (100 ton), ME, El, Ⓔ, Sh, CH, SHOM, ACA, Sh, SM; **Club Nautique de Lorient**, Bar, C (1½ ton), FW, Slip.
City All facilities, ✉, Ⓑ, ⇌, ✈. Ferry: Roscoff.

RIVER ÉTEL   10-17-15
Morbihan 47°39'·60N 03°12'·38W

CHARTS
AC 2352; SHOM 7138, 7032; ECM 545; Imray C38
TIDES
+0505 Dover (UT); ML 3·2m; Duration 0617. See 10.17.14
SHELTER
Excellent at marina (1·5-2m) on E bank 1M up-river from the ent, inside the town quay (FVs). Possible ⚓s S of conspic LB ho, off Le Magouër on the W bank or above town (beware strong streams). Pont Lorois (1·3M N) has 9·5m clearance.
NAVIGATION
WPT 47°38'·38N 03°12'·90W, 219°/039° from/to water tr (off chartlet), 1·47M. Appr only by day, in good visibility, at about HW –1½ on the last of the flood, with conspic water tr bearing 039°. Bar dries approx 0·4m; buoyed/lit chan shifts. For directions in simple French, call *Semaphore d'Etel* Ch 13. If no VHF, pre-notify ETA by ☎; fly ensign at mast-head; then expect visual sigs from Fenoux mast, close NW of ent:
Waggle of semaphore arrow = acknowledged; obey signals:
Arrow vert = maintain present course.
Arrow inclined = alter course in direction indicated.
Arrow horiz = no entry for all vessels; conditions dangerous.
● hoisted = no ent for undecked boats and craft <8m LOA.
R flag = insufficient depth over bar. Once inside, the chan is narrow, but well marked, up to Pte Saint-Germain.
LIGHTS AND MARKS
Lt W side of ent, Oc (2) WRG 6s 13m 9/6M, W022°-064°, R064°-123°, W123°-330°, G330°-022°. No ⚓ within 5ca of this lt. Épi de Plouhinic bn, Fl R 2·5s 7m 2M, marks groyne at ent.
RADIO TELEPHONE
Call *Semaphore d'Etel* VHF Ch 13 16 (see above).
TELEPHONE
Hr Mr 97·55·46·62; Aff Mar 97·55·30·32; Auto 36·65·02·56; CROSS 97·55·35·35; Sig Tr 97·55·35·59; Police 97·55·32·11.
FACILITIES
Marina (180 + 20 visitors) FW, AC, C (6 ton), Slip; **Quay** P & D (cans), CH, El, ME, Sh. **Town** Bar, Dr, R, V, Ⓘ, Bus to ⇌ (Auray 15km) and ✈ (Lorient 32km).

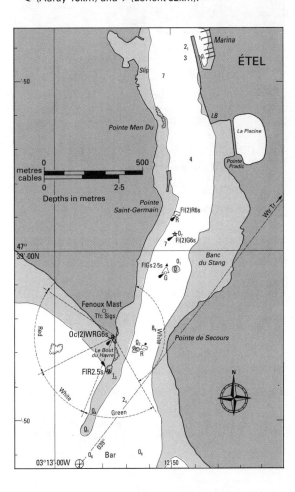

17

LE PALAIS (BELLE ILE)   10-17-16
Morbihan 47°20'·89N 03°08'·98W

CHARTS
AC 2353; Imray C39; SHOM 7142, 7032; ECM 545
TIDES
+0458 Dover; ML 3·1; Duration 0615; Zone –0100

Standard Port BREST (←—)

Times				Height (metres)			
High Water		Low Water		MHWS	MHWN	MLWN	MLWS
0000	0600	0000	0600	6·9	5·4	2·6	1·0
1200	1800	1200	1800				
Differences LE PALAIS							
+0007	–0028	–0025	–0020	–1·8	–1·4	–0·7	–0·3
ILE DE HÖEDIC							
+0010	–0035	–0027	–0022	–1·8	–1·4	–0·7	–0·3

SHELTER
Good, except in strong E winds which cause marked swell. Very crowded in season. Deep draft yachts moor on 3 trots of ⚓s inside Mole Bourdelle; shallow draft on ⚓s to port. Inner hbr mostly dries. Lock into the Bassin à Flot opens HW –1½ to +1 (0600-2200LT), berths on S side (2·5m); thence via lifting bridge into marina (1·7m). See below for Sauzon, 4M WNW.
NAVIGATION
WPT 47°21'·20N 03°08'·00W, 065°/245° from/to Jetée Nord lt, 0·80M. No navigational dangers, but beware high speed ferries. ⚓ between Sauzon and Le Palais is prohib.
LIGHTS AND MARKS
Lts as chartlet. La Citadelle is conspic on N side of hbr.

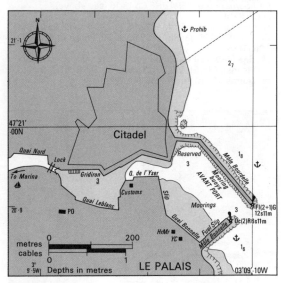

RADIO TELEPHONE
VHF Ch 09.
TELEPHONE
Hr Mr 97·31·42·90; Aff Mar 97·31·83·17; SNSM 97·47·48·49; CROSS 97·55·35·35; ⌗ 97·31·85·95; Auto 36.68.08.56; Police 97·31·80·22; Dr 97·31·40·90; Ⓗ 97·31·48·48; Brit Consul 40·63·16·02.
FACILITIES
Marina ☎ 97·52·83·17, P, D, AC, FW, ME, El, Sh, Access HW–1½ to +1, HJ; **Avant Port** M, AB, P, D, Slip, FW, C (10 & 5 ton). **Town** V, Gaz, R, Bar, ✉, Ⓑ, ⇌ (ferry to Quiberon), ✈. Ferry: Roscoff.

OTHER HARBOUR ON BELLE ILE

SAUZON, Belle Ile, 47°22'·53N 03°12'·93W. AC 2353; SHOM 7142, 7032; ECM 545; HW +0450 on Dover (UT); ML 3·0m; Duration 0615. Small attractive hbr, 4M WNW of Le Palais. Good shelter except in E winds. 12 ⚓s in about 1·5m on W side of Avant Port (FVs moor on E side), or dry out in inner hbr, or ⚓ N of the NW Jetée. Main lt QG 9m 6M. NW Jetée Fl G 4s. SE Jetée Fl R 4s. Facilities: FW on quay; V, R, Bar in village. Hr Mr only operates Jul/Aug.

PORT HALIGUEN   10-17-17
Morbihan 47°29'·40N 03°06'·00W

CHARTS
AC 2353; Imray C38, 39; SHOM 5352, 7032, 7033; ECM 545
TIDES
+0500 Dover; ML 3·1; Duration 0615; Zone –0100

Standard Port BREST (←—)

Times				Height (metres)			
High Water		Low Water		MHWS	MHWN	MLWN	MLWS
0000	0600	0000	0600	6·9	5·4	2·6	1·0
1200	1800	1200	1800				
Differences PORT HALIGUEN							
+0015	–0020	–0015	–0010	–1·7	–1·3	–0·6	–0·3
LA TRINITÉ							
+0020	–0020	–0015	–0005	–1·5	–1·1	–0·5	–0·2

SHELTER
Good, but uncomfortable in strong NW to NE winds. Access H24 at all tides. Marina boat will meet. Visitors usually berth alongside on pontoon K to stbd of ent.
NAVIGATION
WPT 47°29'·80N 03°05'·00W, 060°/240° from/to bkwtr lt, 0·75M. From W or S, appr via Passage de la Teignouse. Banc de Quiberon, marked by NCM and SCM buoys, is shoal (1·5m) at S end. 500m ENE of bkwtr lt in R sector 240°-299°, beware 1·8m shoal, with unlit SCM buoy.
LIGHTS AND MARKS
W sector 246°-252° of Port-Maria Main lt, Q WRG 28m 14/10M, leads N of Banc de Quiberon; W sector 299°-306° of bkwtr lt, Oc (2) WR 6s 10m 12/9M, leads S of it.
RADIO TELEPHONE
VHF Ch 09.
TELEPHONE
Hr Mr 97·50·20·56; Aff Mar 97·50·08·71; ⌗ 97·55·73·46; CROSS 97·55·35·35; SNSM 97·50·14·39; Meteo 97·64·34·86; Auto 36.68.08.56; Police 97·50·07·39; Dr 97·50·13·94.
FACILITIES
Marina (760 + 100 visitors) ☎ 97·50·20·56, Slip, P, D, C (2 ton), BH (13 ton), ME, El, Sh, AC, CH, FW, ▣, SM, Bar, R, V. **Town** (Quiberon) V, Gaz, R, Ice, Bar, ✉, Ⓑ, ⇌, ✈. Ferry: Roscoff.

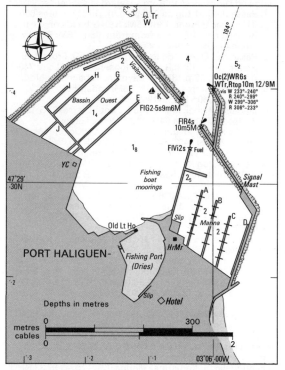

PORT MARIA, Morbihan, 47°28'·65N 03°07'·25W. AC 2353; SHOM 5352, 7032. Tides as 10.17.17. Shelter good in all winds, but busy ferry/FV port; only suitable for yachts as a refuge or in emergency. Access dangerous in strong SE–SW winds. N half hbr dries. E mole reserved for ferries. ⚓ in SW of hbr in approx 2m. Hr Mr/Aff Mar ☎ 97·50·08·71; Facilities: ⌗, C (6 ton), FW at E quay, El, ME, Sh, SHOM.

LA TRINITÉ-SUR-MER   10-17-18

Morbihan 47°34'·06N 03°00'·06W

CHARTS

AC 2358, 2353; Imray C39; SHOM 5352, 7033, 7034; ECM 545, 546

TIDES

+0455 Dover; ML 3·2; Duration 0610; Zone –0100

Standard Port BREST (←). Differences as see 10.17.17.

SHELTER

Very good, except in strong SE/S winds near HW when La Vaneresse sandbank is covered. Access H24 at all tides. Marina boat will meet. No ⚓/fishing in river. Speed limit 5kn.

NAVIGATION

WPT 47°31'·90N 02°59'·63W, 167°/347° from/to front ldg lt, 2·3M. No navigational dangers; the river is well marked by buoys and perches. Best water close to E bank. Beware many oyster beds, marked with perches.

LIGHTS AND MARKS

Conspic daymarks include: Mousker rk, W top; caravan site 3ca NNE; and ✠ spire at La Trinité. Pte de Kernevest ldg lts 347°: Front Q WRG 11m 10/7M (W345°-013°); rear Dir Q 21m 15M, synch, intens 337°-357°. 1M up-river: Dir lt 347°, Oc WRG 4s 9m 13/11M (W346°-348°). S Pier, Oc (2) WR 6s (W293°-300°).

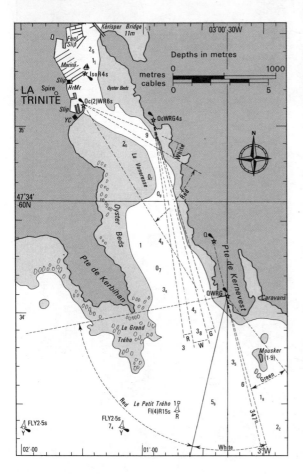

CROUESTY   10-17-19

Morbihan 47°32'·52N 02°54'·03W

CHARTS

AC 2358, 2353; Imray C39; SHOM 6992, 7034, 7033; ECM 546

TIDES

+0505 Dover; ML 3·0; Duration 0555; Zone –0100

Standard Port BREST (←)

Times				Height (metres)			
High Water		Low Water		MHWS	MHWN	MLWN	MLWS
0000	0600	0000	0600	6·9	5·4	2·6	1·0
1200	1800	1200	1800				
Differences PORT NAVALO							
+0030	–0005	–0010	–0005	–2·0	–1·5	–0·8	–0·3

SHELTER

Good, protected from W'lies by Quiberon Peninsula; additional shelter in very large marina which contains 5 large separate basins. Visitors in first basin to stbd.

NAVIGATION

WPT 47°32'·04N 02°55'·21W, 238°/058° from/to front ldg lt, 1·1M. There are no navigational dangers, the ent being well marked and dredged 1·8m. See also Morbihan 10.17.20.

LIGHTS AND MARKS

Ldg lts 058°: both Dir Q 10/27m 19M, intens 056·5°-059·5°. By day, front W vert stripe on R panel; rear grey lt ho. Bkwtr hds: N = Oc (2) R 6s, S = Fl G 4s, plus lead-in buoys.

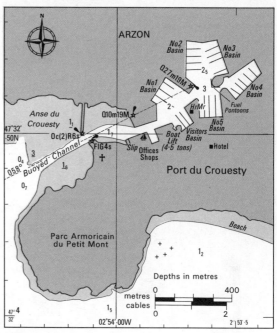

ISLAND HARBOUR IN THE BAIE DE QUIBERON

ÎLE HOUAT, 47°23'·60N 02°57'·25W. AC 2353; SHOM 7033. HW +0505 on Dover (UT); ML 3·1m; Duration 0605. See 10·17·18 (Île Höedic). Good shelter, except from N/NE'lies, at Port St Gildas, near E end of the N coast. Appr from N or NE passing abeam La Vieille rk (conspic 14m). Avoid rks 6m inboard of bkwtr and 15m off lt tr. Moor on double trots; no ⚓ in hbr. S part of hbr dries. Keep clear of ferries and FVs on W and N quays. Lts as 10.17.4. Few facilities.

17

MORBIHAN   10-17-20
Morbihan 47°32'·92N 02°55'·26W

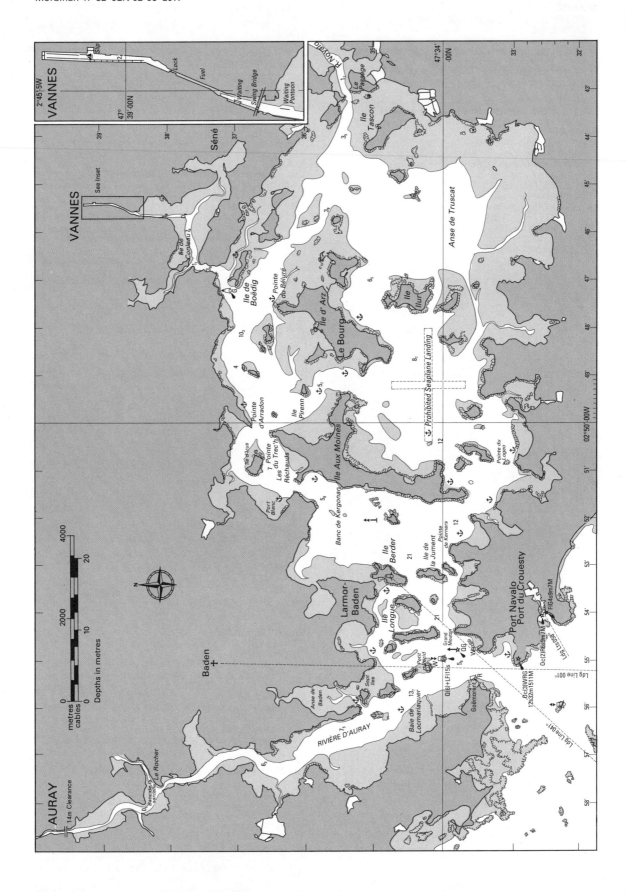

CHARTS
AC 2358, 2353; Imray C39; SHOM 6992, 7034, 7033; ECM 546
TIDES
−0515 Dover; ML 3·0; Zone −0100

Standard Port BREST (←)

Times				Height (metres)			
High Water		Low Water		MHWS	MHWN	MLWN	MLWS
0000	0600	0000	0600	6·9	5·4	2·6	1·0
1200	1800	1200	1800				
Differences AURAY							
+0055	0000	+0020	+0005	−2·0	−1·4	−0·8	−0·2
VANNES							
+0220	+0200	+0200	+0125	−3·6	−2·7	−1·6	−0·5
ARRADON							
+0155	+0145	+0145	+0130	−3·7	−2·7	−1·6	−0·5
LE LOGEO							
+0155	+0145	+0145	+0125	−3·7	−2·7	−1·6	−0·5

The Golfe du Morbihan is an inland sea of about 50sq miles with deep apprs and ent. It is thick with islands, all but two privately owned. The many ⚓s (see chartlet and below) are increasingly restricted by extensive moorings. It is essential to use chain when ⚓ing, unless well out of the tide. Avoid oyster beds and, especially in SE, bird sanctuaries. Much of E & SE dries. See 10.17.21. Vannes.

NAVIGATION
WPT 47°32'·04N 02°55'·21W, 181°/001° from/to Petit Vezid front ldg mark, 2·2M. Beware very strong tides, max 8kn sp, in the ent and in some narrow chans, but easing in the upper reaches. Springs should be avoided for a first visit; it is likely to be impossible for an aux yacht to enter against a sp ebb. HW times become later, the further into the Morbihan one goes, ie HW Vannes is 2 hrs after HW Port Navalo. At the ent the flood divides: a weaker flow into the R Auray; but the main stream buckets NE into the main chan, with a strong set towards Petit and Grand Mouton rks.

To avoid these, keep up to the ldg line until safely past Grand Mouton, but beware shoals to port off Goëmorent R bn tr. Pilotage is not difficult, but due to higher than usual speeds over the ground, it helps to pre-plot the desired trks/distances within the chan; marks can then be more readily identified and track adjusted with ease, especially if beating.

LIGHTS AND MARKS
At the ent ldg daymarks on 001° are: front Petit Vezid W obelisk, rear Baden ✠ spire (3·3M); maintain until abeam Port Navalo lt ho.
Chans and dangers are well marked; the only lts are: Port Navalo Oc (3) WRG 12s 32m 15/11M at ent, W sector 359°-015°. Inside ent: Grand Mouton SHM bn, QG and Le Grégan SCM bn, Q (6) + L Fl 15s. Roguédas SHM bn, Fl G 2·5s, at W end of Ile de Boëdig marks appr to Vannes.

SHELTER AND FACILITIES (clockwise from ent)
PORT NAVALO: ⚓ in bay, but space limited by moorings, and exposed to W/NW winds. Convenient to await the tide. All facilities. ⌗ ☎ 97·41·21·53; Police 97·24·17·17.
LOCMARIAQUER: Drying ⚓ off village quay; ferries use the buoyed chan to jetty. V, R, ME.
SEPT ILES: Small, quiet ⚓; chan leads into Anse de Baden.
LE ROCHER: Good shelter, but almost full of moorings. Further N the river almost dries, but can be navigated on the tide.
BONO: Moor or ⚓ (rky bottom) off Banc de la Sarcelle. **Village**, ME, R, V, Gaz.
AURAY: Access at mid-flood via a bridge, 3ca S of town, with 14m clearance MHWS. Note: this clearance, coupled with little depth of water, may need careful calculations for safe passage by high-masted yachts. Moor in a pool S of the bridge; 12 🅐s or drying AB at St Goustan beyond. Facilities: ME, EI, Sh, SHOM, CH. **Town** R, V, Bar, ✉, ≉.
ILE LONGUE: near SE tip ⚓ out of the stream. No landing.
LARMOR BADEN: good ⚓s to S, but many moorings; Aff Mar ☎ 97·57·05·66; V, R.
ILE BERDER: pleasant ⚓ E of the island; causeway to mainland.
PORT BLANC: Hr Mr ☎ 97·57·01·00. FW, P & D pontoon, but many moorings.
ILE AUX MOINES: a much-frequented, public island. The narrows between the mainland and Les Réchauds rks can

be rough. ⚓ off N end, landing at Pte du Trec'h or pick up 🅐 (see Hr Mr) off Pte des Réchauds where there is a small marina. Water taxi available; call VHF Ch 09 or sound foghorn. Hr Mr ☎ 97·26·30·57, D, FW. Other quieter ⚓s off W side and S tip.
ARRADON: limited ⚓, exposed to S'ly. Hr Mr ☎ 97·26·01·23; M, Slip, FW, ME.
ILE PIRENN: exposed ⚓ in tidal stream.
ILE D'ARZ: a public island. ⚓ NE of Pte du Béluré; E of Le Bourg (good shelter), or to the W, depending on winds. Rudevent village: ME, EI, Sh.
ILE DE BOEDIG: sheltered ⚓ in chan N of the E end of island.
ILE DE CONLEAU: ⚓ or moor in bight just S of village. ME, EI, Sh, R in village.
SÉNÉ: ME.
VANNES: see 10·17·21.
R. NOYALO : ⚓ off Pte du Passage or in Anse de Truscat, 2M to SW of river ent. Depths further up-river are uncertain.
KERNERS: ⚓ off the Anse de Kerners in 3 to 6m.
ILE DE LA JUMENT (also known as Ar Gazek): good shelter to E of island out of the tide; convenient for leaving on the tide.

VANNES   10-17-21
Morbihan 47°38'·45N 02°45'·62W

CHARTS
AC 2358, 2353; Imray C39; SHOM 7034; ECM 546
TIDES/CHARTLET
See under Morbihan 10.17.20. ML 2·0m
SHELTER
Very good, protected from all winds. Access by day only. Waiting pontoons down/upstream of **swing bridge**, which only opens whilst lock gate into wet basin is open, as follows: Bridge will open at H and H+30 in season and at weekends; but only at H out of season (1 Jan-15 Jun and 15 Sep-31 Dec). However, during the first and final ½ hour periods that the lock is open, the bridge may open at any time. Outbound vessels have priority over arrivals. **The lock**, remotely-controlled by Hr Mr, opens HW±2½ (0700-2200LT in season; 0900-1800 Mon-Sat and 0700-2100LT Sun out of season). Note: HW Vannes −2½ just happens to be HW Port Tudy (10.17.13) which is used by the Hr Mr to determine when the lock opens; or write to: Bureau du Port de Plaisance, La Rabine, 56000 Vannes for the free annual timetable of lock hours. Lock sill, 1·3m above CD, retains 2·4m inside wet basin.
Berthing: Marina boat may indicate a vacant finger pontoon, but visitors usually berth N/S on pontoons D and G just before inner foot-bridge (passerelle).
NAVIGATION
WPT: see 10·17·20. Beware very strong streams between Pte de Toulindag and the mainland and in the Conleau chan; also Les Réchauds rks marked by 2 SHM bns. Due to an eddy around Ile d'Irus the stream runs mainly SW between Les Réchauds and Pte d'Arradon. Thereafter passage to Conleau is simple and well marked. Beacon'd appr chan to Vannes is narrow, with min depth 0·7m; only advised near HW.
LIGHTS AND MARKS
Bridge sigs (vert) on main bridge pier are:
2 Ⓡ = no passage; 2 Oc Ⓡ = standby; 2 Ⓖ = proceed;
2 Oc Ⓖ = only transit if committed;
Ⓨ = unmasted boats may transit.
Lock sigs: Ⓖ and Ⓡ = Lock closed; No lts = Lock open.
RADIO TELEPHONE
VHF Ch 09. (Summer 0830-2100; winter HW±2½ and 0900-1200 and 1330-1800).
TELEPHONE
Hr Mr 97·54·16·08; Aff Mar 97·63·40·95; ⌗ 97·63·18·71; CROSS 97·55·35·35; SNSM 97·26·00·56; Meteo 97·64·34·86; Auto 36.68.08.56; Police 97·54·22·56; Dr 97·47·47·25; Ⓗ 97·42·66·42; Brit Consul 40·63·16·02.
FACILITIES
Marina (240+60 visitors), ☎ 97·54·16·08, Fax 97.42.48.80, FF95, Slip, ▣, FW, AC, ME, C (12 ton); P & D @ HW±2½ from pontoon on E side of canal, just S of lock.
Town V, R, Sh, CH, EI, Ⓔ, CH, SM, SHOM, ✉, Ⓑ, ≉, ✈ (Vannes, Lorient or St Nazaire).

17

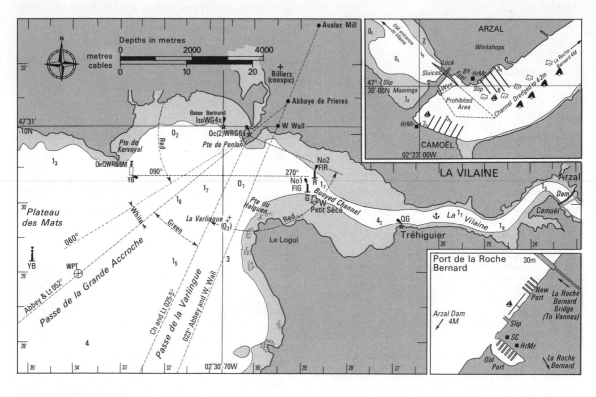

VILAINE RIVER   10-17-22

Morbihan 47°30'·40N02°28'·60W

CHARTS

AC 2353; SHOM 2381, 5418, 7033; ECM 546; Imray C39

TIDES

+0500 Dover; ML (Penerf) 3·3; Duration 0610; Zone –0100

Standard Port BREST (←)

Times				Height (metres)			
High Water		Low Water		MHWS	MHWN	MLWN	MLWS
0000	0600	0000	0600	6·9	5·4	2·6	1·0
1200	1800	1200	1800				
Differences PENERF							
+0020	–0025	–0015	–0015	–1·5	–1·1	–0·6	–0·3

SHELTER

Good shelter up-river: moorings at Tréhiguier; marina above Arzal dam in non-tidal waters, with pontoons at Arzal (N bank) and Camoël (S bank); and 5M upstream at La Roche Bernard on visitors' pontoon between the 2 marinas; also 4½M further up-river at Foleux marina. Yachts with masts can transit the swing bridge at Cran to reach Redon where there is a marina, crane and access to Brittany canals (see 10.15.18).

NAVIGATION

WPT Passe de la Grande Accroche 47°29'·00N 02°33'·90W, 232°/052° from/to Penlan lt, 3·3M. Appr to La Vilaine has a bar (min 0·5m), on which seas break in strong onshore winds esp at sp ebb. Best to enter/leave on last of the flood. River is well buoyed up to Tréhiguier and adequately so up-stream; keep strictly to the buoyed chan as depths may be less than charted due to silting.

The Arzal dam has a lock which opens on the hour, up to 9 times per day, 0700–2200 (LT) in Jul/ Aug; in other months 0800, 0900, 1200, 1400, 1600, 1700, 1900, 2000LT. But these times vary daily; check with Hr Mr VHF Ch 09 or recording ☎ 97·45·01·15. Yachts should avoid the prohib area (Y buoys) below/above the dam by keeping strictly to the buoyed chan. There is room to ⚓ below the dam to await lock opening.

LIGHTS AND MARKS

There are two apprs and ldg lines to river ent:
(1) Passe de la Grande Accroche (Penlan lt ho on with Abbey de Prières at 052°). Marks are reportedly conspic by day.
(2) Passe de la Varlingue: Penlan lt on with Billiers ch tr 023°. This leaves Varlingue Rk (dries 0·3m) close to stbd.

Two principal lts are visible in the approaches:
(1) Basse Bertrand G tr, Iso WG 4s 6m 9/6M, W040°-054°, G054°-227°, W227°-234°, G234°-040°.
(2) Penlan, W tr with R bands Oc (2) WRG 6s 26m 15/11M, R292°-025°, G025°-052°, W052°-060°, R060°-138°, G138°-180°.
At the river mouth Petit Sécé W bn tr is easier to see than No 1 and 2 chan buoys.

RADIO TELEPHONE

Lock VHF Ch 18 (HX); Arzal-Camoël marina Ch 09 (French); no VHF at La Roche Bernard.

TELEPHONE .

Hr Mr (Camoël) 99·90·05·86; Hr Mr (R Bernard) 99·90·62·17; Aff Mar 99·90·32·62; CROSS 97·52·35·35; ⌗ (Vannes) 97·63·18·71; Dr (Arzal) 97·45·01·21; Ⓗ (Vannes) 97·01·41·41; Ⓗ (R Bernard) 99.90.61.20; Dr (R Bernard) 99·90·61·25; Auto 36·68·08·56; Police 17; Brit Consul 40·63·16·02.

FACILITIES

ARZAL/CAMOËL: **Marina** (630 total, inc 25 visitors on each bank) ☎ 99·90·05·86, FF75, FW, AC, Ⓒ, C (15 ton), P, D, Gaz, SM, ME, El, Sh, CH, Ⓔ, R, Bar. Note: all these facilities are at Arzal. Camoël has Hr Mr and showers. **Towns** (both 3km) V, R, Bar, Ⓑ, ✉.
LA ROCHE BERNARD: **Marina (New Port)** (110) ☎ 99·90·62·17, FF65, FW, AC, M, ME, El, Ⓔ, Sh, CH; **Marina (Old Port)** (200), P, D, Ⓒ, C, AC, CH, FW, Slip. **Town** V, Gaz, R, Bar, Ice, ✉, Ⓑ, ⇌ (Pontchateau), ✈ (Nantes or Rennes).
Foleux: ☎ 99·91·80·87. Marina on N bank; buoys off both banks. FW, AC, R.

ADJACENT HARBOUR

PENERF, Morbihan, 47°30'·10N 02°38'·80W, AC 2353; SHOM 5418, 7033. HW +0515 on Dover (UT); ML 3·3m; Duration 0610. See 10.17.22. Shelter good, except in fresh W'lies. SDs and SHOM 5418 are advised. Appr between Penvins PHM By and Borenis SHM By. Ldg marks: Le Pignon PHM lt bn tr on 359° with Le Tour du Parc spire. 3 ents are not easy: Passe de l'Ouest is shoal and ill marked. Passe du Centre is the widest and easiest, ldg 150m W of a drying reef, La Traverse SHM bn, N of which depth is 0·5m; thence 40m E of Le Pignon. In the river head ENE for 1M to ⚓ off Penerf quay. Passe de l'Est has 4m, but is narrower and rks are close to stbd. It leads E of La Traverse and Le Pignon bns to join Passe du Centre. Beware oyster beds in the river. Le Pignon lt, Fl (3) WR 12s 6m 9/6M, W sector 349°-028° covers the appr, but night entry not advised. Facilities: P & D (on quay), Slip, CH, El, ME, Sh. **Village** Bar, Dr, R, V.

LA TURBALLE   10-17-23

Loire Atlantique 47°20′·78N 02°30′·80W

CHARTS
AC 2353; Imray C39, 40; SHOM 6826, 7033; ECM 546

TIDES
As for Le Croisic 10.17.24

SHELTER
Good in all winds, but heavy swell can enter in strong SSW winds. Access H24; inside ent, turn smartly stbd into marina (1·5-2m) in SE corner. Sardine FVs occupy the rest of the hbr.

NAVIGATION
WPT 47°20′·25N 02°32′·35W, 245°/065° from/to W bkwtr lt, 1·15M. Appr from S or W avoiding Plateau du Four, which is well marked/lit. From NW, beware tanker berths (buoyed) off Pte du Castelli, 2·5M WNW of hbr.

LIGHTS AND MARKS
Plateau du Four, Fl 5s 23m 19M, is 5M SW. Hbr is in G sector (136°-345°) of Le Croisic, Iso WG 4s, 2M to S. (Note: WPT is also on Le Croisic ldg line 156°). Appr in W sector (315°-060°) of W bkwtr lt, Fl (4) WR 12s, to pick up ldg lts 065°, both Dir F Vi 11/19m 3M, intens 004°-009°. By day Trescalan ✠ and water tr (conspic), 1M ENE of hbr, lead 070° to just S of ent. R bn tr is 80m off W bkwtr.

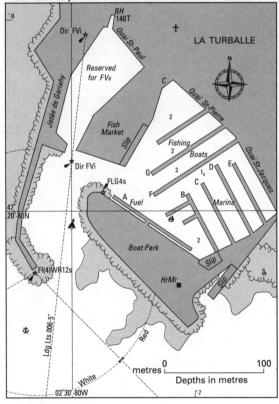

RADIO TELEPHONE
VHF Ch 09.

TELEPHONE
Hr Mr 40·23·41·65; Aff Mar 40·23·33·35; ⌗ 40·23·32·51; Auto 36·68·08·44; SNSM 40·23·42·67.

FACILITIES
Marina (290+20 visitors), ☎ 40·62·80·40, FW, AC, Slip, M, C (16 tons), BH (140 tons), D (H24), P at garage 500m, ME, El, Ⓔ, Sh, CH. Extension to marina is planned.

ADJACENT HARBOUR

PIRIAC, Loire-Atlantique, 47°23′·00N 02°32′·63W, AC 2353; SHOM 7033. HW +0505 on Dover (UT); −0015 and HW ht −1·9m on Brest; ML 3·1m; Duration 0605. A small resort village with drying FV hbr. Access HW±3; 15 ⚓s via Hr Mr ☎ 40·23·52·32 (July-Aug only). Lt Oc (2) WRG 6s 8m 10/6M; W194°-201° leads through hbr ent. Bkwtr lts are Fl G 4s and Fl R 4s. Night ent not advised. Facilities: D, P on quay, CH, Ⓔ, El, ME, Sh.

Ile Dumet, 3·5M WNW of Piriac, has pleasant ⚓ on NE side in 2m, clear of mussel beds. Appr with lt ho brg 215°.

LE CROISIC   10-17-24

Loire Atlantique 47°18′·56N 02°31′·27W

CHARTS
AC 2353; Imray C39; SHOM 6826, 6825, 7033; ECM 546, 547

TIDES
+0450 Dover; ML 3·3; Duration 0605; Zone −0100

Standard Port BREST (←—)

Times				Height (metres)			
High Water		Low Water		MHWS	MHWN	MLWN	MLWS
0000	0600	0000	0600	6·9	5·4	2·6	1·0
1200	1800	1200	1800				
Differences LE CROISIC							
+0015	−0040	−0020	−0015	−1·5	−1·1	−0·6	−0·3

SHELTER
Five drying (1·7m) basins, called *Chambres* are formed by islands *(Jonchères)*. Berth in the last *Chambre*, bows to pontoon or against the wall. Access HW±1. See Hr Mr for mooring or ⚓ in Le Poul which is crowded; tripping line is advised. Safest ⚓ in Pen Bron Creek; streams run hard.

NAVIGATION
WPT 47°19′·00N 02°31′·80W, 336°/156° from/to front ldg lt, 1·2M. Sp tides reach 4kn. Safest ent is HW±1 sp, HW±2 np. Beware the rks at Hergo Tr, SHM, Fl G 2·5s. Note: the W sector (093°-137°) of Tréhic lt, Iso WG 4s, which leads clear of distant dangers, will lead onto close-in dangers. Keep to the ldg lines as appr and hbr dry extensively to the E.

LIGHTS AND MARKS
The sanatorium, hospital and ch belfry are conspic. Outer ldg lts 156°: both Dir Oc (2+1) 12s 10/14m 18M; intens 154°-158°, synch; Y □s on W pylons, rear has G top.

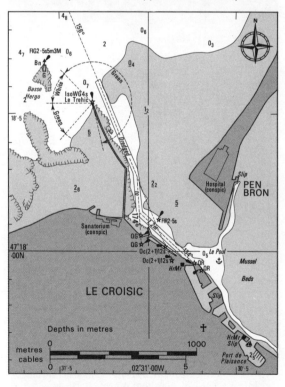

Middle ldg lts 174°: both QG 5/8m 11M; vis 170°-177°; Y □s with G stripe on G & W pylons. Inner ldg lts 134°: both QR; R/W chequered □s on Fish market.

RADIO TELEPHONE
VHF Ch 09 (0800-1200; 1330-2000 in season).

TELEPHONE
Hr Mr 40·23·10·95; Aff Mar 40·23·06·56; CROSS 97·55·35·35; SNSM 40·23·01·17; ⌗ 40·23·05·38; Meteo 40·90·08·80; Auto 36.68.08.44; Police 40·23·00·19; Dr 40·23·01·70; Ⓗ 40·23·01·12; Brit Consul 40·63·16·02.

FACILITIES
Marina (5th Chambre; 220+15 visitors), FW, ME, El, Sh; **Quai** Slip, M, C (10 ton), CH, V, R, Bar, Ⓔ, Divers. **Town** P & D (cans, ½M), V, Gaz, R, Bar, ✉, Ⓑ, ⇌, ✈ (St Nazaire).

17

LE POULIGUEN/PORNICHET
Loire Atlantique   **10-17-25**

CHARTS
AC 3216, 2353; Imray C39; SHOM 6825, 7033, 6797; ECM 547
TIDES
Sp +0435 Dover, Nps +0530 Dover; ML 3·3; Duration Sp 0530, Nps 0645; Zone −0100

Standard Port BREST (←)

Times				Height (metres)			
High Water		Low Water		MHWS	MHWN	MLWN	MLWS
0000	0600	0000	0600	6·9	5·4	2·6	1·0
1200	1800	1200	1800				
Differences LE POULIGUEN							
+0020	−0025	−0020	−0025	−1·5	−1·1	−0·6	−0·3
PORNICHET							
+0020	−0045	−0022	−0022	−1·4	−1·0	−0·5	−0·2

FACILITIES (Le Pouliguen)
Quai (Pontoons 850+30 visitors) ☎ 40·60·03·50, Slip, P, D, AC, L, FW, C (18 ton), M, ME, Sh, CH, Ⓔ, El, Divers, SM; **La Baule YC** ☎ 40·60·20·90 (allocates berths for visitors). **Town** V, Gaz, R, Bar, ✉, Ⓑ, ⇌, ✈ (St Nazaire).

PORNICHET 47°15′·55N 02°21′·05W

SHELTER
A very large artificial marina at the E end of the B de la Baule, with excellent shelter and facilities. Access at all tides for up to 3·5m draft.

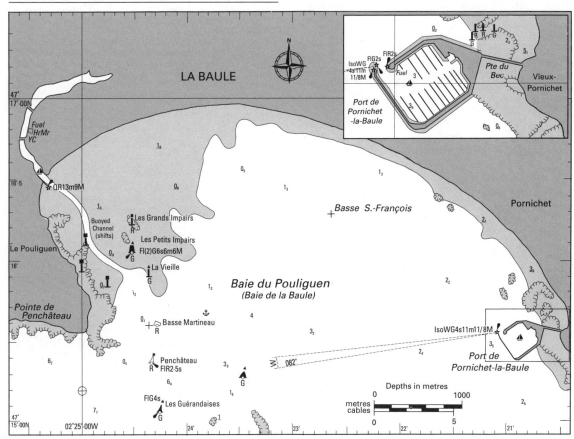

LE POULIGUEN 47°16′·40N 02°25′·40W

SHELTER
Very good, except in SE winds. Visitors berths (30) to stbd at ent. Fixed bridge up-river has only 1m clearance MHWS.
NAVIGATION
WPT 47°15′·20N 02°25′·00W, 250°/070° from/to Penchâteau PHM Fl R 2·5s, 0·58M. Appr from W between Pte de Penchateau and the Grand Charpentier. Best appr HW −1. Beware rks extending SE 4M to the Grand Charpentier lt ho, Q WRG, and breakers in shallow water when wind in S. It is not advisable to enter at night. Beware strong ebb tide.
LIGHTS AND MARKS
From Penchâteau and Basse Martineau, leave La Vieille and Les Impairs to stbd, and three chan bns to port. S jetty QR 13m 9M, vis 171°-081°.
RADIO TELEPHONE
Pouliguen VHF Ch 09.
TELEPHONE
Hr Mr 40·60·37·40; Aff Mar 40·42·32·55; CROSS 97·55·35·35; SNSM 40·61·03·20; ☷ 40·61·32·04; Meteo 40·90·00·80; Auto 36.68.08.44; Police 40·24·48·17; Dr 40·60·51·73.

NAVIGATION
Appr from the W, as for Le Pouliguen (3M), then direct via W sector (082°) of Iso WG 4s bkwtr lt; also from SW, track 035° between Les Evens PHM and Les Troves SHM unlit buoys; or from SSE track 335° from Grand Charpentier lt.
LIGHTS AND MARKS
S bkwtr Iso WG 4s 11m 12/8M, W081°-084° (3°), G084°-081° (357°). Inside ent, R & G Fl 2s 3m 2M define chan.
RADIO TELEPHONE
VHF Ch 09.
TELEPHONE
Hr Mr 40·47·23·71; ☷ 40·61·32·04; Meteo 40·90·08·80; Auto 36·68·08·44; Aff Mar 40·60·56·13; CROSS 97·55·35·35; Ⓗ (St Nazaire) 40·90·60·60; SNSM 40·61·03·20; Dr La Baule 40·60·17·20; Brit Consul 40·63·16·02.
FACILITIES
Marina (1000+150 visitors) ☎ 40·61·03·20, AC, Slip, FW, P, D, BH (24 ton), V, R, Bar, ▣, ME, El, Ⓔ, Sh, CH, SHOM. **Town** Bar, Dr, R, V, Ⓑ, ✉, ⇌, ✈ (St Nazaire).

RIVER LOIRE/ST NAZAIRE

Loire Atlantique
10-17-26

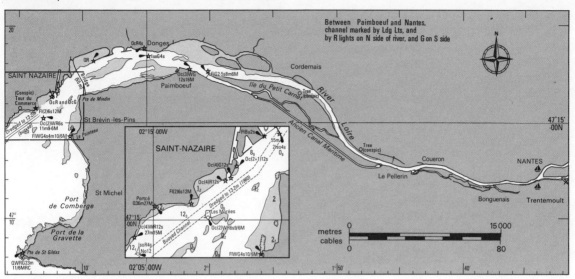

SAINT-NAZAIRE

CHARTS
AC 2985, 2989, 3216; Imray C40; SHOM 6797, 6493, 6260, 6261, 5992, 6854, 6825; ECM 248, 547

TIDES
St Nazaire: Sp +0445 Dover, Nps –0540 Dover; ML 3·6; Duration Sp 0640, Nps 0445; Zone –0100

Standard Port BREST (⟵)

Times				Height (metres)			
High Water		Low Water		MHWS	MHWN	MLWN	MLWS
0000	0600	0000	0600	6·9	5·4	2·6	1·0
1200	1800	1200	1800				
Differences ST NAZAIRE							
+0030	–0040	–0010	–0010	–1·1	–0·8	–0·4	–0·2
LE GRAND CHARPENTIER							
+0015	–0045	–0025	–0020	–1·5	–1·1	–0·6	–0·3
DONGES							
+0040	–0030	0000	0000	–0·9	–0·7	–0·5	–0·4
CORDEMAIS							
+0055	–0005	+0105	+0030	–0·7	–0·5	–0·7	–0·4
LE PELLERIN							
+0110	+0010	+0145	+0100	–0·7	–0·5	–0·9	–0·4
NANTES (Chantenay)							
+0133	+0055	+0215	+0125	–0·6	–0·3	–0·8	–0·1

SHELTER
Hbr is mainly naval and commercial, but yachts can berth at S end of Bassin Penhoet; ent via E lock and Bassin de St Nazaire. ⚓ in Bonne Anse.

NAVIGATION
WPT 47°07'·95N 02°20'·00W, 205°/025° from/to front ldg lt, 7·3M, via S chan. Or appr from W, via N chan, to join dredged chan (13·2m) SE of Grand Charpentier lt Q WRG. In strong W winds the bar (outside chan) is only safe HW –3 to HW. R Loire navigable 28M to Nantes and ent to canals (10.15.18). Tolls may be due above Nantes; see 10.15.8.

LIGHTS AND MARKS
Ldg lts over bar, 025°; both Q 23/27M, intens 022°-028°.

RADIO TELEPHONE
St Nazaire Port VHF Ch **12** 16 06 14 67 69 (H24). Other stns: Donges Ch 12 16 (occas); Nantes Ch 12 16 06 67 69 (0700-1100, 1300-1700, except Sun); water level reports (St Nazaire to Nantes) broadcast on Ch 73 every 15min from H+00.

TELEPHONE
ST NAZAIRE Hr Mr 40·00·45·20; Aff Mar 40·22·46·32; CROSS 97·55·35·35; SNSM 40·61·03·20; ☒ 40·66·82·65; Meteo 40·90·00·80; Auto 36.68.08.44; Police 40·70·55·00; Dr 40·22·15·32; Ⓗ 40·90·60·60.
NANTES Hr Mr 40·44·20·54; Aff Mar 40·73·18·70; ☒ 40·73·39·55; Meteo 40·84·80·19; Auto 36.68.08.44; Dr 40·47·03·19; Ⓗ 40·48·33·33; Brit Consul 40·63·16·02.

FACILITIES
ST NAZAIRE **Quai** P, D, L, FW, C, M, ME, El, Sh, CH, Ⓔ, SHOM. **Town** V, Gaz, R, Bar, ☒, Ⓑ, ⇌, ✈.
NANTES **Quai** FW, C, CH, SHOM, ME, El, Ⓔ; **Trentemoult** AB. **City** all facilities: ☒, Ⓑ, ⇌, ✈. Ferry: St Malo/Roscoff.

MINOR HARBOURS BETWEEN SAINT-NAZAIRE AND POINTE DE SAINT-GILDAS

The following three small hbrs lie NE of Pte de St-Gildas, on the E side of the R Loire estuary; see chartlet above. They are flanked by shellfish beds on rky ledges drying to about 4ca offshore; they are sheltered from W'lies but open to N'lies. Charts are AC 3216; SHOM 6854, 6825; ECM 547. Tidal data may be interpolated from Le Grand Charpentier, St-Nazaire (10.17.26) and Pornic (10.18.9). The bay is shallow. Note: 4M N of Pte de St-Gildas is La Truie rk, drying 2·6m and marked by unlit IDM bn; 1·3M SSW of it is a shoal patch 0·7m.

PORT DE COMBERGE, Loire Atlantique, 47°10'·60N 02°09'·50W; this is position of S bkwtr lt, Oc WG 4s 7m 9/5M, W tr with G top, W123°-140°, G elsewhere. Appr in the W sector or by day on 136° with the bkwtr lt in transit with the disused lt ho beyond. Beware Les Moutons, rk drying 0·4m, 7½ca NW of the bkwtr lt, close to the approach track. The ent is narrow; tiny hbr dries about 2m, access from half-flood. Hr Mr ☎ 40.27.82.85; Facilities: M, FW, YC, Slip, C (6 ton), quay. Other facilities at nearby town of St Michel-Chef-Chef.

PORT DE LA GRAVETTE, Loire Atlantique, 47°09'·71N 02°12'·60W; this is position of the lt on end of the bkwtr, Fl (3) WG 12s 7m 8/5M, W sector 124°-224°, G elsewhere. The hbr is 2·2M NE of Pte de St-Gildas. Daymarks are bkwtr lt in transit 130° with La Treille water tr, 2M inland. Shellfish beds to the W and E are marked by unlit NCM bns. On rounding the 600m long bkwtr, turn stbd between lateral buoys; there is about 1·2m water in the N part of the hbr which dries closer in. Many local moorings, few facilities.

SAINT-GILDAS (Anse du Boucau), Loire Atlantique, 47°08'·45N 02°14'·65W. Make good L'Apcheu, SHM bn, 5ca N of Pte de St Gildas lt ho, Q WRG 23m 11/6M (see 10.17.4). Two SHM buoys, Fl G 2s, are laid May-Oct NW and N of the hbr bkwtr which extends 3ca N and has a large automatic tide gauge at its seaward end. Appr from about 1M N of Pte de St-Gildas on a brg of 177° or at night in its W sector 174°-180°. L'Ilot rky ledge is marked by a PHM bn. Pick up a mooring in 1·5m in the N part of the hbr or dry out further S. Hr Mr ☎ 40.21.60.07. VHF Ch 09. Facilities: Slips, YC, FW, C (5 ton), V at Préfailles 1M to the E.

17

Volvo Penta service

Sales and service centres in area 18
Names and addresses of Volvo Penta dealers in
this area are available from:

France *Volvo Penta France SA*, 1 Rue de la Nouvelle, B. P. 49, 78133 Les
Mureaux Tel 33-1-30912799, Fax 33-1-34746415 Telex 695221 F.
Spain *Volvo Penta Espana SA*, Paeso De La Castellana 130, 28046 Madrid
Tel 010 341 5261500 Fax 010 341 56 22207

Area 18

South Biscay
River Loire to Spanish Border

**VOLVO
PENTA**

18

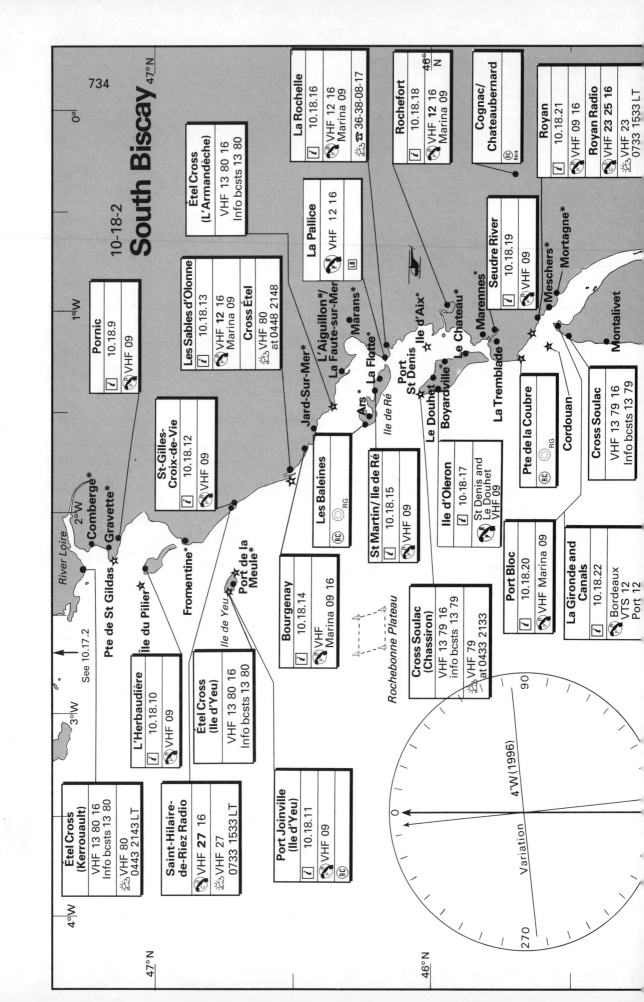

Étel Cross (Kerrouault)

i	VHF 13 80 16
	Info bcsts 13 80
	VHF 80
	0443 2143 LT

Saint-Hilaire-de-Riez Radio

	VHF **27** 16
	VHF 27
	0733 1533 LT

Port Joinville (Ile d'Yeu) — 10.18.11

i	VHF 09
	RC

L'Herbaudière — 10.18.10

i	VHF 09

Étel Cross (Ile d'Yeu)

	VHF 13 80 16
	Info bcsts 13 80

Pornic — 10.18.9

i	VHF 09

St-Gilles-Croix-de-Vie — 10.18.12

i	VHF 09

Les Sables d'Olonne — 10.18.13

i	VHF **12** 16
	Marina 09

Cross Étel

	VHF 80
	at 0448 2148

Étel Cross (L'Armandèche)

	VHF 13 80 16
	Info bcsts 13 80

Bourgenay — 10.18.14

i	VHF
	Marina 09 16

Cross Soulac (Chassiron)

	VHF 13 79 16
	info bcsts 13 79
	VHF 79
	at 0433 2133

La Pallice — La Pallice

	VHF 12 16
	LB

Les Baleines

RC	RG

St Martin/ Ile de Ré — 10.18.15

i	VHF 09

Ile d'Oleron — 10.18.17

i	St Denis and Le Douhet VHF 09

Port Bloc — 10.18.20

i	VHF Marina 09

La Gironde and Canals — 10.18.22

i	Bordeaux VTS 12 Port 12

La Rochelle — 10.18.16

i	VHF 12 16
	Marina 09
	36-38-08-17

Rochefort — 10.18.18

i	VHF **12** 16
	Marina 09

Cognac/ Chateaubernard

RC	Aero

Seudre River — 10.18.19

i	VHF 09

Pte de la Coubre

RC	RG

Cross Soulac

	VHF 13 79 16
	Info bcsts 13 79

Royan — 10.18.21

i	VHF 09 16

Royan Radio

	VHF **23 25** 16
	VHF 23
	0733 1533 LT

Pte de St Gildas
Comberge*
Gravette*
Ile du Pilier
Fromentine*
Port de la Meule*
Ile de Yeu
Jard-Sur-Mer*
L'Aiguillon*/ La Faute-sur-Mer*
Marans*
La Flotte*
Ars*
Ile de Ré
Marennes*
Le Chateau*
Ile d'Aix*
Le Douhet*
Port St Denis
Boyardville*
La Tremblade
Meschers*
Mortagne*
Cordouan
Montalivet
Rochebonne Plateau

River Loire

See 10.17.2

4°W(1996)
Variation

0°W 1°W 2°W 3°W 4°W

47° N 46° N

47°N 46° N

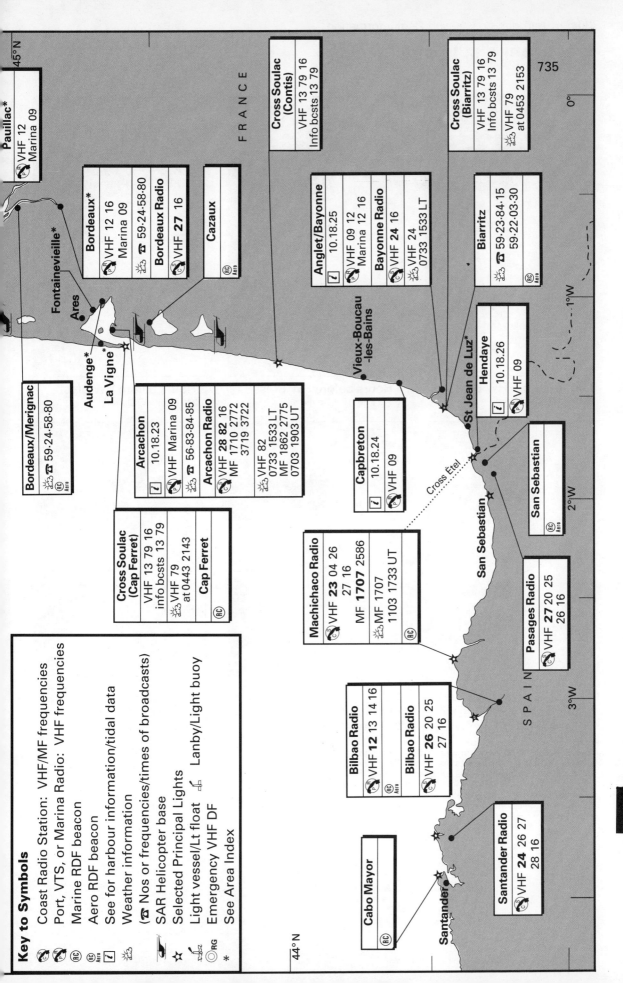

Key to Symbols

Coast Radio Station: VHF/MF frequencies

Port, VTS, or Marina Radio: VHF frequencies

Marine RDF beacon

Aero RDF beacon

See for harbour information/tidal data

Weather information

(☎ Nos or frequencies/times of broadcasts)

SAR Helicopter base

Selected Principal Lights

Light vessel/Lt float   Lanby/Light buoy

Emergency VHF DF

See Area Index

FRANCE

Pauillac*
VHF 12
Marina 09

Bordeaux/Merignac
☎ 59-24-58-80

Fontainevieille*

Ares

Audenge*

La Vigne

Bordeaux*
VHF 12 16
Marina 09
☎ 59-24-58-80
Bordeaux Radio
VHF **27** 16

Cazaux

Cross Soulac (Contis)
VHF 13 79 16
Info bcsts 13 79

Cross Soulac (Biarritz)
VHF 13 79 16
Info bcsts 13 79
VHF 79 at 0453 2153

735

Anglet/Bayonne
10.18.25
VHF 09 12
Marina 12 16
Bayonne Radio
VHF **24** 16
VHF 24
0733 1533 LT

Biarritz
☎ 59-23-84-15
59-22-03-30

Arcachon
10.18.23
VHF Marina 09
☎ 56-83-84-85
Arcachon Radio
VHF **28 82** 16
MF 1710 2772
3719 3722
VHF 82
0733 1533 LT
MF 1862 2775
0703 1903 UT

Cross Soulac (Cap Ferret)
VHF 13 79 16
info bcsts 13 79
VHF 79
at 0443 2143
Cap Ferret

Vieux-Boucau -les-Bains

Capbreton
10.18.24
VHF 09

St Jean de Luz*

Hendaye
10.18.26
VHF 09

Cross Étel

San Sebastian

San Sebastian

Machichaco Radio
VHF **23** 04 26
27 16
MF **1707** 2586
MF 1707
1103 1733 UT

Pasages Radio
VHF **27** 20 25
26 16

SPAIN

Bilbao Radio
VHF **12** 13 14 16

Bilbao Radio
VHF **26** 20 25
27 16

Santander Radio
VHF **24** 26 27
28 16

Cabo Mayor

Santander

44°N

45°N

2°W

3°W

1°W

0°

18

10.18.3 AREA 18 TIDAL STREAMS

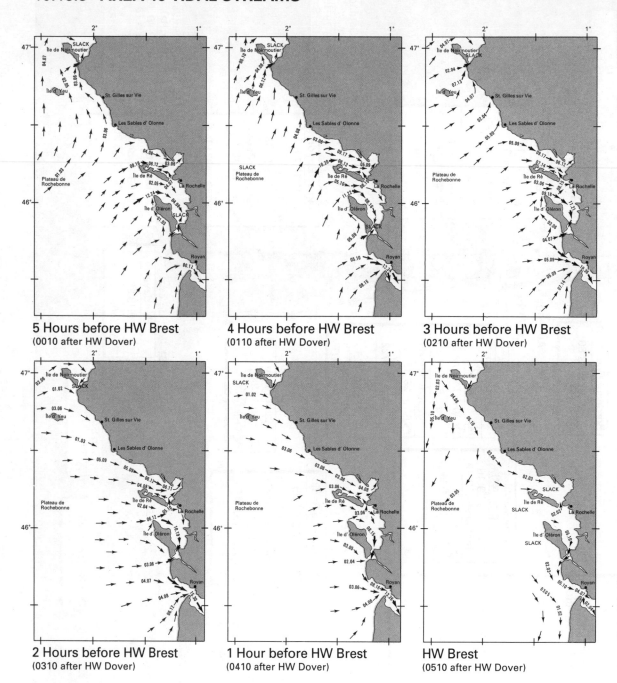

5 Hours before HW Brest
(0010 after HW Dover)

4 Hours before HW Brest
(0110 after HW Dover)

3 Hours before HW Brest
(0210 after HW Dover)

2 Hours before HW Brest
(0310 after HW Dover)

1 Hour before HW Brest
(0410 after HW Dover)

HW Brest
(0510 after HW Dover)

CAUTION: Due to the very strong rates of the tidal streams in some of the areas, many eddies may occur. Where possible some indication of these eddies has been included. In many areas there is either insufficient information or the eddies are unstable. Generally tidal streams are weak offshore and strong winds have a very great effect on the rate and direction of the tidal streams.

Northward 10.17.3

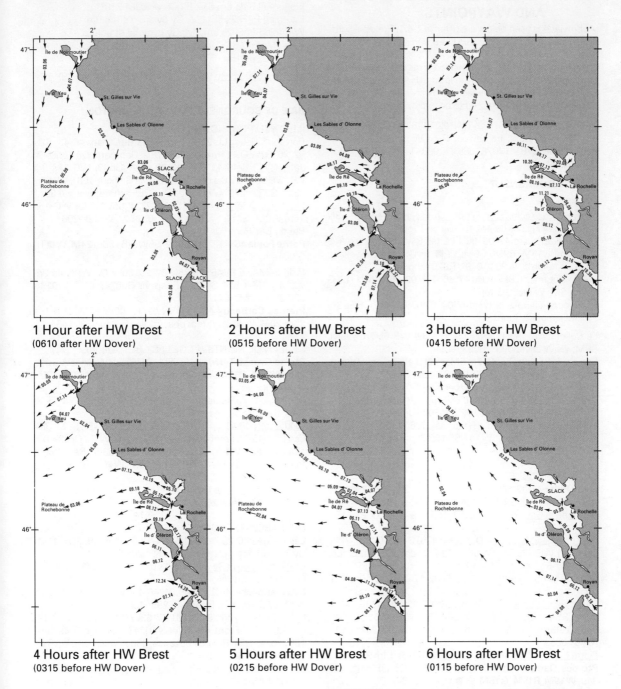

1 Hour after HW Brest
(0610 after HW Dover)

2 Hours after HW Brest
(0515 before HW Dover)

3 Hours after HW Brest
(0415 before HW Dover)

4 Hours after HW Brest
(0315 before HW Dover)

5 Hours after HW Brest
(0215 before HW Dover)

6 Hours after HW Brest
(0115 before HW Dover)

CAUTION: Due to the very strong rates of the tidal streams in some of the areas, many eddies may occur. Where possible some indication of these eddies has been included. In many areas there is either insufficient information or the eddies are unstable. Generally tidal streams are weak offshore and strong winds have a very great effect on the rate and direction of the tidal streams.

18

10.18.4 COASTAL LIGHTS, FOG SIGNALS AND WAYPOINTS

Abbreviations used below are given in 1.4.1. Principal lights are in **bold** print, places in CAPITALS, and light-vessels, light floats and Lanbys in *CAPITAL ITALICS*. Unless otherwise stated lights are white. m – elevation in metres; M – nominal range in miles. Fog signals are in *italics*. Useful waypoints are underlined – use those on land with care. All geographical positions should be assumed to be approximate. See 4.4.1.

Pte de Saint-Gildas 47°08'·10N 02°14'·67W Q WRG 23m W11M, R6M, G6M; framework Tr on W house; vis R264°-308°, G308°-078°, W078°-088°, R088°-174°, W174°-180°, G180°-264°; RC.

BAIE DE BOURGNEUF

PORNIC

Noëveillard Yacht Hbr Digue Ouest Hd   47°06'·53N 02°06'·61W Fl (2) R 6s 4m 4M; B col, T top.
Pte de Noëveillard 47°06'·68N 02°06'·84W Oc (3+1) WRG 12s 22m W13M, R9M, G9M; W ■ Tr, G top, W dwelling; vis G shore-051°, W051°-079°, R079°-shore.
Pte de Gourmalon Bkwtr Hd 47°06'·70N 02°06'·40W Fl (2) G 6s 4m 8M; W mast, G top.
La Bernerie-en-Retz Jetty Hd 47°04'·6N 02°02'·4W Fl R 2s 3m 2M; W structure, R top.

Le Collet 47°01'·80N 01°59'·00W Oc (2) WR 6s 7m W9M, R6M; vis W shore-093°, R093°-shore.
Ldg Lts 118° both QG 4/12m 6M; W■G stripe, on W pylon.
Étier des Brochets 46°59'·90N 02°01'·90W Oc (2+1) WRG 12s 8m W10M, R7M, G7M; G Tr, W band; vis G071°-091°, W091°-102·5°, R102·5°-116·5°, W116·5°-119·5°, R119·5°-164·5°.
Bec de l'Époids 46°56'·40N 02°04'·50W Dir Iso WRG 4s 6m W12M, R9M, G9M; W n Tr, R top; vis G106°-113·5°, R113·5°-122°, G122°-157·5°, W157·5°-158·5°, R158·5°-171·5°, W171·5°-176°.

ÎLE DE NOIRMOUTIER

Île du Pilier 47°02'·62N 02°21'·53W Fl (3) 20s 33m **29M**; Gy ▲ Tr. Auxiliary Lt QR 10m 11M, same Tr; vis 321°-034°.
Passe de la Grise Lt By 47°01'·73N 02°19'·90W Q (6) + L Fl 15s; SCM.
P de l'Herbaudière Jetée Ouest Hd 47°01'·69N 02°17'·79W Oc (2+1) WG 12s 9m W10M, G7M; W col and hut, G top; vis W187·5°-190°, G190°-187·5°.
Ldg Lts 187·5°.   Front 47°01'·65N 02°17'·76W Q 10m 7M; Gy mast. Rear, 310m from front, Q 26m 7M; Gy mast.
Basse du Martroger 47°02'·65N 02°17'·05W Q WRG   10m W9M, R6M, G6M; NCM; vis G033°-055°, W055°-060°, R060°-095°, G095°-124°, W124°-153°, R153°-201°, W201°-240°, R240°-033°.
Pierre Moine 47°03'·43N 02°12'·30W Fl (2) 6s 14m 9M; IDM.
Pte des Dames 47°00'·73N 02°13'·18W Oc (3) WRG 12s 34m **W19M, R15M, G15M**; W■Tr; vis G016·5°-057°, R057°-124°, G124°-165°, W165°-191°, R191°-267°, W267°-357°, R357°-016·5°.
Noirmoutier Jetty Hd 46°59'·30N 02°12'·95W Oc (2) R 6s 6m 7M; W col, R top.
Pte de Devin 46°59'·20N 02°17'·40W Oc (4) WRG 12s 10m W11M, R8M, G8M; W col and hut, G top; vis G314°-028°, W028°-035°, R035°-134°.

FROMENTINE

Pte de Notre Dame-de-Monts 46°53'·30N 02°08'·50W Dir Oc (2) WRG 6s 21m W13M, R10M, G10M; W Tr, B top; vis G000°-043°, W043°-063°, R063°-073°, W073°-094°, G094°-113°, W113°-116°, R116°-175°, G175°-196°, R196°-230°.
Bridge, each side on centre span Iso 4s 32m **18M**; H24.
Tourelle Milieu 46°53'·60N 02°09'·00W Fl (4) R 12s 6m 5M; R ■ on Tr.

ROUTE DU GOIS CAUSEWAY

E shore Fl R 4s 6m 6M; R hut; vis 038°-218°.
E turning Pt Fl 2s 5m 6M; Gy pyramid structure.
W turning Pt Fl 2s 5m 3M; Gy pyramid structure.
Bassotière 46°56'·10N 02°08'·90W Fl G 2s 7m 2M; W tripod, G lantern; vis 180°-000°.

Les Boeufs Lt By 46°55'·10N 02°28'·00W VQ (9) 10s; WCM; *Bell.*

BAIE DE BOURGNEUF TO PERTUIS BRETON

ÎLE D'YEU/PORT JOINVILLE

Port Joinville Ldg Lts 219°. Front, Quai du Canada 46°43'·67N 02°20'·87W QR 11m 6M. Rear, Quai Georgette QR 16m 5M.
Jetty NW Hd 46°43'·83N 02°20'·73W Oc (3) WG 12s 9m W11M, G9M; W 8-sided Tr, G top; vis G shore-150°, W150°-232°, G232°-279°, W279°-285°, G285°-shore; *Horn(3) 30s.*
Les Chiens Perrins 46°43'·65N 02°24'·55W Q (9) WG 15s 16m W8M, G4M; WCM; vis G330°-350°, W350°-200°.
Pte du But *Horn 60s.*
Petite Foule 46°43'·20N 02°22'·85W Fl 5s 56m **24M**; W■Tr, G lantern; RC.

P de la Meule Pt 46°41'·75N 02°20'·60W Oc WRG 4s 9m W9M, R6M, G5M; Gy ■ Tr, R top; vis G007·5°-018°, W018°-027·5°, R027·5°-041·5°.
Pte des Corbeaux 46°41'·45N 02°17'·00W Fl (2+1) R 15s 25m **20M**; W ■ Tr, R top; obsc by Île de Yeu 083°-143°.

ST JEAN DE MONTS /ST GILLES-CROIX-DE-VIE

Pte de Grosse Terre 46°41'·60N 01°57'·84W Fl (4) WR 12s 25m **W17M**, R13M; W truncated conical Tr; vis W290°-125°, R125°-145°.
St Jean de Monts Jetty Hd 46°47'·15N 02°05'·05W Q (2) R 5s 10m 3M; W mast, R top.
Pilours Lt By 46°41'·04N 01°58'·01W Q (6) + L Fl 15s; SCM; *Bell.*
Ldg Lts 043·5°. Front 46°41'·92N 01°56'·67W Dir Oc (3+1) R 12s 7m 13M; W■Tr, R top; intens 033·5°-053·5°. Rear, 260m from front, Dir Oc (3+1) R 12s 28m 13M; W ■ Tr, R top; synch with front; intens 033·5°-053·5°.
Jetée de la Garenne Hd 46°41'·51N 01°57'·18W Q WG 8m, W9M, G6M; *Reed 20s.*

LES SABLES D'OLONNE

Les Barges 46°29'·76N 01°50'·42W Fl (2) R 10s 25m **17M**; Gy Tr, helicopter platform; vis 265°-205°.
La Petite Barge Lt By 46°28'·96N 01°50'·53W Q (6) + L Fl 15s 8m 7M; SCM; *Whis.*
L'Armandèche 46°29'·47N 01°48'·21W Fl (2+1) 15s 42m **24M**; W 6-sided Tr, R top; vis 295°-130°.
Nouch Sud Lt By 46°28'·63N 01°47'·33W Q (6) + L Fl 15s; SCM.
Ldg Lts 033°. **Front** 46°29'·48N 01°46'·28W Iso R 4s 14m **16M**; mast; H24. **Rear La Potence**, 330m from front, Iso R 4s 33m **16M**; W ■ Tr; H24.
Ldg Lts 320°, Jetée des Sables Hd Front 46°29'·49N 01°47'·43W QG 11m 8M; W Tr, G top. Rear, Tour de la Chaume, 465m from front, Oc (2+1) 12s 33m 13M; large Gy ■ Tr, W turret.
Ldg Lts 327°, Front FR 6m 11M; R line on W hut. Rear, 65m from front, FR 9m 11M; R line on W Tr; intens 324°-330°.
Jetée St Nicolas Hd 46°29'·29N 01°47'·44W UQ (2) R 1s 16m 10M; W Tr, R top; vis 143°-094°.

BOURGENAY

Ldg Lts 040°. Front 46°26'·40N 01°40'·50W QG 8M. Rear QG 8M.
Roches du Joanne Lt By 46°25'·35N 01°41'·90W L Fl 10s; SWM.
Digue W Hd 46°26'·37N 01°40'·59W Fl R 4s 9M.

PLATEAU DE ROCHEBONNE (Offshore shoal)

NW Lt By 46°12'·90N 02°31'·60W Q (9) 15s; WCM; *Whis.*
NE Lt By 46°12'·80N 02°24'·80W Iso G 4s; SHM.

SW Lt By 46°10'·15N 02°26'·90W Fl (2) R 6s; PHM.
SE Lt By 46°09'·30N 02°21'·00W Q (3) 10s; ECM; *Bell*.

Les Baleines 46°14'·70N 01°33'·60W Fl (4) 15s 53m **27M**;
Gy 8-sided Tr, R lantern; RC.
Les Baleineaux 46°15'·87N 01°35'·12W Oc (2) 6s 23m 11M;
pink Tr, R top.

PERTUIS BRETON/ÎLE DE RÉ

JARD-SUR-MER/LA TRANCHE-SUR-MER
Jard-sur-Mer S Bkwtr Hd 46°24'·44N 01°34'·77W; PHM.
La Tranche Pier Hd 46°20'·62N 01°25'·50W Fl (2) R 6s 6m
6M; R col.
Pte du Grouin-du-Cou 46°20'·73N 01°27'·75W Fl WRG 5s
29m **W20M, R16M, G16M**; W 8-sided Tr, B top; vis R034°-
061°, W061°-117°, G117°-138°, W138°-034°.

L'AIGUILLON/LA FAUTE-SUR-MER
Le Lay Lt By 46°16'·17N 01°16'·41W Q (6) + L Fl 15s; SCM.
No. 1 By 46°16'·65N 01°16'·20W; SHM.

ANSE DE L'AIGUILLON/MARANS
Pte de L'Aiguillon Lt By 46°15'·80N 01°11'·31W L Fl 10s;
SWM.
Port du Pavé ent 46°18'·21N 01°07'·91W Fl G 4s 9m 7M; W
col, G top.

PORT DU PLOMB
W Môle 46°12'·18N 01°12'·13W Fl R 4s 9m 7M; W col, R top.

LA FLOTTE
La Flotte N Bkwtr Hd 46°11'·38N 01°19'·23W Fl WG 4s 10m
W12M, G9M; W ● Tr, G top; vis G130°-205°, W205°-220°,
G220°-257°; *Horn(3) 30s* (by day HW-2 to HW+2). Moiré effect
Dir Lt 212·5°.
Rivedoux-Plage Ldg Lts 200°. Front, N Pier Hd 46°09'·83N
01°16'·56W QG 6m 6M; W Tr, G top. Rear, 100m from front,
QG 9m 7M; W and G chequered col; synch with front.

St MARTIN DE RÉ
Bkwtr West Hd 46°12'·57N 01°21'·82W Fl R 2·5s 7m 4M;
W post, R top.
On ramparts E of ent 46°12'·50N 01°21'·80W Oc (2) WR 6s
18m W10M, R7M; W Tr, R top; vis W shore-245°, R245°-
281°, W281°-shore.
Mole Hd Iso G 4s 10m 6M; W tripod, G top; obsc by Pte de
Loix when brg less than 124°.

PORT D'ARS-EN-RÉ
Le Fier d'Ars Ldg Lts 265°. Front 46°14'·12N 01°28'·65W Iso
4s 5m 11M; ■ on W hut; vis 141°-025°. **Rear**, 370m from
front, Dir Iso G 4s 13m **15M**; G ■ on dwelling; synch with
front, intens 263°-267°.
Ldg Lts 232°. Front 46°12'·81N 01°30'·50W Q 5m 9M; W hut,
R lantern. Rear, 370m from front, Q 13m 11M; B stripe on W
framework Tr, G top; vis 142°-322°.

ÎLE DE RÉ SOUTH/PERTUIS D'ANTIOCHE/ÎLE D'OLÉRON

ÎLE DE RÉ (SOUTH)
Chanchardon 46°09'·78N 01°28'·33W Fl WR 4s 15m W11M,
R9M; B 8-sided Tr, W base; vis R118°-290°, W290°-118°.
Chauveau 46°08'·09N 01°16'·33W Oc (2+1) WR 12s 23m
W15M, R11M; W ● Tr, R top; vis W057°-094°, R094°-104°,
W104°-342°, R342°-057°.
Pte de Sablanceaux 46°09'·82N 01°15'·08W Q Vi 7m 1M; W
mast and hut, G top.

PERTUIS D'ANTIOCHE/LA ROCHELLE
Chauveau Lt By 46°06'·62N 01°15'·98W VQ (6) + L Fl 10s;
SCM; *Whis*.
Roche du Sud Lt By 46°06'·43N 01°15'·15W Q (9) 15s; WCM.

Le Lavardin 46°08'·15N 01°14'·45W Fl (2) WG 6s 14m
W11M, G8M; vis G160°-169°, W169°-160°; IDM.
La Pallice, Môle d'Escale 46°09'·42N 01°14'·43W Dir Lt 016°.
Dir Q WRG 33m W14M, R13M, G13M; Gy Tr; vis G009°-
014·7°, W014·7°-017·3°, R017·3°-031°. Sig Stn.
Tour Richelieu 46°08'·95N 01°10'·27W Fl (4) R 12s 10m 9M;
R Tr; RC; *Siren (4) 60s* (HW-1 to HW+1).
La Rochelle Ldg Lts 059°. Front 46°09'·42N 01°09'·06W Dir Q
15m 13M; R ●Tr, W bands; intens 056°-062°; by day Fl 4s.
Rear, 235m from front, Q 25m 14M; W 8-sided Tr, G top; synch
with front, vis 044°-074°, obsc 061°-065° by St Nicolas Tr; by
day Fl 4s

Lt By PA 46°05'·69N 01°42'·37W Iso 4s 8m 7M; SWM;
Whis; Ra refl.

ÎLE D'AIX/PASSAGE DE L'EST
Île d'Aix 46°00'·67N 01°10'·60W Fl WR 5s 24m **W24M,
R20M**; two W ● Trs, one for Lt, one to screen R sector;
vis R103°-118°, W118°-103°.
Fort Boyard Lt Tr 46°00'·03N 01°12'·78W Q (9) 15s.

FOURAS
Port Sud Bkwtr Hd 45°59'·03N 01°05'·63W Fl WR 4s 6m 9/6M.
Port Nord Pier Hd 45°59'·88N 01°05'·75W Oc (3+1) WG 12s
9m W11M, G8M; W&G Tr; vis G084°-127°, W127°-084°.

LA CHARENTE/ROCHEFORT
Ldg Lts 115°. Front, **Fort de la Pointe** 45°58'·02N 01°04'·29W
Dir QR 8m **19M**; W ■ Tr, R top. **Rear**, 600m from front, Dir QR
21m **20M**; W ■ Tr, R top; both intens 113°-117°. QR 21m 8M;
same Tr; vis 322°-067° over Port-des-Barques anchorage.
Port-des-Barques Ldg Lts 134·5°. Front, 45°57'·01N
01°04'·09W Iso G 4s 5m 9M. Rear, 490m from front, Iso G
4s 13m 11M; synch with front; intens 125°-145°.
Rochefort No. 1 Basin ent 45°56'·61N 00°57'·21W (unmarked).

ÎLE D'OLÉRON
Pte de Chassiron 46°02'·80N 01°24'·60W Fl 10s 50m, **28M**;
W ● Tr, B bands; part obsc 297°-351°; Sig Stn.
Rocher d'Antioche 46°04'·00N 01°23'·70W Q 20m 11M;
NCM.

ST DENIS
E Jetty Hd 46°02'·16N 01°21'·97W Fl (2) WG 6s 6m W9M
G6M, □ hut; vis G205°-277°, W277°-292°, G292°-165°.
Dir Lt 205° 46°01'·67N 01°21'·84W Dir Iso WRG 4s 14m
W11M, R9M, G9M; vis G 190°-204°, W204°-206°, R206°-
220°.

PORT DU DOUHET/PASSAGE DE L'OUEST
N ent Bn 46°00'·18N 01°19'·10W; SHM.
Chan Lt By 46°00'·45N 01°17'·61W Q; NCM.
Chan Lt By 46°00'·29N 01°15'·26W Q; NCM.
Chan Lt By 45°59'·91N 01°14'·71W Q (3) 10s; ECM.

LE CHÂTEAU D'OLÉRON
Ldg Lts 319°. Front 45°53'·05N 01°11'·45W QR 11m 7M; R
line on W Tr; vis 191°-087°. Rear, 240m from front, QR 24m
7M; W Tr, R top; synch with front.
Tourelle Juliar 45°54'·10N 01°09'·45W Q (3) WG 10s 12m
W11M; G8M; ECM; vis W147°-336°, G336°-147°.

BOYARDVILLE (LA PÉRROTINE)
La Pérrotine By 45°58'·37N 01°13'·20W; SHM.
Mole Hd 45°58'·30N 01°13'·76W Fl (2) R 6s 8m 7M; W Tr,
R top; obsc by Pte des Saumonards when brg less than 150°.

LA SEUDRE
Pont de la Seudre 45°48'·00N 01°08'·25W Q 20m 10M each
side, vis 054°-234° and 234°-054°.
Pte de Mus de Loup 45°47'·90N 01°08'·50W Oc G 4s 8m 6M;
G&W col, W to seaward; vis 118°-147°.

18

LA COTINIÈRE

Dir Lt 048°. 45°54'·45N 01°18'·50W Dir Oc WRG 4s 13m W9M, R7M, G7M; W stripe with B border on W col; vis G033°-046°, W046°-050°, R050°-063°.
Ent Ldg Lts 339°. 45°54'·80N 01°19'·70W Front Dir Oc (2) 6s 6m 13M; W Tr, R top; vis 329°-349°; *Horn (2) 20s* (HW-3 to HW+3). Rear, 425m from front, Dir Oc (2) 6s 14m 12M; W Tr, R bands; synch with front; intens 329°-349°.

ATT Maumusson Lt By 45°47'·00N 01°17'·80W; L Fl 10s; SWM.

LA GIRONDE AND APPROACHES

LA GIRONDE, GRANDE PASSE DE L'OUEST

BXA Lt By 45°37'·60N 01°28'·60W Iso 4s 8m 8M; SWM; Ra refl; *Racon; Whis*.
Pte de la Coubre 45°41'·87N 01°13'·93W Fl (2) 10s 64m **28M**; W ● Tr, R top; RC; Sig Stn. F RG 42m 12M; same Tr; vis R030°-043°, G043°-060°, R060°-110°.
Ldg Lts 081·5°. **Front,** 1·1M from rear, Dir Iso 4s 21m **22M**; W mast on dolphin; intens 080·5°-082·5°; Q (2) 5s 10m 3M; same structure. **La Palmyre, common rear** 45°39'·77N 01°07'·15W Dir Q 57m **27M**; W radar Tr; intens 080·5°-082·5°. Dir FR 57m **17M**; same Tr; intens 325·5°-328·5°.
Ldg Lts 327°. **Terre-Nègre**, Front, 1·1M from rear, Oc (3) WRG 12s 39m **W18M**, R14M, G14M; W Tr, R top on W side; vis R304°-319°, W319°-327°, G327°-000°, W000°-004°, G004°-097°, W097°-104°, R104°-116°.
Pointe de Grave Jetée Nord Hd 45°34'·47N 01°03'·58W, Q 6m 2M; NCM.
Spur 45°34'·38N 01°03'·57W Iso G 4s 5m 2M; vis 173°-020°.

LA GIRONDE, PASSE SUD

Cordouan 45°35'·25N 01°10'·34W Oc (2+1) WRG 12s 60m **22/18M**; W ▲ Tr, dark Gy band and top; vis W014°-126°, G126°-178·5°, W178·5°-250°, W(unintens)250°-267°, R(unintens)267°-294·5°, R294·5°-014°; obsc in estuary when brg more than 285°.
Ldg Lts 063°. **St Nicolas Front** 45°33'·80N 01°04'·93W Dir QG 22m **17M**; W ■ Tr; intens 061·5°-064·5°. **Rear Pte de Grave**, 0·84M from front, Oc WRG 4s 26m **W19M**, R15M, G15M; W ■ Tr, B corners and top; vis W(unintens) 033°-054°, W054°-233·5°, R233·5°-303°, W303°-312°, G312°-330°, W330°- 341°, W(unintens) 341°-025°.
Ldg Lts 041°, **Le Chay Front**, 45°37'·35N 01°02'·30W Dir QR 33m **18M**; W Tr, R top; intens 039·5°-042·5°. **Rear St Pierre**, 0·97M from front, Dir QR 61m **18M**; R water Tr; intens 039°-043°.

PORT BLOC/ROYAN/PAUILLAC/BLAYE

Port Bloc Ent N side 45°34'·20N 01°03'·66W Fl G 4s 8m 6M.
S Pier Hd Iso R 4s 8m 6M.
Royan Jetée Sud 45°37'·08N 01°01'·72W UQ (2) R 1s 11m 12M; *Horn (2) 20s*.
Royan Hbr Nouvelle Jetée Hd ent Oc (2) R 6s 8m 6M.
Pauillac NE Bkwtr 45°12'·02N 00°44'·50W Fl G 4s 7m 5M.
Ent E side 45°11'·89N 00°44'·52W QG 7m 5M.
Blaye Ent N side 45°07'·55N 00°39'·91W Q (3) R 5s 6m 4M.

LA GARONNE/BORDEAUX

Pont d'Aquitaine 44°52'·87N 00°32'·23W 4 F Vi.

LA GIRONDE TO L'ADOUR

Hourtin 45°08'·55N 01°09'·65W Fl 5s 55m **23M**; R ■ Tr.

BASSIN D'ARCACHON

Cap Ferret 44°38'·83N 01°14'·90W Fl R 5s 53m **27M**; W ● Tr, R top; RC. Oc (3) 12s 46m 14M; same Tr; vis 045°-135°.
ATT-ARC Lt By 44°35'·21N 01°18'·63W L Fl 10s; SWM; (frequently shifted); *Whis*.
Émissaire Lt By 44°30'·55N 01°17'·55W Fl (2) 6s 8m 5M; IDM. Ra refl.
La Salie Wharf Hd 44°30'·90N 01°15'·60W Q (9) 15s 19m 10M; WCM.
Arcachon W Bkwtr Hd 44°39'·80N 01°09'·10W QG 6M.
La Vigne 44°40'·50N 01°14'·20W Iso R 4s 7m 4M; (occas).
ZDS Lt By 44°28'·00N 01°19'·30W Fl (3) Y 12s 8m 7M; SPM.
ZDL Lt By 44°12'·90N 01°22'·00W Fl Y 4s; SPM.
Contis 44°05'·70N 01°18'·90W Fl (4) 25s 50m **23M**; W ● Tr, B diagonal stripes.

CAPBRETON

Digue Nord Hd 43°39'·45N 01°26'·80W Fl (2) R 6s 13m 12M; W ● Tr, R top; *Horn 30s*.

L'ADOUR TO BAIE DE FONTARABIE

ANGLET/BAYONNE

BA Lt By 43°32'·66N 01°32'·68W L Fl 10s 8m 8M; SWM.
Digue du large Hd 43°31'·96N 01°31'·92W QR 11m 5M; W Tr, R top.
Digue extérieure Sud 43°31'·60N 01°31'·68W, Q (9) 15s 7M; WCM.
Jetée Sud Hd Iso G 4s 9m 10M; W ■ Tr, G top.
Jetée Nord Hd Oc (2) R 6s 12m 8M; W pylon, R top.
Boucau Ldg Lts 090°. Front 43°31'·88N 01°31'·15W Dir Q 9m **19M**. **Rear**, 250m from front, Dir Q 15m 19M; both W Trs, R tops, both intens 086·5°-093·5°.
Ent Ldg Lts 111·5° (moved as necessary and lit when chan practicable). Front Dir FG 6m 14M. Rear, 149m from front, Dir FG 10m 14M; W Tr, G bands; both intens 109°-114°.
Marina ent W side 43°31'·64N 01°30'·44W Fl G 2s 5m 3M; W Tr, G top.

BIARRITZ

Pte Saint-Martin 43°29'·69N 01°33'·17W Fl (2) 10s 73m **29M**; W Tr, B top.
Biarritz Ldg Lts 174°. 43°29'·15N 01°33'·88W both Fl R 2s 7/19m 2M.
Guethary Ldg Lts 133°. Front 43°25'·65N 01°36'·45W QR 11m; W mast, R top. Rear, 66m from front, QR 33m; W Tr.
Aero Mo (L) 43°28'·45N 01°31'·90W 7·5s 80m.

ST JEAN DE LUZ

Socoa Ldg Lts 138·5°. Front 43°23'·77N 01°41'·12W Q WR 36m W12M, R8M; W ■ Tr, B stripe; vis W shore-264°, R264°-282°, W282°-shore. Rear **Bordagain**, 0·77M from front, Dir Q 67m **20M**; synch with front; intens 134·5°-141·5°.
Ste Barbe Ldg Lts 101°. **Front** 43°24'·03N 01°39'·79W Dir Oc (3+1) R 12s 30m **18M;** W▲; intens 095°-107°. **Rear**, 340m from front, Dir Oc (3+1) R 12s 47m **18M**; B ▲ on W Tr; synch with front; intens 095°-107°.
Digue des Criquas Hd 43°23'·92N 01°40'·59W Iso G 4s 11m 7M; G ■ Tr; *Horn 15s*.
Ldg Lts 150·7°, **Front** 43°23'·32N 01°40'·07W Dir QG 18m **16M**; W ■ Tr, R stripe. **Rear**, 410m from front, Dir QG 27m **16M**; W ■ Tr, G stripe. Both intens 149·5°-152°.

HENDAYE

Cap Higuier 43°23'·59N 01°47'·44W Fl (2) 10s 63m **23M.**
Hendaye Epi Socoburu Hd 43°22'·90N 01°47'·28W L Fl R 10s 7m 8M.
Marina Digue Coude Fl (2) R 6s 6m 2M; vis 294°-114°.

10.18.5 PASSAGE INFORMATION

BAY OF BISCAY (charts 2663, 2664)

The *North Biscay Pilot* (Imray/ICC), South to the Gironde, and *South Biscay Pilot* (Adlard Coles), Gironde to La Coruna, are recommended; as is the Admiralty *Bay of Biscay Pilot*. Larger scale French charts are more suitable for inshore waters. For French Glossary see 1.4.2. Some Breton words are in 10.17.5.

Despite its reputation, weather in the B of Biscay is better than in the English Chan, and the S part generally enjoys a warm and settled climate. The Atlantic swells are higher and longer. Although W winds mostly prevail, NE winds are often experienced with anticyclones over the continent. In summer the wind is seldom from SE or S. Often the wind varies in speed and direction from day to day. Sea and land breezes are well developed in summer months (see 10.17.5). Gales may be expected once a month in summer. Coastal rainfall is moderate, increasing in the SE corner, where thunder is more frequent. Sea fog may be met from May to October, but is less common in winter.

Tidal streams are weak offshore, but can be strong in estuaries and channels, and around headlands. The tidal stream chartlets at 10.18.4 are based on NP 265 (Admiralty Tidal Stream Atlas for France, W Coast) which uses data from actual observations out to 15-25M offshore. The equivalent French Atlas gives more data, but based on computer predictions.

The general direction and rate of the surface current much depends on wind: in summer it is SE, towards the SE corner of B of Biscay, where it swings W along N coast of Spain. In winter with W gales, the current runs E along N coast of Spain, sometimes at 3kn or more. When crossing B of Biscay, allow for a likely set to the E, particularly after strong W winds.

BAIE DE BOURGNEUF (charts 3216, 2646)

B de Bourgneuf is entered between Pte de St Gildas and Pte de l'Herbaudière, the NW tip of Île de Noirmoutier. Within the B the only yacht hbrs are Pornic (10.18.9) and L'Herbaudière (10.18.10). There are minor drying hbrs at La Bernerie-en-Retz, Le Collet, Port des Brochets and Bec de l'Epoids; with a good anch 5ca NE of Pte des Dames. The E and S sides of the B are encumbered with shoals, rks and oyster or mussel fisheries. The Bay is sheltered except in W winds, which can raise a heavy sea on the ebb stream.

From the NW (chart 3216) the approach is simple, but beware La Couronnée (dries 1·8m; buoyed) a rky bank about 2M WSW of Pte de St Gildas. Adjacent to it, Banc de Kerouars (least depth 1m; breaks) extends 3M further E. Approach Pornic in the W sector of Pte de Noveillard lt, ie S of Banc de Kerouars and NW of Notre Dame IDM bn tr, which lies 2M SW of Pornic and marks end of a line of rks extending ESE to La Bernerie. Pierre du Chenal is an isolated rk about 1M SSE of Notre Dame.

At the N end of Île de Noirmoutier, Chenal de la Grise, between Île du Pilier and Pte de l'Herbaudière and in the W sector of Martroger NCM bn lt, carries 3m, and gives access to L'Herbaudière marina. If heading E to Pornic, pass N of Martroger, and clear of Roches des Pères about 1M ENE. Extending 6M to seaward off the NW end of the island, beware Chaussée des Boeufs, buoyed rks, some drying on to which the tide sets. The S ent via Goulet de Fromentine (SHOM 5039; ECM 549) is difficult due to a shifting bar and 8 hrs of W-going stream; the conspic bridge has 24m clearance. Once inside, further progress to NNE is restricted to shoal draft at sp HW±1 by Route du Gois, causeway drying 3m.

ILE D'YEU TO PERTUIS BRETON (AC 2663)

Les Marguerites, rky shoals, lie SSW of Goulet de Fromentine, with the part-drying reef, Pont d'Yeu (SCM buoy), extending midway between the mainland and the Île d'Yeu; here anch is prohib due to underwater cables. The passage along the NE of the island carries 6-7m nearer to the island. The low-lying, wooded Côte de la Vendée continues 40M SE to Pte du Grouin Cou with few dangers more than 1·5M offshore, except near Les Sables d'Olonne.

Île d'Yeu, 30m high, has the main lt ho near the NW end and on the NE coast a very conspic water tr close to Port Joinville (10.18.11), crowded in season . Pte des Courbeaux lt ho is at the low SE end of the island and a lesser lt is at the NW end. The SW coast is steep-to and rky, with a tiny drying hbr at Port de la Meule (best to anch outside) and, further E, anch at Anse des Vieilles, both only tenable in settled conditions.

14M to the E of Île d'Yeu lies St Gilles-Croix-de-Vie (10.18.12). Thence 14M further SE is Les Sables d'Olonne, with Les Barges drying reef (lt) 2·5M W of the ent. Bourgenay (10.18.14) is 6M further SE. The approaches to these secure hbrs are exposed to onshore winds from SE to NW, and susceptible to swell. Jard-sur-Mer is a small drying hbr midway between Bourgenay and Pte du Grouin Cou.

PERTUIS BRETON (chart 2641)

Pertuis Breton is entered between Pte du Grouin du Cou and Pte des Baleines on Île de Ré, (both lit). Beware rky ledges (dry) extending 2·5M NW from Les Baleines. It gives access to the hbrs of Ars-en-Ré, St Martin (10.18.15) and La Flotte on the N shore of Île de Ré which is surrounded by shallows and drying areas. From St Martin to Pte de Sablanceaux there are extensive oyster beds.

On the mainland side, in fresh NW winds against tide a bad sea builds on the bank which extends 8M W of Pte du Grouin du Cou. 1M S of the Pte is Roche de l'Aunis (depth 0·8m). From the Pte sand dunes and mussel beds, with seaward limits marked by SPM buoys, run 8M ESE to the drying ent to Rivière Le Lay, which is fronted by a bar (dries 1m), dangerous in bad weather. The chan to L'Aiguillon/La Faute-sur-Mer (10.18.15) is marked by bns and buoys. 4M further E is entrance to Anse de l'Aiguillon, in which are extensive mussel beds. In NE corner is entrance to Sèvre Niortaise which, after 3·5M, gives access to the canal leading to the port of Marans. Further S is a sheltered route to La Rochelle and Pertuis d'Antioche via Coureau de la Pallice and the road bridge (30m clearance) from the mainland to Île de Ré.

PERTUIS D'ANTIOCHE (chart 2746)

A SWM buoy marks the W approach to Pertuis d'Antioche which runs between Île de Ré and Île d'Oléron, giving access to La Rochelle (10.18.16), Ile d'Aix, La Charente and Rochefort (10.18.18). Its shores are low-lying. Île de Ré forms the N side, fringed by rky ledges extending 2·5M SE from Pte de Chanchardon and nearly 1M from Pte de Chauveau (marked by lt tr and two bns). Off Pte de Chassiron (lt ho, Sig Stn), at the N tip of Île d'Oléron, reefs extend 5ca W, 1·5M N to Rocher d'Antioche (lit), and 1·5M E, and there is often a nasty sea.

Well offshore, 34-40M W of Île de Ré, Plateau de Rochebonne is a large rky plateau on which the sea breaks dangerously. It is steep-to on all sides, has least depth 3·3m and is buoyed.

18

ÎLE D'OLERON (charts 2746, 2663)

On the NE coast of Ile d'Oléron (10.18.17) there are marinas at Port St Denis and Le Douhet at the N end; further S are yacht and fishing hbrs at Boyardville and Le Château. All are sheltered from the prevailing W'lies.

From Pertuis d'Antioche, Grande Rade des Trousses is entered via either Passage de l'Est close to Île d'Aix (10.18.17) or Passage de l'Ouest, which run each side of La Longe le Boyard, an extensive sandbank on which stands Ft Boyard tr. From Grande Rade, where good anch is found except in fresh NW winds, the narrow and shallow Coureau d'Oléron winds between ledges, oyster beds and constantly changing shoals, with buoys moved to conform. About 2M SE of Le Chateau it is crossed by a bridge, clearance 15m; the bridge arch for the navigable chan is marked at road level by W □ boards, with G ▲ or R ■ superimposed, illuminated at night. Just N of bridge is Fort du Chapus, connected to mainland by causeway. SHOM 6335 is needed. S-going stream starts at HW Pte de Grave – 0230, N-going at HW Pte de Grave + 0500, sp rates 2kn. Up the Seudre River (10.18.19) there are anchs and yacht facilities at Marennes.

The W coast, from Pte de Chassiron 15M SSE to Pte de Gatseau, is bounded by drying rks and shoals. In bad weather the sea breaks 4 or 5M offshore. La Cotinière, the only hbr, is much used by fishing boats and is exposed to the Atlantic. Tidal streams are weak, sp rate 1kn, starting NW at HW Pte de Grave + 0300 and SE at HW Pte de Grave – 0505, but often overcome by current due to prevailing wind. The rate however increases towards Pte de Gatseau.

Here Pertuis de Maumusson separates the island from the mainland. Its ent is marked by a SWM buoy about 3M WSW of Pte de Gatseau. Banc de Gatseau and Banc des Mattes, both of which dry in places, lie N and S of the chan, and are joined by a sand bar which usually has a depth of about 1·5m. Depth and position vary, and buoys may not mark the best water. Any swell speedily forms breakers, and the chan is very dangerous then or in any onshore winds, especially on the ebb (sp rate 4kn). In calm weather with no swell, a stout craft and reliable engine, and having gained local advice, enter about HW – 1; ideally follow a local FV with deeper draught.

APPROACHES TO LA GIRONDE (chart 2910)

The Gironde is formed from the rivers Garonne and Dordogne, which join at Bec d'Ambès, 38M above Pte de Grave. BXA lt buoy is moored off the mouth of the estuary, about 11M WSW of Pte de la Coubre. Banc de la Mauvaise, the S end of which dries 5M seaward. Cordouan lt ho is on a large rky bank in the middle of the estuary. Grande Passe de l'Ouest starts about 4M E of BXA buoy and is dredged through Grand Banc, the outer bar of La Gironde. Enter to seaward of buoys Nos. 1 and 2, and keep in buoyed chan with ldg lts. Off Terre-Nègre lt the SE-going stream begins at HW – 0500 (sp 1·5kn), and the NW-going at HW+0130 (sp 2·5kn).

Passe Sud, a lesser chan, is entered at the SWM lt buoy, 9M SW of Pte de Grave, and runs NE past Pte de Grave. There are two sets of Ldg lts; the second lead over Platin de Grave, but it is better to pass NW of this shoal. Both entrance chans are dangerous in strong onshore winds, due to breakers and also the mascaret (bore) on the outgoing stream. Westerly swell breaks on La Mauvaise and around Cordouan, and sandbanks shift constantly. In places tidal streams run 4kn or more, and with wind against tide a dangerous sea can build. For Port Bloc, Royan and Gironde/canals, see 10.18.20 – .22.

LA GIRONDE TO CAPBRETON (charts 1102, 2664)

From Pte de la Négade to Capbreton, the coast is a featureless stretch of 107M broken only by the entrance to Arcachon (10.18.23). It is bordered by sand dunes and pine trees, and is often a lee shore with no shelter from W winds. 5M offshore a current usually sets N at about 0·5kn, particularly with a S wind; in winter this may be stronger after W winds. Within 1M of the coast there may be a S'ly counter-current.

A missile range lies offshore: its N boundary is from 45°28'N 01°04'W to 45°11'N 02°04'W, (245°/38M from Pte de la Négade); the S boundary is from 43°41'N 01°31'W to 43°56'N 02°17'W (295°/40M from Capbreton). The inshore limit is 3M off, but it joins the shore at Hourtin (45°08'·5N); S of Arcachon to ZDS SPM buoy (44°28'N); and in 2 small sectors off Biscarosse (44°20'N) and Lamanchs (44°15'N). The range is divided into blocks 31N and 31S, which are N and S of a clear chan (31B) 8M wide running 270° from Arcachon. 31N and 31S are sub-divided into N/S sectors delineated by distance off the coast. Thus, 31S 2745 means the S block, in a sector 27-45M offshore. Various sectors are activated from 0830LT Mon-Fri; never Sat/Sun. Navigation through active sectors is prohib from the coast to 12M offshore; beyond 12M it is strongly discouraged. Centre d'Essais des Landes broadcasts range activity on VHF Ch 06, after warning on Ch 06 and 16, at 0815 and 1615LT Mon-Thurs, and at 0815 and 1030LT Fri. For more info on request (Mon-Thurs 0800-1700LT; Fri 0800-1100) call Landes VHF Ch 06 or ☎ 58.82.51.97 (same hrs); also recorded data H24 on ☎ 58.82.22.42/43. Other sources of info include: Hr Mr, Aff Maritimes, CROSS Soulac and Sémaphores at La Coubre, Cap Ferret and Socoa; all on request Ch 16, which should be monitored on passage.

The Fosse (or Gouf) de Capbreton, a submarine canyon, runs at right angles to the coast. The 50m depth contour is 3ca W of Capbreton hbr bkwtr and the 100m line is 4ca further W. In strong W winds a dangerous sea breaks along the N and S edges of it. Strong N or W winds and swell make the ent to the large marina at Capbreton (10.18.24) impassable.

CAPBRETON TO SPANISH BORDER (charts 1343, 1102)

There is a marina at Anglet (10.18.25), but few facilities for yachts further up the R. Adour at Bayonne. At L'Adour ent the flood runs E and SE, sp rate 2-4kn; the ebb runs W, sp rate 3-5kn. S of Pte St Martin the coast has mostly sandy beaches and rky cliffs, with offlying rky shoals and Pyrenees mountains inland. In strong W winds the sea breaks over Loutrou shoal; and on Plateau de St Jean-de-Luz, a chain of rky shoals lying 1-4M offshore.

St Jean-de-Luz (chart 1343 and 10.18.25) is best approached first time or in bad weather through Passe d'Illarguita (between Illarguita and Belhara Perdun shoals): follow the 138° transit (Le Socoa lt on with Bordagain lt) until the Ste Barbe ldg lts (101°) are in transit; thence enter by Passe de l'Ouest on the 151° transit of the inner hbr ldg lts.

Baie de Fontarabie, in Spanish Rada de Higuer, lies on the border of France and Spain, and is entered between Pte Ste Anne and Cabo Higuer (a bare, rugged cape with lt ho) 1·75M WNW. Les Briquets (dry) lie 1M N of Pte Ste Anne. Keep to W of Banc Chicharvel and Bajo Iruarri in ent to B. Entry should not be attempted with strong onshore winds or heavy swell. R La Bidassoa is entered between breakwaters in SW corner of the B, giving access to marina at Hendaye-Plage (10.18.26). In the middle of the bay is a neutral area, marked by beacons and shown on chart 1181. To seaward of this area the boundary line (approximately 01°46'·2W) runs N from a white pyramid on the S shore, about 1M SW of Pte Ste Anne.

10.18.6   DISTANCE TABLE

Approximate distances in nautical miles are by the most direct route, whilst avoiding dangers and allowing for Traffic Separation Schemes. Places in *italics* are in adjoining areas; places in **bold** are in 10.0.5, Cross-Channel Distances.

		1	2	3	4	5	6	7	8	9	10	11	12	13	14	15	16	17	18	19	20
1.	*Le Conquet*	**1**																			
2.	*St Nazaire*	145	**2**																		
3.	Pornic	146	16	**3**																	
4.	L'Herbaudière	144	16	10	**4**																
5.	Port Joinville	147	35	30	20	**5**															
6.	St Gilles-C-de-Vie	166	45	40	29	18	**6**														
7.	Sables d'Olonne	181	65	55	40	31	16	**7**													
8.	Bourgenay	190	74	64	49	40	25	9	**8**												
9.	St Martin (I de Ré)	208	92	75	67	55	44	27	20	**9**											
10.	La Rochelle	218	101	92	76	66	51	36	29	12	**10**										
11.	Rochefort	242	126	116	102	84	75	61	54	36	26	**11**									
12.	R La Seudre	242	125	116	100	89	71	58	52	33	24	30	**12**								
13.	Port St Denis	220	103	94	78	59	48	33	30	21	13	26	22	**13**							
14.	Port Bloc/Royan	234	122	115	107	97	85	71	60	56	52	68	27	42	**14**						
15.	Bordeaux	289	177	170	162	152	140	126	115	111	107	123	82	97	55	**15**					
16.	Cap Ferret	274	168	160	153	138	130	113	110	102	98	114	75	88	68	123	**16**				
17.	Capbreton	316	220	215	211	192	186	169	166	165	156	172	131	145	124	179	58	**17**			
18.	Anglet/Bayonne	328	232	223	223	200	195	181	178	177	168	184	143	157	132	187	70	12	**18**		
19.	*Santander*	300	243	237	229	212	210	204	204	206	202	218	184	192	180	235	133	106	103	**19**	
20.	*Cabo Finisterre*	382	404	399	390	377	395	393	394	406	407	423	399	397	401	456	376	370	373	274	**20**

10.18.7 Special Notes for France: see 10.15.8
10.18.8 French Glossary: see 1.4.2

PORNIC   10-18-9

Loire Atlantique 47°06′·55N 02°06′·59W

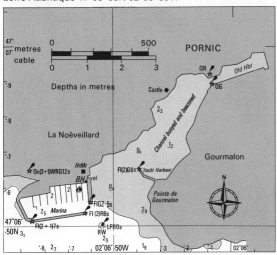

CHARTS
AC 3216, 2646; Imray C40; SHOM 5039, 6854, 6825; ECM 547, 549
TIDES
+0515 Dover; ML 3·6; Duration 0540; Zone –0100

Standard Port BREST (←——)

Times				Height (metres)			
High Water		Low Water		MHWS	MHWN	MLWN	MLWS
0500	1100	0500	1100	6·9	5·4	2·6	1·0
1700	2300	1700	2300				
Differences PORNIC							
–0050	+0030	–0010	–0010	–1·1	–0·8	–0·4	–0·2

SHELTER
Very good in large marina (2m); access HW±5. But no access LW±1 when Coeff >75, nor in winds >F7 from SE to W. Leave the SWM buoy to stbd, especially near LWS. Do not cut the corner round the S bkwtr head due to rky spur. Enter between the SHM pile and 2 PHM piles, on which the ☆s are mounted. A rky spur also extends SW from the head of the E jetty. Visitors berths are on P1, P2 and P3 pontoons (first to stbd). Old hbr dries 1·8m; access HW±2½ via marked, lit drying chan.

NAVIGATION
WPT 47°06′·10N 02°08′·70W, 253°/073° from/to jetty hd, 1·5M. 4-6M WSW of hbr beware Banc de Kerouars, least depth 1m, on which seas break; it is unmarked, but the W sector of Pte de Noëveillard lt clears it by night. From the NW pass between this bank and the mainland. All other hazards are well marked. The S end of B de Bourgneuf is full of oyster beds, and many obstructions.
LIGHTS AND MARKS
Pte de Noëveillard Oc (3+1) WRG 12s 22m 13/9M; G shore-051°, W051°-079°, R079°-shore; the W sector lies between Notre-Dame rk, IDM bn tr, and the E end of Banc de Kerouars. Marina SW elbow Fl (2+1) 7s 4m 3M. Off S jetty head Fl (2) R 6s 4m 4M; off E jetty head Fl G 2·5s 4m 2M. Entry sigs (simplified).
RADIO TELEPHONE
VHF Ch 09 (H24).
TELEPHONE
Hr Mr 40·82·05·40; Aff Mar 40·82·01·69; ⌗ 40·82·03·17; SNSM 40·82·00·47; Auto 36·68·08·44; CROSS 97·55·35·35; Police 40·82·00·29; Dr 40·82·01·80; Brit Consul 40·63·16·02.
FACILITIES
Port-la-Noëveillard Marina (754+165 visitors) ☎ 40·82·05·40, P, D (on pontoon), FW, ME, AC, EI, Sh, BH (20 ton), C (6 ton) CH; **CN de Pornic** ☎ 40·82·34·72; **Services:** ME, EI, Ⓔ, Sh, CH, SM. **Town** Market Sun am. V, Gaz, R, Bar, ✉, Ⓑ, ⇌, ✈ (Nantes). Ferry: Roscoff/St Malo.

18

L'HERBAUDIÈRE   10-18-10

Vendée 47°01'·70N 02°17'·77W

CHARTS

AC 3216, 2646; Imray C40; SHOM 5039, 6825; ECM 547, 549

TIDES

+0500 Dover; ML 3·4; Zone –0100

Standard Port BREST (⟵)

Times				Height (metres)			
High Water		Low Water		MHWS	MHWN	MLWN	MLWS
0500	1100	0500	1100	6·9	5·4	2·6	1·0
1700	2300	1700	2300				
Differences L'HERBAUDIERE							
–0047	+0023	–0020	–0020	–1·4	–1·0	–0·5	–0·2
FROMENTINE							
–0045	+0020	–0015	+0005	–1·7	–1·3	–0·8	–0·1

SHELTER

Good in marina (E side), dredged 1·5m-2·5m; visitors berth pontoon F. FV hbr (W side). ⚓ off Pte des Dames lt, Oc (3) WRG 12s, is exposed to N and E winds.
Or at **Noirmoutier-en-l'Ile**, 4M SE, good shelter and AB but hbr dries 1·8m-2·4m, access HW±1.

NAVIGATION

WPT 47°03'·05N 02°17'·5W, 009°/189° from/to W jetty lt, 1·4M. There are rks and banks to the SW, NW and NE of Pte de l'Herbaudière. Ldg lts and white sector (187·5°-190°) of the W jetty lt both lead into ent chan, dredged to 1·3m and passing close W of two 0·8m patches. Two SHM buoys, Fl G 2s, and a PHM buoy, Fl (2) R 6s, mark the last 2ca of the chan. W bkwtr obscures vessels leaving.
Noirmoutier-en-l'Ile: a long chan marked by bns leads through rks. La Vendette is one of the highest parts of rky ledges, E of ent to Noirmoutier-en-l'Ile.
Fosse de Fromentine: see below.

LIGHTS AND MARKS

Visibility in summer is often poor. Conspic daymarks are R/W radio mast 500m W of hbr and water tr about 1M SE. Ile du Pilier, Fl (3) 20s 33m 29M, is 2·5M WNW of hbr. Appr in any of the 3 W sectors of Basse de Martroger, NCM bn, Dir Q WRG 11m 9/6M, G033°-055°, W055°-060°, R060°-095°, G095°-124°, W124°-153°, R153°-201°, W201°-240°, R240°-033°.
Ldg lts 188°, both grey masts, Q 10/26m 7M, vis 098°-278°, lead over Banc de la Blanche (1·8m) approx 2M N of hbr. L'Herbaudière W jetty, Oc (2+1) WG 12s 9m 10/7M, W187·5°-190° (2½°), G elsewhere. E jetty head Q (2) R 5s 8m 4M; inner head Fl R 2s 3m 1M.

RADIO TELEPHONE

Hr Mr VHF Ch 09 (HO).

TELEPHONE

Hr Mr 51·39·05·05; Aff Mar 51·39·01·64; SNSM 51·39·33·90; CROSS 97·55·35·35; Meteo 40·84·80·19; Auto 36·68·08·85; ⌗ 51·39·06·80; Police 51·39·04·36; Dr 51·39·05·64; Brit Consul 40·63·16·02.

ADJACENT HARBOUR

FROMENTINE, Vendée, 46°53'·60N 02°08'·60W. AC 2646, SHOM 5039, 6853. HW +0550 on Dover (UT); ML 3·2m; Duration 0540. Tides above. Do not appr from Baie de Bourgneuf as there is a road causeway, dries 3m, from Ile de Noirmoutier to the mainland. Enter through Goulet de Fromentine, under the bridge (clearance 27m). The chan is buoyed, moved as necessary, but is very shallow, so dangerous in bad weather. The ebb runs at more than 5kn at sp. Do not attempt night entry. ⚓ W of pier. Coming from N, beware Les Boeufs. Tourelle Milieu lies on the N side of Le Goulet de Fromentine, Fl (4) R 12s 6m 5M, R tr. Pte de Notre Dames-de-Monts Dir lt, Oc (2) WRG 6s 21m 13/10M, W000°-043°, R043°-063°, R063°-073°, W073°-094°, G094°-113°, W113°-116°, R116°-175°, G175°-196°, R196°-230°. Fromentine SWM lt By, Fl 10s + bell, 46°53'·10N 02°11'·50W is about 1·5M WSW of Pte du Notre Dames-de-Monts. Bridge Iso 4s 32m 18M.
Facilities: Aff Mar at Noirmoutier; ⌗ at Beauvois-sur-Mer; **Quay** Slip, C (3 ton), FW; **Cercle Nautique de Fromentine-Barfatre** (CNFB); **Services:** ME, EI, Sh, CH.

FACILITIES

L'HERBAUDIÈRE. **Marina** (442+50 visitors), ☎ 51·39·05·05, Fax 51.39.75.97, FW, P, D, AC, C (25 ton), Slip, ME, SM, ▢, Gas, Gaz, V, R, Bar (July, Aug), Sh, SC; **Quay** Bar, R, ME, Sh, SM, V; **Services:** C, EI, Ⓔ, Sh, CH.
NOIRMOUTIER. **Quay** AB, FW, C (4 ton); **Services:** ME, EI, Ⓔ, Sh, CH, SM.
   Town P, D, V, Gaz, R, Bar, ▢, ✉, Ⓑ, ⇌ (ferry to Pornic, bus to Nantes), ✈ (Nantes). Ferry: Roscoff or St Malo.

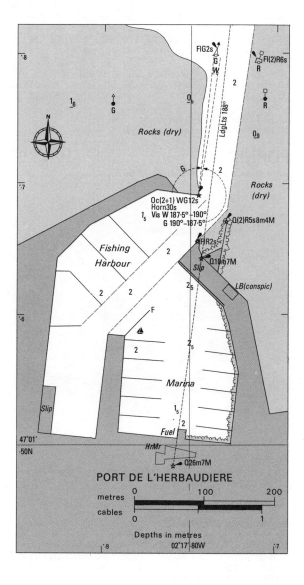

PORT DE L'HERBAUDIERE

Depths in metres
02°17'·80W

PORT JOINVILLE, Ile d'Yeu

Vendée 46°43'·80N 02°20'·75W

10-18-11

CHARTS
AC 3640, 2663; Imray C40; SHOM 6613, 6890, 6853; ECM 549, 1022

TIDES
+0550 Dover; ML 3·1; Duration 0600; Zone –0100

Standard Port BREST (←—)

Times				Height (metres)			
High Water		Low Water		MHWS	MHWN	MLWN	MLWS
0500	1100	0500	1100	6·9	5·4	2·6	1·0
1700	2300	1700	2300				
Differences PORT JOINVILLE (Ile d'Yeu)							
–0025	+0010	–0030	–0030	–1·7	–1·3	–0·6	–0·2

SHELTER
Good in marina, very crowded in season; best to pre-book as it is the only secure hbr on the island. Or yachts can lock into the wet basin (3·7m) HW±1½, mainly for FVs; no pontoons; tfc lts R & G, just S of lock. No ⚓ in outer hbr; swell enters in N/NE winds. If the marina and wet basin are full, yachts can moor between Gare Maritime and the ice factory, keeping clear of ferries to W. A grid to the W of the ice factory is marked by R paint lines on quay wall.

NAVIGATION
WPT Basse Mayence NCM, 46°44'·65N 02°19'·10W, 055°/235° from/to bkwtr lt, 1·4M. Chan dredged 2m, appr with care at LW. Beware Basse du Bouet (dries 0·6m) 3ca NW, La Sablaire shoal to the E and rks along the coast both sides of hbr ent.

LIGHTS AND MARKS
Very conspic high water tr brg 224° leads to hbr. Ldg lts 219°, both QR 11/16m 6M, vis 169°-269°; rear (mast) 85m from front.

NW jetty head Oc (3) WG 12s 9m 11/9M; G shore-150°, W150°-232°, G232°-279°, W279°-285°, G285°-shore; horn (3) 30s, tidal sigs. Quai de Canada hd Iso G 4s 7m 6M unintens 337°-067°. Galiote jetty root Fl R 2·5s 1M.

RADIO TELEPHONE
Yacht Hbr VHF Ch 09 16 (HO).

TELEPHONE
Hr Mr 51·58·38·11; Hbr Office 51·58·51·10; Aff Mar 51·58·35·39; ⌗ 51·55·10·58; CROSS 97·55·35·35; Meteo 51·36·10·78; Auto 36·68·08·85; SNSM 51·58·35·39; Police 51·58·30·05; Dr 51·58·31·70; Ⓗ 51·68·30·23; Brit Consul 40·63·16·02. Note: There are phone-card telephones only.

FACILITIES
Marina (150+30 visitors), FW, AB, P, D, ME, El, Sh; **2nd Tidal Basin** ☎ 51·58·38·11, Slip, L, FW, C (5 ton); **CN Ile d'Yeu** ☎ 51·58·31·50; **Services:** ME, El, Sh, CH, Ⓔ. **Town** V, Gaz, R, Bar, ✉, Ⓑ, ⇌ (St-Gilles-Croix-de-Vie), ✈ (Nantes). Flights from airfield 2M west of Port Joinville to Nantes and (summers only) to Les Sables d'Olonne. Ferry: Roscoff or St Malo. Local ferries to Fromentine, St Gilles and Les Sables-d'Olonne.

ADJACENT HARBOUR ON ILE D'YEU

PORT DE LA MEULE, Ile d'Yeu, Vendée, 46°41'·75N 03°20'·60W. AC 2663; SHOM 6890, 6853. –0050 sp and – 0020 nps on Brest; ML 3·0m. A small, drying fishing hbr on the S side of Ile d'Yeu, only safe in settled offshore weather; untenable in S winds. Many FVs inside hbr; best to ⚓ outside ent. Between Pte de la Père to the W and Pte de la Tranche to the SE, appr brg 034° on W chapel; then 022° towards W square patch on Gy ☐ lt tr, R top, Oc WRG 4s 9m 9/6/5M, vis G007°-018°, W018°-028°, R028°-042°. (Night ent not advised). Within 1ca of ent beware rks, first to port, then to stbd. Few facilities: Slips, R, Bar; V 1½ miles.

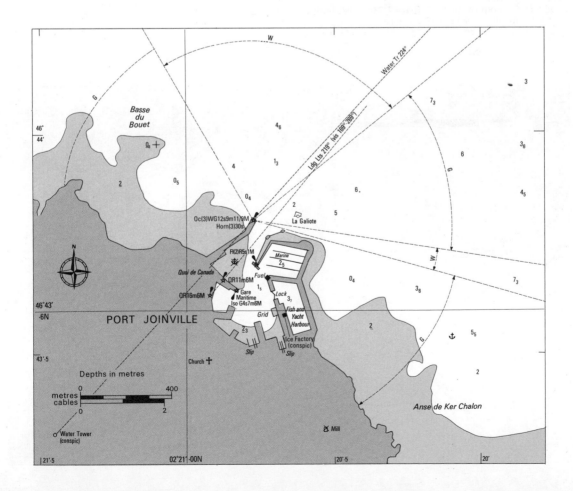

ST GILLES-CROIX-DE-VIE

Vendée 46°41'·60N 01°57'·05W   **10-18-12**

CHARTS
AC 3640, 2663; Imray C40; SHOM 6613, 6853, 6523;
ECM 1022, 549
TIDES
+0500 Dover; ML 3·2; Duration 0600; Zone –0100

Standard Port BREST (←—)

Times				Height (metres)			
High Water		Low Water		MHWS	MHWN	MLWN	MLWS
0500	1100	0500	1100	6·9	5·4	2·6	1·0
1700	2300	1700	2300				
Differences ST GILLES-CROIX-DE-VIE							
–0032	+0013	–0033	–0033	–1·8	–1·3	–0·6	–0·3

SHELTER
Good shelter, and easy access except in strong SW
winds or swell when breakers form off ent. Chan (⚓
prohib) dredged 1·5m, but very shallow near bkwtr hds
due to silting. Best arr/dep HW –2 to HW, to avoid strong
ebb. On N bank are: small yacht basin inside Grand Môle;
two tidal FV basins; beyond them the marina nominally
dredged to 1·5m. If full, pick up ⚓ or yachts can lie
alongside quay (dries) on E bank below bridge. In good
weather ⚓ off ent, close SE of ldg line.
NAVIGATION
WPT Pill'Hours SCM, Q (6) +L Fl 15s, Bell, 46°41'·05N
01°58'·00W, 231°/051° from/to Jetée de la Garenne lt,
0·75M. Beware Rocher Pill'Hours (2·8m) and drying
reefs extending 1ca (180m) SE. Tide runs very strongly
in ent, particularly on ebb.
LIGHTS AND MARKS
Landmarks are Pte de Grosse-Terre (rky hdland) with lt
ho, W truncated conical tr; the rear ldg lt structure; and
two spires NE of the marina.
Pte de Grosse Terre Fl (4) WR 12s 25m 17/13M, vis
W290°-125°, R125°-145°.
Ldg lts 043°: both Dir Oc (3+1) R 12s 7/28m 13M; both W
☐ trs, R top; intens 033·5°-053·5°, synch.
SE mole hd, QWG 8m 9/6M, vis G045°-335°, W335°-
045°, Reed 20s.
NW mole hd, Fl (2) WR 6s 8m 10/7M, R045°-225°, W225°-045°.

RADIO TELEPHONE
VHF Ch 09 (season 0600-2200; out of season 0800-1200,
1400-1800LT).
TELEPHONE
Hr Mr Port de Plaisance 51·55·30·83; Aff Mar 51·55·10·58;
⌗ 51·55·10·58; CROSS 97·55·35·35; SNSM 51·55·01·19;
Meteo 51·36·10·78; Auto 36·68·08·85; Police 51·55·01·19;
Dr 51·55·11·93; Brit Consul 40·63·16·02.
FACILITIES
Port la Vie Marina (800+60 visitors) ☎ 51·55·30·83, Fax
51.55.31.43, Access H24, P, D, FW, AC, ME, El, CH, Gaz,
SM, BH (26 ton), Slip, R, V, Bar; **Quay** Slip, FW, C (6 ton);
CN de Havre de Vie ☎ 51·55·87·91;
Services: ME, El, Sh, CH, Ⓔ, C (15 ton), SM, SHOM.
Town V, Gaz, R, Bar, ⊠, Ⓑ, ⇌. A ferry runs to Ile d'Yeu.
Ferry: Roscoff or St Malo.

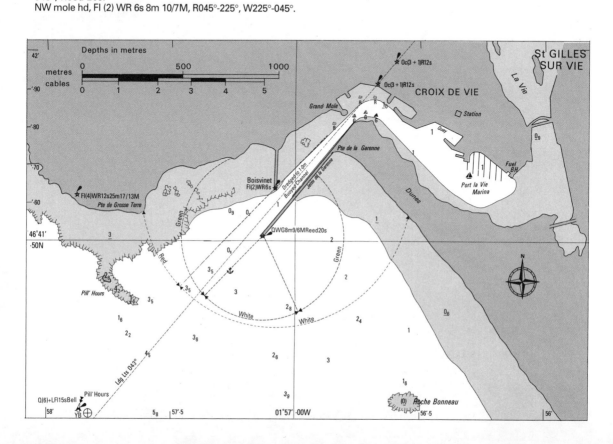

LES SABLES D'OLONNE   10-18-13

Vendée 46°29'·40N 01°47'·40W

CHARTS
AC 3640, 2663; Imray C40; SHOM 6551, 6522, 6523; ECM 1022

TIDES
+0530 Dover; ML 3·2; Duration 0640; Zone –0100

Standard Port BREST (←)

Times				Height (metres)			
High Water		Low Water		MHWS	MHWN	MLWN	MLWS
0500	1100	0500	1100	6·9	5·4	2·6	1·0
1700	2300	1700	2300				
Differences LES SABLES D'OLONNE							
–0030	+0015	–0035	–0035	–1·7	–1·3	–0·6	–0·3

SHELTER
Access at all tides; entry is easy except in winds from SE to SW when apprs get rough. Sailing is prohib in the entry chan to hbr. Commercial and FV Basins prohib to yachts. Access to marina (1·5 - 3·5m) H24. Visitors check in at pontoon port side, by Capitainerie. Pontoon L, at NE end, is for visitors and multihulls; or berth as directed.

NAVIGATION
WPT Nouch Sud SCM, Q (6)+L Fl 15s, 46°28'·63N 01°47'·35W, 220°/040° from/to front ldg lt 033°, 1·2M. To the W, beware Les Barges d'Olonne, extending 3M W of Pte de Aiguille. There are 2 appr chans: the SW chan with La Potence lts 033°, which lead into SE chan on ldg line 320°. In bad weather use the SE chan. Le Noura and Le Nouch are two isolated rks on shallow patches S of Jetée St Nicolas. Further SE, Barre Marine breaks, even in moderate weather. A buoyed wk (dries) lies off hbr ent, to E of 320° ldg line. At hbr ent, dredged chan (2m) initially favours the E side, then mid-chan.

LIGHTS AND MARKS
Les Barges lt ho, Fl (2) R 10s 25m 17M, gy tr, 2M W of ent.
L'Armandèche lt ho, Fl (2+1) 15s 42m 24M, 6ca W of ent.
SW Chan ldg lts 033°: both Iso R 4s 14/33m 16M; rear, 330m from front (both H24).
SE Chan ldg lts 320°: front QG 11m 8M; rear, 465m from front, Oc (2+1) 12s 33m 13M.
St Nicolas jetty hd, UQ (2) R 1s 16m 10M vis 143°-094°; Horn (2) 30s. Inner ldg lts 327°, both FR 6/9m 11M; R/W vert stripes difficult to see by day.

RADIO TELEPHONE
Port VHF Ch 12 16 (0800-1800). Marina Ch 09 16 (0600-2400LT in season; 0800-2000LT out of season).

TELEPHONE
Hr Mr Port de Plaisance 51·32·51·16; Aff Mar 51·21·01·80; CROSS 97·55·35·35; Meteo 51·36·10·78; Auto 36·68·08·85; ⌗ 51·32·02·33; SNSM 51·21·20·55; Police 51·33·69·91; Dr 51·95·14·47; Ⓗ 51·21·06·33; Brit Consul 56·52·28·35.

FACILITIES
Port Olona Marina (1100+110 visitors), ☎ 51·32·51·16, Fax 51.32.37.13, Slip, P, D, FW, ME, El, AC, Sh, ◎;
Services: El, Sh, CH, BH (27 ton), Ⓔ, SHOM, SM, Divers.
Town P, D, V, Gaz, R, Bar, ⊠, Ⓑ, ⇌, ✈. Ferry: Roscoff or St Malo.

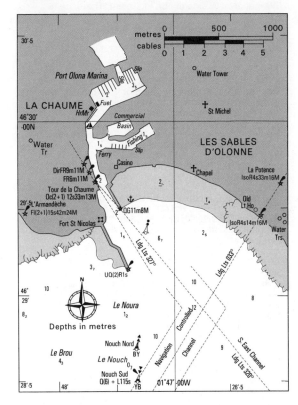

BOURGENAY   10-18-14

Vendée 46° 26'·38N 01° 40'·57W

CHARTS
AC 2663; Imray C41; SHOM 6522; ECM 1022

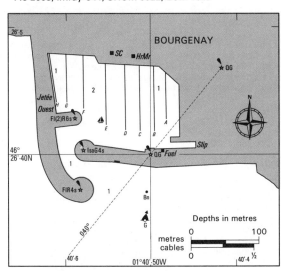

TIDES
+0600 Dover; ML 3·1; Duration 0640; Zone –0100. Use Differences LES SABLES D'OLONNE (10.18.13), 5·5M NW.

SHELTER
Good in the marina (2m). Caution: even in moderate weather, & especially with SW winds, a big swell can break at the ent.

NAVIGATION
WPT Fairway buoy SWM, L Fl 10s, 46°25'·35N 01°41'·90W, 220°/040° from/to pier head, 1·35M. Beware Roches de Joanne, 600m ENE of WPT, (dangerous in bad weather) and shoal patch to E of ent, marked by unlit SHM buoy and bn. Ent chan, dredged 1·0m, has two 90° turns marked by luminous chevrons; 3kn speed limit.

LIGHTS AND MARKS
Ldg lts 040°: both QG 8M; front W hut with G □, vis 020°-060°; rear W pylon, W □ with G border, vis 010°-070°. The Iso G 4s 5M and Fl (2) R 6s 5M are not vis from seaward.

RADIO TELEPHONE
VHF Ch 09 16 (office hrs; in summer 0800-2100LT).

TELEPHONE
Hr Mr/SNSM 51·22·20·36, Fax 51.22.29.45; CROSS Etel 97·55·35·35; Auto 36·68·08·85; ⌗ 51·32·02·33; Aff Mar 51·21·81·71; Police 51·90·60·07; Dr 51·90·62·68; Ⓗ 51·96·00·41; Brit Consul 56·52·28·35.

FACILITIES
Marina (470+90 visitors) ☎ 51·22·20·36, FW, AC, P, D, Slip;
Association Nautique de Bourgenay (ANB) ☎ 51·22·02·57;
Services: CH, C (15 ton), Gaz.
Town R, ◎, V, Bar, ⊠, Ⓑ, ⇌ (Les Sables d'Olonne), ✈ (La Lande, Chateau d'Olonne). Ferry: Roscoff or St. Malo.

18

MINOR HARBOURS IN PERTUIS BRETON

JARD-SUR-MER, Vendée, 46°24′.45N 01°34′.75W. AC 2641, 2663; SHOM 6522. HW +0600 on Dover (UT); −0010 on Brest (zone −0100); HW ht −2·0m on Brest; ML 3·1m; Duration 0640. Small drying hbr, access HW±2, 4·5m max at HW. Moorings inside bkwtr, inc 7 Y **Ⓐ**s. Hr Mr's office with blue roof and adjacent bldgs are conspic from afar. W daymarks 4ca (740m) E of hbr lead 038° via narrow ent between the drying Roches de l'Islatte and Roches de la Brunette, marked by buoys. Then pick up 293° transit of RW marks on W side of hbr, ldg to ent. There are no lights. Hr Mr ☎ 51·33·40·17; ⌗ ☎ 51·95·11·33; Facilities: **Jetty** FW, C (5 ton); **Services:** CH, Divers.

L'AIGUILLON/LA-FAUTE-SUR-MER, Vendée, 46°20′·00N 01°18′·60W. AC 2641, 2663; SHOM 6521. HW +0535 on Dover (UT); −0030 on Pte de Grave (Zone −0100); HW ht +0·6m on Pte de Grave; ML 3·4m. Shelter good in two yacht hbrs, but avoid in strong S or W winds; ent only safe in fine weather with off-shore winds. Access HW±2½. Beware mussel beds with steel piles which cover at HW; also oyster beds. The area is very flat and, being shallow, waves build up quickly in any wind. The bar to seaward dries and is dangerous in bad weather. Ent can best be identified by a conspic transformer on a hill, La Dive, opposite side of chan to Pointe d'Arcay. Enter at Le Lay SCM buoy, Q (6) + L Fl 15s, with transformer brg 033°. ⚓ in R Lay or berth at L'Aiguillon (NE bank); or in drying tidal basin at La Faute (SW bank). Hr Mrs (L'Aiguillon) ☎ 51.97.06.57; (La Faute) ☎ 51·56·45·02; Aff Mar ☎ 51·56·45·35; CROSS ☎ 56·09·82·00; Dr ☎ 51·56·46·17; Facilities: **Club Nautique Aiguillonais et Fautais (CNAF)** ☎ 51·97·04·60; **Services:** ME, CH.

MARANS, Vendée, 46°19′·00N 01°00′·00W. AC 2641, 2663; SHOM 6521; ECM 551. Tides: see L'Aiguillon above; HW at Brault lock = HW La Rochelle + 0020. Good shelter in non-tidal hbr approx 10M from SWM buoy, L Fl 10s, abeam Pte de l'Aiguillon with 10m high B bn. Buoyed chan, dries 1m, leads NE past Pavé jetty, Fl G 4s, thence 3½M up-river to Brault lifting bridge and 5ca to lock, open HW±2 sp, HW±1 np. Best arrival at HW. Waiting buoys before bridge; pontoon inside vast lock which has small swing bridge at far end. Straight 3M canal to stbd side pontoon. Brault lock ☎ 46.01.53.77; Facilities: **Quay** ☎ 46.01.10.36, AB (40+10 visitors), FW, C (3 tons), P & D (cans); **Services:** BY, ME, Sh, SM. **Town** V, R, Bar.

OTHER HARBOURS ON ILE DE RÉ

LA FLOTTE, Ile de Ré, Charente Maritime, 46°11′·35N 01°19′·25W. AC 2641, 2746; SHOM 6668, 6521. HW +0535 on Dover (UT). La Flotte lies 2M SE of St Martin (see 10·18·15). From NW keep clear of Le Couronneau; from E, keep N of bn off Pte des Barres. Appr on 215° in W sector of La Flotte lt ho, W tr with G top, Fl WG 4s 10m 12/9M; vis G130°-205°, W205°-220°, G220°-257°; horn (3) 30s by day HW±2. Moiré indicator shows vert B line for on course 215°, or chevrons to regain course. Waiting Bys outside. Avant port is sheltered by mole and dries 2·4m; inner hbr dries 2·7m. Access HW±2. There is an ⚓ off La Flotte in 3m, sheltered from S and W. Hr Mr on Quai Senac Ouest; Aff Mar and ⌗ at St Martin; Facilities: **Quay** FF75, Slip, FW, **Ⓥ** berth on N Jetty; **Cercle Nautique de la Flotte-en-Ré (CNLF)** (open Jul-15 Sep); **Services:** ME.

ARS-EN-RÉ, Ile de Ré, Charente Maritime, 46°12′·70N 01°30′·62W. AC 2641; SHOM 6521, 6333. HW +0540 on Dover (UT); −0045 on Pte de Grave (Zone −0100); HW ht +0·6m; ML 3·7m. Port d'Ars is at the head of a chan in the SW corner of the bay Le Fier d'Ars, the ent obstructed by drying rks. There is an ⚓ close S of Pte du Fier with min depth of 2·4m; most of the bay dries. Chan is marked by buoys and bns; access HW±3.
Ldg lts to Fiers d'Ars 265°: front, Iso 4s 5m 11M W □ on hut, vis 141°-025°; rear, 370m from front, Dir Iso G 4s 13m 15M, G □ tr on dwelling (synch with front and intens 264°-266°). Port d'Ars ldg lts 232°: front, Q 5m 9M, W □ with R lantern; rear, 370m from front, Q 13m 11M, B □ on W framework tr, G top, vis 142°-322°. Church spire, B & W, is conspic.
There are two sheltered marinas: The first, Bassin de la Criée (2m), is on NW side of chan approx 600m before town; access over sill 2.5m CD, visitors berth port side on pontoon H. The second, Bassin de chasse, is at head of chan. It dries 2·9m, access HW ±2½ via gate which is left open; visitors berths to stbd. Or drying AB on NW quay in mud. VHF Ch 09. Hr Mr ☎ 46·29·25·10; Aff Mar and ⌗ at St Martin (see 10·18·15); SNSM ☎ 46·29·41·49; **Marinas** FF95, Slip, FW, C (6 ton); **Cercle Nautique d'Ars-en-Ré** ☎ 46·29·23·04 (Apl to Nov); **Services:** ME, El, Sh.

ST MARTIN, Ile de Ré   10-18-15

Charente Maritime 46°12'·56N 01°21'·84W

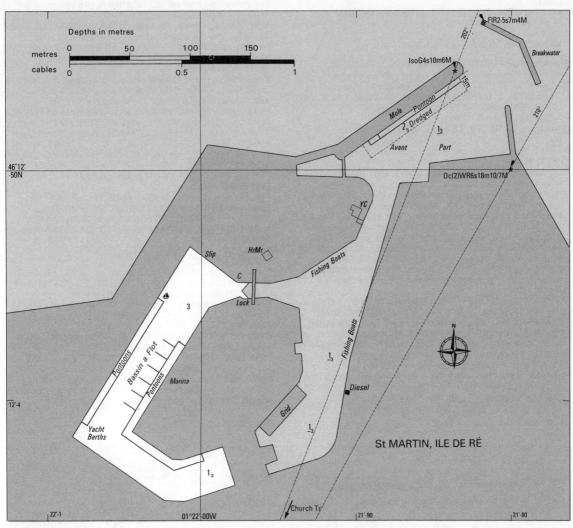

CHARTS
AC 2641, 2746; Imray C41; SHOM 6668, 6521; ECM 551, 1022
TIDES
+0535 Dover; ML 3·7; Zone –0100

Standard Port POINTE DE GRAVE (→)

Times				Height (metres)			
High Water		Low Water		MHWS	MHWN	MLWN	MLWS
0000	0600	0500	1200	5·4	4·4	2·1	1·0
1200	1800	1700	2400				
Differences ST. MARTIN, Ile de Ré							
+0007	–0032	–0030	–0025	+0·5	+0·3	+0·2	–0·1

SHELTER
Complete shelter in non-tidal marina (depth 3m); often very crowded with queue to enter. 4 W waiting buoys off ent. Avant port is protected by mole on NW side, and bkwtr close to the NE. Access HW–3 to +2 via chan (dries 1·5m) to drying basin for FVs. Inside mole a waiting pontoon (summer only) is dredged 2·3m. Marina gates open about HW±1, with sill 0·8m above CD. Berth as directed by Hr Mr.
NAVIGATION
WPT Rocha NCM By, Q, 46°14'·75N 01°20'·80W, 020°/200° from/to St Martin mole hd, 2·4M.
From the NW, pass N and E of Le Rocha, a rky bank extending 2½M ENE from Pte du Grouin.
From SE, pass well N of unlit NCM bn, about ¾M NE of ent, marking Le Couronneau drying ledge in R sector (245°-281°) of St Martin lt ho Oc (2) WR 6s.

By day appr with lt ho and ⊕ □ tr in line 210°, or mole hd lt in transit 202° with ⊕ tr; the lt ho is easier to see.
LIGHTS AND MARKS
Citadelle is conspic 3ca E of hbr ent. Lt ho, Oc (2) WR 6s 18m 10/7M, vis W shore-245°, R245°-281°, W281°-shore, is on ramparts at SE side of ent. Mole hd, Iso G 4s 10m 6M, is obscured by Pte du Grouin when brg <124°.
RADIO TELEPHONE
VHF Ch 09 (0800-1900LT in summer).
TELEPHONE
Hr Mr 46·09·26·69; Aff Mar 46·09·68·89; ⌗ 46·09·21·78; Meteo 46·41·29·14; Auto 36·68·08·17; CROSS 56·09·82·00; Police 46·09·21·17; Dr 46·09·20·08; Ⓗ 46·09·20·01; Brit Consul 56·52·28·35.
FACILITIES
Marina (135+50 visitors), FF90, P, D, FW, AC, ME, El, Sh;
Quay FW, C (4 ton); **YC St Martin** ☎ 46·09·22·07;
Services: ME, El, Ⓔ, Sh, CH, SHOM.
Town P, D, V, Gaz, R, Bar, ✉, Ⓑ, ⇌, ✈ (La Rochelle).
Ferry: Roscoff or St Malo.

18

LA ROCHELLE   10-18-16

Charente Maritime 46°09'·40N 01° 09'·15W

CHARTS
AC 2743, 2746, 2641; Imray C41; SHOM 6468, 6333/4;
ECM 551, 1022

TIDES
+0515 Dover; ML 3·8; Zone −0100

Standard Port POINTE DE GRAVE (→)

Times				Height (metres)			
High Water		Low Water		MHWS	MHWN	MLWN	MLWS
0000	0600	0500	1200	5·4	4·4	2·1	1·0
1200	1800	1700	2400				

Differences LA ROCHELLE and LA PALLICE

+0015	−0030	−0025	−0020	+0·6	+0·5	+0·3	−0·1

SHELTER
Excellent in **Port des Minimes**, a very large marina with
3·5m depth (max LOA 25m); in the Vieux Port, and in the
Inner Basin. The large non-tidal **Bassin des Chalutiers**
has pontoons on the N/NE sides for visitors >16m LOA.
Vieux Port, in the old town, is entered beyond the two trs
of St Nicolas and La Chaine. It has a tidal basin (dredged
1·3m) with 100+ berths for smaller yachts. On the E side a
non-tidal **Inner Basin** (3m) is entered by a lock with sill
1·2m above CD, opens HW−2 to HW+½; night ent by prior
arrangement ☎ 46.41.32.05. Note: La Pallice is strictly a
commercial/FV port 3M W, with no yacht facilities.

NAVIGATION
WPT 46°06'·63N 01°15'·98W, Chauveau SCM By, VQ (6) +
L Fl 10s, 240°/060° from/to Tour Richelieu, 4·6M. Appr
from about 1M S of Le Lavardin lt tr on ldg line 059°. Off
Pte des Minimes (SW of marina) drying rks extend ¼M
offshore; further S there is a firing danger area marked
by 5 SPM buoys. Shallow appr chan needs care at MLWS.
Tour Richelieu (with tide gauge) marks a drying rky spit
to the N of the chan; least depth in chan 0·2m. Ent to Port
des Minimes is 1ca past Tour Richelieu, marked by WCM
and 2 PHM buoys, all unlit; but mole heads are lit.

For Vieux Port stay on 059° ldg line in chan (35m wide),
leaving 4 PHM buoys well to port.
Note: Passage under the bridge (30m clearance) between
Ile de Ré and the mainland must be made N-bound
between piers Nos 13 and 14, and S-bound between
piers Nos 10 and 11. These passages are buoyed/lit.

LIGHTS AND MARKS
Ldg lts 059°: Front, Q 15m 14M (Fl 4s by day), R ○ tr, W
bands; rear, Q 25m 14M (Fl 4s by day), W octagonal tr, G
top; synch, obsc 061°-065° by St Nicolas tr.
Le Lavardin, rky shoal 3M WSW of Tr Richelieu, Fl (2) WG
6s 14m 11/8M, B tr, R band, vis G160°-169°, W169°-160°.
Tour Richelieu, Fl (4) R 12s 10m 9M, conspic R tr, RC,
siren (4) 60s.
Port des Minimes: W mole hd Fl G 4s; E mole hd Fl (2) R 6s.

RADIO TELEPHONE
Port des Minimes Ch 09 (H24). Hbr Ch 06 11 12.

TELEPHONE
Port des Minimes Hr Mr 46.44.41.20, Vieux Port Hr Mr
46.41.68.73; Aff Mar 46.41.43.91; CROSS 56.09.82.00;
Meteo 46.41.29.14; ⌗ 46.42.64.64; Auto 36.68.08.17; Dr
46.42.19.22; Police 46.34.67.55; Ⓗ 46.27.33.33; Brit Consul
56.52.28.35.

FACILITIES
PORT DES MINIMES
Marina (2,800+250 visitors on pontoons 14 and 15), FF95,
☎ 46.44.41.20, Fax 46.44.36.49, Gaz, AC, Slip, C (10 ton), P,
D, FW, BH (50 ton), R. Hourly water bus to the town.
Société des Régates Rochellaises ☎ 46.44.62.44;
Services: ME, Sh, CH, Ⓔ, El, SHOM, SM.
VIEUX PORT
Quay FF95, Slip, FW, C (10 ton), BH (300 ton), SM, ME, Sh,
CH, no toilets/showers, may be noisy.
Inner Basin (100) ☎ 46.41.32.05 (3m), FF95, Access HW −2
to HW+½. **Bassin des Chalutiers** FW, AC.
Town P, D, V, Gaz, R, Bar, ✉, Ⓑ, ⇌, ✈. Ferry to Ile de Ré;
internal air services (and to London in season) from Laleu
airport (2½km N of port). Ferry: Roscoff or St Malo.

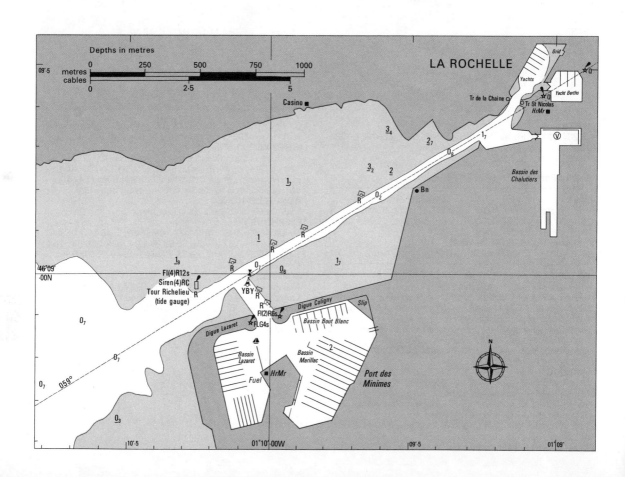

ILE D'OLÉRON   10-18-17
Charente Maritime

CHARTS
AC 2746, 2663; SHOM 6914, 6913, 6912, 6334, 6335; ECM 552
TIDES
+0545 Dover; ML 3·9; Duration 0540; Zone −0100

Standard Port POINTE DE GRAVE (→)

Times				Height (metres)			
High Water		Low Water		MHWS	MHWN	MLWN	MLWS
0000	0600	0500	1200	5·4	4·4	2·1	1·0
1200	1800	1700	2400				
Differences LE CHAPUS							
+0015	−0040	−0025	−0015	+0·6	+0·6	+0·4	+0·2
POINTE DE GATSEAU							
+0005	−0005	−0015	−0025	−0·1	−0·1	+0·2	+0·2

HARBOURS
Port St Denis and Le Douhet are in the N of the island, both with dedicated marinas. Boyardville and Le Chateau on the E coast are mainly for FVs, but have small marinas. La Cotinière, on the W coast, suffers from almost constant Atlantic swell and is much used by FVs. Beware fishing nets with very small floats especially near Port St Denis.

PORT ST DENIS 46°02'·16N 01°21'·97W.

SHELTER
Very good in large marina. Access HW±3½ for 2m draft over sill 1·5m CD. Max depth 2·5m. 3 W waiting buoys approx 700m E of ent in 0·7 - 1m.

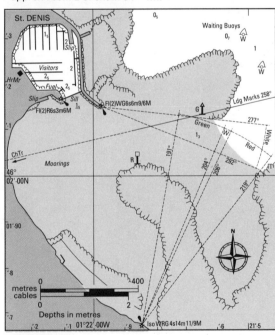

NAVIGATION
WPT 46°03'·27N 01°20'·75W, 025°/205° from/to chan ent, 1·35M. Appr chan dries about 1·1m. Daymarks lead 258° to ent. By night 2 Dir lts lead 205° and 284° in sequence.
LIGHTS AND MARKS
Pte de Chassiron, Fl 10s 50m 28M, 1·9M WNW. Rocher d'Antioche bn, Q 20m 11M, 2·2M NNW. Daymarks: SHM perch on with church tr 258°. Dir lt, ½M S of hbr ent, Iso WRG 4s, W sector 204°-206°, leads 205° to pick up second Dir lt Fl (2) WG 6s on N pier; W sector 277°-292°, leads 284°.
RADIO TELEPHONE
VHF Ch 09.
TELEPHONE
Hr Mr 46·47·97·97; Yacht Club Océan 46·47·80·50; Aff Mar 46·47·60·01; SNSM 46·47·06·33; Ⓗ (12km) 46·47·00·86; Auto 36·68·08·17.
FACILITIES
Marina (600+70 visitors) ☎ 46·47·97·97, Fax 46.47.88.23, FF80, FW, AC, P, D, Slip, BH (10 ton); **YCO** ☎ 46·47·90·50.

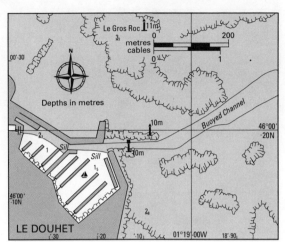

LE DOUHET 46°00'·15N 01°19'·18W.

SHELTER
Very good in marina; access HW −3½ to HW +3 for 1·5m draft, over two sills 2·5m CD. Caution inside ent, training wall to port protects pontoons.
NAVIGATION
WPT 46°00'·54N 01°17'·61W, NCM By Q, 068°/248° from/ to ent 1·1M. Unlit, buoyed appr chan dries about 1·5m to approx 0·35M offshore.
LIGHTS AND MARKS
No lts/ldg marks; bkwtrs marked by perches.
RADIO TELEPHONE
VHF Ch 09.
TELEPHONE/FACILITIES
Hr Mr 46.76.71.13, Fax 46.76.78.26; **Marina** (305+45 visitors), FF70, FW, AC, Max LOA 15m; V at St Georges d'Oléron and La Brée.

OTHER HARBOURS ON ILE D'OLÉRON

BOYARDVILLE, Ile d'Oléron, Charente Maritime, 45°58'·30N 01°13'·76W. AC 2746, 2663; SHOM 6913/4, 6334/5; ECM 552. HW +0545 on Dover (UT); tides as for Ile d'Aix (see overleaf). Fishing port, with good shelter in non-tidal marina (2m), but berths are usually taken and multiple rafting is the norm. Access HW±2 to drying appr chan and into marina to stbd via automatic lock, open approx HW±2. From La Perrotine SHM By steer 263° for 4ca to S bkwtr lt, Fl (2) R 6s 8m 5M. Six W waiting buoys ½M N of chan or ⌁ in 3m. VHF Ch 09. Hr Mr ☎ 46·47·23·71. **Marina** (165+45 visitors) FF70, AC, FW C (10 ton), Slip, P & D on quay; **YCB** ☎ 46·47·05·82. **Services:** ME, El, Sh, CH.

LE CHATEAU, Ile d'Oléron, Charente Maritime, 45°52'·95N 01°11'·30W. AC 2663; SHOM 6913, 6334, 6335; ECM 552. HW +0545 on Dover (UT); tides as for Ile d'Aix (overleaf), ML 3·8m, duration 0540. Mainly occupied by oyster FVs; yachts are tolerated, rather than welcomed. Possible drying berth on NE quay. Access HW±3. From N, appr via Chenal Est, to SCM bn marking Grand Montanne and ent to appr chan. From S, appr via Coureau d'Oléron, under mainland bridge (clnce 18m), thence 1M to ent chan. Ldg lts 319°, QR 11/24m 7M synch. Hr Mr ☎ 46·47·00·01. Facilities: Slip, L, FW, C (25 ton).

18

ROCHEFORT   10·18·18

Charente Maritime 45°56'·60N 00°57'·20W

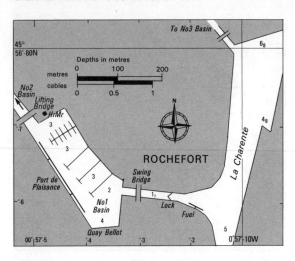

CHARTS
AC 2748, 2746; SHOM 4333, 6334; ECM 552
TIDES
+0610 Dover; Zone –0100

Standard Port POINTE DE GRAVE (→)

Times				Height (metres)			
High Water		Low Water		MHWS	MHWN	MLWN	MLWS
0000	0600	0500	1200	5·4	4·4	2·1	1·0
1200	1800	1700	2400				
Differences ROCHEFORT							
+0020	–0020	+0040	+0115	+1·0	+0·7	+0·1	+0·4
ILE D'AIX							
+0015	–0040	–0030	–0025	+0·7	+0·5	+0·3	–0·1

SHELTER
Rochefort is on N bank of La Charente, about 10M from
Port-des-Barques. Entry advised on late flood, as bar
breaks on ebb. ⌕ out of chan at Soubise or Martrou; or
lock into Port de Plaisance on W bank. Bassin No 1 (access
HW La Rochelle ±1; at nps access can be only HW±¼);
waiting and fuel pontoon, just outside lock, dries to soft
mud. Beware very strong currents here, other than at HW
or LW. Bassin No 2 is entered from No 1, via lifting bridge.
No 3 Bassin, 400m N, is for commercial craft only. The
river is navigable 3·5M on to Tonnay-Charente.
NAVIGATION
WPT Les Palles NCM, Q, 45°59'·58N 01°09'·53W, 293°/
113° from/to front ldg lt 115°, 4·0M. Stream in river runs
about 2kn (4kn in narrows), and at sp there is a small
bore. Beware wk just S of WPT. When WSW of Fouras
pick up second (Port-des-Barques) ldg line (135°). The bar
at Fouras carries about 0·5m. From Port-des-Barques
follow the alignment of lettered pairs (RR to AA) of unlit
ldg bns. Fixed bridge, 32m clearance, is 2M downriver of
Basin No 1.
LIGHTS AND MARKS
Ile d'Aix Fl WR 5s 24m 24/20M; twin W trs with R tops;
vis R103°-118°, W118°-103°. Ldg lts 115°, both QR, intens
113°-117°, W □ trs with R tops. Port Sud de Fouras, pier
hd, Fl WR 4s 6m, 9/6M, vis R117°-177°, W177°-117°. Port-
des-Barques ldg lts 135°, both Iso G 4s synch, intens
125°-145°, W □ trs; rear has B band on W side.
RADIO TELEPHONE
Port VHF Ch 12 16. Marina Ch 09 (HW±1).
TELEPHONE
Hr Mr 46·83·99·96; Aff Mar 46·84·22·67; CROSS 56·09·82·00;
⌗ 46·99·03·90; Meteo 46·41·11·11; Auto 36.68.08.17; Dr
46·99·61·11; Police 46·87·26·12; Brit Consul 56·52·28·35.
FACILITIES
Marina (380+20 visitors) in Basins 1 & 2 ☎ 46·83·99·96,
FF56, FW, ME, El, Sh, D & P (outside lock), AC, C (30 ton);
Port Neuf Slip, FW; **Club Nautique Rochefortais**
☎ 46·87·34·61, Slip; **Services:** ME, El, Ⓔ, Sh, CH. **Town** P,
D, V, Gaz, R, Bar, ✉, Ⓑ, ⇌, ✈ (La Rochelle). Ferry:
Roscoff or St Malo.

ADJACENT ANCHORAGE AT MOUTH OF LA CHARENTE

ILE D'AIX, Charente Maritime, 46°01'·00N 01°10'·00W. AC
2746, 2748; SHOM 6914, 6334. HW +0545 on Dover (UT);
ML 3·9m. Tides see 10.18.17. Only a fine weather ⌕ or
pick up a buoy off the landing jetty at St Catherine's Pt, Fl
WR 5s 24m 24/20M, the most southerly tip of the island.
Moorings available E of St Catherine's Pt (shallow); four
W buoys to west (deeper) and five SE of the pt. Facilities:
C (1·5 ton), Slip, AB (SE jetty), V, R.

SEUDRE RIVER   10-18-19

Charente Maritime 45°48'·00N 01°08'·50W

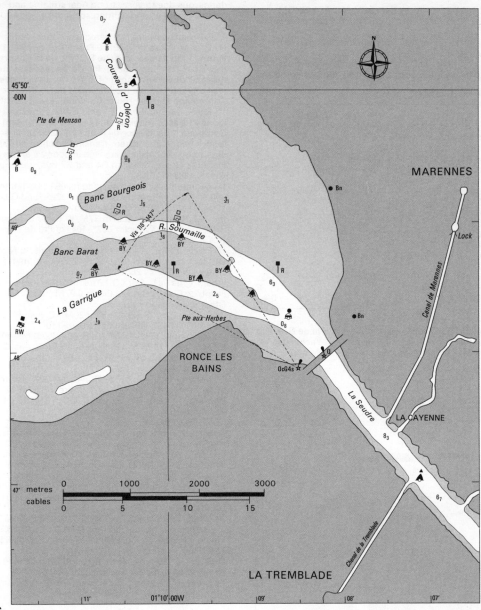

CHARTS
AC 2663; SHOM 6912, 6335; ECM 552
TIDES
+0545 Dover; ML 3·6; Duration Sp 0545, Np 0700

Standard Port POINTE DE GRAVE (→)

Times				Height (metres)			
High Water		Low Water		MHWS	MHWN	MLWN	MLWS
0000	0600	0500	1200	5·4	4·4	2·1	1·0
1200	1800	1700	2400				
Differences LA CAYENNE							
+0030	−0015	−0010	−0005	+0·2	+0·2	+0·3	0·0

SHELTER
Good in the yacht basin (2m) at Marennes. Lock opens about HW±2 sp, HW±1 np; or secure ⚓s at La Cayenne, La Grève (½M upstream), and at ent to Chenal de la Tremblade.
NAVIGATION
WPT 45°55'·88N 01°08'·65W, Chenal Est-Nord WCM buoy, for Chenal Est and Coureau d'Oléron. Best to appr La Seudre from N, through Coureau d'Oléron, and thence via Chenal de la Soumaille (dries about 0·7m). Chenal de la Garrigue carries slightly more water. Both are marked by bns and buoys.

Beware oyster beds. Pont de Seudre has clearance of 18m. Overhead power cables (24m) span Canal de Marennes. La Seudre is navigable to lock at Riberou. Beware: Pertuis de Maumusson is usable only in good weather, at about HW −1; see 10·18·5. In even moderate weather it is **extremely dangerous**, especially with out-going stream or any swell.
LIGHTS AND MARKS
There are no ldg lts/marks. Lights: Pte de Mus de Loup, Oc G 4s 8m 6M, vis 118°-147°. On bridge, between piers 6 and 7, Q 20m 10M, vis up/downstream. Chan marked by W boards.
RADIO TELEPHONE
VHF Ch 09.
TELEPHONE
Marennes: Hr Mr 46·85·02·68; Aff Mar 46·85·14·33; Police 46·85·00·19; Dr 46·85·23·06. La Tremblade: Hr Mr 46·36·00·22; ⌖ 46·47·62·53; Dr 46·36·16·35; Auto 36.68.08.17; Brit Consul 56·36·16·35.
FACILITIES
MARENNES **Basin** ☎ 46·85·15·11, FW, AC, C (6 ton), ME, CH; **Services:** Sh, ME, CH. **Town** Slip, M, P, D, L, FW, V, R, Bar.
LA TREMBLADE **Quay** Slip, P, D, FW, C (5 ton); **Services:** ME, Sh, SM, CH. **Town** Slip, P, D, L, FW, Gaz, V, R, Bar, ✉, Ⓑ, ⇌, ✈ (La Rochelle). Ferry: Roscoff or St Malo.

18

PORT BLOC   10-18-20

Gironde 45°34'·18N 01°03'·64W

CHARTS
AC 2910, 2664, 2916; Imray C42; ECM 553, 554; SHOM
7028, 6335. Note: 7029 & 7030 cover to Bordeaux/Libourne

TIDES
(Pauillac) +0720 Dover; ML 3·0; Duration: Sp 0615; Np
0655; Zone −0100
NOTE: Pte de Grave is a Standard Port; tidal predictions for
each day of the year are given above and apply to Port Bloc

Standard Port POINTE DE GRAVE (→)

Times				Height (metres)			
High Water		Low Water		MHWS	MHWN	MLWN	MLWS
0000	0600	0500	1200	5·4	4·4	2·1	1·0
1200	1800	1700	2400				
Differences RICHARD							
+0018	+0018	+0028	+0033	−0·1	−0·1	−0·4	−0·5
LAMENA							
+0035	+0045	+0100	+0125	+0·2	+0·1	−0·5	−0·3
PAUILLAC							
+0100	+0100	+0135	+0205	+0·1	0·0	−1·0	−0·5
LA REUILLE							
+0135	+0145	+0230	+0305	−0·2	−0·3	−1·3	−0·7
LE MARQUIS							
+0145	+0150	+0247	+0322	−0·3	−0·4	−1·5	−0·9
BORDEAUX							
+0200	+0225	+0330	+0405	−0·1	−0·2	−1·7	−1·0
LIBOURNE (La Dordogne)							
+0250	+0305	+0525	+0540	−0·7	−0·9	−2·0	−0·4

SHELTER
Good shelter. Port Bloc is 4ca (740m) S of Pte de Grave at
the ent to the Gironde. It is dredged to 3m. Yachts use W
side of the hbr on pontoons or moor between buoys.

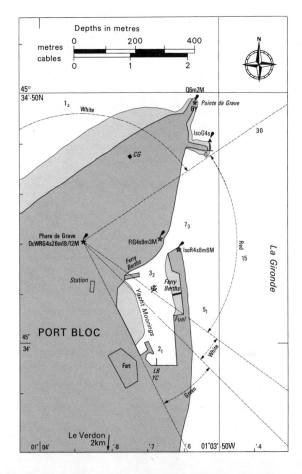

NAVIGATION
WPT BXA SWM buoy, Iso 4s, Whis, Racon, 45°37'·60N
01°28'·60W, 261°/081° from/to Grande Passe de l'Ouest
Nos 1 & 2 buoys, 4·8M. The apprs to the Gironde can be
dangerous due to very strong tidal streams and currents,
extensive shoals and shifting sandbanks, see 10·18·5;
also beware shipping.
The Gironde estuary is entered via 2 appr chans:
(1) Grande Passe de l'Ouest. From BXA buoy 081° on La
Palmyre ldg lts passes close S of Pte de la Coubre;
thence 100° to pass abeam Pte de Terre-Nègre and enter
the river on astern transit of 327°. The chan is deep and
well marked/lit. Give the Mauvaise bank, Banc de la
Coubre and shoals around Cordouan a wide berth.
(2) Passe du Sud. From 'G' unlit SWM buoy track 063° on
the ldg lts at St.Nicolas/Pte de Grave until abeam
Cordouan lt ho; thence 041° on Le Chay/St.Pierre ldg lts
to pick up the 327° astern transit. The chan carries approx
5m through shoals; not advised in poor vis or heavy swell.
Platin de Grave, between G4 and G7 Bys, has only 1·8m.

LIGHTS AND MARKS
(1) Grande Passe de l'Ouest ldg lts 081°, both intens
080·5°-082·5°: Front Dir Iso 4s 21m 22M, and Q (2) 5s
10m 3M same structure, W pylon on dolphin;
rear, La Palmyre ldg Q 57m 27M, W radar tr. From No 9
SHM buoy, use W sector 097°- 104° of Pte de Terre-Nègre,
Oc (3) WRG 12s 39m 18/14M.
(2) Passe du Sud, Outer ldg lts 063°: Front St. Nicolas Dir
QG 22m 16M, intens 061·5°-064·5°, W □ tr; rear, Pte de
Grave Oc WRG 4s 26m 19/15M.
Inner ldg lts 041°, both QR 33/61m 18M, intens 039°-043°:
Front, Le Chay; rear, Ste Pierre 0·97M from front.
Other major lts in estuary:
La Coubre lt ho, Fl (2) 10s 64m 28M RC, also FRG 42m 12/
10M R030°-043°, G043°-060°, R060°-110°.
Courdouan lt Oc (2+1) WRG 12s 60m 22/18M, W014°-
126°, G126°-178·5°, W178·5°-250°, W (unintens) 250°-267°,
R (unintens) 267°-294·5°, R294·5°-014°; obscured in
estuary when brg > 285°.
To enter river NE of Pte de Grave, use 327° astern transit
of Terre-Nègre lt on with La Palmyre, FR 57m 17M.
Port Bloc hbr ent: NW jetty Fl G 4s 9m 3M, SE jetty Iso R
4s 8m 6M.

RADIO TELEPHONE
Bordeaux Traffic and *Radar Verdon* operate a movement
reporting system, compulsory for all vessels, H24 on VHF
Ch 12 16, covering BXA buoy to Bordeaux. Yachts should
listen on Ch 12. Radar assistance in poor vis or by request
to *Radar Verdon* Ch 12. Height of water is broadcast on
Ch 17 every 5 mins, plus a wx bulletin and nav info on
request. Port Bloc marina Ch 09. Ambès Ch 12 (H24).

TELEPHONE
Hr Mr 56·09·63·91; Aff Mar 56·09·60·23; CROSS 56·09·82·00;
≢ 56·09·65·14; Meteo 56·34·20·11; Auto 36.68.08.33;
Police 56·09·60·13; Dr 56·09·60·37; Brit Consul 56·52·28·35.

FACILITIES
Quai FW, C (10 ton); **Moto Yachting Club de la Pte de
Grave** ☎ 56·09·61·58; **Services:** ME, EI, Sh, CH.
Town P, D, AB, Gaz, V, R, ✉ (Verdon), Ⓑ (Verdon), ⇌, ✈
(Bordeaux). Ferry: Roscoff or St Malo.

ROYAN   10-18-21

Charente Maritime 45°37'·20N 01°01'·54W

CHARTS

AC 2910, 2916, 2664; Imray C41, 42; SHOM 7028, 7070;
ECM 553, 554

TIDES

+0530 Dover; ML 3·2; Duration Sp 0615, Np 0655; Zone –
0100

Standard Port POINTE DE GRAVE (→)

Times				Height (metres)			
High Water		Low Water		MHWS	MHWN	MLWN	MLWS
0000	0600	0500	1200	5·4	4·4	2·1	1·0
1200	1800	1700	2400				
Differences ROYAN							
0000	–0005	–0005	–0005	–0·3	–0·2	0·0	0·0

SHELTER

Good. Easy access H24 except with strong W/NW winds.
The ent chan and basins are dredged approx 2·5m; but
beware silting outside head of New Jetty. A good port of
call for Canal du Midi with crane for masts.

NAVIGATION

WPT R1 SHM buoy, Iso G 4s, 45°36'·62N 01°01'·90W, 193°/
013° from/to S Jetty lt, 0·47M. The Gironde apprs can be
dangerous; see 10·18·5 and 10·18·14 for details. The banks
off Royan shift and buoys are consequently altered. Off
hbr ent, there is an eddy, running S at about 1kn on the
flood and 3kn on the ebb. Beware ferries.

LIGHTS AND MARKS

See 10.14.13 for details of appr chans. Other lts as chartlet;
the Iso 4s on end of Quai d'acceuil is a neon sign.

RADIO TELEPHONE

VHF Ch 09 16 (season 0730-2000; otherwise 0900-1800LT).

TELEPHONE

Hr Mr 46·38·72·22; Aff Mar 46·38·32·75; CROSS
56·09·82·00; SNSM 46·38·75·79; ⌖ 46·38·51·27; Meteo
56·34·20·11; Auto 36·68·08·17; Police 46·38·34·22; Dr
46·05·68·69; Ⓗ 46·38·01·77; Brit Consul 56·52·28·35.

FACILITIES

Marina (570 + 60 visitors) ☎ 46·38·72·22, Fax 46.39.42.47,
Slip, P, D, FW, C (6 ton), BH (26 ton), ME, AC, El, Sh; **Les
Régates de Royan** ☎ 46·38·59·64; **Services:** CH, Ⓔ, SM,
SHOM.
Town P, D, V, R, Bar, Gaz, ✉, Ⓑ, ⇌, ✈ (Bordeaux). Ferry:
Roscoff or St Malo.

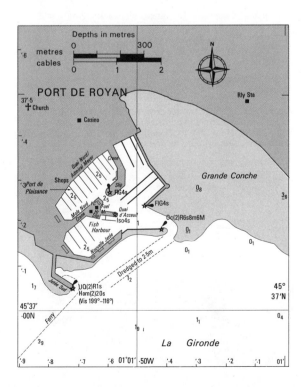

OTHER HARBOURS ON THE GIRONDE

MESCHERS-sur-GIRONDE, Charente Maritime, 45°33'·15N
00°56'·55W. AC 2910, 2916; SHOM 7028; ECM 554. Tides
as for ROYAN, 5M down-river same bank. Good shelter
in all weathers, but access via drying chan is HW–3 to
HW. Appr close to Pte de Meschers between PHM and
SHM unlit perches. Narrow chan has shore close to port
and mudbank close to stbd. Ldg marks/lts 000° are 2 FW
on W posts; entry to hbr is just before the front ldg mark.
To stbd drying marina basin has access HW±3. Dead
ahead an automatic lock gives access over sill 2m CD to a
wet basin HW±2½ by day; waiting pontoons. Hr Mr ☎
46.02.56.89; Auto 36.68.08.17. Facilities: **Marinas** (125 in
drying basin, 123 in wet basin, 18 visitors), FW, AC. **Town**
P & D (cans), R, Bar, V.

MORTAGNE-sur-GIRONDE (La Rive), Charente Maritime,
45°28'·25N 00°48'·75W. AC 2916; SHOM 7028, 7029.
Tides, use RICHARD differences (10.18.20). Good shelter
in marina on E bank of river, 14M from Royan/40M from
Bordeaux (near the 75km mark). Leave the main Gironde
chan at No 18 PHM buoy, Fl (2) R 6s, and head E for 4·5M
to Mortagne appr chan. Ent is marked by large RW stone
dolphin, with ☆ Oc R 2·5s 9m 4M; keep at least 20m clear
SE of it due to concrete debris. Enter chan, 2·5m at mean
tides, on 063°, between 2 unlit perches, for 0·9M across
drying mudbanks to lock which opens HW–2 to HW. VHF
Ch 09. Hr Mr ☎ 46.90.63.15. Facilities: **Marina** (130+20
visitors), 6m depth, FW, AC, Slip, ME, BY, BH (10 ton), V,
Ice; Fuel, Aff Mar, ⌖, and SNSM at Royan; Auto
36.68.08.17.

PAUILLAC, Gironde, 45°11'·88N 00°44'·53W. AC 2916,
2910; SHOM 7029; HW +0620 on Dover (UT); ML 3·0m.
See 10.18.20. Excellent shelter in marina on W bank, 25M
from Le Verdon, and at 47km post from Bordeaux.
Access at all tides (depth 1·5m). Visitors use pontoon A at
ent. Beware current in the river on ent/dep. Lts: Fl G 4s
7m 5M on NE elbow of bkwtr. Ent at S end is marked by
QG and QR. Hr Mr ☎ 56·59·12·16, VHF Ch 09. Aff Mar
56·59·01·58; SNSM/CROSS 56·09·82·00; ⌖ 56·59·04·01;
Meteo 36·68·08·33. Facilities: **Marina** (200+50 visitors),
☎ 56·59·12·16, VHF Ch 09, FW, AC, Slip, ME, El, Sh; **Quay**
FW, D, P (cans), C (14 ton); **CN de Pauillac** ☎ 56·59·12·58;
Services: C for mast step/un-step, CH, Sh.

BLAYE, Charente Maritime, 45°07'·53N 00°39'·90W. AC
2916; SHOM 7029. HW +0715 on Dover (UT); +0145 on
Pte de Grave; HW ht –0·3m on Pte de Grave; ML 2·4m.
Good shelter; access good except in S to SW winds. Ent
is abeam S end of of Ile Nouvelle at 37km post and close
S of La Citadelle (conspic). N quay has Q (3) R 5s 6m 3M,
on R mast. Max stay 24 hours. VHF Ch12 (H24). Hr Mr
☎ 57·42·13·63; ⌖ ☎ 57·42·01·11; Facilities: **Quay** Access
HW±2½, FW, AC, P, D, C (25 ton), Slip, ME.

BORDEAUX, Gironde, 44°52'·80N 00°32'·30W. AC 2916;
SHOM 7029, 7030. HW +0715 on Dover (UT); ML 2·4m.
See 10.18.20. Bordeaux is about 55M up the Gironde
estuary and R Garonne. Beware big ships, strong
currents (up to 5kn when river in spate) and large bits of
flotsam. The chan is well marked and lit. Pte du Jour
marina is 2M from city centre, on W bank close S of Pont
d'Aquitaine suspension bridge (clearance 51m), with 20
visitors berths and de-masting crane, (less handy than
Royan's crane). Berths may also be available, by
arrangement with Hr Mr, 1½M above bridge in No 2
Basin, access HW –1 to HW+½; crane available. Or berth
on wharves between No 1 Basin and Pont de Pierre, but
stream is strong. VHF Ch 12. Hr Mr ☎ 56·52·51·04; Aff
Mar ☎ 56·52·26·23; ⌖ ☎ 56·44·47·10; Meteo ☎ 56·90·91·21;
Facilities: **Marina** ☎ 56·50·84·14 VHF Ch 09; **Sport
Nautique de la Gironde** ☎ 56·50·84·14; **Services:** Slip, C (5
ton), ME, El, Sh, CH, Ⓔ, SHOM.

18

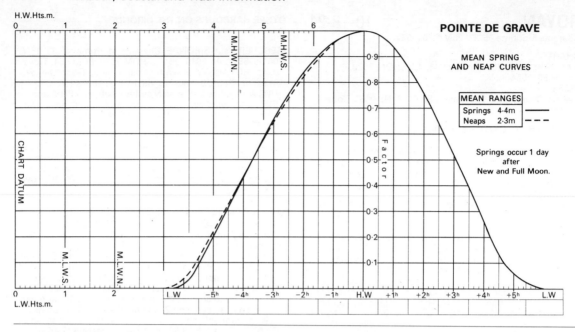

POINTE DE GRAVE

MEAN SPRING
AND NEAP CURVES

MEAN RANGES	
Springs	4·4m
Neaps	2·3m

Springs occur 1 day
after
New and Full Moon.

LA GIRONDE & CANALS   10-18-22

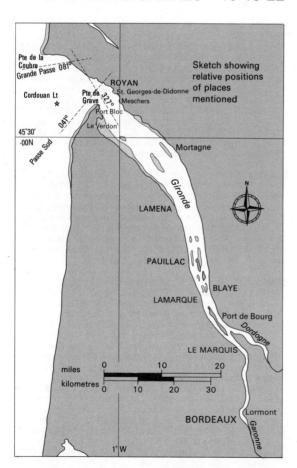

Sketch showing
relative positions
of places
mentioned

The *Canal Latéral à la Garonne* and the *Canal du Midi* provide a popular route to the Med, despite the many locks. The transit can be done in about a week, but 12 days is more relaxed. Masts can be unstepped at Royan, Pauillac or Bordeaux. Leave Bordeaux at LW Pte de Grave for the 30M passage up river to the first lock at Castets. Commercial traffic and W-bound boats have right of way. Most of the locks on the Canal Latéral à la Garonne are automatic. On the Canal du Midi there are many hire cruisers in the summer. Fuel is available by hose at Agen, Castelnaudary and Port de la Robine, and elsewhere by can. V and FW are readily obtained. Further info from: Service de la Navigation de Toulouse, 8 Port St Etienne, 31079 Toulouse Cedex. ☎ 61·80·07·18. Tolls are listed in 10.15.8. *Guide Vagnon No 7* or *Navicarte No 11* are advised.

Canal	From	To	Km/ Locks	Min Depth (m)	Min Height (m)
Lateral à la Garonne	Castets	Toulouse	193/ 53	2·2	3·5
Du Midi	Toulouse	Sete	240/ 65	1·8	3·0
De la Nouvelle	Salleles	Port la Nouvelle	37/ 14	1·8	3·1

Notes: Max LOA 30m; max draft 1·8m; max beam 5·5m. Headroom of 3·3m is to centre of arch; over a width of 4m, clearance is about 2·40m. Speed limit 8km/hr (about 4½kn), but 3km/hr over aqueducts and under bridges.

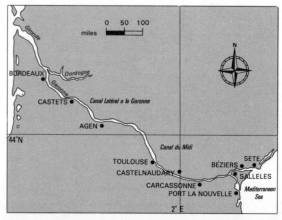

La Gironde is the estuary of the R. Dordogne and Garonne. See 10.18.20 for navigation in the approaches. Yacht hbrs from Royan to Bordeaux* (55M) include St Georges-de-Didonne, Meschers, Mortagne, Pauillac*, Lamarque, Blaye* and Port de Bourg. For *hbrs, see 10·18·21. In the Garonne, the sp flood starts with a small bore and then runs at about 3kn, while the ebb runs at 5kn. In the other rivers at sp the flood reaches 3kn and the ebb 4kn.

TIME ZONE –0100
(French Standard Time)
Subtract 1 hour for UT

For French Summer Time add
ONE hour in non-shaded areas

FRANCE – POINTE DE GRAVE

LAT 45°34′N   LONG 1°04′W

TIMES AND HEIGHTS OF HIGH AND LOW WATERS

YEAR **1996**

JANUARY

Date	Time	m	Time	m	Time	m	Time	m
1 M	0206	4.6	0744	2.0	1425	4.6	2011	2.0
2 TU	0255	4.7	0841	1.9	1514	4.7	2102	1.8
3 W	0335	4.9	0930	1.7	1554	4.9	2146	1.7
4 TH	0411	5.0	1012	1.6	1630	5.0	2225	1.6
5 F ○	0445	5.1	1050	1.5	1705	5.0	2300	1.5
6 SA	0517	5.2	1124	1.4	1738	5.1	2333	1.4
7 SU	0549	5.2	1158	1.4	1809	5.1		
8 M	0007	1.4	0620	5.2	1231	1.4	1841	5.0
9 TU	0040	1.4	0651	5.2	1304	1.4	1913	4.9
10 W	0113	1.5	0722	5.1	1337	1.5	1948	4.8
11 TH	0148	1.5	0800	4.9	1413	1.6	2028	4.7
12 F	0227	1.7	0842	4.8	1453	1.7	2117	4.6
13 SA	0312	1.8	0934	4.6	1542	1.9	2219	4.5
14 SU	0407	1.9	1040	4.5	1644	2.0	2332	4.5
15 M	0514	2.0	1201	4.5	1757	2.0		
16 TU	0047	4.6	0628	1.9	1320	4.6	1910	1.8
17 W	0154	4.8	0739	1.7	1429	4.9	2017	1.6
18 TH	0254	5.1	0846	1.4	1529	5.2	2118	1.3
19 F	0349	5.4	0947	1.1	1622	5.4	2213	1.1
20 SA ●	0441	5.7	1042	0.9	1712	5.6	2305	0.9
21 SU	0531	5.9	1134	0.7	1800	5.7	2354	0.8
22 M	0619	5.9	1221	0.7	1846	5.7		
23 TU	0040	0.7	0705	5.9	1306	0.7	1930	5.5
24 W	0124	0.9	0750	5.7	1349	0.9	2013	5.2
25 TH	0208	1.1	0834	5.4	1432	1.2	2055	4.9
26 F	0253	1.4	0918	5.0	1517	1.5	2142	4.6
27 SA	0344	1.7	1010	4.7	1608	1.8	2246	4.4
28 SU	0443	2.0	1117	4.4	1710	2.1		
29 M	0010	4.3	0554	2.2	1238	4.3	1825	2.2
30 TU	0127	4.3	0709	2.2	1353	4.4	1939	2.2
31 W	0227	4.5	0814	2.1	1451	4.5	2038	2.0

FEBRUARY

Date	Time	m	Time	m	Time	m	Time	m
1 TH	0314	4.7	0907	1.9	1536	4.7	2125	1.8
2 F	0353	4.9	0951	1.7	1614	4.9	2204	1.6
3 SA	0427	5.1	1029	1.5	1648	5.0	2240	1.5
4 SU ○	0459	5.2	1105	1.4	1720	5.1	2315	1.3
5 M	0530	5.3	1139	1.3	1750	5.2	2348	1.2
6 TU	0600	5.3	1212	1.2	1821	5.2		
7 W	0021	1.2	0631	5.3	1244	1.2	1852	5.2
8 TH	0053	1.2	0701	5.3	1316	1.3	1925	5.1
9 F	0127	1.2	0737	5.1	1349	1.3	2001	5.0
10 SA	0203	1.3	0816	5.0	1426	1.5	2044	4.8
11 SU	0244	1.5	0903	4.8	1510	1.6	2139	4.6
12 M	0334	1.7	1006	4.6	1607	1.8	2251	4.5
13 TU	0439	1.9	1131	4.5	1720	2.0		
14 W	0016	4.5	0558	1.9	1300	4.5	1842	1.9
15 TH	0134	4.7	0719	1.8	1415	4.8	1959	1.7
16 F	0241	5.1	0833	1.5	1511	5.4	2105	1.4
17 SA	0338	5.4	0936	1.1	1611	5.4	2201	1.1
18 SU ●	0429	5.7	1030	0.8	1659	5.6	2252	0.8
19 M	0516	5.9	1118	0.7	1743	5.7	2338	0.7
20 TU	0601	5.9	1203	0.6	1825	5.7		
21 W	0022	0.7	0645	5.9	1245	0.7	1904	5.5
22 TH	0103	0.8	0723	5.7	1324	0.9	1940	5.3
23 F	0143	1.0	0800	5.4	1402	1.1	2013	5.0
24 SA	0223	1.3	0836	5.0	1442	1.5	2049	4.7
25 SU	0307	1.6	0918	4.7	1526	1.8	2138	4.4
26 M	0358	1.9	1016	4.4	1621	2.1	2256	4.2
27 TU	0505	2.2	1143	4.2	1735	2.4		
28 W	0034	4.2	0626	2.3	1313	4.2	1858	2.4
29 TH	0150	4.3	0740	2.2	1421	4.3	2006	2.2

MARCH

Date	Time	m	Time	m	Time	m	Time	m
1 F	0244	4.5	0838	2.0	1510	4.6	2056	1.9
2 SA	0327	4.8	0923	1.7	1549	4.8	2138	1.7
3 SU	0403	5.0	1003	1.5	1623	5.0	2215	1.4
4 M	0435	5.2	1039	1.3	1655	5.2	2251	1.3
5 TU ○	0507	5.3	1114	1.1	1726	5.3	2325	1.1
6 W	0538	5.4	1148	1.1	1757	5.3	2359	1.0
7 TH	0609	5.4	1221	1.1	1829	5.4		
8 F	0033	1.0	0642	5.4	1253	1.1	1903	5.3
9 SA	0106	1.0	0717	5.3	1327	1.2	1940	5.2
10 SU	0143	1.1	0758	5.1	1404	1.3	2022	5.0
11 M	0224	1.3	0845	4.9	1448	1.5	2114	4.6
12 TU	0313	1.5	0947	4.6	1544	1.8	2225	4.6
13 W	0417	1.8	1115	4.5	1658	2.0	2355	4.5
14 TH	0540	1.9	1248	4.5	1824	2.0		
15 F	0118	4.7	0707	1.8	1403	4.8	1945	1.8
16 SA	0227	5.0	0821	1.5	1504	5.1	2051	1.4
17 SU	0324	5.3	0921	1.1	1556	5.3	2146	1.1
18 M	0413	5.6	1012	0.9	1641	5.5	2235	0.9
19 TU ●	0458	5.8	1058	0.7	1722	5.6	2319	0.7
20 W	0539	5.8	1140	0.7	1800	5.6		
21 TH	0001	0.7	0617	5.7	1220	0.8	1836	5.5
22 F	0039	0.8	0654	5.6	1256	1.0	1908	5.3
23 SA	0116	1.0	0727	5.3	1331	1.2	1939	5.1
24 SU	0153	1.2	0801	5.0	1408	1.5	2012	4.8
25 M	0232	1.5	0839	4.7	1448	1.8	2049	4.5
26 TU	0318	1.9	0931	4.4	1537	2.1	2157	4.3
27 W	0416	2.2	1048	4.1	1643	2.4	2328	4.1
28 TH	0533	2.3	1224	4.1	1806	2.4		
29 F	0058	4.2	0653	2.3	1339	4.3	1920	2.3
30 SA	0202	4.4	0757	2.0	1433	4.5	2016	2.0
31 SU	0250	4.7	0847	1.8	1515	4.8	2102	1.7

APRIL

Date	Time	m	Time	m	Time	m	Time	m
1 M	0330	4.9	0928	1.5	1551	5.0	2142	1.5
2 TU	0405	5.1	1007	1.3	1625	5.2	2221	1.3
3 W	0439	5.3	1044	1.1	1658	5.4	2258	1.1
4 TH	0513	5.4	1120	1.0	1732	5.5	2335	1.0
5 F	0548	5.5	1156	1.0	1807	5.5		
6 SA	0011	0.9	0624	5.5	1232	1.0	1844	5.5
7 SU	0048	0.9	0702	5.4	1308	1.1	1924	5.3
8 M	0127	1.0	0744	5.2	1348	1.3	2009	5.2
9 TU	0211	1.2	0834	4.9	1434	1.5	2103	4.9
10 W	0302	1.4	0943	4.7	1532	1.8	2213	4.7
11 TH	0407	1.7	1107	4.5	1645	1.9	2340	4.7
12 F	0528	1.8	1234	4.6	1809	1.9		
13 SA	0101	4.8	0651	1.7	1347	4.8	1927	1.7
14 SU	0209	5.0	0803	1.5	1446	5.0	2032	1.5
15 M	0306	5.3	0900	1.2	1536	5.2	2126	1.2
16 TU	0354	5.4	0950	1.0	1619	5.4	2214	1.0
17 W ●	0436	5.5	1034	0.9	1658	5.4	2257	0.9
18 TH	0515	5.6	1115	0.9	1734	5.5	2338	0.9
19 F	0551	5.5	1153	1.0	1808	5.4		
20 SA	0015	0.9	0626	5.4	1228	1.1	1841	5.3
21 SU	0050	1.1	0700	5.2	1302	1.3	1912	5.1
22 M	0125	1.3	0733	5.0	1337	1.5	1947	4.9
23 TU	0202	1.5	0811	4.7	1416	1.7	2022	4.7
24 W	0244	1.8	0858	4.4	1500	2.0	2112	4.5
25 TH	0334	2.0	1001	4.2	1557	2.2	2226	4.3
26 F	0439	2.2	1124	4.1	1708	2.3	2349	4.2
27 SA	0555	2.2	1244	4.2	1822	2.3		
28 SU	0104	4.3	0704	2.1	1344	4.4	1924	2.1
29 M	0201	4.5	0800	1.8	1432	4.7	2016	1.8
30 TU	0248	4.8	0847	1.6	1512	4.9	2103	1.6

18

Chart Datum: 2·93 metres below Lallemand System (Mean Sea Level, Marseilles)

TIME ZONE –0100
(French Standard Time)
Subtract 1 hour for UT
For French Summer Time add ONE hour in non-shaded areas

FRANCE – POINTE DE GRAVE

LAT 45°34′N   LONG   1°04′W

TIMES AND HEIGHTS OF HIGH AND LOW WATERS   YEAR **1996**

MAY

Day		Time	m	Time	m	Time	m	Time	m
1	W	0329	5.0	0930	1.4	1551	5.2	2146	1.3
16	TH	0414	5.2	1010	1.2	1635	5.2	2235	1.1
2	TH	0408	5.2	1011	1.2	1628	5.4	2228	1.1
17	F	0452	5.3	1051	1.1	1710	5.3	● 2315	1.1
3	F / O	0448	5.4	1051	1.0	1707	5.5	2310	0.9
18	SA	0528	5.3	1128	1.2	1745	5.3	2352	1.1
4	SA	0528	5.5	1132	0.9	1747	5.6	2352	0.9
19	SU	0603	5.2	1203	1.2	1818	5.2		
5	SU	0610	5.5	1212	0.9	1829	5.6		
20	M	0027	1.2	0638	5.1	1237	1.3	1851	5.1
6	M	0034	0.9	0654	5.4	1254	1.0	1914	5.5
21	TU	0101	1.3	0712	4.9	1312	1.5	1926	5.0
7	TU	0117	0.9	0742	5.2	1338	1.2	2004	5.3
22	W	0137	1.5	0749	4.7	1349	1.6	1959	4.8
8	W	0204	1.1	0835	5.0	1427	1.4	2100	5.1
23	TH	0215	1.6	0831	4.5	1430	1.8	2043	4.6
9	TH	0257	1.3	0939	4.8	1525	1.6	2206	4.9
24	F	0259	1.8	0922	4.3	1517	2.0	2135	4.4
10	F	0400	1.5	1055	4.6	1633	1.8	2323	4.8
25	SA	0351	2.0	1025	4.2	1615	2.1	2242	4.3
11	SA	0512	1.7	1215	4.6	1749	1.8		
26	SU	0455	2.1	1138	4.2	1722	2.2	2353	4.3
12	SU	0039	4.8	0627	1.6	1325	4.7	1903	1.7
27	M	0604	2.0	1245	4.4	1827	2.1		
13	M	0146	4.9	0737	1.5	1425	4.9	2007	1.5
28	TU	0101	4.4	0706	1.9	1342	4.6	1926	1.9
14	TU	0243	5.1	0835	1.4	1515	5.0	2103	1.3
29	W	0200	4.7	0801	1.7	1431	4.8	2020	1.6
15	W	0332	5.2	0925	1.2	1557	5.2	2151	1.2
30	TH	0251	4.9	0851	1.4	1516	5.1	2111	1.4
31	F	0339	5.1	0938	1.2	1601	5.3	2159	1.1

JUNE

Day		Time	m	Time	m	Time	m	Time	m
1	SA / O	0425	5.3	1024	1.0	1645	5.5	2247	0.9
16	SU	0509	5.0	1107	1.3	1724	5.1	● 2332	1.3
2	SU	0512	5.4	1110	0.9	1731	5.6	2335	0.8
17	M	0545	5.2	1141	1.3	1758	5.1		
3	M	0559	5.5	1156	0.9	1818	5.6		
18	TU	0006	1.3	0619	5.0	1215	1.3	1831	5.1
4	TU	0022	0.8	0647	5.5	1242	0.9	1907	5.6
19	W	0040	1.3	0652	4.9	1249	1.4	1904	5.0
5	W	0110	0.8	0737	5.3	1330	1.1	1959	5.4
20	TH	0114	1.4	0727	4.8	1325	1.5	1937	4.9
6	TH	0158	1.0	0830	5.1	1420	1.2	2053	5.3
21	F	0150	1.5	0804	4.6	1402	1.6	2015	4.7
7	F	0249	1.2	0928	4.9	1514	1.4	2153	5.0
22	SA	0228	1.6	0846	4.5	1443	1.7	2100	4.6
8	SA	0345	1.4	1034	4.7	1615	1.6	2259	4.9
23	SU	0310	1.7	0936	4.4	1530	1.9	2151	4.4
9	SU	0448	1.5	1146	4.6	1723	1.7		
24	M	0401	1.9	1036	4.3	1626	2.0	2252	4.4
10	M	0009	4.8	0556	1.7	1257	4.6	1833	1.7
25	TU	0503	1.9	1144	4.3	1731	2.0		
11	TU	0117	4.7	0705	1.7	1359	4.7	1940	1.6
26	W	0003	4.4	0610	1.9	1250	4.5	1837	1.9
12	W	0217	4.8	0807	1.6	1452	4.8	2038	1.5
27	TH	0113	4.5	0714	1.7	1351	4.7	1939	1.7
13	TH	0309	4.9	0900	1.5	1536	4.9	2129	1.4
28	F	0216	4.7	0813	1.5	1446	5.0	2038	1.4
14	F	0353	4.9	0947	1.4	1614	5.0	2214	1.3
29	SA	0314	5.0	0909	1.3	1537	5.2	2134	1.2
15	SA	0432	5.0	1029	1.3	1650	5.1	2254	1.3
30	SU	0407	5.2	1002	1.1	1627	5.4	2228	0.9

JULY

Day		Time	m	Time	m	Time	m	Time	m
1	M / O	0458	5.4	1053	0.9	1717	5.6	2321	0.8
16	TU	0526	4.9	1122	1.3	1738	5.1	2347	1.3
2	TU	0548	5.5	1142	0.8	1807	5.7		
17	W	0559	4.9	1155	1.3	1810	5.1		
3	W	0011	0.7	0637	5.5	1231	0.8	1857	5.7
18	TH	0020	1.3	0631	4.9	1228	1.3	1840	5.0
4	TH	0059	0.7	0726	5.4	1318	0.9	1947	5.6
19	F	0052	1.3	0702	4.8	1301	1.3	1911	4.9
5	F	0146	0.8	0815	5.2	1406	1.0	2038	5.4
20	SA	0125	1.3	0735	4.8	1335	1.4	1946	4.8
6	SA	0233	1.0	0906	5.0	1456	1.2	2130	5.1
21	SU	0158	1.4	0812	4.6	1411	1.5	2024	4.7
7	SU	0323	1.2	1002	4.7	1550	1.5	2228	4.8
22	M	0235	1.5	0854	4.5	1452	1.6	2110	4.6
8	M	0417	1.5	1108	4.5	1651	1.7	2332	4.6
23	TU	0318	1.7	0947	4.4	1541	1.8	2208	4.4
9	TU	0519	1.7	1221	4.4	1800	1.8		
24	W	0412	1.8	1053	4.3	1642	1.9	2318	4.4
10	W	0043	4.5	0629	1.8	1331	4.5	1910	1.8
25	TH	0520	1.9	1207	4.4	1754	1.9		
11	TH	0150	4.5	0738	1.8	1429	4.6	2014	1.7
26	F	0037	4.4	0633	1.8	1318	4.6	1906	1.7
12	F	0248	4.5	0837	1.7	1517	4.7	2108	1.6
27	SA	0151	4.6	0742	1.6	1422	4.9	2013	1.5
13	SA	0336	4.7	0927	1.6	1556	4.8	2154	1.5
28	SU	0255	4.9	0845	1.4	1520	5.2	2116	1.2
14	SU	0416	4.8	1009	1.5	1632	5.0	2235	1.4
29	M	0352	5.1	0944	1.1	1613	5.4	2213	0.9
15	M	0452	4.8	1047	1.4	1706	5.0	● 2312	1.3
30	TU / O	0444	5.4	1038	0.9	1704	5.7	2307	0.7
31	W	0534	5.5	1129	0.7	1753	5.8	2356	0.6

AUGUST

Day		Time	m	Time	m	Time	m	Time	m
1	TH	0622	5.5	1216	0.7	1841	5.8		
16	F	0605	5.0	1205	1.2	1814	5.1		
2	F	0043	0.6	0707	5.5	1302	0.7	1928	5.7
17	SA	0028	1.2	0635	5.0	1237	1.2	1844	5.1
3	SA	0127	0.7	0752	5.3	1347	0.9	2014	5.4
18	SU	0059	1.2	0706	4.9	1309	1.3	1917	5.0
4	SU	0210	0.9	0836	5.0	1432	1.1	2100	5.1
19	M	0130	1.3	0740	4.8	1342	1.3	1953	4.8
5	M	0255	1.2	0923	4.7	1521	1.4	2149	4.7
20	TU	0204	1.4	0819	4.7	1420	1.5	2036	4.7
6	TU	0343	1.6	1019	4.4	1617	1.7	2249	4.4
21	W	0244	1.6	0908	4.5	1506	1.6	2132	4.5
7	W	0441	1.9	1135	4.3	1724	2.0		
22	TH	0335	1.7	1012	4.4	1604	1.8	2246	4.3
8	TH	0005	4.3	0551	2.1	1257	4.3	1840	2.0
23	F	0440	1.9	1133	4.4	1720	1.9		
9	F	0123	4.2	0707	2.1	1405	4.4	1950	2.0
24	SA	0015	4.3	0600	1.9	1255	4.5	1842	1.8
10	SA	0228	4.3	0813	1.9	1457	4.6	2047	1.8
25	SU	0135	4.5	0719	1.8	1406	4.8	1956	1.5
11	SU	0318	4.5	0905	1.8	1537	4.8	2134	1.6
26	M	0241	4.8	0829	1.5	1505	5.2	2102	1.2
12	M	0357	4.7	0948	1.6	1612	4.9	2214	1.5
27	TU	0338	5.1	0929	1.2	1559	5.5	2159	0.9
13	TU	0432	4.8	1026	1.4	1645	5.0	2250	1.3
28	W / O	0429	5.4	1023	0.9	1648	5.7	2250	0.7
14	W	0505	4.9	1100	1.3	1715	5.1	● 2324	1.3
29	TH	0516	5.5	1112	0.7	1735	5.8	2337	0.6
15	TH	0535	5.0	1133	1.2	1745	5.1	2357	1.2
30	F	0600	5.6	1158	0.6	1819	5.8		
31	SA	0021	0.6	0643	5.5	1241	0.7	1902	5.7

Chart Datum: 2·93 metres below Lallemand System (Mean Sea Level, Marseilles)

TIME ZONE –0100
(French Standard Time)
Subtract 1 hour for UT
For French Summer Time add
ONE hour in non-shaded areas

FRANCE – POINTE DE GRAVE

LAT 45°34′N   LONG 1°04′W

TIMES AND HEIGHTS OF HIGH AND LOW WATERS

YEAR **1996**

SEPTEMBER

Day	Time	m	Time	m		Day	Time	m	Time	m
1 SU	0103 / 1323	0.8 / 0.9	0723 / 1944	5.3 / 5.4		**16** M	0033 / 1245	1.2 / 1.2	0639 / 1852	5.1 / 5.1
2 M	0143 / 1404	1.0 / 1.2	0801 / 2024	5.0 / 5.3		**17** TU	0105 / 1319	1.3 / 1.3	0713 / 1928	5.0 / 5.0
3 TU	0224 / 1449	1.3 / 1.5	0840 / 2107	4.7 / 4.7		**18** W	0139 / 1357	1.4 / 1.4	0752 / 2012	4.9 / 4.8
4 W	0308 / 1539	1.7 / 1.8	0927 / 2203	4.5 / 4.3		**19** TH	0220 / 1442	1.6 / 1.6	0841 / 2111	4.7 / 4.5
5 TH	0401 / 1644	2.0 / 2.1	1039 / 2323	4.2 / 4.1		**20** F	0309 / 1540	1.8 / 1.8	0947 / 2231	4.5 / 4.4
6 F	0509 / 1804	2.3 / 2.3	1214	4.2		**21** SA	0416 / 1659	2.0 / 2.0	1113	4.4
7 SA	0051 / 1332	4.1 / 4.3	0632 / 1921	2.3 / 2.2		**22** SU	0004 / 1240	4.4 / 4.6	0540 / 1827	2.0 / 1.9
8 SU	0201 / 1429	4.2 / 4.5	0744 / 2021	2.2 / 2.0		**23** M	0123 / 1352	4.6 / 4.9	0703 / 1944	1.9 / 1.6
9 M	0252 / 1512	4.5 / 4.7	0838 / 2108	1.9 / 1.7		**24** TU	0228 / 1451	4.9 / 5.2	0814 / 2048	1.6 / 1.3
10 TU	0332 / 1547	4.7 / 4.9	0921 / 2147	1.7 / 1.5		**25** W	0323 / 1543	5.2 / 5.5	0913 / 2142	1.2 / 1.0
11 W	0406 / 1619	4.8 / 5.1	0959 / 2223	1.5 / 1.4		**26** TH	0411 / 1630	5.4 / 5.7	1005 / 2230	1.0 / 0.8
12 TH	0437 / 1649	5.0 / 5.2	1034 / ● 2257	1.2 / 1.3		**27** F	0455 / 1714	5.5 / 5.8	1053 / O 2315	0.8 / 0.7
13 F	0507 / 1719	5.1 / 5.2	1107 / 2330	1.2 / 1.2		**28** SA	0537 / 1755	5.6 / 5.8	1137 / 2357	0.7 / 0.8
14 SA	0537 / 1748	5.2 / 5.2	1140	1.2		**29** SU	0616 / 1835	5.5 / 5.6	1219	0.8
15 SU	0002 / 1213	1.2 / 1.1	0607 / 1818	5.2 / 5.2		**30** M	0037 / 1258	0.9 / 1.0	0653 / 1912	5.3 / 5.3

OCTOBER

Day	Time	m	Time	m		Day	Time	m	Time	m
1 TU	0114 / 1337	1.2 / 1.3	0727 / 1949	5.1 / 5.0		**16** W	0044 / 1302	1.3 / 1.2	0655 / 1915	5.1 / 5.1
2 W	0152 / 1417	1.5 / 1.6	0802 / 2028	4.8 / 4.7		**17** TH	0122 / 1343	1.4 / 1.4	0738 / 2003	5.1 / 4.9
3 TH	0233 / 1503	1.8 / 1.9	0844 / 2120	4.6 / 4.3		**18** F	0204 / 1430	1.6 / 1.6	0830 / 2101	4.9 / 4.6
4 F	0322 / 1601	2.1 / 2.2	0946 / 2237	4.3 / 4.1		**19** SA	0256 / 1530	1.8 / 1.8	0937 / 2226	4.7 / 4.5
5 SA	0425 / 1718	2.4 / 2.4	1118	4.2		**20** SU	0404 / 1648	2.0 / 2.0	1101 / 2355	4.6 / 4.5
6 SU	0010 / 1246	4.1 / 4.2	0546 / 1841	2.5 / 2.3		**21** M	0526 / 1812	2.1 / 1.9	1225	4.7
7 M	0124 / 1350	4.2 / 4.4	0702 / 1945	2.3 / 2.1		**22** TU	0110 / 1335	4.7 / 4.9	0647 / 1927	1.9 / 1.6
8 TU	0217 / 1437	4.4 / 4.6	0800 / 2033	2.1 / 1.9		**23** W	0212 / 1434	4.9 / 5.3	0757 / 2029	1.6 / 1.4
9 W	0258 / 1516	4.7 / 4.9	0846 / 2114	1.9 / 1.6		**24** TH	0305 / 1525	5.2 / 5.5	0855 / 2121	1.3 / 1.1
10 TH	0333 / 1549	4.9 / 5.1	0926 / 2151	1.6 / 1.5		**25** F	0351 / 1611	5.4 / 5.6	0946 / 2208	1.1 / 1.0
11 F	0406 / 1621	5.1 / 5.2	1003 / 2226	1.4 / 1.3		**26** SA	0433 / 1652	5.5 / 5.6	1032 / O 2252	1.0 / 1.0
12 SA	0438 / 1652	5.2 / 5.3	1039 / ● 2301	1.3 / 1.2		**27** SU	0513 / 1732	5.5 / 5.6	1116 / 2333	0.9 / 1.0
13 SU	0509 / 1725	5.3 / 5.4	1115 / 2335	1.2 / 1.2		**28** M	0550 / 1809	5.5 / 5.5	1156	1.0
14 M	0543 / 1759	5.3 / 5.3	1150	1.1		**29** TU	0011 / 1234	1.2 / 1.2	0625 / 1845	5.3 / 5.2
15 TU	0009 / 1225	1.2 / 1.2	0618 / 1833	5.3 / 5.2		**30** W	0047 / 1311	1.3 / 1.3	0659 / 1920	5.2 / 5.0
						31 TH	0123 / 1349	1.6 / 1.6	0734 / 1958	4.9 / 4.7

NOVEMBER

Day	Time	m	Time	m		Day	Time	m	Time	m
1 F	0202 / 1430	1.8 / 1.9	0812 / 2044	4.7 / 4.4		**16** SA	0157 / 1426	1.5 / 1.5	0827 / 2103	5.1 / 4.8
2 SA	0247 / 1520	2.1 / 2.2	0901 / 2150	4.5 / 4.2		**17** SU	0251 / 1525	1.8 / 1.7	0931 / 2217	4.9 / 4.6
3 SU	0341 / 1625	2.3 / 2.4	1015 / 2315	4.3 / 4.1		**18** M	0356 / 1635	1.9 / 1.8	1047 / 2338	4.8 / 4.6
4 M	0450 / 1743	2.5 / 2.4	1141	4.2		**19** TU	0509 / 1750	2.0 / 1.8	1204	4.9
5 TU	0033 / 1256	4.2 / 4.3	0605 / 1854	2.4 / 2.3		**20** W	0051 / 1314	4.7 / 5.0	0625 / 1903	1.9 / 1.7
6 W	0131 / 1352	4.4 / 4.5	0709 / 1949	2.3 / 2.0		**21** TH	0153 / 1415	4.9 / 5.1	0734 / 2006	1.7 / 1.5
7 TH	0217 / 1437	4.6 / 4.8	0801 / 2034	2.0 / 1.8		**22** F	0247 / 1507	5.1 / 5.3	0834 / 2100	1.5 / 1.4
8 F	0257 / 1515	4.9 / 5.0	0847 / 2115	1.8 / 1.6		**23** SA	0333 / 1553	5.2 / 5.4	0926 / 2147	1.3 / 1.3
9 SA	0333 / 1552	5.1 / 5.2	0929 / 2154	1.5 / 1.4		**24** SU	0415 / 1634	5.3 / 5.4	1013 / 2231	1.2 / 1.2
10 SU	0408 / 1628	5.3 / 5.3	1009 / 2232	1.4 / 1.3		**25** M	0453 / 1713	5.4 / 5.4	1056 / O 2311	1.2 / 1.2
11 M	0445 / 1705	5.4 / 5.4	1050 / ● 2310	1.2 / 1.2		**26** TU	0529 / 1749	5.4 / 5.3	1136 / 2349	1.2 / 1.2
12 TU	0522 / 1744	5.5 / 5.4	1130 / 2349	1.1 / 1.2		**27** W	0604 / 1825	5.3 / 5.2	1214	1.3
13 W	0602 / 1826	5.5 / 5.5	1210	1.1		**28** TH	0024 / 1249	1.4 / 1.4	0638 / 1859	5.2 / 5.0
14 TH	0029 / 1252	1.2 / 1.2	0646 / 1911	5.4 / 5.2		**29** F	0059 / 1325	1.6 / 1.6	0712 / 1935	5.1 / 4.8
15 F	0111 / 1337	1.4 / 1.3	0733 / 2002	5.3 / 5.0		**30** SA	0136 / 1403	1.7 / 1.8	0749 / 2016	4.9 / 4.6

DECEMBER

Day	Time	m	Time	m		Day	Time	m	Time	m
1 SU	0217 / 1446	1.9 / 2.0	0825 / 2106	4.7 / 4.4		**16** M	0244 / 1515	1.5 / 1.5	0920 / 2159	5.2 / 4.8
2 M	0302 / 1536	2.1 / 2.2	0915 / 2211	4.5 / 4.2		**17** TU	0341 / 1614	1.7 / 1.7	1026 / 2311	5.0 / 4.7
3 TU	0357 / 1638	2.3 / 2.3	1027 / 2325	4.3 / 4.2		**18** W	0446 / 1721	1.8 / 1.8	1137	4.9
4 W	0502 / 1749	2.4 / 2.3	1143	4.3		**19** TH	0025 / 1248	4.7 / 4.9	0557 / 1833	1.9 / 1.8
5 TH	0034 / 1253	4.3 / 4.4	0609 / 1854	2.3 / 2.2		**20** F	0131 / 1354	4.8 / 4.9	0708 / 1940	1.8 / 1.8
6 F	0130 / 1351	4.5 / 4.6	0710 / 1948	2.1 / 2.0		**21** SA	0229 / 1451	4.9 / 5.0	0813 / 2039	1.7 / 1.6
7 SA	0217 / 1440	4.8 / 4.8	0804 / 2036	1.9 / 1.7		**22** SU	0319 / 1539	5.0 / 5.1	0908 / 2129	1.5 / 1.5
8 SU	0301 / 1524	5.0 / 5.1	0854 / 2122	1.7 / 1.5		**23** M	0401 / 1621	5.1 / 5.1	0957 / 2214	1.4 / 1.4
9 M	0342 / 1607	5.2 / 5.3	0941 / 2206	1.4 / 1.3		**24** TU	0438 / 1659	5.2 / 5.2	1041 / O 2254	1.3 / 1.4
10 TU	0424 / 1650	5.4 / 5.4	1027 / ● 2250	1.2 / 1.2		**25** W	0513 / 1734	5.3 / 5.2	1120 / 2331	1.3 / 1.4
11 W	0508 / 1734	5.6 / 5.5	1113 / 2334	1.1 / 1.1		**26** TH	0547 / 1808	5.3 / 5.1	1156	1.3
12 TH	0553 / 1820	5.7 / 5.5	1159	1.0		**27** F	0005 / 1231	1.4 / 1.4	0620 / 1841	5.2 / 5.0
13 F	0019 / 1245	1.1 / 1.0	0640 / 1908	5.6 / 5.4		**28** SA	0039 / 1304	1.5 / 1.5	0652 / 1914	5.2 / 4.9
14 SA	0104 / 1332	1.2 / 1.1	0729 / 1959	5.6 / 5.2		**29** SU	0114 / 1339	1.6 / 1.6	0725 / 1949	5.1 / 4.8
15 SU	0152 / 1421	1.3 / 1.3	0822 / 2055	5.4 / 5.0		**30** M	0149 / 1415	1.7 / 1.7	0757 / 2028	4.9 / 4.6
						31 TU	0228 / 1455	1.8 / 1.9	0840 / 2114	4.7 / 4.4

18

Chart Datum: 2·93 metres below Lallemand System (Mean Sea Level, Marseilles)

ARCACHON   10-18-23

Gironde 44°39'·83N 01°09'·04W

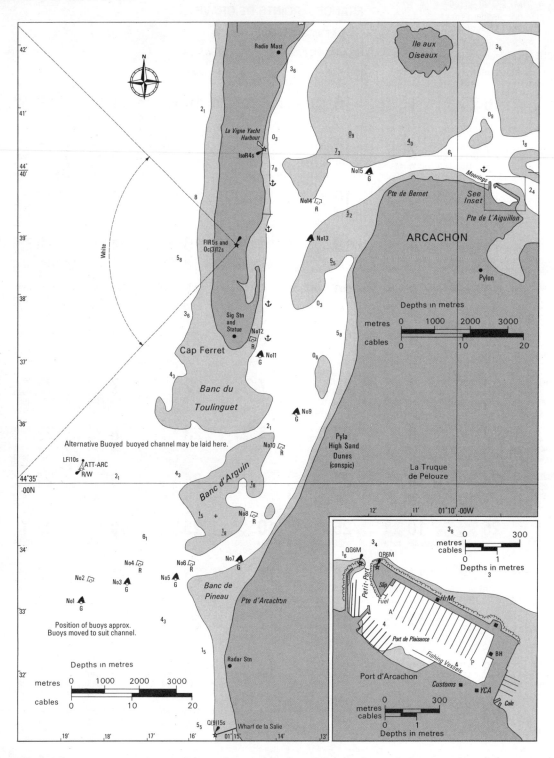

MINOR HARBOURS IN THE ARCACHON BASIN

FONTAINEVIEILLE, Gironde, 44°43'·36N 01°04'·51W. AC 2664; SHOM 6766 (essential); ECM 255. Tides as 10.18.23. Drying marina on NE side of Bassin d'Arcachon, access HW±3 via Chenal de Mouchtalette. Proceed from E0 pile to E8, where fork left onto NNE for 7ca to hbr ent. No lights. Boats dry out at LW on pontoons. Hr Mr ☎ 56.82.17.31; Auto 36.65.08.33. Facilities: **Marina** (178+ 2), FW, Fuel, YC, Slip, ME.

AUDENGE, Gironde, 44°40'·65N 01°01'·50W. AC 2664; SHOM 6766 (essential); ECM 255. Tides as 10.18.23. Drying marina and oyster port 5·5M E of Arcachon, access sp HW–2 to HW, nps HW–1 to HW. Appr from G0 pile via drying Chenal d'Audenge to G8 pile, 5ca short of the ent. Hr Mr ☎ 56.26.88.97. The Old Port (84 berths) is to the N; the New Port has 130 pontoon berths, FW, AC, Fuel, Slip, YC.

ARCACHON *continued*

CHARTS
AC 2664; Imray C42; SHOM 6766, 7070; ECM 255, 1024
TIDES
+0620 Dover; ML 2·5; Zone –0100

Standard Port POINTE DE GRAVE (←→)

Times				Height (metres)			
High Water		Low Water		MHWS	MHWN	MLWN	MLWS
0000	0600	0500	1200	5·4	4·4	2·1	1·0
1200	1800	1700	2400				
Differences ARCACHON							
+0010	+0025	0000	+0020	–1·1	–1·0	–0·8	–0·6
CAP FERRET							
–0015	+0005	–0005	+0015	–1·4	–1·2	–0·8	–0·5

SHELTER
Good in marina (max LOA 15m), but it is impossible to ent Bassin d'Arcachon in strong SW-N winds or at night. If marina full, ‡ off hbr front. Many small drying hbrs around the Bassin (worth exploring) include: on the W, La Vigne*, Le Canon, Piquey and Claouey; on the NE, Port de Lège, Ares, Andernos, Fontainevieille*, Lanton (Cassy) and Audenge*; and on the S, La Teste and Gujan. *see below.
NAVIGATION
WPT 44°30'·15N 01°19'·50W, 258°/078° from/to Wharf de la Salie, WCM bn, Q (9) 15s 19m 10M, 2·9M (off chartlet); the first chan buoys are close N of this WCM bn. Main appr is the S Passe which runs close past Pte d'Arcachon and the dunes (103m); or by the shorter, shallower N Passe (buoyed) between Banc d'Arguin and Banc du Toulinguet. The chans meet close E of Cap Ferret. Between these ent chans beware shifting sand banks on which seas break in any wind, but the chan can be seen through the breakers. Buoys are adjusted frequently. Best time to start appr is HW–1 and no later than HW+1. The S Passe bar (mean depth 4·5m) is impassable from HW+1 until LW, due to the ebb (6kn sp) and it is best to wait until LW+3. Bar may be dangerous when swell higher than 1m. Best time to leave is on the last of the flood; wait in a convenient "lagoon" ‡ near No 10 PHM By in the Banc d'Arguin. For navigation update call *Cap Ferret Semaphore* Ch 16 10 (HJ); or Service de la Marine Gironde ☎ 56·82·32·97. Beware firing ranges between Arcachon and Capbreton, out to 40M offshore; see 10·18·5.
LIGHTS AND MARKS
Cap Ferret Fl R 5s 53m 27M and Oc (3) 12s 46m 14M, vis 045°-135°. La Salie IDM By Fl (2) 6s is about 1M WSW of the S Chan ent and Wharf de Salie WCM bn, Q (9) 15s 19m 10M. ATT-ARC (landfall buoy, SWM) L Fl 10s is moved as necessary to indicate chan ent. Marina: W bkwtr QG, E bkwtr QR. Secondary chans in the Bassin d'Arcachon are marked by piles lettered A to K, plus pile number, clockwise from the North.
RADIO TELEPHONE
VHF Ch 09 16 (H24).
TELEPHONE
Hr Mr 56·83·22·44, Fax 57·52·05·11; Aff Mar 57·52·57·07; ⌗ 56·83·05·89; SNSM 56·83·22·44; CROSS 56·09·82·00; Auto 36·68·08·33; Police 56·83·04·63; Dr 56·83·04·72; Ⓗ 56·83·39·50; Brit Consul 56·52·28·35.
FACILITIES
Marina (2192+ 57 visitors), FF139 (2nd night free), Access HW±3, FW, AC, D, Slip, C (10/20 ton), BH (45 ton); **YC du Bassin d'Arcachon** ☎ 56·83·22·11, P, D, FW, Slip, R, Bar; **Services:** P, D, ME, EI, Ⓔ, SHOM, Sh, CH, SM, ▣. **Town** V, R, Gaz, ⊠, Ⓑ, ⇌, ✈ (Bordeaux). Ferry: Roscoff or St Malo.

MINOR HARBOURS IN THE ARCACHON BASIN (cont)

LA VIGNE, Gironde, 44°40'·50N 01°14'·20W. AC 2664; SHOM 6766; ECM 255. HW time & ht approx as Cap Ferret above; ML 2·4m. Access HW±2. See 10.18.23. Good shelter, but crowded and beware strong currents across hbr ent. 2 perches mark the ent and on the SW point, a lt Iso R 4s 7m 4M. A small bkwtr (unlit) protrudes into the ent from the NE side. Aff Mar ☎ 56·60·52·76. Facilities: **Marina** (268 + 2) ☎ 56·60·54·36, Max LOA 8·5m, AC, Slip, CH, C (2 ton), P, D.

CAPBRETON   10-18-24
Landes 43°39'·42N 01°26'·82W

CHARTS
AC 1102; SHOM 6586, 6557, 6786; ECM 555, 1024
TIDES
+0450 Dover; ML 2·3; Zone –0100

Standard Port POINTE DE GRAVE (←→)

Times				Height (metres)			
High Water		Low Water		MHWS	MHWN	MLWN	MLWS
0000	0600	0500	1200	5·4	4·4	2·1	1·0
1200	1800	1700	2400				
Differences CAPBRETON							
–0030	–0020	0000	0000	–1·4	–0·8	–0·7	–0·5

SHELTER
Good. Appr advised HW–3 to +1; not before LW+2½. Narrow canalised ent dangerous in strong winds from W to N. Do not enter if swell or seas break in mid-chan; they often break on either side. Hbr and chan dredged 1·5m. Visitors' pontoon 'B' (first to stbd of marina ent). There are 3 basins.
NAVIGATION
WPT 49°39'·69N 01°27'·41W, 303°/123° from/to N pier lt, ½M. Bkwtr lts in line 123° lead to hbr ent. Depths shoal rapidly in last 3ca from 50m to 3m; see 10.18.5 for Gouf de Capbreton. No ‡ off ent. Marina is entered through gap in training wall on SE side of Boucarot Chan, abeam conspic Capitainerie bldg.

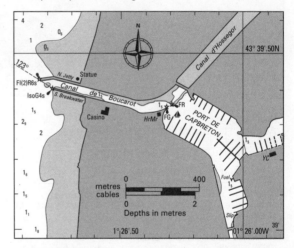

LIGHTS AND MARKS
N pier hd, Fl (2) R 6s 13m 12M, Horn 30s. S bkwtr hd, Fl G 4s 7m 12M. FR/G lts at marina ent. Casino is conspic S of ent.
RADIO TELEPHONE
VHF Ch 09 (0800-1900 in season).
TELEPHONE
Hr Mr 58·72·21·23; Aff Mar 58·72·10·43; ⌗ 59·59·08·29; SNSM 58·72·47·44; CROSS 56·09·82·00; Meteo 56·83·17·00; Auto 36·68·08·40; Ⓗ (Bayonne) 59·44·35·35; Police 58·72·01·18.
FACILITIES
Marina (950+58 visitors), ☎ 58·72·21·23, Fax 58·72·40·35, Slip, BH (28 ton), AC, P, D, FW, ME, EI, C (1·5 ton), Sh, ▣; **Club Nautique Capbreton-Hossegor-Seignone** ☎ 58·72·05·25; **YC Landais; Services:** Sh, CH, SM, Ⓔ; ⇌ Bayonne (17km); ✈ Biarritz (25km).

18

ANGLET/BAYONNE Pyrénées Atlantique 49°31′·95N 01°31′·92W

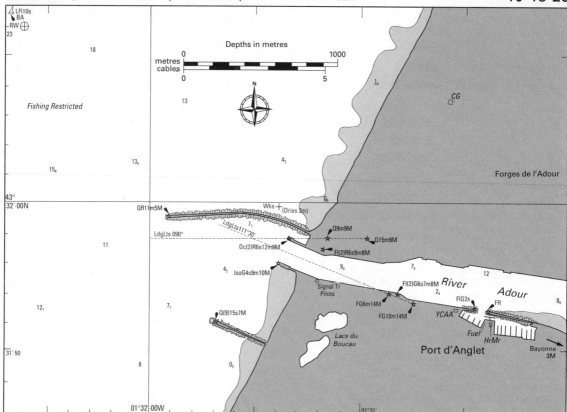

CHARTS
AC 1343, 1102; SHOM 6536, 6557, 6786; ECM 555
TIDES
+0450 Dover (UT); ML 2·5; Zone –0100

Standard Port POINTE DE GRAVE (←—)

Times				Height (metres)			
High Water		Low Water		MHWS	MHWN	MLWN	MLWS
0000	0600	0500	1200	5·4	4·4	2·1	1·0
1200	1800	1700	2400				
Differences L'ADOUR (BOUCAU)							
–0030	–0035	–0025	–0040	–1·2	–1·1	–0·4	–0·3

SHELTER
Very good in Anglet marina, 0·70M from ent, on S bank of R Adour. Possible berths at Bayonne, 3M up river, on S bank below bridge. ‡ prohib in river which is well marked.
NAVIGATION
WPT 43°32′·66N 01°32′·68W, BA SWM buoy, 322°/142° from/to N bkwtr lt, 0·9M. Access good except in strong W winds. Strong tidal stream, max 5kn at sp ebb.
LIGHTS AND MARKS
BA HFP buoy, L Fl 10s (WPT), is NW of ent. Pte St Martin Fl (2) 10s 73m 29M is 2·45M SSW of hbr. Ldg lts 090°, both Q 9/15m 14M, intens 087°-093°. Inside ent, further ldg lts 111°, both QG, moved as required. 3 more sets of ldg lts upriver to Bayonne. Tfc sigs (full code) from sig tr on S side of ent.
RADIO TELEPHONE
Marina Ch 09. Port/pilots 12 16 (0800-1200; 1400-1800LT).
TELEPHONE
Marina 59·63·05·45; Hr Mr Bayonne 59·63·11·57; CROSS 56·09·82·00; ‡ 59·59·08·29; Aff Mar 59·55·06·68; SNSM 59·83·40·50; Ⓗ 59·44·35·35; Meteo 59·23·84·15; Auto 36·65·08·64.
FACILITIES
Marina (367+58 visitors), ☎ 59·63·05·45; P, D, FW, ME, El, AC, C (1·3 ton), Ⓒ, BH (13 ton), Slip, Sh; **Port** C (30 ton), Slip, FW, P, D; **YC Adour Atlantique** ☎ 59·63·16·22; **Services:** CH, Ⓔ, SHOM.
Town ⇌, ✈ (Biarritz). Ferry: Bilboa-Portsmouth.

HARBOURS NEAR THE FRANCO-SPANISH BORDER

ST JEAN-DE-LUZ, Pyrénées Atlantique, 43°23′·92N 01°40′·53W. AC 1343, 1102; SHOM 6526, 6558; ECM 555. HW +0435 on Dover (UT); See 10.18.26. There are 2 hbrs:
St Jean-de-Luz in SE of bay with a small marina at Ciboure, close to rear QG ldg lt; and
Socoa hbr (dries) to the W of the bay.
Approaches: From NE along the coast, keep W of Les Esquilletac, rks ½M N of Pointe St Barbe; not advised. From NW, Passe d'Illarguita (main chan): ldg lts, front (Le Socoa) QWR 12/8M, rear Q 20M lead 138° between Illarguita and Belhara Perdun shoals. Thence, or if approaching from W, join Passe de Belhara Perdun on Ste Barbe ldg lts, both Oc (3+1) R 12s 30/47m 18M, leading 101° S of Belhara Perdun.
Baie de St Jean de Luz: Except in strong NW winds, the bay can be entered at all times via W passage between Digue des Criquas and Digue d'Artha, and good ‡ found in approx 4m. Inner ldg lts, both Dir QG 18/27m 16M intens 149·5°-152°, lead 151° between bkwtrs to port ent. Sailing is prohib in the port. Beware a submerged obstruction in SE corner of the bay. Socoa lt, QWR 36m 12/8M, W shore-264°, R264°-282°, W282°-shore; R sector covers hbr ent. Digue des Criquas Iso G 4s 11m 7M.
Facilities:
ST JEAN-DE-LUZ Hr Mr ☎ 59·47·26·81; Aff Mar ☎ 59·47·14·55; Météo 59·22·03·30. **Quay** FW, AC, P, C; **Services:** Ⓔ, ME, El, Sh, CH.
SOCOA Hr Mr ☎ 59·47·18·44; Aff Mar ☎ 59·47·14·55; ‡ ☎ 59·47·18·44; **Jetty** C (1 ton), FW, P, D, AC; **YC Basque** ☎ 59·47·18·31; **Services:** ME, CH, El, Sh.
Town V, R, Bar, Ⓞ, ✉, Ⓑ, ⇌.

HENDAYE   10-18-26

Pyrénées Atlantique, 43°22´·91N 01°47´·25W

CHARTS
AC 1181, 1102; SHOM 6556, 6558, 6786; ECM 555
TIDES
HW +0450 on Dover (UT); ML 2·3m; Zone −0100

Standard Port POINTE DE GRAVE (←)

Times				Height (metres)			
High Water		Low Water		MHWS	MHWN	MLWN	MLWS
0000	0600	0500	1200	5·4	4·4	2·1	1·0
1200	1800	1700	2400				
Differences ST JEAN DE LUZ (SOCOA) (5M to the E)							
−0040	−0045	−0030	−0045	−1·1	−1·1	−0·6	−0·4

SHELTER
Excellent in marina (3m); access H24. Good ⚓ in river off Fuenterrabia and moorings in the B. de Chingoudy. Note: Hendaye lies on the French bank of the Rio Bidassoa; on the Spanish bank is Fuenterrabia. There is a neutral area in the Baie de Fontarabie.
NAVIGATION
WPT 43°24´·00N 01°46´·50W, 025°/205° from/to W bkwtr hd 1·25M. Beware Les Briquets 8ca N of Pte Ste Anne at E end of the Baie and, near centre of B, keep clear of Bajo Iruarri. River ent is easy except in heavy N'ly swell; sp ebb is very strong. Inshore of Pte des Dunes lt, Fl R 2·5s, hug the E training wall for best water. A spit drying 1·3m (SHM bn, VQ (3) G 5s) off Fuenterrabia narrows the chan to about 100m before marina ent opens up.

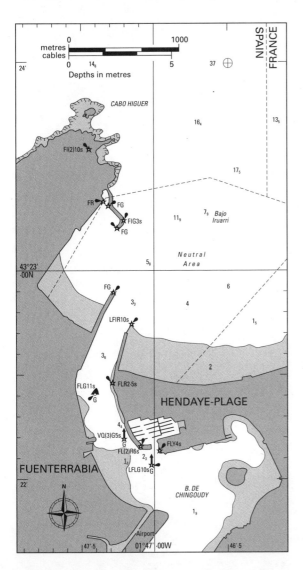

LIGHTS AND MARKS
On W end of bay, Cabo Higuer lt ho , Fl (2) 10s 63m 23M. River ent bkwtrs: East L Fl R 10s 7m 5M; West FG 9m 3M. River dredged to 2m. Marina ent between Fl (2) R 6s 6m 2M on elbow of W bkwtr (hd marked by FR strip lt) and Fl Y 4s 5m 3M at E side; near the latter is a conspic RW TV relay mast (40m).
RADIO TELEPHONE
Marina VHF Ch 09 (H24).
TELEPHONE
Hr Mr 59·48·06·10; ⌗ 59·20·70·82; Aff Mar 59·20·77·67; CROSS 59.09.82.00; Météo 59.24.58.80; Auto 36.68.08.64; SNSM 59.20.60.33; Police 59.20.65.52; Ⓗ 59.20.08.22.
FACILITIES
Marina (600 + 120) ☎ 59.48.06.10, FF160, AC, FW, P, D, BH (30 ton), Slip; Boats > 17m LOA should moor in Baie de Chingoudy; **Club Maritime Hendayais** ☎ 59·20·03·02, Bar; **Services:** CH, Sh, El, Ⓔ, ME.
Town V, R, Bar, Gaz, ✉, Ⓑ, ➾, ✈ (Fuenterrabia or Biarritz). Local ferry from marina to Fuenterrabia. UK ferry from Bilbao/Santander.

TIDAL DIFFERENCES FOR NORTH COAST OF SPAIN   10-18-27

Standard Port POINTE DE GRAVE (←)

Times				Height (metres)			
High Water		Low Water		MHWS	MHWN	MLWN	MLWS
0000	0600	0500	1200	5·4	4·4	2·1	1·0
1200	1800	1700	2400				
Differences PASAJES							
−0050	−0030	−0015	−0045	−1·2	−1·3	−0·5	−0·5
SAN SEBASTIAN							
−0110	−0030	−0020	−0040	−1·2	−1·2	−0·5	−0·4
GUETARIA							
−0110	−0030	−0020	−0040	−1·0	−1·0	−0·5	−0·4
LEQUEITIO							
−0115	−0035	−0025	−0045	−1·2	−1·2	−0·5	−0·4
BERMEO							
−0055	−0015	−0005	−0025	−0·8	−0·7	−0·5	−0·4
ABRA DE BILBAO							
−0125	−0045	−0035	−0055	−1·2	−1·2	−0·5	−0·4
PORTUGALETE (BILBAO)							
−0100	−0020	−0010	−0030	−1·2	−1·2	−0·5	−0·4
CASTRO URDIALES							
−0040	−0120	−0020	−0110	−1·4	−1·5	−0·6	−0·6
RIA DE SANTONA							
−0005	−0045	+0015	−0035	−1·4	−1·4	−0·6	−0·6
SANTANDER							
−0020	−0100	0000	−0050	−1·3	−1·4	−0·6	−0·6
RIA DE SUANCES							
0000	−0030	+0020	−0020	−1·5	−1·5	−0·6	−0·6
SAN VICENTE DE LA BARQUERA							
−0020	−0100	0000	−0050	−1·5	−1·5	−0·6	−0·6
RIA DE TINA MAYOR							
−0020	−0100	0000	−0050	−1·4	−1·5	−0·6	−0·6
RIBADESELLA							
+0005	−0020	+0020	−0020	−1·4	−1·3	−0·6	−0·4
GIJON							
−0005	−0030	+0010	−0030	−1·4	−1·3	−0·6	−0·4
AVILES							
−0100	−0040	−0015	−0050	−1·5	−1·4	−0·7	−0·5
SAN ESTABAN DE PRAVIA							
−0005	−0030	+0010	−0030	−1·4	−1·3	−0·6	−0·4
LUARCA							
+0010	−0015	+0025	−0015	−1·2	−1·1	−0·5	−0·3
RIBADEO							
+0010	−0015	+0025	−0015	−1·4	−1·3	−0·6	−0·4
RIA DE VIVERO							
+0010	−0015	+0025	−0015	−1·4	−1·3	−0·6	−0·4
ORTIGUEIRA							
−0020	0000	+0020	−0010	−1·3	−1·2	−0·6	−0·4
EL FERROL DEL CAUDILLO							
−0045	−0100	−0010	−0105	−1·6	−1·4	−0·7	−0·4
LA CORUNA							
−0110	−0050	−0030	−0100	−1·6	−1·6	−0·6	−0·5
RIA DE CORME							
−0025	−0005	+0015	−0015	−1·7	−1·6	−0·6	−0·5
RIA DE CAMARINAS							
−0120	−0055	−0030	−0100	−1·6	−1·6	−0·6	−0·5

18

Volvo Penta service

Sales and service centres in area 19
Names and addresses of Volvo Penta dealers in
this area are available from:

France *Volvo Penta France SA,* 1 Rue de la Nouvelle, B. P. 49, 78133 Les
Mureaux Tel 33-1-30912799, Fax 33-1-34746415 Telex 695221 F.
Netherlands *Nebim Handelmaatschappij BV,* Postbus 195, 3640 Ad Mijdrecht
Tel 02979-80111, Fax 0279-87364, Telex 15505 NEHA NL.

Area 19

North-East France
Barfleur to Dunkerque

VOLVO PENTA

19

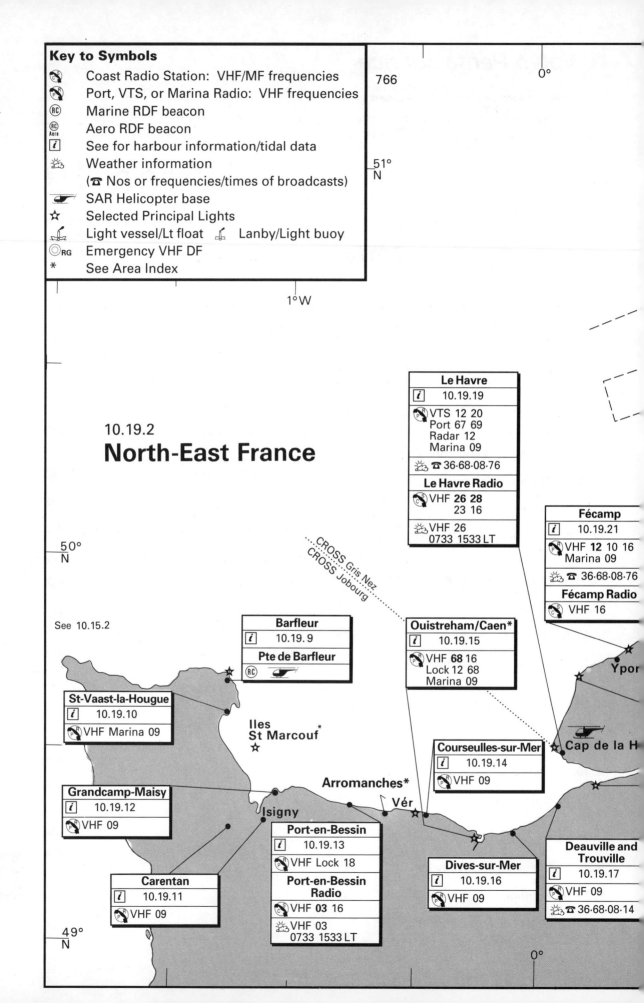

Key to Symbols

📻 Coast Radio Station: VHF/MF frequencies
📻 Port, VTS, or Marina Radio: VHF frequencies
🆁🅲 Marine RDF beacon
🆁🅲 Aero RDF beacon
ⓘ See for harbour information/tidal data
⛅ Weather information
   (☎ Nos or frequencies/times of broadcasts)
🚁 SAR Helicopter base
☆ Selected Principal Lights
⚓ Light vessel/Lt float ⚓ Lanby/Light buoy
Ⓡ🅶 Emergency VHF DF
* See Area Index

766

0°

51°
N

1°W

10.19.2
North-East France

50°
N

See 10.15.2

CROSS Gris Nez
CROSS Jobourg

Le Havre
ⓘ	10.19.19

📻 VTS 12 20
Port 67 69
Radar 12
Marina 09

⛅ ☎ 36·68·08·76

Le Havre Radio
📻 VHF **26 28**
      23 16

⛅ VHF 26
0733 1533 LT

Fécamp
ⓘ	10.19.21

📻 VHF **12** 10 16
Marina 09

⛅ ☎ 36·68·08·76

Fécamp Radio
📻 VHF 16

Barfleur
ⓘ	10.19.9

Pte de Barfleur
🆁🅲   🚁

Ouistreham/Caen*
ⓘ	10.19.15

📻 VHF **68** 16
Lock 12 68
Marina 09

Ypor

St-Vaast-la-Hougue
ⓘ	10.19.10

📻 VHF Marina 09

Iles
St Marcouf*
☆

Courseulles-sur-Mer
ⓘ	10.19.14

📻 VHF 09

🚁 Cap de la H

Arromanches*

Vér

Grandcamp-Maisy
ⓘ	10.19.12

📻 VHF 09

Isigny

Port-en-Bessin
ⓘ	10.19.13

📻 VHF Lock 18

Port-en-Bessin Radio
📻 VHF **03** 16

⛅ VHF 03
0733 1533 LT

Dives-sur-Mer
ⓘ	10.19.16

📻 VHF 09

Deauville and Trouville
ⓘ	10.19.17

📻 VHF 09

⛅ ☎ 36·68·08·14

Carentan
ⓘ	10.19.11

📻 VHF 09

49°
N

0°

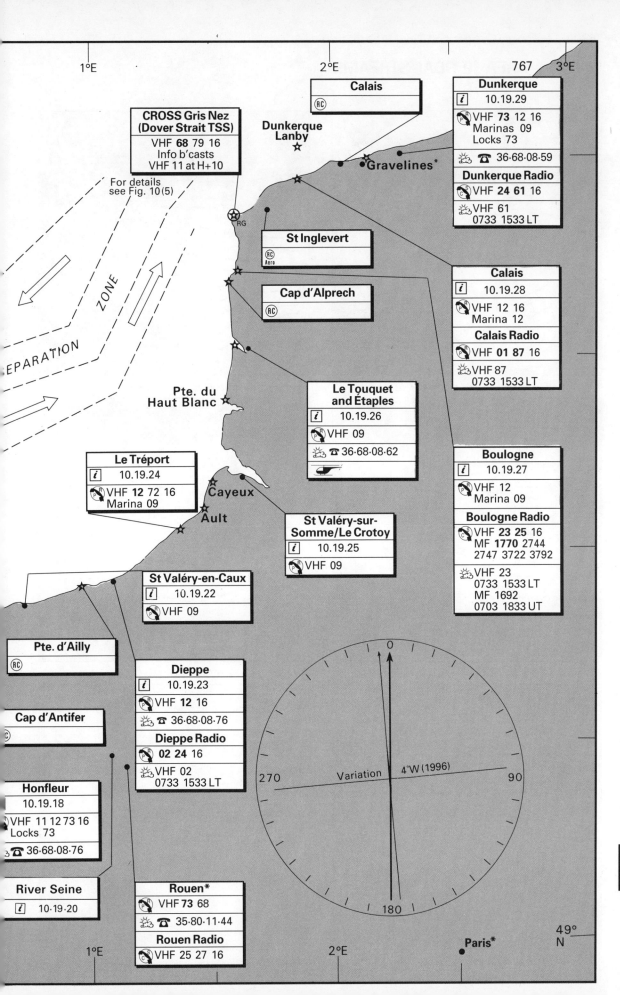

Calais
(RC)

Dunkerque
[i] 10.19.29
VHF **73** 12 16
Marinas 09
Locks 73
☎ 36·68·08·59

Dunkerque Radio
VHF **24 61** 16
VHF 61
0733 1533 LT

CROSS Gris Nez
(Dover Strait TSS)
VHF **68** 79 16
Info b'casts
VHF 11 at H+10

Dunkerque
Lanby ☆

Gravelines*

For details
see Fig. 10(5)

ZONE

SEPARATION

RG

St Inglevert
(RC)
Aero

Cap d'Alprech
(RC)

Calais
[i] 10.19.28
VHF 12 16
Marina 12

Calais Radio
VHF **01 87** 16
VHF 87
0733 1533 LT

Pte. du
Haut Blanc ☆

Le Touquet
and Étaples
[i] 10.19.26
VHF 09
☎ 36·68·08·62

Boulogne
[i] 10.19.27
VHF 12
Marina 09

Boulogne Radio
VHF **23 25** 16
MF **1770** 2744
2747 3722 3792
VHF 23
0733 1533 LT
MF 1692
0703 1833 UT

Le Tréport
[i] 10.19.24
VHF **12** 72 16
Marina 09

Cayeux ☆

Ault ☆

St Valéry-sur-
Somme/Le Crotoy
[i] 10.19.25
VHF 09

St Valéry-en-Caux
[i] 10.19.22
VHF 09

Pte. d'Ailly
(RC)

Cap d'Antifer
(c)

Dieppe
[i] 10.19.23
VHF **12** 16
☎ 36·68·08·76

Dieppe Radio
02 24 16
VHF 02
0733 1533 LT

Honfleur
10.19.18
VHF 11 12 73 16
Locks 73
☎ 36·68·08·76

Variation 4°W (1996)

270   90

0

180

River Seine
[i] 10·19·20

Rouen*
VHF **73** 68
☎ 35·80·11·44

Rouen Radio
VHF 25 27 16

Paris*

19

1°E

2°E

767   3°E

49°
N

1°E

2°E

10-19-3 AREA 19 TIDAL STREAMS

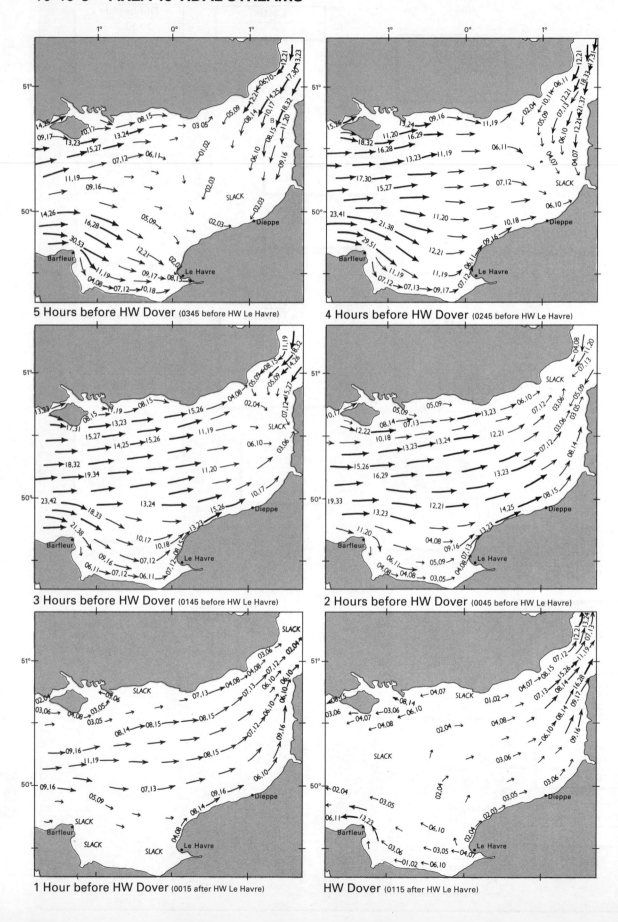

5 Hours before HW Dover (0345 before HW Le Havre)

4 Hours before HW Dover (0245 before HW Le Havre)

3 Hours before HW Dover (0145 before HW Le Havre)

2 Hours before HW Dover (0045 before HW Le Havre)

1 Hour before HW Dover (0015 after HW Le Havre)

HW Dover (0115 after HW Le Havre)

Westward 10.15.3   Northward 10.2.3   North-eastward 10.3.3   Eastward 10.20.3

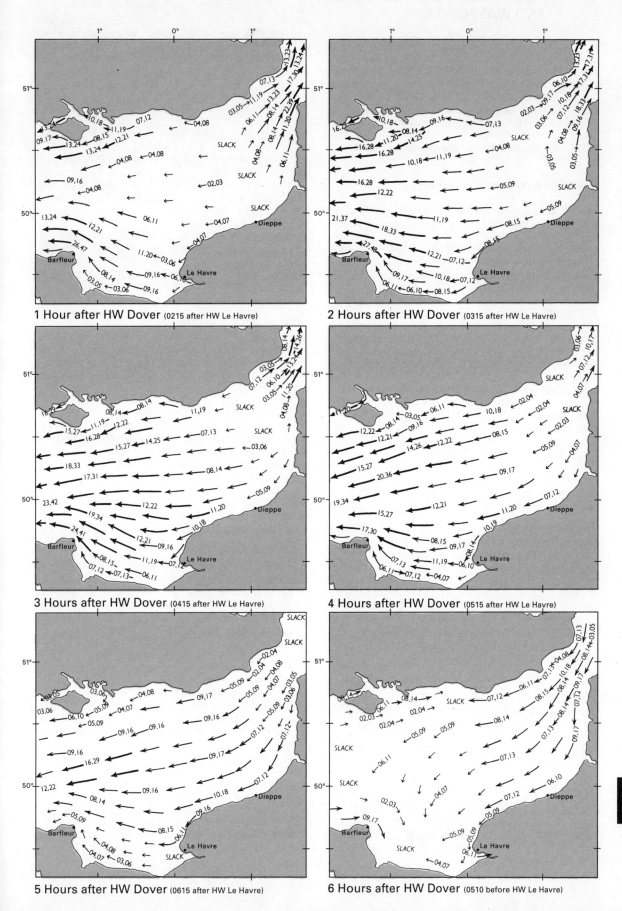

1 Hour after HW Dover (0215 after HW Le Havre)

2 Hours after HW Dover (0315 after HW Le Havre)

3 Hours after HW Dover (0415 after HW Le Havre)

4 Hours after HW Dover (0515 after HW Le Havre)

5 Hours after HW Dover (0615 after HW Le Havre)

6 Hours after HW Dover (0510 before HW Le Havre)

19

10.19.4 COASTAL LIGHTS, FOG SIGNALS AND WAYPOINTS

Abbreviations used below are given in 1.4.1. Principal lights are in **bold** print, places in CAPITALS, and light-vessels, light floats and Lanbys in *CAPITAL ITALICS*. Unless otherwise stated lights are white. m – elevation in metres; M – nominal range in miles. Fog signals are in *italics*. Useful waypoints are underlined – use those on land with care. All geographical positions should be assumed to be approximate. See 4.4.1.

NOTE: For English Channel Waypoints see 10.1.7.

POINTE DE BARFLEUR TO DEAUVILLE

Pte de Barfleur-Gatteville 49°41'·83N 01°15'·87W Fl (2) 10s 72m **29M**; Gy Tr, B top; obsc when brg less than 088°; RC; *Horn (2) 60s*.
La Jamette Bn 49°41'·92N 01°15'·51W; ECM.
La Grotte By 49°41'·12N 01°14'·78W; SHM.
Roche-à-l'Anglais By 49°40'·84N 01°14'·85W; SHM.
Le Hintar By 49°40'·75N 01°14'·76W; PHM.

BARFLEUR
Ldg Lts 219·5°. Front 49°40'·24N 01°15'·53W Oc (3) 12s 7m 10M; W ■ Tr. Rear 288m from front Oc (3) 12s 13m 10M; Gy and W ■ Tr, G top; vis 085°-355°; synch with front.
Jetée Est Hd 49°40'·39N 01°15'·38W Oc R 4s 5m 6M; W hut, R top.
Jetée Ouest Hd Fl G 4s 8m 6M; W pylon, G top.

Pte de Saire Lt Tr 49°36'·44N 01°13'·71W Oc (2+1) 12s 11m 10M; W Tr, G top.

Moulard Bn 49°39'·42N 01°13'·87W; ECM.
Dranguet Bn 49°36'·82N 01°12'·92W; ECM.
Le Vitéquet Bn 49°36'·15N 01°13'·29W; SCM.
Le Gavendest By 49°34'·67N 01°13'·74W; SCM; *Whis*.
La Dent By 49°34'·63N 01°14'·12W; SCM.

ST VAAST-LA-HOUGUE
Jetty Hd 49°35'·25N 01°15'·35W Oc 2 WRG 6s 12m W10M, R7M, G7M; W 8 sided Tr, R top; vis R219°-237°, G237°-310°, W310°-350°, R350°-040°; *Siren Mo(N) 30s*.
NE side Bkwtr Hd Iso G 4s 6m 3M; W tank, G top.
SW side, Groyne Hd Oc (4) R 12s 6m 6M; W hut, R top.
Ldg Lts 267°. Front La Hougue   49°34'·31N 01°16'·30W Oc 4s 9m 10M; W pylon, G top. Rear, Morsalines 1·8M from front, 49°34'·25N 01°18'·95W Oc (3+1) WRG 12s 90m W11M, R8M, G8M; W 8-sided Tr, G top; vis W 171°-316°, G316°-321°, R321°-342°, W342°-355°.

Quineville Lt By 49°31'·85N 01°12'·40W Q (9) 10s; WCM.
S Floxel By 49°30'·75N 01°13'·70W; ECM.
SW Marcouf Lt By 49°29'·80N 01°11'·92W Q (9) 15s; WCM.

ÎLES SAINT-MARCOUF
Île du Large Lt Tr 49°29'·90N 01°08'·70W VQ (3) 5s 18m 8M; ■ Gy Tr, G top.

CARENTAN
CI Lt By 49°25'·30N 01°07'·10W Iso 4s; SWM.
Ldg Lts 209·5°. **Front** 49°20'·55N 01°11'·05W Dir Oc (3) R 12s 6m **18M**; W mast, R top; intens 208·2°-210·7°. Rear, 723m from front, Oc (3) 12s 14m 10M; W gantry, G top; vis 120°-005°; synch with front.
W Channel Ent Bn 49°22'·00N 01°09'·90W Fl (3) G 12s; G △, on G Bn.

ISIGNY-SUR-MER
IS By 49°24'·30N 01°06'30W; NCM.
Ldg Lts 172·5°. **Front** 49°19'·50N 01°06·70W Dir Oc (2+1) 12s 7m **18M**; intens 170·5°-174·5°. **Rear** 625m from front Dir Oc (2+1) 12s 19m **18M**; W pylon, B top; synch with front, intens 170·5°-174·5°.

GRANDCAMP-MAISY
La Maresquerie 49°23'·20N 01°02'·65W Oc 4s 28m 12M; vis 090°-270°.
Jetée Est Hd 49°23'·54N 01°02'·88W Oc (2) R 6s 9m 9M; *Horn Mo(N) 30s*.
Perré 49°23'·40N 01°02'·40W Oc 4s 8m 12M; G pylon on W hut; vis 083°-263°.
Ldg Lts 146°. Front 49°23'·41N 01°02'·93W Dir Q 9m **15M**. Rear, 102m from front, Dir Q 12m **15M**. Both vis: 144·5°-147·5°.

Norfalk Lt By 49°28'·83N 01°03'·40W Q (3) 10s; ECM.
Est du Cardonnet Lt By 49°26'·97N 01°01'·00W VQ (3) 5s; ECM.
Broadsword Lt By 49°25'·39N 00°52'·90W Q (3) 10s; ECM.
Cussy Lt By 49°29'·50N 00°43'·25W VQ (9) 10s; WCM.

PORT-EN-BESSIN/ARROMANCHES
Ldg Lts 204°. Front 49°21'·00N 00°45'·56W Oc (3) 12s 25m 10M; W pylon, G top; vis 069°-339°; *Siren 20s* – sounded over a sector of 90° each side of Ldg line, continuous in the W sector, interrupted in the E (TD 1988). Rear, 93m from front, Oc (3) 12s 42m 11M; W & Gy house; synch with front; vis 114°-294° RC.
Môle Est Hd Oc R 4s 14m 7M; R pylon.
Môle Ouest Hd 49°21'·21N 00°45'·42W Fl WG 4s 14m W10M, G7M; G pylon; vis G065°-114·5°, W114·5°-065°.
Oc (2) R 6s and Fl (2) G 6s mark the pier Hds.
Bombardons By 49°21'·70N 00°39'·15W; WCM.
Roseberry By 49°23'·15N 00°36'·15W; ECM.

Ver 49°20'·47N 00°31'·15W Fl (3) 15s 42m **26M**; W Tr, Gy top; obsc by cliffs of St Aubin when brg more than 275°; RC.
Fosse de Courseulles Lt By 49°21'·33N 00°27'·61W Iso 4s; SWM.

COURSEULLES-SUR-MER
Jetée Ouest Hd 49°20'·47N 00°27'·28W Iso WG 4s 7m W9M, G6M; brown pylon on Dn, G top; vis W135°-235°, G235°-135°; *Horn 30s* sounded from HW±2 hours.

Essarts de Langrune By 49°22'·65N 00°21'·25W; NCM.
Luc By 49°20'·85N 00°18'·20W; NCM.
Lion By 49°20'·80N 00°15'·92W; NCM.

OUISTREHAM/CAEN
Ouistreham Lt By 49°20'·48N 00°14'·73W VQ (3) 5s; ECM.
Merville Lt By 49°19'·71N 00°13'·30W VQ; NCM.
Ouistreham Main Lt 49°16'·85N 00°14'·80W Oc WR 4s 37m **W17M**, R 13M; W Tr, R top; vis W151°-115°, R115°-151°.
Ldg Lts 185°. **Front**, 49°17'·16N 00°14'·72W Jetée Est Hd Dir Oc (3+1) R 12s 10m **17M**; W pylon, R top; Ra refl. **Rear**, 610m from front, Dir Oc (3+1) R 12s 30m **17M**; Tripod, R top; synch with front; intens 183·5°-186·5°.
Enrochements Est Hd (St-Médard) 49°18'·08N 00°14'·54W Oc (2) R 6s 7m 8M; W pylon, R top; Ra refl.
Enrochements Ouest Hd 49°17'·50N 04°14'·74W Iso G 4s 11m 7M; W pylon, G top; Ra refl; *Horn 10s*, (TD 1992).

Viaduc de Calix, Caen 49°11'·23N 00°19'·70W Iso 4s on E and W sides; FG on N side, FR on S side.

DIVES
D1 Lt By 49°18'·78N 00°05'·67W L Fl 10s; SWM.
Dives-sur-Mer 49°17'·85N 00°05'·20W Oc (2+1) WRG 12s 6m W12M, R9M, G9M, R hut; vis G125°-157°, W157°-162°, R162°-194°.

DEAUVILLE/TROUVILLE
Semoy Lt By 49°24'·20N 00°02'·45E VQ (3) 5s; ECM.
Trouville SW Lt By 49°22'·60N 00°02'·64E VQ (9) 10s; WCM.
W Jetty 49°22'·44N 00°04'·17E Fl WG 4s 10m W9M, G6M; B pylon, G top; vis W005°-176°, G176°-005°.
Trouville East 49°22'·28N 00°04'·41E Fl (4) WR 12s 8m W7M, R4M; W pylon, R top; vis W131°-175°, R175°-131°.
Ldg Lts 148°. Front 49°22'·09N 00°04'·57E Oc R 4s 11m 12M; W Tr, R top; vis 330°-150°; *Horn (2) 30s.* Rear, 217m from front, Oc R 4s 17m 10M; W pylon, R top; synch with front vis 120°-170°.

ESTUAIRE DE LA SEINE/LE HAVRE

Ratelets Lt By 49°25'·35N 00°01'·80E Q (9) 15s; WCM.
Ratier S Lt By 49°25'·21N 00°07'·22E VQ (6) + L Fl 10s; SCM.
Ratier NW Lt By 49°26'·85N 00°02'·55E VQ G; SHM.
Ducan-L-Clinch Lt By 49°27'·23N 00°02'·58E VQ (9) 10s; WCM.

CHENAL DE ROUEN
No. 4 Lt By 49°27'·05N 00°02'·64E QR; PHM.
No. 7 Lt By 49°26'·24N 00°04'·82E QG; SHM.
Digue du Ratier Hd "A" 49°25'·97N 00°06'·66E VQ 10m 4M; NCM; Ra refl; tide gauge.
Spillway Lt Bn 49°25'·80N 00°12'·80E VQ (9) 10s 15m 7M; WCM.

HONFLEUR
Falaise des Fonds 49°25'·53N 00°12'·93E Fl (3) WRG 12s 15m **W17M**, R13M, G13M; W ■ Tr, G top; vis G040°-080°, R080°-084°, G084°-100°, W100°-109°, R109°-162°, G162°-260°.
Digue Est Hd 49°25'·73N 00°14'·04E Q 9m 8M; NCM; *Horn (5) 40s.* (Km 356 from Paris).

LA SEINE MARITIME
La Risle, Digue Sud 49°26'·37N 00°22'·07E Iso G 4s 11m 6M; W pylon , G top; Ra refl; (Km 346 from Paris).
Marais-Vernier 49°27'·78N 00°26'·89E Fl G 4s 8m 5M; W Col, R top (Km 340).
Digue Nord, Tancarville 49°28'·81N 00°28'·30E QR 9m 6M; W col, R top; (Km 337).
Quillebeuf 49°28'50N 00°31'·63E QG 12m 8M (Km 332·4).
Caudebec-en-Caux 49°31'·52N 00°43'·78E VQ R (Km 310).
Duclair 49°28'·80N 00°52'·32E QR (Km 278).

ROUEN
Feu de Rouen 49°26'·42N 01°02'·62E Oc (2) R 6s 10m (Km 245·5).

APPROACHES TO LE HAVRE
Spoil Gnd Lt By 49°27'·84N 00°02'·38E Q (9) 15s; WCM.
N du Mouillage Lt By 49°28'·65N 00°01'·36E Fl (4) Y 15s; SPM.
RN Lt By 49°28'·68N 00°01'·10W Fl (2) 6s; IDM.
RNA Lt By 49°28'·70N 00°05'·45W Iso 4s; SWM.
HP Lt By 49°29'·61N 00°03'·70W Fl Y 4s; SPM; *Whis.*
Northgate Lt By 49°30'·40N 00°14'·15W Q; NCM.
***LE HAVRE* Lanby** 49°31'·44N 00°09'·78W Fl (2) R 8s 10m **20M**; W By, R stripes; Racon.
Ldg Lts 106·8°. Front **Quai Roger Meunier** 49°28'·97N 00°06'·58E Dir F 36m **25M**; Gy Tr, G top; intens 106°-108°; (H24). Rear, 0·73M from front, **Quai Joannes Couvert** Dir F 78m **25M**; Gy Tr, G top; intens 106°-108°; (H24); Ra refl.

Cap de la Hève 49°30'·79N 00°04'·24E Fl 5s 123m **24M**; W 8-sided Tr, R top; vis 225°-196°.

LE HAVRE
Digue Sud Hd 49°29'·11N 00°05'·46E VQ (3) G 2s 15m 11M; W Tr, G top.
Digue Nord Hd 49°29'·25N 00°05'·52E Fl R 5s 15m **21M**; W Tr, R top; *Horn 15s.*
Yacht Hbr, Digue Augustin Normand 49°29'·32N 00°05'·63E Q (2) G 5s 5m 2M.

LE HAVRE TO CAP D'ANTIFER
Octeville W Lt By 49°31'·67N 00°01'·90E VQ (6) + L Fl 10s; SCM.
Port du Havre-Antifer 49°39'·59N 00°09'·28E Dir Oc WRG 4s 24m **W15M**, R13M, G13M; W pylon, B top; vis G068·5°-078·5°, W078·5°-088·5°, R088·5°-098·5°.
A17 Lt By 49°41'·60N 00°01'·75E Iso G 4s; SHM.
A18 Lt By 49°42'·07N 00°02'·21E QR; PHM.
Port d'Antifer Ldg Lts 127·5°. **Front** 49°38'·36N 00°09'·20E Dir Oc 4s 105m **22M**; W pylon, G top vis 127°-128°. **Rear**, 430m from front, Dir Oc 4s 124m **22M**; W mast, G top. By day both show FW Lts **33M** vis 126·5°-128·5°; occas.

CAP D'ANTIFER TO POINTE DU HAUT BLANC

Cap d'Antifer 49°41'·07N 00°10'·00E Fl 20s 128m **29M**; Gy 8-sided Tr, G top; vis 021°-222°; RC.
Yport Ldg Lts 166°. Front 49°44'·40N 00°18'·70E Oc 4s 10m, W mast, G top. Rear, 30m from front, Oc 4s 14m, W pylon, G top on house.

FÉCAMP
Jetée Nord 49°45'·99N 00°21'·87E Fl (2) 10s 15m **16M**; Gy Tr, R top; *Horn (2) 30s.*
Lts in line 082°. Front Jetée Sud Hd, 49°45'·95N 00°21'·89E QG 14m 9M; Gy Tr, G top; vis 072°-217°. Rear, Jetée Nord, root, QR 10m 4M; R ● on W mast.

Paluel Lt By 49°52'·20N 00°38'·10E Q; NCM.

SAINT VALÉRY-EN-CAUX
Jetée Ouest 49°52'·40N 00°42'·60E Oc (2+1) G 12s 13m 14M; W Tr, G top. (TE 1993).
Jetée Est Hd 49°52'·35N 00°42'·75E Fl (2) R 6s 8m 4M; W mast.

Roches d'Ailly Lt By 49°56'·58N 00°56'·90E VQ; NCM; *Whis.*
Pointe d'Ailly 49°55'·13N 00°57'·56E Fl (3) 20s 95m **31M**; W ■ Tr, G top; RC; *Horn (3) 60s* (TD 1989).
D1 Lt By 49°57'·11N 01°01'·35E VQ (3) 5s; ECM; *Bell.*
Daffodils Wk Lt By 50°02'·52N 01°04'·10E VQ (9) 10s; WCM.
Berneval Wk By 50°03'·46N 01°06'·62E; WCM.

DIEPPE
Jetée Est Hd 49°56'·22N 01°05'·14E Oc (4) R 12s 12m 8M; R col.
Jetée Ouest 49°56'·19N 01°05'·05E Iso WG 4s 11m W12M, G8M; W Tr, G top; vis W095°-164°, G164°-095°; *Horn 30s.*
Falaise du Pollet 49°55'·98N 01°05'·37E Q R 35m 9M; R & W structure; vis 105·5°-170·5°.

Penly No. 1 Lt By 49°59'·10N 01°11'·47E Fl (3) Y 12s; SPM.
Penly No. 2 Lt By 49°59'·50N 01°12'10E Fl Y 4s; SPM.

LE TRÉPORT
Jetée Ouest Hd 50°03'·94N 01°22'·22E Fl (2) G 10s 15m **20M**; W Tr, G top; *Horn Mo(N) 30s.*
Jetée Est 50°03'·93N 01°22'·30E Oc R 4s 8m 6M; W col, R top. Port signals Fl (5) G 500m SE.

19

Ault 50°06'·32N 01°27'·31E Oc (3) WR 12s 95m **W18M**, R14M, W Tr, R top; vis W040°-175°, R175°-220°.

BAIE DE SOMME/LE CROTOY/ST VALÉRY-SUR-SOMME.
Cayeux-sur-Mer 50°11'·60N 01°30'·80E Fl R 5s 32m **22M**; W Tr, R top.
AT-SO Lt By 50°14'·00N 01°28'·50E VQ; NCM.
Pte du Hourdel Lt Tr 50°12'·85N 01°34'·10E Oc (3) WG 12s 19m W12M, G9M; W Tr, G top; vis W053°-248°, G248°-323°; *Reed (3) 30s.*
Le Crotoy 50°12'·93N 01°37'·45E Oc (2) R 6s 19m 9M; W pylon; vis 285°-135°.
Yacht Hbr, E side 50°13'·02N 01°38'·10E Fl G 2s 4m 2M.
St Valéry-sur-Somme,   Embankment Hd 50°12'·29N 01°35'·92E Q (3) G 6s 2m 2M; G pylon; Ra refl.
W Hd of embankment 50°11'·40N 01°37'·60E Iso G 4s 9m 9M; W pylon, G top; vis 347°-222°.
La Ferté Môle Hd 50°11'·20N 01°38'·70E Fl R 4s 9m 9M; W pylon, R top; vis 000°-250°.

SOMME TO LE TOUQUET
FM By 50°20'·40N 01°31'·00E; WCM.
Pointe du Haut-Blanc (Berck-Plage) 50°23'·90N 01°33'·75E Fl 5s 44m **23M**; W Tr, R bands, G top.
Vergoyer SW Lt By 50°26'·90N 01°00'·10E VQ (9) 10s; WCM.
Bassurelle Lt By 50°32'·70N 00°57'·80E Fl (4) R 15s 6M; Racon (B); R refl; *Whis.*
Écovouga Wk By 50°33'·70N 00°59'·20E; ECM.
Vergoyer W Lt By 50°34'·65N 01°13'·70E Fl G 4s; SHM.
Vergoyer E Lt By 50°35'·75N 01°19'·80E VQ (3) 5s; ECM.
Vergoyer NW Lt By 50°37'·10N 01°18'·00E Fl (2) G 6s; SHM.
Vergoyer N Lt By 50°39'·65N 01°22'·30E VQ; NCM; Racon (C).

LE TOUQUET TO DUNKERQUE

LE TOUQUET
Le Touquet (La Canche) 50°31'·40N 01°35'·60E Fl (2) 10s 54m **25M**; Or Tr, brown band; W and G top.
Mérida Wk By 50°32'·80N 01°33'·30E; WCM.
Camiers, Rivière Canche ent, N side 50°32'·80N 01°36'·40E Oc (2) WRG 6s 17m W10M, R7M, G7M; R pylon; vis G015°-090°, W090°-105°, R105°-141°.

Cap d'Alprech 50°41'·96N 01°33'·83E Fl (3) 15s 62m **23M**; W Tr, B top; RC; FR Lts on radio mast 600m ENE.
Ophélie Lt By 50°43'·91N 01°30'·92E Fl G 4s; SHM.

BOULOGNE
Approaches Lt By 50°45'·36N 01°31'·15E VQ (6) + L Fl 10s 8m 8M; SCM; Ra refl; *Whis.*
Digue (Carnot) 50°44'·48N 01°34'·13E Fl (2+1) 15s 25m **19M**; W Tr, G top; *Horn(2+1) 60s.*
Digue Nord Hd 50°44'·76N 01°34'·27E Fl (2) R 6s 10m 7M; R Tr.
Jetée SW 50°43'·95N 01°35'·19E FG 17m 5M; W col, G top; *Horn 30s.*

ZC1 Lt By 50°44'·94N 01°27'·30E Fl (4) Y 15s; SPM.
Bassure de Baas Lt By 50°48'·50N 01°33'·15E VQ; NCM; *Bell.*
ZC2 Lt By 50°53'·50N 01°31'·00E Fl (2+1) Y 15s; SPM.
Cap Gris-Nez 50°52'·05N 01°35'·07E Fl 5s 72m **29M**; W Tr, B top; vis 005°-232°; RG; *Horn 60s.*
Lt By 50°54'·11N 01°32'·03E Fl (2) 6s; IDM.
Abbeville Lt By 50°56'·05N 01°37'·70E VQ (9) 10s; WCM.
CA3 Lt By 50°56'·80N 01°41'·25E Fl G 4s; SHM; *Whis.*

Sangatte 50°57'·23N 01°46'·57E Oc WG 4s 12m W8M, G6M; W pylon, B top; vis G065°-089°, W089°-152°, G152°-245°.
RCW Lt By 51°01'·20N 01°45'·45E VQ; NCM.
CA2 Lt By 51°00'·91N 01°48'·86E Q; NCM.
CA4 Lt By 50°58'·94N 01°45'·18E VQ (9) 10s 8m 8M; R refl; *Whis.*
CA6 Lt By 50°58'·30N 01°45'·70E VQ R; PHM.
CA5 Lt By 50°57'·70N 01°46'·20E QG; SHM.
CA8 Lt By 50°58'·43N 01°48'·72E QR; PHM; *Bell.*
CA10 Lt By 50°58'·68N 01°50'·00E Fl (2) R 6s; PHM.

CALAIS
Jetée Ouest Hd 50°58'·30N 01°50'·48E Iso G 3s 12m 9M; (in fog Iso 3s); W Tr, G top; *Bell (1) 5s.*
Jetée Est Hd 50°58'·45N 01°50'·54E Fl (2) R 6s 12m **17M**; Gy Tr, R top; *Horn (2) 40s;* Ra refl. (in fog 2 Fl (2) 6s (vert) on request).
Calais 50°57'·73N 01°51'·28E Fl (4) 15s 59m **22M**; W 8-sided Tr, B top; vis 073°-260°.

MPC Lt By 51°06'·17N 01°38'·33E Fl Y 2·5s 10m 6M; SPM.
SANDETTIE Lt F 51°09'·40N 01°47'·20E Fl 5s 12m **24M**; R hull; *Horn 30s;* Racon (T).
Ruytingen SW Lt By 51°04'·99N 01°46'·90E Fl (3) G 12s; SHM; *Whis.*
Ruytingen W Lt By 51°06'·90N 01°50'·60E VQ; NCM.
Ruytingen NW Lt By 51°09'·05N 01°57'·40E Fl G 4s; SHM.
Ruytingen N Lt By 51°13'·12N 02°10'·42E VQ; NCM.
Ruytingen SE Lt By 51°09'·20N 02°09'·00E VQ (3) 15s; ECM.
DUNKERQUE LANBY 51°03'·00N 01°51'·83E Fl 3s 10m **25M**; R tubular structure on circular By; Racon.
RCE Lt By 51°02'·40N 01°53'·20E Iso G 4s; SHM.
Walde 50°59'·57N 01°55'·00E Fl (3) 12s 13m 4M; B pylon on hut.
DKA Lt By 51°02'·59N 01°57'·06E L Fl 10s; SWM.
Dyck E Lt By 51°05'·70N 02°05'·70E Q (3) 10s; ECM.
Haut-fond de Gravelines Lt By 51°04'·10N 02°05'·10E VQ (9) 10s; WCM.
DW5 Lt By 51°02'·20N 02°01'·00E QG; SHM.

GRAVELINES
Jetée Ouest 51°00'·92N 02°05'·56E Fl (2) WG 6s 9m W8M, G8M; Y ● Tr, G top; vis W317°-327°, G078°-085°, W085°-244°.
Jetée Est 51°00'·98N 02°05'·70E Fl (3) R 12s 5m 4M.

DUNKERQUE APPROACHES
DKB Lt By 51°03'·00N 02°09'·34E VQ (9) 10s; WCM.
Port Ouest Ldg Lts 120°. **Front** 51°01'·72N 02°11'·99E Dir FG 16m **21M**; W col, G top; intens 119°-121°. **Rear**, 600m from front, Dir FG 30m **21M**; W col, G top; intens 119°-121°. By day both show F 28M.
Jetée Clipon Hd 51°02'·69N 02°09'·86E Fl (4) 12s 24m 13M; W ● col, R top; vis 278°-243°; *Siren (4) 60s.*
DW23 Lt By 51°03'·60N 02°15'·25E QG; SHM; *Bell.*
DW29 Lt By 51°03'·88N 02°20'·32E Fl (3) G 12s; SHM.

DUNKERQUE PORT EST
Dunkerque 51°02'·98N 02°21'·94E Fl (2) 10s 59m **26M**; W Tr, B top.
Jetée Ouest Hd 51°03'·63N 02°21'·28E Oc (2+1) WG 12s 35m **W15M**, G12M; W Tr, brown top; vis G252°-310°, W310°-252°; Sig Stn; *Dia (2+1) 60s.*
Jetée Est Hd 51°03'·63N 02°21'·28E Fl (2) R 10s 12m **16M**; R □ on W pylon, R top. *Horn (2) 20s;* Fl (2) 10s (in fog).

10.19.5   PASSAGE INFORMATION

For detailed sailing directions refer to: *Normandy and Channel Islands Pilot* (Adlard Coles/Brackenbury), The *Shell Channel Pilot* (Imray/Cunliffe) and *North France Pilot* (Imray/Thompson). Also the Admiralty *Channel Pilot* and *Dover Strait Pilot*, NP 27 and 28.

The coasts of Normandy and Picardy are convenient to hbrs along the S Coast of England – the distance from (say) Brighton to Fécamp being hardly more than an overnight passage. It should be noted however that many of the hbrs dry, so that a boat which can take the ground is an advantage. For details of TSS in the Dover Strait, see Fig. 10 (5). Notes on the English Channel and on cross-Channel passages appear in 10.3.5; see 10.0.5 for cross-Channel distances. For French glossary, see 1.4.2.

The inland waterways system can be entered via the Seine (10.19.20), St Valéry-sur-Somme (10.19.25), Calais, Gravelines (10.19.28), and Dunkerque (10.19.29). See 10.15.8 for tolls.

POINTE DE BARFLEUR TO GRANDCAMP (chart *2613*)

Raz de Barfleur (10.18.5) must be avoided in bad weather. In calm weather it can be taken at slack water (HW Cherbourg –4½ and +2) or the inshore passage used, passing 5ca E of La Jamette ECM bn. Pte de Barfleur marks the W end of B de Seine, which stretches 55M east to C d'Antifer, 12M N of Le Havre. There are no obstructions on a direct course across the Bay, but a transhipment area for large tankers is centred about 10M ESE of Pte de Barfleur. A feature of the Baie de Seine is the stand of tide at HW.

S from Barfleur (10.19.9) the coast runs SSE 4M to Pte de Saire, with rks and shoals up to 1M offshore. 2M S of Pte de Saire is St Vaast-la-Hougue (10.19.10): approach S of Île de Tatihou, but beware drying rks: La Tourelle, 4½ca E of Is; Le Gavendest and La Dent, which lie 6ca SE and SSE of Is and are buoyed.

Îles St Marcouf (10.19.11) lie 7M SE of St Vaast-la-Hougue, about 4M offshore, and consist of Île du Large (lt) and Île de Terre about ¼M apart. Banc de St Marcouf, with depths of 2·4m and many wks, extends 2·5M NW from the islands, and the sea breaks on this in strong N or NE winds. The Banc du Cardonnet, with depths of 5·2m and many wks, extends for about 5M ESE from the islands.

At the head of B du Grand Vey, about 10M S of Îles St Marcouf, are the (very) tidal hbrs of Carentan and Isigny (10.19.11); entry is only possible near HW. The Carentan chan is well buoyed and adequately lit. It trends SSW across sandbanks for about 4M, beyond which it runs between two breakwaters leading to a lock gate, and thence into canal to Carentan. The Isigny chan is deeper, but the hbr dries. Neither chan should be attempted in strong onshore winds.

On E side of B du Grand Vey, Roches de Grandcamp (dry) extend more than 1M offshore, N and W of Grandcamp (10.19.12), but they are flat and can be crossed from the N in normal conditions HW±1½. Three NCM buoys mark the N edge of the shoal. Heavy kelp can give false echo soundings.

GRANDCAMP TO DEAUVILLE (chart 2613)

Between Pte de la Percée and Port-en-Bessin (10.19.13) a bank lies offshore, with drying ledges extending 3ca. A race forms over this bank with wind against tide. Off Port-en-Bessin the E-going stream begins about HW Le Havre – 0500, and the W-going at about HW Le Havre + 0050, sp rates 1·25kn.

From Port-en-Bessin the coast runs east 4M to C Manvieux, beyond which lie remnants of the wartime hbr of Arromanches, where there is occas anch. Between C Manvieux and Langrune, 10M E, Plateau du Calvados lies offshore. Rocher du Calvados (dries 1·6m) lies on the W part of this bank. There are numerous wrecks and obstructions in the area.

Roches de Ver (dry) lie near centre of Plateau du Calvados, extending 8ca offshore about 1M W of Courseulles-sur-Mer (10.19.14). The approach to this hbr is dangerous in strong onshore winds. Les Essarts de Langrune (dry) lie E of Courseulles-sur-Mer, and extend up to 2·25M seaward of Langrune. At their E end lie Roches de Lion (dry), which reach up to 1·5M offshore in places and extend to a point 2·5M W of Ouistreham ferry hbr and marina (10.19.15). Here a canal leads 7M inland to a marina in centre of Caen.

6M E of Ouistreham is R. Dives (10.19.16) with marina. The banks dry for 1M to seaward, and entry is only possible from HW ± 2½, and not in fresh onshore wind conditions.

Deauville/Trouville (10.19.17), 8M ENE of Dives, is an important yachting hbr. The sands dry more than 5ca offshore; in strong W or N winds the entrance is dangerous and the sea breaks between the jetties. In such conditions it is best attempted within 15 mins of HW, when the stream is slack. To the NE beware Banc de Trouville (dries 2m), and shoal water to the N where Les Ratelets dries at the mouth of the Seine.

ESTUAIRE DE LA SEINE/LE HAVRE (charts 2146, 2990)

The Seine est is entered between Deauville and Le Havre, and is encumbered by shallow and shifting banks which extend seawards to Banc de Seine, 15M W of Le Havre. With wind against tide there is a heavy sea on this bank. Here the SW-going stream begins at HW Le Havre + 0400, and the NE-going at HW Le Havre – 0300, sp rates 1·5kn. Between Deauville and Le Havre the sea can be rough in W winds.

Chenal du Rouen is the main chan into R. Seine, and carries much commercial tfc. The S side of the chan is contained by Digue du Ratier, a training wall which extends E to Honfleur (10.19.18). Note that for tidal reasons Honfleur is not a useful staging port when bound up-river. See 10.19.20 for notes on R. Seine, Rouen and Paris; and canals to the Med.

Le Havre (10.19.19) is a large commercial port, as well as a yachting centre. From the NW, the most useful mark is the Le Havre Lanby 9M W of C de la Hève (lt). The appr chan, which runs 6M WNW from the hbr ent, is well buoyed and lit. Strong W winds cause rough water over shoal patches either side of the chan. Coming from the N or NE, there is deep water close off C de la Hève, but from here steer S to join the main ent chan. Beware Banc de l'Éclat (depth 0·1m), which lies on N side of main chan and about 1·5M from harbour ent.

9M N of C de la Hève is Port d'Antifer, a VLCC harbour. A huge breakwater extends about 1·5M seaward, and should be given a berth of about 1·5M, or more in heavy weather when there may be a race with wind against tide. Commercial vessels in the buoyed app chan have priority. Yachts should cross the app chan to the NW of A17/A18 lt buoys; at 90° to its axis; as quickly as possible, and well clear of ships in the chan. Crossing vessels should contact *Vigie Port d'Antifer* and any priority vessel on VHF Ch 16. Off Cap d'Antifer the NE-going stream begins about HW Le Havre – 0430, and the SW-going at about HW Le Havre + 0140. There are eddies close inshore E of Cap d'Antifer on both streams.

CAP D'ANTIFER TO DIEPPE (chart 2451)

From C d'Antifer to Fécamp (10.19.21) drying rks extend up to 2½ca offshore. At Fécamp pierheads the E-going stream begins about HW Le Havre – 0500, and the W-going at about HW Le Havre + 0025, sp rates 2·75kn. Off Pte Fagnet, close NE of Fécamp, lie Les Charpentiers (rks which dry, to almost 2ca offshore).

From Fécamp to St Valéry-en-Caux (10.19.22), 15M ENE, (and beyond to Le Treport and Ault) the coast consists of chalk cliffs broken by valleys. There are rky ledges, extending 4ca offshore in places. The nuclear power station at Paluel 3M W of St Valéry-en-Caux (prohibited area marked by lt buoy) is conspic. Immediately E of St Valéry-en-Caux shallow sandbanks, Les Ridens, with a least depth of 0·6m, extend about 6ca offshore. At St Valéry-en-Caux ent the E-going

19

stream begins about HW Dieppe – 0550, and the W-going stream begins about HW Dieppe – 0015, sp rates 2·75kn. E of the ent a small eddy runs W on the E-going stream.

Between St Valéry-en-Caux and Pte d'Ailly (lt, fog sig, RC) there are drying rks 4ca offshore in places. About 1·5M E of Pte de Sotteville a rky bank (depth 4·2m) extends about 1M NNW; a strong eddy causes a race over this bank.
Drying rks extend 5ca off Pte d'Ailly, including La Galère, a rk which dries 6·8m, about 3ca N of the Pte. Dangerous wks lie between about 1·2M WNW and 1·5M NNW of the lt ho. About 6M N of Pte d'Ailly, Les Ecamias are banks with depths of 11m, dangerous in a heavy sea.
From Pte d'Ailly to Dieppe (10.19.23) the coast is fringed by a bank, drying in places, up to 4ca offshore. E of Pte d'Ailly an eddy runs W close inshore on first half of E-going stream. Off Dieppe the ENE-going stream begins about HW Dieppe – 0505, and the WSW-going at about HW Dieppe + 0030, sp rates 2kn.

DIEPPE TO BOULOGNE

Between Dieppe and Le Tréport (10.19.24), 14M NE, rky banks, drying in places, extend 5ca offshore. A prohib area extends 6ca off Penly nuclear power station and is marked by lt Bys. About 3M NW of Le Tréport, Ridens du Tréport (depth 5·1m) should be avoided in bad weather. Banc Franc-Marqué (depth 3·6m) lies 2M offshore, and about 3M N of Le Tréport.

N of Ault (lt) the coast changes from medium cliffs to low sand dunes. Offshore there are two shoals, Bassurelle de la Somme and Quémer, on parts of which the sea breaks in bad weather. 4·5M NW of Cayeux-sur-Mer the stream is rotatory anti-clockwise. The E-going stream begins about HW Dieppe –0200, and sets 070° 2·5kn at sp : the W-going stream begins about HW Dieppe + 0600, and sets 240° 1·5kn at sp.

B de Somme, between Pte du Hourdel and Pte de St Quentin, is a shallow, drying area of shifting sands. The chan, which runs close to Pte du Hourdel, is buoyed, but the whole est dries out 3M to seaward, and should not be approached in strong W or NW winds. For St Valéry-sur-Somme and Le Crotoy, see 10.19.25.

From Pte de St Quentin the coast runs 17M N to Pte du Touquet, with a shallow coastal bank which dries to about 5ca offshore, except in the approaches to the dangerous and constantly changing Embouchure de l'Authies (about 7M north), where it dries up to 2M offshore.

Le Touquet/Étaples (10.19.26) lies in the Embouchure de la Canche, entered between Pte du Touquet and Pte de Lornel, and with a drying bank which extends 1M seaward of a line joining these two points. Le Touquet-Paris-Plage lt is shown from a conspic tr, 1M S of Pte du Touquet. Off the entrance the N-going stream begins about HW Dieppe – 0335, sp rate 1·75kn; and the S-going stream begins about HW Dieppe + 0240, sp rate 1·75kn.

In the approaches to Pas de Calais a number of shoals lie offshore: La Bassurelle, Le Vergoyer, Bassure de Baas, Le Battur, Les Ridens, and The Ridge (or Le Colbart). In bad weather, and particularly with wind against tide in most cases, the sea breaks heavily on all these shoals. From Pte de Lornel to Boulogne (10.19.27; chart 438) the coast dries up to 5ca offshore. Off Digue Carnot the N-going stream begins HW Dieppe – 0130, and the S-going at HW Dieppe + 0350, sp rates 1·75kn.

BOULOGNE TO DUNKERQUE (charts *2451, 1892, 323*)

Between Boulogne and C Gris Nez (lt, fog sig) the coastal bank dries about 4ca offshore. The NE-bound traffic lane of the TSS Fig. 10 (2) lies only 3M off C Gris Nez. Keep a sharp lookout not only for coastal traffic in the ITZ, but also cross-Channel ferries, particularly very fast hovercraft, jetfoils and catamarans. 1M NW of C Gris Nez the NE-going stream begins at HW Dieppe – 0150, and the SW-going at HW Dieppe + 0355, sp rates 4kn.

In bad weather the sea breaks heavily on Ridens de Calais, 3M N of Calais (10.19.28 and chart 1352), and also on Ridens de la Rade about 1·5M NE of the hbr. The drying hbr of Gravelines (10.19.28), which should not be used in strong onshore winds, is about 3M SW of Dunkerque Port Ouest; this is a commercial/ferry port which yachts should not enter. The old port, Dunkerque Port Est (10.19.29), has good yacht facilities and is 7·5M further E.

Offshore a series of banks lie roughly parallel with the coast: Sandettié bank (about 14M to N), Outer Ruytingen midway between Sandettié and the coast, and the Dyck banks which extend NE'wards for 30M from a point 5M NE of Calais. There are well-buoyed channels between some of these banks, but great care is needed in poor visibility. In general the banks are steep-to on the inshore side, and slope seaward. In bad weather the sea breaks on the shallower parts.

10.19.6   DISTANCE TABLE

Approximate distances in nautical miles are by the most direct route, whilst avoiding dangers and allowing for Traffic Separation Schemes. Places in *italics* are in adjoining areas; places in **bold** are in 10.0.5, Cross-Channel Distances; places underlined are in 10.0.7, Distances across the North Sea.

	1	2	3	4	5	6	7	8	9	10	11	12	13	14	15	16	17	18	19	20
1. *Cherbourg*	1																			
2. Barfleur	20	2																		
3. **St Vaast**	26	10	3																	
4. Carentan	41	26	20	4																
5. Grandcamp-Maisy	39	21	16	13	5															
6. Courseulles	54	39	35	37	25	6														
7. **Ouistreham**	66	46	46	46	35	11	7													
8. Dives-sur-Mer	69	53	49	51	38	17	8	8												
9. **Deauville/Trouville**	76	56	53	56	43	21	14	7	9											
10. Honfleur	82	62	69	62	50	28	24	17	10	10										
11. **Le Havre**	70	56	53	56	45	23	19	13	8	9	11									
12. Fécamp	80	64	63	72	64	40	39	39	32	34	25	12								
13. St Valéry-en-Caux	82	77	78	88	80	55	58	55	44	45	38	15	13							
14. **Dieppe**	108	94	95	105	94	75	68	67	61	63	54	29	16	14						
15. St Valéry-sur-Somme	130	120	120	132	125	103	103	97	95	95	85	62	45	35	15					
16. Étaples	134	124	130	140	130	110	110	117	100	100	90	70	58	50	19	16				
17. **Boulogne**	142	128	133	145	135	118	115	108	108	110	101	76	61	54	30	12	17			
18. **Calais**	160	148	157	170	168	140	138	129	128	130	121	96	81	74	50	32	20	18		
19. Dunkerque	182	170	179	192	190	162	160	151	150	152	143	118	103	96	69	51	42	22	19	
20. *Nieuwpoort*	197	185	194	207	205	177	175	166	165	167	158	133	118	111	84	66	57	37	15	20

10.19.7 English Channel Waypoints: See 10.1.7

10.19.8 Special Notes for France: See 10.15.8.

BARFLEUR   10-19-9

Manche 49°40'·40N 01°15'·40W

CHARTS
AC 1349, 1106, *2613*; SHOM 7090, 5609, 6864; ECM 528; Imray C32; Stanfords 1, 7

TIDES
–0208 Dover; ML 3·9; Duration 0550; Zone –0100

Standard Port CHERBOURG (←)

Times				Height (metres)			
High Water		Low Water		MHWS	MHWN	MLWN	MLWS
0300	1000	0400	1000	6·4	5·0	2·6	1·1
1500	2200	1600	2200				
Differences BARFLEUR							
+0110	+0055	+0052	+0050	+0·1	+0·3	0·0	+0·1

SHELTER
Excellent, but ent difficult in fresh E/NE winds. Hbr dries; access HW ±2½. Yachts berth at SW end of quay, clear of FVs; limited space. Beware rks/shoals in SE of hbr. Safe to ⚓ outside hbr in off-shore winds. See Hr Mr for moorings.

NAVIGATION
WPT 49°41'·30N 01°14'·21W, 039°/219° from/to front ldg lt, 1·35M. In rough weather, esp wind against tide, keep 5M off Pte de Barfleur to clear the Race; see 10.19.5. From the N, identify La Jamette ECM bn and La Grotte SHM buoy. From the S, keep seaward of Pte Dranguet and Le Moulard, both ECM bns. Beware cross currents and Le Hintar rks (buoyed) and La Raie (bn) to E of ldg line. The chan may not be clearly identified until close in. A new spur bkwtr (55m long) is planned, from the ☆ Fl G 4s, halfway across the ent, toward the ☆ Oc R 4s; (date?).

LIGHTS AND MARKS
Pte de Barfleur lt ho is conspic 1½M NNW of hbr, Fl (2) 10s 72m 29M, grey tr, B top, Reed (2) 60s. The church tr is a conspic daymark.
Ldg lts 219°: both Oc (3) 12s 7/13m 10M, W □ trs, synch; not easy to see by day. Buoys are small. Jetée Est Oc R 4s 5m 6M. Jetée Ouest Fl G 4s 8m 6M.

RADIO TELEPHONE
None.

TELEPHONE
Hr Mr 33.54.08.29; Aff Mar 33.23.36.12; CROSS 33.52.72.13; SNSM 33.23.10.10; ⊞ 33.53.79.65; Meteo 33.53.53.44; Auto 36.68.08.50; Police 17; SAMU 15; Dr 33.54.00.02; Brit Consul 33.44.20.13.

FACILITIES
NW Quay (100 + 45 visitors), AB 37FF, M, Slip, L, D, FW, AC (long cable needed); **SC** ☎ 33.54.02.68.
Town Gaz, ME (Montfarville: 1km S), V, R, Bar, ✉, Ⓑ, bus to Cherbourg for ⇌ , ✈, Ferry.

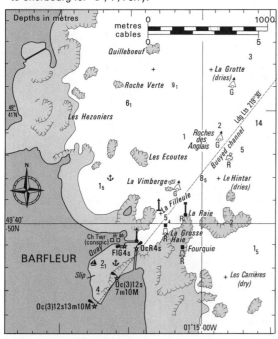

ST VAAST-LA-HOUGUE   10-19-10

Manche 49°35'·25N 01°15'·35W

CHARTS
AC 1349, *2613*; SHOM 7090, 6864, 7056; ECM 527, 528; Imray C32; Stanfords 1, 7

TIDES
–0240 Dover; ML 3·9; Duration 0530; Zone –0100

Standard Port CHERBOURG (←)

Times				Height (metres)			
High Water		Low Water		MHWS	MHWN	MLWN	MLWS
0300	1000	0400	1000	6·4	5·0	2·6	1·1
1500	2200	1600	2200				
Differences ST VAAST-LA-HOUGUE							
+0111	+0056	+0119	+0104	+0·2	+0·4	–0·3	–0·2

SHELTER
Excellent in marina, 2·3m; lock open HW–2¼ to HW+3. Ⓥ pontoons C and outer halves of D & E. Crowded in season. If full, or awaiting lock, ⚓ off in W sector of jetty lt between brgs of 330° and 350°, but untenable in strong E-S winds.

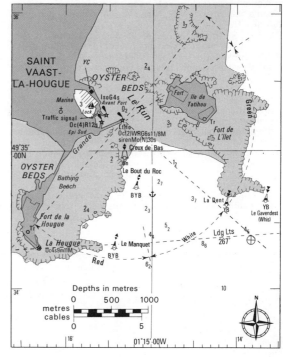

NAVIGATION
WPT 49°34'·40N 01°13'·78W, 130°/310° from/to main jetty lt (Oc 6s) 1·3M. Appr in W sector, leaving La Dent SCM By to stbd and Le Bout du Roc ECM By and Le Creux de Bas ECM bn to port. The ent is wide and well marked. Beware boats at ⚓, cross currents and oyster beds. "Le Run" appr is not advised and should not be attempted >1·2m draft.

LIGHTS AND MARKS
Do not confuse similar towers (conspic) on Ile de Tatihou and La Hougue Pte. From N, Pte de Saire Oc (2+1) 12s 11m 10M. From E, ldg lts 267°: front La Hougue Oc 4s 9m 10M; rear Morsalines Oc (3+1) WRG 12s 90m 11/8M in W sector. Main jetty hd lt, Oc (2) WRG 6s 12m 10/7M, W tr + R top, vis W310°-350°. R/G tfc sigs at lock ent.

RADIO TELEPHONE
VHF Ch 09.

TELEPHONE
Hr Mr 33.54.48.81, Fax 33.54.09.55; Aff Mar 33.54.43.61; ⊞ 33.44.16.00; CROSS 33.52.72.13; SNSM 33.54.42.52; Meteo 33.43.20.24; Auto 36.68.08.50; Police 33.54.23.11; Dr 33.54.43.42; Brit Consul 33.44.20.13.

FACILITIES
Marina (500 + 165 visitors) ☎ 33.54.48.81, FF96, Access HW –2¼ to +3, FW, C (25 ton), AC, D, P, BY, ME, El, Sh, Gaz, CH, Bar, R, 🅾, V, Slip; **Cercle Nautique de la Hougue** ☎ 33.54.55.73, Bar, R, C (3 ton), P, D, CH, FW, V.
Town P, D, V, Gaz, R, Bar, 🅾, ✉, Ⓑ, ⇌ (bus to Valognes), ✈. Ferry (Cherbourg).

19

CARENTAN/ISIGNY   10-19-11

Manche   Calvados

CHARTS
AC *2613*; SHOM 7056; ECM 527; Imray C32; Stanfords 1

TIDES
−0225 Dover; ML Rade de la Capelle 4·3; Duration 0510; Zone −0100

Standard Port CHERBOURG (←)

Use differences RADE DE LA CAPELLE 10.19.12
HW Carentan is HW Cherbourg +0100. See tidal graph for Carentan appr chan (facing page).

SHELTER
Temp ⚓ N of buoyed chans in winds <F5. Ent protected from prevailing S to W winds, but not advised in onshore winds >F5.
At **Carentan** complete shelter in the canal/river and in the locked marina (max/min depths 3·5/2·9m).
At **Isigny** drying pontoons on SW bank ¼M N of town.
In emergency the Iles St Marcouf, conspic 5M N, provide some shelter from NNE, N and W winds (see next col).

NAVIGATION
WPT CI SWM buoy, Iso 4s, 49°25'·30N 01°07'·10W, 034°/214° from/to ent to drying chan, 1·6M for **Carentan**; dep WPT at HW−2 to −1½. Chan is liable to vary in both depth and direction. Graph on facing page gives approx access times, using draft and tidal range at Cherbourg. Least water (drying 3·4m) reported between No 5b and 7 buoys. All buoys have R or G reflective panels; 5 are lit, Fl (3) 12s R/G. After about 4M the chan enters between 2 bkwtrs, marked by bns. 3·5M further on the chan divides into three, forming a small pool. Enter the lock ahead (opens HW −2 to HW +3, tfc sigs); waiting pontoons are on E side above and below lock. Lock-keeper will assign ♥ berth.
Isigny, dep WPT at HW −2½ heading about 150°/1·1M for IS unlit NCM buoy and ent to buoyed chan which is deeper than Carentan's.
Caution: The W end of the Baie de Seine is much affected by floating Sargassum weed; in hbrs from St Vaast to Grandcamp propeller fouling is commonplace.

LIGHTS AND MARKS
Carentan: Bkwtr outer bns are lit, Fl (3)R 12s and Fl (3)G 12s. Ldg Its: Front Oc (3)R 12s 6m 17M and rear Oc (3) 12s 14m 11M, lead 209°30' for 1·6M from the ends of the bkwtrs and immediately outside (not valid within the buoyed chan). From front ldg lt, lock is approx 3M.
Lock sigs: FG = lock open, FR = lock closed.
Isigny: Ldg Its, both Oc (2+1) 12s 7/19m 18M synch & intens 171°-175°, lead 173° for 1·9M between bkwtrs to front ldg lt. Here turn port into R l'Aure for ½M to town.

RADIO TELEPHONE
VHF Carentan Ch 09 (0800-1800LT & in lock opening hrs). Ch 09 also at Isigny (0800-2000).

TELEPHONE
Hr Mr Carentan 33.42.24.44; Lockmaster 33.71.10.85; Hr Mr Isigny 31.22.10.67; Aff Mar 33.44.00.13; ⌗ 33.44.16.00; CROSS 33.52.72.13; Auto 36.68.08.50; Police 33.42.00.17; Ⓗ 33.42.14.12; Dr 33.42.33.21; Brit Consul 33.44.20.13.

FACILITIES
CARENTAN:
Marina (220 + 50 visitors) ☎ 33.42.24.44, FF73, Access HW −2 to HW +3, FW, AC, P & D (0900-1000), Slip, C (50 ton), BH (16 ton);
YC Croiseurs Côtiers de Carentan ☎ 33.42.40.42, Bar;
Services: ME, El, Sh, CH, BY. **Town** Bar, Ⓑ, D, P, ✉, ⇌, R, V, ›› (Cherbourg). Ferry: Cherbourg.
ISIGNY
Quay AB (55+5), FW, AC, P, D, C (8 ton), Slip; **Club Nautique** AB, C, R, Bar; **Services**: ME, El, Sh. **Town** R, V, Bar, Ⓑ, ✉.

ADJACENT ANCHORAGE

ILES ST MARCOUF, Manche, 49°29'·70N 01°08'·70W. AC *2613*; SHOM 7056. Tides, see 10.19.12. The two islands, Ile de Terre and to the N, Ile du Large, look from afar like ships at ⚓. The former is a bird sanctuary and is closed to the public; the latter has a small dinghy hbr on the W side. ⚓ SW or SE of Ile du Large or SE or NE of the Ile de Terre. Ile du Large lt, VQ (3) 5s 18m 9M. Both islands are surrounded by drying rks, uninhabited and lack facilities.

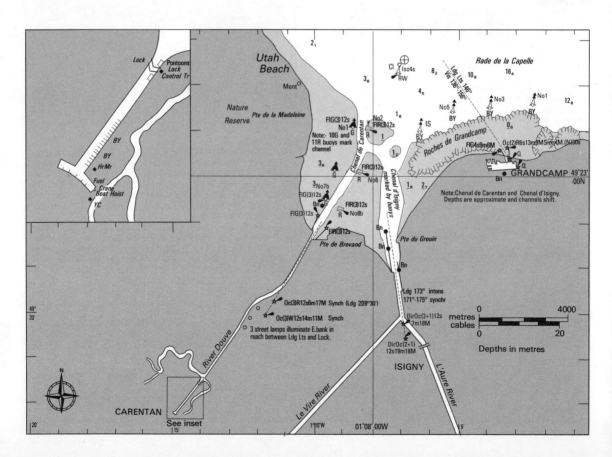

CARENTAN *continued*

CARENTAN TIDAL GRAPH

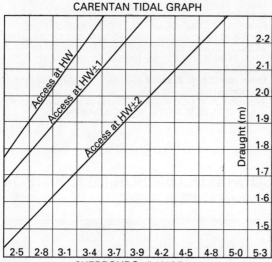

Caution: This graph, based on data from Port-Carentan, includes a safety clearance of 0·5m. Skippers may wish to add an additional margin to cater for depth variations due to shifting of the channel and/or meteorological conditions.

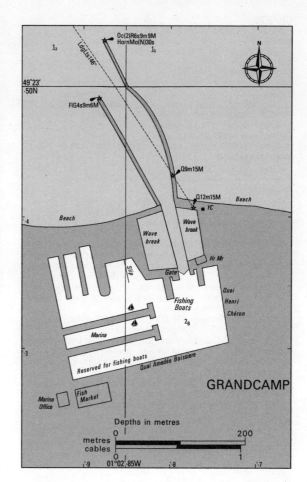

GRANDCAMP

GRANDCAMP-MAISY   10-19-12

Calvados 49°23'·50N 01°02'·87W

CHARTS
AC *2613*; SHOM 7056; ECM 527; Imray C32; Stanfords 1
TIDES
−0220 Dover; ML Rade de la Capelle 4·4; Duration 0510; Zone −0100

Standard Port CHERBOURG (←—)

Times				Height (metres)			
High Water		Low Water		MHWS	MHWN	MLWN	MLWS
0300	1000	0400	1000	6·4	5·0	2·6	1·1
1500	2200	1600	2200				
Differences RADE DE LA CAPELLE (3M to NW)							
+0116	+0052	+0128	+0115	+0·8	+0·9	+0·1	+0·2
ILES SAINT MARCOUF							
+0118	+0052	+0125	+0112	+0·6	+0·7	+0·1	+0·1

SHELTER
Access day & night, but difficult in NW to NE winds > F6. Safe appr sp HW ±2, nps HW ±1.5. Gate into wet basin, with marina to the W, opens at LW Dunkerque (10.19.29) and closes at HW Dunkerque, ie approx local HW ±2½. **Ⓥ** on N pontoon at E end. SW corner of basin is very dirty.
NAVIGATION
WPT 49°25'·00N 01°04'·60W, 326°/146° from/to front ldg lt 2·0M. Large flat rks, Les Roches de Grandcamp, extend about 1½M out from the hbr and dry approx 1·5m; heavy kelp cover can cause echosounders to under-read.
LIGHTS AND MARKS
3 NCM Bys, numbered 1, 3 and 5, mark the seaward limit of Les Roches de Grandcamp. Appr between Nos 3 & 5. E pier hd lt, Oc (2) R 6s, on a RW col. Ldg lts 146°: both Dir Q 9/12m 15M (vis 144·5°-147·5°). Two other ldg lts: Oc 4s 8/28m 12M, to E and S of hbr, lead 221°.

RADIO TELEPHONE
VHF Ch 09.
TELEPHONE
Hr Mr 31.22.63.16; Aff Mar 31.22.60.65; CROSS 33.52.72.13; SNSM 31.22.67.12; Meteo 21.33.25.26; Auto 36.68.08.14; Police 31.22.00.18; Dr 31.22.60.44; Ⓗ Bayeux 31.51.51.51; Brit Consul 35.42.27.47.
FACILITIES
Marina (268 + 25 visitors) ☎ 31.22.63.16, FF55, El, FW, BH (5 ton), Bar, V, AC; **Services:** ME, El, ✉, Sh, CH, Gaz, C. **Town** P & D (cans), Gaz, ✉, Ⓑ, ⇌ (Carentan), ✈ (Caen). Ferry: Cherbourg, Ouistreham.

ANCHORAGE BETWEEN PORT-EN-BESSIN AND COURSEULLES-SUR-MER

ARROMANCHES, Manche, 49°21'·80N 00°37'·20W. AC *2613*; SHOM 6927. HW is −0040 on Le Havre; see Port-en-Bessin (10.19.13). Strictly a fair weather ⚓, with little shelter from the WW II Mulberry caissons which are conspic esp at LW. Rocher du Calvados dries 1·6m, 7ca ENE of ent. There are many wrecks offshore; 3 to the W and N are marked by a WCM and two ECM buoys. The most N'ly ECM buoy (Roseberry, 49°23'·2N 00°36'·1W) bears approx 025°/1·5M from the ent (lat/long as line 1) which is marked by a small unlit PHM and SHM buoy. Enter on about 245° for ⚓ in 3m to S of the caissons, or sound closer inshore. Caution rky plateau off the beach and obstructions to SE of ent, marked by four W buoys. Facilities: **YC Port Winston** ☎ 31.22.31.01, 2 slips (dinghies).

19

PORT-EN-BESSIN   10-19-13

Calvados 49°21'·22N 00°45'·40W

CHARTS
AC 2613; SHOM 7056; ECM 527; Imray C32; Stanfords 1
TIDES
−0215 Dover; ML 4·4; Duration 0520; Zone −0100

Standard Port LE HAVRE (⟶)

Times				Height (metres)			
High Water		Low Water		MHWS	MHWN	MLWN	MLWS
0000	0500	0000	0700	7·9	6·6	3·0	1·2
1200	1700	1200	1900				
Differences PORT-EN-BESSIN							
−0043	−0039	−0039	−0046	−0·7	−0·7	−0·4	−0·1
ARROMANCHES							
−0044	−0036	−0036	−0039	−0·4	−0·4	−0·1	0·0

SHELTER
Good in 2nd basin; outer hbr dries completely. There is little room for yachts. Basins accessible HW ±2. Contact Hr Mr on arrival. Waiting berths on Quai de L'Epi.
NAVIGATION
WPT 49°22'·00N 00°44'·90W, 024°/204° from/to front ldg lt 204°, 1·1M. ⌕ prohib in outer hbr and 1ca either side of 204° transit. Busy fishing port. Yachts may stay for up to 24 hrs. Ent is difficult with strong N/NE winds and >F8 it is dangerous. Beware submerged jetty (marked by R bn) to port of ent chan. Keep out of G sector of Mole Ouest lt.
LIGHTS AND MARKS
Ldg lts 204°: Front Oc (3) 12s 25m 10M, W pylon, G top, vis 069°-339°; Siren 20s (sounded over 90° each side of ldg line, continuous in W sector, interrupted in E sector); rear, Oc (3) 12s 42m 11M, W and grey house; vis 114°-294°, synch with front; RC. Other lts as chartlet; inner pier hds are Oc (2) R 6s and Fl (2) G 6s.
Entry sigs: Ⓡ over Ⓖ, or R over G flags = basins closed. Bridge has FR lt each side, and FR in the middle when shut. Lock opens HW ±2. When lock open, bridge opens whenever possible to suit yachts and FVs.

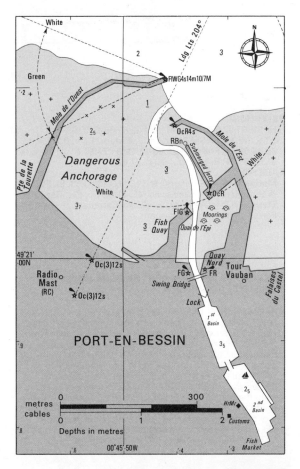

RADIO TELEPHONE
VHF Ch 18 (HW ±2) for lock opening.
TELEPHONE
Hr Mr 31.21.70.49; Aff Mar 31.21.71.52; ⌗ 31.21.71.09; CROSS 33.52.72.13; Semaphore/SNSM 31.21.81.51; Auto 36.68.08.14; Lock 31.21.71.77; Police 31.21.70.10; Dr 31.21.74.26; Ⓗ 31.51.51.51; Brit Consul 35.42.27.47.
FACILITIES
Outer Hbr Slip, L; **Bassin II** Slip, M, L, FW, AB, C (4 ton); **Services:** CH, El, Ⓔ, ME, Sh.
Town P, AB, V, Gaz, R, Bar, ⊠, Ⓑ, ⇌ (bus to Bayeux), ✈ (Caen, ☎ 31.26.58.00). Ferry: See Ouistreham.

COURSEULLES-SUR-MER 10-19-14

Calvados 49°20'·48N 00°27'·27W

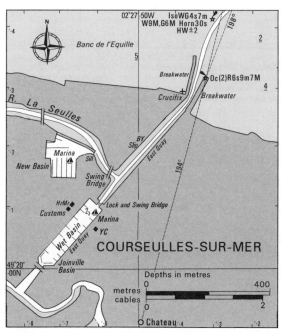

CHARTS
AC 1349, 2613; SHOM 5598, 6927; ECM 526, 527; Imray C32; Stanfords 1
TIDES
−0300 Dover; ML 4·6; Duration No data; Zone −0100

Standard Port LE HAVRE (⟶)

Times				Height (metres)			
High Water		Low Water		MHWS	MHWN	MLWN	MLWS
0000	0500	0000	0700	7·9	6·6	3·0	1·2
1200	1700	1200	1900				
Differences COURSEULLES-SUR-MER							
−0025	−0015	−0020	−0025	−0·5	−0·5	−0·2	−0·1

SHELTER
Good except in strong W to NE winds. Avant Port dries 2·5m; best entry is at HW −1. Lock into Bassin Joinville (3m) opens HW ±2. Alternatively consider New Basin marina (2m), if LOA <9m; cross sill (dries 3m) HW ±3. Swing bridges to both marinas open on request.
NAVIGATION
WPT 49°22'·00N 00°28'·70W, 314°/134° from/to landfall By SWM Iso 4s, 1.0M. Plateau du Calvados extends 2M seaward and banks dry for 0.6M. Outer ldg marks: front Bernières-sur-mer church tr on with La Delivrande church twin spires (partly obscd by trees), lead 134° close to landfall buoy. Beware rks awash at CD either side of ldg line. Maintain 134° for 0.55M until ent bears 198°.

COURSEULLES *continued*

LIGHTS AND MARKS
W bkwtr lt, Iso WG 4s 7m 9/6M (stay in W sector); also marked by SHM bns and conspic crucifix at root. E bkwtr marked by PHM bns and Oc (2) R 6s 9m 7M at root. This lt in transit with Chateau (conspic) leads 194° to hbr ent.

RADIO TELEPHONE
VHF Ch 09, 0900-1200LT and HW±3.

TELEPHONE
Hr Mr 31.37.51.69; Control tr 31.37.46.03; Aff Mar 31.37.46.19; CROSS 33.52.72.13; SNSM 31.37.45.47; ⌗ West Quai, no ☎; Météo 31.26.28.11; Auto 36.68.08.14; Police 31.37.07.13; Dr 31.37.45.24; Brit Consul 35.42.27.47

FACILITIES
Joinville Basin ☎ 31.37.51.69, FF100, Slip, P & D (cans), FW, AC, Sh, C (10 ton), CH; **Marina** (New Basin) ☎ 31.37.46.03, P, D, FW, ME, EI, Sh; **Sté des Régates de Courseulles** ☎ 31.37.47.42, Bar. **Services:** BY, ME, EI, Ⓔ, Sh, CH, M, SM. **Town** P, D, V, Gaz, R, Bar, ✉, Ⓑ, ⇌ (bus to Caen), ✈ (Caen). Ferry: See Ouistreham.

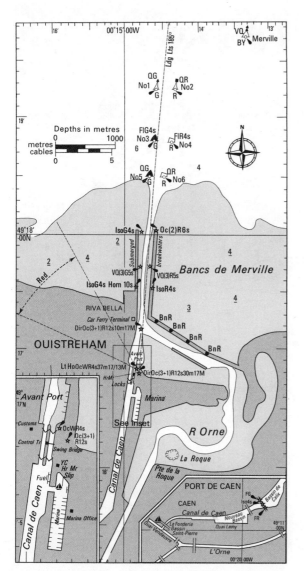

OUISTREHAM   10-19-15
Calvados 49°16'·88N 00°14'·81W (E lock)

CHARTS
AC 1349, *2613*; SHOM 7055, 6927, 6928; ECM 526; Imray C32; Stanfords 1

TIDES
−0118 Dover; ML 4·6; Duration 0525; Zone −0100

Standard Port LE HAVRE (→)

Times				Height (metres)			
High Water		Low Water		MHWS	MHWN	MLWN	MLWS
0000	0500	0000	0700	7·9	6·6	3·0	1·2
1200	1700	1200	1900				
Differences OUISTREHAM							
−0007	−0007	−0005	−0005	−0·3	−0·3	−0·3	−0·3

Note: There is a double HW at Ouistreham (also at Dives and Trouville). The HW differences, when referred to the start of the stand at Le Havre, give the time of the first HW.

SHELTER
Very good in marina (depth 3·5m and access HW±3), 1ca S of locks on E side. Waiting pontoon on E of Avant Port.

NAVIGATION
WPT ECM buoy, VQ (3) 5s, 49° 20'·48N 00° 14'·73W, 352°/172° from/to No 1 & 2 buoys, 1·26M. Training walls, with bns, mark the ent chan. Enter canal by locks either side of control tr; yachts normally use E lock. Beware turbulence in locks. Lock opens for arrivals at HW−2½*, −1½, +2¼ and +3¼* ; and for departures at HW−3, −2, +1¾ and +2¾*. * denotes extra openings (0700–2000LT) mid Jun-mid Sep; also at weekends and public hols only, from 1 Apr-mid Jun and mid Sep-31 Oct.

LIGHTS AND MARKS
From WPT, pick up ldg lts 185°, both Dir Oc (3+1) R 12s 10/30m 17M, synch, intens 183·5°–186·5°. Chan has lt bys. Main lt ho, W + R top, conspic, Oc WR 4s 37m 17/13M. IPTS (full code) shown from control tr. Yachts may only enter when Ⓦ shows to port or stbd of lowest main tfc lt, indicating E or W lock. Three Fl R 4s on waiting pontoon.

RADIO TELEPHONE
Call *Ouistreham Port* VHF Ch **68** 16; Lock Ch 12 68 (HW −2 to HW +3). Sté des Régates Ch 09 (office hours).

TELEPHONE
Hr Mr/Lock 31.97.14.43; Port de Plaisance 31.97.13.05; Aff Mar 31.97.18.65; CROSS 33.52.72.13; SNSM 31.97.14.43; Ferry terminal 31.96.80.80; ⌗ 31.86.61.50; Météo 31.26.68.11; Auto 36.68.08.14; Police 31.97.13.15; Dr 31.97.18.45; Brit Consul 35.42.27.47; Taxi 31.97.35.67.

FACILITIES
Marina (600 + 65 visitors) ☎ 31.97.13.05, FF130, Slip, FW, ME, EI, Sh, CH, AC, BH (8 ton), Gas, Gaz, Kos, SM, Bar, P, D, (Fuel pumps open ½hr before outbound lock opening); **Société des Régates de Caen-Ouistreham** (SRCO) ☎ 31.97.13.05, FW, ME, EI, Sh, CH, V, Bar; **Services:** BY, Sh, EI, Ⓔ, ME, CH, SM, SHOM. **Town** V, Gaz, R, Bar, ✉, Ⓑ, ⇌ (bus to Caen), ✈ (Caen). Ferry: to Portsmouth. (May-Sept, also to Poole).

CAEN 49°11'·03N 00°21'·13W.

Passage and Facilities:
The 8M canal passage is simple and takes approx 1¾hrs. Bridges will open free for yachts which transit at the posted times; at other times fees (at least FF81) are due. Daily transit times are posted at the SRCO YC: S-bound is usually pm and N-bound am. It is important to be *at the first bridge* at/before the posted transit time; allow ½hr from Ouistreham to Pegasus bridge. Depths 2·5m to 10m; max speed 7kn; transit only permitted by day; no overtaking. Outbound vessels have right of way. Keep listening watch on Ch 68.
Four moving bridges at: Bénouville (Pegasus) (2½M from locks), Colombelles (5M), Calix (6½M) and La Fonderie (8M); each shows Ⓖ when passage clear.
Turn stbd after La Fonderie bridge for marina at Bassin St Pierre in city centre. VHF *Caen Port* Ch 12 68. Hr Mr ☎ 31.52.12.88; Aff Mar ☎ 31.85.40.55; ⌗ ☎ 31.86.61.50; Facilities: **Marina** (64 visitors) ☎ 31.95.24.47, FF80, P & D (cans), ME, Sh, EI, AB, FW; **Services:** ME, EI, Sh, SM, CH. **City** Ⓑ, Bar, Ⓗ, ✉, R, V, ⇌, ✈ (Carpiquet).

19

DIVES-SUR-MER   10-19-16
Calvados 49°17'·86N 00°05'·13W

CHARTS
AC 2146; SHOM 6928; ECM 526; Imray C32; Stanfords 1
TIDES
−0135 Dover; ML 5·1m; Duration; Zone −0100

Standard Port LE HAVRE (→)

Times				Height (metres)			
High Water		Low Water		MHWS	MHWN	MLWN	MLWS
0000	0500	0000	0700	7·9	6·6	3·0	1·2
1200	1700	1200	1900				

Differences DIVES-SUR-MER

−0020	−0010	0000	0000	+0·3	+0·2	+0·1	0·0

Note: There is a double HW at Dives (also at Ouistreham and Trouville). The HW differences, when referred to the start of the stand at Le Havre, give the time of the first HW.

SHELTER
Good, but appr dries to 1M offshore and can be difficult in NW/NE > F5. Marina ent 400m W of Dir lt, off shallow R La Dives. Access HW±3 (HW±2½ for draft >1·5m) via single gate. Sill below gate is 2·5m above CD; gate opens when tide 4·5m above CD. Or follow river chan to berth on YC pontoon (2 🟦) below footbridge (max draft 1·5m).
NAVIGATION
WPT 49°18'·78N 00°05'·67W, Landfall buoy "DI", L Fl 10s, 339°/159° from/to No 1 and 2 Bys, 4ca. (Note: buoy "DI" is off chartlet). Two waiting Bys (untenable in WNW F4) are reported close to WPT in 3m. Beware sandbanks (drying 4·2m) each side of buoyed chan; keep well clear of two large SHM bns on W side. After last chan buoys, hug the shore to G (R horiz band) Division buoy and 4 G perches marking submerged training wall leading to marina ent.
LIGHTS AND MARKS
By day ent is seen at W end of densely wooded hills behind Houlgate.
Dir lt 159° Oc (2+1) WRG 12s 7m 12/9M, R hut opposite Pte de Cabourg, vis G125°-157°, W157°-162°, R162°-194°. W sector covers chan only up to Nos 3/4 marks; thence follow the chan buoys/bns. 4 PHM and 2 SHM buoys, all unlit, are moved to suit shifting chan; Nos 3 and 5 SHMs are bns, lit QG 12m 4M and Fl G 4s 13m 4M respectively. Close E of marina ent a Division buoy, IQG (2+1), indicates preferred chan to port and marks shoals to N. Caution: Buoys/bns may not be numbered; positions are approximate due to the lack of large-scale charts.
RADIO TELEPHONE
VHF Ch 09, H24.
TELEPHONE
Hr Mr 31.24.48.00; CROSS 35.52.72.13; Meteo = via Hr Mr; Auto 36.68.08.14; Police 31.24.85.00; Dr 31.91.05.44.

FACILITIES
Marina (Port Guillaume) (545+55 visitors) ☎ 31.24.48.00, Fax 31.24.73.02, AC, FW, P, D, 🅟, Slip, BH (30 ton); C (1·5 ton); **Cabourg YC** ☎ 31.91.23.55, Bar; **Services:** BY, ME, EI, CH, Sh.
Town V, R, Bar, Ⓑ, ✉, ✈ (Deauville). Ferry: Ouistreham.

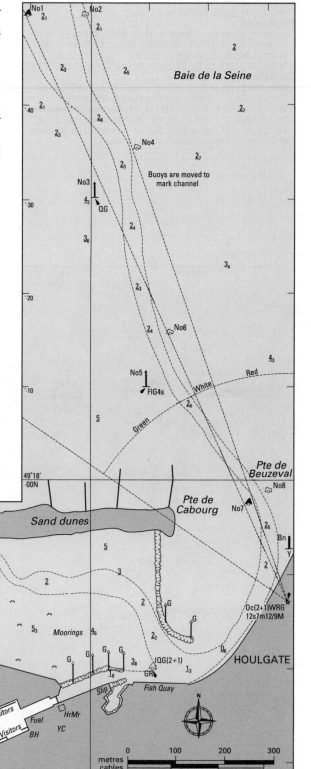

DEAUVILLE/TROUVILLE   10-19-17
Calvados 49°22'·44N 00°04'·23E

CHARTS
AC 1349, 2146, *2613*; SHOM 6928, 6736; ECM 526, 1012; Imray C32; Stanfords 1

TIDES
−0130 Dover; ML 5·1; Duration 0510; Zone −0100

Standard Port LE HAVRE (→)

Times				Height (metres)			
High Water		Low Water		MHWS	MHWN	MLWN	MLWS
0000	0500	0000	0700	7·9	6·6	3·0	1·2
1200	1700	1200	1900				
Differences TROUVILLE							
−0033	−0013	−0002	−0010	−0·2	−0·2	−0·2	−0·1

Note: There is a double HW at Trouville (also at Ouistreham and Dives). The HW differences, when referred to the start of the stand at Le Havre, give the time of the first HW.

SHELTER
Good in marina and Yacht Hbr, but ent to chan difficult in NW/N winds > force 6. Chan and river dry 2·4m; no access LW±2½, for 2m draft. Marina lock opens H24, if enough water outside. Yacht Hbr gate open HW −2 to HW +2½.

NAVIGATION
WPT 49°23'·00N 00°03'·70E, 328°/148° from/toW bkwtr lt Fl WG 4s, 0·65M. Semoy ECM, VQ (3) 5s, marks wreck 2·2M from ent, on ldg line. Do not appr from E of N due to Les Ratelets and Banc de Trouville. Trouville SW buoy, WCM, VQ (9) 10s, is 1M WNW of ent.

LIGHTS AND MARKS
Casino is conspic on Trouville side. Ldg lts 148°, both Oc R 4s synch. Yacht Hbr ent sigs (vert): 3 Ⓡ = closed; 3 Ⓖ = passage one way; 2 Ⓖ over Ⓦ = passage both ways.

RADIO TELEPHONE
Marina and Yacht Hbr VHF Ch 09.

TELEPHONE
Hr Mr Marina 31.98.30.01; Marina lock 31.8895.96; Hr Mr Yacht Hbr 31.98.50.40; Yacht Hbr lock 31.88.36.21; Aff Mar 31.88.36.21; SNSM 31.89.28.09; CROSS 33.52.72.13; ⌗ 31.88.35.29; Auto (local) 36.68.08.14; Auto (regional) 36.68.08.76; Police 31.88.13.07; Dr 31.88.23.57; Ⓗ 31.88.14.00; Brit Consul 35.42.27.47.

FACILITIES
Port Deauville (Marina) (800 + 100 visitors) ☎ 31.98.30.01, Fax 31.88.70.55, FF106, D, AC, FW, ME, El, Sh, C (6 ton), BH (45 ton), Slip, CH, SM, R, Bar; **Deauville Marina Club**.
Yacht Hbr (320+80 visitors) ☎ 31.98.50.40, FF97, FW, AC, Slip, D (pump S end of Bassin Morny), P (cans, 20m); **Deauville YC** ☎ 31.88.38.19, L, FW, C (8 ton), AB, CH, Bar; **Services:** CH, ME, El, Sh.
Both towns P (cans), V, Gaz, R, Bar, ✉, Ⓑ, BY, CH, Slip, Sh, ME, El, Ⓔ, ⇌, ✈ Deauville. Ferry: See Le Havre and Ouistreham.

22·5

Ldg Lts 148°

White ✦ FIWG4s 12/9M Green

G

G

G

2·4

✦ Fl(4)WR12s8m7/4M Red

1·5

G

G

✦ IsoG4s 5M

G

Dredged 1m above CD

Recommended Course R

R

R

R

QG

Obsc. Red OcR4s12MHorn(2)30s

Diesel

Boat Lift 45T

Lock

Visitors 3

YC

49°22' ·00N

HrMr

Wooden Piers

Oc R 4s vis 120°-170°

TROUVILLE

YC(CNTH)

N

metres
cables

0   200

0   1

Depths in metres

Casino (Conspic)

Fish Quay

Slip

PORT-DEAUVILLE (MARINA)

Slip

Gate

La Touques

Yacht Harbour

Hr Mr

DEAUVILLE

Bassin Morny

Slip

Club House DYC

Co

00°04'·50E

0°5'

19

HONFLEUR 10-19-18

Calvados 49° 25'·75N 00° 13'·93E

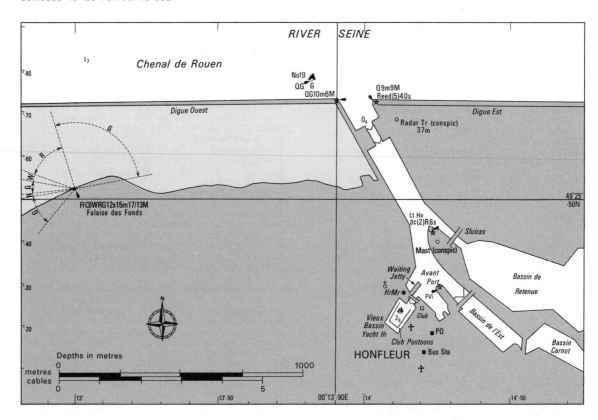

CHARTS
AC 2994, 2146, *2613*; SHOM 6796, 6683; ECM 1012; Imray C31; Stanfords 1

TIDES
−0135 Dover; ML 5·1; Duration 0540; Zone −0100

Standard Port LE HAVRE (→)

Times				Height (metres)			
High Water		Low Water		MHWS	MHWN	MLWN	MLW
0000	0500	0000	0700	7·9	6·6	3·0	1·2
1200	1700	1200	1900				

Differences HONFLEUR

| −0138 | −0137 | +0006 | +0040 | −0·1 | −0·2 | −0·1 | +0·2 |

There is a HW stand of about 2hrs 50 mins. Differences are for the beginning of the stand.

SHELTER
Excellent in the Vieux Bassin. Visitors raft on pontoon at NW quay. Ask YC if hoping to berth on YC finger pontoons. Larger yachts can enter Bassin de l'Est; see Hr Mr.

NAVIGATION
WPT Ratier NW SHM buoy, VQG, 49°26'·63N, 00°03'·41E, at ent to well buoyed Chenal de Rouen. Appr at HW ±3, keeping between the Digue Nord, marked by posts, and the PHM chan buoys to avoid shipping. Ent between No 19 SHM buoy and very conspic radar tr. Beware strong currents across ent.

The **outer lock** (fitted with recessed bollards and ladders, but no pontoons) operates H24 and is open at H, every hour for arrivals; and every H+30 for departures. Access H24 for 1·5m draft; but for 2m draft no access LW±1.

At the Vieux Bassin the old lock gate is permanently open. The **road bridge** lifts as shown below (LT). Note these times were on trial in 1995, and may change in 1996. Yachts leaving have priority over arrivals.

Mid season (1 Mar-31 May; 16 Sept-31 Oct)
Weekdays: 0730, 1030, 1530, 1830.
Sat/Sun/Hols: 0730, 0830, 0930, 1030, 1730, 1830, 1930, 2030.

High Season (1 Jun-15 Sept)
Every day: same as Sat/Sun/National holidays in mid-season.

Low season (1 Nov-28 Feb)
Weekdays: as mid season.
Sat/Sun/Hols: 0730, 0830, 0930, 1030, 1530, 1630, 1730, 1830.

LIGHTS AND MARKS
Falaise des Fonds lt, 0·75M W of ent Fl (3) WRG 12s 15m, 17/13M, W □ tr, vis G040°-080°, R080°-084°, G0084°-100°, W100°-109°, R109°-162°, G162°-260°. E mole Q 9m 9M, Y metal framework tr with B top, Reed (5) 40s. W mole QG 10m 6M, G framework tr.

Traffic signals (all vert, from the top) at lock:

3 ⓡ	=	Closed; no passage
3 ⓖ	=	One way passage
ⓖⓖⓦ	=	Two way passage
ⓖⓦⓖ	=	Passage only allowed with special instructions.

Note: The new Pont de Normandie, 1·7M E of Honfleur ent, has 52m clearance and a pile lt, Fl Y 2·5s 3m, on N side of chan.

RADIO TELEPHONE
VHF Ch **73** 11 12 16 (H24).

TELEPHONE
Hr Mr 31.89.20.02, Fax 31.89.42.10; Lock 31.89.22.57; Aff Mar 31.89.20.67; CROSS 33.52.72.13; SNSM 31.88.11.13; Auto (regional) 36.68.08.76; Auto (offshore) 36.68.08.08; ⌗ 31.89.12.13; Police 31.89.21.24; Dr 31.89.34.05; Ⓗ 31.89.07.74; Brit Consul 35.42.27.47.

FACILITIES
Vieux Bassin Yacht Hbr (120+30 visitors, max LOA 20m) ☎ 31.89.01.85, AB, FW, AC; **Cercle Nautique d'Honfleur** ☎ 31.89.87.13, M; **Services:** BY, Sh, Ⓔ, C (10 ton), Slip.
Town P & D (cans), V, R, Bar, ⊘, Gaz, ✉, Ⓑ, ⇌, ✈
Deauville. Ferry: Le Havre.

TIME ZONE –0100
(French Standard Time)
Subtract 1 hour for UT
For French Summer Time add ONE hour in non-shaded areas

FRANCE – LE HAVRE

LAT 49°29′N   LONG 0°07′E

TIMES AND HEIGHTS OF HIGH AND LOW WATERS   YEAR **1996**

JANUARY

Day		Time	m	Time	m	Time	m	Time	m
1	M	0136	2.8	0728	6.8	1417	2.7	2000	6.7
2	TU	0242	2.7	0827	7.0	1518	2.5	2055	6.9
3	W	0339	2.5	0914	7.2	1610	2.2	2139	7.1
4	TH	0427	2.2	0952	7.3	1654	1.9	2217	7.3
5	F	0509	2.0	1027	7.5	1733	1.7	O 2251	7.4
6	SA	0548	1.9	1059	7.6	1810	1.6	2324	7.5
7	SU	0624	1.8	1132	7.6	1845	1.6	2357	7.5
8	M	0656	1.8	1205	7.6	1917	1.6		
9	TU	0031	7.5	0729	1.8	1238	7.6	1948	1.6
10	W	0104	7.4	0800	1.9	1311	7.5	2020	1.8
11	TH	0139	7.3	0834	2.0	1348	7.3	2052	2.0
12	F	0217	7.1	0908	2.2	1427	7.1	2127	2.2
13	SA	0258	7.0	0949	2.5	1512	6.9	2210	2.5
14	SU	0347	6.8	1038	2.7	1606	6.7	2305	2.7
15	M	0450	6.7	1141	2.8	1721	6.6		
16	TU	0017	2.7	0613	6.8	1300	2.7	1849	6.7
17	W	0143	2.6	0727	7.0	1426	2.3	2001	7.0
18	TH	0301	2.1	0830	7.4	1537	1.8	2103	7.4
19	F	0407	1.7	0927	7.7	1640	1.3	2159	7.8
20	SA	0508	1.3	1019	8.0	1740	0.9	● 2250	8.0
21	SU	0606	1.0	1109	8.2	1834	0.6	2339	8.1
22	M	0657	0.8	1157	8.3	1923	0.5		
23	TU	0026	8.2	0743	0.8	1243	8.2	2005	0.6
24	W	0111	8.0	0825	1.0	1327	8.0	2045	0.9
25	TH	0154	7.8	0903	1.3	1410	7.7	2120	1.4
26	F	0236	7.5	0939	1.8	1453	7.4	2151	1.9
27	SA	0319	7.1	1016	2.3	1540	7.0	2229	2.4
28	SU	0409	6.8	1102	2.7	1638	6.6	2320	2.9
29	M	0515	6.5	1204	3.1	1756	6.3		
30	TU	0036	3.2	0639	6.4	1325	3.1	1926	6.3
31	W	0158	3.1	0756	6.6	1441	2.8	2032	6.6

FEBRUARY

Day		Time	m	Time	m	Time	m	Time	m
1	TH	0308	2.8	0850	6.8	1543	2.5	2119	6.9
2	F	0404	2.4	0932	7.1	1633	2.1	2157	7.1
3	SA	0451	2.1	1006	7.3	1716	1.8	2231	7.3
4	SU	0532	1.8	1040	7.5	1754	1.5	O 2304	7.5
5	M	0608	1.6	1113	7.6	1828	1.4	2337	7.6
6	TU	0640	1.5	1146	7.7	1900	1.3		
7	W	0010	7.6	0712	1.4	1219	7.7	1931	1.3
8	TH	0043	7.6	0744	1.5	1253	7.7	2003	1.4
9	F	0118	7.6	0817	1.6	1329	7.6	2035	1.6
10	SA	0154	7.4	0850	1.8	1406	7.4	2108	1.8
11	SU	0231	7.2	0926	2.1	1446	7.1	2145	2.2
12	M	0314	7.0	1009	2.4	1536	6.9	2233	2.5
13	TU	0411	6.8	1107	2.6	1648	6.6	2341	2.8
14	W	0537	6.7	1226	2.7	1825	6.6		
15	TH	0113	2.7	0704	6.9	1401	2.4	1945	6.9
16	F	0241	2.3	0814	7.2	1519	1.9	2052	7.3
17	SA	0352	1.7	0915	7.6	1628	1.3	2148	7.7
18	SU	0458	1.3	1007	7.8	1729	0.9	● 2237	8.0
19	M	0555	0.9	1055	8.1	1825	0.6	2323	8.1
20	TU	0643	0.7	1140	8.2	1906	0.5		
21	W	0006	8.1	0725	0.7	1223	8.2	1945	0.6
22	TH	0047	8.1	0802	0.8	1304	8.1	2019	0.9
23	F	0126	7.9	0835	1.2	1343	7.8	2050	1.3
24	SA	0203	7.5	0906	1.6	1421	7.4	2114	1.9
25	SU	0239	7.2	0936	2.1	1501	7.0	2149	2.4
26	M	0320	6.7	1012	2.7	1550	6.5	2231	2.9
27	TU	0417	6.4	1009	3.1	1703	6.2	2335	3.3
28	W	0541	6.2	1225	3.3	1840	6.1		
29	TH	0108	3.4	0714	6.2	1357	3.1	1959	6.3

MARCH

Day		Time	m	Time	m	Time	m	Time	m
1	F	0232	3.0	0819	6.5	1509	2.7	2051	6.7
2	SA	0336	2.5	0904	6.9	1605	2.2	2130	7.0
3	SU	0426	2.1	0941	7.2	1651	1.8	2205	7.3
4	M	0509	1.7	1015	7.5	1731	1.5	2239	7.5
5	TU	0546	1.5	1050	7.6	1806	1.3	O 2313	7.7
6	W	0619	1.3	1124	7.8	1838	1.1	2347	7.7
7	TH	0651	1.2	1159	7.8	1911	1.1		
8	F	0021	7.8	0726	1.1	1234	7.8	1944	1.1
9	SA	0056	7.8	0759	1.2	1311	7.7	2017	1.3
10	SU	0133	7.6	0834	1.4	1350	7.5	2051	1.6
11	M	0211	7.4	0909	1.7	1431	7.2	2127	2.0
12	TU	0254	7.1	0951	2.1	1521	6.9	2215	2.4
13	W	0351	6.8	1046	2.5	1636	6.6	2322	2.7
14	TH	0519	6.6	1206	2.6	1813	6.6		
15	F	0056	2.7	0648	6.8	1344	2.4	1933	6.9
16	SA	0227	2.3	0800	7.1	1504	1.9	2039	7.3
17	SU	0340	1.8	0901	7.5	1614	1.4	2133	7.7
18	M	0445	1.3	0951	7.8	1714	0.9	2219	7.9
19	TU	0538	0.9	1037	8.0	1802	0.7	● 2302	8.0
20	W	0623	0.8	1120	8.1	1843	0.6	2343	8.1
21	TH	0701	0.7	1200	8.1	1919	0.7		
22	F	0021	8.0	0736	0.9	1239	8.0	1950	1.0
23	SA	0057	7.8	0807	1.2	1316	7.7	2019	1.4
24	SU	0132	7.6	0857	1.6	1353	7.4	2044	1.9
25	M	0206	7.2	0902	2.0	1429	7.0	2114	2.4
26	TU	0241	6.9	0934	2.5	1512	6.6	2151	2.9
27	W	0328	6.4	1020	3.0	1614	6.2	2249	3.3
28	TH	0443	6.1	1132	3.3	1748	6.0		
29	F	0019	3.5	0619	6.1	1303	3.2	1911	6.2
30	SA	0145	3.2	0733	6.3	1422	2.8	2010	6.6
31	SU	0254	2.7	0826	6.7	1523	2.3	2055	7.0

APRIL

Day		Time	m	Time	m	Time	m	Time	m
1	M	0349	2.2	0908	7.1	1614	1.9	2133	7.3
2	TU	0435	1.8	0946	7.4	1657	1.5	2209	7.5
3	W	0515	1.5	1023	7.6	1736	1.3	2245	7.7
4	TH	0552	1.2	1059	7.8	1812	1.1	O 2321	7.8
5	F	0628	1.0	1136	7.9	1848	1.0	2357	7.9
6	SA	0705	0.9	1215	7.9	1924	1.0		
7	SU	0035	7.9	0742	1.0	1255	7.8	2000	1.2
8	M	0114	7.7	0819	1.2	1337	7.6	2036	1.5
9	TU	0156	7.5	0857	1.5	1422	7.3	2116	1.9
10	W	0242	7.2	0940	1.9	1516	7.0	2205	2.3
11	TH	0342	6.9	1037	2.3	1632	6.7	2314	2.6
12	F	0507	6.7	1201	2.5	1801	6.7		
13	SA	0045	2.6	0631	6.8	1328	2.3	1917	7.0
14	SU	0210	2.3	0742	7.1	1445	1.9	2021	7.3
15	M	0321	1.8	0842	7.4	1553	1.5	2113	7.6
16	TU	0424	1.4	0932	7.6	1650	1.2	2158	7.8
17	W	0515	1.1	1016	7.8	1736	1.0	● 2239	7.9
18	TH	0557	1.0	1058	7.9	1815	1.0	2318	7.9
19	F	0634	1.0	1137	7.9	1849	1.1	2355	7.8
20	SA	0707	1.1	1215	7.8	1920	1.2		
21	SU	0030	7.7	0738	1.3	1252	7.6	1950	1.5
22	M	0104	7.5	0808	1.6	1328	7.3	2017	1.9
23	TU	0138	7.2	0836	1.9	1404	7.0	2047	2.3
24	W	0212	6.9	0906	2.3	1443	6.7	2122	2.7
25	TH	0252	6.6	0946	2.7	1533	6.3	2212	3.1
26	F	0348	6.2	1046	3.0	1649	6.2	2324	3.3
27	SA	0514	6.1	1205	3.1	1816	6.2		
28	SU	0048	3.2	0637	6.2	1323	2.9	1920	6.5
29	M	0158	2.8	0738	6.6	1429	2.5	2012	6.9
30	TU	0258	2.3	0828	6.9	1525	2.0	2055	7.2

19

Chart Datum: 4·72 metres below Lallemand System (Mean Sea Level, Marseilles)

TIME ZONE –0100
(French Standard Time)
Subtract 1 hour for UT
For French Summer Time add ONE hour in non-shaded areas

FRANCE – LE HAVRE

LAT 49°29′N   LONG 0°07′E

TIMES AND HEIGHTS OF HIGH AND LOW WATERS

YEAR **1996**

MAY

#	Time	m	#	Time	m
1 W	0350 0911 1614 2136	1.9 7.2 1.4 7.5	**16** TH	0446 0956 1705 2217	1.5 7.5 1.5 7.7
2 TH	0437 0952 1700 2215	1.6 7.5 1.4 7.7	**17** F ●	0528 1038 1744 2255	1.4 7.6 1.4 7.7
3 F O	0521 1033 1743 2254	1.3 7.7 1.2 7.8	**18** SA	0606 1116 1819 2330	1.3 7.6 1.4 7.7
4 SA	0604 1114 1825 2334	1.0 7.8 1.0 7.9	**19** SU	0640 1153 1853	1.3 7.6 1.5
5 SU	0646 1157 1906	0.9 7.9 1.0	**20** M	0005 0713 1230 1925	7.6 1.4 7.5 1.7
6 M	0016 0728 1241 1947	7.9 0.9 7.8 1.1	**21** TU	0040 0745 1306 1954	7.5 1.6 7.3 1.9
7 TU	0059 0808 1327 2028	7.8 1.0 7.7 1.4	**22** W	0114 0815 1342 2027	7.3 1.8 7.1 2.2
8 W	0145 0851 1416 2112	7.6 1.3 7.4 1.8	**23** TH	0148 0846 1418 2101	7.1 2.1 6.8 2.5
9 TH	0235 0937 1512 2204	7.4 1.7 7.1 2.2	**24** F	0224 0921 1500 2142	6.8 2.4 6.6 2.8
10 F	0335 1034 1624 2310	7.1 2.0 6.9 2.4	**25** SA	0310 1007 1553 2238	6.6 2.7 6.4 3.0
11 SA	0451 1147 1741	6.9 2.2 6.9	**26** SU	0409 1110 1706 2347	6.4 2.9 6.4 3.1
12 SU	0029 0607 1305 1852	2.5 6.9 2.2 7.0	**27** M	0526 1220 1822	6.3 2.8 6.5
13 M	0146 0717 1417 1956	2.2 7.0 2.0 7.2	**28** TU	0103 0641 1329 1922	2.9 6.5 2.6 6.8
14 TU	0254 0819 1522 2050	2.0 7.2 1.8 7.4	**29** W	0203 0741 1433 2014	2.5 6.8 2.2 7.1
15 W	0355 0911 1619 2135	1.7 7.4 1.6 7.6	**30** TH	0303 0834 1531 2100	2.1 7.1 1.9 7.4
			31 F	0359 0922 1625 2145	1.7 7.4 1.5 7.6

JUNE

#	Time	m	#	Time	m
1 SA O	0452 1008 1716 2230	1.3 7.6 1.3 7.8	**16** SU ●	0539 1059 1753 2309	1.6 7.4 1.7 7.5
2 SU	0542 1055 1805 2315	1.0 7.8 1.1 7.9	**17** M	0617 1134 1830 2344	1.5 7.4 1.7 7.5
3 M	0630 1142 1853	0.8 7.9 1.0	**18** TU	0652 1210 1905	1.5 7.4 1.7
4 TU	0001 0718 1230 1939	8.0 0.8 7.9 1.1	**19** W	0018 0725 1246 1937	7.5 1.6 7.3 1.9
5 W	0048 0804 1319 2025	7.9 0.8 7.8 1.2	**20** TH	0052 0757 1320 2010	7.4 1.7 7.2 2.0
6 TH	0136 0850 1409 2112	7.8 1.1 7.6 1.5	**21** F	0125 0827 1354 2042	7.2 1.9 7.1 2.2
7 F	0227 0937 1503 2203	7.5 1.4 7.3 1.8	**22** SA	0200 0900 1431 2117	7.1 2.1 6.9 2.4
8 SA	0323 1029 1604 2259	7.3 1.7 7.1 2.1	**23** SU	0240 0937 1514 2200	7.0 2.4 6.8 2.6
9 SU	0427 1128 1710	7.0 2.0 7.0	**24** M	0327 1023 1606 2253	6.7 2.6 6.7 2.8
10 M	0003 0535 1233 1818	2.3 6.9 2.2 7.0	**25** TU	0424 1122 1711 2358	6.6 2.7 6.6 2.8
11 TU	0112 0645 1341 1925	2.3 6.9 2.2 7.0	**26** W	0535 1231 1825	6.5 2.7 6.7
12 W	0218 0753 1445 2024	2.2 7.0 2.2 7.2	**27** TH	0109 0652 1344 1930	2.6 6.7 2.5 7.0
13 TH	0320 0850 1542 2113	2.0 7.1 2.0 7.3	**28** F	0223 0757 1453 2026	2.3 6.9 2.1 7.3
14 F	0414 0938 1632 2156	1.9 7.3 1.9 7.4	**29** SA	0326 0854 1555 2119	1.8 7.2 1.7 7.6
15 SA	0459 1021 1714 2234	1.7 7.4 1.8 7.5	**30** SU	0426 0948 1653 2209	1.4 7.5 1.4 7.8

JULY

#	Time	m	#	Time	m
1 M O	0523 1039 1749 2259	1.1 7.8 1.1 8.0	**16** TU O	0558 1115 1812 2323	1.6 7.4 1.7 8.0
2 TU	0618 1129 1842 2348	0.8 7.9 1.0 8.1	**17** W	0634 1149 1847 2357	1.5 7.4 1.7 7.5
3 W	0710 1219 1932	0.6 8.0 0.9	**18** TH	0707 1223 1919	1.5 7.4 1.7
4 TH	0036 0758 1307 2020	8.1 0.6 8.0 1.0	**19** F	0030 0739 1256 1951	7.5 1.5 7.4 1.8
5 F	0125 0844 1356 2105	8.0 0.8 7.8 1.2	**20** SA	0103 0809 1329 2022	7.4 1.7 7.3 1.9
6 SA	0213 0927 1444 2149	7.7 1.1 7.6 1.6	**21** SU	0137 0840 1404 2054	7.3 1.8 7.2 2.1
7 SU	0302 1011 1535 2236	7.4 1.6 7.3 2.0	**22** M	0213 0912 1442 2131	7.1 2.1 7.0 2.3
8 M	0356 1058 1631 2329	7.1 2.0 7.0 2.3	**23** TU	0255 0950 1526 2215	6.9 2.3 6.9 2.5
9 TU	0458 1154 1736	6.8 2.4 6.8	**24** W	0343 1038 1620 2311	6.7 2.6 6.7 2.7
10 W	0032 0609 1300 1849	2.5 6.7 2.6 6.8	**25** TH	0446 1142 1732	6.6 2.7 6.7
11 TH	0141 0726 1408 1959	2.6 6.7 2.6 6.9	**26** F	0023 0610 1303 1853	2.7 6.6 2.7 6.8
12 F	0246 0831 1509 2054	2.4 6.8 2.5 7.1	**27** SA	0153 0729 1425 2000	2.4 6.8 2.3 7.1
13 SA	0344 0922 1604 2138	2.2 7.0 2.2 7.2	**28** SU	0302 0834 1533 2059	2.0 7.2 1.9 7.5
14 SU	0434 1005 1651 2216	2.0 7.2 2.0 7.4	**29** M	0406 0932 1636 2153	1.5 7.5 1.4 7.8
15 M ●	0518 1041 1733 2250	1.7 7.3 1.9 7.5	**30** TU O	0508 1025 1736 2245	1.1 7.8 1.1 8.1
			31 W	0607 1116 1832 2334	0.7 8.0 0.8 8.2

AUGUST

#	Time	m	#	Time	m
1 TH	0659 1204 1921	0.5 8.1 0.7	**16** F	0647 1158 1858	1.4 7.6 1.5
2 F	0021 0745 1250 2006	8.2 0.5 8.1 0.8	**17** SA	0006 0717 1230 1930	7.7 1.4 7.6 1.6
3 SA	0107 0827 1335 2047	8.1 0.7 8.0 1.0	**18** SU	0039 0747 1303 2000	7.6 1.5 7.5 1.6
4 SU	0152 0906 1418 2126	7.9 1.0 7.7 1.5	**19** M	0113 0818 1337 2033	7.5 1.6 7.4 1.8
5 M	0236 0943 1502 2204	7.5 1.6 7.3 1.9	**20** TU	0149 0850 1414 2107	7.3 1.9 7.2 2.1
6 TU	0322 1027 1550 2248	7.1 2.1 7.0 2.4	**21** W	0228 0924 1454 2146	7.1 2.2 7.0 2.4
7 W	0417 1102 1650 2347	6.7 2.6 6.7 2.8	**22** TH	0313 1007 1544 2237	6.8 2.5 6.8 2.6
8 TH	0529 1215 1807	6.4 3.0 6.5	**23** F	0415 1106 1656 2348	6.6 2.8 6.7 2.8
9 F	0102 0658 1332 1932	2.9 6.4 3.0 6.6	**24** SA	0545 1232 1828	6.5 2.8 6.7
10 SA	0214 0812 1441 2033	2.8 6.6 2.8 6.8	**25** SU	0128 0712 1405 1942	2.6 6.8 2.5 7.1
11 SU	0317 0905 1541 2119	2.4 6.9 2.5 7.1	**26** M	0244 0821 1517 2044	2.0 7.2 1.9 7.5
12 M	0412 0946 1622 2155	2.1 7.1 2.1 7.3	**27** TU	0351 0919 1622 2139	1.5 7.6 1.4 7.9
13 TU	0457 1020 1715 2228	1.8 7.3 1.9 7.5	**28** W O	0455 1011 1723 2229	1.0 7.9 1.0 8.1
14 W ●	0538 1052 1753 2301	1.6 7.5 1.7 7.6	**29** TH	0552 1058 1817 2316	0.7 8.1 0.8 8.3
15 TH	0614 1125 1827 2333	1.5 7.5 1.6 7.6	**30** F	0642 1144 1903	0.5 8.2 0.7
			31 SA	0001 0725 1227 1944	8.3 0.5 8.2 0.8

Chart Datum: 4·72 metres below Lallemand System (Mean Sea Level, Marseilles)

TIME ZONE –0100
(French Standard Time)
Subtract 1 hour for UT

For French Summer Time add
ONE hour in non-shaded areas

FRANCE – LE HAVRE

LAT 49°29′N   LONG 0°07′E

TIMES AND HEIGHTS OF HIGH AND LOW WATERS   YEAR **1996**

SEPTEMBER

Day	Time	m	Day	Time	m
1 SU	0044 / 0803 / 1309 / 2021	8.2 / 0.7 / 8.0 / 1.0	16 M	0015 / 0724 / 1237 / 1939	7.7 / 1.3 / 7.7 / 1.4
2 M	0126 / 0838 / 1348 / 2056	7.9 / 1.2 / 7.7 / 1.5	17 TU	0050 / 0756 / 1312 / 2013	7.7 / 1.5 / 7.6 / 1.6
3 TU	0207 / 0910 / 1427 / 2129	7.6 / 1.7 / 7.3 / 2.0	18 W	0128 / 0830 / 1350 / 2048	7.5 / 1.8 / 7.4 / 1.9
4 W	0249 / 0939 / 1509 / 2206	7.1 / 2.3 / 7.0 / 2.5	19 TH	0208 / 0904 / 1431 / 2126	7.2 / 2.1 / 7.1 / 2.2
5 TH	0338 / 1023 / 1603 / 2257	6.7 / 2.8 / 6.6 / 3.0	20 F	0256 / 0947 / 1522 / 2216	6.9 / 2.5 / 6.9 / 2.6
6 F	0447 / 1122 / 1722	6.3 / 3.3 / 6.3	21 SA	0359 / 1046 / 1636 / 2328	6.6 / 2.8 / 6.7 / 2.8
7 SA	0016 / 0622 / 1254 / 1855	3.2 / 6.2 / 3.3 / 6.3	22 SU	0534 / 1214 / 1812	6.6 / 2.9 / 6.7
8 SU	0141 / 0744 / 1412 / 2005	3.1 / 6.4 / 3.1 / 6.6	23 M	0107 / 0659 / 1351 / 1927	2.6 / 6.8 / 2.6 / 7.1
9 M	0249 / 0839 / 1515 / 2052	2.7 / 6.7 / 2.6 / 6.9	24 TU	0229 / 0807 / 1504 / 2030	2.1 / 7.3 / 2.0 / 7.5
10 TU	0344 / 0919 / 1606 / 2129	2.2 / 7.1 / 2.2 / 7.2	25 W	0337 / 0904 / 1608 / 2123	1.5 / 7.7 / 1.4 / 7.9
11 W	0431 / 0953 / 1651 / 2202	1.8 / 7.4 / 1.8 / 7.5	26 TH	0438 / 0953 / 1706 / 2211	1.1 / 8.0 / 1.1 / 8.1
12 TH ●	0512 / 1025 / 1729 / 2235	1.6 / 7.5 / 1.6 / 7.6	27 F ○	0532 / 1038 / 1756 / 2256	0.8 / 8.1 / 0.8 / 8.2
13 F	0549 / 1058 / 1802 / 2308	1.4 / 7.7 / 1.5 / 7.7	28 SA	0619 / 1121 / 1840 / 2339	0.7 / 8.2 / 0.8 / 8.2
14 SA	0621 / 1130 / 1834 / 2341	1.3 / 7.7 / 1.4 / 7.8	29 SU	0659 / 1202 / 1918	0.7 / 8.1 / 0.9
15 SU	0652 / 1204 / 1907	1.3 / 7.7 / 1.4	30 M	0020 / 0735 / 1241 / 1953	8.1 / 1.0 / 8.0 / 1.2

OCTOBER

Day	Time	m	Day	Time	m
1 TU	0100 / 0807 / 1318 / 2025	7.9 / 1.4 / 7.7 / 1.6	16 W	0031 / 0738 / 1251 / 1956	7.8 / 1.4 / 7.7 / 1.5
2 W	0139 / 0834 / 1355 / 2055	7.5 / 1.9 / 7.4 / 2.0	17 TH	0112 / 0814 / 1331 / 2034	7.6 / 1.7 / 7.5 / 1.7
3 TH	0219 / 0907 / 1433 / 2128	7.1 / 2.4 / 7.0 / 2.6	18 F	0156 / 0851 / 1416 / 2114	7.3 / 2.1 / 7.3 / 2.1
4 F	0304 / 0944 / 1510 / 2213	6.7 / 2.9 / 6.6 / 3.0	19 SA	0246 / 0936 / 1510 / 2205	7.0 / 2.5 / 7.0 / 2.4
5 SA	0406 / 1039 / 1633 / 2324	6.3 / 3.4 / 6.2 / 3.3	20 SU	0353 / 1037 / 1625 / 2316	6.8 / 2.8 / 6.8 / 2.7
6 SU	0535 / 1206 / 1805	6.1 / 3.5 / 6.2	21 M	0524 / 1204 / 1755	6.7 / 2.9 / 6.8
7 M	0055 / 0700 / 1333 / 1922	3.3 / 6.3 / 3.3 / 6.4	22 TU	0051 / 0643 / 1335 / 1908	2.5 / 7.0 / 2.5 / 7.1
8 TU	0210 / 0800 / 1439 / 2015	2.9 / 6.6 / 2.8 / 6.8	23 W	0211 / 0749 / 1447 / 2011	2.1 / 7.3 / 2.0 / 7.5
9 W	0308 / 0844 / 1532 / 2056	2.4 / 7.0 / 2.4 / 7.1	24 TH	0318 / 0845 / 1549 / 2104	1.6 / 7.7 / 1.5 / 7.8
10 TH	0357 / 0920 / 1618 / 2132	2.0 / 7.4 / 1.9 / 7.4	25 F	0416 / 0932 / 1644 / 2152	1.3 / 7.9 / 1.2 / 8.0
11 F	0440 / 0954 / 1658 / 2207	1.7 / 7.6 / 1.7 / 7.6	26 SA ○	0508 / 1016 / 1732 / 2236	1.1 / 8.0 / 1.1 / 8.1
12 SA ●	0518 / 1028 / 1734 / 2242	1.5 / 7.7 / 1.5 / 7.8	27 SU	0552 / 1057 / 1814 / 2318	1.0 / 8.1 / 1.0 / 8.1
13 SU	0552 / 1103 / 1808 / 2317	1.3 / 7.8 / 1.3 / 7.8	28 M	0631 / 1137 / 1851 / 2358	1.3 / 8.0 / 1.1 / 8.0
14 M	0626 / 1137 / 1844 / 2353	1.3 / 7.8 / 1.3 / 7.8	29 TU	0705 / 1214 / 1925	1.3 / 7.9 / 1.3
15 TU	0702 / 1213 / 1919	1.3 / 7.8 / 1.3	30 W	0036 / 0738 / 1250 / 1957	7.8 / 1.6 / 7.7 / 1.6
			31 TH	0114 / 0806 / 1326 / 2027	7.5 / 2.0 / 7.4 / 2.0

NOVEMBER

Day	Time	m	Day	Time	m
1 F	0153 / 0839 / 1402 / 2059	7.1 / 2.4 / 7.1 / 2.5	16 SA	0147 / 0845 / 1406 / 2109	7.5 / 1.9 / 7.5 / 1.8
2 SA	0234 / 0914 / 1443 / 2138	6.8 / 2.9 / 6.7 / 2.9	17 SU	0240 / 0933 / 1501 / 2201	7.2 / 2.3 / 7.2 / 2.2
3 SU	0325 / 1001 / 1539 / 2234	6.4 / 3.2 / 6.3 / 3.2	18 M	0345 / 1033 / 1612 / 2307	7.0 / 2.6 / 7.0 / 2.4
4 M	0439 / 1110 / 1702 / 2352	6.2 / 3.5 / 6.2 / 3.3	19 TU	0504 / 1149 / 1731	6.9 / 2.7 / 6.9
5 TU	0602 / 1233 / 1824	6.3 / 3.4 / 6.3	20 W	0028 / 0617 / 1311 / 1843	2.4 / 7.0 / 2.5 / 7.1
6 W	0112 / 0708 / 1347 / 1926	3.1 / 6.5 / 3.0 / 6.6	21 TH	0145 / 0724 / 1423 / 1948	2.2 / 7.3 / 2.1 / 7.3
7 TH	0218 / 0759 / 1447 / 2015	2.7 / 6.9 / 2.6 / 6.9	22 F	0252 / 0822 / 1525 / 2045	1.9 / 7.5 / 1.8 / 7.5
8 F	0313 / 0842 / 1537 / 2057	2.3 / 7.2 / 2.2 / 7.2	23 SA	0351 / 0912 / 1620 / 2134	1.7 / 7.7 / 1.5 / 7.7
9 SA	0400 / 0920 / 1621 / 2137	1.9 / 7.5 / 1.8 / 7.5	24 SU	0442 / 0956 / 1708 / 2218	1.5 / 7.8 / 1.4 / 7.8
10 SU	0442 / 0958 / 1703 / 2215	1.6 / 7.7 / 1.5 / 7.7	25 M ○	0526 / 1037 / 1749 / 2300	1.5 / 7.9 / 1.3 / 7.8
11 M ●	0522 / 1035 / 1743 / 2254	1.5 / 7.8 / 1.3 / 7.8	26 TU	0604 / 1115 / 1826 / 2338	1.5 / 7.9 / 1.3 / 7.8
12 TU	0602 / 1113 / 1823 / 2334	1.3 / 7.9 / 1.2 / 7.9	27 W	0639 / 1151 / 1901	1.6 / 7.8 / 1.4
13 W	0642 / 1152 / 1851 / 2358	1.3 / 7.9 / 1.1 / 8.0	28 TH	0016 / 0713 / 1226 / 1934	7.7 / 1.7 / 7.7 / 1.6
14 TH	0016 / 0723 / 1234 / 1944	7.8 / 1.4 / 7.8 / 1.3	29 F	0053 / 0759 / 1302 / 2006	7.5 / 2.0 / 7.4 / 1.9
15 F	0100 / 0804 / 1318 / 2026	7.7 / 1.6 / 7.7 / 1.5	30 SA	0129 / 0817 / 1336 / 2037	7.2 / 2.3 / 7.2 / 2.2

DECEMBER

Day	Time	m	Day	Time	m
1 SU	0206 / 0851 / 1412 / 2111	7.0 / 2.6 / 6.9 / 2.6	16 M	0231 / 0932 / 1450 / 2153	7.5 / 1.9 / 7.5 / 1.8
2 M	0246 / 0929 / 1453 / 2152	6.7 / 2.9 / 6.6 / 2.9	17 TU	0329 / 1024 / 1551 / 2248	7.3 / 2.2 / 7.2 / 2.1
3 TU	0336 / 1019 / 1549 / 2248	6.5 / 3.2 / 6.4 / 3.1	18 W	0434 / 1125 / 1700 / 2356	7.1 / 2.4 / 7.0 / 2.3
4 W	0446 / 1123 / 1704 / 2356	6.4 / 3.3 / 6.3 / 3.1	19 TH	0543 / 1236 / 1811	7.0 / 2.5 / 6.9
5 TH	0604 / 1239 / 1824	6.5 / 3.2 / 6.4	20 F	0110 / 0653 / 1351 / 1922	2.4 / 7.1 / 2.4 / 7.0
6 F	0109 / 0707 / 1345 / 1927	3.0 / 6.7 / 2.9 / 6.7	21 SA	0221 / 0758 / 1458 / 2026	2.3 / 7.2 / 2.2 / 7.2
7 SA	0217 / 0759 / 1448 / 2019	2.6 / 7.0 / 2.5 / 7.0	22 SU	0323 / 0853 / 1556 / 2119	2.1 / 7.4 / 1.9 / 7.4
8 SU	0315 / 0845 / 1543 / 2106	2.2 / 7.3 / 2.0 / 7.3	23 M	0417 / 0939 / 1646 / 2205	2.0 / 7.5 / 1.8 / 7.5
9 M	0407 / 0928 / 1633 / 2150	1.9 / 7.6 / 1.7 / 7.6	24 TU ○	0502 / 1020 / 1728 / 2245	1.8 / 7.6 / 1.6 / 7.6
10 TU ●	0455 / 1010 / 1720 / 2234	1.6 / 7.8 / 1.3 / 7.8	25 W	0541 / 1057 / 1805 / 2322	1.7 / 7.7 / 1.5 / 7.6
11 W	0542 / 1052 / 1807 / 2318	1.4 / 7.9 / 1.1 / 7.9	26 TH	0618 / 1132 / 1841 / 2357	1.7 / 7.7 / 1.5 / 7.6
12 TH	0628 / 1136 / 1853	1.2 / 8.0 / 1.0	27 F	0654 / 1206 / 1915	1.7 / 7.7 / 1.5
13 F	0004 / 0714 / 1222 / 1939	7.9 / 1.2 / 8.0 / 1.0	28 SA	0032 / 0727 / 1240 / 1948	7.5 / 1.8 / 7.5 / 1.7
14 SA	0051 / 0759 / 1309 / 2023	7.9 / 1.3 / 7.9 / 1.2	29 SU	0106 / 0758 / 1313 / 2018	7.4 / 2.0 / 7.4 / 1.9
15 SU	0140 / 0844 / 1358 / 2106	7.7 / 1.6 / 7.7 / 1.4	30 M	0140 / 0830 / 1345 / 2048	7.2 / 2.2 / 7.2 / 2.2
			31 TU	0213 / 0902 / 1419 / 2120	7.0 / 2.5 / 7.0 / 2.4

19

Chart Datum: 4·72 metres below Lallemand System (Mean Sea Level, Marseilles)

LE HAVRE

Seine Maritime 49°29'·18N 00°05·51E

10-19-19

LIGHTS AND MARKS
Ldg Its 107° both Dir FW 36/78m 25M; grey trs, G tops; intens 106°-108° (H24). 2 chys, RW conspic, on ldg line.

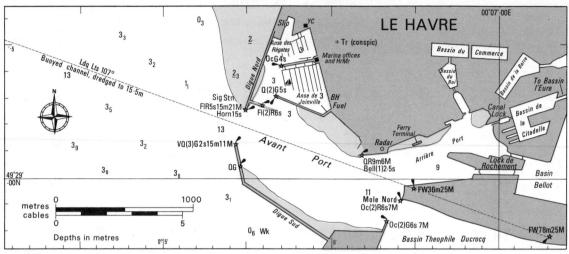

CHARTS
AC 2990, 2146, *2613*; SHOM 6683, 6796, 6736; ECM 526, 1012; Imray C31; Stanfords 1

TIDES
−0103 Dover; ML 4·9; Duration 0543; Zone −0100.
Le Havre is a Standard Port; tidal predictions are given above. There is a stand at HW of about 3 hours.

SHELTER
Excellent in the marina, access H24. Ⓥ berth pontoon O. Or request Hr Mr for long stay in Bassin du Commerce.

NAVIGATION
WPT 49°31'·05N 00°04'·00W, 287°/107° from/to bkwtrs, 6·4M. ‡ prohib in and to the N of the fairway; it is also prohib to cross the fairway E of buoys LH7 and LH8. Banc de l'Éclat, awash at LW, lies N of appr chan and lobster pots close each side. Obey IPTS at end of Digue Nord.

RADIO TELEPHONE
Call: *Havre Port* Control tr VHF Ch 12 20 (or 2182 kHz). Port Ops Ch 67 69 (H24). Radar Ch 12. Marina Ch 09.

TELEPHONE
Hr Mr 35.22.72.72; Hr Mr Port de Plaisance 35.21.23.95; Aff Mar 35.22.41.03; CROSS 33.52.72.23; ⌗ 35.41.33.51; SNSM 35.22.41.03; Meteo 35.42.21.06; Auto 36.68.08.76; Dr 35.41.23.61; Ⓗ 35.73.32.32; Brit Consul 35.42.27.47.

FACILITIES
Marina (973 + 41 visitors) ☎ 35.21.23.95, Fax 35.22.72.72, FF92, AC, BH (16 ton), C (6 ton), CH, Slip, P & D (cash in working hrs; credit card at other times), El, FW, Gas, Gaz, R, Ⓡ, V; **YC Sport Nautique (SNH)** ☎ 35.21.01.41, Bar; **Sté des Régates du Havre (SRH)** ☎ 35.42.41.21, R, Bar; **Services:** Ⓔ, ME, El, Sh, CH, SHOM, ACA.
City All needs. Ferry: Portsmouth.

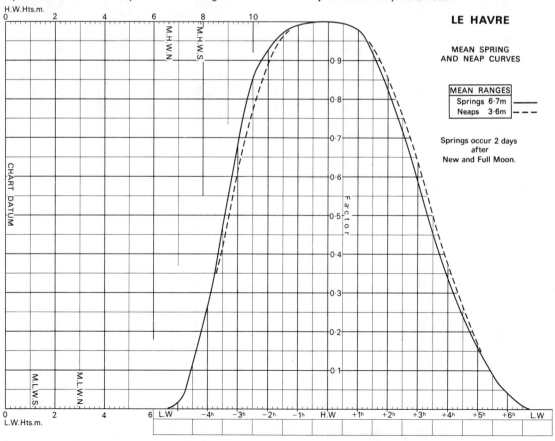

LE HAVRE

MEAN SPRING AND NEAP CURVES

MEAN RANGES	
Springs 6·7m	—
Neaps 3·6m	---

Springs occur 2 days after New and Full Moon.

RIVER SEINE   10-19-20

CHARTS
AC 2880, 2994, 2146, *2613*; SHOM 6796, 6117; Imray C31

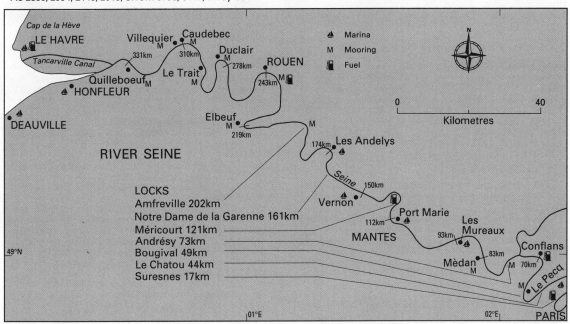

TIDES

Standard Port LE HAVRE (←) Zone –0100

Times				Height (metres)			
High Water		Low Water		MHWS	MHWN	MLWN	MLWS
0000	0500	0000	0700	7·9	6·6	3·0	1·2
1200	1700	1200	1900				

Differences TANCARVILLE*

–0107	–0100	+0106	+0138	–0·1	–0·1	–0·2	+1·0
QUILLEBOEUF*							
–0044	–0051	+0122	+0200	0·0	0·0	0·0	+1·4
VATTEVILLE*							
+0004	–0022	+0223	+0250	0·0	–0·1	+0·6	+2·3
CAUDEBEC*							
+0020	–0013	+0230	+0300	–0·3	–0·2	+0·7	+2·4
ROUEN							
+0438	+0413	+0523	+0525	–0·2	–0·1	+1·4	+3·6

*HW differences refer to the start of the stand, which lasts about 2¾ hrs up to Vatteville and about 1¾hrs at Duclair.

It is important to study the tides. The flood stream starts progressively later as a boat proceeds upriver. So even a 4kn boat leaving the estuary at LW can carry the flood for the 78M (123km) to Rouen. But going down river on the ebb a boat will meet the flood. Rather than ⚓ for about 4 hrs, in a fast boat it is worth continuing, because the ebb starts sooner the further downstream one gets. Between Quilleboeuf (335km) and La Mailleraye (303km) the Seine bore (*mascaret*) still runs at HWS if the river is in flood.
NAVIGATION: The Seine gives access to Paris and central France, and to the Mediterranean via the canals (below). But there is a constant traffic of barges (*péniches*), and in the tidal section (below Amfreville) the strong stream and ships' wash make it dangerous to moor alongside and uncomfortable to ⚓. Masts can be lowered at Deauville, Le Havre (marina) and Rouen. Yacht navigation is prohib at night, and ⚓s are scarce. A good ⚓ Ⓦ light is needed, and it is useful to have a radar reflector and a VHF aerial, even with the mast lowered. Listen on Ch 73.
ENTRY is usually via the dredged/buoyed Chenal de Rouen, which can be rough in a strong W'ly wind and ebb tide. Care is needed, especially near the mouth where there are shifting banks and often morning fog.
ENTRY VIA THE CANAL DE TANCARVILLE may be preferred if sea conditions are bad, but with 3 locks and 9 bridges delays must be expected. To enter the Canal at Le Havre transit the lock Quinette de Rochemont (E of the front ldg lt) into Bassin Bellot. At the E end transit the

Vétillart lock; thence via 3 bridges through Garage de Graville, Bassin de Despujols, and across the N end of Bassin de Lancement, which leads into the canal proper with 3 more bridges. Exit into the Seine (at 338km) via locks close E of Tancarville suspension bridge (50m).
LOCKS: Locks are as shown above. Call VHF Ch 18† or 22. Above Amfreville the current is about 1kn in summer, but more in winter.
FACILITIES: The most likely places for mooring and fuel are shown above. For Rouen and Paris see below.
REFERENCE: For detailed information see *A Cruising Guide to the Lower Seine* (Imray).

ROUEN, Seine Maritime, 49°26'·63N 01°03'·00E. AC 2880, 2994; SHOM 6117. HW +0330 on Dover (UT); ML 6·2m; Duration 0400. Yacht navigation prohib SS+½ to SR–½. Use pontoon SE side Bassin St Gervais (N bank) for mast unstep/restep (max stay 48 hrs); or mast step at Darse des Docks 250km. Berth in La Halte de Plaisance NE side of Ile Lacroix. VHF call *Rouen Port Capitainerie* Ch **73** 68. Hr Mr 35.52.54.56; Aff Mar 35.98.53.98; ⌗ 35.98.27.60; Meteo 35.80.11.44; Facilities: **Bassin St Gervais** C (3 to 25 ton), FW; **La Halte de Plaisance** (50) ☎ 35.88.00.00, FW, AC, Slip, C (30 ton), BH (4 ton); **Rouen YC** ☎ 35.66.52.52; **Services:** ME, El, Sh, P, D, CH, Ⓔ.

PARIS. The Touring Club de France ☎ 42.65.90.70, Fax 42.65.11.31, has AB, AC, FW on the N bank near Place de la Concorde, but noise and wash intrude. The **Port de Paris-Arsenal**, the first basin of the Canal St Martin, has complete shelter for 112 + 65 visitors; depth 1·9m. Ent is on the NE bank 170m before Pont d'Austerlitz at lock 9, which, with air clearance of 5·2m, is remotely controlled by Hr Mr (0800-2345LT); waiting pontoon (with intercom to Hr Mr) upstream. VHF Ch 09. Caution strong current if river in flood. Hr Mr ☎ 43.41.39.32, Fax 44.74.02.66; AC, FW, C (7 ton), D & P (cans), Ⓠ, plus city amenities; Aff Mar ☎ 42.73.55.05; River Police 47.07.17.17; Metro stns: Quai de la Rapée and Bastille (lines 1, 5), RER, ⇄, ✈.

CANALS TO THE MEDITERRANEAN
The quickest route is Le Havre/Paris/St Mammes/canal du Loing/canal du Briare/canal Latéral à la Loire/canal du Centre/Saône/Rhône, approx 1318km (824M), 182 locks. Max dimensions: LOA 38·5m, beam 5m, draft 1·8m, air draft 3·5m. Further info and dates of closures (*chomages*) are available every March from the French Tourist Office, 178 Piccadilly, London, W1V OAL, ☎ 0171 629-2869, Fax 0171 493-6594. Tolls are due; see 10.15.8.

19

FÉCAMP   10-19-21

Seine Maritime 49°45'·97N 00°21'·85E

CHARTS
AC 1352; SHOM 7207, 6765, 6824; ECM 1012; Imray C31; Stanfords 1

TIDES
−0044 Dover; ML 4·9; Duration 0550; Zone −0100

Standard Port DIEPPE (⟶)

Times				Height (metres)			
High Water		Low Water		MHWS	MHWN	MLWN	MLWS
0100	0600	0100	0700	9·3	7·3	2·6	0·8
1300	1800	1300	1900				
Differences FÉCAMP							
−0015	−0016	−0033	−0040	−0·9	−0·5	+0·3	+0·4
ETRETAT							
−0020	−0026	−0048	−0050	−1·2	−0·7	+0·3	+0·4
ANTIFER							
−0046	−0039	−0051	−0100	−1·3	−0·6	+0·4	+0·5

SHELTER
Excellent in basins, but in even moderate W/NW winds a considerable surf runs off the ent and the Avant Port (visitors at C pontoon) can be uncomfortable; or lock into Bassin Bérigny (HW −2 to HW). Access best at HW +1. Chan dredged 1·5m, but subject to silting; best water in ent chan is close to N jetty. Boats < 1·2m draft can enter at any tide and in most weathers.

NAVIGATION
WPT 49°46'·10N 00°21'·12E, 282°/102° from/to Jetée Nord lt, 0·50M. Beware the Charpentier Rks off Pte Fagnet. Strong cross currents occur, depending on tides.

LIGHTS AND MARKS
Ent lies SSW of conspic ✠, sig stn and TV mast on Pte Fagnet cliff. N jetty Fl (2) 10s 15m 16M, grey tr, R top; horn (2) 30s sounded HW −2½ to HW +2; root QR 10m 4M. Jetée Sud hd, QG 14m 9M; obscd by cliff when brg more than 217°. QR and QG lead 085° to ent. IPTS on tr by Avant Port show when Bassin Bérigny lock is open.

RADIO TELEPHONE
VHF Ch **12** 10 16 (HW −3 to HW + 1). Ch 09 Marina and Berigny lock (0800-1200; 1400-2000LT).

TELEPHONE
Hr Mr 35.28.25.23; Aff Mar 35.28.16.35; ⌗ 35.28.19.40; SNSM 35.28.00.91; CROSS 21.87.21.87; Auto 36.68.08.76; Police 35.28.16.69; Ⓗ 35.28.05.13; Brit Consul 35.42.27.47.

FACILITIES
Marina (500 + 30 visitors) ☎ 35.28.13.58, FF105, FW, AC, D, C (Mobile 36 ton); **Bassin Bérigny** AB, M, D, L, FW, CH, Slip; **Sté des Régates de Fécamp** ☎ 35.28.08.44, AB, FW; **Services:** Slip, M, ME, El, Ⓔ, Sh, Gaz, C (30 ton), CH. **Town** EC Mon; P, D, V, Gaz, R, Bar, ✉, Ⓑ, ⇌, ✈ (Le Havre).

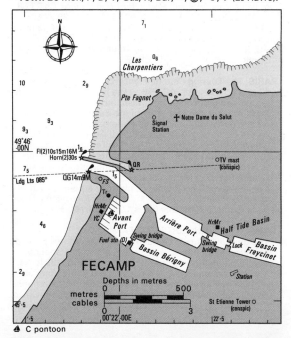

▲ C pontoon

ST VALÉRY-EN-CAUX   10-19-22

Seine Maritime 49°52'·44N 00°42'·54E

CHARTS
AC *2451*; SHOM 6794; ECM 1012; Imray C31; Stanfords 1

TIDES
−0044 Dover; ML 4·6; Duration 0530; Zone −0100

Standard Port DIEPPE (⟶)

Times				Height (metres)			
High Water		Low Water		MHWS	MHWN	MLWN	MLWS
0100	0600	0100	0700	9·3	7·3	2·6	0·8
1300	1800	1300	1900				
Differences ST VALÉRY-EN-CAUX							
−0008	−0013	−0002	−0009	−0·5	−0·2	−0·2	+0·2

SHELTER
Good. Avant Port dries 3m; access from HW −3. Lock opens HW ±2¼ by day; by night, at HW±½ (bridge opens H and H+30 during these periods). Ⓥ pontoon to stbd, past lock.

NAVIGATION
WPT 49°53'·00N 00°42'·50E, 000°/180° from/to Jetée Ouest lt, 0·50M. Ent is easy, but in strong N/E winds seas break across ent. Coast dries to approx 150m off the pier hds. Inside the pier hds, wave-breaks (marked by posts each side) dampen the swell. Shingle builds up against W wall; hug the E side. W waiting buoys N of lock.

LIGHTS AND MARKS
Hbr is difficult to see between high chalk cliffs. From N or W the nuclear power stn at Paluel is conspic 3M W of ent. Conspic white bldg E of ent. W pier lt Oc (2 + 1) G 12s 13m 14M; E pier lt, Fl (2)R 6s 8m 4M. Tfc sigs at the bridge/lock are coordinated to seaward/inland:
Ⓖ = ent/exit; Ⓡ = no ent/ exit; Ⓡ + Ⓖ = no movements.

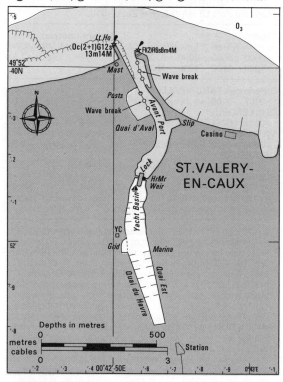

RADIO TELEPHONE
VHF Ch 09.

TELEPHONE
Hr Mr 35.97.01.30; Aff Mar 35.28.16.35; ⌗ 35.28.19.40; CROSS 21.87.21.87; SNSM 35.97.09.03; Meteo 21.31.52.23; Auto 36.68.08.76; Police 35.97.05.27; Dr 35.97.20.13; Ⓗ 35.97.06.21; Brit Consul 35.42.27.47.

FACILITIES
Marina (580 + 20 visitors) ☎ 35.97.01.30, Fax 35.97.90.73, FF100, AC, FW, C (6 ton), CH, El, Gaz, ME, Sh, SM, V, Bar; **Club Nautique Valeriquais** ☎ 35.97.10.88; **Services:** M, Ⓔ. **Town** EC Mon (all day); P, D, CH, V, Gaz, R, Bar, ✉, Ⓑ, ⇌, ✈ (Dieppe). Ferry: Dieppe.

TIME ZONE –0100
(French Standard Time)
Subtract 1 hour for UT

For French Summer Time add ONE hour in non-shaded areas

FRANCE – DIEPPE

LAT 49°56′N   LONG 1°05′E

TIMES AND HEIGHTS OF HIGH AND LOW WATERS

YEAR **1996**

JANUARY

Day	Time	m	Day	Time	m
1 M	0227 / 0818 / 1508 / 2052	2.5 / 7.6 / 2.3 / 7.5	**16** TU	0108 / 0703 / 1354 / 1942	2.4 / 7.6 / 2.3 / 7.6
2 TU	0335 / 0920 / 1611 / 2148	2.3 / 7.8 / 2.1 / 7.8	**17** W	0232 / 0820 / 1515 / 2055	2.2 / 8.0 / 1.9 / 8.1
3 W	0432 / 1009 / 1702 / 2234	2.1 / 8.2 / 1.8 / 8.2	**18** TH	0349 / 0926 / 1624 / 2158	1.7 / 8.5 / 1.4 / 8.6
4 TH	0519 / 1050 / 1745 / 2313	1.8 / 8.4 / 1.5 / 8.4	**19** F	0454 / 1025 / 1727 / 2256	1.3 / 9.0 / 0.9 / 9.1
5 F ○	0600 / 1127 / 1823 / 2348	1.6 / 8.6 / 1.4 / 8.6	**20** SA ●	0554 / 1120 / 1826 / 2348	0.9 / 9.5 / 0.5 / 9.5
6 SA	0637 / 1201 / 1900	1.4 / 8.8 / 1.2	**21** SU	0651 / 1211 / 1920	0.6 / 9.8 / 0.3
7 SU	0022 / 0713 / 1235 / 1934	8.7 / 1.4 / 8.9 / 1.2	**22** M	0038 / 0743 / 1259 / 2009	9.7 / 0.4 / 9.9 / 0.2
8 M	0056 / 0746 / 1308 / 2007	8.8 / 1.4 / 8.9 / 1.2	**23** TU	0124 / 0830 / 1344 / 2054	9.8 / 0.4 / 9.8 / 0.3
9 TU	0129 / 0818 / 1341 / 2038	8.8 / 1.4 / 8.8 / 1.3	**24** W	0208 / 0913 / 1428 / 2133	9.6 / 0.6 / 9.6 / 0.6
10 W	0202 / 0849 / 1414 / 2108	8.7 / 1.5 / 8.7 / 1.4	**25** TH	0251 / 0951 / 1511 / 2209	9.3 / 1.0 / 9.1 / 1.0
11 TH	0236 / 0922 / 1448 / 2141	8.5 / 1.7 / 8.4 / 1.6	**26** F	0332 / 1028 / 1553 / 2245	8.9 / 1.4 / 8.6 / 1.6
12 F	0311 / 0958 / 1526 / 2218	8.3 / 1.9 / 8.2 / 1.9	**27** SA	0415 / 1108 / 1639 / 2325	8.3 / 1.9 / 7.9 / 2.1
13 SA	0351 / 1040 / 1610 / 2302	8.0 / 2.1 / 7.9 / 2.1	**28** SU	0503 / 1156 / 1735	7.7 / 2.4 / 7.3
14 SU	0439 / 1132 / 1705 / 2358	7.8 / 2.3 / 7.6 / 2.3	**29** M	0019 / 0606 / 1301 / 1848	2.6 / 7.2 / 2.8 / 6.9
15 M	0542 / 1235 / 1818	7.6 / 2.4 / 7.4	**30** TU	0131 / 0728 / 1419 / 2014	2.9 / 7.0 / 2.8 / 7.0
			31 W	0251 / 0848 / 1536 / 2123	2.8 / 7.2 / 2.5 / 7.3

FEBRUARY

Day	Time	m	Day	Time	m
1 TH	0402 / 0946 / 1636 / 2212	2.4 / 7.7 / 2.1 / 7.8	**16** F	0328 / 0910 / 1607 / 2147	1.9 / 8.2 / 1.5 / 8.4
2 F	0456 / 1030 / 1724 / 2253	2.0 / 8.1 / 1.7 / 8.2	**17** SA	0439 / 1014 / 1714 / 2245	1.4 / 8.9 / 0.9 / 9.0
3 SA	0540 / 1107 / 1805 / 2329	1.7 / 8.5 / 1.4 / 8.5	**18** SU ●	0542 / 1107 / 1814 / 2336	0.9 / 9.4 / 0.5 / 9.5
4 SU ○	0619 / 1142 / 1842	1.4 / 8.7 / 1.2	**19** M	0639 / 1158 / 1907	0.6 / 9.7 / 0.2
5 M	0003 / 0655 / 1216 / 1917	8.8 / 1.2 / 8.9 / 1.0	**20** TU	0023 / 0728 / 1243 / 1953	9.7 / 0.4 / 9.9 / 0.1
6 TU	0036 / 0729 / 1249 / 1950	8.9 / 1.1 / 9.0 / 0.9	**21** W	0105 / 0808 / 1325 / 2033	9.8 / 0.3 / 9.9 / 0.2
7 W	0109 / 0801 / 1322 / 2021	9.0 / 1.1 / 9.1 / 0.9	**22** TH	0146 / 0851 / 1405 / 2108	9.7 / 0.5 / 9.6 / 0.5
8 TH	0142 / 0833 / 1355 / 2052	9.0 / 1.1 / 9.0 / 1.0	**23** F	0224 / 0924 / 1443 / 2138	9.4 / 0.8 / 9.2 / 0.9
9 F	0214 / 0905 / 1428 / 2123	8.9 / 1.2 / 8.8 / 1.2	**24** SA	0300 / 0955 / 1521 / 2207	9.0 / 1.3 / 8.7 / 1.5
10 SA	0248 / 0938 / 1504 / 2156	8.7 / 1.4 / 8.6 / 1.5	**25** SU	0336 / 1027 / 1559 / 2241	8.4 / 1.8 / 8.0 / 2.1
11 SU	0325 / 1015 / 1544 / 2235	8.5 / 1.7 / 8.2 / 1.8	**26** M	0416 / 1107 / 1646 / 2328	7.7 / 2.3 / 7.3 / 2.6
12 M	0408 / 1101 / 1633 / 2325	8.1 / 2.0 / 7.8 / 2.1	**27** TU	0509 / 1205 / 1752	7.1 / 2.8 / 6.7
13 TU	0504 / 1201 / 1742	7.7 / 2.3 / 7.5	**28** W	0035 / 0629 / 1325 / 1926	3.1 / 6.7 / 3.1 / 6.6
14 W	0033 / 0624 / 1320 / 1914	2.4 / 7.5 / 2.3 / 7.4	**29** TH	0204 / 0804 / 1454 / 2050	3.1 / 6.8 / 2.8 / 7.0
15 TH	0202 / 0755 / 1451 / 2037	2.4 / 7.7 / 2.0 / 7.8			

MARCH

Day	Time	m	Day	Time	m
1 F	0326 / 0915 / 1603 / 2144	2.7 / 7.3 / 2.3 / 7.5	**16** SA	0314 / 0858 / 1554 / 2135	2.0 / 8.1 / 1.5 / 8.4
2 SA	0426 / 1002 / 1655 / 2226	2.2 / 7.8 / 1.8 / 8.1	**17** SU	0426 / 1002 / 1701 / 2231	1.4 / 8.7 / 0.9 / 9.0
3 SU	0513 / 1042 / 1739 / 2303	1.7 / 8.3 / 1.4 / 8.5	**18** M	0529 / 1054 / 1759 / 2320	0.9 / 9.3 / 0.6 / 9.4
4 M	0554 / 1118 / 1818 / 2339	1.4 / 8.7 / 1.1 / 8.8	**19** TU ●	0622 / 1141 / 1847	0.6 / 9.6 / 0.6
5 TU ○	0631 / 1153 / 1854	1.1 / 9.0 / 0.9	**20** W	0003 / 0708 / 1223 / 1930	9.6 / 0.4 / 9.7 / 0.3
6 W	0013 / 0707 / 1227 / 1928	9.1 / 0.9 / 9.2 / 0.8	**21** TH	0043 / 0749 / 1303 / 2006	9.7 / 0.4 / 9.7 / 0.4
7 TH	0046 / 0741 / 1300 / 2001	9.3 / 0.8 / 9.3 / 0.7	**22** F	0120 / 0824 / 1340 / 2039	9.6 / 0.6 / 9.5 / 0.6
8 F	0119 / 0814 / 1334 / 2033	9.3 / 0.8 / 9.3 / 0.7	**23** SA	0155 / 0856 / 1416 / 2107	9.3 / 0.8 / 9.2 / 1.0
9 SA	0152 / 0847 / 1409 / 2105	9.2 / 0.8 / 9.1 / 0.9	**24** SU	0229 / 0924 / 1450 / 2135	9.0 / 1.2 / 8.7 / 1.5
10 SU	0227 / 0921 / 1446 / 2139	9.0 / 1.0 / 8.9 / 1.2	**25** M	0303 / 0954 / 1526 / 2206	8.4 / 1.7 / 8.1 / 2.0
11 M	0305 / 0957 / 1526 / 2217	8.7 / 1.4 / 8.5 / 1.6	**26** TU	0338 / 1029 / 1606 / 2247	7.8 / 2.2 / 7.4 / 2.6
12 TU	0347 / 1042 / 1615 / 2306	8.3 / 1.7 / 7.9 / 2.0	**27** W	0422 / 1118 / 1702 / 2346	7.2 / 2.7 / 6.8 / 3.1
13 W	0442 / 1141 / 1724	7.8 / 2.1 / 7.5	**28** TH	0530 / 1229 / 1829	6.7 / 3.1 / 6.5
14 TH	0013 / 0604 / 1301 / 1859	2.4 / 7.4 / 2.3 / 7.4	**29** F	0109 / 0708 / 1400 / 2001	3.2 / 6.6 / 3.0 / 6.8
15 F	0145 / 0740 / 1436 / 2026	2.4 / 7.6 / 2.0 / 7.8	**30** SA	0237 / 0830 / 1517 / 2103	2.9 / 7.0 / 2.5 / 7.4
			31 SU	0343 / 0924 / 1615 / 2150	2.3 / 7.6 / 2.0 / 8.0

APRIL

Day	Time	m	Day	Time	m
1 M	0435 / 1008 / 1736 / 2231	1.8 / 8.2 / 1.1 / 8.5	**16** TU	0509 / 1035 / 1736 / 2258	1.0 / 9.0 / 0.8 / 9.2
2 TU	0520 / 1048 / 1745 / 2309	1.4 / 8.6 / 1.1 / 8.8	**17** W ●	0600 / 1120 / 1822 / 2339	0.8 / 9.3 / 0.7 / 9.4
3 W	0601 / 1125 / 1824 / 2345	1.1 / 8.9 / 0.9 / 9.1	**18** TH	0643 / 1200 / 1901	0.7 / 9.4 / 0.6
4 TH ○	0640 / 1201 / 1902	0.9 / 9.2 / 0.7	**19** F	0017 / 0721 / 1238 / 1937	9.4 / 0.7 / 9.4 / 0.7
5 F	0020 / 0717 / 1237 / 1938	9.3 / 0.7 / 9.3 / 0.6	**20** SA	0053 / 0755 / 1314 / 2009	9.3 / 0.7 / 9.3 / 0.9
6 SA	0055 / 0754 / 1313 / 2013	9.4 / 0.6 / 9.4 / 0.6	**21** SU	0128 / 0828 / 1349 / 2039	9.2 / 0.9 / 9.0 / 1.1
7 SU	0131 / 0831 / 1351 / 2049	9.4 / 0.6 / 9.3 / 0.8	**22** M	0201 / 0858 / 1424 / 2108	8.9 / 1.2 / 8.6 / 1.5
8 M	0209 / 0907 / 1431 / 2125	9.2 / 0.8 / 9.0 / 1.1	**23** TU	0235 / 0927 / 1459 / 2139	8.4 / 1.6 / 8.2 / 2.0
9 TU	0250 / 0947 / 1515 / 2207	8.9 / 1.2 / 8.6 / 1.5	**24** W	0309 / 1000 / 1537 / 2216	7.9 / 2.0 / 7.6 / 2.4
10 W	0335 / 1033 / 1607 / 2258	8.4 / 1.6 / 8.1 / 1.9	**25** TH	0349 / 1042 / 1624 / 2307	7.4 / 2.5 / 7.1 / 2.8
11 TH	0433 / 1133 / 1719	7.9 / 1.9 / 7.6	**26** F	0444 / 1140 / 1733	6.9 / 2.8 / 6.8
12 F	0006 / 0555 / 1252 / 1848	2.3 / 7.5 / 2.1 / 7.5	**27** SA	0015 / 0604 / 1257 / 1859	3.1 / 6.7 / 2.9 / 6.8
13 SA	0135 / 0725 / 1421 / 2010	2.3 / 7.6 / 1.9 / 7.9	**28** SU	0135 / 0729 / 1417 / 2011	2.9 / 6.9 / 2.6 / 7.2
14 SU	0259 / 0842 / 1537 / 2117	1.9 / 8.1 / 1.5 / 8.4	**29** M	0247 / 0842 / 1522 / 2105	2.5 / 7.4 / 2.1 / 7.8
15 M	0409 / 0944 / 1641 / 2212	1.4 / 8.6 / 1.1 / 8.9	**30** TU	0346 / 0927 / 1616 / 2152	2.0 / 8.0 / 1.7 / 8.3

19

Chart Datum: 4·89 metres below Lallemand System (Mean Sea Level, Marseilles)

TIME ZONE –0100
(French Standard Time)
Subtract 1 hour for UT

For French Summer Time add ONE hour in non-shaded areas

FRANCE – DIEPPE

LAT 49°56′N   LONG 1°05′E

TIMES AND HEIGHTS OF HIGH AND LOW WATERS   YEAR **1996**

MAY

Day	Time	m	Time	m	Time	m	Time	m
1 W	0437	1.5	1012	8.4	1705	1.1	2234	8.8
2 TH	0525	1.2	1054	8.8	1750	1.0	2314	9.1
3 F ○	0610	0.9	1134	9.1	1834	0.8	2353	9.3
4 SA	0653	0.7	1214	9.3	1915	0.7		
5 SU	0032	9.4	0735	0.5	1255	9.4	1955	0.6
6 M	0113	9.5	0816	0.5	1338	9.4	2035	0.7
7 TU	0156	9.3	0858	0.7	1422	9.1	2117	1.0
8 W	0241	9.0	0942	0.9	1510	8.8	2202	1.4
9 TH	0331	8.6	1031	1.3	1606	8.3	2255	1.7
10 F	0431	8.1	1130	1.7	1713	7.9		
11 SA	0002	2.0	0544	7.8	1242	1.9	1828	7.8
12 SU	0120	2.1	0702	7.8	1359	1.8	1944	7.9
13 M	0235	1.9	0816	8.0	1510	1.6	2051	8.3
14 TU	0343	1.5	0919	8.4	1614	1.3	2147	8.6
15 W	0442	1.3	1012	8.7	1708	1.2	2234	8.9
16 TH	0533	1.1	1058	8.9	1753	1.1	2316	9.0
17 F ●	0616	1.0	1138	9.0	1832	1.0	2353	9.0
18 SA	0653	1.0	1216	9.0	1908	1.0		
19 SU	0029	9.0	0729	1.0	1251	9.0	1942	1.1
20 M	0103	8.9	0803	1.1	1327	8.8	2016	1.3
21 TU	0138	8.8	0836	1.2	1402	8.6	2047	1.5
22 W	0212	8.5	0907	1.5	1437	8.3	2118	1.8
23 TH	0246	8.1	0938	1.8	1513	7.9	2153	2.2
24 F	0324	7.7	1016	2.2	1555	7.5	2236	2.5
25 SA	0409	7.3	1103	2.5	1647	7.2	2331	2.7
26 SU	0508	7.1	1203	2.6	1754	7.1		
27 M	0036	2.7	0622	7.0	1312	2.6	1908	7.3
28 TU	0146	2.5	0736	7.3	1423	2.3	2014	7.7
29 W	0253	2.1	0839	7.7	1527	1.9	2109	8.1
30 TH	0353	1.7	0932	8.2	1624	1.5	2158	8.6
31 F	0448	1.3	1021	8.6	1716	1.1	2244	9.0

JUNE

Day	Time	m	Time	m	Time	m	Time	m
1 SA ○	0540	1.0	1108	9.0	1806	0.9	2329	9.3
2 SU	0631	0.7	1154	9.3	1854	0.7		
3 M	0014	9.4	0719	0.5	1240	9.4	1941	0.6
4 TU	0059	9.5	0806	0.4	1327	9.5	2027	0.7
5 W	0146	9.5	0853	0.5	1415	9.3	2113	0.8
6 TH	0235	9.2	0939	0.7	1505	9.0	2200	1.1
7 F	0326	8.9	1028	1.0	1558	8.7	2251	1.4
8 SA	0421	8.4	1122	1.3	1656	8.3	2349	1.7
9 SU	0523	8.1	1222	1.6	1759	8.0		
10 M	0054	1.9	0630	7.8	1327	1.8	1908	7.9
11 TU	0202	1.9	0742	7.8	1435	1.8	2018	8.0
12 W	0310	1.8	0850	8.0	1539	1.7	2119	8.2
13 TH	0411	1.6	0948	8.2	1636	1.6	2210	8.4
14 F	0504	1.5	1036	8.4	1724	1.5	2254	8.6
15 SA	0549	1.4	1118	8.6	1805	1.4	2332	8.7
16 SU ●	0629	1.2	1156	8.7	1844	1.3		
17 M	0008	8.8	0707	1.2	1232	8.7	1921	1.3
18 TU	0043	8.8	0743	1.2	1307	8.7	1956	1.3
19 W	0117	8.7	0817	1.2	1342	8.6	2028	1.5
20 TH	0152	8.6	0849	1.4	1417	8.5	2059	1.6
21 F	0226	8.4	0919	1.6	1451	8.2	2132	1.9
22 SA	0301	8.1	0953	1.8	1527	8.0	2209	2.1
23 SU	0339	7.8	1033	2.1	1609	7.7	2254	2.3
24 M	0425	7.5	1120	2.3	1700	7.5	2348	2.4
25 TU	0522	7.3	1218	2.4	1803	7.4		
26 W	0050	2.4	0633	7.3	1325	2.4	1916	7.5
27 TH	0200	2.2	0748	7.5	1438	2.1	2024	7.9
28 F	0311	1.9	0854	8.0	1545	1.7	2123	8.4
29 SA	0415	1.4	0952	8.5	1646	1.3	2217	8.8
30 SU	0514	1.1	1046	8.9	1742	1.0	2308	9.2

JULY

Day	Time	m	Time	m	Time	m	Time	m
1 M ○	0611	0.7	1137	9.2	1837	0.7	2358	9.5
2 TU	0706	0.5	1228	9.5	1929	0.6		
3 W	0048	9.6	0758	0.3	1317	9.6	2019	0.5
4 TH	0136	9.6	0847	0.3	1405	9.6	2107	0.6
5 F	0225	9.5	0933	0.4	1453	9.4	2152	0.8
6 SA	0312	9.2	1017	0.7	1540	9.0	2237	1.2
7 SU	0401	8.7	1102	1.2	1629	8.6	2325	1.6
8 M	0454	8.3	1151	1.6	1724	8.1		
9 TU	0019	1.9	0553	7.8	1248	2.0	1827	7.7
10 W	0122	2.2	0703	7.5	1353	2.2	1940	7.6
11 TH	0232	2.2	0819	7.5	1502	2.2	2050	7.7
12 F	0340	2.1	0925	7.7	1606	2.0	2148	8.0
13 SA	0438	1.8	1018	8.0	1700	1.8	2235	8.3
14 SU	0527	1.6	1101	8.3	1744	1.6	2315	8.5
15 M ●	0609	1.4	1139	8.5	1824	1.4	2350	8.6
16 TU	0648	1.3	1214	8.7	1902	1.3		
17 W	0024	8.7	0724	1.2	1248	8.7	1937	1.3
18 TH	0058	8.8	0759	1.2	1322	8.8	2009	1.3
19 F	0131	8.8	0830	1.2	1355	8.7	2040	1.4
20 SA	0204	8.6	0900	1.3	1427	8.6	2111	1.5
21 SU	0237	8.5	0931	1.5	1500	8.4	2144	1.7
22 M	0312	8.2	1005	1.7	1537	8.1	2223	2.0
23 TU	0351	7.9	1045	2.0	1619	7.8	2309	2.2
24 W	0439	7.6	1135	2.3	1713	7.6		
25 TH	0005	2.3	0542	7.4	1238	2.4	1824	7.5
26 F	0116	2.3	0703	7.4	1356	2.3	1945	7.7
27 SA	0236	2.1	0823	7.8	1515	1.9	2055	8.2
28 SU	0349	1.6	0930	8.3	1622	1.5	2157	8.7
29 M	0454	1.1	1029	8.8	1724	1.0	2253	9.2
30 TU ○	0556	0.7	1124	9.3	1823	0.7	2345	9.5
31 W	0654	0.4	1215	9.6	1918	0.5		

AUGUST

Day	Time	m	Time	m	Time	m	Time	m
1 TH	0035	9.8	0746	0.2	1303	9.8	2008	0.4
2 F	0122	9.8	0834	0.1	1349	9.8	2053	0.4
3 SA	0208	9.7	0917	0.3	1432	9.6	2135	0.7
4 SU	0252	9.4	0956	0.7	1515	9.2	2214	1.1
5 M	0335	8.9	1033	1.2	1558	8.7	2254	1.6
6 TU	0421	8.3	1114	1.7	1646	8.1	2339	2.1
7 W	0514	7.7	1204	2.3	1743	7.5		
8 TH	0038	2.5	0621	7.2	1310	2.6	1857	7.2
9 F	0152	2.6	0745	7.0	1426	2.7	2021	7.3
10 SA	0309	2.5	0902	7.3	1539	2.4	2127	7.6
11 SU	0414	2.1	0958	7.8	1637	2.0	2216	8.0
12 M	0506	1.7	1042	8.2	1725	1.7	2255	8.4
13 TU	0549	1.4	1119	8.5	1805	1.4	2330	8.6
14 W ●	0628	1.2	1153	8.7	1842	1.3		
15 TH	0004	8.8	0704	1.1	1226	8.9	1916	1.2
16 F	0036	8.9	0737	1.1	1258	8.9	1948	1.2
17 SA	0109	9.0	0808	1.1	1330	8.9	2018	1.2
18 SU	0140	8.9	0838	1.1	1401	8.9	2049	1.3
19 M	0212	8.8	0908	1.3	1433	8.7	2121	1.5
20 TU	0246	8.5	0939	1.5	1508	8.4	2155	1.7
21 W	0323	8.2	1015	1.9	1547	8.1	2237	2.0
22 TH	0408	7.8	1101	2.2	1636	7.8	2331	2.3
23 F	0507	7.5	1202	2.5	1745	7.5		
24 SA	0042	2.4	0631	7.3	1324	2.5	1916	7.5
25 SU	0211	2.2	0801	7.6	1453	2.1	2036	8.0
26 M	0331	1.7	0914	8.3	1606	1.5	2142	8.6
27 TU	0439	1.1	1016	8.9	1709	1.0	2239	9.2
28 W ○	0542	0.7	1110	9.4	1809	0.7	2331	9.6
29 TH	0639	0.3	1159	9.7	1903	0.4		
30 F	0018	9.9	0729	0.2	1244	9.9	1950	0.4
31 SA	0103	9.9	0813	0.2	1327	9.8	2032	0.4

Chart Datum: 4·89 metres below Lallemand System (Mean Sea Level, Marseilles)

TIME ZONE –0100
(French Standard Time)
Subtract 1 hour for UT

For French Summer Time add
ONE hour in non-shaded areas

FRANCE – DIEPPE

LAT 49°56′N   LONG   1°05′E

TIMES AND HEIGHTS OF HIGH AND LOW WATERS   YEAR **1996**

SEPTEMBER

Time	m	Time	m
1 0145 / 0853 / SU 1407 / 2110	9.8 / 0.4 / 9.6 / 0.7	**16** 0115 / 0814 / M 1335 / 2027	9.1 / 1.0 / 9.1 / 1.1
2 0226 / 0927 / M 1446 / 2144	9.4 / 0.8 / 9.2 / 1.1	**17** 0149 / 0845 / TU 1408 / 2100	9.0 / 1.2 / 9.0 / 1.3
3 0305 / 0959 / TU 1525 / 2218	8.9 / 1.3 / 8.7 / 1.6	**18** 0224 / 0918 / W 1444 / 2134	8.8 / 1.4 / 8.7 / 1.6
4 0346 / 1034 / W 1606 / 2258	8.3 / 1.9 / 8.0 / 2.2	**19** 0302 / 0953 / TH 1523 / 2215	8.4 / 1.8 / 8.3 / 1.9
5 0433 / 1120 / TH 1657 / 2352	7.6 / 2.5 / 7.4 / 2.7	**20** 0347 / 1039 / F 1613 / 2309	8.0 / 2.2 / 7.8 / 2.3
6 0535 / 1224 / F 1810	7.0 / 3.0 / 6.9	**21** 0447 / 1141 / SA 1723	7.5 / 2.5 / 7.4
7 0108 / 0705 / SA 1348 / 1944	3.0 / 6.7 / 3.1 / 6.9	**22** 0021 / 0615 / SU 1306 / 1858	2.5 / 7.3 / 2.6 / 7.5
8 0234 / 0833 / SU 1508 / 2059	2.8 / 7.0 / 2.7 / 7.3	**23** 0155 / 0748 / M 1439 / 2021	2.3 / 7.7 / 2.2 / 8.0
9 0345 / 0931 / M 1610 / 2149	2.4 / 7.6 / 2.2 / 7.8	**24** 0318 / 0918 / TU 1552 / 2128	1.7 / 8.3 / 1.6 / 8.6
10 0439 / 1014 / TU 1658 / 2229	1.9 / 8.1 / 1.8 / 8.3	**25** 0425 / 1001 / W 1655 / 2224	1.1 / 8.9 / 1.0 / 9.2
11 0522 / 1051 / W 1739 / 2304	1.5 / 8.6 / 1.4 / 8.7	**26** 0526 / 1053 / TH 1752 / 2314	0.7 / 9.4 / 0.7 / 9.6
12 0601 / 1126 / TH 1816 / ● 2338	1.2 / 8.8 / 1.2 / 8.9	**27** 0619 / 1139 / F 1842 / ○ 2359	0.4 / 9.7 / 0.5 / 9.8
13 0637 / 1159 / F 1851	1.1 / 9.0 / 1.1	**28** 0706 / 1222 / SA 1927	0.4 / 9.8 / 0.5
14 0011 / 0711 / SA 1231 / 1923	9.1 / 1.0 / 9.1 / 1.0	**29** 0041 / 0748 / SU 1302 / 2007	9.8 / 0.4 / 9.8 / 0.6
15 0043 / 0743 / SU 1303 / 1955	9.1 / 1.0 / 9.2 / 1.0	**30** 0121 / 0824 / M 1340 / 2042	9.7 / 0.7 / 9.5 / 0.8

OCTOBER

Time	m	Time	m
1 0159 / 0857 / TU 1416 / 2114	9.3 / 1.0 / 9.2 / 1.2	**16** 0128 / 0826 / W 1347 / 2043	9.2 / 1.1 / 9.2 / 1.1
2 0236 / 0926 / W 1452 / 2145	8.9 / 1.5 / 8.6 / 1.7	**17** 0207 / 0902 / TH 1426 / 2121	9.0 / 1.4 / 8.9 / 1.4
3 0314 / 0958 / TH 1530 / 2220	8.3 / 2.1 / 8.0 / 2.3	**18** 0248 / 0941 / F 1509 / 2204	8.6 / 1.7 / 8.4 / 1.8
4 0356 / 1040 / F 1615 / 2308	7.6 / 2.6 / 7.4 / 2.8	**19** 0336 / 1028 / SA 1601 / 2258	8.1 / 2.1 / 8.0 / 2.1
5 0451 / 1138 / SA 1720	7.0 / 3.1 / 6.8	**20** 0439 / 1131 / SU 1714	7.7 / 2.5 / 7.6
6 0017 / 0613 / SU 1301 / 1851	3.2 / 6.6 / 3.3 / 6.7	**21** 0010 / 0605 / M 1255 / 1844	2.4 / 7.5 / 2.6 / 7.6
7 0146 / 0746 / M 1426 / 2015	3.1 / 6.8 / 3.0 / 7.0	**22** 0141 / 0732 / TU 1424 / 2004	2.2 / 7.8 / 2.2 / 8.0
8 0303 / 0851 / TU 1531 / 2111	2.7 / 7.4 / 2.5 / 7.6	**23** 0301 / 0843 / W 1536 / 2110	1.7 / 8.3 / 1.6 / 8.6
9 0400 / 0938 / W 1622 / 2154	2.1 / 8.0 / 1.9 / 8.2	**24** 0407 / 0942 / TH 1637 / 2206	1.3 / 8.9 / 1.1 / 9.1
10 0447 / 1018 / TH 1705 / 2233	1.6 / 8.5 / 1.5 / 8.6	**25** 0505 / 1032 / F 1732 / 2254	0.9 / 9.3 / 0.9 / 9.4
11 0528 / 1054 / F 1745 / 2309	1.3 / 8.9 / 1.3 / 8.9	**26** 0556 / 1117 / SA 1819 / ○ 2338	0.7 / 9.5 / 0.7 / 9.5
12 0606 / 1129 / SA 1822 / ● 2344	1.1 / 9.1 / 1.1 / 9.1	**27** 0640 / 1158 / SU 1901	0.7 / 9.6 / 0.7
13 0642 / 1203 / SU 1858	1.0 / 9.2 / 1.0	**28** 0018 / 0719 / M 1236 / 1939	9.5 / 0.8 / 9.5 / 0.8
14 0018 / 0717 / M 1237 / 1933	9.2 / 1.0 / 9.3 / 0.9	**29** 0056 / 0754 / TU 1313 / 2014	9.4 / 0.9 / 9.4 / 1.0
15 0052 / 0752 / TU 1311 / 2008	9.3 / 1.0 / 9.3 / 1.0	**30** 0133 / 0827 / W 1348 / 2046	9.2 / 1.2 / 9.1 / 1.3
		31 0210 / 0858 / TH 1424 / 2117	8.8 / 1.6 / 8.6 / 1.7

NOVEMBER

Time	m	Time	m
1 0246 / 0930 / F 1500 / 2150	8.3 / 2.1 / 8.1 / 2.2	**16** 0241 / 0935 / SA 1502 / 2200	8.8 / 1.5 / 8.7 / 1.5
2 0325 / 1006 / SA 1541 / 2230	7.8 / 2.6 / 7.5 / 2.6	**17** 0332 / 1025 / SU 1557 / 2254	8.4 / 1.9 / 8.2 / 1.8
3 0412 / 1056 / SU 1634 / 2325	7.2 / 3.0 / 7.0 / 3.0	**18** 0434 / 1125 / M 1705	8.0 / 2.2 / 7.9
4 0517 / 1203 / M 1748	6.8 / 3.3 / 6.7	**19** 0001 / 0548 / TU 1241 / 1823	2.1 / 7.8 / 2.3 / 7.8
5 0041 / 0640 / TU 1325 / 1912	3.2 / 6.8 / 3.2 / 6.9	**20** 0120 / 0706 / W 1401 / 1939	2.1 / 7.9 / 2.1 / 8.0
6 0202 / 0756 / W 1438 / 2020	2.9 / 7.2 / 2.7 / 7.3	**21** 0236 / 0817 / TH 1512 / 2046	1.8 / 8.2 / 1.7 / 8.3
7 0309 / 0852 / TH 1535 / 2112	2.4 / 7.8 / 2.2 / 7.9	**22** 0342 / 0918 / F 1614 / 2144	1.5 / 8.6 / 1.4 / 8.7
8 0402 / 0938 / F 1624 / 2156	1.9 / 8.3 / 1.7 / 8.4	**23** 0441 / 1010 / SA 1709 / 2234	1.3 / 9.0 / 1.2 / 9.0
9 0449 / 1019 / SA 1709 / 2237	1.5 / 8.7 / 1.4 / 8.7	**24** 0531 / 1055 / SU 1756 / 2318	1.1 / 9.2 / 1.0 / 9.1
10 0532 / 1058 / SU 1751 / 2316	1.3 / 9.0 / 1.1 / 9.0	**25** 0614 / 1136 / M 1837 / ○ 2358	1.1 / 9.3 / 1.0 / 9.2
11 0613 / 1135 / M 1832 / ● 2354	1.1 / 9.2 / 1.0 / 9.2	**26** 0652 / 1214 / TU 1914	1.1 / 9.3 / 1.0
12 0652 / 1213 / TU 1912	1.0 / 9.4 / 0.9	**27** 0035 / 0728 / W 1250 / 1950	9.1 / 1.2 / 9.2 / 1.1
13 0032 / 0732 / W 1251 / 1952	9.3 / 0.9 / 9.4 / 0.8	**28** 0112 / 0803 / TH 1325 / 2024	9.0 / 1.3 / 9.0 / 1.3
14 0113 / 0811 / TU 1332 / 2033	9.3 / 0.9 / 9.3 / 0.9	**29** 0148 / 0836 / F 1401 / 2056	8.8 / 1.6 / 8.7 / 1.6
15 0155 / 0851 / F 1415 / 2114	9.2 / 1.2 / 9.1 / 1.2	**30** 0223 / 0908 / SA 1436 / 2127	8.4 / 1.9 / 8.3 / 1.9

DECEMBER

Time	m	Time	m
1 0300 / 0940 / SU 1512 / 2201	8.1 / 2.3 / 7.9 / 2.3	**16** 0326 / 1021 / M 1550 / 2248	8.8 / 1.5 / 8.7 / 1.4
2 0339 / 1020 / M 1554 / 2243	7.6 / 2.6 / 7.4 / 2.6	**17** 0421 / 1115 / TU 1648 / 2344	8.4 / 1.8 / 8.2 / 1.8
3 0427 / 1111 / TU 1649 / 2339	7.3 / 2.9 / 7.1 / 2.9	**18** 0523 / 1218 / W 1754	8.1 / 2.1 / 7.9
4 0530 / 1214 / W 1759	7.0 / 3.0 / 6.9	**19** 0050 / 0632 / TH 1329 / 1906	2.0 / 7.9 / 2.1 / 7.8
5 0047 / 0646 / TH 1327 / 1916	2.9 / 7.1 / 2.9 / 7.1	**20** 0201 / 0744 / F 1441 / 2018	2.1 / 8.0 / 2.0 / 7.9
6 0201 / 0756 / F 1437 / 2022	2.7 / 7.5 / 2.5 / 7.5	**21** 0312 / 0852 / SA 1548 / 2122	1.9 / 8.2 / 1.8 / 8.2
7 0309 / 0853 / SA 1538 / 2116	2.3 / 7.9 / 2.1 / 8.0	**22** 0414 / 0949 / SU 1646 / 2216	1.7 / 8.5 / 1.5 / 8.5
8 0406 / 0942 / SU 1632 / 2204	1.9 / 8.4 / 1.6 / 8.5	**23** 0507 / 1037 / M 1735 / 2301	1.6 / 8.7 / 1.3 / 8.7
9 0457 / 1027 / M 1722 / 2249	1.5 / 8.8 / 1.2 / 8.9	**24** 0552 / 1119 / TU 1817 / ○ 2342	1.4 / 8.9 / 1.2 / 8.8
10 0545 / 1110 / TU 1810 / 2333	1.2 / 9.2 / 1.0 / 9.2	**25** 0631 / 1157 / W 1855	1.3 / 9.0 / 1.1
11 0631 / 1153 / W 1856	1.0 / 9.4 / 0.8	**26** 0018 / 0708 / TH 1232 / 1931	8.9 / 1.3 / 9.0 / 1.1
12 0017 / 0717 / TH 1237 / 1941	9.4 / 0.9 / 9.5 / 0.6	**27** 0053 / 0744 / F 1306 / 2006	8.9 / 1.3 / 8.9 / 1.2
13 0102 / 0802 / F 1322 / 2027	9.5 / 0.8 / 9.5 / 0.7	**28** 0128 / 0818 / SA 1341 / 2038	8.8 / 1.4 / 8.8 / 1.4
14 0148 / 0849 / SA 1409 / 2112	9.4 / 0.9 / 9.4 / 0.8	**29** 0202 / 0849 / SU 1414 / 2107	8.7 / 1.6 / 8.6 / 1.6
15 0236 / 0933 / SU 1457 / 2158	9.2 / 1.2 / 9.1 / 1.1	**30** 0236 / 0918 / M 1447 / 2137	8.4 / 1.9 / 8.3 / 1.8
		31 0309 / 0951 / TU 1522 / 2211	8.1 / 2.1 / 7.9 / 2.1

19

Chart Datum: 4·89 metres below Lallemand System (Mean Sea Level, Marseilles)

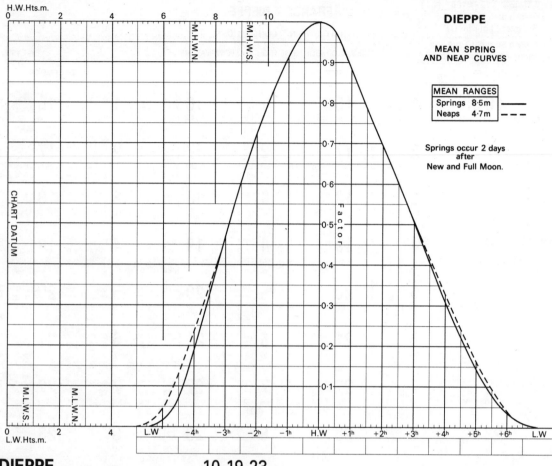

DIEPPE

MEAN SPRING AND NEAP CURVES

MEAN RANGES	
Springs	8·5m
Neaps	4·7m

Springs occur 2 days after New and Full Moon.

DIEPPE   10-19-23

Seine Maritime 49°56'·36N 01°05'·08E

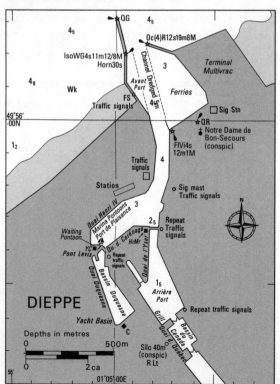

DIEPPE

Depths in metres

CHARTS
AC 2147, *2451*; SHOM 7317, 7083, 6824; ECM 1011, 1012; Imray C31; Stanfords 1
TIDES
–0011 Dover; ML 4·9; Duration 0535; Zone –0100
NOTE: Dieppe is a Standard Port. Tidal predictions for each day of the year are given above.

SHELTER
Very good. Access at all tides, but chan is exposed to winds from NW to NE, causing a heavy scend. The ferry terminal is at the E side of ent. The marina is in the Avant Port at Quai Henri IV. Or yachts can lock into the Bassin Duquesne HW –2 to +1; bridge opens H and H+30 during each period; berth in NW corner. No yachts in Arrière Port.
NAVIGATION
WPT 49°56'·48N 01°04'·60E, 298°/118° from/to W jetty extension, 0·35M. Ent to hbr is simple, but beware strong stream across ent. ⚓ is prohib in a zone 5ca off pierhead. Ent chan and Avant Port are dredged 5m. Dieppe is a busy port; ent/exit are controlled during ferry movements. Due to restricted visibility, yachts **must** request entry on Ch 12, 2M before hbr ent; also 10 mins before leaving.
LIGHTS AND MARKS
ECM buoy (DI), VQ (3) 5s, bell, is 2·5M WNW of hbr ent. W jetty, Iso WG 4s 11m 12/8M, W095°-164°, G164°-095°; horn 30s. QG lt marks N end of W jetty extension. In low vis, horn 5s = no entry.
E jetty, Oc (4) R 12s 19m 8M.
IPTS (full code) shown from stns at root of W jetty and on W side of hbr; repeated (simplified code) where shown on chartlet. Extra sigs combined with IPTS:
Ⓖ to right = Ferry entering; Ⓡ to right = Ferry leaving.
Ⓦ to left = Bassin Duquesne lock gates open.
ⓇⓇ (hor) to right = Dredger in chan.

DIEPPE *continued*

Lock sigs at Bassin Duquesne:
Request bridge and lock to open = Sound 2 blasts;
Ⓖ = Enter, no exit; Ⓡ = Exit, no entry
Request will not be met unless Flag P (Ⓦ at night) is
flying from pier hd and dock.

RADIO TELEPHONE
Call: *Dieppe Port* VHF Ch **12** (HO) 16 (H24). See Navigation.

TELEPHONE
Hr Mr 35.84.10.55; Hr Mr (Port de Plaisance) 35.84.32.99;
Aff Mar 35.06.96.70; CROSS 21.87.21.87; ⌗ 35.82.24.47;
SNSM 35.84.30.76; Meteo 21.31.52.23; Auto 36.68.08.76;
Police 35.06.96.74; Ⓗ 35.06.76.76; Brit Consul 35.42.27.47.

FACILITIES
Quai Henri IV Marina (320, inc visitors) FW, AC; **Bassin
Duquesne** (130, inc visitors) ☎ 35.84.34.95, FW, AC, BH
(30 ton), Slip, C, D, CH; **Cercle de la Voile de Dieppe** ☎
35.84.32.99, D, FW, C (3 ton), AB, R, Bar; **Services:** ME, EI,
Ⓔ, Sh, CH, Sh.
Town P, D, FW, V, Gaz, R, Bar, ✉, Ⓞ, Ⓑ, ⇌, ✈, Ferry:
Dieppe - Newhaven.

LE TRÉPORT   10-19-24
Seine Maritime 50°03'·95N 01°22'·24E

CHARTS
AC 1352, 2147, 2612, *2451*; SHOM 7207, 7083, 6824; ECM
1011; Imray C31; Stanfords 1

TIDES
–0025 Dover; ML4·9; Duration 0530; Zone –0100

Standard Port DIEPPE (←)

Times				Height (metres)			
High Water		Low Water		MHWS	MHWN	MLWN	MLWS
0100	0600	0100	0700	9·3	7·3	2·6	0·8
1300	1800	1300	1900				
Differences LE TRÉPORT							
+0005	0000	+0005	+0010	+0·1	+0·1	–0·2	–0·1
CAYEUX							
+0005	+0005	+0013	+0013	+0·9	+0·6	+0·1	+0·3

SHELTER
Good in marina at S side of first S Basin (3·7m), E of FVs.
But ent chan and most of Avant Port dry; S side is dredged
1·5m, but prone to silting. Lock opens HW ±3. Port de
Commerce is only used by yachts as an overflow.
Note: Swing/lifting bridge to be built at E end of marina.

NAVIGATION
WPT 50°04'·30N 01°21'·70E, 315°/135° from/to ent, 0·52M.
Coast dries to approx 300m off the pier hds. Shingle spit
extends NW from E pier hd; keep well to the W. Entry
difficult in strong on-shore winds which cause scend in
Avant Port.

LIGHTS AND MARKS
Le Tréport is identified between high chalk cliffs, with
crucifix (lit) above town and conspic church S of hbr. No
ldg lts/marks. IPTS were due to be installed 1995. W jetty
Fl (2) G 10s 15m 20M. E jetty Oc R 4s 8m 6M. Lock sigs
shown from head of dredged/piled chan to S Basin: Ⓖ =
enter lock; Ⓡ = no entry.

RADIO TELEPHONE
Call: *Capitainerie Le Tréport* VHF Ch 12 16 (HW ±3).
Marina Ch 12 for tidal information.

TELEPHONE
Hr Mr 35.86.17.91, Fax 35.86.60.11; Lock (to marina)
35.50.63.06; Port de Commerce 35.86.27.67; Aff Mar
35.06.96.70; SNSM 35.86.10.91 CROSS 21.87.21.87; ⌗
35.86.15.34; Auto 36.68.08.76; Police 35.86.12.11; Dr
35.86.16.23; Brit Consul 21.96.33.76.

FACILITIES
Marina (130+10) FF99.90, AC, FW; **Avant Port** M; **Port de
Commerce** C (10 ton); **YC de la Bresle** ☎ 35.86.19.93, C,
Bar; **Services:** ME, CH, EI, Ⓔ, P, D, Gaz.
Town P, D, V, Gaz, R, Bar, ✉, Ⓑ, ⇌, ✈ (Dieppe). Ferry:
Dieppe.

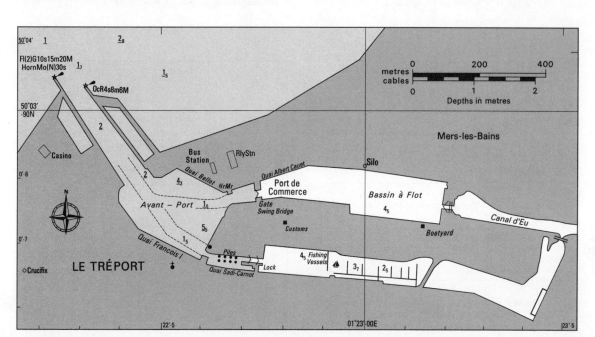

ST VALÉRY-SUR-SOMME/ LE CROTOY   10-19-25

Somme

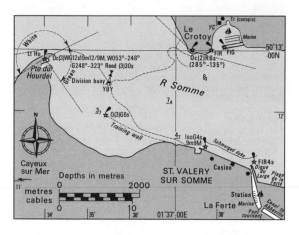

CHARTS
AC 2451; SHOM 7084; ECM 1011; Imray C31; Stanfords 1
TIDES
–0020 Dover; ML —; Zone –0100

Standard Port DIEPPE (←—)

Times				Height (metres)			
High Water		Low Water		MHWS	MHWN	MLWN	MLWS
0100	0600	0100	0700	9·3	7·3	2·6	0·8
1300	1800	1300	1900				
Differences ST VALÉRY-SUR-SOMME							
+0037	+0044	No data		+0·7	+0·7	No data	
LE HOURDEL							
+0031	+0028	No data		+0·7	+0·6	No data	

SHELTER
The B de Somme is open to W and can be dangerous in onshore winds >F6. All 3 very well sheltered hbrs (ie Le Hourdel, Le Crotoy and St Valéry-sur-Somme) are FV ports; small cargo vessels very occasionally berth at St Valéry town quay. Yachts can:
(1) dry out on hard sand at Le Hourdel; access HW±1½.
(2) enter Le Crotoy marina when tidal range at Dover >4·4m (approx Coefficient 85) with max. draft 1·5m.
(3) enter (HW ±1) St Valéry marina (max. draft 2·5m).
(4) enter Abbeville Canal at St Valéry (max. draft 3m up to Abbeville) by prior arrangement and daylight only.
NAVIGATION
WPT 'ATSO' NCM By, VQ, 50°14'·00N 01°28'·50E, about 1M W of buoyed chan (shifts). From N, beware being set by the flood onto shoals off Pte St Quentin. The whole estuary dries up to 3M seaward of Le Hourdel. The sands build up in ridges offshore, but inside Pte du Hourdel are generally flat, except where R Somme and minor streams scour their way to the sea. If Dover tidal range >4·4m, at HW ±1 there is sufficient water over the sands inside Pte du Hourdel for vessels <1·5m draft.
Start appr from 'ATSO' at HW –2. Chans are ever-shifting but buoys are moved as required. Follow chan with lateral buoys numbered S1 to S50 (some lit), in strict order (no corner-cutting) to small unlit WCM Division buoy, in variable position E of Pte du Hourdel; then see below. Departure from Le Hourdel/Le Crotoy is not possible before HW –2; St Valéry HW–1.
LIGHTS AND MARKS
Only landmark is Cayeux-sur-Mer lt ho (W with R top) Fl R 5s 32m 22M (off chartlet to SSW). Pte du Hourdel lt ho Oc (3) WG 12s 19m 12/9M. Le Crotoy Oc (2) R 6s 19m 9M.

LE HOURDEL: Chan unmarked; follow 'S' buoys, then head SW toward end of shingle spit; hug the shingle.
LE CROTOY: From Division By chan runs N & E with lateral Bys C1 to C10. Enter hbr very close to FV stages (port-side). Secure at last FV stage and ask YC for berth. Tidal hbr badly silted (1995), with 2 drying pontoons.
ST VALÉRY-SUR-SOMME: From Division buoy, buoyed chan continues with SHMs becoming bns on submerged training wall, the seaward end of which is lit, Q (3) G 6s 2m 2M; then four bns on end of groynes. Iso G 4s 9m 9M marks beginning of tree-lined promenade; submerged dyke opposite marked with PHM bns. W tr on head of Digue du Large, Fl R 4s 9m 9M, leads into marina, dredged 2m, and town quay.
RADIO TELEPHONE
VHF Ch 09 (St Valéry HW ±2; Le Crotoy YC Jul/Aug only).
TELEPHONE
St Valéry Hr Mr 22.26.91.64; Le Crotoy 22.27.83.11 (Port de plaisance); Aff Mar 22.27.81.44; ⌗ 22.24.04.75; Lock (canal) 22.60.80.23; CROSS 21.87.21.87; Auto 36.68.08.80; Police 22.60.82.08; Dr 22.26.92.25; Brit Consul 21.96.33.76.
FACILITIES
ST VALÉRY
Marina and YC Sport Nautique Valéricain (250 + 30) ☎ 22.26.91.64, FW, C (6 ton), Slip, R, ▣, Bar; Access HW ±1; **Services:** ME, El, CH, Ⓔ, charts.
Town EC Mon; P, D, CH, V, Gaz, R, Bar, ✉, Ⓑ, ⇌ and ✈ (Abbeville). Ferry: See Boulogne.
LE CROTOY
Marina (280) ☎ 22.27.83.11, FW, C (6 ton), Slip; **YC Nautique de la Baie de Somme** ☎ 22.27.83.11, Bar.
Town EC Mon; Ⓑ, Bar, D, P, ✉, R, ⇌, V.

LE TOUQUET/ÉTAPLES
10-19-26

Pas de Calais

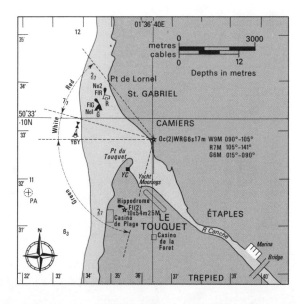

CHARTS
AC 2451; SHOM 7085; ECM 1011; Imray C31; Stanfords 1, 9
TIDES
–0010 Dover; ML 5·3; Duration 0520; Zone –0100

Standard Port DIEPPE (←—)

Times				Height (metres)			
High Water		Low Water		MHWS	MHWN	MLWN	MLWS
0100	0600	0100	0700	9·3	7·3	2·6	0·8
1300	1800	1300	1900				
Differences LE TOUQUET (ÉTAPLES)							
+0008	+0016	+0033	+0030	+0·3	+0·4	+0·4	+0·4
BERCK							
+0008	+0011	+0033	+0025	+0·6	+0·7	+0·5	+0·5

SHELTER
Good, except in strong W'lies. Drying moorings to stbd off Le Touquet YC. At Étaples, access HW±2 to small marina (1m) close downstream of low bridge; beware strong current.

LE TOUQUET/ETAPLES *continued*

NAVIGATION
WPT 50°35'·00N 01°31'·80E, 308°/128° from/to Camiers lt,
3·8M. Appr & ent are not easy; estuary dries 2M offshore.
Best ent is at HW –1. In even moderate W winds the sea
breaks heavily a long way out and entry should not be
attempted. The chan is always shifting and buoys, some
lit, are moved accordingly. Beware drying wreck 2M NW
of Le Touquet lt ho, marked by unlit WCM buoy.

LIGHTS AND MARKS
Le Touquet is at the S end of the Terres de Tourmont, a
conspic range 175m high, visible for 25M.
Appr between Pte de Lornel and Pte du Touquet, where
La Canche lt ho is conspic Or tr, brown band, W & G top,
Fl (2) 10s 54m 25M.
Camiers lt Oc (2) WRG 6s 17m 9/6M (R pylon hard to see
by day) is on NE side of estuary. Chan ent usually lies in
lt's R sector (105°-141°), but may lie in G sector, (015°-
090°) ie S of the WCM wreck buoy, which is in turn
covered by the W sector (090°-105°). Canche No 2 PHM
buoy, Fl (2) R 6s, is first lateral chan buoy; take care not
to cut corners.
R Canche to marina is flanked by sunken training walls,
lit by Fl R 4s on head of NE wall and marked by posts.

RADIO TELEPHONE
VHF Ch 21 16.
TELEPHONE
Hr Mr Le Touquet 21.05.12.77; Hr Mr Etaples 21.94.54.33;
Aff Mar Étaples 21.94.61.50; Auto 36.68.08.62;
⌗ 21.05.01.72; CROSS 21.87.21.87; Police 21.94.60.17;
Dr 21.05.14.42; Brit Consul 21.96.33.76.
FACILITIES
LE TOUQUET
Cercle Nautique du Touquet ☎ 21.05.12.77, M, P, Slip,
ME, D, FW, C, CH, R, Bar; **Services:** BY, Sh, SM. **Town** P,
D, V, Gaz, R, Bar, ⊠, Ⓑ, ⇌, ✈.
ETAPLES
Marina (115 + 15 visitors), FF85, FW, C (3 ton), AC, P, D;
Quay C (3 ton), FW, Slip; **Centre Nautique YC** ☎
21.94.74.26, Bar, Slip; **Services:** CH, El, Ⓔ, M, ME, Sh, D.
Town Ⓑ, Bar, D, P, ⊠, R, ⇌, V. Ferry: Boulogne-Folkestone.

BOULOGNE-SUR-MER   10-19-27
Pas de Calais 50°44'·56N 01°34'·13E

CHARTS
AC 438, *1892, 2451*; SHOM 7247,7323, 7085; ECM 1010,
1011; Imray C31, C8; Stanfords 1, 9
TIDES
0000 Dover; ML 4·9; Duration 0515; Zone –0100

Standard Port DIEPPE (←—)

Times				Height (metres)			
High Water		Low Water		MHWS	MHWN	MLWN	MLWS
0100	0600	0100	0700	9·3	7·3	2·6	0·8
1300	1800	1300	1900				
Differences BOULOGNE							
+0015	+0026	+0037	+0036	–0.4	0.0	+0.2	+0.4

SHELTER
Good, except in strong NW'lies. Ent possible at all tides
and in most weather. Very busy ferry and FV port; beware
wash from FVs. Marina pontoons (2·9m) are on SW side
of tidal basin alongside Quai Chanzy. Max LOA 10m
(>10m apply before arrival or berth on Quai Gambetta).
When R Liane in spate beware turbulent water.
NAVIGATION
WPT 50°44'·50N 01°33'·00E, 270°/090° from/to S bkwtr
(Digue Carnot) lt, 0·72M. Fairway buoy SCM, VQ (6) + L Fl
10s, is 295°/2·1M from S bkwtr lt. Cap d'Alprech Lt Ho, Fl
(3) 15s 62m 23M, is 2·5M S of hbr ent. E side of hbr dries.
Obey IPTS from SW jetty (see below). No navigational
dangers and ent is easily identified and well marked, but
keep W and S of Digue Nord lt tr, Fl (2) R 6s, as outer half
of bkwtr covers at HW.
LIGHTS AND MARKS
Monument tr is conspic 2M E of hbr ent. Cathedral dome
is conspic, 0·62M E of marina. St Nicolas Ch spire leads
123° through Avant Port. Ldg lts 123°: front 3 FG in ▽;
rear Dir FR, intens 113°-133°, lead towards marina. 2 Bu
lts (hor) upriver of marina = sluicing from R Liane.
IPTS are shown from SW jetty hd (FG ☆), and from Quai
Gambetta, opposite ☆ 3FG ▽ (chartlet), visible from
marina. One Ⓡ (below IPTS) = dredger working (this
does not prohibit movements).
RADIO TELEPHONE
VHF Ch **12** (H24). Marina Ch 09.
TELEPHONE
Hr Mr 21.80.72.00; Hr Mr Plaisance 21.31.70.01; Control Tr
21.31.52.43; Aff Mar 21.30.53.23; CROSS 21.87.21.87;
SNSM 21.31.42.59; ⌗ 21.30.14.24; Meteo 21.31.52.23;
Auto 36.68.08.62; Police 21.31.75.17; Ⓗ 21.31.92.13; Brit
Consul 21.30.25.11.

FACILITIES
Marina (114 + 17 visitors) ☎ 21.31.70.01, FW, Slip, AC, P,
D, C (20 ton); **Quai Gambetta** M, P, D, FW, AB, V, R, Bar;
YC Boulonnais ☎ 21.31.80.68, C, Bar;
Services: Ⓔ, ME, El, Sh, M, CH, Divers, SHOM;
Town P, D, V, Gaz, R, Bar, ⊠, Ⓑ, ⇌, ✈ (Le Touquet/
Calais). Ferry to Folkestone.

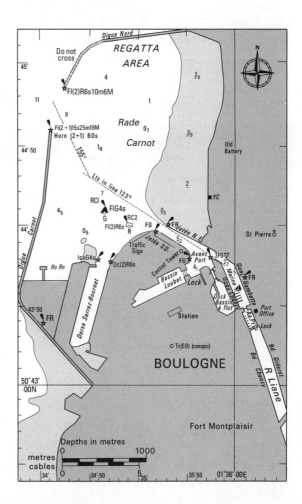

CALAIS   10-19-28

Pas de Calais 50°58'·34N 01°50'·50E

CHARTS
AC 1352, *1892, 323*; SHOM 6474, 6651; ECM 1010; Imray C8; Stanfords 1

TIDES
+0048 Dover; ML 4·0; Duration 0525; Zone –0100

Standard Port DIEPPE (←––)

Times				Height (metres)			
High Water		Low Water		MHWS	MHWN	MLWN	MLWS
0100	0600	0100	0700	9·3	7·3	2·6	0·8
1300	1800	1300	1900				
Differences CALAIS							
+0043	+0057	+0105	+0054	–2·2	–1·3	–0·5	+0·2

SHELTER
Very good, especially in the marina at Bassin de l'Ouest (3-6m). R waiting buoys outside lock (times below). Ent is rough with heavy swell in strong NW to NE winds; access H24. Enter Bassin Carnot only if bound for the canals.

NAVIGATION
WPT 50°58'·50N 01°49'·90E, 298°/118° from/to Jetée Ouest lt, 0·43M. Beware the Ridens de la Rade, about 4ca N of ent, a partly drying (0·6m) sandbank on which seas break. From the E it may be best to keep seaward of this bank until able to round CA8 PHM lt By and appr from 1M W of hbr. Byelaws require yachts to have engine running (even if sailing) and not to impede ferries/commercial vessels. Ent is relatively easy and well marked but there is much shipping.

LIGHTS AND MARKS
Cap Blanc-Nez and Dover Patrol monument are conspic 5·5M WSW of hbr ent. Several churches and bldgs in the town are conspic. From a position ¼M SE of CA 10 PHM buoy, Fl (2) R 6s, the main lt ho (conspic), Fl (4) 15s, leads 141° through ent. The intens sector (115·5°-121·5°) of Dir FR 14m 14M at Gare Maritime leads close past the W jetty Iso G 3s. Hbr Control is conspic, pyramidal bldg on port-side as Arrière Port is entered.
IPTS (full code) are shown from Hbr Control. If no sigs are shown (ie no ferries under way), yachts may enter/leave. They may also follow a ferry entering /leaving, keeping to the stbd side of the fairway. Supplementary traffic sigs, shown alongside the upper IPTS lt, are:
Ⓡ = ferry leaving; no movements.
Ⓖ = ferry entering; no movements.
One Ⓡ (alongside lower IPTS lt) = dredger working, (this does not prohibit movements).
Bassin de l'Ouest: Lock gates and bridge open HW –1½, HW and HW +½. (Sat and Sun HW –2, HW and HW +1).
Ⓨ = 10 mins before lock opens.
Ⓡ = All movements prohib.
Ⓖ = Movement authorised.
4 blasts = Request permission to enter.
Prior to leaving, best to tell bridge operator your ETD.
Bassin Carnot: Gates open HW –1½ to HW +¾. Lock sigs:
ⓇⓇ (hor) = Enter.
ⓇⓇ (hor) = Do not enter.
Ⓖ = Exit from basin permitted.
Ⓡ = Do not exit from basin.
2 blasts = Request permission to enter.

RADIO TELEPHONE
Whilst underway in appr's and hbr, keep a close listening watch on Ch **12** 16 (H24) *Calais Port Traffic* and marina. Carnot lock Ch 12 (occas). Hoverport Ch 20 (occas). Cap Gris Nez, Channel Navigation Info Service (CNIS), call: *Gris Nez Traffic* Ch 11 16 (H24). Info broadcasts in English and French on Ch 11, at H + 10, and also at H + 25 when vis is < 2M. CROSS Ch 11 16.

TELEPHONE
Hr Mr (Marina) 21.34.55.23; Hr Mr (Port) 21.96.31.20; Aff Mar 21.34.52.70; CROSS 21.87.21.87; SNSM 21.96.31.20; ∰ 21.34.75.40; Meteo 21.33.24.25; Auto 36.68.08.62; Police 21.96.74.17; Ⓗ 21.46.33.33; Brit Consul 21.96.33.76.

FACILITIES
Marina (350 + 400 visitors) ☎ 21.34.55.23, AB pontoon: 47FF summer, 39FF winter; AB wall: 24FF summer, 20FF winter. D, P (cans), FW, C (6 ton), BH (3 ton), AC, CH, Gaz, R, Ⓖ, Sh, SM, V, Bar; Access HW –1½ to HW +½; **YC de Calais** ☎ 21.97.02.34, M, P, Bar; **Services:** CH, SM, ME.
Town CH, V, Gaz, R, Bar, ✉, Ⓑ, ⇌, ✈. Ferry: Dover.

ADJACENT HARBOUR
GRAVELINES, Nord, 51°00'·90N 02°05'·75E, AC 1350, *323*; SHOM 7057, 6651. HW +0045 on Dover (UT); +0100 on Dieppe (zone –0100); HW ht –2·8m on Dieppe; ML 3·3m; Duration 0520. See 10.19.29. Good shelter, but chan dries 1·5m. Safest entry HW –1; do not attempt it in strong onshore winds. Appr to bkwtrs, with old lt ho (unlit, conspic B/W spiral) in transit with wtr tr 142°. Nuclear power stn 1M NE. Beware strong E going stream across ent at HW. Keep to W on entry and to E when inside. Hbr dries (soft mud). Yachts may take the ground or enter Bassin Vauban via lock open HW ±1½; waiting pontoon outside. E jetty lt, Fl (3) R 12s 5m 4M. W jetty, Fl (2) WG 6s 9m 10/7M, vis W317°-327°, G078°-085°, W085°-244°. VHF Ch 09 (HO). Aff Mar ☎ 28.23.06.12. Facilities: **Bassin Vauban** (410+40) ☎ 28.23.13.42, FW, AC, BH (12 ton), C (3 ton); **YC Gravelines** ☎ 28.23.14.68, M, C (10 ton); **Services:** CH, EI, M, ME, Sh. **Town** Ⓑ, Bar, D, P, ✉, R, ⇌, V, Ⓖ.

AGENTS WANTED

If you are interested in becoming our agent for any of the following ports, please write to: The Editor, Edington House, Trent, Sherborne, Dorset DT9 4SR, England – and get your free copy of the almanac annually. You do not have to live in a port to be the agent, but at least a fairly regular visitor.

River Exe	Grandcamp-Maisy
Port Ellen (Islay)	Port-en-Bessin
Glandore/Union Hall	Courseulles
River Rance/Dinan	Boulogne
Lampaul	Dunkerque
Port Tudy	Terneuzen/Westerschelde
River Etel	Oudeschild
Le Palais (Belle Ile)	Lauwersoog
Le Pouliguen/Pornichet	Dornumer-Accumersiel
L'Herbaudière	Hooksiel
St Gilles-Croix-de-Vie	Langeoog
River Seudre	Bremerhaven
Royan	Helgoland
Anglet/Bayonne	Büsum
Hendaye	

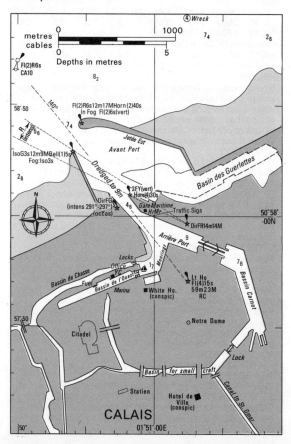

CALAIS

DUNKERQUE   10-19-29

Nord 51°03'·67N 02°21'·10E

CHARTS
AC 1350, *323*, 1872; SHOM 7057, 6651; ECM 1010; Imray
C30; Stanfords 1

TIDES
+0050 Dover; ML 3·2; Duration 0530; Zone –0100

Standard Port DIEPPE (⟵)

Times				Height (metres)			
High Water		Low Water		MHWS	MHWN	MLWN	MLWS
0100	0600	0100	0700	9·3	7·3	2·6	0·8
1300	1800	1300	1900				

Differences DUNKERQUE

+0050	+0122	+0121	+0108	–3·5	–2·4	–1·1	–0·1

SHELTER
Good; hbr accessible at all tides and weather, but fresh
NW–NE winds cause heavy seas at ent and scend in hbr.
This is a busy commercial port; yachts must use E hbr, **not**
the W hbr. Choice of 2 tidal marinas, either side of Port
d'Echouage, ¾M down E side of hbr; or enter non-tidal
marinas in Bassin du Commerce and Bassin de la Marine
via Ecluse Trystram or Wattier and three swing bridges.

NAVIGATION
WPT (E hbr) 51°03'·90N 02°21'·00E, 355°/175° from/to
Jetée Ouest lt, 0·20M. From the W, fetch the Dunkerque
Lanby (Fl 3s), 5M N of Calais, thence to DKA SWM buoy
(L Fl 10s), and then via series of DW lt buoys past W hbr
to DW 29 SHM buoy, ½M WNW of ent. From the E, via
Nieuwpoort Bank WCM buoy, Q (9) 15s, the E1-12 buoys
lead S of Banc Hills. Strong currents reach about 3½kn.

LIGHTS AND MARKS
Main lt ho Fl (2) 10s 59m 28M, W tr with B top. Ldg lts:
Outer (both F Vi) lead 179° through ent. A second pair,
with common rear, lead 185°. (Both pairs are "Big Ship").
Inner, both Oc (2) 6s, lead 137° toward marinas.
IPTS (full) shown from head of Jetée Ouest.
Lock sigs (H24), shown at Ecluse Watier, consist of three
horiz pairs disposed vertically. Middle pair refer to Ecluse
Watier and lowest pair to Ecluse Trystram:

Ⓖ Ⓖ	=	lock open
Ⓡ Ⓡ	=	lock closed

Lock sigs at each lock:

Ⓖ Ⓖ	=	lock ready;
Ⓖ + Fl Ⓖ	=	enter and secure on side of Fl Ⓖ.
Ⓦ	=	enter lock; slack water, both gates
Ⓖ Ⓖ		open.
Ⓡ Ⓡ	=	lock in use, no entry.

RADIO TELEPHONE
VHF Ch 12 16 **73** (H24). Locks Ch 73. Marinas Ch 09.

TELEPHONE
Hr Mr 28.29.72.62; Port Control 28.29.72.87; Aff Mar
28.66.56.14; CROSS 21.87.21.87; SNSM 28.63.23.60; ⌗
28.65.14.73; Meteo 28.66.45.25; Auto 36.68.08.59; Police
28.64.51.09; Ⓗ 28.66.70.01; Brit Consul 28.66.11.98.

FACILITIES
Port du Grand Large (185+25 visitors) ☎ 28.63.23.00, Fax
28.66.66.62, FF65, H24 access (3m), FW, AC, YC, Bar;
YC Mer du Nord Marina (180+70 visitors) ☎ 28.66.79.90,
FF95, approx 2m, Slip, D, P, FW, C (4½ ton), BH (15 ton),
AC, ME, SM, R, Bar;
Access H24 via Ecluse Trystram or Wattier to:
Bassin du Commerce (136) YC de Dunkerque (YCD)
marina (4m) ☎ 28.66.11.06, M, D, L, FW, CH; and to:
Port du Bassin de la Marine (250) , FW, AC, YC.
Services: SHOM, P, D, M, ME, El, Ⓔ, Sh, CH. **Town** P, D,
V, Gaz, R, Bar, ✉, Ⓑ, ⇌, ✈ (Lille). Ferry: Ramsgate.

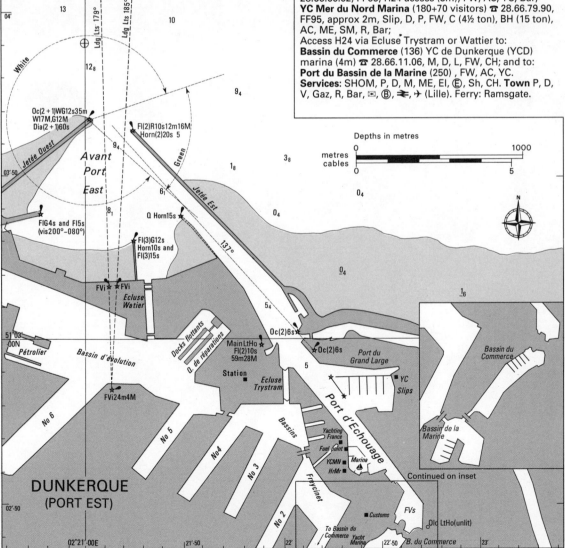

Volvo Penta service

Sales and service centres in area 20
Names and addresses of Volvo Penta dealers in
this area are available from:
Netherlands Nebim Handelmaatschappij BV, Postbus 195, 3640 Ad Mijdrecht
Tel 02979-80111, Fax 0279-87364, Telex 15505 NEHA NL.

**VOLVO
PENTA**

Area 20

Belgium and the Netherlands
Nieuwpoort to Delfzijl

20

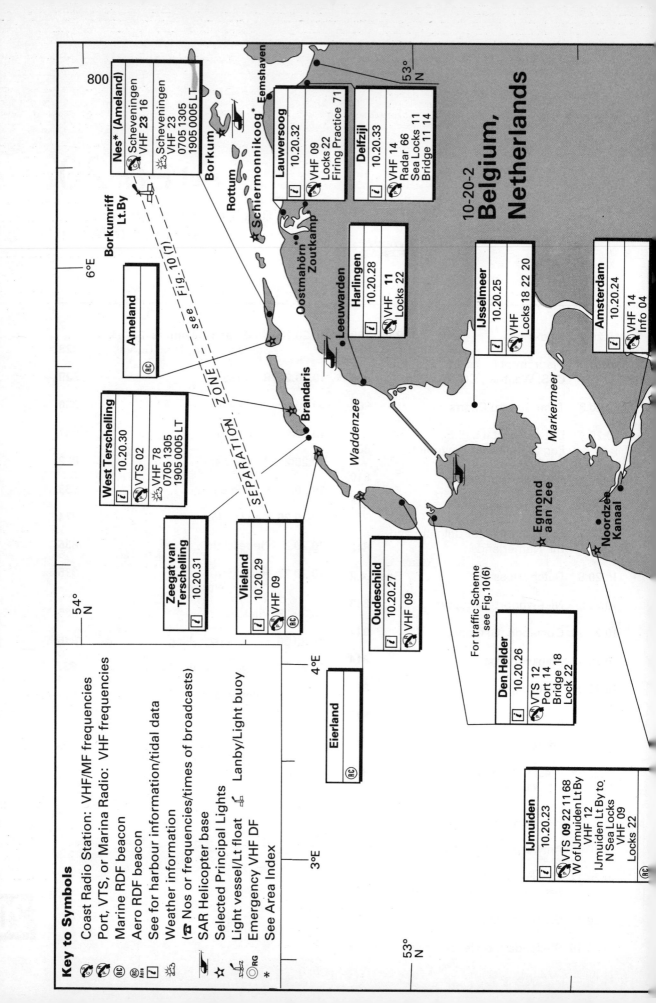

Key to Symbols

Coast Radio Station: VHF/MF frequencies
Port, VTS, or Marina Radio: VHF frequencies
Marine RDF beacon
Aero RDF beacon
See for harbour information/tidal data
Weather information
(☎ Nos or frequencies/times of broadcasts)
SAR Helicopter base
Selected Principal Lights
Light vessel/Lt float   Lanby/Light buoy
Emergency VHF DF
See Area Index

54°
N

6°E

800

Nes* (Ameland)
Scheveningen
VHF **23** 16
Scheveningen
VHF 23
0705 1305
1905 0005 LT

Borkumriff
Lt.By

Borkum

Rottum

Eemshaven

Schiermonnikoog*

Lauwersoog
10.20.32
VHF 09
Locks 22
Firing Practice 71

Delfzijl
10.20.33
VHF 14
Radar 66
Sea Locks 11
Bridge 11 14

53°
N

10-20-2
**Belgium,
Netherlands**

Ameland
ⓇC

see Fig. 10 (7)

Oostmahörn*
Zoutkamp

Harlingen
10.20.28
VHF **11**
Locks 22

Leeuwarden

West Terschelling
10.20.30
VTS 02
VHF 78
0705 1305
1905 0005 LT

Brandaris

Waddenzee

IJsselmeer
10.20.25
VHF
Locks 18 22 20

Amsterdam
10.20.24
VHF 14
Info 04

Markermeer

**Zeegat van
Terschelling**
10.20.31

Vlieland
10.20.29
VHF 09
ⓇC

SEPARATION

ZONE

Oudeschild
10.20.27
VHF 09

Egmond
aan Zee

Noordzee
Kanaal

4°E

Eierland
ⓇC

For traffic Scheme
see Fig.10(6)

Den Helder
10.20.26
VTS 12
Port 14
Bridge 18
Lock 22

3°E

53°
N

IJmuiden
10.20.23
VTS **09** 22 11 68
W of IJmuiden Lt By
VHF 12
IJmuiden Lt By to.
N Sea Locks
VHF 09
Locks 22
ⓇC

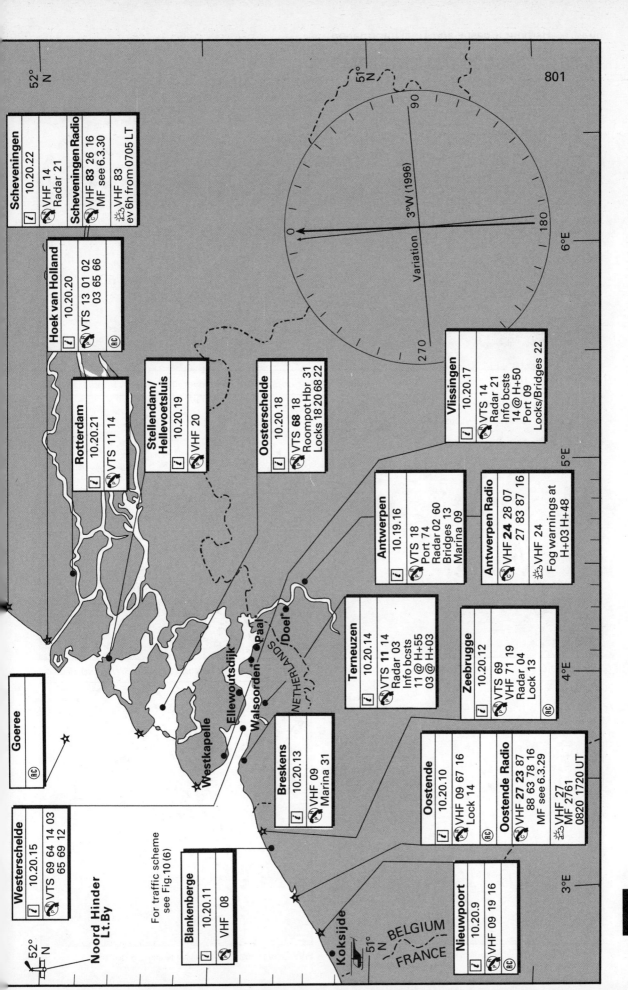

801

20

Scheveningen 10.20.22
ℹ️ VHF 14
Radar 21

Scheveningen Radio
VHF **83** 26 16
MF see 6.3.30
VHF 83
ev 6h from 0705 LT

Hoek van Holland 10.20.20
ℹ️ VTS 13 01 02
03 65 66

Rotterdam 10.20.21
ℹ️ VTS 11 14

Stellendam/ Hellevoetsluis 10.20.19
ℹ️ VHF 20

Oosterschelde 10.20.18
ℹ️ VTS **68** 18
Roompot Hbr 31
Locks 18 20 68 22

Vlissingen 10.20.17
ℹ️ VTS 14
Radar 21
Info bcsts
14 @ H+50
Port 09
Locks/Bridges 22

Antwerpen 10.19.16
ℹ️ VTS 18
Port 74
Radar 02 60
Bridges 13
Marina 09

Antwerpen Radio
VHF **24** 28 07
27 83 87 16
VHF 24
Fog warnings at
H+03 H+48

Terneuzen 10.20.14
ℹ️ VTS **11** 14
Radar 03
Info bcsts
11 @ H+55
03 @ H+03

Zeebrugge 10.20.12
ℹ️ VTS 69
VHF 71 19
Radar 04
Lock 13

Goeree
®ⓒ

Westerschelde 10.20.15
ℹ️ VTS 69 64 14 03
65 69 12

Noord Hinder Lt.By

For traffic scheme
see Fig.10(6)

Blankenberge 10.20.11
ℹ️ VHF 08

Breskens 10.20.13
ℹ️ VHF 09
Marina 31

Oostende 10.20.10
ℹ️ VHF 09 67 16
Lock 14

Oostende Radio
VHF **27 23** 87
88 63 78 16
MF see 6.3.29
VHF 27
MF 2761
0820 1720 UT

Nieuwpoort 10.20.9
ℹ️ VHF 09 19 16

NETHERLANDS
Doel*
Paal*
Walsoorden*
Ellewoutsdijk*
Westkapelle
Koksijde
BELGIUM
FRANCE

52° N
51° N
52°
51°

Variation 3°W (1996)
0
90
180
270

6°E
5°E
4°E
3°E

10-20-3   AREA 20 TIDAL STREAMS

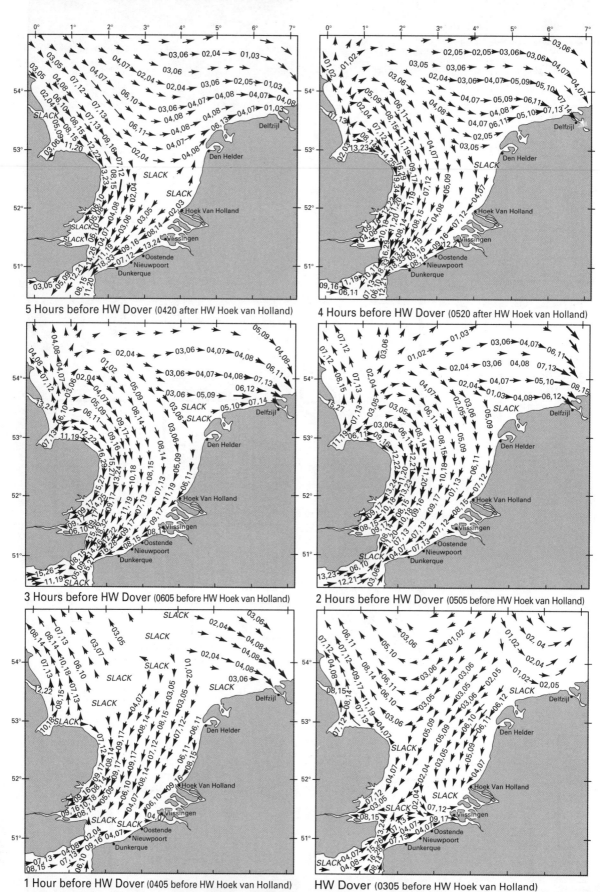

5 Hours before HW Dover (0420 after HW Hoek van Holland)

4 Hours before HW Dover (0520 after HW Hoek van Holland)

3 Hours before HW Dover (0605 before HW Hoek van Holland)

2 Hours before HW Dover (0505 before HW Hoek van Holland)

1 Hour before HW Dover (0405 before HW Hoek van Holland)

HW Dover (0305 before HW Hoek van Holland)

South-westward 10.19.3   North-westward 10.4.3   North-eastward 10.21.3

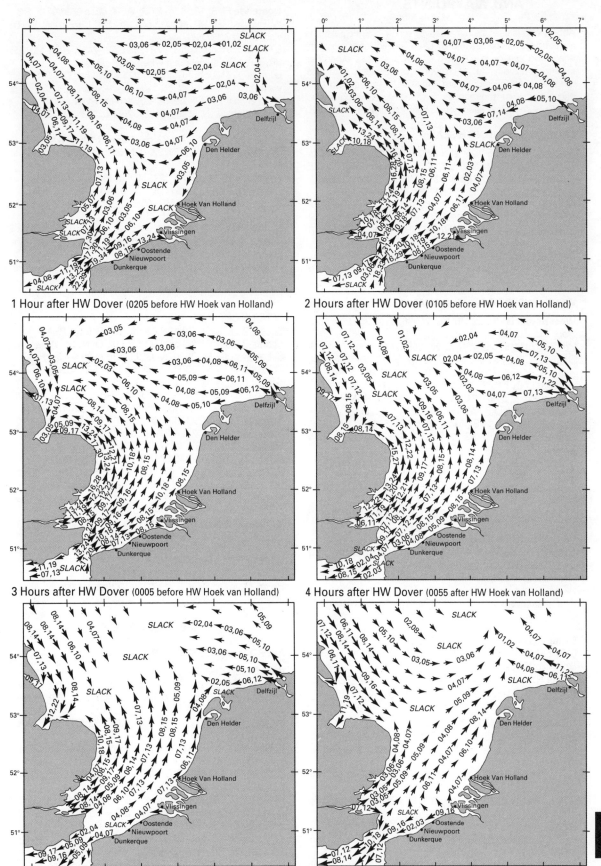

1 Hour after HW Dover (0205 before HW Hoek van Holland)

2 Hours after HW Dover (0105 before HW Hoek van Holland)

3 Hours after HW Dover (0005 before HW Hoek van Holland)

4 Hours after HW Dover (0055 after HW Hoek van Holland)

5 Hours after HW Dover (0155 after HW Hoek van Holland)

6 Hours after HW Dover (0255 after HW Hoek van Holland)

20

10.20.4 COASTAL LIGHTS, FOG SIGNALS AND WAYPOINTS

Abbreviations used below are given in 1.4.1. Principal lights are in **bold** print, places in CAPITALS, and light-vessels, light floats and Lanbys in *CAPITAL ITALICS*. Unless otherwise stated lights are white. m – elevation in metres; M – nominal range in miles. Fog signals are in *italics*. Useful waypoints are underlined – use those on land with care. All geographical positions should be assumed to be approximate. See 4.4.1.

CROSSING THE NORTH SEA

Garden City Lt By 51°29'·20N 02°17'·90E Q (9) 15s; WCM.
Twin Lt By 51°32'·10N 02°22'·62E Fl (3) Y 9s; SPM.
Birkenfels Lt By 51°39'·05N 02°32'·05E Q (9) 15s; WCM.
Track Ferry Lt By 51°33'·80N 02°36'·50E Fl Y 5s; SPM.
NHR-SE Lt By 51°45'·50N 02°40'·00E Fl G 5s; SHM; Racon (N).
NHR-S Lt By 51°51'·40N 02°28'·75E Fl Y 10s; SPM; *Bell*.
Noordhinder Lt By 52°00'·20N 02°51'·50E Fl (2) 10s; Racon (T); SWM
NHR-N Lt By 52°10'·90N 03°05'·00E L Fl 8s; Racon (K); SWM.

BELGIUM

WEST HINDER TO SCHEUR CHANNEL

West Hinder Lt 51°23'·36N 02°26'·36E Fl (4) 30s 23m 13M; *Horn Mo(U) 30s.*
WH Zuid Lt By 51°22'·75N 02°26'·36E Q (6) + L Fl 15s; SCM.
Oost-Dyck Lt By 51°21'·55N 02°31'·20E QG; SHM; *Whis.*
A-Zuid Lt By 51°21'·50N 02°37'·00E Fl (3)G 10s; SHM.
A-Noord Lt By 51°23'·50N 02°37'·00E Fl (4) R 20s; PHM.
Kwintebank Lt By 51°21'·75N 02°43'·00E Q; NCM; *Whis.*
Middelkerke Bk Lt By 51°18'·25N 02°42'·80E Fl G 5s; SHM.
Middelkerke Bk N Lt By 51°20'·87N 02°46'·40E Q; NCM.
Akkaert SW Lt By 51°22'·33N 02°46'·42E Q (9) 15s; WCM; *Whis* .
Mid Akkaert Lt By 51°24'·23N 02°53'·50E VQ (3) 5s; ECM.
Scheur 1 Lt By 51°23'·18N 03°02'·00E Fl G 5s; SHM.
Goote Bank Lt By 51°27'·00N 02°52'·72E Q (3)10s; ECM; *Whis.*
BT Ratel Lt By 51°11'·62N 02°28'·00E Fl (4) R 15s; PHM.

NIEUWPOORT AND APPROACHES

Trapegeer Lt By 51°08'·46N 02°34'·45E Fl G 10s; SHM; *Bell.*
Den Oever Wreck Lt By 51°09'·20N 02°39'·50E Q; NCM.
Nieuwpoort Bk Lt By 51°10'·21N 02°36'·16E Q (9) 15s; WCM; *Whis.*
Weststroombank Lt By 51°11'·39N 02°43'·15E Fl (4) R 20s; PHM.

E Pier near root Fl (2) R 14s 26m **21M**; R Tr, W bands.
E Pier Hd FR 11m 10M; W Tr; vis 025°-250°, 307°-347°; *Horn Mo(K) 30s.*
W Pier Hd FG 11m 9M; W Tr; vis 025°-250°, 284°-324°; RC; *Bell (2) 10s.*

OOSTENDE AND APPROACHES

Zuidstroombank Lt By 51°12'·33N 02°47'·50E Fl R 5s; PHM.
Middelkerke S Lt By 51°14'·78N 02°42'·00E Q (9) R 15s; PHM.
Oostendebank W Lt By 51°16'·25N 02°44'·85E Q (9) 15s; WCM; *Whis.*
Oostendebank E Lt By 51°17'·36N 02°52'·00E Fl (4) R 20s; PHM.
Nautica Ena Wk Lt By 51°18'·12N 02°52'·85E Q; NCM.
Wenduinebank W Lt By 51°17'·28N 02°52'·87E Q (9) 15s; WCM; *Whis.*
Buitenstroombank Lt By 51°15'·20N 02°51'·80E Q; NCM; *Whis.*

Binnenstroombank Lt By 51°14'·50N 02°53'·73E Q (3) 10s; ECM.
Oostende Fl (3) 10s 63m **27M**; W Tr; obsc 069°-071°; RC.
W Pier Hd 51°14'·36N 02°55'·12E FG 12m 10M; W Tr; vis 057°-327°; *Bell (1) 4s.*
E Pier Hd FR 13m 12M; W Tr; vis 333°-243°; *Horn Mo(OE) 30s.* QY Lt at signal mast when chan closed.
Ldg Lts 128°, both FR 4M on W framework Trs, R bands; vis 051°-201°.
A1 Lt By 51°21'·72N 02°58'·20E Iso 8s; SWM; *Whis.*
Oostendebank N Lt By 51°21'·25N 02°53'·00E Q; NCM; *Whis.*
A1 bis Lt By 51°21'·70N 02°58'·10E L Fl 10s; SWM; *Whis.*
SW Wandelaar Lt By 51°22'·00N 03°01'·00E Fl (4) R 20s; PHM.
Wenduine Bk N Lt By 51°21'·50N 03°02'·71E QG; SHM.
Wenduine Bk E Lt By 51°18'·85N 03°01'·70E QR; PHM.
A2 Lt By 51°22'·50N 03°07'·05E Iso 8s; SWM; *Whis.*

BLANKENBERGE

Comte Jean Jetty 51°18'·78N 03°06'·95E Fl (2) 8s 30m **20M**; W Tr, B top; vis 065°-245°.
W Mole Hd FG 14m 11M; W Tr; intens 065°-290°, unintens 290°-335°.
E Pier Hd FR 12m 11M; W Tr; vis 290°-245°; *Bell (2) 15s.*

SCHEUR CHANNEL

Scheur 2 Lt By 51°23'·40N 02°58'·15E Fl R 5s; PHM.
Scheur 3 Lt By 51°24'·35N 03°02'·90E Q; NCM; *Whis.*
Scheur 4 Lt By 51°25'·07N 03°02'·93E Fl (4) R 10s; PHM.
Scheur 5 Lt By 51°23'·73N 03°05'·90E Fl G 5s; SHM.
Scheur 6 Lt By 51°24'·25N 03°06'·00E Fl R 5s; PHM.
Droogte van Schooneveld (MOW 5) 51°25'·50N 03°09'·00E Fl (5) Y 20s 12m 2M; measuring Bn with platform; Ra refl.
Scheur 7 Lt By 51°24'·02N 03°10'·40E Fl G 5s; SHM.
Scheur 8 Lt By 51°24'·48N 03°10'·50E Fl (4) R 10s; PHM.
Scheur 9 Lt By 51°24'·45N 03°15'·05E QG; SHM.
Scheur 10 Lt By 51°24'·92N 03°15'·07E Fl R 5s; PHM.
Scheur 12 Lt By 51°24'·67N 03°18'·30E Fl (4) R 10s; PHM.
Scheur-Wiel Lt By 51°24'·26N 03°18'·00E Q; NCM.

ZEEBRUGGE AND APPROACHES

Scheur-Zand Lt By 51°23'·68N 03°07'·68E Q (3) 10s; ECM.
Zand Lt By 51°22'·52N 03°10'·16E QG; SHM.
W Outer Bkwtr Hd 51°21'·8N 03°11'·3E Oc G 7s 31m 7M; vis 057°-267°, *Horn (1+3) 90s.*
E Bkwtr Oc R 7s 31m 7M; vis 087°-281°.
Heist, Mole Hd Oc WR 15s 22m, **W20M, R18M**; Gy Tr; vis W068°-145°, R145°-212°, W212°-296°; *Horn (3+1) 90s.*

NETHERLANDS

APPROACHES TO WESTERSCHELDE

WIELINGEN CHANNEL
Wielingen Zand Lt By 51°22'·60N 03°10'·80E Q (9) 15s; WCM.
Bol van Heist Lt By 51°23'·15N 03°12'·05E Q (6) + L Fl R 15s; PHM.
MOW3 Tide Gauge 51°23'·45N 03°12'·00E Fl (5) Y 20s; Racon (S); SPM; *Whis*; .
Wielingen Lt By 51°23'·30N 03°15'·00E Fl (3) G 15s; SHM.
W1 Lt By 51°23'·50N 03°18'·00E Fl G 5s; SHM.
W2 Lt By 51°24'·64N 03°21'·58E Iso R 8s; PHM.
W3 Lt By 51°24'·03N 03°21'·58E Iso G 8s; SHM.
W4 Lt By 51°24'·92N 03°24'·48E L Fl R 5s; PHM.
W5 Lt By 51°24'·33N 03°24'·48E L Fl G 5s; SHM.
W6 Lt By 51°25'·15N 03°27'·25E L Fl R 8s; PHM.
W7 Lt By 51°24'·65N 03°27'·30E L Fl G 8s; SHM.
W8 Lt By 51°25'·48N 03°30'·15E L Fl R 5s; PHM.
W9 Lt By 51°24'·97N 03°30'·13E L Fl G 5s; SHM.
W10 Lt By 51°25'·80N 03°33'·00E QR; PHM.

Wave observation post 51°22'·84N 03°22'·82E Fl (5) Y 20s.
Kruishoofd 51°23'·73N 03°28'·36E Iso WRG 8s 14m W8M, R6M, G5M; W ■ Tr, B post; vis R074°-091°, W091°-100°, G100°-118°, W118°-153°, R153°-179°, W179°-198°, G198°-205°, W205°-074°.
Nieuwe Sluis on embankment 51°24'·49N 03°30'·33E *Horn (3) 30s.* 51°24'·48N 03°31'·38E Oc WRG 10s 27m W14M, R11M, G10M; B 8-sided Tr, W bands; vis R055°-086°, W086°-091·5°, G091·5°-134°, W134-140·5°, G140·5°-144·5°, W144·5°-236·5°, G236·5°-243°, R243°-260°, G260°-263·5, R263·5-292°, W292°-055°.

APPROACHES TO BRESKENS
Songa Lt By 51°25'·34N 03°33'·78E QG; SHM.
SS-VH Lt By 51°24'·75N 03°34'·00E Q; NCM.

BRESKENS FERRY HARBOUR
W Mole Hd 51°24'·40N 03°33'·23E FG 8m 4M; B & W mast; in fog FY; Ra refl; Fog Det Lt.
E Mole Hd FR 8m 5M; B & W mast; in fog FY; Ra refl.

BRESKENS
W Mole Hd 51°24'·09N 03°34'·12E F WRG 6m; Gy mast; vis vis R090°-128°, W128°-157°, G157°-169·5°, W169·5°-173°, R173°-194°, G194°-296°, W296°-300°, R300°-320°, G320°-090°; in fog FY; Horn Mo(U) 30s.
E Mole Hd FR 5m; Ra refl.

WESTKAPELLE TO VLISSINGEN
Noorderhoofd Ldg Lts 149·5°, NW Hd of dyke. Front, 0·73M from rear, Oc WRG 10s 18m W13M, R10M, G10M; R Tr, W band; vis R353°-008°, G008°-029°, W029°-169°.
Westkapelle, Common rear Fl 3s 48m **28M**; Tr, R top; obsc on certain brgs.
Zoutelande Ldg Lts 326°, Front 1·8M from rear FR 21m 12M; R ■ Tr; vis 321°-352°.
Molenhoofd 51°31'·61N 03°26'·07E Oc WRG 6s 9m; W mast R bands; vis R306°-328°, W328°-347°, R347°-008°, G008°-031°, W031°-035°, G035°-140°, W140°-169°, R169°-198°.
Kaapduinen, Ldg Lts 130°. Front 51°28'·5N 03°31'·0E Oc 5s 26m 13M; Y ■ Tr, R bands; vis 115°-145°. Rear, 220m from front, Oc 5s 36m 13M; Y ■ Tr, R bands; synch with front; vis 108°-152°.
Fort de Nolle 51°27'·00N 03°33'·20E Fl WRG 2·5s 11m W6M, R4M, G4M; W col, R bands; vis R293°-309°, W309°-324·5°, G324·5°-336·5°, R336·5°-027°, G027°-044°, R044°-090°, G090°-110·5°, W110·5°-114·5°, G114·5°-119°, R119-130°.

VLISSINGEN
Ldg Lts 117°. Leugenaar causeway, front Oc R 5s 5m 7M; W&R pile; intens 108°-126°.
Sardijngeul rear, 550m from front, Oc WRG 5s 8m W12M, R9M, G8M; R △ with W bands on R & W mast; synch; vis R245°-271°, G271°-285°, W285°-123°, R123°-147°.
Koopmanshaven, W Mole root 51°26'·40N 03°34'·58E Iso WRG 3s 15m W12M, R10M, G9M; R pylon; vis R253°-270°, W270°-059°, G059°-071°, W071°-077°, R077°-101°, G101°-110°, W110°-114°.
E Mole Hd FG 7m.
Buitenhaven E Mole Hd FG 4M; 7M; in fog FY.
Buitenhaven W Mole Hd 51°26'·44N 03°36'·12E FR 10m 5M; also Iso WRG 4s; B mast; vis W072°-021°, G021°-042°, W042°-056°, R056°-072°; tfc sigs; *Horn 15s.*
Schone Waardin 51°26'·60N 03°37'·95E Oc WRG 9s 10m W13M, R10M, G9M; R mast, W bands; vis obscd 083°-248°, R326°-341°, G260°-270°, W270°-282°, G282°-325°, W325°-341°, G341°-023°, W023°-024°, G024°-054°, R054°-066°, W066°-076°, G076°-094°, W094°-248°.

VLISSINGEN OOST
W Mole Hd FR 8m 5M; W col; in fog FY; *Horn (2) 20s.*
E Mole Hd FG 8m 4M; W col.
Ldg Lts 023°. Front Oc R 8s 7m 8M; G post. Rear, 100m from front, Oc R 8s 12m 8M; G mast; synch with front, both vis 015°-031°.
Flushing E Hbr Dir Lt 305° 51°27'·93N 03°40'·62E Dir F WRG; vis 303·5°-304·9°. W304·9°-305·1°, G305·1°-306·5°.

WESTERSCHELDE
BORSSELE-NOORDNOL
Pier Hd 51°25'·55N 03°42'·80E Oc WRG 5s; 9m; R mast, W bands; vis R305°-331°, W331°-341°, G341°-000°, W000°-007°, R007°-023°, G023°-054°, W054°-057°, G057°-113°, W113°-128°, R128°-155°, W155°-305°.
Borssele, Total Jetty NW end 51°24'·85N 03°43'·61E Iso WR 4s; vis R133°-141·5°, W141·5°-133°.
Borssele-Everingen 51°24'·73N 03°44'·20E Iso WRG 4s 9m; W structure, R band; vis R021°-026°, G026°-080°, W080°-100°, R100°-137°, W137°-293°, R293°-308°, W308°-344°, G344°-357°, W357°-021°.

ELLEWOUTSDIJK
W Pier Hd (unlit) 51°23'·14N 03°49'·12E.

BRAAKMANHAVEN
Ldg Lts 191°. Front 51°20'·3N 03°45'·8E Iso 4s 10m; B pile, W bands. Rear, 60m from front, Iso 4s 14m; B pile, W bands; synch with front, showing over hbr mouth.
Ldg Lts 211·5°, both Oc G 4s, 10/14m synch, showing middle of turning basin.
W side 51°21'·0N 03°45'·9E FG; G pile, W bands; Ra refl.
E side 51°21'·1N 03°46'·3E FR; R mast, W bands; Ra refl, tfc sigs.
Braakman 51°21'·03N 03°46'·31E Oc WRG 8s 7m W7M, R5M, G4M; B pedestal, W band; vis R116°-132°, W132°-140°, G140°-202°, W202°-116°.

TERNEUZEN
Nieuw Neuzenpolder Ldg Lts 125°. Front Oc 5s 5m 13M; W col, B bands; intens 117°-133°. Rear, 365m from front, Oc 5s 16m 13M; B&W Tr; synch with front; intens 117°-133°.
Dow Chemical Jetty, 4 dolphins showing Fl 3s and Fl R 3s; *Horn 15s.*
Veerhaven W Jetty Oc WRG 5s 14m W9M, R7M, G6M; B&W Tr; vis R090°-115°, W115°-238·5°, G238·5°-248°, W248°-279°, R279°-004°.
W Mole Hd 51°20'·62N 03°49'·7E FG 6m; Gy mast; in fog FY.
E Mole Hd FR 7m; tfc signals.

HOEDEKENSKERKE
De Val 51°25'·20N 03°55'·08E Iso WRG 2s 5m W8M, R5M, G4M; R Tr, W band; vis R008°-034°, W034°-201°, R201°-206°, W206°-209°, G209°-328. W328°-008°.

HANSWEERT
W Mole Hd 51°26'·45N 04°00'·50E Oc WRG 10s 9m W9M, R7M, G6M; R Tr, W band; vis R288°-310°, W310°-334°, G334°-356·5°, W356·5°-044°, R044°-061·5°, W061·5°-073°, G073°-089°, R089°-101·5°, G101·5°-109°, W109°-114·5°, R114·5°-127·5°W127·5°-288°; in fog FY.
E side Pier Hd FG 6m; Gy col; *Horn (4) 30s.*

WALSOORDEN
Ent N Mole Hd FG 5m; Gy col; in fog FY.
Ent S Mole Hd 51°22'·96N 04°02'·18E FR 5m; Gy col.

20

PAAL APPROACHES
Speelmansgat Lt Bn 51°22'·03N 04°06'·26E Fl (5) Y 20s.

ZANDVLIET
Ldg Lts 118°. Front 51°20'·70N 04°16'·40E Oc WRG 5s
11m W9M, R7M, G6M; vis R shore-350°, W350°-017°,
G017°-019°, W019°-088°, G088°-109°, W109°-125°, R125°-
shore. Rear, 200m from front, Oc 5s 18m 9M.

DOEL/LILLO/ANTWERPEN (Belgium)
Ldg Lts 185·5°. Front 51°18'·5N 04°16'·2E Fl WRG 3s 5m
W9M, R7M, G6M; vis Rshore-175°, W175°-202°, G202°-
306·5°, W306·5°-330·9°, R330·9°-shore. Rear, 260m from
front, Fl 3s 14m 9M; synch with front. By day vis 183°-185°.
Doel Jetty Hd 51°18'·72N 04°16'·18E Oc WR 5s 9m W9M,
R7M; Y □, B stripes on Tr; vis R downstream-185°, W185°-
334°, R334°-upstream shore.

LILLO/ANTWERPEN
Lillo Pier SE end 51°18'·20N 04°17'·28E Oc WRG 10s 5m
W9M, R7M, G6M; R □ W band on B Bn; vis Rshore-303·1°,
W303·1°-308·2°, G308·2°-096·5°, W096·5°-148°, R148°-
shore.
No. 109 Lt By 51°14'·04N 04°23'·80E Iso G 8s; SHM.
Antwerp Nic Marina Lock ent 51°13'·85N 04°23'·72E
Yacht Hbr F WR 9m 3M; vis Wshore-283°-R283°-shore.

APPROACHES TO OOSTERSCHELDE

OUTER APPROACHES
Wave observation post VR 51°30'·35N 03°14'·53E Fl Y 5s.
SW Thornton Lt By 51°31'·01N 02°51'·00E Iso 8s; SWM.
Thornton Bank B Lt By 51°34'·45N 02°59'·15E Q; NCM.
Westpit Lt By 51°33'·70N 03°10'·00E Iso 8s; SWM.
Rabsbank Lt By 51°38'·30N 03°10'·00E Iso 4s; SWM.
Middelbank Lt By 51°40'·90N 03°18'·30E Iso 8s; SWM.
Schouwenbank Lt By 51°45'·00N 03°14'·40E Mo (A) 8s;
SWM; Racon (O).
Buitenbank Lt By 51°51'·20N 03°25'·80E Iso 4s; SWM.

WESTGAT/OUDE ROOMPOT (selected marks)
WG1 Lt By 51°38'·05N 03°26'·30E L Fl G 5s; SHM.
WG Lt By 51°38'·25N 03°28'·90E Q; NCM.
WG4 Lt By 51°38'·60N 03°28'·80E L Fl R 8s; PHM.
Wave observation post OS11 51°38'·63N 03°28'·95E L Fl R
8s; R pile.
WG7 Lt By 51°39'·45N 03°32'·75E L Fl G 5s; SHM.
WG 8/OR Lt By 51°39'·75N 03°32'·60E VQ (6) + L Fl 10s;
SCM.
OR2 Lt By 51°39'·48N 03°33'·70E L Fl R 5s; PHM.
OR5 Lt By 51°38'·60N 03°35'·45E L Fl G 8s; SHM.
OR8 Lt By 51°38'·20N 03°37'·35E L Fl R 8s; PHM.
OR11 Lt By 51°37'·05N 03°38'·50E L Fl G 5s; SHM.
OR12 Lt By 51°37'·35N 03°39'·30E L Fl R 5s; PHM.

Roompotsluis Ldg Lts 073·5°. Front Oc G 5s. Rear, 280m
from front, Oc G 5s; synch.
N Bkwtr Hd FR 6m; Horn(2) 30s.
S Bkwtr Hd FG 6m.
Inner Mole Hd QR.

COLIJNSPLAAT
E Jetty Hd 51°36'·25N 03°51'·15E FR 3m 3M; Horn.
W Jetty Hd FG 5m 3M.
Zeeland Bridge. N and S passages marked by FY Lts, 14m.

KATS
N Jetty Hd FG 5m 5M.
S Jetty Hd 51°34'·44N 03°53'·72E Oc WRG 8s 5m 5M;
vis W344°-153°, R153°-165°, G165°-202°, W202°-211°,
G211°-256°, W256°-259°, G259°-313°, W313°-331°.

SAS VAN GOES
S Mole Hd 51°32'·34N 03°55'·95E FR.
N Mole Hd FG.

WEMELDINGE
W Jetty Hd 51°31'·34N 04°00'·25E FG.
E Jetty Hd FR, FY in fog.
W Hd new ent 51°31'·20N 04°00'·90E Oc WRG 5s 7m W9M,
R7M, G7M; vis R 105·5°-114°, W114°-124°, G124°-140·5°,
W140·5°-144°, G144°-192°, W192°-205°, R205°-233·5°,
W233·5°-258·5°, R258·5°-296·5°. R & G Lts mark canal.

YERSEKE
O25/Sv 12 Lt By 51°31'·40N 02°02'·42E Q; xxx
Ldg Lts 155° (through Schaar van Yerseke). Front Iso 4s 8m;
in fog FY. Rear, 180m from front, Iso 4s 13m; synch; in fog
2FY. FG and FR mark mole Hds.

Tholensche Gat. Strijenham 51°31'·40N 04°08'·91E Oc WRG
5s 9m W8M, R5M, G5M; R n, W bands, on mast; vis W shore-
298°, R298°-320°, W320°-052°, G052°-069°, W069°-085°,
R085°-095°, W095°-shore.

Gorishoek 51°31'·57N 04°04'·68E Iso WRG 8s 7m W6M,
R4M, G4M; R pedestal, W bands; vis R260°-278°, W278°-
021°, G021°-025°, W025°- 071°, G071°-085°, W085°-103°,
R103°-120°, W120°-260°.

STAVENISSE
E Mole Hd 51°35'·73N 04°00'·35E Oc WRG 5s 10m W12M,
R9M, G8M; B pylon; W075°-090°, R090°-105·5°, W105·5°-
108°, G108°-118·5°, W118·5°-124°, G124°-155°, W155°-158°,
G158°-231°, W231°-238·5°, R238·5°-253°, W253°-350°.

ST ANNALAND
Entrance W side 51°36'·32N 04°06'·60E FG.
E side FR.

ZIJPE/ANNA JACOBAPOLDER
N Mole Hd Iso G 4s.
St Philipsland, on dyke Oc WRG 4s 9m W8M, R5M, G4M;
pylon on B ● col; vis W051°-100°, R100°-144°, W144°-146°,
G146°-173°.
Zijpsche Bout Oc WRG 10s 9m W12M, R9M, G8M; mast on
R col; vis R208°-211°, W211°-025°, G025°-030°, W030°-
040°, R040°-066°.
Tramweghaven S mole Iso R 4s 7m; Gy Bn.
N Mole FG.
Stoofpolder Iso WRG 4s 10m W12M, R9M, G8M; B Tr,
W bands; vis W147°-154°, R154°-226·5°, G226·5°-243°,
W243°-253°, G253°-259°, W259°-263°, G263°-270°, R270°-
283°, W283°-008°.

Hoek Van Ouwerkerk Ldg Lts 009·2°. Front 51°36'·92N
03°58'·27E Iso WRG 6s; vis R267°-306°, W306°-314°, G314°-
007·5°, W007·5°-011·5°, G011·5°-067°, W067°-068·5°,
G068·5°-085°, W085°-102·5°, G102·5°-112·5°, R112·5°-
121·5°. Rear, 300m from front, Iso 6s.

DE VAL
Engelsche Vaarwater Ldg Lts 019°. Front 51°37'·92N
03°58'·27E Iso WRG 6s 7m W6M, R4M, G4M; R pedestal, W
band; vis R290°-306°, W306°-317°, G317°-334°, W334°-
336°, G336°-017°, W017°-026°, G026°-090°, R090°-108°,
W108°-290°. Rear, 300m from front, Iso 3s 15m 6M; R ■ on
W mast, R bands.

ZIERIKZEE
W Jetty Hd 51°37'·95N 03°53'·45E Oc WRG 6s 10m W6M,
R4M, G4M; R pedestal, W band; vis G060°-107°, W107°-
133°, R133°-156°, W156°-278°, R278°-304°, G304°-314°,
W314°-331°, R331°-354°, W354°-060°.

W Mole Hd FR.
E Mole Hd FG.

FLAUWERSPOLDER
<u>W Mole Hd</u> 51°40'·70N 03°50'·86E Iso WRG 4s 7m W6M, R4M, G4M; W daymark, B band on pylon; vis R303°-344°, W344°-347°, G347°-083°, W083°-086°, G086°-103°, W103°-110°, R110°-128°, W128°-303°.

HAMMEN
<u>E Breakwater Hd</u> 51°41'·28N 03°48'·79E Fl (2) 10s 8m.

BURGHSLUIS
<u>S Mole Hd</u> 51°40'·59N 03°45'·56E F WRG 9m W8M, R5M, G4M; mast on R col; vis W218°-230°, R230°-245°, W245°-253·5°, G253·5°-293°, W293°-000°, G000°-025·5°, W025·5°-032°, G032°-041°, R041°-070°, W070°-095°.

APPROACHES TO STELLENDAM AND HARINGVLIET

<u>Hinder Lt By</u> 51°54'·60N 03°55'·50E Q (9) 15s; WCM.
<u>Ha10</u> 51°51'·80N 03°51'·80E Fl Y 5s; Y pile.
<u>SG Lt By</u> 51°52'·00N 03°51'·50E Iso 4s; SWM.
<u>SG 2 Lt By</u> 51°51'·80N 03°53'·50E Iso R 2s; PHM.
<u>SG 5 Lt By</u> 51°50'·97N 03°55'·45E L Fl G 8s; SHM.
<u>SG 9 Lt By</u> 51°50'·90N 03°57'·30E L Fl G 8s; SHM.
<u>SG 19 Lt By</u> 51°51'·24N 04°00'·02'·1E Iso G 2s; SHM.
<u>G 1 Lt By</u> 51°50'·23N 04°02'48E L Fl G 8s; SHM.

STELLENDAM
N Mole Hd 51°49'·90N 04°02'·1E FG; *Horn (2) 15s.*

HELLEVOETSLUIS
51°49'·2N 04°07'·7E Iso WRG 10s 16m W11M, R8M, G7M; W Tr, R cupola; vis G shore-275°, W275°-294°, R294°-316°, W316°-036°, G036°-058°, W058°-095°, R095°-shore.
W Mole Hd FR 6m.
E Mole Hd FG 6m; in fog FY.
Hoornsche Hoofden, watchhouse on dyke, 51°48'·3N 04°11'·0E Oc WRG 5s 7m W7M, R5M, G4M; vis W288°-297°, G297°-313°, W313°-325°, R325°-335°, G335°-345°, W345°-045°, G045°-055°, W055°-131°, R131°-shore.

HARINGVLIET
Heliushaven, W Jetty 51°49'·3N 04°07'·2E FR 7m 4M.
E Jetty FG 7m 3M; *Horn (3) 20s.*

MIDDELHARNIS
W Pier Hd F WRG 5m W8M, R5M, G4M; vis W144°-164·5°, R164·5°-176·5°, G176·5°-144°.
E Pier Hd FR 5m 5M; in fog FY.

Nieuwendijk. Ldg Lts 303.5°. Front 51°45'·1N 04°19'·5E Iso WRG 6s 8m W9M, R7M, G6M; B framework Tr; vis G093°-100°, W100°-103·5°, R103·5°-113°, W113°-093°. Rear, 450m from front F 11m 9M; B framework Tr.

VOLKERAK
Noorder Voorhaven. W Mole Hd 51°42'·08N 04°25'·88E FG 6m 4M; R lantern on pedestal; in fog FY.

APPROACHES TO EUROPOORT

Noord Hinder Lt By 52°00'·15N 02° 51'·20E Fl (2) 10s 16m **27M**; Racon (T); *Horn(2) 30s.*
<u>Euro Platform</u> 51°59'·99N 03°16'·55E Mo (U) 15s; W structure, R bands; helicopter platform; *Horn Mo(U) 30s.*
Goeree 51°55'·53N 03°40'·18E Fl(4) 20s 32m **28M**; R and W chequered Tr on platform; RC; helicopter platform; Racon (T); *Horn (4) 30s.*

Westhoofd 51°48'·83N 03°51'·90E Fl (3) 15s 55m **30M**; R ■ Tr.

Kwade Hoek 51°50'·3N 03°59'·1E Iso WRG 4s 8m W12M, R9M, G8M; B mast, W bands; vis W 235°-068°, R068°-088°, G088°-108°, W108°-111°, R111°-142°, W142°-228°, R228°-235°. FR on radio mast 4·2M NE.

<u>OS14</u> 51°43'·30N 03°40'·60E Fl Y 5s; Y pile.
<u>BG2</u> 51°46'·10N 03°37'·20E Fl Y 5s; Y pile.
West Schouwen 51°42'·58N 03°41'·60E Fl (2+1)15s 58m **30M**; Gy Tr, R diagonal stripes on upper part.
<u>Ooster Lt By</u> 51°47'·97N 03°41'·32E Q (9) 15s; WCM.
<u>BG5 Lt By</u> 51°49'·50N 03°45'·83E Fl Y 5s; SPM.
<u>Adriana Lt By</u> 51°56'·13N 03°50'·63E VQ (9)10s; WCM.

<u>Maas Center Lt By</u> 52°01'·18N 03°53'·57E Iso 4s; SWM; Racon (M).
<u>Indusbank N Lt By</u> 52°02'·92N 04°03'·73E Q; NCM.

HOEK VAN HOLLAND
Maasvlakte 51°58'·25N 04°00'·94E Fl (5) 20s 66m **28M**; B 8-sided Tr, Y bands; vis 340°-267°.
<u>Nieuwe Noorderdam Hd</u> 51°59'·71N 04°02'·92E FR 24m 10M; Or Tr, B bands; helicopter platform; in fog Al Fl WR 6s, vis 278°-255°.
<u>Nieuwe Zuiderdam Hd</u> 51°59'·19N 04°02'·58E FG 24m 10M; Y Tr, B bands; helicopter platform; in fog Al Fl WG 6s, vis 330°-307°; *Horn 10s.*

Maasmond Ldg Lts 112° Ldg Lts 107° **Front** 51°58'·6N 04°07'·6E Iso R 6s 29m **18M**; R Tr, W bands; vis 100°-115°. **Rear** 450m from front Iso R 6s 43m **18M**; vis 100°-115°, synch.

EUROPOORT
Calandkanaal Entrance Ldg Lts 116°. **Front** Oc G 6s 29m ; W Tr, R bands; vis 108°-124°, synch with **Rear**, 550m from front Oc G 6s 43m **16M**; W Tr, R bands; vis 108·5°-123·5°.
Beerkanaal Ldg Lts 192·5°. Front Iso G 3s 20m 2M. Rear, 50m from front, Iso G 3s 23m 2M.

HOEK VAN HOLLAND TO DEN HELDER

SCHEVENINGEN
<u>SCH Lt By</u> 52°07'·80N 04°14'·20E Iso 4s; SWM.
Scheveningen 52°06'·3N 04°16'·2E Fl (2) 10s 48m **29M**; brown Tr; vis 014°-244°.
Ldg Lts 156°. Front Iso 4s 17m 14M. Rear 100m from front Iso 4s 21m 14M; synchronised with front.
<u>SW Mole Hd</u> 52°06'·28N 04°15'·22E FG 11m 9M; B 6-sided Tr, Y bands, R lantern; *Horn (3) 30s.*
NE Mole Hd FR 11m 9M; B 6-sided Tr, Y bands, R lantern.

Noordwijk-aan-Zee 52°15'·00N 04°26'·10E Oc (3) 20s 32m **18M**; W ■ Tr.
Survey platform 52°16'·4N 04°17'·9E FR and Mo (U) 15s; *Horn Mo(U) 20s.*
<u>Eveline Lt By</u> 52°25'·55N 04°25'·15E VQ (9) 10s; WCM.

IJMUIDEN
<u>IJmuiden Lt By (IJM)</u> 52°28'·50N 04°23'·87E Mo (A) 8s; SWM; Racon; (also known as Verkenningston).
Ldg Lts 100°. **Front** F WR 30m **W16M**, R13M; dark R Tr; vis W050°-122°, R122°-145°; W145°-160°; RC. By day F 4m vis 090·5°-110·5°. **Rear,** 560m from front, Fl 5s 52m **29M**; dark R Tr; vis 019°-199°.
S Bkwtr Hd 52°27'·86N 04°32'·00E FG 14m 10M; in fog Fl 3s; *Horn (2) 30s.*
N Bkwtr Hd FR 14m 10M.
N Pier Hd QR 11m 9M; vis 263°-096°; in fog F.
S Pier Hd QG 11m 9M; vis 096°-295°; in fog F.

20

NOORDZEE KANAAL
Ø Km mark 52°27'·86N 04°35'·64E.
20 Km mark 52°25'·21N 04°51'·94E

AMSTERDAM
Yacht Hbr 52°23'·02N 04°53'·77E F & FR.

IJMUIDEN TO TEXEL
BP3 Lt By
CP-Q8-A Platform 52°35'·75N 04°31'·80E Mo (U) 15s.
Egmond-aan-Zee 52°37'·20N 04°37'·40E Iso WR 10s 36m
W18M, R14M; W Tr; vis W010°-175°, R175°-188°.
Petten Lt By 52°47'·38N 04°36'·80E VQ (9) 10s; WCM.

ZEEGAT VAN TEXEL
TX1 Lt By 52°48'17N 04°15'·60E Fl G 5s; SHM.
TX3 Lt By 52°58'·60N 04°22'·60E Fl (3) G 9s; SHM.
ZH (Zuider Haaks) Lt By 52°54'·70N 04°34'·84E VQ (6)
+ L Fl 10s; SCM.
MR (Middelrug) Lt By 52°56'·80N 04°33'·90E Q (9) 15s;
WCM.
NH (Noorder Haaks) Lt By 53°00'·30N 04°35'·45E VQ; NCM.
Grote Kaap Oc WRG 10s 31m W11M, R8M, G8M; vis G041°-
088°, W088°-094°, R094°-131°.

Schulpengat. Ldg Lts 026·5°. **Front** 53°00'·9N 04°44'·5E Iso
4s **18M**; vis 024·5°-028·5°. Rear, **Den Hoorn** 0·83M from
front Oc 8s **18M**; church spire; vis 024°-028°.
Huisduinen 52°57'·20N 04°43'·37E F WR 27m W14M, R11M;
■ Tr; vis W070°-113°, R113°-158°, W158°-208°.

Kijkduin, Rear 52°57'·35N 04°43'·60E Fl (4) 20s 56m **30M**;
brown Tr; vis except where obsc by dunes on Texel.
Ldg Lt 253° with Den Helder, Harssens Is (QG).

SCHULPENGAT
SG Lt By 52°52'·95N 04°38'·00E Mo (A) 8s; Racon (Z); SWM.
S1 Lt By 52°53'·57N 04°38'·88E Iso G 4s; SHM.
S2 Lt By 52°53'·87N 04°38'·02E Iso R 4s; PHM.
S3 Lt By 52°54'·48N 04°39'·62E Iso G 8s; SHM.
S4 Lt By 52°54'·65N 04°39'·53E Iso R 8s; PHM.
S5 Lt By 52°55'·40N 04°40'·30E Iso G 4s; SHM.
S6 Lt By 52°55'·55N 04°39'·78E Iso R 4s; PHM.
S7 Lt By 52°56'·30N 04°40'·99E Iso G 8s; SHM.
S6A Lt By 52°56'·57N 04°40'·60E QR; PHM.
S8 By 52°57'·12N 04°41'·10E (unlit); PHM.
S9 By 52°56'·90N 04°42'·15E (unlit); SHM.
S10 Lt By 52°57'·65N 04°41'·65E Iso R 8s; PHM.
S11 Lt By 52°57'·60N 04°43'·35E Iso G 4s; SHM.

MOLENGAT
MG Lt By 53°03'·95N 04°39'·45E Mo (A) 8s; SWM.
MG1 Lt By 53°02'·05N 04°41'·46E Iso G 4s; SHM.
MG2 Lt By 53°02'·18N 04°41'·87E Iso R 4s; PHM.
MG6 Lt By 53°01'·08N 04°41'·83E Iso R 4s; PHM.
MG5 Lt By 53°01'·08N 04°41'·52E Iso G 4s; SHM.
MG9 Lt By 53°00'·07N 04°41'·50E QG; SHM.
MG10 Lt By 53°00'·13N 04°41'·83E Iso R 8s; PHM.
MG13 Lt By 52°59'·17N 04°42'·30E Iso G 8s; SHM.
MG16 Lt By 52°59'·10N 04°42'·86E QR; PHM.
MG 18 By 52°58'·67N 04°43'·70E; PHM.
S14/MG17 Lt By 52°58'·42N 04°43'·40E VQ (6) + L Fl 10s;
SCM.
MG20 Lt By 52°28'·77N 04°44'·40E Iso R 8s; PHM.

MARSDIEP/DEN HELDER
Marinehaven, W Bkwtr Hd (Harssens I) 52°58'·00N 04°46'·84E
QG 12m 8M; *Horn 20s.*
MH6, E side of ent, Iso R 4s 9m 4M; R pile; Ra refl.
Ent W side, Fl G 5s 9m 4M; vis 180°-067° (H24).
Ent E side, QR 9m 4M; (H24).

Ldg Lts 191°. Front Oc G 5s 16m 14M; B △ on bldg; vis 161°-
221°. Rear, 275m from front, Oc G 5s 25m 14M; B ▽ on bldg;
vis 161°-247°, synch.

Schilbolsnol 53°00'·56N 04°45'·78E F WRG 27m **W15M**,
R12M, G11M; G Tr; vis W338°-002°, G002°-035°, W035°-038°
(leading sector for Schulpengat), R038°-051°, W051°-068°.

WADDENZEE

MOK
Mok 53°00'·25N 04°46'·85E Oc WRG 10s 10m W10M, R7M,
G6M; vis R229°-317°, W317°-337°, G337°-112°.
Ldg Lts 284°·5'. Front Iso 2s 7m 6M. Rear, 245m from front,
Iso 8s 10m 6M; both vis 224·5°-344·5°.

Malzwin KM/RA1 52°58'·70N 04°49'·46E Fl (5) Y 20s; post.
Malzwin M5 52°58'·3N 04°49'·9E Iso G 4s; G pile.
Wierbalg W3A 52°58'·1N 04°57'·1E QG; G pile.
Pile 01 52°57'·0N 05°00'·6E Iso G 8s; G pile.
Pile 05 52°56'·9N 05°01'·9E Iso G 4s; G pile.

DEN OEVER
Ldg Lts 131·5°. Front and rear both Oc 10s 7M; vis 127°-137°.
Detached Breakwater N Hd, L Fl R 10s.

Stevinsluizen, E wall, Iso WRG 5s 15m W10, R7, G7; vis
G226°-231°, W231°-235°, R235°-290°, G290°-327°, W327°-
335°, R335°-345°.
W wall, 80m from Hd, Iso WRG 2s; vis G195°-213°, W213°-
227°, R227°-245°.

TEXELSTROOM
T5/MH2 Lt By 52°58'·38N 04°47'·80E Fl (2+1) G 12s; preferred
chan to port.
T11/GvS2 Lt By 52°59'·95N 04°49'·20E Fl (2+1) G 12s;
preferred chan to port.
T17 Lt By 53°01'·20N 04°51'·50E Iso G 8s; SHM.

OUDESCHILD
T14 Lt By 53°02'·62N 04°51'·52E Iso R 8s; PHM.
S Mole Hd 53°02'·37N 04°51'·26E FR 7m; *Horn (2) 30s*
(sounded 0600-2300).
N Mole Hd FG 7m.
Oc 6s 7m Lt seen between FR and FG leads into hbr.
T23 Lt By 53°03'·55N 04°55'·70E Iso G 4s; SHM.

DOOVE BALG
D4 53°02'·7N 05°04'·1E Iso R 8s; R pile; Ra refl.
D3A/J2 53°02'·1N 05°07'·0E Fl (2+1) G 12s; G post, R band.
D14 53°02'·5N 05°09'·2E Iso R 4s; R pile; Ra refl.
D11 53°02'·9N 05°12'·0E Iso G 8s; G pile; Ra refl.

KORNWERDERZAND
W side, 53°04'·0N 05°17'·6E Iso R 4s 9m 4M; Gy pedestal,
R lantern; vis 049°-229°.

Buitenhaven, W Mole Hd FG 9m 7M; *Horn Mo(N) 30s.*
E Mole Hd FR.
Spuihaven Noord, W Mole Hd LFIG 10s 7m 7M.

BOONTJES/APPROACHES TO HARLINGEN
BO11/K2/2 53°05'·0N 05°20'·3E Q; NCM.
BO28 53°07'·9N 05°22'·6E Iso R 8s; R pile.
BO34 53°08'·9N 05°23'·0E Iso R 2s; R pile.
BO39 53°10'·0N 05°23'·4E Iso G 4s; G pile.
BO40 53°10'·0N 05°23'·3E Iso R 4s; R pile.

VLIESTROOM (selected marks)
VL1 Lt By 53°19'·00N 05°08'·80E QG; SHM.
VL2/SG1 Lt By 53°19'·86N 05°09'·15E Fl (2+1) R 12s; preferred
chan to stbd.

VL5 Lt By 53°18'·60N 05°09'·55E L Fl G 8s; SHM.
VL6 By 53°18'·97N 05°11'·00E; PHM.
VL9 Lt By 53°17'·65N 05°10'·10E Iso G 4s; SHM.
VL12/WM1 Lt By 53°17'·20N 05°11'·25E VQ (9) 10s; WCM.
VL14 Lt By 53°16'·50N 05°11'·05E L Fl R 8s; PHM.
VL15 Lt By 53°15'·95N 05°09'·80E L Fl G 8s; SHM.

APPROACH TO HARLINGEN/BLAUWE SLENK
(selected marks)
BS1/IN2 Lt By 53°15'·30N 05°10'·14E Fl 2(+1) G 12s; preferred
chan to port.
BS2 Lt By 53°15'·30N 05°10'·59E QR; PHM.
BS3 Lt By 53°14'·87N 05°10'·54E L Fl G 5s; SHM.
BS4 Lt By 53°14'·96N 05°10'·86E L Fl R 5s; PHM.
BS7 Lt By 53°14'·14N 05°11'·25E L Fl G 8s; SHM.
BS8 Lt By 53°14'·23N 05°11'·53E L Fl R 8s; PHM.
BS11 Lt By 53°13'·63N 05°13'·30E Iso G 4s; SHM.
BS12 Lt By 53°13'·80N 05°13'·30E Iso R 4s; PHM.
BS19 Lt By 53°13'·40N 05°17'·00E QG; SHM.
BS20 Lt By 53°13'·55N 05°17'·10E QR; PHM.
BS27 Lt By 53°11'·95N 05°18'·25E QG; SHM.
BS28 Lt By 53°12'·10N 05°18'·42E QR; PHM.
BS31 Bn 53°11'·60N 05°19'·70E L Fl G 8s; G pile, SHM.
BS32 Lt By 53°11'·72N 05°19'·75E L Fl R 8s; PHM.

POLLENDAM
SHMs: P1 Fl G 2s; P3 Iso G 4s; P5 Fl G 2s.
PHMs: P2 Fl R 2s 7m; P4 Iso R 8s 7m; P6 Iso R 4s 7m, P10
Fl R 2s.

HARLINGEN
Ldg Lts 112°. Front 53°10'·56N 05°24'·42E Iso 6s 8m 4M; vis
097°-127°; and FG 9m 7 Rear 500m from front Iso 6s 19m
13M; both on B masts, W bands; vis 104·5°-119·5° (H24).
N Mole Hd 53°10'·57N 05°24'·42E Iso R 5s 8m 4M; R pedestal.
S Mole Hd ; Horn(3) 30s.

TEXEL TO AMELAND

Eierland N Pt of Texel 53°10'·97N 04°51'·40E Fl (2) 10s 52m
29M; R Tr; RC.

VL CENTER LANBY 53°27'·00N 04°40'·00E Fl 5s; Racon (C);
Horn(2) 30s.
TX 3 Lt By 52°58'·61N 04°22'·50E Fl (3) G 9s; SHM.
VL South Lt By 53°08'·95N 04°26'·63E L Fl Y 10s; SPM.
VL 1 Lt By 53°11'·00N 04°35'·40E Fl (2) G 10s; SHM.
Baden Lt By 53°13'·62N 04°41'·35E Q (9) 15s; WCM.
EG Lt By 53°13'·39N 04°47'·15E VQ (9) 10s; WCM.
Tide gauge 53°11'·33N 04°48'·05E Fl (5) Y 20s 5M.
VL 5 Lt By 53°16'·93N 04°39'·68E Fl (3) G 9s; SHM.
VL 7 Lt By 53°22'·92N 04°43'·98E QG; SHM.
SM Lt By 53°19'·29N 04°55'·71E Iso 4s; SWM.
TG Lt By 53°24'·22N 05°02'·40E Q (9) 15s; WCM.
Otto Lt By 53°24'·70N 05°06'·60E VQ (3) 5s ECM.
VL 9 Lt By 53°25'·50N 04°54'·00E Fl (3) G 9s; SHM.
VL 11 Lt By 53°28'·12N 05°04'·00E L Fl G 10s; SHM.
TE 1 Lt By 53°30'·02N 05°13'·60E Fl (3) G 9s; SHM.
TE 3 Lt By 53°31'·86N 05°23'·00E L Fl G 10s; SHM.
TE 5 Lt By 53°33'·70N -5°32'·63E Fl (3) G 9s; SHM.
Vlieland 53°17'·8N 05°03'·6E Iso 4s 53m **20M**; RC.

ZUIDER STORTEMELK (selected marks)
ZS-Bank Lt By 53°18'·98N 04°57'·95E VQ; NCM.
ZS1 Lt By 53°18'·85N 04°59'·62E Fl G 5s; SHM.
ZS13/VS2 Lt By 53°18'·80N 05°05'·93E Fl (2+1) G 12s; leave
to port for Vlieland and to stbd for Terschelling and Harlingen.

VLIELAND
E Mole Hd 53°17'·73N 05°05'·59E FG.
W Mole Hd 53°17'·72N 05°05'·57E FR.
ZS14 Lt By 53°19'·00N 05°05'·55E L Fl R 8s; PHM.
ZS15 Lt By 53°18'·97N 05°07'·10E L Fl G 5s; SHM.
ZS18 Lt By 53°19'·36N 05°06'·95E L Fl R 5s; PHM.

TERSCHELLING
Ent via Schuitengat (Bys changed frequently).
VL 2/SG 1 Lt By 53°19'·78N 05°09'·18E VQ (9) 10s; WCM.
SG 17 Lt By 53°21'·22N 05°13'·50E
Brandaris Tr 53°21'·67N 05°12'·99E Fl 5s 55m **29M**; Y ■ Tr;
vis except where obsc by dunes on Vlieland and Terschelling.
Ldg Lts 053°, W Hbr Mole Hd, front 53°21'·3N 05°13'·1E FR
5m 8M; R post, W bands, vis ; Horn 15s (TD 1989). **Rear**, on
dyke, 1·1M from front Iso 5s 14m **19M**; vis 045°-061°, intens
045°-052°.
E Pier Hd FG 5m 4M.

TS Lt By 53°28'·20N 05°21'·60E VQ; NCM.

BR Lt By 53°30'·65N 05°33'·60E Q; NCM.
Ameland, W end 53°27'·02N 05°37'·60E Fl (3) 15s 57m **30M**;
brown Tr, W bands; RC.

NES
Nieuwe Veerdam Mole Hd 53°26'·02N 05°46'·53E Iso 6s 2m 8M.

AMELAND TO DELFZIJL

AMELAND TO SCHIERMONNIKOOG
BR Lt By 53°30'·07N 05°33'·60E Q; NCM.
AM Lt By 53°31'·00N 05°44'·80E VQ; NCM.
NAM 21 Lt By 53°31'·20N 05°55'·50E Fl Y; SPM.
WRG Lt By 53°32'·78N 06°01'·75E Q; NCM.
WG Lt By 53°32'·25N 06°06'·11E Iso 8s; SWM.
Schiermonnikoog 53°29'·20N 06°08'·90E Fl (4) 20s 43m
28M; ● Tr, dark R Tr. F WR 28m W15M, R12M; (same Tr)
F WR **W15M** R12M; vis W210°-221°, R221°-230°.
Ferry Pier Hd 53°28'·17N 06°12'·21E 2 F.

LAUWERSOOG
E Mole Hd 53°24'·72N 06°12'·14E FR 4M.
W Mole Hd FG 3M; in fog FY; Horn (2) 30s.

OOSTMAHORN
Ent 53°23'·00N 06°09'·72E FG

ZOUTKAMP
Ent (unlit) 53°20'·42N 06°17'·66E.

DELFZIJL ENTRANCE
W Mole Hd E ent 53°19'·10N 07°00'·38E FG; Ra refl.
E Mole Hd FR, In fog FY; Horn 15s.
Ldg Lts 203°. Front 53°18'·56N 07°00'·16E Iso 2s. Rear,
310m from front; Iso 2s.
Zeehavenkannaal, N side (odd numbered posts); 3 QG;
4 Fl G 2s, 6 Fl G 5s; R Refl.
Zeehavenkannaal, S side (even numbered posts);
1 Fl (2) R 6s;1 Fl R 2s, 5 Fl R 5s, 1 QR; R Refl.
E side ent No. 21 (Marina ent) Fl G 5s; W post on dolphin.

TERMUNTERZIJL
BW 13 Lt By 53°18'·70N 07°02'·37E Fl G 5s; SHM.
Wybelsum 53°20'·20N 07°06'·57E F WR 16m W6M, R5M;
W framework Tr, R bands; radar antenna; vis W295°-320°,
R320°-024°, W024°-049°; Fog Det Lt.
Logum Ldg Lts 075°. Front 53°20'·17N 07°08'·05E Oc (2)
12s 16m 12M; W mast, R bands. Rear, 630m from front,
Oc (2) 12s 28m 12M; W mast, R bands; synch with front.

20

10.20.5   PASSAGE INFORMATION

North Sea Passage Pilot (Imray/Navin) covers the North Sea and Belgian/Dutch coasts to Den Helder. *Cruising Guide to the Netherlands* (Imray/Navin) continues to the Ems. Refer also to *Havengids Nederland* (Vetus) in Dutch, well illustrated.

BELGIUM (chart 1872)

Features of this coast are the long shoals lying roughly parallel to it. Mostly the deeper, buoyed chans run within 3M of shore, where the outer shoals can give some protection from strong W or SW winds. Strong W to NE winds can equally create dangerous conditions especially in wind against tide situations. Approaching from seaward it is essential to fix position from one of the many marks, so that the required chan is correctly identified before shoal water is reached. Shipping is a hazard, but it helps to identify the main routes.

From the SW/W, the natural entry to the buoyed chans is at Dunkerque Lanby. From the Thames, bound for Oostende (10.20.10) or the Westerschelde (10.20.15), identify W Hinder lt. From the N, route via NHR-S and NHR-SE buoys or the N Hinder lt buoy. For TSS see Fig 10 (6).

Off the Belgian coast the E-going stream begins at HW Vlissingen – 0320 (HW Dover – 0120), and the W-going at HW Vlissingen + 0240 (HW Dover + 0440), sp rates 2kn. Mostly the streams run parallel with the coast. Nieuwpoort lies 8M from the French border. From the W (Dunkerque), approach through Passe de Zuydcoote (buoyed with least depth 3·3m) and West Diep. From ENE app through Kleine Rede, the inner road off Oostende which carries a depth of 6m. There are other apprs through the chans and over the banks offshore, but they need care in bad weather.

Sailing E from Oostende, leave about HW Vlissingen – 0300 to carry the E-going stream. If bound for Blankenberge (10.20.11) it is only necessary to keep a mile or two offshore, but if heading E of Zeebrugge (10.20.12) it is advisable to clear the hbr extension by 1M or more. The main route to Zeebrugge for commercial shipping is through Scheur (the deep water chan of the Westerschelde) as far as Scheur-Zand lt buoy, about 3M NW of hbr ent. There is much commercial traffic, and yachts should keep clear (S of) the buoyed chan so far as possible. Beware strong tidal stream and possibly dangerous seas in approaches to Zeebrugge.

NETHERLANDS (charts 325, 110, 2322)

While British Admiralty charts are adequate for through passages, coastal navigation, and entry to the main ports, larger scale Dutch charts are essential for any yacht exploring the cruising grounds along this coast or using any of the smaller hbrs. For Dutch Glossary, see 1.4.2.

There are numerous wrecks and obstructions which lie offshore and in coastal areas. Some of these are marked, but many are not. The Off Texel TSS extends NNE from the TX 1 lt buoy, see Fig.10 (7): the separation zone incorporates the Helder gas field. Some 20–30M N lie the Placid and Petroland fields with production platforms. For general notes on N Sea oil and gas installations, see 10.5.5. The shoals of the North Sea coast and Waddenzee are liable to change due to gales and tidal streams; sea level may also be affected by barometic pressure.

WESTERSCHELDE TO DEN HELDER

The main approach chans to Westerschelde are Scheur/Wielingen and Oostgat, but yachts are required to keep clear of these. From Zeebrugge keep close to S side of estuary until past Breskens (10.20.13) when, if proceeding to Vlissingen (10.20.17), cross close W of By H-SS. From N, use Deurloo/Spleet chans to S side of estuary. The tide runs hard in the estuary, causing a bad sea in chans and overfalls on some banks in strong winds. Vessels under 20m must give way to larger craft; and yachts under 12m are requested to stay just outside the main buoyed chans, including those between Walsoorden and Antwerpen (10.20.16) if navigation permits.

The Oosterschelde (10.20.18 and chart 192) is entered via the Roompotsluis, in the South half of the barrage. Coming from the S, Oostgat runs close to the Walcheren shore. Westkapelle l t ho is conspic near the W end of Walcheren. There are two lesser lts nearby: Molenhoofd 5ca WSW and Noorderhoofd 7ca NNW. Having passed the latter the coast runs NE past Domburg but becomes shallower as the Roompot is approached, so it is necessary to keep near the Roompot chan which here is marked by unlit buoys. It is important to have updated information on the buoyage and the chans.

The Schaar, Schouwenbank, Middelbank and Steenbanken lie off the W approaches to Oosterschelde. Westgat and Oude Roompot are the main channels, both well marked. From the north, Geul van de Banjaard (unlit) leads to Oude Roompot. Further north, the Slijkgat (lit) is the approach chan to Stellendam (10.20.19) and entry to the Haringvliet.

Shipping is very concentrated off Hoek van Holland (10.20.20) at the ent to Europoort and Rotterdam (10.20.21). Maas TSS must be noted and regulations for yachts obeyed, see 10.20.20.

The coast N to Den Helder is low, and not easily visible from seaward, like most of the Dutch coast. Conspic landmarks include: Scheveningen light house and big hotels, Noordwijk aan Zee light, big hotels and breakwaters at Zandvoort, and two lt ho's at IJmuiden, chys of steelworks N of IJmuiden, Egmond aan Zee lt, and chys of nuclear power station 1·5M NNE of Petten. For TSS see Figs 10 (6) & 10 (7). 3M W of IJmuiden (10.20.23) the N-going stream begins at HW Hoek van Holland – 0120, and the S-going at HW Hoek van Holland + 0430, sp rates about 1·5kn. Off ent to IJmuiden the stream turns about 1h earlier and is stronger, and in heavy weather there may be a dangerous sea. At IJmuiden the Noordzeekanaal leads to Amsterdam and the IJsselmeer.

THE WEST FRISIAN ISLANDS (charts 2593)

N from Den Helder (10.20.26), thence E for nearly 150M along the Dutch and German coasts, lies the chain of Frisian Is. They have similar characteristics – being low, long and narrow, with the major axis parallel to the coast. Texel is the largest and, with Vlieland and Terschelling, lies further offshore.

Between the islands, narrow chans (zeegat in Dutch, Seegat in German) give access to/from the North Sea. Most of these chans are shallow for at least part of their length, and in these shoal areas a dangerous sea builds up in a strong onshore wind against the outgoing (ebb) tide. The zeegaten between Den Helder and Texel, between Vlieland and Terschelling and the zeegat of the Ems are safe for yachts up to force 8 winds between SW and NE. All the others are unsafe in strong onshore winds.

The flood stream along this coast is E-going, so it starts to run in through the zeegaten progressively from W to E. Where the tide meets behind each Is, as it flows in first at the W end and a little later at the E end, is formed a bank called a wad (Dutch) or Watt (German). These banks between the Is and the coast are major obstacles to E/W progress inside the Is. The chans are narrow and winding, marked by Bys or by withies (⚑⚑) in the shallower parts, and they mostly dry; so that it is essential to time the tide correctly.

This is an area most suited to shallow-draft yachts, particularly flat bottomed or with bilge keels or centreboards, that can take the ground easily. Whilst the zeegaten are described briefly below, the many chans inside the islands and across the Waddenzee are mentioned only for orientation.

TEXEL TO TERSCHELLING

Zeegat van Texel (chart 191) lies between Den Helder and the Is of Texel, and gives access to the Waddenzee, the tidal part of the former Zuider Zee. Haaksgronden shoals extend 5M seaward, with three chans: Schulpengat on S side, leading into Breewijd; Westgat through centre of shoals, where the stream sets across the chan, is only suitable for passage in good weather and in daylight; and Molengat near the Texel shore. Schulpengat is the well marked main chan, buoys being prefixed with letter 'S'; but strong SW winds cause rough sea against the SW-going (ebb) stream which begins at HW Helgoland – 0330, while the NE-going (flood) stream begins at HW Helgoland + 0325, sp rates 1·5kn. Molengat is marked by buoys prefixed 'MG', but strong winds between W and N cause a bad sea. When coming from the NW or NE the Molengat is always the best route unless the weather is exceptionally bad. Routeing via the Schulpengat involves a southerly deviation of approx 15M and leads W of the very dangerous Zuider Haaks which should be avoided in bad weather. In Molengat the N-going (ebb) stream begins at HW Helgoland – 0145, and the S-going (flood) stream at HW Helgoland + 0425, sp rates 1·25kn. For Oudeschild, see 10.20.27.

E of Den Helder and the **Marsdiep**, the flood makes in three main directions through the SW Waddenzee:
(a) to E and SE through Malzwin and Wierbalg to Den Oever (where the lock into IJsselmeer is only available during daylight hours on working days); thence NE along the Afsluitdijk, and then N towards Harlingen (10.20.28);
(b) to NE and E through Texelstroom and Doove Balg towards the Pollen flats; and (c) from Texelstroom, NE and N through Scheurrak, Omdraai and Oude Vlie, where it meets the flood stream from Zeegat van Terschelling. The ebb runs in reverse. The Kornwerderzand locks (available H24), near NE end of Afsluitdijk, also give access to the IJsselmeer (10.20.25).
Eierlandsche Gat, between Texel and Vlieland, consists of dangerous shoals between which run very shallow and unmarked chans, only used by fishermen.

Zeegat van Terschelling (chart 112 and 10.20.31), between Vlieland (10.20.29) and Terschelling, gives access to the hbrs of Vlieland, West Terschelling (10.20.30) and Harlingen (10.20.28); also to the locks at Kornwerderzand. Shallow banks extend more than 5M seaward; the main chan (buoyed) through them is Zuider Stortemelk passing close N of Vlieland. In this chan the buoys are prefixed by letters 'ZS', and the E-going (flood) stream begins at HW Helgoland + 0325, while the W-going (ebb) stream begins at HW Helgoland – 0230, sp rates 2·5kn. Vliesloot leads to Oost Vlieland hbr. Schuitengat forks ENE to West Terschelling. From Zuider Stortemelk the Vliestroom, a deep well buoyed chan (buoys prefixed by letters 'VL'), runs S about 4M until its junction with Blauwe Slenk and Inschot. Blauwe Slenk runs ESE to Harlingen; and Inschot SE to Kornwerderzand.

AMELAND TO DELFZIJL (charts 2593, 3509, 3510)

Zeegat van Ameland, between Terschelling and Ameland, is fronted by the sandbank of Bornrif extending 3M seaward. Westgat is the main entrance, with buoys prefixed by letters 'WG'. The chan runs close N of Terschelling, and divides into Boschgat and Borndiep. For Nes (Ameland), see 10.20.28. In Westgat the flood stream begins at HW Helgoland + 0425, and the ebb stream at HW Helgoland – 0150, sp rates 2kn. A dangerous sea develops in strong onshore winds.

Friesche Zeegat, between Ameland and Schiermonnikoog (10.20.33), has a main chan also called Westgat and buoys marked 'WG'. In strong winds the sea breaks across the whole passage. Westgat leads S through Wierumer Gronden, past Engelsmanplaat (a prominent sandbank) and into Zoutkamperlaag which is the main chan (marked by buoys prefixed 'Z') to Lauwersoog (10.20.32), where locks give access to the Lauwersmeer and inland waterways.

Further E, the estuary of R Ems (chart 3509) runs seaward past the SW side of the German island of Borkum (10.21.11). It leads to Delfzijl and Termunterzijl (10.20.33), or Emden (10.21.9), see 10.21.5. Hubertgat, which runs parallel to and S of the main Westerems chan, is slightly more direct when bound to/from the W, but in both these well lit chans there is a dangerous sea in strong NW winds over the ebb. The E-going (flood) stream begins at HW Helgoland + 0530, and the W-going (ebb) stream begins at HW Helgoland – 0030, sp rates 1·5kn.

CROSSING NORTH SEA FROM BELGIUM AND SCHELDE
(charts 1406, 323)

Avoid major traffic areas and cross TSS (Fig. 10(6)) at 90° to take departure from either Dunkerque Lanby or W Hinder lt depending on destination. From Dunkerque Lanby make good Ruytingen SW buoy, thence CS4 buoy and S Goodwin lt F (on W-going stream) or E Goodwin lt F (on N-going stream). From W Hinder lt for N Thames Estuary, make good Garden City buoy (on E-going stream) or Twin buoy (on W-going stream) in order to make N or S Galloper buoys and thence Long Sand Head buoy. Avoid shallower patches over W Hinder, Fairy, N Falls and Galloper Banks, particularly in rough weather when under-keel clearance may be reduced. For distances across the North Sea, see 10.0.7.

CROSSING NORTH SEA FROM THE NETHERLANDS
Charts 1406, 1408, 1872, 2449, 3371

From ports S of Hoek van Holland proceed westward across banks avoiding shallower patches to pick up Birkenfels buoy, across N Hinder W TSS (Fig 10 (6)) and thence to N Galloper buoy (for N Thames estuary) or Outer Gabbard buoy (for Lowestoft and North). For ports N of Hoek van Holland passages can be made from coast to coast avoiding TSS areas and crossing DW routes (Figs 10 (6) and (7)) with care.

10.20.6   DISTANCE TABLE

Approximate distances in nautical miles are by the most direct route, whilst avoiding dangers and allowing for Traffic Separation Schemes. Places in *italics* are in adjoining areas; places in **bold** are in 10.0.6, Distances across the North Sea.

		1	2	3	4	5	6	7	8	9	10	11	12	13	14	15	16	17	18	19	20
1.	*Dunkerque*	1																			
2.	**Nieuwpoort**	15	2																		
3.	**Oostende**	26	9	3																	
4.	Blankenberge	35	18	9	4																
5.	**Zeebrugge**	40	23	13	5	5															
6.	**Vlissingen**	55	39	29	21	16	6														
7.	**Roompotsluis**	68	51	40	33	28	24	7													
8.	Stellendam	90	83	72	55	50	45	32	8												
9.	Hook of Holland	92	77	67	59	54	47	48	16	9											
10.	Rotterdam	112	97	87	79	74	67	68	36	20	10										
11.	Scheveningen	106	91	81	73	68	61	50	30	14	34	11									
12.	IJmuiden	131	116	106	98	93	86	87	55	39	59	25	12								
13.	Amsterdam	144	129	110	111	106	99	100	68	52	72	38	13	13							
14.	**Den Helder**	169	154	131	136	131	120	125	93	77	97	63	38	51	14						
15.	Den Oever	180	165	142	147	142	131	136	104	88	108	74	49	*62	11	15					
16.	Harlingen	199	184	161	166	161	150	155	123	107	127	93	68	81	30	21	16				
17.	Vlieland	202	187	164	169	164	153	158	126	110	130	96	71	84	33	33	18	17			
18.	Terschelling	201	186	163	168	163	152	157	125	109	129	95	70	83	39	34	19	7	18		
19.	**Delfzijl**	277	262	239	244	239	228	233	201	185	205	171	146	159	115	110	102	92	85	19	
20.	*Borkum*	257	242	219	224	219	208	213	181	165	185	151	126	139	95	90	80	72	65	22	20

*Amsterdam to Den Oever via IJmuiden and Den Helder = 62M; but via the IJsselmeer = 45M.

20

SPECIAL NOTES FOR BELGIUM AND THE NETHERLANDS   10-20-7

BELGIUM

PROVINCES are given for ports in lieu of UK 'counties'.

CHARTS Those most widely used are the *'Vlaamse Banken'* issued by the Hydrografische Dienst der Kust. Imray C30 is also popular amongst Belgian yachtsmen.

TIME ZONE is –0100, which is allowed for in tidal predictions but no provision is made for daylight saving schemes shown by the non-shaded areas on the tide tables (see 9.1.2).

HARBOURS: Although the Hr Mr ☎ is given for Belgian ports, he is not the key figure for yachtsmen that he is in British ports. Berths and moorings are administered by the local YCs.

SIGNALS IPTS (see colour plate 9) are used at Nieuwpoort, Oostende and Zeebrugge, which are the Ports of entry. In season (early April to late Sept) Blankenberge is also a Port of entry with Customs.
Small craft wind warnings (onshore wind >F3; offshore wind >F4) apply to craft <6m LOA and are shown at these 3 ports and Blankenberge as follows:
Day: 2 black ▼s, points together. By night: Lt Fl Bu.

TELEPHONE To call UK from Belgium, dial 00-44 then the UK area code minus the prefix 0, followed by the number required. To call Belgium from UK, dial 00-32 then the code and number. Dialling codes are 3 digits, followed by a 6 digit subscriber No.

Emergencies: Police 101; Fire, Ambulance and Marine 100. 112 (EC emergency number) is not yet available in Belgium.

MARINE RESCUE CO-ORDINATION CENTRE Oostende, ☎ (059) 70.10.00, 70.11.00, 70.77.01 or 70.77.02. In emergency ☎ 100, or call *Oostende Radio* VHF Ch 16 (☎ 70.24.38). For medical advice call *Radiomédical Oostende* on Ch 16.

PUBLIC HOLIDAYS New Year's Day, Easter Mon, Labour Day (1 May), Ascension Day, Whit Mon, National Day (21 July), Feast of the Assumption (15 Aug), All Saints' Day (1 Nov), Armistice Day (11 Nov), King's Birthday or Fete de la Dynastie (15 Nov), Christmas Day.

RULES: Hbr police are strict about yachts using their engines entering hbr. If sails are used as well, hoist a ▼. Yachts may not navigate within 200m of shore (MLWS).

INLAND WATERWAYS: A "sailing sticker" (*Vaarvignet*), valid only in the Flemish waterways, is obtainable from Bestuur Binnenwateren, 104 Aarlenstraat, 1040 Brussels, ☎ 02/2084530. Boats should fly the 'drapeau de navigation', a R flag with W □ in centre. Foreign yachts can expect to pay between 1000 BeF and 4000 BeF, depending on LOA, boat speed, duration of licence and season of the year. The Belgian authorities are likely to adopt the same Competence requirements as the Dutch (RH col).
Note: More info from Belgian Tourist Office, 29 Princes St, London W1R 7RG, ☎ 0171-6291988, Fax 6290454; or Federation Royale Belge du Yachting, FRYB/KBJV, PB 241 Bouchoutlaan, 1020 Brussels, Belgium.

NETHERLANDS

PROVINCES are given in lieu of 'counties' in the UK.

CHARTS The following Dutch charts are quoted:
a. Zeekaarten (equivalent to AC); issued by the Royal Netherlands Navy Hydrographer, and updated by Dutch Notices to Mariners; available from chart agents.
b. Dutch Yacht Charts (DYC) "Kaarten voor Kust-en Binnenwateren"; issued every March by the Hydrographer in 8 sets, booklet format (54 x 38cm), covering coastal and inland waters.
c. ANWB Waterkaarten (ANWB); 18 charts of inland waterways (lettered A to S, excluding Q).

TIME ZONE is –0100, which is allowed for in tidal predictions, but no provision is made for daylight saving schemes as indicated by the non-shaded areas (see 9.1.2).

HARBOURS The term marina is little used; most yacht hbrs are private clubs or Watersport Associations, hence the prefix VVW (= Vlaamse Vereniging voor Watersport. Gem (Gemeeentelijke) = municipal. It is common (in Belgium also) for berth-holders to show a green tally if berth is available, or a red tally if returning same day. Duty-free fuel (coloured red) is not available for pleasure craft. A tourist tax of f1.00/person/night is often added to hbr dues.

CUSTOMS Main customs/ports of entry are Breskens, Vlissingen, Roompotsluis*, Hoek van Holland, Maassluis, Vlaardingen, Schiedam, Rotterdam, Scheveningen, IJmuiden, Den Helder, Harlingen, Vlieland*, West Terschelling, Lauwersoog and Delfzijl. No entry/customs at Stellendam, Den Oever or Kornwerderzand. *Summer only.

BUOYAGE Buoys are often marked with the abbreviations of the banks or chans which they mark (e.g. ZS = Zuider Stortemelk). A division buoy has the abbreviations of both chans meeting there, eg ZS13-VS2 = as above, plus Vliesloot.
Some chans are marked by withies: SHM bound ⚓; PHM unbound ⚓. On tidal flats (e.g. Friesland) where the direction of main flood stream is uncertain, bound withies are on the S side of a chan and unbound on the N side. In minor chans the buoyage may be moved without notice to accommodate changes.
The SIGNI buoyage system is used in certain inland waters, including the IJsselmeer (see 10.20.25).

SIGNALS Traffic signals The standard French/Belgian system is not used in the Netherlands. Where possible the local system is given.

Sluicing signals The following signals may be shown:
By day: A blue board, with the word 'SPUIEN' on it; often in addition to the night signal of 3 Ⓡ in a △.

Visual storm signals Lt sigs only are shown day and night, as per the International System (see 10.15.8), at Vlissingen, Hoek van Holland, Amsterdam, IJmuiden, Den Helder, West Terschelling, Harlingen, Eierland, Ameland, Oostmahorn, Schiermonnikoog, Zoutkamp and Delfzijl.

Inland waterways
Bridge signals (shown on each side):
To request bridges to open sound 'K' (—•—).
Ⓖ = Bridge open.   Ⓨ = You may pass under this arch.
Ⓡ = Bridge closed (opens on request)
Ⓡ over Ⓖ = Bridge about to open.
2 Ⓡ (vert) = Bridge out of use.
2 Ⓖ (vert) = Bridge open but not in use (you may pass).

Railway bridges
Opening times of railway bridges are in a free annual leaflet *'Openingstijden Spoorwegbruggen'* available from ANWB, L & A/Wat, Postbus 93200, 2509 BA, Den Haag; (send A5 sae with international reply coupon).

RADIO TELEPHONE Keep a listening watch on TSS info broadcasts and make contact on VTS sector channels. See Figs 10 (6) and (7), 10.20.15, 10.20.20 and 10.20.23.
Note: Do not use Ch M in Dutch waters, where it is a salvage frequency. Ch 31 is for Dutch marinas (little used).

TELEPHONE To call UK from the Netherlands, dial 00-44; then the UK area code minus the prefix 0, followed by the number required. To call the Netherlands from the UK dial 00-31 then the area code minus the prefix 0, plus number.
Emergencies: Fire, Police, Ambulance, dial 06-11 or 112.

MARINE RESCUE CO-ORDINATION is the task of the Coast Guard Centre at IJmuiden which keeps watch H24 on VHF Ch 16, 2182Khz and 500Khz; ☎ (0255) 534344; fax 523496.

PUBLIC HOLIDAYS New Year's Day, Easter Mon, Queen's Birthday (30 April), Liberation Day (5 May), Ascension Day, Whit Mon, Christmas and Boxing Days.

INLAND WATERWAYS: All craft must carry a copy of the waterway regulations, *Binnenvaart Politiereglement (BPR)*, as given in the current ANWB publication *Almanak voor Watertoerisme, Vol 1* (written in Dutch).
At present craft >15m LOA or capable of more than 20kph (11kn) must be commanded by the holder of a Certificate of Competence. On lakes, rivers and canals this may be the Helmsman's Overseas Certificate of Competence, but the RYA Coastal Skipper (or higher) Certificate of Competence is required for navigation on the Schelde, Waddensee and IJsselmeer. These requirements are (still) under review.
Note: Further information, including a useful publication 'Watersports Paradise', can be obtained from the Dutch Tourism Board, 25 Buckingham Gate, London, SW1E 6LD, ☎ 0171-931 0707; or the Royal Netherland Embassy, 12a Kensington Palace Gdns, London W8 4QU ☎ 0171-229 1594.

10.20.8 DUTCH GLOSSARY   **See 1.4.2**

NIEUWPOORT
(NIEUPORT)
10-20-9

Belgium, West Flanders 51°09'·40N 02°43'·23E

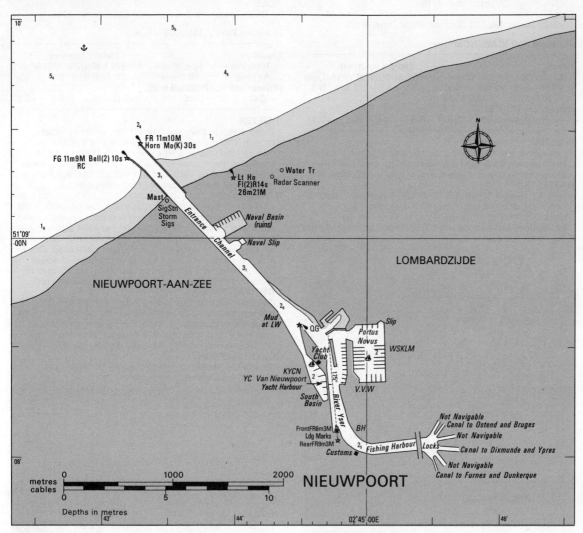

CHARTS
AC 125, 1872, *2449*; Belgian 101, D11; DYC 1801; SHOM 7214; ECM 1010; Imray C30; Stanfords 1, 19

TIDES
+0105 Dover; ML 2·7; Duration 0515; Zone −0100

Standard Port VLISSINGEN (→)

Times				Height (metres)			
High Water		Low Water		MHWS	MHWN	MLWN	MLWS
0300	0900	0400	1000	4·7	3·9	0·8	0·3
1500	2100	1600	2200				
Differences NIEUWPOORT							
−0110	−0050	−0035	−0045	+0·6	+0·5	+0·4	+0·1

SHELTER
Good except in strong NW'lies. There are two yacht hbrs, access H24, run by three YCs: Royal YC of Nieuwpoort (**KYCN**) to the SW gets very full; but there is always room in the Portus Novus, run by the Air Force YC (**WSKLM**) at the N and E side; and **VVW-N**ieuwpoort to the S and centre.

NAVIGATION
WPT 51°10'·00N 02°42'·00E, 308°/128° from/to ent, 0·90M. The bar (1·5m) is liable to silt up but there is usually sufficient water for yachts. At sp the stream reaches 2kn across the ent. The 1M long ent chan to both yacht hbrs is dredged, although levels can drop to about 2m. Note: A firing range E of Nieuwpoort is not used mid-June to end Sept. At other times, call range officer on Ch 67.

LIGHTS AND MARKS
Lt ho Fl (2) R 14s 26m 21M; conspic R tr, W bands. E pier head FR 11m 10M, W tr, vis 025°-250°, 307°-347°, Horn Mo (K) 30s. W pier head, FG 11m 9M, W tr, vis 025°-250°, 284°-324°, Bell (2) 10s, RC.
IPTS from root of W pier, plus: 2 cones, points together or Fl Bu lt = No departure for craft < 6m LOA. Watch out for other tfc sigs, especially STOP sign near exit from Novus Portus, shown in conjunction with IPTS.

RADIO TELEPHONE
VHF Ch 09 19 16 (H24).

TELEPHONE (058)
Hr Mr/Pilots 233000; Hr Mr 235232; Lock 233050; CG/ Marine Police 233045; Marine Rescue Helicopter 311714; ⌗ 233451; Duty Free Store 233433; Police 234246; Ⓗ (Oostende) 707631; Dr 233089; Brit Consul (02) 2179000.

FACILITIES
Berth fees: LOA 7-9m = 360; 9-11m = 450BeF, at all YCs.
KYCN (420 + 80 Ⓥ) ☎ 234413, M, FW, C (10 ton), Slip, CH, Gas, ME, El, Sh, V, D, Ⓓ, R, Bar;
WSKLM (500 + Ⓥ) ☎ 233433, M, L, FW, C (2 ton mobile), CH, R, Bar;
VVW-N (950 + Ⓥ) ☎ 235232, Fax 234058, Slip, FW, BH (45 ton), C (15 ton), AC (meters), CH, D, R, Bar, Free bikes for shopping;
Services: D, L, ME, El, Sh, C (15 ton), Gaz, CH, SM.
Town P, D, V, R, Bar, ⊠, Ⓑ, ⇌, ✈ (Ostend). Ferry: See Ostend. (Fuel can be bought at the hbr by arrangement).

20

OOSTENDE (OSTEND)   10-20-10

Belgium, West Flanders 51°14'·30N 02°55'·18E

CHARTS
AC 125, 325, 1872, *2449*; SHOM 7214; ECM 1010; DYC 1801; Imray C30; Stanfords 1, 19

TIDES
+0120 Dover; ML 2·6; Duration 0530; Zone –0100

Standard Port VLISSINGEN (→)

Times				Height (metres)			
High Water		Low Water		MHWS	MHWN	MLWN	MLWS
0300	0900	0400	1000	4·7	3·9	0·8	0·3
1500	2100	1600	2200				
Differences OOSTENDE							
–0055	–0040	–0030	–0045	+0·4	+0·4	+0·3	+0·1

SHELTER
Very good, esp in the Mercator Yacht Hbr (1·2m); ent via Montgomery Dock and lock. NSYC (2·7m) and ROYC may be uncomfortable due ferries and/or strong W/NW winds.

NAVIGATION
WPT 51°15'·00N 02°53'·97E, 308°/128° from/to ent, 0·98M. Avoid the offshore banks esp in bad weather; appr via West Diep inside Stroombank or from the NW via Kwintebank and buoyed chan. Busy ferry/commercial hbr.

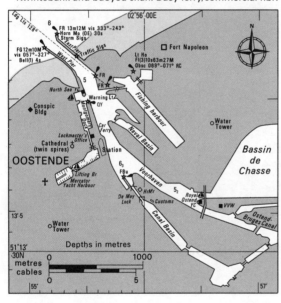

LIGHTS AND MARKS
Europa Centrum bldg (105m) is conspic 3ca SSW of ent. Lt ho Fl (3) 10s 63m 27M, conspic W tr with 2 sinusqidal Blu bands, RC. Ldg lts 128°, both FR 12/18m 4M, both X on W pylons, R bands, vis 051°-201°. W pier, FG 12m 10M, W tr, vis 057°-327°, Bell 4s.
E pier FR 13m 12M, W tr, vis 333°-243°, horn Mo (OE) 30s. IPTS shown from E pier, plus QY lts = keep clear of ent and chan, ferry arr/dep; repeated at Montgomery Dock. 2 ▼, points together or Fl Bu lt = No departure for craft < 6m LOA; (shown at ent to Montgomery dock).

RADIO TELEPHONE
VHF Ch 09 16 67 (H24). Mercator lock & hbr Ch 14 (H24).

TELEPHONE (059)
Hr Mr 705762; Life Saving Service 701100; ⌗ 702009; Police 500925; Ⓗ 707637; Brit Consul (02) 2179000; Weather (no code needed): 1603 (Dutch), 1703 (French).

FACILITIES
Berthing fees: See 10.20.7.
Montgomery Dock (70 + 50 visitors) YC, Bar, R, FW, Slip; **North Sea YC** (at N end of Montgomery Dock) ☎ 702754, L, FW, AB, R, Bar; **Mercator Yacht Hbr** (450+50 visitors) ☎ 705762, FW, AC, D, C, Slip; **Royal Oostende YC** (1M SE up Voorhaven, 160 + 40 visitors) ☎ 321452, Slip, M, L, V, FW, AB, C (½ ton), R, Bar; Note: Access via Achterhaven to the Belgian, Dutch and French canals.
Services: ME, CH, Sh, El, SM. D by tanker ☎ 500874 or at FV hbr. **Town** All amenities, ✉, Ⓑ, ⇌, ✈. Ferry: Ramsgate.

BLANKENBERGE   10-20-11

Belgium, West Flanders 51°18'·95N 03°06'·60E

CHARTS
AC 325, 1872, *2449*; DYC 1801; Imray C30; Stanfords 1, 19

TIDES
+0130 Dover; ML 2·5; Duration 0535; Zone –0100

Standard Port VLISSINGEN (→)

Times		Height (metres)			
High Water	Low Water	MHWS	MHWN	MLWN	MLWS
All times	All times	4·7	3·9	0·8	0·3
Differences BLANKENBERGE					
–0040	–0040	–0·3	–0·1	+0·3	+0·1

SHELTER
Good. Keep to port, past the FV hbr, to the old Yacht Hbr (1·8m); VNZ pontoons are on N side and SYCB to the E. Or turn stbd into new Hbr and marina (1·8m) with 15 pontoons, numbered clockwise I - XV from the N; these are controlled by VNZ, SYCB, VVW and BLOSO. Early Apr to late Sept this is a Port of Entry with Customs.

NAVIGATION
WPT 51°19'·60N 03°05'·40E, 314°/134° from/to piers, 1·0M. Do not attempt entry in strong NW winds. Beware strong tides (and fishing lines) across ent. Ent chan between piers silts, despite dredging to 1·5m (in season only); access HW ±2. Do not try to ent/leave LW±1½ especially at sp. Oct-end May, only ent/leave HW±1, unless depth is pre-checked. Digital panel on E pier lt tr (not visible to departing craft) gives latest depth/drying ht (decimetres) between piers.

LIGHTS AND MARKS
Conspic high-rise blocks E of lt ho, Fl (2) 8s 30m 20M, W tr B top. Ldg lts 134°, both FR 5/8m 3M, (Red X on mast) show the best water. A Water tr is conspic on E side of new Hbr. FS by lt ho shows 2 ▼, points inward, or Fl Bu lt = No departure for craft < 6m LOA (small craft warning).

RADIO TELEPHONE
Marina Ch 08. *Blankenberge Rescue* Ch 08, or relay Ch 16 71 (H24) via Ostend/Zeebrugge.

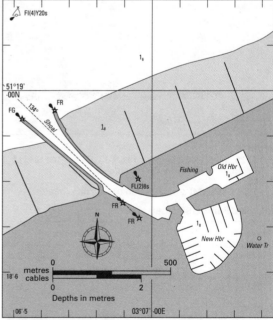

TELEPHONE (050)
Hr Mr 411420; ⌗ Zeebrugge 544223; Police 429842; Dr 333668; Ⓗ 413701; Brit Consul (02) 2179000.

FACILITIES
Berths: Based on beam, ie 3m = 350BeF; 3.5m = 450 BeF; plus 100BeF for every additional 0·25m. **Old Yacht Hbr** (mainly locals): **YC Vrije Noordzeezeilers (VNZ)** ☎ 429150, AC, M, FW, Bar, L, Slip; **Scarphout YC (SYCB)** ☎ 411420, C (10/2½ ton), CH, FW, AC, Slip, Bar, R; **New Hbr** (best for visitors): **Marina (VVW)** ☎ 417536, AC, FW, Bar, ▣, Slip. **Services:** P, D (hose, duty free), ME, Sh, Ⓔ, El, C (20 ton), SM, CH. **Town** Gaz, R, Bar, ✉, Ⓑ, ⇌, ✈ Ostend.

ZEEBRUGGE   10-20-12

Belgium, West Flanders 51°21'·80N 03°11'·60E

CHARTS
AC 97, 325, 1872, *2449*; Zeekaart 1441; DYC 1801, 1803;
Imray C30; Stanfords 1, 19

TIDES
+0110 Dover; ML 2·4; Duration 0535; Zone –0100

Standard Port VLISSINGEN (→)

Times				Height (metres)			
High Water		Low Water		MHWS	MHWN	MLWN	MLWS
0300	0900	0400	1000	4·7	3·9	0·8	0·3
1500	2100	1600	2200				
Differences ZEEBRUGGE							
–0035	–0015	–0020	–0035	+0·1	+0·1	+0·3	+0·1

SHELTER
Very good in the Yacht Hbr, access H24. Zeebrugge is the
port for Brugge, 6M inland by canal. Caution on ent/dep
due to restricted vis and fast FVs; give all jetties a wide berth.
NAVIGATION
WPT Scheur-Zand ECM By, Q (3) 10s, 51°23'·70N 03°07'·68E,
309°/129° from/to ent, 3·1M. Beware strong currents in hbr
apprs (up to 4kn at HW –1) and extensive work in progress in
outer hbr. Zeebrugge is the main Belgian fishing port and a
ferry terminal, so keep clear of FVs and ferries. When LNG-
Gas Tanker is under way all movements prohib in hbr/apprs .
LIGHTS AND MARKS
Heist Oc WR 15s 22m 20/18M, Gy ○ tr, horn (3+1) 90s.
Ldg lts toward Vissershaven for marina at W end:
(1) 136°: Oc 5s 22/45m 8M, vis 131°-141° synch (H24).
(2) 154°: Front Oc WR 6s 20m 3M, R △, W bands; rear
   Oc 6s 34m 3M, R ▽, W bands, synch (H24).
(3) 220°: Front 2FW neon (vert) 30/22m; rear FW neon
   30m. Both W concrete columns, B bands.
(4) 193°: Front 2FR (vert) 30/22; rear FR 29m. Both W
   concrete columns, R bands.
IPTS are shown at NE end of Leopold Dam. A QY lt at S
side of Visserhaven prohibits ent/dep Visserhaven.
RADIO TELEPHONE
VHF Port Ent and Port Control Ch 71 (H24). Locks Ch 13.
TELEPHONE (050)
Hr Mr 543241; Port Control 546867; Lock Mr 543231; CG
545072; Sea Saving Service 544007; ⌗ 54.54.55; Police
544148; Dr 544590; Ⓗ 320832; Brit Consul (02) 2179000.
FACILITIES
Berthing fees: See 10.20.7.
Yacht Hbr (100) ☎ 544903, AB, L, FW, Slip, Sh, CH, D;
Royal Belgian SC ☎ 544903, M, AB; **Alberta** (R, Bar of
RBSC) ☎ 544197; **Services:** ME, EI, CH.
Town P, D, FW, ME, EI, Sh, CH, Gaz, V, R, Bar, ⊠, Ⓑ, ⇥
15 mins to Brugge, Tram to Oostende, ✈ (Ostend).
Ferry: Zeebrugge-Felixstowe/Hull.

BRESKENS   10-20-13

Zeeland 51°24'·02N 03°34'·15E

CHARTS
AC 325, 120; Zeekaart 120, 101; DYC 1801, 1803; Imray
C30; Stanfords 1, 19

TIDES
+0210 Dover; ML no data; Duration 0600; Zone –0100

Standard Port VLISSINGEN (→)

Times				Height (metres)			
High Water		Low Water		MHWS	MHWN	MLWN	MLWS
0300	0900	0400	1000	4·7	3·9	0·8	0·3
1500	2100	1600	2200				
Differences BRESKENS: Use VLISSINGEN figures							
CADZAND (7M WSW)							
–0030	–0025	–0020	–0025	–0·1	–0·3	+0·1	0·0

SHELTER
Good in all winds; access H24, 5m at ent. Ⓥ berth on the N
finger (4m). ⚓ off Plaat van Breskens, in fine weather, not
in commercial/fishing hbr. Beware fast ferries.
NAVIGATION
WPT SS-VH NCM By, Q, 51°24'·75N 03°34'·00E, 353°/173°
from/to W side lt (within W sector), 0·69M. Beware
strong tides across the ent. Do not confuse the ent with
the ferry port ent, 0·7M WNW, where yachts are prohib.
LIGHTS AND MARKS
Large bldg/silo on centre pier in hbr is conspic from afar.
W mole hd F WRG 6m; vis R090°-128°, W128°-157°,
G157°-169·5°, W169·5°-173°, R173°-194°, G194°-296°,
W296°-300°, R300°-320°, G320°-090°; Horn Mo (U) 30s.
E mole hd FR 5m.
Nieuwe Sluis lt, Oc WRG 10s 28m 14/10M, B 8-sided tr, W
bands, is 1·2M W of ferry hbr.
RADIO TELEPHONE
Marina VHF Ch 31.
TELEPHONE (0117)
Hr Mr 381902; ⌗ 382610; Police (0117) 453156; Dr 381566/
381956; Ⓗ (0117) 459000; Brit Embassy (070) 3645800.

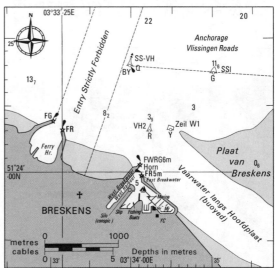

FACILITIES
Marina (Port Scaldis) ☎ 381902, f30, FW, ▨, AC;
YC Breskens ☎ 383278, R, Bar;
Services: SM, CH, D & P (fuel pontoon is in FV hbr), Gaz,
chart agent, BY, C (15 ton), EI, Ⓔ, ME, Sh, Slip.
Town V, R, Bar, ⊠, Ⓑ, Gas, ⇥ (Flushing), ✈ (Ostend or
Brussels). Ferry: See Vlissingen.

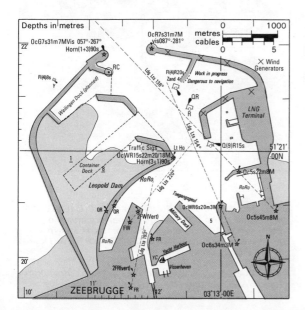

TERNEUZEN   10-20-14

Zeeland 51°20'·62N 03°49'·75E

CHARTS
AC 120; Zeekaart 1443; DYC 1803.2; Imray C30
TIDES
+0230 Dover; ML 2·5; Duration 0555; Zone –0100

Standard Port VLISSINGEN (→)

Times				Height (metres)			
High Water		Low Water		MHWS	MHWN	MLWN	MLWS
0300	0900	0400	1000	4·7	3·9	0·8	0·3
1500	2100	1600	220				
Differences TERNEUZEN							
+0020	+0020	+0020	+0030	+0·4	+0·3	+0·1	0·0

SHELTER
Very good except in strong NW winds. Marina in the
Veerhaven is tidal and exposed to NE. Or enter the E lock
(Oostsluis) and see Lockmaster for berth as on chartlet.
Yachts are prohib in W Hbr and lock (Westsluis).
NAVIGATION
WPT No 18 PHM Buoy, Iso R 8s, 51°20'·95N 03°48'·83E,
299°/119° from/to Veerhaven ent, 0·65M. The Terneuzen-
Gent canal is 17M long with 3 bridges, min clearance
6·5m when closed.
LIGHTS AND MARKS
The Dow Chemical works and storage tanks are conspic
2M W of hbr. For the Veerhaven, the water tr to SE and
the Oc WRG lt on W mole are conspic. When entry
prohib, a second R lt is shown below FR on E mole. Sigs
for Oostsluis: R lts = entry prohib; G lts = entry permitted.
RADIO TELEPHONE
Call: *Havendienst Terneuzen* VHF Ch 11 (H24); also info
broadcasts every H+00 for vessels in the basins & canal.
East lock Ch 18. For Terneuzen-Gent canal call on Ch 11
and keep watch during transit. Contact Zelzate Bridge
(call: *Uitkijk Zelzate*) direct on Ch 11, other bridges
through Terneuzen or, at the S end, *Havendienst Gent*
Ch 05 11 (H24). See also 10.20.15.
TELEPHONE (0115)
Hr Mr 613661; CG 613017 (H24); ⌗ 612377; Police 613017;
Ⓗ 688000; Dr 06-11; Brit Consul (020) 6764343.

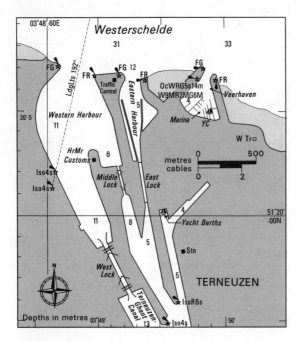

FACILITIES
Yacht Hbr (120) ☎ 697089, Slip, ME, El, Sh, BH (15 ton),
FW, AB; **WSV de Honte YC** ☎ 617633, L, FW, Ⓞ, AB;
Neuzen YC ☎ 14411, M, L, FW, AB;
Services: ME, El, BY, P, D, L, FW, C (40 ton), AB, Sh, Gaz.
Town P, D, CH, V, R, Bar, ✉, Ⓑ, ⇌, ✈ (Ghent). Ferry: See
Vlissingen.

WESTERSCHELDE   10-20-15

Zeeland

CHARTS
AC 120, 139, 325; Zeekaart 1443; DYC 1803; Imray C30
TIDES
+0200 Dover; ML Hansweert 2·6, Westkapelle 2·0, Bath
2·8; Duration 0555; Zone –0100

Standard Port VLISSINGEN (→)

Times				Height (metres)			
High Water		Low Water		MHWS	MHWN	MLWN	MLWS
0300	0900	0400	1000	4·7	3·9	0·8	0·3
1500	2100	1600	2200				
Differences WESTKAPELLE							
–0025	–0015	–0010	–0025	–0·5	–0·5	0·0	0·0
HANSWEERT							
+0100	+0050	+0040	+0100	+0·7	+0·6	+0·1	0·0
BATH							
+0125	+0115	+0115	+0140	+1·1	+0·9	+0·1	0·0

SHELTER AND FACILITIES
Some hbrs for yachts between Terneuzen and Antwerpen
(38M) are listed below in sequence from seaward:
ELLEWOUTSDIJK, 51°23'·00N 03°49'·00E. DYC 1803.2. HW
+0200 and +0·3m on Vlissingen; ML 2·6m. Small, safe hbr;
unlit. Dries, easy access HW ±3; 1·5m at MLWS. Hr Mr ☎
(0113) 548248 FW, D, Gaz; **YC Ellewoutsdijk** ☎ 548446.
HOEDEKENSKERKE, 51°25'·25N 03·55'·00E. DYC 1803.3.
Disused ferry hbr (dries) on N bank, abeam ☆ Iso WRG 2s
R □ tr, W band. Access HW–2½ to +3 for 1m draft. **YC WV
Hoedekenskerke** ☎ (0113) 63x259; Ⓥ berths, P, D, Gaz, FW,
ME. **Town** ✉, Ⓑ, ⇌ (Goes).
HANSWEERT, 51°26'·40N 04°00'·75E. DYC 1803.3. Tidal
differences above. Can be used temporarily, but it is the
busy ent to Zuid Beveland canal. Lt Oc WRG 10s, R lattice
tr, W band, at ent. Waiting berths outside lock on E side.
Ⓥ berths in inner hbr, W side; **Services**: ME, BY, P, D, C
(17 ton), CH, R. **Town** ✉, Ⓑ, ⇌ (Goes).
WALSOORDEN, 51°23'·00N 04°02'·00E. DYC 1803.3. HW is
+0110 and +0·7m on Vlissingen; ML 2·6m. Prone to swell.
SHM buoy 57A, L Fl G 8s, is 1ca N of ent. Ldg lts 220°
both Oc 3s. Hbr ent marked with FG and FR. Yacht basin
dead ahead on ent to hbr, depths 2 to 2·8m. *Zandvliet
Radio* VHF Ch 12. Hr Mr ☎ (0114) 681235, FW, Slip;
Services: Gas, P, D, BY, ME, El. **Town** R, Bar, ✉.
PAAL, 51°21'·30N 04°06'·70E. DYC 1803.3. HW +0120 and
+0·8m on Vlissingen; ML 2·7m. Unlit, drying yacht hbr on
W side at river mouth, ent marked by withy. Appr from
No. 63 SHM buoy, L Fl G 8s, and Tide gauge, Fl (5) Y 20s
across drying Speelmansgat. *Zandvliet Radio* VHF Ch 12.
Hr Mr ☎ (0114) 315548; **Jachthaven** AC, FW; **Services**: V,
P, D, Gaz, ME, El, R.

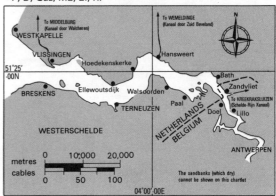

DOEL, Antwerpen, 51°18'·70N 04°16'·15E. DYC 1803.5. HW
+0100 and +0·7m on Vlissingen. Small drying hbr on W
bank. Ldg lts 185·5°: front Fl WRG 3s; rear Fl 3s, synch. N
pier hd lt, Oc WR 5s. Hr Mr ☎ (03) 7733072; **YC de Noord**
☎ 7733669, R, Bar, FW.
LILLO, Antwerpen, 51°18'·24N 04°17'·40E. DYC 1803.5. 1M
SE of Doel on opp bank; small drying hbr for shoal-draft
only; HW±3. Landing stage in river has Oc WRG 10s. Hr
Mr (035) 686456; **YC Scaldis.**

WESTERSCHELDE *continued*

NAVIGATION
WPTs: See Breskens (10.20.13), Terneuzen (10.20.14) and Vlissingen (10.20.17). The Westerschelde chan winds through a mass of well marked sand-banks. It is the waterway to Antwerpen and Gent (via canal), very full of shipping and also of barges (which do not normally conform to the rules; beware unpredictable actions). It is necessary to work the tides, which average 2½kn, more at springs. Yachts should keep to the edge of main chan. Alternative chans must be used with caution, particular going downstream on the ebb.

LIGHTS AND MARKS
The apprs to Westerschelde are well lit by lt ho's: on the S shore at Kruishoofd and Nieuwe Sluis, and on the N shore at Westkapelle and Kaapduinen. See 10.20.4. The main fairway is, for the most part, defined by ldg lts and by the W sectors of the many Dir lts.

RADIO TELEPHONE
Commercial traffic in the Westerschelde must comply with a comprehensive VTS which covers from the N Sea Outer Apprs up-river to Antwerp. Yachts should listen at all times on the VHF Ch for the area in which they are (see next column). Do not transmit, unless called; if you have a problem and need help, state vessel's name, position and the nature of the problem. Dutch is the primary language, English secondary.

If you have an **emergency**, call initially on the working/channel in use; you may then be switched to *Schelde Cordination Centre* (SCC at Vlissingen) Ch 67.

Seven Traffic Centres control the following areas; see also Fig 10 (6) for diagram:

In offshore approaches:
(1) *Wandelaar* Ch 65 (NW of Oostende);
(2) *Zeebrugge* Ch 69 (W, N and E of Zeebrugge);
(3) *Steenbank* Ch 64 (NW of Vlissingen).

Within the Westerschelde:
(4) *Vlissingen* Ch 14 (Vlissingen to E2A/PvN SPR buoys at approx 51°24'N 03°44'E);
(5) *Terneuzen* Ch 03 (thence to Nos 32/35 buoys at approx 51°23'N 03°57'E);
(6) *Hansweert* Ch 65 (thence to Nos 46/55 buoys at approx 51°24'N 04°02'E);
(7) *Zandvliet* Ch 12 (thence to Antwerpen).

Also *Terneuzen* Ch 11 covers the Terneuzen-Gent Canal. In addition, 16 unmanned Radar stns within the 7 Traffic areas provide radar and hbr info on separate VHF Ch's.

Broadcast reports of visibility, met, tidal data and ship movements are made in Dutch and English at:
Every H+50 on Ch 14 by *Vlissingen*;
Every H+05 on Ch 03, and H+55 on Ch 11, by *Terneuzen*;
Every H+35 on Ch 12 by *Zandvliet*.

ANTWERPEN (ANTWERP)   10-20-16

Antwerpen 51°13'·85N 04°23'·77E

CHARTS
AC 139; Zeekaart 1443; DYC 1803

TIDES
+0342 Dover; ML 2·9; Duration 0605; Zone –0100

Standard Port VLISSINGEN (⟶)

Times				Height (metres)			
High Water		Low Water		MHWS	MHWN	MLWN	MLWS
0300	0900	0400	1000	4·7	3·9	0·8	0·3
1500	2100	1600	2200				
Differences ANTWERPEN							
+0128	+0116	+0121	+0144	+1·1	+0·9	0·0	0·0

SHELTER
Excellent in NIC-Haven marina on W bank, 4ca SW of Kattendijksluis and ½M from city centre (via two tunnels). Access by lock HW ±1 (0600-2000). Lock opens in winter only by arrangement. 2 unlit Y waiting Bys N & S of lock.

NAVIGATION
For Westerschelde see 10.20.13/14/15/17. On final 90° river bend to stbd, before marina is a windmill; No. 109 SHM buoy Iso G 8s is 2½ca N of ent.

LIGHTS AND MARKS
Lock sigs at marina:

R flag or ®	=	Ent prohib
G flag or Ⓖ	=	Departure prohib
Bu cone/flag or Bu lt	=	Appr chan closed

Depth sigs at marina:

1 B ● or 1 Ⓦ lt	=	Depth over sill 2·5 – 3·0m
2 B ● or 2 Ⓦ lts	=	Depth over sill 3·0 – 3·5m
3 B ● or 3 Ⓦ lts	=	Depth over sill 3·5 – 3·8m

RADIO TELEPHONE
Antwerpen Havendienst (H24) VHF Ch 74 for Calling and Safety; Radar Ch 02 60; Bridges Ch 13; NIC-Haven Ch 13.

TELEPHONE (03)
Hr Mr 2310680; Marina Lock 2190895; ⌗ 2340840; Police 321840; Ⓗ 2177111.

FACILITIES
NIC-Haven Marina ☎ 2190895, FW, P, D, R, V, Gaz, El, Sh, AC, C (1·5 ton), Slip; **Royal YC van België** ☎ 2192682, Bar, R, M, C (5 ton), D, P, CH, FW, L, Slip; **Kon. Liberty YC** ☎ 2191147; **Services:** By, ME, BH, ACA, DYC Agent.
City All facilities, ⊠, Ⓑ, ≈, ✈. Ferry: See Vlissingen.

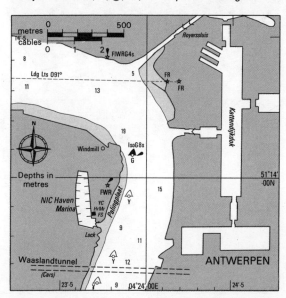

20

VLISSINGEN (FLUSHING)

10-20-17

Zeeland 51°26'·36N 03°34'·70E (Koopmanshaven)

CHARTS

AC 325, 120, 1872; Zeekaart 1442, 1443, 1533; DYC 1801.3, 1803.8; Imray C30; Stanfords 1, 19

TIDES

+0215 Dover; ML 2·3; Duration 0555; Zone –0100
NOTE: Vlissingen is a Standard Port and the tidal predictions for each day of the year are given below.

SHELTER

Very good in both yacht hbrs:

1. **Michiel de Ruyter** marina (2·9m) in the Vissershaven has 6m wide ent, approached from the Koopmanshaven. Storm barrier is open 1 Apr-1 Nov. Sill with 1·0m water at MLWS; check depth gauge on barrier wall. Small swing bridge (pedestrian) is operated by Hr Mr 0800-2000LT, with R/G tfc lts. The bridge is open 2000-0800LT, but only for yachts to leave; ⓇⓇ (vert) tfc lts prohibit arrival from sea, because the marina is not lit.
2. **VVW Schelde** (3m) is near the ent to the Walcheren Canal. Entering the Buitenhaven beware ferries. Keep to port for the locks, close S of ferry terminal; locks operate H24. Marina is to NW, past both Binnenhaven.

NAVIGATION

WPT H-SS NCM buoy, Q, 51°25'·97N 03°37'·54E, 125°/305° from/to Buitenhaven ent, 0·95M. Yachts should keep clear of the main shipping chans: Wielingen from the W and Oostgat from the N.

From the SW there are no dangers. After Zeebrugge, keep S of Wielingen chan past Breskens, and cross to Vlissingen near H-SS buoy.

From N, by day, use Deurloo/Spleet chans to SP4 buoy, then along N edge of Wielingen N anchorage, and close inshore to N of TSS. Yachts are forbidden to sail in the TSS fairways.

Ocean-going ships often transfer pilots off the town. Fast ferries fequently enter/leave the Buitenhaven terminal.

LIGHTS AND MARKS

From NW, ldg lts 117°: Front Leugenaar, Oc R 5s 5m 7M; rear Sardijngeul, 550m from front, Oc WRG 5s 10m 12/8M, R △, W bands on R and W mast. Note: The conspic Radar Tr (SCC on chartlet) shows a Fl Y lt to warn when ships are approaching from the NW, ie around the blind arc from Oostgat/Sardijngeul.

The lt ho at the root of the W bkwtr of Koopmanshaven is brown metal framework tr, Iso WRG 3s 15m 12/9M. On S side of de Ruyter marina is a conspic W metal framework tr (50m), floodlit.

Buitenhaven tfc sigs from mole W side of ent:
R flag or extra Ⓡ near FR on W mole hd = Entry prohib.

RADIO TELEPHONE

Havenschap Vlissingen Ch 09. Lock & bridge info Ch 22. See also Westerschelde (10.20.15) for VTS.

TELEPHONE (0118)

Hr Mr 468080; East Hbr Port Authority 478741; Schelde Tfc Coordination Centre 424790; Buitenhaven Lock 412372; ⚌ 484600; Police 415050; Ⓗ 425000; Dr 412233; Brit Consul (020) 6764343.

FACILITIES

Michiel de Ruyter (100 + 40 visitors) ☎ 414498, f27.42, D, FW, AC, Bar, R, YC;
Jachthaven 'VVW Schelde' (90 + 50 visitors) ☎ 465912, f13.50, AC, Bar, C (10 ton), CH, D, FW, R, Ⓞ, M, Slip, (Access H24 via lock), approx 1km by road from ferry terminal; **Services:** BY, Sh, ME, Sh, SM.
Town P, D, CH, V, R, Bar, ✉, Ⓑ, ⇌, ✈ (Antwerpen).
Ferry: Vlissingen-Breskens.

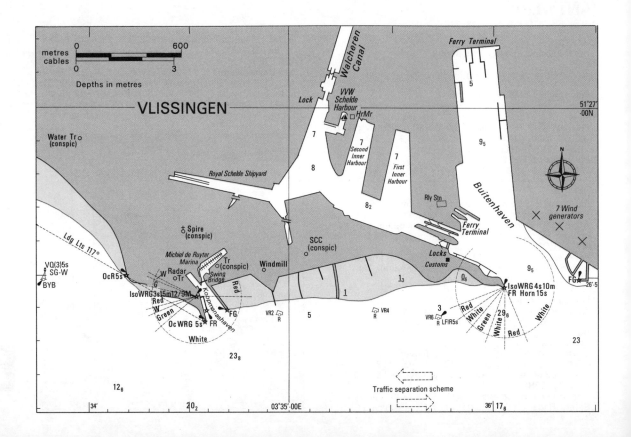

TIME ZONE –0100
(Dutch Standard Time)
Subtract 1 hour for UT
For Dutch Summer Time add
ONE hour in non-shaded areas

NETHERLANDS – VLISSINGEN (FLUSHING)

LAT 51°27′N   LONG 3°36′E

TIMES AND HEIGHTS OF HIGH AND LOW WATERS

YEAR **1996**

JANUARY

Day	Time	m	Day	Time	m
1 M	0434 1049 1731 2329	1.0 4.0 0.7 4.1	**16** TU	0315 0945 1559 2222	0.9 4.1 0.7 4.2
2 TU	0544 1151 1826	0.9 4.1 0.7	**17** W	0436 1052 1715 2328	0.8 4.2 0.6 4.3
3 W	0025 0640 1245 1900	4.2 0.8 4.2 0.7	**18** TH	0550 1155 1819	0.6 4.5 0.5
4 TH	0112 0719 1328 1935	4.3 0.7 4.3 0.7	**19** F	0026 0652 1246 1915	4.5 0.4 4.7 0.4
5 F O	0149 0758 1405 2010	4.4 0.6 4.4 0.6	**20** SA ●	0115 0749 1336 2007	4.7 0.2 4.9 0.3
6 SA	0221 0836 1435 2042	4.4 0.5 4.5 0.6	**21** SU	0205 0835 1423 2052	4.8 0.1 5.0 0.3
7 SU	0256 0912 1507 2118	4.5 0.4 4.6 0.6	**22** M	0248 0926 1509 2138	4.8 0.0 5.0 0.4
8 M	0326 0945 1538 2156	4.6 0.4 4.6 0.6	**23** TU	0335 1012 1556 2222	4.9 0.0 5.0 0.4
9 TU	0359 1026 1616 2228	4.6 0.4 4.6 0.6	**24** W	0420 1058 1645 2302	4.8 0.0 4.9 0.5
10 W	0431 1055 1646 2300	4.5 0.4 4.5 0.7	**25** TH	0506 1139 1736 2348	4.8 0.1 4.7 0.6
11 TH	0506 1130 1720 2337	4.4 0.5 4.5 0.7	**26** F	0555 1226 1826	4.6 0.2 4.5
12 F	0537 1206 1757	4.3 0.5 4.4	**27** SA	0035 0645 1305 1919	0.7 4.4 0.4 4.2
13 SA	0016 0626 1250 1849	0.8 4.2 0.5 4.2	**28** SU	0125 0742 1406 2026	0.8 4.1 0.6 4.0
14 SU	0106 0720 1339 2006	0.8 4.1 0.6 4.1	**29** M	0224 0849 1509 2146	1.0 3.9 0.8 3.7
15 M	0206 0836 1450 2112	0.9 4.0 0.7 4.1	**30** TU	0350 1015 1625 2300	1.0 3.8 0.9 3.8
			31 W	0516 1126 1746	1.0 3.9 0.9

FEBRUARY

Day	Time	m	Day	Time	m
1 TH	0006 0626 1226 1836	3.9 0.8 4.0 0.8	**16** F	0535 1138 1806	0.6 4.3 0.6
2 F	0052 0706 1316 1916	4.1 0.7 4.2 0.7	**17** SA	0008 0640 1236 1902	4.3 0.4 4.6 0.4
3 SA	0131 0742 1346 1950	4.2 0.6 4.3 0.7	**18** SU ●	0102 0736 1325 1952	4.5 0.2 4.8 0.3
4 SU O	0206 0818 1415 2022	4.3 0.5 4.5 0.5	**19** M	0149 0826 1409 2036	4.7 0.0 4.9 0.3
5 M	0230 0850 1445 2058	4.5 0.4 4.6 0.5	**20** TU	0233 0908 1453 2120	4.8 -0.1 5.0 0.3
6 TU	0302 0926 1515 2136	4.6 0.3 4.7 0.5	**21** W	0316 0953 1536 2202	4.9 -0.1 5.0 0.3
7 W	0335 1006 1549 2205	4.7 0.2 4.7 0.5	**22** TH	0359 1035 1622 2242	4.9 0.0 4.9 0.4
8 TH	0405 1035 1620 2239	4.6 0.2 4.7 0.5	**23** F	0442 1113 1707 2326	4.8 0.1 4.7 0.4
9 F	0439 1112 1655 2315	4.6 0.3 4.6 0.5	**24** SA	0526 1152 1748	4.7 0.3 4.5
10 SA	0515 1146 1735 2356	4.5 0.3 4.5 0.6	**25** SU	0006 0609 1229 1838	0.5 4.5 0.4 4.2
11 SU	0556 1226 1822	4.5 0.4 4.4	**26** M	0045 0700 1315 1925	0.7 4.2 0.9 3.9
12 M	0038 0646 1316 1919	0.6 4.3 0.6 4.2	**27** TU	0146 0755 1426 2029	0.9 3.8 0.9 3.6
13 TU	0132 0752 1416 2036	0.7 4.1 0.6 4.0	**28** W	0306 0926 1546 2225	1.0 3.6 1.0 3.5
14 W	0246 0916 1530 2151	0.8 4.0 0.7 3.9	**29** TH	0425 1055 1654 2336	1.0 3.6 1.0 3.7
15 TH	0404 1028 1655 2305	0.8 4.1 0.7 4.0			

MARCH

Day	Time	m	Day	Time	m
1 F	0540 1201 1806	0.9 3.9 0.9	**16** SA	0520 1126 1756 2357	0.6 4.2 0.7 4.1
2 SA	0026 0646 1245 1850	3.9 0.7 4.1 0.7	**17** SU	0632 1225 1850	0.3 4.5 0.5
3 SU	0105 0714 1319 1925	4.1 0.5 4.3 0.6	**18** M	0045 0722 1309 1935	4.4 0.1 4.7 0.4
4 M	0138 0756 1352 2001	4.3 0.4 4.5 0.5	**19** TU ●	0132 0805 1353 2020	4.6 0.0 4.9 0.3
5 TU O	0206 0825 1418 2036	4.5 0.1 4.7 0.2	**20** W	0213 0850 1435 2100	4.8 -0.1 4.9 0.2
6 W	0236 0900 1449 2108	4.6 0.2 4.8 0.3	**21** TH	0255 0930 1516 2140	4.9 -0.1 4.8 0.2
7 TH	0307 0935 1523 2146	4.7 0.1 4.8 0.3	**22** F	0335 1010 1559 2218	4.9 0.0 4.8 0.3
8 F	0340 1013 1556 2222	4.7 0.1 4.8 0.3	**23** SA	0416 1048 1639 2258	4.8 0.2 4.6 0.3
9 SA	0415 1052 1636 2301	4.8 0.2 4.7 0.4	**24** SU	0457 1119 1719 2335	4.7 0.3 4.4 0.5
10 SU	0450 1126 1713 2336	4.7 0.2 4.6 0.4	**25** M	0538 1158 1800	4.5 0.5 4.2
11 M	0533 1211 1759	4.6 0.3 4.4	**26** TU	0016 0619 1236 1846	0.6 4.2 0.7 3.9
12 TU	0022 0621 1257 1855	0.5 4.4 0.5 4.1	**27** W	0106 0715 1335 1935	0.8 3.9 0.9 3.6
13 W	0118 0730 1356 2012	0.6 4.2 0.6 3.9	**28** TH	0235 0826 1506 2044	0.9 3.6 1.1 3.3
14 TH	0230 0855 1510 2132	0.7 4.0 0.8 3.8	**29** F	0346 0955 1615 2250	0.9 3.5 1.0 3.5
15 F	0356 1016 1635 2256	0.7 4.0 0.8 3.9	**30** SA	0456 1115 1725 2348	0.8 3.8 0.9 3.7
			31 SU	0600 1208 1816	0.7 4.1 0.7

APRIL

Day	Time	m	Day	Time	m
1 M	0030 0645 1245 1856	4.0 0.5 4.3 0.6	**16** TU	0028 0705 1256 1920	4.4 0.1 4.6 0.4
2 TU	0101 0726 1317 1930	4.3 0.4 4.5 0.5	**17** W ●	0112 0748 1336 2000	4.6 0.0 4.8 0.3
3 W	0136 0755 1347 2006	4.5 0.3 4.7 0.4	**18** TH	0155 0827 1416 2040	4.7 0.0 4.8 0.2
4 TH O	0206 0830 1422 2046	4.7 0.1 4.9 0.3	**19** F	0235 0907 1456 2120	4.8 0.0 4.8 0.2
5 F	0238 0908 1458 2122	4.8 0.1 4.9 0.2	**20** SA	0313 0946 1536 2201	4.8 0.1 4.7 0.2
6 SA	0316 0951 1535 2205	4.9 0.1 4.9 0.2	**21** SU	0353 1020 1616 2238	4.8 0.2 4.6 0.3
7 SU	0353 1028 1613 2246	4.9 0.1 4.8 0.2	**22** M	0430 1056 1655 2317	4.6 0.4 4.4 0.4
8 M	0431 1110 1655 2325	4.8 0.2 4.6 0.3	**23** TU	0512 1125 1729 2350	4.4 0.6 4.2 0.5
9 TU	0516 1156 1742	4.7 0.3 4.4	**24** W	0552 1205 1815	4.2 0.7 3.9
10 W	0016 0607 1239 1841	0.3 4.5 0.5 4.1	**25** TH	0023 0640 1256 1906	0.7 3.9 0.9 3.7
11 TH	0109 0715 1346 2000	0.4 4.2 0.7 3.9	**26** F	0156 0745 1414 2005	0.8 3.7 1.0 3.5
12 F	0226 0842 1453 2118	0.5 4.1 0.8 3.8	**27** SA	0306 0853 1535 2136	0.8 3.6 1.0 3.4
13 SA	0346 1000 1625 2235	0.6 4.1 0.8 3.9	**28** SU	0405 1014 1635 2256	0.8 3.7 0.9 3.6
14 SU	0516 1109 1746 2339	0.5 4.3 0.7 4.1	**29** M	0516 1119 1724 2346	0.6 4.0 0.7 3.9
15 M	0615 1207 1835	0.3 4.5 0.5	**30** TU	0554 1208 1816	0.5 4.3 0.6

20

Chart Datum: 2·32 metres below Normaal Amsterdams Peil

TIME ZONE –0100
(Dutch Standard Time)
Subtract 1 hour for UT
For Dutch Summer Time add
ONE hour in non-shaded areas

NETHERLANDS – VLISSINGEN (FLUSHING)

LAT 51°27′N   LONG   3°36′E

TIMES AND HEIGHTS OF HIGH AND LOW WATERS   YEAR **1996**

MAY

Day	Time	m	Day	Time	m
1 W	0021 / 0642 / 1246 / 1856	4.2 / 0.3 / 4.5 / 0.4	16 TH	0056 / 0725 / 1321 / 1940	4.5 / 0.2 / 4.6 / 0.3
2 TH	0057 / 0719 / 1317 / 1938	4.5 / 0.2 / 4.7 / 0.3	17 F ●	0137 / 0803 / 1402 / 2020	4.6 / 0.2 / 4.7 / 0.3
3 F O	0133 / 0802 / 1356 / 2019	4.7 / 0.2 / 4.9 / 0.2	18 SA	0215 / 0839 / 1441 / 2058	4.7 / 0.2 / 4.6 / 0.2
4 SA	0213 / 0843 / 1433 / 2102	4.8 / 0.1 / 4.9 / 0.2	19 SU	0257 / 0918 / 1519 / 2140	4.7 / 0.3 / 4.6 / 0.2
5 SU	0253 / 0926 / 1515 / 2145	4.9 / 0.1 / 4.9 / 0.1	20 M	0335 / 0956 / 1555 / 2221	4.7 / 0.4 / 4.5 / 0.2
6 M	0334 / 1008 / 1556 / 2230	4.9 / 0.1 / 4.8 / 0.1	21 TU	0412 / 1036 / 1635 / 2301	4.6 / 0.5 / 4.4 / 0.3
7 TU	0415 / 1056 / 1642 / 2318	4.8 / 0.2 / 4.6 / 0.1	22 W	0449 / 1105 / 1710 / 2335	4.4 / 0.6 / 4.2 / 0.4
8 W	0503 / 1138 / 1732	4.7 / 0.4 / 4.4	23 TH	0530 / 1140 / 1745	4.2 / 0.7 / 4.1
9 TH	0008 / 0559 / 1230 / 1835	0.2 / 4.5 / 0.5 / 4.2	24 F	0004 / 0616 / 1215 / 1836	0.6 / 4.1 / 0.9 / 3.9
10 F	0105 / 0716 / 1325 / 1948	0.3 / 4.3 / 0.6 / 4.0	25 SA	0045 / 0705 / 1304 / 1930	0.7 / 3.9 / 1.0 / 3.7
11 SA	0216 / 0826 / 1446 / 2101	0.3 / 4.2 / 0.8 / 3.9	26 SU	0221 / 0816 / 1445 / 2036	0.7 / 3.8 / 1.0 / 3.7
12 SU	0330 / 0940 / 1605 / 2209	0.4 / 4.2 / 0.8 / 4.0	27 M	0326 / 0918 / 1545 / 2146	0.7 / 3.9 / 0.9 / 3.7
13 M	0456 / 1049 / 1720 / 2315	0.4 / 4.3 / 0.7 / 4.1	28 TU	0416 / 1025 / 1645 / 2251	0.6 / 4.0 / 0.8 / 3.9
14 TU	0557 / 1148 / 1815	0.3 / 4.4 / 0.5	29 W	0510 / 1120 / 1736 / 2339	0.5 / 4.3 / 0.6 / 4.2
15 W	0009 / 0641 / 1235 / 1900	4.3 / 0.2 / 4.6 / 0.4	30 TH	0600 / 1207 / 1819	0.4 / 4.5 / 0.5
			31 F	0026 / 0645 / 1247 / 1908	4.5 / 0.3 / 4.7 / 0.3

JUNE

Day	Time	m	Day	Time	m
1 SA O	0105 / 0736 / 1330 / 1956	4.7 / 0.2 / 4.8 / 0.2	16 SU ●	0206 / 0818 / 1427 / 2042	4.5 / 0.4 / 4.5 / 0.3
2 SU	0148 / 0821 / 1413 / 2046	4.8 / 0.1 / 4.9 / 0.1	17 M	0245 / 0855 / 1505 / 2119	4.6 / 0.4 / 4.5 / 0.2
3 M	0232 / 0905 / 1457 / 2130	4.9 / 0.2 / 4.8 / 0.1	18 TU	0319 / 0929 / 1539 / 2200	4.6 / 0.5 / 4.5 / 0.2
4 TU	0316 / 0950 / 1543 / 2218	4.9 / 0.2 / 4.7 / 0.1	19 W	0355 / 1008 / 1616 / 2240	4.6 / 0.5 / 4.4 / 0.3
5 W	0403 / 1035 / 1630 / 2310	4.9 / 0.3 / 4.6 / 0.0	20 TH	0428 / 1046 / 1648 / 2315	4.6 / 0.6 / 4.4 / 0.4
6 TH	0453 / 1120 / 1726 / 2359	4.8 / 0.4 / 4.5 / 0.0	21 F	0506 / 1120 / 1726 / 2350	4.4 / 0.7 / 4.2 / 0.5
7 F	0547 / 1216 / 1825	4.6 / 0.5 / 4.4	22 SA	0546 / 1149 / 1759	4.2 / 0.8 / 4.1
8 SA	0056 / 0655 / 1316 / 1928	0.1 / 4.5 / 0.6 / 4.2	23 SU	0025 / 0625 / 1224 / 1846	0.5 / 4.1 / 0.8 / 4.0
9 SU	0155 / 0806 / 1415 / 2032	0.2 / 4.4 / 0.7 / 4.1	24 M	0105 / 0720 / 1314 / 1946	0.6 / 4.0 / 0.9 / 3.9
10 M	0254 / 0916 / 1530 / 2139	0.3 / 4.3 / 0.8 / 4.1	25 TU	0216 / 0826 / 1424 / 2055	0.6 / 4.0 / 0.9 / 3.9
11 TU	0420 / 1019 / 1656 / 2246	0.4 / 4.3 / 0.7 / 4.1	26 W	0316 / 0930 / 1534 / 2156	0.6 / 4.1 / 0.8 / 4.0
12 W	0531 / 1126 / 1750 / 2346	0.4 / 4.3 / 0.6 / 4.2	27 TH	0426 / 1031 / 1645 / 2300	0.5 / 4.2 / 0.7 / 4.2
13 TH	0620 / 1215 / 1840	0.3 / 4.4 / 0.5	28 F	0520 / 1132 / 1745 / 2355	0.4 / 4.4 / 0.5 / 4.4
14 F	0038 / 0702 / 1306 / 1926	4.4 / 0.3 / 4.5 / 0.4	29 SA	0621 / 1223 / 1845	0.3 / 4.6 / 0.4
15 SA	0120 / 0739 / 1345 / 2006	4.4 / 0.4 / 4.5 / 0.3	30 SU	0043 / 0710 / 1309 / 1935	4.6 / 0.3 / 4.7 / 0.2

JULY

Day	Time	m	Day	Time	m
1 M O	0131 / 0758 / 1356 / 2028	4.8 / 0.2 / 4.8 / 0.1	16 TU	0229 / 0832 / 1446 / 2106	4.5 / 0.6 / 4.5 / 0.3
2 TU	0216 / 0846 / 1443 / 2115	4.9 / 0.2 / 4.8 / 0.0	17 W	0301 / 0908 / 1519 / 2140	4.6 / 0.5 / 4.5 / 0.3
3 W	0303 / 0933 / 1528 / 2207	5.0 / 0.3 / 4.8 / 0.0	18 TH	0336 / 0945 / 1552 / 2215	4.6 / 0.5 / 4.6 / 0.3
4 TH	0350 / 1022 / 1616 / 2257	5.0 / 0.4 / 4.8 / –0.1	19 F	0408 / 1020 / 1622 / 2251	4.6 / 0.6 / 4.5 / 0.3
5 F	0438 / 1105 / 1705 / 2345	4.9 / 0.4 / 4.7 / 0.0	20 SA	0437 / 1051 / 1655 / 2326	4.5 / 0.7 / 4.4 / 0.4
6 SA	0536 / 1156 / 1758	4.8 / 0.5 / 4.6	21 SU	0511 / 1126 / 1727 / 2356	4.4 / 0.7 / 4.3 / 0.5
7 SU	0035 / 0635 / 1246 / 1858	0.2 / 4.6 / 0.7 / 4.4	22 M	0546 / 1154 / 1806	4.3 / 0.8 / 4.2
8 M	0125 / 0731 / 1345 / 1958	0.2 / 4.4 / 0.7 / 4.3	23 TU	0036 / 0629 / 1246 / 1856	0.5 / 4.3 / 0.8 / 4.1
9 TU	0225 / 0835 / 1456 / 2105	0.3 / 4.3 / 0.8 / 4.1	24 W	0120 / 0730 / 1336 / 2000	0.5 / 4.2 / 0.8 / 4.0
10 W	0329 / 0950 / 1555 / 2215	0.5 / 4.1 / 0.8 / 4.1	25 TH	0215 / 0846 / 1450 / 2116	0.6 / 4.1 / 0.8 / 4.0
11 TH	0456 / 1057 / 1726 / 2325	0.6 / 4.1 / 0.8 / 4.1	26 F	0335 / 0956 / 1605 / 2225	0.6 / 4.1 / 0.8 / 4.1
12 F	0556 / 1159 / 1814	0.6 / 4.2 / 0.6	27 SA	0445 / 1102 / 1720 / 2327	0.6 / 4.3 / 0.6 / 4.4
13 SA	0021 / 0646 / 1256 / 1906	4.2 / 0.6 / 4.3 / 0.5	28 SU	0556 / 1202 / 1825	0.6 / 4.4 / 0.4
14 SU	0116 / 0722 / 1335 / 1951	4.4 / 0.6 / 4.4 / 0.4	29 M	0025 / 0649 / 1256 / 1926	4.6 / 0.6 / 4.6 / 0.3
15 M ●	0151 / 0758 / 1411 / 2025	4.4 / 0.6 / 4.5 / 0.4	30 TU O	0116 / 0746 / 1342 / 2016	4.8 / 0.3 / 4.8 / 0.1
			31 W	0202 / 0833 / 1426 / 2103	5.0 / 0.3 / 4.9 / 0.0

AUGUST

Day	Time	m	Day	Time	m
1 TH	0247 / 0917 / 1513 / 2149	5.0 / 0.3 / 4.9 / –0.1	16 F	0307 / 0920 / 1522 / 2150	4.7 / 0.5 / 4.7 / 0.3
2 F	0333 / 1002 / 1558 / 2238	4.7 / 0.4 / 4.9 / –0.1	17 SA	0338 / 0956 / 1555 / 2225	4.7 / 0.5 / 4.7 / 0.3
3 SA	0420 / 1046 / 1645 / 2322	5.0 / 0.4 / 4.9 / 0.0	18 SU	0408 / 1031 / 1625 / 2301	4.7 / 0.6 / 4.6 / 0.4
4 SU	0509 / 1132 / 1732	4.8 / 0.5 / 4.7	19 M	0441 / 1106 / 1657 / 2330	4.6 / 0.7 / 4.6 / 0.4
5 M	0005 / 0557 / 1215 / 1820	0.1 / 4.6 / 0.6 / 4.6	20 TU	0515 / 1136 / 1735	4.6 / 0.7 / 4.5
6 TU	0055 / 0655 / 1306 / 1919	0.3 / 4.4 / 0.7 / 4.4	21 W	0006 / 0556 / 1216 / 1815	0.5 / 4.4 / 0.7 / 4.4
7 W	0146 / 0755 / 1405 / 2026	0.5 / 4.2 / 0.8 / 4.1	22 TH	0045 / 0645 / 1306 / 1915	0.6 / 4.3 / 0.8 / 4.2
8 TH	0245 / 0909 / 1514 / 2146	0.7 / 3.9 / 0.9 / 3.9	23 F	0142 / 0759 / 1409 / 2035	0.7 / 4.1 / 0.8 / 4.1
9 F	0416 / 1036 / 1645 / 2259	0.8 / 3.9 / 0.9 / 4.0	24 SA	0300 / 0920 / 1535 / 2156	0.8 / 4.0 / 0.9 / 4.1
10 SA	0526 / 1139 / 1753	0.8 / 4.0 / 0.8	25 SU	0420 / 1035 / 1655 / 2306	0.8 / 4.1 / 0.7 / 4.3
11 SU	0006 / 0620 / 1236 / 1849	4.1 / 0.8 / 4.2 / 0.6	26 M	0536 / 1146 / 1815	0.7 / 4.3 / 0.5
12 M	0058 / 0706 / 1319 / 1929	4.3 / 0.7 / 4.3 / 0.5	27 TU	0007 / 0636 / 1237 / 1910	4.6 / 0.6 / 4.5 / 0.3
13 TU	0138 / 0738 / 1356 / 2006	4.4 / 0.7 / 4.4 / 0.5	28 W O	0059 / 0725 / 1325 / 2000	4.8 / 0.5 / 4.8 / 0.1
14 W ●	0210 / 0809 / 1426 / 2046	4.5 / 0.6 / 4.5 / 0.3	29 TH	0145 / 0813 / 1408 / 2045	5.0 / 0.4 / 4.9 / 0.0
15 TH	0240 / 0841 / 1452 / 2111	4.6 / 0.6 / 4.6 / 0.3	30 F	0229 / 0858 / 1451 / 2130	5.1 / 0.4 / 5.0 / 0.0
			31 SA	0313 / 0942 / 1536 / 2216	5.1 / 0.4 / 5.0 / 0.0

Chart Datum: 2·32 metres below Normaal Amsterdams Peil

TIME ZONE –0100
(Dutch Standard Time)
Subtract 1 hour for UT
For Dutch Summer Time add ONE hour in non-shaded areas

NETHERLANDS – VLISSINGEN (FLUSHING)

LAT 51°27′N   LONG 3°36′E

TIMES AND HEIGHTS OF HIGH AND LOW WATERS   YEAR **1996**

SEPTEMBER

	Time	m		Time	m
1 SU	0358 1023 1619 2256	5.0 0.4 5.0 0.1	**16** M	0343 1005 1556 2230	4.9 0.5 4.8 0.3
2 M	0443 1103 1706 2335	4.8 0.5 4.8 0.3	**17** TU	0415 1035 1633 2306	4.8 0.6 4.8 0.4
3 TU	0529 1146 1750	4.6 0.6 4.6	**18** W	0450 1116 1708 2346	4.7 0.6 4.7 0.5
4 W	0016 0616 1230 1839	0.5 4.4 0.7 4.4	**19** TH	0531 1157 1751	4.5 0.7 4.5
5 TH	0054 0716 1336 1946	0.7 4.1 0.9 4.1	**20** F	0026 0626 1245 1848	0.6 4.3 0.7 4.3
6 F	0200 0820 1446 2054	0.9 3.8 1.0 3.8	**21** SA	0120 0736 1355 2016	0.8 4.0 0.8 4.1
7 SA	0314 1001 1605 2236	1.1 3.6 1.0 3.8	**22** SU	0236 0856 1513 2138	0.9 3.9 0.9 4.1
8 SU	0445 1116 1731 2346	1.0 3.8 0.9 4.0	**23** M	0355 1015 1646 2256	1.0 3.9 0.8 4.3
9 M	0557 1209 1825	0.9 4.1 0.7	**24** TU	0520 1126 1800 2355	0.8 4.2 0.5 4.5
10 TU	0028 0640 1256 1904	4.3 0.8 4.3 0.6	**25** W	0619 1217 1855	0.7 4.5 0.3
11 W	0116 0715 1325 1946	4.4 0.7 4.4 0.5	**26** TH	0042 0710 1305 1942	4.8 0.5 4.7 0.1
12 TH ●	0141 0745 1355 2016	4.5 0.7 4.5 0.4	**27** F ○	0126 0748 1348 2025	5.0 0.4 4.9 0.1
13 F	0209 0818 1426 2046	4.7 0.6 4.7 0.4	**28** SA	0210 0838 1430 2106	5.0 0.4 5.0 0.1
14 SA	0237 0852 1452 2121	4.8 0.5 4.8 0.3	**29** SU	0253 0920 1513 2148	5.0 0.4 5.0 0.1
15 SU	0308 0926 1525 2156	4.9 0.5 4.8 0.3	**30** M	0335 1002 1555 2228	5.0 0.4 5.0 0.3

OCTOBER

	Time	m		Time	m
1 TU	0416 1039 1635 2306	4.8 0.5 4.8 0.5	**16** W	0353 1021 1609 2246	4.9 0.5 4.9 0.4
2 W	0501 1120 1719 2346	4.6 0.6 4.6 0.7	**17** TH	0431 1100 1651 2326	4.7 0.5 4.8 0.6
3 TH	0546 1206 1805	4.3 0.7 4.4	**18** F	0515 1145 1737	4.6 0.6 4.6
4 F	0014 0629 1244 1855	0.9 4.0 0.8 4.0	**19** SA	0011 0608 1236 1835	0.7 4.3 0.7 4.3
5 SA	0125 0726 1416 2010	1.1 3.8 1.0 3.8	**20** SU	0106 0715 1346 1954	0.9 4.0 0.8 4.1
6 SU	0245 0839 1526 2145	1.2 3.5 1.1 3.7	**21** M	0216 0838 1506 2115	1.0 3.9 0.8 4.1
7 M	0406 1036 1635 2306	1.2 3.6 1.0 3.9	**22** TU	0333 0955 1630 2231	1.0 3.9 0.7 4.3
8 TU	0505 1132 1745 2356	1.1 3.9 0.8 4.1	**23** W	0505 1101 1742 2335	0.9 4.1 0.5 4.5
9 W	0559 1215 1836	0.9 4.1 0.7	**24** TH	0605 1159 1838	0.8 4.4 0.3
10 TH	0036 0646 1252 1910	4.4 0.8 4.3 0.6	**25** F	0027 0656 1246 1925	4.7 0.6 4.6 0.2
11 F	0108 0715 1322 1939	4.6 0.7 4.5 0.5	**26** SA ○	0109 0736 1326 2003	4.8 0.5 4.8 0.2
12 SA ●	0138 0747 1352 2015	4.7 0.6 4.7 0.4	**27** SU	0153 0817 1410 2045	4.9 0.4 4.9 0.2
13 SU	0207 0822 1422 2048	4.9 0.5 4.8 0.4	**28** M	0235 0858 1452 2123	4.9 0.4 5.0 0.3
14 M	0240 0900 1456 2126	5.0 0.5 4.9 0.3	**29** TU	0316 0940 1533 2202	4.8 0.4 4.9 0.5
15 TU	0316 0940 1533 2206	4.9 0.5 4.9 0.4	**30** W	0357 1018 1615 2236	4.7 0.5 4.8 0.6
			31 TH	0435 1101 1656 2316	4.5 0.6 4.6 0.8

NOVEMBER

	Time	m		Time	m
1 F	0516 1135 1735 2344	4.3 0.7 4.4 0.9	**16** SA	0505 1135 1725 2356	4.6 0.4 4.7 0.7
2 SA	0555 1225 1825	4.1 0.8 4.1	**17** SU	0557 1236 1829	4.3 0.5 4.4
3 SU	0029 0646 1325 1926	1.1 3.9 1.0 3.8	**18** M	0056 0706 1336 1945	0.8 4.1 0.6 4.3
4 M	0156 0746 1445 2036	1.3 3.6 1.0 3.7	**19** TU	0155 0816 1450 2058	1.0 4.0 0.6 4.2
5 TU	0315 0906 1546 2206	1.3 3.5 1.0 3.7	**20** W	0316 0925 1606 2210	1.0 4.0 0.6 4.3
6 W	0416 1036 1644 2311	1.2 3.7 0.9 4.0	**21** TH	0435 1038 1720 2310	1.0 4.1 0.6 4.4
7 TH	0505 1131 1746 2356	1.0 3.9 0.8 4.3	**22** F	0546 1138 1816	0.9 4.3 0.4
8 F	0559 1208 1830	0.9 4.2 0.6	**23** SA	0007 0636 1225 1906	4.5 0.7 4.5 0.4
9 SA	0030 0640 1246 1906	4.5 0.7 4.5 0.5	**24** SU	0055 0718 1310 1942	4.7 0.6 4.6 0.3
10 SU	0105 0716 1318 1940	4.7 0.6 4.7 0.4	**25** M ○	0137 0758 1355 2022	4.7 0.5 4.7 0.4
11 M ●	0140 0756 1353 2020	4.9 0.5 4.9 0.3	**26** TU	0221 0840 1436 2100	4.7 0.4 4.8 0.4
12 TU	0216 0835 1433 2100	4.9 0.4 5.0 0.3	**27** W	0302 0922 1515 2135	4.7 0.4 4.8 0.5
13 W	0255 0920 1513 2142	4.9 0.4 5.0 0.4	**28** TH	0337 0959 1555 2212	4.6 0.4 4.7 0.6
14 TH	0336 1006 1553 2226	4.8 0.4 4.9 0.4	**29** F	0417 1039 1637 2251	4.5 0.4 4.6 0.8
15 F	0416 1050 1636 2311	4.7 0.4 4.8 0.6	**30** SA	0455 1115 1715 2325	4.4 0.5 4.4 0.9

DECEMBER

	Time	m		Time	m
1 SU	0536 1206 1756 2354	4.2 0.7 4.2 1.0	**16** M	0545 1226 1815	4.5 0.3 4.6
2 M	0615 1234 1846	4.0 0.8 4.0	**17** TU	0035 0646 1320 1921	0.7 4.3 0.4 4.4
3 TU	0034 0701 1334 1939	1.1 3.9 0.9 3.9	**18** W	0135 0749 1414 2032	0.8 4.2 0.5 4.3
4 W	0200 0806 1450 2045	1.2 3.7 1.0 3.8	**19** TH	0235 0858 1530 2140	1.0 4.1 0.6 4.2
5 TH	0325 0912 1550 2156	1.2 3.7 0.9 3.9	**20** F	0355 1008 1645 2247	1.0 4.1 0.6 4.2
6 F	0420 1026 1645 2300	1.1 3.8 0.8 4.1	**21** SA	0516 1115 1756 2349	0.9 4.2 0.6 4.3
7 SA	0515 1120 1746 2346	0.9 4.1 0.7 4.4	**22** SU	0615 1208 1840	0.8 4.3 0.5
8 SU	0600 1207 1826	0.8 4.4 0.5	**23** M	0041 0705 1258 1926	4.4 0.6 4.5 0.5
9 M	0031 0645 1247 1916	4.6 0.6 4.6 0.5	**24** TU ○	0129 0746 1345 1959	4.5 0.5 4.6 0.5
10 TU	0112 0729 1331 1955	4.8 0.5 4.8 0.4	**25** W	0208 0826 1425 2038	4.6 0.4 4.6 0.5
11 W	0155 0818 1411 2038	4.9 0.4 4.9 0.3	**26** TH	0247 0905 1502 2115	4.6 0.4 4.7 0.6
12 TH	0236 0906 1455 2125	4.9 0.3 4.9 0.4	**27** F	0325 0941 1538 2149	4.6 0.3 4.7 0.6
13 F	0318 0955 1538 2210	4.8 0.2 5.0 0.4	**28** SA	0359 1022 1616 2225	4.6 0.4 4.6 0.7
14 SA	0405 1039 1626 2256	4.8 0.2 4.9 0.5	**29** SU	0432 1100 1652 2305	4.5 0.4 4.5 0.8
15 SU	0456 1129 1716 2345	4.6 0.2 4.8 0.6	**30** M	0506 1135 1725 2329	4.4 0.4 4.3 0.8
			31 TU	0545 1206 1806	4.2 0.6 4.2

Chart Datum: 2·32 metres below Normaal Amsterdams Peil

20

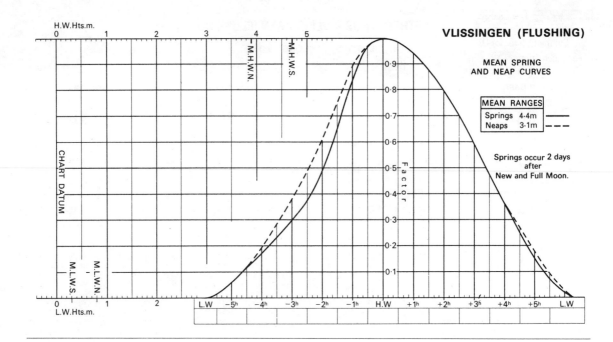

VLISSINGEN (FLUSHING)

MEAN SPRING
AND NEAP CURVES

MEAN RANGES	
Springs	4·4m
Neaps	3·1m

Springs occur 2 days
after
New and Full Moon.

OOSTERSCHELDE   10-20-18

Zeeland 51°37'·30N 03°40'·20E (Roompotsluis)

CHARTS

AC 192, 120, 110; Zeekaart 1448; DYCs 1805, 1801; Imray C30; Stanfords 19

TIDES

+0230 Dover Zone −0100; ML Sas van Goes 2·0, Zierikzee 1·8; Duration Sas van Goes 0615, Zierikzee 0640

Standard Port VLISSINGEN (⟵)

Times				Height (metres)	
High Water		Low Water		MHW	MLW
0300	0900	0400	1000		
1500	2100	1600	2200		
Time Differences				**Actual heights**	
ROOMPOTSLUIS (outside)					
+0002	+0002	−0004	−0004	4·1	1·2
ROOMPOTSLUIS (inside)					
+0119	+0119	+0101	+0101	3·9	1·4
WEMELDINGE					
+0133	+0133	+0110	+0110	4·2	1·1
KRAMMER LOCKS					
+0135	+0135	+0105	+0105	4·2	1·2
BERGSEDIEP LOCK					
+0133	+0133	+0113	+0113	4·3	1·1

SHELTER

Good shelter in many hbrs at any tide; see facing page. Veerse Meer is a non-tidal waterway with moorings; enter from Oosterschelde via Zandkreekdam lock. The Schelde-Rijn Canal can be entered at Bergsediepsluis near Tholen; and the S Beveland Canal at Wemeldinge.

NAVIGATION

WPT WG1 SHM buoy, QG, 51°38'·05N 03°26'·30E at ent to Westgat/Oude Roompot buoyed chan. There are several offshore banks, see 10.20.5. Not advised to enter in strong W/NW'lies, and only from HW −6 to HW +1½ Zierikzee. All vessels must use the Roompotsluis (lock). The areas each side of the barrier are very dangerous due to strong tidal streams and many obstructions. Passage is prohib W of Roggenplaat. Zeelandbrug has 12·2m clearance at centre of arch in buoyed chans. Clearance (m) is indicated on some of bridge supports. If wind < F 7, bascule bridge near N end lifts at H & H+30, Mon-Fri 0700-2130; Sat/Sun from 0900.

LIGHTS AND MARKS

See 10.20.4. Roompotsluis ldg lts 073·5° both Oc G 5s; Ent: N side FR, S side FG; depth 5m.

RADIO TELEPHONE

VHF-fitted craft must monitor Ch 68 in the Oosterschelde. Ch 68 broadcast local forecasts at H+15. *Verkeerspost Wemeldinge* Ch 68 MUST be called if entering canal; also for radar guidance in poor vis. Call *Zeelandbrug* Ch 18 for opening times and clearance. Locks: *Roompotsluis* Ch 18. *Krammersluizen* Ch 22 (H24). Zandreek *Sluis Kats* Ch 18; *Sluis Grevelingen* Ch 20; Bergse Diepsluis Ch 18.

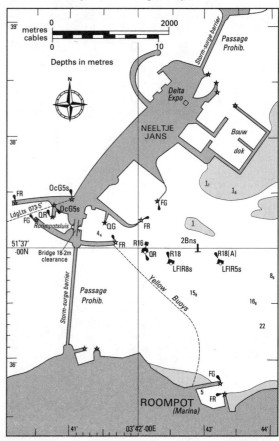

HARBOURS AND FACILITIES

The following are some of the more important of the many hbrs (anti-clockwise from the Roompotsluis):

ROOMPOT MARINA: (150 + 80 visitors) ☎ (0113) 374225, f30.75, AC, D, P, Slip, FW, Gas, Gaz, Ⓞ, R, V, Bar, Ⓑ, Dr ☎ 372565.

COLIJNSPLAAT: Hr Mr ☎ (0113) 695762; **YC WV Noord Beveland** f19.50, AC, Slip, FW, Ⓞ; secure at first floating jetty and report arrival by loudspeaker or at hbr office; beware strong current across hbr ent; **Services:** P, D, BH (40 ton), ME, SM, Sh. **Town** Dr ☎ 695304, V, R, Bar, Gaz, ✉, Ⓑ, ⇌ (Goes), ✈ (Rotterdam).

KATS: Hr Mr ☎ (0113) 600270; **Rest Nautic BV** f13.50, AC, ME, BH (35 ton), FW, SM, Ⓞ; uncomfortable in strong E winds.

SAS VAN GOES: Lock ☎ (0113) 216744, VHF Ch 18; opens Mon-Fri 0600-2200, Sat/Sun 0800-2100. **Jachthaven Het Goese Sas** ☎ 223944, f16.60, AC, FW, D, ME, Slip, BH (12 ton), Ⓞ.

GOES: The canal to Goes starts at Sas van Goes (lock); no facilities at Wilhelminadorp; bridge operates same hrs as lock. Outskirts of Goes: **YC WV De Werf** ☎ (0113) 216372, f16.95, AC, FW, C (3½ ton), P, D; **Marina Stadshaven** in centre: ☎ 216136, f16.95, AC, FW; **Services:** ME, El, Sh, Ⓞ, Gaz, Dr ☎ 227451, Ⓗ ☎ 227000. **Town** V, R, ✉, Ⓑ, ⇌, ✈ (Antwerpen).

WEMELDINGE: Hr Mr ☎ (0113) 622093. Yachts transit the Kanaal door Zuid Beveland via a new section 1km E of the town. Use the former ent (via R/G tfc lts) to berth at the municipal yacht hbrs in the Voorhaven or Binnenhaven; in the former a larger marina is planned. SHM buoy O21 to N of the E mole marks a shoal. **Services:** ME, SM, AC, C (6·5 ton) ME, FW, P, D, Dr ☎ 6227451, Ⓗ ☎ 6227000. **Town** V, R, ✉, Ⓑ, ⇌, ✈ (Antwerpen).

YERSEKE: Leave to port the preferred chan buoy at hbr ent. The two marinas are S of the outer FV hbr. Hr Mr Ch 09; **Prinsess Beatrix Haven** ☎ (0113) 571726, f20.70, 1·6m, FW, D, BH (10 ton); **Services:** SM, Sh, El, Dr ☎ 571444. **Town** V, R, ✉, Ⓑ, ⇌ (Kruiningen), ✈.

STAVENISSE: Hr Mr ☎ (0166) 692815; **Marina** at end of hbr canal (only 1m at LW), f11.80, Slip, FW; **Services:** P & D (cans), Sh, C (4·5 ton), Dr ☎ 692400. **Town** V, Gaz.

ST ANNALAND: **WV St Annaland** Hr Mr ☎ (0166) 652783, (office on YC ship "Buutengaets"), f13.50, AC, FW; **YC** ☎ 652634, Ⓞ, Bar, R; **Services:** ME, A, D, Sh, El, CH, BH (25 ton), Gaz, BY, Dr ☎ 652400. **Town** Gaz, V, R, Ⓑ, ✉, ⇌ (Bergen op Zoom), ✈ (Antwerpen).

BRUINISSE: through lock (Ch 20) to Grevelingenmeer: **WV 'Bru'** Hr Mr ☎ 481506, f15.30, FW; **Jachthaven Bruinisse** Hr Mr ☎ 481485, f18.00, FW, AC, Slip, P, D, Ⓞ, Gaz, Bar, V; **Services:** ME, Sh, C (16 ton). MHW = NAP + 1.53m; Dr ☎ 481280. **Town** ✉, Ⓑ, ✈ (Rotterdam).

ZIJPE: **Vluchthaven**, berth in SW corner; free for 3 days, but yacht must not be left unattended.

ZIERIKZEE: Hr Mr ☎ (0111) 413174; **Haven 't Luitje** and **Nieuwe Haven: WV Zierikzee** Hr Mr ☎ 414877, f17.10, FW, AC; Note: For yachts >15m LOA pre-arrange berth with Hr Mr, Jun-Aug; **Services:** P, D, Gaz, C (18 ton), ME, Sh, SM, CH. **Town** Dr 412080, Ⓗ 416900, Ⓞ, V, R, ✉, Ⓑ, ✈ (Rotterdam).

BURGHSLUIS: Hr Mr ☎ (0111) 651302; **Jachthaven** f13.85, FW, AC, C (6 ton), ME. Facilities at Burg-Haamstede P, D, Gaz, ✉, Ⓑ, ⇌, ✈ (Rotterdam).

NEELTJE JANS: Delta Expo worth visiting; AB available.

TOWNS ON THE VEERSE MEER (non-tidal). Free mooring at many of the islands; normal dues at towns below:

KORTGENE: Hr Mr and **Delta Marina** ☎ (0113) 301315 f20.25, P, D, FW, AC, CH, El, Ⓞ, ME, R, Sh, SM, V, C (16 ton). **Town** Dr ☎ 301319, V, R, Bar, Ⓑ, ⇌ (Goes), ✈ (Rotterdam).

WOLPHAARTSDIJK: WV Wolphaartsdijk (WVW) Hr Mr ☎ (0113) 581565, f12.05, P & D, C (20 ton); & **Royal YC Belgique (RYCB)** ☎ 581496, f10.25, P & D; **Services:** Sh.

DE PIET: Haven has 72m of pontoons for small craft; there are 4 other little havens around De Omloop. No charges.

ARNEMUIDEN: Jachthaven Oranjeplaat Hr Mr ☎ (0118) 501248, f13.20, Slip, P & D, C (12 ton).

VEERE: Yacht berths at: **Jachtclub Veere** in the Stadshaven, very busy, ☎ (0118) 501246, f15.20, FW, AC; **Marina Veere** on the canal side, ☎ 501553, f19.70, FW, AC; **Jachtwerf Oostwatering**, ☎ 501665, f15.20, FW, AC, Ⓞ; **WV Arne**, at Oostwatering – report at ⓥ jetty, ☎ 501484/501929, f12.50, FW, AC. **Town** Dr ☎ 501271, V, R, Bar, ✉, Ⓑ, ⇌ (Middelburg), ✈ (Rotterdam).

MIDDELBURG: (This town is about 3M S of Veere on the Walcheren canal to Vlissingen). No mooring in Kanaal door Walcheren. All bridges & Veere lock: Ch 22. **WV Arne** in the Dockhaven, ☎ (0118) 627180, f14.70, FW, AC, ME, El, Gaz, CH, BY, AC, Sh, Slip. **Services:** D, Gaz, CH, BY, AC, Sh, Slip. **Town** Dr ☎ 612637; Ⓗ ☎ 625555; V, R, Bar, ✉, Ⓑ, ⇌, ✈ (Rotterdam).

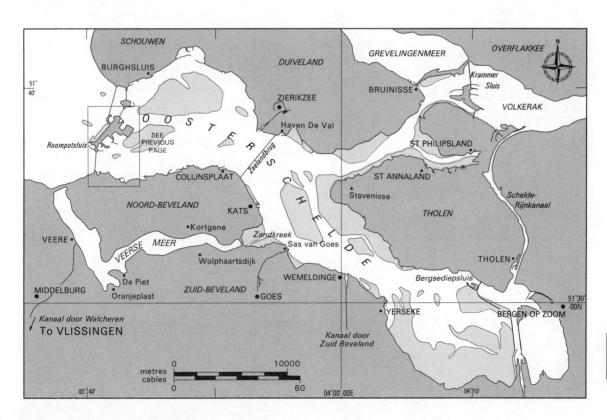

STELLENDAM & HELLEVOETSLUIS

Zuid Holland 50°49'·88N 04°02'·10E

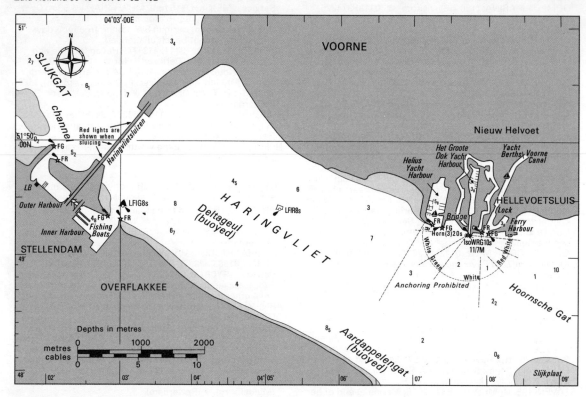

CHARTS
AC 2322; Zeekaart 1447, 1448; DYC 1801.5, 1807.6; Imray C30; Stanfords 19

TIDES
+0300 Dover; ML 1·2; Duration 0510; Zone −0100

Standard Port VLISSINGEN (←)

Times				Height (metres)			
High Water		Low Water		MHWS	MHWN	MLWN	MLWS
0300	0900	0400	1000	4·7	3·9	0·8	0·3
1500	2100	1600	2200				
Differences HARINGVLIETSLUIZEN							
+0015	+0015	+0015	−0020	−1·7	−1·6	−0·4	0·0

NOTE: Double LWs occur. The rise after the 1st LW is called the Agger. Water levels on this coast are much affected by weather. Prolonged NW gales can raise levels by up to 3m.

SHELTER
No shelter at Stellendam for yachts in the outer hbr; the marina is now closed. Once through the lock, shelter in FV hbr just beyond lock or go 3M to Hellevoetsluis for one of the 3 yacht hbrs: Heliushaven (1·9-5m); via lifting bridge into Het Groote Dok (2-4m); and via lock into the Voorne canal (2·8-4·8m).
In the Haringvliet there are about 6 large pontoons (vlot on the DYC) equipped for barbecue picnics; but they are prone to wash and only useable in calm conditions. Within 10M upstream of Hellevoetsluis there are good yacht facilities on the S bank at Middelharnis, Stad aan't Haringvliet and Den Bommel; on the N bank at YC De Put (Vuile Gat) and Hitsertse Kade. If bound for Rotterdam, proceed via Spui or Dordrecht.

NAVIGATION
WPT Slijkgat SG SWM buoy, Iso 4s, 51°52'·00N 03°51'·50E, 290°/110° from/to Kwade Hoek lt, 5·0M. From the N, the Gat van de Hawk chan to Stellendam lock is no longer buoyed and is dangerous due to long-term WIP south of Maasvlakte. It is therefore best to take the well buoyed/lit Slijkgat chan along the Goeree shore, but it is dangerous to enter Slijkgat in strong W/NW winds.
Beware a shoal about 5ca from the lock, marked by SHM buoys. Keep clear of dam during sluicing.

Lock and lifting bridge operate:
Mon-Thurs   H24.   Fri   0000-2200LT
Sat, Sun, Hols 0800-2000LT
Note: Going from Haringvliet to sea, last locking is about ½hr before the final lock times above.
Within the Haringvliet the 3M leg to Hellevoetsluis is well marked by 10 PHM buoys (DG2 to DG18 and HV2); only DG16 is lit as on chartlet. The SW side of the Haringvliet has 6 SHM buoys (DG1-11) leading to the well buoyed, but unlit Aardappelengat chan (S of Slijkplaat) and the ent to Middelharnis.

LIGHTS AND MARKS
Haringvlietsluizen sluicing sigs: 3 Ⓡ in △, shown from pier heads on dam; danger area marked by small Y buoys. Hellevoetsluis lt Iso 10s 16m 11/7M, W stone tr, R cupola. G shore-275°, W275°-294°, R294°-316°, W316°-036°, G036°-058°, W058°-095°, R096°-shore.

RADIO TELEPHONE
Call: Goereese Sluis VHF Ch 20.

TELEPHONE (0187)
Hr Mr Stellendam 491000, Hellevoetsluis 4930911;
⌗ Rotterdam (010) 4298088 or Vlissingen (0118) 484600;
Police 492444; Dr 491425, Dr Hellevoetsluis 4912435;
Brit Consul (020) 6764343.

FACILITIES
STELLENDAM
Inner Hbr free AB or alongside FVs.
Town V, R, Bar, ✉ (2½ km), ✈ (Rotterdam).
HELLEVOETSLUIS
Marina, Het Groote Dok ☎ 4912166, f18.25, bridge lifts every H in daylight from 0800 summertime; waiting pontoons are downstream. El, Gaz, FW, ME, CH;
Helius Haven YC ☎ 4915868, AB, P, D, FW;
Voorne Canal YC ☎ 4915476, AB, P, D, FW;
Services: CH, El, ME.
Town P, D, V, R, Bar, ✉, Ⓑ, ✈ (Rotterdam).
Ferry: Hook of Holland-Harwich; or Rotterdam-Hull.

TIME ZONE –0100
(Dutch Standard Time)
Subtract 1 hour for UT

For Dutch Summer Time add
ONE hour in non-shaded areas

NETHERLANDS – HOEK VAN HOLLAND

LAT 51°59'N   LONG 4°07'E

TIMES AND HEIGHTS OF HIGH AND LOW WATERS

YEAR **1996**

JANUARY

Date	Time	m	Time	m	Time	m	Time	m
1 M	0645	0.4	1129	1.8	1715	0.3		
2 TU	0004	1.9	0820	0.4	1224	1.9	1804	0.3
3 W	0053	1.9	0926	0.3	1314	1.9	1854	0.3
4 TH	0148	2.0	0954	0.3	1353	2.0	1950	0.4
5 F	0223	2.0	0755	0.3	1434	2.0	○ 2025	0.4
6 SA	0304	2.0	0824	0.2	1508	2.1	2117	0.4
7 SU	0335	2.0	0854	0.2	1537	2.2	2240	0.4
8 M	0405	2.0	0925	0.2	1615	2.2	2325	0.4
9 TU	0434	2.0	0953	0.2	1648	2.2		
10 W	0014	0.4	0509	2.0	1036	0.2	1717	2.1
11 TH	0115	0.4	0534	1.9	1110	0.1	1754	2.1
12 F	0155	0.4	0614	1.9	1144	0.1	1835	2.1
13 SA	0220	0.4	0654	1.9	1234	0.1	1924	2.0
14 SU	0205	0.4	0805	1.8	1355	0.1	2032	2.0
15 M	0244	0.4	0915	1.8	1500	0.1	2155	1.9
16 TU	0350	0.4	1024	1.8	1605	0.2	2254	1.9
17 W	0455	0.4	1129	1.9	1716	0.2		
18 TH	0005	2.0	0545	0.3	1229	2.0	1804	0.3
19 F	0058	2.0	0636	0.2	1321	2.2	1855	0.3
20 SA	0147	2.1	0716	0.2	1406	2.3	● 1935	0.3
21 SU	0234	2.1	0755	0.1	1454	2.3	2019	0.4
22 M	0321	2.1	0840	0.1	1538	2.4		
23 TU	0006	0.4	0406	2.1	0921	0.0	1624	2.3
24 W	0044	0.4	0454	2.1	1009	0.0	1711	2.3
25 TH	0155	0.4	0537	2.1	1105	0.0	1757	2.2
26 F	0235	0.4	0624	2.0	1206	0.0	1855	2.1
27 SA	0104	0.4	0718	2.0	1310	0.1	1954	1.9
28 SU	0145	0.4	0814	1.9	1414	0.1	2105	1.8
29 M	0254	0.4	0923	1.8	1534	0.2	2224	1.7
30 TU	0420	0.3	1055	1.7	1644	0.3	2345	1.7
31 W	0513	0.3	1158	1.8	1745	0.3		

FEBRUARY

Date	Time	m	Time	m	Time	m	Time	m
1 TH	0044	1.8	0615	0.3	1259	1.8	1845	0.3
2 F	0134	1.8	0934	0.2	1345	1.9	2147	0.4
3 SA	0219	1.9	1025	0.2	1413	2.0	2014	0.3
4 SU	0242	1.9	0805	0.2	1444	2.1	○ 2057	0.4
5 M	0307	2.0	0824	0.2	1518	2.1	2220	0.4
6 TU	0345	2.0	0855	0.1	1550	2.2	2314	0.3
7 W	0410	2.1	0925	0.1	1624	2.2		
8 TH	0016	0.3	0445	2.0	0959	0.1	1656	2.2
9 F	0056	0.3	0514	2.0	1035	0.1	1734	2.1
10 SA	0124	0.3	0547	2.0	1116	0.1	1810	2.1
11 SU	0155	0.3	0631	2.0	1159	0.0	1857	2.0
12 M	0019	0.3	0713	1.9	1305	0.1	1954	1.9
13 TU	0225	0.3	0829	1.9	1434	0.1	2115	1.8
14 W	0314	0.3	0949	1.8	1545	0.2	2229	1.8
15 TH	0415	0.3	1107	1.9	1654	0.3	2344	1.8
16 F	0525	0.2	1208	2.0	2046	0.3		
17 SA	0044	1.8	0609	0.2	1304	2.1	2135	0.3
18 SU	0137	1.9	0656	0.1	1354	2.2	● 2204	0.3
19 M	0224	2.0	0738	0.0	1438	2.3	2256	0.4
20 TU	0306	2.1	0818	0.0	1521	2.3	2346	0.4
21 W	0350	2.1	0906	0.0	1606	2.3		
22 TH	0036	0.3	0431	2.1	0945	0.0	1650	2.2
23 F	0126	0.3	0514	2.1	1406	0.0	1735	2.1
24 SA	0216	0.3	0514	2.1	1124	0.1	1825	2.0
25 SU	0010	0.3	0640	2.0	1235	0.1	1908	1.9
26 M	0114	0.3	0735	1.9	1350	0.1	2009	1.7
27 TU	0215	0.2	0834	1.8	1507	0.2	2114	1.6
28 W	0406	0.2	0953	1.6	1635	0.3	2315	1.5
29 TH	0506	0.2	1128	1.7	1725	0.3		

MARCH

Date	Time	m	Time	m	Time	m	Time	m
1 F	0014	1.6	0555	0.2	1223	1.8	1840	0.3
2 SA	0103	1.7	0639	0.2	1314	1.9	2117	0.3
3 SU	0154	1.8	0955	0.2	1355	1.9	2155	0.3
4 M	0224	1.8	1015	0.2	1420	2.0	2245	0.3
5 TU	0244	1.9	0755	0.2	1450	2.1	2228	0.3
6 W	0314	2.0	0826	0.1	1524	2.2	2304	0.3
7 TH	0344	2.1	0858	0.1	1556	2.2	2344	0.2
8 F	0416	2.1	0932	0.1	1631	2.2		
9 SA	0035	0.2	0449	2.1	1010	0.0	1708	2.2
10 SU	0115	0.2	0526	2.1	1049	0.0	1751	2.1
11 M	0115	0.2	0608	2.1	1139	0.0	1834	2.0
12 TU	0001	0.2	0657	2.0	1255	0.1	1935	1.8
13 W	0150	0.2	0804	1.9	1424	0.1	2054	1.7
14 TH	0245	0.2	0936	1.8	1535	0.2	2203	1.6
15 F	0355	0.2	1043	1.8	1634	0.3	2323	1.6
16 SA	0459	0.2	1159	1.9	2017	0.2		
17 SU	0030	1.7	0856	0.1	1255	2.0	2105	0.3
18 M	0124	1.8	0635	0.1	1336	2.1	2144	0.3
19 TU	0206	1.9	0718	0.0	1421	2.2	● 2225	0.3
20 W	0246	2.0	0800	0.0	1504	2.2	2305	0.3
21 TH	0326	2.1	0839	0.0	1545	2.2		
22 F	0006	0.2	0408	2.1	1235	0.0	1626	2.1
23 SA	0101	0.2	0447	2.1	1336	0.1	1707	2.1
24 SU	0146	0.2	0528	2.1	1415	0.1	1755	1.9
25 M	0226	0.2	0615	2.0	1236	0.2	1835	1.8
26 TU	0034	0.2	0654	1.9	1328	0.2	1925	1.7
27 W	0140	0.2	0805	1.8	1450	0.2	2018	1.5
28 TH	0340	0.2	0915	1.6	1610	0.3	2134	1.4
29 F	0446	0.1	1044	1.6	1704	0.3	2339	1.5
30 SA	0524	0.1	1205	1.7	1805	0.3		
31 SU	0023	1.6	0614	0.1	1245	1.8	2045	0.2

APRIL

Date	Time	m	Time	m	Time	m	Time	m
1 M	0103	1.7	0900	0.2	1313	1.9	2135	0.2
2 TU	0145	1.8	0956	0.1	1348	2.0	2226	0.2
3 W	0208	2.0	0725	0.1	1420	2.1	2250	0.2
4 TH	0240	2.0	0800	0.1	1454	2.2	○ 2300	0.2
5 F	0315	2.1	0829	0.1	1531	2.2	2346	0.2
6 SA	0349	2.1	1608	2.2				
7 SU	0020	0.2	0428	2.1	0946	0.1	1648	2.1
8 M	0106	0.2	0506	2.1	1029	0.1	1730	2.0
9 TU	0135	0.2	0547	2.1	1130	0.1	1818	1.9
10 W	0105	0.1	0641	2.0	1334	0.1	1919	1.7
11 TH	0135	0.1	0742	1.9	1414	0.2	2045	1.6
12 F	0224	0.1	0919	1.8	1525	0.3	2205	1.5
13 SA	0335	0.1	1039	1.8	1845	0.3	2325	1.6
14 SU	0440	0.1	1145	1.9	2004	0.2		
15 M	0019	1.7	0835	0.1	1234	2.0	2100	0.2
16 TU	0104	1.8	0914	0.1	1324	2.1	2124	0.3
17 W	0144	1.9	0659	0.0	1405	2.1	● 2155	0.3
18 TH	0228	2.0	0739	0.0	1446	2.1	2256	0.2
19 F	0308	2.1	0826	0.1	1526	2.1	2340	0.2
20 SA	0348	2.1	1155	0.1	1607	2.0		
21 SU	0036	0.1	0426	2.1	1305	0.1	1648	2.0
22 M	0116	0.1	0507	2.1	1346	0.2	1724	1.9
23 TU	0156	0.1	0544	2.0	1327	0.2	1805	1.8
24 W	0010	0.1	0624	1.9	1327	0.2	1844	1.7
25 TH	0054	0.1	0713	1.8	1418	0.3	1944	1.6
26 F	0307	0.1	0824	1.7	1545	0.3	2043	1.5
27 SA	0415	0.1	0939	1.6	1640	0.3	2158	1.4
28 SU	0455	0.1	1053	1.7	1735	0.2	2334	1.5
29 M	0554	0.1	1154	1.8	1950	0.2		
30 TU	0025	1.6	0816	0.1	1239	1.9	2106	0.2

20

Chart Datum: 0·84 metres below Normaal Amsterdams Peil

TIME ZONE –0100
(Dutch Standard Time)
Subtract 1 hour for UT
For Dutch Summer Time add ONE hour in non-shaded areas

NETHERLANDS – HOEK VAN HOLLAND

LAT 51°59′N   LONG   4°07′E

TIMES AND HEIGHTS OF HIGH AND LOW WATERS   YEAR 1996

MAY

Day	Time	m	Day	Time	m
1 W	0053 / 0916 / 1314 / 2150	1.8 / 0.1 / 2.0 / 0.1	16 TH	0128 / 0644 / 1347 / 2137	1.9 / 0.1 / 2.0 / 0.3
2 TH	0135 / 0655 / 1348 / 2230	1.9 / 0.1 / 2.1 / 0.2	17 F	0210 / 0725 / 1430 / ● 1955	2.0 / 0.1 / 2.0 / 0.2
3 F O	0208 / 0736 / 1426 / 2254	2.0 / 0.1 / 2.2 / 0.2	18 SA	0247 / 0814 / 1509 / 2325	2.0 / 0.2 / 2.0 / 0.2
4 SA	0246 / 0805 / 1506 / 2029	2.1 / 0.1 / 2.2 / 0.2	19 SU	0327 / 1107 / 1554	2.1 / 0.2 / 2.0
5 SU	0325 / 0845 / 1548 / 2110	2.2 / 0.1 / 2.1 / 0.1	20 M	0005 / 0404 / 1220 / 1634	0.1 / 2.1 / 0.2 / 1.9
6 M	0406 / 0930 / 1632 / 2149	2.2 / 0.1 / 2.1 / 0.1	21 TU	0055 / 0445 / 1257 / 1709	0.0 / 2.1 / 0.2 / 1.9
7 TU	0450 / 1245 / 1714 / 2239	2.2 / 0.2 / 1.9 / 0.1	22 W	0125 / 0520 / 1317 / 1745	0.0 / 2.0 / 0.3 / 1.8
8 W	0534 / 1320 / 1807 / 2345	2.1 / 0.2 / 1.8 / 0.0	23 TH	0135 / 0605 / 1340 / 1819	0.1 / 1.9 / 0.3 / 1.7
9 TH	0628 / 1335 / 1903	2.1 / 0.2 / 1.7	24 F	0030 / 0644 / 1410 / 1904	0.1 / 1.8 / 0.3 / 1.6
10 F	0054 / 0733 / 1420 / 2029	0.0 / 1.9 / 0.2 / 1.6	25 SA	0104 / 0744 / 1515 / 2014	0.1 / 1.8 / 0.3 / 1.6
11 SA	0210 / 0853 / 1715 / 2139	0.0 / 1.9 / 0.3 / 1.6	26 SU	0205 / 0849 / 1604 / 2115	0.1 / 1.7 / 0.3 / 1.5
12 SU	0305 / 1019 / 1825 / 2255	0.0 / 1.9 / 0.2 / 1.6	27 M	0446 / 0954 / 1655 / 2214	0.1 / 1.8 / 0.3 / 1.6
13 M	0701 / 1125 / 1955 / 2354	0.0 / 1.9 / 0.2 / 1.7	28 TU	0530 / 1052 / 1757 / 2325	0.1 / 1.8 / 0.2 / 1.6
14 TU	0755 / 1218 / 2045	0.0 / 2.0 / 0.2	29 W	0617 / 1143 / 2026	0.2 / 1.9 / 0.2
15 W	0044 / 0905 / 1305 / 2120	1.8 / 0.1 / 2.0 / 0.2	30 TH	0015 / 0835 / 1237 / 2115	1.8 / 0.1 / 2.0 / 0.2
			31 F	0058 / 0630 / 1318 / 2206	1.9 / 0.1 / 2.1 / 0.2

JUNE

Day	Time	m	Day	Time	m
1 SA O	0144 / 0705 / 1401 / 1935	2.0 / 0.1 / 2.2 / 0.2	16 SU ●	0234 / 0820 / 1504 / 2024	2.0 / 0.3 / 2.0 / 0.1
2 SU	0224 / 0750 / 1444 / 2009	2.1 / 0.1 / 2.1 / 0.1	17 M	0314 / 0940 / 1538 / 2105	2.0 / 0.3 / 1.9 / 0.1
3 M	0305 / 0829 / 1530 / 2055	2.2 / 0.2 / 2.1 / 0.1	18 TU	0347 / 1058 / 1614	2.1 / 0.3 / 1.9
4 TU	0350 / 0916 / 1616 / 2136	2.2 / 0.2 / 2.0 / 0.1	19 W	0014 / 0424 / 1208 / 1648	0.1 / 2.1 / 0.3 / 1.9
5 W	0434 / 1247 / 1704 / 2225	2.2 / 0.3 / 1.9 / 0.0	20 TH	0044 / 0500 / 1250 / 1725	0.1 / 2.0 / 0.3 / 1.8
6 TH	0521 / 1325 / 1757 / 2325	2.1 / 0.3 / 1.9 / 0.0	21 F	0125 / 0533 / 1315 / 1754	0.1 / 2.0 / 0.3 / 1.8
7 F	0615 / 1430 / 1852	2.1 / 0.3 / 1.8	22 SA	0205 / 0615 / 1404 / 1828	0.1 / 1.9 / 0.3 / 1.7
8 SA	0034 / 0724 / 1545 / 2015	0.0 / 2.0 / 0.3 / 1.7	23 SU	0025 / 0655 / 1437 / 1913	0.1 / 1.9 / 0.3 / 1.7
9 SU	0145 / 0839 / 1644 / 2115	-0.1 / 2.0 / 0.3 / 1.7	24 M	0125 / 0754 / 1516 / 2034	0.1 / 1.9 / 0.3 / 1.7
10 M	0244 / 0944 / 1800 / 2225	0.0 / 1.9 / 0.3 / 1.7	25 TU	0215 / 0905 / 1620 / 2135	0.1 / 1.9 / 0.3 / 1.7
11 TU	0355 / 1059 / 1904 / 2324	0.1 / 1.9 / 0.3 / 1.8	26 W	0309 / 1005 / 1725 / 2237	0.1 / 1.9 / 0.3 / 1.7
12 W	0715 / 1159 / 2020	0.1 / 1.9 / 0.2	27 TH	0415 / 1104 / 1810 / 2335	0.1 / 1.9 / 0.3 / 1.8
13 TH	0025 / 0544 / 1243 / 2104	1.8 / 0.2 / 2.0 / 0.2	28 F	0514 / 1205 / 1754	0.2 / 2.0 / 0.2
14 F	0108 / 0645 / 1338 / 1904	1.9 / 0.2 / 2.0 / 0.2	29 SA	0029 / 0605 / 1255 / 2135	1.9 / 0.2 / 2.1 / 0.2
15 SA	0154 / 0724 / 1425 / 1943	2.0 / 0.2 / 2.0 / 0.2	30 SU	0117 / 0656 / 1340 / 1911	2.1 / 0.2 / 2.1 / 0.2

JULY

Day	Time	m	Day	Time	m
1 M O	0205 / 0731 / 1428 / 1951	2.2 / 0.2 / 2.1 / 0.1	16 TU	0253 / 0854 / 1522 / 2035	2.0 / 0.4 / 1.9 / 0.1
2 TU	0248 / 0816 / 1515 / 2031	2.2 / 0.3 / 2.1 / 0.1	17 W	0330 / 1010 / 1553 / 2115	2.1 / 0.4 / 2.0 / 0.1
3 W	0334 / 1155 / 1559 / 2118	2.3 / 0.4 / 2.0 / 0.0	18 TH	0405 / 1130 / 1629 / 2145	2.1 / 0.4 / 2.0 / 0.1
4 TH	0418 / 1245 / 1646 / 2208	2.3 / 0.4 / 2.0 / 0.0	19 F	0438 / 1224 / 1658	2.1 / 0.3 / 1.9
5 F	0508 / 1325 / 1738 / 2254	2.3 / 0.4 / 1.9 / 0.0	20 SA	0054 / 0515 / 1304 / 1728	0.1 / 2.1 / 0.3 / 1.9
6 SA	0557 / 1424 / 1827 / 2359	2.2 / 0.3 / 1.9 / 0.0	21 SU	0140 / 0544 / 1356 / 1758	0.1 / 2.0 / 0.3 / 1.9
7 SU	0654 / 1530 / 1923	2.1 / 0.3 / 1.9	22 M	0216 / 0618 / 1415 / 1834	0.1 / 2.0 / 0.4 / 1.8
8 M	0109 / 0758 / 1420 / 2035	0.0 / 2.0 / 0.4 / 1.8	23 TU	0015 / 0658 / 1428 / 1924	0.1 / 2.0 / 0.4 / 1.8
9 TU	0214 / 0903 / 1504 / 2145	0.0 / 1.9 / 0.3 / 1.8	24 W	0135 / 0753 / 1434 / 2039	0.1 / 1.9 / 0.3 / 1.8
10 W	0324 / 1035 / 1614 / 2254	0.1 / 1.9 / 0.3 / 1.8	25 TH	0235 / 0925 / 1524 / 2155	0.1 / 1.9 / 0.3 / 1.8
11 TH	0434 / 1134 / 1705 / 2358	0.2 / 1.9 / 0.3 / 1.9	26 F	0334 / 1025 / 1625 / 2305	0.2 / 1.9 / 0.3 / 1.9
12 F	0534 / 1234 / 2050	0.2 / 1.9 / 0.3	27 SA	0444 / 1135 / 1724	0.2 / 1.9 / 0.3
13 SA	0055 / 0624 / 1328 / 2134	1.9 / 0.3 / 1.9 / 0.2	28 SU	0005 / 0544 / 1235 / 1805	2.0 / 0.3 / 2.0 / 0.2
14 SU	0145 / 0715 / 1412 / 1946	1.9 / 0.3 / 1.9 / 0.2	29 M	0057 / 0640 / 1324 / 1851	2.1 / 0.3 / 2.0 / 0.2
15 M ●	0224 / 0810 / 1453 / 2015	2.0 / 0.4 / 1.9 / 0.2	30 TU O	0147 / 0719 / 1411 / 1935	2.2 / 0.3 / 2.1 / 0.1
			31 W	0231 / 0755 / 1458 / 2015	2.3 / 0.4 / 2.1 / 0.0

AUGUST

Day	Time	m	Day	Time	m
1 TH	0315 / 1146 / 1542 / 2058	2.3 / 0.4 / 2.1 / 0.0	16 F	0344 / 1057 / 1604 / 2109	2.2 / 0.4 / 2.1 / 0.2
2 F	0402 / 1236 / 1628 / 2146	2.3 / 0.4 / 2.1 / 0.0	17 SA	0415 / 1154 / 1627 / 2145	2.2 / 0.4 / 2.1 / 0.2
3 SA	0445 / 1326 / 1714 / 2236	2.3 / 0.4 / 2.1 / 0.0	18 SU	0445 / 1246 / 1705 / 2215	2.2 / 0.4 / 2.0 / 0.2
4 SU	0536 / 1404 / 1804 / 2329	2.2 / 0.4 / 2.0 / 0.1	19 M	0515 / 1314 / 1730 / 2256	2.2 / 0.4 / 2.0 / 0.2
5 M	0627 / 1455 / 1855	2.1 / 0.4 / 2.0	20 TU	0547 / 1400 / 1807 / 2336	2.1 / 0.4 / 2.0 / 0.1
6 TU	0040 / 0725 / 1340 / 1955	0.1 / 2.0 / 0.4 / 1.9	21 W	0630 / 1144 / 1854	2.1 / 0.4 / 2.0
7 W	0155 / 0829 / 1434 / 2105	0.1 / 1.9 / 0.3 / 1.8	22 TH	0024 / 0724 / 1350 / 1949	0.1 / 2.0 / 0.4 / 1.9
8 TH	0304 / 0934 / 1544 / 2213	0.2 / 1.8 / 0.3 / 1.8	23 F	0215 / 0845 / 1444 / 2114	0.2 / 1.9 / 0.3 / 1.9
9 F	0420 / 1115 / 1654 / 2332	0.3 / 1.7 / 0.3 / 1.8	24 SA	0326 / 0955 / 1554 / 2235	0.3 / 1.8 / 0.3 / 1.9
10 SA	0524 / 1214 / 1755	0.3 / 1.8 / 0.3	25 SU	0424 / 1104 / 1654 / 2344	0.3 / 1.8 / 0.3 / 2.0
11 SU	0034 / 0624 / 1315 / 2131	1.9 / 0.4 / 1.9 / 0.2	26 M	0535 / 1214 / 1755	0.3 / 1.9 / 0.2
12 M	0128 / 0950 / 1358 / 2210	2.0 / 0.4 / 1.9 / 0.2	27 TU	0040 / 0916 / 1308 / 1835	2.1 / 0.4 / 2.0 / 0.2
13 TU	0203 / 1020 / 1434 / 1955	2.0 / 0.4 / 1.9 / 0.2	28 W O	0128 / 0945 / 1356 / 1911	2.2 / 0.4 / 2.0 / 0.1
14 W ●	0233 / 0830 / 1504 / 2014	2.1 / 0.5 / 2.0 / 0.2	29 TH	0214 / 1024 / 1441 / 1956	2.3 / 0.5 / 2.1 / 0.1
15 TH	0304 / 0917 / 1528 / 2039	2.1 / 0.5 / 2.0 / 0.2	30 F	0255 / 0818 / 1524 / 2035	2.4 / 0.5 / 2.2 / 0.1
			31 SA	0342 / 1215 / 1606 / 2119	2.4 / 0.5 / 2.2 / 0.1

Chart Datum: 0·84 metres below Normaal Amsterdams Peil

TIME ZONE –0100
(Dutch Standard Time)
Subtract 1 hour for UT
For Dutch Summer Time add ONE hour in non-shaded areas

NETHERLANDS – HOEK VAN HOLLAND

LAT 51°59′N   LONG 4°07′E

TIMES AND HEIGHTS OF HIGH AND LOW WATERS

YEAR **1996**

SEPTEMBER

Day		Time	m	Time	m	Time	m	Time	m
1	SU	0426	2.3	1306	0.4	1650	2.2	2205	0.1
16	M	0414	2.3	1215	0.4	1631	2.2	2150	0.2
2	M	0515	2.2	1356	0.4	1735	2.2	2254	0.2
17	TU	0450	2.2	1255	0.4	1709	2.1	2226	0.2
3	TU	0554	2.1	1435	0.4	1818	2.1	2355	0.2
18	W	0526	2.2	1045	0.4	1744	2.2	2305	0.2
4	W	0649	2.0	1250	0.4	1914	2.0		
19	TH	0606	2.1	1125	0.3	1824	2.1	2354	0.3
5	TH	0115	0.3	0745	1.9	1345	0.4	2015	1.9
20	F	0659	2.0	1224	0.3	1925	2.0		
6	F	0240	0.3	0854	1.7	1530	0.3	2145	1.8
21	SA	0200	0.3	0804	1.8	1414	0.3	2044	1.9
7	SA	0355	0.4	1039	1.6	1640	0.3	2315	1.8
22	SU	0254	0.4	0923	1.7	1535	0.3	2215	1.9
8	SU	0504	0.4	1155	1.7	1725	0.3		
23	M	0404	0.4	1043	1.7	1630	0.3	2324	2.0
9	M	0014	1.9	0605	0.4	1248	1.8	1826	0.3
24	TU	0747	0.4	1158	1.8	2025	0.3		
10	TU	0109	2.0	0907	0.4	1345	1.9	2145	0.3
25	W	0024	2.1	0844	0.4	1254	1.9	1809	0.2
11	W	0138	2.1	0954	0.4	1408	1.9	2220	0.4
26	TH	0114	2.2	0924	0.4	1337	2.0	1851	0.1
12	TH ●	0207	2.1	1027	0.4	1434	2.0	1949	0.3
27	F O	0155	2.3	0954	0.5	1419	2.1	1936	0.1
13	F	0237	2.2	0814	0.5	1453	2.1	2009	0.2
28	SA	0240	2.4	0755	0.5	1505	2.2	2015	0.1
14	SA	0314	2.3	1040	0.5	1528	2.1	2045	0.2
29	SU	0324	2.3	0835	0.5	1545	2.3	2100	0.2
15	SU	0344	2.3	1114	0.4	1600	2.2	2116	0.2
30	M	0404	2.3	1236	0.4	1626	2.3	2145	0.3

OCTOBER

Day		Time	m	Time	m	Time	m	Time	m
1	TU	0446	2.2	1326	0.4	1706	2.2	2206	0.3
16	W	0429	2.3	0945	0.4	1646	2.3	2206	0.3
2	W	0155	0.3	0530	2.1	1416	0.4	1747	2.1
17	TH	0506	2.2	1025	0.3	1726	2.3	2255	0.3
3	TH	0235	0.4	0614	2.0	1155	0.4	1839	2.1
18	F	0550	2.1	1116	0.3	1811	2.2	2344	0.4
4	F	0100	0.4	0715	1.8	1310	0.3	1923	1.9
19	SA	0637	1.9	1214	0.3	1904	2.1		
5	SA	0200	0.4	0805	1.7	1504	0.3	2044	1.8
20	SU	0145	0.4	0755	1.8	1345	0.3	2023	1.9
6	SU	0334	0.5	0913	1.6	1604	0.3	2223	1.7
21	M	0250	0.5	0915	1.7	1506	0.3	2205	1.9
7	M	0435	0.5	1124	1.6	1716	0.3	2345	1.8
22	TU	0605	0.5	1035	1.7	1554	0.3	2309	2.0
8	TU	0544	0.5	1214	1.7	1754	0.3		
23	W	0740	0.4	1144	1.8	2006	0.2		
9	W	0035	2.0	0824	0.4	1259	1.8	1835	0.3
24	TH	0009	2.1	0846	0.4	1234	1.9	2055	0.3
10	TH	0109	2.1	0914	0.4	1328	1.9	2124	0.3
25	F	0054	2.2	0915	0.4	1317	2.0	1831	0.2
11	F	0145	2.1	0954	0.4	1354	2.0	1915	0.3
26	SA O	0137	2.3	0935	0.5	1401	2.2	1916	0.3
12	SA ●	0208	2.2	0739	0.4	1424	2.1	1946	0.3
27	SU	0221	2.3	1039	0.4	1444	2.2	1959	0.3
13	SU	0238	2.3	0809	0.4	1458	2.2	2015	0.2
28	M	0304	2.3	0819	0.4	1525	2.3	2045	0.3
14	M	0315	2.3	0840	0.4	1535	2.2	2050	0.2
29	TU	0346	2.2	1215	0.3	1604	2.3	2125	0.4
15	TU	0352	2.3	0904	0.4	1606	2.3	2126	0.3
30	W	0430	2.1	1015	0.2	1645	2.2		
31	TH	0125	0.4	0514	2.0	1340	0.3	1727	2.2

NOVEMBER

Day		Time	m	Time	m	Time	m	Time	m
1	F	0200	0.5	0548	2.0	1130	0.3	1808	2.1
16	SA	0536	2.0	1106	0.2	1758	2.2		
2	SA	0040	0.5	0635	1.9	1224	0.3	1853	2.0
17	SU	0130	0.4	0627	1.9	1244	0.2	1854	2.1
3	SU	0127	0.5	0725	1.8	1314	0.3	1958	1.8
18	M	0147	0.5	0733	1.8	1324	0.2	2025	2.0
4	M	0300	0.5	0824	1.6	1545	0.3	2103	1.7
19	TU	0224	0.5	0854	1.8	1435	0.2	2135	2.0
5	TU	0415	0.5	0928	1.6	1634	0.3	2234	1.8
20	W	0545	0.5	1009	1.7	1546	0.3	2244	2.0
6	W	0514	0.5	1113	1.6	1735	0.3	2354	1.9
21	TH	0707	0.5	1114	1.8	1924	0.2	2344	2.1
7	TH	0724	0.5	1215	1.7	1830	0.3		
22	F	0805	0.4	1210	1.9	2035	0.2		
8	F	0029	2.0	0846	0.4	1244	1.9	2035	0.3
23	SA	0034	2.1	0900	0.4	1300	2.0	1819	0.3
9	SA	0105	2.1	0936	0.4	1313	2.0	2146	0.3
24	SU	0121	2.2	0649	0.5	1344	2.1	1905	0.3
10	SU	0135	2.2	1004	0.4	1355	2.1	1915	0.3
25	M O	0207	2.2	0729	0.4	1426	2.2	1956	0.3
11	M ●	0207	2.3	0746	0.4	1427	2.2	1949	0.3
26	TU	0254	2.2	0809	0.3	1507	2.2	2040	0.4
12	TU	0248	2.3	0815	0.4	1507	2.3	2025	0.3
27	W	0335	2.1	0845	0.3	1547	2.3	2115	0.4
13	W	0326	2.3	0850	0.3	1545	2.3	2105	0.3
28	TH	0414	2.1	1236	0.3	1626	2.2		
14	TH	0411	2.2	0925	0.3	1629	2.3	2156	0.4
29	F	0055	0.4	0455	2.0	1315	0.2	1704	2.2
15	F	0451	2.1	1015	0.2	1712	2.3	2245	0.4
30	SA	0056	0.5	0524	2.0	1055	0.2	1744	2.1

DECEMBER

Day		Time	m	Time	m	Time	m	Time	m
1	SU	0050	0.5	0604	1.9	1144	0.2	1829	2.0
16	M	0140	0.5	0617	2.0	1144	0.1	1844	2.2
2	M	0120	0.5	0649	1.8	1244	0.2	1925	1.9
17	TU	0206	0.5	0725	1.9	1254	0.1	1955	2.1
3	TU	0200	0.5	0734	1.7	1334	0.3	2014	1.8
18	W	0204	0.5	0829	1.8	1405	0.1	2105	2.0
4	W	0330	0.5	0845	1.7	1604	0.3	2135	1.8
19	TH	0305	0.5	0934	1.8	1505	0.2	2214	2.0
5	TH	0425	0.5	0943	1.7	1655	0.3	2228	1.9
20	F	0640	0.5	1044	1.8	1620	0.2	2325	2.0
6	F	0535	0.5	1059	1.7	1800	0.3	2323	1.9
21	SA	0750	0.4	1143	1.9	2000	0.3		
7	SA	0657	0.4	1155	1.8	2005	0.3		
22	SU	0025	2.0	0856	0.4	1240	2.0	1815	0.3
8	SU	0013	2.1	0855	0.4	1245	2.0	1819	0.3
23	M	0110	2.0	0935	0.4	1330	2.0	1905	0.3
9	M	0105	2.2	0946	0.3	1321	2.1	1855	0.3
24	TU O	0157	2.0	0725	0.3	1414	2.1	1945	0.4
10	TU ●	0144	2.2	0714	0.3	1405	2.2	1935	0.3
25	W	0244	2.1	0816	0.3	1455	2.2	2034	0.4
11	W	0226	2.2	0755	0.3	1446	2.3	2015	0.3
26	TH	0323	2.1	0845	0.2	1535	2.2	2147	0.4
12	TH	0310	2.2	0832	0.2	1528	2.4	2055	0.4
27	F	0405	2.1	0915	0.2	1615	2.2	2338	0.4
13	F	0354	2.2	0916	0.2	1615	2.4	2135	0.4
28	SA	0439	2.0	0954	0.2	1649	2.2		
14	SA	0437	2.1	0955	0.1	1659	2.3		
29	SU	0028	0.4	0508	2.0	1035	0.2	1725	2.1
15	SU	0054	0.4	0524	2.0	1049	0.1	1746	2.3
30	M	0100	0.4	0544	1.9	1120	0.2	1753	2.0
31	TU	0130	0.5	0612	1.9	1205	0.2	1834	2.0

20

Chart Datum: 0·84 metres below Normaal Amsterdams Peil

HOEK VAN HOLLAND   10-20-20
(HOOK OF HOLLAND)

Zuid Holland 51°59'·50N 04°02'·78E (Ent)

CHARTS
AC 132, 122; Zeekaart 1540, 1349, 1350, 1449; DYC 1809, 1801; Imray C30, Y5; Stanfords 19

TIDES
+0251 Dover; ML 0·9; Duration 0505; Zone –0100.
HOEK VAN HOLLAND is a Standard Port; predictions for every day of the year are given above. Double LWs occur, more obviously at sp; in effect a LW stand. Predictions are for the *lower* LW. The 1st LW is about 5½ hrs after HW and the 2nd LW about 4¼ hrs before the next HW. The slight rise after the first LW is called the Agger. Water levels on this coast are much affected by the weather. Prolonged NW gales can raise the levels by up to 3m.

SHELTER
Ent safe except in strong on-shore winds when heavy seas/swell develop. Berghaven hbr is closed to yachts; better shelter at Maassluis (3m), 6M up river (km 1019).

NAVIGATION
WPTs From S: MV-N NCM lt By, Q, 51°59'·65N 04°00'·30E, 288°/108° from/to Nieuwe Zuiderdam lt, 1·5M. From N: Indusbank NCM lt By, Q, 52°02'·93N 04°03'·72E, 010°/190° from/to Nieuwe Noorderdam lt, 3·2M. There are no real navigational dangers but it is a very busy waterway with a constant stream of ocean-going and local ships. Keep clear of ships manoeuvering whilst transferring pilots.

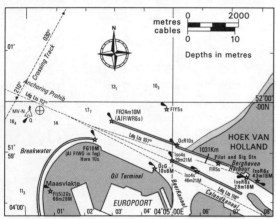

Crossing the Entrance: To cross the Maasgeul (seaward of the bkwtrs), yachts should call *Maas Ent* Ch 03, with position and course, and keep watch on Ch 03. Cross under power on a track, 030°/210°, close W of line joining buoys MV (51°57'·50N 03°58'·50E), MV-N (51°59'·65N 04°00'·30E) and Indusbank N (52°02'·93N 04°03'·72E). Beware the strong tidal set across the ent.
Rules for Yachts (in Nieuwe Waterweg): Comply with VTS (see R/T). Keep to stbd bank, not too close due to sunken debris. No tacking/beating; no ⚓. Eng ready for instant start. Able to motor at 3.24kn (6km/hr). Hoist a radar reflector, esp in poor vis or at night. Cross chan quickly at 90°. Docks, inc the Calandkanaal/Beerkanaal (Europoort), are prohib to yachts, except for access to a marina.

LIGHTS AND MARKS
Maasvlakte Fl (5) 20s 66m 28M; B 8-sided tr, Or bands; vis 340°-267° (H24).
Nieuwe Noorderdam, hd FR 24m 10M; Or tr, B bands, helipad; in fog Al Fl WR 6s.
Nieuwe Zuiderdam, hd FG 24m 10M; Or tr, B bands, helipad; in fog Al Fl WG 6s; Horn 10s.
Ldg lts 107° (for Nieuwe Waterweg): Both Iso R 6s 29/43m 18M; R trs, W bands; vis 100°-114° (H24); synch.
Traffic Sigs from Pilot/Sig Stn, which has RDF bn HH 288, (N side of Nieuwe Waterweg, close W of Berghaven):
Ⓡ Ⓡ Ⓡ
Ⓦ   =   No entry to, or exit from, Maas Estuary
Ⓡ Ⓡ Ⓡ
Nieuwe Waterweg:
Ⓡ Ⓡ   Ⓡ Ⓡ
Ⓦ   =   No entry.   Ⓦ   =   No exit
Ⓡ Ⓡ   Ⓡ Ⓡ
Patrol vessels show a Fl Bu lt. If such vessels show a Fl R lt, it means 'Stop'.

RADIO TELEPHONE
The Hook-Rotterdam VTS (H24) covers from approx 38M W of the Hook to central Rotterdam; see Fig 10 (6).
3 main **Traffic Centres**, each on Ch 13, with their radar sub-sectors (*italics*) on a dedicated VHF Ch, are as follows:
(1)   **Traffic Centre Hoek van Holland (VCH)**
Maas Approach Ch 01, (Outer apps, from 38M W of Hook);
Pilot Maas Ch 02, (from approx 11M in to 4M W of Hook);
Maas Ent Ch 03, (from 4M inward to km 1031);
Waterweg Ch 65, (Nieuwe Waterweg to km 1023);
(2)   **Traffic Centre Botlek (VCB)**
Maassluis Ch 80, (km 1023 to km 1017);
Botlek Ch 61, (km 1017 to km 1011);
(3)   **Traffic Centre Stad (VCS)**
Eemhaven Ch 63, (km 1011 to km 1007);
Waalhaven Ch 60, (km 1007 to km 1003);
Note: Hartel and Maasboulevard Tfc Centres, and their radar sectors, have been omitted because yachts would not often enter their areas. The Hbr Coordination Centre (HCC) administers Rotterdam port on Ch 11.
Yachts should **first report** to *Maas Approach* or *Pilot Maas* (or to *Maas Ent* if using the ITZ), stating name/type of vessel, position & destination; then obey instructions, listening on the appropriate VHF Ch's as shown by W □ signboards on the river banks. (Km signs are similar).
Info broadcasts (weather, vis, tfc and tidal) by Traffic Centres and radar stns on request.
Other stations: Oude Maas Ch 62; Spijkenisserbrug and Botlekbrug Ch 18; Brienenoordbrug Ch 20; Bridge at Alblasserdam Ch 22; Dordrecht Ch 10, 13, 19 (H24).

TELEPHONE (010)
Port Authority (HCC) 4251400; Pilot (Hook) 4251422; Police 4141414; Ⓗ Rotterdam 4112800; Brit Consul (020) 6764343.

FACILITIES
Maassluis ☎ 5912277, AB, CH, El, FW.
Services: BY, ME, Sh.
Town P, D, V, R, Bar, ✉, Ⓑ, ⇌, ✈ (Rotterdam).
Ferry: Hook-Harwich; Rotterdam Europoort-Hull.

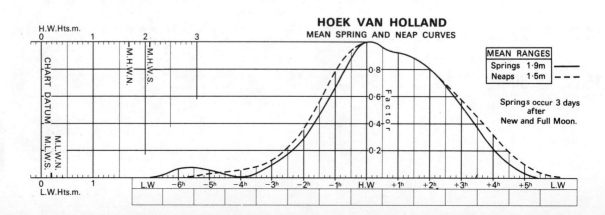

HOEK VAN HOLLAND
MEAN SPRING AND NEAP CURVES

MEAN RANGES	
Springs	1·9m
Neaps	1·5m

Springs occur 3 days after New and Full Moon.

ROTTERDAM 10-20-21

Zuid Holland 51°54'·00N 04°28'·00E

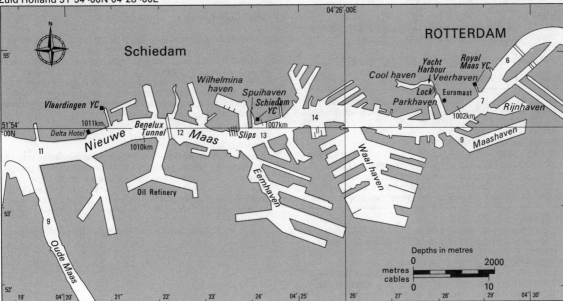

CHARTS
AC 133, 132, 122; Zeekaart 1540/1/2; DYC 1809; Stanfords 19

TIDES
+0414 Dover; ML 0·9; Duration 0440; Zone −0100

Standard Port VLISSINGEN (←—)

Times				Height (metres)			
High Water		Low Water		MHWS	MHWN	MLWN	MLWS
0300	0900	0400	1000	4·7	3·9	0·8	0·3
1500	2100	1600	2200				
Differences MAASSLUIS							
+0125	+0100	+0110	+0255	−2·7	−2·2	−0·5	0·0
VLAARDINGEN							
+0150	+0125	+0135	+0320	−2·7	−2·2	−0·5	0·0

NOTE 1: Maasluis and Vlaardingen are both referenced to Vlissingen, as shown above, in British Admiralty Tables. The Dutch *Guide to the Netherlands and Belgian coasts* (HP11) shows the following time differences relative to HW and the first LW at Hoek van Holland:

	HW	LW
Maasluis	+0113	+0038
Vlaardingen and Schiedam	+0114	+0112
Rotterdam	+0123	+0352

These figures, plus the tidal curves, take account of local river conditions. The Dutch Tables (HP33) do not include Secondary Port differences; in effect all the major ports, including Rotterdam, are regarded as Standard Ports and full daily predictions are published.
NOTE 2: Double LWs occur. The rise after the first LW is called the Agger. See 10.20.20.

SHELTER
Good in the yacht hbrs, but in the river there is always a considerable sea and swell due to constant heavy traffic; Europoort/Rotterdam is the world's largest port complex. All but local yachts are discouraged from using the Nieuwe Maas.

NAVIGATION
See 10.20.20. There are no navigational dangers other than the amount of heavy sea-going traffic. Berghaven to Rotterdam is about 19M. 7M before the centre of Rotterdam, the Oude Maas joins (km 1013); same rules apply as in 10.20.20. Min speed 3.24kn (6km/hr).
Note: Special regulations apply to yachts in the Rhine. These are given in a French booklet *Service de la Navigation du Rhin* obtainable from 25 Rue de la Nuée Bleu, 6700 Strasbourg.

LIGHTS AND MARKS
Marks to locate Yacht Havens:
(1) Ent to Vlaardingen YC (2·7m) is on N bank by Delta Hotel, between km posts 1010-1011.
(2) 2M on, just above the ent to Wilhelmina Haven is the Spuihaven (1·8-2·3m); N bank by km 1007.
(3) Parkhaven and the lock into Coolhaven Yacht Hbr are clearly identified on the N bank by the huge Euromast in the park (km 1002·5).
(4) The Royal Maas YC at the Veerhaven (3·3m), a centre for traditional yachts, is on the N bank (km 1001·5).

RADIO TELEPHONE
The VTS Ch's for central Rotterdam are 63, 60, 81 and 21; see 10.20.20. Call HCC Ch 11 for emergencies. English is official second language.

TELEPHONE (010)
Hbr Coordination Centre (HCC) 4251400, also Emergency; ⊞ 4298088; Police 4141414; Ⓗ 4112800; Brit Consul (020) 6764343.

FACILITIES
Vlaardingen YC (Oude Haven via lock/bridge), M, BY, ME, SM, FW, P, D, Gaz; **Hr Mr** ☎ 4346786.
Schiedam YC (Spuihaven) ☎ 4267765, D, L, FW, ME, El, Sh, CH, AB;
Coolhaven Yacht Hbr ☎ 4738614, Slip, M, P, D, L, FW, ME, El, Sh, C, CH, AB, V, R, Bar;
Royal Maas YC ☎ 4137681, D, L, FW, ME, El, SH, CH, AB;
YC IJsselmonde ☎ 482833, AB (1·2-1·8m), AC, FW; on S bank at km 994, opposite the Hollandsche IJssel fork (off chartlet).
Services: P, D, ME; Gaz, ACA, DYC Agent.
City all facilities, ⊠, Ⓑ, ⇌, ✈, Ferry: Rotterdam - Hull, also Hook-Harwich.

20

SCHEVENINGEN 10-20-22

Zuid Holland 52°06'·28N 04°15'·35E

CHARTS
AC 122, 2322; Zeekaart 1035, 1349, 1350, 1449; DYC 1801;
ANWB H/J; Imray Y5; Stanfords 19

TIDES
+0320 Dover; ML 0·9; Duration 0445; Zone −0100

Standard Port VLISSINGEN (←—)

Times				Height (metres)			
High Water		Low Water		MHWS	MHWN	MLWN	MLWS
0300	0900	0400	1000	4·7	3·9	0·8	0·3
1500	2100	1600	2200				
Differences SCHEVENINGEN							
+0105	+0100	+0220	+0245	−2·5	−2·1	−0·5	−0·1

NOTE: Double LWs occur. The rise after the 1st LW is called
the Agger. Water levels on this coast can be much affected
by the weather. Prolonged NW gales can raise levels by up
to 3m, whilst strong E winds can lower levels by 1m.

SHELTER
Good, but ent can be difficult in on-shore NW winds >F6.
The yacht marina in the Second Hbr gives very good
shelter. Access H24.

NAVIGATION
WPT SCH (SWM) buoy, Iso 4s, 52°07'·80N 04°14'·20E,
336°/156° from/to ent, 1·6M. Strong tidal streams running
NE/SW across the ent can cause problems. Strong winds
from SW to N cause a scend in the outer hbr. Beware
large ships entering and leaving.

LIGHTS AND MARKS
Outer ldg lts, Iso 4s, 156°; Inner Oc G 5s 131°.
Tfc signals (from Semaphore Mast):
Ⓡ over Ⓦ = Entry prohib. Ⓦ over Ⓡ = Exit prohib.
Fl Ⓨ = entry difficult due to vessels leaving.
Q Ⓨ is shown by ent to First Hbr (W side) when vessels
are entering or leaving port.
Tide signals:
Ⓖ over Ⓦ = tide rising. Ⓦ over Ⓖ = tide falling.
Ⓡ = less than 5m in entry chan.

RADIO TELEPHONE
Call: *Scheveningen Haven* VHF Ch 14 (H24) prior to entry/
dep to de-conflict from ferries. Radar Ch 21.

TELEPHONE (070)
Hr Mr 3527701; Marina Hr Mr 3520017; Traffic Centre
3527721; ✚ 3514481; Police 3104911; Dr 3455300;
Ambulance 3222111; Brit Consul (020) 6764343.

FACILITIES
YC Scheveningen (223 + 100 visitors) ☎ 3520017, AC,
Bar, C (15 ton), CH, D, El, FW, ME, R, ▣, Sh, SM; **Club-
house** ☎ 3520308; **Hbr** Slip, FW, ME, Sh, C (60 ton), CH,
R, Bar; **Services:** ME, El, Sh, CH, SM, DYC Agent.
Town P, D, V, R, Bar, ✉, Ⓑ, ⇌, ✈ Rotterdam/Amsterdam.
Ferry: See Rotterdam or Hook.

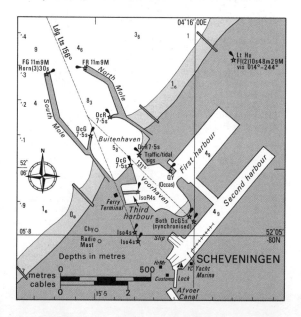

Depths in metres

SCHEVENINGEN

Small Craft Cookery

The art of successful cookery in the confined space of a
yacht's galley depends more on the native ingenuity of the
operator than on any hard and fast rules and recipes. It must
be kept as simple as possible, yet there must be plenty of
variety, or the crew will be perpetually hankering after the
fleshpots of the shore; the preparation of the food should not
need much time, and it should be either cooked quickly or not
need attention during the process.

The basic methods of cooking are outlined, and a few
skeleton (sic) recipes given which can be adapted to the
materials available.

Elaborate schedules of quantity are useless when one has
neither scales nor measures. All that can be done is to give the
"general idea" and leave the individual cook to learn by
experiment, hoping that the rest of the crew will not suffer too
much in the process. All the dishes described can be cooked
on a Primus or oil stove, though some of them need an oven.

Cruising and Ocean Racing: 1935, Seeley Service.

AGENTS WANTED

If you are interested in becoming our agent for any of the
following ports, please write to: The Editor, Edington House,
Trent, Sherborne, Dorset DT9 4SR, England – and get your
free copy of the almanac annually. You do not have to live in
a port to be the agent, but at least a fairly regular visitor.

River Exe	Grandcamp-Maisy
Port Ellen (Islay)	Port-en-Bessin
Glandore/Union Hall	Courseulles
River Rance/Dinan	Boulogne
Lampaul	Dunkerque
Port Tudy	Terneuzen/Westerschelde
River Etel	Oudeschild
Le Palais (Belle Ile)	Lauwersoog
Le Pouliguen/Pornichet	Dornumer-Accumersiel
L'Herbaudière	Hooksiel
St Gilles-Croix-de-Vie	Langeoog
River Seudre	Bremerhaven
Royan	Helgoland
Anglet/Bayonne	Büsum
Hendaye	

IJMUIDEN   10-20-23

Noord Holland 52°28'·03N 04°32'·00E

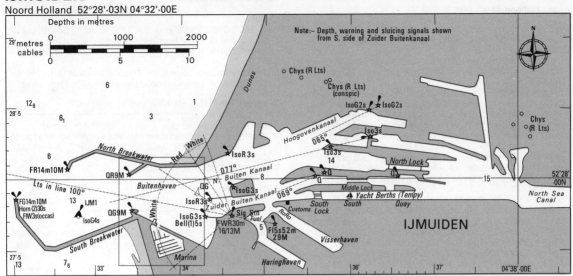

CHARTS
AC 2322, 124; Zeekaart 1450, 1543, 1035, 1350; DYC 1801;
Imray Y5; Stanfords 19

TIDES
+0400 Dover; ML 1·0; Zone –0100

Standard Port VLISSINGEN (←)

Times				Height (metres)			
High Water		Low Water		MHWS	MHWN	MLWN	MLWS
0300	0900	0400	1000	4·7	3·9	0·8	0·3
1500	2100	1600	2200				
Differences IJMUIDEN							
+0145	+0140	+0305	+0325	–2·6	–2·2	–0·5	–0·1

SHELTER
Very good at SPM marina (5·5m - 3m depths) on S side of
Buitenhaven, close E of S bkwtr QG (see chartlet). There
are also temp (24hrs) berths at canal locks. There are
small marinas at IJmond (under lift-bridge in Zijkanaal C,
km 10) and Nauwerna (Zijkanaal D, km 12).

NAVIGATION
WPT IJM (SWM) buoy, Mo (A) 8s, Racon, 52°28'·70N
04°23'·93E, 275°/095° from/to ent, 5·0M. Beware strong
tidal streams across hbr ent, scend inside Buitenhaven
and heavy merchant tfc. There are 4 locks into the
Noordzeekanaal: North, Middle, South and Small; yachts
normally use the Small (Kleine) lock, next to the South.
One in/out cycle per hour, 0600-2100 daily, is scheduled.
Note: the canal level may be above or below sea level.

LIGHTS AND MARKS
Ldg lts 100° into Buitenhaven and Zuider Buitenkanaal:
Front lt ho FWR 30m 16/13M, W050°-122°, R122°-145°,
W145°-160°, RC; rear lt ho, Fl 5s 52m 29M. Both are dark
R trs and show a Ⓦ lt by day.
Marina ent marked by SPM buoy, VQ, "IJM3-SPM", 1ca to
N. Ent sigs: Ⓡ = no entry; Ⓡ+Ⓖ = get ready; Ⓖ = go.
Traffic, tidal, sluicing & storm sigs are shown at/near the
conspic Hbr Ops Centre (HOC) bldg, next to front ldg lt.
Traffic sigs (large frame adjacent to the front ldg lt):
There are 9 lts in a 3 x 3 frame, of which, for **inbound**
yachts, only the 3 right-hand lts normally apply:
Top RH lt (for S Lock) Fl Ⓖ   = wait for lock entry.
                  Ⓖ   = clear to enter.
                  Fl Ⓡ = vessels exiting.
                  Ⓡ   = lock not in use.
Centre RH lt (for Zuider Buiten Kanaal)
                  Fl Ⓡ = vessels exiting.
                  Ⓡ   = traffic prohib.
Bottom RH lt   Ⓡ   = entry prohib, all vessels.
For **outbound yachts** only the top LH lt applies (for
Zuider Buitenkanaal) Fl Ⓡ = vessels entering.
                  Ⓡ   = traffic prohib.
Tidal sigs, from radar tr on HOC bldg:
Ⓖ over Ⓦ = rising tide; Ⓦ over Ⓖ = falling tide.

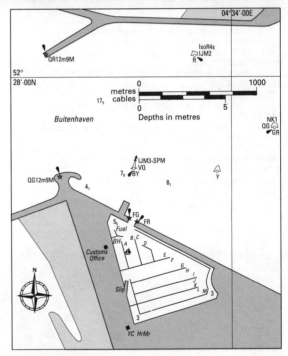

RADIO TELEPHONE
Call the following VTS stns (H24) in sequence for entry:
Traffic Centre IJmuiden   Ch 12 (W of IJM buoy).
IJmuiden Hbr Control (HOC)   Ch 09 (IJM buoy to locks).
(Seaport Marina)   Ch 74).
IJmuiden Locks   Ch 22.
*Traffic Centre Noordzeekanaal*Ch 11 (Lock to km 11·2).
Amsterdam Port Control   Ch 14 (Km 11·2 to A'dam).
Vessels in the roads area, the Buitenhaven and the
Noordzeekanaal should keep watch on the appropriate
Ch, and report to HOC on departure from or arrival at a
port in Noordzeekanaal. Vis broadcasts, when < 1000m,
every H + 00 on Ch 12-14; every H + 30 on Ch 05 -11.

TELEPHONE (0255)
Hr Mr 519027; Pilot 519027; Traffic Centre IJmuiden 534542;
⌗ 523309; Police 535035; Ⓗ 565100; Brit Consul (020) 6764343

FACILITIES
Seaport Marina (SPM) ☎ 33448/Fax 34593 (600 berths inc
visitors), f27, AC, FW, D & P, BH (70 ton), El, Ⓔ, CH, Gas,
Slip, SM, Sh, ME, V, R, Bar, ▣, ⌗, bus to Amsterdam and
Haarlem (summer); **IJmond YC** ☎ 384457, Hr Mr ☎
375003, AB f10.80 inc AC, Bar, BY, C (20 ton), ▣, V, R, D.
Town P, D, Gaz, V, R, Bar, ✉, Ⓑ, ⇌ (bus to Beverwijk), ✈
Amsterdam. Ferry: Hook-Harwich.

AMSTERDAM   10-20-24

Noord Holland 52°23'·00N 04°54'·00E

CHARTS
AC 124; Zeekaart 1543; DYC 1801, 1810; ANWB G, I
TIDES
Amsterdam is between the Noordzeekanaal and the
IJsselmeer, both of which are non-tidal; Zone –0100.
SHELTER
Complete in any of 5 yacht hbrs/marinas (see chartlet &
Facilities). The main one is Sixhaven, on the N bank, NE
of the ⮑ (conspic); it is small, pleasant and well located,
so mostly full by 1800. WV Aeolus is a good alternative.
Twellega is more for the larger yacht; bus to city centre.
Gem. Haven on the S bank, close NW of the Hbr bldg
(conspic), is prone to wash from passing ships and not
recommended. There is a small marina, WV Zuiderzee,
on N bank immediately E of Oranjesluizen.
NAVIGATION
See 10.20.23. The 13·5M transit of the Noordzeekanaal is
simple, apart from the volume of commercial traffic. The
speed limit is 9kn. Schellingwoude bridge (9m), at 500m
E of Oranjesluizen, opens: all year Mon-Fri 0600-0700,
0900-1600, 1800-2200. Sat 0600-2200. Sun & Public hols
from 1 Apr to 1 Nov: 0900-2100; 1 Nov to 1 Apr: closed.
There are waiting pontoons both sides of Oranjesluizen.
Amsterdam gives access to canals running to N & S and
also, via the Oranjesluizen (H24), to the IJsselmeer.
LIGHTS AND MARKS
Both banks of the canal and the ents to branch canals
and basins are lit. The chan E towards the Oranjesluizen
and the Amsterdam-Rijn canal is lit/buoyed.
RADIO TELEPHONE
VHF Ch 14. See also 10.20.23. Oranjesluizen Ch 18.
TELEPHONE (020)
Port Control 6221201; ⌗ 5867511; Emergency 06-11;
Police 5599111; Dr 5555555; Brit Consul: 6764343.
FACILITIES
Marinas: Sixhaven (60 + some visitors) ☎ 6370892, f11.25
inc AC, FW, Bar (weekends);
ZV Aeolus ☎ 6360791, f9.00 inc AC, YC, FW;
Gem. Haven ☎ 5503636, f15.00, no facilities;
Twellega ☎ 6320616, f13.50, AC, FW, Sh, P, C (30 ton);
WV Zuiderzee No ☎, f9.00, YC, AC, FW;
Services: Gaz, Ⓔ, ACA, DYC Agent.
City: All facilities, Ⓑ, ✉, ⮑, ✈. Ferry: See Hook.

IJSSELMEER   10-20-25

CHARTS
AC 1408, 2593; Zeekaart 1351, 1454; DYC 1810 – this chart
is essential to avoid live firing ranges, fishing areas and
other hazards; it also contains many harbour chartlets.
TIDES
The IJsselmeer is non-tidal. Tides at locks at Den Oever
and Kornwerderzand: –0230 Dover; ML 1·2; Zone –0100

Standard Port HELGOLAND (➞)

Times				Height (metres)			
High Water		Low Water		MHWS	MHWN	MLWN	MLWS
0200	0700	0200	0800	2·7	2·3	0·4	0·0
1400	1900	1400	2000				
Differences KORNWERDERZAND							
–0210	–0315	–0300	–0215	–0·5	–0·4	–0·1	+0·2
DEN OEVER							
–0245	–0410	–0400	–0305	–0·8	–0·6	0·0	+0·2

SHELTER
Excellent in the many marinas, some of which are listed
below. Most berths are bows on to a pontoon, stern lines
to piles; there are few ⚓s.
NAVIGATION
The IJsselmeer is the un-reclaimed part of the former
Zuiderzee; it is separated from the Waddenzee by the
20M long Afsluitdijk, completed in 1932. It is divided into
two parts by the Houtribdijk, with locks at Enkhuizen to
the NW and Lelystad in the SE. The SW part is the
Markermeer (20M x 15M, 2-4·5m deep); the rest of the
IJsselmeer is 30M x 20M, 7m max. Three ents via locks:
(1)   IJmuiden, Noordzeekanaal to Oranjesluizen (10.20.24).
(2)   Den Oever (SW end of the Afsluitdijk): Appr from
Waddenzee via well marked/lit chan; ldg lts 132°, both Oc
10s to ent, thence follow Dir Iso WRG 2s, 220° to wait in
Buitenhaven. 2 bridges and locks operate in unison HO.
From IJsselmeer, wait in Binnenhaven; FR/G at ent.
(3)   Kornwerderzand lock (NE end of the Afsluitdijk) H24.
From Waddenzee, via W, NW or NE chans. Ent has FR/G
and Iso G 6s. Wait in Buitenhaven; yachts use the smaller
E lock. From IJsselmeer, ldg lts Iso 4s 348° to FR/G at ent;
wait in Binnenhaven (3·8m).
Standard lock sigs (vert): Ⓡ Ⓡ = not in service; Ⓡ = no
entry; Ⓡ Ⓖ = stand by; Ⓖ = enter.

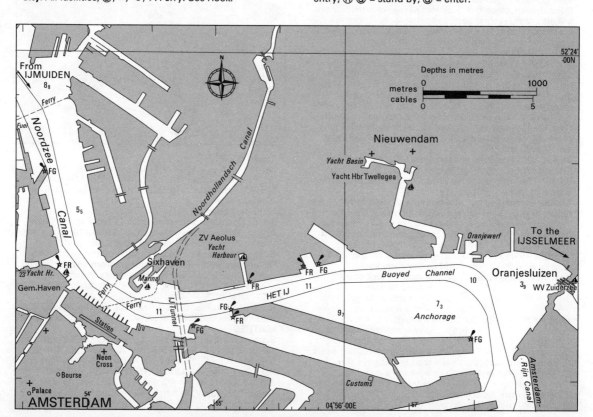

IJSSELMEER *continued*

Speed limits: in buoyed chans and <250m from shore 10·5kn. Hbr limits vary; see ANWB Almanak Vol 2. Strong winds get up very quickly and often cause short seas; they can also raise the water level on a lee shore, or lower it on a weather shore, by 1m or more. Most hbrs have water level gauges which should be checked in bad weather. In non-tidal waters CD usually refers to the level at which the water is kept. In the Netherlands, this may be Kanaalpeil, which is related to Normaal Amsterdams Peil (NAP), which in turn is approx Mean Sea Level.
A firing range, operational Tues to Thurs 1000 - 1900LT, extends S from Breezanddijk (53°01'·0N 05°12'·5E) to 3M N of Medemblik then NNW to Den Oever (DYC 1810.3). Call the range control on Ch 71 *Schietterrein Breezanddijk*. Scheveningen Radio broadcasts firing times on the day of firing after Dutch forecasts, at even hours; also at 1900 the previous day in English Ch 25, 27, 83 after the weather.

BUOYAGE The SIGNI buoyage system is used in the whole of the IJsselmeer. The main features are:
(1) Lateral buoyage as for IALA (Region A).
(2) Supplementary PHM & SHM buoys may be R/W or G/W respectively; they also indicate a least depth of 2m.
(3) At division of chan, a spherical buoy as follows:
a. Chans of equal importance = R & G bands; topmark R and G sphere;
b. Main chan to port = G above R bands; topmark G △ or G △ above a G ○;
c. Main chan to stbd = R above G bands; topmark R □ or R □ above a R ○.

RADIO TELEPHONE

VHF Ch's at locks are: Oranjesluizen 18; Enkhuizen 22; Den Oever 20; Kornwerderzand 18; Lelystad 20.

HARBOURS AND FACILITIES

A useful guide, one of the few in English, is *IJsselmeer Harbours* by Hilary Keatinge (Barnacle Marine 1988). It is essential to have the *Almanac voor Watertoerisme*, Vol I onboard; it contains the BPR (Waterway Code). Some of the many hbrs are listed below (clockwise from the NW):
DEN OEVER: Jachthaven (3m) to port of ent; Hr Mr ☎ (0227) 511789, f13.50, D, P, FW, ⍉.
MAKKUM: Approx 1M SE of Kornwerderzand, a SHM buoy MA7, Iso G4s, marks the 1·2M buoyed chan. FR/FG lts lead 091° into Makkum, Hr Mr ☎ (0515) 231450. To stbd, **Marina Makkum** (2·5m) ☎ (0515) 232828, f11.70, P, D, BY, ME, FW, C (30 ton), BH (30 ton), SM, Gaz. 4 other marinas/YCs are further E. **Town** ⑧, Dr, V, R.
WORKUM: 2·5M N of Hindeloopen; FW ldg lts 081° along buoyed chan to **It Soal Marina** ☎ (0515) 542937, f18.00, BY, ME, C, FW, D, P (cans), Gaz, BH; **Jachthaven Anne Wever** ☎ 542361, f13.50, C (40 ton).
HINDELOOPEN: has 2 marinas, one in town and one 180m to N. **Jachthaven Hindeloopen** (500) Hr Mr ☎ (0514) 531866, f20.00, P, D, FW, AC, ⍉, BH (30 ton), CH, R, Bar; **Old Hbr** f9.00, D, P, FW, ME, El, Sh; **W.V Hylper Haven** Hr Mr ☎ 532009, f9.00, P, D, FW, ME, El, Sh.
STAVOREN: Ent 048° on Dir lt Iso 4s between FR/G. Yacht berths S of ent in Oudehaven; Hr Mr ☎ (0514) 681216; or ent via Nieuwe Voorhaven and lock, about 1km S of Buitenhaven, with FR/G and Fl 5s Dir lt, for **Stavoren Marina** (3m) ☎ 681566, f15.75, BY, ME, C, FW, P, D, SM, Gaz, BH (20 ton). Also 3 other marinas. **Town** ⑧, Dr, V, R, ≋.
LEMMER: has some 14 marinas. Ldg lts 038°, Iso 8s, toward Prinses Margrietkanaal. Next ldg lts 083°, Iso 8s, through Lemstergeul. Lastly FG and Iso G 4s lead 065° into town and marinas. **Gemeente Jachthaven** Hr Mr ☎ (0514) 563331, f12.60; **Services:** AB, BY, ME, C, FW, P, D, Gaz, SM. **Town** ⑧, Dr, V, R, ⊠.
URK: Hbr ent ½M SE of lt ho, Fl 5s 27m 18M. Dir lt Iso G 4s to hbr ent, FR/G. Hbr has 4 basins; keep NNW to berth in Nieuwe Haven, Westhaven or Oosthaven (3·3m), f9.90. Hr Mr ☎ (0527) 681394. FW; **Westhaven** P & D (cans), SM; **Oosthaven** ME, El, Sh, ⒺCH. **Town** EC Tues; ⑧, ⊠, Dr.
KETELHAVEN: Ent Ketelmeer via bridge (12.9m) which lifts at S end; after 4M to By WK1 IsoG 4s, ldg lts Iso 8s 101°/0·7M in buoyed chan. Turn S for unlit marina ent (2·2m). **Marina** (200) f13.50, FW, AC, R. Hr Mr ☎ (0321) 312271. W ent has FG/R lts to Ketelsluis: Hr Mr ☎ 318237 D, P (cans).
LELYSTAD: has 2 marinas: 2M NNE of lock is **Flevo** (550) ☎ (0320) 279800, f21.15, BY, ME, C, FW, AC, P, D, ⍉, BH (50 ton), R, Bar, V. Close N of the lock is **Houtribhaven** (560) Hr Mr ☎ 260198, f13.50, D, CH, V, R, Bar, C (12). Radio mast, R lts, (140m) is conspic; marinas are lit.

MARKERMEER

MUIDERZAND: Ent 1M N of Hollandsebrug at buoys IJM5-JH2/IJM3. **Marina** ☎ (036) 5365151, f20.25, FW, AC, D, P.
NAARDEN: 1M SE of Hollandsebrug (12·9m), ent at GM54 buoy. **Gem Jachthaven** (1000) ☎ (035) 6942106, f13.50, D, P, AC, FW, El, BH, C, CH, V, R, Bar, ≋ (Naarden-Bussum).
MUIDEN: Ldg lts Q 181° into **KNZ & RV Marina** (2·6m), W of ent; home of Royal Netherlands YC (150 berths). Hr Mr ☎ (0294) 261450, f24.75, D, P (cans), CH, FW, Bar, R. On E bank **Stichting Jachthaven** (70) ☎ 261223, f19.00, D, P.
DURGERDAM: Convenient for Oranjesluizen. Ldg lts 337°, both FR. Keep strictly to chan which is ½M E of overhead power lines. Berth to stbd of ent (1·8m), f11.70. ☎ (020) 4904717.
MARKEN (picturesque show piece): Ent Gouwzee from N, abeam Volendam, thence via buoyed chan; Dir FW lt 116° between FR/G at hbr (2·2m). Lt ho, conspic, Oc 8s 16m 9M, on E end of island. Hr Mr ☎ (0299) 603231, f11.25, FW, AC, V, R, ⑧, P & D (cans).
MONNICKENDAM: Appr as for Marken, then W to MO10 Iso R 8s and ldg lts FR at 236°. Hr Mr ☎ (0299) 653939. 4 marinas & facilities: f13.50, ME, C, FW, P (cans), D, Gaz, AC, CH.
VOLENDAM: Berth to stbd (2·4m). Dir lt Fl 5s 313°. FR/G at ent. Hr Mr ☎ (0299) 369620, f8.25, ME, FW, C, P, D, Gaz, SM.
EDAM: Appr via unlit chan keeping Iso W 8s between FG /R at narrow ent; beware commercial traffic. Berth on N side (2·4m); no marina (beware underwater posts). Or lock into the Oorgat and via S canal to Nieuwe Haven. Hr Mr ☎ (0299) 371092, f8.25, ME, El, Sh. **Town** Bar, ⍉, ⊠, Gaz, ⑧.
HOORN: Radio tr (80m) 1·5M ENE of hbr. Iso 4s 15m 10M and FR/G at W Hbr ent. Four options: to port **Stichting Jachthaven Hoorn** (700) Hr Mr ☎ (0299) 415208, f13.50, FW, AC, ⍉, CH, V, ME, El, Sh, C; to stbd ⚓ in **Buitenhaven** (2m); ahead & to stbd **Vluchthaven Marina** f15.30, (100) ☎ 413540 FW; ahead to **Binnenhaven** (2·7m) via narrow lock (open H24) AB f12.15, P, FW.
Town V, CH, ⊠, R, Dr, P & D (cans), ⑧, Gaz, ≋.
ENKHUIZEN: From SW, appr via buoyed chan and ldg lts Iso 4s at 039°; from NE, ldg lts Iso 8s at 230° and FR /G at bkwtrs lead to Krabbersgat lock and hbr. Call lock Ch 22. The 2 marinas and Buitenhaven are NE of the lock:
Compagnieshaven (500) Hr Mr ☎ (0228) 313353 f17.50, P, D, FW, AC, CH, BH (12), Gaz; **Buyshaven** (195) ☎ 315660, f15.25, FW, AC; **Buitenhaven** ☎ 312444 f9.74, FW. **Town** EC Mon; Market Wed; C, Slip, CH, SM, ME, El, Sh, ⑧, Bar, P & D (cans), Dr, ⊠, ≋.   *Continued*

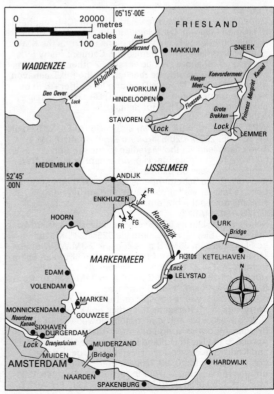

20

IJSSELMEER (WEST)   *Continued*

ANDIJK: Visitors use **Stichting Jachthaven Andijk,** the first
of 2 marinas; (600) ☎ (0228) 593075, f13.50, narrow ent
with tight turn between FR/G lts. ME, C (20), SM, Gaz, ⊙,
D, CH.

MEDEMBLIK: Ent on Dir lt Oc 4s 232° between FR/G. Go via
Oosterhaven (P & D) into Middenhaven (short stay), then
via bridge to Westerhaven. **Pekelharinghaven** (120) Hr Mr
☎ (0227) 542175, f11.50; ent is to port by Castle, CH, Bar,
R; **Middenhaven** Hr Mr ☎ 541686, f11.25, FW; **Stichting
Jachthaven** Hr Mr ☎ 541861 in Westerhaven, f11.25, FW,
AC, ⊙, C. **Town** ⑧, CH, ME, El, SM, Sh, ✉, Dr, Bar, ⊙, R, V.

DEN HELDER   10-20-26

Noord Holland 52°58'·00N 04°47'·35E

CHARTS
AC 191, 2322, 2593; Zeekaart 1454, 1546; DYC 1811.2,
1801; ANWB F; Imray Y5; Stanfords 19

TIDES
−0430 Dover; ML 1·1; Duration No data; Zone −0100

Standard Port HELGOLAND(→)

Times				Height (metres)			
High Water		Low Water		MHWS	MHWN	MLWN	MLWS
0200	0700	0200	0800	2·7	2·3	0·4	0·0
1400	1900	1400	2000				
Differences DEN HELDER							
−0410	−0520	−0520	−0430	−0·9	−0·7	0·0	+0·2

SHELTER
Good in the Naval Hbr, the yacht hbr (KMYC) being hard
to stbd on entering. Den Helder is the main base of the
Royal Netherlands Navy which owns and runs the KMYC
and the Marinehaven Willemsoord. Caution: many FVs,
ferries and off-shore service vessels. 2 other YCs/marinas
both of which can only be reached via the Rijkszeehaven,
Moorman bridge, Nieuwe Diep and lock, offer AB in or
near the Binnenhafen: MWV and YC Den Helder; see
below under FACILITIES for details.

NAVIGATION
WPT Schulpengat SG (SWM) buoy, Mo (A) 8s, 52°52'·95N
04°38'·00E, 206·5°/026·5° from/to Kaap Hoofd, 6·0M.
Two chans lead via the Marsdiep to the hbr ent:
(1) From N, the Molengat is good except in strong NW
winds when seas break heavily.
(2) From S, the Schulpengat is well marked and lit.
Beware fast ferries to/from Texel and strong tidal
streams across the hbr ent.

LIGHTS AND MARKS
Schulpengat: Ldg lts 026·5° on Texel; front Iso 4s 18M;
rear Oc 8s 18M, Ch spire, both vis 025°-028°. Kijkduin lt
ho Fl (4) 20s 56m 30M, R tr, is conspic 2·3M WSW of hbr.
Molengat: ldg lts 141·5°; front Iso 5s 13m 8M; rear, 650m
from front, FW 22m 8M; tr on Ⓗ; both vis 124°-157°.
Hbr ldg lts 191°. Both Oc G 5s 16/25m 14M (synch); front
B ▲ on bldg; rear B ▼ on B framework tr.
A 60m radar tower is conspic on the E side of hbr ent.
Entry sigs, from Harssens hbr office on W side of ent:
ⓇⓌⓇ (vert) = No entry; no traffic allowed within hbr.
Bridges: Moormanbridge operates 7 days a week H24.
Access to the North Holland Canal via the Nieuwe Diep
and Koopvaardersschutsluis.Van Kinsbergenbridge
operated by Hr Mr, 0500-2300 Mon-Fri; 0700-1400 Sat. All
bridges remain closed 0715-0810, 1200-1215, 1245-1300,
Mon-Fri. Also 0830-0910 Mon and 1545-1645 Fri. All LT.

RADIO TELEPHONE
Monitor VTS Ch 12 *Den Helder Traffic* in the apprs and
Marsdiep; weather forecast available on rquest. Port Ch
14 (H24). Koopvaardersschutsluis Ch 22 (H24), which also
operates Burgemeester Vissersbrug by remote control.
Moormanbridge Ch 18 (H24).

TELEPHONE (0223)
Municipal Hr Mr 613955; Hr Mr (Yacht Haven) 637444;
Pilot 617424; Vessel Traffic Centre 652770; Naval
Commander 656822; ⌗ 615182; Police 655700; Ⓗ 611414;
Water Police 616767; Immigration 657515; Brit Consul
(020) 6764343.

FACILITIES
In naval hbr: **KMYC** ☎ 652645, f13.80, FW, D, Bar, R;
In or near Binnenhaven:
MWV YC ☎ 617076, f11.50, P (at garage), D, L, FW, AB;
Yacht Haven Den Helder ☎ 637444, f15.65, ME, El, Sh, C,
CH, Slip, FW, R, Bar; **YC VSOV** ☎ 652173; **YC HWN** ☎
624422;
Services: CH, SM, Floating dock, Gaz.
Town P, CH, V, R, Bar, ✉, ⑧, ⇌, ✈ (Amsterdam).
Ferry: Hook of Holland-Harwich; Rotterdam-Hull.

OUDESCHILD   10-20-27

Texel, 53°02'·39N 04°51'·26E

CHARTS
AC 191, 2593; Zeekaart 1546, 1454; DYC 1811·3
TIDES
–0355 Dover; ML 1·1m; Duration 0625; Zone –0100

Standard Port HELGOLAND (→)

Times				Height (metres)			
High Water		Low Water		MHWS	MHWN	MLWN	MLWS
0200	0700	0200	0800	2·7	2·3	0·4	0·0
1400	1900	1400	2000				
Differences OUDESCHILD							
–0310	–0420	–0445	–0400	–0·9	–0·7	0·0	+0·2

SHELTER
Good in marina (3·5m) in the NE basin. Beware strong cross tides at ent. Not a Port of Entry. Yachts are advised not to ent/dep Mon morning when the entire FV fleet sails.
NAVIGATION
WPT 53°02'·28N 04°51'·72E, 111°/291° from/to hbr ent, 3ca. From seaward, app via Schulpengat or Molengat into Marsdiep (see 10.20.26). Thence from abeam ferry hbr of 't Horntje (Texel) steer NE via Texelstroom for 3·5M to hbr ent, marked by PHM buoy (T14), Iso R 8s. Enter on course 291° with dir lt, Oc 6s, midway between S mole hd FR and N mole hd FG. Speed limit 4kn (7kph).
LIGHTS AND MARKS
Dir lt Oc 6s 14m on G mast. Mole hd lts FR 7m and FG 7m are on R/W and G/W banded poles. Horn (2) 30s on S mole hd, sounded 0600-2300.
RADIO TELEPHONE
Hr Mr VHF Ch 09, 0730-1500LT. Monitor *Den Helder Traffic* (VTS) Ch 12; also wx, vis, tfc, tidal info broadcast at H+05.

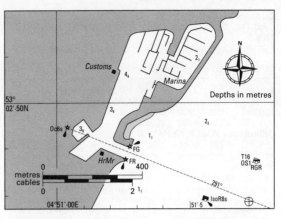

TELEPHONE (0222)
Hr Mr (marina) ☎ 313608 (1100-1130; 1800-1930LT); Port Hr Mr 312710/home 313538; CG 312732; Police 312222; Dr via Hr Mr.
FACILITIES
Marina (200 berths) ☎ 313608, FW, AC, Slip, P, D, Slip, ⊡, Gaz, Bar, R; **YC WV Texel; Services:** CH, ME, BY, Sh, Dry dock, C, SM.
  Village (walking distance), V (supermarket), Ⓑ, ✉, R. Ferry from 't Horntje to Den Helder. UK ferries from Hook/ Rotterdam. ✈ Amsterdam.

HARLINGEN   10-20-28

Friesland 53°10'·63N 05°24'·22E

CHARTS
AC 112, 2593; Zeekaart 1454, 1456; DYC 1811·5; ANWB B; Imray Y5
TIDES
–0210 Dover; ML 1·2; Duration 0520; Zone –0100

Standard Port Helgoland (→)

Times				Height (metres)			
High Water		Low Water		MHWS	MHWN	MLWN	MLWS
0200	0700	0200	0800	2·7	2·3	0·4	0·0
1400	1900	1400	2000				
Differences HARLINGEN							
–0155	–0245	–0210	–0130	–0·4	–0·3	–0·1	+0·2
NES (AMELAND)							
–0135	–0150	–0245	–0225	+0·1	+0·2	+0·2	+0·2

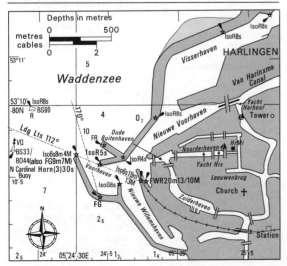

SHELTER
Very good in Noorderhaven, but ent can be rough at HW with W/NW winds. Entering on the flood, beware strong stream across ent. Note: Access to/from Noorderhaven is restricted by the two N/S bridges either end of the Oude Buitenhaven; these open in unison 2 x per hr 0600-2200 in season (on request in winter) and are shut at times of boat trains/ferries. Some berths at Van Harinxma yacht hbr; but only advised if going via the canal on to the lakes.
NAVIGATION
WPT SM buoy from seaward (see 10.20.29). Then follow the buoyed Vliestroom and Blauwe Slenk chans which narrow for the last 2½M. Pleasure craft should use the Hanerak, a buoyed (Nos HR1-23) chan, parallel about 600m S of the Pollendam which is used by ferries. Caution: When training wall is covered, tidal stream sweeps across the Pollendam, marked by lateral lt bns.
LIGHTS AND MARKS
Ldg lts 112°, both Iso 6s. Dir lt F WR 20m 13/10M, R113°-116°, W152°-068°. R 3° sector covers the Pollendam.
RADIO TELEPHONE
VHF Ch 11 (Mon 0000 to Sat 2200LT). Harinxma Canal locks Ch 22.
TELEPHONE (0517)
Hr Mr 413041; CG (Brandaris) (0562) 442341; ⌗ 418750; Police 413333; Ⓗ 499999; Brit Consul (020) 6764343.
FACILITIES
Noorderhaven Yacht Hbr ☎ 415666, FW, El, CH, V, R, Bar, ⊡; **Yacht Hbr Van Harinxma Canal** ☎ 416898, FW, ⊡, C (6 ton); **Services:** CH, El, E, Gaz, Diving/salvage, El, ME (by arrangement), D, P. **Town** EC Mon; LB, D, P, V, R, Bar, SM, ✉, Ⓑ, ⇶, ✈ (Amsterdam). Ferry: See Hook.

NES, AMELAND, Friesland, 53°26'·28N 05°46'·62E. AC 2593, Zeekaart 1458, DYC 1811.6, 1812.2. HW –0055 on Dover; ML 1·6m; Duration 0625. See 10.20.28. Shelter from all but E/S winds. Yacht pontoons at N end of hbr (0·8m) beyond ferry terminal; W side dries to soft mud. Beware sandbanks in the Zeegat van Ameland. Enter from Molengat at MG28-R1 SCM By, VQ(6) + L Fl 10s. Lts: Ameland (W end), Fl (3) 15s 57m 30M, RC. Ferry pier hd Iso 6s 2m 8M. L Fl R 8s and L Fl G 8s piles at ent to yacht hbr ('t Leye Gat, 140 berths), f15.00. Facilities: Gaz, YC. Hr Mr ☎ (0515) 32159.

20

VLIELAND   10-20-29

WEST FRISIAN ISLANDS
Friesland 53°17'·73N 05°05'·57E

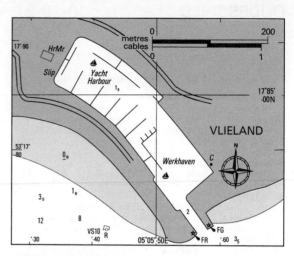

CHARTS
AC 112, 2593; Zeekaart 1456; DYC 1811.4/.5; Imray Y5

TIDES
–0300 Dover; ML 1·4; Duration 0610; Zone –0100

Standard Port HELGOLAND (→)

Times				Height (metres)			
High Water		Low Water		MHWS	MHWN	MLWN	MLWS
0200	0700	0200	0800	2·7	2·3	0·4	0·0
1400	1900	1400	2000				
Differences VLIELAND-HAVEN							
–0250	–0320	–0355	–0330	–0.3	–0.2	+0·1	+0·2

SHELTER
Good; yacht hbr (2m) is very crowded in season. ‡ in 4-9m, about 0·5M W of the hbr (and nearer the village), except in SE/SW winds; but do not ‡ in buoyed chan between hbr and ferry pier (no berthing). From the S a safe ‡ in Fransche Gaatje, SE of Richel, is 6M from hbr.

NAVIGATION
WPT SM (SWM) By, Iso 4s, 53°19'·05N 04°55'·73E, 274°/094° from/to ZS1 and ZS2 Bys, 2·3M (via ZS Bank NCM). See 10.20.31. In fresh W/NW winds a heavy ground swell can raise dangerous seas from the WPT to ZS1/2 Bys. The Zuider Stortemelk is deep, well marked/lit and leads to the Vliestroom. Vliesloot, which forks off to the S, is narrow and in places has only 2·5m at LW sp; keep in mid-chan.

LIGHTS AND MARKS
Main lt ho Iso 4s 53m 20M; R tr, W lantern, R top; RC. Tfc sigs: R Flag or ®® at ent = hbr closed (full).

RADIO TELEPHONE
Hr Mr Ch 09; CG Ch 02 (Brandaris, W. Terschelling). All vessels in the Zeegat van Terschelling and N Waddenzee must monitor Ch 02 for the Brandaris Traffic Centre VTS.

TELEPHONE (0562)
Hr Mr 451729; CG (0562) 442341; ⌗ 451522; Police 451312; Dr 451307; Brit Consul (020) 6764343.

FACILITIES
Yacht Hbr (250) ☎ 451729, FW, ▣; Hbr C (10 ton), P & D (cans, 10 mins); nearest D by hose is at Harlingen.
Village El, CH, Ⓔ, Gaz, V, R, ✉, Ⓑ, ≋ (ferry to Harlingen), ✈ (Amsterdam). Ferry: Hook of Holland-Harwich.

WEST TERSCHELLING   10-20-30

WEST FRISIAN ISLANDS
Friesland 53°21'·40N 05°13'·23E

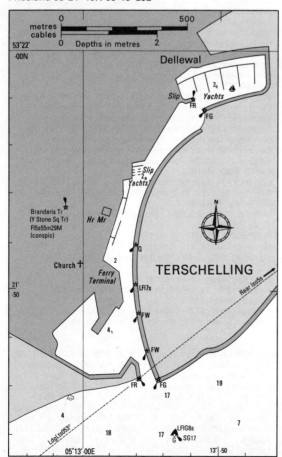

CHARTS
AC 112, 2593; Zeekaart 1456; DYC 1811.4/.5; Imray Y5

TIDES
–0300 Dover; ML 1·4; Duration No data; Zone –0100

Standard Port HELGOLAND (→)

Times				Height (metres)			
High Water		Low Water		MHWS	MHWN	MLWN	MLWS
0200	0700	0200	0800	2·7	2·3	0·4	0·0
1400	1900	1400	2000				
Differences WEST TERSCHELLING							
–0220	–0250	–0335	–0310	–0.4	–0·2	+0·1	+0·2

SHELTER
Good, especially in marina in NE corner of hbr beyond ferry and FV quays. Very crowded in season; considerable commercial traffic in confined waters.

NAVIGATION
WPT: SM buoy from all directions (see 10.20.29 and .31). Thence through Stortemelk to VL2-SG1 buoy, VQ (9) 10s, 53°19'·90N 05°09'·00E, at ent to the Schuitengat which is very narrow and steep-sided at W end. Pick up ldg lts 053° to hbr ent; local advice is desirable. Boomskendiep is no longer buoyed and should not be attempted.

LIGHTS AND MARKS
Brandaris tr (conspic Y ☐ tr), Fl 5s 55m 29M, storm sigs. Ldg lts 053°: front (W mole) FR 5m 5M; R post, W bands; Horn 15s; rear (on dyke 1·1M from front, off chartlet) Iso 5s 14m 19M; vis 045°-061° (intens 045°-052°). Fl (5) Y 20s on tide gauge, close NW of VL2-SG1.

RADIO TELEPHONE
Hr Mr Ch 09. CG Ch 02 04 16 67. Gale warnings, met & tfc broadcasts on Ch 02 at 0730, 0930, 1330 and 1930LT. Yachts in the area must listen on Ch 02 (see 10.20.28).

TELEPHONE (0562)
Hr Mr 442910/442919; CG 442341; ⌗ 442884.

FACILITIES
Marina: Stichting Passantenhaven (500) ☎ 443337, f24.00, C, FW; Hbr Slip, M, FW (in cans), ME, AB; Services: Gaz, ME, SM, Chart agent. Village EC Wed; FW, CH, V, R, Bar, ✉, P & D (cans from village of Midlands, 6km; nearest D by hose is at Harlingen), Ⓑ, ≋ (ferry to Harlingen), ✈ (Amsterdam). Ferry: Hook-Harwich.

ZEEGAT VAN TERSCHELLING

10-20-31

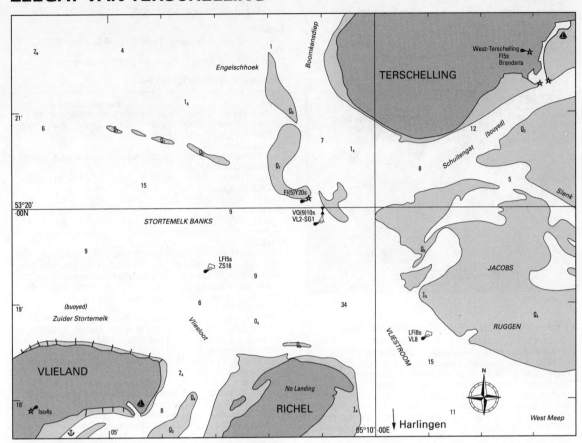

LAUWERSOOG

10-20-32

Friesland, 53°24'·72N 06°12'·10E

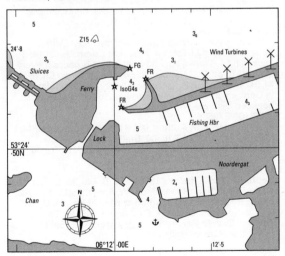

CHARTS

AC 3509, 3761, Zeekaart 1458, DYC 1812.3

TIDES

HW –0150 on Dover; ML 1·7m; Zone –0100

Standard Port HELGOLAND (→)

Times				Height (metres)			
High Water		Low Water		MHWS	MHWN	MLWN	MLWS
0200	0700	0200	0800	2·7	2·3	0·4	0·0
1400	1900	1400	2000				
Differences LAUWERSOOG							
–0130	–0145	–0235	–0220	+0·2	+0·3	+0·3	+0·3

SHELTER

Outer hbr has swell in bad weather. Good shelter in inner FV hbr to await lock. Complete shelter in Noordergat marina 3ca SE of lock; Ⓥs berth on first pontoon (2·4m).

NAVIGATION

Lock operates 0400-2100 Mon-Fri; 0400-1800 Sat; 0900-1000 and 1630-1830LT Sun. Enter the Lauwersmeer and canals from Harlingen to Delfzijl; no need to lower mast.

LIGHTS AND MARKS

W mole FG 3M. E mole FR 4M. Visserhaven mole FR. Lock lead-in jetty Iso 4s. Firing range 1·5m ENE of hbr ent is marked by Fl Y 10s buoys, which alternate W/R when the range is active; info is broadcast on Ch 71.

RADIO TELEPHONE

Hbr VHF Ch 09; Lock Ch 22; Range broadcast Ch 71.

TELEPHONE (0519)

Hr Mr 39023; Lock 39043; Marina 39040.

FACILITIES

Noordergat marina, ☎ 39040, f15.00, Gaz, BY, D, FW; P at ferry terminal (W end of hbr), Bar, R, V, YC.

OTHER HARBOURS IN THE LAUWERSMEER

OOSTMAHORN, Friesland, 53°22'·90N 06°09'·71E. AC 3509, Zeekaarten 1458, DYC 1812·3. Non-tidal hbr on W side of Lauwersmeer; lock in as for Lauwersoog. Floating bns with Y flags mark fishing areas. Main hbr with FR and FG lts at ent has marina (2·2-3·0m). Approx 450m to the SSE the Voorm Veerhaven marina has 1·5-2m. Hr Mr ☎ (0519) 31445/31880; f13.50, most facilities in the marinas.

ZOUTKAMP, Friesland, 53°20'·43N 06°17'·63E. AC 3509, Zeekaarten 1458, DYC 1812·3; non-tidal. Appr down the Zoutkamperril (2·6-4·5m); approx 2ca before lock/bridge, Hunzegat marina (1·5-2·1m) is to port. Beyond the lock and close to port is Oude Binnenhaven marina (2m), f10. FR lts at lock. Facilities: **Hunzegat** (0595) ☎ 402588, AC, FW, SC, Slip. **Oude-Binnenhaven** AC, C, FW; **Services:** ME, El, Sh, C (20 ton), BH. **Town** D, P, SM, Gaz, ✉, R, V, Dr.

20

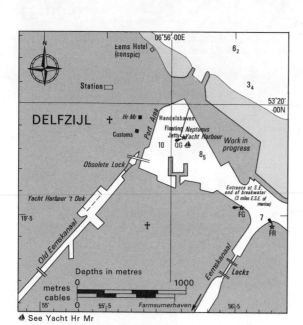

⚓ See Yacht Hr Mr

OTHER HARBOUR ON THE WEST FRISIAN ISLANDS

SCHIERMONNIKOOG, Friesland, 53°28'·12N 06°10'·10E.
AC3509, 3761, Zeekaart 1458, DYC 1812.3. HW −0150 on
Dover. See 10.20.33. Appr via Westgat, buoyed/lit, but in
bad weather dangerous due to shoals (3·8m) at seaward
end. Leave Zoutkamperlaag via Glinder chan (1·5m) to
enter Gat van Schiermonnikoog (buoyed). From GVS16-
R1 buoy a drying chan, marked by perches/withies, runs
1M N to small yacht hbr (1·3-1·5m) about 1M W of the
ferry pier. Access HW −2 to +1, with 1·5m max depth at
HW in apprs. Picturesque, but very full in high season;
not cheap, ie f27.00. Lts: at W end of island, lt ho Fl (4)
20s 43m 28M, R tr; Ferry pier hd lt FW and Fl (5) Y 20s
tide gauge. Hr Mr ☎ (0519) 51544 (May-Sept); Facilities:
FW, AC.

DELFZIJL   10-20-33
Groningen 53°19'·00N 07°00'·50E

CHARTS
AC 3510, 3509; Zeekaart 1555; DYC 1812.6; ANWB A
TIDES
−0025 Dover; ML 2·1; Duration 0605; Zone −0100

Standard Port HELGOLAND (→)

Times				Height (metres)			
High Water		Low Water		MHWS	MHWN	MLWN	MLWS
0200	0700	0200	0800	2·7	2·3	0·4	0·0
1400	1900	1400	2000				
Differences DELFZIJL							
+0020	−0005	−0040	0000	+0·9	+0·9	+0·3	+0·3
SCHIERMONNIKOOG							
−0120	−0130	−0240	−0220	+0·2	+0·3	+0·3	+0·3
KNOCK (R. Ems)							
+0018	+0005	−0028	+0004	+0·6	+0·6	0·0	0·0
EMDEN							
+0041	+0028	−0011	+0022	+0·8	+0·8	0·0	0·0

SHELTER
Good in Neptunus Yacht Hbr (3·5m) at Balkenhaven.
Note: Neptunus is re-located 1994-97 at the Floating Jetty
due to WIP. Berthing (4·5m) also in Farmsumerhaven
(24hr only) via the Eemskanaal lock; or at the N end of
the Old Eemskanaal in Yacht Hbr 't Dok (4m).
NAVIGATION
WPT Huibertgat SWM buoy, Iso 8s, Whis, 53°34'·90N
06°14'·32E, 270°/090° from/to Borkum Kleiner lt, 15·5M, in
W sector. Chan buoys unlit for first 10M.
WPT Westereems SWM buoy, Iso 4s, Racon, 53°36'·97N,
06°19'·48E, 272°/092° from/to Nos 1 and 2 Westereems
chan buoys, 1·6M.
WPT from N & E: Riffgat SWM buoy, Iso 8s, 53° 38'·90N
06° 27'·10E, 312°/132° from/to Westereems chan buoys,
3·2M; and 8·75M to Borkum Kleiner lt (See 10.21.10).
Thence via Ranselgat & Doekegat (well buoyed/lit) to ent
3M ESE of the city of Delfzijl. Beware strong cross tides
at the ent.
LIGHTS AND MARKS
From the river, appr ldg lts 203°, both Iso 4s. Hbr ent, FG
on W arm and FR on E arm (in fog, Horn 15s and FY).
Zeehavenkanaal has Fl G lts to N and Fl R to S.
Entry sigs: 2 R Flags or 2 Ⓡ = No movements, unless
over Ⓖ directed by Hr Mr.
RADIO TELEPHONE
All ships, except recreational craft, must call *Delfzijl
Radar* VHF Ch 66 (H24) for VTS. *Port Control* is Ch 14; Sea
Locks Ch 11. Traffic, wx and tidal info is broadcast every
even H+10 on Ch 14 in Dutch. *Ems Rivier Radio* Ch 18 20
21 (H24) broadcasts every H + 50 weather and tidal info
in German, including gale warnings for coastal waters
between Die Ems and Die Weser.
TELEPHONE (0596)
Hr Mr (Delfzijl Port Authorities) 640477; Neptunus Hr Mr
615004; Hr Mr 't Dok 616560; Sea locks 613293; CG
(Police) 613831; ⌗ 615060; Weather 640477; Police 06-11;
Ⓗ 644444; Brit Consul (020) 6764343.
FACILITIES
Neptunus Yacht Hbr ☎ 615004, f12, D, Bar, M, L, FW;
Yacht Hbr 't Dok AB f10.00, D, FW; **Ems Canal** L, FW, AB;
Motor Boat Club Abel Tasman ☎ 616560 Bar, M, D, FW,
L, Ⓞ, V. **Services**: CH, ACA, DYC Agent, ME, El, Gaz.
Town P, D, V, R, Bar, ✉, Ⓑ, ⇌, ✈ (Groningen/Eelde).
Ferry: See Hook of Holland.

ADJACENT HARBOURS

TERMUNTERZIJL Groningen, 53°18'·21N 07°02'·30E. AC
3510; Zeekaart 1555; DYC 1812. HW −0025 on Dover (UT);
use Differences Delfzijl. Ent (1·3M ESE of Delfzijl ent) is
close to BW13 SHM buoy Fl G 5s (53°18'·70N 07°02'·40E);
thence chan marked by 7 R and 7 G unlit bns. Yachts
berth in Vissershaven (0·9m), stbd of ent, or on pontoons
(1m) to port of ent, f10.00. Hr Mr ☎ (0596) 601891 (Apr-
Sept), VHF Ch 09, FW, AC, Bar, R.

EMDEN see 10.21.9

Area 21

Germany
Emden to Danish border

21

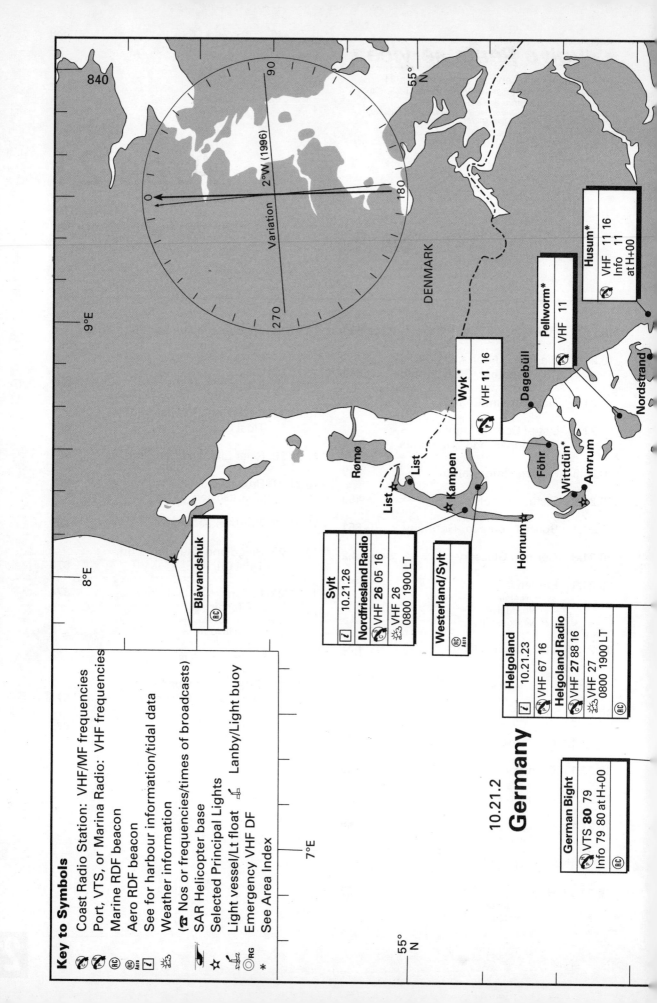

Key to Symbols

- Coast Radio Station: VHF/MF frequencies
- Port, VTS, or Marina Radio: VHF frequencies
- Marine RDF beacon
- Aero RDF beacon
- See for harbour information/tidal data
- Weather information
- (☎ Nos or frequencies/times of broadcasts)
- SAR Helicopter base
- Selected Principal Lights
- Light vessel/Lt float   Lanby/Light buoy
- Emergency VHF DF
- See Area Index

840

2°W (1996)

Variation

DENMARK

55° N

9°E

8°E

7°E

55° N

Blåvandshuk
(RC)

Rømø

List

List

Kampen

Hörnum

Westerland/Sylt
(RC) Aero

Sylt
| ℹ | 10.21.26 |

Nordfriesland Radio
☎ VHF 26 05 16
❄ VHF 26
0800 1900 LT

Helgoland
| ℹ | 10.21.23 |
📞 VHF 67 16

Helgoland Radio
☎ VHF 27 88 16
❄ VHF 27
0800 1900 LT
(RC)

Wyk*
📞 VHF 11 16

Föhr

Wittdün*

Amrum

Dagebüll

Pellworm*
📞 VHF 11

Nordstrand

Husum*
📞 VHF 11 16
Info 11
at H+00

German Bight
📞 VTS **80** 79
Info 79 80 at H+00

10.21.2
Germany

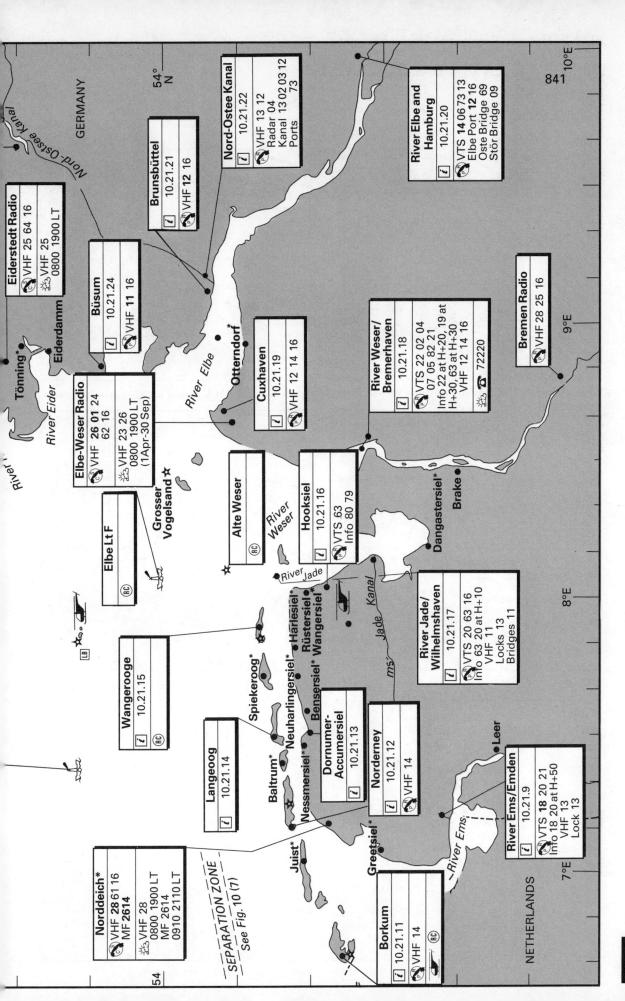

10-21-3   AREA 21 TIDAL STREAMS

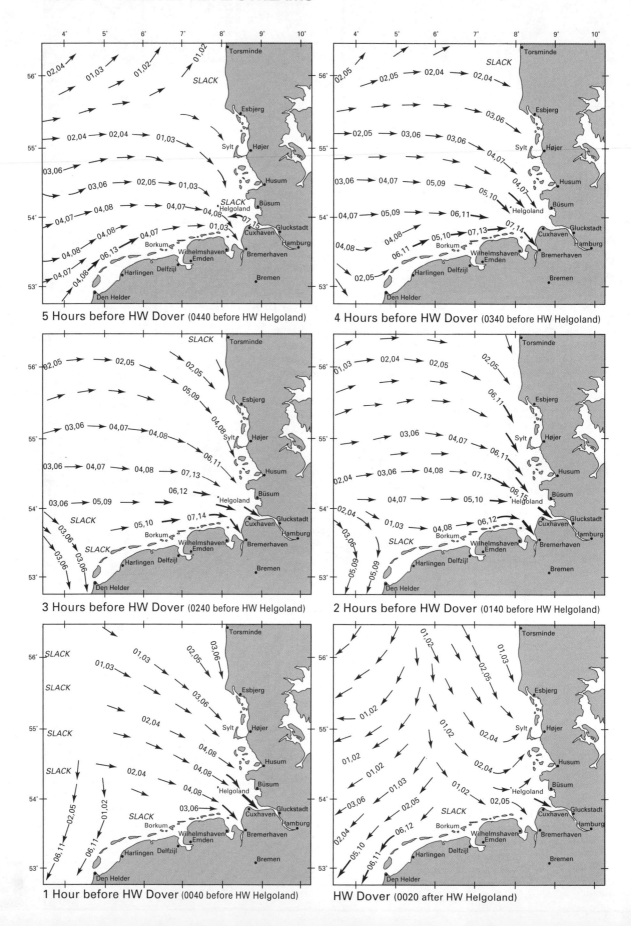

5 Hours before HW Dover (0440 before HW Helgoland)

4 Hours before HW Dover (0340 before HW Helgoland)

3 Hours before HW Dover (0240 before HW Helgoland)

2 Hours before HW Dover (0140 before HW Helgoland)

1 Hour before HW Dover (0040 before HW Helgoland)

HW Dover (0020 after HW Helgoland)

South-westward 10.20.3

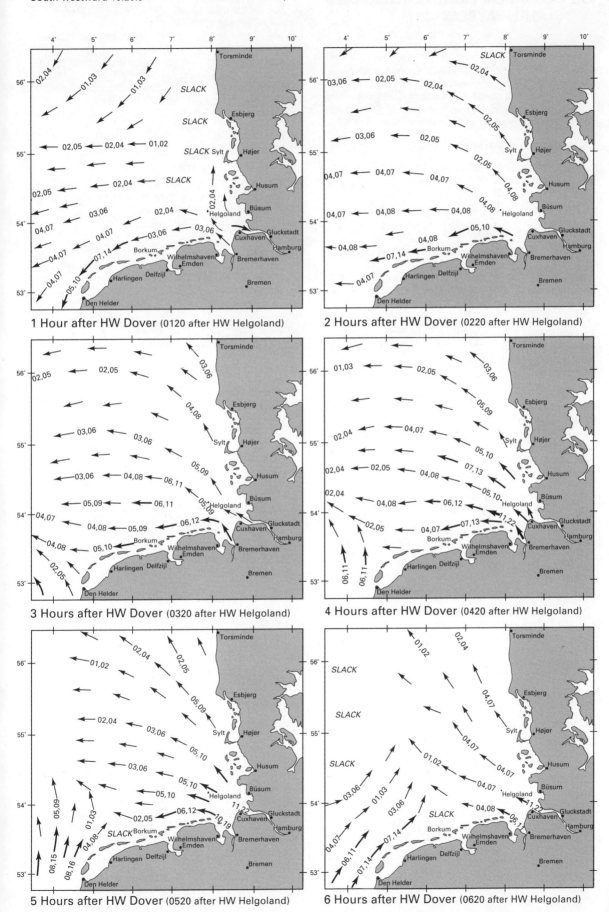

1 Hour after HW Dover (0120 after HW Helgoland)

2 Hours after HW Dover (0220 after HW Helgoland)

3 Hours after HW Dover (0320 after HW Helgoland)

4 Hours after HW Dover (0420 after HW Helgoland)

5 Hours after HW Dover (0520 after HW Helgoland)

6 Hours after HW Dover (0620 after HW Helgoland)

21

10.21.4 COASTAL LIGHTS, FOG SIGNALS AND WAYPOINTS

Abbreviations used below are given in 1.4.1. Principal lights are in **bold** print, places in CAPITALS, and light vessels, light floats and Lanbys in *CAPITAL ITALICS*. Unless otherwise stated lights are white. m – elevation in metres; M – nominal range in miles. Fog signals are in *italics*. Useful waypoints are underlined – use those on land with care. All geographical positions should be assumed to be approximate. See 4.4.1.

CROSSING THE NORTH SEA

GW 12 Lt By 54°13'·30N 07°22'·40E QR; PHM.
GW 8 Lt By 54°12'·90N 06°51'·20E Fl (2) R 9s; PHM.
GW 4 Lt By 54°12'·50N 06°20'·60E QR; PHM.
BG 2 Lt By 53°58'·42N 03°17'·50E L Fl R 10s; PHM.

RIVER EMS AND APPROACHES

Westerems Lt By 53°36'·98N 06°19'·50E Iso 4s; SWM; Racon (G).
Hubert Gat Lt By 53°34'·90N 06°14'·32E Iso 8s; *Whis*; SWM.
Borkum Grosser 53°35'·4N 06°39'·8E Fl (2) 12s 63m **24M**; brown Tr. F RWG 46m **W19M**, R15m, G15M; vis G107·4°-109°, W109°-111·2°, R111·2°-112·6°.

Borkum Kleiner 53°34'·78N 06°40'·08E FW 32m **30M**; R Tr, W bands; FW (intens) 089·9°-090·9° (Ldg sector for Hubertgat); Fl 3s; vis 088°-089·9°; Q (4) 10s; vis 090·9°-093°; RC; Iso Y 4s on tide gauge 420m SW.

BORKUM

Fischerbalje 53°33'·21N 06°43'·00E Oc (2) WRG 16s 15m **W16M**, R12M, G11M; W l Tr, R top and lantern, on tripod; vis R260°-313°, G313°-014°, W014°-068°, (Ldg sector to Fischerbalje), R068°-123°. Fog Det Lt.
Schutzhafen Ent 53°33'·52N 06°45'·11E FG 10m 4M, and FR 8m 4M.
Binnen-Randzel 53°30'·20N 06°49'·95E F WRG 14m W7M, R5M, G4M; B and Gy framework Tr, W tank; vis W 318°-345°, R345°-015·8°, W015·8°-033·5°, R033·5°-077·3°, W077·3°-098°, G098°-122°.

Campen 53°24'·39N 07°01'·00E F 62m **30M**; R framework Tr, 2 galleries, W central col, G cupola; vis 126·5°-127°. Fl 5s (same Tr); vis 126°-127°. Fl (4) 15s (same Tr) vis 127·3°-127·8°.

ALTE EMS

H11 By 53°34'·65N 06°33'·62E; SHM.
A2a By 53°32'·93N 06°39'·53E; PHM.
A3 By 53°32'·85N 06°39'·25E; SHM.
A5 By 53°31'·81N 06°39'·95E; SHM.
33/ Alte Ems II By 53°27'·80N 06°51'·38E; SHM.

EEMSHAVEN (Netherlands)

W Pier 53°27'·80N 06°50·15E FG 8m 3M.

DUKE GAT

No. 35 Lt By 53°27'·08N 06°52'·88E Fl G 4s; SHM.
No. 37 Lt By 53°26'·00N 06°55'·00E QG; SHM.
No. 41 Lt By 53°24'·32N 06°56'·80E Fl (2) G 9s; SHM.
No. 45 By 53°22'·05N 06°58'·57E; SHM.
No. 49 Lt By 53°20'·02N 06°59'·75E Oc (2) G 9s; SHM.

KNOCK

K4 Lt Buoy 53°19'·87N 07°00'·82E QR; PHM.
Knock 53°20'·37N 07°01'·50E F WRG 28m W12M, R9M, G8M; Gy Tr, four galleries, broad top, radar antenna; vis W270°-299°, R299-008·3°, G008·3°-023°, W023°-026·8°, R026·8°-039°, W039°-073°, R073°-119°, W119°-154°; Fog Det Lt.

DELFZIJL ENTRANCE (Netherlands)

W Mole Hd E ent 53°19'·10N 07°00'·38E FG; Ra refl.
E Mole Hd FR, In fog FY; *Horn 15s*.
Ldg Lts 203°. Front 53°18'·68N 07°00'·26E Iso 4s. Rear, 310m from front; Iso 4s.
Zeehavenkannaal, N side (odd numbered posts); 3 QG; 4 Fl G 2s, 6 Fl G 5s; R Refl.
Zeehavenkannaal, S side (even numbered posts); 1 Fl (2) R 6s; 1 Fl R 2s, 5 Fl R 5s, 1 QR; R Refl.
E side ent No. 21 (Marina ent) Fl G 5s; W post on dolphin.

TERMUNTERZIJL (Netherlands)

BW 13 By 53°18'·70N 07°03'·37E; SHM.
Wybelsum 53°20'·20N 07°06'·57E F WR 16m W6M, R5M; W framework Tr, R bands; radar antenna; vis W295°-320°, R320°-024°, W024°-049°; Fog Det Lt.

EMDEN

Logum Ldg Lts 075·2°. Front 53°20'·17N 07°08'·05E Oc (2) 12s 16m 12M; W mast, R bands. Rear, 630m from front, Oc (2) 12s 28m 12M; W mast, R bands; synch with front.
Ldg Lts 087·6°. Front 53°20'·07N 07°12'·15E Oc 5s 14m 14M; intens on Ldg line. Rear, 0·8M from front, Oc 5s 30m 14M; synch with front, intens on Ldg line.
Outer Hbr E pier Hd FG 7m 5M; Ra Refl.
W Pier Hd 53°20'·10N 07°10'·57E FR 10m 4M; Ra Refl; *Horn Mo (ED) 30s*.

RIVER EMS TO RIVER JADE, INCLUDING EAST FRISIAN ISLANDS.

OUTER LIMIT OF INSHORE TRAFFIC ZONE

TG1/Ems Lt By 53°43'·38N 06°22'·40E IQ. G 13s; SHM.
TG3 Lt By 53°44'·65N 06°31'·20E Fl (2) G 9s; SHM.
TG 5 Lt By 53°45'·90N 06°40'·10E Oc (3) G 12s; SHM.
TG 7 Lt By 53°47'·35N 06°49'·78E Fl (2) G 9s; SHM.
TG 9 Lt By 53°48'·45N 06°57'·80E Oc (3) G 12s; SHM.
TG11 Lt By 53°49'·64N 07°06'·60E Fl (2) G 9s; SHM.
TG13 Lt By 53°51'·00N 07°15'·50E Oc (3) G 12s; SHM.
TG15 Lt By 53°52'·20N 07°24'·35E Fl (2) G 9s; SHM.
TG17/JW 1 Lt By 53°53'·47N 07°33'·22E IQ 13s; SHM.
TG19/JW 2 Lt By 53°55'·10N 07°44'·60E Oc (3) G 12s; SHM.

BORKUMRIFF Lt By 53°47'·50N 06°22'·13E Oc (3) 15s; SWM; Racon.
GW/EMS Lt F 54°10'·00N 06°20'·80E Iso 8s 12m **17M**; *Horn Mo (EM) 30s*; Racon.

INSHORE ROUTE EMS TO JADE

Riffgat Lt By 53°38'·90N 06°27'·10E Iso 8s; SWM.
Oosterems Lt By 53°41'·94N 06°36'·20E Iso 4s; *Whis*; SWM.
Juisterriff -N Lt By 53°42'·90N 06°45'·82E Q; NCM.
Juist - N Lt By 53°43'·90N 06°55'·40E VQ; NCM.
53°40'·95N 07°03'·50E Aero Fl 5s 14m (occas).
Schluchter Lt By 53°44'·70N 07°04'·22E Iso 8s; SWM.
Dovetief Lt By 53°45'·38N 07°09'·80E Iso 4s; SWM.
Platform 54°42'·1N 07°10'·0E Mo(u) 15s 24m 9M; R platform, Y stripes; *Horn Mo(U) 30s*.
Norderney N Lt By 53°46'·10N 07°17'·22E Q; NCM.
Accumer Ee Lt By 53°46'·90N 07°24'·99E Iso 8s; SWM; *Bell*; (frequently moved).
Otzumer Balje Lt By 53°47'·95N 07°36'·20E Iso 4s; SWM (frequently moved).
Harle Lt By 53°49'·28N 07°49'·00E Iso 8s; SWM.
Juisterriff-N Lt By 53°42'·90N 06°45'·82E Q; NCM.

GREETSIEL
Meßstation Lt Bn 53°32'·97N 07°02'·22E Fl Y 4s 15m 3M.

JUIST
Training Wall, S end 53°39'·70N 06°59'·92E; pile; SCM.
Juist 53°41'·9N 07°03'·5E Aero Fl 5s 14m.
Schluchter Lt By 53°44'·70N 07°04'·22E Iso 8s; SWM.

NORDDEICH
W training wall, Hd 53°38'·7N 07°09'·0E FG 8m 4M;
G framework Tr, W lantern; vis 021°-327°.
E training wall Hd FR 8m 4M; R & W s on R Tr; vis 327°-237°.
Fog Lt.
Ldg Lts 144°. Front Iso WR 6s 6m W6M, R4M; B mast;
vis 078°-122°, W122°-150°. Rear, 140m from front, Iso 6s 9m
6M; B mast; synch with front.

NORDERNEY
Norderney 53°42'·6N 07°13'·8E Fl (3) 12s 59m **23M**; R 8
sided Tr; unintens 067°-077° and 270°-280°.
Fish Hbr Ldg Lts 274·5°. Front, W Mole Hd 53°41'·9N 07°09'·9E
Oc WR 4s 10m W7M, R4M; R&W Tr; vis W062°-093°, R093°-
259·5°, W259·°-289·5°, R289·5°-062°. Rear. 460m from front,
Oc 4s 18m 7M; Gy mast; synchronised with front.
Norderney–N Lt By 53°46'·10N 07°17'·22E Q; NCM.

BALTRUM
Baltrum groyne Hd 53°43'·3N 07°21'·7E Oc WRG 6s 7m
W6M, R4M, G3M; vis G 074·5°-090°, W090°-095°, R095°-
074·5°.

NESSMERSIEL
Mole N Hd 53°41'·9N 07°21'·7E Oc 4s 6m 5M; G mast.
Accumer Ee Lt By 53°46'·90N 07°24'·99E Iso 8s; SWM;
(frequently moved).

LANGEOOG
W Mole Hd 53°43'·42N 07°30'·13E Oc WRG 6s 8m W7M,
R5M, G4M; R basket on R mast; vis G 064°-070°, W070°-
074°, R074°-326°, W326°-330°, G330°-335°, R335°-064°;
Horn *Mo (L) 30s* (0730-1800LT).

DORNUMER-ACCUMERSIEL
W Bkwtr Hd 53°41'·25N 07°29'·40E.

BENSERSIEL
E training wall Hd 53° 41'·84N 07°32'·90E Oc WRG 6s 6m
W5M, R3M, G2M; vis G110°-119°, W119°-121°, R121°-
110°.
Ldg Lts 138°. Front Iso 6s 7m 9M. Rear, 167m from front,
Iso 6s 11m 9M. Both intens on Ldg line.

Otzumer Balje Lt By 53°47'·95N 07°36'·20E Iso 4s SWM
(frequently moved).

SPIEKEROOG
Spiekeroog 53°45'·0N 07°41'·3E FR 6m 4M; R mast;
vis 197°-114°.

NEUHARLINGERSIEL
Training wall Hd 53°43'·22N 07°42'·30E Oc 6s 6m 5M;
G mast.

HARLESIEL
Harle Lt By 53°49'·28N 07°49'·00E Iso 8s; SWM.
Carolinensieler Balje. Leitdamm 53°44'·13N 07°50'·10E
L Fl 8s 7m 6M; G mast.
N Mole Hd 53°42'·63N 07°48'·70E Iso R 4s 6m 7M.

WANGEROOGE
Wangerooge W end 53°47'·45N 07°51'·52E Fl R 5s 60m
23M; R Tr, 2 W bands; same Tr; F WRG 24m **W22M, W15M,
R17M,** R11M, **G18M,** G10M; vis R002°-011°, W011°-023°,
G023°-055°, W055°-060·5°, R060·5°-065·5°, W065·5°-071°,
G(18M) 119·4°-1138·8°, W(22M) 138·8°-152·2°, Ldg sector,
R (17M) 152·2°-159·9°; RC.
E Mole Hd 53°46'·50N 07°52'·17E FG.

RIVER JADE AND APPROACHES

JW5/Jade 1 Lt By 53°52'·47N 07°44'·10E Oc G 4s; SHM.
Weser 1/Jade 2 Lt By 53°52'·13N 07°47'·36E Fl (2+1) G 15s;
Racon (T); SHM.
Mellumplate 53°46'·35N 08°05'·60E F 27m **24M**; R □ Tr,
W band; vis 116·1°-116·4°; Ldg sector for outer part of
Wangerooger Fahrwasser. The following Lts are shown
from the same Tr over sectors indicated. Fl 4s **23M**; vis 114°-
115·2°. Fl (4) 15s; vis 117·2°-118·4°. Oc WRG 29m W14M,
R11M, G10M; vis R000°-006°, W006°-037·6°, G037·6°-114°,
R118·4°-168°, W168°-183·5°, R183·5°-212°, W212°-266°,
R266°-280°, W280°-000°. Mo(A) 7·5s; vis 115·2°-116·1°.
Ldg sector. Mo(N) 7·5s; vis116·4°-117·2°; Ldg sector.
Helicopter platform.
No. 7/Lt By 53°50'·30N 07°51'·24E Oc (3) G 12s; SHM.
No.11/Lt By 53°49'·23N 07°55'·08E Fl G 4s; SHM.
No.15/Blaue Balje Lt By 53°48'·13N 07°58'·88E IQ. G 13s;
SHM.
No.19 Lt By 53°47'·02N 08°01'·97E QG; SHM.
No.23 Lt By 53°45'·21N 08°02'·81E Oc (3) G 12s; SHM.
Minsener Oog, Buhne A N end 53°47'·30N 08°00'·45E
F WRG 16m W13M, R10M, G9M; □ Tr; vis R050°-055°,
W055°-132·6°, G132·6°-140·6°, W140·6°-158°, R158°-176°,
W176°-268°, G268°-303°, W303°-050°.
Oldoog, Buhne C 53°45'·40N 08°01'·35E Oc WRG 4s 25m
W13M, R10M, G9M; B col, W bands, Radar Tr (55m);
vis W153°-180°, G180°-203°, W203°-232°, R232°-274°,
W274°-033°; Fog Det Lt.
Schillig 53°41'·85N 08°01'·78E Oc WR 6s 15m **W15M,**
R12M; B pylon, W band; vis W195·8°-221°, R221°-254·5°,
W254·5°-278.3°.

Hooksielplate Cross Lt 53°40'·20N 08°09'·00E Oc WRG 3s
25m W7M, R5M, G4M, Radar Tr (55m), R bands; vis R345°-
358·8°, W358·8°-001·8°, G001·8°-012·4°, W012·4°-020·5°,
R020·5°-047·3°, W047·3°-061·9°, G061·9°-079·7°, W079·7°-
092·5°, R092·5°-110.5°; Fog Det Lt.
No. 31/Reede/W Siel 1 Lt By 53°41'·59N 08°04'·50E Oc (3) G
12s; SHM.

WANGERSIEL
No.37/Hooksiel Lt By 53°39'·38N 08°06'·63E IQ G 13s; SHM.

HOOKSIEL
H3 By 53°38'·68N 08°05'·42E; SHM.
Voslap Ldg Lts 164°35'. **Front** 53°37'·19N 08°06'·88E Iso
6s 15m **24M**; R Tr, W bands, R lantern; R Refl; intens on Ldg
line. **Rear,** 2·35M from front Iso 6s 60m **27M;** W Tr, R bands.
Same structure, Cross light F RWG 20m W9M, R6M, G5M;
vis W200°-228°, G228°-248°, W248°-269°, R269°-310°.
Tossens. Ldg Lts 146°. **Front** 53°34'·56N 08°12'·42E Oc 6s
15m **20M**; B Tr, W stripes, R lantern. **Rear,** 2M from front,
Oc 6s 51m **20M;** R Tr, W stripes, 3 galleries; Helicopter
platform.

WILHELMSHAVEN
Eckwarden Ldg Lts 154°. **Front, Solthörner Watt** 53°32'·45N
08°13'·09E Iso WRG 3s 15m **W19M,** W12M, R9M, G8M;
R Tr, W bands; vis R346°-348°, W348°-028°, R028°-052°;
W (intens) 052°-054° Ldg sector, G054°-067·5°, W067·5°-
110°, G110°-152·6°; W (intens) 152·6° across fairway, with

undefined limit on E side of Ldg line. **Rear**, 1·27M from front, Iso 3s 41m **21M;** R Tr & lantern; synch with front.
Neuer Vorhaven Ldg Lts 207°48'. Front Iso 4s 17m 11M; B mast, R lantern. Rear, 180m from front, Iso 4s 23m 11M; Y bldg; intens on Ldg line.
W Mole Hd Oc G 6s 15m 4M.
E Mole Hd Oc R 6s 5M.
Fluthaffen N Mole Hd 53°30'·91N 08°09'·40E F WG 9m W6M, G3M; G Tr; vis W216°-280°, G280°-010°, W010°-020°, G020°-130°.
Flutmole Hd FR 6m 5M.
Arngast Dir Lt 53°28'·91N 08°10'·97E F WRG 30m **W21M,** W10, **R16M, G17M,** G7M; R I Tr, W bands; vis: W135°-142°, G142°-150°, W150°-152°, G152°-160·3°, G168·8°-174·6°, R180·5°-191°, W191°-198·3°, W198·8°-213°, R213°-225°, W(10M) 286°-303°, G(7M) 303°-314°. Same structure Fl WG 3s **W20M,** vis: G174·6°-175·5°, W175·5°-176·4°. Same structure Fl (2) W 9s; vis: 177·4°-180·5°. Same structure Oc 6s; vis: 176·4°-177·4°.

DANGAST
Lock 53°26'·85N 08°06'·60E.

VARELER SIEL
Lock 53°24'·65N 08°11'·40E.

RIVER WESER AND APPROACHES

Weser Lt By 53°54'·25N 07°50'·00E Iso 5s 12m **17M;** SWM; Racon.
Schlüsseltonne Lt By 53°56'·30N 07°54'·87E Iso 8s; SWM.
Alte Weser 53°51'·85N 08°07'·72E F WRG 33m **W22M, R19M, G17M;** R Tr, 2 W bands, B base, floodlit; vis W288°-352°, R352°-003°, W003°-017°, Ldg sector for Alte Weser, G017°-045°, W045°-074°, G074°-118°, W118°-123°, Ldg sector for Alte Weser, R123°-140°, G140°-175°, W175°-183°, R183°-196°, W196°-238°; Fog Det Lt; RC; *Horn Mo (AL) 60s.*
Tegeler Plate, N end 53°47'·90N 08°11'·50E Oc (3) WRG 21m **W21M, R17M, G16M;** R Tr, gallery, W lantern, R roof; vis W329°-340°, R340°-014°, W014°-100°, G100°-116°, R119°-123°, G123°-144°, R147°-264°; same structure, Oc 6s **21M**; vis 116°-119°; Ldg sector for Neue Weser R119°-123°. Ldg sector for Alte Weser 147°-264°; Fog Det Lt.
Hohe Weg, NE part 53°42'·80N 08°14'·65E F WRG 29m **W19M, R16M, G15M;** R 8 sided Tr, 2 galleries, G lantern; vis W102°-138·5°, G138·5°-142·5°, W142·5°-145·5°, R145·5°-184°, W184°-278·5°; Fog Det Lt.
Robbennordsteert 53°42'·20N 08°20'·45E FWR 11m W10M, R7M; R column on tripod; vis W324°-004°, R004°-090°, W090°-121°.
Robbenplate Ldg Lts 122·3°. **Front**, 53°40'·92N 08°23'·06E Oc 15m **17M;** R tripod; intens on Ldg line. **Rear**, 0·54M from front, Oc 6s 37m **18M;** R Tr, 3 galleries, G lantern; vis 116°-125·5°; synch with front; Fog Det Lt.
Wremerloch Ldg Lts 140·1°. Front 53°38'·41N 08°25'·10E Iso 6s 15m12M; vis 132°-166°. Rear, 0·57M from front, Iso 6s 31m 14M; synch with front; Ra Refl.
Dwarsgat Ldg Lts 320·1°. Front 53°43'·15N 08°18'·55E Iso 6s 16m **15M**. **Rear** Iso 6s 31m **15M;** synch with front (same Ldg Line as Wremer Loch).
Langlütjen Ldg Lts 304·6°. Front 53°39'·50N 08°23'·07E   Oc 6s 15m 12M; B mast, B & W gallery; vis 288°-310°; Ra Refl. **Rear**, 0·5M from front, Oc 6s 31m **15M;** synch with front.
Imsum Ldg Lts 124·6°. Front 53°36'·42N 08°30'·59E Oc 6s 15m 13M; R tripod with gallery; **Rear,** 1·02M from front, Oc 6s 39m **16M;** synch with front.
Solthorn Ldg Lts 320·6°. Front 53°38'·34N 08°27'·39E Oc 6s 15m 13M; R&W mast. **Rear**, 700m from front, Iso 4s 31m **17M;** synch with front.

Fischeriehafen Ldg Lts 150·8°. **Common front** 53°31'·93N 08°34'·60E Oc 6s 17m **18M**, R J on W mast. **Rear**, 0·68M from front, Oc 6s 45m 18M 2 R Js on W mast, R bands; synch with front.
No. 61 Lt By 53°32'·28N 08°34'·04E QG; SHM; Km 66·0.

BREMERHAVEN
Vorhafen N Pier Hd 53°32'·19N 08°34'·57E FR 15m 5M.
S Pier Hd 53°32'·14N 08°34'·57E FG 15m 5M.

Nordenham Hafen N ent 53°28'·10N 08°29'·14E FG; Km 56·0.
Hafen von Brake Dir Lt 53°18'·88N 08°29'·27E Dir Iso WRG 4s 15m W9M, R7M, G7M; vis R345°-352·5°, W(intens) 352·5°-356°, G356°-360°; Km 40·5.
Hunte 1 Lt By 53°15'·50N 08°28'·95E IQG; SHM; Km 32·7.

BREMEN
Hasenbüren Sporthafen 53°07'·51N 08°40'·02E 2 FY (vert); Km 11·6.

GERMAN BIGHT

GERMAN BIGHT Lt F 54°10'·70N 07°26'·01E Iso 8s 12m **17M**; R hull marked D-B; RC; Racon; *Horn Mo (DB) 30s.*
D-B Weser Lt By 54°02'·42N 07°43'·05E Oc (3) R 12s; PHM; Racon.

HELGOLAND
Restricted area Helgoland-W By 54°10'·65N 07°48'·29E; WCM.
Helgoland-O Lt By 54°09'·00N 07°53'·57E Q (3) 10s; ECM; *Whis.*
Helgoland Lt Ho Fl 5s 82m **28M**; brown ■ Tr, B lantern, W balcony. FR on radio masts 180m SSE and 740m NNW. Cable Area Oc (3) WG 8s 18m W6M, G4M; W mast, R bands; vis W239°-244°, G244°-280°, W280°-285°.

Vorhafen. Ostmole, S elbow Oc WG 6s 5m W7M, G4M; G post; vis W203°-250°, G250°-109°; Fog Det Lt.
Ostmole Hd FG 7m 4M; vis 289°-180°; *Horn (3) 30s.*
Sudmole Hd Oc (2) R 12s 7m 4M; Gy post, R lantern; vis 101°-334°.
Binnenhafen Ldg Lts 302°. W Pier, Front Oc R 6s 8m 7M. Rear, 50m from front, Oc R 6s 10m 7M; synch with front.

DÜNE
Düne -S Lt By 54°09'·57N 07°56'·04E Q (6) + L Fl 15s; SCM. Ldg Lts 020°. Front Iso 4s 11m 8M; intens on Ldg line. Rear, 120m from front, Iso WRG 17m W11M, R10M, G10M; synch with front; vis G010°-018·5°, W018·5°-021°, R201°-030°, G106°-125°, W125°-130°, R130°-144°.
Sellebrunn -W Lt By 54°14'·43N 07°49'·83E Q (9) 15s; WCM; *Whis.*
Nathurn-N By 54°13'·40N 07°49'·05E; NCM.

RIVER WESER TO RIVER ELBE

Nordergründe-N Lt By 53°57'·08N 08°00'·17W VQ; NCM.
Westertill-N Lt By 53°58'·18N 08°06'·82E Q; NCM.
Scharnhörnriff-W Lt By 53°58'·53N 08°08'·80E Q (9) 15s; WCM.
Scharnhörnriff-N Lt By 53°58'·99N 08°11'·25E Q; NCM.

RIVER ELBE AND APPROACHES

ELBE 1 Lt F 54°00'·00N 08°06'·58E Iso 10s 12m **17M**; R hull and Lt Tr; RC; Racon (T); *Horn Mo(R) 30s;* H24.
Grosser Vogelsand 53°59'·78N 08°28'·68E Fl (3) 12s 39m **25M**; helicopter platform on R ● Tr, W bands; vis 085·1°-087·1°; Fog Det Lt. Same Tr, Iso 3s **26M**; vis 087·1°-091·1°. Oc 6s **26M**; vis 091·1°-095·1°. Fl (4) 15s **19M**; vis 095·1°-101·9°. Fl (4) R 15s 12M; vis 101·9°-105·1°. Fl R 3s **15M**; vis 113°-270°. Oc (4) R 18s 9M; vis 322·5°-012°; Fog Det Lt; *Horn Mo (VS) 30s.*

Neuwerk, S side 53°54'·95N 08°29'·85E L Fl (3) WRG 20s 39m **W16M**, R12M, G11M; vis G165·3°-215·3°, W215·3°-238·8°, R238·8°-321°, R343°-100°.
No.1 Lt By 53°59'·27N 08°13'·30E QG; SHM.
No.5 Lt By 53°59'·35N 08°19'·08E QG; SHM.
No.19 Lt By 53°57'·83N 08°34'·48E QG; SHM.
No.25 Lt By 53°56'·67N 08°38'·32E QG; SHM.

CUXHAVEN
Ldg Lts 151·2°. **Baumrönne**, front 53°51'·25N 08°44'·24E 1·55M from rear, Fl 3s 25m **17M**; W Tr, B band on gallery; vis 143·8°-149·2°. Same Tr, Iso 4s **17M**; vis 149·2°-154·2°. Fl (2) 9s **17M**; vis 154·2°-156·7°. **Altenbruch, common rear**, 53°49'·83N 08°45'·50E Iso 4s 58m **21M**; intens on Ldg line; synch with front. Same structure, Iso 8s 51m **22M**; synch with front. Crosslight Oc WR 44m W7M, R5M; vis 201·9°-232·8°, R232·8°-247·2°, W247·2°-254·6°.
Altenbruch Ldg Lts 261°. **Common front**, 53°50'·08N 08°47'·75E Iso 8s 19m **19M**; W Tr, B bands. Same structure, Iso WRG 8s W8M, R9M, G8M; vis G117·5°-124°, W124°-135°, R135°-140°. Rear, Wehldorf Iso 8s 31m 11M; W Tr, B bands; synch with front.
No.35 Lt By 50°50'·73N 08°45'·86E Oc (2) G 9s; SHM.
No.43 Lt By 53°50'·27N 08°52'·30E Oc (2) G 9s; SHM.

OTTERNDORF
Medem. Hadelner Kanal ent 53°50'·20N 08°53'·93E Fl (3) 12s 6m 5M; B △, on B col.

Balje Ldg Lts 130·8°. **Front** 53°51'·33N 09°02'·70E Iso 8s 24m **17M**; W Tr, R bands; vis G shore-080·5°, W080·5°-shore. **Rear** 1·35M from front, Iso 8s 54m **21M**; W Tr, R bands; intens on Ldg line; synch with front.
Zweidorf 53°53'·42N 09°05'·69E Oc R 5s 9m 3M; R □ on W pylon; vis 287°-107°.
No.51 Lt By 53°51'·07N 09°00'·22E QG; SHM.
No.57 Lt By 53°52'·55N 09°06'·38E QG SHM.

BRUNSBÜTTEL
Ldg Lts 065·5°. Front **Schleuseninsel** Iso 3s 24m **16M**; R Tr, W bands; vis North of 063·3°. Rear **Industriegebiet**, 0·9M from front, Iso 3s 46m **21M**; R Tr, W bands; synch with front.
Alterhaven N Mole (Mole 4) Hd 53°53'·29N 09°07'·59E F WR (vert) 15m W10M, R8M; vis R275·5°-079°, W079°-084°.

NORD-OSTSEE KANAL (KIEL CANAL), RENDSBURG/KIEL-HOLTENAU
No. 2/Obereider 1 Lt By 54°18'·95N 09°42'·71E Fl (2+1) R 15s; PHM.
Kiel Nordmole 54°21'·83N 10°09'·18E Oc (2) WR 9s 23m.
Tiessenkal Oc (3) WG 12s 22m.

FRIEBURG
Entrance Bn (unlit) 53°50'·25N 09°18'·90E; SHM.
Rhinplatte Nord 53°48'·09N 09°23'·36E Oc WRG 6s 11m W6M. R4M, G3M; vis: G122°-144°, W144°-150°, R150°-177°, W177°-122°; Ra refl.
STÖRLOCH/BORSFLETH, STÖR/BEIDENFLETH
Stör Ldg Lts 093·8°. Front 53°49'·29N 09°23'·91E Fl 3s 7m 6M; △ on R ● Tr. Rear, 200m from front, Fl 3s 12m 6M; synch with front.

GLÜCKSTADT
Glückstadt Ldg Lts 131·8° **Front** Iso 8s 15m **19M**; W Tr, R bands; intens on Ldg line. **Rear**, 0·68M from front, Iso 8s 30m **21M**; W Tr, R bands; intens on Ldg line.
N Mole Oc WRG 6s 9m W8M R6M, G5M; W Tr with gallery; vis R330°-343°, W343°-346°, G346°145°, W145°-150°,°, R150°-170°.
N Pier Hd 53°47'·15N 09°24'·58E FR 5m 4M. (FG on South Mole Hd).

Pagensand Ldg Lts 134·2° 53°42'·15N 09°30'·30E. Front Oc WRG 4s 18m W12M, W9M, R6M, G5M; W Tr, R bands; vis: R345°-356·5°, W356·5°-020°, G020°-075°. Rear, 500m from front, Oc 4s 35m 13M; Synch with front; intens on Ldg line.

STADE
Stadersand 53°37'·74N 09°31'·72E Iso 8s 20m 14M.

HAMBURG

HAMBURGER YACHT HAFEN, WEDEL
No. 122 Lt By 53°34'·20N 09°40'·68E Oc (2) R 9s; PHM.
E Ent E Pier Hd 53°34'·30N 09°40'·87E FG 3M.
(Both ent show FR & FG May to Oct).

SCHULAU
No. 123 Lt By 53°33'·90N 09°42'·05E Fl G 4s; SHM.
E Ent E Pier Hd 53°34'·14N 09°42'·05E FG.

NEUENSCHLEUSE
119/HN 1 LT By 53°34'·08N 09°39'·49E QG; SHM.

MÜHLENBERG
Ent E Pier Hd 53°33'·22N 09°49'·48E (unmarked).

TEUFELSBRÜCK
Ent Bkwtr Hd 53°32'·88N 09°52'·12E (unmarked).

RÜSCHKANAL
East Ent 53°32'·63N 09°51'·10E FR 8m 5M.

CITY SPORTHAFEN
Brandenburger Hafen ent 53°32'·56N 09°58'·88E Iso Or 2s.

RIVER ELBE TO DANISH BORDER

INSHORE ROUTE RIVER ELBE TO SYLT

Süderpiep Lt By 54°06'·00N 08°21'·90E Iso 8s; SWM; *Whis.*
Ausseneider Lt By 54°14'·04N 08°18'·21E Iso 4s; SWM.
Hever Lt By 54°20'·45N 08°18'·80E Oc 4s; SWM; *Whis.*
Rütergat Lt By 54°31'·02N 08°12'·00E Iso 8s; SWM.
Amrum Bank-S Lt By 54°32'·00N 08°04'·95E Q (6) + L Fl 15s; SCM.
Vortrapptief Lt By 54°35'·00N 08°12'·20E Oc 4s; SWM.
Amrum Bank -W Lt By 54°38'·00N 07°55'·40E Q (9) 15s; WCM.
Theeknobs -W Lt By 54°43'·52N 08°09'·95E Q (9) 15s; WCM.
Amrum Bank -N Lt By 54°45'·00N 08°07'·00E Q; NCM.
Lister Tief Lt By 55°05'·38N 08°16'·88E Iso 8s; SWM *Whis.*

BÜSUM
Süderpiep Lt By 54°06'·00N 08°21'·90E Iso 8s; SWM; *Whis.*
Büsum 54°07'·65N 08°51'·55E Oc (2) WRG 16s 22m **W17M**, R14M, G13M; vis W248°-317°, R317°-024°, W024°-084°, G084°-091·5°, W091·5°-093·5° Ldg sector for Süder Piep, R093·5°-097°, W097°-148°.
W Mole Hd Oc (3) R 12s 10m 4M; R Tr; FW Fog Det Lt.
E Mole Hd 54°07'·21N 08°51'·70E Oc (3) G 12s 10m 4M; G Tr; vis 260°-168°.
Ldg Lts 355°. Front 54°07'·53N 08°51'·58E Iso 4s 9m 13M; B mast, W bands. Rear, 110m from front, Iso 4s 12m 13M; synch with front.

RIVER EIDER
Ausseneider Lt By 54°14'·04N 08°18'·21E Iso 4s; SWM.
St Peter 54°17'·30N 08°39'·15E L Fl (2) WRG 15s 23m **W15M**, R13M, G11M; R Tr, B lantern; vis R271°-294°, W294°-325°, R325°-344°, W344°-035°, G035°-056·5°, W056·5°-068°, R068°-091°, W091°-113°, G113°-115°, W115°-116°, Ldg sector for Mittelhever, R116°-130°.

Eiderdamm Lock, N Mole, W end Oc (2) R 12s 8m 5M; W Tr.
S Mole, W end Oc G 6s 8m 5M: W Tr, gy top.

TÖNNING
W Mole Hd FR 5m 4M; R col.
Quay 54°18'·95N 08°57'·12E FG 5m 4M; G col.

RIVER HEVER
Hever Lt By 54°20'·45N 08°18'·80E Oc 4s; SWM; *Whis*.
No. 3 Lt By 54°20'·69N 08°23'·12E Fl G 4s; SHM.
No. 8 Lt By 54°21'·39N 08°27'·11E Fl R 4s; PHM.
Norderhever Lt By 54°22'·52N 08°30'·80E Fl (2+1) R 15s; PHM.
Westerheversand 54°22'·45N 08°38'·50E Oc (3) WR 15s
41m **W21M**, **R16M**; R Tr, W bands; vis W012·2°-089°, R089°-
107°, W107°-155·5°, R155·5°-169°, W169°-206·5°, R206·5°-
218·5°, W218.5°-233°, R233°-248°.

HUSUM
Husumer Al Outer Ldg Lts 106·5°.   Front 54°28'·57N
09°00'·78E Iso R 8s 8m 5M; R mast, W bands; intens on Ldg
line. Rear, 0·52M from front, Iso R 8s 17m 6M; Y mast; synch
with front.
Inner Ldg Lts 090°. Front 54°28'·79N 09°00'·32E Iso G 8s 7m
3M; R mast, W bands; intens on Ldg line. Rear, 40m from
front, Iso G 8s 9m 3M; intens on Ldg line; synch with front.

NORDSTRAND
Strucklahnungshörn, W Mole Hd 54°30'·00N 08°48'·5E Oc G
6s 8m 2M.

PELLWORM
Pellworm S side Ldg Lts 041°. **Front** 54°29'·82N 08°40'·05E
Oc WR 5s 14m **W20M**, W11M, R8M. Intens on Ldg line;
vis W303·5°-313·5°, R313.5°-316·5°. **Rear**, 0·8M from front,
Oc 5s 38m **20M**; R Tr, W band; synch with front. Same Tr as
rear Lt, Cross Light Oc WR 5s 38m W14M, W9M, R11M,
R6M; vis R(11M) 122·6°-140°, W(14M) 140°-161·5°, R(11M)
161·5°-179·5°, W(14M) 179·5°-210·2°, R(6)M 255°-265·5°,
W9M 265·5°-276°, R(6)M 276°-297°, W(9)M 297°-307°.

WITTDÜN, AMRUM
Rütergat Lt By 54°31'·02N 08°12'·00E Iso 8s; SWM.
Amrum Hafen Ldg Lts 272·9°. Front 54°37'·88N 08°22'·92E
Iso R 4s 11m 10M; W mast, R stripe; intens on Ldg Line.
Rear, 0·9M from front, Iso R 4s 33m **15M**.
Amrum 54°37'·90N 08°21'·36E Fl 7·5s 63m **23M**; R Tr,
W bands.
Wriakhorn Cross Lt 54°37'·62N 08°21'·22E L Fl (2) WR 15s
26m W9M, R7M; vis W297·5°-319°, R319°-343°, W343°-
014°, R014°-034°.
Nebel 54°38'·75N 08°21'·75E Oc WRG 5s 16m **W20M**,
R15M; **G15M**; R Tr, W band; vis R255·5°-258·5°, W258·5°-
260·5°, G260·5°-263·5°.
Norddorf 54°40'·19N 08°18'·60E Oc WRG 6s 22m **W15M**,
R12M, G11M; W Tr, R lantern; vis W009-032°, G032-034°,
W034°-036·8°. Ldg sector, R036·8°-099°, W099°-156°, R156°-
176·5°, W176·5-178·5°, G178·5°-188°, G(unintens) 188°-202°,
W(partially obscd) 202°-230°.

LANGENESS
Nordmarsch 54°37'·58N 08°31'·85E F WR 13m W14M,
R11M; Dark Brown Tr; vis W268°-279°, R279°-306°,
W306°-045°, R045°-070°, W070°-218°.

OLAND
Near W Pt 54°40'·51N 08°41'·28E F WRG 12m W13M,
R10M, G9M; R Tr; G086°-093°, W093°-160°, R160°-172°.

SCHLÜTTSIEL
Schl No. 20 By 54°40'·83N 08°44'·60E; PHM.
Harbour ent, S side 54°40'·89N 08°45'·10E; SHM.

WYK, FÖHR
Nieblum 54°41'·10N 08°29'·20E Oc (2) WRG 10s 11m
W19M, R15M, G15M; R Tr, W band; vis G028°-031°, W031°-
032·5°, R032·5°-035·5°.

DAGEBÜLL
Dagebüllhaven 53°43'·82N 08°41'·43E Iso WRG 8s 23m
W18M, **R15M**, **G15M**; G mast; vis G042°-043°, W043°-
044·5°, R044·5°-047°.
FW Lts shown on N and S mole Hd.

SYLT
Theeknobs-W Lt By 54°43'·52N 08°09'·95E Q (9) 15s; WCM.
Hörnum Odde Lt By 54°44'·20N 08°18'·00E QR; PHM.
Hörnum Ldg Lts 012·5°. Front 54°44'·82N 08°17'·45E Iso 8s
20m 14M; R Tr, W band; intens on Ldg line. **Rear, Hörnum**
54°45'·29N 08°17'·60E Iso 8s 45m **15M**; R Tr, W band; synch
with front; intens on Ldg line. Same Tr Fl (2) 9s 48m **20M**.
N Pier Hd FG 6m 3M; vis 024°-260°.
South Mole Hd 54°45'·57N 08°17'·97E FR 7m 4M; R mast.
Kampen, Rote Kliff 54°56'·87N 08°20'·50E Oc (4) WR 15s
62m **W20M**, R16M, W Tr, B band; vis W193°-260°,
W(unintens) 260°-339°, W339°-165°, R165°-193°.
Lister Tief Lt By 55°05'·38N 08°16'·88E Iso 8s; SWM *Whis*.

Ellenbogen N end, List West 55°03'·25N 08°24'·19E Oc
WRG 6s 19m W14M, R11M, G10M; W Tr, R lantern; vis
R040°-133°, W133°-196°, R196°-210°, W210°-227°, R227°-
266·4°, W266·4°-268°, G268°-285°, W285°-310°, W(unintens)
310°-040°.
N side, List Ost 55°03'·00N 08°26'·70E Iso WRG 6s 22m
W14M, R11M, G10M; W Tr, R band; vis W(unintens) 010·5°-
098°, W098°-262°, R262°-278°, W278°-296°, R296°-323·3°,
W323·3°-324·5°, G324·5°-350°, W350°-010·5°, Q 4M on Tr
9·4M NNE shown when firing takes place.

List Land 55°01'·07N 08°26'·47E Oc WRG 3s 13m W12M,
R9M, G8M; W mast, R band; vis W170°-203°, G203°-212°,
W212°-215·5°, R215·5°-232·5°, W232·5°234°, G234°-243°,
W243°-050°.

List Hafen N Mole Hd 55°01'·03N 08°26'·52E FG 5m 3M;
G mast; vis 218°-038°.
S Mole 55°01'·01N 08°26'·51E FR 5m 4M; R mast; vis 218°-
353°.

10.21.5 PASSAGE INFORMATION

Refer to: Admiralty Pilot *North Sea (East); Cruising Guide to Germany and Denmark* (Imray/Navin) and *Frisian Pilot* (Adlard Coles/Brackenbury). For German Glossary, see 1.4.2.

RIVER EMS (charts 3509, 3510)

The River Ems forms the boundary between Netherlands and Germany, and is a major waterway leading to Eemshaven, Delfzijl (10.20.33), Emden (10.21.13), Leer and Papenburg. Approach through Hubertgat or Westerems, which join W of Borkum; the latter is advised at night. Both are well buoyed but can be dangerous with an ebb stream and a strong W or NW wind. The flood begins at HW Helgoland + 0530, and the ebb at HW Helgoland – 0030, sp rates 1·5kn.

From close SW of Borkum the chan divides: Randzel Gat to the N and Alte Ems running parallel to it to the S – as far as Eemshaven on the S bank. About 3M further on the chan again divides. Bocht van Watum is always varying so keep in main chan, Ostfriesisches Gatje, for Delfzijl and beyond. Off Eemshaven the stream runs 2-3kn.

Osterems is the E branch of the estuary of R. Ems, passing between Borkum and Memmert. It is poorly marked, unlit and much shallower than Westerems. It also gives access to the Ley chan, leading to the hbr of Greetsiel (10.21.9). But it is not advised except with local knowledge and in ideal weather.

RIVER EMS TO RIVER JADE (chart 3761)

The route to seaward of the Frisian Is from abeam Borkum to the E end of Wangerooge is about 50 miles. This is via the ITZ, S of the Terschellinger-German Bight TSS, Fig. 10 (7), the E-going lane of which is marked on its S side by SHM buoys lettered DB1, DB3, DB5 etc. About 4M S of this line of buoys the landward side of the ITZ is marked by landfall buoys showing the apprs to the eight main seegaten between the East Frisian Is. There are major lts on Borkum, Norderney and Wangerooge. Near the TSS the E-going stream begins at HW Helgoland – 0500, and the W-going at HW Helgoland + 0100, sp rates 1·2kn. Inshore the stream is influenced by the flow through the seegaten.

THE EAST FRISIAN ISLANDS (chart 3761)

The East Frisian Is have fewer facilities for yachtsmen than the Dutch Is to the W, and most of them are closer to the mainland. For general notes, see 10.20.5 and 10.21.10. For navigating inside the islands, in the so-called watt chans, it is essential to have the large scale pleasure craft charts and to understand the system of channel marking. Withies, unbound (⚲ with twigs pointing up) are used as PHMs, and withies which are bound (⚵ with twigs pointing down) as SHMs. Inshore of the Is the *conventional direction of buoyage is always from West to East*, even though this may conflict with the actual direction of the flood stream in places.

Borkum (10.21.11 and chart 3509) lies between Westerems and Osterems, with high dunes each end so that at a distance it looks like two separate islands. Round the W end of Borkum are unmarked groynes, some extending 2¾ca offshore. Conspic landmarks include Grosse bn and Neue bn, a water tr, Borkum Grosser lt ho, Borkum Kleiner lt ho, and a disused lt ho; all of which are near the W end of the island.

Memmert on the E side of Osterems is a bird sanctuary, and landing is prohibited. There are Nature Reserves (entry prohibited) inshore of Baltrum, Langeoog and the W end of Spiekeroog (chart 1875). **Juist** (10.21.10) is the first of the chain of similar, long, narrow and low-lying islands. Most have groynes and sea defences on their W and NW sides. Their bare sand dunes are not easy to identify, so the few conspic landmarks must be carefully selected. Shoals extend seaward for 2M or more in places. The seegaten between the islands vary in position and depth, and all of them are dangerous on the ebb tide, even in a moderate onshore wind. Norderneyer Seegat is a deep chan close W of **Norderney**,

but it is approached across dangerous offshore shoals, through which lead two shallow buoyed channels, Dovetief and Schluchter. Dovetief is the main chan, but Schluchter is more protected from the NE. Depths vary considerably and at times the chans silt up. Neither should be used in strong winds. Further inshore, Norderneyer Seegat leads round the W end of the island to the harbour of Norderney (10.21.12). Beware groynes and other obstructions along the shore.

SW of Norderney, Busetief leads in a general S direction to the tidal hbr of Norddeich (10.21.9), which can also be approached with sufficient rise of tide from Osterems through the Norddeich Wattfahrwasser with a depth of about 2m at HW. Busetief is deeper than Dovetief and Schluchter, and is buoyed. The flood begins at HW Helgoland – 0605, and the ebb at HW Helgoland – 0040, sp rates 1kn.

Baltrum (10.21.10) is about 2·5M long, very low in the E and rising in the W to dunes only about 15m high. With local knowledge and only in good weather it could be approached through Wichter Ee, a narrow unmarked channel between Norderney and Baltrum; but it is obstructed by drying shoals and a bar and is not advised. A small pier and groyne extend about 2ca from the SW corner of Baltrum. The little hbr dries, and is exposed to the S and SW. Southwards from Wichter Ee, the Nessmersiel Balje, with buoys on its W side prefixed by 'N', leads to the sheltered hbr of Nessmersiel (10.21.9).

Proceeding E, the next major chan through the islands is Acummer Ee between Baltrum and **Langeoog**. Shoals extend 2M offshore, depths in chan vary considerably and it is prone to silting; it is marked by buoys prefixed with 'A', moved as necessary. In onshore winds the sea breaks on the bar and the chan should not be used. Apart from Langeoog (10.21.14), Accumer Ee gives access to the mainland hbrs of Dornumer-Accumersiel (10.21.13) and Bensersiel (10.21.15).

Between Langeoog and **Spiekeroog**, the buoyed Westerbalje and Otzumer Balje chans lead inward. The latter is normally the deeper (0·7m–2·0m) but both chans may silt up and should be used only in good weather and on a rising tide.

Harle chan (buoys prefixed by 'H') leads W of **Wangerooge** (10.21.15), but beware Buhne H groyne which extends 7½ca WSW from end of Is to edge of fairway. Dove Harle (buoys prefixed by 'D') leads to the hbr. In bad weather Harlesiel, 4M S on the mainland shore, is a more comfortable berth.

Blau Balje leads between the E end of Wangerooge and **Minsener Oog**. Although marked by buoys (prefixed 'B' and moved as necessary) this chan is dangerous in N winds and there is a prohib area (15 May–31 Aug) S of the E end of Wangerooge for the protection of seals.

RIVER JADE (charts 3368, 3369)

To the E of Wangerooge and Minsener Oog lie the estuaries of R. Jade and R. Weser. Although not so hazardous as R. Elbe, the outer parts of both rivers can become very rough with wind against tide, and are dangerous on the ebb in strong NW winds. The Jade is entered from Jade 1 buoy via the Wangerooger Fahrwasser (buoyed) which leads SSE past Wangersiel and the yachting centre of Hooksiel (10.21.16) to Wilhelmshaven (10.21.17). To the S of Wilhelmshaven, the Jadebusen is a large, shallow area of water, through which chans run to the small hbrs of Dangastersiel and Vareler Siel.

RIVER WESER (charts 3368, 3405, 3406, 3407)

The River Weser is an important waterway leading to the ports of Bremerhaven, Nordenham, Brake and Bremen which in turn connect with the inland waterways. The upper reaches, *Unterweser*, run from Bremen to Bremerhaven (10.21.17) and below Bremerhaven the *Aussenweser* flows into a wide estuary split by two main chans, Neue Weser and Alte Weser. The position and extent of sandbanks vary: on the W side they tend to be steep-to, but on the E side there are extensive shoals (e.g. Tegeler Plate).

Weser lt buoy marks the approach from NW to Neue Weser (the main fairway) and Alte Weser which are separated by Roter Sand and Roter Grund, marked by the disused Roter

21

Sand lt tr (conspic). Both chans are well marked and they join about 3M S of Alte Weser lt tr (conspic). From this junction Hohewegrinne (buoyed) leads inward in a SE direction past Tegeler Plate lt tr (conspic) on the NE side and Hohe Weg lt tr (conspic) to the SW; here it is constrained by training walls. In the Aussenweser the stream, which runs over 3kn at sp, often sets towards the banks and the branch chans which traverse them.

The Weser-Elbe Wattfahrwasser is a demanding, but useful inshore passage between R. Weser and R. Elbe. It leads NNE from the Wurster Arm (E of Hohe Weg), keeping about 3M offshore; SE of Neuwerk and around Cuxhaven training wall. It normally requires two tides, but there are suitable anchs.

RIVER ELBE (charts 3261, 3262, 3266, 3268)

Yachts entering the Elbe are probably bound for the Nord-Ostsee Kanal ent at Brunsbüttel (10.21.21). See 10.21.19 for Cuxhaven and 10.21.20 for for up-river to Hamburg. From E end of TSS the chan is well marked by buoys and bn trs. Commercial traffic is very heavy. At Elbe 1 lt Float the E-going (flood) stream begins at HW Helgoland – 0500, and the W-going (ebb) stream at HW Helgoland + 0500, sp rates 2kn. The stream runs harder N of Scharnhörn, up to 3·5kn on the ebb, when the Elbe estuary is dangerous in strong W or NW winds.

ELBE TO NORTH FRISIAN ISLANDS (charts 1875, 3767)

The W coast of Schleswig-Holstein is flat and marshy, with partly-drying banks extending 5-10M offshore. Between the banks and Is, the chans change frequently. Süderpiep and Norderpiep lead to Büsum (10.21.24) and Meldorfer Hafen, joining S of Blauort. Norderpiep has a bar (depth 3m) and is unlit; Süderpiep is deeper and preferable in W'lies. Landmarks from seaward are Tertius bn and Blauortsand bn, and a conspic silo at Büsum.

Approaching R. Eider from seaward, find the Ausseneider lt buoy, about 6M W of the buoyed ent chan. The ent can be rough in W winds, and dangerous in onshore gales. St Peter lt ho is conspic on N shore. Here the estuary winds up to the Eiderdamm, a storm barrage with a lock (H24) and sluices. Tönning is about 5M up-river. The upper Eider parallels the Nord-Ostsee Kanal which it joins at Gieselau.

The R. Hever consists of several chans on the N side of Eiderstedt Peninsula, and S of the North Frisian Islands of **Süderoogsand** and **Pellworm**. Mittelhever is the most important of the three buoyed chans through the outer grounds, all of which meet SE of Süderoogsand before they separate once more into Heverstrom leading to Husum (10.21.24), and Norderhever which runs NE between Pellworm and Nordstrand into a number of watt channels. Schmaltief and Rütergat give access to **Amrum** (hbr on SE side), to Wyk on the E side of **Fohr** and to Dagebüll.

Sylt (10.21.26) is the largest of the N Frisian Islands, almost 20M long from S to N. It has a straight seaward coast, and a peninsula on its E side connects by Hindenburgdamm to the mainland. Vortrapptief is the chan inward between Amrum and Sylt, leading to Hörnum Hafen. It has a depth of about 4m (subject to frequent change) and is buoyed and lit. The area should not be approached in strong W winds. The flood (ESE-going) stream begins at HW Helgoland – 0350, and the ebb (WNW-going) at HW Helgoland + 0110, sp rates 2·5kn.

Lister Tief is the chan between the N end of Sylt and the Danish island of **Romo**; it gives access to List Roads and hbr as well as to Danish hbrs. Lister Tief is well buoyed, with a least depth over the bar of about 4m. In relative terms it is the safest chan on this coast (after Süderpiep), available for yachts seeking anch under the lee of Sylt in strong W winds (when however there would be a big swell over the bar on the ebb). Beware buoyed obstructions (ODAS), 18M WSW of List West lt ho.

FROM GERMAN BIGHT TO UK (charts 2182A, 1405, 3761, 2593, 1505)

From the Elbe, Weser and Jade estuaries, skirt the E ends of TSS to take departure from Helgoland (10.21.23). Thence parallel the N side of TSS, Fig 10 (7), towards Botney Ground (BG2 buoy) if heading to ports north of the Humber. If bound for the Thames Estuary or down Channel, it is advisable to follow the ITZ westwards until well S of Texel (TX 1 lt buoy); thence take departure westward from the Netherlands (see 10.20.5). The edges of the TSS are well marked by lt buoys. Avoid areas of offshore industrial activity (10.5.5). West of German Bight streams run approx E/W, spring rates under 1kn. For distances across the N. Sea, see 10.0.7.

10.21.6   DISTANCE TABLE

Approximate distances in nautical miles are by the most direct route, whilst avoiding dangers and allowing for Traffic Separation Schemes. Places in *italics* are in adjoining areas; places in **bold** are in 10.0.7, Distances across the North Sea.

		1	2	3	4	5	6	7	8	9	10	11	12	13	14	15	16	17	18	19	20
1.	*Den Helder*	1																			
2.	*Delfzijl*	115	2																		
3.	Borkum	95	22	3																	
4.	Emden	125	10	32	4																
5.	Norderney	115	41	31	47	5															
6.	Langeoog	130	56	46	63	18	6														
7.	Wangerooge	148	65	55	80	29	21	7													
8.	**Helgoland**	153	81	67	85	44	35	24	8												
9.	Hooksiel	150	83	71	97	44	34	19	35	9											
10.	**Wilhelmshaven**	159	89	80	106	53	43	27	43	9	10										
11.	**Bremerhaven**	180	100	88	115	62	47	38	44	36	45	11									
12.	Cuxhaven	175	105	95	120	69	60	42	38	47	56	58	12								
13.	**Brunsbüttel**	192	120	110	137	84	77	55	51	64	70	78	17	13							
14.	Kiel/Holtenau	245	173	163	190	137	130	108	104	117	123	131	70	53	14						
15.	Hamburg	229	159	104	174	81	114	61	88	101	110	81	54	37	90	15					
16.	Husum	198	127	105	137	85	77	52	47	73	82	82	66	76	129	113	16				
17.	Hörnum Lt (Sylt)	192	119	97	129	77	72	60	38	69	78	80	63	75	128	112	48	17			
18.	*Esbjerg*	187	155	133	165	123	119	109	83	116	125	127	110	126	179	163	95	47	18		
19.	*Thyboron*	322	222	200	232	186	204	178	154	301	310	201	200	196	249	233	163	120	90	19	
20.	*Skagen*	378	327	305	342	291	308	283	259	405	414	306	304	301	231	338	268	225	195	104	20

SPECIAL NOTES FOR GERMANY   10-21-7

LANDS are given in place of the 'counties' in the UK.

CHARTS: German charts are issued by the Bundesamt für Seeschiffahrt und Hydrographie (BSH), Hamburg. In this almanac those prefixed 'D' are standard German nautical charts. The BSH prefix refers to the 3000 Series of charts for pleasure craft. These are a convenient size (42 x 59cm) and are stowed in a clear polythene envelope; each set has up to 16 sheets at medium/large scale. All charts are corrected by Nachrichten für Seefahrer (NfS) = Notices to Mariners. Where possible the AC, Imray and Dutch chart numbers are also quoted.

TIME ZONE is –0100, which is allowed for in the tidal predictions, but no provision is made for daylight saving schemes which are indicated by the non-shaded areas on the tide tables (see 9.1.2).

LIGHTS: In coastal waters particular use is made of light sectors. A ldg or Dir sector (usually W, and often intens) may be flanked by warning sectors to show the side on which the vessel has deviated: If to port, a FR lt or a Gp Fl W lt with an even number of flashes; if to stbd, a FG lt or a Gp Fl W lt with an odd number of flashes. Crossing lts with R, W and G sectors may indicate the limits of roadsteads, turning points in chans etc.

SIGNALS: Local port, tidal, distress and traffic signals are given where possible:

Light signals

Ⓡ Ⓡ	= Passage/entry prohib.
Ⓡ	= Be prepared to pass or enter.
Ⓦ Ⓡ Ⓡ	= Bridge closed or down; vessels which can pass under the available clearance may proceed, but beware of oncoming tfc which has right of way.
Ⓦ Ⓦ Ⓡ Ⓡ	= Lift bridge will remain at first step; vessels which can pass under the available vertical clearance may proceed.
Ⓖ Ⓖ	= Passage/entry permitted; oncoming tfc stopped.
Ⓦ Ⓖ Ⓖ	= Passage permitted, but beware of oncoming traffic which may have right of way.
Ⓡ Ⓡ	= Bridge, lock or barrage closed to navigation.
Ⓡ	= Exit from lock prohib.
Ⓖ	= Exit from lock permitted.

Visual storm signals in accordance with the International System (see 10.14.7) are shown at: Borkum, Norderney, Norddeich, Accumersiel, Bensersiel, Bremerhaven, Brunsbüttel, Die Oste, Glückstadt, Stadersand, Hamburg, Büsum, Tönning, Husum, Wyk, List and Helgoland.

Signals hoisted at masts

By day	By night	Meaning
R cylinder	Ⓦ Ⓡ Ⓦ Ⓡ	= Reduce speed to minimize wash.
● ● ▼	Ⓦ Ⓡ Ⓡ Ⓖ	= Fairway obstructed.
● ▼ ▲ (or R board with W band)	Ⓡ Ⓖ Ⓦ	= Chan permanently closed.

When motoring under sail, always display a motoring ▼. Rule 25e is strictly enforced and non-compliance will incur a fine.

HARBOURS: There are no commercially run marinas. Most yacht hbrs are owned by the state or community and run by a local Yacht Club (as in Belgium and the Netherlands).

BROADCASTS: Information broadcasts by VTS centres and associated communications, see Fig 10 (7).

TELEPHONES: To call UK from Germany, dial 00 44; then the UK area code, but omitting the prefix 0, followed by the number required.
To call Germany from UK, dial 00-49 and desired number.

EMERGENCIES: Police: dial 110. Fire, Ambulance: dial 112.

MARINE RESCUE CO-ORDINATION CENTRES: Coast station, Elbe-Weser Radio ☎ (04721) 22066. Kiel Radio, ☎ (0431) 39011. Norddeich Radio, ☎ (04931) 1831.

WEATHER FORECASTS: Similar to the British Marinecall; from 1 April –30 Sept, forecast and outlook are available by dialling 0190 1160 plus two digits for the following areas:

-40 = Inland pleasure craft;
-45 = North Frisian Islands and Helgoland;
-46 = R Elbe from Elbe 1/Cuxhaven to Hamburg;
-47 = Weser estuary and Jade Bay;
-48 = East Frisian Islands and Ems estuary;
-53 = For foreign pleasure craft;
-54 = Denmark;
-55 = Netherlands.

For year round weather synopsis, forecast and outlook, dial 0190 1169 plus two digits as follows:
-20 = General information;
-21 = North Sea and Baltic;
-22 = German Bight and SW North Sea;
-31 = 5 day bulletin for North Sea and Baltic, containing an outlook and forecasts of wind, sea state, air and water temperature, plus warnings of fog, thunderstorms etc.

Strong wind (>F6) and storm warnings for the German North Sea coast may be obtained from ☎ 040 3 196628 (H24); if no warnings are in force, a wind forecast is given.

PUBLIC HOLIDAYS: New Year's Day, Good Friday, Easter Monday, Labour Day (1 May), Ascension Day, Whit Monday, Day of German Unity (3 Oct), Christmas Day and Boxing Day.

NATIONAL WATER PARKS exist in the Wadden Sea areas (tidal mud flats) of Lower Saxony, (excluding the Jade and Weser rivers and the Ems-Dollart estuary), and along the west coast of Schleswig-Holstein. Conservation of the ecology is the prime aim. The Parks (shown on AC & BSH charts) are divided into 3 zones with certain rules:
Zone 1 comprises the most sensitive areas (about 30%) where yachts must keep to buoyed chans, except HW±3. Speed limit 8kn.
Zone 2: A buffer zone.
Zone 3: The remainder. No special constraints exist in Zones 2 and 3.

CUSTOMS: Entry hbrs are Borkum, Norderney, Norddeich, Wilhelmshaven, Bremerhaven, Cuxhaven. Not Helgoland.

GAS: Sometimes Calor gas bottles can be re-filled. German 'Flussig' gas can be used with Calor regulators.

CURRENCY: 1 Deutsche Mark = 100 Pfennig.

USEFUL ADDRESSES: German National Tourist Office, 65 Curzon St, London W1Y 7PE; ☎ 0891 600100 (recorded info); Fax 0171-495 6129. German Embassy, 23 Belgrave Sq, Chesham Place, London SW1X 8PX (☎ 0171-235 5033).

10.21.8 GERMAN GLOSSARY: See 1.4.2.

EMDEN 10-21-9

Niedersächsen, Ostfriesland, 53°20'·10N 07°10'·80E

CHARTS
AC 3510; BSH 90, 91, 3012 sheets 5 & 6

TIDES
HW +0022 on Dover (UT); ML 1·9m; Zone – 0100

Standard Port HELGOLAND (⟶)

Times				Height (metres)			
High Water		Low Water		MHWS	MHWN	MLWN	MLWS
0200	0700	0200	0800	2·7	2·3	0·4	0·0
1400	1900	1400	2000				
Differences EMDEN							
+0041	+0028	–0011	+0022	+0·8	+0·8	0·0	0·0
EMSHÖRN							
–0037	–0041	–0108	–0047	+0·1	+0·2	0·0	0·0
KNOCK (R. Ems)							
+0018	+0005	–0028	+0004	+0·6	+0·6	0·0	0·0

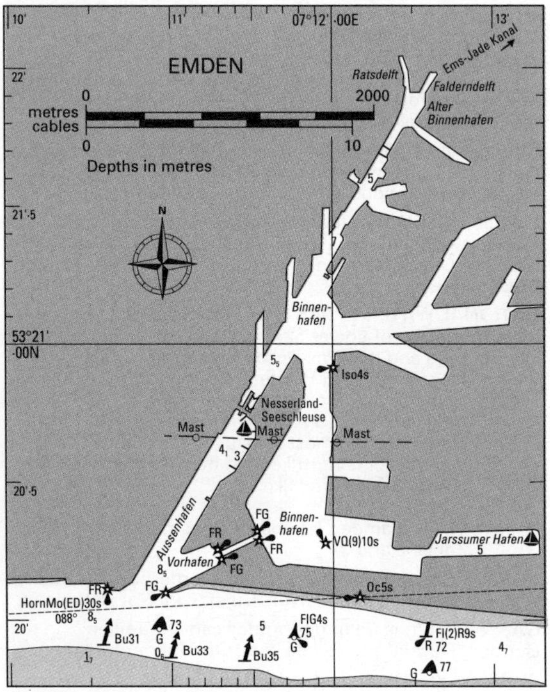

SHELTER
Good shelter, except in SW winds, in Außenhafen (3m) at yacht hbr on E side just before Nesserlander Lock. If full, lock into Binnenhafen, sheltered in all winds; Jarßumer Hafen (5m) in SE corner is mainly for locals and far from city. Possible AB at Alter Binnenhafen (4·5m), Ratsdelft (3m) and Falderndelft (3m) in city centre, if requested to lock-keeper. Lock hrs 0700-1900LT (0700-1530 Sun). For opening sound M (– –). Exceptionally, Binnenhafen can be entered via Vorhafen and Grosse Seeschleuse (H24).

NAVIGATION
See Delfzijl (10.20.33) and Borkum (10.21.11) for outer approaches via well buoyed/lit R Ems to abeam Knock lt ho. Thence 6M via Emder Fahrwasser which has drying banks and training walls close outboard of chan buoys. 3 conspic HT pylons (101m) help identify Außenhafen.

LIGHTS AND MARKS
Fahrwasser ldg lts 075°, both Oc (2) 12s 16/28m 12M. Ldg lts 088°, both Oc 5s 14/30m 12M, lead to hbr ent, marked by FR and FG lts. City centre bears 030°/2M.

RADIO TELEPHONE
VHF Ch 13 (H24) for locks. Info broadcasts H+50 Ch 15 18.

TELEPHONE (04921)
Hr Mr ☎ 897260/897265 (H24); Nesserlander lock ☎ 897-270; Weather ☎ 21458; Tourist Info 20094; Police 110; Fire/Ambulance 112.

FACILITIES
Yacht Club ☎ 26020 FW, AC, AB 11DM; all amenities in city (1M). Ferry to Borkum.
Note: The Ems-Jade canal, 39M to Wilhelmshaven, can be used by yachts with lowering masts & max draft 1·7m. Min bridge clearance 3·75m. It has 6 locks. Speed limit 4kn.

OTHER MAINLAND HARBOURS BETWEEN RIVERS EMS AND JADE

GREETSIEL, Niedersächsen, 53°32'·90N 07°02'·15E. AC 3509, 3761; BSH 89, 3012, 3015.5 & .2. HW –0400 on Dover (UT), –0010 on Helgoland (zone –0100); ML 2·6m. Buoyed chan leads from Osterems 3M SE, then NE to Ley bn, Fl Y 4s, tide gauge. Dir lt 165°, F WRG 10m 8M, leads between 1M long bkwtrs to lock; access HW–4 to +3. Yachts berth on marina pontoons (3m). A canal connects Greetsiel to Emden. There are a few facilities: Hr Mr ☎ (04926) 760; # ☎ (04931) 2764. **Village** R, V, ≹.

NORDDEICH, Niedersächsen, 53°38'·75N 07°08'·98E. AC 3761, BSH 3012.1, 3015.5. HW –0030 on Dover (UT); See 10.21.11. Very good shelter in hbr, reached by chan 50m wide, 2m deep and over 1M long between two training walls which cover at HW and are marked by stakes. Hr divided by central mole; yachts berth in W hbr. Lts on W training wall hd FG 8m 4M, vis 021°-327°. On E training wall hd FR 8m 4M, vis 327°-237°. Ldg lts 144°: front, Iso WR 6s 6m 6/4M; rear, 140m from front, Iso W 6s 9m 6M synch. Ldg lts 350°: front Iso WR 3s 5m 6/4M; rear, 95m from front, Iso W 3s 8m 6M. Ldg lts 170°: front Iso W 3s 12m 10M; rear, 420m from front, Iso W 3s 23m 10M, synch. Hr Mr VHF Ch 14, ☎ 8060; # ☎ 2735; YC ☎ 3560; Facilities: AB, C (5 ton), D ☎ 2721, FW, Slip, CH, BSH agent. **Town** Ⓑ, Bar, Dr, ✉, R, ≹, V, Gaz. Ferry to Juist and Norderney.

NESSMERSIEL, Niedersächsen, 53°41'·80N 07°21'·73E. AC 1875, 3761; BSH 3015.6, D89; HW –0040 on Dover (UT); –0020 on Helgoland (zone –0100); HW ht –0·2m on Helgoland. Good shelter in all weathers. Appr down the Nessmersieler Balje, chan marked by SHM buoys and bns leading to end of Leitdamm. Here, a lt bn, Oc 4s 5M, together with unlit bns mark the course of the Leitdamm on W; ‡ mark the E side of chan. Leitdamm covers at HW. Beyond ferry berth is a Yachthafen (1½M); secure to pontoons S of Ferry Quay. Hbr dries (2m at HW). Hr Mr ☎ 2981; # ☎ 2735. Facilities: **Nordsee YC Nessmersiel**; no supplies except FW. **Village** (1M to S) has limited facilities. Ferry to Baltrum.

EAST FRISIAN ISLANDS   10-21-10

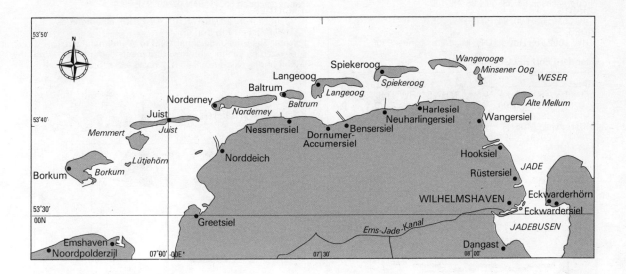

THE EAST FRISIAN ISLANDS

THE EAST FRISIAN ISLANDS off the North Sea coast of Germany and the North Frisian Islands off Schleswig-Holstein and Denmark together comprise the German Frisian Islands. The East Frisian Islands run from the Ems estuary to the Jade Bay with two small islands in the Elbe estuary. They lie between 3 and 20M off-shore and were, at one time, the north coast. The area between the low-lying islands and the present coastline which is now flooded by the sea is called the Watten. The islands are known locally as the Ostfriesischen and the inhabitants speak a patois known as Fries, a language with a close resemblance to English.

TIDES: The gaps between the islands are known as Seegats and the watersheds (where the tide meets having swept both ways round the island, usually about ⅓ the way from the E end of the S side) are known as Watts. Tidal streams are very slack over the watts but very strong in the Seegats, especially on the sp ebb. In strong W/NW winds, the sea level may rise over 0.25m.

BUOYAGE: Deep water chans are buoyed but shallow chans are marked by withies (pricken in German). Withies the natural way up ⥾ are to be taken as PHMs and withies inverted thus ⥿ are to be taken as SHMs. As stated in 10.21.5, the conventional direction of buoyage is always from West to East inside the islands, so leave PHMs to the N whichever way the stream is flowing.

BRIEF NOTES:
   BORKUM (14 sq. miles): The largest island, see 10.21.11.
   LUTJEHORN: Bird sanctuary; landing prohib.
   MEMMERT: Bird sanctuary; landing prohib. Lt on stone tr with G cupola, Oc (2) WRG 14s 15m 17/12M.
   JUIST (6½ sq. miles): No yacht hbr. See next column.
   NORDERNEY (10 sq. miles): Lt on R octagonal tr, Fl (3) W 12s 59m 23M. See 10.21.12.
   BALTRUM (3 sq. miles): Pretty island with small town and hbr at W end. See next column.
   LANGEOOG (7 sq. miles): See 10.21.14.
   SPIEKEROOG (5 sq. miles): See next column.
   WANGEROOGE (2 sq. miles): See 10.21.15.
   MINSENER OOG: Large bn. Beware groynes and overfalls in strong NW winds.
   ALTE MELLUM: Bird sanctuary; landing prohib.
   SCHARNHÖRN (2 sq. miles): Between Alte Mellum and Neu Werk; (off chartlet, in Elbe estuary). Uninhabited.
   GROSSES KNECHTSAND: Between Alte Mellum and Neu Werk; Bird sanctuary; landing prohib; (off chartlet).
   NEUWERK (off chartlet, in Elbe estuary): Island only inhabited by LB crew and lt ho men. Lt in ☐ brick tr with B cupola, L Fl (3) WRG 20s 38m 16/12M. On W side there is a conspic W radar tr and landing stage. Ferry to Cuxhaven.

OTHER HARBOURS IN THE EAST FRISIAN ISLANDS

JUIST, Niedersächsen, 53°39'·70N 07°00'·00E. AC 3509; BSH 90, 3015.4. HW −0105 on Dover (UT); −0035 on Helgoland (zone −0100); HW ht +0·1 on Helgoland (both differences valid at Memmert). Ent through narrow chan running N in the centre of the S side of island, marked by withies to port. To the W of these is the long (5ca) landing pier. Conspic marks are: West bn, on Haakdünen at W end of island, Juist water tr in centre and East bn, 1M from E end of island. Aero lt Fl W 5s 14m (occas) at the airfield. There is no yacht hbr, but yachts can dry out on soft mud alongside quay in ferry hbr. ⚓ 1ca S of W part of town ½M E of steamer pier or at E end of island. Hr Mr ☎ 724; ⌗ ☎ 351. Facilities: FW, Slip, C; villages of Oosdorp, Westdorp and Loog in centre of island have limited facilities, V, R, Bar, Gaz. Ferry to Norddeich.

BALTRUM, Niedersächsen, 53°43'·30N 07°21'·80E. AC 1875, 3761; BSH 3015.6/7. HW −0040 on Dover (UT); Use differences Langeoog 10.21.14. Shelter is good except in SW winds. Without detailed local knowledge and ideal conditions, the appr via the unmarked, drying Wichter Ee Seegat is not recommended. Better appr is at HW via the Norderneyer Wattfahrwasser running S of Norderney (which also gives access to Neßmersiel). Hbr partly dries. Yacht moorings in the Bootshafen at the E end of hbr. Lt at the groyne head Oc WRG 6s 7m 6/3M G082·5°-098°, W098°-103°, R103°-082·5°. Hr Mr ☎ (04939) 448. Facilities: Hbr AB, FW; **Baltrumer Bootsclub YC. Village** (¼M NNE) V, R, Bar. No fuel. Ferry from Neßmersiel.

SPIEKEROOG, Niedersächsen, 53°45'·00N 07°40'·40E. AC 3368, 1875, 3761; BSH 89, 3015.8. HW −0008 on Dover (UT); ML 1·3m; Duration 0555. See differences 10.21.14. Good shelter except in S/SW winds which cause heavy swell. Small ferry hbr (1.6m) on S side of Spiekeroog with yacht pontoons is reached by marked chan, dredged 1·2m. Lt on R mast, FR 6m 4M, vis 197°-114°. Hr Mr ☎ (04976) 235. Facilities: 60+40 visitors, 14DM, C (15 ton), town is ½M from hbr. Ferry from Nieuharlingersiel.

BORKUM   10-21-11
EAST FRISIAN ISLANDS
Niedersächsen 53°33'·50N 06°45'·10E

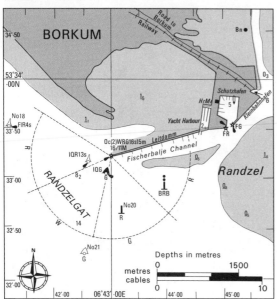

CHARTS
AC 3509, 3761; BSH 3015/2, D90; DYC 1812; ANWB A
TIDES
–0105 Dover; ML 1·4; Duration 0610; Zone –0100

Standard Port HELGOLAND (→)

Times				Height (metres)			
High Water		Low Water		MHWS	MHWN	MLWN	MLWS
0200	0700	0200	0800	2·7	2·3	0·4	0·0
1400	1900	1400	2000				
Differences BORKUM (FISCHERBALJE)							
–0048	–0052	–0124	–0105	0·0	0·0	0·0	0·0
EMSHÖRN							
–0037	–0041	–0108	–0047	+0·1	+0·2	0·0	0·0

SHELTER
Good in the yacht hbr (1·8 - 2·5m), which is preferred to the Schutzhafen (5 - 7·5m) close to the E; access to both H24 with good facilities. To the NE is the tiny triangular Kleinbahnhafen (ferry hbr) prohib to yachts. Note: The S part of the island is a Nature Reserve. Borkum town is 7km NW.
NAVIGATION
WPT Riffgat (SWM) buoy, Iso 8s, 53°38'·90N 06°27'·10E, 302°/122° from/to Fischerbalje lt, 11M. See also 10.20.33. There are many groynes extending up to 2¾ca (500m) off shore. From any direction, pick up the Fischerbalje lt at the end of the Leitdamm. Beware strong currents across the buoyed Fischerbalje chan. Speed limit in hbrs 5kn.
LIGHTS AND MARKS
Landmarks: Water tr, Grosse and Kleine lt ho's at Borkum town; 2 wind turbines 3ca NNE of yacht hbr ent. From the Fischerbalje lt the chan up to the hbr is well buoyed/lit. Yacht hbr ent is abeam F7 SHM buoy, Oc (3) G 12s. Schutzhafen ent shows FR on W and FG on E moles. Fischerbalje lt, Oc (2) WRG 16s 15m 16/11M, W tr with R top and lamp on tripod; R260°-313°, G313°-014°, W014°-068°. Initial app in sector R068°-123° until abm. Fog det lt.
RADIO TELEPHONE
Hr Mr VHF Ch 14 (In season Mon-Fri 0700-2200; Sat 0800-2100; Sun 0700-2000). See also Delfzijl, 10.20.30.
TELEPHONE (04922)
Hr Mr 2420; CG Borkum Kleiner Lt Tr; ⊞ 2287; Police 3950; Ⓗ 813; Brit Consul (040) 446071.
FACILITIES
Yacht Hbr (30 + 170 visitors) ☎ 3380, AB, FW, Slip, D, R, Bar, AC, C (6 ton), V, R; **Kleinbahnhof** C (hand), AB.
Town P, ME, El, Gaz, V, R, Bar, ✉, Ⓑ, ⇌ (ferry to Emden), ✈ (to Emden and Bremen). Ferry: Hamburg-Harwich.

NORDERNEY   10-21-12
EAST FRISIAN ISLANDS
Niedersächsen 53°41'·94N 07°09'·93E

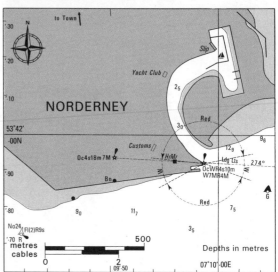

CHARTS
AC 3761; DYC 1812; Zeekarten 1353; BSH 3015, 3012, D89
TIDES
–0042 Dover; ML 1·4; Duration 0605; Zone –0100

Standard Port HELGOLAND (→)

Times				Height (metres)			
High Water		Low Water		MHWS	MHWN	MLWN	MLWS
0200	0700	0200	0800	2·7	2·3	0·4	0·0
1400	1900	1400	2000				
Differences NORDERNEY (RIFFGAT)							
–0024	–0030	–0056	–0045	+0·1	0·0	0·0	0·0
NORDDEICH HAFEN							
–0018	–0017	–0029	–0012	+0·2	+0·2	0·0	0·0
MEMMERT							
	No data		No data	+0·1	+0·1	0·0	0·0

SHELTER
Good; the hbr is accessible H24. Yacht hbr is at the NE of the hbr, where yachts lie bow to pontoon, stern to posts; or AB on W wall of hbr, as crowded in Jul/Aug. Hbr speed limit 3kn.
NAVIGATION
WPT Schlucter SWM buoy, Iso 8s, 53°44'·90N 07°04'·30E, 321°/141° from/to S1 SHM buoy, Oc (2) G 9s, 1·44M. Ent through the Schlucter (see 10.21.5) is well buoyed but the bar can be dangerous in on-shore winds and following seas which break on it, especially on an ebb tide. Follow the buoyed chan closely around W tip of island. Ent via the Dovetief is not advised; it has less water, is more exposed to the NE and buoys are moved more often. Ent at night is dangerous. Note: Tidal streams run across the Schlucter and Dovetief, not along it. Beware merchant shipping.
LIGHTS AND MARKS
Land marks: in centre of island Norderney lt ho, 8-sided R brick tr, Fl (3) 12s 59m 23M. Water tr in town (conspic). Ldg lts, Oc 4s, in line at 274°, synch.
RADIO TELEPHONE
VHF Ch 14 (Mon 0700-1200, 1230-1730; Tues 0900-1200, 1230-1900; Wed – Sun 0700-1200, 1230-1900).
TELEPHONE (04932)
Hr Mr 2850; CG 2293; ⊞ 2386; Weather 549; Police 788; Ⓗ 477 and 416; Brit Consul (040) 446071.
FACILITIES
M, L, FW, C (10 ton), V, R, CH, SM, Slip, ME, El, Sh, P, D, Gaz; **Yacht Club** Bar.
Town V, R, Bar, ✉, Ⓑ, ⇌ (ferry to Norddeich), ✈ (to Bremen). Ferry: Hamburg-Harwich.

DORNUMER-ACCUMERSIEL
10-21-13
Niedersächsen 53°41'·40N 07°29'·40E

CHARTS
AC 1875, 3761; BSH 3015, Sheet 7, D89
TIDES
–0040 Dover; ML 1·4; Duration 0600; Zone –0100

Standard Port HELGOLAND (→)

Use Differences LANGEOOG (10.21.13)

SHELTER
The marina provides complete shelter in all winds; depth 3m, access HW ±4. Ent is narrow; keep to W of chan on entering. Marina is fenced so obtain a key before leaving.
NAVIGATION
Appr through Accumer Ee (see 10.21.5 and 10.21.13) leading into Accumersieler Balje and to AB3 SHM buoy, IQ G 13s. From here keep four withies ‡ to stbd, clear of the Leitdamm. Note warnings on German chart D89.

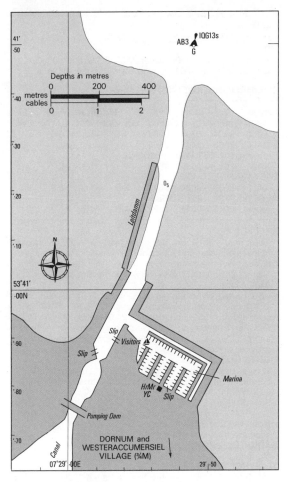

LIGHTS AND MARKS
None.
RADIO TELEPHONE
None.
TELEPHONE (04933)
Hr Mr 1732; Deputy Hr Mr 441; ⌗ (04971) 7184; Lifeboat (04972) 247; Weather Emden 21458; Police 2218; Ⓗ 011502; Brit Consul (040) 446071.
FACILITIES
Dornumer Yacht Haven (250) All facilities; pontoons are lifted out of season, FW, R, Slip, Gaz, D, YC, ME, El, Sh.
Town V, R, Bar, ⌧, Ⓑ, ⇌ (Harlesiel), ✈ (Bremen or Hamburg). Ferry: Hamburg-Harwich.

LANGEOOG
10-21-14
EAST FRISIAN ISLANDS
Niedersächsen 53°43'·42N 07°30'·20E

CHARTS
AC 1875, 3761; ANWB A; BSH 3015, Sheet 7, D89
TIDES
–0010 Dover; ML No data; Duration 0600; Zone –0100

Standard Port HELGOLAND (→)

Times				Height (metres)			
High Water		Low Water		MHWS	MHWN	MLWN	MLWS
0200	0700	0200	0800	2·7	2·3	0·4	0·0
1400	1900	1400	2000				
Differences LANGEOOG							
+0003	–0001	–0034	–0018	+0·3	+0·3	0·0	0·0
SPIEKEROOG							
+0003	–0003	–0031	–0012	+0·4	+0·4	+0·1	0·0
NEUHARLINGERSIEL							
No data		No data		+0·5	+0·5	0·0	0·0

SHELTER
Hbr is well sheltered by 20m high sand dunes, but it is open to the S. The E side of hbr dries; chan to yacht pontoons is marked by ‡ withies.
NAVIGATION
WPT Accumer Ee (see 10.21.5) (SWM) buoy, Iso 8s, Bell, 53°46'·82N 07°24'·25E, 337°/157° from/to A1 chan buoy, SHM, Oc (2) G 9s, 0·90M; thence via buoyed chan to A9/B26 SHM lt buoy. W sector of W mole lt leads 072° to ent.

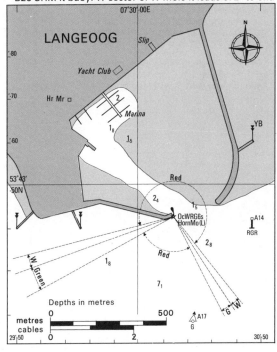

Ice protectors extend about 40m E of E mole, awash at HW, marked by withies.
LIGHTS AND MARKS
Lt bn on W mole, Oc WRG 6s 8m 7/4M; G064°-070°, W070°-074°, R074°-326°, W326°-330°, G330°-335°, R335°-064°, Horn Mo (L) 30s (sounded 0730-1800LT). Daymarks: Langeoog ch and water tr 1·5M to NNW.
RADIO TELEPHONE
None.
TELEPHONE (04972)
Hr Mr 502; Lifeboat CG 247; ⌗ 275; Weather Emden 21458; Police 810; Dr 589; Brit Consul (040) 446071.
FACILITIES
Langeoog Marina (70 + 130 visitors) ☎ 552, Slip, FW, C, (12 ton), El, Bar, R; **Segelverein Langeoog YC**.
Village (1½ M) P, D, V, R, Gaz, Bar, ⌧, Ⓑ, ⇌ (ferry to Norddeich), ✈ (to Bremen). Ferry: Hamburg-Harwich. NOTE: Motor vehicles are prohib on the island. Village is 1½M away; go by foot, pony and trap or train. Train connects with ferries to Bensersiel.

21

OTHER MAINLAND HARBOURS BETWEEN RIVERS EMS AND JADE

BENSERSIEL, Niedersächsen, 53°41'·80N 07°32'·90E. AC 1875, 3761; BSH 3015.7. HW –0024 on Dover (UT); +0005 on Helgoland (zone –0100); HW ht +0·4m on Helgoland. Very good shelter in the yacht hbr (dries). Ent chan from Rute 1·5M between training walls with depth of 1·5m. Walls cover at HW. Yacht hbr to SW just before hbr ent (2m); also berths on the SW side of main hbr.
Lights: E training wall hd Oc WRG 6s 6m 5/2M, G110°-119°, W119°-121°, R121°-110°. W mole hd FG; E mole hd FR. Ldg lts 138°, both Iso W 6s 7/11m 9M (intens on line), synch. Hr Mr VHF Ch 14, ☎ (04971) 2502; ✂ ☎ (04421) 42031; Facilities: FW, C (8 ton), D (on E pier), P (cans), El, Slip, ME, Sh.
Town Ⓑ, Bar, ✉, R, ⇌, V, Gaz. Ferry to Langeoog.

NEUHARLINGERSIEL, Niedersächsen, 53°43'·20N 07°42'·40E. AC 3368, 1875, 3761; BSH 3015.8. HW 0000 on Dover (UT); see differences under 10.21.14. Appr chan well marked from Bakledge N end of Leitdamm, Oc 6s. Beware strong tidal streams across the ent. Chan runs close E of Leitdamm which is marked by stakes with ⚓. It covers at HW. Yachts lie in NE corner of hbr; where there are many poles. Visitors berths very limited. Hr Mr ☎ (04974) 289.
Facilities: **Quay** FW, D.
Village (picturesque) V, R, Bar. Ferry to Spiekeroog (35 mins).

HARLESIEL, Niedersächsen, 53°44'·10N 07°50'·10E. AC 3369, 3368; BSH 3015.8. HW –0100 on Dover (UT); –0005 on Helgoland (zone –0100); HW ht +0·5m on Helgoland. Excellent shelter S of lock which opens approx HW ±1. Yacht berths (120) on pontoons to W by village or at BY to E after passing through lock on W side of dyke. River navigable up to Carolinensiel. Hr Mr ☎ (04464) 1472, berthing fees similar to Wangerooge; ✂ ☎ 249; YC ☎ 1473; Facilities: BY, C, V, R, Slip, P, D, FW.
Town El, ME, Gaz, ✉, V, ✈ and ferry to Wangerooge.

WANGEROOGE   10-21-15
EAST FRISIAN ISLANDS
Niedersächsen 53° 46'·50N 07° 52'·18E

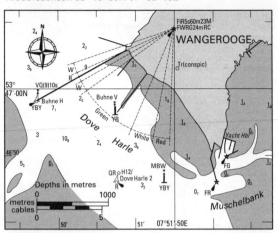

CHARTS
AC 3368, 1875; BSH D2, 3015 Sheet 8
TIDES
E Wangerooge, –0009 Dover; ML 1·9. Duration 0600
W Wangerooge, –0014 Dover; ML 1·5. Zone –0100

Standard Port WILHELMSHAVEN(→)

Times				Height (metres)			
High Water		Low Water		MHWS	MHWN	MLWN	MLWS
0200	0800	0200	0900	4·3	3·7	0·6	0·0
1400	2000	1400	2100				
Differences WEST WANGEROOGE							
–0101	–0058	–0035	–0045	–1·1	–0·9	–0·2	0·0
EAST WANGEROOGE							
–0058	–0053	–0024	–0034	–1·0	–0·8	–0·1	0·0
ALTE WESER LIGHT HOUSE							
–0055	–0048	–0015	–0029	–1·0	–0·9	–0·2	0·0

SHELTER
Good in all winds, but SW gales, and S'lies at HW, cause heavy swell and difficult conditions in hbr. Best access HW±2. Yachts on marina pontoons at E side of hbr have 1·3 to 1·8m depth. The W jetty is for ferries only.
NAVIGATION
WPT Harle (SWM) By, Iso 8s, 53°49'·28N 07°49'·00E, 351°/ 171° from/to Buhne H WCM buoy, VQ (9) 10s, 2·4M. From seaward the Harle chan (see 10.21.5) leads inward between Spiekeroog and Wangerooge; it varies in depth and position, and care is needed. Beware Buhne H groyne, extending 7½ca, buoyed.
LIGHTS AND MARKS
Wangerooge lt ho Fl R 5s 60m 23M; R ○ tr with two W bands; same structure: Dir lt, F WRG 24m 22/10M, R002°-011°, W011°-023°, G023°-055°, W055°-060·5°, R060·5°-065·5°, W065·5°-071°, G (18M) 119·4°-138·8°, W (22M) 138·8°-152·2° (ldg sector), R152·2°-159·9°, RC. Note: the last 3 GWR sectors above lead in from seaward; they are not shown on the chartlet.
RADIO TELEPHONE
None.
TELEPHONE (04469)
Hr Mr 630; ✂ 223; Weather Bremerhaven 72220; Police 205; Ambulance 588; Brit Consul (040) 446071.
FACILITIES
Wangerooge YC ☎ 364, 11.10DM, FW, L, El, M, Gaz.
Village El, V, P and D (cans), CH, ▣, Ⓑ, ⇌ (ferry to Harlesiel), ✈ (to Harle and Helgoland). Ferry: Hamburg-Harwich.

HOOKSIEL   10-21-16

Niedersächsen 53°38'·85N 08°05'40E

CHARTS
AC 3369; BSH 3015 Sheet 10, D7

TIDES
+0034 Dover; ML no data; Duration 0605; Zone –0100

Standard Port WILHELMSHAVEN (→)

Times				Height (metres)			
High Water		Low Water		MHWS	MHWN	MLWN	MLWS
0200	0800	0200	0900	4·3	3·7	0·6	0·0
1400	2000	1400	2100				
Differences HOOKSIEL							
–0023	–0022	–0008	–0012	–0·5	–0·4	–0·1	0·0
SCHILLIG							
–0034	–0029	–0009	–0016	–0·6	–0·5	–0·1	0·0

SHELTER
Temp AB in the Vorhafen (approx 1m at MLWS) but it is very commercial and uncomfortable in E winds. Beyond the lock there is complete shelter in the Binnentief, 2M long and approx 2·8m deep. Best berths for visitors in Alter Hafen Yacht Hbr in the town. Max draught 2m; bigger yachts go to YCs; see Lockmaster.

NAVIGATION
WPT No 37/Hooksiel 1 (SHM) buoy, IQ G 13s, 53°39'·38N 08°06'·63E 227°/047° from/to ent 1·1M. See also 10.21.16 for outer appr's. Ent is marked by H3 SHM buoy, approx 1M W of main Innenjade chan. Appr to lock through Vorhafen, enclosed by two moles. Depth in chan 2·5m. Lock opens Mon - Fri 0800-1900, Sat/Sun 0900-2000 (LT); actual times on board at lock. Secure well in lock. Caution: tanker pier and restricted area to SE of ent.

LIGHTS AND MARKS
Ldg lts 164°, both Iso 6s 15/24m 24/27M, synch & intens, lead W of the WPT. Conspic chys of oil refinery 1·7M S of lock, which is in the W047°-062° sector of Hooksielplate Cross lt, Oc WRG 3s. There is a street lamp on the N mole and L Fl R 6s on dayglo R pile on S mole. Usual R/G tfc sigs at lock.

RADIO TELEPHONE
VHF Ch 63. VTS Centre, *German Bight Traffic* Ch 80 79 broadcasts info every H in German/English; *Jade Revier* broadcasts info in German every H+10 Ch 20 63.

TELEPHONE (04425)
Hr Admin 95800; Lockmaster 430; ⌗ (0441) 42031; CG (0421) 5550555; Weather (0571) 72220; Police, see under Wilhelmshaven; Ⓗ (04421) 2080; Dr 1080; Brit Consul (040) 446071.

FACILITIES
Visitors Yacht Hr (50) AB, based on LOA x beam = m²: 15 - 20m² = 11DM; 20 - 30 m² = 12DM; 30 - 40m² = 15DM. AC, FW, BH (25 ton), Slip, Bar, **Alter Hafen** AB, FW, V, R, Bar; **Wilhemshaven YC** ☎ 285.
Town BY, SM, ME, El, CH, P, D, Gaz, V, R, Bar, Ⓑ, ✉, ⇌ (Wilhelmshaven), ✈ (Wilhelmshaven or Bremen). Ferry: Hamburg-Harwich.

ADJACENT HARBOURS ON THE RIVER JADE

WANGERSIEL, Niedersächsen, 53°41'·00N 08°01'·60E. AC 3369; BSH 3015.9/10. HW –0100 on Dover (UT); use SCHILLIG differences 10.21.16; ML 3·3m. From spar buoy W2 (PHM) besom perches mark the N side of the chan to the hbr. Best water 10 to 20m from perches. Depth at ent, 1·3m. Chan keeps shifting especially at E end. Boats drawing 1·5m can cross the bar HW ±2½. Most of hbr dries. Berth on N quay. YC and FW are in the NW corner. Hr Mr ☎ 238. Facilities: No fuel. At Horumersiel (¼M) V, R, Bar.

RÜSTERSIEL, Niedersächsen, 53°33'·74N 08°09'·33E. AC 3369; BSH 3015.12. Tides approx as Wilhelmshaven, 3M to the S. Appr from No 47 SHM buoy, IQ G 13s; SW for 9ca to Maadesiel, close N of NWO oil pier and tanks. A conspic factory chy (275m) is 4ca N of ent. The outer hbr dries; access HW±2 via sluice gate. The small marina (3m) is 8ca up the Maade river; or continue 1M, via opening bridge (0700-1700 Mon-Fri), to berth on N quay at Rüstersiel.

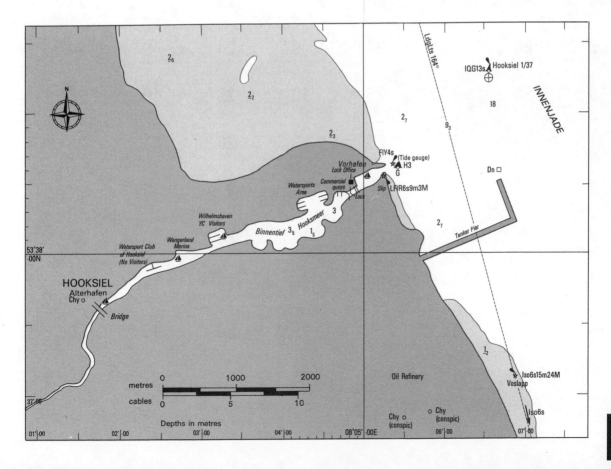

TIME ZONE –0100
(German Standard Time)
Subtract 1 hour for UT
For German Summer Time add ONE hour in non-shaded areas

GERMANY – WILHELMSHAVEN

LAT 53°31′N   LONG 8°09′E

TIMES AND HEIGHTS OF HIGH AND LOW WATERS

YEAR **1996**

JANUARY

Time	m		Time	m
1 0230 0859 M 1511 2135	0.7 3.9 0.6 3.8	**16**	0108 0735 TU 1346 2022	0.6 3.8 0.5 3.7
2 0344 1009 TU 1618 2240	0.6 3.9 0.6 3.9	**17**	0228 0857 W 1509 2140	0.6 3.8 0.4 3.8
3 0453 1110 W 1717 2335	0.6 3.9 0.5 4.1	**18**	0352 1018 TH 1629 2252	0.4 3.9 0.4 4.0
4 0550 1200 TH 1807	0.5 4.0 0.5	**19**	0508 1129 F 1740 2354	0.3 4.0 0.3 4.1
5 0021 0637 F 1243 O 1850	4.2 0.4 4.0 0.4	**20**	0614 1230 SA 1841 ●	0.1 4.1 0.1
6 0100 0716 SA 1322 1928	4.2 0.3 4.0 0.3	**21**	0049 0711 SU 1325 1935	4.3 0.0 4.1 0.1
7 0135 0752 SU 1357 2002	4.2 0.2 4.0 0.2	**22**	0140 0804 M 1418 2026	4.4 –0.1 4.1 0.0
8 0209 0826 M 1430 2034	4.3 0.2 4.0 0.2	**23**	0231 0856 TU 1509 2114	4.4 –0.1 4.1 0.0
9 0241 0857 TU 1500 2104	4.3 0.2 4.0 0.2	**24**	0320 0944 W 1553 2156	4.4 –0.1 4.0 0.0
10 0311 0926 W 1530 2131	4.2 0.2 3.9 0.2	**25**	0404 1026 TH 1632 2232	4.4 0.0 4.0 0.1
11 0342 0956 TH 1604 2203	4.2 0.2 3.8 0.2	**26**	0445 1103 F 1710 2308	4.4 0.1 3.9 0.2
12 0417 1029 F 1643 2239	4.1 0.1 3.8 0.2	**27**	0525 1140 SA 1749 2345	4.2 0.2 3.8 0.3
13 0454 1104 SA 1723 2317	4.0 0.1 3.7 0.3	**28**	0608 1218 SU 1834	4.0 0.4 3.7
14 0535 1142 SU 1808	3.9 0.2 3.6	**29**	0029 0700 M 1305 1930	0.5 3.8 0.5 3.7
15 0003 0626 M 1235 1907	0.5 3.8 0.4 3.6	**30**	0130 0807 TU 1411 2043	0.6 3.7 0.7 3.7
		31	0250 0926 W 1530 2201	0.6 3.7 0.7 3.8

FEBRUARY

Time	m		Time	m
1 0414 1041 TH 1643 2309	0.6 3.7 0.6 3.9	**16**	0325 1000 F 1607 2234	0.3 3.7 0.3 3.9
2 0524 1139 F 1742	0.4 3.8 0.4	**17**	0451 1119 SA 1725 2342	0.1 3.9 0.2 4.1
3 0000 0615 SA 1224 1827	4.1 0.3 3.9 0.3	**18**	0602 1223 SU 1829 ●	0.0 3.9 0.1
4 0040 0654 SU 1303 O 1906	4.1 0.2 3.9 0.2	**19**	0039 0700 M 1316 1923	4.2 –0.2 4.0 –0.1
5 0117 0731 M 1339 1943	4.1 0.1 4.0 0.1	**20**	0129 0751 TU 1405 2012	4.3 –0.2 4.0 –0.1
6 0151 0805 TU 1411 2016	4.2 0.0 4.0 0.0	**21**	0216 0838 W 1450 2056	4.4 –0.2 4.0 –0.1
7 0223 0837 W 1441 2045	4.2 0.0 4.0 0.0	**22**	0301 0923 TH 1530 2135	4.4 –0.2 4.1 –0.1
8 0253 0907 TH 1512 2114	4.2 0.0 3.9 0.0	**23**	0344 1002 F 1607 2210	4.3 –0.1 4.0 –0.1
9 0326 0938 F 1548 2148	4.1 0.0 3.9 0.0	**24**	0422 1036 SA 1641 2242	4.3 0.0 4.0 0.0
10 0403 1013 SA 1627 2224	4.1 –0.1 3.8 0.0	**25**	0458 1106 SU 1714 2313	4.2 0.1 3.9 0.1
11 0440 1046 SU 1703 2257	4.0 –0.1 3.8 0.0	**26**	0534 1135 M 1749 2346	4.0 0.3 3.8 0.3
12 0515 1116 M 1739 2333	3.9 0.0 3.7 0.2	**27**	0616 1212 TU 1838	3.7 0.5 3.7
13 0557 1157 TU 1829	3.8 0.3 3.6	**28**	0037 0717 W 1312 1949	0.5 3.5 0.7 3.6
14 0028 0702 W 1304 1944	0.4 3.7 0.4 3.6	**29**	0154 0838 TH 1436 2116	0.6 3.5 0.7 3.7
15 0151 0829 TH 1434 2112	0.4 3.7 0.4 3.7			

MARCH

Time	m		Time	m
1 0327 1003 F 1602 2234	0.5 3.5 0.6 3.8	**16**	0312 0952 SA 1553 2223	0.2 3.7 0.3 3.9
2 0449 1112 SA 1710 2332	0.3 3.7 0.4 3.9	**17**	0440 1111 SU 1712 2330	0.0 3.8 0.1 4.0
3 0546 1200 SU 1758	0.2 3.8 0.2	**18**	0548 1211 M 1813	–0.1 3.9 0.0
4 0013 0626 M 1238 1838	4.0 0.0 3.9 0.1	**19**	0025 0642 TU 1300 ● 1905	4.2 –0.2 4.0 –0.1
5 0051 0702 TU 1314 O 1916	4.1 –0.1 3.9 0.0	**20**	0113 0730 W 1345 1952	4.3 –0.2 4.0 –0.2
6 0127 0737 W 1348 1952	4.1 –0.1 4.0 –0.1	**21**	0158 0815 TH 1426 2033	4.3 –0.2 4.1 –0.2
7 0201 0811 TH 1420 2025	4.1 –0.1 4.0 –0.1	**22**	0240 0856 F 1503 2110	4.3 –0.1 4.1 –0.1
8 0234 0844 F 1453 2058	4.1 –0.1 4.0 –0.2	**23**	0320 0933 SA 1539 2144	4.3 0.0 4.1 –0.1
9 0310 0920 SA 1531 2133	4.1 –0.2 3.9 –0.2	**24**	0357 1004 SU 1611 2216	4.2 0.0 4.1 0.0
10 0349 0957 SU 1609 2210	4.1 –0.2 3.9 –0.2	**25**	0431 1032 M 1642 2245	4.1 0.1 4.0 0.1
11 0428 1030 M 1645 2242	4.0 –0.2 3.8 –0.1	**26**	0504 1058 TU 1713 2313	3.9 0:2 3.9 0.2
12 0503 1059 TU 1720 2316	3.9 –0.1 3.8 0.0	**27**	0540 1130 W 1755 2354	3.7 0.4 3.8 0.4
13 0545 1136 W 1810	3.8 0.2 3.7	**28**	0633 1222 TH 1900	3.5 0.6 3.6
14 0010 0648 TH 1243 1925	0.3 3.6 0.4 3.7	**29**	0103 0748 F 1341 2024	0.4 3.4 0.7 3.6
15 0133 0817 F 1417 2057	0.3 3.6 0.4 3.7	**30**	0233 0915 SA 1510 2147	0.5 3.4 0.7 3.7
		31	0401 1030 SU 1625 2251	0.3 3.6 0.4 3.9

APRIL

Time	m		Time	m
1 0504 1123 M 1718 2336	0.1 3.7 0.2 4.0	**16**	0527 1151 TU 1748	–0.2 3.9 0.0
2 0547 1204 TU 1802	–0.1 3.9 0.0	**17**	0004 0617 W 1237 ● 1839	4.1 –0.2 4.0 –0.1
3 0016 0625 W 1243 1844	4.0 –0.1 3.9 –0.1	**18**	0053 0705 TH 1321 1928	4.2 –0.1 4.1 –0.1
4 0057 0704 TH 1321 O 1924	4.1 –0.2 4.0 –0.1	**19**	0138 0749 F 1401 2010	4.3 –0.1 4.2 –0.1
5 0136 0743 F 1357 2002	4.1 –0.2 4.0 –0.2	**20**	0219 0828 SA 1436 2045	4.3 0.0 4.2 –0.1
6 0214 0821 SA 1434 2040	4.1 –0.2 4.1 –0.2	**21**	0256 0901 SU 1510 2117	4.2 0.0 4.2 –0.1
7 0253 0900 SU 1512 2119	4.1 –0.2 4.1 –0.2	**22**	0331 0932 M 1543 2149	4.1 0.1 4.2 0.0
8 0335 0939 M 1552 2156	4.1 –0.2 4.0 –0.3	**23**	0406 1001 TU 1614 2220	4.0 0.1 4.1 0.1
9 0416 1014 TU 1631 2232	4.0 –0.1 4.0 –0.2	**24**	0439 1029 W 1645 2249	3.8 0.2 4.0 0.2
10 0457 1048 W 1712 2312	3.9 –0.1 3.9 –0.1	**25**	0513 1100 TH 1724 2325	3.7 0.3 3.9 0.3
11 0544 1132 TH 1806	3.7 0.1 3.8	**26**	0557 1145 F 1818	3.5 0.5 3.8
12 0009 0649 F 1239 1920	0.1 3.6 0.3 3.8	**27**	0021 0700 SA 1250 1930	0.4 3.4 0.6 3.7
13 0132 0814 SA 1409 2048	0.2 3.6 0.4 3.9	**28**	0138 0818 SU 1411 2048	0.4 3.4 0.5 3.7
14 0305 0943 SU 1541 2210	0.1 3.7 0.3 4.0	**29**	0301 0935 M 1527 2156	0.2 3.6 0.4 3.8
15 0427 1056 M 1653 2313	–0.1 3.8 0.1 4.1	**30**	0409 1036 TU 1629 2250	0.1 3.7 0.2 3.9

Chart Datum: 2·26 metres below Normal Null (German reference level)

TIME ZONE –0100
(German Standard Time)
Subtract 1 hour for UT

For German Summer Time add
ONE hour in non-shaded areas

GERMANY – WILHELMSHAVEN

LAT 53°31′N   LONG   8°09′E

TIMES AND HEIGHTS OF HIGH AND LOW WATERS

YEAR **1996**

MAY

Day	Time	m	Day	Time	m
1 W	0500 / 1124 / 1721 / 2338	-0.1 / 3.9 / 0.1 / 4.0	**16** TH	0548 / 1211 / 1812	-0.1 / 4.0 / 0.0
2 TH	0545 / 1208 / 1810	-0.1 / 4.0 / 0.0	**17** F	0030 / 0637 / 1256 / ●1904	4.2 / 0.0 / 4.1 / 0.0
3 F ○	0025 / 0631 / 1251 / 1856	4.1 / -0.2 / 4.1 / -0.1	**18** SA	0117 / 0723 / 1337 / 1948	4.2 / 0.0 / 4.3 / 0.0
4 SA	0110 / 0715 / 1332 / 1939	4.2 / -0.2 / 4.2 / -0.1	**19** SU	0158 / 0801 / 1411 / 2022	4.2 / 0.1 / 4.3 / 0.0
5 SU	0153 / 0758 / 1413 / 2021	4.2 / -0.2 / 4.2 / -0.2	**20** M	0233 / 0833 / 1444 / 2054	4.2 / 0.1 / 4.3 / 0.0
6 M	0237 / 0841 / 1455 / 2104	4.2 / -0.2 / 4.2 / -0.3	**21** TU	0308 / 0904 / 1518 / 2126	4.1 / 0.1 / 4.3 / 0.1
7 TU	0323 / 0923 / 1537 / 2146	4.1 / -0.2 / 4.2 / -0.3	**22** W	0342 / 0935 / 1551 / 2159	4.0 / 0.1 / 4.2 / 0.1
8 W	0408 / 1003 / 1621 / 2228	4.0 / -0.1 / 4.1 / -0.2	**23** TH	0415 / 1006 / 1623 / 2231	3.9 / 0.2 / 4.1 / 0.1
9 TH	0454 / 1044 / 1709 / 2316	3.9 / 0.0 / 4.1 / -0.1	**24** F	0449 / 1039 / 1659 / 2305	3.8 / 0.3 / 4.0 / 0.2
10 F	0547 / 1134 / 1806	3.8 / 0.2 / 4.0	**25** SA	0528 / 1117 / 1743 / 2348	3.7 / 0.4 / 3.9 / 0.3
11 SA	0016 / 0651 / 1240 / 1915	0.0 / 3.7 / 0.3 / 4.0	**26** SU	0618 / 1207 / 1840	3.6 / 0.4 / 3.8
12 SU	0130 / 0807 / 1400 / 2033	0.1 / 3.7 / 0.4 / 4.1	**27** M	0047 / 0722 / 1312 / 1947	0.3 / 3.5 / 0.5 / 3.8
13 M	0251 / 0924 / 1520 / 2148	0.1 / 3.8 / 0.3 / 4.1	**28** TU	0157 / 0834 / 1426 / 2056	0.2 / 3.6 / 0.4 / 3.8
14 TU	0404 / 1030 / 1626 / 2250	0.0 / 3.8 / 0.1 / 4.1	**29** W	0307 / 0942 / 1536 / 2200	0.2 / 3.7 / 0.3 / 3.9
15 W	0500 / 1124 / 1720 / 2341	-0.1 / 3.9 / 0.0 / 4.1	**30** TH	0409 / 1040 / 1638 / 2259	0.0 / 3.9 / 0.2 / 4.1
			31 F	0506 / 1132 / 1736 / 2353	0.0 / 4.1 / 0.1 / 4.2

JUNE

Day	Time	m	Day	Time	m
1 SA ○	0600 / 1221 / 1828	-0.1 / 4.2 / 0.0	**16** SU	0056 / 0659 / 1314 / ●1926	4.2 / 0.2 / 4.3 / 0.1
2 SU	0044 / 0650 / 1307 / 1916	4.2 / -0.1 / 4.3 / -0.1	**17** M	0137 / 0738 / 1350 / 2003	4.2 / 0.2 / 4.4 / 0.1
3 M	0133 / 0737 / 1352 / 2004	4.2 / -0.1 / 4.3 / -0.2	**18** TU	0213 / 0811 / 1423 / 2035	4.1 / 0.1 / 4.4 / 0.0
4 TU	0223 / 0825 / 1440 / 2054	4.2 / -0.1 / 4.3 / -0.3	**19** W	0247 / 0844 / 1457 / 2108	4.1 / 0.1 / 4.3 / 0.0
5 W	0314 / 0912 / 1527 / 2141	4.1 / -0.1 / 4.3 / -0.3	**20** TH	0320 / 0916 / 1530 / 2140	4.0 / 0.1 / 4.3 / 0.1
6 TH	0403 / 0957 / 1614 / 2227	4.1 / -0.1 / 4.3 / -0.2	**21** F	0352 / 0946 / 1602 / 2212	3.9 / 0.2 / 4.2 / 0.1
7 F	0451 / 1042 / 1704 / 2317	4.0 / 0.0 / 4.3 / -0.1	**22** SA	0425 / 1019 / 1637 / 2245	3.9 / 0.2 / 4.1 / 0.1
8 SA	0542 / 1133 / 1800	3.9 / 0.2 / 4.3	**23** SU	0502 / 1054 / 1715 / 2323	3.8 / 0.2 / 4.1 / 0.1
9 SU	0014 / 0641 / 1232 / 1901	0.0 / 3.8 / 0.3 / 4.2	**24** M	0544 / 1135 / 1759	3.7 / 0.3 / 4.0
10 M	0117 / 0744 / 1338 / 2008	0.2 / 3.8 / 0.4 / 4.2	**25** TU	0006 / 0634 / 1225 / 1853	0.2 / 3.7 / 0.4 / 3.9
11 TU	0224 / 0851 / 1447 / 2117	0.2 / 3.8 / 0.3 / 4.1	**26** W	0102 / 0736 / 1329 / 1959	0.2 / 3.7 / 0.4 / 3.9
12 W	0329 / 0955 / 1554 / 2221	0.1 / 3.9 / 0.2 / 4.1	**27** TH	0208 / 0846 / 1443 / 2111	0.2 / 3.8 / 0.4 / 3.9
13 TH	0429 / 1054 / 1654 / 2318	0.1 / 4.0 / 0.1 / 4.1	**28** F	0319 / 0954 / 1556 / 2221	0.2 / 3.9 / 0.3 / 4.1
14 F	0522 / 1146 / 1749	0.1 / 4.1 / 0.1	**29** SA	0428 / 1056 / 1704 / 2325	0.1 / 4.1 / 0.2 / 4.2
15 SA	0008 / 0613 / 1233 / 1841	4.1 / 0.2 / 4.2 / 0.1	**30** SU	0532 / 1153 / 1805	0.1 / 4.2 / 0.1

JULY

Day	Time	m	Day	Time	m
1 M ○	0023 / 0630 / 1245 / 1859	4.2 / 0.0 / 4.3 / -0.1	**16** TU	0117 / 0718 / 1330 / 1944	4.1 / 0.2 / 4.4 / 0.1
2 TU	0117 / 0723 / 1336 / 1952	4.3 / 0.0 / 4.4 / -0.2	**17** W	0154 / 0754 / 1405 / 2019	4.1 / 0.2 / 4.4 / 0.1
3 W	0211 / 0815 / 1427 / 2045	4.2 / -0.1 / 4.5 / -0.3	**18** TH	0228 / 0827 / 1438 / 2051	4.1 / 0.1 / 4.4 / 0.1
4 TH	0305 / 0906 / 1517 / 2137	4.2 / -0.1 / 4.5 / -0.3	**19** F	0258 / 0857 / 1508 / 2120	4.1 / 0.1 / 4.3 / 0.1
5 F	0355 / 0952 / 1605 / 2223	4.1 / -0.1 / 4.5 / -0.2	**20** SA	0327 / 0926 / 1539 / 2150	4.0 / 0.1 / 4.3 / 0.1
6 SA	0440 / 1035 / 1652 / 2310	4.1 / 0.0 / 4.5 / 0.1	**21** SU	0400 / 0958 / 1614 / 2224	4.0 / 0.1 / 4.2 / 0.1
7 SU	0526 / 1121 / 1742 / 2359	4.0 / 0.2 / 4.4 / 0.1	**22** M	0438 / 1034 / 1652 / 2300	3.9 / 0.2 / 4.1 / 0.0
8 M	0615 / 1211 / 1835	4.0 / 0.3 / 4.3	**23** TU	0517 / 1111 / 1729 / 2335	3.8 / 0.2 / 4.0 / 0.1
9 TU	0049 / 0708 / 1305 / 1932	0.2 / 3.9 / 0.4 / 4.2	**24** W	0556 / 1149 / 1811	3.8 / 0.3 / 4.0
10 W	0143 / 0807 / 1407 / 2037	0.3 / 3.9 / 0.4 / 4.1	**25** TH	0017 / 0646 / 1242 / 1910	0.2 / 3.8 / 0.4 / 3.9
11 TH	0246 / 0913 / 1517 / 2148	0.4 / 3.9 / 0.4 / 4.0	**26** F	0117 / 0753 / 1355 / 2027	0.3 / 3.8 / 0.4 / 3.9
12 F	0354 / 1022 / 1628 / 2254	0.4 / 4.0 / 0.3 / 4.0	**27** SA	0235 / 0911 / 1518 / 2149	0.4 / 3.9 / 0.4 / 4.0
13 SA	0458 / 1123 / 1731 / 2350	0.3 / 4.1 / 0.3 / 4.1	**28** SU	0356 / 1026 / 1637 / 2303	0.3 / 4.0 / 0.3 / 4.1
14 SU	0552 / 1212 / 1823	0.3 / 4.2 / 0.2	**29** M	0511 / 1131 / 1748	0.2 / 4.2 / 0.1
15 M	0036 / 0639 / 1254 / ●1906	4.1 / 0.2 / 4.3 / 0.2	**30** TU	0008 / 0616 / 1229 / ○1848	4.2 / 0.1 / 4.3 / 0.0
			31 W	0106 / 0714 / 1322 / 1943	4.2 / 0.0 / 4.5 / -0.2

AUGUST

Day	Time	m	Day	Time	m
1 TH	0200 / 0807 / 1413 / 2035	4.2 / 0.0 / 4.5 / -0.2	**16** F	0203 / 0807 / 1414 / 2029	4.1 / 0.1 / 4.3 / 0.1
2 F	0251 / 0856 / 1503 / 2125	4.2 / -0.1 / 4.5 / -0.2	**17** SA	0233 / 0836 / 1444 / 2057	4.1 / 0.0 / 4.3 / 0.1
3 SA	0338 / 0940 / 1549 / 2210	4.2 / -0.1 / 4.5 / -0.1	**18** SU	0302 / 0905 / 1515 / 2127	4.1 / 0.0 / 4.3 / 0.1
4 SU	0420 / 1020 / 1633 / 2252	4.1 / 0.0 / 4.5 / 0.0	**19** M	0335 / 0937 / 1551 / 2202	4.0 / 0.1 / 4.2 / 0.1
5 M	0500 / 1100 / 1717 / 2332	4.1 / 0.1 / 4.4 / 0.2	**20** TU	0413 / 1015 / 1629 / 2238	4.0 / 0.1 / 4.1 / 0.1
6 TU	0541 / 1142 / 1801	4.0 / 0.3 / 4.3	**21** W	0450 / 1050 / 1704 / 2308	3.9 / 0.2 / 4.0 / 0.1
7 W	0012 / 0625 / 1226 / 1850	0.3 / 4.0 / 0.4 / 4.1	**22** TH	0524 / 1122 / 1740 / 2342	3.9 / 0.2 / 4.0 / 0.3
8 TH	0056 / 0717 / 1321 / 1952	0.5 / 3.9 / 0.6 / 3.9	**23** F	0607 / 1206 / 1834	3.8 / 0.4 / 3.8
9 F	0156 / 0825 / 1434 / 2109	0.6 / 3.9 / 0.6 / 3.8	**24** SA	0038 / 0713 / 1319 / 1954	0.5 / 3.8 / 0.5 / 3.8
10 SA	0313 / 0944 / 1557 / 2227	0.7 / 3.9 / 0.5 / 3.9	**25** SU	0202 / 0838 / 1451 / 2126	0.5 / 3.8 / 0.4 / 3.8
11 SU	0431 / 1057 / 1711 / 2330	0.6 / 4.1 / 0.4 / 4.0	**26** M	0335 / 1003 / 1621 / 2249	0.5 / 4.0 / 0.3 / 4.0
12 M	0533 / 1152 / 1805	0.4 / 4.2 / 0.1	**27** TU	0458 / 1115 / 1736 / 2356	0.4 / 4.2 / 0.1 / 4.1
13 TU	0017 / 0619 / 1232 / 1846	4.1 / 0.3 / 4.3 / 0.0	**28** W ○	0605 / 1213 / 1838	0.2 / 4.3 / 0.0
14 W	0055 / 0658 / 1307 / ●1922	4.1 / 0.2 / 4.3 / 0.1	**29** TH	0053 / 0702 / 1305 / 1930	4.2 / 0.1 / 4.4 / -0.1
15 TH	0130 / 0734 / 1342 / 1957	4.1 / 0.1 / 4.3 / 0.1	**30** F	0143 / 0754 / 1355 / 2019	4.2 / 0.0 / 4.5 / -0.1
			31 SA	0230 / 0840 / 1442 / 2106	4.2 / 0.0 / 4.6 / -0.1

Chart Datum: 2·26 metres below Normal Null (German reference level)

21

TIME ZONE –0100
(German Standard Time)
Subtract 1 hour for UT

For German Summer Time add ONE hour in non-shaded areas

GERMANY – WILHELMSHAVEN

LAT 53°31′N   LONG 8°09′E

TIMES AND HEIGHTS OF HIGH AND LOW WATERS

YEAR **1996**

SEPTEMBER

Day	Time	m	Time	m	Time	m	Time	m
1 SU	0313	4.2	0922	0.0	1527	4.5	2148	0.0
2 M	0352	4.2	0959	0.0	1609	4.5	2226	0.1
3 TU	0429	4.2	1035	0.1	1648	4.3	2300	0.3
4 W	0504	4.1	1110	0.3	1726	4.2	2332	0.5
5 TH	0541	4.0	1146	0.5	1808	3.9		
6 F	0009	0.6	0627	3.9	1234	0.7	1905	3.8
7 SA	0104	0.8	0734	3.8	1346	0.8	2023	3.7
8 SU	0225	0.9	0859	3.8	1516	0.8	2149	3.7
9 M	0353	0.8	1021	4.0	1641	0.6	2301	3.9
10 TU	0505	0.6	1122	4.1	1741	0.4	2350	4.0
11 W	0553	0.4	1203	4.2	1819	0.2		
12 TH ●	0025	4.1	0630	0.3	1237	4.2	1852	0.2
13 F	0059	4.1	0706	0.2	1311	4.2	1927	0.1
14 SA	0134	4.1	0740	0.1	1346	4.2	2001	0.1
15 SU	0206	4.1	0813	0.1	1419	4.3	2033	0.1
16 M	0238	4.1	0845	0.1	1452	4.2	2105	0.1
17 TU	0311	4.1	0919	0.1	1529	4.2	2140	0.1
18 W	0348	4.1	0955	0.1	1607	4.1	2214	0.2
19 TH	0424	4.0	1029	0.1	1642	4.0	2243	0.2
20 F	0458	3.9	1101	0.2	1720	3.9	2318	0.4
21 SA	0542	3.8	1146	0.4	1815	3.8		
22 SU	0015	0.6	0648	3.8	1300	0.5	1937	3.7
23 M	0143	0.7	0817	3.8	1437	0.5	2111	3.8
24 TU	0322	0.6	0946	4.0	1610	0.3	2236	3.9
25 W	0446	0.5	1059	4.2	1724	0.2	2341	4.0
26 TH	0549	0.3	1155	4.3	1821	0.0		
27 F O	0033	4.1	0643	0.2	1245	4.4	1911	0.0
28 SA	0120	4.2	0733	0.1	1334	4.5	1958	0.0
29 SU	0204	4.1	0819	0.1	1419	4.5	2041	0.1
30 M	0244	4.3	0859	0.1	1501	4.5	2120	0.2

OCTOBER

Day	Time	m	Time	m	Time	m	Time	m
1 TU	0321	4.3	0934	0.1	1541	4.4	2155	0.3
2 W	0356	4.3	1007	0.2	1618	4.2	2225	0.4
3 TH	0428	4.2	1039	0.3	1653	4.0	2253	0.5
4 F	0501	4.1	1111	0.5	1731	3.8	2327	0.7
5 SA	0543	3.9	1152	0.7	1821	3.7		
6 SU	0017	0.9	0643	3.8	1257	0.9	1932	3.6
7 M	0132	1.1	0805	3.8	1424	0.9	2057	3.6
8 TU	0300	1.0	0929	3.9	1553	0.7	2215	3.7
9 W	0418	0.8	1036	4.0	1659	0.5	2310	3.9
10 TH	0513	0.5	1122	4.1	1741	0.3	2348	4.0
11 F	0553	0.4	1158	4.1	1814	0.2		
12 SA ●	0024	4.1	0632	0.3	1237	4.1	1852	0.2
13 SU	0101	4.1	0712	0.2	1316	4.2	1930	0.1
14 M	0138	4.1	0749	0.2	1353	4.2	2007	0.2
15 TU	0213	4.2	0825	0.2	1430	4.2	2044	0.2
16 W	0248	4.2	0901	0.1	1508	4.2	2119	0.2
17 TH	0324	4.2	0937	0.1	1547	4.1	2152	0.2
18 F	0401	4.1	1011	0.2	1626	4.0	2225	0.3
19 SA	0440	4.0	1050	0.2	1710	3.8	2305	0.5
20 SU	0530	3.9	1141	0.4	1809	3.7		
21 M	0006	0.7	0637	3.9	1255	0.5	1928	3.7
22 TU	0132	0.8	0802	4.0	1427	0.5	2057	3.7
23 W	0306	0.7	0928	4.1	1555	0.4	2217	3.9
24 TH	0426	0.5	1038	4.2	1703	0.2	2318	4.0
25 F	0526	0.4	1133	4.3	1756	0.2		
26 SA O	0008	4.1	0618	0.3	1223	4.3	1846	0.2
27 SU	0054	4.2	0709	0.3	1311	4.4	1933	0.3
28 M	0137	4.3	0756	0.3	1355	4.4	2015	0.3
29 TU	0215	4.3	0834	0.3	1435	4.4	2050	0.4
30 W	0250	4.4	0908	0.3	1513	4.3	2123	0.4
31 TH	0324	4.3	0940	0.3	1549	4.1	2152	0.4

NOVEMBER

Day	Time	m	Time	m	Time	m	Time	m
1 F	0357	4.2	1011	0.4	1624	3.9	2221	0.5
2 SA	0429	4.1	1042	0.5	1659	3.8	2253	0.7
3 SU	0507	4.0	1119	0.7	1742	3.6	2336	0.9
4 M	0558	3.9	1211	0.8	1840	3.6		
5 TU	0038	1.0	0706	3.8	1324	0.9	1953	3.6
6 W	0155	1.0	0823	3.8	1446	0.8	2111	3.6
7 TH	0314	0.9	0934	3.9	1558	0.6	2215	3.8
8 F	0418	0.7	1030	4.0	1651	0.4	2304	3.9
9 SA	0510	0.5	1117	4.1	1733	0.3	2346	4.1
10 SU	0557	0.4	1202	4.1	1817	0.2		
11 M ●	0028	4.1	0642	0.3	1246	4.2	1900	0.2
12 TU	0109	4.2	0724	0.3	1328	4.2	1942	0.2
13 W	0148	4.3	0804	0.2	1409	4.2	2022	0.2
14 TH	0227	4.3	0845	0.2	1452	4.2	2102	0.4
15 F	0307	4.3	0925	0.1	1535	4.1	2139	0.3
16 SA	0347	4.2	1003	0.1	1618	4.0	2216	0.4
17 SU	0431	4.2	1047	0.2	1706	3.9	2301	0.5
18 M	0524	4.1	1142	0.4	1806	3.8		
19 TU	0001	0.7	0628	4.1	1250	0.5	1917	3.7
20 W	0117	0.8	0743	4.1	1410	0.5	2034	3.8
21 TH	0241	0.8	0901	4.1	1528	0.4	2147	3.8
22 F	0356	0.6	1011	4.2	1634	0.3	2249	3.9
23 SA	0458	0.5	1109	4.2	1729	0.3	2341	4.0
24 SU	0553	0.4	1201	4.2	1820	0.4		
25 M O	0029	4.2	0646	0.4	1250	4.3	1908	0.4
26 TU	0112	4.3	0733	0.4	1333	4.3	1949	0.5
27 W	0149	4.4	0811	0.4	1411	4.3	2023	0.5
28 TH	0223	4.4	0844	0.4	1447	4.2	2055	0.4
29 F	0258	4.4	0917	0.3	1524	4.1	2126	0.4
30 SA	0332	4.3	0949	0.4	1558	3.9	2156	0.5

DECEMBER

Day	Time	m	Time	m	Time	m	Time	m
1 SU	0404	4.2	1020	0.4	1631	3.8	2227	0.6
2 M	0439	4.1	1052	0.5	1707	3.7	2303	0.7
3 TU	0519	4.0	1132	0.6	1752	3.6	2349	0.8
4 W	0611	3.9	1225	0.7	1850	3.6		
5 TH	0049	0.9	0714	3.8	1333	0.7	2000	3.6
6 F	0202	0.9	0824	3.8	1446	0.6	2111	3.7
7 SA	0315	0.8	0932	3.9	1552	0.5	2214	3.9
8 SU	0421	0.6	1033	4.0	1650	0.4	2307	4.0
9 M	0519	0.5	1128	4.1	1742	0.3	2356	4.1
10 TU ●	0611	0.4	1218	4.2	1831	0.3		
11 W	0041	4.2	0658	0.3	1305	4.2	1918	0.2
12 TH	0125	4.3	0744	0.2	1353	4.2	2004	0.2
13 F	0209	4.3	0832	0.1	1441	4.2	2051	0.2
14 SA	0255	4.4	0918	0.0	1528	4.1	2134	0.2
15 SU	0339	4.4	1001	0.1	1614	4.0	2214	0.3
16 M	0425	4.3	1046	0.2	1701	3.9	2258	0.4
17 TU	0516	4.3	1138	0.3	1755	3.8	2351	0.5
18 W	0614	4.2	1237	0.4	1855	3.8		
19 TH	0054	0.6	0718	4.1	1341	0.5	2001	3.8
20 F	0204	0.7	0828	4.1	1450	0.5	2109	3.8
21 SA	0317	0.6	0940	4.1	1558	0.5	2216	3.9
22 SU	0427	0.5	1046	4.1	1700	0.4	2316	4.0
23 M	0530	0.5	1143	4.1	1755	0.5		
24 TU O	0008	4.2	0625	0.4	1232	4.1	1845	0.5
25 W	0051	4.3	0712	0.4	1315	4.2	1926	0.4
26 TH	0129	4.4	0750	0.4	1352	4.2	2001	0.4
27 F	0203	4.4	0824	0.3	1427	4.1	2035	0.4
28 SA	0238	4.4	0858	0.3	1502	4.0	2106	0.3
29 SU	0312	4.3	0930	0.3	1534	3.9	2135	0.3
30 M	0343	4.2	0959	0.3	1605	3.8	2203	0.4
31 TU	0415	4.1	1028	0.3	1638	3.8	2235	0.4

Chart Datum: 2·26 metres below Normal Null (German reference level)

WILHELMSHAVEN   10-21-17

Niedersächsen 53°31'·00N 08°09'·00E

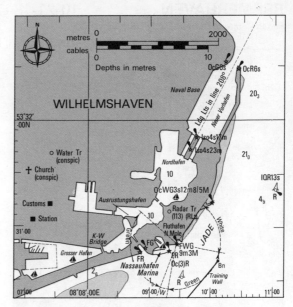

CHARTS
AC 3369; BSH 3015 Sheet 12, D7

TIDES
+0050 Dover; ML 2·3; Duration 0615; Zone –0100
WILHELMSHAVEN is a Standard Port. Predictions above.

SHELTER
Good in the yacht hbrs at Großer Hafen and Nordhafen, inside the sea lock, the latter rather remote. Sea lock operates Mon-Thur: 0600-1830; Fri: 0600-1700; Sat, Sun and hols: 0800-1600 (all LT). The tidal yacht hbr in Nassauhafen is better for a short stay.

NAVIGATION
WPT JW5/Jade 1 SHM buoy, Oc G 4s, 53°52'·42N 07°44'·10E, 296°/116° from/to Mellumplate lt, 14·2M. From abeam this lt, it is approx 15M to Wilhelmshaven, a busy commercial port, via the deep, wide and well marked fairway.

Note: The Ems-Jade canal, 39M to Emden, is usable by yachts with lowering masts and max draft 1·7m. Min bridge clearance 3·75m. It has 6 locks. Speed limit 4kn.

LIGHTS AND MARKS
R Jade is well marked/lit; for principal lts see 10.21.4. Ldg lts 208° into Neuer Vorhafen both Iso 4s. Fluthafen N mole FWG 9m 6/3M (sectors on chartlet); S arm, hd FR.

RADIO TELEPHONE
Port Ch 11 16 (H24). Sea lock Ch 13. Bridge opening Ch 11.

TELEPHONE (04421)
Hr Mr 291256; Port Authority 4800-20; Sea Lock 186480; VTS 489381/2; ∰ 480723; Weather Bremerhaven 72220; Water Police 942358; Ⓗ 8011; Brit Consul (040) 446071.

FACILITIES
Nassauhafen Marina (28 + 100 visitors) ☎ 41439 Slip, BY, ME, P, D, AC, Bar, FW, SM, R; **Wiking Sportsboothafen** (30) ☎ 41301 AC, Bar, CH, El, FW, Gaz, ME, R, SM, V, Sh; **Hochsee YC Germania** ☎ 44121.
Town BY, SM, ME, CH, El, P, D, Gaz, V, ✉, Ⓑ, ⇌, ✈.
Ferry: Hamburg-Harwich.

ADJACENT HARBOUR IN JADEBUSEN

DANGAST, Niedersächsen, 53°27'·00N 08°07'·00E. AC 3369; BSH 3015.13. HW +0055 on Dover (UT); –0007 on Helgoland (zone –0100). 4M S of Wilhelmshaven, drying hbr in the wide bay of Jadebusen, which mostly dries. Appr via Stenkentief, marked on NW side by stakes, thence SW into Dangaster Aussentief (0·5m at LWS). Unlit, other than Arngast lt, F WRG (not visible from SW), R tr, W bands, in the middle of Jadebusen. Yacht hbr (dries) on W side just before lock into Dangaster Tief, access HW ±2. Facilities: usual amenities can be found in the seaside town of Dangast.

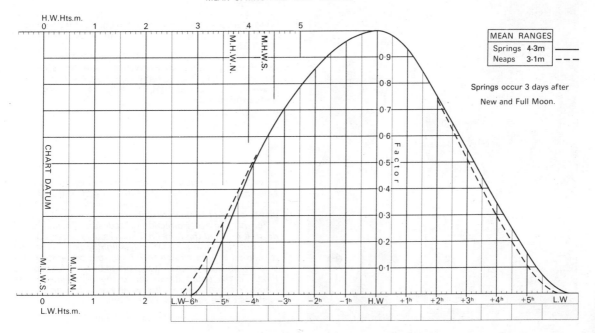

WILHELMSHAVEN
MEAN SPRING AND NEAP CURVES

MEAN RANGES	
Springs	4·3m —
Neaps	3·1m - - -

Springs occur 3 days after New and Full Moon.

BREMERHAVEN   10-21-18
Federal State of Bremen 53°32'·16N 08°34'·57E

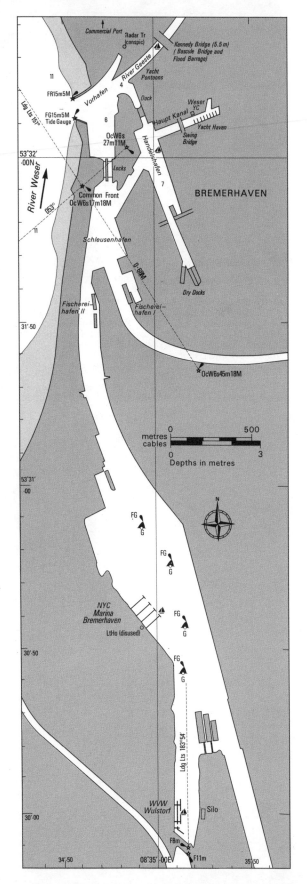

CHARTS
AC 3406, 3405; BSH 3011 Sheets 7, 8 & 10, D4.
TIDES
+0051 Dover; ML 2·0; Duration 0600; Zone −0100

Standard Port WILHELMSHAVEN (←)

Times				Height (metres)			
High Water		Low Water		MHWS	MHWN	MLWN	MLWS
0200	0800	0200	0900	4·3	3·7	0·6	0·0
1400	2000	1400	2100				
Differences BREMERHAVEN							
+0029	+0046	+0033	+0038	−0·3	−0·1	−0·1	0·0
NORDENHAM							
+0051	+0109	+0055	+0058	−0·2	−0·1	−0·3	−0·1
BRAKE							
+0118	+0119	+0140	+0151	−0·2	−0·2	−0·4	−0·2
ELSFLETH							
+0130	+0131	+0200	+0210	−0·1	−0·1	−0·3	0·0
VEGESACK							
+0200	+0156	+0245	+0249	−0·2	−0·2	−0·6	−0·2
BREMEN							
+0207	+0204	+0307	+0307	−0·1	−0·1	−0·6	−0·2

SHELTER
Yachts may enter R Geeste, uncomfortable in SW/W winds, or one of the 3 YC/marinas in the most southerly basin, entered via Vorhafen, close S of conspic 112m radar tr : The Weser YC Yacht Haven to E of Handelshafen; the Nordseeyachting Marina (NYC or Bremerhaven Marina) in Fischereihafen II, 1·3M S of locks on W side (3m); & the Wassersportverein Wulstorf Marina (WVW) 0·5M beyond. There are also yacht hbrs further up the R Weser at Nordenham, Rodenkirchen, Brake and on the R Hunte at Elsfleth and Oldenburg.

NAVIGATION
WPT Alte Weser: Schlüsseltonne (SWM) buoy, Iso 8s, 53°56'·30N 07°54'·87E, 300°/120° from/to Alte Weser lt, 9M. For R Weser (very well marked) see 10.21.5. Leave R Weser at lt buoy 61. Beware much commercial shipping and ferries using R Geeste.

LIGHTS AND MARKS
Ldg lts, both Oc 6s 17/45m 18M, synch, lead 151° down main chan (R Weser). Vorhafen ent FR & FG 15m 5M. To enter Schleusenhafen, sound Q (−−·−) and ent on Ⓖ.

RADIO TELEPHONE
Bremerhaven Port Ch 12 16 (H24). Bremerhaven Weser Ch 14 16 (H24). Info broadcasts in German at H + 20 by: *Alte Weser Radar* Ch 22; *Hohe Weg Radar I & II* Ch 02; *Robbenplate Radar I & II* Ch 04; and *Blexen Radar* Ch 07; also at H + 30 on Ch 19 78 81 by *Bremen-Weser Traffic* and on Ch 63 by *Hunte Traffic*. *Brake Lock* Ch 10 (H24). *Hunte Bridge Radio* Ch 73 (HJ). *Oslebshausen Lock Radio* (Bremen) Ch 12. *Bremen Port Radio* Ch 03 14 16 (H24).

TELEPHONE (0471)
Hr Mr 481260; Weser YC Hafen 23531; NYC Marina 77555 WVW Marina 73268; Fischereihafen Lock 4811; Weather 72220; Police 47011; Ⓗ 42028; Brit Consul (040) 446071.

FACILITIES
Weser YC ☎ 23531 C, AC, FW, R, Bar; **NYC Marina** ☎ 77555 P, D, C, Slip, AC, FW; **WVW Marina** ☎ 73268, FW, Slip, C, El, P, D; **Datema** ☎ 199815 ACA; **Town** all facilities: Gaz, V, R, Bar, ✉, Ⓑ, ⇌, ✈. Ferry: Hamburg-Harwich.

The yacht lay with a very slight heel (thanks to a pair of small bilge-keels on her bottom) in a sort of trough she had dug for herself, so that she was still ringed with a few inches of water, as it were with a moat.

    For miles in every direction lay a desert of sand. To the north it touched the horizon, and was only broken by the blue dot of Neuwerk Island and its lighthouse. To the east it seemed also to stretch to infinity, but the smoke of a steamer showed where it was pierced by the stream of the Elbe. To the south it ran up to the pencil-line of the Hanover shore. Only to the west was it broken by any vestiges of the sea it had arisen from.

Riddle of the Sands: Erskine Childers

CUXHAVEN   10-21-19

Niedersächsen 53°52'·48N 08°42'·56E (Marina ent)

CHARTS
AC 3261; BSH 3010 Sheet 1

TIDES
+0103 Dover; ML 1·7; Duration 0535; Zone −0100
CUXHAVEN is a Standard Port; predictions are below

Standard Port CUXHAVEN (→)

Times				Height (metres)			
High Water		Low Water		MHWS	MHWN	MLWN	MLWS
0200	0800	0200	0900	3·3	2·9	0·4	0·0
1400	2000	1400	2100				
Differences SCHARHÖRN (11M to NW)							
−0045	−0047	−0057	−0059	0·0	0·0	0·0	0·0

SHELTER
Good in the YC marina (4m). Yachts > 20m LOA may be allowed in the Alter Hafen or Alter Fischerei-Hafen. For **Otterndorf** see under 10.21.22.

NAVIGATION
WPT No 31 SHM buoy, Fl G 4s, 53°53'·97N 08°41'·27E, 332°/152° from/to marina ent, 1·7M. From No 23 SHM buoy, appr is in W sector (144°-149°) of Baumrönne ldg lt Fl 3s. Chan well marked/lit, see 10.21.4, .5 and .19. Ebb runs up to 5kn off Cuxhaven. Much commercial shipping.

LIGHTS AND MARKS
Ent to YC Marina is close NW of conspic radar tr, and N of main lt ho (dark R with copper cupola) FWR, Fl (4) 12s, Oc 6s and Fl (5) 12s (for sectors see chartlet). YC marina ent, N side FWG; S side FWR, shown 1 Apr-31 Oct. Tide sigs (lit G by day, Y at night) from radar tr. Upper panel: ∧ = flood tide; ∨ = ebb tide; horiz line below ∨ = level below CD. Lower panel shows ht of tide in dm above CD.

RADIO TELEPHONE
Radar coverage of the Elbe from Elbe lt float to lt buoy No 55 in sequence on Ch 65, 19, 18, 05, 21 and 03; also, in the same area, *Cuxhaven Elbe Traffic* broadcasts nav/weather info in English and German every H + 55 on Ch 71. *Cuxhaven Radar* Ch 21 from lt buoys 27 to 41. *Cuxhaven Elbe Port* Ch **12** 16 (H24). Port/lock work Ch 69.

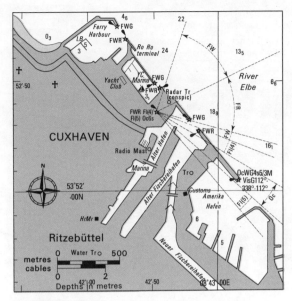

TELEPHONE (04721)
Hr Mr 34111 (Apr-Oct); CG 38011; LB 34622 and Ch 16; Weather 36400; Port Authority 501450; ⌗ 21085; British Cruising Assn and Little Ship Club 35820; Police 110; Dr 112; Brit Consul (040) 446071.

FACILITIES
Cuxhaven YC Marina (Segler-Vereinigung) ☎ 34111 (summer only), 18DM, Slip, FW, P & D (cans), C (10 ton), AC, BY, ME, El, Sh, CH, SM, Gaz, chart agent, Ⓔ, R, Bar, ▣, ⌗; **Little Ship Club** ☎ 35820. **CG and LB** (Ch 16). **City** All facilities, ≈, ✈ (Bremen, Hamburg, Hanover). Ferry: Hamburg -Harwich.

CUXHAVEN
MEAN SPRING AND NEAP CURVES

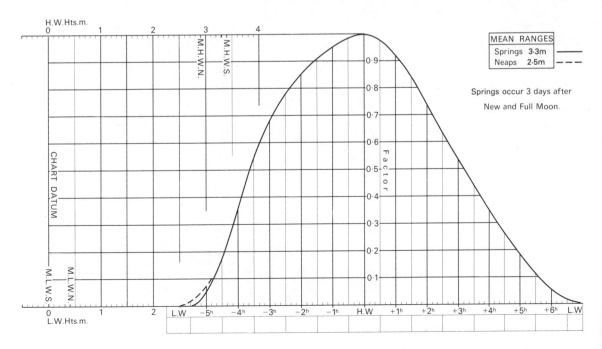

MEAN RANGES	
Springs	3·3m
Neaps	2·5m

Springs occur 3 days after
New and Full Moon.

TIME ZONE –0100
(German Standard Time)
Subtract 1 hour for UT
For German Summer Time add ONE hour in non-shaded areas

GERMANY – CUXHAVEN

LAT 53°52′N   LONG 8°43′E

TIMES AND HEIGHTS OF HIGH AND LOW WATERS

YEAR **1996**

MAY

Day		Time	m	Time	m	Time	m	Time	m
1	W	0555	-0.2	1133	2.9	1815	0.0	2348	3.1
16	TH	0640	-0.1	1218	3.1	1904	0.0		
2	TH	0640	-0.2	1215	3.1	1904	-0.1		
17	F ●	0036	3.2	0728	0.0	1303	3.2	1954	0.0
3	F O	0032	3.2	0725	-0.2	1256	3.1	1948	-0.1
18	SA	0123	3.3	0813	0.1	1344	3.3	2037	0.0
4	SA	0116	3.2	0807	-0.2	1335	3.2	2030	-0.2
19	SU	0204	3.3	0850	0.1	1418	3.4	2112	0.0
5	SU	0158	3.3	0848	-0.2	1414	3.2	2113	-0.2
20	M	0240	3.3	0923	0.1	1450	3.4	2145	0.1
6	M	0241	3.2	0931	-0.2	1456	3.3	2157	-0.3
21	TU	0315	3.2	0956	0.1	1524	3.3	2217	0.0
7	TU	0326	3.2	1015	-0.2	1541	3.2	2240	-0.3
22	W	0351	3.1	1026	0.1	1600	3.3	2250	0.0
8	W	0413	3.1	1056	-0.1	1627	3.2	2323	-0.3
23	TH	0426	3.0	1056	0.1	1635	3.2	2321	0.1
9	TH	0501	3.0	1138	-0.1	1717	3.1		
24	F	0502	2.9	1129	0.2	1712	3.1	2357	0.1
10	F	0012	-0.2	0555	2.9	1229	0.1	1817	3.1
25	SA	0543	2.8	1208	0.3	1756	3.0		
11	SA	0112	0.0	0702	2.8	1335	0.2	1928	3.1
26	SU	0041	0.2	0634	2.7	1300	0.3	1854	2.9
12	SU	0227	0.0	0820	2.8	1456	0.2	2046	3.1
27	M	0142	0.2	0738	2.7	1407	0.3	2001	2.9
13	M	0348	0.0	0936	2.9	1617	0.1	2159	3.1
28	TU	0254	0.1	0849	2.7	1522	0.2	2110	2.9
14	TU	0459	-0.1	1041	2.9	1722	0.0	2258	3.2
29	W	0404	0.0	0954	2.8	1631	0.2	2213	3.0
15	W	0553	-0.2	1132	3.0	1814	-0.1	2347	3.2
30	TH	0505	-0.1	1049	3.0	1732	0.1	2310	3.1
31	F	0600	-0.1	1139	3.1	1829	0.0		

JUNE

Day		Time	m	Time	m	Time	m	Time	m
1	SA O	0002	3.2	0653	-0.1	1226	3.3	1921	0.0
16	SU ●	0105	3.2	0749	0.2	1323	3.4	2016	0.1
2	SU	0050	3.3	0741	-0.1	1311	3.3	2008	-0.1
17	M	0146	3.3	0828	0.2	1357	3.5	2053	0.1
3	M	0138	3.2	0827	-0.1	1355	3.4	2056	-0.2
18	TU	0222	3.2	0902	0.1	1431	3.5	2126	0.1
4	TU	0227	3.3	0916	-0.1	1443	3.4	2146	-0.3
19	W	0256	3.2	0935	0.1	1505	3.4	2159	0.1
5	W	0317	3.2	1004	-0.1	1531	3.4	2234	-0.3
20	TH	0330	3.1	1006	0.1	1539	3.4	2231	0.1
6	TH	0407	3.1	1050	-0.1	1620	3.4	2321	-0.2
21	F	0403	3.1	1036	0.1	1614	3.3	2303	0.1
7	F	0457	3.1	1135	0.0	1712	3.4		
22	SA	0438	3.0	1109	0.2	1649	3.2	2337	0.1
8	SA	0012	-0.1	0552	3.0	1226	0.1	1810	3.3
23	SU	0517	2.9	1146	0.2	1728	3.1		
9	SU	0109	0.0	0653	2.9	1325	0.2	1914	3.3
24	M	0015	0.1	0600	2.8	1226	0.2	1813	3.0
10	M	0211	0.1	0758	2.9	1432	0.3	2021	3.2
25	TU	0100	0.1	0651	2.8	1317	0.3	1909	3.0
11	TU	0317	0.1	0905	3.0	1543	0.2	2129	3.2
26	W	0156	0.1	0752	2.8	1423	0.3	2014	3.0
12	W	0424	0.1	1007	3.0	1650	0.1	2231	3.2
27	TH	0304	0.1	0901	2.9	1537	0.2	2125	3.0
13	TH	0522	0.0	1104	3.1	1748	0.1	2326	3.2
28	F	0415	0.1	1006	3.0	1650	0.2	2233	3.1
14	F	0613	0.1	1156	3.2	1841	0.1		
29	SA	0523	0.1	1106	3.2	1757	0.1	2335	3.3
15	SA	0017	3.2	0702	0.1	1242	3.3	1932	0.1
30	SU	0625	0.1	1200	3.3	1858	0.0		

JULY

Day		Time	m	Time	m	Time	m	Time	m
1	M O	0030	3.3	0721	0.0	1252	3.4	1952	-0.1
16	TU	0129	3.2	0809	0.2	1339	3.4	2035	0.1
2	TU	0124	3.3	0813	0.0	1341	3.5	2044	-0.2
17	W	0205	3.2	0845	0.1	1414	3.5	2110	0.1
3	W	0217	3.3	0906	-0.1	1432	3.5	2137	-0.2
18	TH	0238	3.2	0917	0.1	1447	3.4	2142	0.1
4	TH	0310	3.2	0957	-0.1	1522	3.5	2228	-0.2
19	F	0308	3.2	0947	0.1	1518	3.4	2210	0.1
5	F	0359	3.2	1043	-0.1	1610	3.5	2315	-0.1
20	SA	0339	3.1	1015	0.1	1550	3.3	2241	0.1
6	SA	0447	3.2	1126	0.0	1700	3.5		
21	SU	0413	3.1	1049	0.1	1626	3.2	2316	0.1
7	SU	0001	0.0	0536	3.1	1212	0.2	1752	3.5
22	M	0451	3.0	1126	0.1	1705	3.1	2353	0.0
8	M	0050	0.1	0629	3.1	1303	0.2	1848	3.4
23	TU	0532	2.9	1202	0.1	1743	3.1		
9	TU	0140	0.2	0724	3.0	1358	0.3	1947	3.3
24	W	0028	0.1	0613	2.9	1240	0.2	1827	3.0
10	W	0235	0.3	0823	3.0	1501	0.4	2052	3.1
25	TH	0110	0.2	0704	2.9	1334	0.3	1927	3.0
11	TH	0339	0.3	0928	3.0	1612	0.3	2201	3.1
26	F	0212	0.3	0811	2.9	1450	0.3	2042	3.0
12	F	0447	0.3	1035	3.1	1722	0.3	2306	3.1
27	SA	0331	0.3	0926	3.0	1614	0.3	2203	3.1
13	SA	0549	0.3	1135	3.2	1822	0.2		
28	SU	0452	0.2	1039	3.1	1733	0.2	2316	3.2
14	SU	0002	3.2	0642	0.2	1224	3.3	1913	0.2
29	M	0605	0.2	1143	3.3	1842	0.1		
15	M ●	0048	3.2	0729	0.2	1304	3.4	1957	0.2
30	TU O	0018	3.3	0708	0.1	1238	3.4	1941	0.0
31	W	0113	3.3	0805	0.0	1330	3.5	2034	-0.1

AUGUST

Day		Time	m	Time	m	Time	m	Time	m
1	TH	0206	3.3	0857	0.0	1419	3.6	2125	-0.2
16	F	0215	3.2	0857	0.1	1425	3.4	2119	0.1
2	F	0257	3.3	0946	-0.1	1508	3.6	2215	-0.2
17	SA	0244	3.2	0926	0.1	1455	3.4	2147	0.1
3	SA	0344	3.2	1030		1555	3.6	2300	-0.1
18	SU	0314	3.1	0955	0.1	1526	3.3	2218	0.1
4	SU	0427	3.2	1109	0.0	1641	3.6	2341	0.1
19	M	0347	3.1	1029	0.1	1603	3.2	2254	0.1
5	M	0511	3.2	1150	0.2	1728	3.5		
20	TU	0426	3.0	1107	0.1	1643	3.2	2330	0.1
6	TU	0021	0.2	0556	3.1	1233	0.3	1815	3.3
21	W	0505	3.0	1142	0.1	1719	3.1		
7	W	0101	0.4	0642	3.1	1318	0.4	1906	3.2
22	TH	0001	0.1	0541	3.0	1213	0.2	1757	3.0
8	TH	0146	0.5	0736	3.0	1413	0.5	2009	3.0
23	F	0035	0.3	0626	2.9	1300	0.3	1852	2.9
9	F	0248	0.6	0844	3.0	1528	0.5	2125	3.0
24	SA	0133	0.4	0733	2.9	1416	0.4	2012	2.9
10	SA	0406	0.5	1002	3.0	1651	0.4	2243	3.0
25	SU	0259	0.4	0857	2.9	1550	0.3	2143	2.9
11	SU	0524	0.5	1113	3.2	1804	0.3	2346	3.1
26	M	0432	0.3	1021	3.1	1719	0.2	2304	3.1
12	M	0625	0.4	1206	3.3	1857	0.3		
27	TU	0553	0.3	1130	3.2	1831	0.1		
13	TU	0032	3.1	0710	0.3	1244	3.3	1938	0.2
28	W O	0009	3.2	0658	0.2	1226	3.4	1930	0.0
14	W ●	0108	3.2	0749	0.2	1318	3.4	2014	0.1
29	TH	0102	3.2	0753	0.1	1315	3.5	2020	-0.1
15	TH	0142	3.2	0825	0.1	1353	3.4	2048	0.1
30	F	0151	3.3	0843	0.0	1402	3.6	2108	0.0
31	SA	0238	3.3	0928	0.0	1449	3.6	2154	0.0

Chart Datum: 1·66 metres below Normal Null (German reference level)

TIME ZONE –0100
(German Standard Time)
Subtract 1 hour for UT

For German Summer Time add
ONE hour in non-shaded areas

GERMANY – CUXHAVEN

LAT 53°52′N   LONG 8°43′E

TIMES AND HEIGHTS OF HIGH AND LOW WATERS   YEAR **1996**

JANUARY

Day	Time	m	Day	Time	m
1 M	0328 / 0918 / 1608 / 2155	0.5 / 3.0 / 0.5 / 2.9	**16** TU	0204 / 0754 / 1445 / 2040	0.4 / 2.9 / 0.3 / 2.8
2 TU	0442 / 1027 / 1715 / 2259	0.5 / 3.0 / 0.4 / 3.0	**17** W	0327 / 0915 / 1608 / 2157	0.4 / 2.9 / 0.3 / 3.0
3 W	0549 / 1127 / 1813 / 2353	0.5 / 3.0 / 0.4 / 3.2	**18** TH	0452 / 1034 / 1727 / 2307	0.3 / 3.0 / 0.2 / 3.1
4 TH	0644 / 1217 / 1902	0.4 / 3.1 / 0.4	**19** F	0607 / 1143 / 1836	0.2 / 3.1 / 0.2
5 F O	0037 / 0731 / 1300 / 1945	3.2 / 0.3 / 3.1 / 0.3	**20** SA ●	0007 / 0712 / 1241 / 1935	3.2 / 0.0 / 3.2 / 0.1
6 SA	0114 / 0810 / 1337 / 2022	3.3 / 0.2 / 3.1 / 0.2	**21** SU	0100 / 0807 / 1334 / 2028	3.3 / -0.1 / 3.2 / 0.0
7 SU	0148 / 0846 / 1411 / 2055	3.3 / 0.2 / 3.1 / 0.2	**22** M	0150 / 0859 / 1427 / 2119	3.4 / -0.1 / 3.2 / -0.1
8 M	0221 / 0919 / 1444 / 2127	3.3 / 0.1 / 3.1 / 0.1	**23** TU	0239 / 0950 / 1517 / 2207	3.5 / -0.2 / 3.1 / -0.1
9 TU	0254 / 0951 / 1515 / 2156	3.3 / 0.1 / 3.1 / 0.1	**24** W	0327 / 1038 / 1602 / 2248	3.5 / -0.1 / 3.1 / 0.0
10 W	0324 / 1020 / 1545 / 2225	3.3 / 0.1 / 3.0 / 0.1	**25** TH	0412 / 1119 / 1643 / 2324	3.5 / 0.0 / 3.1 / 0.1
11 TH	0356 / 1050 / 1620 / 2259	3.2 / 0.1 / 2.9 / 0.1	**26** F	0455 / 1156 / 1723	3.4 / 0.1 / 3.0
12 F	0431 / 1124 / 1659 / 2335	3.1 / 0.1 / 2.8 / 0.2	**27** SA	0001 / 0538 / 1232 / 1805	0.2 / 3.3 / 0.2 / 3.0
13 SA	0509 / 1200 / 1740	3.0 / 0.1 / 2.8	**28** SU	0040 / 0624 / 1309 / 1851	0.2 / 3.1 / 0.3 / 2.9
14 SU	0012 / 0552 / 1239 / 1826	0.2 / 3.0 / 0.1 / 2.8	**29** M	0125 / 0717 / 1358 / 1949	0.3 / 3.0 / 0.4 / 2.8
15 M	0058 / 0645 / 1332 / 1927	0.3 / 2.9 / 0.3 / 2.8	**30** TU	0227 / 0824 / 1506 / 2102	0.4 / 2.8 / 0.5 / 2.8
			31 W	0347 / 0943 / 1627 / 2219	0.4 / 2.8 / 0.5 / 2.9

FEBRUARY

Day	Time	m	Day	Time	m
1 TH	0511 / 1057 / 1741 / 2325	0.4 / 2.8 / 0.4 / 3.0	**16** F	0426 / 1015 / 1706 / 2249	0.1 / 2.8 / 0.2 / 3.0
2 F	0619 / 1155 / 1838	0.3 / 2.9 / 0.3	**17** SA	0551 / 1132 / 1822 / 2355	0.0 / 2.9 / 0.1 / 3.1
3 SA	0015 / 0709 / 1239 / 1924	3.1 / 0.2 / 3.0 / 0.2	**18** SU ●	0659 / 1232 / 1924	-0.1 / 3.0 / -0.1
4 SU O	0053 / 0750 / 1316 / 2002	3.2 / 0.1 / 3.0 / 0.1	**19** M	0048 / 0755 / 1323 / 2016	3.3 / -0.2 / 3.1 / -0.1
5 M	0128 / 0825 / 1350 / 2037	3.2 / 0.0 / 3.0 / 0.0	**20** TU	0136 / 0844 / 1411 / 2103	3.3 / -0.2 / 3.1 / -0.2
6 TU	0202 / 0859 / 1422 / 2108	3.3 / 0.0 / 3.1 / 0.0	**21** W	0221 / 0930 / 1456 / 2147	3.4 / -0.2 / 3.1 / -0.2
7 W	0234 / 0930 / 1452 / 2137	3.3 / 0.0 / 3.0 / -0.1	**22** TH	0306 / 1014 / 1537 / 2226	3.4 / -0.2 / 3.1 / -0.1
8 TH	0303 / 1000 / 1522 / 2208	3.3 / 0.0 / 3.0 / -0.1	**23** F	0349 / 1053 / 1616 / 2301	3.4 / -0.1 / 3.1 / -0.1
9 F	0335 / 1032 / 1558 / 2243	3.2 / -0.1 / 2.9 / -0.1	**24** SA	0430 / 1126 / 1652 / 2335	3.4 / 0.0 / 3.1 / 0.0
10 SA	0413 / 1108 / 1638 / 2320	3.1 / -0.1 / 2.9 / -0.1	**25** SU	0508 / 1156 / 1727	3.2 / 0.1 / 3.0
11 SU	0451 / 1141 / 1716 / 2352	3.0 / -0.1 / 2.8 / 0.0	**26** M	0006 / 0546 / 1225 / 1804	0.1 / 3.0 / 0.2 / 2.8
12 M	0528 / 1211 / 1753	3.0 / 0.0 / 2.8	**27** TU	0039 / 0630 / 1302 / 1854	0.2 / 2.8 / 0.3 / 2.8
13 TU	0027 / 0612 / 1252 / 1846	0.1 / 2.9 / 0.1 / 2.8	**28** W	0129 / 0732 / 1405 / 2006	0.3 / 2.7 / 0.5 / 2.7
14 W	0125 / 0717 / 1402 / 2001	0.1 / 2.8 / 0.3 / 2.8	**29** TH	0249 / 0854 / 1533 / 2132	0.4 / 2.6 / 0.5 / 2.8
15 TH	0251 / 0844 / 1534 / 2128	0.2 / 2.8 / 0.2 / 2.9			

MARCH

Day	Time	m	Day	Time	m
1 F	0424 / 1019 / 1700 / 2249	0.3 / 2.7 / 0.3 / 2.9	**16** SA	0413 / 1005 / 1653 / 2236	0.0 / 2.7 / 0.1 / 3.0
2 SA	0545 / 1126 / 1807 / 2345	0.2 / 2.8 / 0.2 / 3.0	**17** SU	0539 / 1122 / 1809 / 2341	-0.2 / 2.9 / 0.0 / 3.1
3 SU	0642 / 1213 / 1855	0.0 / 2.9 / 0.1	**18** M	0644 / 1219 / 1907	-0.3 / 2.9 / -0.1
4 M	0025 / 0722 / 1249 / 1935	3.1 / -0.1 / 3.0 / -0.1	**19** TU ●	0032 / 0736 / 1306 / 1957	3.2 / -0.3 / 3.0 / -0.2
5 TU O	0101 / 0757 / 1323 / 2011	3.1 / -0.1 / 3.0 / -0.1	**20** W	0117 / 0822 / 1350 / 2042	3.3 / -0.3 / 3.1 / -0.2
6 W	0136 / 0831 / 1356 / 2044	3.2 / -0.2 / 3.0 / -0.2	**21** TH	0202 / 0905 / 1432 / 2123	3.4 / -0.2 / 3.2 / -0.2
7 TH	0210 / 0904 / 1427 / 2116	3.2 / -0.2 / 3.0 / -0.2	**22** F	0244 / 0945 / 1510 / 2200	3.4 / -0.1 / 3.2 / -0.2
8 F	0241 / 0937 / 1500 / 2151	3.2 / -0.2 / 3.0 / -0.2	**23** SA	0325 / 1022 / 1546 / 2235	3.3 / -0.1 / 3.2 / -0.1
9 SA	0316 / 1012 / 1537 / 2228	3.2 / -0.2 / 3.0 / -0.2	**24** SU	0403 / 1054 / 1621 / 2307	3.3 / 0.0 / 3.2 / -0.1
10 SU	0355 / 1050 / 1617 / 2305	3.1 / -0.2 / 2.9 / -0.2	**25** M	0440 / 1122 / 1653 / 2336	3.1 / 0.1 / 3.1 / 0.0
11 M	0435 / 1124 / 1655 / 2338	3.0 / -0.2 / 2.9 / -0.2	**26** TU	0514 / 1148 / 1726	3.0 / 0.2 / 3.0
12 TU	0512 / 1152 / 1732	2.9 / -0.1 / 2.8	**27** W	0004 / 0553 / 1220 / 1809	0.1 / 2.8 / 0.3 / 2.9
13 W	0012 / 0555 / 1231 / 1823	-0.1 / 2.8 / 0.0 / 2.8	**28** TH	0045 / 0647 / 1314 / 1915	0.2 / 2.6 / 0.4 / 2.8
14 TH	0107 / 0701 / 1340 / 1940	0.0 / 2.7 / 0.2 / 2.8	**29** F	0156 / 0804 / 1437 / 2039	0.3 / 2.5 / 0.4 / 2.7
15 F	0234 / 0831 / 1516 / 2112	0.1 / 2.7 / 0.2 / 2.8	**30** SA	0330 / 0930 / 1608 / 2201	0.3 / 2.6 / 0.3 / 2.8
			31 SU	0458 / 1044 / 1723 / 2303	0.1 / 2.7 / 0.2 / 2.9

APRIL

Day	Time	m	Day	Time	m
1 M	0600 / 1135 / 1815 / 2348	-0.1 / 2.8 / 0.0 / 3.0	**16** TU	0621 / 1159 / 1842	-0.3 / 2.9 / -0.1
2 TU	0643 / 1213 / 1858	-0.2 / 2.9 / -0.1	**17** W ●	0010 / 0709 / 1243 / 1931	3.2 / -0.3 / 3.0 / -0.2
3 W	0026 / 0720 / 1250 / 1939	3.1 / -0.3 / 3.0 / -0.2	**18** TH	0056 / 0756 / 1327 / 2018	3.2 / -0.2 / 3.1 / -0.1
4 TH O	0105 / 0758 / 1327 / 2017	3.1 / -0.2 / 3.0 / -0.2	**19** F	0142 / 0839 / 1407 / 2100	3.3 / -0.1 / 3.3 / -0.1
5 F	0143 / 0835 / 1401 / 2054	3.2 / -0.2 / 3.1 / -0.2	**20** SA	0223 / 0916 / 1443 / 2135	3.3 / 0.0 / 3.3 / -0.1
6 SA	0219 / 0912 / 1437 / 2132	3.2 / -0.2 / 3.1 / -0.3	**21** SU	0301 / 0951 / 1516 / 2208	3.3 / 0.0 / 3.3 / -0.1
7 SU	0257 / 0952 / 1515 / 2211	3.2 / -0.2 / 3.1 / -0.3	**22** M	0338 / 1023 / 1550 / 2241	3.2 / 0.0 / 3.3 / -0.1
8 M	0339 / 1031 / 1556 / 2250	3.1 / -0.2 / 3.1 / -0.3	**23** TU	0413 / 1051 / 1624 / 2311	3.1 / 0.1 / 3.2 / 0.0
9 TU	0422 / 1107 / 1638 / 2327	3.0 / -0.2 / 3.0 / -0.3	**24** W	0448 / 1119 / 1657 / 2340	2.9 / 0.1 / 3.1 / 0.1
10 W	0504 / 1142 / 1721	2.9 / -0.1 / 2.9	**25** TH	0526 / 1150 / 1736	2.8 / 0.2 / 3.0
11 TH	0009 / 0553 / 1227 / 1817	-0.2 / 2.8 / 0.0 / 2.9	**26** F	0016 / 0612 / 1236 / 1831	0.2 / 2.7 / 0.3 / 2.9
12 F	0107 / 0700 / 1336 / 1933	0.0 / 2.7 / 0.2 / 2.9	**27** SA	0114 / 0716 / 1344 / 1944	0.2 / 2.6 / 0.4 / 2.8
13 SA	0230 / 0827 / 1508 / 2101	0.0 / 2.7 / 0.2 / 3.0	**28** SU	0234 / 0834 / 1508 / 2102	0.2 / 2.6 / 0.3 / 2.8
14 SU	0404 / 0955 / 1639 / 2221	-0.1 / 2.8 / 0.1 / 3.1	**29** M	0358 / 0948 / 1625 / 2209	0.1 / 2.7 / 0.2 / 2.9
15 M	0524 / 1106 / 1749 / 2322	-0.2 / 2.9 / -0.1 / 3.1	**30** TU	0506 / 1047 / 1725 / 2302	-0.1 / 2.8 / 0.1 / 3.0

Chart Datum: 1·66 metres below Normal Null (German reference level)

21

TIME ZONE –0100
(German Standard Time)
Subtract 1 hour for UT
For German Summer Time add ONE hour in non-shaded areas

GERMANY – CUXHAVEN

LAT 53°52′N   LONG 8°43′E

TIMES AND HEIGHTS OF HIGH AND LOW WATERS   YEAR **1996**

SEPTEMBER

Day	Time	m	Day	Time	m
1 SU	0321 / 1010 / 1534 / 2236	3.3 / 0.0 / 3.6 / 0.1	**16** M	0249 / 0937 / 1503 / 2156	3.2 / 0.1 / 3.3 / 0.1
2 M	0402 / 1048 / 1618 / 2314	3.3 / 0.1 / 3.5 / 0.2	**17** TU	0323 / 1011 / 1540 / 2231	3.2 / 0.1 / 3.3 / 0.1
3 TU	0441 / 1125 / 1700 / 2348	3.3 / 0.2 / 3.4 / 0.3	**18** W	0400 / 1048 / 1620 / 2306	3.1 / 0.1 / 3.2 / 0.1
4 W	0520 / 1201 / 1741	3.2 / 0.3 / 3.3	**19** TH	0438 / 1122 / 1657 / 2337	3.1 / 0.1 / 3.1 / 0.2
5 TH	0021 / 0559 / 1238 / 1826	0.4 / 3.1 / 0.4 / 3.1	**20** F	0515 / 1155 / 1737	3.0 / 0.2 / 3.0
6 F	0058 / 0647 / 1325 / 1924	0.6 / 3.0 / 0.6 / 2.9	**21** SA	0012 / 0601 / 1242 / 1834	0.3 / 2.9 / 0.3 / 2.9
7 SA	0156 / 0755 / 1438 / 2043	0.7 / 3.0 / 0.6 / 2.8	**22** SU	0111 / 0710 / 1359 / 1957	0.5 / 2.9 / 0.4 / 2.8
8 SU	0319 / 0920 / 1611 / 2210	0.7 / 3.0 / 0.6 / 2.9	**23** M	0242 / 0839 / 1537 / 2131	0.5 / 3.0 / 0.4 / 2.9
9 M	0449 / 1041 / 1736 / 2321	0.7 / 3.1 / 0.5 / 3.0	**24** TU	0421 / 1007 / 1709 / 2254	0.5 / 3.1 / 0.2 / 3.0
10 TU	0559 / 1140 / 1834	0.5 / 3.2 / 0.3	**25** W	0542 / 1117 / 1819 / 2356	0.3 / 3.2 / 0.1 / 3.1
11 W	0008 / 0646 / 1218 / 1912	3.1 / 0.4 / 3.3 / 0.2	**26** TH	0643 / 1210 / 1913	0.2 / 3.4 / 0.0
12 TH ●	0041 / 0723 / 1250 / 1945	3.1 / 0.2 / 3.3 / 0.1	**27** F ○	0045 / 0734 / 1256 / 2001	3.2 / 0.1 / 3.5 / 0.0
13 F	0113 / 0758 / 1324 / 2018	3.2 / 0.1 / 3.3 / 0.1	**28** SA	0130 / 0822 / 1343 / 2046	3.3 / 0.1 / 3.5 / 0.1
14 SA	0146 / 0832 / 1359 / 2051	3.2 / 0.1 / 3.3 / 0.1	**29** SU	0214 / 0907 / 1428 / 2128	3.3 / 0.1 / 3.6 / 0.2
15 SU	0218 / 0904 / 1431 / 2123	3.2 / 0.1 / 3.3 / 0.1	**30** M	0255 / 0947 / 1511 / 2208	3.4 / 0.2 / 3.5 / 0.2

OCTOBER

Day	Time	m	Day	Time	m
1 TU	0333 / 1024 / 1552 / 2244	3.4 / 0.2 / 3.5 / 0.3	**16** W	0259 / 0954 / 1520 / 2211	3.3 / 0.1 / 3.3 / 0.2
2 W	0409 / 1058 / 1631 / 2314	3.4 / 0.3 / 3.3 / 0.4	**17** TH	0337 / 1030 / 1600 / 2245	3.2 / 0.1 / 3.2 / 0.2
3 TH	0444 / 1130 / 1709 / 2343	3.3 / 0.4 / 3.2 / 0.5	**18** F	0415 / 1106 / 1641 / 2319	3.2 / 0.1 / 3.1 / 0.3
4 F	0520 / 1202 / 1749	3.2 / 0.5 / 3.0	**19** SA	0457 / 1145 / 1727	3.1 / 0.2 / 2.9
5 SA	0017 / 0604 / 1243 / 1843	0.6 / 3.1 / 0.6 / 2.8	**20** SU	0001 / 0549 / 1238 / 1828	0.4 / 3.0 / 0.3 / 2.8
6 SU	0108 / 0706 / 1349 / 1956	0.8 / 3.0 / 0.7 / 2.7	**21** M	0103 / 0659 / 1353 / 1950	0.5 / 3.0 / 0.4 / 2.8
7 M	0226 / 0828 / 1519 / 2122	0.9 / 2.9 / 0.7 / 2.8	**22** TU	0231 / 0825 / 1527 / 2119	0.6 / 3.1 / 0.4 / 2.9
8 TU	0358 / 0952 / 1650 / 2238	0.8 / 3.0 / 0.6 / 2.9	**23** W	0406 / 0950 / 1654 / 2237	0.6 / 3.2 / 0.3 / 3.0
9 W	0516 / 1057 / 1755 / 2331	0.6 / 3.1 / 0.4 / 3.0	**24** TH	0524 / 1057 / 1800 / 2336	0.4 / 3.3 / 0.1 / 3.1
10 TH	0609 / 1141 / 1835	0.4 / 3.2 / 0.3	**25** F	0621 / 1149 / 1850	0.3 / 3.3 / 0.1
11 F	0006 / 0648 / 1215 / 1909	3.1 / 0.3 / 3.2 / 0.2	**26** SA ○	0023 / 0710 / 1236 / 1937	3.2 / 0.2 / 3.4 / 0.2
12 SA ●	0039 / 0726 / 1252 / 1945	3.1 / 0.2 / 3.2 / 0.1	**27** SU	0107 / 0816 / 1323 / 2022	3.3 / 0.2 / 3.5 / 0.3
13 SU	0115 / 0804 / 1330 / 2022	3.2 / 0.2 / 3.3 / 0.1	**28** M	0150 / 0845 / 1407 / 2102	3.4 / 0.3 / 3.5 / 0.3
14 M	0150 / 0841 / 1407 / 2058	3.2 / 0.2 / 3.3 / 0.2	**29** TU	0229 / 0923 / 1448 / 2139	3.5 / 0.3 / 3.5 / 0.3
15 TU	0224 / 0917 / 1442 / 2135	3.3 / 0.2 / 3.3 / 0.2	**30** W	0304 / 0958 / 1526 / 2213	3.5 / 0.3 / 3.4 / 0.4
			31 TH	0338 / 1032 / 1604 / 2244	3.4 / 0.3 / 3.2 / 0.4

NOVEMBER

Day	Time	m	Day	Time	m
1 F	0413 / 1103 / 1641 / 2313	3.4 / 0.4 / 3.1 / 0.5	**16** SA	0401 / 1059 / 1632 / 2311	3.3 / 0.1 / 3.1 / 0.3
2 SA	0448 / 1134 / 1719 / 2345	3.3 / 0.5 / 2.9 / 0.6	**17** SU	0447 / 1143 / 1722 / 2357	3.3 / 0.2 / 3.0 / 0.4
3 SU	0528 / 1211 / 1805	3.1 / 0.6 / 2.8	**18** M	0542 / 1238 / 1824	3.2 / 0.3 / 2.9
4 M	0028 / 0620 / 1304 / 1905	0.7 / 3.0 / 0.7 / 2.7	**19** TU	0058 / 0648 / 1347 / 1938	0.5 / 3.2 / 0.4 / 2.9
5 TU	0132 / 0730 / 1419 / 2020	0.8 / 3.0 / 0.7 / 2.7	**20** W	0215 / 0805 / 1507 / 2057	0.6 / 3.2 / 0.4 / 2.9
6 W	0252 / 0847 / 1544 / 2136	0.8 / 3.0 / 0.6 / 2.8	**21** TH	0339 / 0923 / 1627 / 2208	0.6 / 3.2 / 0.3 / 3.0
7 TH	0412 / 0957 / 1656 / 2238	0.7 / 3.0 / 0.4 / 2.9	**22** F	0455 / 1031 / 1732 / 2307	0.4 / 3.3 / 0.2 / 3.0
8 F	0516 / 1052 / 1747 / 2324	0.5 / 3.1 / 0.3 / 3.0	**23** SA	0554 / 1126 / 1824 / 2358	0.3 / 3.3 / 0.2 / 3.1
9 SA	0606 / 1137 / 1829	0.4 / 3.2 / 0.2	**24** SU	0646 / 1216 / 1913	0.3 / 3.3 / 0.3
10 SU	0003 / 0652 / 1219 / 1912	3.1 / 0.3 / 3.2 / 0.2	**25** M ○	0045 / 0737 / 1304 / 1959	3.3 / 0.4 / 3.4 / 0.4
11 M ●	0043 / 0736 / 1301 / 1953	3.2 / 0.3 / 3.3 / 0.4	**26** TU	0127 / 0823 / 1348 / 2038	3.4 / 0.4 / 3.4 / 0.4
12 TU	0121 / 0816 / 1342 / 2033	3.3 / 0.2 / 3.3 / 0.3	**27** W	0204 / 0900 / 1426 / 2113	3.5 / 0.4 / 3.4 / 0.5
13 W	0159 / 0857 / 1422 / 2114	3.3 / 0.2 / 3.3 / 0.2	**28** TH	0237 / 0935 / 1503 / 2147	3.5 / 0.4 / 3.3 / 0.4
14 TH	0238 / 0938 / 1504 / 2155	3.4 / 0.1 / 3.3 / 0.2	**29** F	0311 / 1009 / 1540 / 2219	3.5 / 0.3 / 3.2 / 0.4
15 F	0319 / 1019 / 1548 / 2233	3.4 / 0.1 / 3.2 / 0.2	**30** SA	0347 / 1041 / 1615 / 2248	3.4 / 0.3 / 3.1 / 0.4

DECEMBER

Day	Time	m	Day	Time	m
1 SU	0422 / 1112 / 1651 / 2319	3.3 / 0.4 / 3.0 / 0.5	**16** M	0439 / 1141 / 1715 / 2352	3.4 / 0.1 / 3.0 / 0.3
2 M	0458 / 1145 / 1730 / 2355	3.2 / 0.5 / 2.9 / 0.6	**17** TU	0532 / 1233 / 1812	3.4 / 0.2 / 3.0
3 TU	0540 / 1225 / 1817	3.1 / 0.5 / 2.8	**18** W	0046 / 0632 / 1331 / 1915	0.4 / 3.3 / 0.3 / 2.9
4 W	0042 / 0633 / 1320 / 1916	0.7 / 3.0 / 0.6 / 2.7	**19** TH	0149 / 0738 / 1436 / 2022	0.5 / 3.3 / 0.4 / 2.9
5 TH	0145 / 0738 / 1430 / 2026	0.7 / 2.9 / 0.5 / 2.8	**20** F	0301 / 0848 / 1546 / 2130	0.5 / 3.2 / 0.4 / 2.9
6 F	0259 / 0848 / 1544 / 2134	0.7 / 2.9 / 0.4 / 2.8	**21** SA	0416 / 0958 / 1655 / 2235	0.5 / 3.2 / 0.3 / 3.0
7 SA	0413 / 0955 / 1650 / 2234	0.6 / 3.0 / 0.3 / 3.0	**22** SU	0525 / 1103 / 1756 / 2334	0.4 / 3.2 / 0.3 / 3.1
8 SU	0517 / 1054 / 1747 / 2324	0.5 / 3.1 / 0.3 / 3.1	**23** M	0624 / 1159 / 1849	0.4 / 3.2 / 0.4
9 M	0615 / 1146 / 1838	0.4 / 3.2 / 0.3	**24** TU ○	0025 / 0717 / 1248 / 1937	3.3 / 0.4 / 3.3 / 0.4
10 TU ●	0010 / 0706 / 1233 / 1925	3.2 / 0.3 / 3.3 / 0.2	**25** W	0107 / 0803 / 1331 / 2018	3.4 / 0.4 / 3.3 / 0.4
11 W	0053 / 0753 / 1318 / 2009	3.3 / 0.2 / 3.3 / 0.2	**26** TH	0143 / 0841 / 1408 / 2052	3.5 / 0.3 / 3.3 / 0.3
12 TH	0136 / 0838 / 1405 / 2056	3.4 / 0.1 / 3.3 / 0.2	**27** F	0216 / 0916 / 1443 / 2126	3.5 / 0.3 / 3.2 / 0.3
13 F	0221 / 0925 / 1453 / 2144	3.4 / 0.1 / 3.3 / 0.2	**28** SA	0251 / 0950 / 1517 / 2158	3.5 / 0.3 / 3.2 / 0.3
14 SA	0307 / 1012 / 1540 / 2227	3.4 / 0.0 / 3.2 / 0.2	**29** SU	0324 / 1022 / 1550 / 2226	3.4 / 0.3 / 3.1 / 0.3
15 SU	0352 / 1056 / 1626 / 2308	3.4 / 0.1 / 3.1 / 0.3	**30** M	0357 / 1050 / 1622 / 2256	3.3 / 0.3 / 3.0 / 0.3
			31 TU	0431 / 1121 / 1657 / 2329	3.2 / 0.3 / 2.9 / 0.3

Chart Datum: 1·66 metres below Normal Null (German reference level)

RIVER ELBE/HAMBURG   10-21-20
Niedersächsen/Schleswig-Holstein

CHARTS
AC 3262, 3266, 3268; BSH 3010 Sheets 1 to 12 (as shown below), D46, D47, D48

TIDES

Glückstadt	ML 1·2 Duration 0515	Zone −0100
Brunshausen	ML 1·1 Duration 0510	
Hamburg	ML 1·3 Duration 0435	

Standard Port CUXHAVEN (←—)

Times				Height (metres)			
High Water		Low Water		MHWS	MHWN	MLWN	MLWS
0200	0800	0200	0900	3·3	2·9	0·4	0·0
1400	2000	1400	2100				
Differences GLÜCKSTADT							
+0205	+0214	+0220	+0213	−0·2	−0·2	−0·1	+0·1
STADERSAND							
+0241	+0245	+0300	+0254	−0·1	0·0	−0·2	+0·1
SCHULAU							
+0304	+0315	+0337	+0321	+0·1	+0·1	−0·2	+0·1
HAMBURG							
+0338	+0346	+0421	+0406	+0·3	+0·3	−0·3	0·0

NAVIGATION
Distances: Elbe lt float to Cuxhaven = 24M; Cuxhaven to Wedel Yacht Haven = 45M; Wedel to City Sport Hafen = 11·5M. The river has 13m up to Hamburg and is tidal to Geesthacht, 24M above Hamburg. Strong W winds can raise the level by as much as 4m. Entry should not be attempted with strong W/NW winds against the ebb. It is a very busy waterway and at night the many lights can be confusing. Yachts should keep to stbd, preferably just outside the marked chan. Elbe VTS (not mandatory for yachts) offers radar guidance and broadcasts met, nav & tidal info; see 10.21.19 & .21 and R/TELEPHONE below.

SHELTER AND FACILITIES
Some of the better hbrs are listed below, but it is not a particularly salubrious yachting area:

FREIBURG: 7M above Brunsbüttel on the SW bank. Small vessels can enter at HW and there is excellent shelter at Freiburg Reede. ML 2·2m. Hr Mr ☎ (04779) 8314.
Facilities: ME, EI, Sh, C, FW, Slip, YC; **Jugendheim & YC Klubheim** V, R, Bar. (Sheet 4).

STÖRLOCH/BORSFLETH: Ent approx 600m above locks on E bank. ML 2·8m. Hr Mr ☎ (04124) 71437 Facilities: FW, YC. Stör Bridge VHF Ch 09, 16. (Sheet 4).

STÖR/BEIDENFLETH: ML 2·8m (Sheet 4). **Langes Rack YC**.

GLÜCKSTADT: on the NE bank, 2½M above mouth of R. Stör. Good shelter; inner and outer hbrs have 2m depth. Lock into inner hbr opens HW −2 to +½. VHF Ch 11. Hr Mr ☎ (04124) 2087; ⌗ ☎ 2171. YC, FW, C, D, V, R, ⊙, Bar. (Sheet 5).

WISCHHAFEN: Hr Mr ☎ (04770) 334; ⌗ 3014 FW, M, Slip, P, D, ML 2·7m. (Sheet 5).

RUTHENSTROM: Ldg marks into hbr, two bns with △ topmarks on 197°. ML 2·6m. Hr Mr ☎ (04143) 5282; C, Slip, FW, ME, EI, Sh. (Sheet 6).

KRÜCKAUMÜNDUNG JACHTHAFEN: ☎ (04125) 1521 Slip, FW. ML 2·7m. ⌗ ☎ 20551. (Sheet 6).

PINNAUMÜNDUNG JACHTHAFEN: Ent via lock gate on N bank after passing through main locks. ML 2·5m. Hr Mr ☎ (04101) 22447 Slip, M, FW, YC, C. (Sheet 10).

PINNAU-NEUENDEICH: Marina 1½M up the Pinnau from main locks and another at approx 2M. (Sheet 6).

ABBENFLETH: Ent marked by two bns in line 221° with △ topmarks. (Sheets 6/7).

HASELDORF Hafen: Hr Mr ☎ (04129) 268 Slip, FW, V, YC.

R.SCHWINGE on SW bank, 12M up-river from Glückstadt:
   BRUNSHAUSEN (04141) 3085
   HÖRNE/WÖHRDEN ML 2·8m
   STADE (04141) 101275 C, YC, V; Access HW ±2.
Very good shelter in scenic town. ⌗ ☎ 3014. (Sheets 7/8).

LÜHE: Hafen in town of Lühe. (Sheet 8).

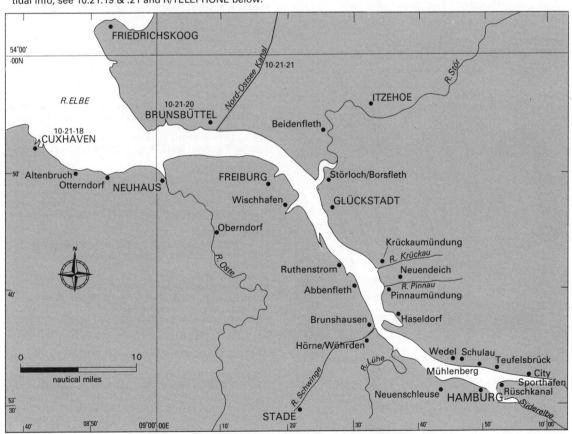

HAMBURG

A busy commercial port with several marinas. Visitors berth at Wedel in Hamburger Yachthafen or in the City Sporthafen, in city centre esp for visitors (see below) .

WEDEL: on N bank, 12M downstream from Hamburg, very good shelter available H24; **Hamburger Yachthafen**, 10DM, (1800 berths) with 2 ents (23m wide) marked by FR and FG lts. A conspic 20m high radar tr is at W corner of hbr. Hr Mr ☎ (04103) 4438 (office), 5632 (Hr Mr east), 88608 (Hr Mr west); ⌗ ☎ 2688; D & P, Bar, BH (16 ton), BY, C, CH, El, Ⓔ, FW, ME, SC, Sh, Slip, SM. (Sheets 8/9).

SCHULAU: Good shelter, 7ca E of Wedel. Beware strong tidal streams across ent, marked by FR and FG lts. Hr Mr ☎ 2422, Slip, C, P, D, ME, Ⓗ, CH, SC. (Sheet 8/9).

NEUENSCHLEUSE: opposite Wedel. (Sheet 9).

MÜHLENBERG: N bank, (250), Slip, FW, SC. Small boats only; 0·6m above CD. (Sheets 9/10).

TEUFELSBRÜCK: small hbr on N bank. Good shelter, sandbar at ent. Bar, FW, SC. (Sheets 9/10).

RÜSCHKANAL: on S bank in Finkenwerder, C, CH, El, FW, ME, Slip, Sh, with 4 SCs and nearby resort area.

CITY SPORTHAFEN: (80+50) ☎ 364297, 20DM, D, P, FW, AC; Ent on N bank beyond St Pauli-Landungsbrücken.

RADIO TELEPHONE

Elbe VTS: see 10.21.18 for VHF and radar coverage up to buoy No 53. Thereafter listen on Ch 68 up to buoy No 122 (Wedel ent). From 2M E of Wedel listen to *Hamburg Port Radio* Ch 06 13 **14** 73 (H24); also Hbr Control vessel Ch 14. *Hamburg Radar* service may be requested in vis <1M. Süderelbe: Kattwyk bridge and Harburg lock Ch 13 (H24). All stns monitor Ch 16.

TELEPHONE (040)

Met 3190 8801, or 0190-116456 Auto; Brit Consul 446071.

FACILITIES

City all facilities, ACA, ✉, Ⓑ, ⇌, ✈. Ferry: Hamburg-Harwich.

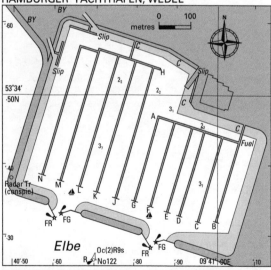

HAMBURGER YACHTHAFEN, WEDEL

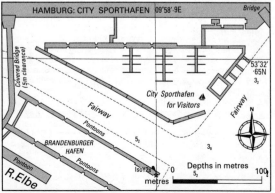

HAMBURG: CITY SPORTHAFEN

BRUNSBÜTTEL   10-21-21

Schleswig-Holstein 53°53'·28N 09°07'·85E

CHARTS

AC 2469, 3262; BSH 3010 Sheet 3

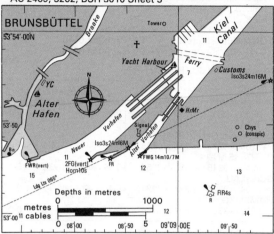

TIDES

+0203 Dover; ML 1·4; Duration 0520; Zone –0100

Standard Port CUXHAVEN (⟵)

Times				Height (metres)			
High Water		Low Water		MHWS	MHWN	MLWN	MLWS
0200	0800	0200	0900	3·3	2·9	0·4	0·0
1400	2000	1400	2100				
Differences BRUNSBÜTTEL							
+0057	+0105	+0121	+0112	–0·2	–0·2	–0·1	0·0

SHELTER

Good shelter in drying yacht hbr, access HW ±3, outside the locks to the W in the Alter Hafen. Waiting posts are close E of FWG ☆ at ent to Alter Vorhafen. The stream sets strongly across ents to locks. Very good shelter in yacht hbr inside, immediately NW of Neue locks.

NAVIGATION

No navigational dangers in the near apprs, but commercial traffic is heavy. Yachts usually use the smaller SE locks.

LIGHTS AND MARKS

Ldg lts 065°, both Iso 3s 24/46m 16/21M, synch, for locks. Ldg lts 012°, both Oc (3) R, for Alter Hafen. For lock sigs see 10.21.21.

RADIO TELEPHONE

Call: *Brunsbüttel Elbe Port* Ch **12** 16 (H24). See 10.21.22 Nord-Ostsee Kanal for entry procedures. Info broadcasts in English and German by *Brunsbüttel Elbe Traffic* every H + 05 on Ch 68 from buoy 55 to 122; (see also Cuxhaven 10.21.19).

TELEPHONE (04852)

Hr Mr 8011 ext 360; CG 8444; ⌗ 87241; Weather 36400; Police 112; Ⓗ 601; Brit Consul (040) 446071.

FACILITIES

Alter hafen ☎ 3107, Slip, SC, AC, C (20 ton), FW, R; **Kanal-Yachthafen** ☎ 8011, FW, AC, ⌗, Bar. **Town** P, D, ME, El, Sh, Gaz, V, R, LB, Ⓗ, Bar, ✉, Ⓑ, ⇌, ✈ (Hamburg). Ferry: Hamburg-Harwich. KIEL: **Nautischer Dienst** (0431) 331772 ACA.

HARBOUR ON SOUTH BANK OF THE ELBE

OTTERNDORF, Niedersachsen, 53°50'·20N 08°54'·00E. AC 3261, 3262; BSH 3014.11. HW +0100 on Dover (UT); +0120 on Helgoland (zone –0100); HW ht +0·5 on Helgoland; ML 2·9m; Duration 0525. Ent marked by Medem lt bn Fl (3) 12s 6m 5M and perches. Chan (0·6m) from Elbe divides and yachts can take the W branch to Kutterhafen (0·9m) or the canal to E, through lock then turn sharp stbd to yacht hbr. Lockmaster ☎ (04751) 2190; Yacht hbr ☎ 13131 C, AC, FW, Bar.

Town (3km) ME, Gaz, V, ✉. Note: The Hadelner and Geeste Kanals (1·5m depth and air draft 2·7m) link Otterndorf to Bremerhaven (32M) and Bederkesa.

NORD-OSTSEE KANAL
(Kiel Canal)   10-21-22
Schleswig-Holstein

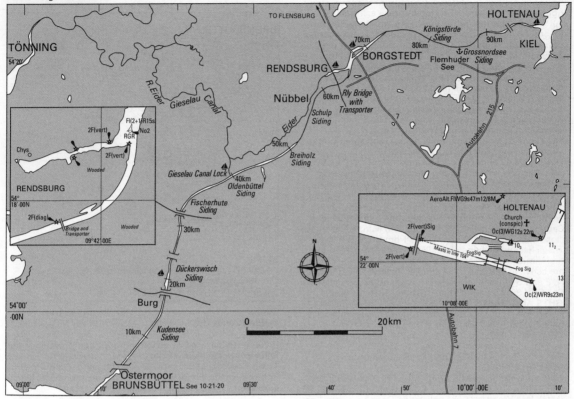

CHARTS
AC 2469, 696 (Kieler Förde); BSH 3009, Sheets 1-4
NAVIGATION
The Canal runs from Brunsbüttel (10.21.21) to Kiel-Holtenau, 53·3M (98·7 km). Km posts start from Brunsbüttel. Width is 103 to 162m on the surface, and depth 11m. Yachts may only use the Canal and its ents by day and good vis. (This does not apply to craft going to the Inner or Old Hbrs at Brunsbüttel, or to the yacht berths at Holtenau). Speed limit is 8kn. All 6 bridges have 40m clearance. Fly flag 'N' (no pilot). Sailing, except motor sailing is prohib; yachts must then display a B ▼, or a B pennant. Canal dues are paid at the Holtenau locks at the 'Dues Office' (N bank). Yachts purely in transit are not usually troubled by the Customs Authority; they should fly the third substitute of the International Code.
SHELTER
The principal port along the canal is Rensburg, between km posts 60 and 67, with all facilities including 3 yacht hbrs in the Obereidersee. Rensburg is linked to Tönning (see under 10.21.24) by the R Eider and Gieselau Canal. There are 9 passing places (sidings or *weichen*). Yachts are to regulate their passage so as to reach their planned berthing places during daylight. These may be at:
1) Brunsbüttel (km 0);
2) Kudensee siding (km 9·5);
3) Dückerswisch siding (km 20·7);
4) Fischerhütte siding (km 35);
5) Oldenbüttel siding (km 40), at ent to Gieselau Canal;
6) Breiholz siding (km 48);
7) Schülp siding (km 57);
8) The Obereidersee (Rendsburg), ent at km 66;
5) The Borgstedter See, ent at km 70;
10) Königsförde siding (km 80);
11) Grossnordsee siding (km 85), or ⚓ in Flemhuder See;
12) Schwartenbek siding (km 92);
12) Kiel-Holtenau (km 98·7).
Kiel-Holtenau, at the Baltic end of the canal, is a major port with a Yacht Hbr on the N bank (E of locks); all usual facilities. Two pairs of locks (yachts usually use the N pair) lead into the Kieler Förde which is practically tideless and at almost the same level as the canal.

SIGNALS
Lock signals (shown at signal tr and centre pier of lock):

Ⓡ	= no entry.
Ⓦ over Ⓡ	= prepare to enter.
Ⓦ	= yachts may enter (berth on pontoons).
Ⓦ over Ⓖ	= enter without pilot (yachts follow ships flying Flag N); secure to middle wall.
Ⓖ	= enter with pilot; secure to middle wall.
Ⓦ over Ⓦ and Ⓖ	= enter with pilot and secure by Ⓦ lt.

In the canal, the only traffic sig applicable to yachts is :

3 Ⓡ (vert)   = STOP. Keep to stbd; give way to large vessel approaching.

RADIO TELEPHONE
Before entering, yachts should report as follows (all H24): at Brunsbüttel to *Kiel Kanal I* on Ch 13; or at Holtenau to *Kiel Kanal IV* on Ch 12. When exiting (W-bound) call *Brunsbüttel Radar I* Ch 04. Ports: Ostermoor (Brunsbüttel to Burg) Ch 73; Breiholz (Breiholz to Audorf) Ch 73.
Canal. Maintain listening watch as follows:
Kiel Kanal I   (Brunsbüttel ent and locks) Ch 13;
Kiel Kanal II   (Brunsbüttel to Breiholz) Ch 02;
Kiel Kanal III (Breiholz to Holtenau) Ch 03;
Kiel Kanal IV   (Holtenau ent and locks) Ch 12.
Info broadcasts by *Kiel Kanal II* on Ch 02 at H+15, H+45; and by *Kiel Kanal III* on Ch 03 at H+20, H+50. Vessels should monitor these broadcasts and not call the station if this can be avoided.
FACILITIES
A BP fuel barge is on the N bank, close E of the Holtenau locks. At Wik (S side of locks) **Nautischer Dienst** (Kapt Stegmann & Co) ☎ 0431 331772 are ACA & BSH Agents. The **British Kiel YC** is 5ca NNW of Stickenhörn ECM buoy, Q (3) 10s, 1M NNE of the locks. It is part of a military centre with no commercial facilities; but AB (about 18DM) may well be available for visitors to whom a friendly welcome is extended. Call *Sailtrain* VHF Ch 67 or ☎ (0431) 398833.

21

HELGOLAND   10-21-23

Schleswig-Holstein 54°10'·30N 07°54'·00E

CHARTS
AC 126, 1875; D3, 88; BSH 3013, 3014.2 & .3, 3015

TIDES
–0030 Dover; ML 1·4; Duration 0540; Zone –0100
Helgoland is a Standard Port and tidal predictions for each
day of the year are given below.

SHELTER
Good in safe artificial hbr (5m); yachts should berth on
pontoons on the NE side of the Südhafen which gets very
crowded. Or ⚓ in the SW part of the Vorhafen, sheltered
except in SE'lies. Also possible AB in Binnenhafen, S side.
Yachts are prohib from the Nordost hbr, the Dünen hbr
and from landing on Düne Island.
NOTE: Helgoland is not a port of entry into Germany.
Customs in Helgoland are for passport control. Duty free
goods are obtainable; hence many day-trippers by ferry.

NAVIGATION
WPT Helgoland ECM buoy, Q (3) 10s, Whis, 55°09'·00N
07°53'·57E, 202°/022° from/to Düne front ldg lt, 2·1M.
Beware the Hogstean shoal, 4ca S of Sudmole head lt, and
other rky shoals either side of chan. The S chan and ent
are used by ferries. Beware lobster pots around Düne Is.
Caution: Entry is prohib at all times into Nature Reserves
close either side of the appr chans from SSW and NW.
These Reserves extend about 2M NE and SW of Helgoland;
their limits are marked by Cardinal buoys. Marine police
are active in this respect. A smaller Reserve, lying to the
N, E and S of Dune, is a prohib ⚓, with other restrictions.
See BSH 3014.2 and AC 126, 3761 and 1875 for limits.

LIGHTS AND MARKS
Helgoland lt ho, Fl 5s 82m 28M; brown ▢ tr, B lantern, W
balcony; RC.
Düne ldg lts 020°: front Iso 4s 11m 8M; rear Dir Iso WRG
4s 17m 11/10M synch, W sector 018·5°–021°.
Binnenhafen ldg lts 302°: both Oc R 6s, synch.

RADIO TELEPHONE
Helgoland Port Radio Ch 67 16 (Mon-Fri: 0700-1800; Sat
0800-1700; Sun 0800-1000LT). Coast Radio Ch 03 16 27 88
(H24). Info broadcasts in English and German every H on
Ch 79 80 by *German Bight Traffic* (at Helgoland lt ho) for
26M radius of Helgoland.

TELEPHONE
Hr Mr 504; CG 210; ⌗ 304; Met (04725) 606; Police 607; Dr
7345; Ⓗ 8030; LB 210; SAR 524; Brit Consul (040) 446071.

FACILITIES
Vorhafen L, AB; **Südhafen** ☎ 504, AB 11DM, D, FW, ME,
CH, C (mobile 12 ton), V, R, Bar; **Binnenhafen** ☎ 504, P, D,
FW, ME, CH, AB, V, R, Bar; **Wasser Sport Club** ☎ 585 Bar,
R, M, C (12 ton), D, P, CH, ME, El, Sh, FW, Ⓞ, V.
Town Gaz, V, R, Bar, ✉, Ⓑ, ⇌ (ferry Cuxhaven), ✈ (to
Bremen, Hamburg and Cuxhaven). Ferry: Hamburg-
Harwich.

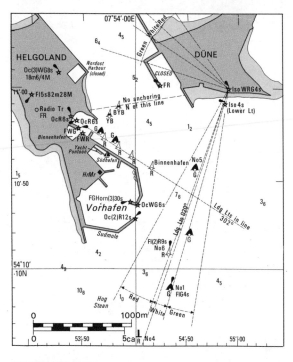

AGENTS WANTED

If you are interested in becoming our agent for any of the
following ports, please write to: The Editor, Edington House,
Trent, Sherborne, Dorset DT9 4SR, England – and get your
free copy of the almanac annually. You do not have to live in
a port to be the agent, but at least a fairly regular visitor.

River Exe	Grandcamp-Maisy
Port Ellen (Islay)	Port-en-Bessin
Glandore/Union Hall	Courseulles
River Rance/Dinan	Boulogne
Lampaul	Dunkerque
Port Tudy	Terneuzen/Westerschelde
River Etel	Oudeschild
Le Palais (Belle Ile)	Lauwersoog
Le Pouliguen/Pornichet	Dornumer-Accumersiel
L'Herbaudière	Hooksiel
St Gilles-Croix-de-Vie	Langeoog
River Seudre	Bremerhaven
Royan	Helgoland
Anglet/Bayonne	Büsum
Hendaye	

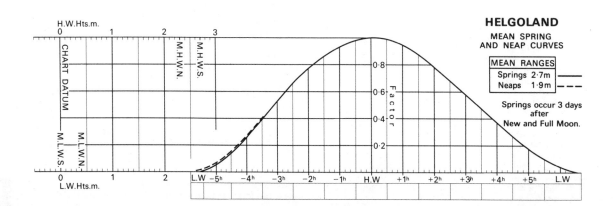

HELGOLAND

MEAN SPRING
AND NEAP CURVES

MEAN RANGES
Springs 2·7m ——
Neaps 1·9m - - -

Springs occur 3 days
after
New and Full Moon.

TIME ZONE –0100
(German Standard Time)
Subtract 1 hour for UT
For German Summer Time add
ONE hour in non-shaded areas

GERMANY – HELGOLAND

LAT 54°11′N   LONG 7°53′E

TIMES AND HEIGHTS OF HIGH AND LOW WATERS   YEAR 1996

JANUARY

	Time	m		Time	m
1 M	0213 0804 1451 2041	0.5 2.5 0.5 2.4	**16** TU	0051 0642 1330 1924	0.4 2.4 0.3 2.3
2 TU	0326 0913 1555 2144	0.4 2.5 0.4 2.5	**17** W	0213 0802 1450 2042	0.4 2.4 0.3 2.4
3 W	0430 1013 1648 2238	0.4 2.5 0.4 2.6	**18** TH	0334 0920 1606 2153	0.3 2.5 0.2 2.5
4 TH	0522 1103 1735 2324	0.4 2.6 0.4 2.7	**19** F	0446 1028 1713 2256	0.1 2.6 0.1 2.7
5 F O	0607 1146 1818	0.3 2.6 0.3	**20** SA	0548 1127 1811 2349	0.0 2.6 0.1 2.7
6 SA	0002 0645 1224 1855	2.7 0.2 2.6 0.2	**21** SU	0642 1219 1902	–0.1 2.6 0.0
7 SU	0037 0719 1258 1928	2.7 0.2 2.6 0.2	**22** M	0038 0733 1311 1952	2.8 –0.1 2.6 0.0
8 M	0111 0751 1330 2000	2.7 0.1 2.5 0.1	**23** TU	0126 0824 1401 2039	2.8 –0.2 2.6 –0.1
9 TU	0144 0823 1401 2030	2.7 0.1 2.5 0.1	**24** W	0215 0912 1446 2121	2.9 –0.1 2.6 0.0
10 W	0213 0853 1432 2100	2.7 0.1 2.5 0.1	**25** TH	0300 0953 1527 2200	2.9 0.0 2.5 0.1
11 TH	0244 0926 1506 2136	2.7 0.1 2.4 0.1	**26** F	0343 1032 1608 2240	2.8 0.1 2.5 0.1
12 F	0318 1003 1544 2215	2.6 0.1 2.3 0.2	**27** SA	0425 1111 1650 2322	2.7 0.2 2.4 0.2
13 SA	0357 1040 1625 2254	2.5 0.1 2.3 0.2	**28** SU	0511 1152 1738	2.6 0.3 2.3
14 SU	0439 1121 1712 2343	2.5 0.2 2.3 0.3	**29** M	0011 0604 1244 1836	0.3 2.4 0.4 2.3
15 M	0533 1216 1811	2.4 0.3 2.3	**30** TU	0117 0712 1354 1949	0.4 2.3 0.5 2.4
			31 W	0239 0830 1513 2106	0.4 2.3 0.5 2.4

FEBRUARY

	Time	m		Time	m
1 TH	0359 0944 1622 2212	0.4 2.3 0.4 2.5	**16** F	0315 0900 1549 2135	0.1 2.3 0.2 2.4
2 F	0502 1042 1716 2302	0.3 2.4 0.3 2.6	**17** SA	0434 1017 1702 2243	0.0 2.4 0.1 2.6
3 SA	0548 1127 1800 2341	0.2 2.4 0.2 2.6	**18** SU ●	0538 1117 1801 2337	–0.1 2.5 –0.1 2.7
4 SU O	0626 1203 1838	0.1 2.5 0.1	**19** M	0632 1208 1852	–0.2 2.5 –0.1
5 M	0017 0700 1237 1912	2.6 0.0 2.5 0.0	**20** TU	0024 0720 1254 1937	2.7 –0.2 2.5 –0.2
6 TU	0051 0732 1308 1943	2.7 0.0 2.5 0.0	**21** W	0108 0806 1339 2020	2.8 –0.2 2.5 –0.2
7 W	0123 0803 1338 2013	2.7 0.0 2.5 –0.1	**22** TH	0153 0850 1421 2101	2.8 –0.2 2.6 –0.1
8 TH	0152 0834 1409 2045	2.6 0.0 2.4 –0.1	**23** F	0236 0928 1459 2138	2.7 –0.1 2.5 –0.1
9 F	0223 0908 1443 2122	2.6 –0.1 2.4 –0.1	**24** SA	0316 1002 1536 2213	2.7 0.0 2.5 0.0
10 SA	0259 0945 1521 2200	2.5 –0.1 2.3 –0.1	**25** SU	0354 1034 1612 2247	2.6 0.1 2.5 0.1
11 SU	0337 1020 1559 2234	2.5 –0.1 2.3 0.0	**26** M	0432 1107 1651 2327	2.5 0.2 2.4 0.1
12 M	0414 1052 1637 2312	2.4 0.0 2.3 0.1	**27** TU	0517 1150 1741	2.3 0.3 2.3
13 TU	0459 1138 1730	2.4 0.2 2.3	**28** W	0025 0619 1257 1853	0.3 2.2 0.4 2.2
14 W	0014 0605 1251 1845	0.2 2.3 0.2 2.3	**29** TH	0148 0741 1425 2019	0.4 2.1 0.4 2.2
15 TH	0142 0731 1422 2013	0.2 2.3 0.2 2.3			

MARCH

	Time	m		Time	m
1 F	0319 0906 1548 2137	0.3 2.1 0.4 2.4	**16** SA	0305 0849 1539 2121	0.0 2.2 0.1 2.4
2 SA	0433 1013 1649 2233	0.2 2.2 0.2 2.5	**17** SU	0425 1005 1651 2227	–0.1 2.3 0.0 2.5
3 SU	0523 1100 1735 2313	0.1 2.3 0.1 2.5	**18** M	0525 1103 1746 2319	–0.2 2.4 –0.1 2.6
4 M	0601 1135 1814 2348	0.0 2.4 0.0 2.5	**19** TU ●	0615 1150 1834	–0.3 2.4 –0.2
5 TU O	0635 1208 1849	–0.1 2.4 –0.1	**20** W	0005 0701 1232 1918	2.7 –0.3 2.5 –0.2
6 W	0023 0707 1240 1922	2.6 –0.2 2.4 –0.2	**21** TH	0048 0742 1313 1959	2.7 –0.2 2.6 –0.2
7 TH	0056 0739 1312 1954	2.6 –0.2 2.5 –0.2	**22** F	0129 0822 1353 2037	2.7 –0.1 2.6 –0.2
8 F	0128 0813 1345 2029	2.6 –0.2 2.4 –0.2	**23** SA	0210 0858 1429 2113	2.7 –0.1 2.6 –0.1
9 SA	0202 0849 1421 2107	2.6 –0.2 2.4 –0.2	**24** SU	0248 0930 1505 2147	2.6 0.0 2.6 –0.1
10 SU	0240 0927 1459 2145	2.5 –0.2 2.4 –0.2	**25** M	0324 1000 1538 2218	2.5 0.1 2.5 0.0
11 M	0320 1002 1536 2219	2.5 –0.2 2.3 –0.1	**26** TU	0359 1030 1612 2252	2.4 0.2 2.4 0.1
12 TU	0357 1034 1615 2258	2.4 –0.1 2.3 –0.1	**27** W	0439 1108 1656 2341	2.2 0.3 2.3 0.2
13 W	0441 1119 1708 2358	2.3 0.1 2.3 0.1	**28** TH	0534 1207 1801	2.1 0.4 2.2
14 TH	0547 1233 1825	0.0 2.2 0.2	**29** F	0056 0651 1331 1925	0.3 2.0 0.4 2.2
15 F	0128 0716 1408 1956	0.1 2.2 0.2 2.3	**30** SA	0228 0817 1500 2048	0.3 2.0 0.3 2.3
			31 SU	0349 0930 1609 2151	0.1 2.2 0.2 2.4

APRIL

	Time	m		Time	m
1 M	0445 1021 1658 2235	0.0 2.3 0.1 2.5	**16** TU	0504 1040 1722 2254	–0.3 2.4 –0.1 2.6
2 TU	0524 1059 1739 2312	–0.1 2.4 –0.1 2.5	**17** W ●	0550 1125 1810 2342	–0.2 2.4 –0.1 2.6
3 W	0600 1134 1819 2349	–0.2 2.4 –0.1 2.5	**18** TH	0636 1208 1856	–0.2 2.5 –0.1
4 TH O	0637 1210 1856	–0.2 2.4 –0.2	**19** F	0027 0717 1249 1937	2.7 –0.1 2.6 –0.1
5 F	0027 0713 1245 1932	2.6 –0.2 2.5 –0.2	**20** SA	0108 0753 1326 2013	2.7 0.0 2.7 –0.1
6 SA	0104 0750 1322 2011	2.6 –0.2 2.5 –0.2	**21** SU	0145 0827 1401 2048	2.7 0.0 2.7 –0.1
7 SU	0142 0830 1400 2051	2.6 –0.2 2.5 –0.3	**22** M	0221 0859 1436 2121	2.6 0.0 2.6 –0.1
8 M	0223 0909 1440 2131	2.5 –0.2 2.5 –0.3	**23** TU	0257 0929 1510 2152	2.5 0.1 2.6 0.0
9 TU	0305 0946 1520 2211	2.5 –0.2 2.4 –0.3	**24** W	0332 1000 1544 2226	2.4 0.2 2.5 0.1
10 W	0348 1025 1604 2256	2.4 –0.1 2.4 –0.2	**25** TH	0410 1037 1623 2308	2.2 0.2 2.4 0.2
11 TH	0438 1115 1702 2358	2.3 0.0 2.3 0.0	**26** F	0458 1127 1717	2.1 0.3 2.3
12 F	0545 1229 1818	2.2 0.2 2.3	**27** SA	0010 0603 1238 1830	0.3 2.1 0.4 2.3
13 SA	0123 0710 1400 1945	0.0 2.2 0.2 2.4	**28** SU	0130 0719 1400 1948	0.2 2.0 0.3 2.3
14 SU	0256 0837 1527 2104	–0.1 2.2 0.1 2.5	**29** M	0251 0833 1514 2056	0.1 2.1 0.2 2.3
15 M	0411 0947 1632 2205	–0.2 2.3 0.0 2.5	**30** TU	0353 0931 1610 2148	0.0 2.2 0.1 2.4

Chart Datum: 1·68 metres below Normal Null (German reference level)

21

TIME ZONE –0100
(German Standard Time)
Subtract 1 hour for UT
For German Summer Time add ONE hour in non-shaded areas

GERMANY – HELGOLAND

LAT 54°11′N   LONG 7°53′E

TIMES AND HEIGHTS OF HIGH AND LOW WATERS   YEAR **1996**

MAY

Day	Time / m	Day	Time / m
1 W	0439 −0.1 / 1016 2.4 / 1658 0.0 / 2232 2.5	16 TH	0522 −0.1 / 1059 2.5 / 1745 0.0 / 2319 2.6
2 TH	0522 −0.2 / 1058 2.5 / 1745 −0.1 / 2316 2.5	17 F ●	0608 0.0 / 1145 2.6 / 1834 0.0
3 F O	0604 −0.2 / 1139 2.5 / 1828 −0.1 / 2358 2.6	18 SA	0007 2.7 / 0651 0.0 / 1227 2.7 / 1916 0.0
4 SA	0646 −0.2 / 1219 2.6 / 1909 −0.2	19 SU	0048 2.7 / 0727 0.1 / 1303 2.8 / 1950 0.0
5 SU	0040 2.6 / 0727 −0.2 / 1300 2.6 / 1952 −0.2	20 M	0123 2.6 / 0800 0.1 / 1337 2.7 / 2024 0.0
6 M	0124 2.6 / 0811 −0.2 / 1342 2.6 / 2037 −0.3	21 TU	0158 2.6 / 0832 0.1 / 1411 2.7 / 2057 0.0
7 TU	0209 2.5 / 0853 −0.2 / 1425 2.6 / 2121 −0.3	22 W	0234 2.5 / 0904 0.1 / 1446 2.6 / 2130 0.1
8 W	0256 2.5 / 0935 −0.1 / 1510 2.6 / 2207 −0.2	23 TH	0310 2.4 / 0937 0.2 / 1521 2.6 / 2205 0.1
9 TH	0344 2.4 / 1021 0.0 / 1600 2.5 / 2259 −0.2	24 F	0347 2.3 / 1013 0.2 / 1557 2.5 / 2243 0.2
10 F	0439 2.3 / 1116 0.1 / 1700 2.5	25 SA	0428 2.2 / 1056 0.3 / 1641 2.4 / 2331 0.3
11 SA	0001 0.0 / 0545 2.3 / 1226 0.2 / 1811 2.5	26 SU	0520 2.2 / 1150 0.3 / 1738 2.4
12 SU	0116 0.0 / 0701 2.3 / 1346 0.2 / 1928 2.5	27 M	0034 0.2 / 0620 2.1 / 1259 0.3 / 1846 2.3
13 M	0237 0.0 / 0817 2.3 / 1503 0.1 / 2040 2.6	28 TU	0145 0.1 / 0731 2.2 / 1412 0.2 / 1955 2.4
14 TU	0346 −0.1 / 0921 2.3 / 1605 0.0 / 2139 2.6	29 W	0253 0.1 / 0835 2.3 / 1518 0.2 / 2057 2.4
15 W	0437 −0.1 / 1012 2.4 / 1655 0.0 / 2229 2.6	30 TH	0350 0.0 / 0931 2.4 / 1616 0.1 / 2153 2.5
		31 F	0442 0.0 / 1021 2.5 / 1710 0.0 / 2244 2.6

JUNE

Day	Time / m	Day	Time / m
1 SA O	0532 −0.1 / 1110 2.6 / 1801 −0.1 / 2332 2.7	16 SU ●	0627 0.2 / 1206 2.7 / 1855 0.1
2 SU	0620 −0.1 / 1155 2.7 / 1847 −0.1	17 M	0030 2.6 / 0705 0.1 / 1243 2.8 / 1930 0.1
3 M	0019 2.7 / 0707 −0.1 / 1241 2.7 / 1936 −0.2	18 TU	0106 2.6 / 0738 0.1 / 1317 2.8 / 2004 0.1
4 TU	0109 2.6 / 0755 −0.1 / 1328 2.7 / 2027 −0.3	19 W	0140 2.6 / 0812 0.1 / 1352 2.8 / 2037 0.1
5 W	0200 2.6 / 0843 −0.1 / 1416 2.7 / 2116 −0.3	20 TH	0214 2.5 / 0843 0.1 / 1425 2.7 / 2109 0.1
6 TH	0250 2.5 / 0928 −0.1 / 1503 2.7 / 2204 −0.2	21 F	0247 2.5 / 0915 0.1 / 1458 2.7 / 2143 0.1
7 F	0340 2.5 / 1016 0.0 / 1554 2.7 / 2256 −0.1	22 SA	0322 2.4 / 0951 0.2 / 1533 2.6 / 2220 0.1
8 SA	0434 2.4 / 1110 0.1 / 1652 2.7 / 2354 0.0	23 SU	0400 2.4 / 1031 0.2 / 1612 2.5 / 2259 0.1
9 SU	0534 2.4 / 1212 0.2 / 1756 2.7	24 M	0443 2.3 / 1113 0.2 / 1656 2.5 / 2346 0.1
10 M	0057 0.1 / 0639 2.4 / 1319 0.3 / 1902 2.6	25 TU	0532 2.2 / 1206 0.3 / 1751 2.4
11 TU	0204 0.1 / 0745 2.4 / 1429 0.2 / 2009 2.6	26 W	0044 0.1 / 0632 2.2 / 1313 0.3 / 1857 2.4
12 W	0310 0.1 / 0847 2.4 / 1534 0.1 / 2111 2.6	27 TH	0152 0.1 / 0739 2.3 / 1425 0.3 / 2008 2.4
13 TH	0406 0.1 / 0943 2.5 / 1631 0.1 / 2207 2.6	28 F	0300 0.1 / 0845 2.4 / 1535 0.2 / 2115 2.5
14 F	0455 0.1 / 1035 2.6 / 1723 0.1 / 2259 2.6	29 SA	0404 0.1 / 0947 2.6 / 1639 0.1 / 2216 2.6
15 SA	0543 0.1 / 1124 2.7 / 1812 0.1 / 2348 2.6	30 SU	0504 0.1 / 1044 2.7 / 1738 0.0 / 2311 2.7

JULY

Day	Time / m	Day	Time / m
1 M O	0600 0.0 / 1137 2.7 / 1831 −0.1	16 TU	0011 2.6 / 0647 0.2 / 1225 2.8 / 1911 0.1
2 TU	0004 2.7 / 0652 0.0 / 1227 2.8 / 1923 −0.2	17 W	0048 2.6 / 0721 0.1 / 1259 2.8 / 1945 0.1
3 W	0057 2.6 / 0743 −0.1 / 1317 2.8 / 2016 −0.2	18 TH	0121 2.6 / 0753 0.1 / 1333 2.8 / 2016 0.1
4 TH	0151 2.6 / 0833 −0.1 / 1406 2.9 / 2108 −0.2	19 F	0152 2.6 / 0823 0.1 / 1403 2.8 / 2046 0.1
5 F	0241 2.6 / 0919 −0.1 / 1454 2.9 / 2155 −0.2	20 SA	0222 2.5 / 0854 0.1 / 1434 2.7 / 2118 0.1
6 SA	0327 2.5 / 1004 0.0 / 1542 2.9 / 2242 0.0	21 SU	0255 2.5 / 0929 0.1 / 1508 2.6 / 2155 0.1
7 SU	0416 2.5 / 1053 0.1 / 1634 2.8 / 2332 0.1	22 M	0333 2.4 / 1009 0.1 / 1546 2.6 / 2232 0.0
8 M	0509 2.5 / 1145 0.2 / 1729 2.7	23 TU	0412 2.4 / 1046 0.1 / 1625 2.5 / 2308 0.1
9 TU	0023 0.2 / 0604 2.4 / 1242 0.3 / 1827 2.6	24 W	0452 2.3 / 1125 0.2 / 1709 2.5 / 2353 0.2
10 W	0119 0.3 / 0703 2.4 / 1347 0.3 / 1932 2.6	25 TH	0542 2.3 / 1222 0.3 / 1809 2.4
11 TH	0224 0.3 / 0808 2.4 / 1459 0.3 / 2041 2.5	26 F	0058 0.3 / 0648 2.3 / 1338 0.3 / 1924 2.4
12 F	0332 0.3 / 0914 2.5 / 1607 0.2 / 2146 2.5	27 SA	0216 0.2 / 0804 2.4 / 1501 0.3 / 2043 2.5
13 SA	0432 0.3 / 1014 2.6 / 1705 0.2 / 2242 2.6	28 SU	0334 0.2 / 0919 2.5 / 1616 0.2 / 2156 2.6
14 SU	0522 0.2 / 1105 2.7 / 1753 0.2 / 2330 2.6	29 M	0444 0.2 / 1025 2.7 / 1722 0.0 / 2258 2.6
15 M ●	0607 0.2 / 1147 2.7 / 1835 0.1	30 TU O	0546 0.1 / 1123 2.8 / 1819 −0.1 / 2353 2.7
		31 W	0641 0.0 / 1215 2.8 / 1911 −0.1

AUGUST

Day	Time / m	Day	Time / m
1 TH	0045 2.7 / 0731 0.0 / 1303 2.9 / 2002 −0.2	16 F	0056 2.6 / 0732 0.1 / 1309 2.8 / 1952 0.1
2 F	0136 2.6 / 0819 −0.1 / 1351 2.9 / 2052 −0.2	17 SA	0126 2.6 / 0802 0.0 / 1339 2.7 / 2021 0.1
3 SA	0223 2.6 / 0903 −0.1 / 1438 2.9 / 2136 −0.1	18 SU	0156 2.6 / 0832 0.0 / 1409 2.7 / 2053 0.1
4 SU	0306 2.6 / 0945 0.0 / 1523 2.9 / 2218 0.1	19 M	0229 2.5 / 0907 0.1 / 1444 2.6 / 2130 0.1
5 M	0349 2.6 / 1028 0.0 / 1609 2.8 / 2300 0.2	20 TU	0306 2.5 / 0946 0.1 / 1523 2.6 / 2207 0.1
6 TU	0435 2.6 / 1113 0.2 / 1656 2.7 / 2341 0.3	21 W	0343 2.5 / 1022 0.1 / 1559 2.6 / 2238 0.1
7 W	0522 2.5 / 1200 0.3 / 1747 2.6	22 TH	0419 2.4 / 1055 0.2 / 1638 2.5 / 2316 0.3
8 TH	0029 0.5 / 0616 2.5 / 1300 0.4 / 1850 2.5	23 F	0504 2.3 / 1146 0.3 / 1734 2.4
9 F	0133 0.5 / 0724 2.4 / 1418 0.5 / 2006 2.4	24 SA	0018 0.4 / 0610 2.3 / 1304 0.3 / 1853 2.4
10 SA	0252 0.5 / 0841 2.5 / 1540 0.4 / 2123 2.4	25 SU	0145 0.4 / 0735 2.4 / 1437 0.3 / 2023 2.4
11 SU	0407 0.4 / 0952 2.6 / 1647 0.3 / 2226 2.5	26 M	0315 0.3 / 0900 2.5 / 1601 0.2 / 2143 2.5
12 M	0504 0.4 / 1046 2.7 / 1736 0.3 / 2312 2.6	27 TU	0432 0.2 / 1012 2.7 / 1709 0.0 / 2248 2.6
13 TU	0548 0.3 / 1127 2.7 / 1814 0.2 / 2350 2.6	28 W O	0534 0.1 / 1109 2.8 / 1805 −0.1 / 2341 2.6
14 W ●	0626 0.2 / 1203 2.7 / 1849 0.1	29 TH	0627 0.1 / 1159 2.9 / 1855 −0.1
15 TH	0024 2.6 / 0701 0.1 / 1237 2.8 / 1922 0.1	30 F	0029 2.7 / 0715 0.0 / 1245 2.9 / 1942 −0.1
		31 SA	0115 2.7 / 0759 0.0 / 1331 2.9 / 2028 −0.1

Chart Datum: 1·68 metres below Normal Null (German reference level)

TIME ZONE –0100
(German Standard Time)
Subtract 1 hour for UT

For German Summer Time add
ONE hour in non-shaded areas

GERMANY – HELGOLAND

LAT 54°11′N   LONG 7°53′E

TIMES AND HEIGHTS OF HIGH AND LOW WATERS   YEAR **1996**

SEPTEMBER

Day	Time	m	Time	m	Time	m	Time	m
1 SU	0159	2.7	0842	0.0	1416	2.9	2110	0.0
16 M	0131	2.6	0811	0.1	1346	2.7	2030	0.1
2 M	0240	2.7	0922	0.0	1500	2.9	2148	0.2
17 TU	0205	2.6	0846	0.1	1421	2.7	2106	0.1
3 TU	0319	2.7	1001	0.1	1541	2.8	2223	0.3
18 W	0241	2.6	0923	0.1	1500	2.6	2141	0.1
4 W	0359	2.7	1039	0.3	1621	2.7	2258	0.4
19 TH	0317	2.6	0959	0.1	1538	2.5	2213	0.2
5 TH	0440	2.6	1120	0.4	1707	2.5	2340	0.6
20 F	0354	2.5	1035	0.2	1619	2.5	2253	0.3
6 F	0529	2.5	1214	0.5	1806	2.4		
21 SA	0441	2.4	1127	0.3	1716	2.4	2357	0.5
7 SA	0042	0.7	0637	2.4	1331	0.6	1925	2.3
22 SU	0550	2.4	1247	0.6	1838	2.3		
8 SU	0206	0.7	0801	2.4	1502	0.6	2050	2.3
23 M	0127	0.5	0719	2.5	1424	0.3	2011	2.4
9 M	0333	0.6	0922	2.5	1620	0.4	2202	2.4
24 TU	0302	0.4	0847	2.6	1550	0.2	2133	2.5
10 TU	0438	0.5	1021	2.7	1712	0.3	2249	2.5
25 W	0419	0.3	0957	2.7	1654	0.1	2234	2.6
11 W	0522	0.3	1101	2.7	1747	0.2	2322	2.6
26 TH	0517	0.2	1051	2.8	1746	0.0	2323	2.6
12 TH	0558	0.2	1134	2.7	1819	0.1	●2354	2.6
27 F	0607	0.1	1139	2.9	1834	0.0	O	
13 F	0634	0.1	1207	2.7	1852	0.1		
28 SA	0008	2.7	0653	0.1	1225	2.9	1918	0.0
14 SA	0027	2.6	0707	0.1	1241	2.7	1924	0.1
29 SU	0052	2.8	0737	0.1	1309	2.9	2000	0.1
15 SU	0059	2.6	0738	0.1	1314	2.7	1956	0.1
30 M	0133	2.8	0818	0.1	1352	2.9	2040	0.2

OCTOBER

Day	Time	m	Time	m	Time	m	Time	m
1 TU	0212	2.8	0856	0.1	1434	2.9	2115	0.3
16 W	0143	2.7	0826	0.1	1402	2.7	2043	0.2
2 W	0249	2.8	0932	0.2	1512	2.7	2147	0.4
17 TH	0220	2.7	0904	0.1	1441	2.6	2119	0.2
3 TH	0325	2.7	1007	0.3	1549	2.6	2219	0.5
18 F	0257	2.6	0943	0.1	1523	2.5	2156	0.3
4 F	0403	2.6	1043	0.4	1631	2.4	2258	0.6
19 SA	0339	2.6	1026	0.2	1610	2.4	2242	0.4
5 SA	0448	2.5	1131	0.6	1726	2.3	2354	0.7
20 SU	0432	2.5	1122	0.3	1712	2.3	2348	0.5
6 SU	0550	2.4	1242	0.7	1839	2.2		
21 M	0542	2.5	1239	0.4	1832	2.3		
7 M	0113	0.8	0712	2.4	1410	0.7	2004	2.3
22 TU	0116	0.6	0706	2.6	1411	0.4	2000	2.4
8 TU	0242	0.8	0835	2.5	1535	0.5	2120	2.4
23 W	0247	0.5	0830	2.6	1534	0.2	2116	2.5
9 W	0355	0.6	0941	2.6	1633	0.4	2212	2.5
24 TH	0400	0.4	0937	2.7	1634	0.1	2214	2.5
10 TH	0444	0.4	1024	2.7	1711	0.3	2247	2.5
25 F	0455	0.3	1030	2.8	1722	0.1	2301	2.6
11 F	0522	0.3	1058	2.7	1743	0.2	2320	2.6
26 SA	0543	0.2	1118	2.8	1809	0.1	O2346	2.7
12 SA	0601	0.2	1135	2.7	1819	0.1	●2355	2.6
27 SU	0631	0.2	1205	2.9	1853	0.2		
13 SU	0638	0.1	1212	2.7	1855	0.1		
28 M	0030	2.8	0715	0.2	1249	2.9	1932	0.3
14 M	0031	2.6	0713	0.1	1248	2.7	1930	0.1
29 TU	0109	2.9	0753	0.3	1329	2.9	2008	0.3
15 TU	0107	2.7	0749	0.1	1324	2.7	2007	0.2
30 W	0146	2.9	0830	0.3	1408	2.8	2043	0.4
31 TH	0222	2.8	0905	0.3	1446	2.7	2115	0.4

NOVEMBER

Day	Time	m	Time	m	Time	m	Time	m
1 F	0257	2.8	0939	0.3	1523	2.5	2147	0.5
16 SA	0246	2.7	0934	0.2	1515	2.5	2147	0.3
2 SA	0333	2.7	1014	0.4	1602	2.4	2224	0.6
17 SU	0331	2.7	1023	0.2	1607	2.4	2237	0.4
3 SU	0414	2.6	1056	0.5	1650	2.3	2312	0.7
18 M	0426	2.7	1121	0.3	1708	2.4	2341	0.5
4 M	0507	2.5	1153	0.6	1751	2.3		
19 TU	0533	2.6	1230	0.4	1821	2.4		
5 TU	0017	0.8	0616	2.5	1309	0.7	1905	2.3
20 W	0059	0.6	0649	2.7	1350	0.5	1939	2.4
6 W	0137	0.8	0733	2.5	1430	0.6	2020	2.3
21 TH	0220	0.5	0805	2.7	1506	0.3	2049	2.4
7 TH	0254	0.7	0843	2.5	1536	0.4	2121	2.4
22 F	0332	0.4	0912	2.7	1608	0.2	2148	2.5
8 F	0353	0.5	0937	2.6	1624	0.3	2206	2.5
23 SA	0429	0.3	1007	2.7	1657	0.2	2238	2.6
9 SA	0441	0.4	1020	2.6	1704	0.2	2245	2.6
24 SU	0520	0.3	1058	2.8	1744	0.3	2326	2.7
10 SU	0526	0.3	1102	2.7	1745	0.2	2324 O	2.7
25 M	0610	0.3	1148	2.8	1829	0.4		
11 M	0609	0.2	1143	2.7	1825 ●	0.2		
26 TU	0010	2.8	0654	0.3	1232	2.8	1907	0.4
12 TU	0004	2.7	0648	0.2	1223	2.7	1905	0.2
27 W	0048	2.9	0731	0.3	1309	2.8	1942	0.4
13 W	0043	2.8	0728	0.2	1305	2.7	1946	0.2
28 TH	0124	2.9	0806	0.3	1346	2.7	2017	0.4
14 TH	0124	2.8	0810	0.1	1347	2.7	2027	0.3
29 F	0159	2.9	0841	0.3	1424	2.6	2050	0.4
15 F	0205	2.8	0852	0.1	1430	2.6	2106	0.2
30 SA	0235	2.8	0916	0.3	1500	2.5	2122	0.4

DECEMBER

Day	Time	m	Time	m	Time	m	Time	m
1 SU	0309	2.7	0950	0.4	1536	2.4	2156	0.5
16 M	0325	2.8	1019	0.1	1600	2.5	2231	0.3
2 M	0346	2.6	1026	0.5	1617	2.4	2237	0.6
17 TU	0418	2.8	1113	0.2	1657	2.4	2328	0.4
3 TU	0428	2.6	1110	0.5	1705	2.3	2326	0.7
18 W	0518	2.7	1213	0.3	1759	2.4		
4 W	0521	2.5	1207	0.6	1803	2.3		
19 TH	0032	0.5	0623	2.7	1318	0.4	1906	2.4
5 TH	0030	0.7	0626	2.4	1316	0.5	1911	2.3
20 F	0144	0.5	0732	2.7	1428	0.4	2014	2.4
6 F	0143	0.7	0736	2.4	1427	0.4	2019	2.3
21 SA	0257	0.4	0842	2.6	1535	0.3	2118	2.5
7 SA	0254	0.6	0842	2.5	1530	0.3	2117	2.5
22 SU	0403	0.3	0945	2.6	1632	0.3	2216	2.6
8 SU	0355	0.5	0940	2.6	1623	0.3	2207	2.6
23 M	0501	0.3	1042	2.7	1722	0.4	2308	2.7
9 M	0450	0.4	1030	2.7	1712	0.2	2254	2.7
24 TU	0552	0.3	1133	2.7	1808	0.4	O2353	2.8
10 TU	0540	0.3	1116	2.7	1758	0.2	●2338	2.7
25 W	0636	0.3	1216	2.7	1848	0.4		
11 W	0626	0.2	1201	2.7	1843	0.2		
26 TH	0031	2.9	0713	0.3	1254	2.7	1923	0.4
12 TH	0022	2.8	0711	0.1	1248	2.7	1930	0.2
27 F	0106	2.9	0747	0.3	1328	2.7	1957	0.3
13 F	0108	2.8	0759	0.1	1337	2.7	2016	0.2
28 SA	0141	2.9	0822	0.3	1403	2.6	2030	0.3
14 SA	0154	2.8	0846	0.0	1425	2.6	2059	0.2
29 SU	0215	2.8	0855	0.3	1437	2.5	2100	0.3
15 SU	0239	2.7	0931	0.0	1511	2.6	2142	0.2
30 M	0247	2.7	0926	0.3	1509	2.4	2133	0.3
31 TU	0319	2.6	1000	0.3	1545	2.4	2209	0.3

Chart Datum: 1·68 metres below Normal Null (German reference level)

21

BÜSUM   10-21-24

Schleswig-Holstein, 54°07'·20N 08°51'·60E

CHARTS
AC 1875, 3767; BSH105, 3014.4
TIDES
HW +0036 on Dover (UT); ML 1·8m; Duration 0625

Standard Port HELGOLAND (←—)

Times				Height (metres)			
High Water		Low Water		MHWS	MHWN	MLWN	MLWS
0100	0600	0100	0800	2·7	2·3	0·4	0·0
1300	1800	1300	2000				
Differences BÜSUM							
+0054	+0049	−0001	+0027	+0·9	+0·9	+0·1	0·0
LINNENPLATE							
+0047	+0046	+0034	+0046	+0·7	+0·6	+0·1	0·0
SÜDERHÖFT							
+0103	+0056	+0051	+0112	+0·8	+0·7	+0·1	0·0

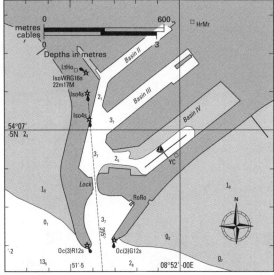

SHELTER
Very good; after lock turn 90° stbd into yacht hbr (2·5m) in Basin IV. Lock manned H24; for opening, call on VHF or sound 1 long blast in appr chan; 2 long blasts on reaching lock if not already open; comply with R/G lts.
NAVIGATION
WPT 54°06'·50N 08°19'·10E, SWM buoy Iso 8s, 270°/090° from/to Süderpiep No 2 PHM buoy, 5M. Appr by 2 well-buoyed chans, Süderpiep and Norderpiep (unlit) each approx 15M long. Beware strong tidal streams across ent and sudden winds over the moles.
LIGHTS AND MARKS
Lt ho Iso WRG 16s 22m 17/14/13M; W091·5°-093·5° leads 092·5° for last 4M of Süderpiep. Hbr lts as chartlet. A high bldg is conspic 9ca NW of hbr; silo is conspic in hbr.
RADIO TELEPHONE
VHF call *Büsum Port* Ch 11 16.
TELEPHONE (04834)
Hr Mr 2183; CG 2025; ⌗ 2376; Dr 2088; YC 2997.
FACILITIES
Yacht hbr AB 13.50DM, AC, EI, FW, M, ME, C, P, D, ▣.
Town CH, V, R, Bar, ✉, Ⓑ, ⇌, Ⓗ, ✈ (Hamburg).
Note: Meldorf yacht hbr is 4M ESE; full yacht facilities.

OTHER HBRS ON W COAST OF SCHLESWIG-HOLSTEIN

TÖNNING, Schleswig-Holstein, 54°18'·92N 08°57'·11E. AC 3767; BSH104, 3014.8. HW +0246 and +0·5m on Helgoland; ML 2·7m. Eiderdamm lock, 5·5M seawards, operates H24. VHF Ch 14 16. Lock N mole Oc (2) R 12s; S mole Oc G 6s. R Eider with the Gieselau Kanal links Tönning with the Kiel Canal (see 10.21.22). Above the dam, R Eider is tidal, depending on operation of sluices HW +3 to HW+½, (beware strong currents). Berth in middle of S quay, 3m at MHW. If heading E up river, bridge (clnce 5·6m) opens on request Mon-Sat 0600-SS. Hr Mr ☎ (04861) 1400; Dr ☎ 389; Ⓗ ☎ 706; Facilities: **Quay** 13.50DM, FW, P, D, BY, C (5 ton), Slip; YC ☎ 754 (all welcome). **Town** Ⓑ, ✉, ⇌, Gaz.

HUSUM, Schleswig-Holstein, 54°28'·78N 09°00'·00E. AC 3767; BSH 105, 3013.12. HW + 0036 on Dover (UT); ML 1·9m; Duration 0555. See 10.21.26. A sluice/lock, 7ca W of rly bridge, is shut when level > 0·3m over MHW, as shown by ℝ. Beware the canal effect when passing big ships in the narrow appr chan. In the outer hbr yachts should turn stbd just before rly bridge for pontoons on S bank, or pass through bridge (clnce 5m when shut) to inner hbr by SC Nordsee; both dry. VHF call *Husum Port* Ch 11. Tfc reports broadcast on Ch 11 every H +00 from HW −4 to HW +2. Outer ldg lts 106° both Iso R 8s, synch & intens on ldg line. Inner ldg lts 090° both Iso G 8s, synch & intens on ldg line. Night entry not advised. Hr Mr ☎ (04841) 667217; Sluice ☎ 2565; **Husum YC** ☎ 65670; **SC Nordsee** ☎ 3436; ⌗ ☎ 61759. AB 13.50DM, P, D, at hbr.

HARBOURS IN THE NORTH FRISIAN ISLANDS

PELLWORM, 54°31'·31N 08°41'·24E. AC 3767; BSH 3013.11. Tides: interpolate Suderoogsand/Husum, opposite. Outer appr via Norderhever; ldg lts 041° Oc 5s. Ent chan from NH18 PHM buoy, Fl (2+1) R 15s, has 0·2m; access near HW. Small yacht hbr 2·8m at MHW; drying on soft mud.

WYK, Island of Föhr, 54°41'·70N 08°34'·80E. AC 3767; BSH107, 3013.6. HW +0107 on Dover (UT); +0137 on Helgoland (zone −0100); ML 2·8. Good yacht hbr (1·5m) to N of ent, sheltered in all winds; visitors berth W side of pontoon 1. Access H24. Also berths on E quay of inner hbr. Ferry hbr (4m). Lts: Oldenhorn (SE point of Föhr), R tr, Oc (4) WRG 15s 10m 13/9M; W208°-250°, R250°-281°, W281°-290°, G290°-333°, W333°-058°, R 058°-080°. S mole Oc (2) WR 12s 12m 7/4M; W220°-322°, R322°-220°. Port VHF Ch **11** 16. Yacht hbr Hr Mr ☎ (04681) 3030; Commercial Hr Mr ☎ 2852; **YC** ☎ 1280; Dr ☎ 8998; ⌗ ☎ 2594; Facilities: **Hbr road** (500m), CH, ▣, P & D (cans); **Yacht Hbr** 18DM, R, V; **W Quay** D.

WITTDÜN, Amrum, 54°37'·85N 08°24'·65E. AC 3767; BSH107, 3013.6. HW +0107 on Dover (UT); +0137 on Helgoland (zone −0100); ML 2·7m; Duration 0540. See 10.21.26. Wittdün is the main hbr of Amrum. Yachts berth S of stone quay, lying bows to pontoon, stern to posts. Good shelter except in E winds. The quay 800m to the E is reserved for ferries only. Chan has 2m and is marked by PHM withies ⌕. Ldg lts 272°: Both Iso R 4s 11/33m 10/15M; W masts, R bands; intens on ldg line. Lt ho Fl 7·5s 63m 23M; R tr, W bands; same location as rear ldg lt. It is not advisable to enter at night. Wriakhörn, Cross lt, is 1M WSW of hbr, L Fl (2) WR 15s 26m 9/7M; W297°-319°, R319°-343°, W343°-014°, R014°-034°. Hr Mr ☎ (04682) 2294; ⌗ ☎ 2026; Dr ☎ 2612; Facilities: AB 18DM, P & D (cans) at Nebel; **Amrum YC** ☎ 2054.

TIDAL DIFFERENCES FOR WEST COAST OF DENMARK   10-21-25

These figures are mean values, to be used with caution.

Standard Port HELGOLAND (←—)

Times				Height (metres)			
High Water		Low Water		MHWS	MHWN	MLWN	MLWS
0300	0700	0100	0800	2·7	2·3	0·4	0·0
1500	1900	1300	2000				
Differences HØJER							
+0247	+0322	No data		−0·3	−0·2	0·0	0·0
RØMØ HAVN							
+0227	+0302	+0221	+0201	−0·8	−0·7	−0·1	0·0
GRADYB BAR							
+0137	+0152	No data		−1·2	−1·1	−0·1	0·0
ESBJERG							
+0307	+0307	+0221	+0221	−1·1	−0·9	−0·2	−0·1
BLAVANDSHUK							
+0147	+0157	+0131	+0121	−0·9	−0·9	−0·1	0·0
TORSMINDE							
+0337	+0357	+0301	+0231	−1·8	−1·6	−0·3	0·0
THYBORON							
+0427	+0537	+0631	+0431	−2·3	−2·0	−0·3	0·0
HANSTHOLM							
+0407	+0647	+0601	+0351	−2·4	−2·0	−0·3	0·0
HIRTSHALS							
+0402	+0627	+0601	+0321	−2·4	−2·0	−0·3	

SYLT   10-21-26

Schleswig-Holstein 54°45'·54N 08°17'·86E (Hörnum)

CHARTS
AC 3767/8; BSH D107, D108, 3013.3 List, 3013.5 Hörnum

TIDES
+0110 Dover; ML 1·8; Duration 0540; Zone −0100

Standard Port HELGOLAND (←)

Times				Height (metres)			
High Water		Low Water		MHWS	MHWN	MLWN	MLWS
0100	0600	0100	0800	2·7	2·3	0·4	0·0
1300	1800	1300	2000				
Differences LIST							
+0252	+0240	+0201	+0210	−0·7	−0·6	−0·2	0·0
HÖRNUM							
+0223	+0218	+0131	+0137	−0·5	−0·3	−0·2	0·0
AMRUM-HAFEN							
+0138	+0137	+0128	+0134	+0·2	+0·2	+0·1	0·0
DAGEBÜLL							
+0226	+0217	+0211	+0225	+0·6	+0·6	−0·1	0·0
SUDEROOGSAND							
+0116	+0102	+0038	+0122	+0·3	+0·4	+0·1	0·0
HUSUM							
+0205	+0152	+0118	+0200	+1·2	+1·1	+0·1	0·0

SHELTER
The island of Sylt is about 20M long, has its capital Westerland in the centre, List in the N and Hörnum in the S. The Hindenburgdamm connects it to the mainland.
LIST: The small hbr is sheltered except in NE/E winds. Ent is 25m wide and hbr 3m deep.

HÖRNUM: Good in the small hbr, approx 370m x 90m, protected by outer mole on SE side and by 2 inner moles. Yacht haven at the N end. Good ⚓ in Hörnum Reede in W and N winds and in Hörnumtief in E and S winds. There are two other hbrs; Rantum (9DM) and Munkmarsch (13.50DM) which both dry; access HW ±3. Large areas of Sylt are nature reserves; landing prohib.

NAVIGATION
LIST WPT: Lister Tief SWM buoy, Iso 8s, 55°05'·37N 08°16'·87E, 292°/112° from/to List Ost lt, 6·1M. Lister Tief (see 10.21.5) is well marked. In strong W/NW winds expect a big swell on the bar (depth 4m) on the ebb, which sets on to Salzsand. NE quay is open construction and not suitable for yachts. Chan buoys through roadstead lead to hbr. Access at all tides, but beware strong tidal streams across ent.

HÖRNUM WPT: Vortrapptief (SWM) buoy, Oc 4s, 54°35'·00N 08°12'·20E, 215°/035° from/to Norddorf lt (Amrum), 6·35M. Appr through Vortrapptief buoyed chan (see below) inside drying banks. In strong W winds the sea breaks on off-lying banks and in the chan. Final appr from NE, keeping mid-chan in hbr ent. Access at all tides.

LIGHTS AND MARKS
LIST See 10.21.4 for List West lt Oc WRG 6s, List Ost Iso WRG 6s, List Land Oc WRG 3s and Kampen Oc (4) WR 15s. Römö church is conspic. N mole hd FG, vis 218°-038°. S mole hd FR, vis 218°-353°.

HÖRNUM Conspic radio mast (5 Fl R lts) 3M N of hbr. Follow W041°-043° sector of Norddorf lt (Oc WRG 6s) to line of Hörnum ldg lts 012°, both Iso 8s. N pier hd FG, vis 024°-260°. Outer mole hd FR (mole floodlit).

RADIO TELEPHONE
None.

TELEPHONE List (04652); Hörnum (04653)
LIST Hr Mr 374; Police 510; Ⓗ (04651) 841; ✚ 413, CG 365; Dr 350;
HÖRNUM Hr Mr 1027; Dr 1016; Police 1510; CG 1256.

FACILITIES
LIST, **Hbr** AB 14DM, FW, ⚒, C (35 ton), Slip, SC. **Village** V, R, Bar, P & D (cans), Ferry to Römö (Denmark).
WESTERLAND CG 85199; Police 7047. **Town** V, R, Bar, P & D (cans), Gaz, ⚒, ✉, Ⓑ, ➤, ✈.
HÖRNUM Sylter YC ☎ 274, AB 18DM, Bar, AC, FW, ▣. **Town** V, R, Bar, ME, ✉, Ⓑ.

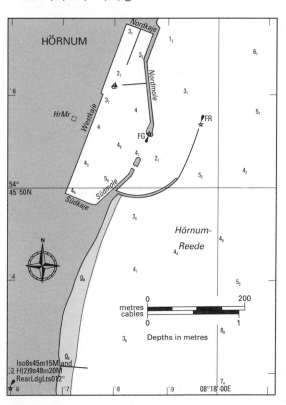

Late corrections

Up to and including *Admiralty Notices to Mariners*, Weekly Edition No. 24/95.

Navigational information in the main body of this Almanac is corrected to *Admiralty Notices to Mariners*, Weekly Edition No. 13/1995. For ease of reference each correction is sequentially numbered, followed by the Almanac page number.

Chapter 4 – Radio Navigational Aids

1.41   4.2.4   Differential GPS.
RH col. Line 22. Amend to read: The charge for this service is £395 per annum (or £890 for 3 years).

2.43   Fig. 4(2) DECCA CHAINS NW EUROPE. Decca chains 4C and 6A serving North-West and Southern Spain have permanently ceased operation. Delete reference to these chains on the map.

RADIOBEACONS.
3.48   **No. 3 Lizard Lt**.
Col. 9 add: DGPS service 284·00 kHz 56M.
No. 29 Girdle Ness.
Col. 9 add: DGPS service 311·50 kHz 40M.

RADAR BEACONS.
4.57   No. 121 **Eilean Glas Lt**.
Amend to: 3 & 10cm and range **16M**.

5.58   NETHERLANDS.
Insert: No. 392 3 & 10cm **Markham Field Platform J6-A** 53°49'·39N 02°56'·75E 000°-180° **M**.
No. 403 3 & 10cm **NAM Field Platform F3-OLT** 54°51'·3N 04°43'·6E 360° **D**.

Chapter 6 – Communications

6.81   LH col. **NAVTEX Message categories.**
Delete code L Navigation warnings additional to letter A.
Insert:
L Navigational warnings additional to letter A, and for the UK only, individual rigmoves.
V Amplifying details of navigation warnings initially broadcast under letter A. The weekly Riglist will also be broadcast using letter V.

6.3.26   UK Coast Radio Stations.
7.82   **Ilfracombe Radio**
Add: Note (1) VHF Ch 07 directed to River Severn.
8.83   **Jersey Radio.**
To Note 6 add: MMSI 002320060.

Niton Radio.
Amend Note (1) to read: VHF Ch 04 directed to the Brighton area.
North Foreland Radio.
Delete: Ch 65 and all reference to MF frequencies.
Humber Radio.
Amend Note (1) to read: VHF Ch 85 directed to the Wash.

9.85   **Fig. 6(2).** North Foreland Radio.
Delete: VHF Ch 65.

10.86   **Anglesey Radio.**
Add: Note (1) VHF Ch 28 directed to River Mersey.

11.97   **Scheveningen Radio** VHF weather bulletins.
RH col. Bottom line.
Delete: 0705. Insert: 0805.

Chapter 7 – Weather

12.106   **7.2.9   Facsimile broadcasts.**
RH col. Selected UK Fax broadcast schedule.
Line 2. Delete: 0300 Northwood.
Insert: 0400 Northwood.

13.107   **7.2.11   Volmet.**
Delete: 4722 and 11200 kHz.
Insert: 4739 and 11178 kHz.

14.114   **7.2.19   Local Radio Stations - Coastal Weather Forecasts.**
Amend as follows:

BBC Radio Devon.
Mon-Fri: Add: **2212 2315**
Sat: Add: 0733
Sun: Delete: 0633.
            Insert: **0633** 0833.
Bold times = Live forecasts from Bristol Weather Centre.

BBC Radio Solent.
Delete times in toto.
Insert:
Mon-Fri: 0500 0530 **0533** 0610 *0635* 0710 *0735* **0745** 0810 *0835* 0850 0904 1004 1104 1204 *1327* 1404 1504 *1525* 1604 *1625* 1710 *1735* 1810 *1835* 1904 2004 2104 2208 *2305*.
Sat: 0604 *0633* 0710 0733 **0745** 0810 0830 0850 0904 1004 1104 1204 *1307* 1404 1504 *1758* 1804.
Sun: 0604 *0633* 0710 0733 **0745** 0810 0904 1004 1104 1204 1309 1404 *1504* 1604 1704 1804.

Bold   = Shipping forecast/tides
Bold italic = Live weather from Southampton Weather Centre.

15.116   **TABLE 7(4)**.
BT SOUTHERN REGION.
North Foreland. Delete: 1707 kHz.

16.121   **NETHERLANDS**.
Scheveningen Radio VHF stations
Col. 3. Weather Messages.
Delete: 0705. Insert: 0805.
Col. 4. Add 24h wind fcsts at 0005 and 1905.

GERMANY.
Norddeutscher Rundfunk Hamburg
(NDR 4).
Col 3. Delete: 0105. Insert: 0930 2320.
Col 6. Delete: 1900.

Chapter 8 – Safety

17.128   RH col. **Digital Selective Calling.**
Line 18. Delete: MMSCI. Insert: MMSI.

Chapter 9 – Tides

18.142   **Tidal Streams**.
LH col. Lines 3/4. Tidal Stream Atlases.
Amend to: NP 218 Edition 5 North coast of
Ireland, West coast of Scotland 1995.

Chapter 10 – Introduction

19.149   FERRY SERVICES, NORTH SEA.
Newcastle to IJmuiden. Delete: To be
announced. Insert: 14 hours; under frequency
column insert: Varies, May-Sep.
IRISH SEA, Rosslare-Pembroke Dock and
Dublin-Holyhead; amend B & I Lines to Irish
Ferries; ☎ Bookings 0345 171717.

20.154/5   Fig.10(3)1 TSS Diagrams.
LH map margin.
SKERRIES.
Delete: 54°30'N. Insert: 53°30'N.
Fig. 10(4)1. TUSKAR ROCK TSS.
RH col. Line 2.
After 52°14'·0N insert: 06°00'·8W.
Fig.10(4)3. OFF SMALLS TSS.
RH map grid margin.
Delete: 51°30'N. Insert: 51°50'N.

Area 1 – South-West England

LIGHTS, FOG SIGNALS & WAYPOINTS.
21.169   LH col. PLYMOUTH SOUND.
Lines 5/7. **Plymouth Bkwtr W Hd**.
Amend to: Plymouth Bkwtr W Hd W12M,
R9M.
Iso W 4s (same Tr). Amend to: 10M and
vis 033°-037°. Amend ◌))) to: *Horn 15s*.
Line 25. Bkwtr E Hd.
Amend to: L Fl WR 10s 9m W8M, R6M etc.

Line 30. Whidbey.
Amend to: Oc (2) WRG 10s 29m W8M,
R6M, G6M

22.186   PLYMOUTH. NAVIGATION.
Lines 11/13. Amend to read: The E'ly of 3
conspic high-rise blocks brg 331° leads
through The Bridge chan. Caution: a charted
depth 1·8m is close SW of No. 3 SHM bn,
Fl (3) G 10s.

23.187   PLYMOUTH, CHARTLET.
Bkwtr West Head ☆: Amend ranges of
Fl WR 10s to 12/9M, and range of Iso 4s to
10M. Delete Bell; insert Horn. Re-draw
pecked lines to show visibility sector of
W Iso 4s light as 033°-037°(4°).
Bkwtr East Head ☆, amend to L Fl WR 10s
8/6M.
LIGHTS & MARKS.
Line 2. Amend 15/12M to 12/9M and 12M
to 10M.
Line 3. Amend 031°-039° to 033°-037°(4°).
Amend Bkwtr E Hd to L Fl WR 10s 9m 8/6M
etc.
Line 8.   After Whidbey (138·5°) insert:
Staddon Pt (044°).

24.188   PLYMOUTH. RADIO TELEPHONE.
Line 5. After Queen Anne's Battery, insert
Sutton Harbour.

25.204   BRIDPORT. SHELTER.
Lines 4/5.   Delete references to Coaster
berths; ditto on Chartlet. (Coasters no longer
call; berths normally used by FV's).

Area 2 – Central Southern England

LIGHTS, FOG SIGNALS & WAYPOINTS.
26.210   RH col. NORTH CHANNEL.
Line 6, After Inner Bkwtr Hd 2 FG (vert) 3M.
Insert: Parkstone Yacht Haven 2 FR (vert)
4m 2M.

27.211   LH col. ASHLETT CREEK.
Fawley Lt By.
Amend pos to: 50°49'·93N 01°19'·33W.

28.212   LH col. PORTSMOUTH & APPROACHES.
Line 3. Saddle Lt By.
Amend pos to: 50°45'·17N 01°04'·89W.
Line 31. Ballast Lt By.
Amend pos to: 50°47'·63N 01°06'·73W.

29.213   PASSAGE INFORMATION.
RH col. W Approaches to Solent, first para,
last line, add: Due to shoaling (1995) on the
ldg line, the SW Shingles lt buoy has been
moved 130m SSE. See 10.2.16.

30.227   POOLE HARBOUR. FACILITIES.
Parkstone Haven, lines 4-6, amend all after
(Fl G 3s) as follows: 2 PHM and 3 SHM unlit
buoys. Ldg daymarks 006°, both Y ◊s; ldg lts,
front Iso Y 4s, rear FY. 2 FG and 2 FR (vert)
on bkwtr hds.

31.234   NEEDLES CHANNEL.
LH col. First para, last line add: Due to
shoaling (1995) on the ldg line, the SW
Shingles lt buoy has been moved 130m SSE.
See 10.2.4.

32.239   SOLENT AREA.
Weather and Navigation Broadcasts by
BBC Radio Solent.
Line 3. Delete all from A to end of daily
broadcast schedule. Substitute:
A   Forecast summary.
B   Shipping forecast and tidal details.
C   Live forecast from Southampton Weather
     Centre.
D   Shipping movements.

Daily Broadcasts (LT)

0500 A (Mon-Fri)	1309 A (Sun)
0530 A (Mon-Fri)	1327 C (Mon-Fri)
0533 B (Mon-Fri)	1404 A
0604 A (Sat/Sun)	1504 A. B on Sun
0610 A (Mon-Fri)	1525 C (Mon-Fri)
0633 B/C (Sat); C (Sun)	1604 A (Mon-Fri & Sun)
0635 B/C (Mon-Fri)	1625 C (Mon-Fri)
0710 A	1704 A (Sun)
0733 A (Sat-Sun)	1710 A (Mon-Fri)
0735 C (Mon-Fri)	1735 C (Mon-Fri)
0745 B	1758 C (Sat only)
0810 A	1804 A (Sat/Sun)
0830 A (Sat)	1810 A (Mon-Fri)
0835 C (Mon-Fri)	1835 C (Mon-Fri)
0850 D (Mon-Sat)	1904 A (Mon-Fri)
0904 A	2004 A (Mon-Fri)
1004 A	2104 A (Mon-Fri)
1104 A	2208 A (Mon-Fri)
1204 A	2305 C (Mon-Fri)
1307 C (Sat)	

SOLENT AREA WAYPOINTS.
33.240   Delete: *Beta (Portsmouth) and *Echo.
Insert:
*Brunswick Gate 50°46'·05N 01°05'·66W.
34.241   **Saddle**. Amend to: 50°45'·17N 01°04'·89W.
*Vail Williams 50°46'·80N 01°07'·25W.

35.258   PORTSMOUTH. NAVIGATION.
Line 1. Amend latitude of No. 4 Bar buoy to
50°46'·98W.

36.261   LANGSTONE HARBOUR.
Langstone Marina has been renamed
Southsea Marina. This correction applies to
both chartlets, Lights & Marks line 4, and
Facilities line 1.

Area 3 – SE England

AREA MAP.
37.267   **North Foreland Radio block**.
📡. Delete: VHF **65** and MF 1707.
📻. Delete: MF 1707.

LIGHTS, FOG SIGNALS & WAYPOINTS.
38.271   RH col. RAMSGATE.
Line 9. W Pier Hd. Delete: tfc sigs.

39.284   FOLKESTONE. RADIO TELEPHONE.
Delete Ch 22. Insert: Ch 15.

40.289   RAMSGATE. LIGHTS & MARKS.
Lines 4/5. Delete IPTS. . . Royal Hbr.
Substitute: At E Pier, IPTS (Sigs 2 & 3)
visible from seaward and from within Royal
Hbr, control appr chan, outer hbr and ent/exit
to/from Royal Hbr. In addition a Fl Y Lt
means a ferry is under way either in the chan
or outer hbr. At W Pier, depth...
CHARTLET. Move caption Watch Ho, SS
(Traffic Signal) from W Pier to E Pier, close
N of ☆ Oc 10s. Delete: Horn (1) 60s.
Insert: Horn 60s after ☆ Oc 10s 8m 4M at root
of N bkwtr.

Area 4 – E England

LIGHTS, FOG SIGNALS & WAYPOINTS.
41.298   RH col. HARWICH CHANNEL.
<u>S Threshold Lt By</u>.
Amend Long to: 01°33'·29E.

42.299   LH col. Line 7, <u>Erwarton Ness Lt Bn</u>.
Amend Lat to: 51°57'·10N.
RH col. LOWESTOFT AND
APPROACHES VIA STANFORD CHAN.
<u>Newcombe Sand Lt By</u>.
Amend pos to: 52°26'·94N 01°47'·23E.
<u>S. Holm Lt By</u>.
Amend pos to: 52°27'·41N 01°47'·34E.

43.302   EAST ANGLIAN WAYPOINTS.
Cork Sand Lt By.
Amend long to: 01°25'·95E.
Newcombe Sand Lt By.
Amend pos to: 52°26'·94N 01°47'·23E.
South Holm Lt By.
Amend pos to: 52°27'·41N 01°47'·34E.

Area 5 – NE England

LIGHTS, FOG SIGNALS & WAYPOINTS.
44.348   RH col. WELLS-NEXT-THE-SEA.
<u>Wells Fairway Lt By.</u>
Amend pos to: 52°59'·92N 00°49'·61E.
RH col. THE WASH.
ROARING MIDDLE Lt F.
Amend pos to: 52°58'·61N 00°21'·15E.

No. 3 Lt By. Amend pos to: 52°54'·52N.
No. 3A Lt By. Amend pos to: 52°53'·64N.
Bar Flat Lt By. Amend pos to: 52°55'·19N
00°16'·51E.

45.349   LH col. BOSTON DEEP.
Wainfleet Roads By. Amend pos to:
53°06'·22N 00°21'·55E.

46.349   RH col. RIVER HUMBER TO WHITBY.
Hornsea Sewer Outfall Lt By.
Amend pos to: 53°55'·02N 00°08'·27E.

47.350   LH col. TEES APPROACH.
Amend pos as follows:
Tees Fairway Lt By to: 54°40'·95N
01°06'·23W.
Tees N (Fairway) Lt By to: 54°40'·33N
01°07'·02W.
Tees S (Fairway) Lt By to: 54°40'·22N
01°06'·87W.

48.361   RIVER HUMBER. NAVIGATION.
After last line add margin Note: Due to
continuous shoaling upriver of No. 26 Lt
buoy (off Hull marina), a new channel has
been marked to the south of Hull Middle
shoal. It starts at No. 20 ECM Lt buoy,
formerly a PHM, and is marked by three
PHM Lt bys, Nos. 20A, 22A and 24A.
There is a least depth of 1·2m near No. 20A
buoy.   Further info to be promulgated by
NMs.

49.373   HOLY ISLAND. CHARTLET.
Delete Slip close S of The Heugh.
LIGHTS & MARKS.
Line 1. Delete white; insert reddish.
TELEPHONE.
Hr Mr insert prefix 3 before 89217.

Area 7 – NE Scotland

50.413   PASSAGE INFORMATION.
RH col. Last para, line 3, after 10.7.24
insert: Recommended Traffic Routes: NW-
bound ships pass to the NE (no closer than
10M to Sumburgh Hd) or SW of Fair Isle;
SE-bound ships pass no closer than 5M off
N Ronaldsay (Orkney).

51.420   WICK. CHARTLET.
Delete: ☆ F Vi on W wall of Inner Hbr.

52.426   LERWICK. LIGHTS & MARKS.
After 23M, insert Cro of Ham, Fl 3s 3M.

Area 8 – NW Scotland

LIGHTS, FOG SIGNALS & WAYPOINTS.
53.437   LH col. BARRA/CASTLEBAY.
Line 8. Sgeir Dubh. Amend vis to:
W280°-117°, G117°-280°.

54.442   CASTLEBAY.
Delete lines 8-10. (Beware . . .7m 8M);
Insert: Beware rks NNW of Sgeir Dubh a
conspic W/G tr, Fl (2) WG 6s 6m 7/5M,
vis W280°-117°, G117°-280°; which leads
283° in transit with Sgeir Liath, Fl 3s 7m
8M. Chan Rk, 2ca to the S is marked by
Fl WR 6s 4m 6/4M.

55.447   LOCH ALSH.
Line 5. After clearance, insert: Call *Bridge
Control* Ch 12.
Penultimate line, after 534167, insert VHF
Ch 11.

56.448   ARISAIG HARBOUR.
3 lines from end. Amend VHF to Ch 16, M.

Area 9 – SW Scotland

57.485   TROON. CHARTLET.
Delete the 2 most SE'ly pontoons. Re-letter
the remaining 5 pontoons as A/B, C/D, E/F,
G/H and I/J.
LIGHTS & MARKS.
Last line. Add: A SHM lt buoy, FG, marks
the chan in the ent to the marina.
FACILITIES.
Line 1. Amend number of berths to 250 + 50
visitors.
Line 3. Insert: Some berths for LOA 36m
x 3m draft at end of pontoons.

Area 10 – NW England

LIGHTS, FOG SIGNALS & WAYPOINTS.
58.492   RH col. RIVER RIBBLE.
Line 6. Delete: El Oso Wreck Lt By.

Area 11 – South Wales and Bristol Channel

LIGHTS, FOG SIGNALS & WAYPOINTS.
LH col. Lines 4/5.
59.520   **St Tudwal's**.
Amend to: Fl WR 15s **W14M**, R10M.

60.521   LH col. Lines 10/11.
Delete: Whitford Lt Tr.

61.522   LH col. PORTISHEAD.
Line 2. Delete: *Horn 15s* . . . expected.

62.526 ABERSOCH. CHARTLET.
Amend St Tudwal's ☆ to Fl WR 15s 46m
14/10M.

63.528 ABERAERON.
Line 10. Amend 7m to 11m.
Last line, amend VHF to 14 16.

64.528 ABERYSTWYTH. SHELTER.
Delete all after dredged.
Substitute: 1·7m. Rest of hbr dries. The
Bar, close off S pier head, and outer hbr have
0·5m least depth; inner hbr 0·3m. Access
approx HW±3.
NAVIGATION.
Delete 4th sentence (The Bar...MLWS).

65.536 BURRY INLET. CHARTLET.
Whiteford Lt Ho (conspic), delete Fl 5s 7m
7M (occas) and ☆ and light flash.
NAVIGATION.
Line 8. After Whiteford Lt Ho insert
(disused).
LIGHTS & MARKS. Line 1. After
Whiteford Lt Ho, amend to: is conspic, but
no longer lit.

Area 12 – South Ireland

LIGHTS, FOG SIGNALS & WAYPOINTS.
66.555 LH col. BALLYCOTTON.
Line 5. Pollock Rk Lt By. Delete: Bell.

67.563 DUN LAOGHAIRE. CHARTLET.
Amend fog signal at light on end of East
Pier, to Horn (30s) or reserve signal of
Bell 6s.

68.570 DUNMORE EAST. CHARTLET.
Delete ⚓ symbol off West Wharf.
SHELTER.
Add Margin Note: In 1995 there was
effectively no space in hbr for yachts due to
heavy FV usage and WIP on W Wharf.
(Marina planned to NW of hbr where Small
Craft Moorings shown).

69.570 WATERFORD. SHELTER.
Line 2, after (9M up the estuary) insert:
Caution, four groynes (marked by SPM lt
buoys) close W of Cheek Point may be a
hazard: quays have silted up.

Area 13 – North Ireland

LIGHTS, FOG SIGNALS & WAYPOINTS.
70.592 LH col. DUNDALK.
Lines 3/4. Pile Lt. Oc G 5s Lt. Amend vis to:
325·5°-328·5°.

71.600 STRANGFORD LOUGH.
Line 2 (below title) amend longitude to
05°30'·85W.

72.601 STRANGFORD LOUGH. CHARTLET.
Inset of Strangford Creek.
Delete pecked leading line 181° and ☆
Oc R 10s at its S end. Amend the front ldg lt
on 256° to read Oc WRG 5s.

73.603 BELFAST LOUGH. TELEPHONE.
Last line, amend: Police (01247) 454444;
Dr 468521.

74.609 LOUGH FOYLE. TIDES.
Line 3. Amend Moville –0350 Dover.
Line 5. Amend Warren Point –0430 Dover.

75.613 WESTPORT. CHARTLET.
Delete Station ■. Note the railway station is
off chartlet to the East; regular daily service
to Dublin.

Area 15– South Brittany

76.652 SPECIAL NOTES FOR FRANCE.
TELEPHONES.
Add Margin Note: With effect from 2300LT
18 Oct 1996, all subscriber numbers will
provisionally become 10 digits by prefixing
the 8 digit numbers with the following 2 digits
for regions:
01 - Ile de France (Paris area)
02 - NW France
03 - NE France
04 - SE France
05 - SW France
All mobile ☎ Nos will be prefixed by 06.
If calling a French number from abroad, omit
the 0 from the above prefixes. The code for
making international calls from France will
change from 19 to 00.
Emergency ☎ Nos will not change.

77.660 CARTERET. LIGHTS & MARKS.
Insert after last line: A PHM and SHM
beacon, respectively Fl (2) R 6s and Fl (2) G
6s, mark the bend in the chan approx 5ca N of
W Jetty head.
CHARTLET.
Insert a PHM and a SHM lt beacon (as above)
at 49°22'·64N 01°47'·15W and 49°22'·61N
01°47'·12W respectively.

Area 16 – North Brittany

78.689 TRÉBEURDEN. LIGHTS & MARKS.
Last sentence. After IPTS, Sigs 2 & 4, amend
to: on PHM bn marking sill gateway; 4 Y
SPM bns mark fixed sill.

79.697   ILE DE MOLENE.
3 lines from end, after 1·5m, insert: 10 ⊘ at inner hbr, FF30.

Area 17 – South Brittany

LIGHTS, FOG SIGNALS & WAYPOINTS.
80.710   LH col. AUDIERNE.
Line 1. Pointe de Lervily.
Amend to: Fl (3) WR 12s etc.

81.717   AUDIERNE. CHARTLET.
Amend Pte de Lervily Lt (approx 48°00'·1N 04°34'·0W) to Fl (3) WR 12s etc.

Area 18 – South Biscay

LIGHTS, FOG SIGNALS & WAYPOINTS.
82.738   LH col. PORNIC.
Noëveillard Yacht Hbr Digue Ouest Hd.
Amend to: Fl (2) R 10s.

83.743   PORNIC. LIGHTS & MARKS.
Amend 7s to 10s.
CHARTLET.
Ditto (Lt at SW elbow of S bkwtr).

Area 19 – NE France

84.773   PASSAGE INFORMATION.
RH col. Estuaire de la Seine, 2nd para, delete 3rd sentence; substitute: With almost 24 hours access/exit, Honfleur is a useful starting port when bound up-river.

85.781   DEAUVILLE. CHARTLET.
W bkwtr lt Fl WG 4s, amend ranges to 9/6M.
E Bkwtr lt Fl (4) WR 12s, insert W against White sector 131°-175° (44°).

86.787   ROUEN. Line 7.
After 68 insert: **82 for height of water**

Area 20 – Belgium and the Netherlands

LIGHTS, FOG SIGNALS & WAYPOINTS.
87.804   LH & RH cols. BELGIUM.
Kwintebank Lt By. Delete: *Whis*.
Akkaert Lt By. Delete: *Whis*.
Trapegeer Lt By. Delete: *Bell*.
Nieuwpoort Bk Lt By. Delete: *Whis*.
Wenduinebank W Lt By. Delete: *Whis*.
Oostendebank N Lt By. Delete: *Whis*.
A1 bis Lt By. Delete: *Whis*.

88.805   LH col. VLISSINGEN.
Lines 16/19. Schone Waardin.

Delete: vis obscd 083°-. . .W094°-248°.
Insert: vis R248°-260·5°, G260·5°-269°, W269°-283°, G283°-326°, R326°-341°, G341°-023°, W023°-024°, G024°-054°, R054°-065°, W065°-075·5°, G075·5°-079·5°, R079·5°-083°.
RH col. BRAAKMANHAVEN.
Line 9. Braakman.
Amend range to: W4M.
RH col. HANSWEERT.
Line 3. Amend vis to: W356·5°-042·5°, R042·5°-061·5°.W061·5°-082·5°, G082·5°-102·5°, W102·5°-114·5°, R114·5°-127·5°, W127·5°-288°.

89.806   LH col. KATS.
Lines 3/4, S Jetty Hd. Amend vis to: W344°-153°,   R153°-165°, G165°-200°, W200°-214°, G214°-258°, W258°-260°, G260°-313°, W313°-331°.
RH col. ZIERIKZEE.
W Jetty Hd. Lines 2/4. Amend vis to: G063°-100°, W100°-133°, R133°-156°, W156°-278°, R278°-306°, G306°-314°, W314°-333°, R333°-350°, W350°-063°.

90.807   RH col. Kwade Hoek. Amend vis to: W235°-068°, R068°-088°, G088°-107°, W107°-113°, R113°-142°, W142°-228°, R228°-235°.
RH col. HOEK VAN HOLLAND.
Line 9. Delete Ldg Lts 112°.
Lines 10/11. Maasmond Ldg Lts 107°. Amend to: **Front**, Iso R 4s 29m **18M**; vis 099·5°-114·5°. **Rear**, Iso R 6s 43m **18M**, vis 099·5°-114·5°. Both sync.

91.809   LH col. POLLENDAM.
Line 1. SHM's. Delete: P1 Fl G 2s.
Insert: P1 53°11'·43N 05°20'·40E Iso G 2s.
Amend P5 to: Iso G 2s.

92.812   SPECIAL NOTES FOR BELGIUM, INLAND WATERWAYS.
Delete the first and third sentences. Substitute: As from May 1995 "licence plates" (*immatriculation/immatriculatieplaat*) are required for all yachts on the Flemish waterways, in lieu of the former *Vaarvignet*. These plates cost 1000Bef (1995) and are obtained from: 2000 ANTWERPEN, Markgravestraat 16. ☎ 03/232.98.05; also from offices in Brussels, Brugge, Charleroi, Gent, Liege, Hasselt and Tournai.

93.818   VLISSINGEN. CHARTLET.
At ✫ Iso WRG 4s (approx 51°26'·5N 03°36'·1E) delete the White and Red sectors

immediately south of the light; the large W sector continues clockwise to abut the Green sector. See also 10.20.4.

94.831   IJMUIDEN. FACILITIES.
Seaport Marina; Amend f27 to f32; Delete V, ⌗. Last line, after Ferry insert: IJmuiden-Newcastle.

Area 21 – Germany

LIGHTS, FOG SIGNALS & WAYPOINTS.
95.844   RH col. *GW/EMS Lt F*.
Amend ◒)) to: *Horn Mo (R) 30s*; Racon (T).

96.845   RH col. **Wangerooge.**
Lines 3/6. Delete: vis . . . to RC.
Insert: vis R358·5°-008°, W008°-018·5°, G018·5°-055°, W055°-060·5°, R060·5°-065·5°, W065·5°-071°, G(18M) 119·4°-138·8°, W(22M) 138·8°-152·2° Ldg sector, R(17M) 152·2°-159·9°. RC.
<u>Hooksielplate Cross Lt.</u>
Amend vis to: R345°-359·3°, W359·3°-002·1°, G002·1°-011·8°, W011·8°-018·5°, R018·5°-098·7°, W098·7°-104·6°, G104·6°-115·3°, W115·3°-119·8°, R119·8°-129·2°.

97.846   LH col. **Arngast** Dir Lt.
Lines 2/4. Delete: vis: G152°-160·3° to G(7M) 303°-314° inclusive.
After W150°-152° Insert: G152°-174·6°, R180·5°-191°, W191°-213°, R213°-225°, W(10M) 286°-303°, G(7M)303°-314°, G174·6°-175·5°, W175·5°-176·4°.
Tegeler Plate. Delete: vis: R119°- to **21M** vis 116°-119° inclusive.
Insert: W116°-119° Ldg sector for Neue Weser, R119°-123°, G123°-144°, W144°-147°.

98.847   RH col. Pagensand Ldg Lts.
Delete present entry.
Substitute: Pagensand Ldg Lts 135°. Front, 53°42'·15N 09°30'·30E, Iso 4s 20m 13M. Rear, 880m from front, Iso 4s 32m 13M.
RIVER EIDER.
Lines 4/5. **St Peter**.
Delete: From W 091° to R116°-130°.
Substitute: W091°-120°.

99.848   LH col. RIVER HEVER.
Lines 6/8. **Westerheversand.**
Amend vis to: W012·2°-069°, G069°-079·5°, W079·5°-080·5°, Ldg sector for Hever, R080·5°-107°, W107°-157°, R157°-169°, W169°-206·5°, R206·5°-218·5°, W218·5°-233°, R233°-248°.

100.851   SPECIAL NOTES FOR GERMANY.
Visual Storm Signals, line 2, amend 10.14.7 to 10.15.8.

101.856   WANGEROOGE. LIGHTS & MARKS.
Line 3.   Delete R002°...G023°-055°.
Substitute: R358·5°-008°, W008°-018·5°, G018·5°-055°.
CHARTLET.
Amend these 3 sectors accordingly.

102.863   CUXHAVEN. SHELTER.
Line 1. Insert: Marina Cuxhaven, close S of radio mast, is entered from Alter Hafen via bridge which opens H and H+30, requested by 2 long blasts.
FACILITIES.
Line 4.   Insert: **Marina Cuxhaven**, ☎ 37363, open all year, 90 berths inc approx 45 for ⍟, usual facilities.

103.874   PELLWORM.
Insert VHF Ch 11.

104.874   WYK.
Lines 7/8. Amend light on SE point of Föhr to: Oc (4) WR 15s 10m 13/10M; W208°-245°, R245°-298°, W298°-333°, R333°-080°.

105.875   LIST. RADIO TELEPHONE.
Delete: None. Insert: VHF Ch 11.

106.875   SYLT. CHARTLET.
In LH col, amend light on SE point of Föhr to: Oc (4) WR 15s 10m 13/10M.

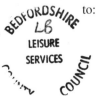
BEDFORDSHIRE
LB
LEISURE
SERVICES
COUNTY COUNCIL

Index

Explanation
Abbreviations are entered under the full word and not the abbreviation.
   For example St Abb's comes under Saint not St.
The prefix C before a page number indicates a Coast Radio Station.
The prefix L before a page number indicates an entry in the lists of Coastal Lights, Fog Signals and Waylights.
The prefix R before a page number indicates a Radio Navigational Aid.

B

C

H

L

Q

Z